Third Edition
# Clinical Pediatric Nephrology

Third Edition

# Clinical Pediatric Nephrology

Edited By

## Kanwal K. Kher

Chairman, Department of Nephrology
Phoenix Children's Hospital
Phoenix, AZ, USA
and Emeritus Professor of Pediatrics
George Washington University
School of Medicine
Washington, DC, USA

## H. William Schnaper

Vice Chair Department of Pediatrics
Northwestern University
Feinberg School of Medicine
and Ann & Robert H. Lurie Children's
Hospital of Chicago
Chicago, IL, USA

## Larry A. Greenbaum

Division Director of Pediatric Nephrology
Marcus Professor of Pediatrics
Emory University School of Medicine
and Children's Healthcare of Atlanta
Atlanta, GA, US

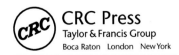

CRC Press
Taylor & Francis Group
Boca Raton   London   New York

CRC Press is an imprint of the
Taylor & Francis Group, an **informa** business

CRC Press
Taylor & Francis Group
6000 Broken Sound Parkway NW, Suite 300
Boca Raton, FL 33487-2742

First issued in paperback 2020

© 2017 by Taylor & Francis Group, LLC
CRC Press is an imprint of Taylor & Francis Group, an Informa business

No claim to original U.S. Government works

Version Date: 20160808

ISBN 13: 978-0-367-57422-2 (pbk)
ISBN 13: 978-1-4822-1462-8 (hbk)

**Visit the Taylor & Francis Web site at**
**http://www.taylorandfrancis.com**

**and the CRC Press Web site at**
**http://www.crcpress.com**

# Contents

# Preface

This third edition of *Clinical Pediatric Nephrology* continues to have as its main goal providing a primer of pediatric nephrology. Its intended audience includes committed medical students and general trainees, as well as pediatric nephrology fellows and pediatric nephrologists. Our focus remains on the clinical diagnosis and management of pediatric renal disorders.

The book has been thoroughly updated, and each chapter has been rewritten. The number of chapters has expanded from 37 to 53. In part, this represents a degree of specialization, with several chapters divided to focus on specific disorders as their pathogenesis has been clarified. The organization of the book has also been changed with an additional emphasis on the physiology of kidney diseases. Sections now cover kidney anatomy and development, diagnostic evaluation, disorders of homeostasis, glomerular and tubular diseases, systemic diseases and the kidney, acute and chronic kidney disease, renal replacement therapies, hypertension, inherited disorders, urologic disorders, and research tools. We believe that this reorganization and the expansion in the number of chapters better reflects the status of pediatric nephrology today. Each chapter includes "Key Points" boxes to emphasize issues that the authors and editors believe are important take-aways in the section, a set of review questions for the reader, and where appropriate a clinical vignette describing how the information in the chapter could be clinically applied in real life.

An important change has been an evolution in the editorship. Dr. Larry Greenbaum has joined the editorial team. He brings immense experience as an academic nephrologist, clinician and a researcher to the editorial team. His role in shaping the content of the third edition is evident in all sections of the book. We also wish to express our sincerest gratitude and thanks to Dr. Sudesh Makker, who guided the editorial work in the first two editions of this book.

We wish to thank all the contributors who worked diligently with us, under tight time-lines, through several revisions of their texts, and who willingly provided elements for the chapters that are unique to this publication. The outstanding editorial, production, and marketing teams at Taylor and Francis have provided support that has been essential to our reaching fruition. We are especially grateful to Our sincerest thanks to Henry Spilberg, who has managed the publication of the second edition and guided us in the concept design of the third edition of this book at Taylor and Francis. Miranda Bromage, who has taken over the reigns, has been an inspiration to work with. She provided her extraordinary skills in guiding the production of the book. Henry and Miranda were instrumental in advocating for an "all-color" book, which has enhanced its content and visual appeal. We thank both of them from the bottom of our hearts. Amy Blalock and Linda Van Pelt provided their superb expertise in copy editing and composing the galleys. Kyle Meyer, at the Boca Raton office of CRC Press-Taylor and Francis worked patiently with us in the editing of galleys of all chapters. Without his help, publication of this book would not have materialized. Figures in this edition were drawn by a very talented pool of artists. They are the unsung heroes of this work. We wish to thank each one of them for their contributions.

We owe a major debt of gratitude to two groups. Our students, residents, nephrology fellows and colleagues have provided inspiration and frequently challenged us on communication of scientific and educational content, as well as the format of this work. Most importantly, our families, who tolerate our busy and often distracting schedules have provided consistent support and a sense of perspective as we undertook this task. They provide an essential foundation for our lives. It is only with their individual commitments that we have succeeded in completing this task. We owe our heartfelt gratitude and appreciation to each one of them.

Kanwal K. Kher
Larry A. Greenbaum
H. William Schnaper

# Contributors

**Sun-Young Ahn, MD**
Medical director, nephrology inpatient services
Children's National Health System,
The George Washington University
Washington DC, USA

**Farah N. Ali, MD, MS**
Assistant Professor of Pediatrics
Ann and Robert H. Lurie Children's Hospital of Chicago
Chicago, Illinois

**Uri S. Alon, MD**
Professor of Pediatrics
University of Missouri, Kansas City School of Medicine
and
Section of Pediatric Nephrology
The Children's Mercy Hospital
Kansas City, Missouri

**Mary Andrich, MD**
Clinical Associate Professor of Radiology
The George Washington University School of Medicine
Washington, DC

**David Askenszi MD, MSPH**
Associate Professor of Pediatrics
Medical Director - Pediatric and Infant Center for Acute
    Nephrology
University of Alabama at Birmingham
Birmingham Alabama , USA

**Meredith Atkinson, MD, MHS**
Associate Professor of Pediatrics
Division of Pediatric Nephrology
Johns Hopkins University School of Medicine
Baltimore, Maryland, USA

**Diego H. Aviles, MD**
Division Chief, Pediatric Nephrology
Children's Hospital of New Orleans
Professor of Clinical Pediatrics
Louisiana State University Health Sciences Center
    New Orleans
New Orleans, Louisiana

**Rossana Baracco, MD**
Assistant Professor of Pediatrics
Children's Hospital of Michigan
Wayne State University
Detroit, Michigan, USA

**Michel Baum, MD**
Sara M. and Charles E. Seay Chair in Pediatric Research
Professor of Pediatrics and Internal Medicine
Department of Pediatrics
University of Texas Southwestern Medical Center
Dallas, Texas

**Detlef Bockenhauer, PhD**
Professor of Paediatric Nephrology
UCL Institute of Child Health and Great Ormond Street
    Hospital for Children
NHS Foundation Trust
London, United Kingdom

**Raed Bou Matar, MD**
Assistant Professor of Pediatrics
Cleveland Clinic Lerner College of Medicine of Case
    Western Reserve University
Center for Pediatric Nephrology
Cleveland, Ohio

**Dorothy Bulas, MD**
Professor of Pediatrics and Radiology
The George Washington University School of Medicine
Children's National Health System
Washington, DC

**Timothy E. Bunchman, MD**
Director Pediatric Nephrology
Children's Hospital of Richmond
and
Professor of Pediatrics
Virginia Commonwealth University School of Medicine
Richmond, Virginia

**Melissa A. Cadnapaphornchai, MD**
Associate Professor of Pediatrics and Medicine
University of Colorado Anschutz Medical Campus
The Kidney Center
Children's Hospital Colorado
Aurora, Colorado

**Stephen Cha, MD**
Clinical Assistant Professor of Pediatrics
Northeast Ohio Medical University
Nephrology & Pediatric Hypertension Center
Akron Children's Hospital
Akron , Ohio

**Akash Deep MD, FRCPCH**
Honorary Lecturer, King's College
Director, Pediatric Intensive Care Unit
King's College Hospital, London, UK

**W. Robert DeFoor, MD, MPH**
Associate Professor of Surgery
University of Cincinnati
and
Director Clinical Research
Division of Pediatric Urology
Cincinnati Children's Hospital Medical Center
Cincinnati, Ohio

**Georges Deschênes, MD, PhD**
Head of Pediatric Nephrology
APHP Robert-Debré, Université Sorbonne-Paris-Cité
Paris, France

**Prasad Devarajan, MD**
Louise M. Williams Endowed Chair
Professor of Pediatrics and Developmental Biology
Director of Nephrology and Hypertension
Cincinnati Children's Hospital Medical Center
University of Cincinnati School of Medicine
Cincinnati, Ohio

**Joseph T. Flynn, MD, MS**
Chief, Division of Nephrology
Seattle Children's Hospital
Professor of Pediatrics
University of Washington School of Medicine
Seattle, Washington

**John W. Foreman, MD**
Chief, Pediatric Nephrology
Department of Pediatrics
Duke University Medical Center
Durham, North Carolina

**Debbie S. Gipson, MD, MS**
Professor of Pediatrics
University of Michigan School of Medicine
Ann Arbor, Michigan , USA

**Caroline Gluck, MD**
Pediatric Nephrology Fellow
Children's Hospital of Philadelphia
Philadelphia, Pennsylvania, USA

**Brittany Goldberg MD, MS**
Adjunct Assistant Professor of Pediatrics
George Washington University School of Medicine
Division of Infectious Diseases
Children's National Health System
Washington, DC

**Stuart L. Goldstein, MD, FAAP, FNKF**
Director, Center for Acute Care Nephrology
Division of Nephrology and Hypertension
The Heart Institute Cincinnati
Children's Hospital Medical Center
Cincinnati, Ohio, United States of America

**Larry Greenbaum, MD, PhD, FAAP**
Marcus Professor of Pediatric Nephrology
Chief, Division of Nephrology
Emory University School of Medicine
and
Children's Healthcare of Atlanta
Atlanta, Georgia USA

**Lisa M. Guay-Woodford, MD**
Hudson Professor of Pediatrics
George Washington University
and
Director, Center for Translational Science
and
Director, Clinical and Translational Institute at
    Children's National
Children's National Health System
Washington, DC

**M. Colleen Hastings, MD, MS**
Associate Professor, Pediatrics and Medicine
University of Tennessee Health Science Center
and
Le Bonheur Children's Hospital
and
Children's Foundation Research Institute
Memphis, Tennessee

**Danniele Gomes Holanda, MD**
Clinical Assistant Professor
Director, Electron Microscopy Laboratory
Department of Pathology
University of Iowa Hospitals and Clinics
Iowa City, Iowa, USA

**Christer Holmberg, MD, PhD**
Professor of pediatrics
Pediatric Nephrology and Transplantation
Children's Hospital
University of Helsinki
Helsinki
Finland

**Franca Iorember, MD, MPH**
Associate Professor of Pediatrics
Clinical Division of Nephrology
Children's Hospital of New Orleans
and
Department of Pediatrics
Louisiana State University Health Sciences Center
    New Orleans
New Orleans, Louisiana

**Sherron M. Jackson, MD**
Associate Professor, Pediatric
Hematology-Oncology
Director of Pediatric Sickle Cell Clinic
Medical University of South Carolina
Charleston, South Carolina USA

**Hannu Jalanko, MD**
Professor, Head of the Department
Pediatric Nephrology and Transplantation
Children's Hospital, University of Helsinki
Helsinki University Central Hospital
Helsinki, Finland

**Barbara Jantausch, MD**
Professor of Pediatrics
George Washington University School of Medicine
and
Division of Infectious Diseases
Children's National Medical Center
Washington, DC

**Kurt E. Johnson, PhD**
Professor of Anatomy and Regenerative Biology
Professor of Obstetrics and Gynecology (Research)
George Washington University School of Medicine  and
Health Sciences
Washington, DC

**Stanley C. Jordan, MD**
Director, Nephrology
Director, HLA and Transplant Immunology Laboratory
Comprehensive Transplant Center
Medical Director, Kidney Transplant Program
Cedars-Sinai Medical Center, Los Angeles, California

**Gaurav Kapur, MD**
Associate Professor, Pediatrics
Director, Pediatric Dialysis
Wayne State University School of Medicine
Children's Hospital of Michigan
Detroit, Michigan, USA

**Clifford E. Kashtan, MD**
Professor of Pediatrics
Chief, Division of Pediatric Nephrology
University of Minnesota Amplatz
Children's Hospital
Minneapolis, Minnesota

**Frederick J. Kaskel, MD, PhD**
Professor and Vice Chair of Pediatrics
Director, Life Course Research Program
Block Institute for Clinical & Translational
Research
Albert Einstein College of Medicine
and
Children's Hospital at Montefiore
Bronx, NY

**Kanwal K. Kher, MD**
Professor Emeritus of Pediatrics
George Washington University School of Medicine
Washington, DC
and
Division Chief, Nephrology and Hypertension
Phoenix Children's Hospital
Phoenix, AZ

**Jeffrey B. Kopp, MD**
Kidney Disease Section
National Institute of Diabetes and Digestive and
Kidney
Bethesda, Maryland

**Martin A. Koyle, MD**
Professor Department of Surgery
University of Toronto
Department Head, Urology
The Hospital for Sick Children
Toronto, Canada

**Craig B. Langman, MD**
The Isaac A Abt MD Professor of Kidney Diseases
Feinberg School of Medicine, Northwestern University
Head, Kidney Diseases
The Ann and Robert H Lurie Children's Hospital of
Chicago
Chicago, Illinois USA

**Armando J. Lorenzo, MD**
Associate Professor
Department of Surgery
University of Toronto
and
Department of Urology.
The Hospital for Sick Children,
Toronto, Canada

**John D. Mahan, MD**
Professor, Department of Pediatrics
Pediatric Nephrology
The Ohio State University College of Medicine
and
Nationwide Children's Hospital
Columbus Ohio

**Massoud Majd**
Professor of Pediatrics and Radiology
The George Washington University School of
Medicine
and
Children's National Health System
Washington, DC

**Robert Mak, MD, PhD**
Pediatric Nephrology
University of California San Diego
La Jolla, California

**Bruce Markle, MD**
Associate Professor of Pediatrics and Radiology
The George Washington University School of Medicine
Children's National Health System
Washington, DC

**Tej K. Mattoo, MD, DCH, FRCP (UK)**
Professor of Pediatrics
Wayne State University School of Medicine
Chief, Pediatric Nephrology and Hypertension
Children's Hospital of Michigan
Detroit, Michigan

**Karen McNiece Redwine, MD, MPH**
Associate Professor of Pediatrics
Pediatric Nephrology
University of Arkansas for Medical Sciences/Arkansas
    Children's Hospital
Little Rock, Arkansas

**Michele Mietus-Snyder, MD**
Associate Professor of Pediatrics
The George Washington University School of Medicine
and
Children's National Health System
Washington, DC

**Eugene Minevich, MD**
Professor of Surgery
Division of Pediatric Urology
Cincinnati Children's Hospital Medical Center
Cincinnati, Ohio

**Kirtida Mistry, MBBCh, DCH, MRCPCH**
Assistant Professor of Pediatrics
Division of Pediatric Nephrology
The George Washington University School of Medicine
and
Medical Director, Dialysis Services
Children's National Medical Center
Washington, DC

**Asha Moudgil, MD**
Professor of Pediatrics
George Washington University School of Medicine
Acting Chief Division of Nephrology
and
Medical Director, Renal Transplantation
Children's National Medical Center
Washington, DC

**Marva Moxey-Mims, MD**
KUH Deputy Director for Clinical Research
Director, Pediatric Nephrology and Renal Centers
    Programs
NIH, NIDDK, DKUH
Bethesda, Maryland

**Raj Munshi, MD**
Seattle Children's Hospital
Seattle, Washington

**Carla M. Nester, MD, MSA**
Assistant Professor
Departments of Internal Medicine and Pediatrics
Division of Nephrology
University of Iowa Hospital and Clinics
Iowa City, Iowa

**Patrick Niaudet, MD**
Pediatric Nephrology
Hôpital Necker-Enfants Malades
Université Paris-Descartes
Paris, France

**Hans G. Pohl, MD, FAAP**
Associate Professor
Urology and Pediatrics
George Washington University
and
Associate Chief, Department of Urology
Children's National Medical Center
Washington, DC

**Raymond Quigley MD**
Division of Pediatric Nephrology
University of Texas Southwestern Medical Center
Dallas, Texas

**Shreya Raman, MBBS, MRCP, MSc, FRCPath**
Specialist Registrar in Histopathology
Royal Victoria Infirmary
Newcastle upon Tyne Hospitals NHS Foundation Trust
Newcastle upon Tyne, United Kingdom

**Michelle N. Rheault, MD**
Assistant Professor of Pediatrics
and
Medical Director of Dialysis
Division of Pediatric Nephrology
University of Minnesota Amplatz Children's Hospital
Minneapolis, Minnesota

**Norman D. Rosenblum MD, FRCPC**
Paediatric Nephrologist
Hospital for Sick Children
Professor of Paediatrics, Physiology, and Laboratory
    Medicine and Pathobiology
Canada Research Chair in Developmental Nephrology
University of Toronto
Peter Gilgan Centre for Research and Learning
Hospital for Sick Children
Toronto, Canada

**Isidro B. Salusky, MD**
Distinguished Professor of Pediatrics
Chief. Division of Pediatric Nephrology
Director, Clinical and Translational Research Center
Associate Dean for Clinical Research
David Geffen School of Medicine at UCLA
Los Angeles, California, USA

**Lisa M. Satlin, MD**
Herbert H. Lehman Professor and Chair
Jack and Lucy Clark Department of Pediatrics
Mount Sinai Medical Center
Pediatrician-in-Chief
Kravis Children's Hospital at Mount Sinai
Icahn School of Medicine at Mount Sinai
New York, New York

**John Sayer, MBChB, PhD, FRCP**
Senior Clinical Lecturer in Nephrology
Institute of Genetic Medicine
International Centre for Life
Newcastle University
Newcastle Upon Tyne, United Kingdom

**H. William Schnaper, MD**
Irene Heinz Given and John Laporte Given Professorship
    in Pediatric Research
Vice Chair, Department of Pediatrics
Northwestern University Feinberg School of Medicine
and
Ann & Robert Lurie Children's Hospital of Chicago
Chicago, Illinois

**George J. Schwartz, MD**
Professor of Pediatrics and Medicine
Chief, Division of Pediatric Nephrology
Department of Pediatrics
University of Rochester School of Medicine
Rochester, New York

**Dave Selewski, MD, MS**
Assistant Professor
Pediatric Nephrology
University of Michigan
Ann Arbor, Michigan

**Eglal Shalaby-Rana, MD**
Assistant Professor of Radiology and Pediatrics
George Washington University School of Medicine
and
Children's National Medical Center
Washington, DC

**Ibrahim F. Shatat, MD, MS**
Associate Professor of Pediatrics
Division of Nephrology and Hypertension
MUSC Children's Hospital
Charleston, South Carolina

**William E. Smoyer, MD**
C. Robert Kidder Endowed Chair
Vice President Clinical and Translational Research
Director, Center for Clinical and Translational Research
The Research Institute at Nationwide Children's Hospital
Professor of Pediatrics
Columbus, Ohio USA

**Shalabh Srivastava, MBBS, MRCP**
Specialist Registrar in Nephrology
Institute of Genetic Medicine
Newcastle University
Newcastle upon Tyne, United Kingdom

**Tarak Srivastava, MD**
Associate Professor of Pediatrics
University of Missouri, Kansas City School of Medicine
and
Director, Nephrology Research Laboratory
Children's Mercy Hospital
Kansas City, Missouri

**Mihail M. Subtirelu, MD**
Adjunct Associate Professor
University of Missouri, Kansas City
Division of Pediatric Nephrology
and
Children's Mercy Hospital
Kansas City, Missouri

**Jordan M. Symons, MD**
Professor of Pediatrics
University of Washington School of Medicine
Attending Nephrologist
Seattle Children's Hospital
Seattle, Washington, USA

**David B. Thomas, MD**
Professor of Pathology
University of Miami Miller School of Medicine
University of Miami Hospital
Miami, Florida

**Shamir Tuchman, MD, MPH**
Assistant Professor of Pediatrics
George Washington University School of Medicine
and
Division of Pediatric Nephrology
Children's National Medical Center
Washington, DC

**Natalie S. Uy, MD**
Assistant Professor of Pediatrics
Pediatric Nephrology
Columbia University Medical Center
New York, NY

**Rudolph P. Valentini, MD**
Chief Medical Officer
Pediatric Nephrology
Children's Hospital of Michigan
Clinical Professor of Pediatrics
Wayne State University School of Medicine
Detroit, Michigan

**Vesa Matti Vehaskari, MD, PhD**
Professor of Pediatrics
LSU Health Sciences Center
Children's Hospital of New Orleans
New Orleans, Louisiana

**Bradley A. Warady, MD**
Professor of Pediatrics
University of Missouri, Kansas City School of Medicine
and
Senior Associate Chairman, Department of Pediatrics
Director, Division of Pediatric Nephrology
Children's Mercy Hospital
Kansas City, Missouri

**Katherine Wesseling-Perry, MD**
Associate Professor of Pediatrics
Division of Pediatric Nephrology
David Geffen School of Medicine at UCLA
University of California, Los Angeles
Los Angeles, California

**Robert J. Wyatt, MD, MS**
Professor of Pediatrics
University of Tennessee Health Science Center
and
Le Bonheur Children's Hospital
Memphis, Tennessee

**Ihor V. Yosypiv, MD**
Associate Professor
Department of Pediatrics
Tulane University Health Sciences Center
New Orleans, Louisiana

# Kidney anatomy and development

# Anatomy and embryology of the urinary tract

KURT E. JOHNSON

Kidneys serve as an important metabolic organ that eliminates nitrogenous waste products, maintains fluid and electrolyte balance, and performs important hormonal functions, such as synthesis of 1-25-dihydroxy vitamin D and erythropoietin. Being paired organs, kidneys have also been used in living organ donation for renal replacement therapy in patients with end-stage renal disease (ESRD). Developmental aspects of kidney have received considerable attention recently and much has now been deciphered about the control of renal and ureteric development. It is also becoming increasingly clear that nephron endowment at birth is an important fetal factor that may determine the development of hypertension and chronic kidney disease (CKD) in adults. This chapter discusses the clinically relevant anatomy and embryogenesis of the kidneys and the urinary tract.

## GROSS STRUCTURE AND RELATIONS

In adults, each kidney is reddish-brown, approximately 11 cm long, 5 cm wide, and 3 cm thick, and weighs approximately 130 g. By renal ultrasound measurement, renal length in healthy newborns has been reported to be 4.21 ± 0.45 cm for the right kidney and 4.32 ± 0.46 cm for the left kidney.[1] Kidneys grow with age and achieve adult length by approximately 18 years of age.[2,3] Interestingly, renal length is greater in obese children, possibly reflecting hypertrophy resulting from hyperfiltration.[4] Both kidneys are more or less similar in shape, with a convex lateral surface and a deep recess at the hilum of the kidney on the medial surface that is called the renal sinus. The renal artery and vein

and some adipose tissue occupy the renal sinus, along with a funnel-shaped expansion of the ureter known as the renal pelvis. Within the kidney, the renal pelvis is divided into two elongated major calyces and several shorter branches called the minor calyces.

### KEY POINT

Newborn kidneys are approximately 4.5 cm long as measured by ultrasound.

The two kidneys lie on the posterior abdominal wall along either side of the vertebral column in the retroperitoneal space, but at slightly different levels. The left kidney has its superior pole at approximately the level of the middle of T11 vertebral body and its inferior pole at approximately the level of the bottom of L2. In contrast, the right kidney lies slightly lower, with its superior pole at the top of T12 and its inferior pole at the top of L3. The superior poles of each kidney are in contact with the diaphragm, and their posterior surfaces are covered by skeletal muscles (from medial to lateral): psoas major, quadratus lumborum, and transversus abdominis.

In a longitudinally cut section, the kidney has a darker cortex, whereas the inner medulla is lighter in color. Each kidney has a collection of triangular renal pyramids, or lobes, with a base bordering the cortex and an apex projecting as renal papillae into the minor calyces (Figure 1.1). Each renal pyramid consists of medullary tissue associated with the corresponding cap of cortical tissue. The distinction

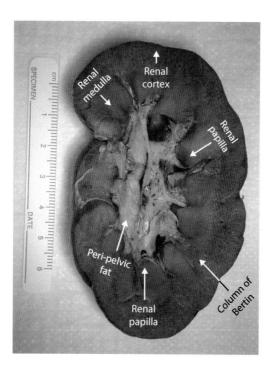

Figure 1.1 Cut surface of normal kidney of a child with anatomic landmarks shown. (Photograph provided by Ronald Przygodzki, MD.)

between cortex and medulla in the kidneys is made difficult by the projection of medullary tissue into the cortex as medullary rays and by the cortical tissue bundled between the renal pyramids, known as the renal columns of Bertin.

The ureters are 25 cm long in an adult but are of variable length in children. The ureter has a thick, fibromuscular wall and a small lumen. Along its descent from the abdominal cavity (upper half) into the lesser pelvis (lower half), the ureter is located retroperitoneally and is closely adherent to the overlying peritoneal lining. Ureters enter the urinary bladder posteriorly. The urinary bladder is a hollow muscular organ located posterior to the symphysis pubis, and its superior surface is covered by a reflection of the peritoneal lining. It is innervated by nerves from the vesical plexus, which has fibers from two distinct sources: (1) sympathetic lumbar nerves through the hypogastric plexus and (2) parasympathetic pelvic splanchnic nerves.

## MICROSCOPIC ANATOMY

The renal parenchyma consists of functional units called uriniferous tubules, each with two distinct components: (1) the nephron and (2) the collecting tubules. The nephron consists of the Bowman capsule, proximal convoluted tubules (PCTs), loop of Henle, and distal convoluted tubules (DCTs). Nephrons have highly variable lengths. In general, the superficial (cortical) nephrons are shorter and the deep (juxtamedullary) nephrons are longer, mostly because of the longer loop of Henle. These long nephrons are important

in the urinary concentrating mechanism (Figure 1.2). Uriniferous units converge to form the apex of the renal pyramids as they enter the minor calyces. Starting at the bases of the renal pyramids, adjacent to the corticomedullary junction, bundles of tubules and associated blood vessels may project toward the surface of the kidney as radially arranged medullary rays.

### KEY POINTS

- Nephrons with glomeruli close to the corticomedullary junction have long loops of Henle. These nephrons participate in the urinary concentration mechanism.
- Superficial or cortical nephrons have shorter loops of Henle.

The most proximal structure of the nephron is the Bowman capsule, a thin-walled, spherical dilation, which is deeply invaginated into a two layered, cup-like structure, with a visceral layer and a parietal layer. The space between these two layers, which is continuous with the lumen of the PCTs, is called the urinary (or Bowman) space. The concave depression in the Bowman capsule is occupied by a network of capillaries known as the glomerulus. The glomerulus and Bowman capsule together constitute a renal corpuscle and comprise the functional filtering units in the kidney.

The PCT receives the glomerular filtrate from the urinary space of Bowman capsule. It is lined by a simple columnar epithelium. Its cells have an abundance of mitochondria that make the cytoplasm intensely acidophilic. Epithelial cells of the PCT have an elaborate apical microvillous brush border, which fills much of the lumen of the PCT, and deep invaginations of the basilar surface membrane. The lateral borders of individual cells are extensively interdigitated, thus giving the individual cells the appearance of a tree stump with elaborate buttressing. These microscopic features play an important role in the reabsorption of tubular water, electrolytes, bicarbonate, phosphate, and amino acids. Proximal tubules also reabsorb and metabolize filtered albumin in proteinuric states and return the amino acids and dipeptides to body's nutrition pool. The PCT leads into a proximal straight tubule, and from there the glomerular filtrate passes into the descending thin limb, the ascending thin limb, and the ascending thick limb of the loop of Henle.

Once the glomerular filtrate has ascended the loop of Henle, it passes into the DCT. A portion of the DCT contacts the vascular pole of the renal corpuscle, where it forms the macula densa of the juxtaglomerular apparatus (JGA). The DCT is lined by simple cuboidal epithelium, although it has a wider lumen than the PCT. There are only scattered apical microvilli in the DCT. The cells in the thin limbs of the loop of Henle are generally flattened and are often frankly

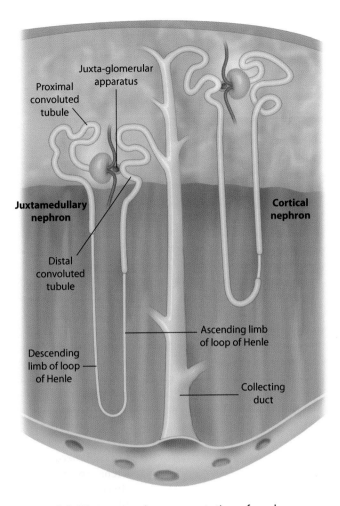

Figure 1.2 Diagrammatic representation of nephrons arranged in the kidney. Juxtaglomerular nephrons have long loops of Henle that dip deep into medulla and are important in the countercurrent urine concentrating mechanism. Cortical nephrons have relatively short loops of Henle. (Figure in the public domain; artwork by Holly Fischer. Reproduced under Creative Commons Attribution 3.0.)

squamous. The collecting tubules, the last component of the nephron, have squamous epithelium, whereas the collecting ducts have taller epithelial cells, starting as cuboidal cells in the cortex but growing taller along the route of descent to the renal papilla, eventually to form tall columnar cells in the walls of the papillary ducts (of Bellini), just before they penetrate the area cribrosa to enter the minor calyx.

## RENAL BLOOD SUPPLY

Blood flow through the kidneys is surprisingly extensive (approximately 25% of cardiac output), with approximately 90% flowing through the cortex and the rest flowing through the medulla. This immense blood supply ensures rapid removal of nitrogenous wastes from the blood by the kidneys. The renal artery enters the renal sinus and divides into anterior and posterior branches, which then form segmental arteries. Segmental arteries branch into lobar arteries for each renal pyramid (lobe), which then branch again, passing in the renal columns, between the renal pyramids as interlobar arteries. Once the interlobar arteries have penetrated to the corticomedullary junction, they branch into arcuate arteries, which run parallel to the surface of the kidney. At regular intervals along the arcuate arteries, interlobular arteries project radially toward the most superficial parts of the cortex. As the interlobular arteries pass from the deep cortex to the superficial cortex, they send out branches called afferent arterioles that supply blood to the glomeruli. After leaving the glomerulus, blood enters the efferent arteriole. From here, the blood follows different pathways for cortical nephrons and juxtamedullary nephrons. In cortical nephrons, with short loops of Henle, blood passes through a complex network of capillaries, some surrounding the PCTs and DCTs (as a cortical peritubular capillary network). In contrast, in juxtamedullary nephrons, with long loops of Henle, the efferent arterioles (vasa recta), follow the loop of Henle to its tip. These blood vessels then drain into interlobular veins, arcuate veins, interlobar veins, and eventually the renal vein.

---

### KEY POINTS

- Efferent arterioles of juxtamedullary nephrons develop anatomically distinct, long vascular channels that dip deep into the medulla along the side of their own nephrons and are called vasa recta.
- Vasa recta are low-flow arteries and are prone to desaturation-induced sickling of red blood cells in patients with sickle cell anemia or sickle cell trait.

---

The spaces between the renal tubules are filled with connective tissue, known as the renal interstitium. It is relatively sparse in the cortex but more abundant in the medulla. The renal interstitium also connects to a distinct connective tissue capsule around the entire kidney, with an inner layer of potentially contractile myofibroblasts and an outer layer of fibroblasts.

## THE RENAL CORPUSCLE

The renal corpuscle is a prominent feature of the renal cortex. It consists of three main structures: (1) the glomerulus, a network of capillaries supplied by the afferent arteriole and drained by the efferent arteriole; (2) the Bowman capsule, an invaginated, balloon-like expansion of the PCT; and, (3) mesangial cells (Figure 1.3). Glomerular capillary endothelial cells have numerous 70- to 100-nm fenestrae

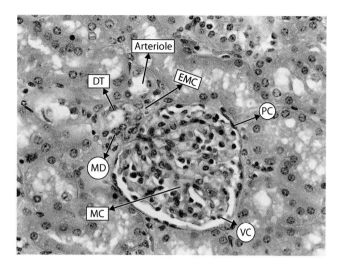

Figure 1.3 Light microscopy showing a glomerulus with the juxtaglomerular apparatus. DT, distal tubule; EMC, extraglomerular mesangial cells MC, mesangial cell with mesangial matrix; MD, macula densa; PC, parietal epithelial cell; and VC, visceral epithelial cells.

(transcellular pores) without diaphragms, and they rest on a basement membrane (Figure 1.4A). The glomerular basement membrane (GBM) is a multilayered structure with a lamina rara interna (adjacent to capillary endothelium), a lamina densa, and a lamina rara externa (adjacent to the podocytes). The laminae rarae are rich in polyanions such as heparan sulfate. These negatively charged macromolecules presumably repel anions that would otherwise cross from the capillary lumen into the urinary space (and vice versa). In addition, the laminae rarae have an abundance of fibronectin, a cell adhesion glycoprotein. Mesangial cells form a

supportive complex between the capillary endothelial cells. They can proliferate and produce a basement membrane–like material and appear to have contractile, secretory, and phagocytic activity.

GBM is one of the thickest and most functionally important basement membranes in the body. The GBM is a complex extracellular matrix that is formed by both capillary endothelial cells and podocytes. It contains type IV collagen, laminin, fibronectin, entactin, and proteoglycan complex with polyanionic glycosaminoglycans such as heparan sulfate. The thickness of the GBM varies with age; it is a mean of 373 nm in men and 326 nm in women.[5] In children, however, GBM is thinner at birth, rapidly increases in size by the second year of life, and reaches adult proportions by 9 to 11 years of age.[6,7] Before 1 year, the thickness of GBM has been reported to be 132 to 208 nm, and it reached 244 to 307 nm by 11 years in one study.[6] Thinned GBM is usually seen in Alport syndrome, thin basement membrane nephropathy (TBMN), and occasionally in immunoglobulin A (IgA) nephropathy.

By electron microscopy, the GBM has a thick, central, electron-dense lamina densa (see Figure 1.4A), with less electron-dense layers adjacent to the capillary endothelial cells (lamina rara interna), and podocytes (lamina rara externa). The collagen is thought to function as a scaffold for the attachment of other glycoproteins and proteoglycans that constitute the rest of the GBM. Type IV collagen consists of three intertwined α-chain monomers, each with three distinct domains: the 7S N-terminus, a middle helical collagenous domain, and a C-terminus noncollagenous (NC1) domain.[8] The GBM also allows attachment of epithelial cells (through cell surface integrin receptors for extracellular matrix molecules such as collagen, laminin, and fibronectin) to itself and one another, and it serves as a part

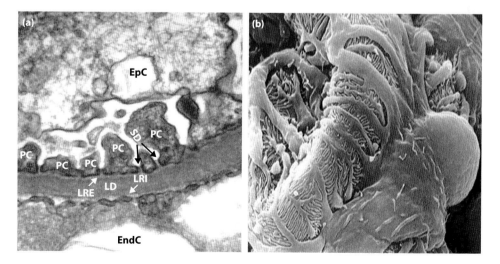

Figure 1.4 (a) Electron micrograph of the basement glomerular capillary. Capillary cross section showing an endothelial cell (EndC), the lamina rara interna (LRT), the lamina rara externa (LRE), the lamina densa (LD), the podocyte foot processes (PC), the epithelial cell cytoplasm (EpC), and the slit diaphragm (SD). (b) Electron micrograph showing extensive interdigitation of the podocyte foot processes around the basement membrane on the external or urinary side.

of the selective filtration barrier between the lumen of the glomerular capillary (the vascular space) and the lumen of the Bowman capsule (the urinary space).

## PODOCYTES

The visceral layer of the Bowman capsule is formed by a sheet of stellate epithelial cells called podocytes, which have a large central cell body containing a nucleus and numerous primary, secondary, and tertiary branches projecting from the cell body. Podocytes have foot processes, which interdigitate extensively and attach the podocytes to the lamina rara externa of the GBM (Figure 1.4B).

The gaps between the adjacent foot processes, known as filtration slits, are covered by a zipper-like slit diaphragm (SD), which forms the second barrier to macromolecular transport after glomerular endothelial and GBM barriers.[8] The structure and function of SDs have been the subject of intense study. Discoveries in this area have provided important insights into the role played by the podocytes in glomerular function. The zipper-like structure of SD is made up of protein molecules from the two adjacent foot-processes that overlie each other in the midline to form the filtration barrier.[9] Of these molecules, nephrin was the first to be identified. Nephrin, which forms the bulk of SD filtration barrier, is a transmembrane protein that is anchored to the cytoplasmic membrane by podocin.[10,11] Neph 1, Neph 2, and Neph3 are other important podocyte-SD proteins that are structurally similar to nephrin and are believed to react with both nephrin and podocin to maintain the cytoskeletal structure and scaffoldings within podocytes.[12-15] The podocyte foot processes are anchored to the GBM by $\alpha_3\beta_1$ integrin.

---

**KEY POINTS**

- Epithelial cells and their foot processes are now recognized as among the most functionally relevant cell types in the glomeruli.
- Alterations in podocytes resulting from gene mutations have been linked to the pathogenesis of several types of nephrotic syndrome in children.
- With aging, podocytes are normally shed in urine.
- Injured podocytes do not regenerate.

---

Mutations in podocytes foot process–associated proteins cause proteinuria and nephrotic syndrome. Nephrin (*NPHS1* gene) mutation in humans result in the Finnish type of congenital nephrotic syndrome, whereas podocin (*NPHS2* gene) mutation also gives rise to steroid-resistant nephrotic syndrome.[15-17] In experimental animals, Neph1-lacking mice develop severe proteinuria that resembles the nephrin mutation in humans.

## THE JUXTAGLOMERULAR APPARATUS

The DCT returns to its parent glomerulus and rests close to the vascular pole, in proximity to the afferent arteriole (see Figure 1.3). This specialized structure is the JGA. The JGA consists of three identifiable microscopic structures: (1) specialized cells of the DCT known as the macula densa, (2) juxtaglomerular (JG) cells in the afferent arteriole, and (3) extraglomerular mesangial (EGM) cells. The JGA is a sensor for sodium delivery to the distal nephron and alters the afferent and efferent arterial tone and blood flow through the locally generated renin-angiotensin system (RAS).

---

**KEY POINTS**

- The JGA is a specialized structure that is essential for renin-angiotensin hormone generation.
- The JGA controls intraglomerular pressure by regulating the relative diameter of the afferent and efferent arterioles.

---

### Macula densa

The macula densa is the collection of columnar epithelial cells in the wall of the DCT in intimate contact with the vascular pole of the Bowman capsule and the JG cells. Here, the nuclei of the tubular epithelial cells are more crowded together than in the rest of the DCT. The apical surfaces of cells in the macula densa have numerous microvilli and a single cilium.

### Juxtaglomerular cells

JG cells are modified smooth muscle like cells in the wall of the afferent arteriole. They are also sometimes found in smaller numbers in the wall of the efferent arteriole. They contain electron-dense granules of renin. As systemic blood pressure falls, the JG cells release their renin granules into the systemic circulation. Renin then cleaves angiotensinogen into the decapeptide angiotensin I. Angiotensin I is converted in pulmonary circulation into angiotensin II by the angiotensin-converting enzyme (ACE) in endothelial cells of alveolar capillaries. Angiotensin II, a potent vasoconstrictor, helps restore blood pressure to the normal range.

### Extraglomerular mesangial cells

EGM cells look like fibroblasts. They provide a communicating connection between the macula densa and the JG cells. Ultrastructural studies reveal that EGM cells have long, thin processes that contact both other elements of the JGA. In addition, there are gap junctions at the tips of these processes where the EGM cells contact other cells, probably thus allowing communication among the three cell types of the JGA.

## RENAL EMBRYOLOGY

Kidney and ureters develop from the intermediate meso-derm, a bulbous ridge of tissue that lies in the intraembryonic mesoderm between the somites and the lateral plate meso-derm. In contrast, bladder and the urethra develop from the urogenital sinus. Renal development occurs in three phases in a cranial to caudal sequence, starting in the fourth week. The first two stages, pronephros and mesonephros, are tran-sitional renal structures, whereas the third stage, the meta-nephros, forms the definitive kidney (Figure 1.5).

The pronephros is the first renal structure, which arises as few solid or vesicular tissue segments in the cervical region at the beginning of the fourth week. It degenerates by the end of the fourth week and leaves no adult remnants. The mesonephric kidney and its associated mesonephric duct form in the urogenital ridge of the intermediate mesoderm from the upper thoracic to the upper lumbar segments. The mesonephric kidney forms rudimentary nephrons and probably functions in humans to produce some dilute urine. Most of the mesonephros degenerates by the end of the eighth week. The mesonephric duct persists in boys and men as the epididymis, the vas deferens, and the seminal vesicle, structures that drain the testis. In girls and women, the mesonephric duct forms vestigial structures such as the epoöphoron and Gartner cysts.

The metanephric kidney is the definitive kidney and the last to develop. It begins to form in the fifth week and is

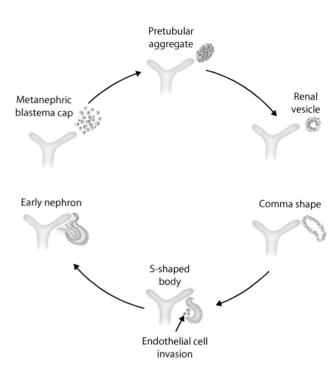

Figure 1.6 Developmental stages of the kidney in the fetus. After the ureteric bud branching, the mesenchymal cells aggregate around the tip of the ureteric bud to form cap-mesenchyme. Next, these cells evolve through the stages of renal vesicle, comma-shaped body, and then S-shaped body. The end of S-shaped body that is clos-est to the ureteric bud fuses with it and becomes part of the distal nephron, whereas the opposite end invaginates to give rise to the glomerular structure. Endothelial cells invade the glomerulus to form glomerular capillaries.

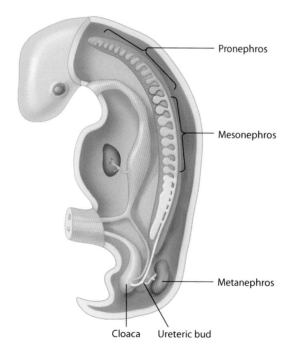

Figure 1.5 A diagrammatic view showing various phases of renal development in the embryo. The pronephros and mesonephros degenerate, whereas the metanephros formed at 5 weeks of gestation gives rise to the definitive kidney.

located in the caudal portion of the urogenital ridge. An evagination of the mesonephric duct, called the ureteric bud, grows into the surrounding mesenchyme of the uro-genital ridge, called the metanephric blastema. By a recipro-cal inductive interaction, the metanephric blastema triggers branching of the ureteric bud, thus ultimately forming the renal pelvis, major calyces, minor calyces, and collecting tubules. Meanwhile, the ureteric bud stimulates formation of blood vessels and nephrons in the metanephric blastema. Transformation of the metanephric blastema into a neph-ron undergoes the developmental stages of renal vesicle, comma-shaped body, and S-shaped body (Figure 1.6). The proximal portion of the S-shaped body invaginates to form the Bowman capsule with a cup-like recess for the develop-ment of glomerular capillaries. The distal potion connects to the branching ureteric bud to form the collecting duct.

## ASCENT OF THE METANEPHROS

The metanephric kidneys originate in the pelvis (S1 to S2 level), but following decurvature of the body axis and lumbar and sacral body growth, the definitive kidneys ascend to the lumbar area (T12 to L3). The metanephric kidney ascends between 6 and 9 weeks of gestation. When the caudal poles of the metanephroi fuse, the ascent of a horseshoe kidney is halted by the inferior mesenteric artery, a branch from the aorta that supplies hindgut derivatives. Initially, the metanephroi are supplied by sacral branches of the aorta, but as they ascend cranially, they take new branches from the dorsal aorta that eventually develop into the renal arteries. The caudal branches usually degenerate, but supernumerary renal arteries sometimes persist, often caudal to the main renal artery. During ascent, the fetal kidneys also rotate medially by 90 degrees, so that the renal hilum, with the ureter and renal vessels, faces medially. In arrested ascent, metanephric kidneys may be formed in the pelvis, either unilaterally or bilaterally, resulting in ectopic or pelvic kidneys.

## CLOACA AND FORMATION OF THE UROGENITAL SINUS

The most caudal portion of the early hindgut is the cloaca. The hindgut precursor and cloaca have a diverticulum, called the allantois, which projects far into the umbilical cord. By the fifth week, the proximal part of the cloaca becomes slightly expanded into a precursor of the urinary bladder. During the fifth week and onward, the urorectal septum divides the cloaca into a posterior anal canal and an anterior urogenital sinus. The urogenital sinus eventually gives rise to major portion of urinary bladder, and the pelvic part that becomes the membranous and prostatic urethra, and phallus. Each ureter enters the urinary bladder more lateral to the midline of the bladder, to form a roughly triangular structure called the trigone of the bladder, which is defined by the two ureteric inlets superiorly and the urethral outlet inferiorly. The proximal ends of the ureters become incorporated into the wall of the urinary bladder, so that it is lined transiently by mesodermally derived epithelium in the trigone. Later, the trigone is overgrown by endodermally derived epithelium from the rest of the bladder.

The distal portion of the allantois eventually degenerates, but the proximal portion persists as a urachal diverticulum that still projects into the umbilical cord. Eventually, the proximal urachal diverticulum forms the median umbilical ligament. Rarely, however, persistent urachus can lead to urachal fistula, wherein urine leaks from the bladder into the umbilicus or urachal cysts in the median umbilical ligament.

## INTRAUTERINE RENAL FUNCTION

In humans, the pronephros is a rudimentary structure. It does not form functional nephrons and involutes in a short time. The human mesonephric kidney forms rudimentary renal corpuscles with a Bowman capsule and glomerulus and associated tubules, but there is little substantiation of its function. Mesonephric nephrons have short loops of Henle, a structure suggesting that the small volume of urine produced in the mesonephros is likely to be dilute. By the 16th week of gestation, the mesonephric kidney loses

its functional capacity, and the metanephric kidney develops into a urine-producing structure, with renal corpuscles and well-differentiated PCTs with microvillous brush borders at the lumen. However, because the loops of Henle are not fully developed, fetal urine is hypotonic with respect to plasma and is slightly acidic. At term, the human fetus voids approximately 450 mL/day into the amniotic fluid. The urethra is patent in the fetus at approximately 8 weeks.

> **KEY POINT**
>
> The urethra is patent by the eighth week of gestation, and urine begins to form a part of amniotic fluid at around that time.

## NEPHRON ENDOWMENT AND FUTURE HEALTH RISKS

Each normal adult kidney has approximately 1 million nephrons, but this estimate is quite variable. Using mature adult kidneys obtained at autopsy, Nyengaard and Bendtsen[18] noted the mean nephron number to be 617,000. A more recent US-Australian, multiethnic autopsy study[19] in adults revealed a significant variation in nephron number, ranging from 210,332 to 1,825,380 in each kidney, with a mean of 870,582 ± 31,062.

Nephron number in human fetuses increases throughout gestation, from a mean of 15,000 at 15 weeks to 740,000 in each kidney by 40 weeks.[20] This number appears to plateau at approximately 36 weeks.[20] Nephrogenesis in full-term fetuses concludes by approximately 34 to 36 weeks of gestation, and new nephrons are not formed after birth.[20,21] Premature infants, conversely, have fewer nephrons, and nephronogenesis may continue after birth for as long as 3 months.[22,23] The clinical impact of low endowed nephron number in premature infants is likely to last a lifetime and is referred to as fetal programming. Indeed, renal length and volume by ultrasonography are known to be significantly lower in young adults who were born prematurely (at less than 32 weeks), a finding suggesting long term adverse renal consequences and risks in these persons.[24] An increased risk for hypertension and CKD associated with prematurity, low birth weight, and intrauterine growth retardation was suggested by Brenner et al.,[25-27] starting in the 1980s. In an Australian study,[28] 18-year-old survivors of extreme prematurity (gestational age less than 28 weeks) had higher

> **KEY POINT**
>
> Poor nephron endowment at birth (fetal programming) affects blood pressure, development of microalbuminuria, and can lead to ESRD in adults.

ambulatory blood pressure readings, thus lending weight to the hypotheses proposed by Brenner and others. A meta-analysis of studies relating prematurity and blood pressure also demonstrated a higher blood pressure in persons who were born prematurely (range, 28.8 to 34.1 weeks).[29]

The link between poor nephron endowment and CKD is plausible, but less well established. Microalbuminuria noted in otherwise healthy nondiabetic adults (46 to 54 years old) has been correlated with low birth weight as a risk factor.[30] Increased prevalence of ESRD in adults born with a birth weight of less than 2.5 kg was noted in one study in the United States, and the odds ratio for ESRD was 1.4 (95% confidence interval [CI], 1.1 to 1.8), as compared with a birth weight of 3 to 3.5 kg.[31] Carmody and Charlton[32] suggested that apart from low nephron endowment in premature infants, other factors that may enhance the risk for CKD include neonatal acute kidney injury, use of nephrotoxic antibiotics, poor nutrition, and hypoxia in early life.

---

## KEY POINTS

Renal risks in premature infants are compounded by:

- Acute kidney injury
- Hypoxia
- Use of nephrotoxic drugs
- Poor nutrition

---

## CONGENITAL ABNORMALITIES OF THE KIDNEY AND URINARY TRACT

The term *congenital abnormalities of the kidney and urinary tract* (CAKUT) denotes developmental urologic and renal abnormalities encountered in children.[32,33] CAKUT, as a term, also emphasizes the shared developmental destiny of the kidney and the urinary tract (Figure 1.7). The CAKUT spectrum encompasses diverse clinical disorders, such as unilateral or bilateral renal agenesis, renal hypodysplasia, multicystic dysplastic kidney (MCDK), ureteropelvic junction obstruction, posterior urethral valves, vesicoureteral reflux (VUR), duplex renal collecting system, ectopic ureters, and megaureter.

---

## KEY POINT

CAKUT, as a concept, reflects a common origin of renal and urologic anomalies in utero.

---

CAKUT occurs in approximately 1 in 500 live births, but severe abnormalities resulting in neonatal death occur less frequently, in approximately 1 in 2000 births.[33,34] By using prenatal ultrasound as the screening method in 709,030 live births, stillbirths, and induced abortions, 1130 infants

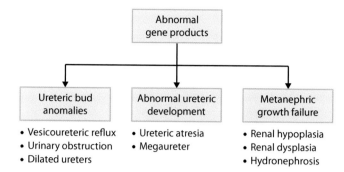

Figure 1.7 Pathogenesis of congenital abnormalities of the kidney and urinary tract. This unifying hypothesis breaks from previously believed concepts that developmental renal defects arise from urinary obstruction. It is now believed that genetic defects disrupt critical signaling processes between the ureteric bud and nephrogenic mesenchyme, eventually leading to uronephrologic developmental disorders. (Based on Ichikawa I, Kuwayama F, Pope JC, 4th, et al. Paradigm shift from classic anatomic theories to contemporary cell biological views of CAKUT. Kidney Int. 2002 61:889–98.)

and fetuses were diagnosed with at least one renal or urologic abnormality, amounting to an incidence of 1.6 in 1000 pregnancies.[35] CAKUT is often encountered as an isolated or sporadic anomaly, but it can also be a clinical feature of numerous syndromes. Additionally, an increased risk of urinary tract anomalies has been reported in the close family members of these patients.[36,37] Some of the common CAKUT malformations are discussed here, as well as in Chapter 2. VUR is discussed in Chapter 48.

## Renal agenesis

Bilateral renal agenesis is an uncommon disorder. Potter described 20 cases of bilateral renal agenesis in 5000 autopsies performed in children and estimated the incidence to be 1 in 3000 to 1 in 4000 births.[38,39] Approximately 25% to 40% of fetuses with bilateral renal agenesis are stillborn. Bilateral renal agenesis can result in the clinical features of Potter sequence as a result of prolonged lack of intrauterine urine and oligohydramnios.[40–42] Potter sequence (or Potter syndrome) is characterized by: bilateral renal agenesis (or severe fetal renal disease), oligohydramnios, pulmonary

---

## KEY POINTS

Potter sequence includes:

- Renal agenesis or severe dysplasia
- Oligohydramnios
- Pulmonary hypoplasia
- Low-set ears
- Clubfeet
- Pointed nose

hypoplasia, clubfeet, micrognathia, a pointed nose, and low-set malformed ears.[40] Potter facies refers to the typical facial features seen in Potter sequence. Potter sequence can result from any fetal disorder that leads to prolonged oligohydramnios. There has been an ongoing speculation that bilateral renal agenesis may be an inherited disorder, primarily because of a significantly higher incidence of occult renal defects in close relatives of index cases.[43] Recessive mutations in the integrin $\alpha_8$-encoding gene *ITGA8* have been described in families with fetal loss secondary to bilateral renal agenesis.[44] Such findings are likely to stimulate investigative pathways to genetic pathogenesis of bilateral renal agenesis.

Accurate information of the incidence of unilateral renal agenesis is difficult to obtain because many of these cases go undetected as a result of compensatory hypertrophy of the contralateral kidney, as well as normal intrauterine and postnatal renal function. Using renal ultrasound screening in healthy school-age children (6 to 15 years), Sheih et al.[45] reported the occurrence of unilateral renal agenesis to be 1 in 290 in the general population of children. European data also suggest the incidence of unilateral renal agenesis to be 1 in 2000 births.[46]

Unilateral renal agenesis is often associated with ipsilateral defects in other genital duct derivatives such as the ductus deferens in boys and the uterine tubes and uterus in girls. VUR is common (approximately 25%) in these patients, and extrarenal malformations affecting the gastrointestinal, cardiac, and musculoskeletal systems are seen in approximately 30% of patients.[46] An increased incidence of renal anomalies in the children and siblings of patients with unilateral renal agenesis has been noted in some studies.[36]

## Pelvic and horseshoe kidneys

Pelvic kidney and horseshoe kidney are related renal malformations that result from failed ascent of the kidneys. In horseshoe kidney, the caudal poles of the metanephric kidney are fused. Horseshoe kidney is one of the most common congenital anomalies of the kidney. On the basis of abdominal CT scan data in 15,320 patients, the incidence of horseshoe kidney was noted to be 1 in 666.[47] Approximately half of the patients diagnosed with horseshoe kidney are asymptomatic; the remainder present for renal stones and ascending urinary tract infections.[48] The Rovsing sign, consisting of nausea, vomiting, and abdominal pain that is accentuated on hyperextension, is seen in a minority of patients with horseshoe kidney.[48] Horseshoe kidney can occur as an isolated congenital birth defect but is more frequent in patients with Turner syndrome and trisomy 18 (Edwards syndrome).[48,49]

## Multicystic dysplastic kidneys

MCDKs are developmental, nonfunctional cystic masses caused by abnormalities in metanephric differentiation. These kidneys are characterized by abnormal and

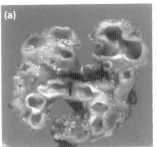
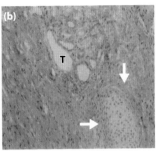

Figure 1.8 **(a)** Cut section of a kidney from a neonate shows cystic dysplasia. Renal architecture is poorly defined, numerous cysts are present, and the corticomedullary differentiation is absent. **(b)** Microscopic section of a kidney with renal dysplasia. Arrows shows the presence of cartilage. Tubulointerstitial tissue is poorly organized, and a large dilated renal tubule (T) is shown. (Photomicrograph courtesy of Arthur Cohen, MD.)

noncommunicating dilated cysts of variable size, with little identifiable renal structure or stroma (Figures 1.8 and 1.9). Renal arterial flow and excretory functions, as demonstrable by mercaptoacetyltriglycine (MAG3) renal scan, are absent.

MCDK is commonly identified by the presence of a unilateral cystic kidney in the fetus during prenatal ultrasound evaluation. Cystic kidneys may involve during gestation in some cases, and the infant is born with a solitary kidney. Other modes of presentation include an abdominal mass noted by the parents or during a clinical examination within few months of birth. In a study of 97 infants with the diagnosis of MCDK, 85% of the cases were detected by prenatal ultrasound evaluation, 4% by the presence of a mass postnatally, and 11% by a postnatal ultrasound examination

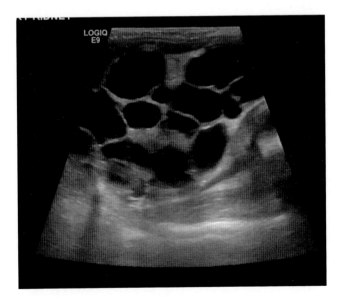

Figure 1.9 Renal ultrasound scan showing multiple large cysts in an infant with multicystic dysplastic kidney disease. Nuclear scan demonstrated no blood flow or excretory function in this kidney.

performed for an unrelated diagnosis.[50] MCDK is slightly more common on the left side in some studies, whereas other investigators have noted a right-sided predominance; these findings suggest that both sides can be equally involved.[38,39] Contralateral kidneys show abnormalities in approximately 40% of cases that include renal agenesis, renal dysplasia or hypoplasia, VUR, hydroureter or pyelectasis, duplex collecting system, and ectopic ureters.[39] In a meta-analysis of the abnormalities in the contralateral system, Schreuder et al.[51] reported VUR in approximately 20% cases: 15% in the contralateral system, ipsilateral VUR in 3.3%, and bilateral VUR in 2.4% cases. Ureteropelvic junction obstruction was the next most common anomaly in the contralateral renal system, accounting for 4.8% cases in this meta-analysis.

Involution of the cystic mass occurs usually occurs over several years, but the rate of involution is variable. Some patients have complete involution of the MCDK in utero and are thus born with a solitary kidney and unilateral agenesis. Complete involution of the MCDK was noted in 34% at 2 years (165 patients), 47% at 5 years (117 patients), and 59% at 10 years (43 patients) in a study from the United Kingdom.[52] The contralateral normal kidney usually undergoes compensatory hypertrophy.

Hypertension has been well documented in patients with MCDK and is believed to be mediated by the RAS.[53] More recent studies, however, point out that the risk of hypertension in MCDK is low. In a review of 29 studies, Narchi et al.[54] reported hypertension to be present in only 6 of the 1115 cases, a finding suggesting the mean probability of developing hypertension in MCDK to be 5.4 in 1000 cases (estimated 95% CI, 1.9 to 11.7 per 1000).

A high risk for Wilms tumor and renal cell carcinoma in the MCDK was suggested in older studies. However, the risk of tumors was very low in several more recent, comprehensive, well-conducted studies.[55,56] Surgical resection of the MCDK, which was often practiced until the late 1980s for the prevention of hypertension and to protect against development of malignant disease, appears to be difficult to justify with the evidence-based results.[54–57]

## WAGR syndrome

Wilms tumor, aniridia, genitourinary abnormalities, and mental retardation (WAGR) was first reported as a distinct clinical disorder by Miller et al.[58] in 1964 (Online Mendelian Inheritance in Man [OMIM] number 194072). It is now well established that the disorder results from deletion in distal band of 11p13 in such a way that *WT1* and *PAX6* genes, which are adjacent to each other, are affected by the deletion.[59] The *WT1* gene deletion results in renal malformations and risk for Wilms tumor; whereas the *PAX6* gene deletion results in aniridia and brain malformations.

The *WT1* gene encodes for Wilms tumor suppressor protein (WT1), a transcription factor containing a DNA binding domain, with four zinc fingers. WT1 transcription factor is essential for the development of the nephron, as well as the gonads, and is thought to be involved in

mesenchymal-epithelial transition in the renal and germ cell lines.[60] With mutations in the *WT1* gene, the development of glomeruli and of the proximal and distal tubules is adversely affected, leading to renal malformations. A propensity for Wilms tumor in WAGR and other syndromes with the *WT1* gene mutation, such as Denys-Drash syndrome, results from the presence of undifferentiated or poorly differentiated mesenchymal cells in the kidneys.[60,61]

The genital malformations seen in WAGR syndrome include cryptorchidism, ambiguous genitalia, hypospadias, streaked ovaries, and hypoplastic uterus. Renal and urinary tract anomalies encountered in WGAR syndrome include hypoplastic kidneys, unilateral renal agenesis, duplicated ureters,, development of focal segmental glomerulosclerosis, nephrogenic rests, nephroblastomatosis, and renal cysts.[62] Aniridia can be partial or complete and results in severe visual impairment. Apart from risk of CKD and ESRD imposed by the development of Wilms tumor, patients with WAGR syndrome are inherently at an increased risk for development of ESRD. The National Wilms Tumor Study Group reports the incidence of ESRD to be 53% in patients with WAGR syndrome.[63,64] Monitoring of kidneys by ultrasound every 3 months until 6 years of age has been recommended in some studies for Wilms tumor surveillance in patients with WAGR syndrome.[62]

## Bladder exstrophy

Bladder exstrophy is an uncommon developmental anomaly seen in newborn infants. It is caused by a ventral body wall, an anterior bladder wall defect, and eversion of the bladder wall mucosa. The term exstrophy, which is derived from the Greek word *ekstriphein*, means "turned inside out." In the newborn infant, the exposed bladder mucosa is bright red and has a raw appearance. The exposed mucosa sometimes undergoes metaplasia, forming colonic epithelium rather than transitional epithelium. Bladder exstrophy is also associated with other congenital abnormalities of the external genitalia such as bifid penis, epispadias, and abnormal scrotal development

Using the Healthcare Cost and Utilization Project Nationwide Inpatient Sample database, Nelson et al.[65] estimated the incidence of bladder exstrophy to be 2.15 in 100,000 live births (or approximately 1 in 40,000 births). The male-to-female ratio was equal in this study, and the congenital malformation appeared to be more common in whites than in nonwhites. Some genetic analyses have demonstrated a higher prevalence of duplication of 22q11.21 in patients with bladder exstrophy.[66]

Surgical repair of bladder exstrophy has evolved since the 1990s. Both early closure and delayed closure of the defect are acceptable surgical options and are generally dictated by technical preference of the surgical team.[67] Postrepair attention to incontinence, recurrent urinary tract infections secondary to associated VUR, and correction of epispadias are common concerns to be addressed during childhood. Many patients require continent urinary diversion procedures, as well as bladder augmentation by cystoplasty. However, lower urinary tract symptoms persist in 80% of patients with exstrophy as they grow into adulthood.[68] Sexual dysfunction is also a concern in adulthood.[69] In addition, adenocarcinomas occur with higher frequency in the exposed bladder mucosa. Surgical intervention and repair can extend the patient's life and ensure normal renal function.

## Angiotensin-converting enzyme fetopathy

Experimental observations indicate that RAS exerts its influence on renal development by promoting the ureteric bud branching process and therefore plays a key role in nephrogenesis.[70,71] The RAS may affect ureteric bud branching and nephrogenesis through its influence on GDNF, the *WT1* gene, and the *PAX2* gene. Disruption of the RAS during nephrogenesis by ACE inhibitors (ACEIs) is well known to cause fetopathy.[70,72] ACEI fetopathy risk is low if the drug is consumed in the first trimester.[72–74] Clinical characteristics of ACEI fetopathy are: oligohydramnios, renal tubular dysgenesis, neonatal anuria, skull defects, intrauterine growth retardation, and patent ductus arteriosus.

---

### KEY POINTS

- The RAS plays a crucial role in nephrogenesis.
- Maternal ACEI use after the first trimester is associated with fetopathy that includes renal dysgenesis.

---

### SUMMARY

A significant advance in our understanding of the signal pathways involved during development of the kidneys and the urinary tract in fetal life has occurred since the 1990s. What has also become obvious is that the renal development is supported by the development of the rest of the urinary tract, especially the ureteric bud. A disruption in any of these developmental processes can lead to abnormalities of renal development and CAKUT. Nephron endowment at birth is beginning to be recognized as an important predictor of CKD and hypertension in adults. Attention to prenatal health and prevention of poor nephron endowment may be ways that kidney disease and hypertension can be prevented in adults.

## REFERENCES

1. Scott JE, Hunter EW, Lee RE, et al. Ultrasound measurement of renal size in newborn infants. Arch Dis Child. 1990;65:361–4.

2. Pantoja Zuzuárregui JR1, Mallios R, Murphy J. The effect of obesity on kidney length in a healthy pediatric population. Pediatr Nephrol. 2009;24:2023–7.

3. Alev Kadioglu. Renal measurements, including length, parenchymal thickness, and medullary pyramid thickness, in healthy children: What are the normative ultrasound values? AJR Am J Roentgenol. 2010;194:509–15.

4. Rosenbaum DM, Korngold E, Teele RL. Sonographic assessment of renal length in normal children. AJR Am J Roentgenol. 1984;142:467–9.

5. Steffes MW, Barbosa J, Basgen JM, et al. Quantitative glomerular morphology of the normal human kidney. Lab Invest. 1983;49:82–6.

6. Vogler C, McAdams AJ, Homan SM. Glomerular basement membrane and lamina densa in infants and children: An ultrastructural evaluation. Pediatr Pathol. 1987;7:527–34.

7. Morita M, White RH, Raafat F, et al. Glomerular basement membrane thickness in children: A morphometric study. Pediatr Nephrol. 1988;2:190–5.

8. Miner JH. Glomerular basement membrane composition and the filtration barrier. Pediatr Nephrol. 2011;26:1413–7.

9. Rodewald R, Karnovsky MJ. Porous substructure of the glomerular slit diaphragm in the rat and mouse. J Cell Biol. 1974;60:423–33.

10. Kestilä M1, Lenkkeri U, Männikkö M, et al. Positionally cloned gene for a novel glomerular protein—nephrin—is mutated in congenital nephrotic syndrome. Mol Cell. 1998;1:575–82.

11. Wartiovaara J, Ofverstedt LG, Khoshnoodi J, et al. Nephrin strands contribute to a porous slit diaphragm scaffold as revealed by electron tomography. J Clin Invest. 2004;114:1475–83.

12. Sellin L, Huber TB, Gerke P, et al. NEPH1 defines a novel family of podocin interacting proteins. FASEB J. 2003;17:115–7.

13. Liu G, Kaw B, Kurfis J, et al. Neph1 and nephrin interaction in the slit diaphragm is an important determinant of glomerular permeability. J Clin Invest. 2003;112:209–21.

14. Garg P, Verma R, Nihalani D, et al. Neph1 cooperates with nephrin to transduce a signal that induces actin polymerization. Mol Cell Biol. 2007;27:8698–712.

15. Grahammer F, Schell C, Huber TB. The podocyte slit diaphragm: From a thin grey line to a complex signalling hub. Nat Rev Nephrol. 2013;9:587–98.

16. Heeringa SF, Vlangos CN, Chernin G, et al. Thirteen novel NPHS1 mutations in a large cohort of children with congenital nephrotic syndrome. Nephrol Dial Transplant. 2008;23:3527–33.

17. Machuca E, Benoit G, Nevo F, Tête MJ, et al. Genotype-phenotype correlations in non-Finnish congenital nephrotic syndrome. J Am Soc Nephrol. 2010;21:1209–17.

18. Nyengaard JR, Bendtsen TF. Glomerular number and size in relation to age, kidney weight, and body surface in normal man. Anat Rec. 1992;232,194–201.

19. Hoy WE, Douglas-Denton RN, Hughson MD, et al. A stereological study of glomerular number and volume: Preliminary findings in a multiracial study of kidneys at autopsy. Kidney Int Suppl. 2003;63, S31–7.

20. Hinchliffe SA, Sargent PH, Howard CV, et al. Human intrauterine renal growth expressed in absolute number of glomeruli assessed by the dissector method and Cavalieri principle. Lab Invest. 1991;64:777–84.

21. Moritz KM, Caruana G, Wintour EM. Development of kidneys and urinary tract. In Rodeck CH, Whittle MF, editors. Fetal Medicine: Basic Science and Clinical Practice, 2nd ed. Philadelphia: Churchill Livingstone; 2009. p. 147.

22. Hinchliffe SA, Lynch MR, Sargent PH, et al. The effect of intrauterine growth retardation on the development of renal nephrons. Br J Obstet Gynaecol. 1992;99:296–301.

23. Mañalich R1, Reyes L, Herrera M, et al. Relationship between weight at birth and the number and size of renal glomeruli in humans: A histomorphometric study. Kidney Int. 2000;58:770–3.

24. Keijzer-Veen MG1, Devos AS, Meradji M, et al. Reduced renal length and volume 20 years after very preterm birth. Pediatr Nephrol. 2010;25:499–507.

25. Brenner BM, Garcia DL, Anderson S. Glomeruli and blood pressure: Less of one, more of the other? Am J Hypertens. 1988;1:335–47.

26. Brenner BM, Mackenzie HS. Nephron mass as a risk factor for progression of renal disease. Kidney Int Suppl. 1997;63 S124–7.

27. Luyckx VA, Bertram JF, Brenner BM, et al. Effect of fetal and child health on kidney development and long-term risk of hypertension and kidney disease. Lancet. 2013 20;382:273–83.

28. Roberts G1, Lee KJ, Cheong JL, et al. Higher ambulatory blood pressure at 18 years in adolescents born less than 28 weeks' gestation in the 1990s compared with term controls. J Hypertens. 2014;32:620–6.

29. de Jong F, Monuteaux MC, van Elburg RM, et al. Systematic review and metaanalysis of preterm birth and later systolic blood pressure. Hypertension. 2012;59:226–34.

30. Yudkin JS, Phillips DI, Stanner S. Proteinuria and progressive renal disease: Birth weight and microalbuminuria. Nephrol Dial Transplant. 1997;12(Suppl 2):10–3.

31. Lackland DT, Bendall HE, Osmond C, et al. Low birth weights contribute to high rates of early-onset chronic renal failure in the Southeastern United States. Arch Intern Med. 2000;160:1472–6.

32. Carmody JB, Charlton JR. Short-term gestation, long-term risk: Prematurity and chronic kidney disease. Pediatrics. 2013;131:1168–79.

33. Ichikawa I, Kuwayama F, Pope JC, 4th, et al. Paradigm shift from classic anatomic theories to contemporary cell biological views of CAKUT. Kidney Int. 2002;61:889–98.

34. Pope JC 4th, Brock JW, 3rd, Adams MC, et al. How they begin and how they end: Classic and new theories for the development and deterioration of congenital anomalies of the kidney and urinary tract, CAKUT. J Am Soc Nephrol. 1999;10:2018–28.

35. Wiesel A, Queisser-Luft A, Clementi M, et al. Prenatal detection of congenital renal malformations by fetal ultrasonographic examination: An analysis of 709,030 births in 12 European countries. Eur J Med Genet. 2005;48:131–44.

36. McPherson E. Renal anomalies in families of individuals with congenital solitary kidney. Genet Med. 2007;9:298–302.

37. Bulum B, Ozçakar ZB, Ustüner E, et al. High frequency of kidney and urinary tract anomalies in asymptomatic first-degree relatives of patients with CAKUT. Pediatr Nephrol. 2013;28:2143–7.

38. Mansoor O, Chandar J, Rodriguez MM, et al. Long-term risk of chronic kidney disease in unilateral multicystic dysplastic kidney. Pediatr Nephrol. 2011;26:597–603.

39. Damen-Elias HA, Stoutenbeek PH, Visser GH, et al. Concomitant anomalies in 100 children with unilateral multicystic kidney. Ultrasound Obstet Gynecol. 2005;25:384–8.

40. Potter EL. Bilateral renal agenesis. J Pediatr. 1946;29:68–76.

41. Potter EL. Normal and Abnormal Development of the Kidney. Chicago: Year Book Medical Publishers; 1972. p. 1–305.

42. Wilson RD, Baird PA. Renal agenesis in British Columbia. Am J Med Genet. 1985;21:153–69.

43. Roodhooft AM, Birnholz JC, Holmes LB. Familial nature of congenital absence and severe dysgenesis of both kidneys. N Engl J Med. 1984;310:1341–5.

44. Humbert C, Silbermann F, Morar B, et al. Integrin alpha 8 recessive mutations are responsible for bilateral renal agenesis in humans. Am J Hum Genet. 2014;94:288–94.

45. Sheih CP, Liu MB, Hung CS, et al. Renal abnormalities in schoolchildren. Pediatrics. 1989;84:1086–90.

46. Westland R, Schreuder MF, Ket JC, et al. Unilateral renal agenesis: A systematic review on associated anomalies and renal injury. Nephrol Dial Transplant. 2013;28:1844–55.

47. Weizer AZ, Silverstein AD, Auge BK, et al. Determining the incidence of horseshoe kidney from radiographic data at a single institution. J Urol. 2003;170:1722–6.

48. Glenn JF. Analysis of 51 patients with horseshoe kidney. N Engl J Med. 1959;261:684–7.

49. Bilge I, Kayserili H, Emre S, et al. Frequency of renal malformations in Turner syndrome: Analysis of 82 Turkish children. Pediatr Nephrol. 2000;14:1111–4.

50. Kuwertz-Broeking E, Brinkmann OA, Von Lengerke HJ, et al. Unilateral multicystic dysplastic kidney: Experience in children. BJU Int. 2004;93:388–92.

51. Schreuder MF, Westland R, van Wijk JA. Unilateral multicystic dysplastic kidney: A metaanalysis of observational studies on the incidence, associated urinary tract malformations and the contralateral kidney. Nephrol Dial Transplant. 2009;24:1810–8.

52. Aslam M, Watson AR, Trent, and Anglia MCDK Study Group. Unilateral multicystic dysplastic kidney: Long term outcomes. Arch Dis Child. 2006;91:820–3.

53. Snodgrass WT. Hypertension associated with multicystic dysplastic kidney in children. J Urol. 2000;164:472–3.

54. Narchi H. Risk of hypertension with multicystic kidney disease: A systematic review. Arch Dis Child. 2005;90:921–4.

55. Narchi H. Risk of Wilms' tumour with multicystic kidney disease: A systematic review. Arch Dis Child. 2005;90:147–9.

56. Eickmeyer AB, Casanova NF, He C, et al. The natural history of the multicystic dysplastic kidney: Is limited follow-up warranted? J Pediatr Urol. 2014;10:655–61.

57. Tilemis S, Savanelli A, Baltogiannis D, et al. Is the risk of hypertension an indication for prophylactic nephrectomy in patients with unilateral multicystic dysplastic kidney? Scand J Urol Nephrol. 2003;37:429–32.

58. Miller RW, Fraumeni JF Jr, Manning MD. Association of Wilms' tumor with aniridia, hemihypertophy and other congenital malformations. N Engl J Med. 1964;270:922–7.

59. Francke U, Holmes LB, Atkins L, Riccardi VM. Aniridia-Wilms' tumor associations: Evidence for specific deletion of 11p13. Cytogenet Cell Genet. 1979;24:185–92.

60. Rauscher FJ. The WT1 Wilms tumor gene product: A developmentally regulated transcription factor in the kidney that functions as a tumor suppressor. FASEB J. 1993;7:896–903.

61. Morrison AA, Viney RL, Saleem MA, et al. New insights into the function of the Wilms tumor suppressor gene WT1 in podocytes. Am J Physiol Renal Physiol. 2008;295:F12–7.

62. Fischbach BV, Trout KL, Lewis J, et al. WAGR syndrome: A clinical review of 54 cases. Pediatrics. 2005;116:984–8.

63. Breslow NE, Norris R, Norkool P, et al. Characteristics and outcomes of children with the Wilms' tumor-aniridia syndrome: A report from the National Wilms' Tumor Study Group. J Clin Oncol. 2003;24:4579–85.

64. Breslow NE, Collins AJ, Ritchey ML, et al. End stage renal disease in patients with Wilms tumor: Results from the National Wilms Tumor Study Group and the United States Renal Data System. J Urol. 2005;174:1972–5.

65. Nelson CP, Dunn RL, Wei JT. Contemporary epidemiology of bladder exstrophy in the United States. J Urol. 2005;173:1728–31.

66. Draaken M, Baudisch F, Timmermann B, et al. Classic bladder exstrophy: Frequent 22q11.21 duplications and definition of a 414 kb phenocritical region. Birth Defects Res A Clin Mol Teratol. 2014;100:512–7.

67. Dickson AP. The management of bladder exstrophy: The Manchester experience. J Pediatr Surg. 2014;49:244–50.

68. Taskinen S, Suominen JS. Lower urinary tract symptoms (LUTS) in patients in adulthood with bladder exstrophy and epispadias. BJU Int. 2013;111:1124–9.

69. Gupta AD, Goel SK, Woodhouse CR, et al. Examining long-term outcomes of bladder exstrophy: A 20-year follow-up. BJU Int. 2014;113:137–41.

70. Yosypiv IV. Renin-angiotensin system in ureteric bud branching morphogenesis: Insights into the mechanisms. Pediatr Nephrol. 2011;26:1499–512.

71. Song R, Spera M, Garrett C, et al. Angiotensin II AT2 receptor regulates ureteric bud morphogenesis. Am J Physiol Renal Physiol. 2010;298:F807–17.

72. Pryde PG, Sedman AB, Nugent CE, Barr M. Angiotensin-converting enzyme inhibitor fetopathy. J Am Soc Nephrol. 1993;3:1575–82.

73. Buttar HS. An overview of the influence of ACE inhibitors on fetal-placental circulation and perinatal development. Mol Cell Biochem. 1997;176:61–71.

74. Anonymous. Post marketing surveillance for angiotensin-converting enzyme inhibitor use during the first trimester of pregnancy: United States, Canada, and Israel, 1987–1995. MMWR Morb Mortal Wkly Rep. 1997;46:240–2.

## REVIEW QUESTIONS

1. The juxtamedullary nephrons have long loops of Henle that participate in:
   a. Sodium reabsorption
   b. Chloride transport
   c. Urine concentrating mechanism
   d. None of the above

2. Nephrin constitutes a structural component of:
   a. Endothelial cytoskeleton
   b. Podocyte cytoskeleton
   c. Slit diaphragm
   d. Bowman capsule

3. Which of the following combinations are transitional embryonic kidneys?
   a. Metanephros and mesonephros
   b. Mesonephros and pronephros
   c. Pronephros and metanephros
   d. None of the above

4. In a premature infant, nephrogenesis can continue up to 3 months after birth:
   a. True
   b. False
5. Characteristic finding on MAG3 renal scan in a patient with multicystic dysplastic kidney (MCDK) is:
   a. Photopenic areas in the affected kidney suggesting cysts
   b. Arterial flow from the surrounding tissue
   c. Adequate blood flow but no excretory function
   d. No demonstrable renal blood flow and no excretory function
6. Vesicoureteral reflux on the same side or contralateral side of MCDK occurs in:
   a. Fewer than 5% cases
   b. 20% cases
   c. 50% cases
   d. Almost always in all patients
7. Wilms tumor, aniridia, genitourinary anomalies, and mental retardation (WAGR) is caused by:
   a. Mutation in WT1 gene
   b. Mutation in PAX6 gene
   c. Mutation in PAX6 and WT1
   d. Mutation in *WT1* and GDNF
8. ACEI-induced fetapathy is more common if the drug exposure occurs in:
   a. First 2 weeks of pregnancy
   b. Six to 12 weeks of pregnancy
   c. Last week of pregnancy
   d. After first trimester of pregnancy
9. Horseshoe kidneys are common in:
   a. Down syndrome
   b. Turner syndrome
   c. WAGR syndrome
   d. Renal coloboma syndrome
10. Low nephron number at birth is associated with:
    a. Future risk of diabetes mellitus
    b. Future risk of cardiac disease
    c. Future risk of hypertension
    d. No associated risk of disease

## ANSWER KEY

1. c
2. c
3. c
4. a
5. d
6. b
7. c
8. d
9. b
10. c

# Molecular basis of developmental renal disease

NORMAN D. ROSENBLUM

Developmental abnormalities of the urinary tract are common and account for 30% to 50% cases of end-stage renal disease in children.[1] Formation of the kidney consists of a complex series of morphogenetic events during intrauterine development that are complete by approximately 34 weeks of gestation. However, growth of kidney cells continues after birth, as does functional development of the kidneys. Renal development is incomplete at birth, even in full-term infants and to a greater extent in preterm infants. Mature levels of renal function are not achieved until approximately 2 years of age. The objectives of this chapter are to supplement the broad concepts of renal embryologic development discussed in Chapter 1 and to explore the molecular events involved in nephrogenesis.

## EARLY FETAL KIDNEY DEVELOPMENT

In mammals, the kidneys develop in three stages, from rostral (head end) to caudal (rump end): the pronephros, the mesonephros, and the metanephros (permanent kidney). The pronephros is rudimentary and nonfunctional. The mesonephros functions briefly and then involutes toward the end of the first trimester. The metanephros does not involute and becomes the permanent kidneys. Metanephric development begins during the fifth week of gestation, and urine excretion is initiated at approximately the 10th week of gestation.

During fetal life, the kidneys are lobulated, but a lobular appearance is present even at birth. Thereafter, the external kidney surface becomes smooth as the kidney grows. It is becoming increasingly apparent that the number of nephrons endowed at birth has an important bearing on the susceptibility to hypertension and chronic kidney disease as adults.[2] Minimizing disruptions in fetal renal development may, indeed, be central to preventing kidney disease in adults.

Initially, the kidneys lie adjacent to each other in the pelvis, and the hilum of each faces ventrally (toward the anterior abdominal wall). As the trunk grows, the kidneys come to lie higher in the abdomen and farther apart. In addition, the hilum rotates almost 90 degrees. By 9 weeks of gestation, the kidneys attain their adult positions. Malrotation and ectopic kidney location are caused by abnormal rotation and ascent, respectively. Failure of the kidneys to migrate upward from the pelvis results in the formation of pelvic kidneys. These kidneys are positioned close to each other and may fuse in some cases to give rise to a *pancake kidney*. In approximately 1 in 500 persons, the inferior poles fuse before ascent, thus generating a *horseshoe kidney*.

---

### KEY POINTS

- The met anephros develops at approximately 5 weeks.
- Urine excretion starts at approximately 10 weeks.

---

### KEY POINTS

- Failure to migrate up (cephalad) from the pelvic location in ectopic kidneys.
- Pancake kidney and horseshoe kidney result from fusion of the fetal kidneys.

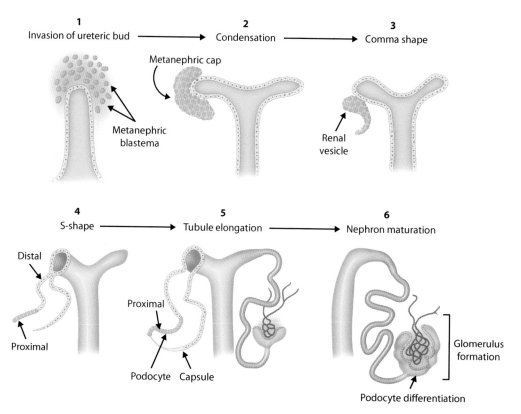

**1**
Invasion of ureteric bud → **2** Condensation → **3** Comma shape

Metanephric cap

Metanephric blastema

Renal vesicle

**4**
S-shape → **5** Tubule elongation → **6** Nephron maturation

Distal

Proximal

Proximal

Podocyte   Capsule

Glomerulus formation

Podocyte differentiation

Figure 2.1 Stages of renal morphogenesis. Ureteric bud outgrowth from the wolffian duct is modulated by factors secreted by the metanephric blastema and the mesoderm surrounding the duct (1). Morphologic intermediates formed during nephrogenesis consist of condensation of the metanephric cap around the ureteric bud branch (2) renal vesicle comma shape (3), S shape (4), elongation of the tubule (5), invasion of blood vessels into the glomeruli, and formation of the glomerular corpuscle (6). (Modified from Chau YY, Hastie ND. The role of Wt1 in regulating mesenchyme in cancer, development, and tissue homeostasis. Trends Genet. 2012;28:515–24.)

At the earliest stage of kidney formation, the renal arteries are derived as branches of the common iliac arteries. As the metanephroi ascend, they receive branches from the distal aorta, then from the abdominal aorta. Normally, the distal branches disappear, and the abdominal branches become the permanent renal arteries. Variations in the arterial supply are common and reflect the changing nature of the arterial supply during fetal life. Although most persons have a single renal artery, approximately 25% have two to four.[3]

## METANEPHRIC DEVELOPMENT

Metanephric induction occurs at 5 weeks of gestation, at a time when the ureteric bud is induced to grow out from the wolffian (mesonephric) duct and invade the metanephric blastema. The blastema is composed of a heterogeneous population of cells, including mesenchymal cells that eventually transform into epithelial, glomerular, tubular progenitors, and stromal cells that support the formation of glomerular and tubular elements.

Under the direction of growth factor–mediated signals elaborated by the metanephric mesenchyme, the ureteric bud undergoes repetitive growth and branching events, a

process termed branching morphogenesis. In general, each branch divides to form two daughter branches that create generations of ureteric bud branches. In reciprocal fashion, the ureteric bud induces the mesenchyme adjacent to each bud tip to develop through a stereotypic sequence of structures consisting of mesenchymal aggregates (known as cap mesenchyme), renal vesicles, and comma-shaped and S-shaped bodies (Figure 2.1). At the distal end of the S-shaped body, a layer of epithelial cells gives rise to future podocytes. The basal aspect of these cells rests on the future glomerular basement membrane. A cleft between the podocytes becomes the glomerulus and the proximal tubule.

### KEY POINTS

- Under the influence of growth factors from metanephric mesenchyme, the ureteric bud undergoes programmed and repetitive divisions or branching morphogenesis.
- Ureteric branching provides the biologic architecture for nephrogenesis.

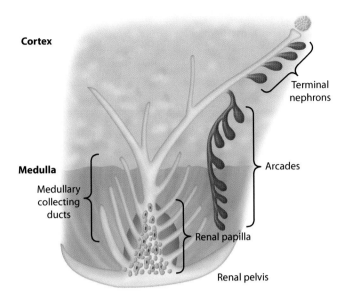

**Figure 2.2** Patterning of the kidney into a cortex and medulla. The cortex consists of nephrons with short and long tubular (Henle) loops and collecting ducts that connect to the distal tubules. The medulla consists of the tubules from long loops of Henle and collecting ducts that terminate in the papillae.

Endothelial and mesangial cells migrate into this cleft. Each branch of the ureteric bud and its daughter collecting ducts induce formation of one nephron.

The formation of 15 generations of ureteric buds and collecting ducts induces an identical number of nephrons. The remaining nephrons are formed by induction of approximately 10 nephrons around the stem of an elongating ureteric bud and collecting duct branch that are initially formed. The connecting tubules of each of these nephrons then attach to the stem of the collecting duct branch in series to form an arcade (Figure 2.2). After formation of arcades, the terminal branch of the 15th generation begins to elongate and to develop a succession of ampullae that also induce nephrons on each side of the terminal branch. During the latter stages of kidney development, tubular segments formed from the first five generations of ureteric bud branching undergo remodeling to form the pelvis and calyces.

## SEQUENCING MOLECULAR EVENTS

During embryogenesis, formation of tissues is controlled by one or more morphogenetic pathways that consist of a hierarchy of control elements integrated within a circuit. An ever-expanding body of knowledge of embryonic renal development has been generated by the study of experimental models, most notably in the mouse, which has kidney development closely resembling that in humans.

Nephron development is initiated by the activity of one or more genes that control the behavior of target cells. These target cells are either those in which the genes are themselves expressed or the neighboring cells. After receiving appropriate signals, the target cells are instructed to engage in a repertoire of activities that include proliferation, programmed cell death (apoptosis), movement, shape change, or alteration in their interactions with extracellular matrices. One or more of these changes in cell behavior will influence the manner in which a particular three-dimensional structure (e.g., a collecting duct) is constructed. In turn, changes in cell behavior and structural architecture affect inducing gene expression, thereby creating a feedback mechanism.

## URETERIC BUD OUTGROWTH

Outgrowth of the ureteric bud from the wolffian duct performs a critical role in nephrogenesis. Development of the ureteric bud from the wolffian duct is controlled by genes expressed in both in the wolffian duct and the metanephric blastema.[4] These genes function within a morphogenetic pathway and tightly regulate the pathways that promote or inhibit ureteric bud development and eventual nephrogenesis.

### KEY POINTS

Key genes regulating ureteric bud growth are:

- *Pax2*: transcription factor
- *Eya1*: transcription factor
- *GDNF*: growth factor
- *RET*: the GDNF receptor

Genes expressed in the metanephric blastema that are required for ureteric bud outgrowth include the transcription factors *Pax2* and *Eya1*, the secreted growth factor glia-derived neurotrophic factor (GDNF), and RET, which is the GNDF cell surface receptor. Genes that function upstream of *Gdnf* either limit or promote its expression, thereby precisely controlling ureteric bud outgrowth. *Pax2* and *Eya1* are positive regulators of *Gdnf* and promote its expression.[5,6] Homozygous deficiency of *Pax2*, *Eya1*, *Gdnf*, or *Ret* in mice causes failure of ureteric bud outgrowth and results in bilateral renal agenesis or severe renal dysgenesis, depending on the gene involved. Identical phenotypes have also been observed in mice deficient in heparan sulfate 2-sulfotransferase, a finding demonstrating a critical role for heparan sulfate in mediating interactions between the ureteric bud and the metanephric blastema.[7]

*Foxc1* (also known as *Mf1*), a forkhead/winged helix transcription factor, is expressed during embryonic development in a metanephric domain similar to that of *Gdnf*. Homozygous *Foxc1*-null mutant mice exhibit renal abnormalities consisting of ureteric duplication, hydroureter, and ectopic ureteric buds, findings suggesting that *Foxc1* negatively controls the domain of *Gdnf* expression.[8] BMP4 (bone

## KEY POINTS

- BMP4, expressed in the mesenchymal cells surrounding the wolffian duct, exerts an inhibitory control by regulating the site from which the ureteric bud would emerge.
- BMP4 prevents development of ectopic ureteric bud sites from emerging.

morphogenetic protein 4) is another inhibitory gene that is expressed in the mesenchymal cells surrounding the wolffian duct. By inhibiting ectopic ureteric budding, *BMP4* regulates the site in the wolffian duct from where the ureteric bud emerges.[9] *Bmp4* heterozygous null mutant mice develop renal and ureteric abnormalities, such as hypodysplastic or dysplastic kidneys, hydroureter, ectopic ureterovesical junction, and double collecting system.[9]

During kidney development, the site of ureteric bud outgrowth is invariant, precisely positioned, and the number of outgrowths is limited to one. It is believed that outgrowth of a single ureteric bud at the appropriate position is controlled by mesenchymal factors that restrict the location of ureteric bud outgrowth (Figure 2.3). Furthermore, the site of ureteric bud outgrowth from the wolffian duct determines the final site of the ureter orifice in the bladder. A more caudal or cranial budding from the wolffian duct can lead to a defective ureterovesical valve, urinary outflow obstruction, and aberrant insertion of the ureteric bud into the metanephric mesenchyme that can result in renal dysplasia.

## COLLECTING DUCT BRANCHING AND ELONGATION

The relatively fixed number and spatial pattern of collecting ducts in the mature kidney suggest that ureteric bud branching morphogenesis is tightly regulated. In mice,

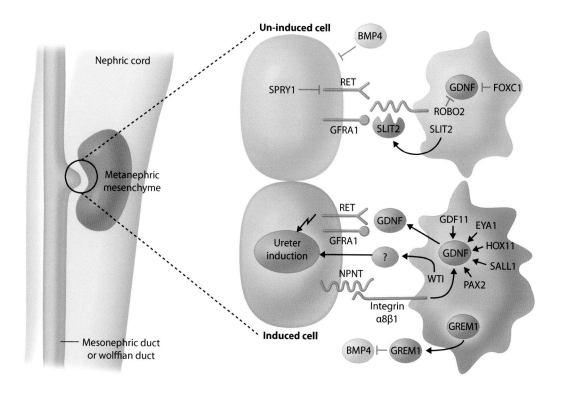

Figure 2.3 Gene products that control cellular events and induction of the ureteric bud in the wolffian duct. Mesenchymal cells at the caudal end of the nephrogenic cord (light blue cell) express various factors that activate expression of glial-derived neurotrophic factor (GDNF). In addition, mesenchymal cells release gremlin-1 (GREM1), an inhibitor of bone morphogenetic protein (BMP) signaling, and other still unidentified factors. Released GDNF binds to RET and GDNF-family receptor $\alpha_1$ (GFRA1) receptors that are on the epithelial cells of the mesonephric duct (wolffian duct). The combination of these signals induces ureteric budding. Mesenchymal cells at a more rostral level (dark blue cell) express forkhead box protein C1 (FOXC1), slit homologue 2 (SLIT2), and its receptor roundabout homologue 2 (ROBO2), leading to a repression of GDNF. In epithelial cells of the mesonephric duct, the tyrosine kinase inhibitor sprouty 1 (*Spry1*) suppresses RET activation. Finally, BMP4 also inhibits ureter outgrowth. EYA1, eyes-absent homologue 1; GDF11, growth differentiation factor-11; HOX11, homeobox protein 11; NPNT, nephronectin; WT1, Wilms tumor transcription factor. (From Schedl A. Renal abnormalities and their developmental origin. Nat Rev Genet. 2007;8:791–802.)

fewer ureteric bud branches are formed in the posterior than in the anterior portion of the kidney. This asymmetry is probably controlled, in part, by *Hox* genes, originally described as regulators of body segmentation in fruit flies.[10] In addition to their critical roles during ureteric bud outgrowth, GDNF and its cognate receptors stimulate ureteric bud branching. In mice, genetic deficiency of *Gdnf* and *Ret* causes decreased ureteric bud branching. RET expression is controlled by members of the retinoic acid receptor (RAR) family of transcription factors. These members, including RAR α and RAR β$_2$, are expressed in stromal cells surrounding *Ret*-expressing ureteric bud branch tips.[11,12] Mice deficient in these receptors exhibit a decreased number of ureteric bud branches and diminished expression of *Ret*.

---

## KEY POINTS

- GDNF plays a critical role in ureteric bud formation, as well as branching of the bud.
- Inhibitory signals and positive gene signals are crucial for programmed ureteric bud branching and renal morphogenesis.

---

Two members of the fibroblast growth factor (FGF) family of signaling peptides stimulate collecting duct morphogenesis in mice. Homozygous null mutations in the *Fgf7* gene result in a reduced number of ureteric bud branches and underdevelopment of the renal papilla.[13] Mice with a homozygous null mutation in *Fgf10* also have kidneys that are smaller than those in wild-type mice and exhibit a decreased number of medullary collecting ducts, medullary dysplasia, and dilatation of the renal pelvis.[14] Thus, a repertoire of signaling pathways promotes renal branching morphogenesis.

Renal branching morphogenesis is also regulated by inhibitory signaling pathways. In mice, BMP signaling through their activin-like kinase (ALK) receptors inhibits branching morphogenesis. Targeted overexpression of ALK3 in the ureteric bud lineage decreases branching morphogenesis and is associated with decreased nephron formation.[15] Deficiency of BMPs and their signaling intermediates is associated with increased branching.[16] Thus, integration of signals from these diverse and opposing pathways by ureteric bud and collecting duct cells controls branching behavior.

Elongation of collecting ducts is noted during later stages of renal development. This is accomplished by cell divisions that are aligned with the long axis of the duct, a process termed oriented cell division. Members of the WNT family of secreted proteins, specifically WNT9b and WNT7b, are required for collecting duct elongation and formation of the medulla and papillae.[17,18] Collecting ducts deficient in WNT9b dilate during embryonic development because of loss of alignment of the mitotic spindle with the long axis

of the tubule, and they develop into large cysts postnatally. Similar abnormalities in the medulla are observed in mice lacking WNT7b.

## FORMATION OF THE CALYCES AND PELVIS

Patterning of the collecting system to form the calyces and pelvis is controlled by sonic hedgehog (SHH), by members of the BMP family, and by angiotensin and its cell surface receptors. SHH is a secreted growth factor that controls cell determination and proliferation in many developmental contexts. In mice, *Shh* deficiency interferes with formation of the smooth muscle layer surrounding the upper ureter and causes dilatation of the pelvis.[19] Loss of *Bmp4* expression appears to be a pathogenetic mechanism in the genesis of hydronephrosis in these mice. Consistent with these observations, a subset of mice with spontaneous and engineered mutations in *Bmp4* and *Bmp5* demonstrates dilatation of the ureters and collecting system (ureterohydronephrosis), and ureteral bifurcation.[20,21] Mutations in the genes encoding components of the renin-angiotensin axis, best known for their role in controlling renal hemodynamics, also cause abnormalities in the development of the renal calyces and pelvis.

---

## KEY POINT

Sonic hedgehog (SHH) and members of the BMP gene family control the patterning of the renal collecting system: the calyces and the pelvis.

---

Mice that are homozygous null for angiotensin receptor-1 (*Agtr1*) demonstrate atrophy of the papillae and underlying medulla.[9] The underlying defect appears to be a decrease in proliferation of the smooth muscle cell layer lining the pelvis that results in decreased thickness of this layer in the proximal ureter. Mutational inactivation of *Agtr2* results in a range of anomalies including vesicoureteral reflux (VUR), a duplex kidney, renal ectopia, ureteropelvic junction stenosis, ureterovesical junction stenosis, renal dysplasia, renal hypoplasia, multicystic dysplastic kidney (MCDK), or renal agenesis.[22] Null mice demonstrate a decreased rate of apoptosis of the cells around the ureter, a finding suggesting that *Agtr2* plays a role in modeling of the ureter. Together, these studies highlight the role of smooth muscle patterning in the formation of the pelvic-ureteric junction.

## FORMATION OF GLOMERULAR AND TUBULAR PRECURSORS

The development of metanephric derivatives begins when the blastema is rescued from apoptosis and is induced to proliferate coincident with the invasion of the ureteric bud. Expression of the Wilms Tumor 1 (Wt1) gene product, a transcription factor, is critical in maintaining viability of the metanephric blastema at this early stage of development.[23] With the invasion of the ureteric bud, the blastemal cells differentiate along distinct pathways. Cells adjacent to the ureteric bud tips aggregate and begin to display morphologic and molecular features characteristic of nephron epithelial cells, a process termed mesenchymal to epithelial transformation (MET). Other metanephric mesenchyme cells, which are stromal cells, give rise to endothelial and mesangial cells and interstitial fibroblasts.

---

### KEY POINT

Morphologic and molecular transformation of mesenchymal cells adjacent to the ureteric bud into various epithelial components of the glomeruli is termed mesenchymal-to-epithelial transformation (MET).

---

## MAINTAINING PROGENITOR CELL POOL

A pool of self-renewing progenitor cells gives rise to nephrons and controls transformation of metanephric mesenchyme cells into cells with specific differentiated characteristics. The molecular mechanisms that control maintenance of this pool are being defined at an ever-increasing level of detail. Before and after invasion of the metanephric mesenchyme by the ureteric bud cells, expression of genes including Wt1, Fgf8 and its cognate receptors, and Bmp7 is required to maintain cell viability.[23–25] In the absence of these gene products, metanephric mesenchyme cells undergo apoptosis, and very few, if any, nephrons form.

The cells that can take part in the formation of any nephron progenitor structure—glomerulus, proximal tubule, and distal tubule—are marked by expression of Six2, a transcription factor. SIX2-positive cells are then further specified to become differentiated cells in proximal or distal nephron segments. Analysis of gene expression in these segments has identified a large number of genes, the expression of which is restricted to either segment.[26,27] Some of these genes are functionally required to define the identity of these segments. For example, distal segments require the expression of Brn1, a transcription factor.[28] In contrast, expression of Lhx1 and NOTCH family members is required for establishment of the proximal tubule.[29,30]

## PODOCYTE AND ENDOTHELIAL DIFFERENTIATION

Several classes of genes are required for formatting podocytes and for directing the migration of endothelial cells into the glomerulus. As nephrogenesis proceeds, Wt1 expression becomes restricted to the podocyte lineage. Transcription of Wt1 results in the formation of multiple isoforms generated by alternative splicing. Mutations in Wt1 that prevent the generation of certain splice forms result in formation of abnormal glomeruli, thereby implicating Wt1 in glomerulogenesis.[31] Lmx1b is a transcription factor mutated in patients with nail-patella syndrome and is expressed in podocytes.[32] Mutational inactivation in mice decreases formation of foot processes and decreases expression of the $\alpha_3$ and $\alpha_4$ chains of type IV collagen. Pod1 is a basic helix-loop-helix class transcription factor that is expressed in podocytes in S-shaped bodies. Pod1 deficiency in mice results in arrest at the single capillary loop stage of glomerular development.[33]

---

### KEY POINTS

- Podocyte and vascular endothelium formation in the glomeruli is controlled by multiple genes.
- The Wt1 gene plays an important role in glomerulogenesis.

---

Kreisler (MafB), a leucine zipper class transcription factor, is expressed in podocytes. Kreisler deficiency in mice results in failure of foot process attachment to the basement membrane.[34] The $\alpha_3$ chain of $\alpha_3\beta_1$ integrin is required for formation of foot processes in mice.[35] Podocalyxin is a sulfated cell surface sialomucin that is expressed on the surface of podocytes. In a podocalyxin-deficient state, foot process and slit diaphragm assembly is abrogated.[36] Podocyte-derived vascular endothelial growth factor A (VEGF-A) and Notch 2 play central roles in directing endothelial cell migration into glomeruli. Inactivation of VEGF-A in podocytes by genetic means in mice disrupts glomerular capillary formation.[37] Similarly, inactivation of Notch2, a member of a family of cell determination genes, results in a similar phenotype.[38]

## GENE FUNCTIONS AND DEVELOPMENTAL RENAL DISORDERS

The human and mouse genome projects have been complementary in generating a rapid expansion of our knowledge of human developmental biology. Although the diversity of human phenotypes projects existence of more than 80 loci associated with renal dysplasia, to date mutations in a much smaller number of genes have been implicated in pathogenesis.[39] The functions of a subset of these genes have been elucidated in genetic mouse models that provide critical insights into the molecular control of normal and abnormal renal development (Table 2.1). Some of the disorders described here are also discussed in Chapters 1 and 46.

Table 2.1  Human gene mutations exhibiting defects in renal morphogenesis

| Primary disease | Gene | Kidney phenotype | References |
|---|---|---|---|
| Alagille syndrome | JAGGED1 | Cystic dysplasia | 49 |
| Apert syndrome | FGFR2 | Hydronephrosis | 50 |
| Beckwith-Wiedemann syndrome | p57KIP2 | Medullary dysplasia | 51 |
| Branchio-oto-renal (BOR) syndrome | EYA1 | Unilateral or bilateral agenesis or dysplasia, hypoplasia, collecting system abnormalities | 52 |
| Campomelic dysplasia | SOX9 | Dysplasia, hydronephrosis | 53 |
| Fraser syndrome | FRAS1 | Agenesis, dysplasia | 54 |
| Hyoparathyroidism, sensorineural deafness, and renal anomalies (HDR) syndrome | GATA3 | Dysplasia | 55 |
| Kallmann syndrome | KAL1 | Agenesis | 56 |
| Mammary-ulnar syndrome | TBX3 | Dysplasia | 57 |
| Meckel Gruber syndrome | MKS1 MKS3 NPHP6 NPHP8 | Cystic dysplasia | 58 |
| Nephronophthisis | CEP290, GLIS2, RPGRIP1L, NEK8, SDCCAG8, TMEM67, TTC21B | Cystic dysplasia | 59 |
| Okihiro syndrome | SALL4 | Unilateral agenesis, VUR, malrotation, cross fused ectopia | 60 |
| Pallister Hall syndrome | GLI3 | Agenesis, dysplasia, hydronephrosis | 61 |
| Renal coloboma syndrome | PAX2 | Hypoplasia, VUR | 62 |
| Renal hypodysplasia, isolated | TCF2, PAX2, EYA1, SIX1, SIX2, SALL1, RET, BMP4, DSTYK | Hypoplasia, VUR | 63–67 |
| Renal tubular dysgenesis | Renin, angiotensinogen, ACE, AT1 receptor | Tubular dysgenesis | 68 |
| Rubinstein-Taybi syndrome | CREBBP | Agenesis, hypoplasia | 69 |
| Simpson-Golabi-Behmel syndrome | GPC3 | Medullary dysplasia | 70 |
| Smith-Lemli-Opitz syndrome | DHCR7 | Hypoplasia, cysts, aplasia | 71 |
| Townes-Brock syndrome | SALL1 | Hypodysplasia, VUR | 72 |
| Zellweger syndrome | PEX1 | Cystic dysplasia | 73 |

ACE, angiotensin-converting enzyme; AT1 receptor, angiotensin I receptor; VUR, vesicoureteral reflux.

## PAX2

Heterozygous mutations in *PAX2* are found in patients with the renal coloboma syndrome (Online Mendelian Inheritance in Man [OMIM] 120330) that is characterized by renal hypoplasia and VUR. Heterozygous *Pax2* mutations in mice result in a similar phenotype.[40] Investigation of *Pax2* suggests that it functions in the ureteric bud to promote cell proliferation and inhibit apoptosis.[41] These results support a model that proposes that *Pax2* controls the number of ureteric bud branches, thereby determining the number of nephrons formed.

## EYA1

*EYA1*, a transcription factor, is mutated in patients with branchio-oto-renal (BOR) syndrome (OMIM 113650) and with unilateral or bilateral renal agenesis, or dysplasia.[42] In mice, the spatial pattern of *Eya1* expression overlaps that of *Gdnf* at the time of ureteric bud outgrowth. Because biallelic inactivation of *Eya1* causes renal agenesis and abrogates *Gdnf* expression, *Eya1* is thought to function upstream of *Gdnf* to control ureteric bud outgrowth.

## SALL1

*SALL1*, a transcription factor, is expressed in the metanephric mesenchyme at the time of induction by the ureteric bud. Mutations in *SALL1* exist in patients with Townes-Brock syndrome (OMIM 107480). In *Sall1*-deficient mice, ureteric bud outgrowth occurs, but the bud fails to invade the metanephric blastema, with resulting renal agenesis. This failure of invasion appears to be caused by a *Sall1*-dependent signal rather than the competence of the metanephric blastema to undergo induction.[43]

## GLI3

The gene encoding GLI3 is mutated in patients with Pallister-Hall syndrome (OMIM 146510) and renal dysplasia. GLI3 is one member among a family of GLI proteins that control gene transcription. Their actions are controlled by SHH. All *GLI3* mutations identified to date result in the expression of a truncated protein that functions as a transcriptional repressor. Investigations in mice provide insight into the biologic significance of this repressor form of GLI3. During inductive stages of kidney development, GLI3 repressor represses the transcription of GLI1 and GLI2, renal patterning genes including *Pax2* and *Sall1,* and genes that modulate the cell cycle (cyclin D1 and N-Myc), resulting in renal aplasia or severe dysplasia.[44] During later stages of renal development, GLI3 repressor plays cell lineage-specific roles; it is required for ureteric branching but abrogates coordinated contraction of the ureter by deleterious effects on renal pacemaker cells.[45,46]

## Glypican-3 and p57$^{KIP2}$

Investigation of the genes mutant in two human overgrowth syndromes, Simpson–Golabi–Behmel syndrome (OMIM 312870) and Beckwith-Wiedemann syndrome (OMIM 13650), provides novel insight into the pathogenesis of medullary renal dysplasia. Patients with Simpson–Golabi–Behmel syndrome have mutations in glypican-3, a glycosyl-phosphotidylinositol (GPI)–linked cell surface heparan sulfate proteoglycan. The pathogenesis of renal medullary dysplasia in *Gpc3*-deficient mice involves massive medullary collecting duct apoptosis preceded by increased ureteric bud proliferation.[47] Thus, *Gpc3* controls collecting duct cell number and survival. A role for control of the cell cycle in the pathogenesis of medullary renal dysplasia is further supported by the finding of medullary renal dysplasia in mice and humans (Beckwith-Wiedemann syndrome) with inactivating mutations in *p57*$^{KIP2}$, a cell cycle regulatory gene that encodes a cyclin-dependent kinase inhibitor.[48]

Table 2.1 lists clinical syndromes that feature renal anomalies and genes associated with these syndromes.[49-73] Identification of genes such as these has provided a basis for screening children with sporadic cases of renal hypodysplasia.[63,64,67,74,75] These investigations have identified mutations in genes including *TCF2, PAX2, EYA1, SIX1, SIX2, SALL1, RET, BMP4, and DSTYK*. Remarkably, mutations in genes previously identified in the context of a particular clinical syndrome have also been identified in patients with no evidence of that syndrome, other than the presence of a renal malformation.

Advances in genetics have generated a revolution in our understanding of congenital malformations of the kidney. Although it has been accepted that an association exists among poorly developed kidneys, renal dysfunction, and urologic abnormalities, a generation ago it was widely held that some sort of obstructive process led to maldevelopment. The discovery of these genetic relationships has led to an understanding that maldevelopment results from failure of programmed genetic control, with the likelihood that VUR and urinary tract obstruction stem from the same failure. As a result, we have come to understand that such disorders may demonstrate familial predisposition that can have clinical relevance.

The three categories of developmental abnormalities that can occur, separately or in concert, are renal hypoplasia, renal dysplasia, and abnormal development of the lower urinary tract.

## HYPOPLASIA

Renal hypoplasia is characterized by a smaller than normal complement of nephrons in the kidney. The nephron structure and the overall renal architecture are well maintained. Hypoplasia can affect one or both kidneys. In hypoplasia, an abnormality in epithelial-mesenchymal interactions leads to decreased or abnormal branching of the ureter. Unless it is associated with other malformations, renal hypoplasia can be asymptomatic. Hypoplasia is often discovered as an incidental finding during an abdominal sonogram or other imaging studies, in which a smaller than normal kidney is detected. Decreased renal function and chronic kidney disease can be seen in patients with severe cases with bilateral disease. Renal hypoplasia has been reported to be a predisposing condition for hypertension later in life.[2]

## MULTICYSTIC DYSPLASTIC KIDNEY

MCDK is reported to be the second most common renal anomaly diagnosed by prenatal ultrasound examination, with a reported prevalence of 1 in 3640 births.[76] MCDK can manifest as a flank mass in newborn infants. Renal ultrasound evaluation shows a large, cystic, nonreniform structure located in the renal fossa. The characteristic and diagnostic finding is absence of any function demonstrated by radionuclide scans. VUR in the contralateral normal kidney is the most common associated urinary tract abnormality and has been reported in approximately 25% of cases.[77] Hypertension can be seen some patients but appears to be less common than previously assumed.[77] Wilms tumor has been reported in patients with MCDK. It has been argued that these cases of apparent malignant degeneration in MCDK may actually result from nephrogenic rests.

Gradual reduction in renal size and eventual resolution of the mass of the MCDK are common. At 2 years, an involution in size by ultrasound examination has been noted in up to 60% of the affected kidneys.[78] Complete disappearance of the MCDK can occur in a minority of patients (3% to 4%) by the time of birth and in 20% to 25% by 2 years. Increase in the size of MCDK can be seen in some cases. The contralateral kidney shows compensatory hypertrophy by ultrasound evaluation.

Management of patients with MCDK has shifted from routine nephrectomy in the past to observation and medical therapy. Because of the risk of associated anomalies in the contralateral kidney, the possibility of VUR should be considered, and clinical follow-up for evolution of hypertension is advised. Renal ultrasound is generally recommended at an interval of 3 months for the first year of life and then every 6 months up to involution of the mass, or at least for up to 5 years. Compensatory hypertrophy of the contralateral kidney is expected and should be followed on ultrasound evaluations. Medical therapy is usually effective in treating hypertension in most patients, but nephrectomy may be curative in resistant cases.

## RENAL DYSPLASIA

Renal dysplasia is characterized by the presence of malformed and disorganized tissue elements, a decreased number of nephrons, collecting ducts surrounded by muscular rings (Figure 2.4), and elements of aberrant development, such as cartilage, or even calcified tissue. Often, dysplasia is accompanied by hypoplasia of the kidney as well. Abnormalities of renal function and development of chronic kidney disease should be expected in patients with severe bilateral renal dysplasia or those with additional urinary tract malformations, such as obstruction. Potter syndrome, which is characterized by oligohydramnios, pulmonary hypoplasia, renal failure, low-set ears, and a beaked nose, may be observed in patients with severe cases of renal dysplasia.

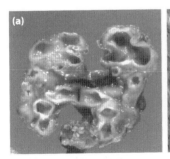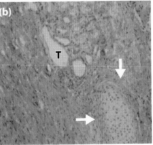

Figure 2.4 Renal dysplasia. **(a)** A cut section of dysplastic kidney with malformed collecting system, lack of well-patterned renal parenchyma, and absence of corticomedullary differentiation. **(b)** Microscopic section of the kidney from the patient demonstrating malformed tubules. Some tubules are widely dilated (T). Arrows show cartilage within the renal parenchyma. (Figure courtesy of Arthur Cohen, MD.)

## SUMMARY

This chapter summarizes the major morphologic features of the developing and mature kidney. The concept of morphogenetic pathways is presented as a means to understand how genes control cellular events that, in turn, build three-dimensional structures. Genetic pathways that control normal renal branching morphogenesis are assuming an important role in understanding nephrogenesis and are likely to be explored in detail. An understanding of genetic mutations associated with renal hypoplasia and dysplasia has begun to appear, and it provides a link to the congenital abnormalities of the kidney and urinary tract (CAKUT) malformations complex. An understanding of the genetics of renal development also highlights the close developmental path that the urinary tract and the kidneys take in their mutual organogenesis. All these discoveries provide a window into our understanding of the pathogenic role played by genetic mutations in clinical disorders of the kidney and the urinary tract encountered by pediatric nephrologists.

## ACKNOWLEDGMENTS

This work was supported by grants from the Canadian Institutes of Health Research, Kidney Foundation of Canada, and Canada Research Chairs Program (to NDR).

## REFERENCES

1. Warady BA, Chadha V. Chronic kidney disease in children: The global perspective. Pediatr Nephrol. 2007;22:1999–2009.
2. Keller G, Zimmer G, Mall G, et al. Nephron number in patients with primary hypertension. N Engl J Med. 2003;348:101–8.
3. Moore KL, Persaud TVN. The Developing Human. 7th ed. Philadelphia: WB Saunders; 2003.
4. Piscione TD, Rosenblum ND. The molecular control of renal branching morphogenesis: Current knowledge and emerging insights. Differentiation. 2002;70:227–46.
5. Brophy PD, Ostrom L, Lang KM, et al. Regulation of ureteric bud outgrowth by Pax2-dependent activation of the glial derived neurotrophic factor gene. Development. 2001;128:4747–56.
6. Xu P-X, Adams J, Peters H, et al. Eya1-deficient mice lack ears and kidneys and show abnormal apoptosis of organ primordia. Nat Genet. 1999;23:113–7.
7. Bullock SL, Fletcher JM, Beddington RSP, et al. Renal agenesis in mice homozygous for a gene trap mutation in the gene encoding heparan sulfate 2-sulfotransferase. Genes Dev. 1998;12:1894–906.

8. Kume T, Deng K, Hogan BLM. Murine forkhead/winged helix genes Foxc1 (Mf1) and Foxc2 (Mfh1) are required for the early organogenesis of the kidney and urinary tract. Development. 2000;127:1387–95.

9. Miyazaki Y, Oshima K, Fogo A, et al. Bone morphogenetic protein 4 regulates the budding site and elongation of the mouse ureter. J Clin Invest. 2000;105:863–73.

10. Patterson LT, Pembaur M, Potter SS. Hoxa11 and Hoxd11 regulate branching morphogenesis of the ureteric bud in the developing kidney. Development. 2001;128:2153–61.

11. Mendelsohn C, Batourina E, Fung S, et al. Stromal cells mediate retinoid-dependent functions essential for renal development. Development. 1999;126:1139–48.

12. Batourina E, Gim S, Bello N, et al. Vitamin A controls epithelial/mesenchymal interactions through Ret expression. Nat Genet. 2001;27:74–8.

13. Qiao J, Uzzo R, Obara-Ishihara T, et al. FGF-7 modulates ureteric bud growth and nephron number in the developing kidney. Development. 1999;126:547–54.

14. Ohuchi H, Kimura S, Watamoto M, et al. Involvement of fibroblast growth factor (FGF)18-FGF8 signaling in specification of left-right asymmetry and brain and limb development of the chick embryo. Mech Dev. 2000;95:55–66.

15. Hu MC, Piscione TD, Rosenblum ND. Elevated Smad1/beta-catenin molecular complexes and renal medullary cystic dysplasia in ALK3 transgenic mice. Development. 2003;130:2753–66.

16. Hartwig S, Hu MC, Cella C, et al. Glypican-3 modulates inhibitory Bmp2-Smad signaling to control renal development in vivo. Mech Dev. 2005;122:928–38.

17. Karner CM, Chirumamilla R, Aoki S, et al. Wnt9b signaling regulates planar cell polarity and kidney tubule morphogenesis. Nat Genet. 2009;41:793–9.

18. Yu J, Carroll TJ, Rajagopal J, et al. A Wnt7b-dependent pathway regulates the orientation of epithelial cell division and establishes the cortico-medullary axis of the mammalian kidney. Development. 2009;136:161–71.

19. Yu J, Carroll TJ, McMahon AP. Sonic hedgehog regulates proliferation and differentiation of mesenchymal cells in the mouse metanephric kidney. Development. 2002;129:5301–12.

20. Miyazaki Y, Oshima K, Fogo A, et al. Bone morphogenetic protein 4 regulates the budding site and elongation of the mouse ureter. J Clin Invest. 2000;105:863–73.

21. Green MC. Mechanism of the pleiotropic effects of the short-ear mutant gene in the mouse. J Exp Zool. 1968;176:129–50.

22. Nishimura H, Yerkes E, Hohenfellner K, et al. Role of the angiotensin type 2 receptor gene in congenital anomalies of the kidney and urinary tract, CAKUT, of mice and men. Mol Cell. 1999;3:1–10.

23. Kreidberg JA, Sariola H, Loring JM, et al. WT-1 is required for early kidney development. Cell. 1993;74:679–91.

24. Grieshammer U, Cebrian C, Ilagan R, et al. FGF8 is required for cell survival at distinct stages of nephrogenesis and for regulation of gene expression in nascent nephrons. Development. 2005;132:3847–57.

25. Dudley AT, Lyons KM, Robertson EJ. A requirement for bone morphogenetic protein-7 during development of the mammalian kidney and eye. Genes Dev. 1995;9:2795–807.

26. Kobayashi A, Valerius MT, Mugford JW, et al. Six2 defines and regulates a multipotent self-renewing nephron progenitor population throughout mammalian kidney development. Cell Stem Cell. 2008;3:169–81.

27. Brunskill EW, Aronow BJ, Georgas K, et al. Atlas of gene expression in the developing kidney at microanatomic resolution. Dev Cell. 2008;15:781–91.

28. Nakai S, Sugitani Y, Sato H, et al. Crucial roles of Brn1 in distal tubule formation and function in mouse kidney. Development. 2003;130:4751–9.

29. Kobayashi A, Kwan KM, Carroll TJ, et al. Distinct and sequential tissue-specific activities of the LIM-class homeobox gene Lim1 for tubular morphogenesis during kidney development. Development. 2005;132:2809–23.

30. Cheng HT, Kim M, Valerius MT, et al. Notch2, but not Notch1, is required for proximal fate acquisition in the mammalian nephron. Development. 2007;134:801–11.

31. Hammes A, Guo JK, Lutsch G, et al. Two splice variants of the Wilms' tumor 1 gene have distinct functions during sex determination and nephron formation. Cell. 2001;106:319–29.

32. Chen H, Lun Y, Ovchinnikov D, et al. Limb and kidney defects in Lmx1B mutant mice suggest an involvement of LMX1B in human nail patella syndrome. Nat Genet. 1998;19:51–5.

33. Quaggin SE, Schwartz L, Cui S, et al. The basic-helix-loop-helix protein pod1 is critically important for kidney and lung organogenesis. Development. 1999;126:5771–83.

34. Sadl V, Jin F, Yu J, et al. The mouse Kreisler (Krml1/MafB) segmentation gene is required for differentiation of glomerular visceral epithelial cells. Dev Biol. 2002;249:16–29.

35. Kreidberg JA, Donovan MJ, Goldstein SL, et al. Alpha 3 beta 1 integrin has a crucial role in kidney and lung organogenesis. Development. 1996;122:3537–47.

36. Doyonnas R, Kershaw DB, Duhme C, et al. Anuria, omphalocele, and perinatal lethality in mice lacking the CD34-related protein podocalyxin. J Exp Med. 2001;194:13–27.

37. Eremina V, Sood M, Haigh J, et al. Glomerular-specific alterations of VEGF-A expression lead to distinct congenital and acquired renal diseases. J Clin Invest. 2003;111:707–16.

38. McCright B, Gao X, Shen L, et al. Defects in development of the kidney, heart and eye vasculature in mice homozygous for a hypomorphic Notch2 mutation. Development. 2001;128:491–502.

39. Reidy KJ, Rosenblum ND. Cell and molecular biology of kidney development. Semin Nephrol. 2009;29:321–37.

40. Porteous S, Torban E, Cho N-P, et al. Primary renal hypoplasia in humans and mice with PAX2 mutations: Evidence of increased apoptosis in fetal kidneys of Pax2$^{1Neu}$ +/- mutant mice. Hum Mol Genet. 2000;9:1–11.

41. Dziarmaga A, Clark P, Stayner C, et al. Ureteric bud apoptosis and renal hypoplasia in transgenic PAX2-Bax fetal mice mimics the renal-coloboma syndrome. J Am Soc Nephrol. 2003;14:2767–74.

42. Abdelhak S, Kalatzis V, Heilig R, et al. A human homologue of the *Drosophila eyes absent* gene underlies branchio-oto-renal (BOR) syndrome and identifies a novel gene family. Nat Genet. 1997;15:157–64.

43. Nishinakamura R, Matsumoto Y, Nakao K, et al. Murine homolog of SALL1 is essential for ureteric bud invasion in kidney development. Development. 2001;128:3105–15.

44. Hu MC, Mo R, Bhella S, et al. GLI3-dependent transcriptional repression of Gli1, Gli2 and kidney patterning genes disrupts renal morphogenesis. Development. 2006;133:569–78.

45. Cain JE, Islam E, Haxho F, et al. GLI3 repressor controls nephron number via regulation of Wnt11 and Ret in ureteric tip cells. PLoS One. 2009;4:e7313–25.

46. Cain JE, Islam E, Haxho F, et al. GLI3 repressor controls functional development of the mouse ureter. J Clin Invest. 2011;121:1199–206.

47. Grisaru S, Cano-Gauci D, Tee J, et al. Glypican-3 modulates BMP- and FGF-mediated effects during renal branching morphogenesis. Dev Biol. 2001;230:31–46.

48. Zhang P, Liégeois NJ, Wong C, et al. Altered cell differentiation and proliferation in mice lacking p57$^{KIP2}$ indicates a role in Beckwith-Wiedemann syndrome. Nature. 1997;387:151–8.

49. Oda T, Elkahloun AG, Pike BL, et al. Mutations in the human Jagged1 gene are responsible for Alagille syndrome. Nat Genet. 1997;16:235–42.

50. Wilkie AOM, Slaney SF, Oldridge M, et al. Apert syndrome results from localised mutations of FGFR2 and is allelic with Crouzon syndrome. Nat Genet. 1996;9:165–72.

51. Hatada I, Ohashi H, Fukushima Y, et al. An imprinted gene p57$^{KIP2}$ is mutated in Beckwith-Wiedemann syndrome. Nat Genetics. 1996;14:171–3.

52. Chang EH, Menezes M, Meyer NC, et al. Branchio-oto-renal syndrome: The mutation spectrum in EYA1 and its phenotypic consequences. Hum Mutat. 2004;23:582–9.

53. Wagner T, Wirth J, Meyer J, et al. Autosomal sex reversal and compomelic dysplasia are caused by mutations in and around the SRY-related gene SOX9. Cell. 1994;79:1111–20.

54. McGregor L, Makela V, Darling SM, et al. Fraser syndrome and mouse blebbed phenotype caused by mutations in FRAS1/Fras1 encoding a putative extracellular matrix protein. Nat Genet. 2003;34:203–8.

55. Van Esch H, Groenen P, Nesbit MA, et al. GATA3 haplo-insufficiency causes human HDR syndrome. Nature. 2000;406:419–22.

56. Franco B, Guioli S, Pragliola A, et al. A gene deleted in Kallmann's syndrome shares homology with neural cell adhesion and axonal path-finding molecules. Nature. 1991;353:529–36.

57. Bamshad M, Lin RC, Law DJ, et al. Mutations in human TBX3 alter limb, apocrine and genital development in ulnar-mammary syndrome. Nat Genet. 1997;16:311–5.

58. Barker AR, Thomas R, Dawe HR. Meckel-Gruber syndrome and the role of primary cilia in kidney, skeleton and central nervous system development. Organogenesis. 2014;10:96–107.

59. Benzing T, Schermer B. Clinical spectrum and pathogenesis of nephronophthisis. Curr Opin Nephrol Hypertens. 2012;21:272–8.

60. Sakaki-Yumoto M, Kobayashi C, Sato A, et al. The murine homolog of SALL4, a causative gene in Okihiro syndrome, is essential for embryonic stem cell proliferation, and cooperates with Sall1 in anorectal, heart, brain and kidney development. Development. 2006;133:3005–13.

61. Kang S, Graham JM, Jr., Olney AH, et al. GLI3 frameshift mutations cause autosomal dominant Pallister-Hall syndrome. Nat Genet. 1997;15:266–8.

62. Sanyanusin P, Schimmenti LA, McNoe LA, et al. Mutation of the PAX2 gene in a family with optic nerve colobomas, renal anomalies and vesicoureteral reflux. Nat Genet. 1995;9:358–63.

63. Weber S, Moriniere V, Knuppel T, et al. Prevalence of mutations in renal developmental genes in children with renal hypodysplasia: Results of the ESCAPE study. J Am Soc Nephrol. 2006;17:2864–70.

64. Weber S, Taylor JC, Winyard P, et al. SIX2 and BMP4 mutations associate with anomalous kidney development. J Am Soc Nephrol. 2008 ;19:891–903.

65. Saisawat P, Tasic V, Vega-Warner V, et al. Identification of two novel CAKUT-causing genes by massively parallel exon resequencing of candidate genes in patients with unilateral renal agenesis. Kidney Int. 2012 ;81:196–200.

66. Thomas R, Sanna-Cherchi S, Warady BA, et al. HNF1B and PAX2 mutations are a common cause of renal hypodysplasia in the CKiD cohort. Pediatr Nephrol. 2011;26:897–903.

67. Skinner MA, Safford SD, Reeves JG, et al. Renal aplasia in humans is associated with RET mutations. Am J Hum Genet. 2008 ;82:344–51.

68. Gribouval O, Gonzales M, Neuhaus T, et al. Mutations in genes in the renin-angiotensin system are associated with autosomal recessive renal tubular dysgenesis. Nat Genet. 2005;37:964–8.

69. Petrij F, Giles RH, Dauwerse HG, et al. Rubinstein-Taybi syndrome caused by mutations in the transcriptional co-activator CBP. Nature. 1995;376:348–51.

70. Pilia G, Hughes-Benzie RM, MacKenzie A, et al. Mutations in GPC3, a glypican gene, cause the Simpson-Golabi-Behmel overgrowth syndrome. Nat Genet. 1996;12:241–7.

71. Nowaczyk MJ, Irons MB. Smith-Lemli-Opitz syndrome: Phenotype, natural history, and epidemiology. Am J Med Genet C Semin Med Genet. 2012;160C:250–62.

72. Salerno A, Kohlhase J, Kaplan BS. Townes-Brocks syndrome and renal dysplasia: A novel mutation in the SALL1 gene. Pediatr Nephrol. 2000;14:25–8.

73. Shimozawa N, Tsukamoto T, Suzuki Y, et al. A human gene responsible for Zellweger syndrome that affects peroxisome assembly. Science. 1992;255:1132–34.

74. Vivante A, Mark-Danieli M, Davidovits M, et al. Renal hypodysplasia associates with a WNT4 variant that causes aberrant canonical WNT signaling. J Am Soc Nephrol. 2013;24:550–8.

75. Sanna-Cherchi S, Sampogna RV, Papeta N, et al. Mutations in DSTYK and dominant urinary tract malformations. N Engl J Med. 2013;369:621–9.

76. James CA, Watson AR, Twining P, et al. Antenatally detected urinary tract abnormalities: Changing incidence and management. Eur J Pediatr. 1998;157:508–11.

77. Sukthankar S, Watson AR. Unilateral multicystic dysplastic kidney disease: Defining the natural history. Anglia Paediatric Nephrourology Group. Acta Paediatr. 2000;89:811–3.

78. Heymans C, Breysem L, Proesmans W. Multicystic kidney dysplasia: A prospective study on the natural history of the affected and the contralateral kidney. Eur J Pediatr. 1998;157:673–5.

## REVIEW QUESTIONS

1. Metanephric induction begins at:
   a. Week 7 of gestation
   b. Week 10 of gestation
   c. Week 5 of gestation
   d. Week 20 of gestation
2. Renal dysplasia is characterized by a decreased number of nephrons, the presence of collecting ducts surrounded by muscular rings, and elements of aberrant development, such as cartilage, or even calcified tissue.
   a. True
   b. False
3. Branchio-oto-renal (BOR) syndrome results from mutation of:
   a. *PAX2*
   b. *PEX1*
   c. *SOX9*
   d. *EYA1*
4. The most common urinary tract abnormality associated with multicystic dysplastic kidney (MCDK) is:
   a. Duplication of the collecting system
   b. Vesicoureteric reflux
   c. Posterior urethral valves
   d. Wilms tumor
5. During renal development, the *WT1* gene is important in:
   a. Glomerulogenesis
   b. Tubulogenesis
   c. Formation of the renal pelvis
   d. Renal ascent
6. BMP4, expressed in the mesenchymal cells surrounding the wolffian duct, exerts a positive control in directing the site from which ureteric bud would emerge.
   a. True
   b. False
7. Patterning of the renal collecting system (renal pelvis and calyces) is controlled by:
   a. Sonic hedgehog (SHH) and BMP gene family
   b. Renin, angiotensinogen genes
   c. *JAGGED1* gene
   d. *SIX1* and *SIX2* genes
8. The characteristic renal phenotype in Alagille syndrome consists of:
   a. Renal dysplasia
   b. Renal aplasia
   c. Multicystic dysplastic kidney
   d. Hypoplasia

## ANSWER KEY

1. c
2. b
3. d
4. b
5. a
6. b
7. a
8. a

# Diagnostic evaluation of kidney diseases

# Urinalysis

## GEORGE J. SCHWARTZ

Urinalysis provides a window into the function and some inflammatory pathologic processes in the kidneys. A carefully conducted urinalysis can reveal underlying renal and systemic disorders. Evaluation of urine has been recorded since ancient times and was commonly practiced by Roman and Greek physicians.[1] Uroscopy (also known as urinoscopy), or visual examination of urine, eventually evolved as a formal science among English and Italian physicians during the Renaissance. The next major contribution to the technique of urinalysis was made by Thomas Addis, who developed the method for quantifying urinary excretion of red blood cells (RBCs) in the diagnosis and prognosis of Bright disease.[2] The science of urinalysis has further evolved in the last several decades, especially with the advent of the dipstick technology, wherein a fairly precise chemical analysis of urine can be ascertained within a few minutes by the bedside or in the clinic facility. This chapter will discuss the urinalysis procedure and its diagnostic utility in nephrology.

## URINE SAMPLE COLLECTION

In general, the most reproducible urine specimen for urinalysis is the one obtained on waking from sleep, because it is not influenced by exercise and can assess urinary concentration after withholding fluid overnight. It is often recommended that parents bring in the first morning urine from home when a child has difficulty urinating on command.

In absence of toilet training, younger children should have urine collected in a plastic bag device attached to the perineum. A patient identifier label should be affixed to the urine container before being handed over to the patient for collection. The container for urinalysis need not be sterile, but it should be clean. In adults, second morning urine is sometimes preferable to the first morning urine sample because of convenience and also because of concern that cellular elements in the urine may undergo autolysis in the bladder overnight.[3]

## PRINCIPLES OF EVALUATION

Collected urine should be evaluated quickly, no later than 2 hours after collection. Routine urinalysis consists of the following three evaluation steps: (1) appearance of the collected urine, (2) chemical analysis, and (3) microscopy of the urine sediment.[4]

### KEY POINTS

- Only a freshly collected urine sample should be used for urinalysis.
- Automated dipstick-based methodologies for chemical analysis have increased the range of tests that can be conducted with a few drops of urine.

In most clinical laboratories the chemical analysis of urine is done with the help of urine test strips, also known as dipsticks. Early versions of this technology were limited to detection of urine glucose and albumin, but current versions are able to test for urine pH, specific gravity, protein, blood, glucose, ketones, urobilinogen, nitrite, and leukocyte esterase. Change of color of the individual test strips after they have been moistened by the urine is used to determine the test results. To automate the urinalysis and standardize the results, several devices are available for clinical use, especially for point-of-care testing.

## APPEARANCE AND CONSTITUENTS

Urine samples should be grossly examined and then routinely tested for pH, specific gravity, protein, blood, glucose, and nitrites using commercially available dipsticks.

## APPEARANCE

Fresh urine generally ranges from pale yellow to deep amber. The color of urine may provide clues to some of the underlying renal and nonrenal disorders (Table 3.1). Red discoloration may be caused by the presence of blood (hematuria), hemoglobin (hemoglobinuria), or myoglobin (myoglobinuria). RBCs are seen only in the urinary sediment of patients with hematuria. Urinary bleeding from the bladder or other parts of the collecting system (urologic hematuria) tends to color the urine pink or red, whereas glomerular bleeding appears rusty brown or the color of cola or tea (Figure 3.1). Red urine also may be seen in patients with porphyrias, as well as after intake of beets, certain food additives, or some drugs.

The urine is usually clear but may be turbid because of the precipitation of phosphates in alkaline urine or uric acid in acid urine, especially on chilling. The presence of leukocytes in the urine also can render the urine cloudy.

## ODOR

The normal odor of urine is mildly aromatic. Bacterial infection may lead to a fetid or ammonia odor. Some disorders of metabolism cause particular odors in the urine. In maple syrup urine, the urine smells like burnt sugar or maple syrup; in phenylketonuria the urine smells musty;

Table 3.1 Causes of abnormal urine color

| Pathologic Causes | Physiologic, foods, drugs |
|---|---|
| **Red-Burgundy-Pink** | **Red-Burgundy-Pink** |
| • Menstrual contamination | • Beets |
| • Gross hematuria | • Blackberries |
| • Papillary necrosis (often with clots) | • Urates |
| • Hemoglobinuria, hemolysis | • Pyridium |
| • Myoglobinuria | • Phenolphthalein |
| • Porphyria | • Anthocyanin |
| • *Serratia marcescens* infection | • Rhodamine B |
| | • Aminopyrine |
| **Dark Brown or Black** | • Phenytoin sodium |
| • Homogentisic aciduria | • Azo dyes |
| • Alkaptonuria | |
| • Methemoglobinemia | **Dark Brown or Black** |
| • Melanin | • Senna |
| • Tyrosinosis | • Cascara |
| | • Aniline |
| **Blue-Green** | • Hydroxyquinone |
| • Obstructive jaundice | • Resorcinol |
| • Hepatitis | • Thymol |
| • Blue diaper syndrome (intestinal tryptophan transport defect) | **Blue-Green** |
| • *Pseudomonas* infections | • Carotene |
| • Phenol poisoning | • Chlorophyll |
| | • Riboflavin |
| **Cloudy-Milky** | • Methylene blue |
| • Urinary tract infection | • Indigo-carmine |
| • Urates, uric acid (acid pH) | • Resorcinol |
| • Calculi, "gravel" (phosphates, oxalates) | • Tetrahydronaphthalene |
| • Chyluria | • Methocarbamol |
| • Nephrotic syndrome | |
| • Radiographic dye (acid pH | |

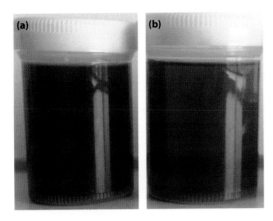

Figure 3.1 **(a)** Visible hematuria in a patient with post-streptococcal glomerulonephritis. The urine is dark coke-colored (glomerular hematuria). **(b)** Visible hematuria in a patient during passage of renal stone showing light pinkish urine color (urologic hematuria).

cystinuria and homocystinuria have sulfur-like odor; and tyrosinemia has an odor similar to that of fish or cabbage.

## PH

Urine pH normally ranges from 4.5 to 8, depending on the acid-base balance, metabolic state, and dietary habits. In general, vegetarians may have a more alkaline urine pH and a high-protein meal may cause the urine pH to be more acidic. Freshly voided urine should be examined for determining pH, because loss of carbon dioxide to air will falsely alkalinize the pH. Bacterial contamination also may change the baseline pH, depending on the metabolism of the particular organism. This dipstick determination of pH is adequate for routine testing, but if a precise urine pH value is to be obtained, it can be done using a pH meter in the laboratory.

## SPECIFIC GRAVITY AND OSMOLALITY

Urine osmolality is the key indicator of urinary concentration and is maximal after an overnight thirst (greater than 870 mOsm/kg in children younger than 2 years).[5] Urine osmolality is a function of the concentration of solutes present in the urine. Determination of the urine specific gravity and osmolality in a urine sample obtained after overnight thirsting can be a useful screening test for the diagnosis of diabetes insipidus. Apart from central and nephrogenic diabetes insipidus, urine specific gravity and osmolality may be decreased in renal insufficiency. Presence of protein, glucose, and osmotic contrast agents may increase urine specific gravity. In these cases, osmolality is the preferred measurement to assess urinary concentration ability.

Urine osmolality is not routinely measured in most clinical laboratories, but it can be approximated from the specific gravity according to the following formula[5]:

$$\text{Osmolality} = (\text{Specific gravity} - 1.000) \times 40{,}000$$

## PROTEIN

Proteinuria is an important indicator of renal disease. Normally, the glomerulus restricts the filtration of proteins based on size and charge. Most proteins that are filtered are reabsorbed by endocytosis of the proximal tubule, and less than 10 mg/dL is found in normal urine. Most of these are low-molecular-weight proteins filtered at the glomerulus. Tamm-Horsfall protein (uromodulin) is a tubular glycoprotein normally secreted by the thick ascending limb of the loop of Henle and forms the matrix of urinary casts.[6]

## Quantification of proteinuria

### DIPSTICK TEST

The urinary dipstick examination for proteinuria is a convenient method for detection of proteinuria. This method is able to provide a semiquantitative estimate of the degree of proteinuria. The test is affected by the urinary concentration and pH level. Concentrated urine may give a positive reading even when the daily protein excretion is normal, whereas a dilute urine may result in a negative or only slightly positive reading, even in the presence of elevated daily protein excretion. False-positive results also may occur if the urine is highly alkaline; false-negative results can be seen in the presence of ingestion of large doses of ascorbic acid.

> **KEY POINTS**
>
> - First morning urine sample is preferred to quantify baseline proteinuria and establish the diagnosis of orthostatic proteinuria in children.
> - Dipsticks are more specific for urinary albumin and are unable to detect globulin or Bence-Jones proteinuria.
> - Very alkaline urine can give a false-positive dipstick test for protein.

### SULFOSALICYLIC ACID TEST

Proteinuria also can be detected by using 10% sulfosalicylic acid, which precipitates urinary protein (Table 3.2). This semiquantitative assessment of the urine's turbidity correlates well with total urinary protein, including albumin. The sulfosalicylic acid test is not affected by urine pH or the presence of ascorbic acid.

> **KEY POINTS**
>
> Proteinuria can be quantified by:
>
> - Dipstick ( semiquantitative)
> - 24-Hour urine collection
> - Ratio of urine protein to urine creatinine

Table 3.2 Semiquantitative estimation of proteinuria using the sulfosalicylic acid precipitation test and the dipsticks

| Sulfosalicylic acid | | | |
|---|---|---|---|
| Degree of turbidity | | Protein (mg/dL) | Dipstick equivalent |
| No turbidity | Negative | No protein | Negative |
| Slight turbidity | Trace | 1–20 | Trace |
| Turbid (newsprint visible) | 1+ | 30 | 1+ |
| White cloud (heavy lines visible) | 2+ | 100 | 2+ |
| Fine precipitate (heavy lines invisible) | 3+ | 300 | 3+ |
| Flocculent precipitate (like yogurt) | 4+ | >500 | 4+ (2000 mg/dL) |

Note: Sulfosalicylic acid test is conducted by adding 10 drops of 10% sulfosalicylic acid to 10 mL of urine. Sulfosalicylic acid detects all urinary proteins, including albumin. A dipstick test is more specific for albumin and does not detect globulins or tubular proteins.

## Timed collection

The gold standard of urinary protein quantitation is the quantitative measurement of protein in a carefully timed urine collection, usually over 24 hours. Normal value for 24-hour urine protein excretion is less than 100 mg/m²/day, and nephrotic range proteinuria exceeds 1000 mg/m²/day, or 40 mg/m²/h.[7] Calculation of the creatinine excretion index in the collected urine is often employed by nephrologists to judge completeness of the collected 24-hour urine sample. The creatinine excretion index, or creatinine excretion per kilogram of body weight (total urinary creatinine ÷ patient's weight), should be 15 to 20 mg/kg/24 h for the urine collection to be considered adequate.

## Protein-to-creatinine ratio

Because of the difficulty in collecting timed urine samples in children, spot urine protein and creatinine estimation is preferred in children and also has been endorsed by the Kidney Disease Outcomes Quality Initiative (KDOQI) clinical practice guidelines.[8] The urine protein-to-creatinine (mg/mg) ratio correlates well with the 24-hour urine protein excretion.[9-13] Normal value for urinary protein-to-creatinine ratio is less than 0.2, but is slightly higher in younger children (Table 3.3). Proteinuria is considered to be of nephrotic range if the protein-to-creatinine ratio exceeds 2.0.[9,10] An approximate value of 24-hour urine protein excretion can

Table 3.3 Urinary protein-to-creatinine ratios showing age-related 95th percentiles

| Age (years) | Protein (mg/mg creatinine) |
|---|---|
| <2 | 0.492 |
| 2–13 | 0.178 |
| >13 | 0.178 |

Source: Data from Houser MJ. Assessment of proteinuria using random urine samples. J Pediatr. 1984;104:845.

be calculated from urine protein and creatinine obtained in a spot sample and using the following formula[11]:

24-Hour urinary protein excretion = Urine protein/urine creatinine × 0.63  (mg/m²/day)

## MICROALBUMINURIA

Microalbuminuria (also known as albuminuria), is used to screen children with diabetes of 5 years or longer of duration and is usually expressed as an albumin-to-creatinine ratio (ACR). Normal ACR is less than 30 mg/g creatinine.[14,15] Urine collections of 24 hours are not necessary in most children, and a spot urine sample estimation is sufficient for screening purposes. Orthostatic proteinuria in children can affect the quantification of ACR; therefore, estimation using the first morning urine sample is recommended.

### KEY POINTS

- In patients with diabetes, urine ACR estimation is used to detect early manifestations of diabetic nephropathy.
- First morning urine should be used for measuring the ACR ratio in children with diabetes.
- Normal ACR is less than 30 mg/g of creatinine.

## BLOOD

Dipsticks detect the presence of hemoglobin in the urine. The reaction relies on the peroxidase-like activity of hemoglobin to catalyze the reaction of a hydroperoxide with tetramethylbenzidine to give a green-blue color. Myoglobin also will give a positive reaction with the dipsticks. Therefore, a positive dipstick test for blood may be the result of hematuria, hemoglobinuria (intravascular hemolysis), or myoglobinuria (muscle injury or disease). Identification of RBCs on urine microscopy establishes the diagnosis of hematuria, and lack of RBCs suggests hemoglobinuria or myoglobinuria. Differentiation between hemoglobinuria and myoglobinuria can be accomplished using immunochemical methods. A negative dipstick test rules out hematuria.

---

### KEY POINTS

A positive test for blood may result from:

- Hematuria
- Myoglobinuria
- Hemoglobinuria

---

## GLUCOSE

Dipstick detection of glucose is based on the oxidation of glucose by glucose oxidase. False-negative results occur if there are large quantities of reducing agents, such as vitamin C, tetracyclines, or homogentisic acid in the urine. False-positive results have not been reported. Glycosuria is seen in patients with diabetes mellitus and those with proximal tubular disorders, such as Fanconi syndrome. Renal glycosuria is an isolated proximal tubular defect of glucose reabsorption and is distinguished from diabetes mellitus by a normal simultaneously obtained serum glucose level and a normal hemoglobin A1C level. Abnormalities in SGLT2, a critical tubular glucose transporter located in the S1 segment of the proximal tubule, has been demonstrated to be associated with familial renal glycosuria.[16]

---

### KEY POINTS

Glucosuria with a normal simultaneously drawn serum glucose level can be the result of:

- Renal glycosuria
- Fanconi syndrome

---

## NITRITE

More than 90% of common urinary pathogens are nitrite-forming bacteria that convert urinary nitrate to nitrite with the help of the enzyme nitrate reductase. Nitrite can be detected in urine using a dipstick containing $p$-arsanilic acid, which reacts with nitrite to generate a diazonium compound that is then converted to 3-hydroxy-1,2,3,4-tetrahydrobenzo-quinolin-3-ol to produce a pink azo dye. Bacteria must be in contact with urine for 2 to 4 hours to allow nitrate conversion to nitrite and result in a positive test. Patients who have urinary frequency associated with the urinary tract infection (UTI) may not allow sufficient bacterial contact time, resulting in a false-negative urine test for nitrite. It is also important to point out that the nitrite test is not able to detect UTIs secondary to *Staphylococcus saprophyticus*, *Pseudomonas*

species or enterococci, all of which lack the enzyme nitrate reductase and are unable to convert nitrate to nitrite.[17] A false-positive reading will occur if bacterial overgrowth is allowed to occur during inappropriate transport of the urine to the laboratory. False-negative results occur in the presence of ascorbic acid. The nitrite test for UTI is highly specific, but its sensitivity is low. Meta-analysis of pediatric studies demonstrated that the specificity of nitrite test was 98% (96% to 99%) and sensitivity was 49% (41% to 57%).[18]

---

### KEY POINTS

- The nitrite test cannot detect infections caused by organisms that do not produce the nitrate reductase.
- Bacterial contact with urine needs to be at least 2 to 4 hours (in the bladder) for the nitrite test to be positive.
- The nitrite test has high specificity (98%) but low sensitivity (50%).

---

## LEUKOCYTE ESTERASE

Leukocyte esterase (LE) has been incorporated into the routine dipstick evaluation of urine for almost a decade. The LE test is a colorimetric test that detects the presence of esterase produced by the polymorphonuclear leukocytes in the urine and is therefore used for the diagnosis of UTI. False-positive results may be seen in contamination of urine with vaginal secretions, tubulointerstitial nephritis, and severe glomerulonephritis. False-negative LE test results can be caused by high urinary protein concentration (nephrotic syndrome) and high urinary ascorbic acid level. Combining the LE and nitrite tests offers a better sensitivity and specificity profile than either of them separately. In a meta-analysis of pediatric studies, the LE test or nitrite-positive dipstick had a specificity of 88% (82% to 91%) and sensitivity of 79% (69% to 87%).[18]

## MICROSCOPIC ANALYSIS

Microscopic examination of the urine is used semiquantitatively to confirm the presence of RBCs, cellular casts, crystals, and bacteria. Urine for microscopy should be freshly obtained, because stored samples are prone to developing autolysis of the cells and casts, rendering the evaluation inaccurate.

---

### KEY POINTS

- Freshly obtained urine samples should be used for microscopy.
- Stored or frozen samples result in disruption of cellular elements.

## Technique

The Clinical and Laboratory Standards Institute recommends that each laboratory should standardize the urine microscopy procedure. A standard urine volume (10, 12, or 15 mL) should be spun for a standard time of 5 minutes.[19] The centrifuge speed should be such as to achieve a relative centrifugal force (RCF) of approximately 400. To calculate RCF from rotations per minute (RPM) for a specific centrifuge, following formula should be used:

$$RCF (g) = 1.18 \times 10^{-5} \times Radius (cm) \times RPM^2$$

After centrifugation, the supernatant is decanted, and the pellet resuspended in the remaining 0.25 to 0.5 mL of urine (Figure 3.2). The sediment is gently resuspended in urine by tapping the pellet in the centrifuge tube, and is then examined under low-power (10 × 10 = 100 ×) and high-power (10 × 40 = 400 ×) microscopy. An examination of five random fields at 40 × throughout the slide permits assessment of the number of cells per high-power field (hpf). Urinary microscopy is generally performed in unstained urinary sediment slides. If a detailed analysis and identification of white blood cells (WBCs) is necessary (e.g., identification of eosinophils in interstitial nephritis), the sediment may be stained by Sternheimer-Malbin stain (Sedi-Stain, Becton, Dickinson, Franklin Lakes, NJ).

## Red blood cells

In healthy children the normal upper limit for the number of RBCs in fresh midstream urine is 2 to 4 per hpf. The morphology of the RBCs should be reviewed in high power to distinguish between glomerular and nonglomerular hematuria. Dysmorphic RBCs with a large variation in size and shape, cell wall blebs, and distribution of hemoglobin content are more likely to be seen with glomerulonephritis (Figure 3.3).[20] The dysmorphic RBCs with a doughnut shape or with one or more blebs are also known as G1 cells. Eumorphic or normal RBCs are observed in nonglomerular urinary bleeding secondary to stones, hypercalciuria, and trauma.[21,22] At times, glomerular hematuria also can have a mixture of eumorphic and dysmorphic RBCs. The value of erythrocyte morphology in the diagnosis of glomerular disease in patients with persistent isolated hematuria was evaluated by Fogazzi et al.[23] In 16 such patients (10 children and 6 adults) classified as having glomerular hematuria, a renal biopsy showed glomerular disease in 14 of the 16 patients (87.5%).

> ### KEY POINTS
>
> - Urine should be centrifuged at standardized speeds for 5 minutes.
> - Unstained specimens provide adequate information for most clinical purposes.
> - Staining the urine sediment may be indicated to identify some cellular elements.

## White blood cells

In healthy children, the upper limit of normal for the number of WBCs in fresh midstream urine is 0 to 4 per hpf, with most of these being neutrophils. Neutrophils are recognizable by the presence of a multilobed nucleus and granular cytoplasm. In UTIs, neutrophils are the dominant type of WBCs noted in the urinary sediment and lymphocytes may be present in large numbers in urine during acute renal transplant rejection. Although eosinophils in the urinary sediment (eosinophiluria) can be seen in allergic interstitial nephritis, they are not pathognomonic of this disorder and can be seen in other inflammatory lesions of the kidneys and the urinary tract.[24]

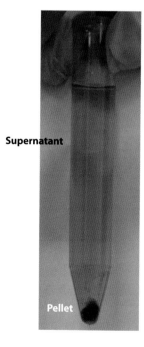

Figure 3.2 Centrifuged urine in a conical tube in a patient with visible hematuria showing the pellet of red blood cells at the bottom and the clear supernatant.

## Renal epithelial cells

Epithelial cells found in urine can come from the renal tubules, collecting system, or bladder, each with distinctive morphologic characteristics. Renal tubular epithelial (RTE) cells are only slightly larger than white cells and have a large central nucleus (Figure 3.4). These are normally present in small numbers in the urinary sediment, but an excessive number may be seen in acute kidney injury (AKI) and acute

Figure 3.3 **(a)** Crenated red blood cells (RBCs) seen in concentrated (hypertonic) urine. These cells are isomorphic RBCs that are deformed in a hypertonic urine (intracellular dehydration). They do not represent glomerular hematuria. **(b)** Dysmorphic RBCs showing margination of hemoglobin and formation of "doughnut-shaped RBCs." **(c and d)** Acanthocytes or G1 cells (RBCs) in glomerular hematuria with cytoplasmic blebs (Mickey Mouse RBCs). Arrows point to the various types of dysmorphic cells in the urinary sediment. ([a] and [c] reproduced with permission from: Fogazzi GB, Verdesca S, Garigali G. Urinalysis: core curriculum 2008. Am J Kidney Dis. 2008;51:1052.)

renal transplant rejection. In nephrotic syndromes, RTEs may appear granular because of the accumulation of proteins or lipids in cytoplasmic vesicles. "Oval fat bodies" is the term reserved for fat-laden RTE cells seen in patients with nephrotic syndrome (Figure 3.5A). When viewed with a polarized light source, birefringence of lipid droplets in the RTE cells results in the Maltese-cross appearance of these cells (Figure 3.5B).

Bladder epithelial cells are three to four times the size of leukocytes, are thin, may appear folded upon themselves along edges, and have a relatively small nucleus. Although normally present in the urinary sediment, an excessive

number may be seen in cystitis and urethritis. Transitional cells originate in the renal pelvis and ureters and are midway between RTE cells and bladder epithelial cells in their cellular characteristics.

## Casts

Casts are cylindrical structures formed in the renal tubules by the precipitation of Tamm-Horsfall protein (uromodulin) and are sometimes overlaid with cellular elements. Hyaline casts are derived entirely from Tamm-Horsfall protein and appear as translucent cylindrical

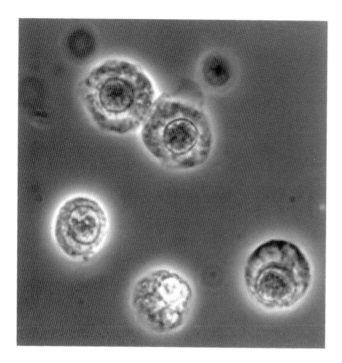

Figure 3.4 Renal tubular cell showing large central nuclei and granular cytoplasm. (Reproduced with permission from: Fogazzi GB, Verdesca S, Garigali G. Urinalysis: core curriculum 2008. Am J Kidney Dis. 51:1052, 2008.)

structures. These may be seen in concentrated urine of normal children, as well as in fever, exercise, dehydration, diuretic use, congestive heart failure, and nephrotic syndrome. Cells may be trapped within the matrix, giving rise to cellular casts. Degeneration of the cellular elements eventually leads to formation of granular casts (Figure 3.6A). Cellular casts are classified according to the dominant cell type included therein (red, white, or epithelial cell). WBC casts can be observed in acute pyelonephritis, glomerular diseases, and transplant rejection. RBC casts appear as round discoid cells embedded in the Tamm-Horsfall matrix and may be further identified by the hemoglobin pigment within the matrix of the cast (Figure 3.6B). RBC casts are pathognomonic of glomerular bleeding, or glomerulonephritis.

Waxy casts are similar to hyaline casts, but are more broad (Figure 3.6C). They are commonly seen in chronic renal diseases. Large waxy casts (broad casts) are often seen in chronic kidney disease (CKD). Broad casts are believed to originate in damaged nephron segments or from the collecting system. Fatty casts result from the incorporation of fat within the Tamm-Horsfall matrix and are common in nephrotic syndrome. Casts made of renal tubular cells can be seen in AKI (Figure 3.6D). A muddy brown cast is a specific type of granular cast seen in AKI that is an intensely brownish color and may be derived from degeneration of tubular epithelial cells. Light brown pigment casts also can be seen in hemoglobinuria and myoglobinuria.

## Bacteriuria

Significant bacteriuria usually can be detected using a 40 × objective. From a standardization perspective, centrifuged urine (10 mL) sediment stained with Gram stain provides the most reproducible results. This method has been reported to have 95% sensitivity with 1 bacterium per oil immersion field and 95% specificity for bacteriuria if more than 5 bacteria are visualized.[25] Being cumbersome and time-consuming, the

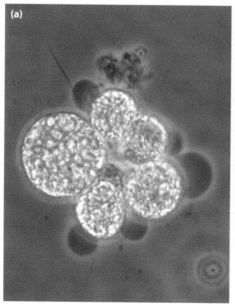

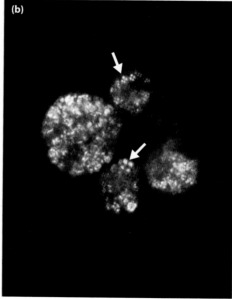

Figure 3.5 (a) "Oval fat bodies" or renal tubular cells packed with lipid droplets. (b) Same sediment viewed with polarized light showing the Maltese crosses (arrows). (Reproduced with permission from: Fogazzi GB, Verdesca S, Garigali G. Urinalysis: core curriculum 2008. Am J Kidney Dis. 2008;51:1052.)

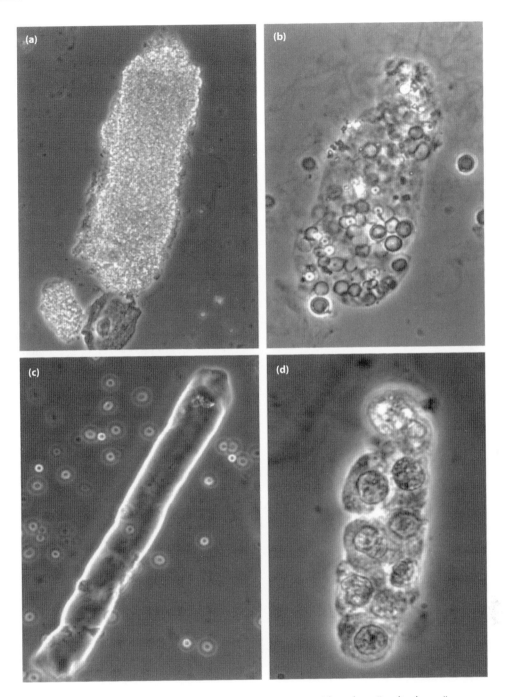

Figure 3.6 **(a)** A finely granular cast. **(b)** A short RBC cast. **(c)** Waxy cast with a clear "melted wax" appearance. **(d)** A renal tubular epithelial (RTE) cell cast. RTE cells are identified by a single large central nucleus. (Reproduced with permission from: Fogazzi GB, Verdesca S, Garigali G. Urinalysis: core curriculum 2008. Am J Kidney Dis. 2008;51:1052.)

test is rarely performed in the office or emergency departments, for which it was primarily intended.

## Crystals

Solutes are normal constituents of urine and can precipitate as crystals if their solubility changes with the decrease in temperature outside the body, especially in a supersaturated state. Although most urinary crystals have no diagnostic significance, excessive amounts of crystals and presence of some distinct types of crystals may be diagnostically relevant.

### AMORPHOUS CRYSTALS

Amorphous crystals are made of either urate or phosphate.[25,26] Amorphous phosphate crystals are found in alkaline urine, and urate crystals are seen in acidic urine. Amorphous phosphate crystals precipitate in the urine tube as a white button on spinning, whereas the urate crystals are brick red (Figure 3.7). Amorphous phosphate precipitate

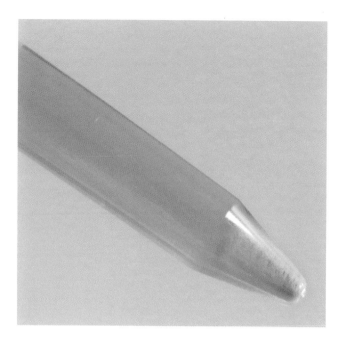

Figure 3.7 Centrifuged urine showing brick-brown sediment that is characteristic of uric acid (urate) crystals in acidic urine.

can be dissolved by addition of acetic acid, and amorphous urate crystals are dissolved by adding a few drops of alkali or by warming the urine tube.

## CALCIUM OXALATE CRYSTALS

Calcium oxalate crystals are envelope-shaped crystals (Figure 3.8A) found in normal urine.[4,26,27] They also can be shaped like dumbbells. Excessive amounts of calcium oxalate crystals can be seen as a result of dietary intake of foods with a high oxalate content, such as spinach, tomatoes, rhubarb, and asparagus. Calcium oxalate crystals may be prominent in hyperoxaluria and some forms of hypercalciuria, particularly in acid urine and in stone formers.

## STRUVITE CRYSTALS

Struvite (magnesium ammonium phosphate) crystals are also known as triple phosphate crystals.[4,26,27] They are often seen are seen in patients with UTIs caused by bacteria, such as *Proteus, Pseudomonas, Klebsiella, Staphylococcus,* and *Mycoplasma* species, that produce the urea-splitting enzyme urease. Struvite crystals are transparent and rectangular, giving the appearance of a coffin lid. These are more common in alkaline urine.

## URIC ACID CRYSTALS

Uric acid crystals can have multiple shapes, such as amorphous plates, diamonds, and trapezoids, and often appear yellow or orange under the microscope (Figure 3.8B).[4,26,27] Uric acid crystals are more commonly seen if the urine has been left standing for an extended period at room temperature, especially if the urine is acidic. Although they are normally seen, the presence of uric acid crystals in a fresh urine sample may indicate the presence of a stone. Other conditions in which uric acid crystals can be found are tumor lysis syndrome, leukemic children undergoing chemotherapy, and the rare genetic disorder Lesch-Nyhan syndrome.

## AMMONIUM URATE CRYSTALS

Ammonium urate crystals are commonly seen when urine is left standing for a prolonged period and the action of urea-splitting bacteria produces free ammonia. These crystals appear in various shapes, ranging from needle-like to the characteristic "thorn apple" shape.[4,26,27]

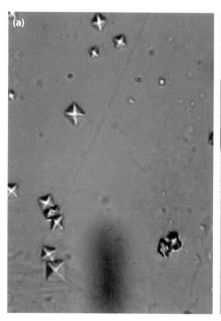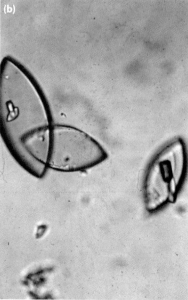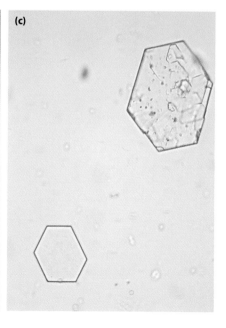

Figure 3.8 Urinary crystals in unstained urinary sediment. **(a)** Envelope-shaped square crystals of calcium oxalate. **(b)** Uric acid discoid-shaped crystals. **(c)** Hexagonal clear crystals of cystinuria. (Figure courtesy of Uri Alon, MD.)

## CYSTINE CRYSTALS

The hexagonal crystals of cystinuria (Figure 3.8C) in acid urine are characteristic of cystinuria, a genetic disorder of renal cysteine transport that results in recurrent cystine stones. Cystine crystals are not seen in normal urine.

## DRUG CRYSTALS

Many drugs have been associated with crystalluria, which can sometimes cause AKI by precipitation within the tubules. Compiling the list of such drugs continues; the well-known ones are amoxicillin, sulfonamides, ciprofloxacin, acyclovir, ganciclovir, indinavir, atazanavir, and triamterene.[28-34] Crystals of each of these drugs have a characteristic microscopic appearance. Some drugs, such as furosemide, can cause hypercalciuria and may cause crystalluria, nephrocalcinosis, or even renal stones.[34] Drug-induced crystalluria can cause renal tubular obstruction and AKI.

## SUMMARY

Urinalysis provides an important insight into renal physiology and also can provide diagnostic clues into many pathologic states. It is often the first investigation in the evaluation of patients with renal disease. The technology of urinalysis has been evolving over the years, especially with the development of chemical analysis using dipsticks. Screening for proteinuria, hematuria, and UTI in the emergency department and physician offices has been particularly facilitated by these developments. Microscopic analysis of the urine sediment requires knowledge and the experience of having viewed the sediment in physiologic as well as disease states. Use of stock images for determining the formed urinary sediment components is evolving but is an imperfect technique at this stage.

## REFERENCES

1. Pardalidis N, Kosmaoglou E, Diamantis A, et al. Uroscopy in Byzantium (330–1453 AD). J Urol. 2008;179:1271–6.
2. Addis T. A clinical classification of Bright's diseases. JAMA. 1925;85:163–7.
3. The European Confederation of Laboratory Medicine (ECLM). European urinalysis guidelines: Summary. Scand J Clin Lab Invest. 2000;60:1–96.
4. Fogazzi GB, Verdesca S, Garigali G. Urinalysis: Core curriculum 2008. Am J Kidney Dis. 2008;51:1052–67.
5. Edelmann CM Jr, Barnett HL, Stark H, et al. A standardized test of renal concentrating capacity in children. Am J Dis Child. 1967;114:639–44.
6. Iorember FM, Vehaskari VM. Uromodulin: Old friend with new roles in health and disease. Pediatr Nephrol. 2014;29:1151–8.
7. International Study of Kidney Disease in Children. Nephrotic syndrome in children: Prediction of histopathology from clinical and laboratory characteristics at time of diagnosis. Kidney Int. 1978;13:159–65.
8. National Kidney Foundation. KDOQI clinical practice guidelines for chronic kidney disease: Evaluation, classification and stratification. Am J Kidney Dis. 2002;39(Suppl 1):S1–266.
9. Ginsberg JM, Chang BS, Matarese RA, et al. Use of single voided urine samples to estimate quantitative proteinuria. N Engl J Med. 1983;309:1543–6.
10. Houser M. Assessment of proteinuria using random urine samples. J Pediatr. 1984;104:845–8.
11. Abitbol C, Zilleruelo G, Freundlich M, et al. Quantitation of proteinuria with urinary protein/creatinine ratios and random testing with dipsticks in nephrotic children. J Pediatr. 1990;116:243–7.
12. Bangstad H-J, Dahl-Jorgensen K, Kjaersgaard P, et al. Urinary albumin excretion rate and puberty in non-diabetic children and adolescents. Acta Paediatr. 1993;82:857–62, 1993.
13. Morgenstern BZ, Butani L, Wollan P, et al. Validity of protein-osmolality versus protein-creatinine ratios in the estimation of quantitative proteinuria from random samples of urine in children. Am J Kidney Dis. 2003;41:760–66.
14. Hogg RJ, Furth S, Lemley KV, et al. National Kidney Foundation's kidney disease outcomes quality initiative clinical practice guidelines for chronic kidney disease in children and adolescents: Evaluation, classification, and stratification. Pediatrics. 2003;111:1416–21.
15. Assadi FK. Quantitation of microalbuminuria using random urine samples. Pediatr Nephrol. 2002;17:107–10.
16. Santer R, Calado J. Familial renal glucosuria and SGLT2: From a mendelian trait to a therapeutic target. Clin J Am Soc Nephrol. 2010;5:133–41.
17. Nys S, van Merode T, Bartelds AI, et al. Urinary tract infections in general practice patients: Diagnostic tests versus bacteriological culture. J Antimicrob Chemother. 2006;57:955–8.
18. Williams GJ, Macaskill P, Chan SF, et al. Absolute and relative accuracy of rapid urine tests for urinary tract infection in children: A meta-analysis. Lancet Infect Dis. 2010;10:240–50.
19. Rabinovitch A, Sarewitz SJ, Woodcock SM et al. Urinalysis and Collection, Transportation, and Preservation of Urine Specimens. Approved Guideline, 2 ed. Clinical and Laboratory Standards document GP16-A2. Wayne, PA: National Committee for Clinical Laboratory Standards; 2001.

20. Fairley KF, Birch DF. Hematuria: A simple method for identifying glomerular bleeding. Kidney Int. 1984;21:105–8.
21. Stapleton FB, Roy SI, Noe HN, et al. Hypercalciuria in children with hematuria. N Engl J Med. 1984;310:1345–8.
22. Andres A, Praga M, Bello I, et al. Hematuria due to hypercalciuria and hyperuricosuria in adult patients. Kidney Int. 1989;36:96–9.
23. Fogazzi GB, Edefonti A, Garigali G, et al. Urine erythrocyte morphology in patients with microscopic haematuria caused by a glomerulopathy. Pediatr Nephrol. 2008;23:1093–100.
24. Nolan CR, Kelleher SP. Eosinophiluria. Clin Lab Med. 1988;8:555–65.
25. Jenkins RD, Fenn JP, Matsen JM. Review of urine microscopy for bacteriuria. JAMA 1986;255:3397–403.
26. Graff L. A Handbook of Routine Urinalysis. St. Louis: JB Lippincott; 1983.
27. Fogazzi GB. Crystalluria: A neglected aspect of urinary sediment analysis. Nephrol Dial Transplant. 1996;11:379–87.
28. Hess B. Drug-induced urolithiasis. Curr Opin Urol. 1998;8:331–4.
29. Saltel E, Angel JB, Futter NG, et al. Increased prevalence and analysis of risk factors for indinavir nephrolithiasis. J Urol. 2000;164:1895–7.
30. Chopra N, Fine PL, Price B, Atlas I. Bilateral hydronephrosis from ciprofloxacin induced crystalluria and stone formation. J Urol. 2000;164:438.
31. Lyon AW, Mansoor A, Trotter MJ. Urinary gems: Acyclovir crystalluria. Arch Pathol Lab Med. 2002;126:753–4.
32. Fogazzi GB, Cantù M, Saglimbeni L, et al. Amoxicillin: A rare but possible cause of crystalluria. Nephrol Dial Transplant. 2003;18:212–4.
33. Nasr SH, Milliner DS, Wooldridge TD, et al. Triamterene crystalline nephropathy. Am J Kidney Dis. 2014;63:148–52.
34. Hufnagle KG, Khan SN, Penn D, et al. Renal calcifications: A complication of long-term furosemide therapy in preterm infants. Pediatrics. 1982;70:360–3.

## REVIEW QUESTIONS

1. Urine was collected on your 3-year-old febrile patient at home and was stored at room temperature for 18 hours. Urinalysis showed specific gravity 1.015, pH 6.5, protein negative, blood negative, nitrite positive, and leukocyte esterase negative. Your recommendation is:
   a. Patient has a UTI, obtain a urine culture and start on antibiotics.
   b. Patient does not have a UTI, but a culture should be obtained.
   c. Patient does not have a UTI, and nothing more needs to be done.
   d. Patient does not have a UTI, and a urine culture does need to be obtained. Obtain a urinalysis in freshly obtained urine in the clinic.
2. You need to evaluate urinary sediment in a patient with suspected glomerulonephritis who has had visible hematuria for 1 week but is improving, with only faintly pink urine. You are unable to evaluate the urinary sediment for the next 4 hours. Your laboratory technician labeled the urine sample and froze it at –20° C, with the hope of preserving the casts and cellular elements for you to evaluate later. When you evaluated the urine sediment later in the day after thawing it, you found unclear cell types and no clearly identifiable casts were present. Choose the *best* interpretation of these findings.
   a. Patient does not have glomerulonephritis.
   b. Patient's cellular elements and casts were likely disrupted by freezing.
   c. Patient has glomerulonephritis, but there is no evidence of it in the urinary sediment.
   d. Patient's urine sample may have been labeled incorrectly.
3. A 3+ positive test for heme on dipstick is diagnostic for the presence of:
   a. Blood in urine
   b. Myoglobin in urine
   c. Hemoglobinuria secondary to intravascular hemolysis
   d. All of the above
4. A meta-analysis of pediatric studies has indicated that urine nitrite test for UTI:
   a. Correlates best with a randomly obtained urine.
   b. Has low specificity and high sensitivity.
   c. Has high specificity and low sensitivity.
   d. Correlates poorly with UTI.
5. Drug-induced crystalluria can result in:
   a. Acute kidney injury
   b. Renal stone formation
   c. Nephrocalcinosis
   d. All of above
6. Which of the following correlates highly with significant bacteria in the urine of a patient with UTI?
   a. 1 bacterium/HPF seen in uncentrifuged urine under 40× magnification
   b. 1 bacterium/oil immersion field seen in centrifuged urine stained with Gram stain

c. 1 bacterium/HPF seen in centrifuged urine stained with Gram stain

d. 1 bacterium/oil immersion field seen in centrifuged urine stained with Sedi-Stain

7. Urine obtained for urinalysis needs to be collected in a clean container that does not have to be sterile.

a. True

b. False

8. A 10-year-old male patient in septic shock is noted to have a serum creatinine level of 2.0 mg/dL. Although the patient has good urine output, the intensive fellow wants a nephrology consult. Urinalysis shows specific gravity 1.010, pH 6.5, blood 3+, protein 2+. Microscopic analysis shows TNTC RBCs, a few granular casts, an occasional muddy brown cast, and many renal tubular epithelial cells. Your interpretation of the patient's urinalysis, given the clinical picture is:

a. Patient has prerenal azotemia.

b. Patient has acute kidney injury.

c. Patient has glomerulonephritis.

d. Patient has acute interstitial nephritis.

9. Dipstick detection for detection of proteinuria is:

a. Specific for tubular proteinuria

b. Nonspecific and detects all types of urinary proteins

c. Able to detect microalbuminuria

d. Specific for albuminuria

10. UTI caused by *Proteus, Pseudomonas, Klebsiella, Staphylococcus,* and *Mycoplasma* that produce the urea-splitting enzyme urease can result in crystalluria and renal stones.

a. True

b. False

## ANSWER KEY

1. d
2. b
3. d
4. c
5. d
6. b
7. a
8. b
9. b
10. a

# Clinical assessment of renal function

## GEORGE J. SCHWARTZ

The kidney plays a central role in the maintaining fluid and electrolyte balance, acid-base homeostasis, systemic blood pressure, and erythrocyte production through erythropoietin, as well as maintaining bone and mineral metabolism. Clinical evaluation and interpretation of these complex functions can be categorized into tests for glomerular functions, tubular functions, and hormonal functions (Table 4.1). Clinicians use broad sets of evaluation tools to judge renal function in adults and children. Such evaluation requires testing blood and urine, and it may include injection of exogenous substances to measure glomerular filtration rate (GFR). Dynamic radiologic tests, such as radionuclide renal scans, to evaluate renal perfusion and excretion functions are equally important in evaluation of renal functions. Estimated GFR (eGFR) determination with mathematical formulas using either creatinine (Cr) or cystatin C (Cys-C) has been an important step in early discovery and clinical follow-up of renal dysfunction in children and adults. This chapter discusses the pathophysiology, test methodology, and interpretation of clinically useful renal function tests.

## GLOMERULAR FILTRATION RATE

GFR provides the most common and best estimate of overall functioning renal mass. Knowledge of GFR enables the clinician to determine progression of the renal disease, predict the development of end-stage disease, adjust medications excreted by the kidney, and rationally prescribe fluids and solutes. Because of the importance and clinical utility of GFR, several different approaches have been used to estimate or determine it.

## PHYSIOLOGY OF GLOMERULAR FILTRATION

Approximately 20% of the cardiac output flows through the approximately 2 million glomerular capillary units.[1] The glomerulus consists of a tuft of capillaries interposed between the afferent and efferent arterioles. The glomerular capillary wall, through which the filtrate must pass, is made up of three layers: the fenestrated endothelial cell, the glomerular basement membrane (GBM), and the epithelial cell (podocyte) (Figure 4.1). The epithelial cells are attached to the GBM by discrete foot processes. The pores between the foot processes are slit pores, which are covered by a thin membrane called a slit diaphragm.[1-3] The GBM is derived from material produced by endothelial and epithelial cells, including type IV collagen, laminin, nidogen, and heparan sulfate proteoglycans. Laminin and nidogen form a tight complex to promote cell adhesion. The anionic heparan sulfate proteoglycans serve to form the charge barrier to the filtration of anionic macromolecules.[1,2]

One of the major functions of the glomerulus is to allow the filtration of small solutes such as sodium and urea and water while restricting the passage of larger molecules. This action permits the kidney to maintain homeostasis by excreting the daily solute load derived from dietary intake, but preserving the larger proteins. Solutes up to the size of inulin (molecular weight [MW] 5200) are freely filtered, whereas myoglobin (MW 17,000) is filtered less completely than inulin, and albumin (MW 69,000) is filtered only to a minor degree. Filtration is also limited for ions or drugs that are bound to albumin.

Table 4.1 Laboratory investigations used in clinical investigations of kidney functions

| Test category | Test name |
|---|---|
| Glomerular function | Glomerular filtration rate |
| | Urinary protein excretion and microalbuminuria |
| Tubular function | Urinary concentrating ability |
| | Urinary acidification |
| | Enzymuria and abnormal tubular proteinuria |
| Hormonal function | Erythropoietin production and anemia |
| | Vitamin D and bone health regulation |
| | Renin-aldosterone control of salt and blood pressure |

## Starling forces

GFR is determined by two factors: the filtration rate in each nephron (single nephron GFR or SNGFR); and the number of filtering nephrons (nephron mass), which are approximately 1 million units per kidney in humans at birth. Blood entering through the afferent arteriole passes through the glomerular capillary tuft and exits through

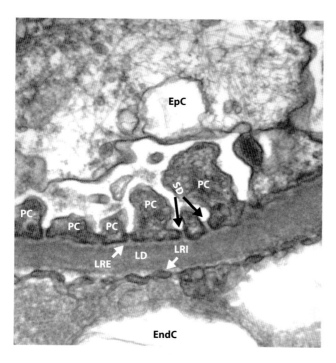

Figure 4.1 Electron micrograph of a normal glomerulus showing ultrastructure of the filtration barrier. EndC, endothelial cell; EpC, epithelial cell; LD, lamina densa; LRE, lamina rara externa; LRI, lamina rara interna; PC, epithelial cell podocytes; SD, slit diaphragm. (Courtesy of Dr. Bhaskar Kallakuri, Department of Pathology, Georgetown University Hospital, Washington, DC.)

the efferent arteriole. Along the glomerular capillary tuft, a portion of the glomerular filtrate is ultrafiltered into the Bowman space (urinary space). This ultrafiltrate is processed by the renal tubules and collecting duct and eventually leaves the kidney as urine. Fluid movement across the glomerulus is governed by Starling forces, which are proportional to the permeability of the glomerular capillary wall and to the balance between hydraulic and oncotic pressure gradients:

$$\text{SNGFR} = L_pS \, (\Delta \text{ hydraulic pressure} - \Delta \text{ oncotic pressure})$$
$$= L_pS \, [(P_{gc} - P_{bx}) - s(\pi_p - \pi_{bs})]$$

where $L_p$ is the unit permeability (or porosity) of the capillary wall, S is the surface area available for filtration, $P_{gc}$ and $P_{bs}$ are the hydraulic pressures in the glomerular capillary and the Bowman space, $\pi_p$ and $\pi_{bs}$ are the oncotic pressures in the plasma entering the glomerulus and in the Bowman space, and s is the reflection coefficient of proteins across the capillary wall (ranging from 0 [completely permeable] to 1 [completely impermeable]).

With the filtrate being essentially protein free, $\pi_{bs}$ is 0, and s is 1, so that:

$$\text{SNGFR} = L_pS \, (P_{gc} - P_{bs} - \pi_p).$$

The $L_pS$ in the glomerular capillary is 50 to 100 times that of a muscle capillary, and the capillary hydraulic pressure (and mean gradient favoring filtration [$P_{gc} - P_{bs} - \pi_p$]) is much greater in the glomerulus than in a muscle capillary.[3,4] These factors contribute to the high rate of glomerular filtration in the kidney.

The plasma oncotic pressure ($\pi_p$) rises in response to the ultrafiltration of protein-free fluid. After the filtration of 20% of the nephron plasma flow, filtration equilibrium is normally achieved. Further filtration at the same plasma flow does not occur because the plasma oncotic pressure equals the hydraulic pressure, and there is no net ultrafiltration pressure. Thus, the presence of filtration equilibrium indicates that renal plasma flow is a major determinant of GFR.[2-4]

## Size selectivity

The glomerular barrier filters molecules based on size and charge. Both the GBM and the slit diaphragms contribute to size selectivity.[1,2,5] The size limitation in the GBM represents functional pores in the spaces between the tightly packed cords of type IV collagen.[2] There is also an important role for cellular elements and slit diaphragms in limiting the passage of macromolecules.[1,2,6] Most pores of the glomerular capillary wall are relatively small (mean radius, ~4.2 nm). They partially restrict the filtration of albumin (mean radius, 3.6 nm) but allow the passage of smaller solutes and water. The endothelial cells do not contribute to size selectivity because the endothelial fenestrae are relatively wide open and do not begin to restrict the passage of macromolecules with a radius of less than approximately 40 nm.[7] However, endothelial cells do contribute to charge selectivity (see later). Modeling of the glomerular filtration barrier suggests that the major portion of the capillary wall functions as an isoporous membrane, but a very small fraction of the filtrate passes through larger pores.[5]

## KEY POINTS

- Permeability of the glomerular capillaries is 50 to 100 times greater than that of capillaries in muscles, thus allowing for filtration to occur.
- Starling forces in the glomerular capillary favor ultrafiltration up to the limit of 20% of nephron plasma flow.
- Both size selectivity and charge selectivity appear to be important in preventing macromolecular transport (e.g., plasma proteins) across the GBM.

## Charge selectivity

Molecular charge is the second major determinant of filtration across the GBM.[1,2,6] The inhibitory effect of charge results from the electrostatic repulsion by anionic heparan sulfate proteoglycans, in both the endothelial fenestrae and the GBM.[1,2,8] Filtration of albumin amounts to only approximately 5% of filtration rate of neutral dextran of a similar molecular radius. Thus, charge is considered important in limiting the filtration of albumin.

## CLINICAL ASSESSMENT OF GLOMERULAR FILTRATION RATE

### Concept of clearance

Given that the total kidney GFR is equal to the sum of the SNGFRs in each of the functioning nephrons, the total GFR can be used as an index of functioning renal mass. A decline

## KEY POINTS

- Determination of GFR provides the best estimate of overall kidney function.
- GFR can be measured by classical renal clearance or plasma disappearance techniques.
- GFR can also be estimated from endogenous biomarkers such as Cr and Cys-C

in the GFR may be the only clinical recognizable sign of renal disease, even when urinalysis results and serum electrolyte composition are relatively normal. Serial monitoring of GFR can be used to estimate severity and to monitor the course of kidney disease. Measurement of GFR is also useful in determining the appropriate dose of drugs that are excreted through the kidney.

The most common measurement of GFR is based on the concept of clearance, which is defined as the equivalent volume of plasma from which a substance would have to be totally removed to account for its rate of excretion in urine per unit of time. The renal clearance of a substance x ($C_x$) is calculated as follows:

$$C_x = \frac{U_x \cdot V}{P_x}$$

where V is urine flow rate (mL/min) and $U_x$ and $P_x$ are the urine and plasma concentrations of substance x, respectively. $C_x$ is expressed as mL/min and is usually normalized to a standard 1.73 $m^2$, idealized adult body surface area (BSA) ($C_x$ in mL/min/1.73 $m^2$) by the factor 1.73 / BSA, where BSA is the BSA (in $m^2$) of the examined subject.

For the plasma clearance to reflect GFR accurately, the marker used must be freely permeant across the glomerular capillary, uncharged, biologically inert, and neither secreted nor reabsorbed by the renal tubule. In the case of an ideal marker (Table 4.2), the renal excretory rate of substance x equals the rate of marker x filtered across the glomerulus:

$$P_x \, GFR = U_x \, V$$

Or

$$GFR = \frac{U_x V}{P_{x,}}$$

Properties of biologic or pharmaceutical markers commonly employed for determination of GFR in children and adults are listed in Table 4.3.

Table 4.2 Characteristics of an ideal marker for estimation of glomerular filtration rate

1. Nontoxic
2. Biologically inert
3. Not protein bound in plasma
4. Exclusively and freely filtered by the glomeruli
5. Not reabsorbed by the renal tubules
6. Not secreted by the renal tubules
7. No extrarenal excretion
8. Assay highly sensitive and reliable
9. Clearance not affected by concentration in plasma over a wide range

Table 4.3 Commonly used markers for determining glomerular filtration rate

**Endogenous Markers**
- Creatinine
- Cystatin C
- Blood urea nitrogen

**Exogenous Markers**
- Inulin
- Iothalamate
- Iohexol
- Radionuclide agents
  - DTPA
  - EDTA
  - Iothalamate

*Abbreviations:* DTPA, diethylene triamine penta-acetic acid; EDTA, ethylene diamine tetra-acetic acid.

## Inulin clearance

GFR is measured indirectly through the concept of clearance discussed earlier. The gold standard for measuring GFR is clearance of inulin, a fructose polysaccharide, which has a mean molecular radius of 1.5 nm and an MW of approximately 5200 daltons. Inulin is freely filtered and not protein bound, and is not reabsorbed, secreted or metabolized by the kidney. Therefore, in the case of inulin as a marker, the $C_x = C_{In} = GFR$.[9]

The classical (standard) inulin clearance requires an intravenous priming dose followed by a constant infusion to establish a steady-state inulin plasma concentration.[10] After equilibration for approximately 45 min, serial urine samples are collected every 10 to 20 min through an indwelling bladder catheter. Under current practice, the insertion of a bladder catheter for renal functional measurement alone is not justifiable, and therefore urine collections are obtained every 20 to 30 min, as dictated by the urge of the patient to urinate. In this case, urine flow is maintained high by providing an initial oral fluid load of 500 to 800 mL water/$m^2$ and replacing urine output with intake of water (mL for mL).[11] Inulin is assayed in the timed

> **KEY POINTS**
>
> - Clearance of a substance is the volume of plasma from which it would be completely removed in a unit of time.
> - Inulin clearance, considered the "gold standard," is seldom performed in clinical circumstances.

urine collection, as well as in the serum. GFR is calculated using the clearance formula given earlier. GFR by inulin clearance methodology in newborns, infants, and children is given in Table 4.4.

The use of inulin clearances in children is limited by several concerns. First, some children may not be toilet trained and are unable to provide accurate collections of timed urine. Second, urologic problems are common causes of chronic kidney disease (CKD) in infants and young children, some of whom may have significant vesicoureteral reflux, neurogenic bladders, and bladder dysynergias.[12] Collecting timed urine samples in such patients is problematic and fraught with error. Technical difficulties encountered in performing inulin infusions, reaching a steady state of inulin distribution, and accurately measuring inulin concentrations in plasma are added concerns. In addition, the inulin assay is not very specific, and it can be potentially hazardous (boiling acid reagents). These problems have rendered the standard inulin clearance impractical for use in children.

## Constant infusion technique without urine collection

Despite previously stated concerns, understanding the principles behind inulin clearance is helpful in comprehending the rationale of using clearance of various molecules for determining GFR. The clearance of a substance denotes its removal from the blood. Therefore, it is possible to determine the plasma clearance by infusing the substance at a constant rate until a steady state is achieved.

Table 4.4 Properties of markers commonly used to determine glomerular filtration rate

|  | Inulin | Creatinine | Iothalamate | DTPA | EDTA | Iohexol |
|---|---|---|---|---|---|---|
| MW (Da) | 5,200 | 113 | 636 | 393 | 292 | 821 |
| Elimination half-life (min) | 70 | 200 | 120 | 110 | 120 | 90 |
| Protein binding (%) | 0 | 0 | <5 | 5 | 0 | <2 |
| Space distribution | ECW | TBW | ECW | ECW | ECW | ECW |

*Source:* Adapted from Rahn KH, Heidenreich S, Bruckner D. How to assess glomerular function and damage in humans. J Hypertens. 1999;17:309–17.
*Abbreviations:* Da, daltons; DTPA, diethylene thiamine penta-acetic acid; ECW, extracellular water; EDTA, ethylene diamine tetra-acetic acid; MW, molecular weight; TBW, total body water.

This constant infusion technique has used inulin, although other markers, especially radionuclide tagged tracers, also can be used (discussed later). After equilibration of the marker in its distribution space, the excretion rate equals the infusion rate. The renal clearance of the molecule can then be calculated from the rate of infusion and the concentration in plasma.[13]

$$C_x = \frac{I_x R}{S_x}$$

where $I_x$ is infusion concentration of substance x, R is infusion rate (mL/min), $S_x$ is the serum concentration of x, and $C_x$ is the clearance in mL/min/1.73 m². 

The constant infusion method will overestimate GFR if steady concentration of the marker is not achieved.

## Endogenous creatinine clearance and the use of cimetidine

Because of the difficulties with administering and measuring inulin, endogenous Cr clearances have been used to estimate GFR. Clearance of Cr provides a useful clinical tool, albeit less precise than inulin clearance, for estimation of GFR. Cr clearance is determined by the following formula:

$$C_{cr} = \frac{U_{cr} V}{S_{cr}}$$

where $C_{cr}$ is Cr clearance, $U_{cr}$ is urine Cr concentration, V is flow rate of urine in mL/min, and $S_{cr}$ is serum Cr, and the calculation is normalized to BSA by multiplying by the factor 1.73 / BSA in m². 

Adequacy of urine collection is essential for this test. The relative constancy of Cr production and its urinary excretion in the steady state helps one analyze for completeness of the collection. Historically, Cr clearance is derived from a 24-h urine collection. On the day of the test, the child is asked to void and empty the bladder in the morning (7 a.m.), the urine is discarded, and the time is noted as the start of the collection. All urine voided in the next 24 h is collected in the container as part of this collection. At the end of 24 h (7 a.m. on the next day), the bladder is emptied, and the last void is deposited in the container as the final part of the collection. The volume of urine is noted accurately, and the urine is analyzed for Cr concentration. Blood (for serum Cr) is drawn during the urine collections. Urinary Cr excretion (Cr index) should generally exceed 15 to 20 mg/kg/day in children older than 3 years of age and is 20% higher than that for pubertal adolescent boys.[14–16] Lower Cr index values generally indicate urine collection of less than 24 h or loss of some urine. Nevertheless, daily variation in urinary Cr excretion results in a standard deviation of 10% to 15%.[17]

Averaging several short clearance periods (~30 min) after water loading tends to minimize errors in urine collection and improve supervision of the study.[18–20] Large variations in urine Cr excretion often indicate significant vesicoureteral reflux or inadequate bladder emptying, and they may warrant bladder catheterization to improve accuracy of the test. In addition, Cr concentration is affected, to a small extent, by dietary intake of meat, exercise, and pyrexia. More importantly, it is well known that Cr is secreted by the renal tubules; this secretory component accounts for approximately 10% of the urinary Cr excretion in normal individuals.[20] Therefore, Cr clearance exceeds inulin clearance, by at least 10%, particularly at low levels of GFR.[10]

Whereas in the steady state, Cr production equals its urinary excretion, Cr production is not constant during growth, by more than doubling from term infancy to adolescence.[14,21] The consequence of the increasing Cr production with growth is the steady increase in plasma Cr as a function of age, with an additional increase resulting from the increment in muscle mass in male adolescents (Figure 4.2).[22]

The administration of cimetidine to patients with renal disease causes a decrease in renal tubular Cr secretion that results in a reduction in Cr clearance to the level of actual GFR.[23] A protocol for cimetidine treatment developed for use in children has similarly equated Cr clearance to the level of GFR.[19] This requires that cimetidine be given for 3 days at a dose of 20 mg/kg/day, divided into two doses, to a maximum of 1600 mg per day (with a sliding scale reduction for decreases in GFR).[19] After an oral load of 7 to 8 mL/kg of fluids, four urinary collection periods of approximately 30 min each

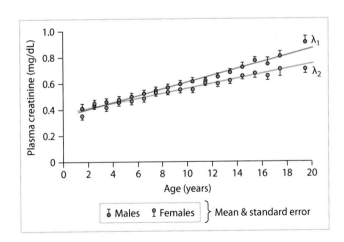

Figure 4.2 Serum creatinine as a function of age in boys (red circles) and girls (blue circles) with 1 standard error estimate, taken from 772 boys and girls females. Creatinine was measured using a modification of the Technicon Autoanalyzer Jaffe assay. (From Schwartz GJ, Haycock GB, Spitzer A. Plasma creatinine and urea concentration in children: normal values for age and sex. J Pediatr. 1976;88:828–30.)

follow, with urine replaced milliliter for milliliter during this time. Although the cimetidine protocol is a convenient and an inexpensive procedure for estimating GFR, there are likely to be inaccuracies in children with severe reflux, neurogenic bladders, and bladder dyssynergias.

## Serum creatinine

Cr is produced by enzymatic degradation of creatine that is primarily synthesized in the skeletal muscles. The urinary excretion of Cr is determined by muscle catabolism and is hence an index of muscle mass.[16] In the steady state, serum Cr correlates well with the muscle mass, but several physiologic, pharmacologic, and pathologic states can affect its serum concentration (Table 4.5).[20,24] Cr has an MW of 113 daltons. It is eliminated from the body exclusively by the kidneys, primarily by glomerular filtration, but also to a small extent by tubular secretion. Whereas urinary Cr contributed by tubular secretion does not normally exceed 10%, this fraction rises greatly in chronic renal insufficiency, so Cr clearance may greatly exceed GFR.[20] Diffusion of Cr into the gut with subsequent catabolism may also interfere with the accuracy of its clearance in uremic patients.[25] GFR

### KEY POINTS

- Growth and development lead to increased muscle mass and therefore elevated serum Cr concentration.
- Height factored by serum Cr ($ht/S_{cr}$) provides an accurate estimate of GFR in most children.

Table 4.5 Factors that influence serum creatinine level

| Increase serum creatinine | Decrease serum creatinine |
| --- | --- |
| Hyperglycemia (Jaffe) | Malnutrition |
| Ketotic states (Jaffe) | Dietary protein restriction |
| Cephalosporins (Jaffe) | Bilirubin (Jaffe) |
| Flucytosine (enzymatic method) | Advanced liver disease |
| Cimetidine (block tubular secretion) | Female sex |
| Trimethoprim (block tubular secretion) | Advanced age (adults) |
| Vigorous exercise | |
| Cooked meat | |
| Creatine nutritional supplement | |

*Source:* Rosner MH, Bolton WK. Renal function testing. Am J Kidney Dis. 2006;47:174–83.

Table 4.6 Glomerular filtration rate in normal infants and children, assessed by inulin clearance

| Age | Mean GFR ± SD (mL/min/1.73 m²) |
| --- | --- |
| **Preterm babies** | |
| 1–3 days | 14.0 ± 5[*] |
| 1–7 days | 18.7 ± 5.5[†] |
| 4–8 days | 44.3 ± 9.3[‡] |
| 3–13 days | 47.8 ± 10.7[§] |
| 8–14 days | 35.4 ± 13.4[†] |
| 1.5–4 mo | 67.4 ± 16.6[§] |
| **Full-term babies** | |
| 1–3 days | 20.8 ± 5.0[†] |
| 3–4 days | 39.0 ± 15.1[¶] |
| 4–14 days | 36.8 ± 7.2[#] |
| 6–14 days | 54.6 ± 7.6[**] |
| 15–19 days | 46.9 ± 12.5[†] |
| 1–3 mo | 85.3 ± 35.1[¶] |
| 0–3 mo | 60.4 ± 17.4[††] |
| 4–6 mo | 87.4 ± 22.3[††] |
| 7–12 mo | 96.2 ± 12.2[††] |
| 1–2 yr | 105.2 ± 17.3[††] |
| **Children** | |
| 3–4 yr | 111.2 ± 18.5[††] |
| 5–6 yr | 114.1 ± 18.6[††] |
| 7–8 yr | 111.3 ± 18.3[††] |
| 9–10 yr | 110.0 ± 21.6[††] |
| 11–12 yr | 116.4 ± 18.9[††] |
| 13–15 yr | 117.2 ± 16.1[††] |
| 2.7–11.6 yr | 127.1 ± 13.5[‡] |
| 9–12 yr | 116.6 ± 18.1[¶] |
| **Young adults** | |
| 16.2–34 yr | 112 ± 13[‡‡] |

[*] Data from reference 89.
[†] Data from reference 90.
[‡] Data from reference 91.
[§] Data from reference 92.
[¶] Data from reference 93.
[#] Data from reference 94.
[**] Data from reference 95.
[††] Data from reference 96.
[‡‡] Data from reference 97.

based on Cr clearance in infants, children, and adolescents is listed Table 4.6.

## Creatinine-based estimated glomerular filtration rate

The close relationship between Cr clearance and GFR on the one hand and Cr production and muscle mass on the other has led to the concept of estimating GFR (eGFR) from serum Cr and some parameter of body habitus. This has been detailed by Schwartz et al.,[26] using the following formula:

$$eGFR\ (ml/min/1.73\ m^2) = \frac{kL}{S_{cr}}$$

where eGFR is estimated GFR in mL/min/1.73 m², k is a constant determined empirically by Schwartz et al.,[21] L is height in cm, and $S_{cr}$ is serum Cr in mg/dL.

This formula is also based on the relationship that Cr clearance is reciprocally proportional to serum Cr. A dimensional analysis of k (mg Cr/100 min × cm × 1.73 m²) indicates that k is equal to $U_{Cr}V / L$, which is directly related to urinary Cr excretion that, in turn, is proportional to lean body mass.[14,21].

Using Cr, the value of k was determined Schwartz et al. to be 0.45 for term infants during the first year of life,[14] 0.55 for children and adolescent girls,[26] and 0.7 in adolescent boys.[15] eGFR, using Schwartz's formula, generally provides a good estimate of GFR (r ~ 0.9) when compared with Cr and inulin clearance data.[19,26]. Interestingly, at high values of GFR, the variation between inulin clearance and GFR estimated by the Schwartz formula was approximately 20%, but it was much smaller at lower levels of GFR.[19,26]. There was no explanation for this finding. The eGFR Schwartz formula can be rewritten as follows:

$$GFR(ml/min/1.73m^2) = \frac{Height\ in\ centimeters}{Serum\ creatinine(mg/dL)} \times k$$

Where k = constant based on age:
0.70 in adolescent boys
0.55 in adolescent girls and children
0.45 in full-term newborns
0.33 in preterm infants

The foregoing given constants were generated using Cr measured using a modification of the Technicon Autoanalyzer (Seal Analytical, Mequon, WI), which relied on a modification of the Jaffe chromogen reaction to determine Cr. The newer generation of autoanalyzers determine serum Cr enzymatically, using the creatinase methods. Although the enzymatic Cr method appears to agree with "true" Cr obtained from the Jaffe reaction after Fuller earth absorption, some manufacturers use calibration factors (bias) to produce Jaffe-comparable results. This bias is not linear and therefore is unlikely to improve the accuracy of serum Cr determination in children. Without the bias, the enzymatic Cr generally runs 10% to 20% lower than those measured by the Jaffe method.[27] Therefore, one would anticipate that k values should be comparably smaller than those listed earlier.

The Schwartz formula for eGFR was revised to overcome the approximately 20% bias of overestimation of GFR.[28] The modified Schwartz formula used a single value of k for children with mild to moderate CKD who were 1.5 to 18 years of age:

$$eGFR(mL/min/1.73m^2) = \frac{Height\ in\ centimeters}{Serum\ creatinine\ (mg/dL)} \times 0.413$$

If using SI units:

$$GFR(mL/min/1.73m^2) = \frac{Height\ in\ centimeters}{Serum\ creatinine\ (\mu mol/L)} \times 36.2$$

The modified Schwartz formula has been validated only in patients with CKD; it may not be applicable to patients with acute kidney injury (AKI). Additionally, this formula mandates using enzymatic serum Cr measurement that is calibrated to reference standards of isotope dilution mass spectroscopy (IDMS), but not to "Jaffe" (alkaline picrate) methods.[29] Staples et al.[30] successfully extended the updated Schwartz formula to adolescents with higher levels of GFR. Whereas some clinical laboratories can mathematically convert the results from the Jaffe method to IDMS-traceable results by instrument-specific factors provided by the manufacturers of equipment for assaying serum Cr; this black box approach may be flawed by the magnitude of correction required for children with low levels of serum Cr.

Counahan et al.[31] generated a similar formula for estimating GFR using "near-true" Cr determinations, and the resulting k in their study was 0.43. This value of k is lower than the original Schwartz formula's value and may reflect the lower value of Cr after removal of non-Cr chromogen with an ion exchange resin. However, this k represents a value that is very close to the updated value of 0.413 obtained in the Chronic Kidney Disease in Children (CKiD) study of children with CKD.[28] Indeed, this k is approximately 20% lower than the original k obtained from the modified Technicon Autoanalyzer and is in keeping with the expected reduction in apparent serum Cr concentration with the "true" method.

These eGFR formulas must be used with caution and may not be accurate in cases of severe obesity, malnourishment, or limb amputation because in these patients body height may not accurately reflect muscle mass.[21] Additionally, these estimate formulas are not accurate when GFR is rapidly changing, such as in patients with AKI or those in the intensive care unit.[32]

The Cockcroft-Gault equation, used to estimate GFR in adults, may also be useful in children older than 12 years of age.[33]

$$eGFR = (140 - age)\ (body\ weight\ in\ kg)/(72 \times S_{cr})$$

where eGFR is the estimated GFR using the Cockcroft-Gault equation in boys; in girls, a correction factor of 0.85 is used.

This formula has limited utility in pediatrics because of the inaccuracies in children 8 years old or younger. Whereas there is good overall agreement with standard inulin clearances in children, the correlation with GFR is less consistent than with the Schwartz estimate, and the scatter appears larger.[34] In general, the Modification of Diet in Renal Disease (MDRD) eGFR equation is not useful in children.[34]

## Cystatin C

Cys-C is a low-MW protein (13 kDa) that is produced by all nucleated cells.[35] Cys-C is filtered by the glomeruli and is reabsorbed in the proximal tubules by megalin-facilitated endocytosis.[36] Cys-C is catabolized in the proximal tubule, and an insignificant amount may be recovered in urine.[37] Because megalin is also involved in the endocytosis of albumin present in the glomerular filtrate, saturation of megalin in proteinuric states may result in increased urinary Cys-C excretion without affecting the serum concentration.[38,39]

Cys-C has been proposed as an endogenous marker for GFR that could be more accurate in detecting more subtle decrements of GFR.[40] The advantage of Cys-C over serum Cr as an marker for GFR lies in the finding that serum Cys-C levels fluctuate very little beyond the first year of life and are not largely influenced by age, gender, and body weight.[41,42] However, several clinical conditions can alter serum Cys-C level and need to be considered in estimation of Cys-C–based GFR (Table 4.7).[43–54] In addition, because Cys-C is almost entirely reabsorbed and metabolized in the proximal renal tubules, it cannot be used to measure GFR by traditional clearance techniques (e.g., Cr clearance). Therefore, Cys-C GFR can be estimated only by mathematically derived formulas or eGFR calculations. In AKI,

Table 4.7 Clinical conditions and pharmacologic therapies that affect serum cystatin C level

| Serum cystatin c level | Clinical conditions |
| --- | --- |
| Increase | Obesity |
| | High-dose methylprednisone |
| | Kidney transplant |
| | Hyperthyroidism |
| | Amyotrophic lateral sclerosis |
| | Malignant disease |
| | Bone marrow transplant |
| | Asthma |
| | Elevated C-reactive protein |
| | Cigarette smoking |
| | Cardiac disease (atherosclerotic) |
| Decrease | Nephrotic syndrome (related to urinary loss) |
| | Hypothyroidism |
| | Cyclosporine |
| | Hypertriglyceridemia |
| No effect | Age |
| | Gender |
| | Body weight |
| | Moderate-dose prednisone or methylprednisolone |
| | Mycophenolate mofetil |
| | Azathioprine |

Table 4.8 Serum cystatin C level (mg/L) in neonates of varying gestational ages obtained postnatally at 0 to 3 days and at 22 to 30 days

| Gestational age | Postnatal day 0–3 | Postnatal day 22–30 |
| --- | --- | --- |
| <28 wk | 1.60 ± 0.21 (range, 1.2–2.1) | 2.02 ± 0.42 (range, (1.4–2.5) |
| 29–32 wk | 1.56 ± 0.28 (range, 0.3–2.1) | 1.84 ± 0.27 (range, 1.4–2.3) |
| 33–36 wk | 1.67 ± 0.25 (range, 1.2–2.5) | 1.64 ± 0.23 (range, 1.3–2.1) |
| >37 wk | 1.64 ± 0.32 (range, 0.9–2.9) | 1.56 ± 0.39 (range, 1.0–2.4) |

Source: Data from Lee JH, Hahn WH, Ahn J, et al. Serum cystatin C during 30 postnatal days is dependent on the postconceptional age in neonates. Pediatr Nephrol. 2013;28:1073–8.

however, the presence of Cys-C in urine may be used as an early indicator of proximal tubular injury.

Serum Cys-C levels are high in full-term neonates and gradually decline in the first 4 months of life. Serum Cys-C levels are even higher in preterm infants and appear to be inversely influenced by gestational age (Table 4.8).[55–57] One criticism of the normative Cys-C data in preterm infants is that many children in this cohort have other medical conditions that may directly influence their serum Cys-C levels. Near-adult serum levels of Cys-C are reached by 1 year of age (Table 4.9). Beyond the first year, the constancy of Cys-C is relatively stable and is largely independent of muscle mass, gender, body composition, and age.[48] In an analysis of National Health and Nutrition Examination Survey III (NHANES III) data, Groesbeck et al.,[58] however, noted that serum Cys-C levels in girls and women 12 to 19 years of age are lower than in boys and men. Similarly, obesity has also been noted to influence serum Cys-C level.[45]

### KEY POINTS

- Because Cys-C is reabsorbed and metabolized by the proximal renal tubule, its urinary excretion is nearly zero. Therefore, traditional clearance methods of determining GFR with Cys-C are not applicable, and only eGFR calculations are valid.
- Combining plasma Cys-C with serum Cr in estimation of GFR formulas greatly enhances the accuracy of eGFR.

Several eGFR calculations using serum Cys-C level have been validated in adults and children, and these calculations correlate well with traditional GFR measurements by inulin clearance, Cr clearance, or radionuclide GFR.[59–62] However, these calculations are generally more complex for bedside clinical use than the Schwartz eGFR calculations. Because

Table 4.9 Serum cystatin C reference ranges in infants, children, and adolescents

| Age group | Mean and range |
| --- | --- |
| 0–3 mo | 1.37 (range, 1.81–2.32) |
| 4–11 mo | 0.98 (range, 0.65–1.49) |
| 1–3 yr | 0.79 (range, 0.50–1.25) |
| 4–8 yr | 0.80 (range, 0.49–1.11) |
| 9–17 yr | 0.82 (range, 0.53–1.29) |
| 12–17 yr (NHANES III data) | Male patients: 0.89 |
| | Female patients: 0.79 |

*Source:* Data from Finney H, Newman DJ, Thakkar H, et al. Reference ranges for plasma cystatin C and creatinine measurements in premature infants, neonates, and older children. Arch Dis Child. 2000;82:71–5. National Health and Nutrition Examination Survey III (NHANES III) data from Groesbeck D, Köttgen A, Parekh R, et al. Age, gender, and race effects on cystatin C levels in US adolescents. Clin J Am Soc Nephrol. 2008;3:1777–85.

serum Cys-C levels are known to be elevated in patients with renal transplants and to underestimate the true GFR in these patients, a correction factor of 1.2 has been suggested by Zappitelli et al.[61] to be applied to Cys-C–based GFR in transplant recipients.

Additional accuracy in estimating GFR can be derived from formulas that incorporate both serum Cr and Cys-C. Such formulas, by Bouvet et al., Zappitelli, and Schwartz, are capable of estimating 80% of determinations within 30% of measured GFR and nearly 40% within 10% of measured GFR.[29,61-63] Modification of the Schwartz equation using immunonephelometric measurements of Cys-C was derived from the CKiD population of children with mild to moderate CKD and proved very accurate, with 91% of estimates falling within 30% of measured GFR and 45% within 10% of measured GFR.[62] Table 4.10 lists the eGFR calculations using serum Cr, Cys-C and the combination of Cys-C and Cr.

Table 4.10 Estimated glomerular filtration rate calculation formulas using serum creatinine, serum cystatin C and the combination of serum creatinine and cystatin C

| Reference source | Formula |
| --- | --- |
| **Serum creatinine** | |
| Schwartz et al. (1976)[26] | $$GFR(ml/min/1.73m^2) = \frac{Height\ in\ centimeters}{Serum\ creatinine(mg/dL)} \times k$$ Where k = constant based on age 0.70 in adolescent boys 0.55 in adolescent girls and children 0.45 in full-term newborns 0.33 in preterm infants |
| Schwartz et al. (2009)[28] (IDMS-traceable creatinine based Schwartz GFR formula, or modified Schwartz formula) | $$eGFR(ml/min/1.73m^2) = \frac{Height\ in\ centimeters}{Serum\ creatinine\ (mg/dL)} \times 0.413$$ If using SI units: $$eGFR(mL/min/1.73m^2) \times \frac{Height\ in\ centimeters}{Serum\ cretinine\ (\mu mol/L)} \times 36.2$$ |
| Counahan et al. (1976)[31] | $$eGFR\ (ml/min/1.73\ m^2) = \frac{0.43 \times Height\ in\ cm}{Serum\ cretinine\ (mg/dL)}$$ |
| Cockcroft and Gault (1976)[33] | eGFR = (140 − age) (body weight in kg) / (72 × $S_{cr}$) |
| **Serum cystatin C** | |
| Bökenkamp et al. (1999)[59] | GFR (mL/min/1.73 m²) = 137/Cys-C − 20.4 |
| Hoek et al. (2003)[60] | GFR (mL/min/1.73 m²) = −4.32 + 80.35 (Cys-C)$^{-1}$ |
| Zappitelli et al. (2006)[61] | GFR (mL/min/1.73 m²) = 75.94 / [Cys-C$^{1.17}$] If renal transplant patient, multiply by a factor of 1.2 |
| Schwartz et al. (2012)[62] | GFR (mL/min/1.73 m²) = 70.69 (Cys-C)$^{-0.931}$ |
| **Serum creatinine and cystatin C** | |
| Schwartz et al. (2012)[62] | GFR (mL/min/1.73 m²) = 39.8 (height/$S_{cr}$)$^{0.456}$ × (1.8 / Cys)$^{0.418}$ × (30 / BUN)$^{0.079}$ × (1.076$^{male}$) × (height/1.4)$^{0.179}$ |
| Bouvet et al. (2006)[63] | GFR (mL/min/1.73 m²) = 63.2 × (1.2/Cys-C)$^{0.56}$ × [($S_{cr}$ × 88.4/96)]$^{-0.35}$ × (weight/45)$^{0.30}$ × (age/14)$^{0.40}$ |
| Zappitelli et al. (2006)[61] | GFR (mL/min/1.73 m²) = (43.82 × e$^{0.003 \times height}$) (Cys-C$^{-0.635}$) × ($S_{cr}^{-0.547}$) |

*Abbreviations:* BUN, blood urea nitrogen; Cys-C, cystatin C; GFR, glomerular filtration rate; eGFR, estimated glomerular filtration rate; IDMS, isotope dilution mass spectroscopy; $S_{cr}$, serum creatinine.

## Single injection clearance techniques

The renal clearance of a substance that is not metabolically produced or degraded and that is excreted from the body totally or almost totally in the urine can be calculated from compartmental analysis by monitoring its rate of disappearance from the plasma following a single intravenous injection.[64] The mathematical model for the disappearance curve is an open two-compartment system. The GFR marker is injected in the first compartment, equilibrates with the second compartment, and is excreted from the first compartment by glomerular filtration. Initially, the concentration falls rapidly but at a progressively diminishing rate because of diffusion of the marker in its distribution volume as well as its renal excretion. Thereafter, the slope of the decline of plasma concentration reflects predominately its renal excretion rate. This latter decrease occurs at the same exponential rate in the compartments wherein it is distributed.

Indeed, the plasma disappearance curve can be resolved into two exponential decay curves by plotting the log of the plasma concentration as a function of time and applying the technique of curve stripping (Figure 4.3). The terminal slow (renal) portion of the curve (line A) is extrapolated back to zero time, and its Y intercept (A) and slope ($\alpha$) are determined. When the values along line A are subtracted from the original curve, a second linear function (line B) is obtained. Its Y intercept (B) and slope ($\beta$) are also noted. The clearance of the substance, taken as GFR, can be calculated as follows[64]:

$$GFR = Dose \times 0.693 / [(exp\ (A)/\alpha + (exp\ (B) / \beta)],$$

where Dose is the administered amount of GFR marker, and GFR is normalized to 1.73 $m^2$ by multiplying by 1.73 / BSA.

Thus, to obtain an accurate plasma disappearance curve, several blood samples are required. Extension of sampling to 5 h is essential to ensure accuracy at low levels of GFR.

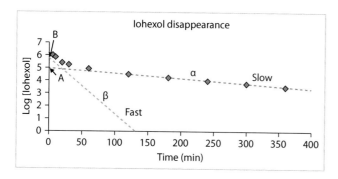

Figure 4.3 Disappearance of iohexol as a function of time after injection into the blood. The natural log of the iohexol concentration is plotted against the time in minutes. The curve can be stripped into two components: the slow or renal curve with slope $\alpha$ and intercept A. When those points are subtracted from the initial curve, a straight line with a steeper slope $\beta$ defines the fast or distribution curve with intercept B.

Excellent and comparable results may also be obtained using the one-compartment (renal curve) model, by which samples are obtained 2 to 5 h after injection, as described by Brochner-Mortensen[65]:

$$GFR = C1 \times GFR\ (A) + C2 \times [GFR\ (A)]^2$$

where GFR (A) = Dose / [exp (A)/$\alpha$], and C1 = 0.9908 and C2 = 0.001218, as generated by Brochner-Mortensen in adults by comparing to plasma disappearance curves for chromium-51–ethylene diamine tetra-acetic acid (EDTA).

Recently, Ng et al.[66] have developed a universal equation to calculate GFR from the slow renal disappearance curve in children and adults.

$$GFR = slowGFR / [1 = 0.12 * (slowGFR / 100)]$$

where slowGFR is the GFR calculated from the iohexol dose divided by the area under the renal (slow) curve.

Such an equation has allowed the CKiD cohort to use a two-point plasma disappearance GFR by sampling at 120 and 300 min after iohexol infusion. Such an equation can be applied universally and is not dependent on the dose of infused iohexol. The results obtained were superior to those generated from the pediatric and adult forms of the Brochner-Mortensen one-compartment models noted earlier.

## Diethylene triamine penta-acetic acid, ethylene diamine tetra-acetic acid, and iothalamate

Historically, the plasma disappearance curve was most often used when assessing GFR with radionuclides. Even with single injection techniques, radioactive markers are best avoided in small children. Moreover, families are reluctant to approve of repeated use of radioactivity to monitor the course of CKD. Diethylene triamine penta-acetic acid (DTPA) has an MW of 393 daltons and is excreted primarily by glomerular filtration. GFR can be measured in each kidney by using a scintillation camera and the technetium-99m ($^{99m}$Tc)–DTPA complex; however, the correlation with 24-h Cr clearances is only fair.[67] The plasma clearance of $^{99m}$Tc-DTPA significantly exceeds the urinary clearance.[68,69] Conversely, the plasma clearance of $^{99m}$Tc-DTPA correlates well with the renal clearance of inulin.[68] Failure to measure GFR accurately may reflect the findings that $^{99m}$Tc can dissociate from DTPA during the study and there can be variations in protein binding depending on the ligand attached to DTPA.[70] Some preparations with calcium-sodium-DTPA gave results comparable to those with chromium-51–EDTA, whereas others underestimated GFR by 7% to 22%.[70] Thus, the accuracy of $^{99m}$Tc-DTPA may depend on the commercial source.

EDTA is another marker for determining GFR. It has an MW of 292 daltons and is used as a chelate of chromium- 51–, primarily in Europe. Its plasma clearance exceeds its urinary clearance by approximately 6 mL/min, particularly in patients with reduced renal function.[68] However, plasma clearance of chromium-51–EDTA ($^{51}$Cr-EDTA) agrees well with that of renal inulin clearance, a finding indicating that it is a good marker for GFR. Values of $^{51}$Cr-EDTA plasma clearances increase from birth to age 18 months and plateau thereafter.[68] The absolute numbers agree well with measurements performed using inulin clearances given in Table 4.5.

Iothalamate sodium has an MW of 637 daltons. It has been used as iodine-125 ($^{125}$I) radiolabeled or without a radioactive label, and its plasma concentration is measured by x-ray fluorescence, high-performance liquid chromatography (HPLC), or capillary electrophoresis. In a comparison of agents, the plasma clearance of $^{125}$I-iothalamate was 13% higher than that of $^{51}$Cr-EDTA.[71] The difference was reduced by pretreatment of the patients with probenecid, an organic anion secretory inhibitor. Extensive laboratory studies have shown unambiguously that iothalamate is actively secreted by renal proximal tubular cells, and it may also undergo some tubular reabsorption.[71] The renal clearance of iothalamate significantly exceeds that of inulin in patients with normal renal function,[72] and any reported agreement with inulin clearance may reflect a fortuitous cancellation of errors between tubular excretion and protein binding.[73,74] Thus, iothalamate cannot be recommended as an ideal marker for measuring GFR.

## Iohexol

A reliable alternative to inulin clearance avoids both the use of radioactivity and the problems related to timed urination and continuous infusion of the marker. Iohexol is a non-ionic, low-osmolar, x-ray contrast medium (Omnipaque) that is safe and nontoxic. Iohexol is used for angiographic and urographic procedures and is eliminated from plasma exclusively by glomerular filtration.[74] Iohexol has an MW of 821 daltons and a plasma elimination half-time of approximately 90 min; it is distributed into the extracellular space and has less than 2% plasma protein binding.[74–76] Iohexol is excreted completely unmetabolized in the urine with 100% recovery within 24 h after injection.[76] Because iohexol can be quantified in small samples, capillary and venous sampling can be employed.[77] Extrarenal elimination of iohexol in a setting of reduced GFR is negligible.[78] Iohexol is measured in deproteinized plasma or serum by HPLC or x-ray fluorescence. The commercially available preparations contain two isomers of iohexol, both of which are handled similarly by the body.[77,79] In practice, the major peak, eluting at approximately 5 min, is used for determining serum and plasma concentrations.[79] Most studies indicate close agreement between GFR (measured by inulin clearance) and clearance of iohexol, measured as standard renal clearance or plasma disappearance.[76,79–82] There is not only a very good correlation between plasma iohexol clearance and that of chromium-51–EDTA, but also no difference between the methods by Bland-Altman analysis.[83] Direct comparison

with iothalamate indicates that the iothalamate clearance exceeds that of iohexol by 19%.[84]

Modeling of plasma disappearance of iohexol indicates that its excretion conforms to a two-compartment open

---

### KEY POINTS

- Iohexol (Omnipaque) closely approximates inulin clearance as a marker for GFR determination.
- Iothalamate clearance exceeds inulin clearance by nearly 20%.

---

system.[76,79] In a pilot study for the National Institutes of Health-supported CKiD study, we found that even with low GFR, serum iohexol concentrations decrease exponentially along the slow (renal) curve within 60 to 120 min of injection.[84] GFR measured after 5 h was comparable to that after 6 h, but shortening to 4 h in children resulted in a significant 3% overestimation of GFR.[85] Such studies have demonstrated the accuracy of GFR measurement obtained from two- and three-point blood sampling during the renal disappearance curve. The clearance of iohexol (GFR) may also be calculated from the slow (renal) plasma disappearance curve (one-compartment system approximation beginning 120 min after injection) according to the method of Brochner-Mortenson (see earlier), or by applying the Chantler correction, which assumes a correction factor of 0.87.[65,86,87] However, the Ng calculation is more accurate, is better correlated, and provides smaller bias and root mean square error.[66]

The collection of urine without urinary catheters (using various methods to establish that the bladder is empty after voiding) does not add significant accuracy to the clearance estimate.[85,86] The 24-h urine determinations may vary by as much as 10% to 15% from one day to another, and a similar phenomenon is noted when averaging multiple short urine collections.[17] Therefore, a fair correlation with standard inulin clearance is perhaps the best that can be expected, especially because bladder catheterization is considered more than minimal risk. The plasma disappearance of a marker that is excreted only by glomerular filtration may in fact be the gold standard that replaces the standard inulin clearance.

## Determination of glomerular filtration rate by radionuclide scan

Estimation of GFR by use of radioisotopes is a commonly used technique in children, particularly with the limited availability of inulin and difficulties in collecting accurate timed urines in children. Commonly used radioisotopes are $^{99m}$Tc-DTPA, $^{131}$I or $^{125}$I-Hippuran (a solution containing iodohippurate sodium), and $^{99m}$Tc-MAG-3 (mercaptoacetyltriglycine). Only the first is useful for GFR measurement. One method calculates GFR from the uptake of labeled tracer in each kidney and allows determination of separate assessment of each kidney separately (split functions).[67] A second method uses the disappearance of the labeled marker from the plasma, and, as noted earlier, DTPA is variably accurate as a marker of GFR.[87]

Hippuran is secreted and thus does not give a measure of GFR, but rather of renal blood flow. Because of protein binding, Hippuran is not as accurate as p-aminohippurate for this purpose. Yet, it has been used as a dynamic radionuclide renographic determinant of renal function that complements the predominantly anatomic information provided by most other imaging techniques. MAG-3 has now supplanted hippuran for this purpose because of its higher extraction ratio, which results in improved renal images.[88]

---

### KEY POINT

When corrected for body surface area, GFR reaches adult levels by the second year of life.

---

## GLOMERULAR FILTRATION RATE TREND DURING CHILDHOOD

As seen in Table 4.4, full-term newborn infants have a very low GFR of 20.8 ± 5 mL/min/1.73 m$^2$ at birth, and by 19 days the GFR increases to 46.9 ± 12.5 mL/min/1.73 m$^2$.[89-97] Preterm babies, conversely, have even lower GFR, with a mean of 14.0 ± 5 mL/min/1.73 m$^2$ at 1 to 3 days. An increasing trend in GFR is, however, noticeable in the first 8 weeks in both full-term and preterm infants. Vieux et al.[98] reported GFR determined by 12-h Cr clearance methodology in very preterm infants, ranging from 27 to 31 weeks of gestation. An inverse relationship of GFR to the gestational age was noted in this series, with most preterm infants having the lowest median GFR. Mathematical derivation of median expected GFR in the very preterm infants can be calculated by the formulas proposed by these authors (Table 4.11).[98] Improvement in GFR is noted throughout infancy. When corrected for body surface area, GFR reaches adult levels by 2 years of age.

---

### KEY POINTS

- Kidney tubular functions are responsible for reabsorbing filtered solutes and regulating serum concentrations of electrolytes, divalent ions, and neutral solutes; various transporters are expressed by the kidney to perform these functions.
- Clearance studies and urine collection under specific conditions enable physicians to assess such tubular functions globally.

---

Table 4.11 Calculation of expected median glomerular filtration rate in very preterm infants at day 7 to 28 of postnatal life

| Postnatal day | Median GFR (mL/min/1.73 m²) |
| --- | --- |
| Day 7 | −63.57 + (2.85 × GA) |
| Day 14 | −60.73 + (2.85 × GA) |
| Day 21 | −58.97 + (2.85 × GA) |
| Day 28 | −55.93 + (2.85 × GA) |

Source: Data from Vieux R, Hascoet JM, Merdariu D, et al. Glomerular filtration rate reference values in very preterm infants. Pediatrics. 2010; 125:e1186–92.

Example: In a 27 week gestation baby at 7 days of age the median expected GFR is: −63.57 + (2.85 × 27), or 13.38 mL/min/1.73m2.

Abbreviations: GA, gestational age in weeks; GFR, glomerular filtration rate.

The presence of low GFR in newborns, especially in very preterm babies, indicates that the doses of all drugs, especially those excreted by the kidneys, must be appropriately adjusted to avoid drug toxicities.

---

## TESTS FOR TUBULAR FUNCTIONS

The renal tubules transport solutes, hydrogen ions, organic ions, and water to maintain fluid, electrolyte, and acid-base homeostasis. Targeted evaluation of renal tubular functions may be necessary if there is suspicion of specific transport defects such as renal bicarbonate wasting, persistent metabolic acidosis, a concentrating defect, or a specific electrolyte transport disorder. Tests exploring specific aspects of the renal tubular functions under conditions in which the renal tubules must develop an adaptive response may uncover disorders that are not readily apparent under basal conditions.

Renal regulation of acid-base balance requires the reclamation of bicarbonate that is filtered at the glomerulus, primarily in proximal tubular function. Failure to reabsorb the filtered bicarbonate results in proximal renal tubular acidosis (PRTAs, or Type 2 RTA), a well-known cause of failure to thrive. Children with PRTA exhibit significant urinary bicarbonate loss. A second major renal function in maintaining acid-base homeostasis comprises the excretion of protons (H$^+$) and the generation of new bicarbonate to replenish the bicarbonate pool in the body. This function is primarily attributable to the distal nephron, predominately the cortical and medullary collecting ducts. The tests described in the

---

### KEY POINT

Bicarbonate is reabsorbed quantitatively up to a threshold level, primarily by proximal tubular function.

next sections help characterize functions of the renal tubular segments. These tests have been functionally categorized as dealing with bicarbonate reabsorption, hydrogen ion excretion, water reabsorption, and solute reabsorption.

## TESTS FOR RENAL BICARBONATE HANDLING

### Renal bicarbonate threshold

Edelmann et al.[99] defined the renal threshold for bicarbonate as the point at which urinary excretion of bicarbonate exceeded 0.01 to 0.02 mmol/dL GFR, and this corresponded to a urine pH between 6.5 and 7.0. Oetliker and Rossi[100] considered urinary pH higher than 6.8 as a criterion for renal threshold. The bicarbonate titration is usually conducted after determining that the urine pH is less than 5.8 and therefore contains very little bicarbonate. At that point, the serum bicarbonate concentration is considered to be below the renal threshold.

---

### KEY POINTS

- Synthesis and secretion of ammonia provide a major buffer for the excretion of acids and maintenance of acid-base homeostasis during acidosis.
- There is a maturational rise in the ability to concentrate and dilute the urine, and specific tests for these functions are given in this chapter.
- Urinary handling of a variety of solutes demonstrates maturational decreases in the excretion of sodium, potassium, calcium, phosphate, magnesium, and oxalate.

---

A baseline arterialized capillary blood sample or arterial blood is sampled for measurement of total carbon dioxide ($tCO_2$), pH, and partial pressure of $CO_2$ ($pCO_2$). Then, an intravenous solution of 0.2 to 0.5 M sodium bicarbonate ($NaHCO_3$) is infused at a rate anticipated to raise serum bicarbonate by approximately 2 mEq/L/h. Renal bicarbonate threshold is the serum bicarbonate level at which urine pH reaches between 6.5 and 7. Bicarbonate thresholds are 20 to 22 mM in infants, 22 to 24 mM in children, and higher than 24 mM in adolescents, but they are substantially reduced in children with PRTA.[73,100] In early investigative works, GFR with inulin was simultaneously obtained to evaluate bicarbonate filtered load and the serum threshold. However, endogenous Cr to calculate GFR and fractional excretion of bicarbonate ($FE_{HCO3}$) at the normal bicarbonate threshold is considered adequate.[101] The bicarbonate infusion is often doubled after the bicarbonate threshold is determined. This is to provide an additional alkali load for the purpose of calculating urine-blood $pCO_2$ (U-B $pCO_2$) to assess distal nephron function (discussed later). Clearly, this test must be done without significant volume expansion,

which is known to lower serum bicarbonate threshold and raise $FE_{HCO3}$, thus necessitating a slow infusion rate.

Because of its complex procedure, the bicarbonate threshold test is not generally performed in most clinical cases. Other easily performed clinical tests that provide similar diagnostic evidence are preferred over this test.

### Fractional excretion of bicarbonate

The fraction of filtered bicarbonate excreted in urine is negligible in normal individuals. However, large amounts of filtered bicarbonate are lost in the urine of patients with PRTA. The fractional excretion of bicarbonate ($FE_{HCO3}$) test determines the fraction of filtered bicarbonate excreted in urine and can be used to differentiate PRTA from other types of RTA. The $FE_{HCO3}$ is calculated from the following formula:

$$FE_{HCO3} = \frac{U_{HCO3} \times S_{crea}}{S_{HCO3} \times U_{creat}} \times 100$$

where $U_{HCO3}$ is urine bicarbonate, $S_{crea}$ is serum Cr, $S_{HCO3}$ is serum bicarbonate, and $U_{creat}$ is urine Cr.

Whereas serum bicarbonate, serum Cr,, and urine Cr can be easily assayed in most clinical laboratories, urine bicarbonate assay requires the use of blood gas machine. The conventional blood gas machines measure pH and $pCO_2$ and then mathematically calculate the bicarbonate value, using the Henderson-Hasselbalch equation. The output results from the blood gas machine are mathematically final data points, and no further calculations are necessary. Many clinical laboratories, however, do not feel comfortable in allowing the use of urine samples in the same blood gas machines as used for testing blood. The lack of harm to the machines or to the validity of the urine bicarbonate test results was convincingly demonstrated by Gonzalez et al.[102] Mathematically, urine $HCO_3^-$ can be calculated from the Henderson–Hasselbalch equation:

$$HCO_3^- = \alpha CO_2 \times pCO_2 \times 10^{pH-pK}$$

where $\alpha$ is the solubility coefficient of urinary $pCO_2$ (0.0309).

$$pH = pK + \log (HCO_3^- / 0.03 \times pCO_2)$$

where pK is corrected for cation concentrations using the formula:

$$\frac{6.33 - 0.5}{\times \sqrt{\text{urine sodium (mmol/L)} + \text{urine potassium (mmol/L)}}}$$

The expected $FE_{HCO3}$ at a normal level of serum bicarbonate is less than 5% in distal RTA (DRTA), greater than 15% in PRTA, and between 5% and 15% in type IV hyperkalemic RTA.[103] Apart from the diagnostic information, calculation of $FE_{HCO3}$ at the normal level of serum bicarbonate threshold also provides guidance in determining the appropriate initial dosage of bicarbonate therapy in children with RTA.

## TESTS FOR URINARY ACIDIFICATION

The proton secretory capability of the distal nephron is tested to diagnose RTA in the presence of observed metabolic acidosis. Distal tubular secreted protons are present in solution, as determined by urine pH, or bound to two major urinary buffers, the phosphate and to a greater extent with ammonia. Titratable acid refers to the amount of alkali needed to raise the urine pH to 7.4. Urinary net acid excretion equals the sum of titratable acid and ammonium, minus bicarbonate.

### Urine pH

Urine pH is a screening tool for distal tubular proton secretion. By examining the pH of the second fasting urine of the morning, one can exclude the possibility of incomplete or minor forms of DRTA if the pH is less than 6.0. The range of urine pH in early morning urine of normal children is 5.16 to 7.07, with a median pH of 6.0.[104] This clearly demonstrates the low specificity of urine pH as a screening test. Children who cannot concentrate the urine may also be unable to decrease urine pH adequately. Similarly, in patients with decreased extracellular volume, the urinary acidification defect may be a result of lack of sodium at the luminal side of the distal nephron. Other conditions causing high urine pH during metabolic acidosis include the following:

- Urinary infections with urea-splitting organisms
- Severe potassium depletion stimulating ammoniagenesis and generating excessive ammonia to buffer all free luminal protons
- Gastrointestinal losses producing avid salt retention with decreased distal sodium delivery, leading to an abnormal distal luminal electrochemical gradient and subsequent increased urinary pH[105,106]

Therefore, it is important also to measure urinary sodium and osmolality in addition to pH and ammonium, because a low pH associated with reduced ammoniuria does not exclude defective distal acidification, and contrarily, high ammoniuria may cause urine pH not to decrease to less than 5.5.

### Urine-blood partial carbon dioxide pressure

Urine minus blood $pCO_2$ (U-B $pCO_2$) is an extension of bicarbonate threshold test discussed earlier, or it can be performed as a stand-alone test. In the setting of alkaline urine (and a higher driving force) resulting from bicarbonate

loading, increased secretion of protons ($H^+$) is also favored distally. The secreted protons combine with filtered bicarbonate to generate carbonic acid. Because of the limited carbonic anhydrase activity in the luminal side of the medullary collecting duct, the carbonic acid dehydrates very slowly into $CO_2$ and water.[107] This medullary trapping of $CO_2$ and the unfavorable surface-to-volume ratio of the lower urinary tract limit the diffusion of $CO_2$ out of the tubular lumen. Thus, the partial pressure of urinary $CO_2$ (U $pCO_2$) remains elevated with ongoing proton secretion, and this can be used as a reliable index of distal nephron proton secretion in conjunction with bicarbonate titration test.[108]

The U-B $pCO_2$ in the setting of alkaline urine (pH >7.5) is capable of detecting subtle defects of distal nephron acidification.[109,110] The normal value for U-B $pCO_2$ is greater than 20 mm Hg.[110,111] In DRTA, this value is less than 20 mm Hg.

> ### KEY POINTS
>
> - Patients with DRTA (Type 1 RTA) are unable to maximally decrease urine pH and increase net acid excretion up to normal values.
> - In PRTA (Type 2 RTA), minimal urine pH and normal net acid excretion are achieved once serum bicarbonate falls to less than the renal threshold.
> - Patients with type IV RTA show normal ability to decrease urinary pH but defective excretion of ammonium and titratable acid.

### Ammonium chloride loading test

Renal proton excretion (distal tubular function) is tested by measuring urinary ammonium excretion in response to an acid load. The acid load is usually given as ammonium chloride at a dose of 75 to 150 mEq/m², usually by oral route dissolved in lemon juice and sugar, or as enteric-coated capsules given over an hour. This regimen generally results in a state of moderate metabolic acidosis with blood pH lower than 7.33 and serum bicarbonate approximately 16 to 18 mEq/L. Normal subjects lower urine pH to less than pH 5.5 and increase net acid excretion to more than 70 µEq/min/1.73 m² (Table 4.12).[110,112] Patients with DRTA cannot

> ### KEY POINTS
>
> - Protons are secreted primarily by the distal nephron and result in decreased urinary pH.
> - Failure to secrete protons results in DRTA.
> - Furosemide increases distal sodium delivery and facilitates proton secretion.
> - Failure to secrete protons results in urinary pH exceeding pH 5.5.

Table 4.12 Maturational changes of the renal response to an acute acid load seen in infants and children*

| Age | UpH | Titratable acid | Ammonium | Net acid excretion |
|---|---|---|---|---|
| Preterm (1–3 wk)[†] | 6.0 ± 0.1[‡] | 25 ± 4[‡] | 29 ± 2[‡] | 54 ± 6[‡] |
| Preterm (4–6 wk)[†] | 5.2 ± 0.4 | 36 ± 9 | 40 ± 8[‡] | 76 ± 13[‡] |
| Preterm (3–4 mo)[§] | 5.2 ± 0.2 | 54 ± 20 | 37 ± 10[‡] | 90 ± 24[‡] |
| Term (1–3 wk)[†] | 5.0 ± 0.2 | 32 ± 8[‡] | 56 ± 9[‡] | 88 ± 8[‡] |
| Infants (1–16 mo) | 4.9 ± 0.1 | 62 ± 16 | 57 ± 14[‡] | 119 ± 30 |
| Children (7–12 yr) | 4.9 ± 0.2 | 50 ± 10 | 80 ± 12 | 130 ± 14 |

*Solution:* Data from Edelmann CM, Jr., Rodriguez-Soriano J, Boichis H, et al. Renal bicarbonate reabsorption and hydrogen ion excretion in infants. J Clin Invest. 1967;46:1309–17.

* Mean ± SD; minimum urine pH (UpH); maximal titratable acid, ammonium, and net acid excretion in timed urine collections given as ± Eq/min per 1.73 m². Acute acid load was $NH_4Cl$ given orally at 3.9 to 5 mEq/kg (75 to 100 mEq per m²) for infants and 5.4 mEq/kg (150 mEq per m²) for children.
† Data from [1]Svenningsen NW. Renal acid-base titration studies in infants with and without metabolic acidosis in the postneonatal period. Pediatr Res. 1974;8:659–72.
‡ Significantly different ($P < 0.05$) from values in children by Tukey's test.
§ Data from Schwartz GJ, Haycock GB, Edelmann CM, Jr., et al. Late metabolic acidosis: a reassessment of the definition. J Pediatr. 1979; 95:102–7.

decrease urine pH to less than 5.5 or increase net acid excretion to more than 70 μEq/min/1.73 m². In PRTA, these levels are achieved once serum bicarbonate falls to less than the reduced renal threshold. Patients with type IV RTA have a normal ability to decrease urine pH but defective excretion of ammonium and net acid. Like the bicarbonate titration test, the ammonium chloride loading test is seldom performed in clinical practice, and it has been replaced by other indirect measures of urinary ammonium excretion.

## Urinary net charge

Urinary ammonium assay is not routinely performed in most clinical laboratories, and the ammonium chloride loading test is difficult to perform in clinical circumstances. Urinary net charge (UNC) or urinary anion gap is used as one of the surrogate tests for urinary ammonium excretion.[110,113–115] UNC is calculated from the urinary electrolytes obtained in a spot urine sample using the following formula:

$$UNC = UNa^+ + UK^+ - UCl^-$$

where UNa⁺ is urinary sodium, UK⁺ is urinary potassium, and UCl⁻ is urinary chloride.

A negative UNC is the appropriate response to chronic metabolic acidosis, indicating that urinary ammonium is present; a positive value suggests an absence of urinary ammonium and a defect in distal urinary acidification. The UNC cannot be used in high serum anion gap acidosis (because of excessive urinary organic anions) or in severe volume depletion with avid sodium retention (because of

decreased distal delivery). Caution should be used when interpreting the UNC in neonates.[116]

If excessive unmeasured urinary anions are suspected, urinary ammonium concentration can also be estimated from the difference between measured and calculated urine osmolalities.[115,117]

$$Urine\ NH_4^+ = 0.5 \times Osmolality - [2(Na^+ + K^+) + urea / 2.8 + glucose / 18]$$

where ammonium ($NH_4^+$), Na⁺, and K⁺ are in mM; urea and glucose are in mg/dL.

A value lower than 20 mM is anticipated in a patient with DRTA.

## Furosemide test

Furosemide increases distal sodium delivery, which generates an electronegative lumen potential, thus favoring proton secretion. This observation has been used to test distal tubular acidification. Within 2 h of furosemide administration (dose, 1 mg/kg) intravenously or orally, normal subjects excrete urine with pH lower than 5.2 and with kaliuresis. In a study of 20 children given 1 mg/kg furosemide, the mean urine pH recorded was 4.96, and fractional excretion of potassium ($FE_K$) was 35.4%.[118]

Patients with DRTA who have an intrinsic defect in the proton pump cannot maximally decrease urine pH in response to furosemide. Conversely, patients with type IV RTA and those with subnormal distal proton secretion secondary to low distal delivery of sodium (i.e., nephrotic syndrome) or reversible impairment of sodium distal reabsorption (i.e., sickle cell anemia or lithium administration) respond normally.

## Acetazolamide test

The acetazolamide test is an extension of the U-B $pCO_2$ test and bicarbonate loading test to evaluate distal proton secretion capacity.[119] Acetazolamide inhibits carbonic anhydrase and reduces proximal tubular reabsorption of bicarbonate with resultant bicarbonaturia and alkaline urine. Acetazolamide simulates a bicarbonate load presented to the distal nephron. After oral acetazolamide administration at a dose of 15 to 20 mg/kg, $pCO_2$ is measured in blood and urine. A normal response shows an increase in urine $pCO_2$, suggesting increased proton secretion in the distal nephron, and U-B $pCO_2$ reaches to more than 20 mm Hg. Children with primary defects of the distal proton pump do not increase urine $pCO_2$.

## TESTS FOR GLUCOSE HANDLING

The glucose loading test evaluates the glucose transport capacity of the proximal tubule. This test can be helpful in patients with a suspected diagnosis of Fanconi syndrome or PRTA. Filtered glucose is reabsorbed in the proximal tubule, and below a threshold level, all filtered glucose is reabsorbed and none is present in the urine. Once the filtered glucose saturates the proximal tubular transport systems, the maximal rate of reabsorption is attained. From that point onward, the urinary glucose excretion equals the filtered load of glucose. This test determines the serum glucose level at which the proximal tubular glucose transport is fully saturated.

To test the proximal tubular reabsorption of glucose, the patient should be in a fasting state so that the urine is free of glucose. The patient is hydrated by providing a water load (5 mL/kg). A 30% glucose solution is infused at a starting rate of 1.6 mL/m² per min, and the infusion rate is progressively increased to provide an increasing glucose load.[120] After a 20-min equilibration period, two or three 15-min collections of urine are obtained. Accurate urine collections may require bladder catheterization in young children. Serum samples are obtained at the midpoint of each urine collection period. The titration curve can be generated from the obtained data.

The normal serum glucose threshold is 180 mg/dL; the maximal tubular reabsorption of glucose normalized to 1.73 m² body surface area averages $213 \pm 73$ mg/min for infants 2.5 to 24 weeks old and $362 \pm 96$ mg/min for children 1.5 to 13 years old.[111] When it is normalized to GFR, there is no difference in maximum tubular glucose reabsorption ($294 \pm 74$ mg/dL GFR for infants and $283 \pm 47$ mg/dL GFR for children).[121] Patients with Fanconi syndrome and PRTA have reduced thresholds for glucose reabsorption and have persistent glycosuria as a part of their symptom complex. The presence of glucose in the urinalysis should prompt the physician to the possibility of proximal tubular dysfunction.

## TESTS FOR URINARY CONCENTRATING ABILITY

The ability to concentrate urine is an important evolutionary function of the kidneys. Difficulty in concentrating urine can be seen in many clinical conditions and may lead to repeated episodes of dehydration in infants if the condition is not recognized early. The simplest way to test urinary concentrating ability is to measure urinary osmolality after withholding fluids overnight. If frank diabetes insipidus is suspected, there is a significant risk of dehydration with this maneuver. In such cases, the water deprivation test should be performed during daytime under careful observation and over shorter a period of 6 to 8 h. A loss of 3% of body weight should be set as a trigger to terminate the test.

The overnight fluid withholding water derivation test involves giving a normal noon meal on the test, followed by a dry evening meal for dinner. The child does not ingest any water or food until the test is completed by the next morning. The bladder is emptied at bedtime, and all urine passed from bedtime to 7 a.m. is pooled as an overnight collection. Two subsequent urine collections are made in the morning for osmolality. Urine osmolality increases after 12 h of water deprivation. In healthy children older than 2 years of age, the mean value of urinary osmolality in the first and second urine samples voided after the overnight collection is greater than 1000 mOsm/kg (Table 4.13).[122,123] Infants during the first month of life concentrate the urine to approximately 60% of levels in older children. Maximal urinary concentration in these newborns can actually be enhanced to almost mature levels by ingesting a very high-protein diet (8 g/day/kg) while restricting in fluids to 120 mL/kg.[124]

In the absence of heavy proteinuria or radiocontrast material in the urine, osmolality can be approximated from urine specific gravity by multiplying the last two digits of the refractometric measurement by 40.[122] For example, a specific gravity of 1.027 corresponds to an osmolality of 1080 mOsm/kg, which denotes a normal concentrating capacity.

A longer period of fluid restriction may be required in patients with primary polydipsia because of hypotonic

Table 4.13 Urinary concentrating capacity in infants and children*

| Age | Urinary osmolality |
| --- | --- |
| 7–40 days[†] | $657 \pm 115$ |
| 2 mo–3 yr[‡] | $416 \times$ log (age days) $+ 63 \pm 145$ |
| 3–15 yr[‡] | $1,069 \pm 128$ |
| 2–16 yr[§] | $1,089 \pm 110$ |

* Data represented as mean ± SD.
† Data from Edelmann CM. *Renal concentrating mechanisms in newborn infants: effect of dietary protein and water content, role of urea, and responsiveness to antidiuretic hormone. J Clin Invest.* 1960;39:1062–9.
‡ Data from Winberg J. Determination of renal concentration capacity in infants and children without renal disease. *Acta Paediatr.* 1959;48:318–28. (Data from Winberg's subjects obtained after overnight thirst combined with intramuscular pitressin tannate.)
§ Data from Edelmann CM, Jr., Barnett HL, Stark H, et al. A standardized test of renal concentrating capacity in children. *Am J Dis Child.* 1967;114:639–44.

medullary interstitium in these patients. In such cases, a progressive reduction in fluid intake over days to weeks may be required before exposing the child to a concentrating test.

## Vasopressin stimulation test

If a concentrating defect is demonstrated or suspected, the sensitivity of the kidney to exogenous antidiuretic hormone (ADH) is necessary to determine responsiveness to the hormone and to differentiate nephrogenic diabetes insipidus from a deficiency of ADH (central diabetes insipidus). Although vasopressin can be used, the agent used most commonly is 1-desamino-8-D-arginine vasopressin (desmopressin, DDAVP), which can be given intranasally or orally at doses of 10 µg in infants and 20 µg in children.[123] In infants, the usual fluid intake is restricted by 50% in the 12 h following DDAVP administration to prevent water retention and development of hyponatremia. Osmolality is measured in the individual urine samples over the 6 to 8 h after DDAVP administration. Assessing urinary concentration capacity by giving DDAVP at bedtime and collecting first morning urine sample the following morning also yields reliable results in children.[125]

## TESTS FOR URINARY DILUTION ABILITY

When challenged with excess water, kidneys are able to excrete additional urine volume and rebalance the fluid status. This is an important homeostatic function that may be impaired in some patients and thus lead to fluid overload. Excretion of dilute urine requires the following important prerequisites: (1) ADH secretion must be completely, or nearly completely, suppressed; and (2) the nephron segments responsible for water free solute reabsorption (the ascending limb of the loop of Henle and the proximal portion of the distal convoluted tubule) must be morphologically and functionally intact. Inadequate free water clearance by the kidneys can result in inappropriate water retention and hyponatremia. Evaluation of renal water excretion, therefore, is important in the assessment of patients with true hyponatremia.

## Osmolar and free water clearance

To understand the concept of water clearance more thoroughly, it is important to conceptualize that water excretion in urine consists of two separate compartments: (1) a vehicle for removal of daily solute load removal in an iso-osmotic state, the osmolal clearance ($C_{osm}$); and (2) water excretion that is not associated with any solute excretion, or free water clearance ($C_{H_2O}$). Of the two theoretical subparts, the volume of water excreted as $C_{osm}$ (in mL) is determined by the solute content in diet. Water excretion as $C_{H_2O}$ (in mL), conversely, represents the fraction that needs to be excreted to maintain a neutral fluid balance.

Total urinary water excretion (V) in mL = $C_{osm}$ (mL) + $C_{H_2O}$ (in mL)

Rewriting the formula:

$$C_{H_2O} \text{ (in mL)} = V \text{ (mL)} - C_{osm} \text{ (mL)}$$

Osmolar clearance is calculated by the following formula:

$$C_{osm} \text{(in mL/min)} = \frac{\text{Urine Osmolality } (U_{osm}) \times \text{Urine Volume in mL}(V)}{\text{Plasma Osmolality } P_{osm}}$$

Therefore,

$$C_{H_2O}\text{(in mL)} = V\text{(mL)} - \frac{U_{osm}\text{(mL)} \times V\text{(mL)}}{P_{osm}}$$

Or

$$C_{H_2O}\text{(in mL)} = V\text{(mL)} \times \left[1 - \frac{U_{osm}\text{(mL)}}{P_{osm}}\right]$$

### EXAMPLE

Urine volume = 4 mL/min

Urine osmolality = 150 mOsm/kg

Plasma osmolality = 285 mOsm/kg

Free water clearance or $C_{H_2O}$ (in mL/min) = $4 \times \left[1 - \frac{150}{285}\right]$

Or 4 × [1 − 0.52]

Or 4 × 0.48 = 1.92 mL/min

### INTERPRETATION

Calculating free water clearance ($C_{H_2O}$) is used a tool to judge fluid status and responsiveness to ADH in patients with hyponatremia and other hypo-osmolar states. A $C_{H_2O}$ of zero means that the kidneys are excreting sufficient water to maintain a balanced volume status. A positive $C_{H_2O}$ value reflects that more free water is being removed than ingested and that the body is in a net negative state of water balance. A negative $C_{H_2O}$ value, which is also known as tubular reabsorption of water ($T^r_{H_2O}$), suggests that kidneys are retaining water in an amount greater than ingested, as would be the case in the syndrome of inappropriate antidiuretic hormone (SIADH), or volume depletion.

## Water loading test

The water loading test is rarely performed in clinical circumstances, but it may be necessary in a patient with hyponatremia. This test provides information on whether kidneys are excreting appropriate amount of free water to maintain homeostasis. The intent of the test is to suppress vasopressin and aldosterone maximally and to determine the following:

1. Measure the percentage of intake fluid volume excreted in a defined time.
2. Calculate indices of free water clearance and osmotic clearance.
3. Because renal free water is generated by reabsorption of solute without accompanying water in the diluting segment of the tubule (ascending limb of loop of Henle and proximal part of distal convoluted tubule), water load can also provide an indirect estimate of solute reabsorption in these segments of the nephron.[126]

## PROCEDURE

The water loading test (also referred to as the Chaimovitz test) consists of providing an initial oral load of water at 20 mL/kg, followed by a constant intravenous infusion of 2000 mL/1.73 m² of 0.45% saline, administered over 2 h.[126] Urine and serum samples collected every 20 min and midpoint serum samples are also obtained for the next 4 h. Total volume of intake of fluids and urine excreted in 4 h is documented.[126,127] Calculations for osmolar clearance

($C_{osm}$) and free water clearance ($C_{H2O}$) are performed at the peak of sustained diuresis, by using the formulas given earlier. Both infants (1 to 15 months old) and children (2 to 12 years old) are able to lower the urinary osmolality to 51.8 ± 12.8 mOsm/kg and 54.1 ± 13.3 mOsm/kg, respectively.[127,128] Clearances of solute (x), such as sodium, potassium, and chloride, are performed using the previously discussed clearance formula:

$$C_x = \frac{U_x \times V}{S_x}$$

## INTERPRETATION

Normal individuals, including children, are able to excrete the entire volume or more of the fluid intake in 4 h of the test. Excretion of less than 80% of fluid intake as urine indicates an abnormally elevated amount of ADH, such as in SIADH.

Tubular sodium transport has been studied using the water loading test. To produce maximally dilute urine, sodium transport in the diluting tubular segments is enhanced. In patients with impaired sodium transport in these segments, decreased sodium absorption can be calculated from the obtained test data. Indeed, the water loading test was important in characterizing the site of sodium and chloride transport defects in Bartter syndrome.[126] Although the computed indices given in Table 4.14 can provide

Table 4.14 Urinary indices in normal infants and children undergoing maximal free water clearance*

| Parameter | Infants | Children |
|---|---|---|
| Urine osmolality (mOsm/kg) | 51.8 ± 12.8 | 54.1 ± 13.3 |
| Urine volume (mL/dL GF) | 22.8 ± 3.6 | 17.2 ± 2.7[†] |
| Osmolar clearance (mL/dL GF) | 4.3 ± 1.3 | 3.2 ± 0.7[†] |
| Free water clearance (mL/dL GF) | 18.5 ± 2.9 | 14.0 ± 2.6[†] |
| Sodium clearance (mL/dL GF) | 1.9 ± 0.8 | 1.4 ± 0.4[†] |
| Potassium clearance (mL/dL GF) | 19.9 ± 12.0 | 12.9 ± 5.2[†] |
| Distal delivery (water + sodium, mL/dL GF) | 20.4 ± 2.9 | 15.3 ± 2.6[†] |
| Percentage of sodium reabsorbed distally (%) | 90.8 ± 4.5 | 90.9 ± 3.3 |
| Creatinine clearance (mL/min/1.73 m²) | 88.5 ± 27.1 | 124.8 ± 25.2[†] |

*Source:* Data from Rodriguez-Soriano J, Vallo A, Castillo G, et al. Renal handling of water and sodium in infancy and childhood: a study using clearance methods during hypotonic saline diuresis. Kidney Int. 1981;20:700–4.

* Data are mean ± SD. Data obtained at peak values of sustained water diuresis, resulting from an oral water load of 20 mL/kg over 30 min plus 0.45% saline at 1000 mL/h/1.73 m² over 2 h. N = 22 for infants (0.25 to 15 mo), 17 for children (2 to 12 years old). GF, glomerular filtrate; glomerular filtration rate is approximated by endogenous creatinine clearance.

† Significantly different from infants (P < 0.05).

*Notes:* Standard clearance formula: Cx = Ux × V/Px and is corrected to glomerular filtrate or 1.73 m² body surface area. Free water clearance, $C_{H2O}$ = Volume – Osmolar clearance, and it provides an estimate of sodium reabsorption by the diluting segments. Distal delivery = free water clearance + sodium clearance; in the absence of bicarbonaturia or hyperkaluria, distal delivery is nearly identical when using sodium or chloride clearance. Percentage of sodium reabsorbed distally = free water clearance / (free water + sodium clearances).

useful information about tubular transport, several theoretic assumptions used in the test model require interpretation with caution.[127]

## TESTS FOR URINARY SOLUTE EXCRETION

The kidneys refine the homeostasis of electrolytes by varying their urinary excretion. Most of these solutes are freely filtered and are either secreted or reabsorbed by the tubules. The urinary excretion of such solutes thus reflects tubular transport functions of the kidney. The following section briefly summarizes the normal handling of a variety of such electrolytes and their clinical interpretation.

### Sodium, chloride, and potassium

On a normal Western diet, children excrete approximately 3 to 4 mmol/kg/ day of sodium. Water and salt homeostasis requires independent regulation of sodium and water because the intake of each may vary independently. Thus, the concentration of sodium in the urine depends on the degree of concentration or dilution, in addition to intake. For this reason, the excretion of urinary solutes is frequently normalized to that of Cr. Under conditions of severe volume contraction, sodium can be undetectable in the urine. Normal sodium/Cr ratios are depicted in Table 4.15.

The handling of sodium is often expressed as a fractional excretion rate. The fractional excretion of sodium ($FE_{Na}$) is calculated as follows:

$$FE_{Na} = \frac{U_{Na}/S_{Na}}{U_{Cr}/S_{Cr}} \times 100$$

$FE_{Na}$ ranges from 0.3% to 1.6% depending on salt intake.[129] In patients with prerenal acute renal failure, $FE_{Na}$ is less than 1%, whereas it is greater than 3% in acute tubular necrosis.

Chloride is handled similarly to sodium. The measurement of urinary chloride is useful in the diagnosis of metabolic alkalosis. A urinary chloride concentration greater than 10 mM indicates metabolic alkalosis of renal origin, whereas lower concentrations of urinary chloride suggest volume contraction as the cause of metabolic alkalosis.

Urinary potassium excretion is approximately 1 to 2 mmol/kg/day, and regulation of this process occurs in the distal nephron under the influence of aldosterone and the amount of salt and water delivered to the distal nephron. The renal ability to conserve potassium is not as effective as for sodium, such that urinary potassium excretion does not decrease to less than 15 mM. Normal potassium/Cr ratios are depicted in Table 4.15. Normal fractional potassium excretion in children ranges from 10% to 30%.[101]

### Transtubular potassium gradient

The transtubular potassium concentration gradient (TTKG) is a semiquantitative estimation of potassium secretory process in the distal nephron, primarily cortical collecting duct.[130] The test is useful in evaluating the appropriateness of the potassium secretory process in the presence of hypokalemia and hyperkalemia.[131] Two important assumptions for the test are as follows: (1) urine is not dilute, and urine osmolality should exceed that of plasma (>300 mOsm/kg); and (2) urinary sodium is greater than 25 mmol/L, so distal potassium exchange is not limited by low distal sodium delivery.

TTKG is calculated in a spot urine sample by the following formula:

$$TTKG = \left[ \frac{U_K}{S_K} \div \frac{U_{osm}}{S_{osm}} \right]$$

Where $U_K$ is urine potassium, $S_K$ is serum potassium, $U_{osm}$ is urine osmolality, and $S_{osm}$ is serum osmolality.

Table 4.15. Age-dependent fifth and ninety-fifth percentiles for urinary solute/creatinine ratios*

| Solute/Cr (mol/mol) | Age (yr) | | | | | | | | | | | | | | | |
|---|---|---|---|---|---|---|---|---|---|---|---|---|---|---|---|---|
| | 0.1–1 | | 1–2 | | 2–3 | | 3–5 | | 5–7 | | 7–10 | | 10–14 | | 14–17 | |
| | 5% | 95% | 5% | 95% | 5% | 95% | 5% | 95% | 5% | 95% | 5% | 95% | 5% | 95% | 5% | 95% |
| Na/Cr | 2.5 | 54 | 4.8 | 58 | 5.9 | 56 | 6.6 | 57 | 7.5 | 51 | 7.5 | 51 | 6 | 35 | — | 28 |
| K/Cr | 11 | 74 | 9 | 68 | 8 | 63 | 6.8 | 48 | 5.4 | 33 | 4.5 | 22 | 3.4 | 15 | — | 13 |
| Ca/Cr | 0.09 | 2.2 | 0.07 | 1.5 | 0.06 | 1.4 | 0.05 | 1.1 | 0.04 | 0.8 | 0.04 | 0.7 | 0.04 | 0.8 | 0.04 | 0.7 |
| P/Cr | 1.2 | 19 | 1.2 | 14 | 1.2 | 12 | 1.2 | 8 | 1.2 | 5 | 1.2 | 3.6 | 0.8 | 3.2 | 0.8 | 2.7 |
| Mg/Cr | 0.4 | 2.2 | 0.4 | 1.7 | 0.3 | 1.6 | 0.3 | 1.3 | 0.3 | 1 | 0.3 | 0.9 | 0.2 | 0.7 | 0.2 | 0.6 |
| Ox/Cr | 0.06 | 0.2 | 0.05 | 0.13 | 0.04 | 0.1 | 0.03 | 0.08 | 0.03 | 0.07 | 0.02 | 0.06 | 0.02 | 0.06 | 0.02 | 0.06 |
| Ur/Cr | 0.75 | 1.55 | 0.5 | 1.4 | 0.47 | 1.3 | 0.4 | 1.1 | 0.3 | 0.8 | 0.26 | 0.56 | 0.2 | 0.44 | 0.2 | 0.4 |

*Source:* Data from references 73, 134, and 140.
*Abbreviations:* Ca, calcium; Cr, creatinine; K, potassium; Mg, magnesium; Ox, oxalate; P, phosphate; Ur, urate.
* For conversion to mg units, 1 mmol = 113 mg Cr; 23 mg Na; 39 mg K; 40 mg Ca; 32 mg P; 24 mg Mg; 90 mg Ox; and 168 mg Ur.

## INTERPRETATION

Indirectly, TTKG tests the action of aldosterone in the distal nephron. TTKG in normal infants (1 to 12 months old) has been shown to be higher (median, 7.8 months) than in children 1 to 15 years old (median, 6.0 years).[132] This may reflect a higher level of serum aldosterone level in infants, as compared with children and adults. In hyperkalemia, TTKG is expected to be high, usually greater than 10. A low TTKG in presence of hyperkalemia in such cases suggests hypoaldosteronism or pseudohypoaldosteronism.[118,132] Rodriguez-Soriano et al.[132] noted that in children with hyporeninemic hypoaldosteronism and pseudohypoaldosteronism, TTKG ranged between 1.9 and 4.1. Normal response in patients with hypokalemia, conversely, is expected to be a low TTKG. Elevated TTKG in such circumstances indicates a mineralocorticoid excess state, either endogenously or when mineralocorticoids (fludrocortisone) are administered exogenously.[133]

## Calcium, phosphate, and magnesium

Urinary calcium excretion is often examined as a cause of hematuria and kidney stones. The excretion of calcium depends not only on diet but also on age, with higher rates of calcium excretion in infants.[134,135] In a southern Italian study, the urinary excretion of calcium ranged from 3 to 4 mg/kg per day in children 3 to 5 years old and decreased to 1.5 to 2.5 mg/kg per day in children 15 to 16 years old.[136] In children older than 5 years of age, hypercalciuria is usually defined as the excretion of more than 4 mg/kg/day or a urine calcium/Cr ratio greater than 0.2, and it constitutes a risk factor for the development of kidney stones or nephrocalcinosis.[137,138]

Urinary phosphate excretion decreases with maturation.[139] Older children normally excrete 15 to 20 mg/kg per day, compared with 35 to 40 mg/kg per day in young children.[136] After age 4 years, the fractional excretion of phosphate is approximately 7% ± 3%.[96]

Urinary magnesium excretion also shows a maturational decrease, as shown by the magnesium/Cr ratios (see Table 4.15). Older children excrete 1.5 to 2.0 mg/kg per day, compared with 2.3 to 2.6 mg/kg per day in younger children.[136] The fractional excretion of magnesium is normally approximately 5%, but it decreases to less than 1% in the setting of magnesium deprivation.[139]

## Uric acid, oxalate, and citrate

Elevated concentrations of uric acid and oxalate and low levels of urinary citrate are also risk factors for the development of kidney stones. Both oxalate and uric acid show maturational decreases in urinary excretion.[140–146] Uric acid excretion decreases from 10 to 20 mg/kg/day in 3- to 5-year old Italian children to 5 to 10 mg/kg/day in older children.[136] Brazilian children show a decrease from 5 to 15 mg/kg/day (mean, 10.5 ± 5.0 mg/kg/day) in preschoolers to 4 to 10 mg/kg per day (mean, 7.0 ± 3.0 mg/kg/day) in adolescents.[143] Hyperuricosuria is also diagnosed by examining urine uric acid concentration factored by Cr clearance ($U_{urate} \times S_{creat} / U_{creat}$, each in mg/dL); hyperuricosuria is defined by a value greater than 0.54 to 0.56 mg/dL of glomerular filtrate.[138,144] Alternatively, hyperuricemia is defined as excretion of uric acid greater than 815 mg/24 h/1.73 m$^2$.[145]

Urinary oxalate excretion ranges from 1 to 2 mg/kg per day in Italian children 3 to 5 years of age and decreasing to 0.3 to 0.7 mg/kg/day in older children.[136] Table 4.15 shows the decrease in urine oxalate/Cr ratios with age.[140] Hyperoxaluria is also defined as urinary oxalate exceeding 0.5 mmol (45 mg)/24 h/1.73 m$^2$, or 0.048 mg oxalate/mg Cr (0.06 mol/mol) in children older than 5 years of age.[140]

Urinary citrate excretion normally averages 0.03 mmol (6.3 mg)/kg/24 h.[146] The range of urinary excretion of citrate does not show maturational changes, but it is clear that girls excrete more urinary citrate than do boys.[147] Hypocitraturia predisposes to kidney stone formation. Hypocitraturia is defined as a urinary citrate/Cr ratio less than 300 mg/g (0.176 mol/mol) in girls and 128 mg/g (0.074 mol/mol) in boys.[147]

## NOVEL BIOMARKERS OF RENAL FUNCTION

Assessment of renal function in patients with AKI is challenging in the context of a very sick child in the intensive care unit undergoing multiple confounding pharmacologic interventions. A rise in serum Cr, which is the most readily available clinical marker of renal function, is a late event marker that rises after more than 50% of the renal function has been lost, making it unsuitable for early detection of renal disease.[148] Serum, Cys-C level, conversely, has been shown to rise before detectable changes in serum Cr are seen.[149] In addition, Cr- or Cys-C–based GFR equations have not been validated in patients with AKI, but these equations may provide a "guesstimate" of the GFR at given point in time for therapeutic considerations in patients.

The last decade has seen a sizable effort toward development of biologic markers that may help in early detection and follow-up of renal function in acutely sick individuals.[150] The role of the novel proteomic biomarkers includes early diagnosis of AKI, concordance with GFR, and allowance of an assessment of therapeutic interventions by monitoring progression. Although several biomarkers have been proposed (Figure 4.4), none is able to predict GFR under the mandated clinical conditions.

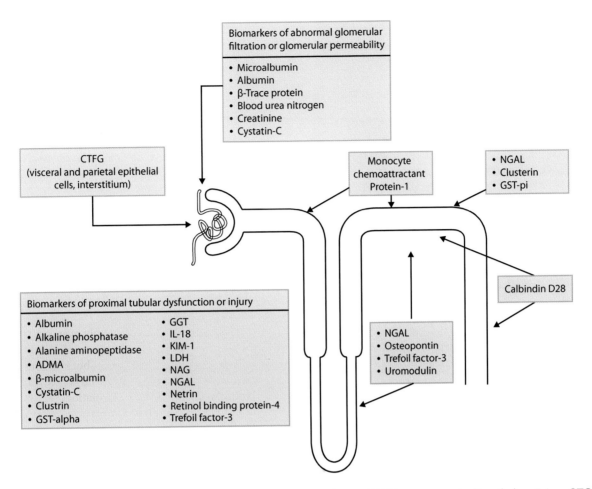

Figure 4.4 Anatomic localization of novel biomarkers along the nephron. ADMA, asymmetric dimethyl arginine; CTGF, connective tissue growth factor; GGT, γ-glutamyl transpeptidase; GST, glutathione-S-transferase; IL-18, interleukin-18; KIM-1, kidney injury molecule-1; LDH, lactate dehydrogenase; NAG, N-acetyl glucosaminidase; NGAL, neutrophil gelatinase-associated lipocalin. (From McMahon GM, Waikar SS. Biomarkers in nephrology: core curriculum 2013. Am J Kidney Dis. 2013;62:165–78.)

Many of the novel proteomic markers for evaluation of renal function can be assayed in urine and blood. Although urinary markers have many advantages, such as being close to the site of injury and potential early detection of abnormalities, potential disadvantages, such as variability resulting from urinary concentration and hydration status, also exist. Broadly, the proposed novel markers of renal injury can be classified into two subgroups[148]:

1. Preformed and upregulated in renal injury
2. Induced by renal injury

Preformed biomarkers are normally present in renal tissue and are released into circulation or urine by renal injury. Examples include: N-acetyl-γ-glucosaminidase (NAG), γ-glutamyl transpeptidase (GGT), kidney injury molecule-1 (KIM-1), and lactate dehydrogenase (LDH). In other cases, the preformed biomarkers may be freely filtered at the glomerulus and are normally reabsorbed by the tubules. In case of renal cell injury, these markers fail to become reabsorbed by their respective tubular segments and are excreted in urine. Examples of this category of preformed biomarkers include: β$_2$-macroglobulin, microalbuminuria, urinary Cys-C, and retinol binding protein-4 (RBP-4). The second class of biomarkers comprises those induced by renal injury or inflammation. Examples of this class of biomarkers include neutrophil gelatinase–associated lipocalin (NGAL), interleukin-18 (IL-18), and osteopontin (OPN).

The utility of biomarkers in the diagnosis and follow up of renal injury is evolving. At this time, no clear gold standard biomarkers have been established. It is likely that a panel of biomarkers will provide a better measure of renal injury in AKI, by evaluating multiple sites of tubular injury in the nephron. The utility of biomarkers in the diagnosis of AKI is also discussed in Chapter 30.

## SUMMARY

Clinical care of children with acute and chronic kidney diseases requires an assessment of renal function from both diagnostic and follow-up perspectives. GFR is long established as the best indicator of overall human renal function. Estimation of GFR by clearance methodology, using exogenously administered and endogenous markers, has been the mainstay of evaluations over the past several decades. An estimation of GFR from endogenous biomarkers by various mathematical equations has been attempted since the 1980s, and many of these methods are available for clinical use. Because of a lack of steady state for Cr as well as Cys-C in AKI, application of the GFR equations cannot be advocated. Indeed, to predict early renal injury in AKI, especially when surgical interventions are necessary or nephrotoxic treatments are planned, several novel markers of renal function are being evaluated. So far, no gold standard markers have been established, and it is likely that a panel of such markers may be clinically relevant. For the near future, to obtain an accurate appraisal of renal function, GFR may require direct measurement by plasma or renal clearance techniques.

## REFERENCES

1. Kanwar YS, Venkatachalam MA. Ultrastructure of glomerulus and juxtaglomerular apparatus. In: Windhager EE, editor. Handbook of Physiology, Section 8: Physiology. New York: Oxford University Press; 1992. p. 3–40.
2. Kanwar YS. Biophysiology of glomerular filtration and proteinuria. Lab Invest. 1984;51:7–21.
3. Rose BD, Post TW. Renal circulation and glomerular filtration rate. In: Wonsiewicz M, McCullough K, Davis K, editors. Clinical Physiology of Acid-Base and Electrolyte Disorders. New York: McGraw-Hill; 2001. p. 21–70.
4. Brenner BM, Humes HD. Mechanics of glomerular ultrafiltration. N Engl J Med. 1977;297:148–54.
5. Deen WM, Lazzara MJ, Myers BB. Structural determinants of glomerular permeability. Am J Physiol Renal Physiol. 2001;281:F579–96.
6. Brenner BM, Hostetter TH, Humes HD. Molecular basis of proteinuria of glomerular origin. N Engl J Med. 1978;298:826–33.
7. Latta H. An approach to the structure and function of the glomerular mesangium. J Am Soc Nephrol. 1992;2:S65–73.
8. Abrahamson DR. Structure and development of the glomerular capillary wall and basement membrane. Am J Physiol Renal Physiol. 1987;253:F783–94.
9. Schwartz GJ. Does kL/$P_{Cr}$ estimate GFR, or does GFR determine k? Pediatr Nephrol. 1992;6:512–5.
10. Arant BS, Jr., Edelmann CM, Jr., Spitzer A. The congruence of creatinine and inulin clearances in children: Use of the Technicon AutoAnalyzer. J Pediatr. 1972;81:559–61.
11. Dalton RN, Haycock GB. Laboratory investigation. In: Barratt TM, Avner ED, Harmon WE, editors. Pediatric Nephrology, 4th ed. Baltimore: Lippincott Williams & Wilkins; 1999. p. 343–64.
12. US Renal Data System, USRDS 2002 Annual Data Report: Atlas of End-Stage Renal Disease in the United States. Bethesda, MD: National Institutes of Health, National Institute of Diabetes and Digestive and Kidney Diseases; 2002.
13. Cole BR, Giangiacomo J, Ingelfinger JR, Robson AM. Measurement of renal function without urine collection. N Engl J Med. 1972;287:1109–14.
14. Schwartz GJ, Feld LG, Langford DJ. A simple estimate of glomerular filtration rate in full-term infants during the first year of life. J Pediatr. 1984;104:849–54.
15. Schwartz GJ, Gauthier B. A simple estimate of glomerular filtration rate in adolescent boys. J Pediatr. 1985;106:522–6.
16. Talbot NB. Measurement of obesity by the creatinine coefficient. Am J Dis Child. 2005;55:42–50.
17. Greenblatt DJ, Ransil BJ, Harmatz JS, et al. Variability of 24-hour urinary creatinine excretion by normal subjects. J Clin Pharmacol. 1976;16:321–8.
18. Richardson JA, Philbin PE. The one-hour creatinine clearance rate in healthy men. JAMA. 1971;216:987–90.
19. Hellerstein S, Berenbom M, Alon US, Warady BA. Creatinine clearance following cimetidine for estimation of glomerular filtration rate. Pediatr Nephrol. 1998;12:49–54.
20. Doolan PD, Alpen EL, Theil GB. A clinical appraisal of the plasma concentration and endogenous clearance of creatinine. Am J Med. 1962;32:65–79.
21. Schwartz GJ, Brion LP, Spitzer A. The use of plasma creatinine concentration for estimating glomerular filtration rate in infants, children, and adolescents. Pediatr Clin North Am. 1987;34:571–90.
22. Schwartz GJ, Haycock GB, Chir B, Spitzer A. Plasma creatinine and urea concentration in children: Normal values for age and sex. J Pediatr. 1976;88:828–30.
23. van Acker BAC, Koomen GCM, Koopman MG, et al. Creatinine clearance during cimetidine administration for measurement of glomerular filtration rate. Lancet. 1992;340:1326–9.
24. Schutte JE, Longhurst JC, Gaffney FA, et al. Total plasma creatinine: an accurate measure of total striated muscle mass. J Appl Physiol. 1981;51:762–6.
25. Jones JD, Burnett PC. Implication of creatinine and gut flora in the uremic syndrome: induction of "creatininase" in colon contents of the rat by dietary creatinine. Clin Chem. 1972;18:280–4.

26. Schwartz GJ, Haycock GB, Edelmann CM, Jr., Spitzer A. A simple estimate of glomerular filtration rate in children derived from body length and plasma creatinine. Pediatrics. 1976;58:259–63.

27. Drion I, Cobbaert C, Groenier KH, et al. Clinical evaluation of analytical variations in serum creatinine measurements: why laboratories should abandon Jaffe techniques. BMC Nephrol. 2012;13:133.

28. Schwartz GJ, Muñoz A, Schneider MF, et al. New equations to estimate GFR in children with CKD. J Am Soc Nephrol. 2009;20:629–37.

29. Schwartz GJ, Kwong T, Erway B, et al. Validation of creatinine assays utilizing HPLC and IDMS traceable standards in sera of children. Pediatr Nephrol. 2009;24:113–19.

30. Staples A, Leblond R, Watkins S, et al. Validation of the revised Schwartz estimating equation in a predominantly non-CKD population. Pediatr Nephrol. 2010;25:2321–6.

31. Counahan R, Chantler C, Ghazali S, et al. Estimation of glomerular filtration rate from plasma creatinine concentration in children. Arch Dis Child. 1976;51:875–8.

32. Fong J, Johnston S, Valentino T, et al. Length/serum creatinine ratio does not predict measured creatinine clearance in critically ill children. Clin Pharmacol Ther. 1995;58:192–7.

33. Cockcroft DW, Gault MH. Prediction of creatinine clearance from serum creatinine. Nephron. 1976;16:31–41.

34. Pierrat A, Gravier E, Saunders C, et al. Predicting GFR in children and adults: a comparison of the Cockcroft-Gault, Schwartz, and modification of diet in renal disease formulas. Kidney Int. 2003;64:1425–36.

35. Grubb A. Diagnostic value of analysis of cystatin C and protein HC in biological fluids. Clin Nephrol. 1992;38:S20–7.

36. Kaseda R, Iino N, Hosojima M, et al. Megalin-mediated endocytosis of cystatin C in proximal tubule cells. Biochem Biophys Res Commun. 2007;357:1130–4.

37. Roald AB, Aukland K, Tenstad O. Tubular absorption of filtered cystatin-C in the rat kidney. Exp Physiol. 2004;89:701–7.

38. Tkaczyk M, Nowicki M, Lukamowicz J. Increased cystatin C concentration in urine of nephrotic children. Pediatr Nephrol. 2004;19:1278–80.

39. Nejat M, Hill JV, Pickering JW, et al. Albuminuria increases cystatin C excretion: implications for urinary biomarkers. Nephrol Dial Transplant. 2012;27:(Suppl 3) 96–103.

40. Madero M, Sarnak MJ, Stevens LA. Serum cystatin C as a marker of glomerular filtration rate. Curr Opin Nephrol Hypertens. 2006;15:610–6.

41. Fischbach M, Graff V, Terzic J, et al. Impact of age on reference values for serum concentration of cystatin C in children. Pediatr Nephrol. 2002;17:104–6.

42. Bökenkamp A, Domanetzki M, Zinck R, et al. Reference values for cystatin C serum concentrations in children. Pediatr Nephrol. 1998;12:125–9.

43. Knight EL, Verhave JC, Spiegelman D, et al. Factors influencing serum cystatin C levels other than renal function and the impact on renal function measurement. Kidney Int. 2004;65:1416–21.

44. Fricker M, Wiesli P, Brändle M, et al. Impact of thyroid dysfunction on serum cystatin C. Kidney Int. 2003;63:1944–7.

45. Chew-Harris JS, Florkowski CM, George PM, et al. The relative effects of fat versus muscle mass on cystatin C and estimates of renal function in healthy young men. Ann Clin Biochem. 2013;50:39–46.

46. Xu H, Lu Y, Teng D, et al. Assessment of glomerular filtration rate in renal transplant patients using serum cystatin C. Transplant Proc. 2006;38:2006–8.

47. Kos J, Štabuc B, Cimerman N, Brunner N. Serum cystatin C, a new marker of glomerular filtration rate, is increased during malignant progression. Clin Chem. 1998;44:2556–7.

48. Stevens LA, Schmid CH, Greene T, et al. Factors other than glomerular filtration rate affect serum cystatin C levels. Kidney Int. 2009;75:652–60.

49. Witzel SH, Butts K, Filler G. Elevated triglycerides may affect cystatin C recovery. Clin Biochem. 2014;47:676–8.

50. Cimerman N, Brguljan PM, Krasovec M, et al. Serum cystatin C, a potent inhibitor of cysteine proteinases, is elevated in asthmatic patients. Clin Chim Acta. 2000;300:83–95.

51. Lertnawapan R, Bian A, Rho YH, et al. Cystatin C is associated with inflammation but not atherosclerosis in systemic lupus erythematosus. Lupus. 2012;21:279–87.

52. Demirtaş S, Akan O, Can M, et al. Cystatin C can be affected by nonrenal factors: a preliminary study on leukemia. Clin Biochem. 2006;39:115–8.

53. Deveci K, Gokakin AK, Senel S, et al. Cystatin C in serum as an early marker of renal involvement in familial Mediterranean fever patients. Eur Rev Med Pharmacol Sci. 2013;17:253–60.

54. Wilson ME, Boumaza I, Lacomis D, Bowser R (2010) Cystatin C: a candidate biomarker for amyotrophic lateral sclerosis. PLoS One. 2010;5:e15133.

55. Finney H, Newman DJ, Thakkar H, et al. Reference ranges for plasma cystatin C and creatinine measurements in premature infants, neonates, and older children. Arch Dis Child. 2000;82:71–5.

56. Lee JH, Hahn WH, Ahn J, et al. Serum cystatin C during 30 postnatal days is dependent on the postconceptional age in neonates. Pediatr Nephrol. 2013;28:1073–8.

57. Filler G, Lepage N. Cystatin C adaptation in the first month of life. Pediatr Nephrol. 2013;28:991–4.

58. Groesbeck D, Köttgen A, Parekh R, et al. Age, gender, and race effects on cystatin C levels in US adolescents. Clin J Am Soc Nephrol. 2008;3:1777–85.

59. Bökenkamp A, Domanetzki M, Zinck R, et al. Cystatin serum concentrations underestimate glomerular filtration rate in renal transplant recipients. Clin Chem. 1999;45:1866–8.

60. Hoek FJ, Kemperman FA, Krediet RT. (2003). A comparison between cystatin C, plasma creatinine and the Cockcroft and Gault formula for the estimation of glomerular filtration rate. Nephrol Dial Transplant. 2003;18:2024–31.

61. Zappitelli M, Parvex P, Joseph L, et al. Derivation and validation of cystatin C–based prediction equations for GFR in children. Am J Kidney Dis. 2006;48:221–30.

62. Schwartz GJ, Schneider MF, Maier PS, et al. Improved equations estimating GFR in children with chronic kidney disease using an immunonephelometric determination of cystatin C. Kidney Int. 2012;82:445–53.63. Bouvet Y, Bouissou F, Coulais Y, et al. GFR is better estimated by considering both serum cystatin C and creatinine levels. Pediatr Nephrol. 2006;21:1299–306.

64. Sapirstein LA, Vidt DG, Mandel MJ, et al. Volumes of distribution and clearances of intravenously injected creatinine in the dog. Am J Physiol. 1955;181:330–6.

65. Brochner-Mortensen J. A simple method for the determination of glomerular filtration rate. Scand J Clin Lab Invest. 1972;30:271–4.

66. Ng DK, Schwartz GJ, Jacobson LP, et al. Universal GFR determination based on two time points during plasma iohexol disappearance. Kidney Int. 2011;80: 423–30.

67. Piepsz A, Denis R, Ham HR, et al. A simple method for measuring separate glomerular filtration rate using a single injection of $^{99m}$Tc-DTPA and the scintillation camera. J Pediatr. 1978;93:769–74.

68. Rehling M, Moller ML, Thamdrup B, et al. Simultaneous measurement of renal clearance and plasma clearance of $^{99m}$Tc-labelled diethylenetriaminepenta-acetate, $^{51}$Cr-labelled ethylenediaminetetra-acetate and inulin in man. Clin Sci. 1984;66:613–9.

69. LaFrance ND, Drew HH, Walser M. Radioisotopic measurement of glomerular filtration rate in severe chronic renal failure. J Nucl Med. 1988;29:1927–30.

70. Carlsen JE, Moller ML, Lund JO, et al. Comparison of four commercial Tc-99m(Sn)DTPA preparations used for the measurement of glomerular filtration rate: concise communication. J Nucl Med. 1980;21:126–9.

71. Odlind B, Hällgren R, Sohtell M, et al. Is $^{125}$I iothalamate an ideal marker for glomerular filtration? Kidney Int. 1985;27:9–16.

72. Perrone RD, Steinman TI, Beck GJ, et al. Utility of radioisotopic filtration markers in chronic renal insufficiency: simultaneous comparison of $^{125}$I-iothalamate, $^{169}$Yb-DTPA, $^{99m}$Tc-DTPA, and inulin. Am J Kidney Dis. 1990;16:224–35.

73. Guignard J-P, Santos F. Laboratory investigations. In: Avner ED, Harmon WE, Niaudet P, editors. Pediatric Nephrology, 5th ed. Philadelphia: Lippincott Williams, & Wilkins; 2004. p. 399–424.

74. Back SE, Krutzen E, Nilsson-Ehle P. Contrast media as markers for glomerular filtration: a pharmacokinetic comparison of four agents. Scand J Clin Lab Invest. 1988;48:247–53.

75. Krutzen E, Back SE, Nilsson-Ehle I, et al. Plasma clearance of a new contrast agent, iohexol: a method for the assessment of glomerular filtration rate. J Lab Clin Med. 1984;104:955–61.

76. Olsson B, Aulie A, Sveen K, et al. Human pharmacokinetics of iohexol: a new nonionic contrast medium. Invest Radiol. 1983;18:177–82.

77. Krutzen E, Back SE, Nilsson-Ehle P. Determination of glomerular filtration rate using iohexol clearance and capillary sampling. Scand J Clin Lab Invest. 1990;50:279–83.

78. Nilsson-Ehle P, Grubb A. New markers for the determination of GFR: Iohexol clearance and cystatin C serum concentration. Kidney Int Suppl. 1994;46:S17–19.

79. Gaspari F, Perico N, Ruggenenti P, et al. Plasma clearance of nonradioactive iohexol as a measure of glomerular filtration rate. J Am Soc Nephrol. 1995;6:257–63.

80. Brown SCW, O'Reilly PH. Iohexol clearance for the determination of glomerular filtration rate in clinical practice: evidence for a new gold standard. J Urol. 1991;146:675–9.

81. Erley CM, Bader BD, Berger ED, et al. Plasma clearance of iodine contrast media as a measure of glomerular filtration rate in critically ill patients. Crit Care Med. 2001;29:1544–50.

82. Rahn KH, Heidenreich S, Bruckner D. How to assess glomerular function and damage in humans. J Hypertens. 1999;17:309–17.

83. Brändström E, Grzegorczyk A, Jacobsson L, et al. GFR measurement with iohexol and $^{51}$Cr-EDTA: a comparison of the two favoured GFR markers in Europe. Nephrol Dial Transplant. 1998;13:1176–82.

84. Schwartz GJ, Furth S, Cole SR, Warady B, Muñoz A. Glomerular filtration rate via plasma iohexol disappearance: Pilot study for chronic kidney disease in children. Kidney Int. 2006 Jun;69(11):2070-7.

85. Schwartz GJ, Abraham AG, Furth SL, et al. Optimizing iohexol plasma disappearance curves to measure the glomerular filtration rate in children with chronic kidney disease. Kidney Int. 2010;77:65–71.

86. Chantler C, Barratt TM. Estimation of glomerular filtration rate from plasma clearance of 51-chromium edetic acid. Arch Dis Child. 1972;47:613–7.

87. Fleming JS, Zivanovic MA, Blake GM, et al. Guidelines for the measurement of glomerular filtration rate using plasma sampling. Nucl Med Commun. 2004;25:759–69.

88. Maisey M. Radionuclide renography: a review. Curr Opin Nephrol Hypertens. 2003;12:649–52.

89. Brion LP, Fleischman AR, McCarton C, A simple estimate of glomerular filtration rate in low birth weight infants during the first year of life: noninvasive assessment of body composition and growth. J Pediatr. 1986;109:698–707.

90. Guignard JP, Torrado A, Da Cunha O, et al. Glomerular filtration rate in the first three weeks of life. J Pediatr. 1975;87:268–72.

91. Barnett HL, McNamara H, Shultz S, et al. Renal clearances of sodium penicillin G, procaine penicillin G, and inulin in infants and children. Pediatrics. 1949;3:418–22.

92. Henry L. Barnett, W. Kendrick Hare, et al. Influence of postnatal age on kidney function of premature infants. Exp Biol Med (Maywood). 1948;69:55–5.

93. Richmond JB, Kravitz H, Segar W, et al. Renal clearance of endogenous phosphate in infants and children. Exp Biol Med (Maywood). 1951;77:83–7.

94. Broberger U. Determination of glomerular filtration rate in the newborn: comparison between results obtained by the single injection technique without collection of urine and the standard clearance technique. Acta Paediatr. 1973;62, 625–8.

95. McCrory WW, Forman CW, McNamara H, et al. Renal excretion of inorganic phosphate in newborn infants. J Clin Invest. 1952;31:357–66.

96. Brodehl J, Gellissen K, Weber HP. Postnatal development of tubular phosphate reabsorption. Clin Nephrol. 1982;17:163–71.

97. Gibb DM, Dalton NR, Barratt MT. Measurement of glomerular filtration rate in children with insulin-dependent diabetes mellitus. Clin Chim Acta. 1989;82:131–9.

98. Vieux R, Hascoet JM, Merdariu D, et al. Glomerular filtration rate reference values in very preterm infants. Pediatrics. 2010;125:e1186–92.

99. Edelmann CM, Jr., Rodriguez-Soriano J, Boichis H, et al. Renal bicarbonate reabsorption and hydrogen ion excretion in infants. J Clin Invest. 1967;46:1309–17.

100. Oetliker O, Rossi E. The influence of extracellular fluid volume on the renal bicarbonate threshold: a study of two children with Lowe's syndrome. Pediatr Res. 1969;3:140–8.

101. Schwartz GJ. Potassium and acid-base. In: Barratt TM, Avner ED, Harmon WE, editors. Pediatric Nephrology, 4th ed. Baltimore: Williams & Wilkins; 1999. p. 155–89.

102. Gonzalez SB, Voyer LE, Corti S, et al. Determination of urinary bicarbonate with the Henderson-Hasselbalch equation: comparison using two different methods. Pediatr Nephrol. 2004;19:1371–4.

103. McSherry E. Renal tubular acidosis in childhood. Kidney Int. 1981;20:799–809.

104. Skinner R, Cole M, Pearson ADJ, et al. Specificity of pH and osmolality of early morning urine sample in assessing distal renal tubular function in children: results in healthy children. BMJ. 1996;312:1337–8.

105. Smulders YM, Frissen PHJ, Slaats EH, et al. Renal tubular acidosis: pathophysiology and diagnosis. Arch Intern Med. 1996;156:1629–36.

106. Gregory MJ, Schwartz GJ. Diagnosis and treatment of renal tubular disorders. Semin Nephrol. 1998;18:317–29.

107. Alpern RJ, Stone DK, Rector FC, Jr. Renal acidification mechanisms. In: Brenner BM, Rector FC, Jr., editors. The Kidney, 5th ed. Philadelphia: WB Saunders; 1996. p. 408–71.

108. DuBose TD, Jr., Pucacco LR, Green JM. Hydrogen ion secretion by the collecting duct as a determinant of the urine to blood $pCO_2$ gradient in alkaline urine. J Clin Invest. 1981;69:145–56.

109. Strife CF, Clardy CW, Varade WS, et al. Urine-to-blood carbon dioxide tension gradient and maximal depression of urinary pH to distinguish rate-dependent from classic distal renal tubular acidosis in children. J Pediatr. 1993;122:60–5.

110. Donckerwolcke RA, Valk C, van Wijngaarden-Penterman MJG, et al. The diagnostic value of the urine to blood carbon dioxide tension gradient for the assessment of distal tubular hydrogen secretion in pediatric patients with renal tubular disorders. Clin Nephrol. 1983;19:254–8.

111. Lin J-Y, Lin J-S, Tsai C-H. Use of the urine-to-blood carbon dioxide tension gradient as a measurement of impaired distal tubular hydrogen ion secretion among neonates. J Pediatr. 1995;126:114–7.

112. Edelmann CM, Jr., Boichis H, Rodriguez-Soriano J, Stark H. The renal response of children to acute ammonium chloride acidosis. Pediatr Res. 1967;1:452–60.

113. Rodriguez-Soriano J, Vallo A. Renal tubular acidosis. Pediatr Nephrol. 1990;4:268–75.

114. Batlle DC, Hizon M, Cohen E, et al. The use of the urinary anion gap in the diagnosis of hyperchloremic metabolic acidosis. N Engl J Med. 1988;318:594–9.

115. Carlisle EJF, Donnelly SM, Halperin ML. Renal tubular acidosis (RTA): recognize the ammonium defect and pHorget the urine pH. Pediatr Nephrol. 1991;5:242–8.

116. Sulyok E, Guignard J-P. Relationship of urinary anion gap to urinary ammonium excretion in the neonate. Biol Neonate. 1990;57:98–106.

117. Dyck RF, Asthana S, Kalra J, et al. A modification of the urine osmolal gap: an improved method for estimating urine ammonium. Am J Nephrol. 1990;10:359–62.

118. Rodriguez-Soriano J, Vallo A. Renal tubular hyperkalaemia in childhood. Pediatr Nephrol. 1988;2:498–509.

119. Alon U, Hellerstein S, Warady BA. Oral acetazolamide in the assessment of (urine-blood) $pCO_2$. Pediatr Nephrol. 1991;5:307–11.

120. Goldsmith DI. Clinical and laboratory evaluation of renal function. In: Edelmann CM, Jr., editor. Pediatric Kidney Disease, 2nd ed. Boston: Little, Brown & Company; 1992. p. 213–24.

121. Brodehl J, Franken A, Gellissen K. Maximal tubular reabsorption of glucose in infants and children. Acta Paediatr Scand. 1972;61:413–20.

122. Edelmann CM, Jr., Barnett HL, Stark H, et al. A standardized test of renal concentrating capacity in children. Am J Dis Child. 1967;114:639–44.

123. Aronson PS, Svenningsen NW. DDAVP test for estimation of renal concentrating capacity in infants and children. Arch Dis Child. 1974;49:654–9.

124. Edelmann CM, Jr., Barnett HL, Troupkou V. Renal concentrating mechanisms in newborn infants: effect of dietary protein and water content, role of urea, and responsiveness to anti-diuretic hormone. J Clin Invest. 1960;39:1062–9.

125. Marild S, Rembratt A, Jodal U, et al. Renal concentrating capacity test using desmopressin at bedtime. Pediatr Nephrol. 2001;16:439–42.

126. Chaimovitz C, Levi J, Better OS, et al. Studies on the site of renal salt loss in a patient with Bartter's syndrome. Pediatr Res. 1973;7:89–94.

127. Rodriguez-Soriano J, Vallo A, Castillo G, et al. Renal handling of water and sodium in infancy and childhood: a study using clearance methods during hypotonic saline diuresis. Kidney Int. 1981;20:700–4.

128. Schnieden H. Water diuresis in children aged 1-3 years. Arch Dis Child. 1957;32:189–92.

129. Rossi R, Danzebrink S, Linnenburger K, et al. Assessment of tubular reabsorption of sodium, glucose, phosphate and amino acids based on spot urine samples. Acta Paediatr.1994;83:1282–6.

130. West ML, Marsden PA, Richardson RM, et al. New clinical approach to evaluate disorders of potassium excretion. Miner Electrolyte Metab. 1986;12:234–8.

131. Choi MJ, Ziyadeh FN. The utility of the transtubular potassium gradient in the evaluation of hyperkalemia. J Am Soc Nephrol. 2008;19:424–6.

132. Rodriguez-Soriano J, Ubetagoyena M, Vallo A. Transtubular potassium concentration gradient: a useful test to estimate renal aldosterone bio-activity in infants and children. Pediatr Nephrol. 1990;4:105–10.

133. Ethier JH, Kamel KS, Magner PO, et al. The transtubular potassium concentration in patients with hypokalemia and hyperkalemia. Am J Kidney Dis. 1990;15:309–15.

134. Matos V, van Melle G, Boulat O, et al. Urinary phosphate/creatinine, calcium/creatinine, and magnesium/creatinine ratios in a healthy pediatric population. J Pediatr. 1997;131:252–7.

135. Sargent JD, Stukel TA, Kresel J, et al. Normal values for random urinary calcium to creatinine ratios in infancy. J Pediatr. 1993;123:393–7.

136. De Santo NG, Di Iorio B, Capasso G et al. Population based data on urinary excretion of calcium, magnesium, oxalate, phosphate and uric acid in children from Cimitile (southern Italy). Pediatr Nephrol. 1992;6:149–57.

137. Stapleton FB, Noe HN, Roy SI, et al. Hypercalciuria in children with urolithiasis. Am J Dis Child. 1982;136:675–8.

138. Stapleton FB. Hematuria associated with hypercalciuria and hyperuricosuria: a practical approach. Pediatr Nephrol. 1994;8:756–61.

139. Sutton RA, Domrongkitchaiporn S. Abnormal renal magnesium handling. Miner Electrolyte Metab. 1993;19:232–40.

140. Matos V, van Melle G, Werner D, et al. Urinary oxalate and urate to creatinine ratios in a healthy pediatric population. Am J Kidney Dis. 1999;34:1–6.

141. Kaufman JM, Greene ML, Seegmiller JE. Urine uric acid to creatinine ratio: a screening test for inherited disorders of purine metabolism. J Pediatr. 1968;73:583–92.

142. Barratt TM, Kasidas GP, Murdoch I, et al. Urinary oxalate and glycolate excretion and plasma oxalate concentration. Arch Dis Child. 1991;66:501–3.

143. Penido MG, Diniz JS, Guimarães MM, et al. Urinary excretion of calcium, uric acid and citrate in healthy children and adolescents. J Pediatr (Rio J). 2002;78:153–60.

144. La Manna A, Polito C, Marte A, et al. Hyperuricosuria in children: clinical presentation and natural history. Pediatrics. 2001;107:86–90.

145. Stapleton FB, Linshaw MA, Hassanein K, et al. Uric acid excretion in normal children. J Pediatr. 1978;92:911–4.

146. Goretti M, Penido MG, Silvério J, et al. Urinary excretion of calcium, uric acid and citrate in healthy children and adolescents. J Pediatr (Rio J). 2002;78:153–60.

147. Norman ME, Feldman NI, Cohn RM, et al. Urinary citrate excretion in the diagnosis of distal renal tubular acidosis. J Pediatr. 1978;92:394–400.

148. Endre ZH, Pickering JW, Walker RJ. Clearance and beyond: the complementary roles of GFR measurement and injury biomarkers in acute kidney injury (AKI). Am J Physiol Renal Physiol. 2011;301:F697–707.

149. Briguori C, Visconti G, Rivera N, et al. Cystatin C and contrast-induced acute kidney injury. Circulation. 2010;121:2117.

150. Vaidya VS, Ferguson MA, Bonventre JV. Biomarkers of acute kidney injury. Annu Rev Pharmacol. 2008;48:463–93.

## REVIEW QUESTIONS

1. A 5-year-old boy was admitted with the diagnosis of acute lymphoblastic leukemia. After induction chemotherapy he was noted to be hyponatremic, with a serum sodium concentration of 131 mmol. Normal saline was given as maintenance solution. Five days later he developed generalized tonic-clonic seizures. His serum electrolytes were as follows: glucose, 107 mg/dL; sodium, 122 mmol/L; chloride, 82 mmol/L; potassium, 3.5 mmol/L; and bicarbonate, 22 mmol/L. BUN was 16 mg/dL, and creatinine was 0.6 mg/dL. A

diagnosis of SIADH was entertained. The calculated serum osmolality of this patient is:

a. 244
b. 122
c. 256
d. 287

2. In a 10-year-old girl who had her right leg amputated at the hip 6 months ago for osteosarcoma, the Schwartz formula and modified Schwartz formula do not predict GFR accurately, and loss of limb needs to be accounted for.

a. True
b. False

3. Accuracy of predicting GFR by formulas based on serum cystatin C and serum creatinine is:

a. No better than each one alone
b. Less accurate than each one alone
c. Better than each one alone
d. Cystatin C alone is always better.

4. Cystatin C is an ideal marker for determining GFR. However, classic clearance methodology for clearance, by using a timed collection of urine and serum concentration, cannot be used with cystatin C because:

a. It is not produced at a constant rate.
b. It is freely filtered by glomeruli but is entirely reabsorbed in the loop of Henle.
c. It is freely filtered by glomeruli but is entirely metabolized in the proximal renal tubule.
d. It is not freely filtered by the glomeruli.
e. It cannot be assayed in urine.

5. The modified Schwartz eGFR formula mandates using enzymatic serum creatinine measurement that is calibrated to reference standards by isotope dilution mass spectroscopy (IDMS), but not to "Jaffe" (alkaline picrate) methods.

a. True
b. False

6. Urea splitting organisms, such as *Proteus, Pseudomonas, Klebsiella, Staphylococcus,* and *Mycoplasma* hydrolyze urea to ammonium and lead to the following changes:

a. Decreased urine pH
b. No change in urine pH
c. Raised urine and blood pH
d. Raised urine pH only

7. Evaluate this statement: "When $C_{H2O}$ is a positive number, it indicates increased free water clearance and a diuretic state."

a. True
b. False

8. Novel biomarkers of renal function are useful for:

a. Early detection of AKI
b. Indicating the onset of AKI after cardiovascular surgery or contrast use
c. Providing information on the potential site of tubular injury in AKI
d. All of the above

9. A 2½ year old white boy presented with a large right abdominal mass of 2 weeks' duration. He also had decreased appetite. Laboratory studies on presentation were as follows (in mmol/L): serum sodium, 130; potassium, 3.9; chloride, 92; and bicarbonate, 21. BUN and creatinine were 10 mg/dL and 0.4 mg/dL, respectively. The patient weighed 13.7 kg and was 92.5 cm tall. He underwent an open biopsy of the abdominal mass that documented the diagnosis of rhabdoid tumor of the right kidney. Regional lymph nodes and lungs had metastases. Right nephrectomy was followed by chemotherapy. He also underwent right flank and whole lung radiation. DTPA nuclear GFR was 48 mL/min/1.73 m² at 6 months. Serum creatinine was 0.6 mg/dL at 6 months, and the serum cystatin C level was 1.03 mg/L. His height and weight at 6 months postoperatively (2.5 years of age) were 13.6 kg and 95.7 cm, respectively. Calculated GFR by various formulas at 6 months was as follows: 104.5 mL/min/1.73 m² (original Schwartz), 65 mL/min/1.73 m² (IDMS-traceable Schwartz GFR formula), and 65.8 mL/min/1.73 m² (CKiD). The patient's estimated GFR is best reflected by all, *except:*

a. CKiD formula
b. Schwartz original eGFR
c. DTPA nuclear GFR
d. IDMS-traceable creatinine based Schwartz GFR

10. In the case given in question 9, a poor correlation of DTPA nuclear GFR and serum creatinine–based eGFR is *best* explained by:

a. Patient's receiving radiation therapy
b. Fluid volume retention
c. Chemotherapy causing renal toxicities
d. Loss of muscle mass resulting from poor nutrition

11. A 30-kg male patient has a 2-day history of gross hematuria and left flank pain. He is treated with intravenous fluids, analgesics, and a blocker agents in the emergency department. He passes a stone in the urine. A 24-h urine study shows the following: volume, 1200 mL; citrate, 400 mg/g creatinine; oxalate, 0.05 mg/mg creatinine; and Ca/Cr ratio, 0.45. The stone passed is *most likely* to be:

a. Uric acid
b. Calcium phosphate
c. Calcium oxalate
d. Struvite

## ANSWER KEY

1. c
2. a
3. c
4. c
5. a
6. d
7. a
8. d
9. b
10. d
11. c

# 5

# Normal and abnormal kidney function in neonates

DAVE T. SELEWSKI AND DAVID J. ASKENAZI

The neonatal period represents a period of rapid changes in renal blood, glomerulogenesis, and physiology that impacts kidney function. This chapter reviews the timing of glomerular development and the physiologic changes that occur following birth, with a particular focus on the pathophysiology associated with perturbation in these processes. This includes a discussion of the impact of prematurity on processes such as tubular function, glomerulogenesis, and glomerular filtration. Finally, this chapter focuses on acute kidney injury (AKI), including definition, high risk populations, and the implication for both short-term and long-term outcomes.

## RENAL PHYSIOLOGY FOLLOWING BIRTH

### RENAL BLOOD FLOW

Changes in renal blood flow shortly after birth drive changes in the neonatal glomerular filtration rate (GFR). There are marked changes in the proportion of cardiac output distributed to the kidneys throughout development and immediately following birth. The blood flow to the fully mature adult kidneys typically accounts for 20% to 30% of the cardiac output. This is in stark contrast to the developing fetal kidney, which receives 2.5% to 4% of cardiac output.[1] In the first 24 hours after birth, this increases to 6% of the cardiac output and continues to increase to 10% of the cardiac output at 1 week of life[2,3] and to 15% to 18% of the cardiac output at 6 weeks.[4] The dynamic changes in renal blood flow that occur following birth are driven by increased renal perfusion pressure and decreased renal vascular resistance.

---

**KEY POINT**

There are dynamic changes in renal blood flow following birth, with increase in the percentage of cardiac output delivered to the kidney from 2.5% to 4% in the fetal kidney to 6% of the cardiac output at 24 hours of life, 10% of the cardiac output at 1 week of life, and to 15% to 18% of the cardiac output at 6 weeks.

---

The increased renal perfusion pressure in the neonatal period results from an increased systemic blood pressure secondary to increased cardiac output and changes in systemic vascular resistance. Following birth there is an increase in the cardiac index, resulting in increased cardiac output in neonates. At the time of birth, the placenta typically receives approximately 40% of the cardiac output. The act of clamping the placenta leads to a significant increase in systemic vascular resistance following birth. Consequently, there is a steady increase in systemic blood pressure during the neonatal period. Although these factors contribute to increases in renal blood flow, the largest contribution results from changes in the renal vascular resistance.[5]

Renal vascular resistance and peripheral vascular resistance both remain high following birth, but renal vascular resistance begins to decrease at 24 hours of life. The decrease in renal vascular resistance occurs at a time when systemic vascular resistance is increasing. As shown in animal models, the decrease in renal vascular resistance is the major contributor to increased renal blood flow in neonates.[5] The decreased renal vascular resistance is driven by a number of factors, including a redistribution of renal blood flow within the kidney, changes in the number of vascular channels, and factors affecting glomerular arteriolar resistance.[6]

The distribution of renal blood flow in the fetal and newborn kidney is different from that in an adult kidney. In the newborn kidney, renal blood flow is preferentially directed toward the renal medulla and the inner cortex. This is reflective of the fetal development of the kidney. Following birth, there is increased renal blood flow to the outer cortex. The change of distribution of renal blood flow matures over the first 3 months of life. The increased distribution of blood to the outer cortex contributes to the decreased renal vascular resistance and subsequent increases in renal blood flow following birth.

---

### KEY POINT

Renal blood flow in the fetal and newborn kidney is distributed differentially throughout the kidney relative to an adult kidney, with blood flow preferentially directed toward the renal medulla and inner cortex.

---

A potential determinate of renal blood flow is the cumulative diameter of vessels. This can be increased by changes in individual diameter and by an increase in the number of vessels. The increased number of vessels is driven by nephrogenesis. In the developing fetus, nephrogenesis is complete by 34 to 36 weeks. The extent to which premature infants complete their potential nephrogenesis after birth has yet to be determined. The degree to which nephrogenesis continues will determine overall renal vascular resistance.[5] Conversely, in a term infant, an increase in vessel number does not make a significant contribution to changes in renal blood flow.

The primary factor determining renal blood flow after birth is changes in the arteriolar resistance driven by the response of small arteries to neurohormonal stimuli. The afferent and efferent arterioles remain the primary determinants of individual glomerular blood flow and contribute to overall renal vascular resistance. The primary drop in renal vascular resistance following birth occurs at the afferent arteriole pole, which allows for increased flow as cardiac output increases.

## CONTROL OF RENAL BLOOD FLOW IN THE NEWBORN

### Autoregulation

The mature kidney has an intricate ability to maintain renal blood flow and GFR despite hemodynamic changes. Two components of this regulation are the myogenic reflex and tubuloglomerular feedback (TGF). The myogenic reflex is an element that is intrinsic to the vascular smooth muscle. In response to increased stretch representing increased flow, the afferent arterioles contract, maintaining a constant renal blood flow and GFR. This phenomenon has been demonstrated in isolated renal vessels. The role of the myogenic reflex in the fetal and neonatal kidney remains unclear.

The second regulatory mechanism is TGF, which describes the phenomenon by which the cells of the macula densa sense the distal tubular fluid flow. This system seeks to maintain a constant flow distally. A number of vasoactive substances are involved in TGF, including angiotensin II (ATII), adenosine, endothelin, and nitric oxide (NO).

### Renin-angiotensin system

The renin-angiotensin system (RAS) is active throughout fetal development and contributes significantly to renal vascular resistance during the fetal and neonatal period through its vasoconstrictive activity. In the fetal and early neonatal period, the circulating levels of renin, angiotensin-converting enzyme (ACE), and angiotensin are frequently higher than adult levels.[7,8] During fetal development, renin production occurs in areas outside of the juxtaglomerular apparatus.[2,9,10] Renin levels are elevated throughout fetal development and remain high in neonates relative to adult values.[11] Following birth, renin production decreases throughout the kidney until it is found only in the juxtaglomerular apparatus.[12] ACE levels remain low throughout fetal life, with slight increases noted approaching term. Levels sharply increase following birth and peak at levels greater than adult values.[8] ATII levels are elevated during the fetal period and remain elevated in the neonatal period.

As part of the maturation of the RAS, there are changes in the types of angiotensin receptors. There are two forms of the angiotensin receptor, AT-1 and AT-2, which are expressed differentially in the fetus and neonate. The AT-1 receptors are coupled to G-proteins, and activation results in increased intracellular calcium and diacylglycerol. The AT-2 receptors are not associated with a G-protein, but instead activate an intracellular phosphatase, decreasing levels of cyclic adenosine monophosphate (cAMP). The AT-2 receptor is expressed in the fetal kidney and plays an important role in kidney development. The expression of AT-2 receptors decreases significantly following birth, but remains present at low levels in adult tissues.[13] The AT-1 receptor is initially at low levels in the developing fetus, but increases rapidly during hemodynamic development of the kidney and after birth.[14] The AT-1 receptor primarily mediates vasoconstriction. In animal models, disruption of either AT-1 or AT-2 receptors is capable of causing congenital malformations of the kidneys and genitourinary tract.

ATII is the effector of the RAS and is highly active in the newborn. ATII acts as a vasoconstrictor on both the afferent and efferent arterioles, leading to increased renal vascular resistance via the AT-1 receptor. ATII is capable of increasing the GFR because the relative diameter of the efferent arteriole is smaller than that of the afferent arteriole, resulting in a greater increase in resistance and increased GFR. ATII also acts in the proximal tubule to increase sodium reabsorption by increasing expression of a number of sodium cotransporters.

## Prostaglandins

Prostaglandins (PGs) are potent vasodilators and increase renal blood flow by causing vasodilatation of the afferent arteriole.[15] $PGE_2$ and $PGI_2$ are the major PGs involved in the regulation of renal blood flow. Under basal conditions there are low levels of PGs present in the neonatal kidneys. PGs become important to maintain renal perfusion during times of stress, including the neonatal period. During critical illness, PGs counterbalance the effects of ATII, catecholamines, and other vasoconstrictive substances elicited by a stress response.

PGs are increased when vasoconstrictive hormones activate phosphatidylinositol turnover, resulting in the production of diacylglycerol, which, following cleavage, leads to the production of PGs.[16] This damps the vasoconstriction of the afferent arteriole, preserving renal blood flow and maintaining GFR. This likely explains the decrease in urine output that can occur with neonatal exposure to inhibitors of PG formation (e.g., indomethacin or ibuprofen).

## Nitric oxide

NO is produced by NO synthetase in vascular endothelial cells. NO is a potent vasodilator of the microcirculation, leading to vasodilatation by activation of cyclic guanosine monophosphate (cGMP). NO is released in response to a number of physiologic stimuli that result from increased vasoconstriction. NO plays a critical role maintaining renal blood flow in the developing kidney and following birth by dampening the effects of potent vasoconstrictors such as AT-2.[17] In animal models, blockade of NO late in fetal

development resulted in significantly increased renal vascular resistance and decreased renal blood flow.[18]

## Bradykinin

Bradykinin is a product of the kallikrein-kinin system and is the major vasodilator produced by this system. Bradykinin elicits vasodilatation by inducing NO and PG production, leading to increased renal blood flow and natriuresis.[19] Blockade of the bradykinin receptors during fetal development can have an impact on nephrogenesis in animal models and predispose to salt-sensitive hypertension.[20,21]

## Endothelin

Endothelin is known to be a potent vasoconstrictor produced by endothelial cells of the renal vasculature, distal tubular cells, and mesangial cells. Endothelin production is regulated by bradykinin, AT-2, catecholamines, and shear stress. Endothelin causes both afferent and efferent arteriolar vasoconstriction, but there is a greater effect on the afferent arteriole, leading to decreased renal blood flow and GFR.[22]

## Adenosine

Adenosine is a breakdown product of adenosine triphosphate and plays an important role in TGF. The effects of adenosine depend on which receptors are activated. Through its action on AT-1 receptors, adenosine causes constriction of the afferent arteriole; binding to AT-2 receptors causes dilation of the afferent and efferent arterioles. Adenosine therefore plays a role in renal blood flow and the distribution of blood flow throughout the kidney. During stress, adenosine predominately causes dilation of the arterioles. Theophylline is nonspecific antagonist of adenosine and has been shown to ameliorate hypoxia-induced renal damage in rabbit models.[23,24] In high-risk neonates with oliguric kidney injury, theophylline has been shown to improve urine output and GFR.[25] Subsequent randomized clinical trials have shown improved renal function and urine output in high-risk neonates treated with theophylline.[26-28]

## Renal nerves

The renal nerves act to control renal vascular resistance primarily by the release of catecholamines and their subsequent action on the afferent arteriole mediated through the $\alpha_1$ adrenoceptor.[29,30] Catecholamines also increase renin release. Around the time of birth, there is an initial rise in catecholamine levels that contributes to increased renal vascular resistance. Over the first couple days of life these levels fall significantly,[31] likely contributing to decreased renal vascular resistance.

## GLOMERULOGENESIS

Renal development commences during the fifth week of gestation with partially functional temporary organs (the pronephros and metanephros), and the first nephrons are formed by approximately the eighth week of gestation. Urine output commences at approximately 12 weeks of gestation. The number of glomerular generations increases during gestation, with 4 generations at 14 weeks and 12 or 13 generations at 36 weeks. The juxtamedullary nephrons develop initially, with superficial ones following. Nephrogenesis continues until 34 to 36 weeks of gestation, at which time the number of nephrons, 1.6 to 2.4 million, approximates that of an adult.[32] Autopsy studies suggest that the extrauterine environment is not amenable to neoglomerulogenesis, leading to low nephron number in premature infants.[33]

Lower nephron number can result in single-nephron hyperfiltration. This enhances GFR such that individuals with a low nephron number can have a GFR that is comparable to that in individuals with normal nephron numbers. The impact of low nephron endowment may become problematic over time as single nephron hyperfiltration may cause dynamic changes leading to glomerulosclerosis and progressive loss of kidney function.

## RENAL TUBULAR FUNCTION

The proximal tubule is responsible for the bulk of solute reabsorption that occurs in the kidney, including bicarbonate, glucose, phosphate, and amino acids. The driving force for much of the absorptive processes in the proximal tubules and throughout the nephron is the gradient created by the $Na^+$-$K^+$-ATPase.[34] The $Na^+$-$K^+$-ATPase is on the basolateral membrane of tubular cells. The $Na^+$-$K^+$-ATPase maintains the low intracellular sodium concentration and negative electrochemical potential that drive a number of reabsorptive processes.[35] $Na^+$-$K^+$-ATPase activity is lower in neonates and increases significantly in the proximal tubule and each segment of the nephron after birth.[36,37]

## SODIUM BALANCE

In the immediate neonatal period, there is a significant natriuresis, which can be profound in preterm infants.[38] This natriuresis is mediated by atrial natriuretic peptide.[39] Following birth, urine sodium excretion is high and is inversely proportional to the maturity of the neonate.[40] In premature infants, fluid losses over the first week of life may be desirable because high fluid intake can be associated with patent ductus arteriosus, bronchopulmonary dysplasia, cardiac failure, necrotizing enterocolitis, and intraventricular hemorrhage.[41]

The inhibition of sodium transport peaks at 4 days following birth and is followed by a shift to conserve sodium, which is needed for growth. This shift toward sodium conservation is driven by maturational changes of sodium transport across multiple nephron segments. In the proximal tubule, there is an increase in activity of the $Na^+$-$H^+$ exchanger, the renal sodium/phosphate type 2 (NaPi-2) transporter, and sodium cotransporters (with glucose, amino acids, and phosphate) driven by maturation of the basolateral the $Na^+$-$K^+$-ATPase. The thick ascending limb of the loop of Henle undergoes significant maturational changes, which at birth has 20% of the adult capacity to transport sodium.[42] This is due to low activity of the $Na^+$2$Cl^-$$K^+$ cotransporter and $Na^+$-$K^+$-ATPase. Following birth, there is significantly increased activity of both transporters. Furthermore, maturational changes occur in the sodium chloride cotransporter in the distal tubule and the epithelial sodium channel in the collecting duct.

## POTASSIUM BALANCE

In older children and adults, there is a neutral potassium balance. During the period following birth, the neonate requires a positive potassium balance to sustain rapid growth.[43] However, even with potassium loading, term infants are able to excrete high amounts of potassium. The capacity to excrete potassium is lower in premature infants, which increases the risk for hyperkalemia. Some have suggested that 25% of infants with extremely low birth weight (less than 1000 g) develop at least one episode of hyperkalemia.[44] Consequently, term and preterm infants frequently have higher potassium levels than older children.[45]

The proximal tubule reabsorbs 50% to 65% of filtered potassium.[43,46,47] As mentioned previously, the mechanisms for the reabsorption of potassium in the loop of Henle are immature following birth; this increases the amount of potassium delivered to the distal nephron.[43,46] The distal nephron is responsible for the final modulation of potassium excretion. There are two channels that are the rate-limiting steps in potassium secretion in the distal nephron. The renal outer medullary potassium channel, found on the principal cells, is responsible for the basal secretion of potassium. The maxi-$K^+$ channel, located on the principal and intercalated cells, is responsible for flow-dependent potassium secretion.[48] In contrast, reabsorption of potassium occurs in the distal tubule by an H-$K^+$-ATPase, which is abundant during the neonatal period. The potassium-retaining characteristics of the neonatal kidney result from a paucity of apical secretory potassium channels and a predominance of the apical H-$K^+$-ATPase.[43]

## ACID-BASE BALANCE

The proximal tubule is responsible for reabsorption of approximately 80% of the filtered bicarbonate. The tubular acidification that drives this process is accomplished by two transporters responsible for $H^+$ excretion: the $Na^+$-$H^+$ exchanger and $H^+$-ATPase. In the adult kidney, the $Na^+$-$H^+$ exchanger is responsible for the majority (approximately two-thirds) of $H^+$ excretion.[49,50] Newborns have a lower bicarbonate level than adults. In term neonates the average bicarbonate level is 22 mEq/L, and in premature infants it may be as low as 15 mEq/L.[51,52] This results from decreased $H^+$ secretion into the proximal tubule. There is decreased activity of the $Na^+$-$H^+$ exchanger (approximately one-third of adult) in neonates, which increases by several-fold following birth. $H^+$-ATPase is virtually undetectable in the proximal tubule at birth, and then increases substantially.[53,50]

## GLUCOSE REABSORPTION

Glucose reabsorption occurs exclusively in the proximal tubule. In healthy adults, the proximal tubule is responsible for reabsorption of 100% of the filtered glucose, but glycosuria occurs if the blood glucose exceeds the normal threshold. Glucose is reabsorbed in a sodium-dependent manner by two transporters in the proximal tubule. In the S1 segment, there is a high activity–low affinity transporter (SGLT-2) that removes the majority of filtered glucose. Abnormalities in this transporter are responsible for benign familial glycosuria. In the S3 segment of the proximal tubule, there is a low activity–high affinity transporter (SGLT-1). Abnormalities in this transporter are responsible for hereditary glucose-galactose malabsorption. Early studies demonstrated that neonatal rabbits transported glucose at approximately one-third the rate of adult rabbits.[54] Consequently, premature infants are more susceptible to renal glycosuria.[55]

## PHOSPHATE BALANCE

In the growing neonate, phosphate is necessary for bone growth, along with many enzymatic activities. As a result, reabsorption of phosphate during the neonatal period is very high. The serum phosphate in neonates is higher than in adults.[56,57] Human and animal studies have shown that the fractional reabsorption of phosphate is much higher in neonates than in adults.[58-60] In fact, neonates reabsorb up to 99% of the filtered phosphate on the first day of life and 90% by the end of the first week of life.[57,61] Multiple factors in the neonatal period contribute to the increased reabsorption of phosphate, including a decreased responsiveness to parathyroid hormone,[62,63] maturational changes in NaPi II transporters,[64] and contributions from growth hormone and thyroid hormone.[65] Additives to breast milk and special formulas have been designed for premature infants to assist them in maintaining positive calcium and phosphorus balance.

## AMINO ACIDS TRANSPORT

Amino acids are actively resorbed by sodium-dependent active transport on the luminal side and transported across the basolateral membrane by facilitated diffusion in the proximal tubule. Transporters exist for amino acids with similar properties, including neutral, acidic, and basic amino acids. Neonates are known to have a generalized aminoaciduria that is worsened with prematurity.[66,67]

### KEY POINTS

- The proximal tubule is responsible for the bulk of solute reabsorption that occurs in the kidney, including bicarbonate, glucose, phosphate, and amino acids. Immature function can lead to lowered serum bicarbonate, glycosuria, and aminoaciduria during the neonatal period.
- During the neonatal period there is a drive to maintain a positive potassium and phosphate balance to ensure growth. As a result, term and preterm infants are known to have higher potassium and phosphate levels.

## GLOMERULAR FUNCTION RATE

GFR is the most useful measurement of kidney function. GFR is measured indirectly through the concept of clearance (the equivalent volume of plasma from which a substance would have to be totally removed to account for its rate of excretion in urine per unit of time). Clearance is calculated by dividing the excretion rate of a substance by its plasma concentration ($C_x = U_x \times V/P_x$); where $U_x$ and $P_x$ are urine and plasma concentrations of substance x, and V is urine flow rate. $C_x$ is expressed as milliliters per minute and is usually normalized to a standard body surface area of 1.73 $m^2$.[68] GFR is the best clinical test to estimate a functional renal mass, which can assist the clinician in prescribing fluids and electrolytes, determine disease progression, and appropriately prescribe medications excreted by the kidney.

The gold standard method for GFR measurement is inulin clearance. Table 5.1 shows the GFR measured by inulin

Table 5.1 Inulin clearance glomerular filtration rate in healthy premature infants

| Age | mL/min/1.73 m² |
| --- | --- |
| 1–3 days | 14.0 ± 5[70] |
| 1–7 days | 18.7 ± 5.5[112] |
| 4–8 days | 44.3 ± 9.3[113] |
| 3–13 days | 47.8 ± 10.7[113] |
| 1.5–4 mo | 67.4 ± 16.6[113] |
| 8 years | 103 ± 12[114] |

*Source:* Adapted from Schwartz GJ, Furth SL. Glomerular filtration rate measurement and estimation in chronic kidney disease. Pediatr Nephrol. 2007;22:1839–48.

clearance in preterm infants. Depending on degree of prematurity, GFR steadily improves from 10 to 20 mL/min/1.73 m² during the first week of life to 30 to 40 mL/min/1.73 m² by 2 weeks following birth, concomitant with alterations in renal blood flow. Thereafter, GFR improves steadily over the first few months of life.[69,70]

Although inulin clearance is the gold standard, it is not commonly used in clinical or research studies as a continuous inulin infusion and frequent laboratory measurements are needed. Other methods that approximate this gold standard include single-injection clearance techniques in which evaluation of the rate of disappearance from the plasma is used to approximate overall clearance. For example, a single injection of iohexol is an accurate alternative to inulin clearance and does not require a radioactive tracer.[69]

Serum creatinine (SCr) is the most common method to monitor renal function, but has significant shortcomings:

- SCr concentrations may not change until 25% to 50% of the kidney function has already been lost.

- At lower GFR, SCr overestimates renal function because of the tubular secretion of creatinine.
- SCr varies by muscle mass, hydration status, sex, age, and gender.
- Different methods (Jaffe reaction vs. enzymatic) produce different values, and medications and bilirubin can affect SCr measurements by the Jaffe method.[71,72]
- Once a patient receives dialysis, SCr can no longer be used to assess kidney function, because SCr is easily dialyzed.

Additional problems with using SCr in neonates include:

- SCr in the first few days of life reflects maternal kidney function and not the infant's renal function.
- Overall GFR in term and preterm infants is very low, and there is a very wide distribution of normal SCr values, which vary greatly depending on level of prematurity and age[73] (Figure 5.1).
- Bilirubin levels in premature infants are normal at birth, rise in the first several days, and return to normal after a few weeks. If the Jaffe method of measuring SCr is used, this may have tremendous impact on the interpretation of SCr.[71] Similarly, cephalosporins, histamine-2–receptor blockers, trimethoprim/sulfa, and other medications can affect SCr measurements. SCr-based estimations of GFR in neonates have suggested the following formula for children younger than 1 year of age.[74]

$$k * SCr/ht;$$

where k = 0.33 for infants with low birth weight and 0.45 for infants with normal birth weight

However, caution should be used in extrapolating this into clinical practice for several reasons. This formula represents an estimate, and the true GFR may be off in either

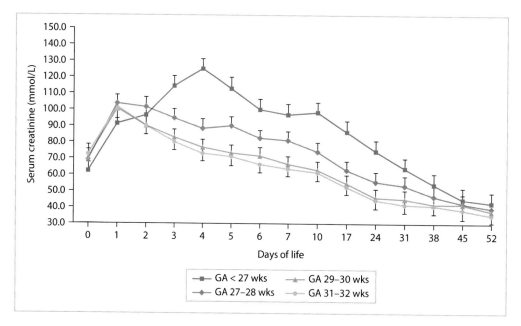

Figure 5.1 Change in serum creatinine during the first 52 days of gestation based on gestational age. (Reproduced with permission from: Gallini F, Maggio L, Romagnoli C, et al. Progression of renal function in preterm neonates with gestational age < or = 32 weeks. Pediatr Nephrol. 2000;15:119–24.)

direction by 20% or more. In addition, these formulas were derived using the Jaffe calorimetric method to measure SCr. The enzymatic method has replaced the Jaffe method at most hospitals; thus, these formulas may no longer be applicable.

Cystatin C, an endogenous proteinase inhibitor has been extensively studied as a measure to estimate GFR and as a marker of AKI. Because cystatin C is not influenced by the maternal level and is highest at birth, it may be superior to SCr for estimating GFR in neonates. Cystatin C concentrations significantly decrease from day 1 to day 3 of life and are independent of gestational age, birth weight, and maternal renal function in infants with very low birth weight.[75] Cystatin C does not differ between males and females. Thus, cystatin C seems to have many of the theoretical advantages needed to be an ideal marker of renal function.[76] However, there are limited data on cystatin c in neonates, including a lack of studies linking levels of Cystatin C levels with short-term and long-term outcomes.

> ### KEY POINT
>
> Depending on the degree of prematurity, GFR steadily improves from 10 to 20 mL/min/1.73 m$^2$ during the first week of life to 30 to 40 mL/min/1.73 m$^2$ by 2 weeks.

## NEONATAL ACUTE KIDNEY INJURY

Historically, neonatal AKI has been classically defined by oliguria, anuria, a persistent SCr of 1.5 mg/dL or greater, or all of these. We[77-81] and others[82-85] have used contemporary categorical definitions that require a rise in SCr to make the diagnosis of AKI, similar to definitions published by the Acute Kidney Injury Network (AKIN) groups in 2007[86] and more recently in 2012 by KDIGO. A neonatal AKI definition (Table 5.2) has been adapted for neonates from the 2012 KDIGO definition. The following modifications have been made to account for specific issues.

- Because SCr normally declines over the first week of life,[73] each SCr is compared to the lowest previous value.
- As SCr of 2.5 mg/dL represents GFR less than 10 mL/min/1.73 m$^2$ in neonates, this cutoff is used to define stage 3 AKI (as opposed to 4.0 mg/dL in adults).

> ### KEY POINT
>
> Neonatal acute kidney injury can be defined by adapting the 2012 KDIGO definition based on absolute rise in creatinine from a previous trough.

## NEONATAL ACUTE KIDNEY INJURY OUTCOME

AKI is associated with mortality in critically ill children[87,88] and adults,[89-93] even after controlling for medical comorbidities, severity of illness scores, and patient demographics. Over the past few years, epidemiologic studies in several high-risk groups of neonates have been performed. These studies add to the sparse literature on the incidence and outcomes of AKI by focusing on specific neonatal groups. In addition, researchers are no longer relying on arbitrary, binary definitions of neonatal AKI (e.g., SCr of 1.5 mg/dL or greater) and instead are using contemporary, categorical AKI frameworks such as modifications of the AKIN[94] staging system and the risk, injury, failure, loss, and end-stage renal disease (RIFLE) classification[87,89] that allow for improved diagnosis and staging of AKI by severity.

Recent epidemiology studies in infants with very low birth weight, sick near-term and term infants admitted to level 2 or 3 neonatal intensive care units (ICUs), term infants with severe perinatal asphyxia who undergo therapeutic hypothermia, infants who receive extracorporeal membrane oxygenation (ECMO), and infants who undergo cardiopulmonary bypass (CPB) surgery confirms that AKI is common in high-risk newborns and that those with AKI have significantly worse outcome. Although larger studies will be needed to determine the contribution of AKI to neonatal morbidity and mortality, these single-center studies

Table 5.2 Definition of acute kidney injury in the neonate

| Stage | SCr criteria | Urine output (UOP criteria) |
|---|---|---|
| 0 | No change or rise < 0.3 mg/dL | UOP > 1 cc/kg/h (over previous 24 h) |
| 1 | ↑ SCr of ≥ 0.3 mg/dL or ↑ SCr to 150-199% of baseline | UOP > 0.5 cc/kg/h and ≤ 1 cc/kg/h (over previous 24 h) |
| 2 | ↑ SCr to 200%–299% of baseline | UOP > 0.1 cc/kg/h and ≤ 0.5 cc/kg/h (over previous 24 h) |
| 3 | ↑ SCr to ≥ 300% of baseline or SCr ≥ 2.5 mg/dL or Receipt of dialysis | UOP ≤ 0.1 cc/kg/h (over previous 24 h) |

Source: Adapted from Jetton JG, Askenazi DJ. Update on acute kidney injury in the neonate. Curr Opin Pediatr. 2012; 24:191-6.
Note: Baseline SCr is defined as the lowest previous SCr value.

suggest that AKI is independently associated with mortality, when controlling for potentially confounding demographics, comorbidities, and interventions.

## INFANTS WITH VERY LOW BIRTH WEIGHT

In 2011, Koralkar et al.[95] published a prospective study on 229 infants with very low birth weight (birth weight between 500 and 1500 g) infants. They categorized each infant according to a modified AKIN definition (see Table 5.2). Using this framework, 41 of 229 (18%) of the cohort developed AKI (stage 1, 10; stage 2, 10; stage 3, 21). Infants with AKI were more likely to have lower birth weight, younger gestational age, and lower Apgar scores, as well as higher rates of assisted ventilation and inotropic support. In the AKI group, 42% (17 of 41) died, compared with 5% (9 of 188) in the non-AKI group (hazard ratio [HR], 9.3; 95% confidence interval [CI], 4.1 to 21.0; $P < 0.01$). Those with AKI had higher mortality independent of multiple adjusted confounders (adjusted HR, 2.3; 95% CI, 0.9 to 5.8; $P = 0.06$).

In 2012, Viswanathan et al.[96] published a retrospective analysis on 472 infants with extremely low birth weight (<1000 g). Using a cutoff of SCr of 1.5 mg/dL or greater to define AKI, the incidence of AKI was 59 of 472 (12.5%). They then performed a matched case-control study (matching for time period, birth weight (±10%), and gestational age (±1 week). Mortality in those with AKI was 33 of 46 (70%) compared to 10 of 46 (22%) in those without AKI ($P < 0.001$).

## SICK NEAR-TERM AND TERM INFANTS

In 2013, Askenazi et al.[97] published on 58 neonates with birth weight greater than 2000 g and 5-minute Apgar score of 7 or less admitted to a level 2/3 neonatal intensive care unit (NICU). AKI occurred in 9 of 58 (16%) infants. All infants without AKI survived, whereas 2 of 9 (22%) of those with AKI died ($P < 0.001$).

## INFANTS WITH PERINATAL ASPHYXIA TREATED WITH HYPOTHERMIA

In 2012, Selewski et al.[98] published a retrospective study on 96 infants who received hypothermia. Using the AKIN definition for AKI, they found that 36 of 96 (38%) infants developed AKI. Only 1 of 58 (2%) infants without AKI died compared to 5 of 36 (14%) with AKI ($P = 0.1$). Those with AKI had longer NICU stays ($P < 0.02$), longer hospitalizations ($P < 0.01$), and longer duration on mechanical ventilation ($P < 0.001$).

## INFANTS ON EXTRACORPOREAL MEMBRANE OXYGENATION

In a large retrospective cohort study using data from the Extracorporeal Life Support Organization registry,

Askenazi et al.[99] evaluated the impact of AKI and renal support therapy (RST) in infants who receive ECMO for noncardiac reasons. AKI was defined as SCr of 1.5 mg/dL or greater at any point in the hospitalization. Of the 7941 neonates in their cohort, 27.4% died. Nonsurvivors had higher rates of AKI than survivors (19% vs. 3.9%; $P < 0.0001$), and more nonsurvivors received RST than survivors (39.7% vs. 16%; $P < 0.0001$). After adjusting for numerous confounding variables, neonates with AKI had 3.2 higher odds of death than those without AKI ($P < 0.0001$); neonates who received RST had 1.9 higher odds of death ($P < 0.0001$) than those who did not receive RST.

Two smaller studies had similar findings. In a retrospective chart review of infants with congenital diaphragmatic hernia requiring ECMO, Gadepalli et al.[100] found 48 of 68 patients (71%) had AKI by the RIFLE classification. Patients with AKI "failure" (300% rise in SCr) had increased time on ECMO, decreased ventilator-free days, and decreased survival (27.3% with "failure" vs. 80% without AKI; $P = 0.001$). Shuhaiber et al.[101] also found higher rates of AKI in nonsurvivors versus survivors (80% vs. 40%; $P = 0.03$) in a small sample of patients (n = 20; 75% neonates) requiring more than one ECMO run after congenital heart surgery.

## INFANTS UNDERGOING CARDIOPULMONARY BYPASS SURGERY

Outcomes after AKI in infants undergoing CPB surgery have been reported. Blinder et al.[102] conducted a retrospective chart review of 430 infants (<90 days, median age 7 days) who had CPB. Using a modified AKIN definition (which included urine output criteria), they documented AKI in 225 of 430 (52%) infants (stage 1, 133, stage 2, 60, stage 3, 30). Postoperative AKI of all stages was associated with longer ICU stay; AKI stages 2 and 3 were associated with increased risk for prolonged mechanical ventilation and need for postoperative inotropic therapy. The mortality rate in those with AKI was higher than in those without (27 of 225 [12%] vs. 6 of 205 [3%]; $P < 0.001$). Moreover, risk for death increased with AKI severity (stage 2 OR, 5.1; 95% CI, 1.7 to 15.2; $P = 0.004$; and stage 3 OR, 9.5; 95% CI, 2.9 to 30.7; $P = 0.0002$).

Krawczeski et al.[103] evaluated 374 patients (including 35 neonates) undergoing CPB surgery. They defined AKI as an absolute increase in SCr of 0.3 mg/dL or greater from baseline within 48 hours of surgery and found that 8 of 35 (23%) had AKI by median 1 day after CPB. No differences in mortality were seen between the neonates with AKI and those without in this small neonatal subset.

In 2013, Alabbas et al.[104] published a retrospective study on 122 infants who received CBS. Using the AKIN definition, the incidence of AKI incidence was 76 of 122 (62%) (AKI stage 1, 22; stage 2, 19; stage 3, 33). Severe stage 3 AKI was associated with increased mortality (OR, 6.7; 95% CI, 1.08 to 41.5) and longer ICU stay (HR, 9.1; 95% CI, 1.3 to 61.0).

## KEY POINT

AKI in the neonatal population has been shown to be associated with clinically significant outcomes in multiple neonatal populations, including infants with low birth weight, near-term and term infants, newborns with perinatal asphyxia treated with therapeutic hypothermia, newborns undergoing ECMO, and newborns following CPB.

## RISK FOR CHRONIC KIDNEY DISEASE IN NEONATES

Premature infants are at high risk for death and other morbidities, including AKI during their initial hospitalization. With the increasing survival of premature infants over the last few decades, focus is now turning toward reducing long-term morbidities. Growing evidence suggests that premature infants are at risk for chronic kidney disease (CKD). A recent meta-analysis showed that premature infants are more likely to have albuminuria, end-stage renal disease, and lower estimated GFR compared to their term peers.[105] Among the 489 children in the Chronic Kidney Disease in Children (CKiD) study sponsored by the National Institutes of Health, there was a high rate of abnormal birth history (low birth weight, less than 2500 g) (17%), prematurity (<13%), small for gestational age (15%), and admission to an ICU (41%), and these factors were associated with decreased stature.[106] Thus, as more extremely premature infants survive and live into adulthood, the impact of CKD on premature infants is a significant long-term concern.

The reasons why premature infants are at risk for developing CKD remain unclear. One explanation is that because nephrogenesis continues until 34 weeks after conception and premature infants are born with a paucity of nephrons.[32] The extrauterine environment may not be amenable to neoglomerulogenesis and proper glomerular development.[33] Another explanation is that premature infants are at risk for acute hypoxic, hyperoxic, ischemic, septic, and nephrotoxic events between birth and termination of glomerulogenesis. The concept that AKI leads to CKD has been clearly elucidated in animal,[107] pediatric,[108,109] and adult[110] cohorts, such that we now know that AKI is a strong risk factor for CKD. Although the pathogenesis from AKI to CKD continues to be explored, most experts believe that endothelial damage leads to nephron dropout and interstitial fibrosis.[111] AKI during ongoing nephrogenesis may play an important role in limiting renal endowment and contribute to reduced renal function.

## KEY POINT

The long-term renal function of neonates, particularly premature neonates and neonates with AKI, is unknown and warrants further study.

## CONCLUSION

The care of the neonate with kidney dysfunction requires consideration of the dramatic changes in kidney function during the neonatal period. There is significant concern about the long-term consequences of AKI in the neonate, even when kidney function appears to normalize. AKI in the premature infant appears to increase the risk for CKD.

## SUMMARY

Neonates are exposed to a variety of stressors that may lead to AKI. Moreover, AKI in neonates may lead to CKD, or even ESRD, as illustrated in Clinical Vignette 5.1. Decreasing kidney size has an ominous prognosis and is usually associated with development of ESRD, albeit not always immediately.

### Clinical Vignette 5.1

A male infant was born via emergent cesarean section after the mother fell and had placental abruption. Apgar scores at 1, 5, and 10 minutes were 1, 4, and 8, respectively. The infant's blood urea nitrogen (BUN)/creatinine steadily rose to 50 mg/dL and 4.0 mg/dL during the first week of life. A peritoneal dialysis catheter was placed in anticipation for the need of dialysis. Because he maintained adequate urine output to keep up with intake, renal replacement therapy was not initiated at that time. By week 2 of life, BUN increased to 110 mg/dL and SCr rose to 6.3 mg/dL and the infant was less alert. His renal ultrasound showed bilateral hyperechoic kidneys with poor corticomedullary differentiation, measuring 4.5 and 4.6 cm on the left and right, respectively. Dialysis was initiated with hourly cycles of the peritoneal dialysis solution Dianeal (Baxter, Newbury, UK). Dwell volumes were advanced slowly, and the number of cycles was diminished. Two months after the initiation of peritoneal dialysis, a renal ultrasound showed that the kidneys were shrinking (now at 4.1 and 3.6 cm). Peritoneal dialysis was held for a 48-hour period to determine if the infant's native kidney function had improved. The BUN and creatinine rose sharply, and thus the child was restarted on peritoneal dialysis. At age 3 months, a similar trial off dialysis showed that he continued to have a sharp increase in BUN and creatinine, and thus his diagnosis changed from AKI to end-stage renal disease (ESRD). At 12 months, he continues on peritoneal dialysis. He weighs 10.2 kg (50th percentile for age) and his length is 72 cm (10th percentile for age). He is achieving neurodevelopmental milestones appropriate for his age. He has been placed on the kidney transplant waiting list and is on six medications to manage his CKD.

# REFERENCES

1. Rudolph AH, Heymann MA, Teramo M, et al. Studies on the circulation of the previable fetus. Pediatr Res. 1971;5:452–65.
2. Jose PA, Fildes RD, Gomez RA, et al. Neonatal renal function and physiology. Curr Opin Pediatr. 1994;6:172–7.
3. Yao LP, Jose PA. Developmental renal hemodynamics. Pediatr Nephrol. 1995;9:632–7.
4. Paton JB, Fisher DE, DeLannoy CW, Behrman RE. Umbilical blood flow, cardiac output, and organ blood flow in the immature baboon fetus. Am J Obstet Gynecol. 1973;117:560–6.
5. Gruskin AB, Edelmann CM Jr, Yuan S. Maturational changes in renal blood flow in piglets. Pediatr Res. 1970;4:7–13.
6. Evan AP Jr, Stoeckel JA, Loemker V, Baker JT. Development of the intrarenal vascular system of the puppy kidney. Anat Rec. 1979;194:187–99.
7. Wolf G. Angiotensin II and tubular development. Nephrol Dial Transplant. 2002;17(Suppl 9):48–51.
8. Yosipiv IV, El-Dahr SS. Developmental biology of angiotensin-converting enzyme. Pediatr Nephrol. 1998;12:72–9.
9. Gomez RA. Role of angiotensin in renal vascular development. Kidney Int Suppl. 1998;67:S12–6.
10. Gomez RA, Lynch KR, Sturgill BC, et al. Distribution of renin mRNA and its protein in the developing kidney. Am J Physiol 1989;257:F850-8.
11. Stalker HP, Holland NH, Kotchen JM, Kotchen TA. Plasma renin activity in healthy children. J Pediatr. 1976;89:256–8.
12. Celio MR, Groscurth P, Inagami T. Ontogeny of renin immunoreactive cells in the human kidney. Anat Embryol (Berl). 1985;173:149–55.
13. Grady EF, Sechi LA, Griffin CA, et a. Expression of AT2 receptors in the developing rat fetus. J Clin Invest. 1991;88:921–33.
14. Tufro-McReddie A, Harrison JK, Everett AD, Gomez RA. Ontogeny of type 1 angiotensin II receptor gene expression in the rat. J Clin Invest. 1993;91:530–7.
15. Gleason CA. Prostaglandins and the developing kidney. Semin Perinatol 1987;11:12–21.
16. Exton JH. Calcium signalling in cells: Molecular mechanisms. Kidney Int Suppl. 1987;23:S68–81.
17. Solhaug MJ, Wallace MR, Granger JP. Nitric oxide and angiotensin II regulation of renal hemodynamics in the developing piglet. Pediatr Res. 1996;39:527–33.
18. Solhaug MJ, Ballevre LD, Guignard JP, et al. Nitric oxide in the developing kidney. Pediatr Nephrol. 1996;10:529–39.
19. Siragy HM, Jaffa AA, Margolius HS. Bradykinin B2 receptor modulates renal prostaglandin E2 and nitric oxide. Hypertension. 1997;29:757–62.
20. El-Dahr SS, Dipp S, Meleg-Smith S, et al. Fetal ontogeny and role of metanephric bradykinin B2 receptors. Pediatr Nephrol. 2000;14:288–96.
21. Schanstra JP, Duchene J, Praddaude F, et al. Decreased renal NO excretion and reduced glomerular tuft area in mice lacking the bradykinin B2 receptor. Am J Physiol Heart Circ Physiol. 2003;284:H1904–8.
22. Naicker S, Bhoola KD. Endothelins: Vasoactive modulators of renal function in health and disease. Pharmacol Ther. 2001;90:61–88.
23. Prevot A, Mosig D, Rijtema M, Guignard JP. Renal effects of adenosine A1-receptor blockade with 8-cyclopentyl-1,3-dipropylxanthine in hypoxemic newborn rabbits. Pediatr Res. 2003;54:400–5.
24. Gouyon JB, Guignard JP. Theophylline prevents the hypoxemia-induced renal hemodynamic changes in rabbits. Kidney Int. 1988;33:1078–83.
25. Huet F, Semama D, Grimaldi M, et al. Effects of theophylline on renal insufficiency in neonates with respiratory distress syndrome. Intensive Care Med. 1995;21:511–4.
26. Jenik AG, Ceriani Cernadas JM, Gorenstein A, et al. A randomized, double-blind, placebo-controlled trial of the effects of prophylactic theophylline on renal function in term neonates with perinatal asphyxia. Pediatrics. 2000;105:E45.
27. Bakr AF. Prophylactic theophylline to prevent renal dysfunction in newborns exposed to perinatal asphyxia: A study in a developing country. Pediatr Nephrol. 2005;20:1249–52.
28. Bhat MA, Shah ZA, Makhdoomi MS, Mufti MH. Theophylline for renal function in term neonates with perinatal asphyxia: A randomized, placebo-controlled trial. J Pediatr. 2006;149:180–4.
29. DiBona GF, Kopp UC. Neural control of renal function. Physiol Rev. 1997;77:75–197.
30. Johns EJ, Kopp UC, DiBona GF. Neural control of renal function. Compr Physiol. 2011;1:731–67.
31. Eliot RJ, Lam R, Leake RD, et al. Plasma catecholamine concentrations in infants at birth and during the first 48 hours of life. J Pediatr. 1980;96:311–5.
32. Abrahamson DR. Glomerulogenesis in the developing kidney. Semin Nephrol. 1991;11:375–89.

33. Rodriguez MM, Gomez AH, Abitbol CL, et al. Histomorphometric analysis of postnatal glomerulogenesis in extremely preterm infants. Pediatr Dev Pathol. 2004;7:17–25.

34. Quigley R. Developmental changes in renal function. Curr Opin Pediatr. 2012;24:184–90.

35. Garg LC, Knepper MA, Burg MB. Mineralocorticoid effects on Na-K-ATPase in individual nephron segments. Am J Physiol. 1981;240:F536–44.

36. Schmidt U, Horster M. Na-K-activated ATPase: Activity maturation in rabbit nephron segments dissected in vitro. Am J Physiol. 1977;233:F55–60.

37. Schwartz GJ, Evan AP. Development of solute transport in rabbit proximal tubule. III. Na-K-ATPase activity. Am J Physiol. 1984;246:F845–52.

38. Hansen JD, Smith CA. Effects of withholding fluid in the immediate postnatal period. Pediatrics. 1953;12:99–113.

39. Tulassay T, Seri I, Rascher W. Atrial natriuretic peptide and extracellular volume contraction after birth. Acta Paediatr Scand. 1987;76:444–6.

40. Siegel SR, Oh W. Renal function as a marker of human fetal maturation. Acta Paediatr Scand. 1976;65:481–5.

41. Bell EF, Acarregui MJ. Restricted versus liberal water intake for preventing morbidity and mortality in preterm infants. Cochrane Database Syst Rev. 2001;(3):CD000503.

42. Horster M. Loop of Henle functional differentiation: In vitro perfusion of the isolated thick ascending segment. Eur J Physiol. 1978;378:15–24.

43. Gurkan S, Estilo GK, Wei Y, Satlin LM. Potassium transport in the maturing kidney. Pediatr Nephrol. 2007;22:915–25.

44. Lorenz JM, Kleinman LI, Markarian K. Potassium metabolism in extremely low birth weight infants in the first week of life. J Pediatr. 1997;131:81–6.

45. Wilkins BH. Renal function in sick very low birthweight infants. III. Sodium, potassium, and water excretion. Arch Dis Child. 1992;67:1154–61.

46. Lelievre-Pegorier M, Merlet-Benichou C, Roinel N, de Rouffignac C. Developmental pattern of water and electrolyte transport in rat superficial nephrons. Am J Physiol. 1983;245:F15–21.

47. Giebisch G. Renal potassium transport: Mechanisms and regulation. Am J Physiol. 1998;274:F817–33.

48. Pacha J, Frindt G, Sackin H, Palmer LG. Apical maxi K channels in intercalated cells of CCT. Am J Physiol 1991;261:F696–705.

49. Koeppen BM SB, editor. Renal Physiology. Philadelphia: Elsevier; 2007.

50. Baum M. Developmental changes in rabbit juxtamedullary proximal convoluted tubule acidification. Pediatr Res. 1992;31:411–4.

51. Baum M, Quigley R. Ontogeny of proximal tubule acidification. Kidney Int. 1995;48:1697–704.

52. Schwartz GJ, Haycock GB, Edelmann CM Jr, Spitzer A. Late metabolic acidosis: A reassessment of the definition. J Pediatr. 1979;95:102–7.

53. Baum M. Neonatal rabbit juxtamedullary proximal convoluted tubule acidification. J Clin Invest. 1990;85:499–506.

54. Schwartz GJ, Evan AP. Development of solute transport in rabbit proximal tubule. I. HCO-3 and glucose absorption. Am J Physiol. 1983;245:F382–90.

55. Wilkins BH. Renal function in sick very low birthweight infants. IV. Glucose excretion. Arch Dis Child. 1992;67:1162–5.

56. Connelly J, Crawford J, Watson J. Neonatal hyperphosphatemia. Pediatrics. 1963;1:155–6.

57. Connelly JP, Crawford JD, Watson J. Studies of neonatal hyperphosphatemia. Pediatrics. 1962;30:425–32.

58. Johnson V, Spitzer A. Renal reabsorption of phosphate during development: Whole-kidney events. Am J Physiol. 1986;251:F251–6.

59. Neiberger RE, Barac-Nieto M, Spitzer A. Renal reabsorption of phosphate during development: Transport kinetics in BBMV. Am J Physiol. 1989;257:F268–74.

60. Brodehl J, Gellissen K, Weber HP. Postnatal development of tubular phosphate reabsorption. Clin Nephrol. 1982;17:163–71.

61. Hohenauer L, Rosenberg TF, Oh W. Calcium and phosphorus homeostasis on the first day of life. Biol Neonate. 1970;15:49-56.

62. Imbert-Teboul M, Chabardes D, Clique A, Montegut M, Morel F. Ontogenesis of hormone-dependent adenylate cyclase in isolated rat nephron segments. Am J Physiol. 1984;247:F316–25.

63. Spitzer A, Barac-Nieto M. Ontogeny of renal phosphate transport and the process of growth. Pediatr Nephrol. 2001;16:763–71.

64. Woda C, Mulroney SE, Halaihel N, et al. Renal tubular sites of increased phosphate transport and NaPi-2 expression in the juvenile rat. Am J Physiol Regul Integr Comp Physiol. 2001;280:R1524–33.

65. Corvilain J, Abramow M, Bergans A. Some effects of human growth hormone on renal hemodynamics and on tubular phosphate transport in man. J Clin Invest. 1962;41:1230–5.

66. Brodehl J, Gellissen K. Endogenous renal transport of free amino acids in infancy and childhood. Pediatrics. 1968;42:395–404.

67. Jones DP, Chesney RW. Development of tubular function. Clin Perinatol. 1992;19:33–57.

68. Schwartz GJ. Alvaro Muñoz MF, Schneider MS, et al. New Equations to Estimate GFR in Children with CKD. J Am Soc Nephrol. 2009 Mar; 20(3):629-637.

69. Schwartz GJ, Furth SL. Glomerular filtration rate measurement and estimation in chronic kidney disease. Pediatr. Nephrol (Berl). 2007;22:1839–48.

70. Brion LP, Fleischman AR, McCarton C, Schwartz GJ. A simple estimate of glomerular filtration rate in low birth weight infants during the first year of life: Noninvasive assessment of body composition and growth. J Pediatr. 1986;109:698–707.

71. Lolekha PH, Jaruthunyaluck S, Srisawasdi P. Deproteinization of serum: Another best approach to eliminate all forms of bilirubin interference on serum creatinine by the kinetic Jaffe reaction. J Clin Lab Anal. 2001;15:116–21.

72. Rajs G, Mayer M. Oxidation markedly reduces bilirubin interference in the Jaffe creatinine assay. Clin Chem. 1992;38:2411–3.

73. Gallini F, Maggio L, Romagnoli C, et al. Progression of renal function in preterm neonates with gestational age < or = 32 weeks. Pediatr Nephrol (Berl). 2000;15:119–24.

74. Schwartz GJ, Feld LG, Langford DJ. A simple estimate of glomerular filtration rate in full-term infants during the first year of life. J Pediatr. 1984;104:849–54.

75. Demirel G, Celik IH, Canpolat FE, et al. Reference values of serum cystatin C in very low-birthweight premature infants. Acta Paediatr. 2013;102:e4–7.

76. Kandasamy Y, Smith R, Wright IM. Measuring cystatin C to determine renal function in neonates. Pediatr Crit Care Med. 2013;14:318–22.

77. Askenazi DJ, Koralkar R, Hundley HE, et al. Fluid overload and mortality are associated with acute kidney injury in sick near-term/term neonate. Pediatr Nephrol (Berl). 2013;28:661–6.

78. Selewski DT, Jordan BK, Askenazi DJ, et al. Acute kidney injury in asphyxiated newborns treated with therapeutic hypothermia. J Pediatr. 2013;162:725–9.

79. Askenazi DJ, Koralkar R, Hundley HE, et al. Urine biomarkers predict acute kidney injury in newborns. J Pediatr. 2012;161:270–5.

80. Askenazi DJ, Montesanti A, Hunley H, et al. Urine biomarkers predict acute kidney injury and mortality in very low birth weight infants. J Pediatr 2011;159:907–12.

81. Koralkar R, Ambalavanan N, Levitan EB, et al. Acute kidney injury reduces survival in very low birth weight infants. Pediatr Res. 2011;69:354–8.

82. Phelps CM, Eshelman J, Cruz ED, Pan Z, Kaufman J. Acute kidney injury after cardiac surgery in infants and children: Evaluation of the role of angiotensin-converting enzyme inhibitors. Pediatr Cardiol. 2012;33:1–7.

83. Aydin SI, Seiden HS, Blaufox AD, et al. Acute kidney injury after surgery for congenital heart disease. Ann Thorac Surg. 2012;94:1589-–95.

84. Jetton JG, Askenazi DJ. Update on acute kidney injury in the neonate. Curr Opin Pediatr. 2012;24:191–6.

85. Li S, Krawczeski CD, Zappitelli M, et al. Incidence, risk factors, and outcomes of acute kidney injury after pediatric cardiac surgery: A prospective multicenter study. Crit Care Med. 2011;39:1493–9.

86. Bagga A, Bakkaloglu A, Devarajan P, et al. Improving outcomes from acute kidney injury: Report of an initiative. Pediatr Nephrol (Berl). 2007;22:1655–8.

87. Akcan-Arikan A, Zappitelli M, Loftis LL, et al. Modified RIFLE criteria in critically ill children with acute kidney injury. Kidney Int. 2007;71:1028–35.

88. Zappitelli M, Parikh CR, Akcan-Arikan A, et al. Ascertainment and epidemiology of acute kidney injury varies with definition interpretation. Clin J Am Soc Nephrol. 2008;3:948–54.

89. Ricci Z, Cruz D, Ronco C. The RIFLE criteria and mortality in acute kidney injury: A systematic review. Kidney Int. 2008;73:538–46.

90. Cuhaci B. More data on epidemiology and outcome of acute kidney injury with AKIN criteria: Benefits of standardized definitions, AKIN and RIFLE classifications. Crit Care Med. 2009;37:2659–61.

91. Uchino S. Outcome prediction for patients with acute kidney injury. Nephron Clin Pract. 2008;109:c217–23.

92. Macedo E, Castro I, Yu L, et al. Impact of mild acute kidney injury (AKI) on outcome after open repair of aortic aneurysms. Ren Fail. 2008;30:287–96.

93. Bagshaw SM, George C, Bellomo R. Changes in the incidence and outcome for early acute kidney injury in a cohort of Australian intensive care units. Crit Care. 2007;11:R68.

94. Mehta RL, Kellum JA, Shah SV, et al. Acute Kidney Injury Network: Report of an initiative to improve outcomes in acute kidney injury. Crit Care 2007;11:R31.

95. Koralkar R, Ambalavanan N, Levitan EB, et al. Acute kidney injury reduces survival in very low birth weight infant. Pediatr Res. 2011;69:354–8.

96. Viswanathan S, Manyam B, Azhibekov T, Mhanna MJ. Risk factors associated with acute kidney injury in extremely low birth weight (ELBW) infants. Pediatr Nephrol (Berl). 2012;27:303–11.

97. Askenazi DJ, Koralkar R, Hundley HE, et al. Fluid overload and mortality are associated with acute kidney injury in sick near-term/term neonate. Pediatr Nephrol (Berl). 2013;28:661–6.

98. Selewski DT, Jordan BK, Askenazi DJ, et al. Acute kidney injury in asphyxiated newborns treated with therapeutic hypothermia. J Pediatr. 2013;162:725–9.

99. Askenazi DJ, Griffin R, McGwin G, et al. Acute kidney injury is independently associated with mortality in very low birthweight infants: A matched case-control analysis. Pediatr Nephrol (Berl). 2009;24:991–7.

100. Gadepalli SK, Selewski DT, Drongowski RA, Mychaliska GB. Acute kidney injury in congenital diaphragmatic hernia requiring extracorporeal life support: An insidious problem. J Pediatr Surg 2011;46:630–5.

101. Shuhaiber J, Thiagarajan RR, Laussen PC, et al. Survival of children requiring repeat extracorporeal membrane oxygenation after congenital heart surgery. Ann Thorac Surg. 2011;91:1949–55.

102. Blinder JJ, Goldstein SL, Lee VV, et al. Congenital heart surgery in infants: Effects of acute kidney injury on outcomes. J Thorac Cardiovasc Surg. 2012;143:368–74.

103. Krawczeski CD, Woo JG, Wang Y, et al. Neutrophil gelatinase-associated lipocalin concentrations predict development of acute kidney injury in neonates and children after cardiopulmonary bypass. J Pediatr 2011;158:1009–15.

104. Alabbas A, Campbell A, Skippen P, et al. Epidemiology of cardiac surgery-associated acute kidney injury in neonates: A retrospective study. Pediatr Nephrol (Berl). 2013;28:1127–34.

105. White SL, Perkovic V, Cass A, et al. Is low birth weight an antecedent of CKD in later life? A systematic review of observational studies. Am J Kidney Dis. 2009;54:248–61.

106. Greenbaum LA, Munoz A, Schneider MF, et al. The association between abnormal birth history and growth in children with CKD. Clin J Am Soc Nephrol. 2011;6:14–21.

107. Basile DP. The endothelial cell in ischemic acute kidney injury: Implications for acute and chronic function. Kidney Int. 2007;72:151–6.

108. Askenazi DJ, Feig DI, Graham NM, et al. 3-5 year longitudinal follow-up of pediatric patients after acute renal failure. Kidney Int. 2006;69:184–9.

109. Mammen C, Al Abbas A, Skippen P, et al. Long-term risk of CKD in children surviving episodes of acute kidney injury in the intensive care unit: A prospective cohort study. Am J Kidney Dis. 2012;59:523–30.

110. Coca SG, Singanamala S, Parikh CR. Chronic kidney disease after acute kidney injury: A systematic review and meta-analysis. Kidney Int. 2012;81:442–8.

111. Basile DP. Rarefaction of peritubular capillaries following ischemic acute renal failure: A potential factor predisposing to progressive nephropathy. Curr Opin Nephrol Hypertens. 2004;13:1–7.

112. Guignard JP, Torrado A, Da Cunha O, Gautier E. Glomerular filtration rate in the first three weeks of life. J Pediatr. 1975;87:268–72.

113. Barnett HL, Hare K, McNamara H, Hare R. Measurement of glomerular filtration rate in premature infants. J Clin Invest. 1948;27:691–9.

114. Vanpee M, Blennow M, Linne T, et al. Renal function in very low birth weight infants: Normal maturity reached during early childhood. J Pediatr. 1992;121:784–8.

## REVIEW QUESTIONS

1. Which of the following factors is the *most* important contributor to the increase in renal blood flow following birth?
   a. Increased cardiac output
   b. Increased renal vascular resistance
   c. Decreased renal vascular resistance
   d. Increased circulating plasma volume
   e. Changes in systemic resistance

2. Which of the following statements about the renin-angiotensin system is *not true*?
   a. Fetal renin levels are higher than adult levels.
   b. Neonatal angiotensin-converting enzyme levels are higher than adult levels.
   c. There is a shift from a predominance of angiotensin receptor type 2 to angiotensin receptor type 1 following birth.
   d. Disruptions of the angiotensin type 1 or type 2 receptors are capable of causing congenital malformations of the kidney.
   e. AT-2 receptors are coupled to G-proteins.

3. Fetal urine output begins at what week during gestation?
   a. 5th week
   b. 8th week
   c. 12th week
   d. 20th week
   e. 36th week

4. Nephrogenesis is completed at:
   a. 28 week s of gestation
   b. 36 weeks of gestation
   c. 40 weeks of gestation
   d. 2 weeks following birth
   e. 2 years of age

5. Which of the following statements about neonatal sodium homeostasis is *not true*?
   a. There is an increase in activity of the $Na^+$-$H^+$ exchanger in the proximal tubules after birth.
   b. There is an initial natriuresis that affects term and preterm neonates equally.
   c. There is a shift toward sodium conservation at day 4 of life.
   d. The loop of Henle has 20% of the adult capacity to transport sodium.
   e. There are maturational changes in the distal tubule handling of sodium after birth.

6. When compared to older infants, neonates can be expected to have a lower level of which of the following?
   a. Serum potassium
   b. Serum phosphorus
   c. Serum bicarbonate
   d. Urine glucose
   e. Urine amino acids

7. Which is *true* of the definition of neonatal acute kidney injury?
   a. Oliguria should be the only criterion because all neonates with AKI are oliguric.
   b. An absolute serum creatinine greater than 1.5 mg/dL is the best approach.
   c. There are currently no large prospective studies that have tested different definitions against hard clinical outcomes.
   d. Because SCr is stable over the first week of life,

looking at an absolute rise in SCr from baseline provides the best definition of neonatal AKI.

 e. The need for dialysis should serve as the definition of AKI.

8. Acute kidney injury has been shown to be associated with adverse outcomes in which neonatal populations?

 a. Infants with very low birth weight

 b. Near term/term infants

 c. Newborns with perinatal asphyxia treated with therapeutic hypothermia

 d. Newborns undergoing extracorporeal membrane oxygenation

 e. Newborns following cardiopulmonary bypass

 f. All of the above

9. Compared to the adult kidney, fetal renal blood flow is typified by which of the following?

 a. Low renal vascular resistance

 b. Greater flow to the renal cortex

 c. Greater flow to the renal medulla

 d. A larger percentage of the cardiac output

## ANSWER KEY

1. c
2. e
3. c
4. b
5. b
6. c
7. c
8. f
9. c

# Diagnostic imaging of the urinary tract

EGLAL SHALABY-RANA, BRUCE MARKLE, AND DOROTHY BULAS

Radiologic imaging plays a vital role in the evaluation of the urinary tract in children. Multiple imaging modalities are available for the diagnostic workup of renal disorders in children, including voiding cystourethrography (VCUG), ultrasonography, computed tomography (CT), and magnetic resonance imaging (MRI). Ultrasonography is particularly useful in the evaluation of the structure of the kidneys and bladder without the use of ionizing radiation. Fetal ultrasound examination has been instrumental in the identification of urologic abnormalities long before they become clinically evident. CT and MRI, with their excellent spatial resolution, are useful in the evaluation of the kidneys and vascular structures. These imaging modalities are often complementary, each with its clinical indications and applications, as well as limitations.

## VOIDING CYSTOURETHROGRAPHY

## INDICATIONS

Voiding cystourethrography (VCUG) is performed for the detection of vesicoureteral reflux (VUR), and for delineating the anatomy of the urinary bladder and urethra. Common indications for a VCUG are urinary tract infection (UTI), and the presence of hydronephrosis, hydroureter, or both. Assessing for VUR before renal transplantation is another use of the VCUG.

## TECHNIQUE

The VCUG needs no specific patient preparation except for explanation of the procedure to the child if age-appropriate.

The presence of parents, a child-life specialist, or both can facilitate the procedure in an apprehensive child. However, if the patient is extremely anxious and not allowing the study to be performed, oral sedation with midazolam, in anxiolytic doses, can be used with the added benefit of amnestic effect of this medication.[1] This may be the case in an older child, typically 3 years of age and older. If sedation is to be used, the study needs to be scheduled in advance, with the child maintained fasting for the appropriate length of time.

An initial scout abdomen radiograph (kidney-ureter-bladder [KUB]) is taken to assess for the presence of calculi along the urinary tract, as well as examine the spine for dysraphism (spina bifida). The stool burden also can be assessed. Subsequently, using sterile technique, the bladder is catheterized with a feeding tube. A urine specimen is usually obtained and sent to the laboratory for culture.

Radioiodinated contrast (Cystoconray, Mallinckrodt Pharmaceuticals, St. Louis, MO) is then instilled into the bladder under gravity drip. An early filling image is taken to evaluate for bladder filling defects, such as ureterocele, which may be obscured by a contrast-filled bladder. Expected bladder filling volume can be approximated by the formula:

$$\text{Bladder volume (mL)} = (\text{Age in years} + 2) \times 30$$

One can also observe for signs of a full bladder, including slowing of the contrast drip, patient discomfort and crying, and upturning of the toes. Images are taken of the full bladder, each ureterovesical junction, the kidney fossae, and the urethra.

Complications of VCUG include UTI, chemical cystitis, vasovagal attack from an extremely full bladder, and retrograde spread of infection leading to acute pyelonephritis

## KEY POINTS

- Contrast VCUG allows delineation of anatomy and an accurate grading of VUR.
- Contrast VCUG is preferred in males to evaluate urinary tract anatomy and VUR reflux.
- Nuclear cystogram allows only a semiquantitative estimation of VUR and does not allow anatomic evaluation with accuracy. Nuclear cystograms may be used to follow progress of VUR.

## INTERPRETATION

The normal urinary bladder is a smooth-walled globular structure centrally placed in the bony pelvis. Urethral walls are smooth, and the posterior urethra is visualized as a nondistended, smooth-walled passage. The urethral passage is subdivided into the anatomic areas of anterior urethra and posterior urethra. In males, the anterior urethra consists of the penile urethra and the bulbous urethra. The posterior urethra begins at the bladder neck and encompasses prostatic urethra and the membranous urethra (Figure 6.1). The female urethra, on the other hand, is a short tube and does not have the complex anatomy of the male urethra. Ureterocele is an abnormal congenital dilatation of the distal portion of the ureter, which herniates into the bladder. Ureteroceles are commonly seen in the duplex collecting system, usually in association with the upper moiety. Because of the narrowing of its ureteral orifice into the bladder, the

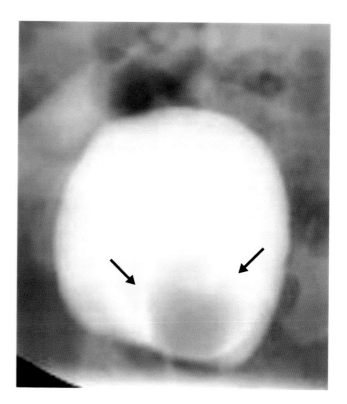

Figure 6.2 Contrast VCUG showing a ureterocele (arrows).

ureterocele often causes obstruction of its ureter resulting in hydronephrosis and hydroureter. Ureterocele is recognized as a filling defect low in the bladder during the early bladder-filling image (Figure 6.2). Bladder wall trabeculation (Figure 6.3) occurs as a result of functional

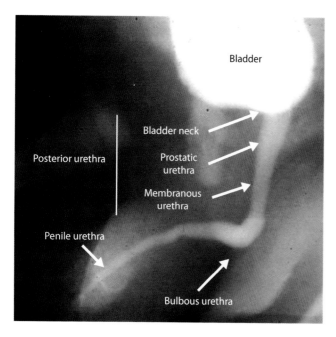

Figure 6.1 Contrast voiding cystourethrography showing normal radiologic anatomy of the male urethra.

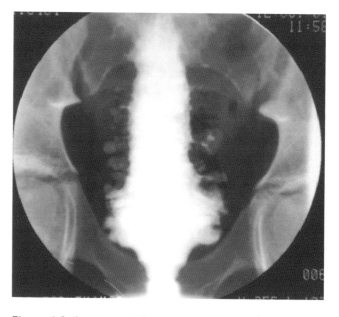

Figure 6.3 Contrast voiding cystourethrography in a patient with spina bifida with a trabeculated elongated bladder (Christmas tree bladder), consistent with a neuropathic bladder.

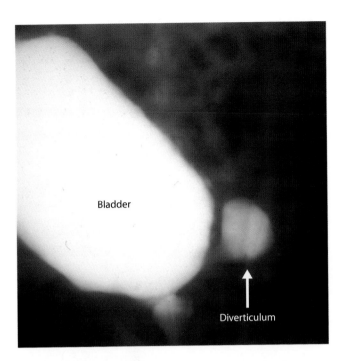

Figure 6.4 Contrast voiding cystourethrography demonstrating a bladder diverticulum (arrow).

(neuropathic bladder) or mechanical bladder outlet obstruction (posterior urethral valve). Diverticula of the bladder (Figure 6.4) also can be seen in the previously mentioned clinical circumstances or may be associated with VUR. Posterior urethral valves (PUVs), which are seen exclusively in boys, result in a dilated posterior urethra with obstructed flow of contrast below the level of the valve (Figure 6.5).

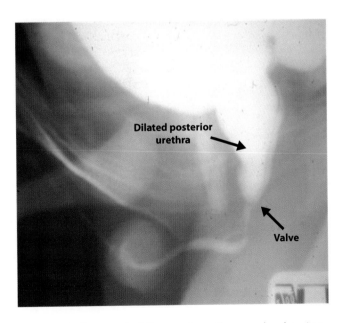

Figure 6.5 Contrast voiding cystourethrography showing posterior urethral valve. Characteristic dilatation of the prostatic urethra by the posterior urethral valve is seen (arrows).

Table 6.1 International Reflux Study in Children grading of vesicoureteric reflux[2]

| | |
|---|---|
| Grade I: | Reflux into the ureter only. |
| Grade II: | Reflux into the collecting system without blunting of calyces. |
| Grade III:t | Reflux into the collecting system with mild blunting of calyces with preservation of papillary impressions; ureter may be mildly dilated. |
| Grade IV: | Reflux into the collecting system with moderate blunting of calyces with some loss of papillary impressions with occasional complete loss of papillary impressions (clubbing); ureter dilated and tortuous. |
| Grade V: | Clubbing of most of calyces. Ureter is dilated and tortuous. |

## CLASSIFICATION OF VESICOURETERAL REFLUX

VUR, if present, can be classified into five grades according to the International Reflux Study in Children grading (Table 6.1).[2] Figure 6.6 shows the VCUG features of these five grades of reflux. Intrarenal reflux may be sometimes seen in association with the high grade VUR (IV and V). In the duplicated collected system, wherein the upper moiety is obstructed, the lower moiety is filled with the contrast and shows an inferior and a lateral displacement of the opacified lower pole moiety. This configuration is referred to as the "drooping lily" sign (Figure 6.7) and should suggest a duplicated collecting system with VUR on the affected side.

## RENAL ULTRASOUND

Ultrasound is an ideal modality for the evaluation of the genitourinary system of fetuses, children, and adults. It is typically inexpensive, does not involve the use of ionizing radiation, does not require sedation, can assess organs in multiple planes, and can evaluate arterial and venous flow with the use of Doppler ultrasound. Ultrasonography can evaluate renal size, position, anatomy, urinary bladder masses, anomalies, and prevoid and postvoid bladder volume. Ultrasound also provides useful information about structures around the urinary tract that may obstruct the kidney and bladder.

Limitations of ultrasound investigative procedures include the inability to penetrate gas or bone. Resolution also may be restricted in crying infants and obese patients. Ultrasound is operator dependent and requires expertise for appropriate technical performance and interpretation.

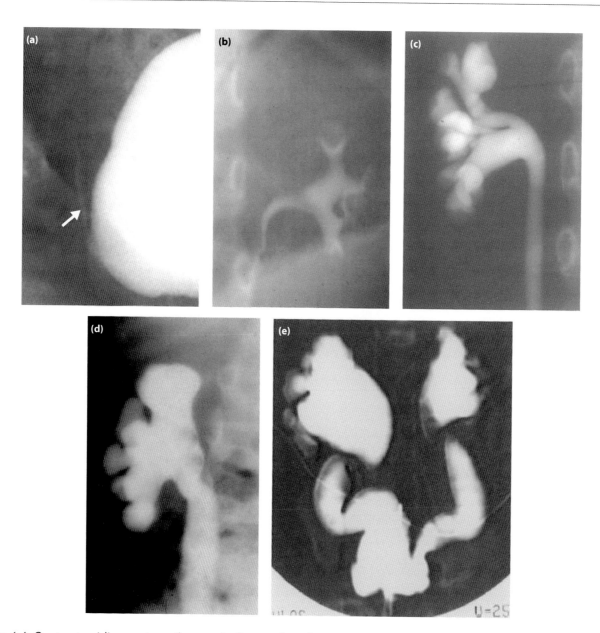

Figure 6.6 Contrast voiding cystourethrography five grades of vesicoureteric reflux. **(a)** Grade 1 vesicoureteral reflux (arrow). Contrast flows into the lower part of the ureter. **(b)** Grade II vesicoureteral reflux. Calyces are sharp, with deep papillary impressions. **(c)** Grade III vesicoureteral reflux. Calyces are blunted, but papillary impressions are preserved. **(d)** Grade IV vesicoureteral reflux. Calyces are significantly blunted, with very shallow papillary impressions. Ureter is also dilated. **(e)** Grade V vesicoureteral reflux. Ureters are dilated and tortuous ureter and clubbing of most calyces are seen.

Despite these limitations, ultrasound is a cornerstone in the evaluation of renal and bladder anatomy.

## RENAL SIZE

Ultrasonographic evaluation of the kidney begins with an assessment of size. Normal data for renal size in children are available for birth through adolescence (Figure 6.8).[3,4] Abnormalities in renal size can be observed in numerous disorders, listed in Table 6.2. Regression equation for determining renal size based on the observations of Rosenbaum et al.[3] is as follows.

For children older than 1 year:

$$\text{Renal length (cm)} = 6.79 + 0.22 \times \text{age (years)}$$

For younger than 1 year:

$$\text{Renal length (cm)} = 4.98 + 0.155 \times \text{age (months)}$$

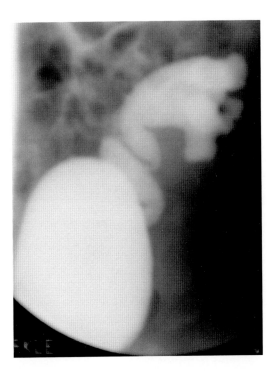

Figure 6.7 Contrast voiding cystourethrography showing vesicoureteral reflux into the lower pole moiety of a duplex system. Downward displacement and lateral position of the collecting system result in the so-called "drooping lily" appearance.

Table 6.2 Causes of abnormal renal size

**Small Kidney(s)**
- Renal hypoplasia and dysplasia
- Renal arterial stenosis
- Reflux nephropathy
- Chronic kidney disease

**Unilateral Nephromegaly**
- Acute pyelonephritis
- Renal vein thrombosis
- Renal tumor
- Hematoma (renal or perirenal)
- Renal abscess
- Urinary tract obstruction, hydronephrosis
- Beckwith-Weidemann syndrome

**Bilateral Nephromegaly**
- Polycystic kidney disease
- Acute glomerulonephritis
- Bladder outlet obstruction, hydronephrosis
- Bilateral Wilms tumor
- Glycogen storage diseases
- Acute lymphatic leukemia (leukemic infiltrates)
- Lymphoma

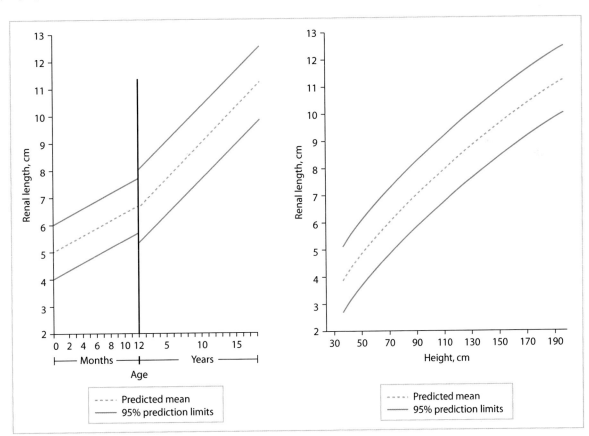

Figure 6.8 Renal size in children as determined by sonography. Age is represented in years unless specified otherwise. (Reproduced from Han BK, Babcock DS. Sonographic measurements and appearance of normal kidneys in children. Am J Roentgenol. 1985;145: 611–6.)

# EVALUATION OF RENAL ARCHITECTURE

Location and configuration of the kidneys are important in the identification of pelvic, horseshoe, and duplex kidneys. Renal parenchyma is assessed for masses, cysts, calcifications, and echogenicity. Loss of corticomedullary differentiation, sometime referred to as "medical renal diseases" (MRDs), is a nonspecific radiologic sign that can be seen in a variety of disorders, such as acute tubular necrosis, infections, glomerulonephritis, glomerulosclerosis, and autosomal recessive polycystic kidney disease (ARPKD).

> ## KEY POINT
>
> Renal ultrasound provides a radiation-free imaging modality that allows evaluation of renal size, architecture, blood flow, and hydronephrosis.

# EVALUATION OF RENAL VESSELS

Using duplex, color, and power Doppler imaging, renal ultrasound can characterize renal vascular flow. The renal arteries and veins, as well as smaller arcuate vessels, can be assessed for renal artery stenosis, renal vein thrombosis, or renal transplant rejection.

## Fetal Urogenital Ultrasonography

Congenital anomalies of the urogenital tract are found in 3% to 4% of the population.[5] Lethal urinary tract anomalies account for 10% of spontaneous pregnancy losses.[6] A systematic prenatal sonographic approach includes evaluation of the amniotic fluid volume, characterization of genitourinary anomalies, and search for associated abnormalities such as the VACTERL association (vertebral anomalies, anal atresia, cardiac defects, tracheoesophageal fistula, and renal and radial limb anomalies).

In their early development, fetal kidneys are located close to the sacral area in the pelvic region and eventually ascend to their lumbar location at approximately the 6th to 9th week. Fetal kidneys are visualized by ultrasound at approximately the 12th to 13th week, and their characteristic fetal architecture can be discerned by the 20th week.[7] The normal fetal kidney has a lobulated appearance with distinct hypoechoic pyramidal structures and variable corticomedullary differentiation (Figure 6.9).

## Amniotic fluid

Although urine production begins at approximately 5 to 8 weeks of gestation, contribution of urine to

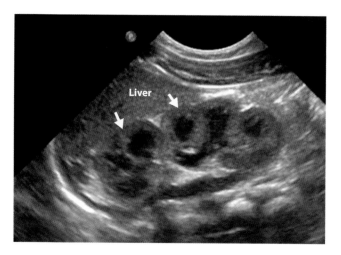

Figure 6.9 Renal ultrasound in a normal term infant. Fetal lobulations (arrows) are seen on the surface of the kidney. The renal cortex is more echogenic than the liver, and the prominent renal pyramids are hypoechoic.

amniotic fluid is minor before the 16th week of gestation. Lack of fetal urine output after 16 gestational weeks, however, results in a rapid decline in amniotic fluid volume. Under these circumstances, the fetus develops the classic Potter sequence, which includes low-set ears, flat nose, clubfeet and hands, and growth restriction. Pulmonary hypoplasia is common in these patients and is often the cause of significant neonatal morbidity and mortality. Lethal genitourinary anomalies are associated with minimal or no urine production. These include renal agenesis, bilateral multicystic dysplastic kidneys, autosomal recessive infantile polycystic kidney disease, and severe posterior urethral valves.

## Antenatal hydronephrosis

Antenatal dilatation of the renal collecting system is a common finding in the fetus. Most cases of pelviectasis noted

> ## KEY POINTS
>
> - Fetal ultrasound allows prenatal diagnosis of urogenital tract abnormalities.
> - The SFU has provided guidelines for grading antenatal hydronephrosis in the fetus.
> - Guidelines for postnatal evaluation of antenatal hydronephrosis will require consensus development.
> - More than 50% of infants with antenatal hydronephrosis demonstrate resolution over 12 to 18 months of postnatal follow-up with ultrasound.

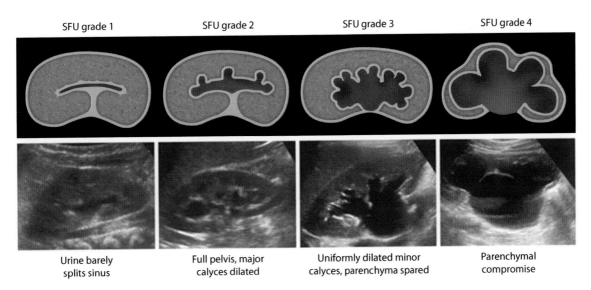

Figure 6.10 Society of Fetal Urology classification of antenatal hydronephrosis. (Reproduced with permission from: Timberlake MD, Herndon CDA. Mild to moderate postnatal hydronephrosis: grading systems and management. Nat Rev Urol. 2013;10: 649–5.)

on routine ultrasound evaluation in early gestation resolve during pregnancy, and only approximately 20% persist into the postnatal period.[7] Measurement of the anteroposterior pelvic diameter (APD) is commonly used to assess fetal hydronephrosis and is a surrogate for potential urinary tract pathology. The fetal APD normally measures less than 3 mm, but its measurement can be affected by gestational age, maternal hydration, and fullness of the fetal bladder.[7,8] There is little consensus on the minimal threshold for APD at various gestational ages that is predictive of urinary tract pathology.[7] Calyceal or ureteral dilatation should always be regarded as an abnormal sonographic finding in a fetus, regardless of the renal pelvic size.

The Society of Fetal Urology (SFU) has developed a grading system for antenatal hydronephrosis. According to this classification, antenatal hydronephrosis is classified into four grades (Figure 6.10), which provide a uniform set of diagnostic criteria for clinical care.[7] It is important to recognize that sonography is unable to differentiate between a dilated urinary collecting system resulting from urinary obstruction and a nonobstructed dilated system secondary to abnormal ureteric muscle development or VUR. Apart from the severity of antenatal hydronephrosis, it is also important to determine if the renal parenchyma is thinned and the calyces and ureters are dilated. If both kidneys are affected and the parenchyma is thinned, echogenic, or has cortical cysts (SFU grade III or IV), close prenatal follow-up is necessary because of the risk for oligohydramnios.

Postnatal imaging protocols for patients with antenatal hydronephrosis continue to evolve.[9] Sonography should be avoided on the first day of life, because the neonate may be in a state of dehydration, which can underestimate the degree of hydronephrosis and result in a false-negative ultrasound study.[10] Need for a VCUG in such patients is less clear. Following these patients by ultrasound evaluation reduces the need for VCUG to less than 50%.[9] In the presence of a strong suspicion of urinary obstruction, MAG-3 renal scan with furosemide (diuretic renal scan) may provide the needed diagnostic information.

### KEY POINT

Ultrasound evaluation of antenatal hydronephrosis on day 1 of life may give a false-negative result because of low urine flow.

## OBSTRUCTIVE UROPATHY

Obstruction at the ureteropelvic junction (UPJ) is the most common form of urinary tract obstruction noted in children. Sonographically, the central pelvis and calyces are dilated with varying degrees of cortical thinning (Figure 6.11). The ureter is normal in size and usually not visualized. Obstruction at the ureterovesical junction (UVJ) can be due to a stricture, ureteroceles (Figure 6.12),

### KEY POINTS

- UPJ obstruction is the most common type of urinary obstruction noted in children.
- Bilateral hydronephrosis in a male infant should raise the suspicion of PUV.
- Febrile UTI may be the initial manifestation of patients with ureteral obstruction.

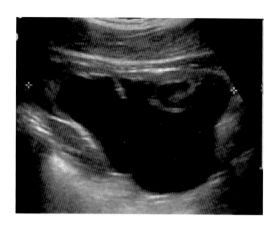

Figure 6.11 Ureteropelvic junction obstruction. Renal ultrasound showing significant pelvic and calyceal dilatation, and cortical thinning resulting from ureteropelvic junction obstruction.

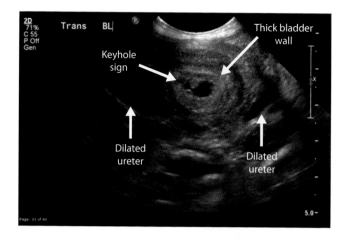

Figure 6.13 Fetal ultrasound demonstrating "key-hole sign." Ureters are dilated bilaterally, bladder wall is thickened, and inferiorly dilated posterior urethra gives the impression of a key hole.

or an ectopic ureteric insertion. Bilateral hydronephrosis may result from lower urinary tract obstruction, such as PUV, urethral stenosis, or atresia. Renal ultrasound in patients with PUV may demonstrate a thick-walled bladder and a dilated prostatic urethra below it, resulting in the so-called "keyhole sign" (Figure 6.13). A thick trabeculated bladder wall noted on ultrasonography (Figure 6.14) is usually suggestive of neurogenic bladder.

## CYSTIC DISEASES

Multicystic dysplastic kidney (MCDK) is a distinct disorder characterized by a nonfunctional cystic kidney. Sonographically, MCDK is diagnosed by the presence of

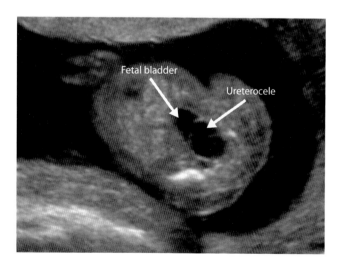

Figure 6.12 Prenatal ultrasound at 24 weeks of gestation demonstrates a transverse image of bladder containing a cyst consistent with a ureterocele.

multiple noncommunicating cysts of varying sizes with minimal surrounding echogenic tissue (Figure 6.15). MCDK is associated with contralateral renal anomalies in up to 25% of cases.[11] VUR in the contralateral (normal kidney) is seen in 20% to 25% of patients with MCDK and may need to be ruled out if the patient develops a UTI.[11] To differentiate MCDK from severe UPJ obstruction in the affected kidney, additional imaging to determine renal blood flow and function, such as with MAG-3 renal scan, is necessary. The diagnostic feature of MCDK is absence of any renal blood flow and lack of excretory activity on the affected side. Regression of the cysts in MCDK is common over several years.[12]

---

### KEY POINTS

- MCDK presents as a multicystic mass without any functional renal tissue.
- Cysts are noncommunicating.
- MAG-3 renal scan shows no perfusion or excretion in the affected kidney.
- Contralateral kidney may have VUR or other abnormalities in approximately 25% of cases.
- Involution of the cystic mass is common.

---

Autosomal recessive polycystic kidney disease (ARPKD) has a wide spectrum of clinical presentations, ranging from perinatal severe renal disease to the juvenile form with minimal renal disease and dominant hepatic fibrosis. Kidneys are enlarged and are echogenic as a result of microcysts, and corticomedullary differentiation is poor (Figure 6.16). Prenatal ultrasound diagnosis of ARPKD may be delayed

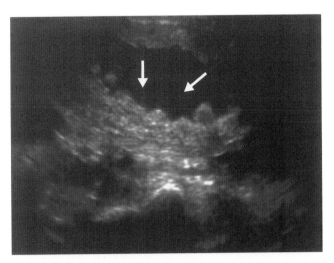

Figure 6.14 Ultrasound image of the urinary bladder showing thickened bladder wall and trabeculations of the mucosa (arrows) in a patient with neurogenic bladder.

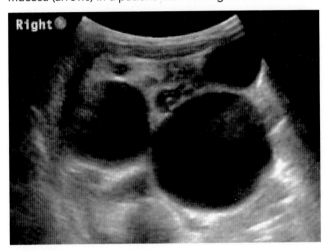

Figure 6.15 Transverse image of the right kidney in a patient with multicystic dysplastic kidney demonstrating multiple cysts of varying size that do not connect with each other. No normal renal parenchyma is present.

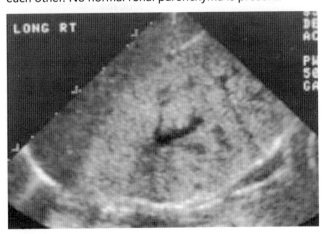

Figure 6.16 Renal ultrasound in an infant with autosomal recessive polycystic kidney disease. Longitudinal view of the kidney demonstrates an echogenic kidney with poor corticomedullary differentiation. No clear evidence of cysts is present.

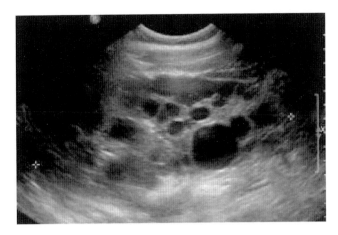

Figure 6.17 Renal ultrasound showing multiple cysts scattered throughout the renal parenchyma in a patient with autosomal dominant polycystic kidney disease.

until the third trimester because kidneys may appear normal earlier in gestation.

Autosomal dominant polycystic kidney disease (ADPKD) is characterized by presence of cysts in the kidney, liver, and some other organs, such as the pancreas and spleen. Prenatally, the kidneys may appear normal or large and echogenic with the variable presence of cysts. Multiple cysts scattered throughout the parenchyma are the hallmark of ADPKD (Figure 6.17). Hemorrhage and calcifications can develop within larger cysts that appear heterogeneous sonographically. A variety of inherited syndromes and genetic and chromosomal disorders that are associated with renal cystic disease are discussed further in Chapter 43.

## RENAL NEOPLASMS

Mesoblastic nephroma, also known as fetal renal hamartoma, may manifest prenatally or neonatally as a solid unilateral vascular mass. This benign tumor cannot be differentiated from a Wilms tumor radiographically, and nephrectomy is generally recommended.[13]

Wilms tumor, also known as nephroblastoma, usually manifests as a large mass distorting the collecting system and the renal capsule. By ultrasound, the mass is typically solid, hyperechoic, and homogeneous. The mass may obstruct the collecting system, and the renal tissue may be severely compressed into a thin rim. Hemorrhage and necrosis may make the tumor heterogeneous in appearance, and cystic components have been reported. Doppler ultrasound study is particularly useful in assessing spread of the tumor into the renal vein and the inferior vena cava.

Cystic nephroma is a rare lesion seen in children that is considered to be benign. It is composed of multiple cysts of varying size. This mass is difficult to distinguish from a cystic Wilms tumor, because both may appear well circumscribed, with multiloculated cysts and septations.

## COMPUTED TOMOGRAPHY AND MAGNETIC RESONANCE IMAGING

CT and MRI are well-established cross-sectional imaging techniques used for diagnosis of renal and retroperitoneal disease in children. Both methods yield relatively high spatial resolution images of the kidneys and the surrounding retroperitoneal structures. Thin-section data sets are now routinely obtained by rapidly scanning multidetector CT systems. CT systems should be optimized for age-appropriate exposure parameters.

Radiation exposures from CT and all radiation-based methods should be included in the clinician's and radiologist's considerations regarding appropriateness of imaging studies. Non–radiation-based imaging as alternative methods should be considered before CT. Wherever possible, imagers should use techniques such as automatic exposure control and lower dose acquisitions combined with noise-reducing "iterative reconstruction" methodologies.[14] CT radiation exposure data should be included in the image data set, and CT reports should document exposure parameters. Data obtained with CT can be used to reconstruct coronal, sagittal, and oblique imaging planes. Three-dimensional surface renderings also can be obtained when large density differences allow separation of various tissues—for example, contrast-enhanced renal vessels, or contrast-enhanced collecting systems.

CT is most commonly used in detection of urinary calculi (without contrast material) and for rapid evaluation of renal neoplasms, particularly at the time of presentation. CT is also capable of demonstrating intra-abdominal spread of the neoplasms and vascular invasion. CT provides a superior technique for demonstration of metastatic disease in lungs, an important staging parameter in the renal neoplasms.

### KEY POINTS

- Both CT and MRI are high-resolution imaging modalities.
- Radiation dose in CT needs to be minimized in children.
- MRI takes longer for image acquisition than CT.

MRI has the advantage of acquiring sectional images directly in virtually any anatomic plane without any ionizing radiation exposure, but the examination time is considerably longer for MRI. Whereas CT scan acquisition time can be a few seconds, MRI acquisition sets take several minutes per acquisition, and a complete MRI examination entailing multiple sequences can take 30 to 45 minutes or more. Sedation is frequently necessary for MRI in children younger than 8 years of age. Preparatory desensitization to the MRI gantry environment can reduce the need for sedation in some patients, particularly when combined with preparatory counseling by child-life specialists in advance of the actual scan date.

A single CT acquisition gives a single phase of vascular and renal contrast enhancement. Multiple phases require additional acquisitions, incurring an additional radiation exposure, ideally avoided to minimize overall radiation exposure.[15,16]

## CONTRAST NEPHROTOXICITY IN COMPUTED TOMOGRAPHY AND MAGNETIC RESONANCE IMAGING

The intravenous contrast agents used in CT can cause nephrotoxicity. This risk is enhanced in patients with acute kidney injury (AKI), chronic kidney disease (CKD), dehydration, diabetes, compromised systemic perfusion, and concurrent use of other nephrotoxic drugs.[17,18]

Ionic, high-osmolality contrast agents have osmolality in the range of 1400 to 2070 mOsm/kg, and "low" osmolality, nonionic agents range from 700 to 800 mOsm/kg. Iso-osmolar agents are also now available. Current recommendations for contrast administration include the use of low-osmolality and iso-osmolar agents, adequate hydration, urine alkalinization, and administration of the lowest possible contrast dose necessary for an adequate examination. $N$-acetyl cysteine, an antioxidant, may be used to ameliorate the nephrotoxic effects of the contrast drugs, but its efficacy is controversial.[19]

### KEY POINTS

- Contrast agents used for CT and MRI can be nephrotoxic.
- Nephrotoxicity is enhanced in states of dehydration, diabetes mellitus, concurrent use of other nephrotoxins, and use of high osmolality contrast agents.

## GADOLINIUM CONTRAST AGENTS AND NEPHROGENIC SYSTEMIC FIBROSIS

Nephrogenic systemic fibrosis (NSF) is a rare but painful, debilitating, and sometimes fatal disorder seen in the setting of renal insufficiency and administration of gadolinium-based contrast agents (GBCAs).[20-23] NSF has been generally reported in patients with advanced CKD (GFR less than 30 mL/min/1.73 m$^2$), with many patients being on dialysis. Patients with CKD III (GFR 30 to 60 mL/min/1.73 m$^2$) and AKI also should be considered at risk for developing NSF. The need for GBCA administration should be examined carefully in such patients. Presence of metabolic acidosis at the time of receiving GBCA is also considered a potential risk factor in developing NSF.[21]

Clinical manifestations of NSF consists of swelling, induration, and tightening of the skin, often with a peau d'orange appearance in the lower and upper extremities.[21,22] In some patients the clinical picture can simulate scleroderma. Involvement of deep soft tissues also occurs in NSF; this can include the skeletal muscle and myocardium.[23] NSF has been reported in several pediatric patients.[24] Progressive worsening of symptoms is usual, and there is no known therapy. Risk for NSF has been reported to be 2.4% with each exposure of GCCA in presence of advanced CKD or end-stage renal disease.[25]

The pathogenesis of NSF is not fully understood. The GBCA metabolites are primarily excreted in urine, and retention of GBCA metabolites in renal failure is thought to result in eventual dissociation of gadolinium ion from the carrier ligand. Free gadolinium (a toxic metal species) has poor solubility and is precipitated in various tissues in conjunction with other ions, such as phosphate or carbonate.[21,26] The gadolinium precipitates are thought to incite an inflammatory response in the deposition sites.[26,27] Macrophage and fibroblast proliferation is common at these sites.[21]

## LIMITATIONS OF MAGNETIC RESONANCE IMAGING

The dominant limitation of MRI imaging arises from the longer overall imaging time required for a complete study. In addition, longer imaging times introduce a significant element of artifact, engendered by physiologic motion from respiration, from gastrointestinal peristalsis, and even from cardiovascular pulsations. Recently updated MRI pulse sequences have improved but not eliminated respiratory motion-based artifacts. Bowel motion is generally uncompensated, but imaging plane selection can ameliorate its effects.

## ASSESSING RENAL FUNCTION WITH COMPUTED TOMOGRAPHY AND MAGNETIC RESONANCE IMAGING

Although nuclear medicine studies have forged the early path to clinical application of imaging for determination of renal function, the dynamic studies of renal perfusion and function also have been performed using MRI and CT.[28-30] CT use is limited because of the high radiation exposure required for serial sampling of the kidneys during passage of contrast through the kidneys. In MRI imaging, serial sampling of signal intensity of kidneys can yield time-signal intensity curves of the transit of the contrast from which the glomerular filtration rate (GFR) can be calculated.[31]

## COMPUTED TOMOGRAPHY AND MAGNETIC RESONANCE IMAGING ANGIOGRAPHY

Rapid thin-section imaging, improved data reconstruction techniques, and rapid contrast injections have made it possible to create angiographic images from cross-sectional data sets. This allows relatively low-risk performance of CT and MR angiograms. The spatial resolution and temporal resolution of these methods do not, however, approach that of traditional catheter-based angiography. Demonstration of the aorta and central, first- and second-order branch vessels can be achieved reasonably well with CT and MR angiography. However, because many cases of renovascular hypertension in children are due to small segmental artery lesions or small accessory renal artery lesions, the role of screening CT angiography and MR angiography in such patients remains controversial.

CT angiography involves a rapid intravenous injection of radiographic contrast material, combined with rapid spiral volume acquisition. This is typically done in sedated, free-breathing infants and young children. Older children and adolescents can be coached to breath-hold, producing more accurate data with less bulk motion artifact. Three-dimensional images of the vessels are created from the acquired data. Limitations to the anatomic accuracy include uncompensated bulk motion, intrinsic pulsatile vascular motion, and some intrinsic CT artifacts.

MR angiography is a highly developed technique in imaging adult patients and is used for evaluation of intrinsic aortic disease and evaluation of patients with possible renovascular hypertension.[32] With a rapid intravenous injection of GBCA, three-dimensional images of the central arterial and venous structures can be obtained (Figure 6.18). The small size of the vessels of small children is more difficult

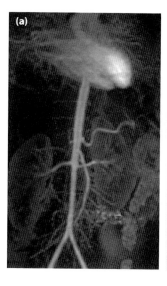 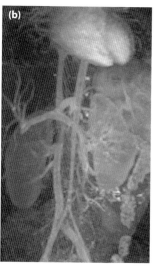

Figure 6.18 Magnetic resonance angiogram. (a) An arterial-phase image in a 4-year-old child showing the major central vascular structures of the abdominal arterial tree. (b) Filling of the venous structures and a general opacification of the parenchymal organs.

to image compared to imaging in adults. Nonetheless, parenchymal perfusion defects can be well demonstrated in smaller lobar and segmental vascular territories. More recently, noncontrast MRI sequences have been developed for evaluation of central renal arteries.

## COMPUTED TOMOGRAPHY AND MAGNETIC RESONANCE UROGRAPHY

The urine-filled collecting system also can be imaged for combined anatomic and physiologic information in dilated and obstructed systems and in dilated and non-obstructed systems by performing MRI urography.[33,34] Noncontrast anatomic images can be generated, taking advantage of long T2 dephasing characteristics of urine (in a fashion similar to that used for MR cholangiopancreatography). This allows demonstration of the fluid-filled renal collecting systems, showing anatomic sites of urinary obstruction and fluid-filled structures such as genitourinary tract cysts, ureteral stricture, ureteroceles, and ureteral ectopia. Anatomic demonstration of the overall anatomy of the abdomen and pelvis is displayed as well.

Physiologic urinary dynamics can be examined using contrast-enhanced MR urography. Following injection of gadolinium and its excretion into the urinary tract, T1-weighted images show a strong signal from the collecting systems while most other tissues show moderate or low signal intensity (Figure 6.19). Thus, the collecting systems can be imaged from the calyces to the level of urinary bladder. Differential uptake in the two kidneys, excretion, and clearance of the contrast can be demonstrated with rapid serial image sequences.

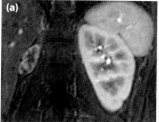 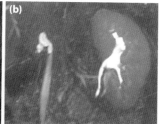

Figure 6.19 Magnetic resonance imaging, nephrogram, and urographic phases. (a) The early nephrogram is visible in this patient with small scarred right kidney secondary to reflux nephropathy and left renal compensatory hypertrophy. (b) The calyces, pelvis, and proximal ureters in the normal left kidney are well seen on the urographic phase as the gadolinium contrast agent is concentrated in the collecting system, and as the nephrogram fades.

## COMPUTED TOMOGRAPHY AND MAGNETIC RESONANCE IMAGING IN RENAL INFECTIONS

CT and MRI are infrequently used modalities for diagnosis of UTIs, but may be useful in selected cases as a sensitive method for detecting acute pyelonephritis and renal scarring. Ischemic focal defects in the renal parenchyma associated with acute pyelonephritis can be demonstrated with contrast-enhanced CT (Figure 6.20), as well as with contrast-enhanced MRI (Figure 6.21). A wedge-shaped parenchymal defect in renal cortex representing ischemic parenchyma can be seen in acute pyelonephritis. MRI has been shown to have diagnostic accuracy in detecting changes in acute pyelonephritis similar to that of cortical scintigraphy (dimercaptosuccinic acid [DMSA] renal scan) in experimental and clinical studies.[35,36] Renal scarring of the kidney associated with chronic pyelonephritis also can be delineated by MRI

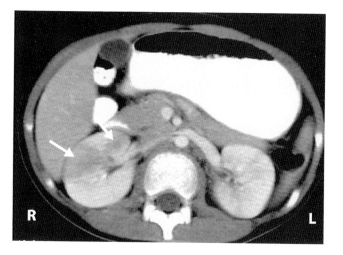

Figure 6.20 Contrast-enhanced computed tomography in a patient with acute pyelonephritis showing the characteristic wedge-shaped defects in the right kidney. Subtle defects are present in the left kidney, in addition.

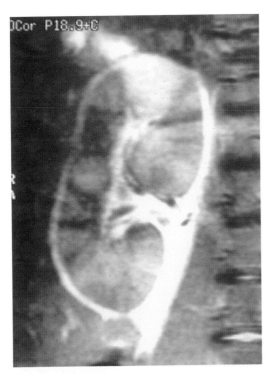

Figure 6.21 Gadolinium-enhanced inversion recovery magnetic resonance imaging showing numerous wedge-shaped zones of abnormal high signal intensity throughout the right kidney. The abnormal perirenal, peripelvic, and periureteric high signal indicates perirenal inflammation.

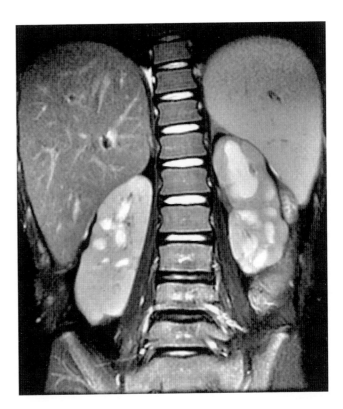

Figure 6.22 Magnetic resonance imaging coronal T2-weighted images showing irregularly dilated and clubbed calyces adjacent to adjacent focal zones of thinned renal parenchyma in a patient with renal scarring.

(Figure 6.22). Severe acute pyelonephritis may occasionally give rise to swelling and a sizeable mass lesion in the kidney, sometimes referred to as lobar nephronia, which may mimic a neoplasm. The mass can be seen as arising from the renal cortex with variable contrast-enhancement patterns.

Renal abscess is recognized by CT as a poorly enhancing mass with a necrotic center. Diffuse bacterial or fungal microabscesses or miliary renal infection may be difficult to diagnose with CT or MRI. The kidneys may be enlarged but show a poor degree of enhancement. Small, discrete parenchymal lesions (microabscesses) may not be evident on CT or MRI in the early stage of development.

# DIAGNOSIS OF MASS LESIONS BY COMPUTED TOMOGRAPHY AND MAGNETIC RESONANCE IMAGING

Most patients with a known, palpable, or suspected abdominal mass lesion undergo CT or MRI cross-sectional imaging following preliminary anatomic triage provided by ultrasonography. This serves to separate hydronephrosis and recognizable cystic lesions from solid lesions, mixed cystic and solid lesions, and lesions arising from perirenal tissues.

## Tumors

Both CT and MRI provide a global anatomic view of the entire abdomen, as well as delineation of bowel, vascular

structures, and normal renal parenchyma as distinct from pathologic renal tissue. Demonstration of bilateral renal masses or the presence of one dominant lesion with additional foci of parenchymal nodules suggests the presence of rests of metanephric blastema or nephroblastomatosis (Figure 6.23). These are important diagnostic clues for early detection and risk assessment for Wilms tumor, because

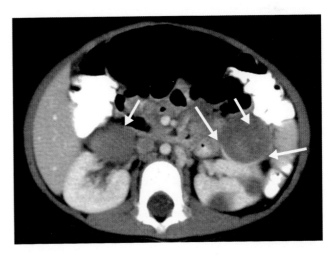

Figure 6.23 Wilms tumor and nephroblastomatosis. CT shows multiple renal masses. One exophytic lesion present in each kidney represents nephroblastomatosis (arrow).

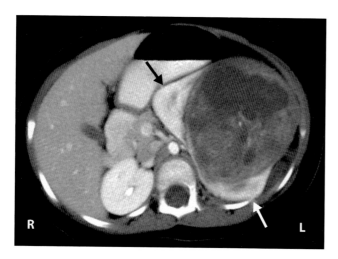

Figure 6.24 Contrast-enhanced computed tomography scan in a patient with Wilms tumor showing a necrotic but well-circumscribed mass arising from in the left abdomen. The mass expands the normal renal tissue creating a "claw" appearance at the boundary between mass and the normal renal tissue.

nephrogenic rests are considered to be precursors of Wilms tumor.[37-39] CT and MRI in Wilms tumor usually demonstrate a renal mass that often compresses the surrounding tissue. Bilateral lesions may be present, and areas of hemorrhage or cyst formation may be seen within the tumor (Figure 6.24). Both CT and MRI provide important information about Wilms tumor and its extension into the surrounding tissues. CT also provides a "one-stop" investigation of the thoracic and abdominal cavities for detection of metastases.

---

### KEY POINTS

- CT and MRI in renal mass lesions provide a comprehensive imaging modality.
- Vascular extension of tumors can be assessed by CT or MRI.
- CT of the lungs done at the same time as CT of the primary renal tumor provides information for tumor staging.

---

## Renal cysts

CT and MRI play an important role in the evaluation of cystic masses of the kidney.[40,41] The dominant imaging feature of a benign or simple cyst is that it is smooth and has a thin wall with a discrete outline. There are usually no internal debris, septations, or mural nodularity within the cyst. On CT or MRI studies there is a homogeneous internal fluid character. Simple cyst fluid has a CT attenuation of less than 20 Hounsfield units on noncontrast images. Mural enhancement following intravenous injection of contrast agents is either minimal or completely absent. Very slight enhancement may represent

compressed normal renal parenchyma around the wall of the cyst or may result from imaging artifacts, such as partial volume effect within adjacent tissue. Following any acute hemorrhage, simple cysts may develop internal debris and subsequently a single thin internal septation.

Some cystic masses may communicate with the renal collecting system. These are diagnosed when contrast agents opacify the cyst on delayed images, indicating a calyceal diverticulum or a pyelogenic cyst (which communicates directly via the renal pelvis). A nonenhancing cystic mass at the renal pelvis indicates a parapelvic cyst, which is an encysted lymphatic collection that often follows trauma or surgery. Developmental effect of an embryonic rest is also an etiologic possibility.

In autosomal recessive forms of polycystic kidney disease (ARPKD), CT and MRI also play a largely supportive imaging role following ultrasonography. The characteristic pattern of ARPKD consists of diffusely enlarged kidneys with uniformly high signal intensity on T2-weighted images. In ARPKD, CT and MRI provide a more global anatomic view of the kidney and associated hepatic disease (hepatic fibrosis).

Multiple renal cysts may be the primary renal manifestation of important heritable multiorgan disorders, such as ADPKD, tuberous sclerosis, Von-Hippel–Lindau disease, Jeune syndrome, Zellweger syndrome, and congenital fibropolycystic disease of the liver. Whereas ultrasound may demonstrate only a few lesions in early ADPKD, CT and MRI may provide information on the full extent of the renal lesions. For example, a patient with a single small, "simple" cyst shown on ultrasonography may demonstrate multiple lesions on CT or MRI, because the sonographic window can be obscured by ribs and bowel gas at times. In addition, CT and MRI also allow global visualization of pancreatic, splenic, or hepatic abnormalities associated with ADPKD. Although the liver demonstrates diffuse and moderate-to-large cystic lesions in ADPKD, fusiform dilatation of the intrahepatic ducts is usually noted in Caroli disease.[42] A "central dot sign," corresponding to the portal vein branch protruding into the lumen of a dilated bile duct also may be seen in Caroli disease.

---

### SUMMARY

A host of radiologic modalities, including ultrasound, VCUG, CT, and MRI, are available for the imaging workup of urinary tract disorders in children. Imaging can assist in the diagnosis of abnormalities, beginning in intrauterine life through childhood. The spectrum of disease ranges from congenital anomalies to infections and tumors. At times, multiple imaging modalities are used in a complementary fashion to make the diagnosis as well as to guide the management.

# REFERENCES

1. Herd D. Anxiety in children undergoing VCUG: Sedation or no sedation? [Review article.] Adv Urol. 2008;498614.
2. Lebowitz RL, Olbing H, Parkkulainen KV, et al. International system of radiographic grading of vesicoureteric reflux. International Reflux Study in Children. Pediatr Radiol. 1985;15:105–9.
3. Rosenbaum DM, Korngold E, Teele RL. Sonographic assessment of renal length in normal children. AJR Am J Roentgenol. 1984;142:467–9.
4. Han BK, Babcock DS. Sonographic measurements and appearance of normal kidneys in children. Am J Roentgenol. 1985;145:611–16.
5. Moore KI, Persaud TVE. The urogenital system. In: Moore KI, editor. The Developing Human: Clinically Oriented Embryology, 6th ed. Philadelphia: WB Saunders; 1998. p. 303.
6. Thoman DFM. Prenatally detected uropathies: Epidemiological considerations Br J Urol Int. 1998;81:8–12.
7. Nguyen HT, Herndon CD, Cooper C, et al. The Society for Fetal Urology consensus statement on the evaluation and management of antenatal hydronephrosis. J Pediatr Urol. 2010; 6:212–31.
8. Bassanese G, Travan L, D'Ottavio G, et al. Prenatal anteroposterior pelvic diameter cutoffs for postnatal referral for isolated pyelectasis and hydronephrosis: More is not always better. J Urol. 2013;190:1858–63.
9. St. Aubin M, Willihnganz-Lawson K, et al. Society for Fetal Urology recommendations for postnatal evaluation of prenatal hydronephrosis: Will fewer voiding cystourethrograms lead to more urinary tract infections? J Urol. 2013;190:1456–61.
10. Laing FC, Burke VD, Wing VW, et al. Postpartum evaluation of fetal hydronephrosis: Optimal timing for follow up sonography. Radiology. 1984;153:423–4.
11. Eickmeyer AB, Casanova NF, He C, et al. The natural history of the multicystic dysplastic kidney: Is limited follow-up warranted? J Pediatr Urol. 2014;10:655–61.
12. Strife JL, Souza AS, Kirks DR, et al. Multicystic dysplastic kidney in children: US follow up. Radiology. 1993;186:785–8.
13. England RJ, Haider N, Vujanic GM, et al. Mesoblastic nephroma: A report of the United Kingdom Children's Cancer and Leukaemia Group (CCLG). Pediatr Blood Cancer. 2011;56:744–8
14. Biester M, Kolditz D, Kalender WA. Iterative reconstruction methods in X-Ray CT. Phys Med. 2012;28:94–108.
15. Miglioretti DL, Johnson E, Williams A, et al. The use of computed tomography in pediatrics and the associated radiation exposure and estimated cancer risk. JAMA Pediatr. 2013;167:700–7.
16. Boone JM, Hendee WR, Mcnitt-Gray MF, et al. Seltzer SE. Radiation exposure from CT scans: How to close our knowledge gaps, monitor and safeguard exposure—Proceedings and recommendations of the Radiation Dose Summit, sponsored by NIBIB, February 24–25, 2011. Radiology. 2012;265:544–54.
17. Aspelin P, Laskey WK, Hermiller JB, et al. Nephrotoxic effects in high risk patients undergoing angiography. N Engl J Med. 2003;348:491–9.
18. Asif A, Epstein M. Prevention of radiocontrast-induced nephropathy. Am J Kidney Dis. 2004;44:12–24.
19. Emch TM, Haller NA. A randomized trial of prophylactic acetylcysteine and theophylline compared with placebo for the prevention of renal tubular vacuolization in rats after iohexol administration. Acta Radiol. 2003;10:514–9.
20. Grobner T. Gadolinium: A specific trigger for the development of nephrogenic fibrosing dermopathy and nephrogenic systemic fibrosis? Nephrol Dial Transplant. 2006;21:1104–08.
21. Grobner T, Prischl FC. Gadolinium and nephrogenic systemic fibrosis. Kidney Int. 2007;72:260–4.
22. Markova A, Lester J, Wang J, et al. Diagnosis of common dermopathies in dialysis patients: A review and update. Semin Dial. 2012;25:408–18.
23. Cowper SE, Robin HS, Steinberg SM, et al. Scleromyxoedema-like cutaneous diseases in renal-dialysis patients. Lancet. 2000;356:1000–1.
24. Nardone B, Saddleton E, Laumann AE, et al. Pediatric nephrogenic systemic fibrosis is rarely reported: A RADAR report. Pediatr Radiol. 2014;4:173–80.
25. Deo A, Fogel M, Cowper SE. Nephrogenic systemic fibrosis: A population study examining the relationship of disease development to gadolinium exposure. Clin J Am Soc Nephrol 2007;2:264–7.
26. Boyd AS, Zic JA, Abraham JL. Gadolinium deposition in nephrogenic fibrosing dermopathy. J Am Acad Dermatol 2007;56:27–30.
27. MacNeil S, Bains S, Johnson C, et al. Gadolinium contrast agent associated stimulation of human fibroblast collagen production. Invest Radiol. 2011;46: 711–7.
28. Vallee JP, Lazeyras F, Khan HG, et al. Absolute renal blood flow quantification by dynamic MRI and Gd-DTPA. Eur Radiol. 2000;10:1245–52.
29. Huang AJ, Lee VS, Rusinek H. Functional renal MR imaging. Magn Reson Imaging Clin N Am. 2004;12:469–86.
30. Grenier N, Cornelis F, Le Bras Y, et al. Perfusion imaging in renal diseases. Diagn Interv Imaging. 2013;94:1313–22.
31. Jones RA, Perez-Brayfield MR, Kirsch AJ, et al. Renal transit time with MR urography in children. Radiology. 2004;233:41–50.

32. Zhang H, Prince MR. Renal MR angiography. Magn Reson Imaging Clin N Am. 2004;12:487–503.
33. Leyendecker JR, Barnes CE, Zagoria, RJ. MR urography: Techniques and clinical applications. Radiographics. 2008;28:23–48.
34. Grattan-Smith JD, Jones RA. MR urography in children. Pediatr Radiol. 2006;36:1119–32.
35. Majd M, Nussbaum Blask AR, et al. Acute pyelonephritis: Comparison of diagnosis with 99mTc-DMSA, SPECT, spiral CT, MR imaging, and power Doppler US in an experimental pig model. Radiology. 2001;218:101–8.
36. Lonergan GJ, Pennington DJ, Morrison JC, et al. Childhood pyelonephritis: Comparison of gadolinium-enhanced MR imaging and renal cortical scintigraphy for diagnosis. Radiology. 1998;207:377–84.
37. Goske MJ, Mitchell C, Reslan WA. Imaging of patients with Wilms' tumor. Semin Urol Oncol. 1999;17:11–20.
38. Glylys-Morin V, Hoffer FA, Kozakewich, et al. Wilms tumor and nephroblastomatosis: Imaging characteristics at gadolinium-enhanced MR Imaging. Radiology. 1999;188:517–21.
39. Hennigar RA, O'Shea PA, Grattan-Smith JD. Clinicopathologic features of nephrogenic rests and nephroblastomatosis. Adv Anat Pathol 2001;8:276–89.
40. El-Merhi FM, Bae, KT. Cystic renal disease. Magn Reson Imaging Clin N Am. 2004;12:449–67.
41. Strand WR, Rushton HG, Markle BM, et al. Autosomal dominant polycystic kidney disease in infants: Asymmetric disease mimicking a unilateral renal mass. J Urol. 1989;141:1151–3.
42. Brancatelli G, Federle MP, Vilgrain V, et al. Fibropolycystic Liver disease: CT and MR imaging findings. Radiographics. 2006;26:659–70.

## REVIEW QUESTIONS

1. All of the following are indications for a VCUG except:
   a. Urinary tract infection
   b. Hydronephrosis/hydroureter
   c. To determine kidney function
   d. Preoperative renal transplantation
2. Regarding vesicoureteral reflux, which of the following is false?
   a. There are five grades of reflux.
   b. Grade I reflux indicates contrast material in the calyces.
   c. Intrarenal reflux may be seen with higher grades of reflux.
   d. The ureter is often dilated in grades IV and V reflux.
3. Regarding the procedure of the VCUG, all statements are true, except:
   a. The bladder needs to be catheterized.
   b. Oral sedation with midazolam is available in cases of extreme anxiety.
   c. Infection is not a complication of performing VCUG.
   d. Parents and child-life specialist may help facilitate the study.
4. Regarding interpretation of the contrast VCUG, the International Reflux Study classifies VUR into:
   a. 4 grades of reflux
   b. 5 grades of reflux
   c. Mild, moderate, and severe grades of VUR
   d. Grade I, Grade II, Grade III
5. Ultrasound is the best modality to evaluate for severity of renal obstruction.
   a. True
   b. False
6. Echogenic kidneys with loss of corticomedullary differentiation are specific findings for glomerulonephritis.
   a. True
   b. False
7. At 20 weeks of gestation, routine ultrasound demonstrates mild pelviectasis (4 to 7 mm) in the fetus. What is the likelihood of pyelectasis persisting after birth in the baby?
   a. 20%
   b. 40%
   c. 60%
   d. 80%
8. A good-quality CT scan of the kidneys should include which of the following?
   a. Intravenous contrast material administration
   b. A three-phase study including delayed excretion images
   c. Multiplanar reconstructions of source images
   d. Catheter drainage of the bladder
   e. Hydration and diuretic administration
9. All the following may contribute to potential radiographic contrast material nephrotoxicity except:
   a. Acidosis
   b. Dehydration
   c. N-acetyl cysteine therapy
   d. Diabetes mellitus
   e. Prior contrast material administration
10. Which of the following is true regarding nephrogenic systemic fibrosis (NSF)?
    a. It is not a risk for pediatric-age patients who are not dehydrated.
    b. The serum creatinine is a satisfactory screen for administration of gadolinium-based MRI contrast agents (GBCAs).

c. A history of dialysis is the only determining factor.

d. There are a few GBCA agents that are considered safe for patients with renal failure (GFR less than 30).

e. Dissociation of free gadolinium ion from the contrast agent ligand plays a role.

11. Which imaging modality is best for screening for recessive polycystic kidney disease?

a. x-ray of the abdomen

b. Radionuclide renal cortical scan

c. CT scan of abdomen

d. Ultrasonography

e. Noncontrast MRI

## ANSWER KEY

1. c
2. b
3. c
4. b
5. b
6. b
7. a
8. c
9. c
10. e
11. d

# Radionuclide renal imaging

EGLAL SHALABY-RANA, MARY ANDRICH, AND MASSOUD MAJD

The chief advantage of radionuclide imaging in pediatric nephrology over other imaging modalities is its ability to provide quantitative functional data. These imaging techniques include renal scintigraphy and radionuclide cystography. Pharmacologic interventions, such as the administration of furosemide or captopril in association with renal imaging, can further improve diagnostic accuracy. Additionally, overlying gas, stool, or plastic tubing does not hamper acquisition of imaging data. In some radionuclide imaging procedures, the ionizing radiation exposure is significantly less compared to other radiographic procedures.

## RADIOPHARMACEUTICALS

Several different $^{99m}$Tc-labeled radiopharmaceuticals are currently available for imaging of the kidneys, ureters, and bladder. The clinical indication determines which of the following radiopharmaceuticals is used.

1. $^{99m}$Tc-DMSA (dimercaptosuccinic acid): Approximately 60% of $^{99m}$Tc-DMSA is taken up by the proximal tubular cells from the peritubular capillaries by active anion transport, and 40% percent is filtered by the glomerulus and excreted in urine. Selective tubular uptake and absence of interference from pelvicalyceal activity makes $^{99m}$Tc-DMSA an ideal imaging agent for demonstration of focal parenchymal abnormalities in acute pyelonephritis, renal scarring, and infarcts.
2. $^{99m}$Tc-MAG3 (mercaptoacetyltriglycine): $^{99m}$Tc-MAG3 is primarily cleared by tubular secretion, allowing excellent visualization of the collecting systems, ureters and bladder, and renal parenchyma. This is used in diuresis renography in the evaluation of hydronephrosis and hydroureter. It is also the agent of choice to evaluate renovascular hypertension using captopril renography. In addition, renal transplants can be well evaluated with this agent.
3. $^{99m}$Tc-DTPA (diethylenediamine pentaacetic acid): $^{99m}$Tc-DTPA is filtered by the glomeruli, allowing visualization of the collecting systems, ureters, and bladder. $^{99m}$Tc-DTPA is used in the determination of glomerular filtration rate (GFR).
4. $^{99m}$Tc-pertechnetate: This radionuclide is used in bladder filling for radionuclide cystography to evaluate for vesicoureteral reflux (VUR) in children with urinary tract infection (UTI). Pertechnetate is the radionuclide of choice; however, in patients with an augmented bladder, Tc-sulfur colloid should be used to avoid absorption of radionuclide causing additional radiation dose to the patient.

## RENAL CORTICAL IMAGING

Renal cortical scans are primarily used for the diagnosis of acute pyelonephritis and renal cortical scars in patients with febrile UTI. A less common indication of dimercaptosuccinic acid (DMSA) scintigraphy may be to search for a small ectopic kidney that may be difficult to detect by sonography and for follow-up evaluation after renal trauma.

After intravenous administration of $^{99m}$Tc-DMSA in a dose of 0.05 mCi/kg (minimum dose 0.5 mCi and maximum

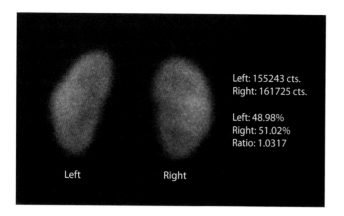

Figure 7.1 Normal DMSA renal scan. Posterior parallel-hole image demonstrating normal uptake in the cortex and normal photopenic medullary pyramids. Quantitative data show symmetric differential renal function.

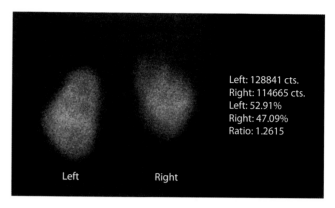

Figure 7.2 DMSA renal scan in acute pyelonephritis. Posterior parallel-hole image demonstrates photopenic defects in the right upper pole without associated parenchymal volume loss, consistent with acute pyelonephritis. Quantitative data show symmetric differential renal function.

3 mCi), renal cortical images are obtained at 1.5 to 2 hours.[1] A high-resolution collimator is used to acquire posterior and posterior oblique images of each kidney. Use of pinhole magnification improves the resolution of the images, improving diagnostic accuracy (Figure 7.1). An alternative imaging technique is the use of single-photon emission computed tomography (SPECT). Because of the length of the study and image acquisition time, sedation may be necessary for children under the age of 4 years.

## ACUTE PYELONEPHRITIS

The diagnosis of acute pyelonephritis may not always be reliably made on the basis of clinical criteria alone.[2] Under such clinical circumstances, cortical scintigraphy or DMSA scan has been shown to be a useful adjunct in the diagnosis of acute pyelonephritis.[3,4] The accuracy of DMSA scan in the diagnosis of acute pyelonephritis has been noted to be comparable to that of both computed tomography (CT) and magnetic resonance imaging (MRI).[5] DMSA scans are able to provide information on the renal parenchymal location of acute pyelonephritis, as well as the extent of renal tissue involvement.

The scintigraphic features of acute pyelonephritis consist of the decreased uptake of tracer (photopenic defects) without associated volume loss of the renal tissue (Figure 7.2). Three different patterns of photopenia can be seen: focal, multifocal, and the infrequently seen diffuse type. Focal defects are not specific for acute pyelonephritis and may be seen with renal masses, infarcts, or traumatic lesions. These defects must be interpreted within the clinical context.

## RENAL SCARRING

Renal scars may develop in patients who have had acute pyelonephritis and may have an impact on management of children with UTI.[6,7] Renal scars are identified on the DMSA scan by the presence of photopenic defects associated with renal parenchymal volume loss (Figure 7.3). When a DMSA scan shows evidence of acute pyelonephritis, consideration should be given to a repeat study in 6 to 12 months to assess for scarring. Approximately 60% of all foci

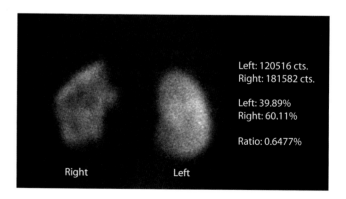

Figure 7.3 DMSA scan in multifocal renal scars. Posterior parallel-hole image demonstrates multiple photopenic defects in the left kidney with volume loss consistent with focal scars. Quantitative data show smaller left kidney with decreased renal function.

---

### KEY POINTS

- DMSA scanning is a useful adjunct in the diagnosis of acute pyelonephritis and detection of renal scars following acute pyelonephritis.
- Acute pyelonephritis is characterized by photopenia in the area of infection.
- Pyelonephritic scars, on the other hand, are characterized by renal parenchymal volume loss, in addition to photopenia.

of acute pyelonephritis, in the absence of high-grade VUR, resolve without scar formation.[7]

## ECTOPIC KIDNEY

Cortical scintigraphy is helpful in the detection of a small ectopic kidney in girls who present with urinary incontinence.[8,9] DMSA can be instrumental in localizing an ectopic kidney associated with an ectopic ureteral insertion. Such an ectopic kidney is typically small, is situated in the anterior pelvis, and may be difficult to locate by sonography because of overlying bowel loops. Although the function is usually poor, the ectopic kidney can be easily detected by anterior planar or SPECT imaging.

## RENAL FUNCTIONAL IMAGING

## DIURESIS RENOGRAPHY

Diuresis renography uses furosemide in conjunction with $^{99m}$Tc-MAG3 scan to evaluate patients with hydronephrosis and hydroureter who may be suspected to have urinary tract obstruction. Apart from assessment of renal function and the diagnosis of the site, diuresis renography can also determine the degree of obstruction and may play an important role in the management of hydronephrosis and hydroureter in infants and children.

### KEY POINTS

- Diuretic renography is helpful in the diagnosis of urinary obstruction. It effectively replaces intravenous pyelography in children.
- Neonates presenting with hydronephrosis may require serial diuretic renography.

### Technique

The most commonly used technique of diuresis renography, recommended by the Society for Fetal Urology and the Pediatric Nuclear Medicine Council, involves administration of furosemide 20 to 30 minutes after injection of $^{99m}$Tc-MAG3.[10] Alternative techniques are to administer furosemide either at the time of ("F-0") or 15 minutes before ("F-15") injection of $^{99m}$Tc-MAG3.[11]

The parents are instructed to maintain the child's normal hydration status, and feedings are not withheld before the study. An intravenous catheter is placed, and hydration with 5% dextrose in one-third normal saline is administered over the course of the entire examination. Infused fluid volume is usually 15 to 20 mL/kg. Placement of an indwelling bladder catheter is recommended to eliminate the effect of increased intravesical pressure on postdiuresis drainage. In addition, the catheter serves to alleviate patient discomfort, decrease the likelihood of VUR, and reduce gonadal radiation exposure from radioactive urine. $^{99m}$Tc-MAG3 in a dose of 0.05 mCi/kg (minimum 1 mCi) is then injected, and a conventional renal scan is obtained for the first 30 minutes. When the dilated system is completely filled with the tracer, furosemide (1 mg/kg; maximum dose 40 mg) is injected intravenously and sequential dynamic images are obtained for an additional 30 minutes. Urine output is recorded during the 30 minutes after diuretic administration to assess adequacy of response by the kidneys.

After completion of the imaging, time-activity curves are generated from the diuresis renogram and washout half-time $(t_{1/2})$ is calculated for each kidney. The half-time $(t_{1/2})$ represents the time needed for half of the activity to clear from the collecting system after administration of the diuretic. If significant residual tracer is noted in the dilated collecting system after the diuresis renogram, static posterior images of the kidneys are obtained, before and after the patient is held upright for 15 minutes, to assess the effect of gravity on drainage. The percentage of clearance is then calculated.[12]

### Interpretation

Interpretation is made by examining the images in conjunction with the quantitative data, including washout half-times, residual tracer activity, the shape of the curve and post upright clearance. Factors affecting the shape of the renogram curve and the rate of washout of tracer from the kidney include the degree of obstruction, renal function, capacity and compliance of the dilated system, state of hydration, bladder fullness, dose and timing of diuretic injection, and patient position.

A flat or rising scintigraph curve, with no significant improvement in drainage on postupright positioning, cortical retention, or both (Figure 7.4) is highly suggestive of urinary obstruction. In neonates, hydronephrosis may be dynamic, changing over time, therefore the diagnosis of urinary obstruction may be difficult to establish based on a single study. However, the initial study provides a baseline for follow-up evaluation of postdiuresis drainage.[13]

## CAPTOPRIL-ENHANCED RENOGRAPHY

Captopril-enhanced renography is a provocative test for the diagnosis of renovascular hypertension in children and adults. The original work on captopril renal scan in children

### KEY POINTS

- Captopril-enhanced renography may be helpful in the screening evaluation of suspected renovascular hypertension.
- If the scan is positive, patients will require an angiographic confirmation.

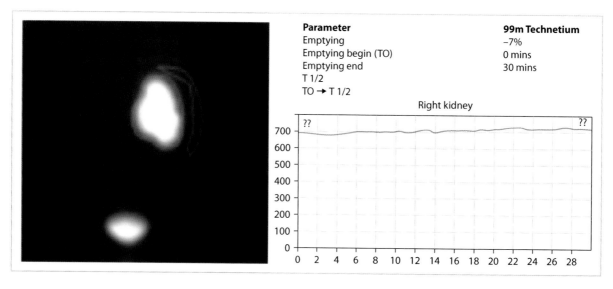

| Parameter | 99m Technetium |
|---|---|
| Emptying | –7% |
| Emptying begin (TO) | 0 mins |
| Emptying end | 30 mins |
| T 1/2 | |
| TO → T 1/2 | |

Right kidney

Figure 7.4 Diuresis renal scan in ureteropelvic junction obstruction. Image demonstrates tracer accumulation in a dilated right collecting system and normal clearance on the left. A flat washout curve after furosemide scan is consistent with high-grade obstruction.

was done using $^{99m}$Tc-DTPA,[14,15] but $^{99m}$Tc-MAG3 is currently the preferred radiopharmaceutical agent because of its more efficient extraction, especially in patients with azotemia.[16] The uptake of $^{99m}$Tc-MAG3, which is handled by tubular secretion, is independent of GFR. However, its clearance from the cortex depends on adequate GFR. Therefore, in the presence of renal artery stenosis, GFR is maintained by constriction of the efferent arterioles, mediated by angiotensin II, which can be verified in a precaptopril MAG-3 scan. Following administration of an angiotensin-converting enzyme inhibitor (ACEI), such as captopril, both the afferent and efferent arterioles dilate, resulting in a decrease in glomerular capillary hydrostatic pressure, decrease in GFR, and decrease in clearance of tracer from the renal cortex, seen visually as renal cortical retention.

## Technique

A baseline precaptopril renal scan is obtained with $^{99m}$Tc-MAG3. For blockade of the renin-angiotensin system, either captopril (1 mg/kg; maximum dose 50 mg, given orally), or enalaprilat (0.03 to 0.04 mg/kg, given intravenously) may be used. A repeat renal scan is then obtained 1 hour after oral administration of captopril or 10 minutes after intravenous administration of enalaprilat. Renogram curves are generated for both the pre-ACEI and post-ACEI scans. A commonly used adaptation in adults is to do a post-ACEI scan first, and, if normal, the examination is finished. If any abnormality is seen, the patient returns at a later time for repeat scan after the patient has been off of the ACEI for at least 2 days. Use of calcium channel–blocking agents at the time of the study may cause false-positive or false-negative results. Therefore, this class of antihypertensive medications should be discontinued before the study.[17]

## Interpretation

The scintigraphic manifestation of decreased renal function is prolonged cortical retention of tracer. A positive study is strongly suggestive of renovascular hypertension and requires further investigation by arteriography (Figure 7.5). A negative study result after a single dose of ACEI does not necessarily exclude the diagnosis of renovascular hypertension. In patients in whom there is a strong clinical suspicion, the scan may be repeated after the patient has been on ACEI for several days. Occasionally, the follow-up scan may become positive after 3 to 4 days of ACEI therapy.

## RENAL TRANSPLANT EVALUATION

Ultrasonography is the study of choice for imaging renal transplant kidneys. It is able to assess the perfusion and the architecture of the transplanted kidney, as well as assess for hydronephrosis.[18] However, if renal function information is needed, radionuclide imaging using $^{99m}$Tc-MAG3 provides an accurate, noninvasive, and non-nephrotoxic technique for evaluation of function of the transplanted kidney. Perfusion is also well evaluated with this technique[19] (Figure 7.6).

## Acute kidney injury

Scintigraphically, acute kidney injury (AKI) is characterized by adequate blood flow to the renal allograft; excretory function is diminished or absent. This is manifested by progressive parenchymal tracer accumulation and delay in excretion, and in severe cases by lack of any urine excretion

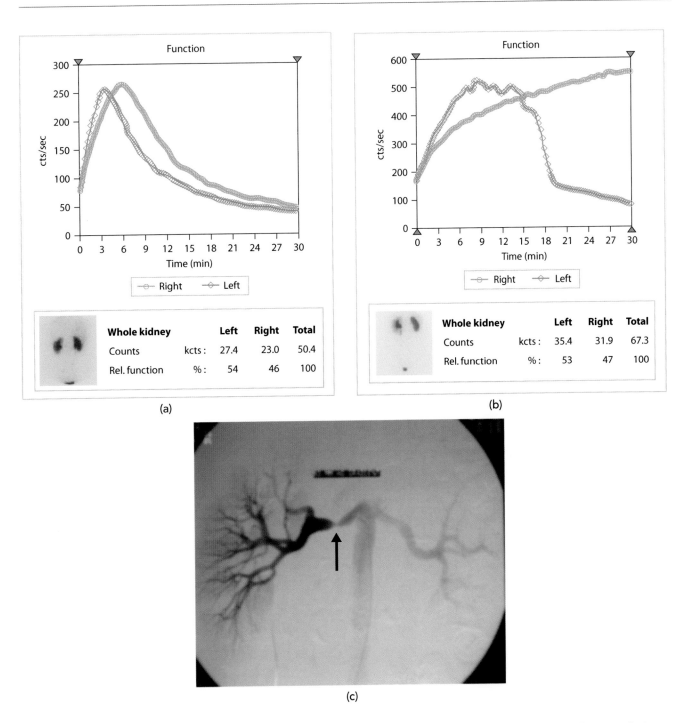

Figure 7.5 Captopril renal scan in right renal artery stenosis. **(a)** Precaptopril image showing normal renal scan with time-activity curve demonstrating normal and symmetric clearance from both kidneys. **(b)** Postcaptopril image shows significant cortical retention on the right side and normal clearance on the left side. Time-activity curve shows rising curve on the right side, also indicative of cortical tracer retention. **(c)** Renal arteriogram demonstrates stenosis of the main right renal artery (arrow).

over the 30-minute imaging sequence (Figure 7.7) Toxicity from immunosuppressant drugs may cause similar scintigraphic changes. The distinguishing feature is the time of onset, being much later (2 to 3 weeks postoperative) with drug-induced toxicity, and the immediate post-transplant period in the case of acute tubular necrosis.

## Vascular compromise

Absence of flow in the initial post-transplant scan indicates either vascular obstruction (arterial or venous) or hyperacute rejection. These entities cannot be distinguished on renal scan, although hyperacute rejection is almost nonexistent

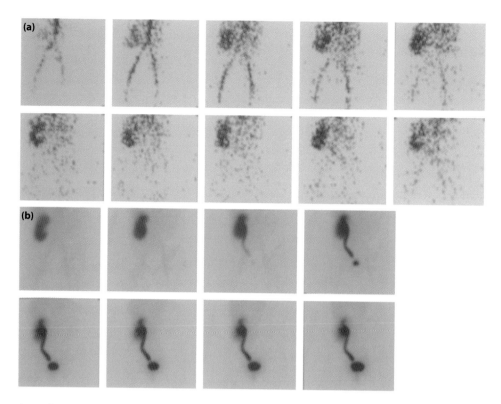

Figure 7.6 Normal renal transplant MAG-3 renal scan. **(a)** Flow images (1-second images) show prompt flow to the kidney, within two frames of the aorta. **(b)** Dynamic functional images demonstrate good parenchymal extraction, excretion, and drainage. Note good cortical clearance of tracer.

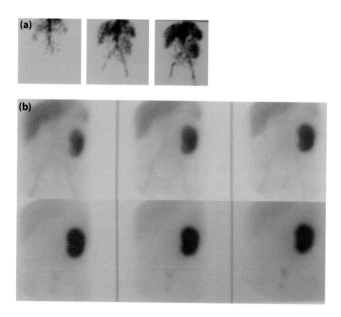

Figure 7.7 Acute kidney injury of renal transplant MAG-3 renal scan. **(a)** Normal flow images (1-second images). **(b)** Dynamic functional images show good cortical uptake with almost no excretion of tracer by 30 minutes and significant cortical retention. Minimal tracer is seen in the ureter and bladder in the last three frames.

now because of the extensive preoperative testing of the recipient.

## Allograft rejection

The scintigraphic findings of acute allograph rejection are decreased perfusion and decreased function. This contrasts with the findings in AKI, in which renal perfusion is well preserved. AKI and acute allograft rejection may coexist, and differentiation may be difficult. Chronic rejection is characterized by gradual evolution of chronic kidney disease and unique allograft biopsy findings. Serial renal scans demonstrate a gradual decrease in perfusion and function.

## Perinephric fluid collection

Perinephric fluid collections leading to partial obstruction of the urinary tract or compression of the vascular pedicle can occur in renal transplants and are frequently identified on ultrasonography. On the early $^{99m}$Tc-MAG3 scintigraphic images (first 30 minutes), perinephric fluid collections appear as a photopenic defect surrounding the kidney or in its vicinity. Delayed imaging is useful in distinguishing photopenia in the case of a hematoma or lymphocele from accumulation of tracer in a urinoma, which also can present as a fluid-filled mass around the renal allograft on ultrasonography.

## GLOMERULAR FILTRATION RATE

Assessment of the GFR in patients receiving nephrotoxic chemotherapy is the primary indication for radionuclide determination of the GFR. The use of radionuclide techniques eliminates the need for urine collection and is the method of choice for determining an accurate GFR in infants and children. The radioactive tracers used for the determination of GFR are: carbon-14 ($^{14}$C) inulin, iodine-125 ($^{125}$I) iothalamate, chromium-51 ($^{51}$Cr) ethylenediaminetetraacetic acid (EDTA), and $^{99m}$Tc-DTPA. $^{51}$Cr EDTA is commonly used in Europe, but $^{99m}$Tc-DTPA is the most widely used tracer in the United States. DTPA meets the criteria for an ideal GFR agent, except for the fact that 5% to 10% of the injected dose is protein-bound.

Several radionuclide-imaging techniques are available for calculating GFR.[20-22] The most commonly used method in children involves injection of a radiotracer, followed by posterior imaging of the kidneys for 20 minutes. Two or three blood samples are drawn 2 to 3 hours after injection of the radiotracer. These blood samples are centrifuged to yield plasma, and radioactivity is counted in the samples, using a well counter. Calculation of GFR is based on plasma clearance of the tracer. Another method uses volume distribution to calculate GFR in children. This technique uses a single plasma sample taken 2 hours after the injection of a dose of $^{51}$Cr-EDTA.[23]

## RADIONUCLIDE CYSTOGRAPHY

Radionuclide cystography (RNC) is used to diagnose VUR. Although VUR is often evaluated by the fluoroscopic voiding cystourethrogram (VCUG), RNC is an alternative method, especially in girls. Similar to the VCUG, the bladder is catheterized except that radioisotope and saline are infused, instead of radio-opaque contrast media. Imaging is begun immediately at the start of filling and continues through the end of voiding. Therefore, reflux that occurs at any time during the examination (filling or voiding) is identified (Figure 7.8). As with the VCUG, if a patient is extremely anxious and unable to cooperate for the radionuclide cystogram, oral midazolam in anxiolytic doses may be used. This medication has the added benefit of providing an amnestic effect for the procedure.[24]

RNC offers several advantages over the VCUG. By far the greatest of these is the significantly lower gonadal radiation dose, less than 5 mrads in girls and less than 2 mrads in boys.[25] Because of the continuous monitoring, the RNC may be more sensitive than the VCUG in the detection of reflux.[26]

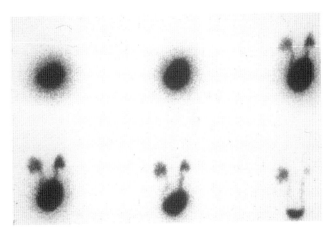

Figure 7.8 Radionuclide cystogram demonstrates vesicoureteral reflux into the collecting systems, bilaterally.

The major disadvantage of RNC, because of its limited spatial resolution, is the inability to evaluate the urethra and grade reflux accurately. Bladder wall abnormalities, such as diverticula and ureteroceles, may remain undetected but are easily seen on ultrasound studies.

The RNC is best suited for the initial diagnostic workup of VUR in girls, in whom urethral anomaly is rare. However, it is not recommended for the initial evaluation in boys because of the inability to evaluate the urethra with this technique. Because of its relatively low radiation burden,[27] RNC is the imaging method of choice for follow-up in patients undergoing serial evaluations, such as children with known VUR. This is applicable for both female and male patients after an initial VCUG in a boy excludes a posterior urethral valve.

---

## KEY POINTS

- Radionuclide cystography, because of its high sensitivity for VUR and its low radiation burden, is recommended when serial follow-up studies are required.
- Radionuclide cystography is not adequate for providing information on urinary tract anatomy, such as posterior urethral valve.

---

## SUMMARY

Nuclear imaging techniques are a useful adjunct to other diagnostic imaging modalities in the management of pediatric nephrology patients. Diuresis renography provides critical information about conditions such as obstructive uropathy. Renal cortical scanning demonstrates the extent of parenchymal involvement in pyelonephritis and scarring. Radionuclide studies offer an opportunity to view the results from a functional perspective. Together with anatomic imaging, they assist the pediatric nephrologist in the care of patients

## REFERENCES

1. Gelfand MJ, Parisi MT, Treves ST. Pediatric Nuclear Medicine Dose Reduction Workgroup. Pediatric radiopharmaceutical administered doses: 2010 North American consensus guidelines. J Nucl Med. 2011;52:318–22.
2. Majd M, Rushton HG, Jantausch B, et al. Relationship among vesicoureteral reflux, p-fimbriated E. coli and acute pyelonephritis in children with febrile urinary tract infection. J Pediatr. 1991;119:578–85.
3. Rushton HG, Majd M, Chandra R, et al. Evaluation of 99m-technetium-dimercaptosuccinic acid renal scans in experimental acute pyelonephritis in piglets. J Urol. 1988;140:1169–74.
4. Parkhouse HF, Godley ML, Cooper, J et al. Renal imaging with 99mTc-labelled DMSA in the detection of acute pyelonephritis: An experimental study in the pig. Nucl Med Commun. 1989;10:63–70.
5. Majd M, Blask ARN, Markle BM, et al. Acute pyelonephritis: Comparison of diagnosis with 99mTc-DMSA SPECT, spiral CT, MR imaging, and power Doppler US in an experimental pig model. Radiology. 2001;218:101–8.
6. Arnold AJ, Brownless SM, Carty HM, et al. Detection of renal scarring by DMSA scanning: An experimental study. J Pediatr Surg. 1990;25:391–3.
7. Rushton HG, Majd M, Jantausch B, et al. Renal scarring following reflux and nonreflux pyelonephritis in children: Evaluation with 99mTechnetium-dimercaptosuccinic acid scintigraphy. J Urol. 1992;147:1327–32,
8. Patteras JG, Rushton HG, Majd M. The role of 99mTechnetum dimercapto-succinic acid renal scans in the evaluation of occult ectopic ureters in girls with paradoxical incontinence. J Urol. 199;162:821–5.
9. Gharagozloo AM, Leibowitz RL. Detection of a poorly functioning malpositioned kidney with single ectopic ureter in girls with urinary dribbling: Imaging evaluation in 5 patients. Am J Radiol. 1995;164:957–61.
10. Society of Fetal Urology, Pediatric Nuclear Medicine Council, Society of Nuclear Medicine. The "well-tempered" diuretic renogram: A standard method to examine the asymptomatic neonate with hydronephrosis or hydroureteronephrosis. Report from combined meetings. J Nucl Med. 1992;33:2047–51.
11. Adeyoju AAB, Burke D, Atkinson C, et al. The choice of timing for diuresis renography: The F+0 method. BJU Int. 2001;88:1–5.
12. Wong DC, Rossleigh MA, Farnsworth RH. Diuretic renography with the addition of quantitative gravity-assisted drainage in infants and children. J Nucl Med. 2000;41:1030–6.
13. Ozcan Z, Anderson PJ, Gordon I. Prenatally diagnosed unilateral renal pelvic dilatation: A dynamic condition on ultrasound and diuretic renography. J Urol. 2004;172:1456–9.
14. Majd M, Potter BM, Guzzetta PC, et al. Effect of captopril on the efficacy of renal scintigraphy in the detection of renal artery stenosis [Abstract]. J Nucl Med. 1983;24:23–8.
15. Lagomarsino E, Orellanna P, Munoz J, et al. Captopril scintigraphy in the study of arterial hypertension in pediatrics. Pediatr Nephrol. 2004;19:66–70.
16. Taylor A. Renovascular hypertension: Nuclear medicine techniques. Q J Nucl Med. 2002;46:268–82.

17. Ludwig V, Martin WH, Delbeke D. Calcium channel blockers: A potential cause of false-positive captopril renography. Clin Nucl Med. 2003;28:108–12.

18. Sharfuddin A. Imaging evaluation of kidney transplant recipients. Semin Nephrol. 2011;31:259–71.

19. Heaf JG, Iversen J. Uses and limitations of renal scintigraphy in renal transplantation monitoring. Eur J Nucl Med. 2000;27:871–9.

20. Dubovsky EV, Russell C. Quantitation of renal function with glomerular and tubular agents. Semin Nucl Med. 1982;12:308–29.

21. Mulligan JS, Blue PW, Hasbargen JA. Methods of measuring GFR with 99mTc-DTPA: An analysis of several common methods. J Nucl Med. 1990;31:1211–9.

22. Cohen ML. Radionuclide clearance techniques. Semin Nucl Med. 1974;4:23–8.

23. Piepsz A, Pintelon H, Ham HR. Estimation of normal chromium-51 ethylene diamine tetra-acetic clearance in children. Eur J Nucl Med. 1994; 21:12–6.

24. Herd D. Anxiety in children undergoing VCUG: Sedation or no sedation? Adv Urol. 2008:498614.

25. Majd M, Belman AB. Nuclear cystography in infants and children. Urol Clin North Am. 1979;6:395–407.

26. Conway JJ, King LR, Belman AB, et al. Detection of vesicoureteral reflux with radionuclide cystography: A comparison study with roentgenographic cystography. Am J Roentgenol Radium Ther Nucl Med. 1972;115:720–7.

27. Majd M. Radionuclide imaging in clinical pediatrics. Pediatr Ann. 1976;15:396–402.

## REVIEW QUESTIONS

1. A six-month-old female infant is hospitalized with a febrile urinary tract infection. The radiopharmaceutical to be used for assessment for acute pyelonephritis imaging is:
   a. $^{99m}$Tc-MAG3
   b. $^{99m}$Tc-pertechnetate
   c. $^{99m}$Tc-DMSA
   d. $^{99m}$Tc-DTPA

2. For the patient in question 1, renal cortical imaging demonstrates multiple areas of photopenia, without loss of volume, involving both the upper and lower poles of the right kidney. The diagnosis is:
   a. Renal scarring
   b. Multifocal acute pyelonephritis
   c. Normal study

3. Clinical indications for DMSA renal cortical scintigraphy include:
   a. Urinary tract infection
   b. Search for a small ectopic kidney
   c. Follow-up in renal trauma
   d. All of the above.

4. A 2-month-old male infant was diagnosed to have pre-natal hydronephrosis in one kidney. Left-side hydronephrosis was confirmed by a postnatal ultrasound recently. There was no evidence of VUR on the VCUG. You should schedule this baby for a:
   a. DMSA renal scan
   b. Captopril renal scan
   c. Radionuclide cystogram
   d. Diuretic renogram

5. The initial imaging on the patient in question 4 demonstrates prompt and symmetric renal function with pooling of activity in the dilated left renal collecting system and prolonged washout half-time. Drainage on the right side is normal. Renal function is normal bilaterally. Which of the following would be the *best* investigative recommendation?
   a. MRI of the abdomen
   b. Repeat diuretic renography in 6 months
   c. Radionuclide cystogram in 6 months
   d. DMSA renal scan

6. All of the statements regarding captopril-enhanced MAG-3 renal scan are true *except*:
   a. The primary use is in the diagnosis of obstructive uropathy.
   b. The primary use is in the diagnosis of renal artery stenosis.
   c. Calcium channel–blocking medication should be discontinued for at least 2 days before the study.
   d. Either captopril or enalaprilat may be used for ACE blockade.

7. To assess the function of the transplanted kidney, the *best* choice of radionuclide investigation is:
   a. $^{99m}$Tc-DTPA
   b. $^{99m}$Tc-pertechnetate
   c. $^{99m}$Tc-DMSA
   d. $^{99m}$Tc-MAG3

8. The *main* indication for obtaining a $^{99m}$Tc-DTPA renal scan is:
   a. Evaluate for obstructive uropathy
   b. Evaluate for vesicoureteral reflux
   c. Determine the glomerular filtration rate
   d. There are no current indications for obtaining a $^{99m}$Tc-DTPA renal scan

9. The following are correct regarding radionuclide cystography *except*:
   a. Oral midazolam may be used for anxiolysis as necessary.
   b. The radiotracer used is $^{99m}$Tc-pertechnetate.
   c. It is indicated in the evaluation of vesicoureteral reflux.
   d. The bladder does not need to be catheterized.

10. Which one of the following statements *best* compares and contrasts the VCUG and the radionuclide cystogram (RNC)?
   a. The VCUG has higher resolution allowing delineation of anatomy and more accurate grading of reflux

compared to the RNC, which has higher sensitivity for detecting reflux and offers less radiation burden.

b. The RNC has higher resolution allowing delineation of anatomy and more accurate grading of reflux compared to the VCUG which has higher sensitivity for detecting reflux and offers less radiation burden.

c. The RNC and VCUG are very similar to each other, one simply a radionuclide study and the other a fluoroscopic study.

d. None of the above.

## ANSWER KEY

1. c
2. b
3. d
4. d
5. b
6. a
7. d
8. c
9. d
10. a

# Renal biopsy

NATALIE S. UY, MIHAIL M. SUBTIRELU, AND FREDERICK J. KASKEL

Renal biopsy is an important tool for establishing the morphologic diagnosis and prognosis, as well as guiding therapy of renal disease in children and adults. Although a renal biopsy can be performed by an open surgical procedure, the percutaneous method is the preferred manner of obtaining the renal biopsy sample in most children. Although percutaneous renal biopsy of palpable tumors was first performed in 1934 by Ball, the use of percutaneous renal biopsy for the diagnosis of medical disease was introduced by Iversen and Brun in 1951.[1,2] Since then, the technique has been continuously enhanced by better guidance and instruments. The advent of real-time ultrasound and automated biopsy needles during the last two decades has simplified the procedure and further improved its success and safety.[3]

## INDICATIONS FOR RENAL BIOPSY

Broadly, indications of renal biopsy include establishing the morphologic nature of the renal disease, assist in predicting prognosis and disease evolution, and in developing an appropriate therapy plan. Renal biopsy may also be used to monitor the response to therapy and disease progression. The value of renal biopsy in influencing management of patients with renal disease is well known.[4]

A common indication for renal biopsy in children is poorly responsive nephrotic syndrome. Corticosteroid-responsive nephrotic syndrome in children is considered to be due to minimal change disease (MCD), and a renal biopsy is not necessary in such patients.[5] On the other hand, a diagnostic renal biopsy is generally recommended in patients with corticosteroid-nonresponsive or corticosteroid-resistant nephrotic syndrome, or where an underlying glomerulonephritis is suspected to be the cause of nephrotic syndrome.[5,6] Focal segmental glomerulosclerosis (FSGS) is a common form of glomerulonephritis encountered in such patients.[7] Renal biopsy is also commonly performed for histologic diagnosis of persistent non-orthstatic proteinuria, which may be indicative of an underlying primary glomerulonephritis, such as FSGS, membranous glomerulonephritis (MGN), or membranoproliferative glomerulonephritis (MPGN).

Another common indication for renal biopsy is persistent isolated hematuria when the diagnosis of Berger disease or immunoglobulin A nephropathy (IgAN), Alport syndrome, or thin basement membrane disease is being considered.[6] Renal biopsy is also recommended in children with acute glomerulonephritis who exhibit a rapidly progressive clinical course. Renal biopsy in such cases should be considered an urgent diagnostic procedure and used to guide therapy. Renal biopsy is generally not considered in patients with non-complicated acute postinfectious glomerulonephritis.

Renal biopsy can be of immense diagnostic value in patients with acute kidney injury (AKI), where intrinsic renal diseases, such as rapidly progressive glomerulonephritis, interstitial nephritis, and vasculitis are suspected to be the etiology. On the other hand, in AKI of hemodynamic or nephrotoxic origin, a renal biopsy is generally unnecessary. In children with chronic renal insufficiency of

Table 8.1 Indications for renal biopsy in children

**Absolute Indications**
- Rapidly progressive glomerulonephritis
- Acute renal failure with nephrotic or nephritic syndrome
- Steroid-resistant nephrotic syndrome
- Persistent, nonorthostatic proteinuria
- Persistent glomerular hematuria, suggestive of active glomerulonephritis
- Atypical or nonresolving acute glomerulonephritis
- Systemic diseases with renal involvement (systemic lupus erythematosus, vasculitis, metabolic diseases such as Fabrey disease)
- Chronic kidney disease of unclear etiology, if kidneys are normal in size
- Renal transplant dysfunction

**Relative Indications**
- Monitoring response to therapy
- Monitoring drug nephrotoxicity
- Protocol biopsies of renal allograft

Table 8.2 Contraindications to percutaneous renal biopsy

**Absolute Contraindications**
- Uncontrolled coagulation abnormalities
- Uncontrolled severe hypertension
- Uncooperative patient (under conscious sedation)
- Acute pyelonephritis

**Relative Contraindications**
- Severe azotemia or end-stage renal failure
- Anatomic abnormalities of the kidney
- Solitary kidney (not transplant)
- Coagulopathy
- Concurrent use of drugs affecting coagulation (e.g., aspirin, dipyridamole)
- Chronic pyelonephritis
- Concurrent urinary tract infection
- Tumors
- Pregnancy
- Extreme obesity

unknown etiology, a renal biopsy may be able to establish the underlying diagnosis. This information is especially relevant in assessing the risk for recurrence of the original disease after renal transplantation. In advanced renal disease, the kidneys may be small and densely echogenic on ultrasound evaluation, and a renal biopsy may only demonstrate atrophic renal tissue and glomerulosclerosis, often referred to as "end-stage kidney."

Renal biopsy is routinely used for the evaluation of renal transplant allograft dysfunction, which may be due to acute and chronic allograft rejection, drug toxicity, recurrence of original disease, or de novo renal disease. Protocol renal allograft biopsies are useful for the diagnosis and post-treatment monitoring of acute rejection and for the surveillance of chronic allograft nephropathy.[8] Table 8.1 presents a list of common indications for renal biopsy.

## CONTRAINDICATIONS TO PERCUTANEOUS RENAL BIOPSY

Percutaneous renal biopsy is an invasive, elective procedure, with well-defined risks. Absolute contraindications to percutaneous renal biopsy (Table 8.2) include clinical conditions associated with high risk of complications. Relative contraindications to renal biopsy (Table 8.2), on the other hand, are clinical circumstances that adversely impact the safety or technical performance of the procedure, and increase the potential for complications. An open surgical diagnostic renal biopsy may be considered if the patient has well-established contraindications to the percutaneous procedure.

## PREPARING THE PATIENT

Adequate preparation for the renal biopsy is the key for a successful and safe procedure. It should start with a thorough prebiopsy evaluation consisting of four elements: history taking, physical examination, laboratory evaluation, and ultrasonographic evaluation of the kidneys. Important elements of the history are bleeding diathesis (personal or family history); allergies to agents used during the renal biopsy; use of aspirin, nonsteroidal anti-inflammatory drugs, or other anticoagulation therapy; and history of severe hypertension. Key elements of the physical examination are blood pressure evaluation, biopsy site assessment, and assessment of anatomic abnormalities that may interfere with imaging or positioning the patient during the biopsy. Laboratory evaluation should include a complete blood count and platelet count, biochemical profile, coagulation profile, type and screen, and urinalysis. A complete ultrasonographic evaluation of the kidneys should be done in advance to evaluate for anatomic abnormalities that might constitute absolute or relative contraindication for a percutaneous renal biopsy.[3]

The procedure needs to be scheduled in advance to ensure a collaboration of the teams involved (nephrology, ultrasonography, pathology). Depending on the institutional practices and prevailing patient needs, the patient

Table 8.3 Prebiopsy order set

- Nothing by mouth for 6 hours before biopsy
- Obtain consent for the procedure
- Send and follow results for:
  - Complete blood count with platelet count
  - Basic metabolic panel for renal function
  - Coagulation profile (prothrombin time, partial thromboplastin time)
  - Bleeding time, if clinically indicated
  - Urinalysis
- Type and hold one unit of packed red blood cells
- Place an intravenous line
- Start intravenous maintenance fluids

may be admitted overnight before the procedure or come on the morning of the procedure. Medications that may affect coagulation must be interrupted for an appropriate duration to ensure a safe procedure. The patient must be instructed to take nothing by mouth (NPO) for 6 hours before the biopsy.

The renal biopsy procedure is generally done in a radiology procedure room that is appropriate for anesthesia and conscious sedation support. Current clinical practice is to guide the renal biopsy with a real-time ultrasound probe. This requires the help of a renal ultrasound technician in the procedure. The pathology department must be notified in advance so the biopsy specimen can be processed in a timely fashion. An intravenous access is placed before the procedure, and maintenance intravenous fluid appropriate for age is provided. An informed consent, appropriate for the patient's age, needs to be obtained before the procedure. The type of sedation and the premedication vary according to institutional protocol. A young or uncooperative patient may require general anesthesia. This is prearranged with the anesthesiologist. Continuous cardiorespiratory monitoring should be started before the procedure and continued until the recovery phase. In absence of any complications, patients are returned to their rooms for postbiopsy care. Table 8.3 provides prebiopsy orders.

## BIOPSY IMAGING

Since the introduction of the percutaneous renal biopsy more than 50 years ago, the safety and use of the procedure have been enhanced by the technologic advancements in imaging and guidance instruments. Intravenous pyelogram with fluoroscopy, the initial modality to image the kidney for the biopsy, was largely replaced by ultrasound in the mid-1980s.[3,9] The 1990s witnessed the introduction of automated ultrasound-guided biopsy devices.[10,11] Real-time ultrasound is the favored method in most centers, but other imaging modalities, such as computed tomography (CT),

also can be used for guidance when localization by ultrasound is unsatisfactory (i.e., obese patient or focal lesions).

## BIOPSY INSTRUMENTS

## VIM-SILVERMAN NEEDLE

In the mid-1950s, Kark et al. and Muehrcke et al. revolutionized the field by using a new technique for percutaneous renal biopsy.[12–14] Besides changing the patient's position from sitting to prone, they replaced the aspiration needle used by Iversen and Brun[2] with a Franklin modified Vim-Silverman needle (Figure 8.1). Their technique increased the success rate of the biopsy from less than 40% to above 90% and significantly decreased the associated morbidity.[3]

The Franklin modified Vim-Silverman needle consists of a trocar, a fitting obturator, and a cutting needle with prongs. The trocar and the fitting obturator are introduced together into the renal cortex after which the obturator is removed, and the cutting needle with prongs is introduced through the trocar. The cutting needle is advanced into the renal parenchyma followed quickly by the trocar. While the relative position of its components is maintained, the biopsy needle is quickly removed. The biopsy core is collected between the prongs of the cutting needle. The Vim-Silverman needle is not disposable and has now been abandoned because of the development of automatic biopsy needles.

## TRUE-CUT NEEDLE

The True-Cut needle (Baxter Healthcare Corporation, Valencia, CA) (Figure 8.2) became popular in the late 1970s and 1980s. This was the first semiautomatic disposable needle introduced for renal biopsy procedures. The True-Cut needle consists of a cutting needle encased into a trocar. The cutting needle slides into the trocar to a preset depth. The trocar and the cutting needle are introduced together into the renal cortex. Once in the renal tissue, the cutting needle is advanced rapidly into the renal parenchyma,

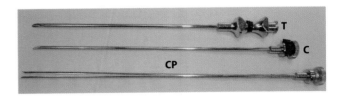

Figure 8.1 Franklin modified Vim-Silverman biopsy needle. The obturator (C) fits into the trocar (T). The cuttings prongs (CP) are shown separately.

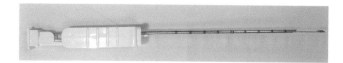

Figure 8.2 Disposable True-Cut biopsy needle (Baxter Healthcare, Valencia, CA).

followed by the trocar. The needle and trocar are removed together, and the biopsy core is collected from the cutting needle.

## SPRING-LOADED AUTOMATED BIOPSY DEVICES

Automatic biopsy devices were introduced in late the 1980s.[15] Several variations of the automated devices are available for clinical use today (Figures 8.3 to 8.6). These devices, when used with real-time ultrasound guidance, have diminished the operator error and improved the success of the procedure.[3,16,17] The automated systems were initially partially reusable (disposable needle and reusable spring-loaded

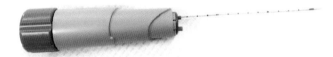

Figure 8.3 Bard Monopty Biopsy Instrument (C. R. Bard, Covington, GA).

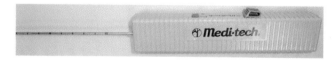

Figure 8.4 Meditech ASAP (Meditech, Boston Scientific, Watertown, MA).

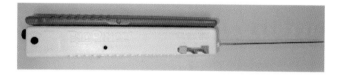

Figure 8.5 Bio-Pince biopsy needle (Ascendia AB, Sollentuna, Sweden).

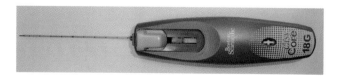

Figure 8.6 Easy-Core biopsy needle (Boston Scientific, Natick, MA).

device), but the currently available devices are fully automatic, for single use, and disposable. The instrument consists of a trocar encasing a cutting needle. Both are mounted on a spring-loaded handle. The needle is armed into the trocar, introduced till the renal cortex is reached, and advanced by releasing the loaded spring with the push of a button or a release switch. One of the disadvantages of the automatic biopsy needles is that the length of the cutting core cannot be adjusted, making it hazardous to use these devices in very small infants, especially those with a thin cortical core. Bio-Pince (Argon Medical Devices, Plano, TX) (see Figure 8.6) is the only commercially available biopsy needle that allows adjustment of the stroke length (also known as "throw") of the cutting core from 13 to 33 mm.

## BIOPSY PROCEDURE

The patient is brought to the procedure room accompanied by a nurse and with continuous cardiorespiratory monitoring. The patient is placed in the prone position on the biopsy table, with a roll of sheets placed under the abdomen to stabilize and push the kidney toward the operator.[12,13] The lower pole of the left kidney, the optimal biopsy area, is localized by ultrasound, and the corresponding point is marked on the skin on the back of the patient (Figure 8.7). The distance from the skin to the renal capsule is recorded from the ultrasound data. The anesthesiology support personnel administer conscious sedation to the patient.

The biopsy area is prepped with povidone-iodine and draped. Local skin anesthesia is done with 1% lidocaine. A spinal tap needle is used to anesthetize the biopsy tract and confirm orientation of the biopsy needle by ultrasound. A small incision of the skin, sufficient to allow the passage of

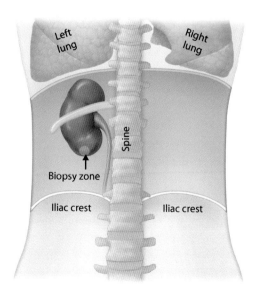

Figure 8.7 Diagram showing landmarks for localization of renal biopsy site in the left kidney.

- Technical advances in imaging and instruments have made the percutaneous renal biopsy a safe diagnostic procedure.
- Percutaneous renal biopsy is usually performed with real-time ultrasound guidance and advanced instruments, which have diminished operator error and improved the success of the procedure.

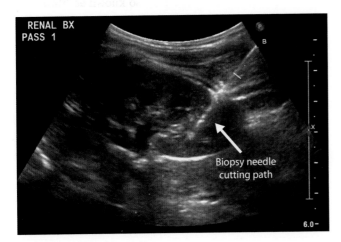

RENAL BX
PASS 1

Biopsy needle cutting path

Figure 8.8 Renal ultrasound of the kidney capturing the moment as the biopsy cutting edge (arrow) enters the kidney for retrieving the renal tissue core.

the biopsy needle, is made using a scalpel. Under real-time ultrasound guidance the biopsy needle is introduced and advanced, using the recorded angle and length of passage, until it reaches the outer kidney cortex (Figure 8.8). If possible, the patient is instructed to hold the breath, and the maneuver to obtain the core of tissue is performed (depending on the biopsy instrument used). The biopsy needle containing the tissue core is quickly removed.

The biopsy tissue obtained is immersed in normal saline and observed under a dissecting microscope for quality and glomerular content. Usually two cores are sufficient to obtain an appropriate biopsy sample. A successful renal biopsy brings at least 20 glomeruli. The biopsy core is then divided and prepared for light microscopy, immunofluorescence, and electron microscopy.

## BIOPSY IN A RENAL TRANSPLANT

The presence of a single kidney allograft in the renal transplant is not a contraindication for percutaneous renal biopsy. The kidney allograft is usually located in an anterior position, in the right or left lower quadrant, and is easily palpable. In preparation for the procedure, the patient is placed in the supine position. Depending on the position,

usually the upper pole is located by ultrasound and marked on the skin and the depth from skin to the renal capsule is recorded. The rest of the procedure is essentially the same. Caution is necessary because the fibrous tissue (capsule) of the kidney allograft may be firm and difficult to penetrate. If the kidney allograft is located in an unusual or inaccessible position, percutaneous biopsy by an interventional radiologist or open biopsy is generally indicated. In highly experienced centers, percutaneous renal biopsies of allografts placed extraperitoneally or intraperitoneally have been reported to have similar complication rates.[17]

## POSTRENAL BIOPSY CARE

Once the percutaneous renal biopsy is completed, the kidney is examined by ultrasound in search for hematomas. This examination may be postponed or repeated later in appropriate cases to increase the chance of detecting a hematoma.[3] Once the ultrasound is completed, the skin is cleaned with povidone-iodine and a pressure dressing is applied. The patient is positioned on the back and transported to an observation area, accompanied by a nurse and with continuous cardiorespiratory monitoring.

The postbiopsy procedure observation orders should be instituted immediately, especially for monitoring the vital signs for any evidence of hypovolemia (Table 8.4). The observation period is needed for the immediate detection of any complications, particularly hemorrhage and anesthesia-related events. The length of postbiopsy hospital

Table 8.4 Postbiopsy order set

- Place patient flat on the back for 6 hours without bathroom privileges
- Continuous cardiorespiratory monitoring until awake from sedation
- Monitor vital signs:
  - Every 15 minutes for 1 hour
  - Every 30 minutes for 2 hours
  - Every 1 hour for 4 hours
- Check biopsy site with each set of vital signs
- Inform physician if:
  - Changes in vital signs outside set parameters
  - Back pain
  - Abdominal pain
  - Active bleeding at the biopsy site
  - Visible urinary bleeding or passage of clots
- Obtain hemoglobin and hematocrit at 4 hours postbiopsy
- Strict intake and output monitoring
- Inform physician if no urine output for 6 hours
- Normal diet once the patient is awake; encourage oral fluid intake
- Discharge patient after 6 to 8 hours, if stable

stay is debatable. There is evidence to point that a shorter observation period (8 hours) with same-day discharge from the hospital is sufficient in selected patients and is more economical.[19-22]

## COMPLICATIONS FOLLOWING RENAL BIOPSY

Complications following a renal biopsy can be separated into minor, major, and severe categories. Technical advancements in both imaging techniques and biopsy needles have kept the complication rate low. Although the incidence of minor complications are common and may reach 100%, major complications have been reported in 5% to 10% of cases.[6] Severe complications are rare. Depending on the era of studies, the reported complication rate is variable. Most complications are the result of bleeding into the collecting system with subsequent hematuria or at the biopsy entry point into renal cortex resulting in perinephric hematoma. Significant postbiopsy bleeding may occasionally result in a drop in hematocrit, with the need for transfusion, surgical intervention, or both. Severe bleeding with the need for nephrectomy is an extremely rare occurrence. In a literature review of 19,459 percutaneous renal biopsies, need for nephrectomy was reported in 13 cases (0.06%).[23] Death directly attributable to renal biopsy is exceptionally rare, with a reported frequency of up to 0.08% in older reviews and 0.02% in the more recent sreviews.[3,23] Table 8.5 and Table 8.6 list complications associated with kidney biopsy.[24-63]

---

### KEY POINTS

- Minor complications such as microscopic or gross hematuria and perinephric hematoma are common, but severe complications are rare.
- The success and safety of the renal biopsy in children requires a knowledgeable and experienced nephrologist familiar with the technique.

---

The main factor associated with higher complication rate is a lower estimated glomerular filtration rate (chronic kidney disease stages 3 to 5), which may be related to platelet dysfunction in the uremic state.[60] Other various conditions that increase the risk for complications include obesity, pregnancy, solitary or small kidney, multiple needle passes, and thrombocytopenia. Most complications occur within 8 hours of the biopsy, but even in those with later complications, readmission rates are not high, suggesting that hospital admission may not be required routinely in all patients who had percutaneous renal biopsy.

Table 8.5 Complications following kidney biopsy

1. Minor
   - Microscopic hematuria
   - Macroscopic hematuria (transient)
   - Perirenal hematoma (not clinically significant)
2. Major
   - Macroscopic hematuria (requiring observation or intervention)
   - Perirenal hematoma (clinically significant)
   - Arteriovenous fistula
   - Renal artery pseudoaneurysm
3. Severe
   - Need for a major surgical intervention
   - Death

Strategies to reduce the complications include efforts to minimize bleeding, including obtaining a complete blood cell count and coagulation profile before the procedure, and identifying patients at higher risk (i.e., thrombocytopenia) for bleeding. Cessation of medications that increase the risk for bleeding (i.e., aspirin) before the procedure is warranted in at-risk patients. Adequate control of hypertension before the procedure is essential because elevated blood pressure is a risk factor for bleeding after the procedure.

### Microscopic hematuria

Microscopic hematuria is the most common complication of renal biopsy and occurs in almost all patients.[3] It usually resolves without intervention and has no clinical significance.

### Macroscopic hematuria

The incidence of macroscopic hematuria after native or allograft biopsies in children is ranging from 2.7% to 26.6%.[22] Macroscopic hematuria usually is not clinically significant and resolves spontaneously within 24 to 48 hours. Rarely, macroscopic hematuria may produce a significant drop in hematocrit, with need for transfusion. The need for an intervention (radiographic or surgical) to stop the bleeding is extremely rare. Infrequently, significant gross hematuria may result in formation of clots with subsequent urinary tract obstruction (Figure 8.9). In most patients, observation and good intravenous hydration may be sufficient, as well as beneficial, in preventing the formation of large clots.

### Perinephric hematoma

The reported incidence of perinephric hematoma following renal biopsy depends on the modality of evaluation. Before the advent of ultrasound and computed tomography, the reported incidence of clinically detectable perinephric hematoma was 1.4%.[46] A recent pediatric study

Table 8.6  Incidence of complications following kidney biopsy

| Complication | | Incidence (%) | References |
|---|---|---|---|
| Microscopic hematuria | | 100 | 3 |
| Macroscopic hematuria | | 2.7-26.6 | 22, 24-36, 59, 60, 61, 63 |
| Urinary tract obstruction secondary to blood clots | | 0.5-5 | 37-45 |
| Perirenal hematoma | Clinical examination | 1.4 | 46 |
| | Ultrasound | 6-70 | 3 |
| | CT scan | 57-91 | 3 |
| Renal arteriovenous fistula | | 5-18 | 47-53, 60, 63 |
| Clinically significant drop in hematocrit requiring blood transfusion | | 0.9-4.1 | 31, 34, 36, 54 |
| Nephrectomy for complications of renal biopsy | | 0.06 | 23 |
| Death directly attributable to renal biopsy | | 0.02-0.08 | 3, 23 |

reported the incidence of postbiopsy hematomas to be 8.1%.[60] It is well known that the incidence of perinephric hematoma, assessed by CT, can be up to 91%.[3] Most perinephric hematomas are clinically insignificant and self-limiting (Figure 8.10). Flank pain or abdominal pain may be encountered in some patients with a perinephric hematoma.

### KEY POINTS

- Microscopic hematuria occurs in almost all patients after a renal biopsy.
- Visible hematuria has been reported in 2.7% to 26.6% patients.
- Need for nephrectomy is uncommon for renal biopsy complications (0.06%).
- Death attributable to renal biopsy procedure has been reported in 0.02% to 0.08% of cases.

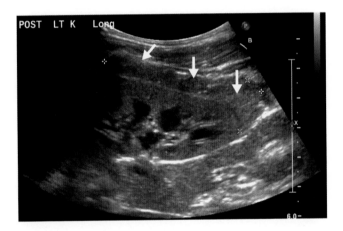

Figure 8.10  Renal ultrasound of a patient showing perirenal hematoma following native kidney biopsy. Hematoma is marked by the arrows. The hematoma measured 5.6 × 1.7 cm.

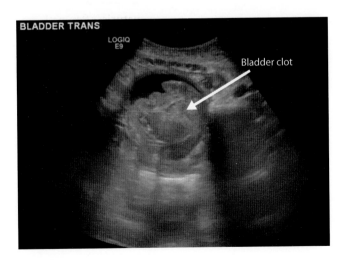

Figure 8.9  Bladder ultrasound examination showing a large hematoma in the bladder following a renal biopsy procedure. The patient had nephrotic syndrome with poor urinary flow, allowing the urinary bleeding to remain in the bladder for a sufficient period and develop into a clot.

## Arteriovenous fistula

Renal arteriovenous fistula (AVF) is a well-recognized complication of percutaneous renal biopsy (Figure 8.11). The reported incidence of AVF following renal biopsy is 6% to 18%, as diagnosed by angiography and 5% to 12%, as diagnosed by color Doppler ultrasound.[47-53] Development of hypertension, hematuria, and abdominal bruit after renal biopsy are clinical clues to the presence of an AVF. Most AVFs are found within 1 month of renal biopsy, but diagnosis can be delayed for years depending on imaging follow-up and clinical symptoms. Renal transplant and multiple needle passes are associated with a higher incidence of AVF.[63] AVFs can cause steal syndrome with relative ischemia of the renal parenchyma outside the lesion, which may induce secondary arterial hypertension, GFR deterioration, or heart failure secondary.[63] Most of these fistulas resolve spontaneously within 1 year, but it is recommended that even small asymptomatic AVFs should be followed by color Doppler ultrasound because of potential for complications.[3] Gradual

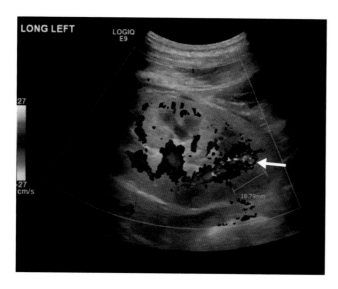

Figure 8.11 Color Doppler evaluation of the kidney demonstrating an arteriovenous fistula following a renal biopsy procedure. The fistula is marked by the area showing the admixture of blue and red blood flow pattern (arrow).

enlargement of an AVF can lead to late bleeding, resulting in renal rupture. Large, symptomatic AVFs may need to be managed by radiologic or surgical intervention, such as coil embolization or stent graft.[3, 63]

## Miscellaneous complications

Infectious complications, such as bacteremia, sepsis, perirenal abscesses, fistulas, and gastrointestinal tract injury, as well as severe hemorrhage and death resulting from injury to the lumbar artery have also been described.[40,54,57,58]

---

### SUMMARY

The technical advances in imaging and instruments have made the percutaneous renal biopsy a safe diagnostic procedure. Use of real-time ultrasound guidance and advanced instruments are the standard of care in our days. In spite of all the advancements, there are still a group of well-defined contraindications for a percutaneous renal biopsy that the clinician must consider carefully. Finally, the success and safety of the percutaneous renal biopsy in children require a knowledgeable and experienced pediatric nephrologist familiar with the technique.

---

## REFERENCES

1. Pirani CL. Renal biopsy. An historical perspective. In: Silva FG, D'Agati VD, Nadasdy T, editors. Renal Biopsy Interpretation, Churchill Livingstone: New York; 1996:1–19.
2. Iversen P, Brun C. Aspiration biopsy of the kidney. Am J Med. 1951;11:324–30.
3. Korbet SM. Percutaneous renal biopsy. Semin Nephrol. 2002;22:254–67.
4. Richards NT, Darby S, Howie AJ, et al. Knowledge of renal histology alters patient management in over 40% of cases. Nephrol Dial Transplant. 1994;9:1255–9.
5. Hogg RJ, Portman RJ, Milliner D, et al. Evaluation and management of proteinuria and nephrotic syndrome in children: Recommendations from a pediatric nephrology panel established at the National Kidney Foundation conference on proteinuria, albuminuria, risk, assessment, detection, and elimination (PARADE). Pediatrics. 2000;105:1242–49.
6. Fogo AB. Renal pathology. In: Avner ED, Niaudet P, Harmon WE, editors. Pediatric Nephrology, 5th ed. Philadelphia: Lippincott Williams & Wilkins, 2003; p. 475.
7. Filler G, Young E, Geier P, et al. Is there really an increase in non-minimal change nephrotic syndrome in children? Am J Kidney Dis. 2003;42:1107–13.
8. Birk PE, Stannard KM, Konrad HB, et al. Surveillance biopsies are superior to functional studies for the diagnosis of acute and chronic renal allograft pathology in children. Pediatr Transplant. 2004;8:29–38.
9. Birnholz JC, Kasinath BS, Corwin HL. An improved technique for ultrasound guided percutaneous renal biopsy. Kidney Int. 1985;27:80–2.
10. Wiseman DA, Hawkins R, Numerow LM, Taub KJ. Percutaneous renal biopsy utilizing real time, ultrasonic guidance and a semiautomated biopsy device. Kidney Int. 1990;38:347–9.
11. Donovan KL, Thomas DM, Wheeler DC, et al. Experience with a new method for percutaneous renal biopsy. Nephrol Dial Transplant. 1991;6:731–3.
12. Kark RM, Muehrcke RC. Biopsy of the kidney in the prone position. Lancet 1954;1:1047–49.
13. Muehrcke RC, Kark RM, Pirani CL. Technique of percutaneous renal biopsy in the prone position. J Urol. 1955;74:267–77.
14. Kark RM, Muehrcke RC, Pollak VE, et al. An analysis of 500 percutaneous renal biopsies. Arch Intern Med. 1958;101:439–351.
15. Komaiko MS, Jordan SC, Querfeld et al. A new percutaneous renal biopsy device for pediatric patients. Pediatr Nephrol. 1989;3:191–3.
16. Burstein DM, Korbet SM, Schwartz MM. The use of the automatic core biopsy system in percutaneous renal biopsies: A comparative study. Am J Kidney Dis. 1993;22:545–52.
17. Feneberg R, Schaefer F, Zieger B, et al. Percutaneous renal biopsy in children: A 27-year experience. Nephron. 1998;79:438–46.

18. Vidhun J, Masciandro J, Varich L, et al. Safety and risk stratification of percutaneous biopsies of adult-sized renal allografts in infant and older pediatric recipients. Transplantation. 2003;76:552–7.

19. Chesney DS, Brouhard BH, Cunningham RJ. Safety and cost effectiveness of pediatric percutaneous renal biopsy. Pediatr Nephrol. 1996;10:493–5.

20. Davis ID, Oehlenschlager W, O'Riordan MA, Avner ED. Pediatric renal biopsy: Should this procedure be performed in an outpatient setting? Pediatr Nephrol. 1998;12:96–100.

21. Simckes AM, Blowey DL, Gyves KM, Alon US. Success and safety of same-day kidney biopsy in children and adolescents. Pediatr Nephrol. 2000;14:946–52.

22. Hussain F, Watson AR, Hayes J, Evans J. Standards for renal biopsies: Comparison of inpatient and day care procedures. Pediatr Nephrol. 2003;18:53–6.

23. Schow DA, Vinson RK, Morrisseau PM. Percutaneous renal biopsy of the solitary kidney: A contraindication? J Urol. 1992;147:1235–7.

24. Dodge WF, Daeschner CW Jr, Brennan JC, et al. Percutaneous renal biopsy in children. I. General considerations. Pediatrics. 1962;30:287–96.

25. White RH. Observations on percutaneous renal biopsy in children. Arch Dis Child. 1963;38:260–6.

26. Karafin L, Kendall AR, Fleisher DS. Urologic complications in percutaneous renal biopsy in children. J Urol. 1970;103:332–5.

27. Altebarmakian VK, Guthinger WP, Yakub YN, et al. Percutaneous kidney biopsies: Complications and their management. Urology. 1981;18:118–22.

28. Chan JC, Brewer WH, Still WJ. Renal biopsies under ultrasound guidance: 100 consecutive biopsies in children. J Urol. 1983;129:103–7.

29. Sweet M, Brouhard BH, Ramirez-Seijas F, et al. Percutaneous renal biopsy in infants and young children. Clin Nephrol. 1986;26:192–94.

30. Alon U, Pery M. Percutaneous kidney needle biopsy in children is less traumatic than in adults. Nephron. 1988;50:57–60.

31. al Rasheed SA, al Mugeiren MM, Abdurrahman MB, Elidrissy AT. The outcome of percutaneous renal biopsy in children: An analysis of 120 consecutive cases. Pediatr Nephrol. 1990;4:600–3.

32. Bohlin AB, Edstrom S, Almgren B. Renal biopsy in children: Indications, technique and efficacy in 119 consecutive cases. Pediatr Nephrol. 1995;9:201–3.

33. Pellegrini C, Cecconi M, Pieroni G, et al. Percutaneous renal biopsy in children: Use of a fine needle. Minerva Urol Nefrol. 1996;48:97–101.

34. Benfield MR, Herrin J, Feld L. Safety of kidney biopsy in pediatric transplantation: A report of the Controlled Clinical Trials in Pediatric Transplantation Trial of Induction Therapy Study Group. Transplantation 1999;67: 544–7.

35. Kamitsuji H, Yoshioka K, Ito H. Percutaneous renal biopsy in children: Survey of pediatric nephrologists in Japan. Pediatr Nephrol. 1999;13:693–6.

36. Sumboonnanonda A, Srajai K, Vongjirad A, et al. Percutaneous renal biopsy in children. J Med Assoc Thai. 2002;85:(Suppl 2)755–61.

37. Proesmans W, Marchal G, Snoeck L, Snoeys R. Ultrasonography for assessment of bleeding after percutaneous renal biopsy in children. Clin Nephrol. 1982;18:257–62.

38. Stegmayr B, Orsten PA. Lysis of obstructive renal pelvic clots with retrograde instillation of streptokinase: A case report. Scand J Urol Nephrol. 1984;18:347–50.

39. Horowitz MD, Russell E, Abitbol C, et al. Massive hematuria following percutaneous biopsy of renal allograft: Successful control by selective embolization. Arch Surg. 1984;119:1430–3.

40. Fruhwald F, Harmuth P, Kovarik J, et al. Bladder obstruction: A rare complication after percutaneous renal biopsy. Eur J Radiol. 1984;4:225–6.

41. Rao KV. Urological complications associated with a kidney transplant biopsy: Report of 3 cases and review of the literature. J Urol. 1986;135:768–70.

42. Schwaighofer B, Fruhwald F, Kovarik J. Sonographically demonstrable changes following percutaneous kidney biopsy. Ultraschall Med. 1986;7:44–7.

43. Bergman SM, Frentz GD, Wallin JD. Ureteral obstruction due to blood clot following percutaneous renal biopsy: Resolution with intraureteral streptokinase. J Urol. 1990;143:113–5.

44. McDonald MW, Sosnowski JT, Mahin EJ, et al. Automatic spring-loaded biopsy gun with ultrasonic control for renal transplant biopsy. Urology. 1993;42:580–2.

45. Mahoney MC, Racadio JM, Merhar GL, First MR. Safety and efficacy of kidney transplant biopsy: Tru-Cut needle vs sonographically guided Biopty gun. AJR Am J Roentgenol. 1993;160:325–6.

46. Diaz-Buxo JA, Donadio JV Jr. Complications of percutaneous renal biopsy: An analysis of 1,000 consecutive biopsies. Clin Nephrol. 1975;4:223–7.

47. Bennett AR, Wiener SN. Intrarenal arteriovenous fistula and aneurysm: A complication of percutaneous renal biopsy. Am J Roentgenol Radium Ther Nucl Med. 1965;95:372–82.

48. Ekelund L, Lindholm T. Arteriovenous fistulae following percutaneous renal biopsy. Acta Radiol Diagn (Stockh). 1971;11:38–48.

49. Jorstad S, Borander U, Berg KJ, Wideroe TE. Evaluation of complications due to percutaneous renal biopsy: A clinical and angiographic study. Am J Kidney Dis. 1984;4:162–5.

50. Rollino C, Garofalo G, Roccatello D, et al. Colour-coded Doppler sonography in monitoring native kidney biopsies. Nephrol Dial Transplant. 1994;9:1260–63.

51. Gainza FJ, Minguela I, Lopez-Vidaur I. Evaluation of complications due to percutaneous renal biopsy in allografts and native kidneys with color-coded Doppler sonography. Clin Nephrol. 1995;43:303–8.

52. Ozbek SS, Memis A, Killi R, et al. Image-directed and color Doppler ultrasonography in the diagnosis of postbiopsy arteriovenous fistulas of native kidneys. J Clin Ultrasound. 1995;23:239–42.

53. Riccabona M, Schwinger W, Ring E. Arteriovenous fistula after renal biopsy in children. J Ultrasound Med. 1998;17:505–8.

54. Gonzalez-Michaca L, Chew-Wong A, Soltero L. Percutaneous kidney biopsy, analysis of 26 years: Complication rate and risk factors. Rev Invest Clin. 2000;52:125–31.

55. Figueroa TE, Frentz GD. Anuria secondary to percutaneous needle biopsy of a transplant kidney: A case report. J Urol. 1988;140:355–6.

56. Rea R, Anderson K, Mitchell D. Subcapsular haematoma: A cause of post biopsy oliguria in renal allografts. Nephrol Dial Transplant. 2000;15:1104–5.

57. Ibarguen E, Sharp HL. Gastrointestinal complications following percutaneous kidney biopsy. J Pediatr Surg. 1989;24:286–8.

58. Wall B, Keller FS, Spalding DM, Reif MC. Massive hemorrhage from a lumbar artery following percutaneous renal biopsy. Am J Kidney Dis. 1986;7:250–3.

59. Hussain F, Malik M, Marks SD, Watson AR. Renal biopsies in children: Current practice and audit of outcomes. Nephrol Dial Transplant. 2010;25:485–9.

60. Tondel C, Vikse BE, Bostad L, et al. Safety and complications of percutaneous kidney biopsies in 715 children and 8573 adults in Norway 1988-2010. Clin J Am Soc Nephrol. 2012;10:1591–97.

61. Hogan JJ, Mocanu M, Berns JS. The Native Kidney Biopsy: Update and Evidence for Best Practice. Clin J Am Soc Nephrol. 2016;11: 354–362.

62. Whittier WL, Korbet SM. Timing of complications in percutaneous renal biopsy. J Am Soc Nephrol. 2004;15:142–47.

63. Franke M, Kramarczyk A, Taylan C, et al. Ultrasound-Guided Percutaneous Renal Biopsy in 295 Children and Adolescents: Role of Ultrasound and Analysis of Complications. PLoS ONE. 2014: 9(12): e114737. DOI:10.1371/journal.pone.0114737.

## REVIEW QUESTIONS

1. Which of the following is *not* considered an *absolute* contraindication for a percutaneous renal biopsy?
   a. Uncooperative patient
   b. Chronic glomerulonephritis
   c. Uncontrolled severe hypertension
   d. Acute pyelonephritis

2. Which of the following statements regarding complications of a renal biopsy is *false*?
   a. Microscopic hematuria is the most common complication.
   b. The incidence of perinephric hematoma following renal biopsy depends on the modality of evaluation.
   c. Most arteriovenous fistulas require surgical intervention.
   d. Macroscopic hematuria usually resolves spontaneously within 24 to 48 hours.
   e. Intravenous hydration is sufficient in most patients to prevent the formation of large clots.

3. The optimal biopsy site for a native kidney is the:
   a. Upper pole of the right kidney
   b. Lower pole of the right kidney
   c. Upper pole of the left kidney
   d. Lower pole of the left kidney

4. Which of the following is *not* an indication for renal biopsy in children?
   a. Rapidly progressive glomerulonephritis
   b. Steroid-resistant nephrotic syndrome
   c. Renal allograft dysfunction
   d. Persistent glomerular hematuria
   e. Steroid responsive nephrotic syndrome

5. Prebiopsy evaluation should include:
   a. Complete blood count
   b. Basic metabolic panel
   c. Ultrasonographic evaluation of the kidneys
   d. Coagulation profile
   e. All of the above

6. A 10-year-old girl underwent a percutaneous renal biopsy and was discharged from the outpatient surgical unit after 6 hours of observation. Next morning the patient complained of left side abdominal pain, which was noted to be 8 on a 10-point scale, and was persistent. Her parent gave her acetaminophen 325 mg orally, but there was no resolution of pain. She is now seen in the emergency room. Patient has been urinating well and the urine color is clear yellow. She was afebrile, and abdominal examination showed tenderness in the left upper quadrant and along the left flank. The biopsy site was very tender to touch. No guarding or rebound tenderness was noted. Your *most likely* initial diagnostic consideration is:
   a. Urinary tract infection
   b. Perforation of the abdominal viscera
   c. Perinephric hematoma
   d. Muscular pain at the biopsy site
   e. Previously undiagnosed renal stone

7. Initial management of the patient should include all *except*:
   a. Renal ultrasound
   b. Obtain a complete blood count
   c. Prescribe intravenous morphine
   d. Prescribe oral codeine and discharge her home

8. You decided to admit the patient and noted that her hematocrit had decreased from prebiopsy value of 39% to 24% in the emergency room (hemoglobin 13 g/dL to 8 g/dL). Patient received morphine intravenously and

was relieved of pain. She had mild tachycardia, pulse 99/min, and BP 105/59 mm Hg. Renal ultrasound demonstrated a large perinephric hematoma. Management of the patient will include all *except:*

a. Observe the patient and continue on IV morphine.
b. Ask for invasive radiology team to evacuate perinephric hematoma.
c. May give 5% albumin intravenously.
d. Arrange for a blood transfusion.
e. Repeat CBC in 2 to 4 hours.

9. Hypertension is a presenting manifestation of the post–renal biopsy arteriovenous fistulas.

a. True
b. False

## ANSWER KEY

1. b
2. c
3. d
4. e
5. e
6. c
7. d
8. b
9. a

# Hematuria and proteinuria

## KANWAL KHER AND MARVA MOXEY-MIMS

Hematuria and proteinuria are the two most common abnormalities in the urinalysis that lead to referral of children to pediatric nephrologists or urologists. Use of automated test strips (dipsticks) in performing screening urinalyses in office practice has further enhanced the rate of detection of these urinary abnormalities. Visible or gross hematuria (GH) can be unnerving for children and their parents, especially if associated symptoms of dysuria or abdominal pain are present. Despite its asymptomatic nature, microscopic hematuria (MH) and low-grade proteinuria may also indicate a serious underlying renal disease. This chapter discusses the epidemiology and clinical evaluation of hematuria in children.

## HEMATURIA

Although hematuria is a common manifestation of many disorders of the kidney and the urinary tract, its mere presence does not necessarily signal a progressive illness. The finding of isolated MH in children may be of minor clinical significance. Concern is warranted when the hematuria is accompanied by proteinuria, hypertension, or renal insufficiency. The presence of associated clinical symptoms, such as dysuria, abdominal pain, or an abdominal mass, also requires prompt attention.

## DEFINITIONS

Hematuria can be an isolated and an asymptomatic event, or it may be associated with symptoms such as dysuria, abdominal pain, or systemic disease. In general, hematuria resulting from urologic causes, such as a lower urinary tract infection, passage of stone, or bladder or renal tumors, may be associated with the foregoing manifestations. Glomerular hematuria, conversely, may not cause any urinary symptoms but may have systemic disease manifestations, such as edema, hypertension, rash, or joint pains.

## Gross hematuria

Visible blood in urine, or GH, depending on the site and type of renal and urinary tract disease, can be rust colored, tea (or cola) colored, bright red, or pink. Rusty urine (cola-colored urine, smoky urine) is usually the result of bleeding from the upper urinary tract, such as in glomerulonephritis. Red or pink urine, in contrast, is usually associated with bleeding in the lower urinary tract, which comprises the bladder and urethra. Apart from the color, timing of visible blood within the micturition cycle is also relevant, and may indicate the site of the bleeding within the urinary tract.

> ### KEY POINTS
>
> - Brownish (rusty, smoky, cola-colored) hematuria is usually of glomerular origin.
> - The presence of proteinuria and RBC casts supports a diagnosis of GH.
> - "Urologic" hematuria is usually pinkish or red.
> - Terminal hematuria, in which a drop of blood is present at the end of micturition, usually suggests lesions in the bulbar or prostatic urethra.

## INITIAL HEMATURIA

The presence of blood at the start of micturition is known as initial hematuria and indicates a lesion in the urethra distal to the external urinary sphincter.

## TOTAL HEMATURIA

The presence of visible blood in urine throughout micturition is considered total hematuria and can be caused by lesions in the kidneys or bladder.

## TERMINAL HEMATURIA

When blood is visible at the end of urination, it is referred to as terminal hematuria, and it usually denotes an injury or disease proximally, in the bulbar or prostatic region of the urethra. Terminal hematuria is often reported as a stain in the patient's underwear or a drop of blood at the end of urination. An example of this type of bleeding is urethrorrhagia seen adolescents who strain and create a high-pressure–associated injury to the posterior urethral mucosa. Although some patients have associated symptoms of dysuria, most patients are asymptomatic. Urethrorrhagia is generally a benign condition that improves with minimal therapeutic intervention.

## Microscopic hematuria

MH is defined as five or more red blood cells (RBC)/high-power field (hpf) of a centrifuged urine specimen. MH is considered persistent if it is present in two to three urinalyses over a 2- to 3-week period.

## DETECTION OF HEMATURIA

RBCs are normal components of urine. Thomas Addis[1] observed that the urinary RBC excretion rate in normal volunteers ranged between 48,900 and 65,600 cells in 12 hours. The urine test strips (or dipstick) used for detection of MH employ paper impregnated with orthotoluidine buffered with organic peroxide. Hemoglobin in the urine or in the RBCs catalyzes the oxidation of orthotoluidine with peroxide to a blue color. The intensity of the color is evaluated against a color chart supplied by the manufacturer of the test strips to quantify the degree of hematuria. In recent years, the process of reading the dipsticks has been automated and is less prone to observer interpretation errors.

The dipstick test detects heme molecules, and a positive test result may indicate hematuria or hemoglobinuria. Demonstrating RBCs in microscopic analysis is essential to differentiate hematuria from the two types of pigmenturia (myoglobinuria and hemoglobinuria). Dipsticks are quite sensitive and may detect as few as two to three RBCs/hpf. A false-positive dipstick result can occur if the urine sample is highly concentrated, contains high concentrations of ascorbic acid, is contaminated with

**Table 9.1 Causes of "red" or dark-colored urine**

Hematuria
Myoglobinuria
Hemoglobinuria
Biologic pigments
- Bilirubin
- Urate crystals
- Melanin

Inborn errors of metabolism
- Alkaptonuria
- Tyrosinosis
- Porphyrinuria

Drugs and food colors
- Foods or dyes
- Beets
- Blackberries
- Rhubarb
- Chloroquine
- Desferroxamine
- Levodopa
- Methyldopa
- Metronidazole
- Nitrofurantoin
- Phenolphthalein
- Phenytoin
- Pyridium
- Rifampin
- Sulfa drugs

cleaning agents such as povidone-iodine, hypochlorite, or has microbial peroxidase. Red discoloration of urine can also result from certain medications, food or vegetable dyes, bilirubin, porphyrins, or inborn errors of metabolism (Table 9.1). Details of testing for hematuria are also discussed in Chapter 3.

## EPIDEMIOLOGY OF HEMATURIA

As compared with MH, visible hematuria or GH is less common during childhood. Over a period of 2 years, Ingelfinger et al.[2] reported that in a walk-in clinic setting, 185 of the 12,395 patients' visits (or 1.3 per 1000 visits) were attributable to a GH event. In a 10-year study of children with hematuria, Greenfield et al.[3] found that GH was predominantly seen in boys older than 3 years of age. In

---

### KEY POINTS

- MH is common is school children.
- It is transient in many cases.

this study, 272 of the 342 patients (80%) were boys. Only 6% of patients were younger than 3 years of age, 199 were 3 to 12 years old (58%), and 36% were 13 to 20 years old.[3]

Dodge et al.,[4] in their landmark study from Texas, reported a new case incidence of MH in 6- to 12-year-old school girls to be 22 per 1000 (2.2%), and 9 per 1000 (0.9%) in boys. More importantly, the study noted that the prevalence of MH decreased by 50% when urinalyses were repeated a second or third time over 2 to 6 weeks.[4] Vehaskari et al.[5] reported that MH was present in 4.1% of 8954 Finnish children 8 to 15 years old. In a national screening of school children extending over 13 years (1974 to 1986), the prevalence rate of MH in Japanese children was found to be to be 0.54% in elementary school children and 0.94% in the junior high school children.[6]

## ETIOLOGY OF HEMATURIA

Bleeding from the urinary tract can be arbitrarily considered in two groupings. The first is glomerular or nephrologic hematuria resulting from diseases that affect the nephron (Table 9.2). The second category is urologic hematuria or bleeding originating from the urinary collecting system, urinary bladder, or urethra (Table 9.3). This classification

Table 9.2 Causes of glomerular hematuria in children

1. Acute post-infectious glomerulonephritis
2. Chronic glomerulonephritis
   - Immunoglobulin A nephropathy
   - Mesangioproliferative glomerulonephritis
   - Membranoproliferative glomerulonephritis
   - Focal segmental glomerulosclerosis
   - Membranous nephropathy
3. Inherited nephropathies
   - Alport syndrome
   - Thin basement membrane nephropathy or benign familial hematuria
   - Nail-patella syndrome
   - Fabry disease
   - Polycystic kidney diseases (usually trauma associated)
   - Medullary cystic disease
4. Systemic disorders
   - Systemic lupus erythematosus
   - Hemolytic uremic syndrome
   - Henoch-Schönlein purpura
   - "Shunt" nephritis
   - Goodpasture syndrome
5. Tubulointerstitial diseases
   - Acute pyelonephritis
   - Nephrocalcinosis
   - Interstitial nephritis
   - Tuberous sclerosis
   - Acute tubular necrosis

Table 9.3 Causes of urologic or nonglomerular hematuria

1. Infections
   - Bacterial cystitis
   - Viral cystitis (immunocompromised patient)
     - BK virus
     - Adenovirus (types 11, 21)
     - Cytomegalovirus
   - Parasitic cystitis
     - Schistosomiasis
   - Pinworm infestation
2. Chemical cystitis
   - Cyclophosphamide
   - Crystal violet
   - Radiation cystitis
3. Stone diseases
   - Urinary calculi
   - Hypercalciuria
4. Urethrorrhagia
5. Urinary tract trauma
   - Accidental
   - Associated with instrumentation (catheterization)
6. Urethral or bladder foreign body
7. Urinary bladder tumors
   - Papilloma
   - Hemangioma
   - Rhabdomyosarcoma
8. Hematologic disorders
   - Sickle cell trait or disease
   - Coagulopathies
9. Vascular disorders
   - Renal vein or artery thrombosis
   - Nutcracker syndrome
   - Loin pain hematuria syndrome
10. Miscellaneous
    - Exercise-induced hematuria

allows clinical distinction and focused investigations in the patient affected by hematuria.

## EVALUATION OF HEMATURIA

The aims of evaluation of hematuria in a pediatric patient are to (1) localize the site of urinary bleeding and (2) determine the cause of hematuria. Historical data and physical examination provide vital insight into the site and potential cause of hematuria.

## HISTORY AND PHYSICAL EXAMINATION

A thorough medical and family history, physical examination, and urinalysis with microscopic evaluation of the sediment are key to determining the origin of hematuria. A directed history, physical examination, and investigation pathway should guide the treating nephrologist in the management of these patients (Table 9.4). Information on the type of hematuria (initial, total, or terminal) and any associated symptoms may be helpful in determining the site and cause of hematuria. As noted previously, terminal hematuria manifests with a drop of blood at the end of micturition, or stained underwear, and is associated with lesions of the bulbar or posterior urethra. Urethrorrhagia is a term used to describe terminal hematuria seen in preadolescent and adolescent boys who are otherwise asymptomatic. Total hematuria can be the result lesions affecting the bladder or kidneys.

---

## KEY POINTS

- Synpharyngitic hematuria occurring 24 to 48 hours after an upper respiratory infection is typical of IgA nephropathy.
- Synpharyngitic GH can also be seen in thin basement membrane nephropathy (TBMN) and Alport syndrome.

---

Abdominal or flank pain associated with hematuria may indicate renal stone passage. Distension of renal pelvis in ureteropelvic junction obstruction can also result in flank pain (Dietl's crisis) but hematuria is uncommon, unless associated with trauma. Development of hematuria within 24 to 48 h of an upper respiratory tract infection (synpharyngitic hematuria) may point to immunoglobulin A (IgA) nephropathy. In contrast, poststreptococcal (postinfectious) glomerulonephritis is characterized by streptococcal pharyngitis (or impetigo) approximately 2 weeks before the onset of GH. The presence of GH in patients with compromised renal function and nephritic urinary sediment should alert the nephrologist to the possibility of glomerulonephritides, such as membranoproliferative glomerulonephritis (MPGN), rapidly progressive glomerulonephritis (RPGN), or Henoch-Schönlein purpura (HSP) nephritis.

A family history of renal disease and deafness are features of Alport syndrome, and a family history of hematuria (usually microscopic) without any history of deafness or renal failure may suggest benign familial hematuria.

Physical examination should include evaluation of blood pressure and documentation of any evidence of edema or rash. The presence of these findings would

Table 9.4 Important aspects of history and physical examination in evaluation of hematuria

**Patient History**
- Timing of hematuria in micturition cycle (throughout/onset/terminal)
- Color of urine, brown or rusty versus red or pink
- Associated urinary symptoms
  - Dysuria
  - Urinary frequency
  - Urinary urgency
  - Suprapubic area pain
  - Abdominal pain, colic
  - Costovertebral angle pain
- Recent upper respiratory infection and relation to onset of hematuria
- Exercise
- Trauma
- Medication
- Muscle or joint pain
- Skin rash
- Stone passage

**Family History**
- Chronic kidney disease
- Hematuria
- Deafness (Alport syndrome)
- Nephrolithiasis
- Sickle trait and sickle disease
- Coagulopathy

**Physical Examination**
- Weight: recent weight gain (edema)
- Blood pressure: hypertension
- Fever
- Evidence of edema
- Rash, purpura
- Swelling of joints, evidence of arthritis
- Suprapubic tenderness
- Costovertebral angle tenderness
- Abdominal mass

support the diagnosis of glomerulonephritis or systemic vasculitis. An abdominal mass in the suprapubic region may indicate a bladder lesion, such as a mass or urinary obstruction, whereas a flank mass could be caused by a renal lesion, such as hydronephrosis, large polycystic kidneys, or a tumor.

## Urine Color

GH of glomerular origin is associated with brownish, tea-colored, or cola-colored urine, as opposed to the pink or bright red color seen with nonglomerular hematuria, or urologic hematuria). The dark color of glomerular hematuria reflects conversion of hemoglobin in the acidic urine to acid hematin (brownish) during transit from the kidneys through the rest of the urinary tract. In patients with visibly red or dark urine without evidence of blood on dipstick testing, other causes of urinary discoloration need to be ruled out (see Table 9.1). Urine that is dipstick positive for blood but without erythrocytes documented on urine microscopy may be due to hemoglobinuria or myoglobinuria (Table 9.5). Pallor and icterus are other clinical findings in hemoglobinuria, whereas a history of severe exercise, myalgia, and demonstration of muscle tenderness suggest myoglobinuria. For diagnostic confirmation of myoglobinuria or hemoglobinuria, urine spectrophotometry is necessary.

Table 9.5 Causes of hemoglobinuria and myoglobinuria

**Hemoglobinuria**
- Hemolytic anemias
- Mismatched blood transfusions
- Mechanical erythrocyte damage (artificial cardiac valves, extracorporeal circulation)
- Sepsis or disseminated intravascular coagulation
- Freshwater near drowning
  - Toxins
  - Carbon monoxide
  - Lead
  - Turpentine
  - Phenol
- Naphthalene

**Myoglobinuria**
- Muscle injury
- Severe exercise
- Prolonged seizures
- Prolonged coma
- Hypokalemia
- Electrical injury
- Thermal injury
- Myositis
  - Viral infections (influenza A and B, Coxsackie B, Epstein-Barr)
  - Collagen-vascular diseases (dermatomyositis, polymyositis)
- Poisons
  - Snake venom
  - Scorpion bite
- Drugs and toxins
  - Statins
  - Colchicine
- Cocaine

## RED DIAPER IN NEONATES

Neonates are sometimes noted to have brick red diaper staining in the first weeks of life as a result of the presence of uric acid crystals in the urine. Test results for hemoglobin in these urine samples are negative. This is a benign and self-limited finding, and no therapy is usually required. Subtle dehydration has been suggested to be the cause of uric acid precipitation in the diapers of these neonates, but the finding may be the consequence of elevated urinary uric acid excretion in these neonates.[7]

Lesch-Nyhan syndrome, in contrast, is a rare X-linked recessive disorder that is characterized by persistent gritty orange-red discoloration of the diapers, with eventual uric acid stones. These patients have self-mutilating behavior, severe developmental delay, and poor muscle tone. Hyperuricemia and hyperuricosuria are present on laboratory evaluation. Lesch-Nyhan syndrome is caused by the deficiency of the enzyme hypoxanthine-guanine phosphoribosyltransferase.

## URINE MICROSCOPY

Establishing the nature of hematuria, whether it is glomerular or nonglomerular, is an important first step in the evaluation of patients with hematuria, and it facilitates a focused evaluation of patients. Urine microscopy of the spun urine sediment can be used to determine whether hematuria is glomerular in origin.[8,9] Glomerular hematuria results from disruption of the glomerular filtration barrier that leads to the formation of dysmorphic erythrocytes, characterized by variability of cell size, irregular outlines, and ringed or doughnut shapes (Figure 9.1). Additional findings of glomerular hematuria in urinalysis include proteinuria and RBC and granular casts. Nonglomerular hematuria, conversely, is characterized by eumorphic erythrocytes (uniform size and shape), absence of casts, and often an absence of accompanying proteinuria. Severe urinary bleeding may, however, be associated with proteinuria because of admixture of plasma with urine. Unusual causes of hematuria include parasitic infections, such as schistosomiasis. A history of travel, microscopic examination of urine

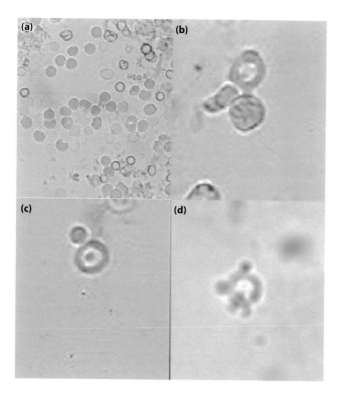

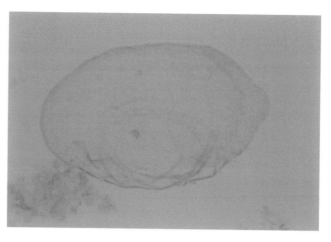

Figure 9.2 Unstained urine sediment of an 8-year-old boy who visited Africa for 2 months and developed gross hematuria on arrival to the United States. The picture shows an egg of *Schistosoma*.

Figure 9.1 Red blood cell (RBC) morphology in hematuria. (a) Eumorphic RBCs; the cell outlines are smooth, and hemoglobin is uniformly distributed in the cells. (b) Dysmorphic RBCs with a doughnut shape; the hemoglobin is marginated toward the periphery of the RBC. (c) Dysmorphic RBC with target shape, hemoglobin is marginated into the center and along the periphery of the RBC. (d) Dysmorphic RBC with an irregular cell wall and margination of hemoglobin in these areas that give rise to a "Mickey Mouse" RBC shape.

(Figure 9.2), and immunologic tests may be necessary for diagnosis in such cases.

## FOCUSED INVESTIGATIONS OF NONGLOMERULAR HEMATURIA

After establishing whether hematuria is glomerular or nonglomerular, the investigational pathways diverge. Patients with nonglomerular hematuria are investigated for urologic and anatomic causes of the condition, whereas patients with the glomerular type of urinary sediment need to be investigated for glomerulonephritis or tubulointerstitial diseases.

The investigative pathway of nonglomerular or urologic hematuria should include urine culture to rule out the possibility of urinary tract infection. A negative urine culture result and persistent symptoms of dysuria and suprapubic tenderness may be seen in patients with viral cystitis. Detection of viral DNA by polymerase chain reaction (PCR) for adenoviruses, BK virus, and JC virus is available in most clinical laboratories and should be sought in patients with a suggestive history, especially those with a kidney or bone

marrow transplant, or those with an immunocompromised clinical state. It is important to note that viral culture of urine requires long incubation periods for the test. Renal and bladder ultrasound scans should be obtained to rule out structural urinary tract anomalies, calculus disease, or tumors. Sickle cell status should be determined in African-American patients, if not done previously. Hypercalciuria is a common cause of nonglomerular MH in children, and it should be ruled out by measuring the calcium/creatinine ratio in a spot urine sample or by a 24-h urine collection. A non-contrast computed tomography (CT) scan and urinary "stone risk analysis" are indicated in patients who are suspected to have urolithiasis. The high radiation dose of CT scans must be carefully considered while determining the benefit of this diagnostic test in any given patient.

Cystoscopy is not generally necessary in most children with hematuria, but it may be warranted if bladder disease such as bladder hemangioma or tumors of the bladder (papilloma, rhabdomyosarcoma) or urethra are suspected as the cause of hematuria. Cystoscopy may also be helpful in localizing the site of GH to one of the ureteral orifices. Further investigations in such cases can then be focused on the anatomic site with documented unilateral hematuria.

## FOCUSED INVESTIGATIONS OF GLOMERULAR HEMATURIA

Hematuria can be the dominant clinical manifestation of several types of glomerulonephritis. In general, because of concerns for long-term renal damage, chronic kidney disease (CKD), and hypertension, investigations and treatment of these patients must be expedited. A history of hematuria in parents suggests a familial type of hematuria, such as benign familial hematuria, also known as thin basement membrane nephropathy (TBMN), or Alport syndrome.

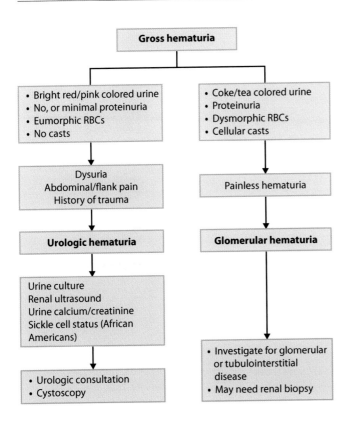

Figure 9.3 Outline of evaluation of gross hematuria. RBCs, red blood cells.

Because postinfectious glomerulonephritis occurs frequently in children, patients with glomerular hematuria should undergo a panel of tests to rule out this diagnosis complement 3 and 4 (C3 and C4), anti–streptolysin O (ASO) titer, and anti-DNAse B titer. Proteinuria should be quantified in all patients considered to have glomerular hematuria. This can be done by determination of the protein/creatinine ratio in a spot sample of urine or by collection of a 24-h urine. Evaluation for systemic lupus erythematosus (SLE) should include screening tests, such as antinuclear activity (ANA) and, anti-dsDNA antibody). Patients suspected to have vasculitis should be tested for the presence of anti–neutrophil cytoplasmic antibodies (ANCAs). A diagnostic renal biopsy may be considered in patients when glomerular hematuria is associated with renal dysfunction, hypertension, and nephrotic syndrome. Flow diagrams of investigation in patients with GH and with MH are shown in Figures 9.3 and 9.4.

## Diagnostic yield

Clinically significant diagnostic yield of investigations in GH is higher compared with MH. For example, of the 228 patients with GH investigated by Bergstein et al.,[10] 53 patients warranted a renal biopsy, and 36 of these patients had IgA nephropathy. Other important diagnoses uncovered in this assessment of GH were 51 cases of hypercalciuria, 3 cases

of Alport syndrome, and 1 case of Wilms tumor. Even after extensive investigations, 37.7% (86) patients in this study had no definable cause of GH. Despite discovery of a few patients with malignant disease, most studies suggest that concern for renal or bladder malignant diseases in children with GH is low.[4,10]

It is reassuring that the published literature on the subject of investigating isolated MH (without proteinuria) suggests a benign outcome in most children. Because of the low yield of clinically significant disorders, Dodge et al.[4] argued against screening for hematuria. This is especially important because hematuria was transient in approximately 50% of patients. Similarly, of the 342 children with MH investigated by Bergstein et al.,[10] no cause was found in 274 (80%). Hypercalciuria comprised the largest single cause of MH in these patients. Feld et al.[11] also demonstrated a lack of serious renal disease in children presenting with isolated MH. The Japanese experience of screening school children has also shed some important light on the absence of serious chronic disease in children with isolated MH. Murakami et al.[6] reported that only 0.009% of screened children were found to have chronic kidney disease (CKD). Commenting on these findings, Stapleton[12] recommended a more restrained approach in investigating children with asymptomatic MH. Although it is true that parents expect clinicians to embark on extensive investigations to map the precise source of the bleeding, discussion and explanation using an evidence-based approach may allow tailoring of investigations.

## KEY POINTS

- Because of the low yield of isolated MH, a restrained approach with limited investigations is recommended.
- Glomerular hematuria, however, should be investigated fully.

## PROTEINURIA

Proteinuria is regarded as an important marker of renal disease. Glomerulonephritis, nephrotic syndrome, tubulointerstitial nephritis, and numerous forms of inherited disorders are characterized by presence of proteinuria. Moreover, proteinuria, by itself, is now considered injurious to the proximal renal tubules (PRTs) and may lead to ongoing tubulointerstitial nephritis. The presence of minute quantities of albumin in urine or microalbuminuria (MA) is well recognized as the forerunner of diabetic nephropathy and has been prognostically linked to cardiac disease and hypertensive renal disease.[13,14]

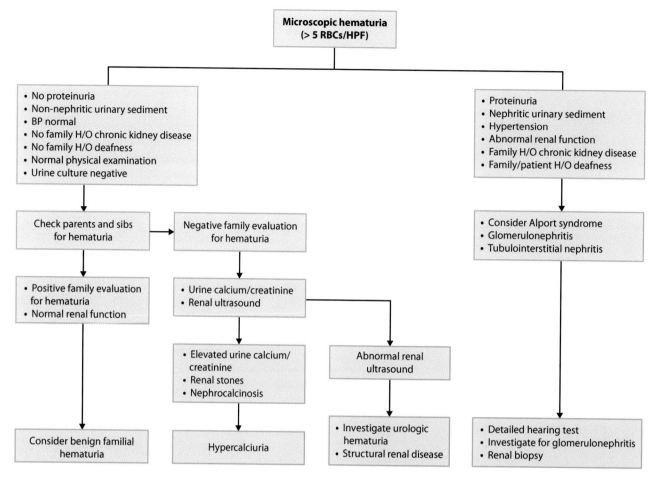

Figure 9.4 Outline of evaluation of microscopic hematuria. BP, blood pressure; H/O, history of; HPF, high-power field; RBC, red blood cell.

## EPIDEMIOLOGY OF PROTEINURIA

Several studies have noted a high prevalence rate of transient proteinuria in children. Vehaskari and Rapola[15] screened 8954 children in Finland and reported that 959 (10.7%) children had proteinuria in a single urinalysis. When two urinalyses were considered, the prevalence declined to 2.5%, and only 0.1% had persistent proteinuria in all four urinalyses performed. The increasing prevalence rate of proteinuria with increasing age in children was well described in this study, as well as that of Dodge et al.[4]

## ETIOLOGY OF PROTEINURIA

A false-positive test result for proteinuria can be caused by urinary tract infection, vulvovaginitis, urethritis, prostatitis, and contamination by menstrual blood. Transient proteinuria can also be seen after exercise, dehydration, or fever.[16,17] Orthostatic or postural proteinuria is a common condition encountered in older children and adolescents. Persistent or "fixed" proteinuria can be a manifestation of nephrotic syndrome, glomerulonephritis, interstitial nephritis, some inherited nephropathies, and CKD). Causes

of proteinuria in children are listed in Table 9.6, and urinary protein excretion in various age groups during childhood is given in Table 9.7.

### KEY POINTS

- Postural or orthostatic proteinuria should be ruled out in children by performing a first morning urine protein/creatinine ratio ($\leq 0.2$).
- Fixed or nonorthostatic proteinuria requires complete evaluation, sometimes including a renal biopsy.

## PATHOPHYSIOLOGY OF PROTEINURIA

The glomerular capillary wall (GCW) is a complex and selective filtration barrier composed of three distinct layers: (1) endothelium with fenestrations and glycocalyx, (2) glomerular basement membrane (GBM), and (3) epithelial cells and the complex network of podocytes (Figure 9.5).

Table 9.6 Causes of proteinuria

**Nonpathologic and Transient Proteinuria**
- Orthostatic proteinuria
- Fever
- Exercise

**Glomerular Disorders (also see Table 9.2)**
- Nephrotic syndrome
- Acute and chronic glomerulonephritis
- Hypertension
- Diabetes mellitus
- HIV nephropathy
- Inherited nephropathies (Alport syndrome, podocytopathies, Fabry disease; also see Table 9.1)

**Tubular Disorders: Inherited**
- Cystinosis
- Wilson disease
- Lowe syndrome
- Dent disease
- Fanconi syndrome

**Tubular Disorders: Acquired**
- Interstitial nephritis
- Reflux nephropathy
- Antibiotics and drug induced
- Antiretroviral therapy induced
- Acute tubular necrosis
- Heavy metal poisoning

**Artifactual Conditions**
- Vulvovaginitis
- Urinary tract infection
- Urethritis
- Prostatitis
- Periurethral infections
- Perineal contact irritation
- Menstrual blood contamination

HIV, human immunodeficiency virus

Table 9.7 Normal 24-h urinary protein excretion in children by age groups

| Age group | Protein excretion (mg/24 h) | Protein excretion (mg/24 h/m² bsa) |
| --- | --- | --- |
| Premature (5–30 days) | 29 (14–60) | 182 (88–377) |
| Full-term (7–30 days) | 32 (15–68) | 145 (68–309) |
| 2–12 mo | 38 (17–85) | 109 (48–244) |
| 2–4 yr | 49 (20–121) | 91 (37–223) |
| 4–10 yr | 71 (26–194) | 85 (31–234) |
| 10–16 yr | 83 (29–238) | 63 (22–181) |

*Source:* Adapted from Miltényi M. Urinary excretion in healthy children. Clin Nephrol. 1979;12:216–21.
BSA, body surface area.

## Endothelial Layer

Endothelium comprises the innermost layer of the glomerular capillary and remains in direct contact with circulating plasma and the cellular constituents of blood. The body of the glomerular endothelial cell rests within the hilum of the capillary loop, in close proximity to mesangial cells. A thin layer of endothelial cytoplasm extends from the endothelial cell and envelops the inner aspect of the capillary lumen. The endothelial cytoplasm has 70- to 100-nm pores known as endothelial fenestrations (EFs). The EFs constitute 30% to 50% of the inner capillary surface.[18]

---

### KEY POINTS

- The role of the endothelial barrier in restricting protein outflow from the glomerular capillary lumen remains unclear.
- The endothelial surface layer, composed of glycocalyx and plasma components, may indeed be important as a barrier.

---

Glomerular capillaries possess hydraulic conductivity (permeability) that permits passage of large volumes of ultrafiltrate and small solutes. Simultaneously, these capillaries also exhibit selective permeability that actively restricts passage of albumin (3800 kDa) and other larger molecules. Low-molecular-weight (LMW) proteins (MW less than 2800 kDa), such as β2-microglobulin and amino acids are relatively easily filtered but are reabsorbed in the PRTs. The role played by the three constituent layers of the GCW in macromolecular transport and proteinuria has been a subject of intense investigations, controversy, and debate. From a functional perspective, and given our current state of knowledge, the three layers seem to be equally important in the macromolecular transport.

Conventional thinking postulates that because of the large pore size of EFs, endothelium does not pose a significant barrier to macromolecular transport. Several other observations suggested that the endothelial cell layer is more complex and provides selective transport characteristic to the GCW.[18,19] Advanced electron microscopy of endothelium demonstrates an additional layer of glycocalyx (Figure 9.6) and plasma components, known as the endothelial surface layer (ESL), that loosely covers the endothelial cell's cytoplasm and EFs. The ESL extends up to 200 nm above the cell surface.[19] The role played by the ESL in protein and other macromolecular transport across the glomerular capillaries is not fully

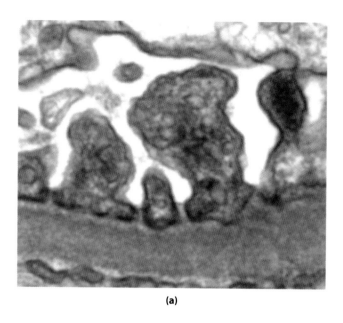

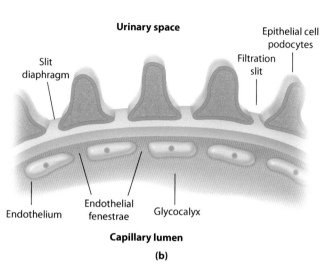

(a)

(b)

Figure 9.5 **(a)** Electron micrograph showing filtration slit with adjacent podocytes (P), slit diaphragm (arrowheads) bridging between the two podocytes and the glomerular basement membrane (GBM). **(b)** Conceptual representation of the glomerular filtration barrier that shows the podocytes resting on the glomerular basement membrane, slit diaphragms between the podocytes, and the endothelial cells lined by the glycocalyx.

understood. Available evidence suggests that apart from regulating many vascular functions, the ESL may be important in bestowing anionic charge to the endothelial barrier and help in preventing protein leak across the GCW.[20-23] Using multiphoton microscopy measurements, Salmon et al.[23] demonstrated that loss of the ESL in aging Munich-Wistar-Frömter rats was associated with proteinuria. These observations, although not proving the role of the ESL in proteinuria and transglomerular capillary transport, do suggest a possible link between the development of proteinuria and endothelial dysfunction. Clearly, more needs to be learned about endothelial functions and their role in glomerular capillary macromolecular transport.

## Glomerular basement membrane

The GBM is an acellular, gel-like structure composed of tightly woven type IV collagen, laminin, heparin sulfate proteoglycans, and nidogen.[24,25] Of these, type IV collagen is the dominant component of the GBM, which comprises more than 50% of the mass of the GBM. In adults, the GBM is 250 to 400 nm thick but it is considerably thinner in children. Ramage et al.[26] reported the thickness of the GBM at 1 year of age to be 194 ± 6.5 nm and at 11 years to be 297 ± 6.0 nm. During embryogenesis and glomerular development, both podocytes and endothelial cells contribute to the development of the GBM. Ultrastructurally, the GBM possesses three distinct layers: the thin lamina rara interna and the lamina rara externa, with the lamina densa sandwiched between them. Nanostructure localization suggests that the GBM consists of highly organized architecture and consists of laminated and possibly interacting proteins, potentially similar to what has now been well described to be the case with podocytes.[27]

The role of the GBM as a barrier to filtration of protein has been widely debated. Transgenic mice lacking laminin in their GBM have been shown to develop proteinuria and secondary podocyte foot process abnormalities.[28] These

Figure 9.6 Electron micrographic visualization of Alcian blue 8GX–stained rat left ventricular myocardial capillary demonstrating glycocalyx. (From van den Berg BM, Vink H, Spaan JA. The endothelial glycocalyx protects against myocardial edema. Circ Res. 2003;92:592–4.)

findings reinforce the view that integrity of GBM plays a critical role in the development of proteinuria in which both size selectivity and charge selectivity play a role.[29,30] An alternate school of thought suggests that the GBM is merely a prefilter with very limited size or charge barrier capability.[31] These investigators believe that slit diaphragms (SDs) of the podocytes are the primary determinants of macromolecular transport and proteinuria, a view referred to as the "two-barriers-in-series" concept.[32,33]

## Podocyte layer

The outermost barrier for the passage of macromolecules and fluid across the GCW is the epithelial cell or the podocyte. Podocytes are large cells that line the urinary space side of the GBM. These specialized cells have branching cytoplasmic extensions known as foot processes that firmly anchor the podocytes to the GBM. The adjacent foot processes do not come in direct contact with each other and are separated by an approximately 40-nm-wide space known as the filtration slit. These filtration slits (see Figure 9.5) are bridged by the slit diaphragm (SD), a membrane-like structure. Important plasma membrane proteins, such as nephrin, NEPH1–3, podocin, Fat-1, P-cadherin, and P-cadherin, reside on the SD.[31,34–36]

---

### KEY POINTS

- Podocytes are emerging as important cells in glomerular functions in disease and health.
- Many important membrane proteins reside in the podocytes and the SDs.
- The SD is important in glomerular filtration and preserving the permselectivity of the glomerular barrier.
- Podocytes do not reproduce, and their loss is permanent.
- Podocytes are thought to be involved in the pathogenesis of a range of diseases, such as minimal change disease, focal segmental glomerulosclerosis, other types of glomerulonephritic and diabetic nephropathy.

---

These proteins are believed to be intimately involved in cell-to-cell signaling and maintaining the normal cytoskeletal structure of podocytes and the associated foot processes. Before the discovery of these proteins in the SD and the podocytes, the importance of this cell and associated structures had been an enigma. It is now well known that the SD plays an important role in providing selective permeability characteristics to the glomerular capillaries.[31,33] The foot processes also contain the contractile protein actin in parallel bundles that constitute podocyte cytoskeleton and maintain its shape, and anchors podocytes to the GBM by transmembrane cell receptors that include integrins.[37]

Gene mutations resulting in abnormalities in the proteins present on SDs lead to specific clinical disorders that are associated with proteinuria or nephrotic syndrome (Table 9.8). Mutation of the nephrin gene *NPHS1* was the first such mutation described and is associated with the Finnish type of congenital nephrotic syndrome.[32]

An important biologic characteristic of podocytes is that these cells are unable to reproduce or replenish themselves in their mature state. Although some shedding of podocytes into the urinary space and excretion in urine is normal, this process can be accelerated by injury and disease states. Urinary loss of podocytes (or podocyturia) can result in a permanent and irreplaceable quantitative deficit of podocytes in the glomeruli (podocytopenia). Indeed, podocyturia and podocytopenia are known to be important findings in many glomerular diseases characterized by proteinuria, such as diabetic nephropathy, focal segmental glomerulosclerosis, membranous nephropathy, and human immunodeficiency virus (HIV) nephropathy.[37-39]

## PERMSELECTIVITY OF THE GLOMERULAR FILTER

Glomerular capillaries possess a unique ability to filter plasma water, electrolytes, and other metabolites while retaining most proteins. The nature of glomerular capillary selective permeability (permselectivity) has been a matter of considerable debate. Based on experimental data and mathematical modeling, glomerular permselectivity has been attributed to (1) molecular size, (2) molecular charge, and (3) molecular configuration. Although it is true that some components of the GCW may be more important in providing size or charge selectivity, the current state of knowledge suggests that all elements of the filtration mechanism must be intact to prevent proteinuria from developing. Glomerular permeability is also discussed in Chapter 10.

---

### KEY POINTS

Permeability of the GBM to macromolecules, such as plasma proteins, depends on:

- Molecular size
- Molecular charge
- Molecular configuration

---

### Size selectivity

Using neutral dextran, passage of molecules has been demonstrated to be almost unrestricted until the molecular size reaches 20 Å. Beyond this molecular size, neutral dextran is progressively excluded from passage across the GCW into the filtrate. At a molecular size of 42 Å, there is negligible clearance of neutral dextran from the glomerular capillaries.[40] Albumin, which has a molecular size of 36 Å

Table 9.8 Genetic causes of proteinuria

| | Chromosomal location | Gene name | Protein | Protein function |
|---|---|---|---|---|
| **Syndromic disorders** | | | | |
| Congenital nephrotic syndrome | 19q13.1 | NPHS1 | Nephrin | Essential component of podocyte SD protein complex |
| Denys-Drash syndrome | 11p13 | WT1 | Wilms tumor 1 | Podocyte-expressed transcription factor |
| Pierson syndrome | 3p21 | LAMB2 | Laminin β2 chain | Subchain of GBM laminin-11 |
| Schimke immunoosseous dysplasia | 2q34-36 | SMARCAL1 | SWI/SNF2-related matrix-associated, actin-dependent regulator of chromatin, subfamily a-like 1 | Gene regulation and replication and DNA repair |
| Nail-patella syndrome | 17q11 | LMX1B | LIM homeobox transcription factor-1β | Podocyte-expressed transcription factor |
| Alport syndrome, X-linked | Xq22.3 | COL4A5 | Type IV collagen, α 5 subchain | Subchain of GBM type IV collagen |
| Alport syndrome, AR | 2q36-q37 | COL4A3 | Type IV collagen, α subchain 3 | Subchain of GBM type IV collagen |
| Alport syndrome, AR | 2q36-q37 | COL4A4 | Type IV collagen, α subchain 4 | Subchain of GBM type IV collagen |
| Mitochondrial cytopathies | 4q21.23 | COQ2 | Parahydroxy-benzoate-polyprenyl-transferase | Biosynthesis of coenzyme Q, involved in mitochondrial respiratory chain electron transport |
| Fechtner syndrome | 22q12.3 | MYH9 | Nonmuscle myosin IIa heavy chain | Actin-binding protein involved in cell motility |
| **Nonsyndromic disorders** | | | | |
| FSGS, AR | 1q25-q31 | NPHS2 | Podocin | Essential SD-associated protein |
| FSGS, AR | 19q13.1 | NPHS1 | Nephrin | Essential component of SD protein complex |
| FSGS, AD | 19q13 | ACTN4 | Alpha-actinin-4 | Actin-binding protein |
| FSGS, AD | 11q21-q22 | TRPC6 | Transient receptor potential channel, subfamily 6 | Podocyte-expressed calcium channel |
| FSGS, AD | 14q32.33 | INF2 | Inverted formin 2 | Actin-regulating protein |
| FSGS, not specified | 6p12 | CD2AP | CD2-associated protein | Actin-binding protein associated with SD protein complex |
| Diffuse mesangial sclerosis, not specified | 10q23 | PLCE1 | Phospholipase C ε 1 | Membrane phospholipid hydrolysis |

Source: Piscione TD, Licht C. Genetics of proteinuria: an overview of gene mutations associated with nonsyndromic proteinuric glomerulopathies. Adv Chronic Kidney Dis. 2011;18:273–89.

Abbreviations: AD, autosomal dominant; AR, autosomal recessive; FSGS, focal segmental glomerulosclerosis; GBM, glomerular basement membrane; SD, slit diaphragm.

(MW 66 kDa), is almost completely prevented from passing through the glomerular capillary barrier. High-MW proteins, such as IgG (MW 150 kDa), IgM (MW 900 kDa), and $\alpha_2$-macroglobulin (MW 725 kDa), are unable to pass through the glomerular filtration barrier. In contrast, LMW proteins, such as $\beta_2$-microglobulin (molecular size 11.8 Å,

MW 12 kDa), and immunoglobulin light chains are readily filtered.[41]

Using mathematical modeling, two distinct types of pore models have been hypothesized within the GCW: (1) the isoporous model and (2) the heteroporous model. The isoporous model suggests that cylindrical pores of the same size

(50 to 55 Å) are distributed throughout the GCW that hold back protein and other macromolecules above this size limit. The heteroporous model is based on the observation that in proteinuric states, such as glomerulonephritis, clearance of dextran greater than 45 Å increases significantly, whereas clearance of smaller molecules changes little, thereby suggesting the existence of a larger pores. The larger pores (>80 Å), which are also known as the "shunt pathway," are believed to be few in number and nonselective in their permeability characteristics.[41-43]

## Charge selectivity

The presence of anionic charge in the components of the GCW has been well established.[44] The role played by this molecular charge in permselectivity and proteinuria has been extensively studied since the 1970s. The first clue about the role of anionic charges in proteinuria was the observation in normal rats that clearance of albumin was significantly lower than that of neutral tracer molecules of dextran of the equal molecular size.[44,45] Similar findings were also noted in nephrotic rats.[46] These observations raise the possibility that molecular size alone may not explain albuminuria and macromolecular transport across the GCW. Extending these observations, it was demonstrated that transport of cationic and neutral tracer molecules was preferentially facilitated across the GCW, as compared with anionic molecules.[47,48] Because plasma proteins possess an anionic surface charge, it has been suggested that the anionic charge of the GCW creates an electrostatic repulsive force that prevents passage of plasma proteins from the glomerular capillary lumen. The primary site for anionic charge in the GCW was initially considered to be the GBM, but the endothelial surface and the epithelial cell surface also have been shown to possess a negative charge.[30,31] Within the GBM, the lamina rara interna and the lamina rara externa demonstrate the most prominent anionic charge sites.[30] Anionic charge in the GBM results from the presence of heparin sulfate proteoglycan and hyaluronic acid.

## Molecular configuration

In addition to size and charge, the shape of filtered molecules is also considered to be an important determinant of macromolecular transport across the GCW. This inference has been drawn from the fractional clearance of dextran and Ficoll (Sigma-Aldrich, St. Louis, MO), both of which have similar effective radius but a different structural configuration. Dextran is a complex branched polysaccharide, a polymer of glucopyranose, with an elongated or sausage-shaped molecular structure. Ficoll, in contrast, is a highly branched, polysaccharide-epichlorohydrin complexed molecule with a globular shape. Bohrer et al.[49] demonstrated that within 24 to 44 Å molecular size range, fractional clearance of dextran was higher than that of Ficoll. This led the investigators

to conclude that molecular configuration was important in macromolecular clearance from the GCW. More flexible molecular configuration of dextran was viewed as preferred over the rigidly structured Ficoll for passage through the GCW. Because most proteins are spherical, it is believed that such rigidly configured protein molecules behave like Ficoll and are prevented from passage across GCW. Findings that Ficoll may actually not be as tightly configured in solution as previously thought has put the role of molecular configuration into question.[50] In addition to configuration, molecular deformability may influence permselectivity of GCW to albumin and other macromolecules.

## FATE OF FILTERED PROTEIN

It has been well known since the early 1950s that plasma proteins filtered from glomeruli are reabsorbed in the PRTs.[51] Micropuncture studies in rats revealed that the glomerular filtrate reaching the PRTs mostly contains LMW proteins and minor amounts of albumin (1 to 3 mg/dL).[52,53] Therefore, in an adult with a glomerular filtration rate (GFR) of 125 mL/min, or 180 L/24 h, the total amount of albumin filtered is 1800 to 5400 mg/day. However, normal urinary protein excretion under physiologic circumstances in an adult is less than 150 mg/24 h, a finding suggesting that renal tubules reabsorb most of the filtered albumin. The mechanism of reabsorption and metabolic pathways of degradation of the absorbed protein in the PRTs has been elucidated more recently.

> ## KEY POINTS
>
> - Most of albumin filtered at the glomerulus is reabsorbed in the PRTs.
> - PRTs take up filtered albumin through cubilin-megalin receptors and metabolize it to dipeptides and amino acids. These are returned to the body's pool along the basolateral surface.

Albumin present in the tubular lumen is reabsorbed in the PRT through active receptor-mediated endocytosis. The albumin molecules in the tubular lumen bind to the cubilin-megalin receptor complex.[54-56] Most of the albumin-receptor binding activity occurs in between the brush-border villi, rather than the tip of the PRT brush border. The albumin-receptor complex is internalized and forms cytoplasmic vesicles. The next step involves acidification of the vesicles, a step facilitated by the chloride channel-5 (ClC-5). This is an important step for albumin to be dissociated from the megalin-cubilin complex and for megalin to be recycled.[57] On dissociating from albumin, the megalin-cubilin complex is processed in the sorting endosomes and is eventually returned to the cell surface through recycling endosomes (Figure 9.7). Albumin, conversely, is passed on to the lysosomes for metabolic digestion to amino acids and dipeptides,

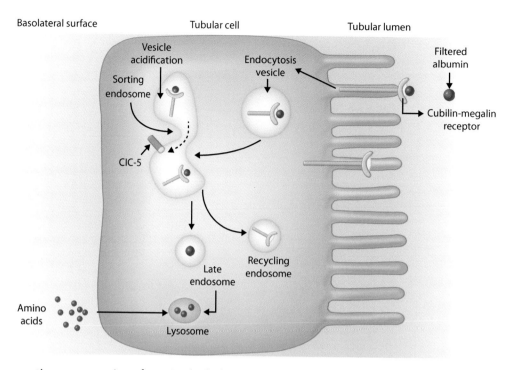

Figure 9.7 Diagrammatic representation of proximal tubular albumin reabsorption. ClC-5, chloride channel-5. See text for details.

which are returned to the body pool through the basolateral surface.[54,56]

## Role of cubilin and megalin in protein reabsorption

Cubilin is an endocytosis receptor that is highly expressed in the PRT brush border, as well as in the intestines. Cubilin is a 460-kDa protein that does not have a transmembrane domain and remains anchored to the brush-border membrane by attaching itself to megalin.[54,55] For all practical purposes, the cubilin-megalin complex is considered to be the receptor for reabsorption of albumin and some LMW proteins from the tubular fluid. Cubilin binds to the albumin molecule, which along with megalin is internalized as an endocytosis vesicle. Cubilin is also present within the gastrointestinal tract, where it is known as the intestinal intrinsic factor-$B_{12}$ receptor (IF-$B_{12}$).

The absence of IF-B12 (cubilin) leads to a rare form of megaloblastic anemia associated with proteinuria, also known as Imerslund-Gräsbeck syndrome.[58] Decreased megalin trafficking in the proximal tubular cells occurs in Dent disease, which is characterized by LMW proteinuria, hypercalciuria, and nephrocalcinosis.[59,60] Dent disease is caused by a mutation in renal ClC-5, which leads to an acidification defect of the endocytic vesicles, an essential step in processing albumin and LMW proteins in the PRT.[57]

## NEPHROTOXICITY OF PROTEINURIA

Proteinuria, irrespective of its origin, in a patient with renal disease, is believed to contribute to ongoing and progressive

deterioration of the kidney disease and function.[61] Several lines of clinical and experimental investigations support the proinflammatory sequence initiated by proteinuria and tubular absorption of protein. Proteinuria is also well known to be an independent risk factor for increased mortality and renal disease progression in both type 1 and type 2 diabetes mellitus.[62] Use of angiotensin-converting enzyme inhibitors (ACEIs) to reduce proteinuria has been shown to improve renal survival in these patients.[63] Self-sustaining interstitial inflammation and fibrosis induced by proteinuria have been shown to be important consequences of proteinuric states, and may serve as the terminal pathway for disease progression in patients with CKD.[62,63] Tubulointerstitial injury in association with proteinuria can arise from several independent and codependent mechanisms. These events are diagrammatically depicted in Figure 9.8 and are discussed here.

---

### KEY POINT

Proteinuria, by itself, may cause renal damage and promote tubulointerstitial inflammation.

---

## Proinflammatory chemokines

Proteinuric states are characterized by an excessive synthesis of a variety of proinflammatory cytokines and chemokines by the tubular cells. The trigger for these chemokines is the generation of nuclear factor κB (NF-kB) in the proximal

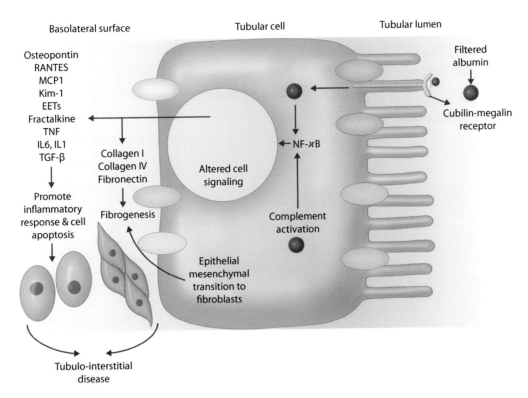

Figure 9.8 Diagrammatic representation of pathogenesis of tubulointerstitial fibrosis resulting from proteinuria. EETs, epoxyeicosatrienoic acids; IL-6, interleukin-6; IL-1, interleukin-1; Kim-1, kidney injury molecule-1; MCP-1, monocyte chemoattractant protein-1; mTOR, mammalian target of rapamycin; PAI-1, plasminogen activator inhibitor; NF-κB, nuclear factor κB; RANTES, Regulated on activation normal T cell expressed and secreted; TGFβ, transforming growth factor-β; TNF, tumor necrosis factor.

tubules in response to protein absorption.[64-66] NF-kB reacts with the mammalian target of rapamycin (mTOR) leading to downstream activation of proinflammatory chemokine genes. These include plasminogen activator inhibitor-1 (PAI-1), which is crucial in fibrogenesis, as well as chemoattractant proteins, such as monocyte chemoattractant protein-1 (MCP-1), RANTES (regulated on activation, normal T cell expressed and secreted), fractalkine, osteopontin, kidney injury molecule-1 (Kim-1), transforming growth factor-β (TGF-β), interleukin-1 (IL-1) and interleukin-6 (IL-6).[65-73] Generating of proinflammatory chemokines and cytokines in the peritubular interstitial space initiates mononuclear cells infiltration, proliferation of fibroblasts in the interstitium, and PRT cell apoptosis.[66,72] The end results of these cellular events are interstitial inflammation, fibrosis, and ongoing tubular cell damage.

## Activation of complement

Complement, as a mediator of injury in proteinuria, has been investigated since the 1980s. Complement components range in size from 80 to 200 kDa, which can be filtered through the GCW in nonselective proteinuric state, but they can also be synthesized locally by the PRT cells and the leukocytes infiltrating the interstitial area.[74] The PRT cell brush border also possesses C3 convertase activity, which can initiate complement cascade events within the tubular lumen and the interstitium. Activation of the complement cascade leads to upregulation of genes for TGF-β and collagen type I, both of which create a profibrotic state in the interstitium.[65,75-77]

## Epithelial-mesenchymal transition

Fibrogenesis is the final pathway in the development of tubulointerstitial fibrosis. The resident fibroblast population, along with its circulating population recruited by various proinflammatory cytokines and complement components, results in the formation of myofibroblasts.[74-77] In addition to these two sources, tubular epithelial cells and pericytes have also been shown to transform into myofibroblasts by a phenomenon known as epithelial-mesenchymal transition (EMT).[78-82] Myofibroblasts lay down collagen matrix and lead to fibrogenesis.

## TYPES OF PROTEINURIA

Proteinuria can be classified into three categories: (1) glomerular proteinuria, (2) tubular proteinuria, and (3) overflow proteinuria.

## Glomerular proteinuria

Proteinuria resulting from diseases of the glomerular ultrafiltration barrier (minimal change, other glomerulonephritides) is referred to as glomerular proteinuria. Urine protein electrophoresis (UPEP) analysis of glomerular proteinuria shows a pattern similar to serum protein analysis, with albumin constituting a dominant fraction (Figure 9.9 (a)). Glomerular proteinuria is detectable by urine dipsticks and can be quantified by usual techniques discussed below.

## Tubular proteinuria

Many inherited tubulopathies (e.g., Fanconi syndrome), and acquired tubular disorders (e.g., nephrotoxins) are characterized by failure to reabsorb the LMW proteins by the PRT cells from the tubular lumen. Proteinuria seen in such clinical circumstances is referred to as tubular proteinuria. In contrast to glomerular proteinuria, urinary dipstick does not detect LMW proteins, and specific analytic methods are necessary to uncover tubular proteinuria. Three markers commonly used as indicators of tubular proteinuria in clinical practice are $\beta_2$-microglobulin, $\alpha_1$-microglobulin, and retinol binding protein. UPEP in tubular proteinuria demonstrates significant $\alpha$ and $\beta$ globulin peaks, in addition to albumin (Figure 9.9 (b)).

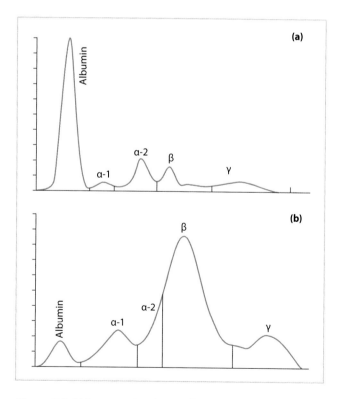

Figure 9.9 Urine protein electrophoresis (UPEP). **(a)** Patient with glomerular proteinuria. Of note is the large albumin peak. The UPEP pattern is similar to that of plasma. **(b)** Patient with tubular proteinuria. Globulin peaks dominate in this type of proteinuria.

> **KEY POINT**
>
> Proteinuria can result from glomerular leak (glomerular proteinuria), failure to reabsorb LMW protein in the PRT (tubular proteinuria), or a high plasma level of certain proteins (overflow proteinuria), and may cause renal damage and promote tubulointerstitial inflammation.

## Overflow proteinuria

This is the least common type of proteinuria found in children. Monoclonal gammopathies characterized by high plasma concentrations of monoclonal immunoglobulin fractions in the serum lead these proteins to appear in the glomerular ultrafiltrate. Once proximal tubular reabsorption capacity of these filtered plasma proteins is exceeded, they begin appear in urine. Such proteinuria is known as overflow proteinuria. Bence-Jones protein, seen in multiple myeloma and other B-cell lymphomas, is an example of such overflow proteinuria. Bence-Jones protein was originally detected by heat precipitation methodology, but immunoelectrophoresis is now generally used to detect the monoclonal (M peaks) urinary protein excretion.

## TAMM-HORSFALL PROTEIN

Another component of normal urine is the glycoprotein called Tamm-Horsfall protein (THP), or uromodulin. THP constitutes approximately 50% of the urinary protein excretion in normal subjects and is produced by the cells of the thick ascending loop of Henle and early distal convoluted tubule.[83] THP is not detected by the routine urinalysis techniques and is measured by immunoassay or high-performance liquid chromatography.

THP forms a gel-like core of the hyaline and other urinary casts. However, its role under physiologic conditions is not fully clear. THP may play a protective role against urinary tract infections by binding to *Escherichia coli*, and it may also protect against stone formation.[84,85] Transiently increased medullary echogenicity seen on ultrasound scans in neonates has been attributed to intratubular gelling of THP in presence of low urine pH.[86]

## QUANTIFICATION OF PROTEINURIA

Urine dipstick provides a convenient method of detection of proteinuria and semiquantitative estimation. The test is affected by the urinary concentration and pH. Concentrated urine may give a positive reading even when the daily protein excretion is normal, whereas dilute urine may result in a negative, or only slightly positive reading even in the presence of elevated daily protein excretion. False-positive results may also occur if the urine is highly alkaline, and false-negative results can be seen after ingestion of large doses of ascorbic acid. Twenty-four-hour collection of urine and the urine protein/creatinine ratio are other, more precise methods to quantify proteinuria. These techniques are further discussed in detail in Chapter 3.

> ## KEY POINTS
>
> - Dipstick ( semiquantitative)
> - 24 hour urine collection
> - Urine protein/urine creatinine ratio

Microalbuminuria (MA) denotes urinary excretion of albumin in quantities less than detected by traditional dipstick and is defined as a persistent elevation of urinary albumin excretion of 30 to 300 mg/day.[87] Persistent MA is considered an early indicator of diabetic nephropathy and a harbinger of renal morbidity in patients with diabetes mellitus. Accumulating evidence suggests that MA also correlates with cardiac morbidity and mortality associated with hypertension, and it may reflect an underlying endothelial cell dysfunction in these patients.[88] MA is prevalent in young adult patients with obesity and metabolic syndrome.[89]

> ## KEY POINTS
>
> - MA is an important marker of early renal disease in diabetes mellitus.
> - MA may also be an indicator of cardiovascular morbidity and mortality associated with hypertension.

## EVALUATION OF PROTEINURIA

Proteinuria can be the only, and sometimes an early, indication of renal disease. Consequently, the purpose of investigations in evaluating a patient with proteinuria is to determine whether any renal disease exists. Orthostatic proteinuria (OP) should be ruled out, especially in adolescents, to avoid extensive and expensive investigations. The recommendation of the expert panel of Pediatric Nephrologists constituted by the National Kidney Foundation provides a framework for evaluation of proteinuria in children.[90]

### History

A thorough history, physical examination, and urinalysis provide a clinical foundation for evaluation of patients with proteinuria. The historical aspects to be established are the duration of documented proteinuria, the presence of any symptoms indicative of nephrotic syndrome, a history of any drug intake or exposure to toxins, and evidence of any primary collagen-vascular disorder characterized by rash, fever, joint pains, or any pulmonary symptoms. A family history of any renal disease must be ascertained to determine whether inherited disorders, such as Alport syndrome, need to be considered.

### Physical examination

The purpose of physical examination is to establish blood pressure, evidence of edema, and any clinical manifestations of rash or joint involvement that may indicate vasculitis or collagen-vascular diseases. The respiratory system, including the sinuses, should be examined for any evidence of clinical disease, sinusitis, or polyps, as seen in Wegener granulomatosis (now reclassified as granulomatosis with polyangiitis).

### Laboratory studies

Once proteinuria has been confirmed, and if it is isolated (i.e., no other urinary abnormalities), the first step should be to rule out the possibility of orthostatis proteinuria (OP). In the absence of OP, the patient can be characterized as having "fixed" proteinuria. Figure 9.10 provides an algorithm for laboratory investigations in these patients. The presence of hematuria, in addition to proteinuria, indicates the possibility of glomerulonephritis, and these patients need to be evaluated along the lines previously indicated in Figure 9.4.

## ORTHOSTATIC PROTEINURIA

The term orthostatic proteinuria (OP) or postural proteinuria denotes documentation of proteinuria when the subject is ambulatory and the absence of any proteinuria in the supine posture. OP is more commonly seen in preteens, teenagers, and young adults. The characteristic feature of OP is mild, selective proteinuria that is seen only when the subject is upright.

The prevalence of OP in children is unclear. Some investigators have estimated it to be as high as 50% to 60% of children with proteinuria. In a published report, 91 children who were 6 to 19 years old were evaluated for diurnal variations in protein excretion, and 20% of them had proteinuria that could be characterized as OP.[91] Boys, those more than 10 years of age and with a body mass index greater than the 85th percentile, were more likely to have OP.

> ## KEY POINTS
>
> - OP is common in children.
> - OP may affect 20% to 50% of children diagnosed to have proteinuria.
> - OP may be associated with nutcracker phenomenon.

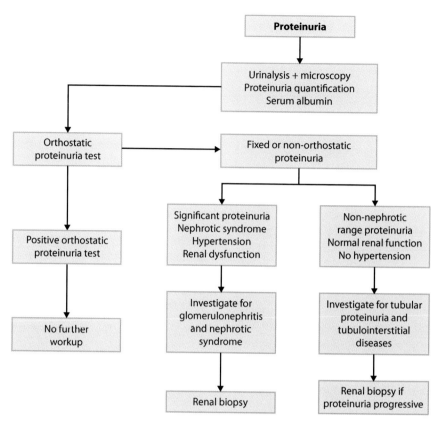

Figure 9.10 Schematic diagram for evaluation of proteinuria.

## Pathogenesis

The cause of OP is unknown. Several case reports have implicated nutcracker phenomenon, or compression of the left renal vein by the aorta and another adjoining vessel, such as the superior mesenteric artery or vertebral artery.[92-94] In an interesting report, a renal transplant donor with OP was noted to have a kink in the renal vein at the time of donor nephrectomy.[94] After nephrectomy, the OP resolved in the transplant donor. The transplant recipient also did not develop proteinuria. The inference drawn by the authors of this report was that a kink in the left kidney was responsible for venous compression in the left renal vein and resultant OP. The role of nutcracker phenomenon as a possible cause of OP was reviewed by Marta et al.[95] The investigators evaluated published studies of OP with imaging data. Of the 229 subjects with OP between the ages of 5.2 to 17 years, these investigators found that 156 or 68% of the subjects had nutcracker phenomenon documented in imaging studies.

## Renal pathologic features

The literature on renal biopsy findings in subjects with OP is scant. Renal biopsy performed in 6 young Air Force recruits with well-documented OP in the in the 1960s demonstrated only slightly thickened basement membranes.[96] A more recent study of 12 subjects with OP demonstrated only subtle and focal increase mesangial matrix, and deposition of

C3 complement and IgG was seen in 10 of the 12 patients.[97] Electron microscopic findings were normal in 11 of the 12 cases, and foot-process fusion was noted in 1 patient. It can be safely concluded that the renal biopsy findings in OP are not profound and may not even be specific.

## Diagnosis

The diagnosis of OP employs a simple test to assess proteinuria during recumbent and upright postures. The principle of the test is to document proteinuria in the upright posture and its absence in recumbent posture. One can obtain differential timed urine collection of 12 h each: while the patient is recumbent and during upright posture. Protein is estimated in each of these urine collections. The diagnosis of OP is established by documenting normal (calculated 24-h) urine protein excretion in the recumbent sample, whereas the upright sample has significant proteinuria.

Alternately, a spot urine collection is obtained after 8 to 10 h of flat overnight rest (first morning void after waking up), and another sample is requested later in the day after 4 to 6 h of ambulation. It is important to remind patients to empty the bladder before sleeping. Both samples of urine are then evaluated for the protein/creatinine ratio. A normal urinary protein/creatinine ratio in the first morning sample (<0.2) and an abnormal protein/creatinine ratio in the afternoon sample suggest OP.

## Prognosis

OP is considered a benign disorder. Rytand and Spreiter[98] provided 50-year follow-up in 6 patients with OP originally diagnosed by Thomas Addis. None of these patients had evidence of renal disease or worsening of their proteinuria. In a 10-year follow-up of 46 Air Force recruits, all were found to have normal renal function, and proteinuria was persistent in 49% cases.[99] Extending these studies to 20 years of follow-up in the same cohort, proteinuria had resolved in all except for 6 cases, and all had normal renal function.[100]

## SCREENING FOR RENAL DISEASE

Although routine urinalysis had been an accepted part of screening for CKD in children previously, the American Academy of Pediatrics no longer recommends routine screening urinalyses.[101,102] Sekhar et al.[103] reported that the cost of each CKD diagnosis by routine urinalysis is $2779.50, thus rendering this screening test to be cost prohibitive. Mass screening for renal disease, with urinalysis as a tool, in school children in Japan and Singapore was also demonstrated to be ineffective.[104,105] Screening of adults in the United States for proteinuria as a marker of CKD was also not found to be cost effective.[106] The American College of Physicians has abandoned urinalysis as screening tool for detection of CKD.[107] Screening of high-risk and selected population groups may result in higher detection rates of renal disease.

## SUMMARY

MH is a relatively common finding in pediatric practice. Evaluation of such patients is generally of low clinical yield and has not been considered cost effective. A higher clinical yield is expected in investigating patients with visible hematuria (GH). All investigations should be focused and conducted within a clinical pathway. Similarly, OP should be ruled out in all children with proteinuria before referral to a pediatric nephrologist. Fixed, or nonorthostatic, proteinuria needs to be investigated for the presence of renal disease and may require a diagnostic renal biopsy.

### Clinical Vignette 9.1

A 15-year-old African-American boy was referred because of persistent proteinuria noted on three separate occasions by his primary care physician. The patient was otherwise asymptomatic. He had no history of swelling of the face of feet or gross hematuria. Physical examination revealed blood pressure of 122/76 mm Hg and was otherwise unremarkable. The primary care physician had obtained the following laboratory studies: 24-h urine protein collection, 520 mg; normal electrolytes; serum creatinine, 1.0 mg/dL; BUN, 22 mg/dL; serum albumin, 4.0 g/dL; total protein, 7.1 g/dL; total cholesterol, 179 mg/dL; complement C3, 94 mg/dL (normal); complement C4, 29 mg/dL (normal). Renal ultrasound findings were normal. Because of the asymptomatic nature of this patient's proteinuria, the diagnosis of orthostatic proteinuria was considered, and a first morning urine for protein and creatinine determination was obtained, which recorded 31/192 = 0.16. The diagnosis of orthostatic proteinuria was confirmed, and the patient was reassured.

### TEACHING POINTS

This case represents a common clinical problem for which children are referred to pediatric nephrologists for consultation. The primary care physician had evaluated the patient extensively and had obtained normal data, except in the 24-h urine protein evaluation. The diagnosis of orthostatic protein was eventually established by the first morning urine protein/creatinine evaluation. If done as the initial evaluation in this asymptomatic patient, urine protein/creatinine could have established the diagnosis, and the expense incurred in the extensive evaluation of this patient could have been avoided. Once orthostatic proteinuria is established, no further evaluations are needed, and the patient can be followed by his or her primary care physician.

In contrast, if this patient did not have orthostatic proteinuria (in other words, if his proteinuria was "fixed"), he would need further evaluation, follow-up, and possibly a renal biopsy. Approximately 30% to 40% patients with focal segmental glomerulosclerosis present clinically with asymptomatic proteinuria, and a biopsy is necessary to confirm the diagnosis in such patients.

## REFERENCES

1. Addis T. The effect of some physiological variables on the number of casts, red blood cells and white blood cells and epithelial cells in the urine of normal individuals. J Clin Invest. 1926;2:417–21.
2. Ingelfinger JR, Davis AE, Grupe WE. Frequency and etiology of gross hematuria in a general pediatric setting. Pediatrics. 1977;59:557.
3. Greenfield SP, Williot P, Kaplan D. Gross hematuria in children: A ten-year review. Urology. 2007;69:166–9.
4. Dodge WF, West EF, Smith EH, et al. Proteinuria and hematuria in school children: Epidemiology and early natural history. J Pediatr. 1976;88:327–47.
5. Vehaskari VM, Rapola J, Koskilnies O, et al. Microscopic hematuria in schoolchildren: Epidemiology and clinicopathologic evaluation. J Pediatr. 1979;95:676–84.

6. Murakami M, Yamamoto H, Ueda Y, et al. Urinary screening of elementary and junior high-school children over a 13-year period in Tokyo. Pediatr Nephrol. 1991;5:50–3.

7. Stapleton FB, Linshaw MA, Hassaneina K, et al. Uric acid excretion in normal children. J Pediatr. 1978;92:911–4.

8. Fairley KF, Birch DF. Hematuria: A simple method for identifying glomerular bleeding. Kidney Int. 1982;21:105–8.

9. Stapleton FB. Morphology of urinary red blood cells: A simple guide to localizing the site of hematuria. Pediatr Clin North Am. 1987;34:561–9.

10. Bergstein J, Leiser J, Andreoli S. The clinical significance of asymptomatic gross and microscopic hematuria in children. Arch Pediatr Adolesc Med. 2005;159:353–5.

11. Feld LG, Meyers KE, Kaplan BS, et al. Limited evaluation of microscopic hematuria in pediatrics. Pediatrics. 1998;102:E42.

12. Stapleton FB. Asymptomatic microscopic hematuria: Time to look the other way? Arch Pediatr Adolesc Med. 2005;159:398–9.

13. Atta MG, Baptiste-Roberts K, Brancati FL, et al. The natural course of microalbuminuria among African Americans with type 2 diabetes: A 3-year study. Am J Med. 2009;122:62–72.

14. Matthew R. Weir. Microalbuminuria and cardiovascular disease. Clin J Am Soc Nephrol. 2007;2:581–90.

15. Vehaskari VM, Rapola J. Isolated proteinuria: Analysis of a school-age population. J Pediatr. 1982;101:661–8.

16. Marks MI, McLaine PN, Drummond KN. Proteinuria in children with febrile illnesses. Arch Dis Child. 1970;45:250–3.

17. Campanacci L, Faccini L, Englaro E, et al. Exercise-induced proteinuria. Contrib Nephrol. 1981;26:31–41.

18. Satchell SC and Braet F. Glomerular endothelial cell fenestrations: An integral component of the glomerular filtration barrier. Am J Physiol Renal Physiol. 2009;296:F947–56.

19. Singh A, Satchell SC, Neal CR, et al. Glomerular endothelial glycocalyx constitutes a barrier to protein permeability. J Am Soc Nephrol. 2007;18:2885–93.

20. Fridén V, Oveland E, Tenstad O, et al. The glomerular endothelial cell coat is essential for glomerular filtration. Kidney Int. 2011;79:1322–30.

21. Ballermann BJ, Stan RV. Resolved: Capillary endothelium is a major contributor to the glomerular filtration barrier. J Am Soc Nephrol. 2007;18:2432–8.

22. Ballermann BJ. Contribution of the endothelium to the glomerular permselectivity barrier in health and disease. Nephron Physiol. 2007;106:19–25.

23. Salmon AHJ, Ferguson JK, Burford JL, et al. Loss of the endothelial glycocalyx links albuminuria and vascular dysfunction. J Am Soc Nephrol. 2012;23:1339–50.

24. Miner JH. Glomerular basement membrane composition and the filtration barrier. Pediatr Nephrol. 2011;26:1413–7.

25. Suh JH, Miner JH. The glomerular basement membrane as a barrier to albumin. Nat Rev Nephrol. 2013;9:470–7.

26. Ramage IJ, Howatson AG, McColl JH, et al. Glomerular basement membrane thickness in children: A stereologic assessment. Kidney Int. 2002;62:895–900.

27. Suleiman H, Zhang L, Roth R, et al. Nanoscale protein architecture of the kidney glomerular basement membrane. eLife 2013;2:e01149.

28. Jarad G, Cunningham J, Shaw AS, et al. Proteinuria precedes podocyte abnormalities in Lamb2 / mice, implicating the glomerular basement membrane as an albumin barrier. J Clin Invest. 2006;116:2272–9.

29. Deen WM. What determines glomerular capillary permeability? J Clin Invest. 2004;114:1412–4.

30. Kanwar YP, Farquhar MG. Anionic sites in the glomerular basement membrane: In-vivo and in-vitro localization to the laminae rarae by cationic probes. J. Cell Biol. 1979;81:137–53.

31. Graham RC, Karnovsky MJ. Glomerular permeability: Ultrastructural cytochemical studies using peroxidases as protein tracers. J Exp Med. 1966;124:1123–34.

32. Tryggvason K. Unraveling the mechanisms of glomerular ultrafiltration: Nephrin, a key component of the slit diaphragm. J Am Soc Nephrol. 1999;10:2440–5.

33. Farquhar MG. The primary glomerular filtration barrier: Basement membrane or epithelial slits? Kidney Int. 1975;8:197–211.

34. Khoshnoodi J, Tryggvason K. Unraveling the molecular make-up of the glomerular podocyte slit diaphragm. Exp Nephrol. 2001;29:355–9.

35. Chugh SS, Kaw B, Kanwar YS. Molecular structure-function relationship in the slit diaphragm. Semin Nephrol. 2003;6:544–55.

36. Greka A, Mundel P. Cell biology and pathology of podocytes. Annu Rev Physiol. 2012;74:299–323.

37. YujiSato, Wharram BL, Lee SK, et al. Urine podocyte mRNAs mark progression of renal disease. J Am Soc Nephrol. 2009;20:1041–52.

38. Wickman L, Afshinnia F, Wang SQ, et al. Urine podocyte mRNAs, proteinuria, and progression in human glomerular diseases. J Am Soc Nephrol. 2013;24:2081–95.

39. Lemley KV. Protecting podocytes: How good do we need to be? Kidney Int. 2012;81:9–11.

40. Brenner BM, Hostetter TH, Humes HD. Glomerular permselectivity: Barrier function based on discrimination of molecular size and charge. Am J Physiol. 1978;234:F455–60.

41. D'Amico G, Bazzi C. Pathophysiology of proteinuria. Kidney Int. 2003;63, 809–25.

42. Chang RLS, Ueki IF, Troy JL et al. Permselectivity of the glomerular capillary wall to macromolecules. II. Experimental studies in rats using neutral dextran. Biophys J. 1975;15:887–906.

43. Deen WM, Bridges CR, Brenner BM, et al. Heteroporous model of glomerular size selectivity: Application to normal and nephrotic humans. Am J Physiol. 1985;249:F374.

44. Rennke HG, Venkatachalam MA. Glomerular permeability: In vivo tracer studies with polyanionic and polycationic ferritins. Kidney Int. 1977;11:44–53.

45. Chang RLS, Deen WM, Robertson CR, et al. Permselectivity of glomerular capillary wall. III. Restricted transport of polyanions. Kidney Int. 1975;8:212–8.

46. Bennett CM, Glassock RJ, Chang RL, et al. Permselectivity of the glomerular capillary wall: Studies of experimental glomerulonephritis in the rat using dextran sulfate. J Clin Invest. 1976;57:1287–94.

47. Rennke, HG, Cotran RS, Venkatachalam MA. Role of molecular charge in glomerular permeability: Tracer studies with cationized ferritins. J Cell Biol. 1975;67:638–46.

48. Guasch A, Deen WM, Myers BD. Charge selectivity of the glomerular filtration barrier in healthy and nephrotic humans. J Clin Invest. 1993;92:2274–82.

49. Bohrer MP, Deen WM, Robertson, J, et al. Influence of molecular configuration on the passage of macromolecules across the glomerular capillary wall. J Gen Physiol. 1979;74:583–93.

50. Venturoli D, Rippe B. Ficoll and dextran vs. globular proteins as probes for testing glomerular permselectivity: Effects of molecular size, shape, charge, and deformability. Am J Physiol Renal Physiol. 2005;288:F605–13.

51. Oliver JO, Moses MJ, Macdowell MC, et al. Cellular mechanisms of protein metabolism in the nephron: The histochemical characteristics of protein absorption droplets. J Exp Med. 1954;99:589–604.

52. Tojo A, Endou H. Intrarenal handling of proteins in rats using fractional micropuncture technique. Am J Physiol. 1992;263:F601–6.

53. Lazzara MJ, Deen WM. Model of albumin reabsorption in the proximal tubule. Am J Physiol Renal Physiol. 2007;292:F430–9.

54. Christensen EI, Birn H. Megalin and cubilin, multifunctional endocytic receptors. Nat Rev Mol Cell Biol. 2002;3:256–66.

55. Verroust PJ, Christensen EI. Megalin and cubilin: The story of two multipurpose receptors unfolds. Nephrol Dial Transplant. 2002;17:1867–71.

56. Christensen EI, Gburek J. Protein reabsorption in renal proximal tubule: Function and dysfunction in kidney pathophysiology. Pediatr Nephrol. 2001;19:714–21.

57. Christensen EI, Devuyst O, Dom G, et al. Loss of chloride channel ClC-5 impairs endocytosis by defective trafficking of megalin and cubilin in kidney proximal tubules. Proc Natl Acad Sci USA. 2003;100:8472–7.

58. Storm T, Emma F, Gesù OB, et al. A patient with cubilin deficiency. N Engl J Med. 2011;364:89–91.

59. Norden AGW, Lapsley M, Igarashi T, et al. Urinary megalin deficiency implicates abnormal tubular endocytic function in Fanconi syndrome. J Am Soc Nephrol. 2002;13:125–133.

60. Lloyd SE, Pearce SH, Günther W, et al. Idiopathic low molecular weight proteinuria associated with hypercalciuric nephrocalcinosis in Japanese children is due to mutations of the renal chloride channel (CLCN5). J Clin Invest. 1997;99:967–74.

61. Zandi-Nejad K, Eddy AA, Glassock RJ, et al. Why is proteinuria an ominous biomarker of progressive kidney disease? Kidney Int Suppl. 2004;66:S76–S89.

62. Amin AP, Whaley-Connell AT, Li S, et al. The synergistic relationship between estimated GFR and microalbuminuria in predicting long-term progression to ESRD or death in patients with diabetes: Results from the Kidney Early Evaluation Program (KEEP). Am J Kidney Dis. 2013:61(Suppl 2):S12–23.

63. Hirst JA, Taylor KS, Stevens RJ, et al. The impact of renin-angiotensin-aldosterone system inhibitors on Type 1 and Type 2 diabetic patients with and without early diabetic nephropathy. Kidney Int. 2012;81, 674–83.

64. Eddy AA. Interstitial nephritis induced by protein-overload proteinuria. Am J Pathol. 1989;135:719–33.

65. Eddy EA, Giachelli CM, Mcculloc L, et al. Renal expression of genes that promote interstitial inflammation and fibrosis in rats with protein-overload proteinuria. Kidney Int. 1995;47:1546–57.

66. Abbate M, Zoja C, Remuzzi G. How does proteinuria cause progressive renal damage? J Am Soc Nephrol. 2006;17:2974–84.

67. Macconi D, Chiabrando C, Schiarea S, et al. Proteasomal processing of albumin by renal dendritic cells generates antigenic peptides. J Am Soc Nephrol. 2009;20:123–30.

68. Zeisberg M, Neilson EG. Mechanisms of tubulointerstitial fibrosis. J Am Soc Nephrol. 2010;21:1819–34.

69. Baines RJ, Brunskill NJ. Molecular interactions between filtered proteins and proximal tubular cells. Nephron Exp Nephrol. 2008;110:e67–e71.

70. Zoja C, Donadelli R, Colleoni S, et al. Protein overload stimulates RANTES production by proximal tubular cells depending on NF-kappa B activation. Kidney Int. 1998;53:1608–15.

71. Reich H, Tritchler D, Herzenberg AM, Kassiri Z, Zhou X, et al. Albumin activates ERK via EGF receptor in human renal epithelial cells. J Am Soc Nephrol. 2005;16:1266–78.

72. Zhuan Cui, Junbao Shi, Yan Liu, et al. Upregulation of soluble epoxide hydrolase in proximal tubular cells mediated proteinuria-induced renal damage. Am J Physiol Renal Physiol. 2013;304:F168–76.

73. Erkan E, Garcia CD, Patterson LT, et al. Induction of renal tubular cell apoptosis in focal segmental glomerulosclerosis: Roles of proteinuria and Fas-dependent pathways. J Am Soc Nephrol. 2005;16:398–407.

74. Zhou W, Marsh JE, Sacks SH. Intrarenal synthesis of complement. Kidney Int. 2001;59:1227–35.

75. Sheerin NS, Sacks SH. Leaked protein and interstitial damage in the kidney: Is complement the missing link? Clin Exp Immunol. 2002;130:1–3.

76. Nangaku M, Pippin J, Couser WG. Complement membrane attack complex (C5b-9) mediates interstitial disease in experimental nephrotic syndrome. J Am Soc Nephrol. 1999;10:2323–31.

77. He C, Imai M, Song H, et al. Complement inhibitors targeted to the proximal tubule prevent injury in experimental nephrotic syndrome and demonstrate a key role for C5b-91. J Immunol. 2005;174:5750–5.

78. Burns WC, Kantharidis P, Thomas MC. The role of tubular epithelial-mesenchymal transition in progressive kidney disease. Cells Tissues Organs. 2007;185:222–31.

79. Kriz W, LeHir M. Pathways to nephron loss starting from glomerular diseases: Insights from animal models. Kidney Int. 2005;67:404–19.

80. Ibrini J, Fadel S, Chana RS, et al. Albumin-induced epithelial mesenchymal transformation. Nephron Exp Nephrol. 2012;120:e91–102.

81. Cook HT. The origin of renal fibroblasts and progression of kidney disease. Am J Pathol. 2010;176:22–4.

82. Humphreys BD, Lin S-J, Kobayashi A, et al. Fate tracing reveals the pericyte and not epithelial origin of myofibroblasts in kidney fibrosis. Am J Pathol. 2010;1:85–97.

83. Serafini-Cessi F, Malagolini N, Cavallone D. Tamm-Horsfall glycoprotein: Biology and clinical relevance. Am J Kidney Dis. 2003;42:658–76.

84. Mo L, Zhu X-H, Huang H-Y, et al. Ablation of the Tamm-Horsfall protein gene increases susceptibility of mice to bladder colonization by type 1-fimbriated Escherichia coli. Am J Physiol Renal Physiol. 2004;286:F795–802.

85. Mo L, Huang H-Y, Zhu X-H, et al. Tamm-Horsfall protein is a critical renal defense factor protecting against calcium oxalate crystal formation. Kidney Int. 2004;66:1159–66.

86. Bouwman A, Verbeke J, Brand M, et al. Renal medullary hyperechogenicity in a neonate with oliguria. Clin Kidney J. 2010;3:176–8.

87. Diabetes and Chronic Kidney Disease Work Group. KDOQI clinical practice guidelines and clinical practice recommendations for diabetes and chronic kidney disease. Am J Kidney Dis. 2007;49(Suppl 2):S1–180.

88. Mahfoud F, Ukena C, Pöss J, et al. Microalbuminuria independently correlates to cardiovascular comorbidity burden in patients with hypertension. Clin Res Cardiol. 2012;101:761–6.

89. Witte EC, Heerspink HJL, de Zeeuw,D, et al. First morning voids are more reliable than spot urine samples to assess microalbuminuria. J Am Soc Nephrol. 2009;20:436–43.

90. Hogg RJ, Portman RJ, Dawn Milliner D, et al. Evaluation and management of proteinuria and nephrotic syndrome in children: Recommendations from a pediatric nephrology panel established at the National Kidney Foundation Conference on Proteinuria, Albuminuria, Risk, Assessment, Detection, and Elimination (PARADE). Pediatrics. 2000;105:1242–9.

91. Brandt JR, Jacobs A, Raissy HH, et al. Orthostatic proteinuria and the spectrum of diurnal variability of urinary protein excretion in healthy children. Pediatr Nephrol. 2010;25:1131–7.

92. Cho BS, Choi YM, Kang HH, et al.: Diagnosis of nutcracker phenomenon using renal Doppler ultrasound in orthostatic proteinuria. Nephrol Dial Transplant. 2001;16:1620–5.

93. Lee SJ, You ES, Lee JE, et al. Left renal vein entrapment syndrome in two girls with orthostatic proteinuria. Pediatr Nephrol. 1997;11:218–20.

94. Devarajan P. Mechanisms of orthostatic proteinuria: Lessons from a transplant donor. J Am Soc Nephrol. 1993;4:36–9.

95. Marta BM, Mazzoni, ML, Simonetti GD, et al. Renal vein obstruction and orthostatic proteinuria: A review. Nephrol Dial Transplant. 2011;26:562–5.

96. Robinson RR, Glover SN, Phillip PJ, et al. Fixed and reproducible orthostatic proteinuria: Light microscopic studies of the kidney. Am J Pathol. 1961;39:405–17.

97. von Bonsdorff M, Tornroth T, Pasternack A. Renal biopsy findings in orthostatic proteinuria. Acta Pathol Microbiol Immunol Scand. 1982;90:11–8.

98. Rytand DA, Spreiter S. Prognosis in postural (orthostatic) proteinuria: Forty to fifty-year follow-up of six patients after diagnosis by Thomas Addis. N Engl J Med. 1981;305:618–21.

99. Thompson AL, Durrett RR, Robinson RR. Fixed and reproducible orthostatic proteinuria. VI. Results of a 10-year follow-up evaluation. Ann Intern Med. 1970;73:235–44.

100. Springberg PD, Garrett LE, Jr., Thompson AL, et al. Fixed and reproducible orthostatic proteinuria: Results of a 20-year follow-up study. Ann Intern Med. 1982;97:516–9.

101. Committee on Practice and Ambulatory Medicine and Bright Futures Steering Committee: Recommendations for preventive pediatric health care. *Pediatrics*. 2007;120:1376.

102. American Academy of Pediatrics. AAP publications reaffirmed and retired. *Pediatrics*. 2011;127:e857.

103. Sekhar DL, Wang L, Hollenbeak CS, et al. A cost-effectiveness analysis of screening urine dipsticks in well-child care. Pediatrics. 2010;125;660–3.

104. Yap HK, Quek CM, Shen Q, et al. Role of urinary screening programs in children in the prevention of chronic kidney disease. Ann Acad Med Singapore. 2005;34:3–7.

105. Murakami M, Hayakawa M, Yanagihara T, et al. Proteinuria screening for children. Kidney Int Suppl. 2005;94:S23–7.

106. Boulware LE, Jaar BG, Tarver-Carr ME, et al. Screening for proteinuria in US adults: A cost-effectiveness analysis. JAMA. 2003;290:3101–14.

107. Qaseem A, Hopkins RH, Jr., Sweet DE, et al. Screening, monitoring, and treatment of stage 1 to 3 chronic kidney disease: A clinical practice guideline from the American College of Physicians. *Ann Intern Med*. 2013;159:835–7.

## REVIEW QUESTIONS

1. Mass screening of children for proteinuria and hematuria is a useful strategy for detection of chronic kidney disease in children.
   a. True
   b. False

2. In a 2-week-old male newborn, parents report that the diaper is occasionally stained red-brown. They are concerned that he has blood in his urine. You reassure the parents with the suggestion that he probably has uric acid crystals in the urine and increasing fluid intake would be helpful. Six weeks later, the patients return, with the symptom that the infant was irritable and that the red-brown staining of the diapers has persisted. Urinalysis of a bagged urine specimen shows no protein or blood. Centrifugation 10 mL of urine shows a large amount of brownish red sediment. Microscopic analysis shows uric acid crystals in the sediment. You would obtain the following investigations:
   a. Urine for spot uric acid
   b. Urine for spot uric acid, spot creatinine
   c. Catheterization of the patient and determining an accurate 24-h urine uric acid
   d. Renal ultrasound, spot urine uric acid, and creatinine

3. Podocyturia and podocytopenia are known to occur in:
   a. Diabetic nephropathy
   b. Focal segmental glomerulosclerosis (FSGS)
   c. Membranous nephropathy
   d. HIV nephropathy
   e. All of the above

4. An 11-year-old white boy developed pink-brown urine following an upper respiratory tract infection. Results of cystoscopy performed in the community hospital were completely normal. His symptoms resolved in about 1 week. Six months later, he again developed fever, nasal stuffiness, and a sore throat, and visible hematuria ensued 2 days later. He was seen in the local emergency department. Urinalysis showed 3+ proteinuria, large (4+) blood, and numerous red blood cell casts in the microscopic examination of the sediment. Serum creatinine, 1.5 mg/dL; BUN, 39 mg/dL; normal electrolytes; ASO titer, normal; C3, 122 mg/dL; C4, 32 mg/dL; ANA, negative. The *least likely* diagnosis is:
   a. Poststreptococcal glomerulonephritis
   b. IgA nephropathy
   c. Thin basement membrane nephropathy
   d. Alport syndrome

5. Proteinuria, by itself, has been proposed to result in tubulointerstitial disease by which of the following mechanisms:
   a. Complement activation
   b. Induction of pro-inflammatory cytokines
   c. Epithelial-mesenchymal transformation
   d. All of the above

6. Mature podocytes can avidly reproduce in case of detachment or loss from the glomerular basement membrane.
   a. True.
   b. False.

7. Terminal hematuria is indicative of:
   a. Urinary tract infection
   b. Balanitis
   c. Posterior urethral or bulbar area lesions
   d. Bladder trauma

8. In the kidneys, cubilin and megalin are involved in:
   a. Proximal tubular phosphate reabsorption
   b. Urinary calcium reabsorption
   c. Reabsorption of urinary albumin and low-molecular-weight proteins
   d. Synthesis of Tamm-Horsfall protein

9. Tubular proteinuria is characterized by:
   a. Failure to reabsorb the low-molecular-weight proteins by the proximal tubular cells
   b. Absence of albumin in the urine protein electrophoresis
   c. Possible assay by determining the microalbumin/creatinine ratio
   d. Detection by a positive dipstick test for urine protein

10. Chloride channel-5 (ClC-5) is required in the reabsorption of tubular albumin at which of the following levels?
    a. Acidification of the endocytosis vesicles and dissociation albumin from the cubilin-megalin receptors complex
    b. Attaching tubular albumin to the cubilin-megalin complex
    c. Transporting of amino acids and dipeptides on the basolateral surface
    d. Transporting the cubilin-megalin complex to the tubular cell surface

## ANSWER KEY

1. b
2. d
3. e
4. a
5. d
6. b
7. c
8. c
9. a
10. a

# Disorders of homeostasis

# Physiology of glomerular filtration

## H. WILLIAM SCHNAPER

The functional unit of the kidney is the *nephron;* each kidney contains approximately 1,000,000 of these structures. Under normal circumstances, the adult human's kidneys filter approximately 150 L/day, more than three times the total body water. Although this system provides a highly efficient means of processing elements dissolved in our fluids, it presents a potential problem of dehydration unless the kidney reabsorbs most of this filtrate. Hence, the nephron has two critical functions: *filtration* and *reabsorption.* Reabsorption is accomplished through a series of highly specific mechanisms that are applied in the renal tubules. Indeed, most of the mass of the kidney is occupied by these structures. Approximately two-thirds of the filtrate is reabsorbed in the proximal tubule (Figure 10.1), with 20% reabsorbed in the loop of Henle and 12% in the distal tubule and cortical collecting duct. This yields 1% of the filtrate in the final urine, or on average approximately 1.5 L/day. How the different parts of the tubule selectively reabsorb elements of the filtrate is the subject of Chapters 11 to 15 of this textbook; this chapter focuses on the regulation of filtration.

## GLOMERULUS

Filtration is accomplished in the *glomerulus,* a structure of capillary loops inside an epithelial capsule. The glomerulus was first described by Marcello Malpighi in the 17th century as a "gland" in the cortical part of the kidney, along with many tubules.[1] Given the kidney's obvious function in producing urine, great controversy raged subsequently regarding whether the glomeruli and tubules were connected. In 1842, William Bowman definitively described such a connection and suggested that the malpighian body was "calculated to favor the escape of water from the blood."[2] Shortly thereafter, Carl Ludwig proposed that hydrostatic pressure is a critical determinant of the passage of water from the glomerular capillary into the urine.[2] Thus, the basic elements of glomerular filtration were drawn conceptually from the renal anatomy.

Like any effectively discriminating filter, the glomerulus has two essential functions: it must permit the passage of certain moieties, and it must restrict the passage of others. The *permissive* function allows the passage of the plasma water and certain, mostly relatively small, substances dissolved within it, from the glomerular capillaries into the urinary space. This property is critical for what we typically consider to be renal function, and its loss is the major determinant of whether renal replacement therapy is required. The *restrictive* function of the glomerulus serves to limit the passage of larger proteins and solid elements (erythrocytes and platelets) into the urine. Its failure does not cause a loss of kidney function as we usually apply the term, but failure of the restrictive component causes significant metabolic derangements such as are seen in the nephrotic syndrome. In addition, the restrictive property is so effective that its failure is a sensitive indicator of pathologic processes in the kidney, through our detection of hematuria or proteinuria. All these disease manifestations are covered in other chapters in this textbook; this chapter is intended to provide a

> ### KEY POINT
>
> The glomerular filter has two key functions: facilitating the passage of small molecules and restricting the passage of larger molecules and solid elements of the blood.

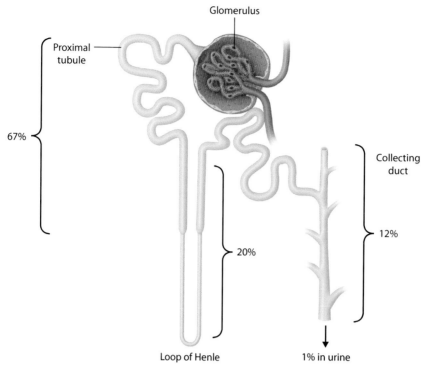

Figure 10.1 Conceptual structure of the nephron. The glomerulus, which comprises approximately 3% of the renal mass, accomplishes filtration. The remaining structure reabsorbs 99% of the glomerular filtrate, thus yielding 1% of the initial filtrate volume as urine. This ratio may change to accommodate variations in fluid intake and environmental conditions, largely accomplished by changes in net reabsorption at the distal tubule. Figures in boxes indicate the approximate fraction of the initial filtrate that is reabsorbed by different parts of the nephron. Note that the distal tubule apposes the entry and exit of the circulation from the glomerulus. (From National Institute of Diabetes and Digestive and Kidney Diseases Image Library, National Institutes of Health, Bethesda, MD.)

perspective on those chapters by focusing on the normal anatomy and physiology of the glomerulus.

## FUNCTIONAL ANATOMY

Unlike the tubule with its myriad, specific transport mechanisms, the glomerulus uses an external force, the cardiac pump, to drive filtration. In the simplest conception, the glomerulus contains a specialized network of capillaries whose walls serve as a filter through which fluid is extruded from the vascular space. This fluid is then collected in the urinary space within the Bowman capsule (Figure 10.2), for subsequent processing by the complex epithelial transport apparatus in the tubule. The endothelial wall of the

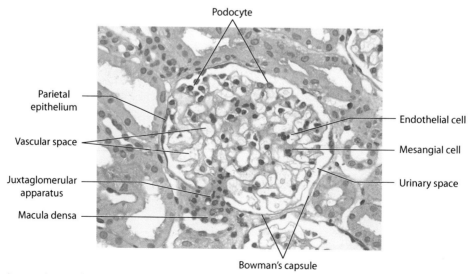

Figure 10.2 The glomerulus. Light microscopy of a glomerulus and surrounding structures. (Courtesy of Shane Meehan, Department of Pathology, University of Chicago, Chicago, IL.)

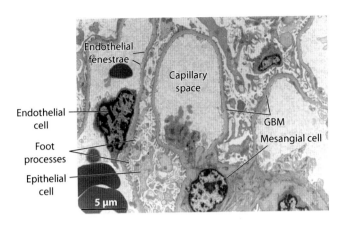

Figure 10.3 The fine structure of the glomerular capillary. Transmission electron micrograph showing the fine structure of the glomerular capillary. Note the discontinuous nature of the endothelial layer resulting from the presence of endothelial fenestrae. GBM, glomerular basement membrane. (Courtesy of Shane Meehan, Department of Pathology, University of Chicago, Chicago, IL.)

Table 10.1 Functions of glomerular cells

**Endothelium**

Fenestrations promote filtration of plasma water
Some restrictive component
Secretion of glycocalyx
Generation of glomerular basement membrane
Regulation of coagulation

**Mesangial cells**

Support structure
Contractile function
Phagocytosis
Cytokine production

**Podocytes**

Regulation of filtration
Generation of slit diaphragm
Generation of glomerular basement membrane
Production of cytokines (VEGF at the slit diaphragm)
Phagocytosis

*Abbreviations:* VEGF, vascular endothelial growth factor.

glomerular capillaries is uniquely fenestrated (Figure 10.3), thereby permitting such passage. The capillaries in each glomerular tuft are supported by a "stalk" consisting of mesangial cells and a small amount of extracellular matrix (ECM) (Figure 10.4), and these vessels are surrounded by podocytes, unique epithelial cells that provide a support structure for the capillaries. Each of these cell types plays an important role in the regulation of glomerular function (Table 10.1).

During filtration, the first barrier encountered by the plasma (Figure 10.5) is the endothelium and its secreted glycocalyx coating composed of glycoproteins, likely derived from both endothelial secretion and plasma molecules.[3] This coating serves to slow the filtration of most molecules and to block the passage of larger ones.[4,5] The next significant component of the filter is the glomerular basement membrane (GBM). This structure, approximately 200 nm thick,[6] is derived from ECM secreted by both the

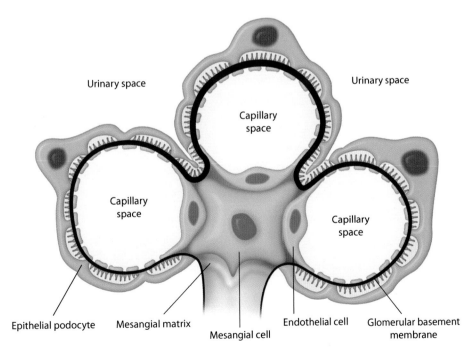

Figure 10.4 The glomerular tuft. An idealized presentation is offered here, with three capillary loops supported by a single cell in the mesangial stalk. Note that a single podocyte may interact with several different capillaries.

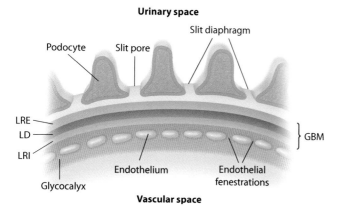

**Urinary space**

Podocyte  Slit pore  Slit diaphragm

LRE
LD  } GBM
LRI

Glycocalyx  Endothelium  Endothelial fenestrations

**Vascular space**

Figure 10.5 The glomerular filtration barrier. During filtration, molecules traverse the fenestrated endothelium with its glycocalyx coating, the glomerular basement membrane (GBM), and the epithelial slit diaphragm. LD, lamina densa; LRE, lamina rara externa; LRI, lamina rara interna. (Modified from Schnaper HW, Kopp JB. Nephrotic syndrome and the podocytopathies: minimal change nephropathy, focal segmental glomerulosclerosis and collapsing glomerulopathy. In: Coffman TM, Falk RJ, Molitoris BM, et al., editors. Schrier's DIseases of the Kidney, 9th ed. Philadelphia: Lippincott Willianms & Wilkins; 2013. p. 1414–521.)

Table 10.2 Podocyte proteins implicated in slit diaphragm form and function

**Cell-Matrix Adhesion Molecules**

$\alpha_3\beta_1$ Integrin
$\beta_4$ Integrin
$\alpha\beta$ Dystroglycan

**Cell-Cell Adhesion Molecules**

Nephrin
P-cadherin
VE-cadherin
ZO1

**Structural Molecules Participating in Slit Diaphragm Stability**

$\alpha$-actinin-4
$CD_2AP$
Fat1
Inverted formin-2 (INF2)
NEPH1-3
Podocalyxin
Podocin

**Signaling Molecules**

Phospholipase C$\epsilon$1
TRPC6 (cation channel)

*Source:* Data from Patrakka J, Tryggvason K. Molecular make-up of the glomerular filtration barrier. Biochem Biophys Res Commun. 2010;396:164–9; and Schnaper HW, Kopp JB. Nephrotic syndrome and the podocytopathies: minimal change nephropathy, focal segmental glomerulosclerosis and collapsing glomerulopathy. In: Coffman TM, Falk RJ, Molitoris BM, et al., editors. Schrier's Diseases of the Kidney, 9th ed. Philadelphia: Lippincott Williams & Wilkins; 2013. p. 1414–521.

endothelium and the podocyte.[7] It provides a significant part of the restrictive component of the glomerular filter, as determined by perfusion studies of decellularized glomeruli, although the cellular layers may be more important for such restriction.[8] The GBM is composed largely of type IV collagen and laminin, with several other ECM components, the two most common being entactin and glycosaminoglycans (GAGs). The GAGs include both heparan sulfate[9] and chondroitin sulfate[10] proteoglycans.

**KEY POINT**

The three main components of the glomerular filter are the fenestrated endothelium and glycocalyx, the GBM, and the epithelial slit diaphragm.

Perhaps the most important restrictive component of the glomerular filter is provided by the podocyte, which, through both its attachment to the GBM and cell-cell adhesions, creates the most selective resistance to the passage of larger molecules. A set of intercellular adhesion molecules, many of which are relatively specific for the podocyte (Table 10.2), creates the *epithelial slit diaphragm* (SD), a porous structure that has been proposed to be the final barrier to molecular passage. The first major component of the SD to be discovered was *nephrin*, a protein with multiple

immunoglobulin-like domains that likely mediate homotypic protein-protein interactions between foot processes of adjacent cells.[11] The result is a latticelike network that provides both a sheetlike structure and openings that permit the transcapillary exit of some molecules.[12] Subsequently, several additional proteins were characterized as contributing to the SD structure, thus stabilizing that structure, fixing it to the cytoskeleton, or regulating cellular signals that promote or inhibit SD functions. These proteins include Neph1, FAT, podocin, $CD_2AP$, $\alpha$-actinin-4, phospholipase C$\epsilon$1, and TRPC6.[13]

Some controversy has arisen regarding whether the SD is the major restrictive component of the glomerular filter. It has been difficult to demonstrate actual trapping of large molecules solely at the level of the SD. Instead, studies using tracers to define the location of macromolecular restriction often have demonstrated localization to the GBM,[14] whereas others have indicated that trapping occurs at both the GBM and the SD.[15] Proponents of a major role for the SD have suggested that other factors such as hemodynamics and electrostatic charge prevent significant macromolecular trapping at the SD (and potential clogging of the slit pore). This issue remains unresolved.

## FACTORS GOVERNING GLOMERULAR FILTRATION

In the average adult, the glomerular filtration rate (GFR) is approximately 100 mL/min. Because we have approximately $10^6$ nephrons, each glomerulus must filter fluid in the range of 10 to 100 nL/min. This estimate was confirmed by studies in Munich-Wistar rats, which have glomeruli on the kidney surface so that direct micropuncture measurements can be taken. These studies were used to determine single nephron GFR (SNGFR). Although there are some minor differences in studies among different rat strains, the data are sufficiently consistent to define principles of glomerular hemodynamics that contribute to determining SNGRF and whole kidney GFR.

## VARIABLES AFFECTING NET FILTRATION

Unlike in the tubule, the "work" of glomerular filtration does not appear to require energy production by the glomerular cells. Instead, the forces governing GFR are supplied by physical properties of the vascular and urinary spaces and their contents. The process of egress across the glomerular filter can be considered as a mass transfer action, not unlike the events that occur with filtration by a dialysis membrane. These events are driven by the Fick laws for the diffusion of mass that, very broadly stated, are as follows: (1) transfer from one compartment to another is driven by gradients; and (2) as equilibration occurs between compartments, the impetus for this transfer decreases. Given that the function of the kidney is to filter the plasma, perfusion of the kidney by the blood stream is a critical force for glomerular filtration, manifested as hydrostatic pressure from within the capillary (Figure 10.6). This pressure is opposed by oncotic

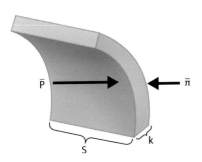

Figure 10.6 Factors governing flux along the glomerular capillary wall. Net hydrostatic pressure (P) is opposed by net oncotic pressure (π). Fluid flux is also a function of the capillary surface available for filtration (S) and the permeability of the filter (k).

pressure resulting from substances that are dissolved in the plasma water. Other forces and factors are mentioned later. This brief discussion is meant to introduce the topic; readers interested in further details are referred to primary sources for more detail.

---

### KEY POINT

The main forces affecting filtration by the glomerulus are blood hydrostatic pressure (outward) and plasma oncotic pressure (inward).

---

Based on the factors that govern glomerular filtration, we can derive a formula that characterizes these factors and can be applied to account for SNGFR. In a single dimension, fluid passage across a point on a capillary wall is proportional to the balance of pressures across the filter at that point. Therefore,

$$J_V \propto P - \pi$$

where $J_V$ represents fluid flux (transfer across the filter), $\propto$ indicates a proportionate relationship, $P$ represents net hydrostatic pressure (outward), and $\pi$ represents net oncotic pressure (inward).

Hydrostatic pressure tends to force fluid out of the capillary, whereas oncotic pressure tends to oppose this movement, so oncotic pressure is subtracted from hydrostatic pressure in this equation. Because the net pressures represent the difference between opposing pressures in the glomerular capillary and in the Bowman space, we can substitute algebraic operations that define these net pressures:

$$J_V \propto (P_{(GC)} - P_{(US)}) - (\pi_{(GC)} - \pi_{(US)})$$

where GC is the glomerular capillary and US is the urinary space.

Because this is a one-dimensional formula, the amount of flux across the capillary in two dimensions must consider the surface area available for filtration, S, so that

$$J_V \propto S[(P_{(GC)} - P_{(US)}) - (\pi_{(GC)} - \pi_{(US)})]$$

Finally, because different filters and membranes have different permeability properties related to thickness, porosity, and other factors, each has a defined hydraulic permeability, k, based on the ability of that particular structure to permit the passage of a fluid. Therefore,

$$J_V = kS[(P_{(GC)} - P_{(US)}) - (\pi_{(GC)} - \pi_{(US)})]$$

Because it is difficult to measure surface area directly, the micropuncturists who defined these relationships inferred both k and S and combined them as $K_f$, so that

$$J_V = K_f[(P_{(GC)} - P_{(US)}) - (\pi_{(GC)} - \pi_{(US)})]$$

Thus, in applying Fick law to glomerular filtration, fluid diffusion across the glomerular filter is determined by the hydraulic permeability of the filter, the surface area available for filtration, and the balance of forces determined by the difference between the net hydrostatic pressure and the net oncotic pressure.

Although this derivation may seem complex, it is critical in considering the application of Fick's second law, which addresses potential changes in this equation resulting from the fact that glomerular filtration represents a dynamic system. Thus, in a child who is dehydrated, $P_{GC}$ may be decreased, lowering SNGFR. This response defines what we call prerenal azotemia. Conversely, under conditions of volume expansion, $P$ may increase, and quite possibly $S$ may be increased by resultant stretching, thereby increasing fluid transfer across the membrane. In another example, a patient who has sepsis, numerous factors involving perfusion pressure ($P$), membrane permeability ($k$), and forces on both sides of the glomerular capillary wall will have significant effects on filtration.

As filtration of the plasma water occurs, and the intact capillary retains protein, the hydrostatic pressure will decrease and oncotic pressure will increase because protein concentration rises as plasma water is lost. Thus, along a hypothetic length of glomerular capillary, the net ultrafiltration pressure will decrease. Theoretically, a point could be reached at which the difference between $P$ and $\pi$ disappears, a point at which the force for ultrafiltration becomes zero and ultrafiltration should cease (Figure 10.7). This point of *filtration equilibrium*[16] would be difficult to demonstrate clinically, but it was critical to the investigators who established the characteristics of glomerular filtration because, by interfering with flow in the proximal tubule, they could cause the pressure in the urinary space to rise to the extent that glomerular filtration ceases. In this way, they could both directly and indirectly measure the forces governing filtration in the glomerulus.

## PHYSIOLOGIC FEEDBACK REGULATING FILTRATION

Of more immediate clinical significance is the concept of *autoregulation*. Because of the importance of $P_{(GC)}$ in SNGFR, a condition in which SNGFR varies directly with systemic blood pressure would be untenable for maintaining steady-state renal function. Instead, autoregulation

### KEY POINTS

- Autoregulation maintains constant pressure for filtration across a span of blood pressures.
- This process is accomplished by both myogenic forces in the vessel wall and active hormonal mechanisms regulating glomerular arteriolar resistance.

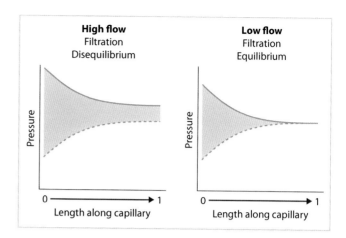

Figure 10.7 Filtration equilibrium. Because of extrusion of plasma water, the outward glomerular capillary hydrostatic pressure (solid line) decreases along the length of an idealized capillary, whereas the increased concentration of protein in the remaining intravascular volume increases the inward force of oncotic pressure (dashed line). Under conditions of high flow, the opposing forces of hydrostatic and oncotic pressure never equalize, so there is a net force for filtration (indicated by shaded area) along the entire length of the capillary. However, under low-flow conditions, the hydrostatic pressure decreases to the extent that, at some point, glomerular capillary hydrostatic pressure equals glomerular capillary oncotic pressure. At this point, there is no net force for filtration, and net flux effectively stops. Any further transfer of solute to the urinary space occurs by diffusion rather than by convection.

maintains $P_{(GC)}$ and SNGFR in a relatively constant manner (Figure 10.8) over a range of at least 40 mm Hg blood pressure.[17] This permits $P_{(GC)}$ to be maintained at a fairly stable value despite moment-to-moment variations in systemic pressure. Autoregulation is effected by a variety of factors, both passive (distensibility of the splanchnic bed, for instance) and active (variations in vascular tone), but the glomerulus benefits from a unique system involving the renin-angiotensin system.[18]

The glomerular circulation is regulated by certain factors that contribute to vasodilation, such as nitric oxide or cyclooxygenase,[19] or vasoconstrictors such as thromboxane

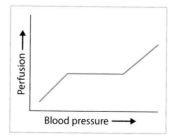

Figure 10.8 Autoregulation. Perfusion pressure and glomerular filtration rate are maintained at a constant value over a range of blood pressures rather than increasing in direct proportion to increases in pressure.

A and 20-hydroxyeicosatetraenoic acid (20-HETE).[20] An important consideration is the regulation of resistance in both the afferent and efferent arterioles of the glomerulus. Because the actual force for filtration is reflected by the drop in blood pressure along the glomerular capillary, the balance between the relative constriction of the two arterioles determines the amount of filtration (Figure 10.9). The net hydrostatic pressure for filtration of fluid is thus determined by the difference in resistance at these points.[21] If arteriolar resistance is very high or very low at both sites, there will be little net filtration pressure (see Figure 10.9). Conversely, constriction of the efferent arteriole but relative relaxation of the afferent arteriole increases filtration.

The distal tubule of the nephron loops back to and touches the vascular pole of the glomerulus, the site of entry and exit of the afferent and efferent arteriole, respectively (see Figure 10.1). Specialized cells in the tubule at this site, termed the *macula densa* (see Figure 10.2), sense distal tubular delivery of solute. Renin produced at this juxtaglomerular apparatus leads ultimately to the production of angiotensin II, a vasoconstrictor that modifies afferent and efferent arteriolar resistance to regulate glomerular capillary blood flow. The rate of tubular fluid flow or the absolute concentration of salt at the macula densa[22,23] determines the level of renin production by the juxtaglomerular apparatus. Vasodilators such as nitric oxide appear to decrease afferent arteriolar resistance preferentially so that, at least at lower levels of renin-angiotensin activity, filtration is increased even in the presence of decreased renal blood flow. Higher levels of renin production constrict both the afferent and efferent vessels sufficiently that glomerular filtration is decreased.[18] In this manner, a feedback system maintains steady production of glomerular ultrafiltrate, somewhat independent of systemic blood pressure but consistent with the potential need to adjust glomerular filtration based on distal delivery of that filtrate. Thus, *tubuloglomerular feedback* regulates glomerular filtration to maintain a balance between glomerular filtration and tubular reabsorption. Other regulators of glomerular flow include vasoconstrictors such as norepinephrine; vasodilators such as histamine, certain prostaglandins, and bradykinin; and molecules that may directly affect $K_f$, such as antidiuretic hormone.

Renal nerve activity has a complex effect on whole organ kidney perfusion and may affect levels of angiotensin activity. However, it does not appear to affect glomerular filtration as strongly as the renin-angiotensin system,[24] and it may influence natriuresis more by altering peritubular blood flow and tubular sodium reabsorption.

## REGULATION OF MACROMOLECULE CLEARANCE

Clearance studies using macromolecules of disperse sizes define a *permselectivity* curve (Figure 10.10), describing the clearance of macromolecules relative to the GFR.[25] Under normal physiologic conditions, such a curve has a sigmoid shape, where clearance of molecules with an effective molecular radius of up to 18 to 20 Å (1.8 to 2 nm) equals the GFR (i.e., such molecules are freely filtered). With increasing size, however, passage of molecules decreases until it is virtually absent at an effective molecular radius of 56 Å.[26] This upper limit defines the functional size of the SD pore and is consistent with studies that have been conducted analyzing the apparent size[27,28] and molecular constitution[12] of the SD. The explanation for the sigmoid curve, rather than an abrupt shutoff of filtration at 56 Å, is straightforward: Once molecules become large enough to interact with the slit pore, even if they are smaller than the pore, they may hit the side of the pore and bounce back into the vascular space, rather than passing through the pore (Figure 10.11).

All molecules, even those that are larger than the apparent molecular size limit of 56 Å, have some likelihood of crossing a semipermeable barrier, by the mechanisms of diffusion and convection. *Diffusion* occurs down a concentration gradient. In the case of protein, the concentration

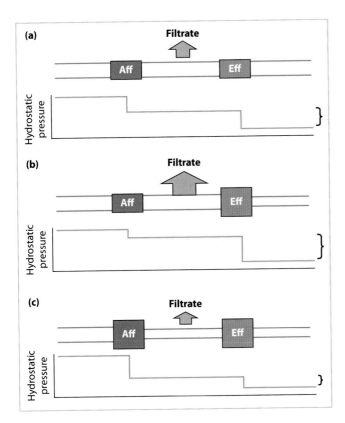

Figure 10.9 Changes in afferent (Aff) and efferent (Eff) glomerular arteriolar resistance modulate the glomerular filtration rate. **(a)** Steady state. **(b)** Increased efferent resistance. **(c)** Increased afferent and efferent resistance. Red and green boxes represent sites of arteriolar smooth muscle where resistance is applied to afferent and efferent arterioles. Box size is proportional to vasoconstrictor tone Brackets show the drop in hydrostatic pressure across the capillary, a major determinant of filtration. The size of the arrow indicates the relative amount of filtrate.

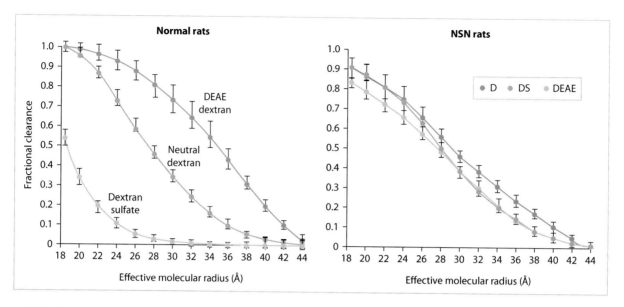

Figure 10.10 Permselectivity curves derived in rats using macromolecules of disperse size. Clearance of molecules at each given size is shown with respect to the clearance of inulin as an indicator of glomerular filtration rate. Note that cations have facilitated clearance at any molecular size, whereas anions have decreased clearance. D, dextran; DEAE, diethylaminoethyl dextran; DS, dextran sulfate. (From Bohrer MP, Bayliss C, Humes HD, et al. Permselectivity of the glomerular capillary wall: facilitated filtration of circulating polycations. J Clin Invest. 1978;61:72–8.)

gradient is so different between the plasma and the urinary space that a small amount of protein always is present in the glomerular filtrate and may appear in the urine. Diffusion accounts for the clearance of large molecules, most commonly when plasma protein concentrations are elevated or filtration equilibrium is reached, as is the case in dehydration. Conversely, *convection* involves the movement of solute along with flow; it sometimes is referred to as "solvent drag." Convection is most likely to increase the amount of protein in the glomerular filtrate with maximal passage of plasma water across the filter, such as occurs in filtration disequilibrium consequent to volume expansion.

broadside). Albumin, which is filtered less than would be anticipated from its size, is a prolate ellipsoid (cigar shaped) and is unlikely to be distensible. Albumin also may be subject to *charge* restrictions. The glycocalyx and the coating of the cells comprising the glomerular filter are negatively charged. Further, the sulfation of GAGs in the GBM contributes to fixed negative charges in the GBM.[30] These electrostatic charges may facilitate the clearance of positively charged macromolecules and inhibit the passage of negatively charged ones[29] (see Figure 10.10). They could play a role in delaying or preventing the passage of some negatively charged proteins, such as albumin, through the glomerular filter, thus accounting for at least some of the restriction

---

### KEY POINTS

- The principal determinant of macromolecular passage through the glomerular filter is steric hindrance (size and shape selectivity).
- Other determinants include electrostatic charge and hemodynamic factors.

---

Several additional factors may influence the passage of macromolecules through the glomerular filter. If the filter has properties of a porous structure, size considerations will be affected by shape and distensibility of the cleared molecule.[29] A long, thin, flexible macromolecule is more likely to pass through a pore than a spherical molecule of the same molecular weight (although this would depend whether the long molecule reached the pore end-on or

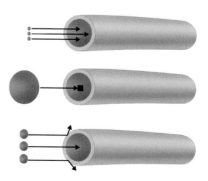

Figure 10.11 Steric hindrance causes a sigmoidal curve in permselectivity. As molecules approach the size where steric hindrance may affect filtration, the macromolecule may strike the edge of a pore in the filter. The larger the molecule, the more likely it is to strike the filter rather than going through the opening.

in clearance of albumin.[26] It has been suggested that this electrostatic hindrance depends not only on the fixed negative charges, but also on the subsequent establishment of a charge gradient across the glomerular filter through a process called "streaming potential,"[31] that acts on larger molecules trapped in the nonlinear flow of the subpodocyte urinary space.[32]

The mechanisms by which the SD is altered to permit the pathologic passage of larger molecules into the urine are discussed elsewhere in this textbook. Briefly, the main cause is likely to be the disruption of podocyte structural integrity. The stability of the SD requires interactions among the cytoskeleton, the cellular adhesion molecules, and accessory molecules that buttress the SD structure and make it relatively rigid. Any change in the interactions among these molecules is likely to cause a change in the size of the slit pore, or even a loss of the diaphragmatic structure, thereby decreasing the restrictive nature of the SD. Loss of charge selectivity may be a maintenance factor for increased clearance of negatively charged molecules in the presence of foot process effacement.[31]

## CELL BIOLOGY OF THE GLOMERULUS

Despite this description of glomerular filtration as a relatively passive process, driven by hydrostatic and oncotic pressure, the three major cells of the glomerulus are active in several ways that contribute to glomerular physiology and function. The capillary endothelium, like all endothelial cells, produces proteins that regulate coagulation and inflammation.[33,34] The podocyte may have phagocytic properties, by absorbing proteins and other molecules such as immunoglobulins that enter the glomerular filter.[35] It serves an important support function in that it helps the capillary resist distending pressure within the vascular space. The loss of the podocyte permits such distention to bring the denuded basement membrane into contact with the Bowman capsule. This contact leads to synechia formation and the extrusion of vascular content directly into the interstitial space, an event implicated by many investigators in the pathogenesis of glomerulosclerosis.[36] Studies have suggested that the podocyte may have a highly mobile phenotype under certain conditions,[37,38] a capability that would futher modulate the podocyte's function in regulating transglomerular passage of macromolecules. Maintenance of the space between podocyte foot processes is essential for optimal glomerular filtration, and foot process effacement may decrease GFR.[39]

The mesangial cell has numerous properties that are similar to those of contractile smooth muscle cells that regulate glomerular perfusion[40] or to those of phagocytic reticuloendothelial cells or inflammatory macrophages,[41-43] although it clearly cannot be characterized as being any one of those cells. The mesangial cell has been described as a pericyte,[44] similar to the Ito cells in the liver. Given its location in an area of the glomerulus where ECM accumulation frequently initiates, the mesangial cell has been considered a critical cell for the synthesis of ECM in glomerulosclerosis.

Communication among the primary cells of the glomerulus represents an important component of glomerular biology. Many investigators propose that vascular endothelial growth factor (VEGF) produced by the podocyte is the stimulus for fenestration of the glomerular endothelial cells.[45] Such a notion appears to contradict the general direction of flow through the glomerular filter, which runs centrifugally from the vascular space toward the urinary space, but more studies suggest that the flow of fluid through the filtration barrier is turbulent rather than streamlined, and paracrine VEGF signaling from the podocyte to the endothelial cell has been implicated in the pathogenesis of transgenic, podocyte-specific VEGF-deletion models.[46] Similarly, proteinuria is a major stimulus of glomerulosclerosis, which appears to initiate in the mesangium. The mechanism by which podocyte dysfunction or proteinuria activates mesangial ECM accumulation is not known, although it is possible that the delivery of large amounts of unanticipated molecules to the ultrafiltrate, inflammation, cell stretch or deformity, altered structure, and abnormal cell-cell communication all may contribute to altered mesangial cell physiology.

Finally, additional cells or cell types reside in the glomerulus. Macrophages are infrequent but present.[47] They appear to have little pathologic significance until normal physiology is perturbed. Additional fibroblasts are likely recruited to the glomerulus from the tubulointerstitium during disease.[48] Attention has focused on the parietal epithelial cells lining the Bowman capsule. It is now thought that these cells, when dedifferentiated, are capable of migrating onto the mesangial stalk to establish or reconstitute the podocyte population.[49]

---

### KEY POINT

The three most important cells of the glomerulus are the podocyte, a specialized epithelial cell; the mesangial cell, a pericyte with contractile and phagocytic properties; and the endothelial cell.

---

### SUMMARY

Together, these cells comprise a complex, synergistic biologic network that plays a critical role in (1) regulating glomerular function, (2) modulating the clearance of solvent and solute from the blood stream, and (3) controlling homeostatic function throughout the kidney. Even a minor disruption of the normal function of these cells can have significant consequences for kidney function and, by extension, total body physiology. The derangements that result are considered more extensively in other chapters of this book.

# REFERENCES

1. Bellomo G. A short history of "glomerulus." Clin Kidney J. 2013;6:250–1.
2. Arendshorst WJ, Gottschalk CW. Glomerular ultrafiltration dynamics: Historical perspective. Am J Physiol. 1985;248:F163–74.
3. Reitsma S, Slaaf DW, Vink H, et al. The endothelial glycocalyx: Composition, functions, and visualization. Pflugers Arch.2007;454:345–59.
4. Ballermann BJ, Stan RV. Resolved: Capillary endothelium is a major contributor to the glomerular filtration barrier. J Am Soc Nephrol. 2007;18:2432–8.
5. Salmon AH, Ferguson JK, Burford JL, et al. Loss of the endothelial glycocalyx links albuminuria and vascular dysfunction. J Am Soc Nephrol. 2012;23:1339–50.
6. Daniels BS, Hauser EB, Deen WM, Hostetter TH. Glomerular basement membrane: In vitro studies of water and protein permeability. Am J Physiol. 1992;262:F919–26.
7. St John PL, Abrahamson DR. Glomerular endothelial cells and podocytes jointly synthesize laminin-1 and -11 chains. Kidney Int. 2001;60:1037–46.
8. Edwards A, Daniels BS, Deen WM. Hindered transport of macromolecules in isolated glomeruli. II. Convection and pressure effects in basement membrane. Biophys J. 1997;72:214–22.
9. van den Heuvel LP, van den Born J, Veerkamp JH, et al. Comparison of heparan sulfate proteoglycans from equine and human glomerular basement membranes. Int J Biochem. 1990;22:903–14.
10. Karasawa R, Nishi S, Suzuki Y, et al. Early increase of chondroitin sulfate glycosaminoglycan in the glomerular basement membrane of rats with diabetic glomerulopathy. Nephron. 1997;76:62–71.
11. Khoshnoodi J, Sigmundsson K, Ofverstedt LG, et al. Nephrin promotes cell-cell adhesion through homophilic interactions. Am J Pathol. 2003;163:2337–46.
12. Wartiovaara J, Ofverstedt LG, Khoshnoodi J, et al. Nephrin strands contribute to a porous slit diaphragm scaffold as revealed by electron tomography. J Clin Invest. 2004;114:1475–83.
13. Patrakka J, Tryggvason K. Molecular make-up of the glomerular filtration barrier. Biochem Biophys Res Commun. 2010;396:164–9.
14. Ghitescu L, Desjardins M, Bendayan M. Immunocytochemical study of glomerular permeability to anionic, neutral and cationic albumins. Kidney Int. 1992;42:25–32.
15. Rennke HG, Cotran RS, Venkatachalam MA. Role of molecular charge in glomerular permeability: Tracer studies with cationized ferritins. J Cell Biol. 1975;67:638–46.
16. Deen WM, Troy JL, Robertson CR, Brenner BM. Dynamics of glomerular ultrafiltration in the rat. IV. Determination of the ultrafiltration coefficient. J Clin Invest. 1973;52:1500–8.
17. Arendshorst WJ, Finn WF, Gottschalk CW. Autoregulation of blood flow in the rat kidney. Am J Physiol. 1975;228:127–33.
18. Kobori H, Nangaku M, Navar LG, Nishiyama A. The intrarenal renin-angiotensin system: From physiology to the pathobiology of hypertension and kidney disease. Pharmacol Rev. 2007;59:251–87.
19. Ichihara A, Imig JD, Navar LG. Cyclooxygenase-2 modulates afferent arteriolar responses to increases in pressure. Hypertension. 1999;34:843–7.
20. Roman RJ. P-450 metabolites of arachidonic acid in the control of cardiovascular function. Physiol Rev. 2002;82:131–85.
21. Arendshorst WJ, Navar LG. Renal circulation and glomerular hemodynamics. In: Coffman TM, Falk RJ, Molitoris BA, et al., editors. Schrier's Diseases of the Kidney, 9th ed. Philadelphia: Lippincott Williams & Wilkins; 2013. p. 74–131.
22. Sipos A, Vargas S, Peti-Peterdi J. Direct demonstration of tubular fluid flow sensing by macula densa cells. Am J Physiol Renal Physiol. 2010;299:F1087–93.
23. Peti-Peterdi J, Harris RC. Macula densa sensing and signaling mechanisms of renin release. J Am Soc Nephrol. 2010;21:1093–6.
24. Johns EJ. Role of the renal nerves in modulating renin release during pressure reduction at the feline kidney. Clin Sci (Lond). 1985;69:185–95.
25. Brenner BM, Hostetter TH, Humes HD. Molecular basis of proteinuria of glomerular origin. N Engl J Med. 1978;298:826.
26. Brenner BM, Hostetter TH, Humes HD. Glomerular permselectivity: Barrier function based on discrimination of molecular size and charge. Am J Physiol. 1978;234:F455.
27. Rodewald R, Karnovsky M. Porous substructure of the glomerular slit diaphragm in the rat and mouse. J Cell Biol. 1974;60:423–33.
28. Gagliardini E, Conti S, Benigni A, et al. Imaging of the porous ultrastructure of the glomerular epithelial filtration slit. J Am Soc Nephrol. 2010;21:2081–9.
29. Bohrer MP, Deen WM, Robertson CR, et al. Influence of molecular configuration on the passage of macromolecules across the glomerular capillary wall. J Gen Physiol. 1979;74:583–93.
30. Latta H, Johnston WH, Stanley TM. Sialoglycoproteins and filtration barriers in the glomerular capillary wall. J Ultrastruct Res. 1975;51:354.
31. Hausmann R, Kuppe C, Egger H, et al. Electrical forces determine glomerular permeability. J Am Soc Nephrol. 2010;21:2053–8.
32. Peti-Peterdi J, Sipos A. A high-powered view of the filtration barrier. J Am Soc Nephrol 2010;21:1835–41.
33. Hertig A, Rondeau E. Role of the coagulation/fibrinolysis system in fibrin-associated glomerular injury. J Am Soc Nephrol. 2004;15:844–53.

34. Iruela-Arispe L, Gordon K, Hugo C, et al. Participation of glomerular endothelial cells in the capillary repair of glomerulonephritis. Am J Pathol. 1995;147:1715–27.

35. Goldwich A, Burkard M, Olke M, et al. Podocytes are nonhematopoietic professional antigen-presenting cells. J Am Soc Nephrol. 2013;24:906–16.

36. Kriz W. The pathogenesis of 'classic' focal segmental glomerulosclerosis-lessons from rat models. Nephrol Dial Transplant. 2003;18(Suppl 6):vi39–44.

37. Hackl MJ, Burford JL, Villanueva K, et al. Tracking the fate of glomerular epithelial cells in vivo using serial multiphoton imaging in new mouse models with fluorescent lineage tags. Nat Med. 2013;19:1661–6.

38. Venkatareddy M, Cook L, Abuarquob K, et al. Nephrin regulates lamellipodia formation by assembling a protein complex that includes Ship2, filamin and lamellipodin. PLoS One. 2011;6:e28710.

39. Bohlin AB. Clinical course and renal function in minimal change nephrotic syndrome. Acta Paediatr Scand. 1984;73:631.

40. Dworkin LD, Ichikawa I, Brenner BM. Hormonal modulation of glomerular function. Am J Physiol. 1983;244:F95–104.

41. Kaur H, Chien A, Jialal I. Hyperglycemia induces Toll like receptor 4 expression and activity in mouse mesangial cells: Relevance to diabetic nephropathy. Am J Physiol Renal Physiol. 2012;303:F1145–50.

42. Merkle M, Ribeiro A, Koppel S, et al. TLR3-dependent immune regulatory functions of human mesangial cells. Cell Mol Immunol. 2012;9:334–40.

43. Suwanichkul A, Wenderfer SE. Differential expression of functional Fc-receptors and additional immune complex receptors on mouse kidney cells. Mol Immunol. 2013;56:369–79.

44. Schlondorff D, Banas B. The mesangial cell revisited: No cell is an island. J Am Soc Nephrol. 2009;20:1179–87.

45. Ballermann BJ. Contribution of the endothelium to the glomerular permselectivity barrier in health and disease. Nephron Physiol. 2007;106:19–25.

46. Sison K, Eremina V, Baelde H, et al. Glomerular structure and function require paracrine, not autocrine, VEGF-VEGFR-2 signaling. J Am Soc Nephrol. 2010;21:1691–701.

47. Lefkowith JB, Schreiner G. Essential fatty acid deficiency depletes rat glomeruli of resident macrophages and inhibits angiotensin II–induced eicosanoid synthesis. J Clin Invest. 1987;80:947–56.

48. Strutz F, Zeisberg M. Renal fibroblasts and myofibroblasts in chronic kidney disease. J Am Soc Nephrol. 2006;17:2992–8.

49. Romagnani P. Parietal epithelial cells: Their role in health and disease. Contrib Nephrol. 2011;169:23–36.

## REVIEW QUESTIONS

1. During glomerular filtration, the passage of larger molecules is restricted by
   a. The glycocalyx
   b. The glomerular basement membrane
   c. The epithelial slit diaphragm
   d. All of the above
2. The podocyte is a differentiated cell that provides a static barrier to filtration.
   a. True
   b. False
3. Increase in which of the following does *not* increase glomerular filtration?
   a. Efferent arteriolar resistance
   b. Glomerular capillary hydrostatic pressure
   c. Glomerular capillary oncotic pressure
   d. Glomerular capillary blood flow
   e. $K_f$
4. Which of the following does *not* increase macromolecular clearance by the glomerulus?
   a. Fever
   b. Shock
   c. Flexible molecules
   d. Hypertrophy
5. Fenestration of the glomerular endothelium is maintained in part by production of
   a. VEGF
   b. TGF-β
   c. COX-2
   d. Endothelin
   e. Glycosaminoglycans

## ANSWER KEY

1. d
2. b
3. c
4. b
5. a

# Sodium and volume homeostasis

## MICHEL BAUM

This chapter will discuss how the kidney functions to maintain a relatively constant extracellular fluid volume and electrolyte composition despite the fact that our intake of salt and water can vary dramatically from day to day. The normal homeostatic mechanisms that preserve a constant *milieu interior* will be presented. The pathophysiology of disturbances in sodium ($Na^+$) composition will be discussed to provide a better understanding of common clinical problems encountered in pediatrics. Salient differences in $Na^+$ handling between the adult and neonatal kidney will also presented.

## BODY FLUID COMPOSITION

Of the weight of an average child, 60% is composed of water, which is distributed between the intracellular and extracellular fluid compartments. As a neonate, 70% of our weight is water, and the fraction of our body weight that is water decreases as we age. Adipose tissue has only 10% water content compared to most organs, which contain 70% to 80% water, and thus excess fat reduces the percentage of body weight that is water. The concept of body composition and maintenance of fluid and electrolyte homeostasis is easily appreciated if we separate these compartments as is shown by the beaker filled with fluid in Figure 11.1. The intracellular compartment comprises 60% of our total body water, with the extracellular compartment making up approximately 40%. The extracellular fluid compartment is predominantly interstitial fluid that bathes cells. A small component of extravascular fluid is in the cerebrospinal fluid, peritoneal and pleural fluid, intraorbital fluid, lymph, and fluid in joint spaces. The intravascular compartment is only one fourth of the extracellular fluid volume. Thus, only approximately 7% to 10% of our total body water is intravascular. Maintenance of the volume and composition of the intravascular fluid space is critical for survival.

The composition of the intracellular and extracellular fluid volume is quite different. The extracellular fluid contains primarily the electrolytes that we are familiar with by measuring serum chemistries. The $Na^+$ concentration in extracellular fluid is 138 mEq/L, which is balanced by chloride anions and to a lesser extent bicarbonate. The electrolyte composition of the intravascular space is comparable to that of the interstitial fluid. In fact, there is a circulation of fluid across the capillary wall because of the hydrostatic pressure on the afferent end causing fluid egress. In the more distal end of capillaries, the hydrostatic pressure decreases as the protein oncotic pressure increases, which results in fluid movement from the interstitial space to the capillary. The forces depicting capillary fluid movement are shown in Figure 11.2.

### KEY POINTS

- Of a child's body weight, 60% is composed of water.
- Intracellular compartment comprises 60% of total body water.
- Extracellular fluid is mostly in the interstitial space.

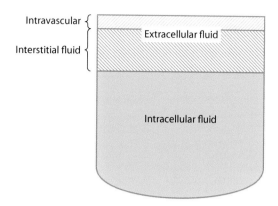

Figure 11.1 Beaker depicting the body fluid compartments. Sixty percent of our body is water. Sixty percent of total body water is in the intracellular compartment, and 40% is in the extracellular fluid compartment. Only 25% of the extracellular fluid compartment is intravascular, the rest being in the interstitial compartment.

The intracellular fluid composition is predominantly made up of potassium (140 mEq/L), whose charge is balanced predominantly by phosphate and negatively charged proteins. The sodium and chloride concentrations inside cells are negligible. The high intracellular potassium and low intracellular sodium concentration is maintained by the Na⁺-K⁺-ATPase on cell membranes. The separation of the electrolytes between cells and the extracellular fluid space is also maintained by the fact that cell membranes are virtually impermeable to electrolytes. Cells have a water channel designated aquaporin 1 that allows free movement of water between the intracellular and extracellular fluid volume. Thus, the osmolality, which is a measure of the number of particles per unit volume, is the same in the intracellular and extracellular fluid spaces.

## CONCEPT OF MAINTENANCE FLUIDS

At this point we will turn back to our beaker of fluid in Figure 11.1 and discuss the concept of fluid and electrolyte balance and administration of maintenance fluids and electrolytes. Maintenance fluids replace the fluids and electrolytes that are normally lost when we are euvolemic under steady-state conditions. Maintenance fluids are often prescribed using the formula shown in Table 11.1.

We administer 1/2 normal saline with 20 mEq/L potassium chloride (KCl) to replace normal losses and maintain the composition of sodium and water unchanged under a basal state. Administration of maintenance fluids replaces the fluid losses from skin and respiration, which is known as *insensible water loss* because we do not realize we are losing this fluid, unlike losses that we know we are having from urine and stool. Insensible water losses are usually 25% of the fluid that is administered using the

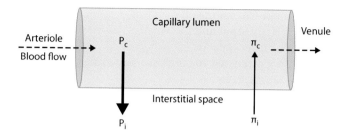

Figure 11.2 Starling forces in the capillary bed. The capillary hydraulic pressure (Pc), on the arterial end of the capillary is higher than the interstitial hydraulic pressure (Pi) and favors movement of fluid from the capillary into the interstitial space. Capillary oncotic pressure (Πc), derived from serum albumin, is higher than interstitial oncotic pressure (Πi), which retards the movement of fluid out of the capillary and into the interstitium. Under normal conditions, the summation of the hydraulic and oncotic forces favors a small movement of fluid (and sodium) out of the capillary into the interstitium. At the venous end the hydraulic pressure is lower and the oncotic pressure has increased as a result of the egress of fluid. The net result is the absorption of interstitial fluid back into the capillary. Some of the remaining interstitial fluid is returned into the general circulation via the lymphatics.

"maintenance" formula. To simplify things, let us take our beaker and fill it to exactly 1 L with 140 mEq/L sodium chloride (NaCl). We come back the next day and find that the volume has decreased to 990 mL and the sodium concentration has increased by 1%. The maintenance for that beaker is 10 mL of water per day. Now let us poke a hole in the beaker and have it drip out 100 mL of 140 mEq/L a day. Maintenance for this new beaker is 10 mL of water for insensible evaporative losses and 100 mL of 140 mEq/L NaCl to replace the visible losses. We are like this beaker. If a patient has no kidneys, it would be necessary to just replace the insensible water losses from skin and respiration (stool losses are negligible). If the patient has kidneys, we go back to our formula—which is a good estimate of the losses of urine for a euvolemic child. If we are dealing with a patient who has impaired renal function, for example, we

Table 11.1 Daily maintenance fluid and solute requirement

| Body weight | Fluid | Sodium | Potassium |
|---|---|---|---|
| 1–10 kg | 100 mL/kg | 5 mEq Na/100 mL | 2 mEq K/100 mL |
| 11–20 kg | 1000 mL+50 mL/kg for each kg > 10 kg | 5 mEq Na/100 mL | 2 mEq K/100 mL |
| > 20 kg | 1500 mL+20 mL/kg for each kg > 20 kg | 5 mEq Na/100 mL | 2 mEq K/100 mL |

can estimate the maintenance for that patient by measuring the urine output and the electrolytes in the urine and adding the insensible water loss to that volume. Note that we have not discussed volume depletion or ongoing losses; this will come later. So when does one use maintenance fluids? Maintenance intravenous fluids should be administered in a euvolemic patient who is not allowed to eat or drink because of an impending procedure—for example, to keep the patient euvolemic. This is a rare event. Under almost all circumstances when we administer intravenous fluids, the patient will be volume depleted and it is usually safer to administer isotonic normal saline.[1]

---

### KEY POINT

Volume-depleted patients should initially receive isotonic fluid replacement.

---

## RENAL REGULATION OF SODIUM

The glomerulus produces an ultrafiltrate of plasma that consists of an essentially protein-free solution with composition identical to that of blood. The adult kidney filters 150 L of fluid per day and delivers this fluid to the renal tubules, where, under normal circumstances, 99% of this fluid is reabsorbed.

The glomerular filtration rate (GFR) is regulated by changes in the relative resistance of the afferent and efferent arterioles. Under conditions of significant volume depletion it is desirable to decrease sodium excretion. In addition to an augmentation in sodium absorption, as described later, the increase in sympathetic nerve activity and angiotensin II secretion results in an increase in both efferent and afferent arteriolar vasoconstriction, as well as contraction of glomerular mesangial cells, which decreases the filtration surface area. These coordinated events result in a decrease in GFR and decrease in the delivery of salt to the kidney. The opposite can occur during volume expansion.

The renal tubules selectively reabsorb the filtered solutes that are needed by the organism while leaving waste products to be excreted in the urine. In addition to this filtration and absorption system, the kidney also secretes many organic anions and cations via specific transporters to increase the efficiency of removal of some protein-bound solutes that are not filtered. Diagrams of the nephron and the transporters involved in sodium and potassium reabsorption are shown in Figure 11.3.

The basic mechanism for sodium absorption by the kidney is the same in every nephron segment.[2] The sodium-transporting cells along the nephron have a basolateral $Na^+$-$K^+$-ATPase that generates an intracellular sodium concentration that is lower (~10 mEq/L) and an intracellular potassium concentration that is higher (~140 mEq/L) than that of the extracellular fluid. The $Na^+$-$K^+$-ATPase transports three sodium ions out of the cell for each two potassium ions it pumps into the cell. The fuel for this process is adenosine triphosphate (ATP). The ion composition gradient between the intracellular and extracellular compartments generated by the $Na^+$-$K^+$-ATPase and the basolateral potassium channel results in a negative potential difference of approximately –60 mV. The low intracellular sodium concentration and the large negative potential difference provide a driving force for apical sodium entry from the tubular lumen into the cell. Thus, most solute transport in the kidney is either directly or indirectly linked to the absorption of sodium. For example, glucose is reabsorbed from the luminal fluid by the proximal tubule via a sodium-dependent process. The energy for glucose absorption is the low intracellular sodium and the negative potential difference generated by the $Na^+$-$K^+$-ATPase. Glucose leaves the cell across the basolateral membrane by facilitated diffusion down its concentration gradient.

## PROXIMAL TUBULAR SODIUM REABSORPTION

The proximal tubule is the work horse of the kidney, where the bulk of reabsorption occurs. The distal nephron is where the fine-tuning occurs. The proximal tubule receives the ultrafiltrate from the glomerulus and reabsorbs approximately 60% of the filtered salt and water filtered in an isosmotic fashion. The proximal tubule reabsorbs all of the filtered glucose and amino acids and the vast majority of the filtered phosphate. Although the proximal tubule is almost 10 mm long, most of the filtered glucose and amino acid absorption occurs in the first 2 mm.[3,4] The proximal tubule also reabsorbs 80% of the filtered bicarbonate and 60% of the filtered chloride.[3] Approximately two-thirds of bicarbonate is reabsorbed via a luminal $Na^+$-$H^+$ exchanger and one-third is via a proton pump.[5,6] The secretion of a proton by either of these two mechanisms results in the formation of carbonic acid ($H_2CO_3$), which dissociates into carbon dioxide ($CO_2$) and water ($H_2O$) with the aid of carbonic anhydrase that is present in the lumen. The $CO_2$ diffuses into the proximal tubule cell and reassociates with $H_2O$ and with the help of carbonic anhydrase, which is also in the cytoplasm of the proximal tubule. The $H_2CO_3$ dissociates back into a proton, which is once again secreted across the apical membrane while the cellular bicarbonate is transported across the basolateral membrane via a $Na(HCO_3)_3$ cotransporter.[7]

The preferential reabsorption of organic solutes and bicarbonate leaves the latter parts of the proximal tubule devoid of organic solutes and with a higher luminal chloride and lower luminal bicarbonate than levels in the peritubular plasma.[2,4] Stated another way, the luminal fluid of the proximal tubule becomes almost isotonic normal saline. This

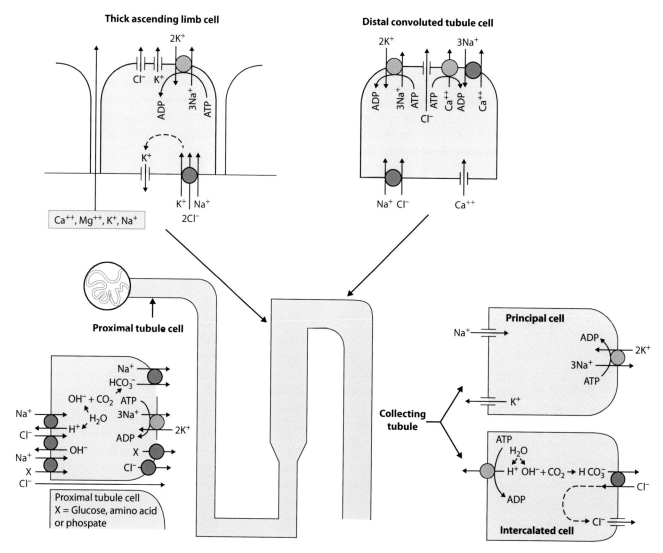

Figure 11.3 Diagram of the nephron showing the transporters present in each nephron segment responsible for NaCl transport.

change in luminal fluid composition provides a gradient for bicarbonate to move from the peritubular plasma into the tubular lumen and chloride to move from the lumen into the peritubular plasma. Because chloride is far more permeable than bicarbonate, the movement of this anion generates a lumen-positive potential that provides a driving force for sodium to move across the paracellular pathway into the peritubular plasma.[4] Thus, the change in solute composition, which occurs in the early proximal tubule, generates a driving force for NaCl absorption without the additional expenditure of energy. Approximately half of NaCl absorption is passive and paracellular.[8] The other half of NaCl transport is active and transcellular. It is mediated by the parallel operation of the $Na^+$-$H^+$ exchanger, which is responsible for bicarbonate reabsorption in the early proximal tubule, and a $Cl^-$-base exchanger results in the net absorption of NaCl and secretion of proton and a base.[9] The nature of the base is unclear. There is evidence that it may be a hydroxyl ion, in which case one $H_2O$ molecule would be secreted for each

NaCl absorbed or a bicarbonate ion, which would then be reabsorbed.[8,10] There is also evidence that the base is a formate molecule, in which case formic acid would be generated and reabsorbed (or recycled) back into the cell.[9]

The coordination between glomerular filtration and proximal tubule reabsorption, where the rate of proximal tubule reabsorption compensates for changes in glomerular filtration, is termed *glomerular-tubular balance*. Glomerular-tubular balance buffers the distal delivery of salt with changes in GFR, preventing a flood of salt with volume expansion with an increase in GFR and the opposite compensation with volume depletion.

Proximal tubule transport is modulated, in part, by peritubular capillary physical factors or Starling forces.[11] The peritubular capillary hydrostatic pressure opposes net proximal tubular sodium reabsorption, and the peritubular capillary oncotic pressure promotes reabsorption. The filtration fraction is the fraction of the renal blood flow filtered, which is regulated predominantly by the resistance of the efferent artery. In the face of volume contraction there is an increase in filtration fraction by preferential contraction of the efferent arteriole to maintain a nearly normal GFR. The fluid entering the peritubular capillaries will have a lower hydrostatic pressure and higher oncotic pressure than under euvolemic conditions, which favors proximal tubule reabsorption. The opposite occurs in volume expansion, which decreases proximal tubule reabsorption.

## SODIUM REABSORPTION IN THE LOOP OF HENLE

The thin limbs of the loop of Henle are able to reabsorb NaCl without expending energy.[2] The thin descending limb is impermeable to NaCl and highly permeable to water. Because the thin limb traverses the hypertonic medulla, water is abstracted and the luminal fluid becomes highly concentrated. At the bend of the loop the permeability properties of the tubule change drastically. The thin ascending limb is impermeable to water and highly permeable to both urea and NaCl. Thus, the concentrated fluid that is progressing upward into a less hypertonic environment has a gradient for NaCl and urea to diffuse out of the lumen into the medullary interstitium. This results in net NaCl absorption and helps generate a hypertonic medulla.

The thick ascending limb reabsorbs approximately 25% of the filtered NaCl. This segment is impermeable to water; thus, this thick ascending limb is in part responsible for creating a hypertonic medulla for urinary concentration. The thick ascending limb is also important for urinary dilution because the fluid that leaves this segment is hypotonic to serum. The apical membrane has a $Na^+$-$K^+$-$2Cl^-$ cotransporter that is inhibited by furosemide and bumetanide. This transporter results in the electroneutral absorption of sodium, potassium, and chloride; the two chloride ions balance the two positive charges from sodium and potassium, so the lumen of this segment is positive because there is an apical potassium channel. Some of the potassium reabsorbed by the $Na^+$-$K^+$-$2Cl^-$ transporter is secreted across the apical membrane into the lumen via this potassium channel. This lumen positive potential is quite important because it generates the driving force for the paracellular absorption of magnesium and calcium in this segment. The paracellular pathway in this segment is quite unique in that it is very permeable to cations. Thus, administration of loop diuretics not only results in a decrease in NaCl absorption but the enhanced excretion of magnesium and calcium, as well as other cations. Sodium, which enters the thick ascending limb leaves via the $Na^+$-$K^+$-ATPase, and the chloride exits the basolateral membrane by either a KCl cotransporter or a chloride channel. Mutations in the $Na^+$-$K^+$-$2Cl^-$ cotransporter, the apical potassium channel (renal outer medullary potassium [ROMK] channel), or the basolateral chloride channel give rise to Bartter syndrome, an inherited familial disease characterized by hypokalemic metabolic alkalosis and associated with elevated renin and aldosterone levels secondary to chronic volume depletion.[12,13] Catecholamines, vasopressin, and renal nerves increase sodium transport in the thick ascending limb.[14,15]

## DISTAL CONVOLUTED TUBULE

The distal convoluted tubule reabsorbs approximately 10% of the filtered sodium by a luminal electroneutral NaCl cotransporter. The NaCl cotransporter is inhibited by thiazide diuretics. All cases of Gitelman syndrome are due to an inactivating mutation of this transporter.[12,16,17] Both the thick ascending limb and the distal convoluted tubule reabsorb salt but are impermeable to water. The osmolality of the fluid that leaves the distal convoluted tubule is 50 mOsm/kg water. If vasopressin (antidiuretic hormone [ADH]) is not secreted to increase the permeability of the collecting tubule to water, the final urine will have an osmolality of 50 mOsm/kg water. In addition to the reabsorption of NaCl, the distal convoluted tubule also reabsorbs a substantial amount of calcium. Unlike in the thick ascending limb, however, the reabsorption of calcium is transcellular. Inhibition of the NaCl cotransporter with thiazide diuretics results in an increase in renal calcium absorption. Thus, whereas loop diuretics cause an increase in calcium excretion, thiazide diuretics decrease calcium excretion. This segment also is responsible for transcellular magnesium reabsorption. Thiazide diuretics result in a substantial amount of magnesium wasting. Sodium transport in the distal convoluted tubule is augmented by angiotensin II and catecholamines.[18,19]

## FINE-TUNING THE URINE CONTENT: THE COLLECTING TUBULE

The collecting tubule is the final segment that adjusts the composition of the urine before urinary excretion. Although this segment reabsorbs only 1% to 3% of the filtered sodium, the collecting tubule nonetheless plays a critical role in regulating salt transport.[2] Sodium is reabsorbed by principal cells in this segment via an apical epithelial sodium channel (ENaC) (Figure 11.3). This leaves the lumen with a negative potential difference compared to the cell. This potential difference provides a driving force for potassium secretion, proton secretion, or the paracellular reabsorption of chloride. The sodium channel is regulated by aldosterone, which causes the sodium channel to insert into the apical membrane, and thus with aldosterone secretion there will be an increase in sodium absorption and potassium or proton secretion. Patients with Liddle syndrome have an overabundance of sodium channels on the apical membrane of the collecting duct, resulting in hypertension and hypokalemic metabolic alkalosis. The sodium channel is inhibited by the diuretics amiloride and triamterene. These diuretics cause an increase in serum potassium because they decrease the lumen negative potential that augments potassium secretion. Sodium absorption in this segment is primarily regulated by aldosterone, which increases the number of ENaC transporters on the apical membrane. Activity of the basolateral $Na^+$-$K^+$-ATPase is also increased by aldosterone, which lowers intracellular sodium and provides a greater driving force for tubular sodium reabsorption. Vasopressin also increases the apical sodium transport, promoting insertion of ENaC in the apical membrane.

Whether the urine is concentrated or dilute compared to blood depends on the presence or absence of vasopressin (ADH). As noted, in the absence of vasopressin the hypotonic urine formed in the thick ascending limb and distal convoluted tubule will be excreted with an osmolality of 50 mOsm/kg water. However, in the presence of vasopressin, water channels (designated aquaporin 2) are shuttled from the cytoplasm into the apical membrane.[20] This increases the permeability of the apical membrane for water. There are also water channels on the basolateral membrane (designated aquaporin 3 and 4) for water to exit the cell. The interstitium is quite hypertonic because the accumulation of salt and urea via mechanisms discussed previously and osmotic equilibration occur. The urine of humans can be concentrated to an osmolality of 1200 mOsm/kg water. This pales by comparison to that of desert rodents, which have very long loops of Henle and can concentrate urine to over 3000 mOsm/kg water.

---

## KEY POINT

During postnatal development there is an increase in the abundance of most renal transporters.

---

## SOLUTE AND WATER TRANSPORT BY THE NEONATAL KIDNEY

The GFR of an adult is approximately 100 mL/min/1.73 $m^2$, whereas that of a term newborn is 2 mL/min. Even if the GFR for an adult's body surface area is factored, the neonate has a GFR of 30 mL/min/1.73 $m^2$. Premature neonates have an even lower GFR. The maturational increase in GFR occurs at the same rate if the baby is still in the womb or is born prematurely.[21,22] The GFR increases to adult values, corrected for surface area, by approximately 12 months of age. The increase in GFR is due to several factors. There is an increase in blood flow to the kidneys, an increase in glomerular filtration pressure, and, if the neonate is born before 34 weeks of gestation, an increase in glomerular number. The most important factor responsible for the postnatal increase in GFR by far is the increase in glomerular capillary surface area with maturation followed by the developmental increase in ultrafiltration pressure.

The principles discussed for solute transport in the adult tubule pertain to the neonate as well. This section will focus on the major differences between the adult and neonatal kidney. The driving force for most active solute transport remains the low intracellular sodium concentration and the negative cell potential difference. The $Na^+$-$K^+$-ATPase generates this low intracellular sodium and potential difference, but the activity of the pump is less in each nephron segment in neonates compared to in adults.[24–26] The lower activity of the pump parallels lower solute transport in each nephron segment in the neonate compared to in the adult.

## NEONATAL PROXIMAL TUBULAR FUNCTION

The maturation of the neonatal proximal tubule keeps pace with the developmental increase in GFR, known as glomerular-tubular balance. Glomerular-tubular balance matches GFR to tubular reabsorption, as discussed previously. The neonatal proximal tubule reabsorbs all of the filtered glucose, the amino acids, and most of the filtered bicarbonate. There are some significant differences that should be noted. First, whereas glomerular-tubular balance is maintained in term neonates, this is not true of premature neonates born before 34 weeks of gestation, who often have proximal tubules that are not able to reabsorb the solutes delivered by glomerular filtration and thus have apparent Fanconi syndrome with glucosuria, amino aciduria, and renal tubular acidosis.[21] Although the rate of all transporters studied is less in the neonate than in the adult, there is one exception. The rate of phosphate transport is higher in the neonatal proximal tubule than in the adult.[27–30] There is an isoform of the apical sodium-phosphate cotransporter in the neonatal proximal tubule responsible for the high rates of phosphate transport, which has very low expression in the adult.[30]

Eighty percent of bicarbonate reabsorption occurs in the proximal tubule, mediated by the $Na^+$-$H^+$ exchanger, which is designated NHE3 in adults. In neonates there is virtually no NHE3 protein or messenger RNA (mRNA) present, but nonetheless there is $Na^+$-$H^+$ exchanger activity.[31] In neonates the predominant $Na^+$-$H^+$ exchanger is NHE8.[32,33] An isoform switch from NHE8 to NHE3 occurs at the time of weaning that is due to the increase in glucocorticoids and thyroid hormone that occurs at that time.[34,37] In the adult proximal tubule the $H^+$-ATPase accounts for one third of proton secretion in the adult segment; however, there is no $H^+$-ATPase activity in the neonatal proximal tubule.[5,6] Thus, not only are there quantitative differences in transport during postnatal maturation, but there are also differences in some of the transporters responsible for neonatal transport. Approximately 60% of the filtered NaCl is reabsorbed by the proximal tubule in the adult. In the adult, NaCl transport from the lumen to the blood is via both transcellular and paracellular mechanisms; however, the permeability of chloride, although high in the adult segment, is zero in the neonate and thus there is no passive chloride transport.[38,39] Finally, water transport deserves note. The abundance of aquaporin 1 is less in the neonate than in the adult segment; however, the permeability of water is actually higher in the neonate.[40] This is due to the fact that the neonatal proximal tubule cytoplasm offers less resistance to water flow than that of the adult segment.

## DISTAL NEPHRON

The distal nephron segments do not have an isoform switch for salt transporters, as has been described in the proximal tubule, but all segments studied have a lower rate of transport in neonates compared to that in adults. The thick ascending limb has been shown to have a lower rate of sodium reabsorption in the neonate than in the adult, which is one factor in the limited capacity of the neonate to produce concentrated urine.[41] The human neonate can concentrate urine to an osmolality of 600 mOsm/kg water. Finally, the neonatal cortical collecting duct has essentially no apical sodium channel and $K^+$ channel activity.[42,43] The maturational increase in apical sodium channel occurs well before that of the $K^+$ channel.[44,45] This paucity of $K^+$ channel occurs despite the fact that there are aldosterone and aldosterone receptors. The lack of $K^+$ channels limits the ability of neonates to excrete potassium and often is an important factor predisposing them to hyperkalemia.

Finally, salt handling and the response to a volume load in neonates and adults should be compared. If the effect of an isotonic volume challenge in a neonate and a comparable volume challenge in an adult are compared, the adult is found to be able to excrete the salt load far more briskly than is the neonate.[46] This is important clinically because neonates are able to be in positive salt balance despite drinking mother's milk, which has a very low salt content. It remains unclear how this occurs, but there is evidence of augmented sodium absorption by the distal convoluted tubule of the neonatal kidney in response to an isotonic fluid load compared to that of an adult.[47] The renin-angiotensin system likely plays a role mediating the increase in sodium absorption in the neonate, because losartan augments natriuresis and diuresis in response to a volume load in neonates.[48] Whereas the term neonate is adept at retaining NaCl, the premature neonate has problems with renal salt wasting because of the immaturity of the transporters in the kidney. This results clinically in hyponatremia and volume depletion unless premature infants have salt supplementation.

## REGULATION OF EXTRACELLULAR FLUID VOLUME—AFFERENT LIMB

Under normal conditions our body is in balance so that the sodium intake is matched by the urinary sodium excretion. If we increase sodium intake by indulging in a very salty meal, we do not develop edema or heart failure if our kidneys and cardiovascular system are intact. We do not become hypernatremic, because we have osmosensors that will cause us to increase water intake. Over the course of a day or so we excrete the extra sodium and return to our old steady state level. The body has multiple afferent pathways to sense the effective fullness of the extracellular fluid volume to protect the organism from volume depletion or volume expansion. The end result of activation of these volume sensors is that signals are relayed to the kidney to regulate salt transport and urinary sodium excretion. There are sensors in both the arterial and venous systems that respond to the fullness of these spaces by responding to stretch to preserve volume homeostasis. Underfilling of the atria results in decreased afferent nerve activity to the hypothalamus and medulla causing an increase in sympathetic nerve activity.[49,50] Distention of the atria as occurs with volume expansion results in natriuresis secondary to an increase in afferent nerve traffic to the brain and a decrease in the afferent sympathetic nerve activity.[49,50] Distention of the atria also results in the release of atrial natriuretic peptide.[51] There is also a brain natriuretic peptide that is synthesized predominantly in the ventricles that produces natriuresis with ventricular distention, as occurs in congestive heart failure.[52]

Important to our survival are baroreceptors that sense volume depletion, located in the carotid sinus and aorta. Baroreceptor activation results in an increase in sympathetic nerve activity, heart rate, activation of the renin-angiotensin system, and, if volume depletion is very severe, secretion of vasopressin. The kidney is able to autoregulate its perfusion pressure to maintain blood flow in response to hypoperfusion. This occurs by a myogenic reflex, as well as a tubuloglomerular feedback mechanism by which salt delivery to the macula densa of the thick ascending limb can affect afferent artery resistance to maintain glomerular filtration. Hypoperfusion of the kidney will result in renin secretion from the juxtaglomerular cells. There are also afferent volume sensors in the intestine and liver. Thus, the body has several systems in the arterial and venous side of the circulation to protect us from volume depletion.

## REGULATION OF RENAL SODIUM TRANSPORT—EFFERENT LIMB

The kidney must regulate sodium reabsorption and excretion in the face of fluctuations in sodium intake or losses such as to maintain sodium homeostasis and defend against changes to the extracellular fluid volume. The afferent system described previously results in alterations in the renin-angiotensin-aldosterone system, sympathetic renal nerve activity, vasopressin secretion, and liberation of other factors that regulate tubular sodium reabsorption to balance sodium and water intake with urinary excretion. The kidney does this by regulating sodium absorption along the nephron. In addition to the kidney, sympathetic nerve activity and the renin-angiotensin system can affect cardiac output and vascular resistance. The changes in the major regulatory factors that occur in the face of a decrease in effective

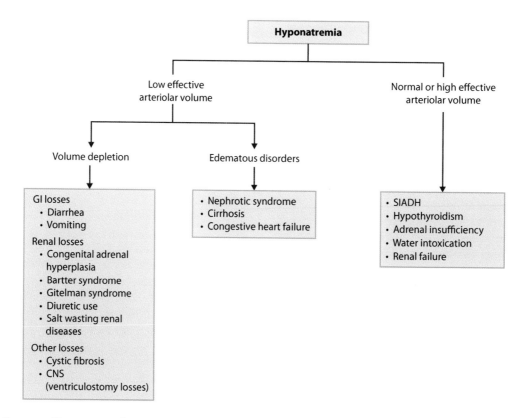

Figure 11.4 Causes of hyponatremia.

arteriolar volume and volume expansion are shown in Figure 11.5A and 11.5B, respectively.

## RENIN-ANGIOTENSIN SYSTEM

The systemic renin-angiotensin system plays an important role in regulation of proximal tubule sodium reabsorption. Renin is secreted by the kidney in response to a decrease in renal perfusion pressure to the juxtaglomerular cells of the afferent arteriole. In addition, the macula densa in the thick ascending limb responds to a decrease in luminal sodium as would be present in volume depletion, by stimulating renin secretion—a response known as tubular glomerular feedback. Third, an increase in renal nerve activity can increase renin secretion. Thus, a decrease in the effective arteriolar volume leads to an increase in plasma angiotensin II levels. angiotensin II preferentially vasoconstricts the efferent arteriole, resulting in an increase in filtration fraction modifying peritubular Starling forces, which will increase proximal

## KEY POINT

With volume depletion there is an increase in angiotensin II, aldosterone, vasopressin, and sympathetic nerve activity to increase tubular transport of salt and water.

tubule reabsorption. The proximal tubule has angiotensin II receptors, and circulating angiotensin II can directly stimulate proximal tubule sodium reabsorption.[53] In addition to the systemic renin-angiotensin system, the proximal tubule contains all of the components of an autonomously functioning intrarenal renin-angiotensin system and secretes angiotensin II into the lumen at concentrations 100-fold higher than that found in the plasma. Both systemic and intraluminal angiotensin II stimulate proximal tubular sodium transport.[54]

## RENAL NERVES

Sympathetic renal nerves innervate the glomerular capillaries and regulate filtration fraction. Sympathetic nerves also directly innervate the proximal tubule and regulate sodium homeostasis.[55,56] During volume contraction, there is an increase in renal nerve activity that stimulates proximal tubule transport. Conversely, renal nerve activity decreases during volume expansion, resulting in a decrease in transport by the proximal tubule. Renal nerves also increase renin secretion and thus contribute to raising systemic angiotensin II and aldosterone levels.

## ALDOSTERONE

Aldosterone acts on the collecting tubule to increase sodium transport. The collecting tubule is responsible for only 1% to 3% of sodium absorption; however, because it is the last segment that transports sodium, it is critical for the final modulation of salt transport. Aldosterone acts by increasing the trafficking of the epithelial sodium channel to the apical membrane of principal cells in the collecting tubule.[57] This will result in a lumen-negative potential difference, which will provide a driving force for potassium or proton secretion. Thus, hyperaldosteronism causes hypertension associated with a hypokalemic metabolic alkalosis. This is seen in Liddle syndrome, in which there is an increase in ENaC on the apical membrane secondary to an inherited defect in ENaC trafficking resulting in increase in apical membrane expression.[58]

## VASOPRESSIN

Vasopressin levels are predominantly regulated by osmolality. However, under conditions of severely reduced effective arteriolar volume, vasopressin secretion is markedly enhanced. Vasopressin is a very potent vasoconstrictor that has direct effects on renal hemodynamics to increase the filtration fraction and secondarily proximal tubule reabsorption by affecting peritubular Starling forces. Vasopressin has a direct effect on the thick ascending limb and collecting duct to increase sodium reabsorption. Finally, vasopressin will increase the insertion of aquaporin 2, resulting in an increase in water absorption from the collecting duct.

## COORDINATION OF REGULATORY PATHWAYS

Under conditions of severe volume contraction there is secretion of catecholamines, angiotensin II, vasopressin, and an increase in renal nerve activity. Left unabated, these factors would cause such intense vasoconstriction as to choke off renal perfusion and excessively reduce the GFR, potentially resulting in renal ischemia. The vasoconstriction would occur at a time when these hormones would be increasing transport and the need for ATP. This is a setup for acute kidney injury (AKI). However, angiotensin II, vasopressin, and catecholamine increase the renal production of prostaglandins. Prostaglandins have little role in regulating glomerular filtration or tubular transport under euvolemic or mild hypovolemia. Under severe volume contraction, prostaglandins are liberated, increasing renal blood flow and filtered sodium, causing vasodilatation of the efferent arteriole resulting in decrease in peritubular forces and decrease in proximal tubule transport . Prostaglandins have a direct effect inhibiting tubular NaCl transport by the thick limb and cortical collecting tubule. The importance of this buffering effect of prostaglandins under conditions of volume depletion is exemplified by the occurrence of AKI following administration of nonsteroidal anti-inflammatory agents (NSAIDs) to volume-contracted patients.[59]

In addition to the previously discussed factors that regulate transport, other hormones play a role. Endothelin inhibits renin release by juxtaglomerular cells.[60,61] Endothelin

has a direct epithelial action to inhibit distal tubular salt transport,[62] Nitric oxide augments sodium excretion under conditions of volume expansion.[63] Atrial natriuretic peptide increases GFR and inhibits renin secretion.[64] Although atrial natriuretic factor does not directly inhibit proximal tubule transport, it blunts the effect of catecholamines and angiotensin II on proximal tubule transport.[65-68] Atrial natriuretic factor has a direct epithelial action to inhibit sodium and water transport by the collecting tubule.[69,70]

## ASSESSMENT AND TREATMENT OF VOLUME AND SODIUM DISTURBANCES

## VOLUME DEPLETION

The diagnosis and management of perturbations in the extracellular volume are an important part of medical care in pediatrics. Most pediatric patients who have volume depletion do so from vomiting and diarrhea. The severity of the problem can be ascertained by asking the frequency of fluid losses and the duration of time that this has been occurring. In children, extracellular volume depletion is quite common. Pertinent history and physical findings are outlined in Table 11.2, but it will be immediately apparent that assessment of volume status is quite crude. Most patients have a recent weight available that can be compared to the present weight that will give an idea of the degree of volume depletion. With mild volume depletion (3% to 5%), patients will be thirsty, have dry mucous membranes, and

Table 11.2 Historical and physical findings in extracellular volume depletion

| Degree of dehydration | History | Physical findings |
| --- | --- | --- |
| Mild (3%–5%) | • Thirst<br>• Decreased urine output | • Dry mucous membranes |
| Moderate (6%–10%) | • Thirst<br>• Decreased urine output<br>• Change in mental status | • Dry mucous membranes<br>• Sunken eyes<br>• Sunken fontanelle<br>• Postural hypotension<br>• Tachycardia |
| Severe (>10%) | • Decreased urine output<br>• Lethargy<br>• Coma | • Dry mucous membranes<br>• Sunken eyes<br>• Sunken fontanelle<br>• Poor perfusion— cool extremities<br>• Hypotension<br>• Tachycardia |

have a decrease in urine output. More moderate degrees of volume depletion (6% to 10%) can result in poor skin turgor, with poor perfusion, sunken eyes or fontanelle, tachycardia and postural changes from decreased blood pressure, and irritability or listlessness. Severe volume depletion (>10%) is associated with lethargy or coma, hypotension, poor skin turgor, and sunken eyes or fontanelle.

Most, if not all, of the fluid losses that occur with acute volume depletion are due to losses from the extracellular fluid volume. The first goal in treating a patient with volume depletion is to stabilize the patient by administering a 10 mL/kg fluid bolus of normal saline. This may need to be repeated based on the severity of the volume depletion and the response to treatment. Once the patient's electrolytes, blood urea nitrogen (BUN), and creatinine have been stabilized, adjustments may be necessary in the subsequent fluids administered. However, most patients will have normal serum sodium levels or be hyponatremic. In patients with volume depletion, it is usually most appropriate to administer normal saline with the addition of potassium once ensuring that renal function is intact and the patient is not hyperkalemic.[1] Administration of hypotonic fluids can precipitate or worsen hyponatremia in the face of volume contraction where vasopressin levels may be elevated. Hypernatremic dehydration is rare, and the urine osmolality must be checked to rule out diabetes insipidus and correct the serum sodium slowly (see later discussion).

## EDEMA FORMATION

Normally, the extracellular fluid volume correlates well with the effective arteriolar volume and an increase in one matches the other, resulting in natriuresis with volume overload. If excessive sodium intake is not matched by natriuresis, the patient is in positive sodium balance and eventually will become edematous. Edema formation can occur if there is primary sodium reabsorption by the kidney, as in acute glomerulonephritis, in which a factor is causing increased tubular sodium reabsorption. We do not know what this factor is, but hypertension, volume overload, and edema can occur even if the GFR is normal. Most edema formation occurs in the face of a decrease of an effective arteriolar volume. In nephrotic syndrome, cirrhosis, and congestive heart failure, sodium intake does not expand the effective arteriolar volume and Starling forces favor fluid distribution into the interstitial space. In nephrotic syndrome and cirrhosis the low oncotic pressure results in an imbalance of capillary fluid egress at the arterial end and fluid reabsorption at the venous end, resulting in expansion of the interstitial space. In congestive heart failure, there is increased venous pressure limiting fluid uptake at the venous end of the capillary. In these edematous disorders the effective arteriolar volume is reduced, resulting in the same response as seen with volume depletion that occurs in augmented renal tubular sodium transport.

---

**KEY POINT**

With volume depletion there is an increase in angiotensin II, aldosterone, vasopressin, and sympathetic nerve activity to increase tubular transport of salt and water.

---

## HYPONATREMIA

Hyponatremia is defined as sodium concentration less than 135 mEq/L.[71] The serum sodium can be factitiously low if the blood is hyperlipidemic or hyperproteinemic and the specimen is measured by flame photometry. However, most modern laboratories measure sodium using ion-selective electrodes that eliminate this source of error. Hyperglycemia can cause a low serum sodium concentration because glucose is an osmotic agent that can cause a shift of water from the intracellular to the extracellular compartment and dilute the serum sodium concentration. For each 100 mg/dL of glucose in the serum above a normal level, the sodium will be lowered by 1.6 mEq/L. In contrast to the patient with true hyponatremia, these patients have a normal serum osmolality.

Three things are necessary to excrete free water and prevent or correct hyponatremia. To excrete free water (a hypotonic urine), there must be adequate delivery of fluid to the diluting segment, the diluting segment (thick ascending limb) must be functioning normally, and ADH) secretion must be suppressed. Problems in one or more of these three steps will result in the inability to excrete free water, which will either predispose the patient to develop hyponatremia or prevent the correction of hyponatremia. Some clinical conditions can interfere with the generation of hypotonic urine; these are outlined in Figure 11.4.

It is helpful to organize the differential diagnosis of hyponatremia based on the volume status of the patient. The most common cause for the inability to excrete free water in children is intravascular volume depletion. This is usually associated with total body volume depletion, but, as shown in Figure 11.4, hyponatremia also can be seen in patients with edema who have decreased effective arteriolar volume resulting from congestive heart failure, cirrhosis, and nephrotic syndrome. During effective arteriolar volume contraction the GFR decreases and the proximal tubule responds to volume contraction by reabsorbing a larger fraction of the filtered load of salt and water. This greatly diminishes the distal delivery of tubular fluid to the thick ascending limb, which is necessary for generating a concentrated medulla. In addition to the decreased distal delivery of fluid to the diluting segment, vasopressin will be secreted if there is significant decrease in effective arteriolar volume resulting in concentrated urine (Figure 11.5A). Finally, volume depletion causes thirst, which leads to the excessive ingestion of hypotonic fluid despite hyponatremia. Extracellular volume expansion, on the other hand, induces adaptations that result in urinary excretion of sodium and water in an attempt to restore the euvolumic state (see Figure 11.5B). Administration of thiazide and loop diuretics such as furosemide is a frequent cause of hyponatremia. In addition to causing sodium loss and decreasing the effective arteriolar volume, they also inhibit transporters responsible for free water generation.

Newborn infants are predisposed to hyponatremia because of their low GFR and consequent low distal delivery of fluid to the diluting segment. If the parent inappropriately dilutes the formula, the infant never becomes satiated and will ultimately take in excessive amounts of hypotonic fluid. Thus, the intake of water will exceed the ability to excrete the free water even though the diluting system is intact and the urine osmolality in a neonate can be as low as in adults (50 mOsm/kg water).

# Inappropriate secretion of antidiuretic hormone.

The syndrome of inappropriate antidiuretic hormone (SIADH) can be due to a number of causes, including carcinomas, pulmonary disorders, increased intracranial pressure, and drugs. Carbamazepine, cyclophosphamide, vincristine, chlorpropamide, narcotics, antipsychotics, antidepressants, and NSAIDs are the drugs most frequently associated with SIADH. The elevated levels of vasopressin lead to the excretion of concentrated urine despite the hypo-osmolality of the serum. The retention of free water leads to hyponatremia and inability to excrete free water to correct the hyponatremia. At the onset of SIADH, the urine osmolality may be quite high, but with time the osmolality can decrease to near isotonic levels.

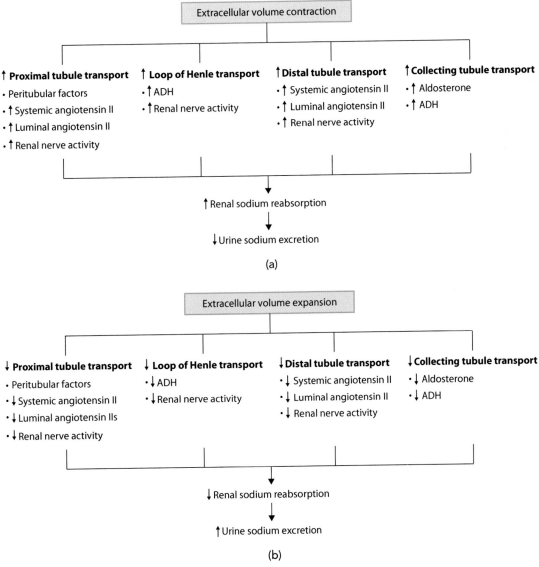

Figure 11.5 Renal response to extracellular volume depletion (a) and extracellular volume expansion (b) are shown. The kidney acts to conserve sodium during states of volume contraction and excrete sodium when there is expansion of the effective arteriolar volume to maintain a constant extracellular fluid volume.

However, the urine is still inappropriately concentrated for the degree of hypo-osmolality. The volume status of these patients is usually normal or slightly elevated. As a result, their BUN and serum uric acid concentrations are usually low and the fractional excretion of sodium (a reflection of the increased effective arteriolar volume status) is usually high. However, occasional patients have SIADH and are volume contracted for other reasons, so a low fractional excretion of sodium does not rule out SIADH. The mainstay of treatment for SIADH is fluid restriction. Ultimately, the cause of SIADH needs to be determined and treated. In some cases, SIADH may become a chronic condition and tolvaptan should be considered (see later discussion).

## KEY POINT

Patients with SIADH are usually euvolemic or slightly volume expanded and should be treated with fluid restriction.

## Treatment of hyponatremia

The treatment of hyponatremia depends on the specific cause and whether the hyponatremia is of acute onset or chronic. Hyponatremia can cause altered mental status, headache, nausea, vomiting, muscle cramps, or seizure. If the patient is having a seizure, hypertonic saline is usually indicated. An increase in serum sodium of only 1 to 3 mEq/L is usually adequate to arrest the seizure activity. For purposes of correction, the amount of sodium to be administered is calculated by the following equation:

$$\text{Na Deficit} = [\text{Na}_{\text{Desired}} - \text{Na}_{\text{observed}}] \times [(\text{Weight in Kg}) \times (0.6)]$$

where $\text{Na}_{\text{Desired}}$ is the desired serum sodium value and $\text{Na}_{\text{Observed}}$ is the actual measured sodium. Administration of 1 to 2 mL/kg of 3% saline with a maximum of 100 mL in an adult will usually stop seizure activity secondary to hyponatremia.[1,72] The serum sodium should never be increased faster than 12 mEq/L in 24 hours or 18 mEq/L in 48 hours because of the risk for developing central pontine myelinolysis or osmotic demyelination syndrome.[72]

The recommendation to administer sodium versus fluid restriction will hinge primarily on the volume status of the patient. If the patient has volume depletion from gastrointestinal or other losses, the volume deficit must be replaced to replenish the patient's extracellular fluid volume, usually with normal saline. After appropriate volume expansion, the patient will be able to regulate free water excretion to correct the serum sodium concentration.

Treatment of patients with euvolemic or hypervolemic hyponatremia is more complex. Patients with SIADH as the cause of hyponatremia need to be fluid restricted. In general, administration of isotonic saline to patients with SIADH

will not be beneficial, because most patients are euvolemic or hypervolemic and will retain water and excrete salt, which can worsen the problem. Fluid restriction remains the treatment of choice unless they are having acute neurologic symptoms. Patients with edematous states, such as in congestive heart failure, cirrhosis, or nephrotic syndrome, should be fluid restricted. Sodium administration to patients with edematous disorders will worsen their edema and may precipitate pulmonary edema in those with cardiovascular disorders. Diuretics will result in the excretion of hypotonic urine, which can be replaced with isotonic normal saline to increase the serum sodium concentration.

Vaptans, which are vasopressin receptor ($V_2$) antagonists, have been used in the treatment of chronic symptomatic hyponatremia. These agents are effective in increasing free water excretion and result in an increase in serum sodium levels.[73-75] Side effects from vaptans include polyuria and thirst. Very few data are available on the use of vaptans in children, and these agents have not been tested and thus cannot be recommended in the treatment of acute symptomatic hyponatremia. However, they may have a role in the treatment of chronic symptomatic hyponatremia secondary to chronic SIADH, congestive heart failure, or cirrhosis in children as in adults.

## HYPERNATREMIA

Outside of the neonatal period, hypernatremia is a rare electrolyte disturbance. When we consume a salty meal, we feel thirsty and will consume enough water to normalize the serum osmolality. Although the kidney can concentrate urine to retain free water,[76] the body's primary defense against hypernatremia is thirst. Very small changes in the serum sodium concentration (and therefore in serum osmolality) result in signals from the thirst center in the hypothalamus to consume water to normalize the serum sodium. Thus, when evaluating a patient with hypernatremia, it is necessary to determine if the thirst center is intact or why the patient did not have access to water.

The concentrating ability of the kidney depends on three major factors: (1) The ability of the hypothalamus and pituitary to synthesize and secrete ADH or vasopressin; (2) the ability of the kidney to generate an osmotic gradient across the collecting duct; and (3) the ability of the collecting duct to respond to ADH. Thus, the inability to maximally concentrate the urine may be due to a defect in one or more of these factors. However, patients who have a defect in the urinary concentrating mechanism will have a normal serum sodium concentration and osmolality as long as they are able to drink water to replace the urinary loss of free water.

Some disorders can impair the kidney's ability to concentrate urine. With *diabetes insipidus* there is either a defect in the production of vasopressin, termed *central diabetes insipidus,* or an inability of the kidney to respond to vasopressin, termed *nephrogenic diabetes insipidus.* A water deprivation test can determine whether a patient has diabetes insipidus and whether it is central or nephrogenic. Water is withheld for a period until either the urine osmolality increases significantly or there is a rise in the serum sodium concentration with no change in the urine osmolality. If the urine osmolality increases significantly, the patient has primary polydipsia. If the patient's serum sodium increases and the urine osmolality remains hypotonic, the patient has diabetes insipidus. To determine if this is due to a central or renal defect, vasopressin is administered. An increase in the urine osmolality with vasopressin indicates that the patient has central diabetes insipidus. It should be pointed out that patients who present with hypernatremia have already been water deprived. At presentation, the urinary osmolality always should be measured to determine if the patient has a urinary concentrating defect. This will obviate the need to perform the water deprivation test in the future. The osmolality should be measured, not the specific gravity. The specific gravity is determined by the weight of solutes in solution, whereas osmolality is determined by the number of particles in solution. So if there is a small amount of protein or glucose, for example, the specific gravity will be very high even if the osmolality of the urine is low. With osmolality, a molecule of protein counts the same as that of glucose or sodium and it is thus a true measure of the number of particles in solution.

## Central diabetes insipidus

Central diabetes insipidus usually results from trauma to the pituitary or a tumor in the hypothalamus or pituitary. Trauma can sometimes be due to neurosurgical procedures. Rarely, central diabetes insipidus is congenital. Some patients with holoprosencephaly have defects in the secretion of vasopressin. Central diabetes insipidus also can be seen with global dysfunction of the pituitary, the panhypopituitary syndrome. The treatment of central diabetes insipidus is to replace vasopressin, usually with DDAVP.

## Nephrogenic diabetes insipidus

Nephrogenic diabetes insipidus results from defects in the collecting duct that prevent the normal response to vasopressin. It can be congenital or acquired. The most common inherited defect is due to a mutation in the vasopressin receptor (V2R) in the collecting duct. Most patients with congenital nephrogenic diabetes insipidus are male because the gene encoding the V2 receptor is on the X chromosome. Patients with nephrogenic diabetes insipidus usually present in the neonatal period with dehydration and fever from the urinary loss of free water. Females rarely can have nephrogenic diabetes insipidus secondary to a mutation in the vasopressin receptor as a result of unequal lyonization. Inherited defects in the AQP2 water channel also have been described. Most of these defects are inherited in the autosomal recessive fashion, but there have been mutations with autosomal dominant transmission.

Nephrogenic diabetes insipidus also can result from an acquired lesion. Obstructive uropathy can damage the cortical collecting duct to the extent that the collecting duct does not respond to vasopressin. Drugs such as lithium, amphotericin, and demeclocycline can impair the effect of vasopressin on the collecting duct. Other causes of acquired nephrogenic diabetes insipidus include hypokalemia and hypercalcemia.

## Treatment of hypernatremia

The principal treatment of hypernatremia is to provide enough free water to correct the elevation in serum sodium concentration. The amount of water needed is known as the "free water deficit" and is calculated by the following equation:

$$Free\ water\ deficit(Liters) = \left[ \frac{Na_{Observed} - Na_{Desired}}{Na_{Desired}} \right] \times \left[ (Weight\ in\ kg) \times (0.6) \right]$$

where $Na_{Desired}$ is the serum sodium value to be achieved and $Na_{Observed}$ is the actual measured sodium. This calculation will give the free water deficit in liters. The serum sodium should be corrected by less than 15 mEq/L per day. Lowering the serum osmolality too quickly will result in cerebral edema with permanent neurologic sequela and potentially death.

One of the difficulties in treating hypernatremic dehydration is determining if the patient has an extracellular fluid volume deficit. Patients with hypernatremic dehydration may appear more volume replete than they actually are. If there was a history of vomiting or diarrhea, the patient may need to receive an isotonic fluid bolus before receiving the free water replacement. Once the extracellular fluid space is expanded, the kidney will be able to excrete the excess sodium. Again, this needs to be done carefully so that the patient's serum sodium does not decrease too rapidly and the patient does not become fluid overloaded.

## SUMMARY

Regulation of fluid balance and electrolyte composition by the kidneys is essential for preserving the internal milieu of the body. Our understanding of the various aspects of ionic and water transport in the tubular cells of the kidney has been exponentially increasing in the last two decades. Discovery of aquaporins, or water channels in the cells, especially in the kidney, has further established mechanisms of movement of water across cellular barriers. A clear understanding of the vasopressin receptors ($V_2$) led to the development of vasopressin receptor ($V_2$) antagonists (vaptans), which are useful in the treatment of chronic symptomatic hyponatremia. Apart from this, a clear understanding of fluid and electrolyte requirement of sick infants and children is relevant from the clinical practice perspective of a pediatrician and pediatric nephrologist. This chapter has attempted to provide a basic outline of the scientific principles that guide clinical management of disorders of sodium and water homeostasis.

### Clinical Vignette 11.1

A 6-month-old child was evaluated by his pediatrician and found to be in good health. The child is exclusively breast fed and has been growing at the 50th percentile for height and weight. Three days after his well-child care visit the child developed profuse diarrhea. The mother continues to breast feed the child; however, after 2 days of diarrhea the mother notes that the child is listless and has a decrease in urine output. She was instructed to go to a local emergency room, where the child looks somewhat lethargic and has sunken eyes although the extremities remain warm and well perfused with good capillary refill. Electrolytes reveal that the child has a serum sodium level of 128 mEq/L, potassium of 5.0 mEq/L, chloride of 111 mEql/L, bicarbonate of 10 mEq/L, BUN of 30 mg/dL, and creatinine of 1.0 mg/dL. Urine was obtained that shows a fractional excretion of sodium of 0.5%.

### TEACHING POINTS

- The patient has hyponatremic dehydration and likely has prerenal azotemia. This is acute dehydration, so essentially all of the volume depletion is from the extracellular fluid volume.
- Multiple homeostatic mechanisms come into play to preserve the extracellular fluid volume. There is an increase in plasma angiotensin II, vasopressin, aldosterone, and renal sympathetic nerve activity, which augments renal tubular salt and water absorption. The high ratio of BUN to creatinine and the low fractional excretion of sodium are consistent with prerenal azotemia, and it is unlikely that severe tubular injury is present.
- The hyponatremia is due the mother feeding the child breast milk, which is hypotonic, and the fact that the volume depletion is severe enough to cause the liberation of vasopressin (ADH), which increases water absorption in the collecting tubule.
- Several findings on physical examination suggest that this patient is approximately 6% to 10% volume depleted. The patient has sunken eyes and is somewhat lethargic. However, all of the physical findings used to assess volume depletion are rather inaccurate. The most accurate way of determining the severity of this child's volume depletion is by comparing the weight at presentation with the weight of the child during the most recent examination by the pediatrician.
- The fluid that should be administered is normal saline. This will expand the extracellular fluid volume and help correct the hyponatremia. The child should be receive at least 10 to 20 mL/kg of normal saline, followed by enough saline to replete the child's volume depletion in addition to maintenance fluids.
- Electrolytes, BUN, and creatinine should be monitored frequently and potassium added to the intravenous fluids once it decreases to the normal range and the BUN and creatinine fall.

## REFERENCES

1. Moritz ML, Ayus JC. New aspects in the pathogenesis, prevention, and treatment of hyponatremic encephalopathy in children. Pediatr Nephrol. 2010;25:1225–38.
2. Moe OW, Baum M, Berry CA, Rector FC. Renal transport of glucose, amino acids, sodium, chloride and water. In: Brenner BM, editor. The Kidney, 7th ed. Philadelphia: Saunders; 2004:413–52.
3. Liu FY, Cogan MG. Axial heterogeneity in the rat proximal convoluted tubule. I. Bicarbonate, chloride, and water transport. Am J Physiol. 1984;247:F816–21.
4. Rector FC, Jr. Sodium, bicarbonate, and chloride absorption by the proximal tubule. Am J Physiol. 1983;244:F461–71.
5. Preisig PA, Ives HE, Cragoe EJ, Jr, et al. Role of the Na+/H+ antiporter in rat proximal tubule bicarbonate absorption. J Clin Invest. 1987;80:970–8.
6. Baum M. Developmental changes in rabbit juxtamedullary proximal convoluted tubule acidification. Pediatr Res. 1992;31:411–4.
7. Moe OW, Preisig PA, Alpern RJ. Cellular model of proximal tubule NaCl and NaHCO3 absorption. Kidney Int. 1990;38:605–11.
8. Baum M, Berry CA. Evidence for neutral transcellular NaCl transport and neutral basolateral chloride exit in the rabbit convoluted tubule. J Clin Invest. 1984;74:205–11.
9. Aronson PS, Giebisch G. Mechanisms of chloride transport in the proximal tubule. Am J Physiol. 1997;273:F179–92.
10. Baum M, Quigley R. Maturation of rat proximal tubule chloride permeability. Am J Physiol Regul Integr Comp Physiol. 2005;289:R1659–64.
11. Reeves BW, Andreoli TE. Tubular sodium transport. In: Schrier RW GC, editor. Diseases of the Kidney, 5th ed. Boston: Little Brown; 1997. pp. 135–7.
12. Scheinman SJ, Guay-Woodford LM, Thakker RV, et al. Genetic disorders of renal electrolyte transport. N Engl J Med. 1999;340:1177–87.
13. Simon DB, Lifton RP. The molecular basis of inherited hypokalemic alkalosis: Bartter's and Gitelman's syndromes. Am J Physiol. 1996;271:F961–6.
14. Baum M. Effect of catecholamines on rat medullary thick ascending limb chloride transport: Interaction with angiotensin II. Am J Physiol Regul Integr Comp Physiol. 2010;298:R954–8.

15. Ares GR, Caceres PS, Ortiz PA. Molecular regulation of NKCC2 in the thick ascending limb. Am J Physiol Renal Physiol. 2011;301:F1143–59.

16. Simon DB, Lifton RP. Mutations in renal ion transporters cause Gitelman's and Bartter's syndromes of inherited hypokalemic alkalosis. Adv Nephrol Necker Hosp. 1997;27:343–59.

17. Simon DB, Nelson-Williams C, Bia MJ, et al. Gitelman's variant of Bartter's syndrome, inherited hypokalaemic alkalosis, is caused by mutations in the thiazide-sensitive Na-Cl cotransporter. Nat Genet. 1996;12:24–30.

18. San-Cristobal P, Pacheco-Alvarez D, Richardson C, et al. Angiotensin II signaling increases activity of the renal Na-Cl cotransporter through a WNK4-SPAK-dependent pathway. Proc Natl Acad Sci USA. 2009;106:4384–9.

19. Sonalker PA, Tofovic SP, Bastacky SI, et al. Chronic noradrenaline increases renal expression of NHE-3, NBC-1, BSC-1 and aquaporin-2. Clin Exp Pharmacol Physiol. 2008;35:594–600.

20. Knepper MA. Molecular physiology of urinary concentrating mechanism: Regulation of aquaporin water channels by vasopressin. Am J Physiol. 1997;272:F3–12.

21. Arant BS, Jr. Developmental patterns of renal functional maturation compared in the human neonate. J Pediatr. 1978;92:705–12.

22. Arant BS, Jr. Postnatal development of renal function during the first year of life. Pediatr Nephrol. 1987;1:308–13.

23. Spitzer A, Schwartz GJ. The kidney during development. In: Windhager EE, editor. The Handbook of Physiology (Renal Physiology), 8th ed. New York: Oxford University Press; 1992:476–544.

24. Rane S, Aperia A. Ontogeny of Na-K-ATPase activity in thick ascending limb and of concentrating capacity. Am J Physiol. 1985;249:F723–28.

25. Schmidt U, Horster M. Na-K-activated ATPase: Activity maturation in rabbit nephron segments dissected in vitro. Am J Physiol. 1977;233:F55–60.

26. Schwartz GH, Evan AP. Development of solute transport in rabbit proximal tubule. III. Na-K-ATPase activity. Am J Physiol. 1984;246:F845–52.

27. Johnson V, Spitzer A. Renal reabsorption of phosphate during development: Whole-kidney events. Am J Physiol. 1986;251:F251–6.

28. Kaskel FJ, Kumar AM, Feld LG, Spitzer A. Renal reabsorption of phosphate during development: Tubular events. Pediatr Nephrol. 1988;2:129-34.

29. Neiberger RE, Barac-Nieto M, Spitzer A. Renal reabsorption of phosphate during development: Transport kinetics in BBMV. Am J Physiol. 1989;257:F268–74.

30. Segawa H, Kaneko I, Takahashi A, et al. Growth-related renal type II Na/Pi cotransporter. J Biol Chem. 2002;277:19665–72.

31. Shah M, Gupta N, Dwarakanath V, et al. Ontogeny of Na+/H+ antiporter activity in rat proximal convoluted tubules. Pediatr Res 2000;48:206–10.

32. Twombley K, Gattineni J, Bobulescu IA, et al. Effect of metabolic acidosis on neonatal proximal tubule acidification. Am J Physiol Regul Integr Comp Physiol. 2010;299:R1360–8.

33. Becker AM, Zhang J, Goyal S, et al. Ontogeny of NHE8 in the rat proximal tubule. Am J Physiol Renal Physiol. 2007;293:F255–61.

34. Baum M, Dwarakanath V, Alpern RJ, et al. Effects of thyroid hormone on the neonatal renal cortical Na+/H+ antiporter. Kidney Int. 1998;53:1254–8.

35. Gattineni J, Sas D, Dagan A, et al. Effect of thyroid hormone on the postnatal renal expression of NHE8. Am J Physiol Renal Physiol. 2008;294:F198–204.

36. Baum M, Quigley R. Prenatal glucocorticoids stimulate neonatal juxtamedullary proximal convoluted tubule acidification. Am J Physiol. 1991;261:F746–52.

37. Baum M, Biemesderfer D, Gentry D, et al. Ontogeny of rabbit renal cortical NHE3 and NHE1: Effect of glucocorticoids. Am J Physiol. 1995;268:F815–20.

38. Sheu JN, Baum M, Bajaj G, et al. Maturation of rabbit proximal convoluted tubule chloride permeability. Pediatr Res. 1996;39:308–12.

39. Quigley R, Baum M. Developmental changes in rabbit proximal straight tubule paracellular permeability. Am J Physiol Renal Physiol. 2002;283:F525–31.

40. Quigley R, Harkins EW, Thomas PJ, et al. Maturational changes in rabbit renal brush border membrane vesicle osmotic water permeability. J Membr Biol. 1998;164:177–85.

41. Horster M. Loop of Henle functional differentiation: In vitro perfusion of the isolated thick ascending segment. Pflugers Arch. 1978;378:15–24.

42. Satlin LM, Palmer LG. Apical K+ conductance in maturing rabbit principal cell. Am J Physiol. 1997;272:F397–404.

43. Satlin LM, Palmer LG. Apical Na+ conductance in maturing rabbit principal cell. Am J Physiol. 1996;270:F391–97.

44. Satlin LM. Postnatal maturation of potassium transport in rabbit cortical collecting duct. Am J Physiol. 1994;266:F57–65.

45. Woda CB, Miyawaki N, Ramalakshmi S, et al. Ontogeny of flow-stimulated potassium secretion in rabbit cortical collecting duct: Functional and molecular aspects. Am J Physiol Renal Physiol. 2003;285:F629–39.

46. Goldsmith DI, Drukker A, Blaufox MD, et al. Hemodynamic and excretory response of the neonatal canine kidney to acute volume expansion. Am J Physiol. 1979;237:F392–7.

47. Aperia A, Elinder G. Distal tubular sodium reabsorption in the developing rat kidney. Am J Physiol. 1981;240:F487–91.

48. Chevalier RL, Thornhill BA, Belmonte DC, et al. Endogenous angiotensin II inhibits natriuresis after acute volume expansion in the neonatal rat. Am J Physiol. 1996;270:R393–7.

49. Paintal AS. Vagal sensory receptors and their reflex effects. Physiol Rev. 1973;53:159–227.

50. Henry JP, Gauer OH, Reeves JL. Evidence of the atrial location of receptors influencing urine flow. Circ Res. 1956;4:85–90.

51. de Bold AJ, Borenstein HB, Veress AT, et al. A rapid and potent natriuretic response to intravenous injection of atrial myocardial extract in rats. Life Sci. 1981;28:89–94.

52. Nagaya N, Nishikimi T, Goto Y, et al. Plasma brain natriuretic peptide is a biochemical marker for the prediction of progressive ventricular remodeling after acute myocardial infarction. Am Heart J. 1998;135:21–8.

53. Cogan MG. Angiotensin II: A powerful controller of sodium transport in the early proximal tubule. Hypertension. 1990;15:451–8.

54. Quan A, Baum M. Regulation of proximal tubule transport by angiotensin II. Semin Nephrol. 1997;17:423–30.

55. Bello-Reuss E. Effect of catecholamines on fluid reabsorption by the isolated proximal convoluted tubule. Am J Physiol. 1980;238:F347–52.

56. Baum M, Quigley R. Inhibition of proximal convoluted tubule transport by dopamine. Kidney Int. 1998;54:1593–1600.

57. Frindt G, Ergonul Z, Palmer LG. Na channel expression and activity in the medullary collecting duct of rat kidney. Am J Physiol Renal Physiol. 2007;292:F1190–6.

58. Schild L, Lu Y, Gautschi I, et al. Identification of a PY motif in the epithelial Na channel subunits as a target sequence for mutations causing channel activation found in Liddle syndrome. EMBO J. 1996;15:2381–7.

59. Krause I, Cleper R, Eisenstein B, et al. Acute renal failure, associated with non-steroidal anti-inflammatory drugs in healthy children. Pediatr Nephrol. 2005;20:1295–8.

60. Moe O, Tejedor A, Campbell WB, et al. Effects of endothelin on in vitro renin secretion. Am J Physiol. 1991;260:E521–5.

61. Rakugi H, Nakamaru M, Saito H, et al. Endothelin inhibits renin release from isolated rat glomeruli. Biochem Biophys Res Commun. 1988;155:1244–7.

62. Ramseyer VD, Cabral PD, Garvin JL. Role of endothelin in thick ascending limb sodium chloride transport. Contrib Nephrol. 2011;172:76–83.

63. Peterson TV, Carter AB, Miller RA. Nitric oxide and renal effects of volume expansion in conscious monkeys. Am J Physiol. 1997;272:R1033–8.

64. Maack T, Atlas SA, Camargo MJ, et al. Renal hemodynamic and natriuretic effects of atrial natriuretic factor. Fed Proc. 1986;45:2128–32.

65. Cogan MG. Atrial natriuretic factor can increase renal solute excretion primarily by raising glomerular filtration. Am J Physiol. 1986;250:F710–4.

66. Garvin JL. ANF inhibits norepinephrine-stimulated fluid absorption in rat proximal straight tubules. Am J Physiol. 1992;263:F581–5.

67. Harris PJ, Thomas D, Morgan TO. Atrial natriuretic peptide inhibits angiotensin-stimulated proximal tubular sodium and water reabsorption. Nature. 1987;326:697–8.

68. Nonoguchi H, Sands JM, Knepper MA. Atrial natriuretic factor inhibits vasopressin-stimulated osmotic water permeability in rat inner medullary collecting duct. J Clin Invest. 1988;82:1383–90.

69. Knepper MA, Lankford SP, Terada Y. Renal tubular actions of ANF. Can J Physiol Pharmacol. 1991;69:1537–45.

70. Nonoguchi H, Sands JM, Knepper MA. ANF inhibits NaCl and fluid absorption in cortical collecting duct of rat kidney. Am J Physiol. 1989;256(1 Pt 2):F179–86.

71. Adrogue HJ, Madias NE. Hyponatremia. N Engl J Med. 2000;342:1581–9.

72. Jovanovich A, Berl T. Mortality and serum sodium in CKD-yet another U-shaped curve. Nat Rev Nephrol. 2012;8:261–3.

73. Berl T, Quittnat-Pelletier F, Verbalis JG, et al. Oral tolvaptan is safe and effective in chronic hyponatremia. J Am Soc Nephrol. 2010;21:705–12.

74. Schrier RW, Gross P, Gheorghiade M, et al. Tolvaptan, a selective oral vasopressin V-2-receptor antagonist, for hyponatremia. N Engl J Med 2006;355:2099–112.

75. Verbalis JG, Adler S, Schrier RW, et al. Efficacy and safety of oral tolvaptan therapy in patients with the syndrome of inappropriate antidiuretic hormone secretion. Eur J Endocrinol. 2011;164:725–32.

76. Adrogue HJ, Madias NE. Hypernatremia. N Engl J Med. 2000;342:1493–9.

## REVIEW QUESTIONS

1. Which nephron segment reabsorbs salt but not water?
   a. Thick ascending limb
   b. Proximal tubule
   c. Cortical collecting duct
   d. Thick descending limb
   e. None of the above

2. A patient with congestive heart failure has intractable hyponatremia. Which drug should be considered in the management?
   a. A nonsteroidal anti-inflammatory agent
   b. Morphine
   c. Tolvaptan
   d. Vasopressin
   e. Dexamethasone

3. In comparison to the adult kidney, the neonatal kidney is characterized by:
   a. Fewer glomeruli
   b. Fewer tubules
   c. Inability to dilute urine
   d. Inability to concentrate urine
   e. None of the above
4. A neonatal patient presents with a serum sodium of 154 mEq/L. You suspect diabetes insipidus. Your initial evaluation should include all of the following *except:*
   a. A family history
   b. Determination of how the child is fed
   c. A water deprivation test
   d. A urine osmolality
   e. An assessment of volume status of the child

5. Which statement about the collecting tubule is *incorrect?*
   a. It is responsive to aldosterone.
   b. It is responsive to vasopressin.
   c. It reabsorbs 1% to 3% of the filtered sodium.
   d. It has a lumen positive potential difference.
   e. It has an apical epithelial sodium channel.

## ANSWER KEY

1. a
2. c
3. e
4. c
5. d

# 12

# Potassium homeostasis

## CAROLINE GLUCK AND LISA M. SATLIN

Potassium ($K^+$) is the most abundant intracellular cation. Approximately 98% of the total body $K^+$ content in the adult is located within cells, primarily muscle, where its concentration ranges from 100 to 150 mEq/L. The remaining 2% of the total body $K^+$ content resides in the extracellular fluid (ECF). In the ECF, the $K^+$ concentration, generally ranging from 3.5 to 5.0 mEq/L in the adult, is tightly regulated by mechanisms that govern the *internal* distribution between the intracellular fluid (ICF) and EFC compartments and *external* balance between intake and output via the kidney and gastrointestinal (GI) tract.

The steep $K^+$ and sodium ($Na^+$) concentration gradients across cell membranes are maintained by the Na-K-adenosine triphosphatase (Na-K-ATPase), an enzyme present on the surface of essentially all eukaryotic cells that pumps three $Na^+$ ions out and two $K^+$ ions into the cell for each molecule of adenosine triphosphate (ATP) hydrolyzed. The unequal cation exchange ratio of the pump creates an electrical gradient across the cell membrane that determines, in large part, the resting membrane potential, which typically ranges from −30 mV to −70 mV (cell interior negative) in most mammalian cells. Pump activity is essential for normal cellular function and, in particular, is critical for the regulation of protein and glycogen synthesis, cell volume, intracellular pH, resting membrane potential, and thus muscle excitability and cardiac function.

## POTASSIUM HOMEOSTASIS

The homeostatic goal of the adult is to remain in zero $K^+$ balance. To this end, approximately 90% to 95% of the typical daily $K^+$ intake of 1 mEq/kg body weight is ultimately eliminated from the body in the urine; the residual 5% to 10% of the daily $K^+$ load is lost through the stool. Normally, the amount of $K^+$ lost through sweat is negligible.

In contrast to the adult, infants older than approximately 30 weeks of gestation must maintain a state of positive $K^+$ balance.[1,2] Net retention of $K^+$ is necessary to ensure the availability of adequate substrate for the increase in cell number and $K^+$ concentration, at least in skeletal muscle, with advancing age.[3-5] The tendency to retain $K^+$ early in postnatal life is reflected in the observation that plasma $K^+$ concentrations in infants (>5 mEq/L), and particularly in premature newborns (>5.5 mEq/L), tend to be higher than in children.[1,2,6,7]

## REGULATION OF POTASSIUM BALANCE BY DIETARY INTAKE AND REDISTRIBUTION

The daily dietary intake of $K^+$ in the adult generally approaches or exceeds the total $K^+$ normally present within the ECF space, which in an individual with an ECF volume of 12 to 14 L and serum $K^+$ concentration of 4 to 5 mEq/L, is approximately 50 to 70 mEq. Approximately 85% of ingested $K^+$ is reabsorbed by the gut in the adult.[8] The urinary excretion of an oral $K^+$ load is sluggish, with only 50% of the $K^+$ eliminated within the first 4 to 6 hours[9]; thus, it can be envisioned that the acute ingestion of 40 mEq of $K^+$ (as may be present in a quart of orange juice) could, if retained exclusively in the ECF compartment, nearly double the plasma $K^+$ concentration and lead to potentially serious consequences.[9] However, life-threatening hyperkalemia is not generally observed during this interval because of the rapid (within minutes) hormonally mediated translocation of most of the ingested $K^+$ into cells, particularly muscle and liver, a response mediated by the $Na^+$-$K^+$-ATPase.[9]

The hormonal, as well as other chemical and physical factors that acutely influence $K^+$ redistribution, are listed in Table 12.1.

## RENAL REGULATION OF POTASSIUM BALANCE

The three processes involved in renal $K^+$ handling include filtration, reabsorption, and secretion. $K^+$ filtered at the glomerulus is reabsorbed almost entirely in proximal segments of the nephron, whereas urinary $K^+$ excretion, at least in the adult, is accomplished by $K^+$ secretion in the distal segments of the aldosterone-sensitive distal nephron (ASDN) (Figure 12.1).

---

### KEY POINT

Net urinary $K^+$ excretion is accomplished by $K^+$ secretion in the ASDN.

---

It is now well established that the neonatal kidney contributes to $K^+$ retention early in life. In newborns, the renal $K^+$ clearance is low, even when corrected for the prevailing low glomerular filtration rate (GFR).[1] The rate of $K^+$ excretion expressed per unit body or kidney weight in infants and young animals subject to exogenous $K^+$ loading is less than that observed in older subjects.[10] However, in response to exogenous $K^+$ loading, infants like adults can excrete $K^+$ at a rate that exceeds its rate of filtration, indicating the capacity for net tubular secretion.[10] In a longitudinal prospective study of premature infants, the fractional excretion of $K^+$ fell by half between 26 and 30 weeks of gestation, a postnatal change that was not accompanied by a significant change in absolute urinary $K^+$ excretion.[1] Given that the filtered load of $K^+$ increased almost three-fold during this same time interval, the constancy of renal $K^+$ excretion was attributed to a developmental increase in the capacity of the kidney for $K^+$ reabsorption.[1]

## Sites of potassium transport along the nephron

$K^+$ is freely filtered at the glomerulus. Studies in both suckling and adult rats indicate that approximately 65% of the filtered load of $K^+$ is reabsorbed along the proximal tubule (Figure 12.2).[11-15] Reabsorption is passive in this segment, closely following reabsorption of filtered $Na^+$ and water. Only approximately 10% of the filtered load of $K^+$ reaches the early distal tubule of the adult, indicating that a significant amount of $K^+$ is reabsorbed in the intervening segments, specifically across the thick ascending limb of the loop of Henle (TALH).[11] In contrast, up to 35% of the filtered load of $K^+$ reaches the distal tubule of the newborn rat.[12] These observations suggest that postnatal maturation of the TALH is characterized by a developmental increase in its capacity for $K^+$ reabsorption, a notion supported by the findings that both the diluting capacity and TALH Na-K-ATPase activity increase after birth.[14,15]

$K^+$ reabsorption in the TALH is mediated by an Na-K-2Cl cotransporter (NKCC2), located on the apical (urinary) membrane, that translocates one $K^+$ ion into the cell accompanied by one $Na^+$ and two chloride ($Cl^-$) ions. Transporter activity is ultimately driven by the basolateral $Na^+$-$K^+$-ATPase, which generates and maintains a low intracellular $Na^+$ concentration and thus a chemical gradient favoring $Na^+$ entry at the apical membrane. Diuretics such as furosemide and bumetanide that inhibit this Na-K-2Cl cotransporter block $K^+$ (as well as $Na^+$) reabsorption at this site and uncover $K^+$ secretion, leading to profound urinary $K^+$ losses (see later discussion of Bartter syndrome).

NKCC2 activity requires the presence of an apical $K^+$ secretory channel, encoded by the *ROMK* (rat outer medullary K channel) gene, to recycle $K^+$ across this membrane, thus ensuring an abundant supply of substrate for the cotransporter.[11,16,17] Loss-of-function mutations in *ROMK* lead to antenatal Bartter syndrome (type 2), also known as the hyperprostaglandin E syndrome, which is characterized by severe renal salt and fluid wasting, consistent with a pattern of impaired TALH function.[18]

Under baseline conditions in the adult, $K^+$ secretion in the ASDN, which includes the distal and connecting tubules and cortical collecting duct (CCD), contributes prominently to urinary $K^+$ excretion.[11] In contrast to the

---

Table 12.1 Factors involved in the regulation of potassium balance

**Redistribution of $K^+$ between the ICF and ECF**
- Insulin
- β-Adrenergic agonists (epinephrine)
- Plasma $K^+$ concentration
- Acid-base balance

**Net $K^+$ excretion from the body**
- Kidney
  - Distal delivery and absorption of $Na^+$
  - Urinary flow rate
  - Aldosterone
- GI tract

*Abbreviations:* ECF, extracellular fluid; ICF, intracellular fluid; GI, gastrointestinal.

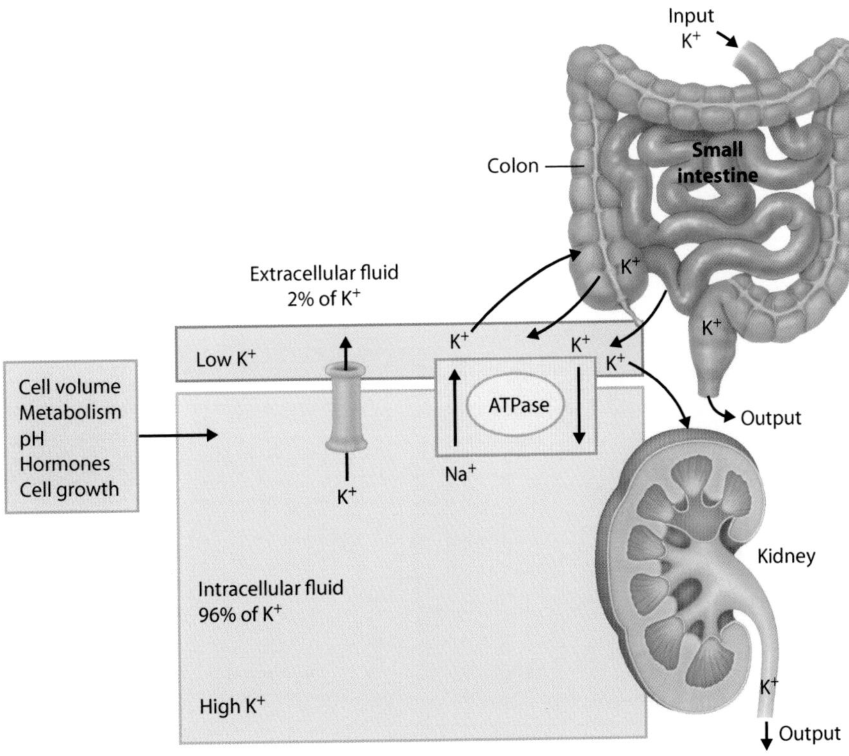

Figure 12.1 Distribution of potassium (K⁺) in the body. Most of K⁺ is located in body cells. Note entry of K⁺ into the small intestine, where it is extensively reabsorbed. K⁺ may be secreted in the colon. The exit of K⁺ from the body is mediated by the kidney and, to a lesser extent, the colon. The distribution of K⁺ between extracellular fluid and intracellular fluid is dependent and regulated by a pump-leak mechanism involving both Na⁺-K⁺-ATPase and membrane K channels. Several factors modify cell K⁺ (see box with brown outline in the diagram). (Reproduced with permission from: Giebisch G, Krapf R, Wagner C. Renal and extrarenal regulation of potassium. Kidney Int. 2007;72:397–410.)

high rate of K⁺ secretion measured in CCDs of adult rabbits and perfused at physiologic flow rates in vitro, segments isolated from neonatal animals show no significant net K⁺ transport until after the third week of postnatal life.[19] By 6 weeks of age, after weaning, the rate of net K⁺ secretion in the CCD is comparable to that observed in the adult.[19] These results indicate that the low rates of K⁺ excretion characteristic of the newborn kidney are due, at least in part, to a low K⁺ secretory capacity of the CCD.

The CCD comprises two cell populations. Principal cells are considered to reabsorb Na⁺ and secrete K⁺, whereas intercalated cells primarily function in acid-base homeostasis but can reabsorb K⁺ in response to dietary K⁺ restriction or metabolic acidosis.[20] The direction and magnitude of net K⁺ transport in the ASDN represents the balance of K⁺ secretion and absorption, opposing processes proposed to be mediated by these two cell types.

## TUBULAR POTASSIUM SECRETION

K⁺ secretion by principal cells in the CCD is accomplished by a two-step process. First, K⁺ is actively taken up into the cell at the basolateral membrane in exchange for Na⁺, a

process mediated by the Na-K-ATPase. The high intracellular K⁺ concentration and lumen-negative voltage within this nephron segment, generated by apical Na⁺ entry across the epithelial Na⁺ channel (ENaC) and its electrogenic basolateral extrusion, create an electrochemical gradient that favors the passive diffusion of cell K⁺ into the luminal fluid through apical K⁺-selective channels. The small conductance secretory K⁺ (SK) channel, encoded by the ROMK gene, is considered to mediate baseline constitutive K⁺ secretion in this nephron segment.[11,21] A high conductance, stretch- and calcium (Ca²⁺)-activated BK (or maxi-K) channel, detected functionally in both principal and intercalated cells, mediates flow-stimulated K⁺ secretion.[21–24] In sum, K⁺ secretion in the CCD requires Na⁺ absorption (to establish a favorable electrochemical gradient) and the presence of K⁺ selective channels in the urinary membrane. Any factor that enhances the electrochemical driving force, such as an increase in tubular flow rate after administration of diuretics, or increases the apical membrane permeability to K⁺ will favor K⁺ secretion.

The limited capacity of the neonatal CCD for baseline net K⁺ secretion appears not to be due to an unfavorable electrochemical gradient.[15,25,26] Cumulative evidence now

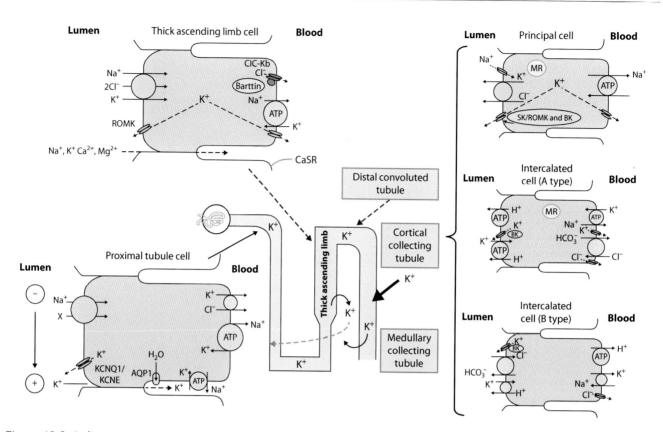

Figure 12.2 A diagramatic representation of K⁺ transport along the nephron. Once filtered by the glomeruli, K⁺ undergoes extensive reabsorption and secretion in the renal tubules. K⁺ is actively secreted in the cortical collection tubules (large arrow). K⁺ reabsortion occurs in the proximal, as well as in the ascending, limb of the loop of Henle. Some of the reabsorbed K⁺ is returned to the descending limb of the loop of Henle via the medullary interstitial recycling. Also shown are the two cell types lining the distal tubule and cortical collecting duct. ATP, adenosine triphosphate; ASDN, aldosterone-sensitive distal nephron; ENaC, epithelial Na⁺ channel; H-K-ATPase, hydrogen, potassium, adenosine triphosphatase; MR, mineralocorticoid receptor; NCC, Na-Cl cotransporter; NKCC, Na-K-2Cl cotransporter; ROMK, rat outer medullary K⁺ channel; SK, = secretory K⁺ (channel).

suggests that the postnatal increase in CCD K⁺ secretory capacity is due to developmental increases in number of apical SK and BK channels, reflecting postnatal upregulation of transcription and translation of functional channel proteins.[27–30]

## KEY POINTS

- K⁺ secretion in the distal nephron requires Na⁺ absorption (to establish a favorable electrochemical gradient) and the presence of K⁺-selective channels in the urinary membrane.
- Any factor that enhances the electrochemical driving force or increases the apical membrane permeability to K⁺ will favor K⁺ secretion.

## Tubular potassium absorption

The distal nephron of K⁺-depleted adults may reabsorb K⁺ via a hydrogen (H⁺), potassium, adenosine triphosphatase (H-K-ATPase), present at the apical membrane of acid-base transporting intercalated cells, that exchanges a single K⁺ (absorption) for a proton (secretion). Significant activity of the apical H-K-ATPase exists in neonatal intercalated cells, suggesting that the ASDN is poised to retain urinary K⁺ early in life.[31] As stated earlier, clearance studies in premature infants younger than 30 weeks gestational age suggest a developmental increase in the capacity of the kidney for K⁺ reabsorption.[1] Similar studies in saline-expanded dogs provide indirect evidence for a diminished secretory and enhanced reabsorptive capacity of the immature distal nephron to K⁺.[32]

## LUMINAL AND PERITUBULAR FACTORS REGULATING RENAL POTASSIUM TRANSPORT

### Sodium delivery and absorption

The magnitude of Na⁺ absorption in the ASDN determines the electrochemical driving force for K⁺ diffusion from the cell into the lumen (i.e., secretion). The dependence of K⁺

secretion on distal Na+ delivery becomes evident at tubular fluid Na+ concentrations of less than 30 mEq/L, a value below which K+ secretion falls sharply.[33,34] In vivo measurements of the Na+ concentration in distal tubular fluid generally exceed 35 mM both in adult and suckling rats and thus would not be expected to limit distal K+ secretion.[35]

---

### KEY POINTS

- K+ secretion in the distal nephron can be enhanced by increasing distal delivery of Na+ or nonreabsorbable anions (e.g., in diabetic ketoacidosis [DKA]), increasing urinary flow rate (e.g., by loop diuretics), activation of the renin-angiotensin-aldosterone system, or a combination of these.
- The normal kidney can reduce urinary K+ excretion to a minimum of approximately 10 mEq/day (vs. urinary Na+, which can be reduced to zero).

---

Extracellular volume expansion or administration of many diuretics (osmotic diuretics, carbonic anhydrase inhibitors, loop and thiazide diuretics) is accompanied by an increase in urinary excretion of both Na+ and K+. The kaliuresis is mediated not only by the increased delivery of Na+ to the distal nephron, but also by the drug-induced increase in tubular fluid flow rate, which maximizes the chemical driving forces favoring K+ secretion, and activates the BK channel in the ASDN. K+-sparing diuretics, such as amiloride and triamterene, block distal Na+ reabsorption, which reduces the electrical potential gradient favoring K+ secretion.

Na+ delivered to the distal nephron is generally accompanied by Cl-. Cl- reabsorption, which occurs predominantly via the paracellular pathway, tends to reduce the lumen negative potential that would otherwise favor K+ secretion. When Na+ is accompanied by an anion less reabsorbable than Cl-, such as bicarbonate ($HCO_3^-$) (as in proximal renal tubular acidosis [RTA]; see later), β-hydroxybutyrate (in DKA) or carbenicillin (during antibiotic therapy), luminal electronegativity is maintained, thereby eliciting more K+ secretion than occurs with a comparable Na+ load delivered with Cl-.

## Tubular fluid (urinary) flow rate

K+ secretion in the CCD of the adult is strongly stimulated by an increase in urinary flow rate, as follows volume expansion or administration of diuretics. The faster the urinary flow rate in the distal nephron, the slower is the rate of rise of tubular fluid K+ concentration as secreted K+ is rapidly diluted in urine of low K+ concentration. Maintenance of a relatively low tubular fluid K+ concentration maximizes the K+ concentration gradient and thus chemical driving force

favoring net K+ secretion. The electrical gradient favoring K+ secretion is further enhanced at fast tubular fluid flow rates by the flow-stimulated increase in ENaC-mediated Na+ absorption.[19,34,36] Finally, increases in luminal flow rate transduce mechanical signals, including circumferential stretch, into increases in cell $Ca^{2+}$ concentration, which in turn, activate apical BK channels.[22]

## Extracellular potassium and potassium intake

An increase in extracellular K+ concentration stimulates K+ secretion by its direct effect on stimulating (1) basolateral Na-K-ATPase–mediated uptake of K+ and (2) aldosterone and insulin secretion.[9,37] However, the changes in plasma K+ concentration and circulating levels of aldosterone following ingestion of a regular meal are relativity insignificant.[38,39] Recent studies provide evidence for a gut factor activated by dietary K+ that increases the renal excretion and extrarenal disposal of K+, independent of plasma K+ concentration.[40]

The adult kidney responds to an increase in K+ intake with an increase in urinary K+ excretion within approximately 1 to 2 days.[41] The adaptation to a high-K+ diet is associated with a rapid (within 6 hours) increase in density of conducting apical SK/ROMK channels in the CCD.[42] Apical ENaC and basolateral Na-K pump activity also increase under these same conditions, changes expected to enhance the electrochemical gradient favoring K+ secretion.[42] Chronic K+ loading also leads to an increase in BK channel protein expression and function in the distal nephron.[43]

Dietary K+ restriction leads to a fall in urinary K+ excretion, an adaptation associated with a reduction in number of active SK/ROMK and BK channels at the apical membrane[42,45] and stimulation of H-K-ATPase–mediated K+ reabsorption by intercalated cells in the ASDN.[42–46] Stimulation of H-K-ATPase activity in intercalated cells results not only in K+ retention, but also urinary acidification and metabolic alkalosis.

## Acid-base status

Disorders of acid-base homeostasis can alter urinary K+ excretion. In acute metabolic acidosis, the net movement of H+ ions into cells from the ECF is associated with the movement of K+ out of the cells, resulting in hyperkalemia. Acidosis leads to a reduction in urine pH, which in turn inhibits apical SK/ROMK channel activity.[47,48] The net effect is a fall in urinary K+ excretion.[49] In chronic metabolic acidosis, K+ secretion is influenced by modifications of the glomerular filtrate (e.g., Cl- and $HCO_3^-$ concentration), tubular fluid flow rate, and circulating aldosterone levels and thus has variable effects on urinary K+ excretion.

Both acute respiratory alkalosis and metabolic alkalosis result in increases in urine pH and $K^+$ excretion. The alkalosis-induced stimulation of $K^+$ secretion reflects two direct effects on principal cells: (1) stimulation of basolateral $K^+$ uptake and (2) an increase in the permeability of the apical membrane to $K^+$ as a result of an increase in activity of SK/ROMK channels.[11]

## Mineralocorticoids

It is well established that aldosterone stimulates $K^+$ secretion in the fully differentiated CCD. This effect of adrenal steroids is considered to be due primarily to an increase in the electrochemical driving force favoring $K^+$ exit across the apical membrane, generated by stimulation of apical $Na^+$ entry and reabsorption.[44]

Aldosterone action requires its initial binding to the mineralocorticoid receptor, followed by translocation of the hormone-receptor complex to the nucleus, where specific genes are stimulated to code for physiologically active proteins. Cellular effects within the fully differentiated CCD include increases in the density of active ENaC channels, as a result of recruitment of intracellular channels to the apical membrane, de novo synthesis of ENaC subunits, and activation of preexisting channels.[50–52] Aldosterone also stimulates Na-K-ATPase activity through both recruitment of intracellular pumps and increased total amounts of Na pump subunits.[53] The net effect of these actions is the stimulation of net $Na^+$ absorption, leading to an increase in the electrochemical gradient facilitating net $K^+$ secretion. The effects of aldosterone on ENaC and, to some extent, the Na-K pump appear to be indirect, mediated by aldosterone-induced proteins.[53]

Plasma aldosterone concentrations in the premature infant and newborn are high compared to those in the adult.[2,54] The density of aldosterone binding sites, receptor affinity, and degree of nuclear binding of hormone receptor appear to be similar in mature and immature rats.[55] Yet, clearance studies in fetal and newborn animals demonstrate a relative insensitivity of the immature kidney to the hormone, presumably because of a postreceptor phenomenon.[2,55,56] Measurements of the transtubular $K^+$ gradient (TTKG; urine-to-plasma $K^+$ concentration divided by the urine-to-plasma osmolality ratio), an index of the $K^+$ secretory capacity of the distal nephron, have been reported to be lower in 27 than 30 weeks gestational age in preterm infants followed over the first 5 weeks of postnatal life.[57] The low TTKG has been attributed to a state of relative hypoaldosteronism but may also reflect the absence of $K^+$ secretory transport pathways (i.e., channel proteins).

## DEVELOPMENTAL ASPECTS OF RENAL POTASSIUM HANDLING

Infants older than approximately 30 weeks gestational age and young children must maintain a state of positive $K^+$ balance for somatic growth. The kidney is the primary organ responsible for regulation of external $K^+$ balance. Kidneys of full-term newborn humans and animals conserve $K^+$. The ASDN is uniquely adapted to retain total body $K^+$ early in life. In contrast to the robust net $K^+$ secretion detected in single CCDs isolated from adult animals, CCDs isolated from newborns show no net $K^+$ secretion during the few weeks of postnatal life. The magnitude and direction of net $K^+$ transport in the CCD reflect the balance of opposing fluxes of $K^+$ secretion and $K^+$ absorption, proposed to be mediated by principal and intercalated cells, respectively. Evidence now indicates that the low capacity of the CCD for $K^+$ secretion early in life is due to a limited capacity of principal cells for $K^+$ secretion, reflecting, at least in part, a relative paucity of conducting $K^+$ (SK/ROMK and BK) channels in the urinary membrane. A relative excess of $K^+$ absorption by adjacent intercalated cells in this nephron segment may further reduce net urinary $K^+$ secretion. Under conditions prevailing in vivo, the balance of fluxes mediated by these two cell types likely contributes to the relative $K^+$ retention characteristic of the neonatal kidney.

## DISORDERS OF POTASSIUM METABOLISM

The estimation of $K^+$ balance depends on the measurement of extracellular (serum or plasma) $K^+$ concentration. Although easily determined, the latter measurements may reflect changes in $K^+$ redistribution between the extracellular and intracellular compartments without net gain or loss of this cation from the total body stores.

## HYPOKALEMIA

Hypokalemia is defined as a serum $K^+$ concentration less than 3.5 mEq/L. Although hypokalemia generally indicates a deficit in total body $K^+$, it also may simply reflect a transcellular shift in $K^+$ from the ECF into cells in the presence of normal body $K^+$ stores. Table 12.2 summarizes the various causes of hypokalemia, which are discussed in the following section.

---

### KEY POINT

The tendency of the neonatal kidney to retain $K^+$ is necessary for growth. Positive potassium balance is due in part to a low $K^+$ secretory capacity of the ASDN.

Table 12.2 Causes of hypokalemia

**Factitious**
- Elevated leukocyte count (e.g., as in leukemia)

**Inadequate intake**
- Dietary/parenteral

**Transcellular shift**
- Metabolic and respiratory alkalosis
- Insulin
- β-Adrenergic agonists (e.g., albuterol, terbutaline, epinephrine), dopamine, theophylline
- Hypokalemic periodic paralysis
- Barium toxicit

**Renal loss**
- Diuretics
  - Thiazides and loop diuretics
  - Osmotic diuretics (mannitol, glucose)
  - Carbonic anhydrase inhibitors
- Excess mineralocorticoid activity
  - Primary hyperaldosteronism (adrenal adenoma/hyperplasia)
  - Activation of renin-angiotensin-aldosterone pathway (renal vascular stenosis, renin producing tumors, or volume depletion)
  - Congenital adrenal hyperplasia (11-hydroxylase deficiency or 17-hydroxylase deficiency)
  - Increased corticosteroid level (Cushing's syndrome, high dose steroids)
  - Excessive licorice ingestion
- Renal tubular defects
  - Type 1 RTA
  - Type 2 RTA
  - Bartter syndrome
  - Gitelman syndrome
  - Liddle syndrome
- Endocrine derangements (thyrotoxicosis, vitamin D intoxication)
- Miscellaneous
  - $Mg^{2+}$ deficiency
  - Drugs (e.g., penicillins, aminoglycosides, polymyxin B, and amphotericin)

**Gastrointestinal loss**
- Vomiting
- Biliary drainage
- Diarrhea
- Laxative or enema abuse
- Villous adenoma
- Ureterosigmoidostomies

**Integumental loss**
- Excessive sweating
- Severe burns

# Clinical disorders of hypokalemia

## FACTITIOUS HYPOKALEMIA

Factitious hypokalemia may be observed in patients with high white blood cells counts (e.g., in leukemia), whose blood samples are stored for prolonged periods at room temperature after collection.[58] The spurious hypokalemia, due to transcellular $K^+$ movement into white blood cells, can be avoided by immediate separation of cells from the plasma after phlebotomy or storage of the sample at 4° C.

## INADEQUATE INTAKE

The response of the adult to a $K^+$-free diet is a reduction in $K^+$ excretion to approximately 10 mEq/day.[59] The inability of the adult kidney to produce a $K^+$-free urine, in light of the obligatory GI loss of $K^+$, can lead to hypokalemia after a prolonged period of inadequate intake. Because almost all foods contain some $K^+$, extreme dietary $K^+$ restriction is achieved in only a few clinical disorders, such as anorexia nervosa and intestinal malabsorption syndromes. Hypokalemia in the latter patient populations may be exacerbated by inappropriately high rates of urinary $K^+$ excretion secondary to magnesium ($Mg^{2+}$) deficiency; intracellular $Mg^{2+}$ normally inhibits $K^+$ secretion through the SK/ROMK channel in the ASDN.[58] Hypokalemia also can be seen in patients who are receiving $K^+$-free parenteral fluids.

## TRANSCELLULAR SHIFT OF POTASSIUM INTO CELLS

### Alkalosis

Both acute metabolic and respiratory alkalosis are frequently accompanied by severe hypokalemia, resulting, in part, from the intracellular uptake of $K^+$ in exchange for $H^+$. Within hours of the onset of an acid-base disturbance, $K^+$ homeostasis is affected not only by the initial effect of pH on cell $K^+$ content, but also by changes in the renal handling of the cation. The profound hypokalemia characteristic of pyloric stenosis, for example, is, in part, due to the alkalemia-induced exchange of extracellular $K^+$ for intracellular $H^+$ and is exacerbated by two additional factors that stimulate renal $K^+$ excretion: volume contraction-induced hyperaldosteronism and delivery of nonreabsorbable anions ($HCO_3^-$) to $K^+$ secretory sites in the ASDN.

### Insulin

Pharmacologic doses of insulin, as administered to patients with DKA, reduce plasma $K^+$ concentration by promoting $K^+$ uptake by muscle and liver cells. This insulin-induced redistribution of $K^+$ is exploited in the treatment of hyperkalemia with insulin with glucose.

### Nonselective β-adrenergic agonists

Nonselective β-adrenergic agonists (e.g., epinephrine, isoproterenol), selective $β_2$-agonists (albuterol, terbutaline), and dopamine directly promote K$^+$ uptake by cells and stimulate insulin release. Theophylline and caffeine indirectly promote cellular K$^+$ uptake by stimulation of sympathetic amine release. The reduction in plasma K$^+$ observed in response to administration of these pharmacologic agents tends to be mild except when a K$^+$ deficit already exists. Thus, for example, a surge in epinephrine secretion during an episode of acute myocardial ischemia can lead to severe hypokalemia in a hypertensive patient on chronic diuretic therapy, thereby increasing the risk for ventricular arrhythmia and sudden death. Treatment of asthmatics with albuterol or theophylline can lead to K$^+$ redistribution and hypokalemia. The latter electrolyte imbalance, if severe, may impair the contractile ability of the respiratory muscles, thereby worsening respiratory status.

## Familial hypokalemic periodic paralysis

In familial hypokalemic periodic paralysis, a rare autosomal dominant disorder, patients experience recurrent, transient episodes associated with a low serum K$^+$ concentration (<2.8 mEq/L), lasting hours to days, that can vary in clinical intensity from mild muscle weakness to flaccid paralysis of the limbs and thorax. Attacks can be precipitated by maneuvers that decrease plasma K$^+$ concentration, including carbohydrate-heavy meals (resulting from the stimulatory effect of insulin on the Na-K pump), rest after strenuous exercise (as K$^+$ released during activity is taken back up into skeletal muscle), or stress. Familial hypokalemic periodic paralysis is associated with mutations in the skeletal muscle voltage-gated Ca$^{2+}$ channel (Ca$_V$1.1) or voltage-gated Na$^+$ channel Na$_V$1.4.[60-62] Oral K$^+$ supplements, spironolactone, and acetazolamide have been used with variable results to prevent recurrent paralytic episodes.[63,64]

## Barium poisoning

Barium poisoning from ingestion or inhalation of large quantities of soluble barium salts, such as barium carbonate used in pesticides, and not the nonabsorbable barium sulfate preparation used in radiologic studies, produces a characteristic muscular paralysis that can lead to respiratory paralysis and death. Barium blocks the K$^+$ conductance of muscle cells, thereby impairing the outward diffusion of K$^+$ pumped into the cell via the Na-K-ATPase.[65] Thus, barium poisoning typically results in a severe fall in serum K$^+$ secondary to the intracellular sequestration of this cation.[66] The clinical picture resembles hypokalemic periodic paralysis (muscle weakness and paralysis) with additional symptoms, including salivation, vomiting, diarrhea, hypertension, ventricular tachycardia, and fibrillation.[67]

## Renal potassium loss

Renal causes of K$^+$ wasting can be subdivided into those that are primarily (e.g., Conn syndrome or Cushing syndrome) or secondarily (e.g., diuretics, RTA) mediated by aldosterone.

## EXCESS MINERALOCORTICOID ACTIVITY

Excess mineralocorticoid activity is well known to lead to renal K$^+$ wasting. Autonomous adrenal aldosterone production (primary aldosteronism), as is observed in adrenal adenoma or bilateral adrenal hyperplasia, should be suspected in any adult who presents with the triad of hypokalemia, hypertension, and metabolic alkalosis.[68,69] Other pathophysiologic causes for activation of the renin-angiotensin-aldosterone pathway, which may lead to hypokalemia in children, include renal vascular disease and renin-producing tumors.

Certain forms of congenital adrenal hyperplasia (CAH) are associated with hypokalemia.[70] Specifically, 11-hydroxylase or 17α-hydroxylase deficiency, resulting from defects in the genes CYP11B1 and CYP17A1, are associated with hypertension and hypokalemic alkalosis. In the former, impaired cortisol production leads to increased adrenocorticotropic hormone secretion, subsequent overproduction of the mineralocorticoid deoxycorticosterone (DOC), and adrenal androgen production; the excessive secretion of DOC leads to hypertension and hypokalemia. The latter form of CAH is also associated with impaired cortisol synthesis, with consequent features of mineralocorticoid excess but also defective production of adrenal androgens.

Some patients with Cushing syndrome (increased cortisol production) or those receiving pharmacologic doses of corticosteroids may present with hypokalemia, presumably a result of the mineralocorticoid effects of these hormones. Plasma levels of the naturally occurring glucocorticoid cortisol, which binds as avidly to the mineralocorticoid receptor, as does aldosterone, are approximately 100-fold greater than circulating levels of aldosterone. The enzyme 11-β-hydroxysteroid dehydrogenase type 2 (11β-HSD2), expressed in the ASDN, metabolizes cortisol to cortisone, which binds to the mineralocorticoid receptor poorly; this reaction is critical in preventing glucocorticoid-dependent activation of the mineralocorticoid receptor. Genetic loss of function or ingestion of inhibitors of 11β-HSD2 can thus lead to inappropriate activation of the mineralocorticoid receptor by cortisol and in turn severe hypertension and hypokalemia. Glycyrrhizic acid, an active ingredient in licorice, inhibits 11β-HSD2; ingestion of excess licorice can manifest with a picture similar to that of primary aldosteronism, but with low levels of aldosterone and plasma renin activity.[71]

## DIURETIC USE (AND ABUSE)

A common cause of hypokalemia is diuretic use. Although the specific mechanism and site of action of each class of diuretic (thiazide, loop, and osmotic diuretics and carbonic anhydrase inhibitors) will determine its associated electrolyte and acid-base, all diuretics cause significant urinary K$^+$ losses resulting from increased volume and Na$^+$ delivery to the distal nephron. Fast tubular fluid flow rates stimulate K$^+$ secretion into the urinary fluid by activation of the BK channel and augmentation of Na+ delivery and absorption in this segment, which enhances the electrochemical gradient favoring K+ secretion. Hyperaldosteronism secondary to a diuretic-induced reduction in effective intravascular volume or concomitant edema (as the cause for administration of the diuretics) may further promote renal K+ secretion; the metabolic alkalosis characteristic of high aldosterone states may enhance cell K+ uptake, which in turn increases the concentration gradient favoring K+ secretion. Finally, some diuretics may enhance distal delivery of nonreabsorbable anions, such as $HCO_3^-$ (carbonic anhydrase inhibitors) to increase luminal electronegativity and K+ secretion in the ASDN.

## RENAL TUBULAR DEFECTS

### Type 1 and 2 RTA

Renal tubular defects can result in renal K+ wasting. Distal (type 1) and proximal (type 2) RTA both result in hypokalemia, albeit by different mechanisms. The mainstay of treatment for RTA is alkali therapy.

Distal RTA (dRTA) is characterized by a defect in H+ secretion into the distal nephron; the failure to secrete positively charged protons into the urinary fluid results in increased luminal electronegativity, enhancing K+ secretion but limiting Na+ absorption. Consequent volume depletion results in secondary hyperaldosteronism, which additionally contributes to K+ loss. Genetic causes of dRTA are due to mutations in acid-base transporting proteins in intercalated cells,[72,73] which secrete H+ into the urinary fluid through apical H+-ATPases functionally coupled to the basolateral $Cl^-/HCO_3^-$ anion exchanger 1 (AE1). Loss-of-function mutations in *ATP6V1B1*, the gene encoding the B1 subtype unit of the apical H+-ATPase, and *ATP6V0A4*, encoding the α subunit, lead to an autosomal recessive dRTA often associated with sensorineural deafness. Mutations in the gene encoding AE1 can manifest as a dominant or recessive dRTA and may be accompanied by erythroid changes. Mutations in the gene encoding AE1 encoding cytosolic carbonic anhydrase II are associated with a recessive mixed proximal-distal RTA, osteopetrosis, and cerebral calcification.

Proximal RTA (pRTA) is characterized by a reduced ability to reabsorb $HCO_3^-$ in the proximal tubule, leading to excessive urinary $HCO_3^-$ losses. The increased delivery of $HCO_3^-$ to the distal nephron again increases the luminal electronegativity, enhancing K+ secretion, whereas urinary wasting of Na+ that escapes proximal reabsorption leads to volume depletion and hyperaldosteronism. The defect in proximal tubule $HCO_3^-$ reabsorption may exist in isolation or as part of Fanconi syndrome, associated with proximal losses of not only $HCO_3^-$ but also of phosphate, glucose, amino acids, uric acid, and low-molecular-weight proteins.[74] Genetic causes of pRTA most often follow an autosomal recessive pattern of inheritance. Loss-of-function mutations in the basolateral Na+-$HCO_3^-$ cotransporter (NBCe1, encoded by *SLC4A4*) lead to a recessive pRTA

with ocular and central nervous system abnormalities.[73] Administration of carbonic anhydrase inhibitors causes isolated proximal $HCO_3^-$ wastage, but more severe Fanconi syndrome can be seen in patients given certain drugs, including ifosfamide, valproic acid, and various antiretrovirals, such as tenofovir.[74] dRTA may occur in association with other renal diseases accompanied by tubular dysfunction (renal transplantation, obstructive uropathy, pyelopnephritis).[75]

Inherited salt-losing tubulopathies, specifically Bartter syndrome and Gitelman syndrome, comprise another category of disorders associated with hypokalemia.[76,77] Patients with Bartter or Gitelman syndrome present with a biochemical profile including hypokalemic, hypochloremic metabolic alkalosis associated with high plasma renin activity and high aldosterone concentration.

## BARTTER SYNDROME AND GITELMAN SYNDROME

In Bartter syndrome, patients typically present early in life with severe urinary salt wasting, polyuria, and hypokalemic alkalosis, a biochemical profile similar to that induced by furosemide. It is now known that Bartter syndrome may be due to mutations in genes encoding proteins critical for transepithelial transport in the TALH, which include the furosemide target NKCC2 (encoded by *SLC12A1*, type 1 Bartter syndrome), the apical SK/ROMK channel (*KCNJ1*, type 2), the basolateral Cl- channel ClC-Kb (*CLCNKB*, type 3), or its associated subunit Barttin (*BSND*, type 4), and the calcium-sensing receptor (*CASR*, type 5).[76] As patients with antenatal Bartter (types 1 and 2) do not establish a transepithelial voltage gradient in the TALH robust enough to drive paracellular $Ca^{2+}$ and $Mg^{2+}$ absorption, these cations are lost in the urine, which predisposes patients to nephrocalcinosis. Typically, patients with Bartter syndrome are born prematurely, with complications that may include polyhydramnios and life-threatening dehydration in the neonatal period. Additional clinical manifestations to those identified previously include failure to thrive and growth failure. Barttin is also located in the cochlea, and patients with mutations in this protein often have deafness.

In Gitelman syndrome, inactivating mutations in the gene (*SLC12A3*) encoding the apical thiazide-sensitive Na-Cl cotransporter (NCC), in the distal convoluted tubule (DCT) lead to a milder salt-losing nephropathy than seen in Bartter syndrome, as would be observed in patients abusing thiazide diuretics.[76] Pediatric patients are often asymptomatic, but may be diagnosed coincidentally during a diagnostic workup for growth retardation, constipation, or enuresis. Because Gitelman syndrome is associated with hypocalciuria, measurement of urinary $Ca^{2+}$ excretion may help distinguish between Gitelman syndrome and Bartter syndrome (which is associated with hypercalciuria).

## LIDDLE SYNDROME

Liddle syndrome is a rare autosomal dominant disorder characterized by early-onset severe hypertension and hypokalemic metabolic alkalosis, low plasma renin activity, and suppressed secretion of aldosterone.[78] The disorder is due to mutations in either the β or γ subunit of ENaC that lead to high constitutive levels of channel activity and $Na^+$ absorption in the distal nephron, enhancing the electrochemical gradient favoring $K^+$ secretion. Treatment of patients with inhibitors of ENaC, including amiloride or triamterene, normalizes blood pressure and hypokalemia.[79-81]

Drugs other than diuretics and miscellaneous disorders associated with hypokalemia secondary to urinary $K^+$ wasting are listed in Table 12.2.

## Extracellular electrolyte Loss

Under normal circumstances, fecal excretion of $K^+$ is approximately 5 to 15 mEq/day. GI tract $K^+$ loss may increase significantly in the face of severe or prolonged diarrhea or laxative abuse. Vomiting and nasogastric suction can lead to volume depletion and metabolic alkalosis, which exacerbates renal $K^+$ loss via activation of the renin-angiotensin-aldosterone system and transcellular shift of $K^+$, respectively. The increased distal delivery of $HCO_3^-$, which serves as a nonreabsorbable anion, in metabolic alkalosis further promotes urinary $K^+$ secretion in the distal nephron.

Under normal circumstances, the concentration of $K^+$ in sweat is only 5 to 10 mEq/L. Integumental loss from either excessive sweating or severe burns may lead to volume contraction and secondary hyperaldosteronism. Of note, in severe burns, hyperkalemia may be seen initially as a result of cell breakdown, which is then followed by hypokalemia secondary to hyperaldosteronism that follows volume contraction.

## Clinical manifestations of hypokalemia

The consequences of $K^+$ depletion affect many organ systems and depend on the magnitude and duration of the deficit. Most prominently affected are the neurologic and cardiovascular systems, muscles, and kidneys.

The ratio of intracellular $K^+$ concentration to that in the ECF is a major determinant of resting membrane potential ($E_m$) across the cell membrane. Alterations in the ICF to ECF $K^+$ concentration ratio will thus affect $E_m$ and neuromuscular excitability. An acute reduction in the extracellular $K^+$ concentration (leading to a high ratio of intracellular to extracellular $K^+$) increases or hyperpolarizes $E_m$, thereby making the cell less excitable. This manifests as neuromuscular weakness and, in severe cases, paralysis. Death may follow from respiratory muscle failure. The effects of hypokalemia on cardiac conduction and rhythm are manifest on the electrocardiogram (ECG) and include ST segment depression, diminished T wave voltage, and appearance of the U wave. These abnormalities typically appear in patients with plasma $K^+$ levels less than 3 mEq/L. Hypokalemia-induced smooth muscle dysfunction is usually manifest as paralytic ileus and diminished ureteral peristalsis.

---

> **KEY POINT**
>
> The most prominent clinical consequences of homeostatic $K^+$ derangements result from the adverse effects on excitable tissues.

$K^+$ depletion also affects renal function. The most common abnormality detected is an inability to maximally concentrate urine. This is due to a reduction in the osmolar gradient in the medullary interstitium as well as impaired activation of renal adenylate cyclase in response to vasopressin.[82,83] In addition to this direct renal effect, $K^+$ depletion stimulates the central thirst center via increased production of angiotensin II (ATII).[84] The resultant polydipsia of severely hypokalemic patients further increases urinary output and exacerbates the concentrating defect.

Hypokalemia may affect carbohydrate and protein metabolism.[85,86] $K^+$ depletion suppresses insulin release, and thereby can result in glucose intolerance. The failure to thrive often seen childhood with severe hypokalemia and total $K^+$ depletion may be due to the disturbance in protein metabolism or insufficient substrate (body $K^+$, the predominant intracellular cation) for cellular growth.[87]

## Diagnostic evaluation of hypokalemia

Diagnostic evaluation should be guided by a thorough history and physical examination. A detailed history should include the assessment of pattern of growth, presence of chronic illness, family history of similar disease, use of medications (e.g., diuretics, laxatives), and symptoms associated with the electrolyte disturbance. Physical examination must include measurement of growth indices, blood pressure, and assessment for edema and altered neuromuscular function.

The initial laboratory evaluation should include a complete blood count (CBC), serum electrolytes including $HCO_3^-$ and $Mg^{2+}$, creatinine and glucose, and a urine analysis. If the laboratory data do not support the diagnoses of pseudohypokalemia or redistribution of $K^+$ from the ECF to ICF space (alkalosis or hypoglycemia), the hypokalemia likely represents total body $K^+$ depletion from GI tract, skin, or renal $K^+$ losses.

If the cause of hypokalemia is not immediately obvious, assessment of urinary $K^+$ excretion can be very helpful.

---

> **KEY POINT**
>
> Elevated or reduced plasma/serum $K^+$ concentrations may not accurately reflect changes in total body $K^+$ content.

A low urinary $K^+$ concentration (<15 mEq/L) in the absence of recent diuretic use implies near maximal urinary $K^+$ conservation, suggesting that the hypokalemia is secondary to inadequate intake, a shift of $K^+$ into cells, or extrarenal losses (GI, skin). The presence of concomitant metabolic acidosis would suggest lower GI losses resulting from diarrhea or laxative abuse.

A high urinary $K^+$ concentration (>15 mEq/L or a urinary $Na^+/K^+$ ratio consistently less than 1 in the absence of renal failure) in a patient with hypokalemia is consistent with renal $K^+$ wasting. Inappropriate urinary $K^+$ wasting associated with hypertension and metabolic alkalosis is a classic finding in hyper-reninemic states, such as renal vascular stenosis and primary hyperaldosteronism. Metabolic acidosis with a high urinary $K^+$ concentration is also seen in DKA or type 1 or type 2 distal RTA. Bartter and Gitelman syndrome should be considered in patients with hypokalemic metabolic alkalosis, salt wasting with volume depletion, and hyper-reninemia and hyperaldosteronism.

## Management of hypokalemia

Management of hypokalemia should be proportional to the severity of $K^+$ depletion. However, $K^+$ replacement should be done cautiously in the presence of complicating factors that affect the transcellular distribution of $K^+$ (e.g., acid-base status), especially in patients with renal or cardiac disease.

Mild hypokalemia will often respond to oral supplementation with foods containing a high $K^+$ content. Oral $K^+$ supplements will be necessary for moderate $K^+$ depletion. Among the oral preparations available in liquid, powder, and slow-release preparations are potassium chloride, potassium citrate, and potassium gluconate; the latter two formulations are ideal for patients with a concomitant acidosis in whom the organic anion provides potential alkali. The adverse effects associated with oral therapy, especially following administration of potassium chloride, include GI irritation, ranging from vomiting to ulceration, and $K^+$ intoxication.

Severe, symptomatic, or both hypokalemia types should be treated with intravenous (IV) potassium chloride. $K^+$ replacement fluid should be formulated in dextrose-free solution to prevent transcellular shifts of $K^+$ as the sugar stimulates insulin secretion. Conventionally, parenteral $K^+$ should be infused in a solution containing no more than 40 mEq/L and infused at a rate not to exceed 0.75 mEq/kg body weight in the first hour of therapy in children or 10 mEq/h in adults. When life-threatening paralysis or ventricular arrhythmias are present, more aggressive $K^+$ replacement may be appropriate in a monitored unit.

In patients with diuretic-induced hypokalemia who require continued use of their diuretic, addition of a $K^+$-sparing diuretic such as amiloride, triamterene, or spironolactone should be considered. Hypomagnesemia can lead to renal $K^+$ wasting and refractoriness to $K^+$ replacement. $Mg^{2+}$ repletion facilitates correction of the coexisting $K^+$ deficit.

## HYPERKALEMIA

Hyperkalemia is defined as a serum $K^+$ concentration greater than 6.0 mEq/L in the newborn and 5.5 mEq/L in the older child and adult. Hyperkalemia is generally due to a shift of $K^+$ from ICF to the ECF or inadequate urinary $K^+$ excretion and may not be accompanied by an increase in total body content of $K^+$. This is particularly evident in patients with DKA, who typically present with hyperkalemia yet are total body $K^+$-depleted. Table 12.3 summarizes the various disorders associated with hyperkalemia, which are discussed in the next section.

> ### KEY POINT
>
> Hyperkalemia is generally not detected in healthy adults subjected to a K+ load due to the efficiency of the initial rapid translocation of K+ that enters the ECF into the vast intracellular reservoirs and the subsequent excretion of the K+ load via the kidneys and GI tract.

## Clinical disorders of hyperkalemia

### PSEUDOHYPERKALEMIA

Pseudohyperkalemia represents an in vitro elevation in serum $K^+$ concentration in the absence of in vivo hyperkalemia, and is due to the transcellular movement of $K^+$ from the cytosol into the ECF during clotting or prolonged storage of a blood sample.[58] The concentration of $K^+$ in the serum is approximately 0.4 mEq/L higher than that in the plasma in samples with normal numbers of blood cells, reflecting release of the cation by leukocytes and platelets during in vitro clotting. Thus, an elevated serum, but not plasma $K^+$ concentration, may be measured in any hematologic disorder associated with marked elevation in number of white blood cells[88] or platelets.[88,89] Red blood cells can also release intracellular $K^+$ (and hemoglobin) via in vitro hemolysis.

Improper phlebotomy techniques may alter serum $K^+$ measurements. Contraction of the forearm muscles during fist clenching can lead to release of $K^+$ from muscle and elevation of the plasma $K^+$ concentration in blood sampled from that extremity.[90] Squeezing an infant's heel or transferring blood vigorously through a small-bore needle may result in hemolysis. Prolonged exposure of blood samples to the cold will inhibit Na-K-ATPase activity and lead to leakage of $K^+$ from the cells.

### INCREASED POTASSIUM LOAD

Hyperkalemia is generally not detected in healthy individuals subject to an exogenous or endogenous $K^+$ load because of the efficiency of the initial rapid translocation of $K^+$ that enters the ECF into the vast intracellular reservoirs and the

Table 12.3 Causes of hyperkalemia

**Pseudohyperkalemia**
- Improper collection of blood
- Hemolysis
- Leukocytosis, thrombocytosis, polycythemia

**Increased load**
- Exogenous (oral vs. parenteral), blood transfusion
- Endogenous (cell breakdown)
  - Intravascular hemolysis
  - Rhabdomyolysis
  - Crush injuries
  - Severe exercise
  - Burns
  - Tumor lysis syndrome
  - Massive GI bleeds
  - Starvation

**Transcellular shift**
- Metabolic acidosis
- Hyperosmolarity
- Insulin deficiency
- Exercise during β adrenergic blockade
- Arginine infusion
- Succinylcholine
- Digoxin overdose
- Familial hyperkalemic periodic paralysis

**Decreased renal excretory capacity**
- Renal failure (acute/chronic)
- Mineralocorticoid deficiency
  - Addison disease
  - Hypoaldosteronism (hyporeninemic vs. defect in 21-hydroxylase or 18-hydroxydehydrogenase activity)
- Impaired tubular secretion without abnormalities in mineralocorticoid production
  - Pseudohypoaldosteronism
  - Obstructive and reflux uropathy
  - Sickle cell disease
  - Renal transplantation
  - Lead nephropathy
  - Systemic lupus erythematosus
  - Papillary necrosis
- Drugs
  - Prostaglandin synthesis inhibitors
  - K+-sparing diuretics
  - ACE inhibitors
  - Miscellaneous

*Abbreviations:* ACE, angiotensin-converting enzyme; GI, gastrointestinal.

subsequent excretion of the $K^+$ load via the kidneys and GI tract. Common sources of exogenous $K^+$ include $K^+$ rich foods, oral or parenteral $K^+$ supplements (including total parenteral nutrition), salt substitutes, high doses of potassium penicillin, and stored blood products.

Endogenous sources of $K^+$ do not increase total body $K^+$ content, but rather cause hyperkalemia through a decrease in the $K^+$ content in the ICF compartment. Cell breakdown leads to release of $K^+$ into the ECF to increase plasma $K^+$ concentration. Significant endogenous $K^+$ release can follow intravascular hemolysis, rhabdomyolysis, crush injuries, severe exercise, burns, tumor lysis syndrome, massive GI bleeds, and starvation.[91] Of note, patients with these conditions often experience concurrent acute kidney injury (AKI) (as follows hypotension or myoglobinuria), volume contraction, or both, conditions that will impair the ability to eliminate the $K^+$ load.

## TRANSCELLULAR SHIFT OF POTASSIUM INTO CELLS

### Metabolic acidosis

In most states of mineral acid metabolic acidosis (uremic acidosis, $NH_4Cl$-induced acidosis), excess hydrogen ions ($H^+$) in the ECF are apparently exchanged for intracellular $K^+$ so that they may be neutralized by intracellular buffers.[92] However, clinical and experimental studies indicate that uncomplicated organic acidemias (including diabetic and alcoholic acidosis, lactic acidosis, acidemias secondary to methylmalonic and isovaleric acid, and ethylene glycol, paraldehyde and salicylate intoxications) do not produce hyperkalemia. Among the complicating factors that may cause hyperkalemia in patients with organic acidemias are volume depletion and renal hypoperfusion, preexisting renal disease, hypercatabolism, diabetes mellitus, and hyperosmolality, hypoaldosteronism, and subsequent therapy. The proposed mechanism(s) underlying the differing effect of mineral and organic acidemias on transcellular movement of $K^+$ suggests that organic anions freely enter into cells without creating a gradient for the $H^+$ ions and, thus, obviate the efflux of intracellular $K^+$.

---

**KEY POINT**

Transcellular shifts in $K^+$ can have large effects on extracellular $K^+$ concentration.

---

### Hormones

Cellular uptake of $K^+$ is stimulated by multiple hormones, including insulin, catecholamines, and mineralocorticoids. Therefore, deficiency in any of these hormones (e.g., in diabetes, adrenal insufficiency) or impairment in their action (e.g., administration of β-blockers or angiotensin converting enzyme inhibitors) can contribute to hyperkalemia, especially if a $K^+$ load is delivered concomitantly.

### Drugs

Certain drugs enhance release of $K^+$ from intracellular compartments, particularly muscle, into the ECF. Arginine hydrochloride, infused during growth hormone stimulation testing, may cause hyperkalemia as the cationic amino acid enters cells and displaces $K^+$.[93] Succinylcholine is a depolarizing muscle relaxant that causes release of $K^+$ from muscles and can be associated with an exaggerated hyperkalemic response in patients with neuromuscular disease, trauma, burns, tetanus, and renal failure.[94-96] In digoxin overdose, the Na-K-ATPase responsible for maintaining the transcellular $Na^+$ and $K^+$ gradients is inhibited, leading to $K^+$ leak from cells and in some cases, marked hyperkalemia.[97]

## Familial hyperkalemic periodic paralysis

In familial hyperkalemic periodic paralysis, an autosomal dominant muscle $Na^+$ channelopathy resulting from a mutation in the SCN4A gene encoding the skeletal muscle voltage-gated channel $Na_v1.4$, disruption of the normal exchange of ions in skeletal muscle results in episodic attacks of flaccid weakness and intermittent myotonia that typically begin in the first decade of life.[98,99] During attacks, individuals may be hyperkalemic or normokalemic. Attacks may be precipitated by exercise, hypothermia, and fasting.

## Nonoliguric hyperkalemia

Nonoliguric hyperkalemia (NOHK), defined as a serum $K^+$ concentration greater than 7.0 mEq/L during the first 72 hours of life in the presence of urinary output of greater than 1 mL/kg/h, is observed in 30% to 50% of infants with very low birth weight.[100,101] This disorder has been proposed to reflect $Na^+$-$K^+$ pump failure, leading to accumulation of $K^+$ in the ECF, as well as a limited renal $K^+$ secretory capacity.[7,102,103] Prenatal steroid treatment may prevent NOHK by stimulating Na-K-ATPase pump activity in the fetus, thereby stabilizing the cell membrane to prevent a shift of $K^+$ out of cells.[104]

### DECREASED RENAL POTASSIUM EXCRETION

## Acute kidney injury

Hyperkalemia is routinely observed in patients with the acute onset of oliguric AKI. The abrupt cessation of renal function leads to an increase in serum $K^+$ concentration of approximately 0.5 mEq/L/day.[105,106] This is due to both the reduction in GFR, which limits the amount of $K^+$ entering the glomerular filtrate, but also diminished urinary flow rates in the $K^+$ secretory sites of the ASDN. The rise in plasma $K^+$ concentration in many patients with renal failure may be exacerbated by endogenous tissue breakdown or administration of exogenous $K^+$ loads, as may accompany blood transfusions.

## Chronic kidney disease

Serum $K^+$ concentration in patients with chronic kidney disease may be maintained within normal limits by a compensatory increase in $K^+$ excretion by surviving nephrons, usually until the GFR is less than 10% of normal. This adaptation may allow excreted $K^+$ to exceed filtered load in patients with major reductions in functional renal mass. However, these patients typically have an impaired ability to excrete an additional acute $K^+$ load. Uremia inhibits the ubiquitous Na-K-ATPase, resulting in impaired cellular uptake of $K^+$.

## Mineralocorticoid deficiency

The renal excretory capacity for $K^+$ also may be limited by mineralocorticoid deficiency, as is observed in primary adrenal insufficiency (Addison disease), hyporeninemic hypoaldosteronism (type 4 RTA), and some forms of CAH that are not accompanied by synthesis of other compounds with mineralocorticoid activity such as DOC. More than 90% of cases of CAH are due to deficiency in 21-hydroxylase, secondary to mutations in CYP21A2, which leads to diminished or loss of mineralocorticoid and glucocorticoid production; these patients present with salt wasting, hyperkalemia, virilization of girls, and failure to thrive.[107] An isolated defect in aldosterone biosynthesis, secondary to aldosterone synthase (corticosterone methyloxidase, CYP11B2) deficiency, can manifest with hyponatremia and hypovolemia, as a result of salt wasting, and hyperkalemia.[108]

## End-organ hyporesponsiveness

Patients may have impaired tubular secretion of $K^+$ as a result of end organ hyporesponsiveness without a deficiency of mineralocorticoid production. Pseudohypoaldosteronism type 1 (PHA1) is a rare inherited disease characterized by resistance to the actions of aldosterone. Infants with PHA1 typically present with failure to thrive, hyperkalemia and salt wasting that does not respond to exogenous mineralocorticoid administration; in fact, they are noted to have elevated levels of aldosterone.[109] Autosomal dominant PHA1 results from inactivating mutations in the gene encoding the mineralocorticoid receptor, whereas the autosomal recessive form of PHA1 is caused by mutations in genes encoding ENaC subunits.[110] Therapy with $Na^+$ supplementation generally corrects the clinical and biochemical abnormalities (except plasma aldosterone levels remain high).[111] Patients with Gordon syndrome, also known as PHAII, and familial hypertension with hyperkalemia, generally present with hyperkalemia, as expected in a state of apparent hypoaldosteronism, but also with hypertension. PHAII is due to mutations in the genes encoding the with-no-lysine (WNK) kinases, a family of kinases that regulate transport proteins in the distal nephron.[112] Type III PHA is typically transient and secondary to nephropathies, including obstructive uropathy, urinary tract infections, sickle cell disease, renal transplantation, and lead nephropathy.[113]

## Drugs

Medications are a common cause of hyperkalemia. Nonsteroidal anti-inflammatory drugs (NSAIDs) have been proposed to induce hyperkalemia by reducing prostaglandin synthesis through cyclo-oxygenase inhibition; prostaglandins increase $K^+$ excretion by stimulating renin secretion (leading to aldosterone secretion), maintaining GFR through preglomerular arteriolar vasodilation, and direct effects on $K^+$ secretory channels sites in the distal nephron.[114,115] Spironolactone, as a competitive inhibitor of aldosterone, and the $K^+$-sparing diuretics triamterene and amiloride block luminal $Na^+$ entry, decreasing the electrochemical gradient favoring K$^+$ secretion, in the distal tubule.

Trimethoprim and pentamidine, frequently prescribed to patients with immunodeficiency, inhibit distal nephron reabsorption of Na$^+$ by blocking apical ENaC in a manner similar to that of the K$^+$-sparing diuretics.[116,117] Angiotensin-converting enzyme (ACE) inhibitors, via suppression of ATII generation, lead to a reduction in aldosterone levels, which may lead to hyperkalemia; combination therapy with an ACE inhibitor and an angiotensin receptor blocker (ARB), compared with monotherapy, is associated with an increased risk for hyperkalemia and acute kidney injury.[118] Hyperkalemia, hypercalciuria, and acidosis often complicate the use of calcineurin inhibitors, immunosuppressive drugs used to prevent organ rejection.[119]

## Clinical manifestations of hyperkalemia

The clinical consequences of hyperkalemia result from the adverse electrophysiologic effects of an altered transmembrane K$^+$ gradient on excitable tissues. Specifically, an increased extracellular K$^+$ concentration shifts the resting membrane potential to a less negative value (e.g., from −90 mV to −80 mV), initially enhancing tissue excitability. Thus, hyperkalemia may manifest as skeletal muscle weakness, paresthesias, and ascending flaccid paralysis.

Although cardiac toxicity generally occurs when the serum K$^+$ concentration rises above 7 mEq/L, treatment should be initiated in any patient with suspected hyperkalemia if ECG abnormalities characteristic of hyperkalemia are noted. The first and most specific ECG abnormality seen with hyperkalemia (usually apparent at serum K$^+$ levels above 7 mEq/L) are tall, peaked T waves. The P-R interval lengthens and the QRS complex then widens. As K$^+$ concentrations rise above 8 mEq/L, the $P$ wave amplitude decreases and may disappear with atrial standstill. As ventricular conduction time continues to lengthen, the QRS complex merges with the peaked T wave, producing a "sine wave" pattern. Finally, ventricular fibrillation or asystole may occur at K$^+$ concentrations above 10 mEq/L.

## Diagnostic evaluation of hyperkalemia

A detailed history should be sought first, with careful documentation of the child's growth pattern, history of chronic illness, and medication review (ACE inhibitors, K$^+$-sparing diuretics, trimethoprim, corticosteroids, β-blockers, and NSAIDs). A physical examination should include measurement of growth indices and blood pressure, and signs of any chronic illness. An ECG must be obtained promptly in any patient with hyperkalemia.

Pseudohyperkalemia should first be excluded by evaluation of plasma (not serum) K$^+$ concentration from a free-flowing venipuncture or vascular access. Additional laboratory tests, including CBC, repeat set of plasma

electrolytes with HCO$_3^-$, creatinine, and glucose and urine analysis, are generally appropriate. Urine electrolytes can provide information about renal K$^+$ conservation. The TTKG provides an indirect estimate of aldosterone bioactivity in the distal nephron and is calculated as described earlier.[57] In adults with normal adrenal and renal function given an oral K$^+$ load, the TTKG increases above 10 within 2 hours, reflecting the stimulated mineralocorticoid activity.[120] Low TTKG values (<6 in adults, <5 in infants and children) are inappropriate in patients with hyperkalemia and may reflect hypoaldosteronism or pseudohypoaldosteronism.[57,121]

## Management of hyperkalemia

Management of hyperkalemia is multipronged and includes measures to (1) reverse the membrane effects of hyperkalemia, (2) enhance the transfer of K$^+$ from the ECF into cells, and (3) remove K$^+$ from the body. The first two measures are only temporizing, so multiple treatments should be initiated concurrently.

> ### KEY POINT
>
> The goal of hyperkalemia management is to stabilize cardiac muscle membrane potential and shift extracellular K$^+$ into the intracellular space until K$^+$ can be removed from the body.

If ECG changes are present, hyperkalemia is severe (>7 mEq/L), or both, the first step in treatment must be the infusion of Ca$^{2+}$ to stabilize the cardiac muscle membrane potential; specifically, Ca$^{2+}$ shifts the threshold potential to a less negative value to restore the difference between the resting and threshold potentials. The effects of intravenous Ca$^{2+}$ occur within 1 to 3 minutes and last for 30 to 60 minutes. Calcium gluconate (10%, 0.6 mL/kg), infused slowly (over 5 to 10 minutes) under continuous electrocardiographic monitoring, is the preferred preparation of intravenous Ca$^{2+}$. Calcium chloride also can be used (10%, 0.2 mL/kg), but because it provides approximately three times the amount of Ca$^{2+}$ per 10-mL dose, caution must be exercised in its administration to avoid potential Ca$^{2+}$ toxicity.[122] Contraindications to administration of Ca$^{2+}$ salts are digoxin intoxication or hypercalcemic states.

Somewhat more long-lasting effects (several hours) can be obtained by transferring extracellular K$^+$ into cells, thereby reestablishing a more physiologic transmembrane potential gradient. The first-line therapy is insulin with glucose,[122,123] the latter not necessary if the patient is already hyperglycemic. Glucose (1 g/kg) plus insulin (0.2 units/g of glucose) may be infused first as a bolus over 15 to 30 minutes and then over an hour until K$^+$ can be eliminated from the body. For example, a 10-kg child would require 10 g dextrose with 2 units of insulin; therefore, 100 mL of $D_{10}W$ to which is added 2 units of insulin would be infused over 30 minutes and then at a rate of 100 mL/h. Of importance, this is an approximation and will need to be adjusted for individual patients based on close blood glucose monitoring. Because supraphysiologic doses of insulin (up to 20 units) are required to elicit a maximal $K^+$ shift in adults, and hyperosmotic glucose infusions alone may exacerbate hyperkalemia through fluid shifts and solvent drag, it may be unwise to treat nondiabetic hyperkalemic patients with glucose alone, expecting endogenous insulin release to adequately reduce plasma $K^+$ concentration.[124] The effect of insulin is seen within 10 to 20 minutes of administration and can last for hours and be expected to decrease $K^+$ levels by 0.5 to 1.5 mEq/L.

Administration of $\beta2$ agonists, and specifically albuterol, may also promote $K^+$ uptake by cells. In 11 children (aged 5 to 18 years) with end-stage renal disease, nebulized salbutamol (2.5 mg if the child weighed less than 25 kg, 5 mg if above) reduced the plasma $K^+$ concentration by 0.6 and 1 mM/L by 30 and 60 min, respectively, with effects lasting for up to 2 hours.[125] Transient side effects associated with this class of drugs include tachycardia, tremor, and mild vasomotor flushing. Caution is recommended for patients on $\beta$-blockers and those with known cardiac disease.

Finally, infusion of sodium bicarbonate ($NaHCO_3$; 8.4%, 1 to 2 mEq/kg IV over 30 minutes) may induce a transcellular shift of $K^+$ in patients with metabolic acidosis. However, it is ineffective in the acute treatment of hyperkalemic patients without acidosis.[124,126] Of note is that $NaHCO_3$ should not be mixed with solutions containing $Ca^{2+}$ because of the possibility of precipitating calcium carbonate. The major toxicities of $HCO_3^-$ therapy include $Na^+$ overload and precipitation of tetany in the face of preexisting hypocalcemia.

Ultimately, in cases of increased total body $K^+$ content, the cation must be removed from the body via renal or gut excretion. Net $K^+$ removal from the body in individuals with good renal function can be accomplished by stimulating flow-dependent $K^+$ secretion in the distal nephron, by volume expansion, administration of loop diuretics, or by a combination of these. Furosemide (1 mg/kg; maximum of 20 mg for patients not chronically on loop diuretics) promotes urinary $K^+$ losses via both its inhibition of NKCC2 in the TALH as well as its effect on increasing urinary flow rates in $K^+$ secretory sites of the distal nephron.[21,122]

However, in patients with renal insufficiency, dialysis may be necessary to reduce the total body $K^+$ burden. The rate of $K^+$ removal from the plasma depends on the gradient between the plasma and dialysate $K^+$ concentrations and can be maximized using a $K^+$-free dialysate. Hemodialysis is considered to be the most efficient means of removing $K^+$ in hyperkalemic patients and is able to remove 50 to 80 mEq/L of $K^+$ in a 4-hour session.[123,124,127] However,

peritoneal dialysis is more widely available and more easily applied to infants than is hemodialysis. Continuous venovenous hemofiltration provides another means of removing total body $K^+$ from hemodynamically compromised patients.

$K^+$ binding resins, such as sodium polystyrene sulfonate (Kayexalate 1 g/kg orally or per rectum), which exchanges bound $Na^+$ for cations including $K^+$, releasing $Na^+$ into the gut for absorption, are no longer recommended to reduce total body $K^+$ in the acute setting. In fact, salbutamol infusion has recently been reported to be more effective, faster, and safer than Kayexalate in the treatment of NOHK in preterm infants.[128] Kayexalate when administered with hypertonic sorbitol has been associated with intestinal obstruction in neonates and, when administered orally or by nasogastric tube to adults, necrosis of the GI tract.[128-130] Oral resin also has been associated with bezoar formation in infants with extremely low birth weights.[129] In addition, stool $K^+$ excretion in adults who received Kayexalate with laxatives was not significantly increased above that measured in patients given laxatives alone.[131]

---

### Clinical Vignette 12.1

A 5-year-old boy with a history of multiple admissions for dehydration presents with vomiting and diarrhea for 1 day. He is afebrile with heart rate (HR) of 130/min, respiration rate of 18/min, blood pressure (BP) of 80/60 mm Hg, and oxygen saturation 100% on room air. His weight is 30 kg. His mother notes that at his last well child check, his BP was 100/70 mm Hg, and his weight was 33 kg. She states that he has always been small for his age. His physical examination is notable for a sleepy but arousable child with dry mucous membranes and diffuse muscle weakness. An IV line is placed, laboratory tests ordered, and he receives a bolus of normal saline. After the bolus, he is more alert, with HR 100/min and BP 85/60 mm Hg, but he still has diffuse muscle weakness. His laboratory chemistry results reveal $Na^+$ 137 mEq/L, $K^+$ 2.0 mEq/L, $Cl^-$ 88 mEq/L, $HCO_3^-$ 30 mEq/L, BUN 11 mEq/L, and creatinine 0.5 mEq/L. Noting his severe hypokalemia, dehydration, and relative hypochloremia, his physician orders urine electrolyte tests, which show $Na^+$ 25 mEq/L, $K^+$ 20 mEq/L, and $Cl^-$ 64 mEq/L.

### TEACHING POINTS

- This patient has severe dehydration, as evidenced by his approximately 10% weight loss and hypotension.
- Despite his dehydrated state, his kidneys fail to maximally conserve $Na^+$. In addition, he is hypokalemic and likely total body $K^+$-depleted, given his muscle weakness, and is wasting $K^+$ in his urine.

- His biochemical profile and urinary losses of $Na^+$, $K^+$, and $Cl^-$ are typical of furosemide administration.
- However, the absence of history of diuretic use should prompt this child's pediatrician to consider a diagnosis of Bartter syndrome, a possibility that is consistent with the boy's medical history of multiple admissions for dehydration and apparent failure to thrive.
- Bartter syndrome is caused by various mutations affecting transport in the TALH, summarized in this chapter. Bartter syndrome types I (loss-of-function mutation in NKCC2) and II (loss-of-function mutation in ROMK) typically manifest in the neonatal period, whereas type III (loss-of-function mutation in CLCNKB) often manifests with episodes of dehydration in a patient who has failure to thrive.
- Bartter syndrome results in reduced absorption of $Na^+$, $K^+$, and $Cl^-$ in the TALH, which is normally responsible for reabsorbing approximately 25% of the filtered load of $Na^+$. As a result, there is increased delivery of NaCl to the distal nephron, which ultimately results in polyuria and volume contraction.
- The urinary $K^+$ wasting seen in this disorder is due to increased distal $Na^+$ delivery and hyperaldosteronism, both of which enhance $Na^+$ reabsorption in the ASDN (thereby increasing the electrochemical gradient favoring $K^+$ secretion), and increased urinary flow in the distal nephron, which activates the BK channel.
- Despite the elevated levels of renin and angiotensin, patients with Bartter syndrome do not have hypertension because of vascular receptor desensitization.
- Other derangements observed in Bartter syndrome include hypocalcemia, hypomagnesemia, metabolic alkalosis, and hyperprostaglandinemia. Hypocalcemia and hypomagnesemia are due to decreased paracellular absorption in the TALH secondary to a reduced lumen positive potential (normally generated by $K^+$ secretion through the SK/ROMK channel).
- Whereas Bartter and Gitelman syndromes can both manifest with hypokalemic metabolic alkalosis, they can be distinguished on the basis of urinary calcium excretion: normocalciuria or hypercalciuria in Bartter syndrome and hypocalciuria in Gitelman syndrome.
- The molecular basis for the hyperprostaglandinemia is unclear; however, NSAIDs are known to improve polyuria and urinary salt wasting in some patients with Bartter syndrome.

## REFERENCES

1. Delgado MM, Rohatgi R, Khan S, et al. Sodium and potassium clearances by the maturing kidney: Clinical-molecular correlates. Pediatr Nephrol. 2003;18:759–67.
2. Sulyok E, Nemeth M, Tenyi I, et al. Relationship between maturity, electrolyte balance and the function of the renin-angiotensin-aldosterone system in newborn infants. Biol Neonate. 1979;35:60–5.
3. Flynn MA, Woodruff C, Clark J, Chase G. Total body potassium in normal children. Pediatr Res. 1972;6:239–45.
4. Butte NF, Hopkinson JM, Wong WW, et al. Body composition during the first 2 years of life: An updated reference. Pediatr Res. 2000;47:578–85.
5. Dickerson JW, Widdowson EM. Chemical changes in skeletal muscle during development. Biochem J. 1960;74:247–57.
6. Rodriguez-Soriano J, Vallo A, Castillo G, Oliveros R. Renal handling of water and sodium in infancy and childhood: A study using clearance methods during hypotonic saline diuresis. Kidney Int. 1981;20:700–4.
7. Lorenz JM, Kleinman LI, Markarian K. Potassium metabolism in extremely low birth weight infants in the first week of life. J Pediatr. 1997;131:81–6.
8. Holbrook JT, Patterson KY, Bodner JE, et al. Sodium and potassium intake and balance in adults consuming self-selected diets. Am J Clin Nutr. 1984;40:786–93.
9. Bia MJ, DeFronzo RA. Extrarenal potassium homeostasis. Am J Physiol. 1981;240:F257–68.
10. Tudvad F, McNamarh NH, Barnett HL. Renal response of premature infants to administration of bicarbonate and potassium. Pediatrics. 1954;13:4–16.
11. Giebisch G. Renal potassium transport: Mechanisms and regulation. Am J Physiol. 1998;274:F817–33.
12. Lelievre-Pegorier M, Merlet-Benichou C, Roinel N, de Rouffignac C. Developmental pattern of water and electrolyte transport in rat superficial nephrons. Am J Physiol. 1983;245:F15–21.
13. Solomon S. Absolute rates of sodium and potassium reabsorption by proximal tubule of immature rats. Biol Neonate. 1974;25:340–51.
14. Zink H, Horster M. Maturation of diluting capacity in loop of Henle of rat superficial nephrons. Am J Physiol. 1977;233:F519–24.
15. Schmidt U, Horster M. Na-K-activated ATPase: Activity maturation in rabbit nephron segments dissected in vitro. Am J Physiol. 1977;233:F55–60.
16. Ho K, Nichols CG, Lederer WJ, et al. Cloning and expression of an inwardly rectifying ATP-regulated potassium channel. Nature. 1993;362:31–8.
17. Zhou H, Tate SS, Palmer LG. Primary structure and functional properties of an epithelial K channel. Am J Physiol. 1994;266:C809–24.
18. Konrad M, Köckerling A, Ziegler A, et al. Mutations in the gene encoding the inwardly-rectifying renal potassium channel, ROMK, cause the antenatal variant of Bartter syndrome: Evidence for genetic heterogeneity. International Collaborative Study Group for Bartter-like Syndromes. Hum Mol Genet. 1997;6:17–26.

19. Satlin LM. Postnatal maturation of potassium transport in rabbit cortical collecting duct. Am J Physiol. 1994;266:F57–65.

20. Gurkan S, Estilo GK, Wei Y, Satlin LM. Potassium transport in the maturing kidney. Pediatr Nephrol. 2007;22:915–25.

21. Woda CB, Bragin A, Kleyman TR, Satlin LM. Flow-dependent K+ secretion in the cortical collecting duct is mediated by a maxi-K channel. Am J Physiol Renal Physiol. 2001;280:F786–93.

22. Liu W, Xu S, Woda C, Kim P, et al. Effect of flow and stretch on the [Ca2+]i response of principal and intercalated cells in cortical collecting duct. Am J Physiol Renal Physiol. 2003;285:F998–1012.

23. Bailey MA, Cantone A, Yan Q, et al. Maxi-K channels contribute to urinary potassium excretion in the ROMK-deficient mouse model of type II Bartter's syndrome and in adaptation to a high-K diet. Kidney Int. 2006;70:51–9.

24. Pacha J, Frindt G, Sackin H, et al. Apical maxi K channels in intercalated cells of CCT. Am J Physiol. 1991;261:F696–705.

25. Constantinescu AR, Lane JC, Mak J, et al. Na+-K+-ATPase-mediated basolateral rubidium uptake in the maturing rabbit cortical collecting duct. Am J Physiol Renal Physiol. 2000;279:F1161–8.

26. Satlin LM, Evan AP, Gattone VH, 3rd, Schwartz GJ. Postnatal maturation of the rabbit cortical collecting duct. Pediatr Nephrol. 1988;2:135–45.

27. Benchimol C, Zavilowitz B, Satlin LM. Developmental expression of ROMK mRNA in rabbit cortical collecting duct. Pediatr Res. 2000;47:46–52.

28. Zolotnitskaya A, Satlin LM. Developmental expression of ROMK in rat kidney. Am J Physiol. 1999;276:F825–36.

29. Satlin LM, Palmer LG. Apical K+ conductance in maturing rabbit principal cell. Am J Physiol. 1997;272:F397–404.

30. Woda CB, Miyawaki N, Ramalakshmi S, et al. Ontogeny of flow-stimulated potassium secretion in rabbit cortical collecting duct: Functional and molecular aspects. Am J Physiol Renal Physiol. 2003;285:F629–39.

31. Constantinescu A, Silver RB, Satlin LM. H-K-ATPase activity in PNA-binding intercalated cells of newborn rabbit cortical collecting duct. Am J Physiol. 1997;272:F167–77.

32. Kleinman LI, Banks RO. Segmental nephron sodium and potassium reabsorption in newborn and adult dogs during saline expansion. Proc Soc Exp Biol Med. 1983;173:231–7.

33. Good DW, Wright FS. Luminal influences on potassium secretion: Sodium concentration and fluid flow rate. Am J Physiol. 1979;236:F192–205.

34. Stokes JB. Potassium secretion by cortical collecting tubule: Relation to sodium absorption, luminal sodium concentration, and transepithelial voltage. Am J Physiol. 1981;241:F395–402.

35. Aperia A, Elinder G. Distal tubular sodium reabsorption in the developing rat kidney. Am J Physiol. 1981;240:F487–91.

36. Morimoto T, Liu W, Woda C, et al. Mechanism underlying flow stimulation of sodium absorption in the mammalian collecting duct. Am J Physiol Renal Physiol. 2006;291:F663–9.

37. Hiatt N, Davidson MB, Bonorris G. The effect of potassium chloride infusion on insulin secretion in vivo. Horm Metab Res. 1972;4:64–8.

38. Rabinowitz L, Sarason RL, Yamauchi H. Effects of KCl infusion on potassium excretion in sheep. Am J Physiol. 1985;249:F263–71.

39. Rabinowitz L, Green DM, Sarason RL, Yamauchi H. Homeostatic potassium excretion in fed and fasted sheep. Am J Physiol. 1988;254:R357–80.

40. Youn JH. Gut sensing of potassium intake and its role in potassium homeostasis. Semin Nephrol. 2013;33:248–56.

41. Rabinowitz L, Sarason RL, Yamauchi H, et al. Time course of adaptation to altered K intake in rats and sheep. Am J Physiol. 1984;247:F607–17.

42. Palmer LG, Frindt G. Regulation of apical K channels in rat cortical collecting tubule during changes in dietary K intake. Am J Physiol. 1999 ;277:F805–12.

43. Najjar F, Zhou H, Morimoto T, et al. Dietary K+ regulates apical membrane expression of maxi-K channels in rabbit cortical collecting duct. Am J Physiol Renal Physiol. 2005;289:F922–32.

44. Palmer LG, Antonian L, Frindt G. Regulation of apical K and Na channels and Na/K pumps in rat cortical collecting tubule by dietary K. J Gen Physiol. 1994;104:693–710.

45. Wei Y, Bloom P, Lin D, et al. Effect of dietary K intake on apical small-conductance K channel in CCD: Role of protein tyrosine kinase. Am J Physiol Renal Physiol. 2001;281:F206–12.

46. Silver RB, Soleimani M. H+-K+-ATPases: Regulation and role in pathophysiological states. Am J Physiol. 1999;276:F799–811.

47. Boudry JF, Stoner LC, Burg MB. Effect of acid lumen pH on potassium transport in renal cortical collecting tubules. Am J Physiol. 1976;230:239–44.

48. Wang WH, Schwab A, Giebisch G. Regulation of small-conductance K+ channel in apical membrane of rat cortical collecting tubule. Am J Physiol. 1990;259:F494–502.

49. Stanton BA, Giebisch G. Effects of pH on potassium transport by renal distal tubule. Am J Physiol. 1982;242:F544–51.

50. Masilamani S, Kim GH, Mitchell C, et al. Aldosterone-mediated regulation of ENaC alpha, beta, and gamma subunit proteins in rat kidney. J Clin Invest. 1999;104:R19–23.

51. Pacha J, Frindt G, Antonian L, et al. Regulation of Na channels of the rat cortical collecting tubule by aldosterone. J Gen Physiol. 1993;102:25–42.

52. Blazer-Yost BL, Liu X, Helman SI. Hormonal regulation of ENaCs: Insulin and aldosterone. Am J Physiol. 1998;274:C1373–9.

53. Thomas W, Harvey BJ. Mechanisms underlying rapid aldosterone effects in the kidney. Annu Rev Physiol. 2011;73:335–57.

54. Van Acker KJ, Scharpe SL, Deprettere AJ, et al. Renin-angiotensin-aldosterone system in the healthy infant and child. Kidney Int. 1979;16:196–203.

55. Stephenson G, Hammet M, Hadaway G, Funder JW. Ontogeny of renal mineralocorticoid receptors and urinary electrolyte responses in the rat. Am J Physiol. 1984;247:F665–71.

56. Aperia A, Broberger O, Herin P, Zetterstrom R. Sodium excretion in relation to sodium intake and aldosterone excretion in newborn pre-term and full-term infants. Acta Paediatr Scand. 1979;68:813–7.

57. Rodriguez-Soriano J, Ubetagoyena M, Vallo A. Transtubular potassium concentration gradient: A useful test to estimate renal aldosterone bio-activity in infants and children. Pediatr Nephrol. 1990;4:105–10.

58. Dalal BI, Brigden ML. Factitious biochemical measurements resulting from hematologic conditions. Am J Clin Pathol. 2009;131:195–204.

59. Squires RD, Huth EJ. Experimental potassium depletion in normal human subjects. I. Relation of ionic intakes to the renal conservation of potassium. J Clin Invest. 1959;38:1134–48.

60. Wu F, Mi W, Hernandez-Ochoa EO, Burns DK, et al. A calcium channel mutant mouse model of hypokalemic periodic paralysis. J Clin Invest. 2012;122:4580–91.

61. Jurkat-Rott K, Lehmann-Horn F, Elbaz A, et al. A calcium channel mutation causing hypokalemic periodic paralysis. Hum Mol Genet. 1994;3:1415–9.

62. Sternberg D, Maisonobe T, Jurkat-Rott K, et al. Hypokalaemic periodic paralysis type 2 caused by mutations at codon 672 in the muscle sodium channel gene SCN4A. Brain. 2001;124:1091–9.

63. Resnick JS, Engel WK, Griggs RC, Stam AC. Acetazolamide prophylaxis in hypokalemic periodic paralysis. N Engl J Med. 1968;278:582–6.

64. Matthews E, Portaro S, Ke Q, et al. Acetazolamide efficacy in hypokalemic periodic paralysis and the predictive role of genotype. Neurology. 2011;77:1960–4.

65. Hermsmeyer K, Sperelakis N. Decrease in K+ conductance and depolarization of frog cardiac muscle produced by Ba++. Am J Physiol. 1970;219:1108–14.

66. Diengott D, Rozsa O, Levy N, Muammar S. Hypokalaemia in barium poisoning. Lancet. 1964;2:343–4.

67. Roza O, Berman LB. The pathophysiology of barium: Hypokalemic and cardiovascular effects. J Pharmacol Exp Ther. 1971;177:433–9.

68. Kassirer JP, London AM, Goldman DM, Schwartz WB. On the pathogenesis of metabolic alkalosis in hyperaldosteronism. Am J Med. 1970;49:306–15.

69. Nicholls MG, Espiner EA, Hughes H, et al. Primary aldosteronism: A study in contrasts. Am J Med. 1975;59:334–42.

70. White PC. Abnormalities of aldosterone synthesis and action in children. Curr Opin Pediatr. 1997;9:424–30.

71. Robles BJ, Sandoval AR, Dardon JD, Blas CA. Lethal liquorice lollies (liquorice abuse causing pseudo-hyperaldosteronism). BMJ Case Rep. 2013; pii. bcr2013201007.doi:10.1136/bcr-2013-201007.

72. Batlle D, Haque SK. Genetic causes and mechanisms of distal renal tubular acidosis. Nephrol Dial Transplant. 2012;27:3691–704.

73. Alper SL. Familial renal tubular acidosis. J Nephrol. 2010;23(Suppl 16):S57–76.

74. Haque SK, Ariceta G, Batlle D. Proximal renal tubular acidosis: A not so rare disorder of multiple etiologies. Nephrol Dial Transplant. 2012;27:4273–87.

75. McSherry E. Renal tubular acidosis in childhood. Kidney Int. 1981;20:799–809.

76. Fremont OT, Chan JC. Understanding Bartter syndrome and Gitelman syndrome. W J Pediatr. 2012;8:25–30.

77. Seyberth HW, Schlingmann KP. Bartter- and Gitelman-like syndromes: Salt-losing tubulopathies with loop or DCT defects. Pediatr Nephrol. 2011;26:1789–802.

78. Warnock DG. Liddle syndrome: An autosomal dominant form of human hypertension. Kidney Int. 1998;53:18–24.

79. Hansson JH, Nelson-Williams C, Suzuki H, et al. Hypertension caused by a truncated epithelial sodium channel gamma subunit: Genetic heterogeneity of Liddle syndrome. Nat Genet. 1995;11:76–82.

80. Shimkets RA, Warnock DG, Bositis CM, et al. Liddle's syndrome: Heritable human hypertension caused by mutations in the beta subunit of the epithelial sodium channel. Cell. 1994;79:407–14.

81. Jeunemaitre X, Bassilana F, Persu A, et al. Genotype-phenotype analysis of a newly discovered family with Liddle's syndrome. J Hypertens. 1997;15:1091–100.

82. Manitius A, Levitin H, Beck D, Epstein FH. On the mechanism of impairment of renal concentrating ability in potassium deficiency. J Clin Invest. 1960;39:684–92.

83. Schwartz WB, Relman AS. Effects of electrolyte disorders on renal structure and function. N Engl J Med. 1967;276:452–8.

84. Berl T, Linas SL, Aisenbrey GA, et al. On the mechanism of polyuria in potassium depletion: The role of polydipsia. J Clin Invest. 1977;60:620–5.

85. Conn JW. Hypertension, the potassium ion and impaired carbohydrate tolerance. N Engl J Med. 1965;273:1135–43.

86. Welt LG, Hollander W, Jr, Blythe WB. The consequences of potassium depletion. J Chronic Dis. 1960;11:213-54.

87. Wilde WS. Potassium. In: Comar C.L. and Bronner F, eds. Mineral Metabolism: An Advanced Treatise. Volume UUB. New York: Academic Press; 1962. pp. 73–107.

88. Bronson WR, DeVita VT, Carbone PP, et al. Pseudohyperkalemia due to release of potassium from white blood cells during clotting. N Engl J Med. 1966;274:369–75.

89. Hartmann RC, Auditore JV, Jackson DP. Studies on thrombocytosis. I. Hyperkalemia due to release of potassium from platelets during coagulation. J Clin Invest. 1958;37:699–707.

90. Seimiya M, Yoshida T, Sawabe Y, et al. Reducing the incidence of pseudohyperkalemia by avoiding making a fist during phlebotomy: A quality improvement report. Am J Kidney Dis. 2010;56:686–92.

91. DeFronzo RA, Bia M, Smith D. Clinical disorders of hyperkalemia. Annu Rev Med. 1982;33:521–54.

92. Aronson PS, Giebisch G. Effects of pH on potassium: New explanations for old observations. J Am Soc Nephrol. 2011;22:1981–9.

93. Hertz P, Richardson JA. Arginine-induced hyperkalemia in renal failure patients. Arch Intern Med. 1972;130:778–80.

94. Cooperman LH. Succinylcholine-induced hyperkalemia in neuromuscular disease. JAMA. 1970;213:1867–71.

95. Walton JD, Farman JV. Suxamethonium hyperkalaemia in uraemic neuropathy. Anaesthesia. 1973;28:666–8.

96. Gronert GA, Theye RA. Pathophysiology of hyperkalemia induced by succinylcholine. Anesthesiology. 1975;43:89–99.

97. Reza MJ, Kovick RB, Shine KI, Pearce ML. Massive intravenous digoxin overdosage. N Engl J Med. 1974;291:777–8.

98. Charles G, Zheng C, Lehmann-Horn F, et al. Characterization of hyperkalemic periodic paralysis: A survey of genetically diagnosed individuals. J Neurol 2013;260:2606–13.

99. Jurkat-Rott K, Lehmann-Horn F. Hyperkalemic periodic paralysis type 1. In: Pagon RA, Adam MP, Bird TD, et al., editors. GeneReviews. Seattle, 1993-2014. http://www.ncbi.nlm.nih.gov/books/NBK1496/. Accessed December 27, 2014.

100. Brion LP, Schwartz GJ, Campbell D, et al. Early hyperkalaemia in very low birthweight infants in the absence of oliguria. Arch Dis Child. 1989;64:270–2.

101. Mildenberger E, Versmold HT. Pathogenesis and therapy of non-oliguric hyperkalaemia of the premature infant. Eur J Pediatr. 2002;161:415–22.

102. Stefano JL, Norman ME, Morales MC, et al. Decreased erythrocyte Na+,K+-ATPase activity associated with cellular potassium loss in extremely low birth weight infants with nonoliguric hyperkalemia. J Pediatr. 1993;122:276–84.

103. Sato K, Kondo T, Iwao H, et al. Internal potassium shift in premature infants: Cause of nonoliguric hyperkalemia. J Pediatr. 1995;126:109–13.

104. Omar SA, DeCristofaro JD, Agarwal BI, et al. Effect of prenatal steroids on potassium balance in extremely low birth weight neonates. Pediatrics. 2000;106:561–7.

105. Lordon RE, Burton JR. Post-traumatic renal failure in military personnel in Southeast Asia: Experience at Clark USAF hospital, Republic of the Philippines. Am J Med. 1972;53:137–47.

106. Strauss MB. Acute renal insufficiency due to lower-nephron nephrosis. N Engl J Med. 1948;239:693–700.

107. Speiser PW, White PC. Congenital adrenal hyperplasia. N Engl J Med. 2003;349:776–88.

108. White PC. Aldosterone synthase deficiency and related disorders. Mol Cell Endocrinol. 2004;217:81–7.

109. Cheek DB, Perry JW. A salt wasting syndrome in infancy. Arch Dis Child. 1958;33:252–6.

110. Furgeson SB, Linas S. Mechanisms of type I and type II pseudohypoaldosteronism. J Am Soc Nephrol. 2010;21:1842–5.

111. Guran T, Degirmenci S, Bulut IK, et al. Critical points in the management of pseudohypoaldosteronism type 1. J Clin Res Pediatr Endocrinol. 2011;3:98–100.

112. Xie J, Craig L, Cobb MH, et al. Role of with-no-lysine [K] kinases in the pathogenesis of Gordon's syndrome. Pediatr Nephrol. 2006;21:1231–6.

113. Bonny O, Rossier BC. Disturbances of Na/K balance: Pseudohypoaldosteronism revisited. J Am Soc Nephrol. 2002;13:2399–414.

114. Harris RC, Breyer MD. Update on cyclooxygenase-2 inhibitors. CJASN. 2006;1:236–45.

115. Flores D, Liu Y, Liu W, et al. Flow-induced prostaglandin E2 release regulates Na and K transport in the collecting duct. Am J Physiol Renal Physiol. 2012;303:F632–8.

116. Schlanger LE, Kleyman TR, Ling BN. K+-sparing diuretic actions of trimethoprim: Inhibition of Na+ channels in A6 distal nephron cells. Kidney Int. 1994;45:1070–6.

117. Kleyman TR, Roberts C, Ling BN. A mechanism for pentamidine-induced hyperkalemia: Inhibition of distal nephron sodium transport. Ann Intern Med. 1995;122:103–6.

118. Fried LF, Emanuele N, Zhang JH, et al. Combined angiotensin inhibition for the treatment of diabetic nephropathy. N Engl J Med. 2013;369:1892–903.

119. Hoorn EJ, Walsh SB, McCormick JA, et al. The calcineurin inhibitor tacrolimus activates the renal sodium chloride cotransporter to cause hypertension. Nat Med. 2011;17:1304–9.

120. Ethier JH, Kamel KS, Magner PO, et al. The transtubular potassium concentration in patients with hypokalemia and hyperkalemia. Am J Kidney Dis. 1990;15:309–15.

121. Choi MJ, Ziyadeh FN. The utility of the transtubular potassium gradient in the evaluation of hyperkalemia. J Am Soc Nephrol. 2008;19:424–6.

122. Hegenbarth MA; American Academy of Pediatrics Committee on Drugs. Preparing for pediatric emergencies: Drugs to consider. Pediatrics. 2008;121:433–43.

123. Lehnhardt A, Kemper MJ. Pathogenesis, diagnosis and management of hyperkalemia. Pediatr Nephrol. 2011;26:377–84.

124. Blumberg A, Weidmann P, Shaw S, et al. Effect of various therapeutic approaches on plasma potassium and major regulating factors in terminal renal failure. Am J Med. 1988;85:507–12.

125. McClure RJ, Prasad VK, Brocklebank JT. Treatment of hyperkalaemia using intravenous and nebulised salbutamol. Arch Dis Child. 1994;70:126–8.

126. Kamel KS, Wei C. Controversial issues in the treatment of hyperkalaemia. Nephrol Dial Transplant 2003;18:2215–8.

127. Morgan AG, Burkinshaw L, Robinson PJ, Rosen SM. Potassium balance and acid-base changes in patients undergoing regular haemodialysis therapy. Brit Med J. 1970 28;1:779–83.

128. Yaseen H, Khalaf M, Dana A, et al. Salbutamol versus cation-exchange resin (Kayexalate) for the treatment of nonoliguric hyperkalemia in preterm infants. J Perinatol. 2008;25:193–7.

129. Ohlsson A, Hosking M. Complications following oral administration of exchange resins in extremely low-birth-weight infants. Eur J Pediatr. 1987;146:571–4.

130. Rashid A, Hamilton SR. Necrosis of the gastrointestinal tract in uremic patients as a result of sodium polystyrene sulfonate (Kayexalate) in sorbitol: An underrecognized condition. Am J Sur Pathol. 1997;21:60–9.

131. Emmett M, Hootkins RE, Fine KD, et al. Effect of three laxatives and a cation exchange resin on fecal sodium and potassium excretion. Gastroenterology. 1995;108:752–60.

## REVIEW QUESTIONS

1. A 16-year-old girl is noted to have a plasma K$^+$ concentration of 7.0 mEq/L with peaked T waves on ECG. The *first* step of management should be:
   a. Administration of IV insulin with glucose
   b. Administration of IV sodium bicarbonate
   c. Administration of nebulized albuterol
   d. Administration of IV calcium gluconate
   e. Administration of IV furosemide

2. Severe hypokalemia *may be* associated with:
   a. Hypotension
   b. Renal concentrating defect
   c. Skeletal muscle weakness
   d. ST depression and appearance of U wave on ECG
   e. All of the above

3. K$^+$ is freely filtered in the glomerulus. The majority of filtered K$^+$ is reabsorbed in the _____, and the net urinary K$^+$ secretion, and thus excretion, occurs in the _____.
   a. TALH; distal nephron (distal convoluted tubule and collecting duct)
   b. Proximal tubule; distal nephron (distal convoluted tubule and collecting duct)
   c. Distal nephron (distal convoluted tubule and collecting duct); TALH
   d. Proximal tubule; TALH
   e. Distal nephron (distal convoluted tubule and collecting duct); proximal tubule

4. A 10-year-old patient with history of acute lymphoblastic anemia is noted to be in septic shock and disseminated intravascular coagulation. She is paralyzed with succinylcholine for intubation and placed on pressors for hypotension. Her sedation is maintained with propofol, and the patient requires multiple units of pRBCs for severe anemia. Arterial blood gas (ABG) reveals that she is acidotic, with an elevated lactate. Her ABG also reveals a K$^+$ of 7.5 mEq/L. The team sends off a sample to verify the K$^+$ result. You are concerned that the value is real because:
   a. Succinylcholine can promote K$^+$ release from muscle cells.
   b. The patient may have sustained acute kidney injury secondary to her hypotension.
   c. The patient received a large K$^+$ load via both intravascular hemolysis and pRBC transfusion.
   d. All of the above.

5. An 8-year-old boy with obstructive uropathy is noted to have chronic hypokalemia and non-gap metabolic acidosis. Despite his acidosis, his urine pH remains 6.0. His urine is negative for glucose and protein. Given his underlying uropathy, the patient *most likely* has:
   a. Type 1 RTA involving the inability of the proximal tubule to reabsorb HCO$_3^-$
   b. Type 1 RTA involving the inability of the distal nephron to secrete H$^+$
   c. Type 2 RTA involving the inability of the proximal tubule to reabsorb HCO$_3^-$
   d. Type 2 RTA involving the inability of the distal nephron to secrete H$^+$

6. A 2-week-old girl is brought to the emergency department for vomiting and lethargy. She is noted to have thready pulses and poor capillary refill. She has not yet regained birth weight. Samples for CBC, chemistry,

VBG, blood culture, urine culture, and CSF culture are sent to the laboratory, and the patient is started on IV antibiotics. Results are significant for acidosis, severe hyponatremia and hyperkalemia. Based on the patient's presumed diagnosis, you expect urine electrolytes to show:

a. FeNa <1%, TTKG > 8
b. FeNa <1%, TTKG > 8
c. FeNa <1%, TTKG < 4
d. FeNa >10%, TTKG < 4
e. FeNa >10%, TTKG > 8
  FeNa = fractional excretion of sodium; TTKG = transtubular potassium gradient.

7. Patients with nephrotic syndrome are predisposed to developing hypokalemia because of:
   a. Treatment with loop diuretics
   b. Impaired reabsorption of filtered $K^+$
   c. Secondary hyperaldosteronism
   d. Increased $K^+$ filtration by the glomerulus
   e. Choices a and c

8. Bartter syndrome is characterized by the following derangements:
   a. Hypernatremia, hypochloremia, hyperkalemia, hyperprostaglandinemia, metabolic alkalosis
   b. Hyponatremia, hyperchloremia, hypokalemia, hypoprostaglandinemia metabolic acidosis
   c. Hyponatremia, hypochloremia, hypokalemia, hyperprostaglandinemia, metabolic alkalosis
   d. Hypernatremia, hyperchloremia, hyperkalemia, hyperprostaglandinemia, metabolic acidosis

## ANSWER KEY

1. d
2. e
3. b
4. d
5. b
6. d
7. e
8. c

# 13

# Disorders of mineral metabolism

## FARAH N. ALI AND CRAIG B. LANGMAN

Mineral metabolism involves a complex interplay of ion and hormonal control by individual organs in support of overall total body homeostasis. The kidney is a vital participant in the maintenance of homeostasis of these essential ions. This chapter presents an overview of regulation of calcium, magnesium, and phosphorus homeostasis in the body and the role played by the kidneys in their regulation. Clinical disorders of the homeostasis affecting these ions and the evaluation and management of these disorders are also discussed.

## CALCIUM METABOLISM

Calcium is a vital ion for many essential cellular metabolic functions and for skeletal development. The regulation of calcium balance is a complex, multicompartmental interplay of the gastrointestinal (GI) tract, kidneys, skeletal system, and numerous hormones. Dietary calcium is absorbed actively from the proximal GI tract, primarily in the duodenum and jejunum. The bioactive form of vitamin D, $1,25(OH)_2D_3$, formed in the kidneys, is the sole hormonal stimulus for intestinal calcium transport. Additionally, passive flux of calcium from intestinal lumen to blood may occur through the concurrent absorption of simple sugars, even in the absence of active vitamin D. The latter process is much less efficient and not well regulated. The skeletal system is the major site of calcium storage (99%); only 1% of calcium is stored in the intracellular and extracellular compartment (Figure 13.1).

Within the plasma, 40% of the calcium is bound to plasma proteins and is not ultrafiltrable across the glomeruli. Approximately 50% of serum calcium is found in the ionized form. The remainder (10%) of the calcium is complexed with anions, such as phosphate or carbonate. Of the plasma protein-bound fraction of calcium, 90% is bound to albumin and the remainder to globulins. Each gram of albumin, at the physiologic pH (7.4), binds 0.8 mg/dL of calcium. In the setting of hypoalbuminemia, the measured serum total calcium value must be corrected to account for low plasma albumin concentration. Corrected total serum calcium can be calculated in hypoalbuminemic patients by the following formula:

Corrected calcium = (4.0 − [plasma albumin] g/dL) × 0.8 + [serum calcium] mg/dL

The acid-base status of the body affects ionized plasma calcium concentration substantially. During acidemia (excess hydrogen ion [$H^+$]), the negatively charged sites on the plasma proteins buffer the excess $H^+$, thus displacing the calcium ions from these sites and raising the ionized calcium level. Alkalemia has the opposite effect, decreasing the ionized calcium level.[1] An important clinical implication of this relationship is that aggressive correction of metabolic

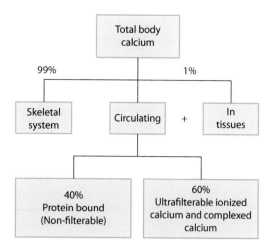

Figure 13.1 Distribution of calcium within various compartments in the body.

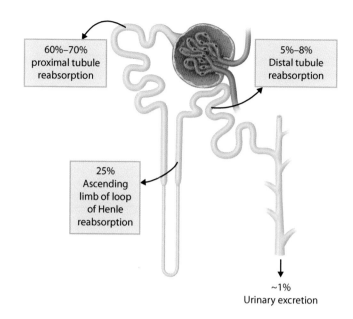

Figure 13.2 Sites of reabsorption of calcium in the nephron.

acidosis in a patient with concomitant mild hypocalcemia can result in symptomatic hypocalcemia.

---

**KEY POINTS**

- Ionized calcium is the biologically active fraction of total body calcium.
- Metabolic alkalosis decreases serum ionized calcium concentration, and metabolic acidosis raises serum ionized calcium concentration.
- Rapid correction of metabolic acidosis in patients with borderline or low serum calcium level can precipitate tetany and cardiac dysrhythmia by lowering serum ionized calcium concentration.

---

## RENAL HANDLING OF CALCIUM

### Calcium homeostasis

Calcium homeostasis is maintained by three key hormones—parathyroid hormone (PTH), calcitonin, and vitamin D—which act on the GI tract, the kidneys, and the skeletal system (Table 13.1). The actions of these hormones are interrelated and interdependent.

### Parathyroid hormone

PTH, an 84-amino acid–containing single-chain polypeptide, is produced by the chief cells of the parathyroid glands. The secretion of PTH from the parathyroid gland is regulated by the extracellular ionized calcium concentration. The cell membranes of the parathyroid gland chief cells have an extracellular calcium-sensing receptor (ECaR) that responds to the plasma ionized calcium.[5,6] A high plasma

calcium activates the ECaR and results in a decrease in PTH, whereas a reduction in plasma calcium inactivates the receptor and increases PTH secretion.

PTH acts on bone to stimulate the osteoclast-mediated release of calcium and phosphorus from the mineral matrix, in addition to providing a trophic action on bone mass accretion. In the kidney, PTH enhances calcium reabsorption in the distal tubular segment. It also inhibits the reabsorption of phosphate in the proximal convoluted tubule, with

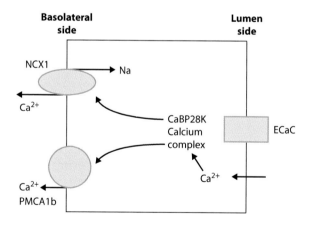

Figure 13.3 Diagrammatic representation of a distal tubular cell showing the mechanisms involved in the active tubular reabsorption of luminal calcium in this segment. The tubular cells in this nephron segment have calcium ($Ca^{2+}$) channels (ECaC) on the apical aspects that facilitate transport of luminal calcium into the cell. Once within the cytosol, calcium combines with the calcium-binding protein calbindin-D28K (CaPB28K) that shuttles it to the basolateral aspect of the tubular cell. The sodium calcium exchanger 1 (NCX1) and the plasma membrane calcium adenosine triphosphatase (ATPase) (PMCA1b) pumps facilitate the transport of calcium out of the tubular cell at the basolateral surface.

resulting phosphaturia (Figure 13.2 and 13.3). In addition, PTH increases the activity of the enzyme 25-hydroxyvitamin D 1-α-hydroxylase in the proximal renal tubule, which mediates conversion of 25(OH) $D_3$ to 1,25(OH)$_2$D$_3$ in the kidney. This is the active form of vitamin D; it increases intestinal calcium absorption. The action of vitamin D on the intestinal tract to increase the plasma calcium concentration takes place over several days. This contrasts with the impact of PTH secretion, which occurs within minutes.

The overall impact of these PTH-dependent processes is to maintain the blood calcium and phosphorus in the normal range. Taking advantage of these discoveries in the control of calcium homeostasis, an allosteric ECaR agonist ("calcimimetic") agent, cinacalcet hydrochloride (Sensipar), has been introduced for the treatment of secondary hyperparathyroidism in patients with chronic kidney disease (CKD).

---

## KEY POINTS

- The extracellular calcium-sensing receptors of the parathyroid glands continuously sense ionized calcium levels in the plasma and respond by altering PTH levels.
- Calcimimetic agents or ECaR agonists are now available to treat patients with secondary hyperparathyroidism in CKD.

---

## Vitamin D

Vitamin D is either ingested in the diet or produced from a common steroid precursor, 7-dehydrocholesterol, in the skin by the action of ultraviolet rays from the sun. Vitamin D ingested in the diet is absorbed in the proximal small intestine. To achieve biologic activation, vitamin D undergoes hydroxylation in the liver at the carbon-25 position by the cytochrome CYP2R1 to form 25(OH)D$_3$ (Figure 13.4). The transformed compound, 25(OH)D$_3$, undergoes further hydroxylation, at the carbon-1 position, in the kidney through the action of 25-hydroxyvitamin D 1-α-hydroxylase, a specific mitochondrial P450 enzyme CYP27A1. Although earlier work had suggested that the proximal renal tubule was the exclusive site of the 1-α-hydroxylase activity,[7,8] further observations using more sensitive probes suggest that the distal convoluted tubule, collecting duct, and papillary epithelia may also possess this enzyme activity.[9] Although 25(OH)D$_3$ represents the largest circulating fraction of vitamin D and serves as the measure of its nutritional status, it does not possess any of the biologic functions of vitamin D.

Following its synthesis in the kidney, 1,25(OH)$_2$D$_3$ and other hydroxylated metabolites of vitamin D are transported in blood by vitamin D–binding protein. The biologic actions of 1,25(OH)$_2$D$_3$ are exerted after it binds the paranuclear vitamin D receptor (VDR) in target cells.[10] This receptor has been found in virtually

---

Table 13.1 Hormonal mediators of calcium and phosphorus balance

| Mediator | Stimulus for secretion | Renal response | Bone response | Gastrointestinal response | Net effect on serum calcium | Net effect on serum phosphorus |
|---|---|---|---|---|---|---|
| Parathyroid hormone (PTH) | Hypocalcemia | Decreased phosphorus reabsorption (phosphaturia) Increased calcium reabsorption Upregulation of 1,25(OH)$_2$D$_3$ production | Osteoclast activation and egress of calcium | Increased calcium absorption through up-regulation of 1,25(OH)$_2$D$_3$ | Increase | Decrease |
| Calcitonin | Hypercalcemia | Increased calcium and phosphorus excretion | Inhibition of osteoclast activity | No effect | Decrease | Decrease |
| 1,25-dihydroxy-vitamin D | Hypocalcemia, Elevated PTH Hypophosphatemia | Increased calcium and phosphorus reabsorption | Increased osteoclast activation (variable) | Increased calcium and phosphorus absorption | Increase | Increase |
| Fibroblast growth factor-23 (FGF-23) | Excesses of dietary phosphorus intake | Decreased phosphate reabsorption (phosphaturia) Inhibition of 25-hydroxyvitamin D-1-α-hydroxylase | | Reduced calcium absorption from effects on vitamin D | Unchanged | Decrease |

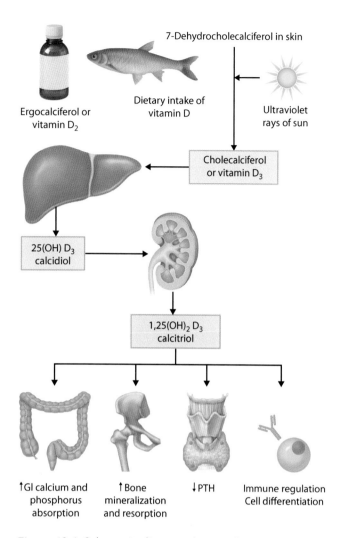

7-Dehydrocholecalciferol in skin

Ergocalciferol or vitamin D$_2$

Dietary intake of vitamin D

Ultraviolet rays of sun

Cholecalciferol or vitamin D$_3$

25(OH) D$_3$ calcidiol

1,25(OH)$_2$ D$_3$ calcitriol

↑GI calcium and phosphorus absorption

↑Bone mineralization and resorption

↓PTH

Immune regulation Cell differentiation

Figure 13.4 Schematic diagram showing bioconversion of vitamin D in the body and its biologic actions. GI, gastrointestinal; PTH, parathyroid hormone.

all cells, although its precise biologic functions in some cells are not fully understood.

### KEY POINTS

- 25(OH) D$_3$ represents the largest circulating fraction of the vitamin D endocrine system and serves as measure of nutritional adequacy.
- To assess nutritional adequacy or overdose of vitamin D, both 25(OH)D$_2$ derived from intake of ergocalciferol (synthetic) and 25(OH)D$_3$ need to be assayed.

## Calcitonin

Calcitonin is a 32-amino acid–containing straight-chain peptide hormone produced by the parafollicular cells (also known as C cells) of the thyroid gland. Calcitonin demonstrates hormonal functions for modulating calcium and phosphorus metabolism, but its role as an important regulatory hormone in calcium metabolism is less than convincing. As with PTH, the primary target organs for the action of calcitonin are the kidney and the bone.[11] Calcitonin is secreted in response to increase in plasma calcium level. Its actions on the bone are to inhibit bone resorption and consequently reduce serum calcium levels. This physiologic action of calcitonin is sometimes used to treat hypercalcemia. In the kidneys, calcitonin increases urinary calcium and phosphorus excretion, but the magnitude of its phosphaturic action is less than seen with PTH.[12,13] Calcitonin also increases the renal production of 1,25(OH)$_2$D$_3$.[14]

### KEY POINT

Calcitonin reduces serum calcium by inhibiting bone resorption, and in a minor role it increases urinary calcium excretion.

## HYPOCALCEMIA

Hypocalcemia is defined as serum total calcium concentration of less than 8.8 mg/dL (2.2 mmol/L) in a patient whose serum albumin concentration is normal, or when the blood ionized value is less than 4.2mg/dL (1.05 mmol/L). Several formulas have been derived to "normalize" the serum total calcium in hypoalbuminemic states, but none is superior to measurement of the blood ionized calcium concentration. Broadly, hypocalcemia can be divided into disorders of parathyroid function, of vitamin D metabolism, or of their receptors. Table 13.2 lists the common causes of hypocalcemia seen in infants and children.

## CLINICAL MANIFESTATIONS

The clinical manifestations of hypocalcemia are varied and are determined by the severity and rapidity of its onset (Table 13.3). Whereas mild hypocalcemia may remain asymptomatic, more severe or rapid-onset hypocalcemia results in neuromuscular irritability and tetany. Alteration of consciousness and seizures may occur in severe cases.

Neuromuscular irritability secondary to hypocalcemia can be elicited by the Chvostek and Trousseau signs. The Chvostek sign is performed by tapping the jaw with a reflex hammer, or by a firm finger tap. A twitch elicited in response

Table 13.2 Causes of hypocalcemia

**Artifactual**
- Low serum albumin
- Use of gadolinium-based MRI contrast agent

**Lack of Vitamin D**
- Nutritional deficiency
- Inadequate sunlight exposure
- Fat malabsorption

**Defective Vitamin D Metabolism**
- Anticonvulsant therapy
- Renal disease
- Hepatic disease

**Vitamin D–Dependent Rickets**
- Type I, 25-hydroxyvitamin D 1$\alpha$-hydroxylase deficiency
- Type II, inactivating mutations of the vitamin D receptor (vitamin D resistance)

**Lack of Parathyroid Hormone**
- Congenital hypoparathyroidism
- Postparathyroidectomy state
- Postthyroidectomy state
- Hypomagnesemia

**Parathyroid Hormone Resistance**
- Pseudohypoparathyroidism

*Abbreviations:* MRI, magnetic resonance imaging.

Table 13.3 Clinical manifestations of hypocalcemia

**Neuromuscular Irritability**
- Paresthesias
- Muscular weakness
- Carpopedal spasms
- Positive Chvostek and Trousseau signs
- Tetany
- Seizures

**Cardiovascular Dysfunction**
- Prolonged QT interval
- Arrhythmias
- Left ventricular dysfunction
- Hypotension
- Cardiomyopathy

**Skeletal System**
- Poor bone mineralization
- Poor dentition

**Miscellaneous**
- Neuropsychiatric disturbances
- Papilledema

denotes a positive sign of neuromuscular irritability. The Chvostek sign is not specific for hypocalcemia. A Trousseau sign is elicited by applying a tourniquet or blood pressure cuff to the arm. A positive sign is indicated by carpal spasm following 3 minutes of inflation of the pressure cuff above the patient's systolic blood pressure. This sign is more specific for hypocalcemic tetany. A prolonged QT interval is noted in most cases of mild to moderate hypocalcemia, but other cardiac arrhythmias can be seen in severe cases of hypocalcemia.[15] Abnormalities of electrocardiogram (ECG) mimicking myocardial infarction have also been reported.[16] Long-standing hypocalcemia can result in digoxin-resistant left ventricular dysfunction and cardiomyopathy.[17,18] With long-standing hypocalcemia, abnormal dentition and cataracts may also be seen.

## DISORDERS OF HYPOCALCEMIA

### Hypoparathyroidism

Hypoparathyroidism or a low circulating level of PTH can be diagnosed in the setting of a normal serum magnesium concentration and results in hypocalcemia and hyperphosphatemia. A transient form of hypoparathyroidism may be seen in newborn infants through the second week of life. Risk factors for transient neonatal hypoparathyroidism include prematurity, low birth weight, infants of diabetic mothers, as well as babies born to mothers with hypercalcemia.[19]

Permanent forms of hypoparathyroidism occur in the velocardiofacial syndrome, which is a spectrum of disorders caused by gene deletions in the chromosome 22q11.[20] These disorders include the DiGeorge anomaly, which is associated with cardiac and facial defects, in addition to thymic and parathyroid hypoplasia of varying degrees. Familial hypoparathyroidism is a rare disorder that may be inherited as an isolated autosomal recessive, autosomal dominant, or X-linked recessive endocrinopathy.[21]

Hypoparathyroidism, sensorineural deafness, and renal dysplasia (HDR) comprise a distinct disorder that is inherited as an autosomal dominant disease. HDR is associated with mutations in dual zinc finger transcription factor, GATA3 (a transcription factor that specifically binds the DNA sequence A/T-GATA-A/G, hence the name GATA).[21,22] GATA3 is a transcription factor for vertebrate embryonal development. The molecular mechanism behind this defect's causing HDR is still undetermined. Activating mutations in the calcium-sensing receptor gene are associated with hypoparathyroidism and hypocalcemia.[21,23]

### Pseudohypoparathyroidism

After PTH attaches to its cellular receptors, it activates guanine nucleotide regulatory proteins (Gs), which in turn mediate activation of cyclic adenosine monophosphate (cAMP) for the cellular effects of PTH to be completed.[6] Pseudohypoparathyroidism is characterized by an end-organ resistance to PTH at any of the foregoing pathways. Findings of elevated circulating levels of PTH and hyperphosphatemia in the absence of renal dysfunction in a hypocalcemic patient are characteristic findings of this disorder. Two types of pseudohypoparathyroidism, with distinct clinical and laboratory markers, have been described.

---

### KEY POINT

PTH level in hypoparathyroidism is low, and in pseudohypoparathyroidism it is elevated.

---

Type I pseudohypoparathyroidism is characterized by an absence of guanine nucleotide regulatory proteins (Gs). Type I pseudohypoparathyroidism includes McCune-Albright osteodystrophy, which is characterized by the clinical features of short stature, skeletal abnormalities, mental retardation, hypothyroidism, and hypogonadotrophism, in addition to end-organ PTH resistance.[1,24] Type II pseudohypoparathyroidism is associated with a yet-unknown defect downstream from activation of cAMP.[25] No characteristic phenotype has been reported. The two types of pseudohypoparathyroidism are distinguished by urinary levels of cAMP in response to exogenous PTH infusion (Ellsworth-Howard test). In type I pseudohypoparathyroidism, urinary cAMP does not increase with stimulation; in type II, the urinary cAMP levels increase in response to PTH.

Magnesium is required for adequate release of preformed PTH from the parathyroid gland under conditions of hypocalcemia.[26] Moderate to severe hypomagnesemia may lead to falsely low PTH levels. Peripheral resistance to the actions of PTH has also been considered a factor in the pathogenesis of hypocalcemia under these circumstances.[27] Correction of hypomagnesemia promptly results in correction of hypocalcemia and parathyroid resistance.

## Vitamin D deficiency states

Vitamin D deficiency results in hypocalcemia, elevated PTH level, hypophosphatemia, and aminoaciduria. Nutritional vitamin D deficiency is common in the developing world. However, it is also recognized increasingly in the Western world, especially in patients with malabsorption of vitamin D resulting from abnormalities of structure or function of the GI tract.[28,29] Liver diseases

with an inability to 25-hydroxylate the parent vitamin D may also lead to vitamin D deficiency rickets and hypocalcemia. Apart from hypocalcemia and hypophosphatemia, diminished levels of 25-hydroxyvitamin D are the hallmarks of vitamin D deficiency rickets. Radiographs of the skeleton demonstrate the characteristic findings of rickets. Treatment consists of providing vitamin D supplements, but patients with liver disease require therapy with $1,25(OH)_2D_3$ (calcitriol). Healing of radiographic skeletal abnormalities can be noted by 6 to 8 weeks.

## Vitamin D–dependent rickets

Vitamin D–dependent rickets (VDDR) is a heterogenous and rare metabolic disorder that is characterized by hypocalcemia and all the clinical and biochemical features of rickets. Two clinical variants of VDDR have been described (Figure 13.5). VDDR type I, also known as pseudovitamin D deficiency rickets, is an autosomal recessive disease associated with markedly diminished or absent synthesis of $1,25(OH)_2D_3$ resulting from deficiency of the

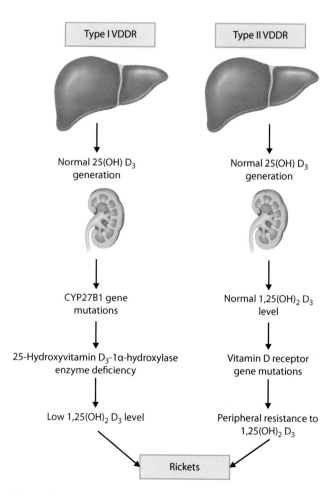

Figure 13.5 Schematic representation of the pathogenesis of type I and type II vitamin D–dependent rickets (VDDR).

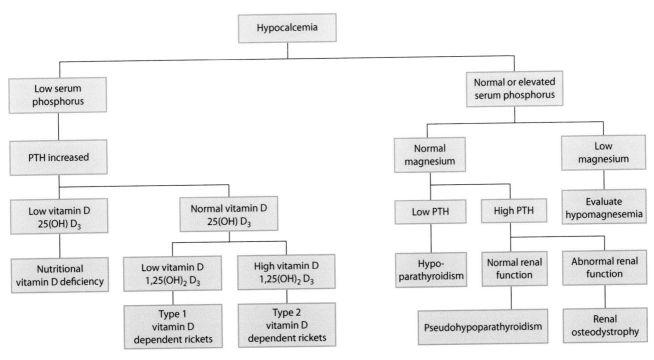

Figure 13.6 A suggested algorithm for evaluation of children with hypocalcemia. PTH, parathyroid hormone.

25-hydroxyvitamin D₃ 1α-hydroxylase enzyme in the kidney. Numerous mutations in the *CYP27B1* gene that encodes 25-hydroxyvitamin D₃ 1α-hydroxylase in the kidney have been described in association with this disorder.[30] Patients with VDDR type I present in early infancy with muscle weakness, bony deformities (rickets), and hypocalcemic seizures.[31] The plasma level of $1,25(OH)_2D_3$ is low or absent, whereas the $25(OH)D_3$ level is elevated or normal. Exogenous administration of a physiologic dose of $1,25(OH)_2D_3$ (calcitriol) corrects the clinical, radiologic, and biochemical abnormalities associated with this disorder.

The clinical features of VDDR type II include bony deformities characteristic of rickets, poor linear growth, early onset of alopecia, and loss of teeth.[32] Some patients do not have alopecia.[33] Apart from hypocalcemia, patients have hyperparathyroidism and a high circulating level of $1,25(OH)_2D_3$. VDDR type II is caused by mutations in the vitamin D receptor gene.[34,35] Patients demonstrate end-organ resistance to vitamin D and are resistant to high-dose vitamin D therapy and supplementation with $1,25(OH)_2D_3$ (calcitriol). Long-term intravenous calcium supplementation has been shown to be effective in the treatment of VDDR.[36]

# EVALUATION OF HYPOCALCEMIA

An evaluation of hypocalcemia should include concurrent measurement of serum ionized calcium, serum phosphorus, serum intact PTH, 25-(OH)D₃, $1,25(OH)_2D_3$, and serum magnesium, as well as an evaluation of acid-base status (free-flowing venous blood is acceptable) and assessment of renal function. Values for urinary excretion of minerals and electrolytes may be needed in some circumstances. Figure 13.7 provides algorithms for evaluation of children and adults with hypocalcemia.

## Serum phosphorus

Determination of serum phosphorus concentration aids in distinguishing the cause of low serum calcium levels beyond the neonatal age. In neonates, the serum phosphorus level is normally higher as a result of the limited ability of the neonatal kidney to excrete phosphorus, and It does not modulate in a fashion similar to that in older children. Hypocalcemia, coupled with hypophosphatemia, often points to an abnormality in vitamin D metabolism, whereas the presence of hyperphosphatemia points to a diagnosis of hypoparathyroidism, pseudohypoparathyroidism, or renal failure.

## Serum magnesium

Magnesium is required for the secretion of PTH and should be evaluated in patients presenting with previously undiagnosed hypocalcemia. Hypomagnesemia is an especially common cause of hypocalcemia in neonates.

## Parathyroid hormone

An elevated serum level of PTH may be seen in pseudohypoparathyroidism, chronic renal failure, vitamin D deficiency, or in abnormalities of vitamin D metabolism. Low levels point to hypoparathyroidism.

## Vitamin D level

Hypocalcemia in the setting of hypophosphatemia, and with elevations of serum PTH and alkaline phosphatase, suggests a disorder of vitamin D metabolism. Measurement of circulating levels of $25(OH)D_3$ and $1,25(OH)_2D_3$ should be performed to identify any nutritional deficiency of vitamin D, or defects in the metabolic pathways of vitamin D.

# MANAGEMENT OF HYPOCALCEMIA

Treatment of hypocalcemia is usually urgent, especially in patients with neuromuscular irritability or seizures. Intravenous calcium therapy is required in these patients, whereas milder hypocalcemia may be amenable to oral treatment. Therapy also needs to be tailored to the underlying origin and pathogenesis of hypocalcemia.

## Calcium supplements

Oral calcium supplements such as carbonate, citrate, and acetate salts of calcium are often used for long-term restoration and maintenance of blood calcium levels. The elemental calcium content of these compounds is variable. The GI calcium absorption rate of calcium is also highly variable, and absorption may be further impeded in vitamin D deficient states. An approximate starting dose for oral calcium supplementation is 5 to 20 mg elemental calcium/kg/dose, but the dose should be titrated by frequent assessment of blood calcium, to avoid hypercalcemia.

## Vitamin D and analogues

The minimum daily requirement of vitamin D is 400 international units for babies and small children. High content of vitamin D is present in only few naturally occurring foods, such as fish (salmon), beef liver, cheese, egg yolks, and fortified dairy products, thus necessitating supplementation in most children. Vitamin D is available as ergocalciferol (vitamin $D_2$), and cholecalciferol (vitamin $D_3$). The two forms of vitamin D are considered bioequivalent. For treatment of nutritional vitamin D deficiency, ergocalciferol and cholecalciferol are the preferred supplemental compounds. For patients with other disturbances of vitamin D metabolism, hypoparathyroidism, or renal osteodystrophy, pharmacologic preparations are available that often bypass the need for kidney activation. Calcitriol,

paricalcitol, and doxercalciferol are available in the United States for such therapy.

## HYPERCALCEMIA

Hypercalcemia is defined as occurring when serum calcium values are greater than 10.6 mg/dL or when the blood ionized calcium is greater than 1.38 mmol/L. Broadly, hypercalcemia can be divided into disorders of parathyroid function, of vitamin D excess, or of their respective receptors. Numerous miscellaneous causes exist as well. Table 13.4 details the causes of hypercalcemia in infants and children.

# CLINICAL MANIFESTATIONS

The symptoms of chronic hypercalcemia include muscle weakness, anorexia, nausea, vomiting, constipation, altered mental status, depression, hypertension, and weight loss. Additionally, polydipsia and polyuria may result from impairment in tubular concentrating ability. Nephrocalcinosis may occur with prolonged hypercalcemia and cause a progressive decrease in renal function. Nephrolithiasis may be present with persistent and long-standing hypercalcemia, and it can manifest with flank pain and hematuria. Skeletal involvement in hyperparathyroidism may lead to fractures. Infants may exhibit poor feeding, failure to thrive, and hypotonia. Some patients, however, may be asymptomatic, presenting only in response to incidental laboratory findings of elevated serum calcium concentrations.

# DISORDERS OF HYPERCALCEMIA

## Hyperparathyroidism

Primary hyperparathyroidism is a rare disorder in children, often manifesting in late childhood or early teens. Median age at presentation in a study was 16.8 years (range, 4 to 18.9 years).[37] Solitary benign adenomas of the parathyroid gland are the most common pathologic findings (65% to 85%), whereas diffuse hyperplasia of the glands accounts for the remaining 15% to 35% cases.[37-39] Among patients with diffuse parathyroid hyperplasia, the disorder can result from

---

**KEY POINT**

Hypophosphatemia and hypercalcemia point to the diagnosis of primary hyperparathyroidism.

Table 13.4 Causes of hypercalcemia

**Artifactual Cause**
- Increased serum albumin

**Hyperparathyroidism**
- Infant of mother with hypoparathyroidism
- Adenoma of parathyroid gland
- Multiple endocrine neoplasia

**Heritable Disorders**
- Calcium-sensing receptor disorders: familial hypocalciuric hypercalcemia
- Severe neonatal hyperparathyroidism
- Williams syndrome
- Jansen syndrome (a form of a metaphyseal dysplasia)
- Hypophosphatasia
- Idiopathic infantile hypercalcemia

**Excess Vitamin D**
- Surreptitious or intentional excess vitamin D intake
- Ectopic vitamin D synthesis:
  - Granulomatous disease (sarcoidosis, tuberculosis)
  - Subcutaneous fat necrosis in neonates

**Malignancy-Associated Causes**
- Paraneoplastic (PTH-rP or 1,25(OH)$_2$D$_3$ excesses)
- Bone metastases with lysis

**Drugs**
- Vitamin D intoxication
- Vitamin A intoxication
- Thiazide diuretics
- Lithium therapy

**Miscellaneous Causes**
- Immobilization
- Hyperalimentation (with inappropriately high calcium)
- Hypophosphatemia
- Adrenal insufficiency
- Thyrotoxicosis
- Milk-alkali syndrome
- Down syndrome

*Abbreviations:* PTH-rp, parathyroid hormone–related peptide.

multiple endocrine neoplasia (MEN) or familial non-MEN. In neonates, hyperparathyroidism can manifest as neonatal severe primary hyperparathyroidism (NSHPT), which is discussed later.

## Familial hypocalciuric hypercalcemia

Familial hypocalciuric hypercalcemia (FHH) is a benign disorder characterized by lifelong hypercalcemia, a normal PTH level, and lack of hypercalciuria. The parathyroid glands are normal in histologic structure, and subtotal parathyroidectomy does not cure the disorder.[40] FHH is inherited as an autosomal dominant disorder and results from heterozygous mutations in one allele for the gene that encodes the extracellular calcium-sensing receptor in the parathyroid gland and in the kidneys.[41] This condition leads to the characteristic findings of reduced urine calcium, despite the systemic hypercalcemia. Patients with FHH are asymptomatic, and no treatment is necessary. This disorder is commonly mistaken for primary hyperparathyroidism, and it is important to avoid unnecessary parathyroidectomy.

---

**KEY POINTS**

- FHH is a benign disorder.
- Inheritance: autosomal dominant.
- Despite hypercalcemia, urinary calcium excretion is low.
- PTH level is normal, and parathyroidectomy is not indicated.

---

## Neonatal severe hyperparathyroidism

Severe hypercalcemia associated with hyperparathyroidism in neonates is caused by homozygous mutation of the calcium-sensing receptor and is termed neonatal severe primary hyperparathyroidism (NSHPT).[42] Whereas heterozygous mutation of the calcium-sensing receptor leads to benign familial hypercalcemia, NSHPT is associated with severe, life-threatening hypercalcemia in the neonatal period.[43] Clinical manifestations consist of feeding difficulties, respiratory distress, hypotonia, failure to thrive, and unexplained fractures. Radiography of the long bones reveals subperiosteal resorption, demineralization, and fractures. Onset in later childhood, and even in adults, has been reported.[43,44] Emergency parathyroidectomy is generally advocated to control severe hypercalcemia, but more conservative management with pamidronate has been reported in some cases.[44]

---

**KEY POINTS**

- NSHPT causes unresponsive hypercalcemia.
- It is caused by homozygous mutation of the calcium sensing receptor.
- PTH level is elevated.
- Parathyroidectomy is indicated.

## Vitamin D excess states

Vitamin D intoxication is rare, but it may result from ingestion of milk products fortified with vitamin D or when excessive vitamin D is used as a supplement in children.[45,46] Other causes of vitamin D–mediated hypercalcemia include disorders causing extrarenal, ectopic production of $1,25(OH)_2D$, the active hormone of the vitamin D endocrine system. The latter category includes granulomatous diseases, such as sarcoidosis or tuberculosis, as well as subcutaneous fat necrosis, in which macrophage production of the active hormone may occur in an unregulated manner.[47–49]

---

### KEY POINTS

- Accidental ingestion or incorrectly compounded vitamin D preparations can cause vitamin D intoxication and hypercalcemia.
- PTH level is low.
- It is important to assay vitamin $D_2$ and $D_3$ concentrations in serum in patients suspected of overdose of vitamin D.

---

Several mechanisms can cause hypercalcemia associated with malignant diseases.[50]. In 1987, the PTH-related peptide (PTH-rP), a gene product that is separate from PTH and causes hypercalcemia, was isolated from carcinoma of the lung.[51] The PTH-rP shares structural homology with the amino terminal portion of the PTH molecule and results in the humoral hypercalcemia of malignancy (HHM).[51,52] PTH-rP has been associated with numerous solid organ and hematologic malignant diseases.

A second cause of hypercalcemia of malignancy involves ectopic $1,25(OH)_2D_3$ production by the malignant cells.[53,54] Increased intestinal calcium absorption, osteoclastic bone resorption, and decreased renal calcium excretion have been implicated in the pathogenesis of hypercalcemia as a result of ectopic $1,25(OH)_2D_3$ production in malignant diseases.[50] A third cause of hypercalcemia of malignancy is tumor cell metastasis to bone, which produces lytic lesions and resultant hypercalcemia.

## SYNDROMES ASSOCIATED WITH HYPERCALCEMIA

### Williams syndrome

Williams syndrome is characterized by supravalvular aortic stenosis, elfin-like facies, and hypercalcemia. The disorder is caused by a 1.5-Mb deletion containing the elastin gene and flanking genes on chromosome 7q11.23.[55] Hypercalcemia is reported in 5% to 15% of patients with Williams syndrome.[56,57] The mechanism of the hypercalcemia remains obscure, but it may involve altered vitamin D metabolism.

### Idiopathic infantile hypercalcemia

Idiopathic infantile hypercalcemia (IIH) is another distinct inherited clinical disorder that is characterized by failure to thrive, hypercalcemia, vomiting, and nephrocalcinosis. IIH results from loss-of-function mutations in the *CYP24A1* gene.[58] This gene regulates downstream catabolism of $1-25(OH)_2D_3$ into calcitroic acid through the enzyme 24-hydroxylase. In patients with IIH, clearance of $1-25(OH)_2D_3$ is dramatically decreased, resulting in high serum $1-25(OH)_2D_3$ levels, hypercalcemia, and suppression of PTH. This syndrome has been described in infants as well as in adults with kidney stones.[58,59]

### Jansen syndrome

Jansen syndrome (metaphyseal dysplasia), which was previously classified as cartilage dysplasia, is also associated with hypercalcemia. Clinically, this disorder is characterized by a rachitic-appearing skeletal structure present from birth. Several mutations in the gene encoding the common PTH/PTH-rP receptor-1 have been associated with this disorder.[60] Hypercalcemia results from ligand-independent, autoactivation of this G-protein–coupled receptor. Despite the findings of hypercalcemia, PTH and PTH-rP are undetectable in this disorder.

## EVALUATION OF HYPERCALCEMIA

### Parathyroid hormone assay

Based on the plasma PTH level, patients with hypercalcemia can be segregated into those with low PTH and those with inappropriately normal or increased levels of PTH. The latter situations are found in primary hyperparathyroidism and in familial hypocalciuric hypercalcemia.

### Vitamin D level

If a suppressed level of PTH is found in the diagnostic workup of a hypercalcemic patient, the differential diagnosis shifts to diseases associated with elevated circulating vitamin D metabolites. Normal levels of vitamin D metabolites, conversely, should prompt investigations of other sources of the hypercalcemia, such as a malignant disease. In the case of malignant disease, measurement of the serum PTH-rP level should be considered.

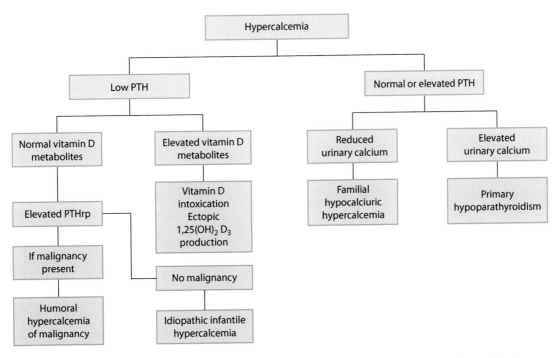

Figure 13.7 A suggested algorithm for evaluation of patients with hypercalcemia. Not all possible etiologies are shown in the algorithm. PTH, parathyroid hormone; PTHrp, parathyroid hormone–related peptide.

## MANAGEMENT OF HYPERCALCEMIA

Treatment of hypercalcemia largely depends on the severity of the abnormality and the symptoms. In mild cases, no treatment may be necessary; serum calcium levels should be followed, and all calcium or vitamin D supplementation should be discontinued. Consideration of the use of a calcium-restricted diet may also be appropriate for treatment of mild hypercalcemia. Moderate hypercalcemia (serum calcium 12 to 14 mg/dL or 3 to 3.5 mmol/L) should be treated with saline diuresis, and calcitonin may also be considered for refractory cases. Hypercalcemic crises (serum calcium greater than 14 mg/dL or 3.5 mmol/L) require urgent attention and therapy.

### Saline diuresis

Treatment of hypercalcemia should begin with hydration, using intravenous fluids appropriate for the child's age. In adults, normal saline is generally the recommended intravenous fluid for inducing diuresis. These patients often are dehydrated as a result of hypercalcemia-induced polyuria, and hydration is an important adjunct in their management. Additionally, volume expansion enhances renal calcium excretion and helps mitigate hypercalcemia. Addition of furosemide further reduces distal renal tubular calcium reabsorption and increases urinary calcium excretion. With diuresis alone, reduction in serum calcium level occurs gradually over several days. In general, fluid volume to be used should be age appropriate at 1.5 to 2 times normal maintenance. Such therapy should, however, be used with caution in infants and younger children because of the risk of inducing hypernatremia and fluid overload.

### Calcitonin

Calcitonin induces hypocalcemia by inhibiting osteoclastic activity in the bones. Subcutaneous injection of calcitonin (Calcimar) results in a rapid decline in serum calcium level. Nasal spray of calcitonin has been approved for treatment of postmenopausal osteoporosis, but it is not yet approved for the purposes of treatment of hypercalcemia. The starting dose of calcitonin is 2 to 4 international units/kg, given every 12 hours, subcutaneously. Actions of calcitonin are short-lived, usually lasting 48 to 72 hours. Gradual resistance to therapy develops after extended use.

### Bisphosphonates

Although bisphosphonates (pamidronate) have been used for of hypercalcemia in neonates and children, data on the long-term safety of these agents are unclear.[44] Bisphosphonates act by adsorbing onto hydroxyapatite of the bones, inhibiting bone resorption, reducing bone turnover, and increasing bone mineral accretion. The usual dose of intravenous pamidronate is 0.5 to 1 mg/kg in 0.9% saline infused over 2 to 4 hours. The therapeutic effect of pamidronate in decreasing serum calcium level is evident in 48 to 72 hours after the infusion is given, and it can last for 3 to 4 months. The drug is most helpful in patients with malignancy-induced hypercalcemia. Transient flulike symptoms consisting of muscle ache, fever, and lymphopenia are common. Other adverse effects include hypocalcemia, hypophosphatemia, hypomagnesemia, and acute kidney injury (AKI).

## Corticosteroids

In the past, use of corticosteroids was advocated for the treatment of hypercalcemia, but the role of these drugs is limited at present. In general, corticosteroids are useful in treating hypercalcemia in conditions such as sarcoidosis or tuberculosis, where abnormal synthesis of 1-25(OH)$_2$D$_3$ by macrophages drives hypercalcemia by enhancing GI calcium absorption.

## Parathyroidectomy

Parathyroidectomy may be indicated in the treatment of recalcitrant hypercalcemia. Hyperparathyroidism caused by an adenoma or hyperplasia is a common indication for parathyroidectomy. The procedure is also indicated in patients with NSHPT or uncontrolled tertiary hyperparathyroidism (e.g., renal transplantation).

## OTHER THERAPIES

Treatment of underlying malignant disease may be necessary for resolution of hypercalcemia in malignancy-associated hypercalcemia. Other therapeutic agents may include corticosteroids or mithramycin. Hemodialysis, using a low-calcium dialysate bath, should be considered for patients who are resistant to therapy or have life-threatening severe hypercalcemia.

## MAGNESIUM METABOLISM

Magnesium is a dominant intracellular cation and is essential for metabolic processes. It is also an important component of bones and teeth. Bone and muscle are the major tissue pools for magnesium within the body. Bone accounts for approximately 60% of the total body magnesium stores, whereas the remaining 40% of magnesium resides intracellularly in soft tissues, with more than half in muscle cells. Liver is also a prominent store of magnesium.

## RENAL HANDLING OF MAGNESIUM

### Magnesium homeostasis

After its absorption from the small intestine, magnesium homeostasis is maintained through excretion by the kidney. Vitamin D, PTH, and increased sodium absorption in the intestine may directly enhance magnesium absorption. Conversely, calcium, phosphate, and increased intestinal motility decrease absorption of magnesium from the GI tract.[62] A small amount of magnesium is secreted into the GI tract normally, and its excretion is increased in diarrhea. Figure 13.8 depicts tubular sites of magnesium reabsorption.

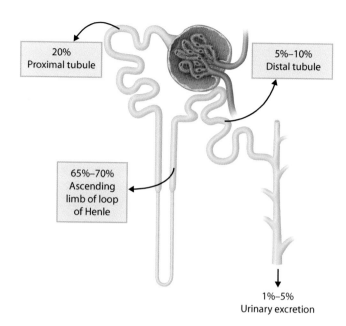

Figure 13.8 Tubular sites of magnesium reabsorption in the nephron.

Chronic or acute metabolic acidosis increases urinary excretion of magnesium, whereas metabolic alkalosis decreases it. Other factors that inhibit renal magnesium reabsorption include expansion of the extracellular fluid volume, glucagon, calcium, low PTH levels, and diuretics. Loop diuretics such as furosemide inhibit the Na-K-2Cl transporter and diminish the paracellular reabsorption of magnesium by reducing the transepithelial voltage. Thiazide diuretics act primarily at the Na-Cl cotransporter in the distal convoluted tubule and may cause small and variable magnesium wasting. Volume contraction, magnesium deficiency, thyrocalcitonin, and elevated PTH levels enhance renal magnesium reabsorption.[61]

### KEY POINT

The primary site of magnesium reabsorption in the renal tubules is in the thick ascending limb of the loop of Henle.

## HYPOMAGNESEMIA

Hypomagnesemia may arise from either diminished intake or excessive excretion by the kidneys or the GI tract. Inadequate intake of magnesium may result from dietary deficiency or when an insufficient amount of magnesium has been provided during prolonged intravenous fluid therapy. Malabsorptive states such as chronic diarrhea or celiac disease may also lead to magnesium deficiency. Excessive urinary excretion of magnesium may result from diuretic therapy, primary aldosteronism, hyperparathyroidism, postobstructive diuresis, acute tubular necrosis, diuresis following renal transplantation, and nephrotoxic agents such as cyclosporine, cisplatinum, aminoglycosides, and amphotericin B. Several inherited disorders characterized by hypomagnesemia have also been identified. Functional deficiency of magnesium may be caused by intracellular shift of magnesium during respiratory alkalosis and treatment of diabetic ketoacidosis with insulin. Postparathyroidectomy "hungry bone syndrome," as well as refeeding of malnourished children, can also result in hypomagnesemia because of the incorporation of this ion into the regenerating tissues. Table 13.5 lists the causes of hypomagnesemia encountered in children.

## CLINICAL MANIFESTATIONS

The symptoms of hypomagnesemia largely consist of increased neuromuscular irritability, including tremors, seizures, tetany, carpopedal spasms, and neuropsychiatric manifestations (Table 13.6). Positive Chvostek and Trousseau signs seen in hypocalcemia may also be elicited in patients with hypomagnesemia. Disorientation, nausea, anorexia, abnormal cardiac rhythm, and ECG changes, such as prolonged QT, U waves, or nonspecific T-wave changes, also may occur.[63] Hypocalcemia and hypokalemia are common biochemical findings encountered in hypomagnesemia. The degree of symptoms does not always correlate with the serum level of magnesium, however, possibly because magnesium is largely an intracellular cation and the serum level may not reflect the total body magnesium content.

Table 13.5 Causes of hypomagnesemia

**Poor Absorption or Intake**
- Protein-calorie malnutrition
- Chronic diarrhea
- Selective defect of magnesium absorption in the intestine

**Magnesium Shift Into Cells**
- Postparathyroidectomy hungry bone syndrome
- Insulin in treatment of diabetic ketoacidosis
- Respiratory alkalosis
- Refeeding in malnutrition

**Renal Magnesium Wasting**
- Inherited disorders
  - Hypomagnesemia with secondary hypocalcemia
  - Isolated familial hypomagnesemia:
    - Autosomal dominant
    - Autosomal recessive
- Familial hypomagnesemia with hypercalciuria and nephrocalcinosis (paracellin-1 mutations)
- Tubular sodium or chloride transport defects:
  - Gitelman syndrome
  - Bartter syndrome
- Drugs
  - Aminoglycosides
  - Cyclosporine
  - Cisplatinum
  - Amphotericin B
  - Dopamine
  - Insulin
  - Loop and thiazide diuretics
- States of diuresis
  - Postobstructive diuresis
  - Acute tubular necrosis: diuretic phase
  - Volume expansion
  - Osmotic diuresis
  - Post-renal transplant diuresis

**Miscellaneous Disorders**
- Hypoparathyroidism
- Phosphate deprivation
- Hypercalcemia
- Hyperthyroidism

Table 13.6 Manifestations of magnesium depletion

**Neuromuscular**
- Muscle weakness
- Positive Chvostek and Trousseau signs
- Spontaneous carpopedal spasm
- Seizures
- Psychosis

**Cardiovascular**
- Prolonged PR interval
- Widened QRS complex
- Inversion of T waves
- Life-threatening ventricular arrhythmias
- Enhanced toxicity of cardiac glycosides

**Metabolic**
- Resistant hypocalcemia
- Resistant hypokalemia
- Increased insulin secretion
- Carbohydrate intolerance

# CLINICAL DISORDERS

## Gitelman syndrome

Gitelman syndrome (see Chapter 41) is an autosomal recessive disorder characterized by metabolic alkalosis, hypokalemia, hypomagnesemia, and hypocalciuria. Other findings include increased urinary loss of magnesium and potassium.[64-66] Gitelman syndrome results from inactivating mutations in the SLC12A3 gene (mapped to chromosome 16q) that encodes the thiazide-sensitive Na-Cl cotransporter present in the distal convoluted tubule of the kidney.[66] These patients usually present during childhood or adolescence and exhibit normal linear growth. Although the disorder is often asymptomatic, transient episodes of weakness and tetany secondary to profound hypomagnesemia can be observed. Variations in phenotype are common, even within the same family with identical gene mutations.[67] Adults with Gitelman syndrome occasionally develop chondrocalcinosis with deposition of calcium pyrophosphate dehydrate crystals.[68]

## Bartter syndrome

## Hypomagnesemia with secondary hypocalcemia

Hypomagnesemia with secondary hypocalcemia is an autosomal recessive disorder that manifests in the newborn period with seizures, tetany, and muscle spasms. This disorder is believed to result from a primary defect in intestinal magnesium transport.[71] Hypocalcemia results from parathyroid failure as a result of sustained magnesium deficiency. Mutations in a novel gene, TRPM6, encoding an ion channel expressed throughout the intestinal tract and within distal convoluted tubule cells, have been reported.[72] This disease can be fatal without the administration of high-dose oral magnesium.

## Isolated familial hypomagnesemia

Isolated familial renal magnesium wasting is a rare but increasingly recognized disorder. The disorder has been reported as a dominantly or recessively inherited condition. In isolated dominant hypomagnesemia (IDH), low serum magnesium is seen in conjunction with renal magnesium wasting and hypocalciuria.[73] This disorder is distinguished from Gitelman syndrome by the absence of hypokalemic metabolic alkalosis. Patients with IDH can present in the neonatal period and early childhood with severe hypomagnesemia. Mutations in the FXYD2 gene located on chromosome 11q23 that result in abnormality in the y subunit of the basolateral $Na^+$-$K^+$-ATPase in the distal convoluted tubule have been proposed to be the abnormality in IDH.[74] Other clinicians have reported the lack of FXYD2 gene mutation, a finding suggesting that IDH may be caused by other genetic mutations.[75] Isolated recessive hypomagnesemia (IRH) also appears in childhood with manifestations of hypomagnesemia, but it is not associated with hypocalciuria.[76] No candidate gene for this disorder has yet been identified.

## Familial hypomagnesemia with hypercalciuria and nephrocalcinosis

Familial hypomagnesemia with hypercalciuria and nephrocalcinosis (FHHN) is an autosomal recessive disorder in which nephrocalcinosis is the cardinal finding. The biochemical abnormalities include hypomagnesemia with hypermagnesuria, and normal serum calcium with hypercalciuria. Some patients may also have findings of partial distal renal tubular acidosis.[77] Patients may present in early childhood with urinary tract infection, nephrolithiasis, polyuria, polydipsia, and failure to thrive. Manifestations of hypomagnesemia such as tetany and seizures are also common. Ocular abnormalities have been reported in these patients and include myopia, nystagmus, and chorioretinitis.[78] Patients with FHHN eventually progress to chronic renal failure in childhood or adolescence, and this feature distinguishes this disorder from other causes of hypomagnesemia such as Gitelman syndrome or isolated familial hypomagnesemia. Hyperparathyroidism, disproportionate to renal insufficiency, has also been reported, and it may be seen before onset of renal dysfunction. Therapy is aimed to reduce the progression of nephrocalcinosis and renal stones with thiazide diuretics. Renal transplantation is curative. Mutations in the gene CLDN16, located on chromosome 3q, which encodes for paracellin-1, a member of the tight junction proteins, have been reported in patients with FHHN.[79]

## Autosomal dominant hypoparathyroidism

Autosomal dominant hypoparathyroidism may manifest in infancy with hypomagnesemia and hypocalcemia, with increased urinary excretion of magnesium and calcium. Defects in the ECaSR gene encoding the calcium/magnesium ($Ca^{2+}$/$Mg^{2+}$)–sensing receptor in the parathyroid gland have been implicated in this disorder.[21] An activating mutation in this gene shifts the set point of the receptor and enhances the affinity of the mutant receptor for extracellular calcium and magnesium, thereby diminishing PTH secretion and reducing the renal tubular reabsorption of magnesium and calcium.

# EVALUATION OF HYPOMAGNESEMIA

A thorough clinical history and examination and evaluation of serum magnesium, calcium, and phosphorus levels should be conducted in patients with hypomagnesemia. The focus of investigations is to determine whether the hypomagnesemia is the result of nutritional inadequacy, GI diseases, or excessive renal wasting. Kidney function and urinary evaluation and measurements of urinary calcium and magnesium excretions, preferably in a 24-hour sample, should be conducted. Fractional excretion of magnesium can be determined on a spot sample of urine, by using the following formula:

$$FEMg\ (\%) = [UMg \times PCr] / [(0.7 \times PMg) \times UCr] \times 100$$

where FEMg is the fractional excretion of magnesium (%), UMg is the urinary magnesium concentration (mg/dL), PMg is the plasma magnesium concentration (mg/dL), PCr is the plasma creatinine concentration (mg/dL), and UCr is the urine creatinine concentration (mg/dL).

Because only 70% of the plasma magnesium is ultrafiltrable (not bound to albumin), the plasma magnesium concentration is multiplied by a factor of 0.7. Fractional excretion of magnesium greater than 2.0% in patients with normal renal function suggests renal magnesium wasting. Patients with extrarenal loss of magnesium, such as with diarrhea or other GI disorders, have fractional excretion of magnesium lower than 1.5%.

---

## KEY POINT

The initial evaluation of hypomagnesemia focuses on determining whether it is the result of GI disorders or renal disease.

---

# MANAGEMENT OF HYPOMAGNESEMIA

## HYPERMAGNESEMIA

Because of excellent renal modulation of magnesium homeostasis, hypermagnesemia rarely occurs in patients with normal renal function, except as an accidental toxic ingestion. Of course, patients with renal insufficiency often develop mild to moderate hypermagnesemia. Hypermagnesemia is defined as a serum magnesium level greater than 2.5 mEq/L. Sources of magnesium loads that may lead to elevated serum magnesium levels include laxatives (Milk of Magnesia), enemas, antacids, intravenous fluids with high magnesium load, accidental overdose with therapy, and neonates born to mothers treated with magnesium sulfate for pre-eclampsia. Addison disease may be associated with mildly elevated serum magnesium. A rare syndrome of decreased renal magnesium excretion and hypermagnesemia has also been reported.[82]

Symptoms of hypermagnesemia include hyporeflexia, flaccidity, respiratory depression, hypotension, disturbances in cardiac atrioventricular conduction, drowsiness, and coma. In addition to careful history taking to elucidate a cause, the evaluation generally includes serum and urinary measurements of calcium and magnesium. Treatment of hypermagnesemia includes intravenous calcium gluconate, exchange transfusion, and diuresis. Dialysis may be necessary for patients with renal failure.

## PHOSPHORUS METABOLISM

Phosphorus is mainly stored in the body within the skeleton and teeth. Besides being a vital constituent of bone mineral, phosphorus is also required for vital intracellular metabolic processes, such as energy metabolism, protein

Table 13.7 Magnesium contents of commercially available supplements

| Magnesium Salt | Brand names | Magnesium (mg/g) | Percent elemental magnesium (%) | Remarks |
|---|---|---|---|---|
| Magnesium oxide | MagOx; many other brands | 603 | 60.3 | Magnesium supplement |
| Magnesium hydroxide | Milk of Magnesia (MOM); other brands | 417 | 41.7 | Used as antacid |
| Magnesium citrate | Citroma; other brands | 162 | 16.2 | Used as bowel cleanser |
| Magnesium chloride | SlowMag; other brands | 120 | 12.0 | Magnesium supplement |
| Magnesium lactate | MagTab; other brands | 120 | 12.0 | Magnesium supplement |
| Magnesium sulfate | Numerous brands | 99 | 9.9 | Bowel cleanser; magnesium supplement; also available as a parenteral preparation |
| Magnesium aspartate | Numerous brands | 75 | 7.5 | Nutritional supplement |
| Magnesium gluconate | Numerous brands | 54 | 5.4 | Nutritional supplement |

Source: Some data from Blaine Pharmaceuticals, Fort Wright, KY. http://www.magox.com/healthcaretypes.htm

phosphorylation, and nucleotide and phospholipid metabolism. Phosphorus, as phospholipids, is an important component of cell membranes. Of the total body phosphorus, approximately 85% resides in the skeletal stores, and the remaining 15% is present in the soft tissues as an intracellular ion. A small fraction of the total phosphorus is found in the extracellular fluid. Within the plasma, phosphorus is present as organic compounds (phospholipids and phosphate esters), as inorganic phosphates (as $HPO_4^{2-}$ or $H_2PO_4^-$), and as complexes with other ions, such as calcium and magnesium ions. Approximately 10% to 15% of plasma inorganic phosphorus is protein bound, and the remaining 85% to 90% is ultrafiltrable by the glomeruli. Whereas the adult phosphorus balance is zero, growing children have a positive phosphorus balance to meet the needs of skeletal growth.[1]

---

## KEY POINTS

- Like calcium, bones are the main repository of phosphorus in the body.
- Phosphorus forms an important component of cellular energy transfer in the form of adenosine triphosphate (ATP).

---

Serum phosphorus is governed by a circadian rhythm, with a rapid decrease in levels early in the morning, a nadir before noon, and a peak after midnight. When measuring the serum phosphorus level, it is best to obtain a specimen in the morning fasting state to minimize the effect of dietary changes on the serum level. The normal serum concentration of phosphorus varies with age, with values higher in infants than in older children and adults (Table 13.8). Other factors that may affect the serum level include metabolic acidosis and intravenous calcium infusion, both of which may increase the serum phosphorus. Decreased serum phosphorus levels may result from intravenous infusion of glucose or insulin, acute respiratory alkalosis, and epinephrine administration.

Between 80% and 97% of the filtered phosphorus is reabsorbed by the renal tubules, mostly by the proximal tubules (70% to 80%), 5% to 10% in the distal tubule, and 2% to 3% in the collecting tubule (Figure 13.9). In the proximal tubule, phosphorus transport is coupled to sodium

Table 13.8 Serum phosphorus level in normal infants and children

| Age group | Serum phosphorus level (mg/dL) |
| --- | --- |
| Infancy | 4.8–7.4 |
| Toddlerhood | 4.5–5.8 |
| Midchildhood | 3.5–5.5 |
| Adolescence to adulthood | 2.4–4.5 |

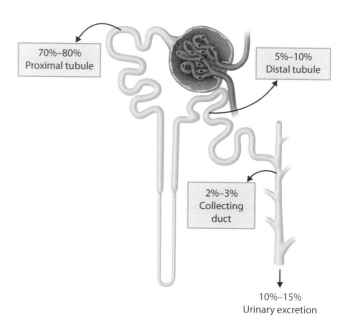

Figure 13.9 Tubular sites of phosphorus reabsorption in the nephron.

transport, being unidirectional, against a gradient, and a transcellular secondary active process. Proximal tubular phosphate transport is mediated by the sodium-phosphate (Na-$P_i$) cotransporter present in the apical brush-border membrane. Three distinct types of Na-$P_i$ cotransporters—type I, type II, and type III—have been described in the renal tubules. Of these, the type IIa Na-$P_i$ cotransporter is believed to be the most significant phosphate reabsorption protein. The Na-$P_i$ cotransporter picks one phosphate ion along with three sodium ions and delivers these into the proximal tubular cells. Phosphorus exits the tubular cell by active basolateral Na-K-ATPase pumps.[83,84]

## PHOSPHORUS HOMEOSTASIS

In adults, dietary intake results in a net intestinal absorption of 60% to 65% of the ingested quantity of phosphorus. In infants, this net absorption is higher and may exceed 90%. Most of the ingested phosphorus is absorbed from the duodenum and jejunum, through passive diffusion by a paracellular pathway. When the luminal concentration is low, phosphorus may also be absorbed actively by a sodium-dependent transcellular process. Once in the extracellular fluid compartment, phosphorus exists in equilibrium with the bone and soft tissue pools.

### Vitamin D

Vitamin D plays an active role in phosphorus homeostasis. Hypophosphatemia causes an increase in renal $1,25(OH)_2D_3$ synthesis.[85,86] This leads to increased phosphorus and calcium absorption from the gut and increased mobilization of calcium and phosphorus from bone. These combined effects elicit an increase in serum calcium and phosphorus. Elevated serum calcium causes a decrease in PTH secretion, which enhances renal phosphorus reabsorption and also increases renal calcium excretion. Hypophosphatemia also directly increases calcium excretion in the kidney. The net result of all these factors is an increase in serum phosphorus concentration, with relatively little change in the serum calcium. Hyperphosphatemia results in opposite effects by decreasing levels of $1,25(OH)_2D_3$ and increasing PTH levels, thereby decreasing the serum phosphorus level.[85,86]

## Parathyroid hormone

PTH inhibits phosphate reabsorption in the proximal tubule by inhibiting phosphate transport by reducing the number of type IIa Na-$P_i$ cotransporters (Na-Pi-IIa) and type IIc Na-$P_i$ cotransporters (Na-Pi-IIc) on the luminal brush border of these cells. In contrast, with an absence of PTH (e.g., after parathyroidectomy), there is an increase in the number of Na-$P_i$ cotransporters.[83] PTH mediates its actions in the proximal tubule through the type 1 PTH receptor.

## Fibroblast growth factor-23

FGF-23 is a phosphaturic hormone distinct from PTH. FGF-23 is derived from osteocytes and osteoblasts in the bone, and its actions are mediated by binding to the FGF receptor -αKlotho complexes.[87,88] Similar to the actions of PTH, FGF-23 inhibits renal phosphate reabsorption by downregulating luminal expression of sodium-phosphate cotransporters type IIa and c (Na-Pi-IIa, Na-Pi-IIc) and sodium-dependent inorganic phosphate transporter (PiT2) in the apical brush-border surface of the proximal tubule.[83,88] FGF-23 also inhibits the synthesis of $1, 25(OH)_2D$ in the kidney.

Missense mutations involving the *FGF23* gene cause autosomal dominant hypophosphatemic rickets. These mutations in *FGF23* result in an inability of FGF-23 to be cleaved and inactivated, thereby leading to phosphaturia and rickets.[88] Similarly, inactivating mutations in the *PHEX* gene, which regulates FGF-23 inactivation, leads to high FGF-23 levels and causes renal phosphate wasting in X-linked hypophosphatemic rickets (XLH).[88] Conversely, FGF-23 deficiency caused by mutations in *FGF23* result in familial tumoral calcinosis (FTC), which is characterized by hyperphosphatemia, elevated $1,25(OH)_2D$ level, and tumoral calcinosis.[89]

---

### KEY POINTS

- FGF-23 and PTH both lead to phosphaturia, but by independent molecular mechanisms.
- Both PTH and FGF-23 downregulate luminal expression of two sodium-phosphate cotransporters: Na-Pi-IIa and Na-Pi-IIc.
- FGF-23 reduces $1-25(OH)_2D$ (calcitriol) synthesis.
- PTH increases $1-25(OH)_2D$ (calcitriol) synthesis.

---

## HYPOPHOSPHATEMIA

Serum phosphorus levels in children vary by age (see Table 13.3), and these variations need to be considered in defining hypophosphatemia in children. Serum phosphorus may not reflect total body phosphorus levels because it is predominantly an intracellular ion. Both primary and secondary hyperparathyroidism may result in phosphaturia and consequent hypophosphatemia. Nonselective urinary phosphate wasting, leading to hypophosphatemia, can be seen in numerous renal diseases, such as Fanconi syndrome, distal renal tubular acidosis, postobstructive diuresis, and the diuretic phase of acute tubular necrosis.

Hypophosphatemia with reduced urinary phosphorus excretion may result from nutritional deficiency of phosphorus, malnutrition, impaired intestinal absorption from phosphorus-binding antacids, or intestinal disorders. Refeeding with a large carbohydrate load after prolonged malnutrition, as well as leukemic blast crisis, in which phosphate is incorporated into the proliferating cells, can lead to hypophosphatemia.[90] Respiratory alkalosis stimulates the formation of intracellular sugar-phosphate moieties and may cause hypophosphatemia with low urinary phosphorus. Intracellular phosphorus shift may also result from infusion of glucose, fructose, lactate and amino acids, exogenous administration of insulin, glucagon, androgens, and β-agonists.[91] Table 13.9 lists the causes of hypophosphatemia seen commonly in infants and children.

## CLINICAL MANIFESTATIONS

Symptoms of low serum phosphorus generally result from decreased intracellular ATP and impaired tissue oxygen delivery, especially in hypophosphatemia of long duration. Symptoms may include anorexia, vomiting, paresthesias, myopathy, rickets, confusion, and seizures (Table 13.10). Life-threatening events, such as cardiac failure, ventricular arrhythmias, hypotension, red blood cell hemolysis, rhabdomyolysis, respiratory failure, and coma, may result from severe phosphorus deficits (less than 1.0 mg/dL).[92]

## CLINICAL DISORDERS OF HYPOPHOSPHATEMIA

### X-linked hypophosphatemic rickets

XLH, also known as familial hypophosphatemic rickets, is characterized by renal phosphate wasting, hypophosphatemia, growth retardation, and clinical manifestations of rickets. Serum calcium and PTH levels are normal, but the vitamin $1,25(OH)_2D_3$ level is low. The disorder is transmitted as an X-linked dominant disease and is caused by inactivating mutations in the *PHEX* gene (phosphate-regulating gene with homologies to endopeptidases on the X chromosome) in affected persons.[93,94] This mutation is believed

Table 13.9 Causes of hypophosphatemia

**Poor Phosphate Intake or Absorption**
- Malnutrition
- Anorexia nervosa
- Phosphate-binding antacids (e.g., calcium carbonate [Tums])
- Malabsorption
- Inadequate phosphate in intravenous hyperalimentation

**Shift of Phosphate Into Cells**
- Rapid infusion of large dose of carbohydrates (glucose, fructose)
- Endogenous or exogenous hormones
  - Insulin for correction of hyperglycemia
  - Catecholamines: epinephrine, dopamine, albuterol
  - Glucagon
  - Calcitonin
- Respiratory alkalosis

**Cellular Incorporation of Phosphate**
- Postparathyroidectomy hungry bone syndrome
- Leukemic blast crises
- Refeeding in malnutrition

**Renal phosphate Wasting (Phosphaturia)**
- Proximal renal tubular acidosis (Fanconi syndrome)
- Primary hyperparathyroidism
- Metabolic acidosis
- Diuretic therapy
- Glucocorticoid therapy
- Mineralocorticoid therapy
- Volume expansion
- Sodium bicarbonate infusion

**Inherited Disorders**
- *PHEX* mutation
  - X-linked hypophosphatemic rickets
- *FGF23* mutation
  - Autosomal dominant hypophosphatemia
- *SLC34A3* mutation
  - Hereditary hypophosphatemia with hypercalciuria
- *ENPP1* mutation
  - Autosomal recessive hypophosphatemic rickets

**Miscellaneous Disorders**
- Postrenal transplant hypophosphatemia
- Continuous renal replacement therapy: insufficient phosphate in the dialysate and/or replacement fluids
- Acute systemic infections

Table 13.10 Clinical and laboratory manifestations of phosphate depletion

**Muscular**
- Proximal myopathy
- Weakness
- Rhabdomyolysis

**Gastrointestinal**
- Dysphagia
- Ileus

**Respiratory**
- Hyperventilation
- Hypoventilation
- Respiratory muscle paralysis

**Hematologic**
- Hemolysis
- Impaired phagocytosis
- Impaired platelet function, thrombocytopenia

**Renal**
- Magnesuria
- Hypercalciuria
- Increased tubular phosphate reabsorption
- Increased $1,25(OH)_2D_3$ synthesis

**Skeletal**
- Bone pain
- Rickets or osteomalacia
- Pseudofractures or fractures

**Neurologic**
- Irritability
- Confusion
- Encephalopathy, coma

to prevent inactivation of FGF-23, a phosphaturic factor. Resultant increased FGF-23 concentration causes phosphaturia and the clinical manifestations of XLH (Figure 13.10). Treatment of XLH includes phosphate and calcitriol supplementation. Improvements in growth have been noted with such therapy, but nephrocalcinosis can be a side effect.[95,96]

## Autosomal dominant hypophosphatemia

Autosomal dominant hypophosphatemia (ADH) is phenotypically a heterogenous disorder. Patients can present either in early childhood (1 to 3 years) or in the adolescent and adult age groups.[88,92,97] Clinical manifestations of children with ADH include muscle weakness, short stature, clinical rickets, and bone pain. Adults presenting with this disorder do not have any skeletal deformities, but they may have short stature, bone pain, and fatigue, and pseudofractures or stress fractures may be seen on radiographs.[97] In women, the disease may first manifest during or after pregnancy. Regression and resolution of hypophosphatemia in

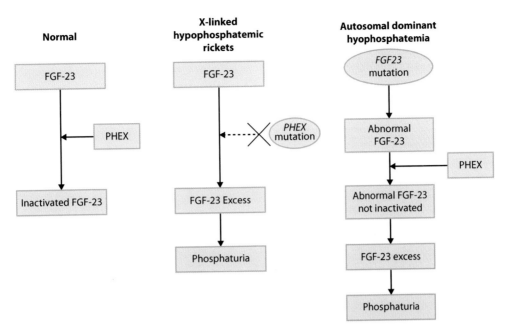

Figure 13.10 Pathogenesis of hypophosphatemia in X-linked hypophosphatemic rickets and autosomal dominant hypophosphatemia. FGF-23, fibroblast growth factor-23; *PHEX*, phosphate-regulating gene with homologies to endopeptidases on the X chromosome.

affected persons have been reported. Serum calcium level is normal, PTH level is normal or marginally elevated, and $1,25(OH)_2D_3$ level is normal or modestly low. ADH is caused by missense mutations in *FGF23* that lead to the formation of a mutant FGF-23 molecule that is resistant to normal cleavage.[88,98,99] Excess FGF-23 accumulates and leads to phosphaturia and hypophosphatemia and the clinical manifestations of ADH.

## Oncogenic osteomalacia

Tumor-induced osteomalacia (TIO), also known as oncogenic osteomalacia, is a paraneoplastic disorder that is characterized by phosphaturia, hypophosphatemia, and inappropriately low serum levels of 1,25-dihydroxyvitamin $D_3$.[100] TIO is caused by excessive production of FGF-23 by tumors, which are often of mesenchymal tissue origin.[101] Patients have severe bone pain and skeletal demineralization. Excision of the tumor is usually curative in TIO.

## Hereditary hypophosphatemia with hypercalciuria

Hereditary hypophosphatemia with hypercalciuria (HHH) is another disorder of selective renal phosphorus wasting.[102] Clinical manifestations of HHH include short stature, phosphaturia, hypophosphatemia, hypercalciuria, nephrolithiasis, and rickets. The serum $1,25(OH)_2D_3$ level is elevated, whereas the PTH level is suppressed. HHH results from homozygous loss-of-function mutations in the *SLC34A3* gene encoding the renal type IIc cotransporter, NaPi-IIc.[103] Treatment with phosphorus supplementation improves rickets, despite ongoing phosphaturia.

## Post–renal transplantation hypophosphatemia

Hypophosphatemia that can persist for up to several months is commonly seen after renal transplantation. Hyperparathyroidism associated with CKD persisting in the early course of transplantation had historically been considered the most likely suspect in the causation of phosphaturia and hypophosphatemia in these patients. It is now clear that persistence of elevated levels of FGF-23 has a major role in hypophosphatemia after renal transplantation.[104] Treatment consists of phosphate supplementation and adequate doses of vitamin D.

## Idiopathic hypercalciuria

Renal phosphate wasting and hypophosphatemia was reported in a small group of children with idiopathic hypercalciuria.[105] Vitamin D levels were elevated in these patients, and phosphorus supplementation reduced calciuria and restored normal serum phosphorus values.

## Hungry bone syndrome

Hungry bone syndrome refers to the transient phenomenon of hypocalcemia and hypophosphatemia seen due to increased avidity of bone for calcium and phosphorus after the resolution of long-standing primary or secondary hyperparathyroidism.[105] This disorder is commonly seen following parathyroidectomy in patients with primary or secondary hyperparathyroidism. Manifestations of hypophosphatemia as well as hypocalcemia can persist for weeks to several months. Oral supplemental calcium and vitamin

D therapy is needed for treatment of most patients with hungry bone syndrome. An occasional patient may require prolonged intravenous calcium supplementation and vitamin D to avoid life-threatening hypocalcemia. Hypophosphatemia is usually responsive to oral supplementation.

# EVALUATION OF HYPOPHOSPHATEMIA

Disorders of hypophosphatemia can be classified as those with renal phosphate wasting and those with reduced urinary phosphorus. If the urinary phosphorus level is elevated, this suggests a phosphaturic mechanism, and serum PTH measurement is essential. Elevated PTH points to disorders of hyperparathyroidism, either primary or secondary. If the serum PTH level is normal or low, then it is necessary to determine whether the urinary losses are selective for phosphorus or whether nonselective phosphorus wasting, such as associated with Fanconi syndrome, may be present. FGF-23 measurement may be indicated in patients who have disorders associated with an increased FGF-23 level, such as TIO, XLH, and ADH. Bone radiography for evidence of osteoporosis and bone densitometry may also help in determining the impact of hypophosphatemia and phosphaturia on bone health. Tests that can be performed to document phosphaturia are discussed here.

## Fractional excretion of phosphorus

Urinary phosphorus excretion and tubular reabsorption of phosphorus can be studied in a spot sample of urine by obtaining fractional excretion of phosphorus, by using the following formula:

$$FEPO_4 (\%) = (UPhos \times PCr) / (PPhos \times UCr) \times 100$$

where $FEPO_4$ is the fractional excretion of phosphate (%), UPhos is the urine phosphorus (mg/dL), PPhos is the plasma phosphorus (mg/dL), PCr is the plasma creatinine (mg/dL), and UCr is the urine creatinine (mg/dL).

The fractional excretion of phosphate in normal children is 15% to 20%, and it is lower in growing infants. A fractional excretion of phosphate of more than 20% indicates phosphaturia.

## Tubular reabsorption of phosphorus

Another derived index of phosphate excretion is tubular reabsorption of phosphate (TRP). TRP represents the percentage of the filtered phosphate that is reabsorbed in the renal tubules, by using the formula:

$$TRP(\%) = 100 - FEPO_{4\,(\%)}$$

Renal tubules reabsorb greater than 80% of filtered phosphate; therefore, TRP is 80% (or 0.8) in normal children. Higher values of TRP are expected in infants and growing children with high phosphorus accrual rates.[106] Both the fractional excretion of phosphate and TRP can be affected by renal function and plasma phosphorus concentration.

## Tubular maximum rate of phosphate reabsorption

An index of renal phosphate excretion considered to be independent of renal function is the ratio of the TRP to the glomerular filtration rate (GFR). This index provides a theoretical lower limit of serum phosphorus below which all filtered phosphate would be reabsorbed. This index can be calculated either from a nomogram (Figure 13.11) or from the following formula[107,108]:

If TRP is 0.86 or lower, then:

$$TmP/GFR = TRP \times Serum\ phosphate$$

If the TRP is greater than 0.86 then:

$$TmP/GFR = 0.3 \times TRP / \{1 - (0.8 \times TRP)\} \times Pp$$

TmP/GFR in normal persons varies with age; it is high in younger children and decreases with age, and it ranges from approximately 4.4 to 5.4 mg/dL in young children and 2.5 to 4.5 mg/dL in adolescents.[108,109] Lower TmP/GFR reflects poor TRP (phosphaturia). Tests of TRP can be done on a spot sample of urine, but a short timed collection (2 to 4 hours) obtained with the patient in a fasting state is usually preferred to avoid variability related to dietary intake. A suggested algorithm for diagnosis of hypophosphatemia is given in Figure 13.12.

# MANAGEMENT OF HYPOPHOSPHATEMIA

Treatment of hypophosphatemia in patients believed to have a normal total body phosphorus concentration may be deferred, unless clinical symptoms are present. Mild hypophosphatemia (greater than 2.5 mg/dL) may be treated with increased phosphate content in the diet. Milk and milk products are particularly high in phosphorus content, and their intake may be encouraged in such patients. Asymptomatic patients with moderate hypophosphatemia (1.5 to 2.5 mg/dL) may be treated with oral phosphorus supplementation (Table 13.11). Care should be taken not to provide calcium supplementation with meals because this may further exacerbate hypophosphatemia through binding of dietary phosphorus with calcium and thereby preventing its absorption.

Intravenous phosphorus infusion therapy is generally reserved for patients with symptomatic hypophosphatemia or a serum phosphorus level lower than 1 mg/dL. Sodium phosphate (phosphorus, 3.0 mmol/mL, and sodium, 4.0 mmol/mL) or potassium phosphate (phosphorus, 3.0 mmol/mL, and potassium, 4.4 mmol/mL) can be used for intravenous phosphate replacement (Table 13.12). It is important to remember that for every 1 mmol of phosphorus ordered as potassium phosphate, the patient will also receive approximately 1.47 mmol of potassium.

The usual dose for elemental phosphate for intravenous use is 0.08 to 0.2 mmol/kg, but higher doses can be used in monitored circumstances, such as in intensive care units.[110] Intravenous phosphate replacement

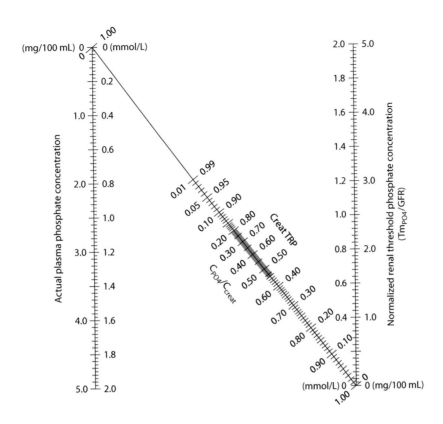

Figure 13.11 Nomogram for the calculation of renal tubular reabsorption of phosphate (TmPO4/GFR) from plasma phosphate concentration and the fractional reabsorption of phosphate (TRP). Inner aspect of the vertical axis on right and the left side represents data in SI units (mmol/L). Outer aspect of the vertical axis on right and the left side represents data in mass units (mg/100 mL). First step in using the graph is to calculate TRP, as detailed in the text. A straight line joining plasma phosphate concentration (left vertical axis), TRP (middle of the nomogram), and the right vertical axis gives the TmPO4/GFR. CCREAT, creatinine clearance; CPO4, phosphate clearance. (Reproduced with permission from: Walton RJ, Bijvoet OL. Nomogram for derivation of renal threshold phosphate concentration. Lancet. 1975;2(7929):309–10.)

is infused over 4 to 6 hours, and the generally recommended rate of infusion is no more than 0.2 mmol/kg/h of elemental phosphorus. The phosphate infusions are formulated in normal saline- or dextrose-containing solutions and may be incorporated in the intravenous hyperalimentation. However, these infusions should not be mixed with calcium-containing solutions such as Ringer lactate, because of the risk of precipitation. Hypocalcemia, hypomagnesemia, and hyperphosphatemia can result following intravenous infusion of phosphate, and patients need close monitoring for these electrolyte abnormalities. Hyperkalemia and consequent cardiac toxicity can result from potassium phosphate infusion, even in patients with normal renal function. Rapid infusions may result in phosphaturia.[111]

## HYPERPHOSPHATEMIA

Chronic hyperphosphatemia is an uncommon clinical disorder, except in patients with CKD. Acute hyperphosphatemia occurs in circumstances of AKI if a high phosphorus dose is administered in the form of intravenous hyperalimentation or as phosphate enema (Fleet phosphate enema: monobasic sodium phosphate 19 g and dibasic sodium phosphate 7 g in 4.7 ounces).[112] Tumor lysis syndrome (TLS) is another frequent cause of acute hyperphosphatemia in children.[113] Endocrinopathies, such as hypoparathyroidism and pseudohypoparathyroidism, are well-known causes of hyperphosphatemia as well. Common causes of hyperphosphatemia in children are listed in Table 13.13.

## CLINICAL MANIFESTATIONS

Patients with elevated serum phosphorus levels are frequently asymptomatic. Acute elevations in phosphorus usually cause hypocalcemia, and patients can become symptomatic with paresthesias, tetany, seizures, or cardiac arrhythmias.[114,115] Hypocalcemia is believed to result from chelation and precipitation of phosphorus and calcium ions in the soft tissues, especially when the calcium times phosphorus product is greater than 70.[114] Suppression of 1-25(OH)$_2$D$_3$ synthesis associated with AKI in these patients has been suggested as the other

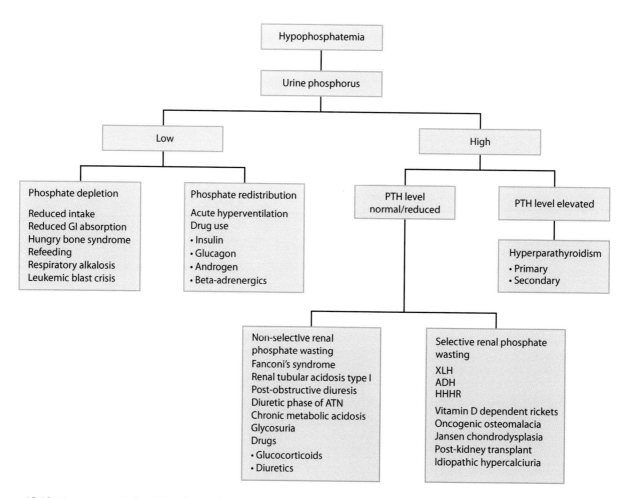

Figure 13.12 A suggested algorithm for evaluation of hypophosphatemia in children. ATN, acute tubular necrosis; ADH, autosomal dominant hypophosphatemia; HHHR, hereditary hypophosphatemia with hypercalciuria and rickets; PTH, parathyroid hormone; XLH, X-linked hypophosphatemic rickets.

possible mechanism of hypocalcemia.[116] Symptoms may also result from metastatic tissue calcification and calciphylaxis syndrome characterized by rapid calcification in subcutaneous fat and small blood vessels, thus leading to painful necrosis.[117]

Table 13.11 Available oral preparations of phosphorus for treatment of hypophosphatemia

| Formulation | Phosphate content | Sodium load | Potassium load |
| --- | --- | --- | --- |
| Neutra-Phos | 250 mg/ pack | 7.1 mmol/ pack | 7.1 mmol/ pack |
| Neutra-Phos K | 250 mg/ capsule | 0 | 14.25 mmol/ pack |
| K-Phos Original | 150 mg/ capsule | 0 | 3.65 mmol/ capsule |
| K-Phos Neutral | 250 mg/ tablet | 13 mmol/ tablet | 1.1 mmol/ tablet |

## CLINICAL DISORDERS

### Kidney disease

Hyperphosphatemia is common in AKI, as well as in CKD. This is especially true if the GFR falls to less than 60 mL/min/1.73 m². Despite enhanced phosphate excretion mediated by elevations in PTH and FGF-23 by functioning nephrons, absolute excretion falls.[118] Hyperphosphatemia is worsened by enhanced dietary phosphorus intake. Whereas hyperphosphatemia is common in the oliguric phase of AKI, hypophosphatemia may be encountered during the nonoliguric phase.

### Cytolytic disorders

Hyperphosphatemia is caused by a rapid release of intracellular phosphate during cellular breakdown; potassium and magnesium levels are also increased as a result of intracellular release. This is seen in TLS, rhabdomyolysis, and severe hemolytic anemia.[113,115] Underlying kidney dysfunction, caused by hyperuricemia or hyperphosphatemia, may be present in these patients.

Table 13.12 Preparations of potassium for parenteral use

| Intravenous preparation | Sodium (mMol/mL) | Phosphorus (mMol/mL) | Potassium (mMol/mL) | Dose mMol/kg | Duration of infusion | Caution |
|---|---|---|---|---|---|---|
| Sodium phosphate, USP | 3 | 4 | 0 | Mild hypophosphatemia: 0.08–0.16<br>Moderate hypophosphatemia: 0.32–0.4<br>Severe hypophosphatemia: 0.6 | Monitored (ICU): 6 h<br>Ward: 24 h | Sodium overload |
| Potassium phosphate, USP | 0 | 3 | 4.4 | Mild hypophosphatemia: 0.08–0.16<br>Moderate hypophosphatemia: 0.32–0.4<br>Severe hypophosphatemia: 0.6 | Monitored (ICU): 6 h<br>Ward: 24 h | Hyperkalemia |

ICU, intensive care unit.

Table 13.13 Causes of hyperphosphatemia

**Artifactual Causes**
- In vitro hemolysis of blood samples
- Hypertriglyceridemia

**Increased Intake**
- Phosphate-containing enemas
- Increased phosphate in intravenous nutrition
- Cows' milk feeding of premature infants

**Endogenously Increased Phosphate Load**
- Tumor lysis
- Malignant hyperthermia
- Rhabdomyolysis
- Hemolysis

**Extracellular Shift of Phosphorus Acidosis**
- Metabolic acidosis
- Respiratory acidosis

**Impaired Renal Excretion**
- AKI
- CKD
- End-stage renal disease

**Hypomagnesemia**

*Endocrinopathies*
- Hypoparathyroidism
- Pseudohypoparathyroidism
- FGF-23 deficiency
- Hypothyroidism
- Acromegaly
- Tumoral calcinosis

**Miscellaneous Causes**
- Hypomagnesemia
- Excess vitamin D intake (especially in renal insufficiency)
- Bisphosphonate therapy

## Tumoral calcinosis

This inherited disorder results from mutations in the *FGF23* gene that cause impaired action of FGF-23 in the renal tubules and an inability to excrete phosphorus, with resultant hyperphosphatemia and widespread ectopic calcifications.[119] The clinical manifestations include periarticular calcifications located along the extensor surfaces of major joints.[117,120] Some cases may be associated with nephrolithiasis and dental abnormalities.[121] Serum calcium concentration is normal, and there is inappropriate lack of suppression of $1,25(OH)_2D_3$, resulting in enhanced renal phosphate reabsorption and hyperphosphatemia.[89,119] Some patients respond to the use of phosphate binders and reduction in dietary calcium and phosphorus.[117]

## EVALUATION OF HYPERPHOSPHATEMIA

The evaluation of hyperphosphatemia should include evaluation of renal function, serum calcium, PTH level, vitamin D status, urinary phosphorus excretion, and serum FGF-23 level (Figure 13.13). Abnormal renal function may point to AKI or CKD as the cause of hyperphosphatemia. Secondary hyperparathyroidism in these patients is noted, especially in patients with CKD. Hypoparathyroidism can be diagnosed by presence of low serum PTH level, whereas PTH level is elevated in pseudohypoparathyroidism. Decreased urinary phosphate excretion denotes either renal impairment or other disorders (e.g., hypoparathyroidism) that are associated with increased renal tubular reabsorption of phosphorus. Because the spectrum of *FGF23* mutations in tumoral calcinosis is still evolving, FGF-23 serum levels may be included in the evaluation of selected cases of hyperphosphatemia.

## MANAGEMENT OF HYPERPHOSPHATEMIA

Treatment of hyperphosphatemia is directed toward managing the underlying cause. Oral calcium salts may

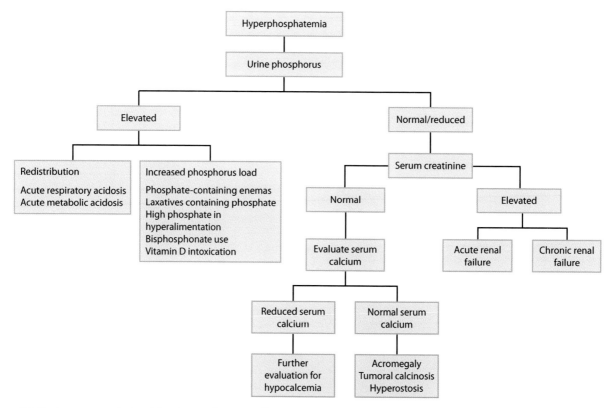

Figure 13.13 A suggested algorithm for evaluation of hyperphosphatemia in children.

assist in binding dietary phosphorus, prevent phosphorus absorption, and thereby lessen hyperphosphatemia. In patients with severely impaired kidney function, dialysis may be the only feasible treatment, but the efficiency of hemodialysis and peritoneal dialysis in removal of phosphorus is limited. Continuous renal replacement therapy (CRRT) with hemodiafiltration is able to remove phosphorus efficiently and may be useful in acutely sick patients, such as those with TLS or acute phosphorus intoxication. Caution should be exercised, as CRRT may also remove the therapeutically essential chemotherapeutic agents from patients undergoing treatment for malignant disease.

## KEY POINTS

- Hyperphosphatemia is a common problem in CKD and AKI.
- Treatment is usually effective with phosphate binders, given orally.
- Hypoparathyroidism and disorders with low FGF-23 can result in hyperphosphatemia.

## SUMMARY

The metabolism of calcium, phosphorus, and magnesium is interdependent and interrelated. The kidney plays an important role in maintaining the homeostasis of all three ions. Advances in our understanding of the hormonal control, cellular actions, and molecular mechanisms of their handling by the kidneys have resulted in a better understanding of many enigmatic clinical disorders (e.g., hypophosphatemic rickets) and the development of newer therapies (e.g., calcitriol). The scientific advance in understanding the biology of FGF-23 is beginning to have a profound impact on the pathogenesis of numerous disorders affecting the metabolism of phosphorus. Indeed, these findings may have significant pharmacotherapeutic applications, including addressing cardiovascular disease relating to aberrant mineral metabolism.

## REFERENCES

1. Lindsay RM, Pierratos A, Lockridge RS. Calcium and phosphorus control. Contrib Nephrol. 2004;145:63–8.

2. Friedman PA, Gesek FA. Cellular calcium transport in renal epithelia: Measurement, mechanisms, and regulation. Physiol Rev. 1995;75:429–71.

3. Hoenderop JG, Willems PH, Bindels RJ. Toward a comprehensive molecular model of active calcium reabsorption. Am J Physiol Renal Physiol. 2000;278:F352–60.

4. Reilly RF, Ellison DH. Mammalian distal tubule, physiology, pathophysiology, and molecular anatomy. Physiol Rev. 2000;80:277–313.

5. Brown EM, MacLeod RJ. Extracellular calcium sensing and extracellular calcium signaling. Physiol Rev. 2001;81:239–97.

6. Houillier P, Paillard M. Calcium-sensing receptor and renal cation handling. Nephrol Dial Transplant. 2003;18:2467–70.

7. Brunette MG, Chan M, Ferriere C, Roberts KD. Site of 1,25-dihydroxyvitamin $D_3$ synthesis in the kidney. Nature. 1978;276:287–9.

8. Kawashima H, Torikai S, Kurokawa K. Localization of 25-hydroxyvitamin $D_3$ 1a-hydroxylase and 24-hydroxylase along the rat nephron. Proc Natl Acad Sci U S A. 1981;78:1199–203.

10. Brown AJ, Dusso A, Slatopolsky E. Vitamin D. Am J Physiol. 1999;277:F157–75.

11. Scarpace PJ, Neuman WF, Raisz LG. Metabolism of radioiodinated salmon calcitonin in rats. Endocrinology. 1977;100:1260–67.

12. Buclin T, Cosma Rochat M, Burckhardt P, et al. Bioavailability and biological efficacy of a new oral formulation of salmon calcitonin in healthy volunteers. J Bone Miner Res. 2002;17:1478–85.

13. Zalups RK, Knox FG. Calcitonin decreases the renal tubular capacity for phosphate reabsorption. Am J Physiol. 1983;245:F345–8.

14. Shinki T, Ueno Y, DeLuca HF, Suda T. Calcitonin is a major regulator for the expression of renal 25-hydroxyvitamin $D_3$-1a-hydroxylase gene in normocalcemic rats. Proc Natl Acad Sci U S A. 1999;96:8253–8.

15. Davis TME, Singh B, Choo KE, et al. Dynamic assessment of the electrocardiographic QT interval during citrate infusion in healthy volunteers. Br Heart J. 1995;73:523–6.

16. Lehmann G, Deisenhofer I, Ndrepepa G, et al. ECG changes in a 25-year-old woman with hypocalcemia due to hypoparathyroidism: Hypocalcemia mimicking acute myocardial infarction. Chest. 2000;118:260–2.

17. Bashour T, Basha HS, Cheng TO. Hypocalcemic cardiomyopathy. Chest. 1980;78:663.

18. Lang RM, Fellner SK, Neumann A, et al. Left ventricular contractility varies directly with blood ionized calcium. Ann Intern Med. 1988;108:524–9.

19. Salle BL, Delvin E, Glorieux F, David L. Human neonatal hypocalcemia. Biol Neonate. 1990;58(Suppl 1):22–31.

20. Driscoll DA, Budarf ML, Emanuel BS. A genetic etiology for DiGeorge syndrome: Consistent deletions and microdeletions of 22q11. Am J Hum Genet. 1992;50:924–33.

21. Thakker RV. Genetics of endocrine and metabolic disorders: Parathyroid. Rev Endocr Metab Disord. 2004;5:37–51.

22. Nesbit MA, Bowl MR, Harding B, et al. Characterization of GATA3 mutations in the hypoparathyroidism, deafness, and renal dysplasia (HDR) syndrome. J Biol Chem. 2004;279:22624–34.

23. Baron J, Winer KK, Yanovski JA, et al. Mutations in the Ca$^{(2+)}$-sensing receptor gene cause autosomal dominant and sporadic hypoparathyroidism. Hum Mol Genet. 1996;5:601–6.

24. Marguet C, Mallet E, Basuyau JP, et al. Clinical and biological heterogeneity in pseudohypoparathyroidism syndrome: Results of a multicenter study. Horm Res. 1997;48:120–30.

25. Elli FM, Bordogna P, de Sanctis L, Giachero F, Verrua E, Segni M, Mazzanti L, Boldrin V, Toromanovic A, Spada A, Mantovani G. Screening of PRKAR1A and PDE4D in a Large Italian Series of Patients Clinically Diagnosed with Albright Hereditary Osteodystrophy and/or Pseudohypoparathyroidism. J Bone Miner Res. 2016 Jan 13. doi: 10.1002/jbmr.2785.

26. Anast CS, Mohs JM, Kaplan SL, Burns TW. Evidence for parathyroid failure in magnesium deficiency. Science. 1972;177:606–8.

27. Rude RK, Oldham SB, Singer FR. Functional hypoparathyroidism and parathyroid hormone end-organ resistance in human magnesium deficiency. Clin Endocrinol (Oxf). 1976;5:209-24.

28. Dusso AS, Brown AJ, Slatopolsky E. Vitamin D. Am J Physiol Renal Physiol. 2005;289:F8–28.

29. Hanley DA, Davison KS. Vitamin D insufficiency in North America. J Nutr. 2005;135:332–37.

30. Kitanaka S, Takeyama K, Murayama A, et al. Inactivating mutations in the 25-hydroxyvitamin $D_3$-1-alpha-hydroxylase gene in patients with pseudovitamin D–deficiency rickets. N Engl J Med. 1998;338:653–61.

31. Prader A, Illig, R., Heierli E. An unusual form of primary vitamin D–resistant rickets with hypocalcemia and autosomal dominant hereditary transmission: Hereditary pseudo-deficiency rickets. Helv Paediat Acta. 1961;16:452–68 [in German].

32. Rosen JF, Fleischman AR, Finberg L, et al. Rickets with alopecia: An inborn error of vitamin D metabolism. J Pediatr. 1979;94:729–35.
33. Marx SJ, Spiegel AM, Brown EM, et al. A familial syndrome of decrease in sensitivity to 1,25-dihydroxyvitamin D. J Clin Endocrinol Metab. 1978;47:1303–10.
34. Feldman D, Chen T, Cone C, et al. Vitamin D resistant rickets with alopecia: Cultured skin fibroblasts exhibit defective cytoplasmic receptors and unresponsiveness to 1,25 (OH)$_2$D$_3$. J Clin Endocrinol Metab. 1982;55:1020–2.
35. Hughes MR, Malloy PJ, Kieback DG, et al. Point mutations in the human vitamin D receptor gene associated with hypocalcemic rickets. Science. 1988;242:1702–5.
36. Balsan S, Garabedian M, Larchet M, et al. Long-term nocturnal calcium infusions can cure rickets and promote normal mineralization in hereditary resistance to 1,25-dihydroxyvitamin D. J Clin Invest. 1986;77:1661–7.
37. Kollars J, Zarroug AE, van Heerden J, et al. Primary hyperparathyroidism in pediatric patients. Pediatrics. 2005;115:974–80.
38. Allo M, Thompson NW, Harness JK, et al. Primary hyperparathyroidism in children, adolescents, and young adults. World J Surg. 1982;6:771–6.
39. Hsu SC, Levine MA. Primary hyperparathyroidism in children and adolescents: The Johns Hopkins Children's Center experience 1984–2001. J Bone Miner Res. 2002;17(Suppl 2):N44–50.
40. Law WM, Jr, Heath H, 3rd. Familial benign hypercalcemia (hypocalciuric hypercalcemia): Clinical and pathogenetic studies in 21 families. Ann Intern Med. 1985;102:511–19..
41. Heath III H, Odelberg S, Jackson CE, et al. Clustered inactivating mutations and benign polymorphisms of the calcium receptor gene in familial benign hypocalciuric hypercalcemia suggest receptor functional domains. J Clin Endocrinol Metab. 1996;81:1312–7.
42. Thakker RV. Diseases associated with the extracellular calcium-sensing receptor. Cell Calcium. 2004;35:275–82.
43. Pearce S, Steinmann B. Casting new light on the clinical spectrum of neonatal severe hyperparathyroidism. Clin Endocrinol (Oxf). 1999;50:691–3.
44. Waller S, Kurzawinski T, Spitz L, et al. Neonatal severe hyperparathyroidism: Genotype/phenotype correlation and the use of pamidronate as rescue therapy. Eur J Pediatr. 2004;163:589–94.
45. Nako Y, Tomomasa T, Morikawa A. Risk of hypervitaminosis D from prolonged feeding of high vitamin D premature infant formula. Pediatr Int. 2004;46:439–43.
46. Barrueto F, Jr, Wang-Flores HH, Howland MA, et al. Acute vitamin D intoxication in a child. Pediatrics. 2005;116:e453–6.
48. Lee CT, Hung KH, Lee CH, et al. Chronic hypercalcemia as the presenting feature of tuberculous peritonitis in a hemodialysis patient. Am J Nephrol. 2002;22:555–9.
49. Dudink J, Walther FJ, Beekman RP. Subcutaneous fat necrosis of the newborn: Hypercalcaemia with hepatic and atrial myocardial calcification. Arch Dis Child Fetal Neonatal Ed. 2003;88:F343–5.
50. Clines GA, Guise TA. Hypercalcaemia of malignancy and basic research on mechanisms responsible for osteolytic and osteoblastic metastasis to bone. Endocr Relat Cancer. 2005;12:549–83.
51. Moseley JM, Kubota M, Diefenbach-Jagger H et al. Parathyroid hormone-related protein purified from a human lung cancer cell line. Proc Natl Acad Sci U S A. 1987;84:5048–52.
52. Mangin M, Webb AC, Dreyer BE, et al. Identification of a cDNA encoding a parathyroid hormone–like peptide from a human tumor associated with humoral hypercalcemia of malignancy. Proc Natl Acad Sci U S A. 1988;85:597–601.
53. Rosenthal N, Insogna KL, Godsall JW, et al. Elevations in circulating 1,25-dihydroxyvitamin D in three patients with lymphoma-associated hypercalcemia. J Clin Endocrinol Metab. 1985;60:29–33.
54. Seymour JF, Gagel RF, Hagemeister FB, et al. Calcitriol production in hypercalcemic and normocalcemic patients with non-Hodgkin lymphoma. Ann Intern Med. 1994;121:633–40.
55. Zhang J, Kumar A, Roux K, et al. Elastin region deletions in Williams syndrome. Genet Test. 1999;3:357–9.
56. Amenta S, Sofocleous C, Kolialexi A, et al. Clinical manifestations and molecular investigation of 50 patients with Williams syndrome in the Greek population. Pediatr Res. 2005;57:789–95.
57. American Academy of Pediatrics. Committee on Genetics 2001 health care supervision for children with Williams syndrome. Pediatrics. 2001;107:1192–204.
58. Schlingmann KP, Kaufmann M, Weber S, et al. Mutations in CYP24A1 and idiopathic infantile hypercalcemia. N Engl J Med. 2011;365:410–21.
59. Dinour D, Davidovits M, Aviner S, et al. Maternal and infantile hypercalcemia caused by vitamin-D-hydroxylase mutations and vitamin D intake. Pediatr Nephrol. 2015;30:145–52.
60. Calvi LM, Schipani E. The PTH/PTHrP receptor in Jansen's metaphyseal chondrodysplasia. J Endocrinol Invest. 2000;23:545-54.
61. Bastepe M, Raas-Rothschild A, Silver J, et al. A form of Jansen's metaphyseal chondrodysplasia with limited metabolic and skeletal abnormalities is caused by a novel activating parathyroid hormone (PTH)/PTH-related peptide receptor mutation. J Clin Endocrinol Metab. 2004;89:3595–600.

62. Dai LJ, Ritchie G, Kerstan D, et al. Magnesium transport in the renal distal convoluted tubule. Physiol Rev. 2001;81:51–84.

63. Konrad M, Schlingmann KP, Gudermann T. Insights into the molecular nature of magnesium homeostasis. Am J Physiol Renal Physiol. 2004;286:F599–605.

64. Flink EB. Magnesium deficiency: Etiology and clinical spectrum. Acta Med Scand Suppl. 1981;647:125–37.

65. Gitelman HJ, Graham JB, Welt LG. A new familial disorder characterized by hyopokalemia and hypomagne semia. Trans Assoc Am Physicians. 1966;79:221–35.

66. Shaer AJ. Inherited primary renal tubular hypokalemic alkalosis: A review of Gitelman and Bartter syndromes. Am J Med Sci. 2001;322:316–32.

67. Sabath E, Meade P, Berkman J, et al. Pathophysiology of functional mutations of the thiazide-sensitive Na-Cl cotransporter in Gitelman disease. Am J Physiol Renal Physiol. 2004;287:F195–203.

68. Lin SH, Cheng NL, Hsu YJ, Halperin ML. Intrafamilial phenotype variability in patients with Gitelman syndrome having the same mutations in their thiazide-sensitive sodium/chloride cotransporter. Am J Kidney Dis. 2004;43:304–12.

69. Ea HK, Blanchard A, Dougados M, Roux C. Chondrocalcinosis secondary to hypomagnesemia in Gitelman's syndrome. J Rheumatol. 2005;32:1840–2.

70. Bartter FC, Pronove P, Gill JR, Jr, et al. Hyperplasia of the juxtaglomerular complex with hyperaldosteronism and hypokalemic alkalosis: A new syndrome. Am J Med. 1962;33:811–28.

71. Jeck N, Konrad M, Peters M, et al. Mutations in the chloride channel gene, CLCNKB, leading to a mixed Bartter–Gitelman phenotype. Pediatr Res. 2000;48:754–8.

72. Skyberg D, Stromme JH, Nesbakken R, et al. Neonatal hypomagnesemia with selective malabsorption of magnesium: A clinical entity. Scand J Clin Lab Invest. 1968;21:355–63.

73. Schlingmann KP, Weber S, Peters M, et al. Hypomagnesemia with secondary hypocalcemia is caused by mutations in TRPM6, a new member of the TRPM gene family. Nat Genet. 2002;31:166–70.

74. Geven WB, Monnens LA, Willems HL, et al. Renal magnesium wasting in two families with autosomal dominant inheritance. Kidney Int. 1987;31:1140–44.

74. Meij IC, Koenderink JB, van Bokhoven H, et al. Dominant isolated renal magnesium loss is caused by misrouting of the Na(+), K(+)–ATPase gamma-subunit. Nat Genet. 2000;26:265–66.

75. Balon TW, Jasman A, Scott S, et al. Genetic heterogeneity in familial renal magnesium wasting. J Clin Endocrinol Metab. 2002;87:612–7.

76. Geven WB, Monnens LA, Willems JL, et al. Isolated autosomal recessive renal magnesium loss in two sisters. Clin Genet. 1987;32:398–402.

77. Michelis MF, Drash AL, Linarelli LG, et al. Decreased bicarbonate threshold and renal magnesium wasting in a sibship with distal renal tubular acidosis. (Evaluation of the pathophysiological role of parathyroid hormone). Metabolism. 1972;21:905–20.

78. Benigno V, Canonica CS, Bettinelli A, et al. Hypomagnesaemia-hypercalciuria-nephrocalcinosis: A report of nine cases and a review. Nephrol Dial Transplant. 2000;15:605–10.

79. Weber S, Schneider L, Peters M, et al. Novel paracellin-1 mutations in 25 families with familial hypomagnesemia with hypercalciuria and nephrocalcinosis. J Am Soc Nephrol. 2001;12:1872–81.

80. Fine KD, Santa Ana CA, Porter JL, et al. Intestinal absorption of magnesium from food and supplements. J Clin Invest. 1991;88:396–402.

81. Firoz M, Graber M. Bioavailability of US commercial magnesium preparation. Magnes Res. 2001;14:257–62.

83. Biber J, Hernando N, Forster I, et al. Phosphate transporters and their function. Annu Rev Physiol. 2013;75:535–50.

84. Tenenhouse HS, Murer H. Disorders of renal tubular phosphate transport. J Am Soc Nephrol. 2003;14:240–8.

85. Hughes MR, Brumbaugh PF, Hussler MR, et al. Regulation of serum $1\alpha$, 25-dihydroxyvitamin $D_3$ by calcium and phosphate in the rat. Science. 1975;190:578–80.

86. Tanaka Y, DeLuca HF. The control of 25-hydroxyvitamin D metabolism by inorganic phosphorus. Arch Biochem Biophys. 1973;154:566–74.

87. Quarles LD. Role of FGF23 in vitamin D and phosphate metabolism: Implications in chronic kidney disease. Exp Cell Res. 2012;318:1040–8.

88. Wagner CA, Rubio-Aliaga I, Biber J, et al. Genetic diseases of renal phosphate handling. Nephrol Dial Transplant. 2014;29(Suppl 4):iv45–54.

89. Sprecher E. Familial tumoral calcinosis: From characterization of a rare phenotype to the pathogenesis of ectopic calcification. J Invest Dermatol. 2010;130:652–60.

90. Skipper A. A systematic review of cases: Refeeding syndrome or refeeding hypophosphatemia. Nutr Clin Pract. 2012;27:134–40.

91. Liamis G, Milionis HJ, Elisaf M. Medication-induced hypophosphatemia: A review. QJM. 2010;103:449–59.

92. Amanzadeh J, Reilly RF, Jr. Hypophosphatemia: An evidence-based approach to its clinical consequences and management. Nat Clin Pract Nephrol. 2006;2:136–48.

93. Econs MJ, Francis F. Positional cloning of the PEX gene: New insights into the pathophysiology of X-linked hypophosphatemic rickets. Am J Physiol Renal Physiol. 1997;273:F489–98.

94. Lee JY, Imel EA. The changing face of hypophosphatemic disorders in the FGF-23 era. Pediatr Endocrinol Rev. 2013;10(Suppl 2):367–79.

95. Hee Y, Cho, Bum H, et al. A clinical and molecular genetic study of hypophosphatemic rickets in children. Pediatr Res. 2005;58:329–3.

96. Vaisbich MH, Koch VH. Hypophosphatemic rickets: Results of a long-term follow-up. Pediatr Nephrol. 2006;21:230–4.

97. Econs MJ, McEnery PT. Autosomal dominant hypophosphatemic rickets/osteomalacia: Clinical characterization of a novel renal phosphate wasting disorder. J Clin Endocrinol Metab. 1997;82:674–81.

98. Alizadeh Naderi AS, Reilly RF. Hereditary disorders of renal phosphate wasting. Nat Rev Nephrol. 2010;6:657–65.

99. ADHR Consortium. Autosomal dominant hypophosphataemic rickets is associated with mutations in FGF23: The ADHR Consortium. Nat Genet. 2000;26:345–8.

100. Farrow EG, White KE. Tumor-induced osteomalacia. Exp Rev Endocrinol Metab. 2009;4:435–42.

101. Shimada T, Mizutani S, Muto T, et al. Cloning and characterization of FGF23 as a causative factor of tumor-induced osteomalacia. Proc Natl Acad Sci U S A. 2001;98:6500–5.

102. Tieder M, Modai D, Samuel R, et al. Hereditary hypophosphatemic rickets with hypercalciuria. N Engl J Med. 1985;312:611–7.

103. Lorenz-Depiereux B, Benet-Pages A, Eckstein G, et al. Hereditary hypophosphatemic rickets with hypercalciuria is caused by mutations in the sodium-phosphate cotransporter gene SLC34A3. Am J Hum Genet. 2006;78:193–201.

104. Han SY, Hwang EA, Park SB, et al. Elevated fibroblast growth factor 23 levels as a cause of early post–renal transplantation hypophosphatemia. Transplant Proc. 2012;44:657–60.

105. Witteveen JE, van Thiel S, Romijn JA, et al. Hungry bone syndrome: Still a challenge in the post-operative management of primary hyperparathyroidism: A systematic review of the literature. Eur J Endocrinol. 2013;168:R45–53.

106. Kruse K, Kracht U, Göpfert G. Renal threshold phosphate concentration (TmPO4/GFR). Arch Dis Child. 1982;57:217–23.

107. Walton RJ, Bijvoet OL. Nomogram for the derivation of renal tubular threshold concentration. Lancet. 1975;2:309–10.

108. Barth JH, Jones RG, Payne RB. Calculation of renal tubular reabsorption of phosphate: The algorithm performs better than the nomogram. Ann Clin Biochem. 2000;37:79–81.

109. Payne RB. Renal tubular reabsorption of phosphate (TmP/GFR): Indications and interpretation. Ann Clin Biochem. 1998;35:201–6.

110. Felsenfeld AJ, Levine BS. Approach to treatment of hypophosphatemia. Am J Kidney Dis. 2012;60:655–61.

111. Scanni R, vonRotz M, Jehle S, et al. The human response to acute enteral and parenteral phosphate loads. J Am Soc Nephrol. 2014;25:2730–9.

112. Domico MB, Huynh V, Anand SK, et al. Severe hyperphosphatemia and hypocalcemic tetany after oral laxative administration in a 3-month-old infant. Pediatrics. 2006;118:e1580–3.

113. Wilson FP, Berns JS. Tumor lysis syndrome: New challenges and recent advances. Adv Chronic Kidney Dis. 2014;21:18–26.

114. Hebert LA, Lemann J, Jr, Petersen JR, et al. Studies of the mechanism by which phosphate infusion lowers serum calcium concentration. J Clin Invest. 1966;45:1886–94.

115. Agarwal B, Walecka A, Shaw S, et al. Is parenteral phosphate replacement in the intensive care unit safe? Ther Apher Dial. 2014;18:31–6.

116. Llach F, Felsenfeld AJ, Haussler MR. The pathophysiology of altered calcium metabolism in rhabdomyolysis-induced acute renal failure: Interactions of parathyroid hormone, 25-hydroxycholecalciferol, and 1,25-dihydroxycholecalciferol. N Engl J Med. 1981;305:117–23.

117 Finer G, Price HE, Shore RM, White KE, Langman CB. Hyperphosphatemic familial tumoral calcinosis: Response to acetazolamide and postulated mechanisms. Am J Med Genet A. 2014 Jun;164A(6):1545-9. doi: 10.1002/ajmg.a.36476

118. Oliveira RB, Cancela AL, Graciolli FG, et al. Early control of PTH and FGF23 in normophosphatemic CKD patients: A new target in CKD-MBD therapy? Clin J Am Soc Nephrol. 2010;5:286–91.

119. Araya K, Fukumoto S, Backenroth R, et al. Fibroblast growth factor (FGF)23 gene as a cause of tumoral calcinosis. J Clin Endocrinol Metab. 2005;90:5523–7.

120. Shah A, Miller CJ, Nast CC, et al. Severe vascular calcification and tumoral calcinosis in a family with hyperphosphatemia: A fibroblast growth factor 23 mutation identified by exome sequencing. Nephrol Dial Transplant. 2014;29:2235–43.

121. Favia G, Lacaita MG, Limongelli L, et al. Hyperphosphatemic familial tumoral calcinosis: Odontostomatologic management and pathological features. Am J Case Rep. 2014;15:569–75.

## REVIEW QUESTIONS

1. All of the following hormones have a net effect of reducing serum phosphorus values except:
   a. Parathyroid hormone
   b. Calcitonin
   c. Calcitriol
   d. FGF-23
2. Which of the following conditions leads to hypocalcemia?
   a. Pseudohypoparathyroidism
   b. Jansen syndrome
   c. Vitamin A intoxication
   d. Thyrotoxicosis
3. When conducting an evaluation of hypocalcemia, which of the following blood levels WILL NOT be affected by recent administration of intravenous calcium therapy?
   a. Parathyroid hormone
   b. 25(OH) vitamin D
   c. Ionized calcium
   d. 1,25(OH)$_2$ vitamin D
4. Hypophosphatemia in Fanconi syndrome leads to which of the following hormonal changes?
   a. Elevated blood FGF-23 levels
   b. Elevated blood cortisol levels
   c. Lowered blood levels of calcitriol
   d. No distinct pattern in calciotropic hormones
   e. Elevated blood levels of calcitonin
5. Which of the following segments of the kidney handle the majority of magnesium homeostasis
   A. Proximal tubule
   B. Thick ascending limb
   C. Thin ascending limb
   D. Distal convoluted tubule
   E. Collecting ducts
      a. D and E
      b. B and D
      c. A and C
      d. A and B
      e. All of the above
6. Which of the following is *not* associated with hypophosphatemia?
   a. Tumoral calcinosis
   b. Refeeding syndrome
   c. XLH
   d. Calcitonin therapy
7. Ionized calcium is the biologically active component of total body calcium and comprises:
   a. 50% of the total body calcium
   b. 1% of the serum calcium
   c. 1% of the total body calcium
   d. 50% of the serum calcium
8. The vast majority of phosphorus handling occurs in this part of the nephron:
   a. Proximal tubule
   b. Loop of Henle
   c. Distal tubule
   d. Collecting duct
9. Which of the following is *not* associated with hypomagnesemia?
   a. Chronic diarrhea
   b. Addison disease
   c. Gitelman syndrome
   d. Loop diuretics
10. When calculating the fractional excretion of magnesium, the plasma magnesium must be multiplied by 0.7 because:
    a. The majority of magnesium is albumin bound.
    b. The majority of magnesium is not ultrafiltrable.
    c. That is the ultrafiltrable percentage of magnesium
    d. That is the percentage of magnesium that is reabsorbed distally.

## ANSWER KEY

1. c
2. a
3. b
4. d
5. d
6. d
7. d
8. a
9. b
10. c

# Acid-base homeostasis

RAYMOND QUIGLEY

Acid-base homeostasis and disturbances can be some of the most complicated and challenging electrolyte problems encountered by the pediatric nephrologist. To assess and correctly treat the disturbances requires knowledge of acid-base chemistry, physiology, and pathophysiology. This chapter will briefly review the fundamentals of acid-base chemistry and physiology. Disturbances in acid-base homeostasis will be reviewed in a systematic approach so that the pathophysiology of the most complex cases can be understood. The historical development of the ideas behind acid-base homeostasis also will be reviewed to help understand how these concepts developed. Finally, the approach to clinical acid-base disorders will be briefly reviewed.

## APPLIED ACID-BASE CHEMISTRY

It is useful to review definitions of some terms used in the discussions related to acid-base balance.[1-3] An acid is defined as a proton donor and a base as a proton acceptor. The following reaction depicts a generalized acid ionization equilibrium:

$$HA \leftrightarrow H^+ + A^- \tag{14.1}$$

where $H^+$ is the proton and $A^-$ is the anion. The reaction kinetics can be summarized by the equation for the equilibrium association constant:

$$Ka = \frac{[H^+] \times [A^-]}{[HA]} \tag{14.2}$$

The anion of the acid is also known as the conjugate base, because it is capable of accepting a proton. The magnitude of the association constant is usually on the order of $10^{-4}$ to $10^{-8}$, so a more convenient way to represent the constant is the pKa ($pKa = -logKa$). Thus, an acid with a Ka of $10^{-4}$ would have a pKa of 4.

The reaction for pure water is:

$$H_2O \leftrightarrow H^+ + OH^-$$

Because the concentration of water is constant, the denominator in calculating the equilibrium constant is left out by convention. Thus, instead of an association constant (Ka), the constant is referred to as Kw:

$$Kw = [H^+] \times [OH^-]$$

The value of Kw is approximately $10^{-14}$ (pKw = 14). Therefore, when water is neutral (i.e., $[H^+] = [OH^-]$), the concentration of $H^+$ ion is equal to that of $OH^-$, or $10^{-7}$ mol/L.

The pH scale is logarithmic and based on the $H^+$ concentration (ph = $-logH^+$). This means that water that is neutral has a pH of 7. In addition, as can be seen in the following derivation, the logarithmic form of Equation 14.2 becomes the Henderson–Hasselbalch equation:

$$log(Ka) = log\left\{\frac{[H^+] \times [A^-]}{[HA]}\right\}$$

$$log(Ka) = log(H^+) + log\left\{\frac{[A^-]}{[HA]}\right\}$$

and because $pH = -\log[H^+]$ and $pKa = -\log(Ka)$, this becomes:

$$pH = pKa + \log\left(\frac{[A^-]}{[HA]}\right) \qquad (14.3)$$

The applied and clinical utility of this equation is further discussed in the section on acid-base physiology.

## KEY POINT

Acids are defined as proton donors and bases as proton acceptors.

Strong acids completely ionize, so that in Equation 14.1 the concentration of HA is nearly zero. Thus, the $H^+$ ion concentration is equal to the amount of acid added to the solution. An example would be HCl. A solution of 1 mmol/L of HCl in water will result in a pH of 3 ($[H^+] = 10^{-3}$ mol/L, thus pH = 3). Weak acids do not completely ionize, so the amount of HA present becomes more significant. An example of a weak acid is lactic acid, which has a pKa of approximately 3.4 at 37° C. It should be pointed out that most weak acids would still be almost completely dissociated at a normal serum pH of 7.4 because their pKa is significantly less than 7.4. For example, lactic acid at a pH of 7.4 would dissociate with a ratio of 10,000 parts of lactate ions to 1 part of H-lactate.

Buffers are weak bases that are capable of binding free protons and thus stabilizing any changes in pH. The number of protons that the buffer can absorb would depend on the concentration of the buffer in the solution as well as the pKa of the buffer. As can be seen by examining Equation 14.3, when the concentrations of the acid form and the anion are equal (i.e., $[A^-] = [HA]$), $\log [A^-]/[HA] = 0$ and the pH of the solution will be equal to the pKa. Thus, buffers will tend to keep the pH of a solution close to the pKa of the buffer.

In mammals, including humans, circulating bicarbonate serves as the primary buffer system.[2] As will be discussed later, the bicarbonate buffer system depends on and is regulated by the respiratory system. The Henderson–Hasselbalch equation will then be expressed as:

$$pH = pKa + \log\left(\frac{[HCO_3^-]}{[H_2CO_3]}\right) \qquad (14.4)$$

One final point in basic acid-base chemistry is the fact that some acids have multiple equilibria. In particular, the phosphate ion can have up to three hydrogen ions attached to it. Each of the dissociation reactions has a different pKa.

$$H_3PO_4 \leftrightarrow H^+ + H_2PO_4^-$$

$$H_2PO_4^- \leftrightarrow H^+ + HPO_4^{-2}$$

$$HPO_4^{-2} \leftrightarrow H^+ + PO_4^{-3}$$

The respective pKa for each of these equilibrium reactions at 37° C is 2, 6.8, and 12. Therefore, at a normal blood pH of 7.4, most of the phosphate ions exist in the forms of $HPO_4^{-2}$ and $H_2PO_4^-$. The ratio of these species in the blood can be determined by the Henderson–Hasselbalch equation as follows:

$$7.4 = 6.8 + \log\left(\frac{HPO_4^{-2}}{H_2PO_4^-}\right)$$

Thus, the ratio of $HPO_4^{-2}/H_2PO_4^-$ is 4:1 (i.e., $10^{0.6}$). The amounts of the other species of phosphate are essentially zero at a pH of 7.4.

## ACID-BASE PHYSIOLOGY

Circulating bicarbonate is the primary buffering system against the threat of acidosis in humans and most mammals. Within normal parameters of bicarbonate and pCO$_2$ the serum pH is maintained at 7.4. This means that the $H^+$ ion concentration is 40 nmol/L ($40 \times 10^{-9}$ mol/L) (see Equation 14.6). With an average adult human weighing 70 kg and having 42 L of total body water, this indicates that there are only approximately 1.68 µmol of $H^+$ ions in the body. Thus, with the generation of acid at approximately 1 to 2 mmol (1000 to 2000 µmol)/kg of body weight per day, there is a very high turnover rate in this very small pool of $H^+$ ions. So, one can see how the pH of the blood can quickly change with addition of acid or base.

## BICARBONATE-CARBON DIOXIDE BUFFER SYSTEM

Bicarbonate in plasma acts as the first line of protection against acidosis by buffering the excess $H^+$ generated. The bicarbonate buffering system in the blood is an "open" system, because it generates carbon dioxide, which can be quickly eliminated by the respiratory system. The relationship between bicarbonate buffering and carbon dioxide is depicted in the following reaction equations:

$$H^+ + HCO_3^- \longleftrightarrow H_2CO_3 \xleftrightarrow{\text{carbonic anhydrase}} H_2O + CO_2 \qquad (14.5)$$

From Equation 14.5 it is clear that the bicarbonate buffering system is closely linked to carbon dioxide production and its eventual elimination through the lungs. It is also evident that alterations in the carbon dioxide concentration will cause the reactions in Equation 14.5 to shift. If the patient hyperventilates and the $pCO_2$ decreases, the concentration of carbonic acid ($H_2CO_3$) will decrease and will lower the $H^+$ concentration, leading to respiratory alkalosis. The opposite is true for respiratory failure when the $pCO_2$ rises, causing an increase in the concentration of carbonic acid and a rise in the proton concentration, resulting in respiratory acidosis. The relationship between the concentrations of dissolved carbon dioxide and carbonic acid at 37° C is constant (in the presence of carbonic anhydrase) and is depicted in the following equation:

$$H_2CO_3 = 0.03 \times pCO_2$$

This is simply the conversion of $pCO_2$ in millimeters of mercury (mm Hg) to carbonic acid in millimoles per liter. Thus, the commonly written form of the Henderson–Hasselbalch equation becomes:

$$pH = pKa + \log\left(\frac{[HCO_3^-]}{[0.03 \times pCO_2]}\right) \quad (14.6)$$

With a normal bicarbonate concentration of 24 mmol/L, $pCO_2$ of 40 mm Hg, and pKa of 6.1, the normal blood pH is 7.4.

To maintain these parameters within the normal range, the body must not only regulate the $pCO_2$ by the respiratory system but also must excrete acid that is generated by metabolic activity. Therefore, long-term homeostasis is determined by a balance between the generation of acid from the diet and from new bone formation and the excretion of acid, primarily through the kidney. In addition, short-term changes in the acid-base homeostasis can occur if the generation or excretion of either acid or base changes abruptly or if the respiratory status changes rapidly. This can lead to accumulation of acid or base, which is excreted, eventually, by the kidneys over time.

## KEY POINTS

- Circulating bicarbonate is the first line of defense against acidosis.
- Respiratory compensation forms the second mechanism of acid-base homeostasis.
- Kidney provides the third and a delayed mechanism in maintaining acid-base homeostasis.
- Other buffer systems include bone and various cellular and circulating proteins.

## GENERATION OF ACID

Our diet consists of a combination of carbohydrates, fats, and proteins.[4,5] In the normal state, carbohydrates and fats are fully metabolized to carbon dioxide and water and therefore do not contribute to an acid load. Most amino acids are also neutral because the acid part of the amino acids is balanced by the amine moiety so that there is no net acid generation. The acid generated from our diet comes primarily from the metabolism of sulfur-containing amino acids (cysteine and methionine) to sulfuric acid. The typical Western diet results in daily generation of approximately 1 to 2 mmol of acid per kilogram of body weight.[4]

## KEY POINTS

- Acid generation from our diet comes from the oxidation of sulfur-containing amino acids.
- Hydroxyapatite from growing bones also adds to acid load in children.

In addition, children generate acid from the production of hydroxyapatite $[(Ca)_{10}(PO_4)_6(OH)_2]$ in growing bone.[6] This adds to their acid generation so that the total amount generated is approximately 2 to 3 mmol of $H^+$ per kilogram of body weight, which is higher than that seen in adults (1 mmol of $H^+$/kg body weight).

## ROLE OF KIDNEYS IN ACID-BASE HOMEOSTASIS

### Renal bicarbonate reabsorption

The kidney is intimately involved in maintaining normal acid-base homeostasis.[7,8] The high filtration rate of the kidney is designed to excrete nitrogenous waste in the form of urea. However, this also means that an enormous amount of filtered bicarbonate would be lost in urine, if it was not reclaimed.[9] The proximal tubule is designed to reabsorb (or reclaim) 80% to 90% of the filtered load of bicarbonate and prevent bicarbonate loss. The mechanisms responsible for this are depicted in Figure 14.1.[10]

## KEY POINT

The proximal tubule and thick ascending limb of Henle reabsorb the bulk of the filtered load of bicarbonate.

The first step in the reabsorption of bicarbonate is the secretion of protons into the proximal tubule lumen. This is achieved primarily by the sodium-proton exchanger ($NHE_3$) located in the luminal membrane, that derives its energy from the low intracellular sodium concentration maintained by the basolateral sodium-potassium ATPase (Na-K-ATPase).

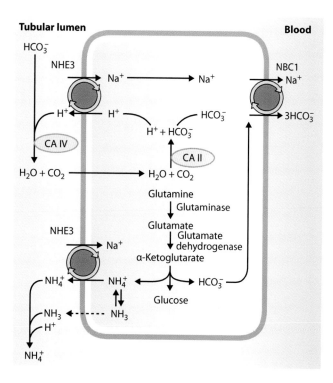

**Figure 14.1** Bicarbonate reabsorption by the proximal tubule involves a number of steps. First, protons are secreted into the tubule lumen by the sodium-proton antiporter (NHE3). The proton combines with bicarbonate to form carbonic acid that is converted by carbonic anhydrase (CA IV) to water and carbon dioxide. These diffuse into the cell and are converted back to carbonic acid that dissociates into a proton and bicarbonate. The bicarbonate is then transported into the blood stream by way of the sodium bicarbonate cotransporter (NBC1). (Reproduced with permission from: Fry AC, Karet FE. Inherited renal acidoses. Physiology (Bethesda). 2007;22:202–11.)

In addition, approximately one-third of the proton secretion is attributed to a luminal proton pump (H[+]-ATPase).[11]

Once the proton is in the tubule lumen, it combines with the filtered bicarbonate to form carbonic acid. In the presence of carbonic anhydrase, it will eventually dissociate into carbon dioxide and water, as shown in Equation 14.5:

$$H^+ + HCO_3^- \longleftrightarrow H_2CO_3 \xleftarrow{\text{carbonic anhydrase}} H_2O + CO_2$$

The water and carbon dioxide molecules can then diffuse into the intracellular compartment of the proximal tubule, where the reverse reaction occurs to form carbonic acid that then ionizes to a proton and bicarbonate. Bicarbonate is then transported across the basolateral membrane, where it can then diffuse into the blood stream and the proton is available to be secreted back into the tubule lumen.

The thick ascending limb of Henle also reabsorbs bicarbonate. It is responsible for reclamation of approximately 10% of the filtered load of bicarbonate.[12,13] Thus, at a point

when tubular fluid reaches the distal nephron, very little of the filtered bicarbonate is present in it.

## Renal acid excretion

To prevent development of an excessive base deficit, the body also needs to excrete the acid that is continually generated from diet and the daily metabolic activities. This is accomplished in the collecting duct, as H[+] ion excretion.[14] The collecting duct is made up of several cell types. Most of the cells in the collecting duct are principal cells that are involved with reabsorption of sodium and excretion of potassium. The other cell types are alpha and beta intercalated cells. In general, there are more alpha intercalated cells that excrete acid, with the remainder beta intercalated cells that secrete bicarbonate into the tubule lumen for elimination.

The mechanism for excretion of acid (H[+]) by the alpha intercalated cell is depicted in Figure 14.2.[10] The proton pump in the luminal membrane uses the energy directly from adenosine triphosphate (ATP) to pump protons into the tubule lumen for excretion. Inside the cell, carbonic anhydrase catalyzes the hydration of carbon dioxide into carbonic acid that ionizes into the proton and a bicarbonate ion (see Equation 14.5). Bicarbonate is transported via the basolateral membrane anion exchanger (AE1) and reabsorbed into the blood stream. The H-K-ATPase depicted in Figure 14.2 is primarily involved in retention of potassium. It is not clear if it plays an important role in the routine excretion of acid, but seems to be upregulated in the setting of potassium deficiency. Thus, the alpha intercalated cell of the collecting duct is responsible for secreting the 1 to 2 mEq/kg body weight of acid that is generated by the metabolism of the body.

---

## KEY POINT

The alpha intercalated cells of the collecting ducts are responsible for actively secreting the acid (H[+]) generated by metabolic activity.

---

## Role of ammonia and phosphate in renal acid excretion

Once the protons (H[+]) are secreted into the tubule lumen, it is critical to have buffers to accept the protons in the tubular luminal fluid (urine). To illustrate this point, consider that typical 70-kg adults must excrete 50 to 100 mmol of protons in their urine per day. If we relied solely on the protons that are dissolved in solution, this would require 5,000 to 10,000 L of urine if the urine pH were 5 (i.e., [H[+]] = 10[-5] mol/L). Urinary buffers allow protons to be excreted without having to lower the pH of the urine or have a large urine

**Tubular lumen**          **Blood**

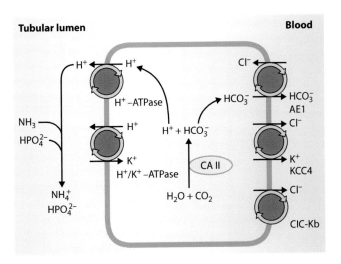

Figure 14.2 Proton secretion in the alpha intercalated cell of the collecting duct is mediated by the proton pump (H⁺-ATPase). Carbonic anhydrase (CAII) converts water and carbon dioxide into carbonic acid to provide the proton for secretion. Bicarbonate is transported into the blood stream by way of the anion exchanger (AE1). (Reproduced with permission from: Fry AC, Karet FE. Inherited renal acidoses. Physiology (Bethesda). 2007;22:202-11.)

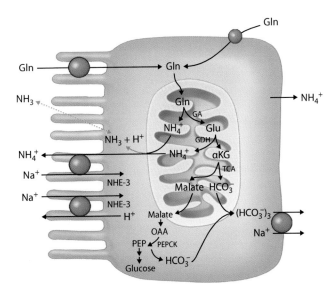

Figure 14.3 Ammoniagenesis in the proximal tubule cell is critical for providing ammonia as a buffer for the excretion of acid. Glutamine (Gln) is taken up across both the apical and basolateral membranes and undergoes metabolism by glutaminase and glutamate dehydrogenase to provide two ammonia molecules for secretion. (Reproduced with permission from: Weiner ID, Hamm LL. Molecular mechanisms of renal ammonia transport. Annu Rev Physiol. 2007;69:317–40.)

volume. The primary buffers in our urine are ammonium ions and phosphate.

## KEY POINT

Ammonia and phosphate are critical buffers in the urine that allow for the excretion of acid in a small amount of urine.

As shown in Figure 14.3, ammonia is generated in the proximal tubules of the kidney.[15-19] Glutamine is taken up by the proximal tubular cells through the apical and basolateral membranes and transported into the mitochondria. There, the enzyme glutaminase converts the glutamine into one glutamate and one ammonia molecule. Glutamate dehydrogenase can then produce a second molecule of ammonia by converting glutamate to α-ketoglutarate. The remaining α-ketoglutarate is then converted into carbon dioxide and water by enzymes in the Krebs cycle. These substrates are provided by the liver and are recycled to continue moving more ammonia precursors to the proximal tubule.

Although it used to be thought that much of the ammonia that is produced in the proximal tubule could move through the cell membrane as a gas, more recent studies have shown that it is secreted into the tubule lumen as ammonia ion by way of the sodium proton antiporter (NHE3).[15,16]

Ammonium is then recycled through the descending limb of Henle and the thick ascending limb in a process that keeps the medullary concentration of ammonium high[16] (Figure 14.4). It appears as though it may move partly as ammonia gas and ammonium ions into the collecting duct, where the protons secreted by the alpha intercalated cells will convert it to ammonium ion.[15] It then is excreted in the urine in the form of ammonium chloride.

The equilibrium reaction for ammonia and ammonium is shown in the following reaction equation:

$$NH_3 + H^+ = NH_4^+$$

The pKa for this reaction is approximately 9.0. Thus, at a pH of 7.4, most of the ammonia is in the form of ammonium. In addition, because the pKa is 9.0, $NH_3$ will tend to raise the pH of the urine. This can sometimes be confusing because the body will increase ammoniagenesis in the setting of acidosis. This can sometimes cause the urine pH to be higher than expected because of the high concentration of $NH_4^+$ in the urine.

The generation of ammonia by the proximal tubule can be upregulated in the presence of acidosis by a factor of as much as 5 to 10 over the baseline rate in adults.[20-23] The ability of the neonatal kidney to upregulate ammonium excretion is somewhat limited and can therefore prolong the recovery phase of acidosis in infants.[24,25] The upregulation of ammonium production and secretion serves as the

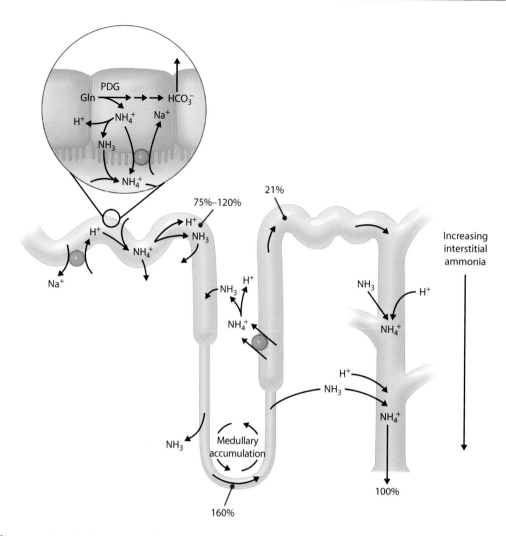

Figure 14.4 After secretion by the proximal tubule, ammonia is trapped in the medulla so that it can then be transported as ammonia and ammonium ions into the collecting duct lumen to act as a buffer for proton secretion. (Reproduced with permission from: Weiner ID, Hamm LL. Molecular mechanisms of renal ammonia transport. Annu Rev Physiol. 2007;69:317–0.)

principal means of correcting acidosis that is due to nonrenal causes of acidosis.

As discussed previously, the phosphate ion exists in several forms depending on the pH of the solution. With a normal blood pH of 7.4, most of the phosphate ion is in the form of $HPO_4^{-2}$. However, as the tubular fluid travels from the glomerulus, through the various tubule segments, its pH becomes lower. This will convert more of the phosphate ion to the $H_2PO_4^-$ form. When the urine pH becomes 4.8, the ratio of $HPO_4^{-2}/H_2PO_4^-$ will then be 1:100. So there is a large potential for excreting acid in the form of phosphate. Phosphate accounts for the bulk of what is termed *titratable acid* in the urine.

## Net acid excretion

The total amount of acid excreted by the kidneys is referred to as the net acid excretion (NAE) and is expressed as:

$$NAE = (U_{NH_4^+} + U_{TA} - U_{HCO_3}) \times V$$

where V is the urine flow rate, $U_{NH_4}$ is the urine ammonium concentration, $U_{TA}$ is the urine titratable acid concentration, and $U_{HCO_3}$ is the urine bicarbonate concentration. Thus, the components of acid secretion can be thought of as bicarbonate reclamation to prevent bicarbonate loss, ammonium excretion, and titratable acid excretion. The titratable acid component is predominately phosphate, but may also contain some sulfate ions. The concept of NAE provides a framework for the approach to evaluating the patient's ability to excrete acid as will be seen below.

## ACID-BASE DISORDERS

Because bicarbonate is the primary buffering system of the blood, the carbonic acid equilibrium reaction serves as a framework for thinking about acid-base disturbances in clinical circumstances.[3,26–28] This is depicted in Equation 14.5:

$$H^+ + HCO_3^- \longleftrightarrow H_2CO_3 \xleftarrow{\text{carbonic anhydrase}} H_2O + CO_2$$

Expressed as the Henderson–Hasselbalch equation (Equation 14. 6):

$$pH = pKa + \log\left(\frac{[HCO_3^-]}{[0.03 \times pCO_2]}\right)$$

where 0.03 represents the conversion factor from $pCO_2$ to $[H_2CO_3]$. Thus, changes in either $pCO_2$ or in the bicarbonate concentration will affect the blood pH.

# CLASSIFICATION OF ACID-BASE DISORDERS

The terms *acidemia* and *alkalemia* refer to the pH values being lower or higher than normal, which is determined by the prevailing $H^+$ ion concentration. The terms *acidosis* and *alkalosis* refer to the *processes* that lead to the abnormal blood pH. These processes (acidosis and alkalosis) can be the result of either metabolic or respiratory disturbances. Therefore, there are four primary acid-base disorders: metabolic acidosis, metabolic alkalosis, respiratory acidosis, and respiratory alkalosis. Because of compensatory responses, primary acid-base disorders rarely exist alone.

# PATIENT EVALUATION

It is critical to obtain a detailed history and physical examination for clues that will help in determining the underlying pathogenesis of the acid-base disorder and aid in developing an appropriate therapeutic plan.

As noted earlier, most acid-base disorders are of mixed nature because of the compensatory changes induced in an intact organism. To illustrate this, we will discuss a patient with diabetic ketoacidosis (DKA). When a patient with diabetes lacks insulin, the metabolism shifts to primarily using fatty acids instead of glucose. The production of ketoacids from this process will quickly exceed the kidney's ability to excrete the acid load, and metabolic acidosis will ensue. The respiratory system will then compensate by decreasing the $pCO_2$ with Kussmaul respirations, resulting in respiratory

---

**KEY POINT**

Metabolic acidosis leads to increased minute ventilation and decreased $pCO_2$ respiratory compensation.

---

alkalosis. In essence, the ratio of bicarbonate to carbonic acid (approximated as $0.03 \times pCO_2$) should remain at 20 to maintain a blood pH of 7.4 (see Equation 14.5). Thus, if the bicarbonate concentration falls by 50% to 12 mEq/L, the $pCO_2$ should decrease from 40 to 20 mm Hg to yield a blood pH of 7.4.

Assessment of acid-base status can be difficult when the correction is not complete, as is often the case. In the earlier example of the patient with DKA, the respiratory compensation is almost never complete. The $pCO_2$ might decrease to 30 mm Hg, and in that case the resulting pH would be 7.22. Thus, the patient would have a primary metabolic acidosis and a compensatory respiratory alkalosis. In some clinical circumstances, more than one acid-base disturbance may inherently exist, even without compensatory responses. The classic example of this is salicylate poisoning, which causes metabolic acidosis but also stimulates the respiratory center directly. The resulting respiratory alkalosis actually can cause the blood pH to be high early in the course of the intoxication.

## Blood gas analysis

The assessment of the patient's acid-base status begins with obtaining a complete set of data that includes not only the serum bicarbonate concentration but also the pH and the $pCO_2$ in the blood. In most blood gas analyzers, the pH and $pCO_2$ are measured and the bicarbonate concentration is then calculated. If the electrolytes are measured using a serum chemistry autoanalyzer, the bicarbonate value might vary from the one obtained in the blood gas analyzer because of the different assay methodologies.[29] It is useful to check that the three pieces of data obtained are agreeable. If one of the values does not agree with the Henderson–Hasselbalch equation, there is a good chance there may be a laboratory error in the data.

## Base deficit

Both the respiratory system and the kidneys regulate the acid-base status, and the contribution of each of them to the underlying acid-base problem must be determined. Clinicians rely on the base deficit calculated by most blood gas analyzers as a way to identify the nonrespiratory component of the acid-base disturbance. Base deficit is defined as the amount of bicarbonate (in milliequivalents per liter) that needs to be added or subtracted from the blood to give a pH of 7.4, when the $pCO_2$ is adjusted to 40 mm Hg.[2] Normal base deficit is –2 to +2 mEq/L. Metabolic acidosis is characterized by a base deficit of greater than 5 mEq/L. The base excess is the same as the base deficit multiplied by –1. These calculations are attempts to identify the primary acid-base disorder by separating the respiratory (carbon dioxide) component from the metabolic (bicarbonate) component.

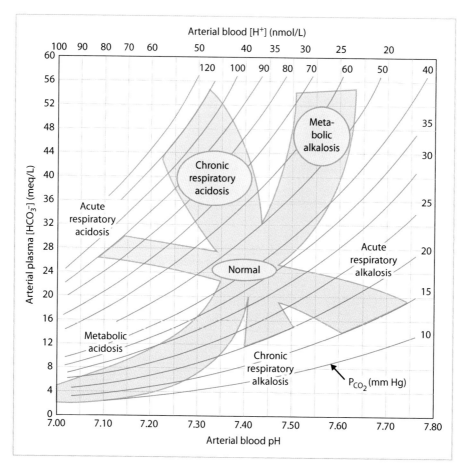

Figure 14.5 Acid-base nomogram. The acid-base nomogram is critical in evaluating the acid-base status of the patient. These nomograms are based on data from animal studies as well as human cases.

## Nomograms

In practice, the best way to understand the acid-base status of the patient is to plot the pH, $pCO_2$, and bicarbonate concentrations on an acid-base nomogram (Figure 14.5). The advantage of this method over relying on the base deficit is that the nomogram data are derived from animal models and actual patients. The nomogram thus provides the clinician with a clearer and a more realistic picture of the acid-base status of the patient. In addition, the acute or chronic nature of the disturbance also becomes evident. As can be seen in Figure 14.5, the areas that correspond to acute and chronic conditions are clearly separated. These nomograms are available on the World Wide Web as well as on mobile platforms (Acid Plus). After the data are plotted

on the nomogram, the primary acid-base disorder as well as evidence of compensation will be much more apparent. Although there are many rules of thumb for helping to determine these disorders, there are numerous exceptions to the rules and these can end up being misleading.

## METABOLIC ACIDOSIS

One of the most common acid-base disturbances that the pediatric nephrologist is asked to evaluate is a patient with metabolic acidosis.[30] Metabolic acidosis occurs either when excess acid is generated or the base is lost at a rate that cannot be corrected by the kidney.[30]

The evaluation of patients with metabolic acidosis includes history as well as physical examination for clinical clues. Nonrenal loss of base (bicarbonate), such as in diarrhea, ingestion of a substance that would result in production of acids, or infusion of aminoacids, such as in total parenteral nutrition, should be looked at in the historical data.

## INITIAL INVESTIGATIONS

It is critical to first assess the complete acid-base status of the patient with a blood gas analysis, so that a true diagnosis

---

## KEY POINTS

- Accurate assessment of the acid-base status of the patient requires measuring the pH, $pCO_2$ and the serum bicarbonate.
- The acid-base status is best understood by plotting these data on an acid-base nomogram.

of acidosis can be ascertained. It is important to recognize that a low serum bicarbonate value may result from acute or chronic respiratory alkalosis. Also, a significant time delay between drawing the blood sample and analysis of the serum may result in the serum bicarbonate concentration to be lower than expected. The advantage of a blood gas analysis is that the sample is usually analyzed shortly after the blood is drawn and laboratory errors are minimized.

## Anion gap

One of the primary tools used in evaluation of patients with metabolic acidosis is the anion gap.[31,32] Although reported in the 1970s, its interpretation has undergone considerable refinement.[33,34] The principle behind the anion gap is that the cations (positive charge) and the anions (negative charge) in the blood must be quantitatively the same to balance the electric charge (Figure 14.6A). The commonly measured cations sodium and potassium account for most of the cations, but there are many more that are termed *unmeasured cations*. These include calcium, magnesium, and gamma-globulin proteins. The commonly measured anions include chloride and bicarbonate. The unmeasured anions consist of primarily albumin but also phosphate, sulfate ions, and organic anions. In addition, there might be other anions present that are produced by the disease process, such as lactate or ketoacids, or from ingestion of a compound such as ethylene glycol.

The usual way to calculate the anion gap is:

$$\text{Anion Gap} = Na^+ - (Cl^- + HCO_3^-)$$

The concentration of potassium is ignored in the calculation of anion gap, because it is small compared to sodium and does not deviate much from approximately 4 mEq/L. The normal range for the anion gap is approximately 8 to 12 mEq/L. However, it is critical to understand how a particular laboratory measures these ions and defines the normal range. Evidence suggests that the newer methodologies for measuring ions with ion-selective electrodes results in higher chloride concentrations than in the previously used method of flame photometry.[35] This means that the normal anion gap range might be lower than previously reported.

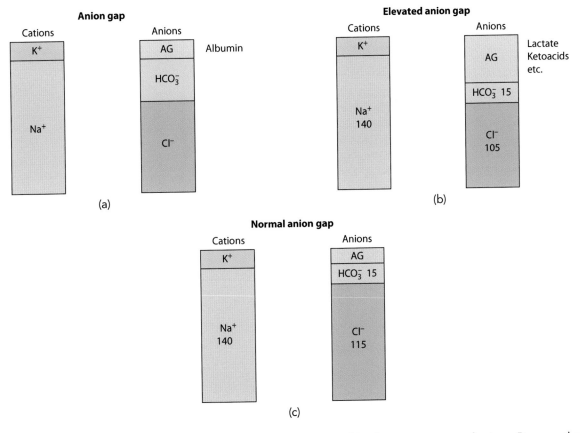

Figure 14.6 **(a)** Normal anion gap in the serum. Cations must be balanced by the same amount of anions. Because the commonly measured ions do not account for all the ions in the blood, there are both unmeasured cations as well as anions in plasma. **(b)** Elevated anion gap metabolic acidosis. There are extra retained anions (e.g., lactate or ketoacids) that cause the chloride concentration to decrease. Thus, the calculated anion gap is increased. **(c)** Normal anion gap metabolic acidosis. As the bicarbonate concentration decreases, the chloride concentration increases to the same degree so that the calculated anion gap remains in the normal range, or from ingestion of a compound.

It is also important to realize that the bulk of the anion gap in normal individuals is made up of serum albumin.[36,37] The isoelectric point of serum albumin is 4.7. Therefore, at a normal serum pH of 7.4, albumin carries many negative charges and hence contributes to the anion gap. If the patient's albumin value is low, such as in nephrotic syndrome, the anion gap also will be low. This will be reflected in a higher than normal chloride concentration. This means that if a patient with nephrotic syndrome presents with a very low albumin value, normal chloride and bicarbonate concentrations and thus normal anion gap, he or she probably has an unmeasured anion that is elevated. In other words, the patient likely has an increased anion gap metabolic acidosis.

---

### KEY POINTS

- Serum albumin constitutes the bulk of anion gap in normal individuals.
- The anion gap is affected by the serum albumin and serum pH.
- Anion gap in uncomplicated nephrotic patients is low.

---

The other effect that albumin has on the anion gap is that its charge will change depending on the pH of the serum.[38] When the patient is acidotic, albumin will contribute fewer negative charges and thus the anion gap will be slightly lower than normal.[38] If the patient is alkalotic, the opposite is true. The albumin molecule will have more negative charges that are not canceled by protons and thus will contribute to an elevated anion gap. It is not uncommon to be misled by a patient with respiratory alkalosis if the bicarbonate concentration is low because of metabolic compensation and the anion gap is elevated secondary to the increased negative charges on the albumin.

## CLASSIFICATION OF METABOLIC ACIDOSIS

Traditionally, metabolic acidosis has been divided into two main categories: conditions with an increase in the anion gap and conditions with a normal anion gap (hyperchloremic acidosis). These are outlined in Tables 14.1 and 14.3. Clinical aspects of some of the more common conditions resulting in metabolic acidosis are discussed in the following section.

## INCREASED ANION GAP METABOLIC ACIDOSIS

Many mnemonics (Table 14.2) can be used for remembering the causes of increased anion gap metabolic acidosis, and

Table 14.1 Causes of increased anion gap metabolic acidosis

**Lactic acidosis**
**Ketoacidosis**
Diabetes
Ethanol ingestion
Starvation
Inborn errors of metabolism

**Intoxications**
Salicylates
Ethylene glycol
Methanol
Paraldehyde, propylene glycol, paregoric
5-Oxoproline (pyroglutamic acid)

**Uremia**

---

there are some common pathophysiologic mechanisms that will be reviewed. Although Table 14.1 contains most of the conditions that lead to high anion gap metabolic acidosis, the list is not exhaustive. With the suggested investigative

Table 14.2 Mnemonics used for recalling causes of increased anion gap metabolic acidosis

**KUSMALE (Misspelled Adolph Kussmaul's Name)**
Ketoacidosis
Uremia
Salicylate poisoning
Methanol
Aldehyde (paraldehyde)
Lactate
Ethylene glycol

**MUD PILES**
Methanol
Uremia
Diabetes
Paraldehyde
Iron and isoniazid
Lactate
Ethylene glycol
Salicylate

**GOLD MARK**
Glycols (ethylene and propylene)
Oxoproline
L-lactate, D-lactate
Methanol
Aspirin
Renal failure
Ketoacidosis

Table 14.3 Causes of normal anion gap acidosis (hyperchloremic acidosis)

Diarrhea

Renal tubular acidosis
- Addition of acid
- Total parenteral nutrition
- Arginine chloride
- Ammonium chloride
- Early uremia (rare)

outline, the clinician should be able to analyze the information on the patient to determine the underlying cause of metabolic acidosis.

---

## KEY POINT

The anion gap increases when unmeasured anions are retained. Often this is due to either volume depletion or some degree of acute kidney injury (AKI).

---

## DIABETIC KETOACIDOSIS

One of the more common causes of an increased anion gap acidosis is DKA.[39] These patients have a lack of insulin that causes their metabolism to shift so that they metabolize fatty acids instead of glucose. This results in the production of ketoacids, acetoacetate, and β-hydroxybutyrate, which increases the anion gap. Acetone is also produced but does not contribute to the anion gap. As the production rate of acid quickly exceeds the kidney's ability to excrete it, the patient develops metabolic acidosis with a low bicarbonate concentration and normal chloride concentration, which results in an elevated anion gap (see Figure 14.6B).

If the patient remains well hydrated and is not volume depleted, the kidney is quite capable of excreting the ketoacids. However, because of the osmotic diuresis generated by the elevated glucose concentration, the patient quickly becomes volume depleted and usually develops some degree of AKI. Under these conditions, the ketoacids are retained and an elevated anion gap develops. Once the patient is volume expanded with normal saline (0.9% saline), the patient will then excrete these ketoacids and normalize the anion gap. With appropriate therapy of DKA, the increased metabolic acidosis may convert to normal anion gap acidosis.[40] The same principle applies to other forms of increased anion gap acidosis as well.

Because of its high glomerular filtration rate, the kidney is capable of excreting large amounts of filtered ions. If the body is retaining the ions and causing an increase in the anion gap, there is almost always volume depletion with or without some degree of acute kidney injury causing their retention.

## LACTIC ACIDOSIS

Lactic acidosis is another of the increased anion gap acidoses, listed in Table 14.1, that deserves some discussion.[41] When glucose is metabolized in the presence of adequate oxygenation, the end products are water and carbon dioxide and there is no production of acid. However, lactic acid is produced in the setting of anaerobic glycolysis. This occurs during times of increased exercise, such as sprinting.[42] Because athletes have good tissue perfusion, the oxygen debt is eventually restored, and lactate is metabolized to water and carbon dioxide.[43,44]

The clinician often encounters lactic acidosis in the intensive care unit in patients with sepsis and multiorgan dysfunction.[45] Lactic acidosis in these patients persists as long as the tissue perfusion remains suboptimal. In these patients, in addition to increased tissue production of lactate, there is often a decreased renal function and compromised clearance of lactate via the kidney, as well. As a result, both enhanced production and retention of lactate result in increased blood lactate level.

Our understanding of lactic acidosis has progressed considerably in recent years. It is important to recognize that lactate itself is not toxic, but just a sign of poor tissue perfusion and cellular utilization of glucose. Thus, it becomes fruitless to try to remove the lactate by using various forms of renal replacement therapy. The lactic acidosis will improve only when the patient's tissue perfusion improves. Some studies suggest that monitoring the serum lactate concentration can provide information on the cardiovascular status of the critically ill patient.[46]

## INBORN ERRORS OF METABOLISM

Another class of diseases that result in an elevated anion gap acidosis in pediatric patients is the inborn errors of metabolism.[47] Many of these diseases result in the production of organic acids that cannot be further metabolized and result in an elevated anion gap. These will usually manifest within the first several days or weeks of life and can sometimes cause hyperammonemia.

## ETHYLENE GLYCOL INGESTION

A number of ingestions result in an increased anion gap acidosis. In particular, ethylene glycol ingestion can cause metabolic acidosis and acute kidney injury and can be lethal.[48] Thus, the recognition of the ingestion and treatment in a timely fashion is imperative. When the patient first ingests ethylene glycol, acidosis does not develop immediately. Because ethylene glycol is an alcohol, it results in the patient having central nervous system depression.

Not being an ion, by itself, ethylene glycol does not contribute to an anion gap. However, when the enzyme alcohol dehydrogenase metabolizes ethylene glycol there is a transient intermediary known as glycolic acid that has been shown to be the anion responsible for the increased anion gap. This new substance is also very toxic to the kidney and other organs. The end product of the metabolism of ethylene glycol is oxalate. Urine of these patients often shows numerous oxalate crystals by microscopic evaluation.

## Osmolar gap

Because the patient does not have an increase in the anion gap on presentation, ethylene glycol poisoning might go undetected until it is too late to treat. The way to determine quickly if there is a substance such as ethylene glycol in the blood is to examine the osmolar gap.[49] This is done by measuring the osmolality of the blood and also determining the calculated osmolality with the following equation:

$$\text{Calculated Osmolality} = 2 \times [Na^+] + \frac{glucose}{18} + \frac{BUN}{2.8}$$

where glucose is the serum glucose concentration in milligrams per deciliter and BUN is the blood urea nitrogen in milligrams per deciliter. Dividing the glucose by 18 and the BUN by 2.8 converts their units to millimoles per liter. Multiplying the sodium concentration by 2 will account for the accompanying anions with the sodium. So, the osmolar gap would then be the difference of the measured osmolality and the calculated osmolality, which is normally on the order of 8 to 12 mOsm/L.

Ethylene glycol and the other alcohols, ethanol, methanol, and isopropyl alcohol, have low molecular weights and would therefore contribute to an increase in the measured osmolality. Because they are not ions, they would not contribute to the calculated osmolality. Thus, an increased osmolar gap is very good evidence that the patient ingested one of these substances.

As the ethylene glycol is metabolized, the osmolar gap decreases and the anion gap will increase because of the formation of glycolic acid. This is also true for methanol (antifreeze poisoning) that is metabolized to formic acid, but ethanol and isopropyl alcohol are not metabolized to anions. Thus, a patient who has ingested ethanol or isopropyl alcohol and develops elevated anion gap acidosis usually has developed either ketoacidosis from starvation or has lactic acidosis as a result of respiratory or cardiac depression.

The treatment of ethylene glycol or methanol ingestion is aimed at reducing the production of the toxic compounds.[50] In the case of ethylene glycol, the toxin is glycolic acid, and in the case of methanol, it is formic acid. The enzyme alcohol dehydrogenase produces these compounds; thus, blocking the enzyme in the early phases of treating these ingestions is critical. Ethanol (alcohol) can be used for this purpose, because its affinity for the enzyme is much higher than that of ethylene glycol and methanol. Unfortunately, it is also a substrate and will need to be given continuously. Another inhibitor, fomepizole, also is used because it is a noncompetitive inhibitor.[49] Dialysis can be used to remove

these compounds because they are low-molecular-weight compounds with a relatively small volume of distribution and have no protein binding.

## 5-OXOPROLINE–INDUCED METABOLIC ACIDOSIS

Another substance that recently has been found to cause increased anion gap acidosis is 5-oxoproline (also known as pyroglutamic acid).[51-53] This molecule is a result of metabolism involving the γ-glutamyl pathway. This is a metabolic pathway involved in the intracellular transport and metabolism of a number of amino acids. Glutathione is involved in these reactions. Although there are rare inherited defects that can result in excess 5-oxoproline, it also can develop in patients who are glutathione deficient and have chronic acetaminophen use.

## NORMAL ANION GAP METABOLIC ACIDOSIS

The normal anion gap acidosis (Table 14.3) is often due to loss of bicarbonate or bicarbonate equivalents in the patients. Diarrheal disease and renal tubular acidosis (RTA) are two common forms of normal anion gap metabolic acidosis in childhood.

## DIARRHEAL DISEASE

The most common diagnosis of normal anion gap metabolic acidosis in children is diarrhea. These patients lose massive amounts of bicarbonate equivalents in the stool, and serum bicarbonate concentration declines quickly. Because of volume depletion and activation of the renin-angiotensin-aldosterone system, the kidney attempts to conserve as much sodium as possible to maintain the volume status of the patient. Because the bicarbonate ions are in low concentration, the sodium is reabsorbed with chloride and the patient develops hyperchloremia. Thus, the anion gap (calculated as $Na^+ - (Cl^- + HCO_3^-)$) remains in the normal range (see Figure 14.6C).

## RENAL TUBULAR ACIDOSIS

Another group of disorders that result in normal anion gap acidosis is RTA. RTA is discussed further in Chapter 42. The basic problem in these disorders is that the kidney cannot excrete the acid generated by normal metabolic activity on a daily basis, resulting in metabolic acidosis.

## Urinary anion gap

Sometimes differentiating metabolic acidosis resulting from diarrheal disease and RTA is difficult. The primary difference in these two forms of normal anion-gap acidosis is the source of bicarbonate loss and the renal response to the acidosis. As discussed earlier, the primary urinary buffer used for the excretion of acid is ammonium. If the patient becomes acidotic from gastrointestinal losses, the kidney has the capacity to increase ammonium excretion by four-fold or five-fold to help correct the acidosis. However, patients with RTA are not able to increase their ability to excrete ammonium.

Therefore, urinary excretion of ammonium can be used to differentiate these two disorders. Currently, most clinical laboratories do not measure urinary ammonium on a routine basis. Therefore, the amount of ammonium in the urine must be extrapolated by examining other ions in the urine. In a manner similar to serum anion gap, one can examine the urine anion gap for this purpose.[54] The principle is that the total cations and the anions in the urine must be equal in terms of their charges. This is summarized in the following equation:

$$Na^+ + K^+ + NH_4^+ = Cl^- + HCO_3^-$$

Because urinary bicarbonate is generally not measured in clinical laboratories, urine pH may be used to reflect the amount of bicarbonate. If the urine pH is less than 6.5, the amount of bicarbonate will be negligible. In addition, there are a number of unmeasured cations and anions such as calcium, magnesium, phosphate, and sulfate and many organic anions that are not accounted for in this calculation. This leaves the urine concentration of sodium, potassium, and chloride as the usual ions that are measured. Thus, the common method of calculating the urinary anion gap is:

$$\text{Urinary anion gap} = ([Na^+] + [K^+]) - [Cl^-]$$

Under normal conditions, the urinary anion gap will be zero. This is due to the fact that the ammonium present in the urine will be equal to the amount of unmeasured anions. However, when a patient has diarrhea, the amount of ammonium (excreted as with chloride) will increase greatly. In this condition, the amount of chloride will be greater than the sum of the sodium and potassium and the urinary anion gap will be negative. If the patient has RTA, the ability of the kidney to excrete ammonium will

## KEY POINT

The evaluation of a patient with a normal anion gap metabolic acidosis needs to include an estimate of the urinary ammonium excretion. This can be done by examining the urinary anion gap.

be limited and the urinary anion gap will be positive (i.e., the sum of sodium and potassium will be greater than the chloride).

This approach has proved to be useful, but also has some limitations. If the patient has ketoacidosis, the amount of anions being excreted will be greatly increased and will cause the sodium and potassium excretion to increase as well. This will yield a positive urinary anion gap in a patient who might have normal renal function. Thus, another approach to estimate the ammonium in the urine is the urinary osmolar gap.[55,56] This can account for other unmeasured anions that could lead to misinterpretation of the urinary anion gap.

## KEY POINT

Mixed acid-base conditions can be understood in many cases by comparing the change in the anion gap to the change in the serum bicarbonate concentration.

## Delta anion gap

In many cases, the patient might have a combination of an increased anion gap acidosis and a normal anion gap acidosis. For example, if patients who have DKA also develop diarrhea, they could present with a mixed picture of a normal anion gap and increased anion gap. This can be somewhat confusing. The approach to take in this setting is to analyze the change in the anion gap and compare it to the change in the bicarbonate concentration. This has been termed the *delta anion gap* or the *delta delta gap*.[57,58]

The underlying concept of *delta anion gap* is that in the setting of an elevated anion gap acidosis, change in the anion gap should be equal to the decrease in the serum bicarbonate concentration. For example, if a patient presents with DKA and has the following electrolyte values: sodium, 132 mEq/L; chloride, 95 mEq/L; and bicarbonate, 12 mEq/L, the anion gap would be 25 mEq/L (132−95−12). If the normal anion gap is considered to be 12, then the delta anion gap (difference of observed and normal) would be 13 mEq/L. The change in bicarbonate would be the same (25 − 12 = 13). So this is clearly a pure increased anion gap acidosis.

Consider a patient with diarrhea as the cause of acidosis. He might present with the following electrolyte values: sodium, 132 mEq/L; chloride, 108 mEq/L; and bicarbonate, 12 mEq/L. This yields an anion gap of 12 mEq/L, which is in the normal range. Analyzing the differences in the observed and normal bicarbonate concentrations and the anion gap, it is clear that the change in bicarbonate (13 mEq/L) is much greater than the change in the anion gap (12 − 12 = 0). This indicates a normal anion gap acidosis.

Now consider the patient with DKA who also has diarrhea. She could present with the following electrolytes values: sodium, 132 mEq/L; chloride, 105 mEq/L; and bicarbonate, 12 mEq/L. This yields an anion gap of 15 mEq/L. The difference in the bicarbonate concentration is 13 mEq/L, but the difference in the anion gap is now only 3. Thus, this would indicate a mixed picture of increased anion gap acidosis and normal anion gap acidosis.

Other conditions in which this approach can prove helpful is in the patient who has respiratory alkalosis in addition to a metabolic acidosis. An example would be the patient who presents with salicylate toxicity. As with any test in clinical medicine, there always will be exceptions to the rules. A recent study indicated that the use of the delta gap might not be as helpful as many investigators thought. The reason for some of the discrepancies might be that the normal range for the anion gap has been changing with the newer methodologies for measuring serum chemistries.[35]

## METABOLIC ALKALOSIS

Metabolic alkalosis is less common in clinical practice than metabolic acidosis. However, alkalosis often can be associated with higher morbidity and mortality. Human physiology is designed to help prevent alkalosis. Recall that we have a high-filtration system for the excretion of urea that normally necessitates the reabsorption of large quantities of bicarbonate to prevent acidosis. A person who ingests a large amount of bicarbonate would quickly excrete the bicarbonate and would not sustain an alkalosis. Thus, one of the key points of metabolic alkalosis is the concept that it occurs in two phases. Metabolic alkalosis requires its generation, and then under conditions that promote the retention of bicarbonate, the alkalosis is maintained.[59] Metabolic alkalosis traditionally has been classified as chloride responsive and chloride nonresponsive and will be discussed along those lines in this chapter, as well.

---

### KEY POINTS

- Metabolic alkalosis first must be generated and then sustained by abnormal clinical events.
- Metabolic alkalosis can be approached as being chloride responsive versus chloride nonresponsive.

---

## PYELORIC STENOSIS AND VOMITING

The classic example of metabolic alkalosis in children is a state of persistent vomiting, such as in patients with pyloric stenosis.[60] These patients lose gastric secretions, resulting in loss of H+ ions (as hydrochloric acid), sodium, chloride, and volume. Under normal conditions, the pancreas secretes

bicarbonate into the lumen of the intestines to neutralize the stomach acid and provide an optimal pH for intestinal and pancreatic enzymes to work. However, with the blockade at the pylorus and without gastric secretions, the unneutralized bicarbonate in the intestine is reabsorbed, leading to metabolic alkalosis. It should be pointed out that because of early diagnosis and prompt treatment of pyloric stenosis today, patients may not have as severe metabolic alkalosis as had been the case in past.[60]

Alkalosis associated with vomiting or prolonged nasogastric suction is also associated with hypokalemia. Hypokalemia results in these patients from two possible mechanisms. First, increased aldosterone secretion as a result of the volume depletion leads to distal tubular K+ and H+ secretion. Interestingly, because of increased distal H+ secretion, sometimes these alkalotic patients may have acidic urine (paradoxical aciduria), with urine pH reaching below 5.5. Second, as enhanced proximal tubular sodium reabsorption is associated with chloride reabsorption, increased bicarbonate delivery to distal nephron promotes distal potassium secretion, to preserve electroneutrality. As a result of total body potassium depletion, patients with pyloric stenosis require careful repletion with potassium ion, in addition to volume.

## ALKALOSIS IN EXTRARENAL CHLORIDE LOSS

Conditions that lead to nonrenal chloride loss also result in metabolic acidosis. Two commonly encountered clinical conditions associated with extrarenal chloride loss are cystic fibrosis and congenital chloride diarrhea.[61-63] As expected, the urinary chloride excretion in these conditions is very low.

## CONTRACTION ALKALOSIS

Metabolic alkalosis can be observed under the conditions of volume depletion, and has been known as contraction alkalosis. Contraction alkalosis represents a classic form of chloride-responsive alkalosis, which is associated with low urinary chloride level. The chloride-responsive metabolic alkalosis seen in children can be seen in numerous clinical states associated with loss of chloride via renal and nonrenal routes. Cannon et al.,[64] who first described "contraction alkalosis," attributed it to sudden extracellular volume contraction. Traditionally, it has been thought that volume contraction promotes proximal tubular sodium and water reabsorption, along with that of bicarbonate, leading to metabolic alkalosis. Chloride depletion is now considered the pathogenic mechanism for contraction alkalosis. Some have even suggested that this condition be reclassified as "chloride depletion," rather than the traditional nomenclature of "contraction alkalosis."[65] Volume expansion and provision of chloride ions in the form of 0.9% saline allows the patient to excrete the excess bicarbonate and thus mitigate alkalosis.

## DIURETICS IN BARTTER AND GITELMAN SYNDROMES

Bartter syndrome and Gitelman syndrome lead to metabolic alkalosis secondary to urinary chloride loss resulting from defects in the thick ascending limb of Henle and the distal convoluted tubule.[66] Loop diuretics (such as furosemide) that cause urinary loss of chloride, often lead to metabolic alkalosis and can mimic Bartter syndrome. Thiazide diuretics inhibit chloride transport in the distal convoluted tubule and also cause alkalosis, but it is usually milder than that seen with the use of the loop diuretics. In these examples, the urine chloride is elevated and response to chloride repletion may be suboptimal.

## CHLORIDE-NONRESPONSIVE METABOLIC ALKALOSIS

Some forms of metabolic alkalosis are termed *chloride unresponsive* because they generally have a high urinary chloride concentration and do not show resolution on volume expansion with 0.9% saline administration. The best example of this is primary hyperaldosteronism. In this condition, the patient is in a volume expanded state because of the retention of sodium in the collecting duct. Because of the high aldosterone concentration, the collecting duct actively secretes protons and potassium ($H^+$ and $K^+$), resulting in alkalosis and hypokalemia.

## HYPOKALEMIC ALKALOSIS

Potassium depletion is a well-known cause of metabolic alkalosis. The pathophysiologic mechanism is complex and includes upregulation of the H-K-ATPase in the collecting duct to help reabsorb potassium as well as complex interactions with ammoniagenesis.

## RESPIRATORY COMPENSATION IN METABOLIC ALKALOSIS

Severe metabolic alkalosis can result in respiratory acidosis, in an attempt to correct metabolic alkalosis by carbon dioxide retention. These patients may have slow and shallow breathing, and respiratory depression from metabolic alkalosis has been reported.[67,68]

## RESPIRATORY ACIDOSIS

Respiratory acidosis occurs when the $pCO_2$ in the blood is elevated (hypercapnia) because of pulmonary disease and poor ventilator functions. Although this sounds fairly simple and straightforward, it can sometimes be difficult to determine if the patient has isolated ventilation problems. In particular, if the patient has chronic respiratory acidosis, the kidney can compensate with metabolic alkalosis, resulting in a mixed acid-base disturbance.

For example, if a patient has a $pCO_2$ of 60 mm Hg, the bicarbonate concentration will increase to 36 mEq/L and the blood pH will be 7.4. Thus, often one of the clues that a patient has chronic respiratory acidosis is the elevated bicarbonate in the absence of vomiting or other causes of metabolic alkalosis. In this example, the patient has a normal blood pH, even though there is significant respiratory failure. If such patients become critically ill and require intubation for respiratory support, they may manifest only metabolic alkalosis. This is because even though the $pCO_2$ can quickly become normalized on ventilator support, correction of bicarbonate will take some time. These patients also run the risk for becoming volume depleted because the urinary elimination of excess bicarbonate will be accompanied by sodium ion and require a large urine output.

Another acid-base disorder is the triple acid-base disorder. In the previous example, the patient has primary respiratory acidosis with a $pCO_2$ of 60 mm Hg. The patient also has metabolic alkalosis to compensate for this, with a bicarbonate concentration of 36 mEq/L. If the patient now develops diarrhea and has metabolic acidosis, there will be three concurrent acid-base disorders. This patient's bicarbonate concentration will be in the normal range of approximately 24 mEq/L (resulting from gastrointestinal loss of bicarbonate). However, the blood gas analysis will show that the patient is acidotic and will have a pH of 7.22 $\{6.1 + \log [24/(0.03 \times 60)]\}$. On the surface this patient may appear to have acute respiratory acidosis, but detailed analysis will reveal a complex acid-base disturbance. The key here is the serum chloride and the anion gap.

## RESPIRATORY ALKALOSIS

Respiratory alkalosis results from excessive removal of $pCO_2$ through lungs by hyperventilation (hypocapnia), induced accidentally or intentionally in a mechanically ventilated patient or due to psychogenic hyperventilation. Respiratory alkalosis can be acute or chronic in time course. Acute respiratory alkalosis is characterized by low $pCO_2$ level and an alkalemic blood pH. In contrast, chronic respiratory alkalosis has low $pCO_2$ level but the blood pH is normal or near normal. In the setting of acute respiratory alkalosis, the kidney has not had time to compensate and reduce the serum bicarbonate concentration. However, over a period of days, the kidney will excrete excess bicarbonate and bring the blood pH to a more normal level. The best way to determine the chronicity of this condition is to examine the acid-base nomogram (see Figure 14.5).

## SUMMARY

As discussed previously, the acid-base homeostasis is determined by respiratory function and metabolic function. The challenge has always been to determine how much of a disturbance is due to the respiratory or the metabolic components. The fundamentals of acid-base physiology were developed during the early to mid-20th century. Much of this information is reviewed by Davenport.[2]

Henderson had expressed the ionization reaction for a general acid using the principle of mass action that had been developed in the late 19th century. Hasselbalch then converted the Henderson equation into the familiar logarithmic form that is well known as the Henderson–Hasselbalch equation. As techniques improved for the measurement of the components of the blood gases (i.e. pH and $pCO_2$) efforts to determine the two components, respiratory versus metabolic, began to develop. The first was the *standard base*. This was measured by taking the sample of blood and allowing it to equilibrate with gas to yield a $pCO_2$ of 40 mm Hg. Thus, a sample with a low standard bicarbonate would indicate a metabolic acidosis.

The concept of base excess was then developed. It is defined as the amount of acid or base needed to titrate the bicarbonate concentration to 24 mEq/L while keeping the $pCO_2$ at 40 mm Hg. The advantage to this approach was that it would also take into account the other buffers present in the blood sample, including hemoglobin. During this time, the approach taken by investigators in Boston was directed at estimating the predicted values of the blood gas determinants to understand the patient's acid-base disturbance, while the approach in Copenhagen was based on the measured base excess. This resulted in the "Great Trans-Atlantic Acid-Base Debate."[69] Currently, most physicians use the base excess approach.

More recently, Stewart reintroduced the concept of the "strong ion difference."[70] This is a more physico-chemical approach to the understanding of acid-base physiology. The merits of this approach continue to be debated.[71-74] Even the more practical tools that are used in the assessment of the patient with acid-base disorders have evolved. The acid-base nomogram (see Figure 14.5) used to be complicated and difficult to use, but mobile platform adoption and computing software are making its clinical applications easier.[75]

The causes of increased anion gap acidosis have shifted over time. The occurrence of paraldehyde overdose is rare, but the finding of 5-oxoproline overdose has been reported several times. Thus, the mnemonic for increased anion gap acidosis, MUDPILES, becomes less relevant. A new mnemonic for the 21st century designated GOLD MARK (see Table 14.2) has been proposed by Mehta and colleagues.[76]

### Clinical Vignette 14.1

A 2-year-old patient with Leigh syndrome (mitochondrial defect) was admitted to the hospital and found to have the following serum electrolyte profile: sodium, 136 mEq/L; potassium 3.5, mEq/L; chloride 113 mEq/L; and bicarbonate 11 mEq/L. An arterial blood gas analysis showed blood pH 7.46, $pCO_2$ less than 16 mm Hg, and bicarbonate (calculated), 11 mEq/L. Urinalysis revealed a urine pH of 8.

### TEACHING POINTS

- Because of a picture consistent with normal anion gap metabolic acidosis, hyperchloremia, and a high urine pH, the clinicians thought that the patient had proximal RTA.
- The treatment plan included starting the patient on bicarbonate replacement therapy.
- A closer look at the blood gas analysis, however, shows that the patient had respiratory alkalosis (alkalemia and low $pCO_2$). The patient had a high urine pH because of renal bicarbonate wasting in an attempt to lower the blood pH and not because of RTA.
- Treating this patient with bicarbonate supplementation would have exacerbated the clinical state, because the kidney would have had to excrete the extra bicarbonate load, along with added need for osmotic diuresis.
- This case highlights the need for complete set of data points for an accurate interpretation of acid-base status in a sick patient.

## REFERENCES

1. Astrup P, Engel K, Jorgensen K, Siggaard-Andersen O. Definitions and terminology in blood acid-base chemistry. Ann N Y Acad Sci. 1966;133:59–65.
2. Davenport HW. The ABC of Acid-Base Chemistry. 6th ed. Chicago: University of Chicago Press; 1974.
3. Gluck SL. Acid-base. Lancet. 1998;352:474–9.
4. Halperin ML, Jungas RL. Metabolic production and renal disposal of hydrogen ions. Kidney Int. 1983;24:709–13.
5. Chan JC. The influence of dietary intake on endogenous acid production: Theoretical and experimental background. Nutr Metab. 1974;16:1–9.
6. Kildeberg P, Engel K, Winters RW. Balance of net acid in growing infants: Endogenous and transintestinal aspects. Acta Paediatr Scand. 1969;58:321–9.
7. Oh MS, Carroll HJ. Whole body acid-base balance. Contrib Nephrol. 1992;100:89–104.
8. Robinson JR. Renal acid-base control. Biochem Clin. 1963;2:115–24.

9. Quigley R. Proximal renal tubular acidosis. J Nephrol. 2006;19(Suppl 9):S41–5.

10. Fry AC, Karet FE. Inherited renal acidoses. Physiology (Bethesda). 2007;22:202–11.

11. Nakhoul NL, Hamm LL. Vacuolar H(+)-ATPase in the kidney. J Nephrol. 2002;15(Suppl 5):S22–31.

12. Good DW. The thick ascending limb as a site of renal bicarbonate reabsorption. Semin Nephrol. 1993;13:225–35.

13. Lee S, Lee HJ, Yang HS, et al. Sodium-bicarbonate cotransporter NBCn1 in the kidney medullary thick ascending limb cell line is upregulated under acidic conditions and enhances ammonium transport. Exp Physiol. 2010;95:926–37.

14. Lee Hamm L, Hering-Smith KS, Nakhoul NL. Acid-base and potassium homeostasis. Semin Nephrol. 2013;33:257–64.

15. Weiner ID, Verlander JW. Renal ammonia metabolism and transport. Compr Physiol. 2013;3:201–20.

16. DuBose TD, Jr, Good DW, Hamm LL, Wall SM. Ammonium transport in the kidney: New physiological concepts and their clinical implications. J Am Soc Nephrol. 1991;1:1193–203.

17. Tannen RL. Ammonia metabolism. Am J Physiol. 1978;235:F265–77.

18. Pitts RF. Renal production and excretion of ammonia. Am J Med. 1964;36:720–42.

19. Weiner ID, Hamm LL. Molecular mechanisms of renal ammonia transport. Annu Rev Physiol. 2007;69:317-40.

20. Seldin DW, Teng HC, Rector FC, Jr. Ammonia excretion and renal glutaminase activity during administration of strong acid and buffer acid. Proc Soc Exp Biol Med. 1957;94:366–8.

21. Halperin ML, Vinay P, Gougoux A, et al. Regulation of the maximum rate of renal ammoniagenesis in the acidotic dog. Am J Physiol. 1985;248:F607–15.

22. Curthoys NP, Moe OW. Proximal tubule function and response to acidosis. Clin J Am Soc Nephrol. 2014;9:1627–38.

23. Curthoys NP, Watford M. Regulation of glutaminase activity and glutamine metabolism. Annu Rev Nutr. 1995;15:133–59.

24. Quigley R. Developmental changes in renal function. Curr Opin Pediatr. 2012;24:184–90.

25. Quigley R, Baum M. Neonatal acid base balance and disturbances. Semin Perinatol. 2004;28:97–102.

26. Carmody JB, Norwood VF. A clinical approach to paediatric acid-base disorders. Postgrad Med J. 2012;88:143–51.

27. Harrison RA. Acid-base balance. Respir Care Clin N Am. 1995;1:7–21.

28. Whittier WL, Rutecki GW. Primer on clinical acid-base problem solving. Dis Mon. 2004;50:122–62.

29. Kumar V, Karon BS. Comparison of measured and calculated bicarbonate values. Clin Chem. 2008;54:1586–7.

30. Kraut JA, Madias NE. Metabolic acidosis: Pathophysiology, diagnosis and management. Nat Rev Nephrol. 2010;6:274–85.

31. Emmett M, Narins RG. Clinical use of the anion gap. Medicine (Baltimore). 1977;56:38–54.

32. Kraut JA, Madias NE. Serum anion gap: Its uses and limitations in clinical medicine. Clin J Am Soc Nephrol. 2007;2:162–74.

33. Kellum JA. Closing the gap on unmeasured anions. Crit Care. 2003;7:219–20.

34. Mehta AN, Emmett JB, Emmett M. GOLD MARK: An anion gap mnemonic for the 21st century. Lancet. 2008;372:892.

35. Sadjadi SA, Manalo R, Jaipaul N, et al. Ion-selective electrode and anion gap range: What should the anion gap be? Int J Nephrol Renovasc Dis. 2013;6:101–5.

36. Oh MS, Carroll HJ. The anion gap. N Engl J Med. 1977;297:814–7.

37. Emmett M. Anion gap, anion gap corrected for albumin, and base deficit fail to accurately diagnose clinically significant hyperlactatemia in critically ill patients. J Intensive Care Med. 2008;23:350.

38. Paulson WD. Effect of acute pH change on serum anion gap. J Am Soc Nephrol. 1996;7:357–63.

39. Halperin ML, Bear RA, Hannaford MC, Goldstein MB. Selected aspects of the pathophysiology of metabolic acidosis in diabetes mellitus. Diabetes 1981;30:781–7.

40. Hammeke M, Bear R, Lee R, et al. Hyperchloremic metabolic acidosis in diabetes mellitus: A case report and discussion of pathophysiologic mechanisms. Diabetes. 1978;27:16–20.

41. Fall PJ, Szerlip HM. Lactic acidosis: From sour milk to septic shock. J Intensive Care Med. 2005;20:255–71.

42. Robergs RA, Ghiasvand F, Parker D. Biochemistry of exercise-induced metabolic acidosis. Am J Physiol Regul Integr Comp Physiol. 2004;287:R502–16.

43. Gladden LB. Lactate metabolism: A new paradigm for the third millennium. J Physiol. 2004;558:5–30.

44. Gladden LB. A lactatic perspective on metabolism. Med Sci Sports Exerc. 2008;40:477–85.

45. Gunnerson KJ, Saul M, He S, Kellum JA. Lactate versus non-lactate metabolic acidosis: A retrospective outcome evaluation of critically ill patients. Crit Care. 2006;10:R22.

46. Bakker J, Nijsten MW, Jansen TC. Clinical use of lactate monitoring in critically ill patients. Ann Intensive Care. 2013;3:12.

47. Seashore MR. The organic acidemias: An overview. In: Pagon RA, Adam MP, Ardinger HH, et al., editors. GeneReviews. Seattle: University of Washington Press; 1993.

48. Ting SM, Ching I, Nair H, et al. Early and late presentations of ethylene glycol poisoning. Am J Kidney Dis. 2009;53:1091–7.

49. Velez LI, Shepherd G, Lee YC, Keyes DC. Ethylene glycol ingestion treated only with fomepizole. J Med Toxicol. 2007;3:125–8.

50. Kraut JA, Kurtz I. Toxic alcohol ingestions: Clinical features, diagnosis, and management. Clin J Am Soc Nephrol. 2008;3:208–25.

51. Fenves AZ, Kirkpatrick HM, 3rd, Patel VV, et al. Increased anion gap metabolic acidosis as a result of 5-oxoproline (pyroglutamic acid): A role for acetaminophen. Clin J Am Soc Nephrol. 2006;1:441–7.

52. Verma R, Polsani KR, Wilt J, Loehrke ME. 5-Oxoprolinuria as a cause of high anion gap metabolic acidosis. Br J Clin Pharmacol. 2012;73:489–91.

53. Moe OW, Fuster D. Clinical acid-base pathophysiology: Disorders of plasma anion gap. Best Pract Res Clin Endocrinol Metab. 2003;17:559–74.

54. Batlle DC, Hizon M, Cohen E, et al. The use of the urinary anion gap in the diagnosis of hyperchloremic metabolic acidosis. N Engl J Med. 1988;318:594–9.

55. Kamel KS, Ethier JH, Richardson RM, et al. Urine electrolytes and osmolality: When and how to use them. Am J Nephrol. 1990;10:89–102.

56. Oh MS, Phelps KR, Lieberman RL, Carroll HJ. Determination of urinary ammonia by osmometry. Anal Chem. 1979;51:2247–8.

57. Wrenn K. The delta (delta) gap: An approach to mixed acid-base disorders. Ann Emerg Med. 1990;19:1310–3.

58. Rastegar A. Use of the DeltaAG/DeltaHCO3– ratio in the diagnosis of mixed acid-base disorders. J Am Soc Nephrol. 2007;18:2429–31.

59. Seldin DW, Rector FC, Jr. Symposium on acid-base homeostasis: The generation and maintenance of metabolic alkalosis. Kidney Int. 1972;1:306–21.

60. Tutay GJ, Capraro G, Spirko B, et al. Electrolyte profile of pediatric patients with hypertrophic pyloric stenosis. Pediatr Emerg Care. 2013;29:465–8.

61. Kennedy JD, Dinwiddie R, Daman-Willems C, et al. Pseudo-Bartter's syndrome in cystic fibrosis. Arch Dis Child. 1990;65:786–7.

62. Bates CM, Baum M, Quigley R. Cystic fibrosis presenting with hypokalemia and metabolic alkalosis in a previously healthy adolescent. J Am Soc Nephrol. 1997;8:352–5.

63. Kere J, Lohi H, Hoglund P. Genetic disorders of membrane transport III: Congenital chloride diarrhea. Am J Physiol. 1999;276:G7–13.

64. Cannon PJ, Heinemann HO, Albert MS, et al. "Contraction" alkalosis after diuresis of edematous patients with ethacrynic acid. Ann Intern Med 62: 979–990, 1965

65. Luke RG, Galla JH. It is chloride depletion alkalosis, not contraction alkalosis. J Am Soc Nephrol. 2012;23:204–7.

66. Shaer AJ. Inherited primary renal tubular hypokalemic alkalosis: A review of Gitelman and Bartter syndromes. Am J Med Sci 2001;322:316–32.

67. Javaheri S, Kazemi H. Metabolic alkalosis and hypoventilation in humans. Am Rev Respir Dis. 1987;136:1011–6.

68. Javaheri S, Shore NS, Rose B, Kazemi H. Compensatory hypoventilation in metabolic alkalosis. Chest. 1982;81:296–301.

69. Severinghaus JW. Siggaard-Andersen and the "Great Trans-Atlantic Acid-Base Debate." Scand J Clin Lab Invest Suppl. 1993;214:99–104.

70. Morgan TJ. The Stewart approach: One clinician's perspective. Clin Biochem Rev. 2009;30:41–54.

71. Kurtz I, Kraut J, Ornekian V, Nguyen MK. Acid-base analysis: A critique of the Stewart and bicarbonate-centered approaches. Am J Physiol Renal Physiol. 2008;294:F1009–31.

72. Kellum JA. Clinical review: Reunification of acid-base physiology. Crit Care. 2005;9:500–7.

73. Siggaard-Andersen O, Fogh-Andersen N. Base excess or buffer base (strong ion difference) as measure of a non-respiratory acid-base disturbance. Acta Anaesthesiol Scand Suppl. 1995;107:123–8.

74. Severinghaus JW. Blood gas calculator. J Appl Physiol. 1966;21:1108-16.

75. Pronicka E, Piekutowska-Abramczuk DH, Popowska E, et al. Compulsory hyperventilation and hypocapnia of patients with Leigh syndrome associated with SURF1 gene mutations as a cause of low serum bicarbonates. J Inherit Metab Dis. 2001;24:707–14.

76. Mehta AN, Emmett JB, Emmett M. GOLD MARK: An anion gap mnemonic for the 21st century. Lancet. 2008; 372:892.

## REVIEW QUESTIONS

1. A 3-year-old boy presents with a 3-week history of progressive eye swelling. He also has some swelling in his legs, and his mom reports his abdomen to be more distended. On examination, his blood pressure is 110/50 mm Hg and heart rate is 85 beats/min. He is afebrile. He has 2+ periorbital edema and 2+ pitting edema of his legs. His cardiac and lung examinations were normal. His urinalysis showed 4+ protein and is negative for blood. His serum chemistries are creatinine, 0.3 mg/dL; sodium, 132 mEq/L; potassium, 4.5 mEq/L; chloride 107 mEq/L; and bicarbonate, 25 mEq/L. This yields an anion gap of zero. Which of the following is the *most* likely cause of the low anion gap?
   a. The laboratory made an error.
   b. The serum calcium must be elevated.

c. His gamma-globulin fraction must be elevated.

d. His serum albumin is very low.

e. He has bromide intoxication.

2. A 1-year-old infant was admitted with a 3-day history of diarrhea. The laboratory analysis on the day of admission revealed sodium, 135 mEq/L; chloride, 115 mEq/L; and bicarbonate 15 mEq/L. After 2 days, the diarrhea has stopped and the patient has been volume expanded with 0.9% saline, the electrolytes were measured again and found to be sodium 138 mEq/L; chloride, 115 mEq/L; and bicarbonate of 17 mEq/L. The urinary electrolytes were found to be sodium of 35 mEq/L; potassium 75 mEq/L; and chloride of 105 mEq/L. The urine pH was 7.0. The *most* likely explanation for these findings is:

a. The patient has distal RTA.

b. The patient has cystinosis.

c. The 0.9% saline has caused dilutional alkalosis.

d. The ability to increase ammoniagenesis is impaired because of the patient's age.

3. A 15-year-old male patient has reportedly attempted suicide by drinking antifreeze containing ethylene glycol. His electrolytes were found to be sodium, 142 mEq/L; chloride, 111 mEq/L; and bicarbonate, 21 mEq/L. Other laboratory findings were glucose, 72 mg/dL, BUN, 28 mg/dL; and serum osmolality, 345 mOsm/kg water. The *best* evidence that he actually drank the ethylene glycol is:

a. The history of drinking antifreeze

b. The elevated anion gap

c. The high osmolar gap

d. No evidence for ethylene glycol ingestion

4. A 14-year-old female presents with a 3-week history of polyuria and polydipsia. The family also reports that she has lost 6 lb during this period. On examination, her blood pressure is 110/59 mm Hg, heart rate is 140 beats/min, and respiratory rate is 26 breaths/min. Serum chemistries demonstrated sodium, 132 mEq/L; potassium, 5.8 mEq/L; chloride, 98 mEq/L; and bicarbonate, 8 mEq/L (anion gap, 26). Her serum glucose was 820 mg/dL. Her urinalysis reveals no protein or blood, but had 4+ glucose. Her anion gap is *most* likely elevated because of:

a. Decreased serum albumin

b. Increased serum acetoacetate

c. Increased serum acetone

d. Increased serum calcium

e. Increased serum lactate

5. The primary source of acid in our diet is:

a. Fatty acids

b. Citric acid

c. Phosphate

d. Ascorbic acid

e. Sulfur-containing amino acids

6. A 10-kg patient generates 10 mEq of $H^+$/day that need to be excreted in her urine. If the patient's urine had no buffers and he made 1 L of urine, what would be the final pH of the urine?

a. 1

b. 2

c. 5

d. 6

e. Cannot calculate with the given information

7. A 6-week-old male infant has had nonbilious emesis for the past 2 days and appears volume depleted. The electrolyte values were sodium, 132 mEq/L; potassium, 2.8 mEq/L; chloride, 88 mEq/L; and bicarbonate 36 mEq/L. The *most* likely source for the loss of his potassium is:

a. Emesis

b. Stool

c. Urine

d. He has not lost any potassium, but it has shifted into the intracellular compartment

e. Sweat

8. A 2-year-old, ex–29-week preterm infant with bronchopulmonary dysplasia is being seen for diarrhea. He has lost 0.6 kg in the past 2 days and now weighs 9.5 kg. His blood pressure is 98/45 mm Hg, and his heart rate is 112 bpm. His respiratory rate is 32 breaths/min, and his lungs have coarse bronchi throughout. His skin turgor is decreased, with positive tenting. Laboratory studies revealed sodium, 136 mEq/L; potassium, 3.6 mEq/L; chloride, 90 mEq/L; and bicarbonate, 24 mEq/L. An arterial blood gas sample showed the pH to be 7.22 and $pCO_2$ to be 60 mm Hg. Serum creatinine is 0.5 mg/dL. The *most* likely explanation for these findings is:

a. The laboratory made an error in the ABG result.

b. The patient has acute respiratory acidosis that is uncompensated.

c. The patient has chronic respiratory acidosis with acute metabolic acidosis.

d. The patient must have had some vomiting.

9. A 3-year-old infant is being evaluated for stridor and hyperventilation. During the workup, serum electrolyte examination results revealed sodium, 138 mEq/L; potassium, 4.3 mEq/L; chloride, 108 mEq/L; and bicarbonate, 15 mEq/L. To assess the concern regarding the low bicarbonate, the *most* appropriate next step would be:

a. Perform a cortisone stimulation test.

b. Obtain arterial blood gas sample to assess pH and $pCO_2$.

c. Collect urine for anion gap.

d. Perform bicarbonate loading to determine transport maximum for bicarbonate.

10. A 13-year-old female presents for the evaluation of hypertension. Her blood pressure is 165/112 mm Hg. Her family history is positive for many individuals with hypertension, including her mother and two uncles. Her physical examination is otherwise normal. Laboratory values showed sodium, 145 mEq/L; potassium, 2.8 mEq/L; chloride, 99 mEq/L; and bicarbonate

36 mEq/L. An arterial blood gas has a pH of 7.5 and $pCO_2$ 50 mm Hg. Her urinary electrolytes were sodium, 78 mEq/L; potassium 56 mEq/L; and chloride, 148 mEq/L. These laboratory values would indicate:
a. She is wasting chloride and should be given extra chloride.
b. She most likely has renal tubular acidosis.
c. She needs to be examined for chronic lung disease.
d. She has chloride-unresponsive alkalosis.

## ANSWER KEY

1. d
2. d
3. c
4. b
5. e
6. b
7. c
8. c
9. b
10. d

# 15

# Water homeostasis

MELISSA A. CADNAPAPHORNCHAI

In *The Origin of Species* (1859),[1] Charles Darwin introduced the scientific theory of evolution, proposing that species continually adapt over time to their environments. Almost a century later, Homer Smith proposed that the concentrating capacity of the mammalian kidney was a major contributor to the evolution of various biologic species including humans.[2] Early protovertebrates resided in a saltwater environment whose composition was similar to that of their own extracellular fluid. Therefore, these animals could ingest salt water without affecting the composition of their *milieu intérieur*.[3] However, as early vertebrates migrated into freshwater streams, the development of a more water-impermeable integument was required to avoid fatal body fluid dilution by the hypoosmotic freshwater environment. A vascular tuft or primitive glomerulus thus developed, enabling the fish to filter excess fluid from the blood. The subsequent development of proximal and distal tubules in vertebrates allowed for the preservation of sodium and the excretion of solute-free water, respectively. Importantly, there was now a means to uncouple sodium and water regulation.

As vertebrates progressed to dry land, conservation of fluid became critical for survival, requiring evolution of a sensitive mechanism to concentrate the urine. Mammals and birds are unique among vertebrates in possessing loops of Henle and in the ability to compensate for water loss by elaborating urine that is more concentrated than blood. Our understanding of water metabolism has greatly advanced in the past few decades with the identification and characterization of aquaporin (AQP) water channels and urea transporters, as well as improved conceptualization of the countercurrent concentrating mechanism. This chapter reviews urinary concentration and dilution

mechanisms, evaluation of disorders of water balance, and management of hyponatremia and hypernatremia in children.

## DETERMINANTS OF URINARY CONCENTRATION AND DILUTION

The mammalian kidney maintains nearly constant plasma osmolality (POsm) and sodium concentration by mechanisms that independently regulate water and sodium excretion. Because fluid intake is typically not continuous, and sodium and its anions are the primary osmotic constituents of plasma, the mechanisms that control fluid and sodium balance must be distinct. Limitation of water intake results in concentration of plasma with production of urine that is hypertonic to plasma. Alternatively, high fluid intake results in dilution of plasma with production of urine that is more dilute than plasma. Thus, urine osmolality (UOsm) varies widely in response to fluid intake, ranging from less than 50 mOsm/kg $H_2O$ to approximately 1400 mOsm/kg $H_2O$ in humans, whereas total urine solute excretion is relatively constant. A comprehensive approach to disordered water metabolism requires a thorough understanding of the physiologic factors that regulate urinary concentrating and diluting capacity.

## GLOMERULAR FILTRATION RATE AND PROXIMAL TUBULAR REABSORPTION

Glomerular filtration rate (GFR) and proximal tubular reabsorption are primarily important in determining the rate of sodium and water delivery to the more distal portions of the nephron where renal concentration and dilution occur. Fluid reabsorption in the proximal tubule is isosmotic; therefore, tubular fluid is neither concentrated nor diluted in the proximal segment of the nephron. Approximately 70% of the glomerular filtrate is reabsorbed in the proximal tubules, with the remaining 30% entering the loop of Henle isotonic to plasma. A decrease in GFR or an increase in proximal tubular reabsorption has the following effects: (1) diminishes the amount of fluid delivered to the distal nephron, thereby limiting renal capacity to excrete free water; and (2) limits the delivery of sodium chloride (NaCl) to the ascending limb, where NaCl is reabsorbed without water to support the hypertonic medullary interstitium, thereby limiting the renal capacity to concentrate urine.

## DESCENDING AND ASCENDING LIMBS OF THE LOOPS OF HENLE AND DISTAL TUBULE

In 1942, Kuhn and Ryffel proposed that a small difference in osmotic concentration (*einzeln effekt* or "single effect") at any point between fluid flowing in opposite directions in two parallel tubes connected in a hairpin manner can be multiplied many times along the length of the tubes.[4] In the kidney, such a gradient would lead to a high osmolar concentration difference between the corticomedullary junction and the hairpin loop at the tip of the papilla, with resulting concentration of the urine (Figure 15.1). Subsequent studies expanded on this concept.[5–7] The process by which the interstitial osmolality of the medulla is increased from iso-osmotic to hyperosmotic is called

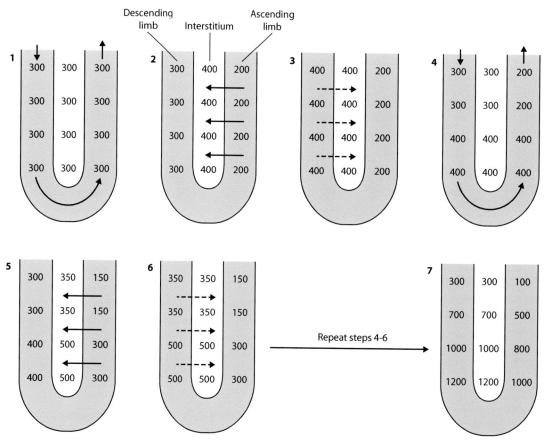

Figure 15.1 The process of countercurrent multiplication. **(1)** At time zero, the fluids in the descending and ascending limbs and the interstitium are isosmotic to plasma. **(2)** Sodium chloride (NaCl) is reabsorbed from the ascending limb into the interstitium until a gradient of 200 mOsm/kg is reached. **(3)** Fluid in the descending limb equilibrates osmotically with the interstitium by water movement out of the tubule. **(4)** The hypertonic fluid is presented to the thick ascending limb with an increased solute concentration in the region near the tip of the system. Again, active NaCl transport along the ascending limb establishes a 200 mOsm/kg gradient increasing interstitial concentrations and by water abstraction descending limb contents. Concentrations near the tip begin to be higher than those near the base. **(5 to 7)** Continued operation of the countercurrent mechanism results in hypertonicity with the highest osmolality observed at the papillary tip. (From Koeppen BM, Stanton BA. Renal Physiology. St. Louis: Mosby; 1992.)

*countercurrent multiplication.* The term "countercurrent" refers to the opposite directions of flow in the descending and ascending limbs associated with the hairpin configuration of the loop of Henle. Critical to this process is the differential permeability to water and solutes occurring along the loop of Henle (Figure 15.2). Specifically, the descending limb is permeable to water, through aquaporin-1 (AQP1) water channels, and to a lesser extent to NaCl and urea. In contrast, NaCl is actively transported into the medullary interstitium from the thick ascending limb by the sodium-potassium–2 chloride (Na-K-2Cl) cotransporter but has minimal permeability to water because of a lack of AQP1.[8]

If we assume a hypothetic time zero when NaCl enters the medullary interstitium from the thick ascending limb, the interstitial osmolality is increased. This induces water movement from the descending limb into the interstitium. Active transport of NaCl into the interstitium continues in the thick ascending limb, thus stimulating further water movement from descending limb to interstitium along an osmotic gradient. As this process continues, interstitial osmolality is "multiplied" (see Figure 15.1). The maximum interstitial osmolality that can be achieved is directly proportional to the lengths of the loops (of Henle) and to the gradient achieved between ascending limb and interstitium. Thus, the majority of countercurrent multiplication occurs in the 30% of long-looped nephrons of the juxtamedullary and midcortical regions.

In humans, the maximal osmolality achieved at the papillary tip is 1200 to 1400 mOsm/kg $H_2O$ and is, therefore, the maximum UOsm possible. However, the final osmolality of the urine is primarily determined by water permeability in the collecting tubules and not by the events in the loop of Henle.

## MEDULLARY BLOOD FLOW

Medullary blood flow also alters the renal capacity to concentrate and dilute the urine. Although medullary blood flow represents only 5% to 10% of total renal blood flow, it is several times faster than tubular flow. Blood that enters the descending vasa recta becomes concentrated as water diffuses out of and solutes diffuse into the descending limb. The hairpin turn of the vasa recta does not allow the high-solute blood to leave the medulla. In the ascending portion of the vasa recta, water diffuses into the vasa recta and solute moves out, thus maintaining medullary hypertonicity. Therefore, circumstances that increase vasa recta flow, such as very high solute load, "wash out" the medullary interstitium and lead to impaired urinary concentrating ability.

## ARGININE VASOPRESSIN

Arginine vasopressin (AVP), or antidiuretic hormone (ADH), is the primary determinant of final UOsm. AVP is

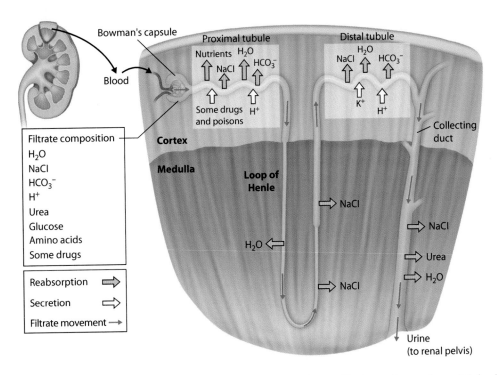

Figure 15.2 Differential permeability to water ($H_2O$) and sodium chloride (NaCl) along the nephron. $H^+$, hydrogen ion; $HCO_3^-$, bicarbonate; $K^+$, potassium; $NH_3$, ammonia. (From: Campbell NA; Reece JB, Taylor MR, et al. Biology: Concepts and Connections, 6th ed. Upper Saddle River, NJ: Pearson Education; 2009. Printed and electronically reproduced by permission of Pearson Education, Inc., Upper Saddle River, New Jersey.)

synthesized in magnocellular neurons of the paraventricular and supraoptic nuclei of the hypothalamus. Axons from these neurons project to the neural lobe of the hypophysis where AVP is stored. The precursor of AVP is a 164-amino acid peptide that is cleaved into three peptides (mature AVP nonapeptide, neurophysin, and copeptin) during its descent along the axons of the pituitary stalk. The hormone and associated peptides are released into the blood in response to several factors, including increased POsm and decreased effective circulating blood volume.[9,10] Copeptin is released into the blood in amounts equimolar to AVP. Because this peptide has a longer half-life and is easier to measure than AVP, copeptin a useful surrogate marker for AVP in research studies.[11]

---

## KEY POINT

AVP or ADH is the primary determinant of final UOsm.

---

POsm is primarily generated by solutes that do not cross cell membranes (e.g., NaCl) and is the most important stimulus for AVP release under physiologic conditions. Osmoreceptor neurons in the circumventricular organum vasculosum of the lamina terminalis and in the anterior wall of the third ventricle sense changes in osmotic pressure that stimulate

magnocellular neurons to secrete AVP and the insular and cingulate cortex to induce thirst. AVP release is stimulated by very small changes in POsm (i.e., less than 1 mOsm/kg $H_2O$), before someone can even sense thirst (Figure 15.3A). This exquisitely sensitive threshold ensures that AVP is almost always present in the plasma, except when fluids are ingested in abundance.[12]

Plasma AVP concentrations in usual conditions of health range from undetectable to 3 pg/mL. However, changes in plasma AVP concentration lower than the lower detectable limit (approximately 0.5 pg/mL) can still have significant effects on UOsm. Arterial stretch, sensed by baroreceptors in the aortic arch and carotid sinus and transmitted to the central nervous system by the vagus and glossopharyngeal nerves, tonically inhibits AVP release. Arterial underfilling, secondary to peripheral vasodilation, decreased cardiac output, or intravascular volume depletion, eliminates this inhibition and leads to nonosmotic AVP release.[13,14] In contrast to POsm, relatively large changes in blood volume are required to stimulate AVP secretion (Figure 15.3B). AVP is also secreted in response to other nonosmotic stimuli such as pain, stress, and nausea, which can have a significant impact on water homoeostasis and serum sodium concentration (SNa).

## AQUAPORIN-2

Similar to the loops of Henle, the cortical and medullary collecting tubules have permeability characteristics that

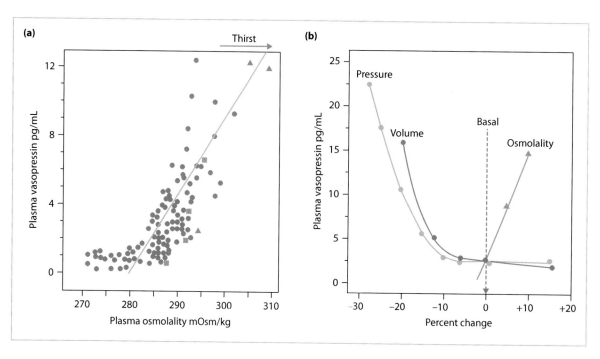

Figure 15.3 **(a)** Relationship of plasma arginine vasopressin concentration with plasma and urine osmolality in healthy adults in varying states of water balance. The level at which thirst begins is noted at the top of the figure. (**(b)** Comparative sensitivity of the osmoregulatory and baroregulatory mechanisms for vasopressin secretion. ((a) From Robertson GL, Athar S, Shelton RL. Osmotic control of vasopressin function. In: Andreoli TE, Grantham JJ, Rector FC Jr, editors. Disturbances in Body Fluid Osmolality. Bethesda, MD: American Physiological Society; 1977. p. 125; (b) from: Robertson GL, Berl T. Pathophysiology of water metabolism. *In* Brenner BM, Rector FC, Jr, editors. The Kidney, 5th ed. Philadelphia: Saunders; 1996.)

regulate the final osmolality of the urine. These segments are impermeable to the passive movement of NaCl; this characteristic is critical for the maintenance of the osmotic gradient of the medullary interstitium and subsequent generation of concentrated urine. The collecting tubule is the principal site of free water reabsorption, which occurs through the water channel AQP2 (Figure 15.4). Circulating AVP binds to its $V_2$ receptor on the basolateral surface of the principal cell of the collecting duct, a process inducing activation of an adenylyl cyclase–cyclic adenosine monophosphate (cAMP)–protein kinase A cascade that exerts dual effects. The short-term effect is phosphorylation of serine-256 of the C-terminal cytoplasmic domain of AQP2 that leads to the exocytosis of water channels from cytosolic storage vesicles and insertion into the apical membrane with subsequent water resorption.

Constitutively present basolateral AQP3 and AQP4 then permit passage of water into the systemic circulation.[15] The long-term effect occurs through phosphorylation of cAMP-response element binding protein in the nucleus, which leads to increased synthesis of AQP2. With resolution of the inciting factor, plasma AVP concentration diminishes, ultimately resulting in reclamation of AQP2 from the apical membrane to the cytoplasm.[16–18] Prostaglandins (e.g., PGE2) may impair the action of AVP; thus, prostaglandin

---

> ## KEY POINT
>
> POsm is primarily generated by solutes that do not cross cell membranes (e.g., NaCl) and is the most important stimulus for AVP release under physiologic conditions.

inhibitors are of benefit in nephrogenic diabetes insipidus (NDI), in which the $V_2$ receptor or AQP2 regulation is defective.

## Urea transporters

Approximately half of the solute present at the papillary tip during antidiuresis is urea. As AVP stimulates water reabsorption from the cortical and outer medullary collecting tubules, the urea concentration in the tubular fluid markedly rises. In contrast, permeability to urea in the innermost segment of the medullary collecting tubule is relatively high in the basal state and is further increased by AVP through insertion of the urea transporters UT-A1 and UT-A3 into the luminal membrane. Therefore, at this site, urea diffuses into the interstitium and increases the interstitial osmolality. Urea accumulation in the medulla also indirectly depends on

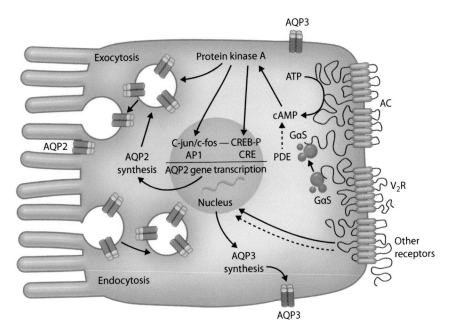

Figure 15.4 Regulation of aquaporin-2 (AQP2) trafficking and expression in collecting duct principal cells. Vasopressin acts on $V_2$ receptors ($V_2R$) in the basolateral plasma membrane. Through the guanosine triphosphate (GTP)–binding protein (Gs), adenylyl cyclase (AC) is activated, which accelerates the production of cyclic adenosine monophosphate (cAMP) from adenosine triphosphate (ATP). cAMP then binds to the regulatory subunit of protein kinase A (PKA), which activates catalytic subunit of PKA. PKA phosphorylates AQP2 in intracellular vesicles. cAMP participates in the long-term regulation of AQP2 by increasing the levels of the catalytic subunit of PKA in the nuclei, which is thought to phosphorylate transcription factors, such as cAMP responsive element (CRE) binding protein (CREB-P) and C-Jun/c-Fos. Binding of these factors is thought to increase gene transcription of AQP2, thus resulting in synthesis of AQP2 protein, which in turn enters the regulated trafficking system. In parallel, AQP3 and AQP4 synthesis and trafficking to the basolateral plasma membrane occur. (From Nielsen S, Knepper MA, Kwon T-H, Frokiaer J: Regulation of water balance: urine concentration and dilution. *In* Schrier RW, editor. Diseases of the Kidney and Urinary Tract, 8th ed. Philadelphia: Lippincott Williams & Wilkins; 2007.)

active transport of NaCl in the ascending limb. The NaCl-driven rise in interstitial osmolality directly increases the activity of UT-A1 by an effect that is independent of AVP. Moreover, loop NaCl reabsorption dilutes the tubular fluid and enhances concentration of the medullary interstitium, thereby creating an osmotic gradient to allow water reabsorption in the collecting tubules. This increase in water reabsorption raises the tubular fluid urea concentration, which enhances the gradient for urea entry into the interstitium. Recirculation of accumulated urea from interstitium to thin ascending limb and descending limb tubular fluid occurs through the urea transporter UT-A2. This process allows the amount of urea in the early distal tubule to be similar to the amount filtered, even though 60% of the filtered urea was reabsorbed in the proximal tubule. Therefore, both urinary and interstitial urea concentrations are high in the presence of AVP. The elevation in medullary interstitial urea leads to increased interstitial osmolality, thereby directly augmenting urinary concentrating capacity, and it also promotes passive sodium reabsorption in the thin descending limb.

To summarize, the excretion of concentrated urine involves the following fundamental steps:

1. Creation of a hypertonic medullary interstitium by reabsorption of NaCl without water in the medullary ascending limb of the loop of Henle and, to a lesser extent, by urea entry into the interstitium from the medullary collecting tubule
2. Secretion of AVP with stimulation of AQP2 water channels in the collecting tubules, with associated reabsorption of free water

Urinary dilution also has two fundamental steps:

1. The reabsorption of NaCl without water in the ascending limb of the loop of Henle decreases the osmolality of the tubular fluid while increasing the osmolality of the interstitium.
2. The relative absence of AVP results in minimal water reabsorption in the collecting duct.

## IMPAIRED URINARY CONCENTRATION AND DILUTION IN INFANTS

Although nephrogenesis is completed by 32 to 34 weeks of gestational age, tubular development continues throughout the first 2 to 3 years of life, and children demonstrate impaired urinary concentrating ability through 1 year of age. The preterm infant can achieve a maximal UOsm of approximately 600 mOsm/kg $H_2O$ and the term infant approximately 800 mOsm/kg $H_2O$. It is well established that total body water is higher in neonates, especially those who are premature.[19,20] Under normal physiologic conditions, term infants excrete this excess water over the first week of life, thus accounting in part for the usual decrease

in weight observed in this interval.[21] Therefore, the ability to maximally concentrate urine is not critical at birth in the otherwise healthy term infant. However, in premature infants or term infants requiring intensive care, impaired urinary concentrating ability is associated with a high risk of water and electrolyte disturbances.[22] Contributing factors include resistance to AVP through reduced generation and increased degradation of cAMP, resulting in decreased expression of AQP2, as well as lower tonicity of the medullary interstitium.[23] Additional contributors include the low dietary solute intake of breast milk and commercially available infant formulas, the high anabolic state with ingested protein used for growth rather than urea synthesis, low sodium transport by the thick ascending limb of the loop of Henle, short loops of Henle, and immaturity of urea transporters leading to diminished medullary tonicity.[24–29] As anticipated, high-protein diets or urea supplements increase urinary concentrating ability in neonates.[30,31]

Impaired urinary dilution is also evident in infants in whom large free water loads (e.g., excessive dilution of formula) can lead to hyponatremia with seizures. Infants have diminished GFR compared with older children and adults. Therefore, there is limited delivery of the free water load to the distal nephron for excretion.

## IMPAIRED URINARY CONCENTRATION AND DILUTION IN CHRONIC RENAL INSUFFICIENCY

As GFR declines, urinary concentrating and diluting abilities are limited by the decreased nephron mass. A higher solute load is imposed on each functioning nephron, and decreased tubular surface area limits medullary hypertonicity. UOsm is similar to that of plasma (isosthenuria). Because solute intake remains relatively constant, the obligate urine volume increases. When water intake exceeds excretion and other losses, hyponatremia and hypo-osmolality ensue.

## CLINICAL ASSESSMENT OF WATER HOMEOSTASIS

Numerous sources of objective clinical and laboratory data are available to aid in the assessment of water balance in children. Perhaps the most important, however, is a detailed history. The history should include a review of fluid balance for the several days preceding clinical presentation, with particular attention to the nature and volume of the patient's usual intake and output and any recent changes. This includes review of formula preparation and administration in patients receiving liquid diets, as well as review of the nature and volume of administered parenteral fluids in hospitalized patients. Consideration of the patient's ability to regulate fluid and solute intake independently is important. For example, an infant who is experiencing new and significant fluid and electrolyte losses through diarrhea relies on an attentive caregiver to provide appropriate enteral support to compensate for the stool losses. Any barriers to fluid intake such as vomiting or refusal to drink should be noted. The type and magnitude of losses, including gastrointestinal (vomiting, diarrhea, or other), urine, and insensible losses, should be assessed. Parents may relay concern for edema or abdominal distention suggestive of "third space" fluid accumulation.

A review of medications that could induce water or sodium loss (e.g., diuretics) or retention, is indicated. Recent brain trauma, surgical procedures or infection, or underlying brain malformations may increase the risk for abnormal regulation and secretion of AVP. Nonosmotic stimuli known to induce AVP secretion, including nausea, pain, or the postoperative state, should be noted. A family history of disordered water metabolism, such as diabetes insipidus (DI), should be reviewed.

The physical examination begins with evaluation of vital signs. Fever or tachypnea is associated with increased insensible water loss. Hypertension may suggest intravascular volume excess, whereas hypotension and tachycardia may indicate diminished effective circulating volume.

## KEY POINT

A detailed history is critical to the accurate evaluation of disordered water homeostasis.

Comparison of the patient's current weight with a recent weight obtained when the patient was well (i.e., euvolemic) can provide invaluable information. Several physical findings alert the physician to the presence of intravascular volume depletion, including decreased skin turgor, sunken eyes or anterior fontanel, lack of tear production, dry mucous membranes, and delayed capillary refill. The degree of alterations correlates with the severity of intravascular volume depletion. These physical findings may not be as striking in the setting of hypernatremic dehydration because extracellular volume is maintained at the expense of intracellular volume. The presence and degree of peripheral edema, ascites, or anasarca should be noted. These findings may represent intravascular volume overload. However, these same clinical findings can occur in the setting of fluid "leak" from intravascular to third space, resulting in intravascular hypovolemia; thus, accurate interpretation of the constellation of physical findings may be necessary to reach an appropriate conclusion regarding the individual patient's volume status.

Strict recording of intake and output and daily weights in the hospitalized patient is necessary. An indwelling urethral catheter is often needed for accurate assessment of urine output, but its risks and benefits need to be considered in a given patient. Serial weight measurements are useful in the hospital setting.

## LABORATORY ASSESSMENT OF WATER HOMEOSTASIS

## URINE OSMOLALITY

UOsm is a measure of the solute concentration in urine. Assessment of UOsm routinely or under artificial conditions (e.g., water deprivation or water loading) provides data on the kidney's ability to maintain tonicity and extracellular fluid balance. Osmotically active particles include chloride, sodium, urea, potassium, and glucose. Glucose can significantly elevate UOsm, such as in uncontrolled diabetes mellitus.

Older children and adults can dilute urine to an osmolality of 40 to 80 mOsm/kg $H_2O$ and can maximally concentrate to osmolality of 800 to 1400 mOsm/kg $H_2O$. Random UOsm is typically 300 to 800 mOsm/kg $H_2O$ in healthy individuals. Urine specific gravity (USG) is another measure of the concentration of solutes in the urine, and it measures the ratio of urine density to water density (1.000). Studies in healthy adults suggest that at pH 7, USG of 1.010 is equivalent to approximately 300 mOsm/kg $H_2O$, and each increase in specific gravity of 0.01 correlates with approximately 200 mOsm/kg $H_2O$ increase in UOsm.[32] Although there is good correlation between USG and UOsm from neonates through adults, the regression equations are significantly different in younger children, and maturation to adult values occurs by approximately 5 years of age.[33]

USG is significantly increased in the presence of high-molecular-weight substances, such as glucose, methanol, ethanol, and ethylene glycol, as well as contrast dye. The presence of these abnormal solutes also increases USG disproportionately in comparison with UOsm. Therefore, although USG provides a quick and an inexpensive assessment of urinary concentration in the generally healthy population, UOsm is more accurate and is preferred for evaluation of disordered water metabolism.

## PLASMA OSMOLALITY

*POsm or serum (SOsm) osmolality* is a measure of the solute concentration per unit plasma or serum. From a practical standpoint, POsm and SOsm are generally very similar, and laboratory preference may dictate use. Osmoles per kilogram water defines osmolality, whereas osmoles per liter of solution defines osmolarity. Osmolality is a technically more precise expression because solute concentration expressed on the basis of weight is temperature independent.[34] However, at physiologic solute concentrations, these two measurements are comparable. Although basal POsm can vary among persons, the range in the general population under conditions of normal hydration is 280 to 295 mOsm/kg $H_2O$.

Total osmolality is not always equivalent to *effective osmolality* (sometimes termed plasma "tonicity"). Only solutes that are impermeable to the cell membrane and remain relatively compartmentalized within the extracellular fluid are "effective" solutes (i.e., they are capable of creating osmotic gradients across cell membranes that can induce movement of water between the extracellular and intracellular fluid compartments). The concentration of effective solutes in plasma should be used to determine whether clinically significant hypo-osmolality is present. Sodium and its accompanying anions (chloride, bicarbonate) are the major effective plasma solutes, so hyponatremia and hypo-osmolality are often, *but not always,* synonymous. Glucose and urea do not greatly affect POsm unless they are present in high amounts. POsm is calculated using the following formula:

$$POsm = [2 \times Na] + [glucose / 18] + [BUN / 2.8]$$

where POsm is measured in mOsm/kg $H_2O$, sodium concentration in mEq/L, and glucose and blood urea nitrogen (BUN) in mg/dL. Sodium concentration is multiplied by 2 to account for the accompanying anions. Glucose and BUN are divided by 18 and 2.8, respectively, to convert mg/dL to mmol/kg.

Toxic alcohols such as methanol, isopropyl alcohol, ethylene glycol, or polyethylene glycol increase POsm. In such cases, there may be a significant discrepancy between measured and calculated osmolality (the osmolal gap) that can provide an early clue to alcohol intoxication.

Hyponatremia is defined as plasma sodium concentration (PNa) or SNa concentration lower than 135 mEq/L. There are two critical pitfalls in the interpretation of PNa. First, PNa is a concentration and not an absolute value. Therefore, hyponatremia could reflect decreased total body sodium content, increased total body water, or both. Second, hyponatremia can occur in the setting of low, normal, or elevated plasma osmolality. It is essential to recognize the association of hyponatremia with normal or elevated POsm because hyponatremia does not require treatment in such situations.

### KEY POINT

Hyponatremia can occur with normal, increased, or decreased POsm. In contrast, hypernatremia is always associated with hyperosmolality.

A marked elevation in plasma lipids or proteins can cause artifactual decreases in PNa in response to the larger relative proportion of plasma volume that is occupied by the excess lipids or proteins. This condition is termed pseudohyponatremia. Because the increased protein or lipid does not significantly alter the total number of solute particles in solution, the directly measured POsm is normal in such cases, and the patient is isotonic rather than hypotonic. This situation is observed in severe hyperlipidemia (e.g., serum triglycerides greater than 1500 mg/dL) and hyperproteinemia (e.g., serum total protein greater than 10 g/dL), which are rarely seen in the pediatric population, and with indirect-reading but not direct-reading ion-selective electrode potentiometry.[35]

In dilutional hyponatremia, effective solutes other than sodium are present in the plasma and induce water movement from intracellular to extracellular compartments; the result is a decrease in the measured sodium concentration with normal or elevated POsm. This condition occurs with hyperglycemia, radiographic contrast agents, and mannitol. In hyperglycemia, for every 100 mg/dL increase greater than normal in serum glucose, a decrease of 1.6 mEq/L is observed in measured SNa.[36] A more recent small study in adults suggested that a correction factor of a 2.4 mEq/L decrease in SNa per 100 mg/dL increase in glucose concentration may provide a better overall estimate of this association than the usual correction factor of 1.6, but this approach has not been widely adopted.[37]

In contrast, hypernatremia (PNa 145 mEq/L or greater) is always associated with hyperosmolality. It is again important to recognize that PNa is a concentration that can reflect increased total body sodium content, free water loss, or both.

## URINE SODIUM CONCENTRATION

Determining urine sodium concentration (UNa) can be useful clinically, but it is influenced by multiple hormonal and other nonrenal factors. Because it is a concentration and not an absolute value, it is also subject to pitfalls in interpretation. For example, a child with NDI may demonstrate low UNa, but when interpreted in light of a urine volume of 10 L/day, the absolute amount of urine sodium excretion may be significant. UNa is affected by diuretics and sodium-containing parenteral fluids. The *fractional excretion of sodium (FENa)* can be used to correct for renal water reabsorption as follows:

$$FENa\ (\%) = Quantity\ of\ Na^+\ excreted/Quantity\ of\ Na^+\ filtered = [(UNa \times SCr) / (SNa \times UCr)] \times 100$$

where sodium concentrations are expressed in mEq/L and creatinine (Cr) concentrations in mg/dL.

Values lower than 3% in neonates or 1% in older children suggest renal sodium conservation, as would be expected in the setting of an appropriate renal response to decreased effective circulating volume.

Elevated uric acid excretion can be observed in syndrome of inappropriate ADH secretion (SIADH) and cerebral salt wasting (CSW). The fractional excretion of uric acid may be useful for diagnosis in such cases, with normal values lower than 10%. It has been further suggested that the fractional excretion of phosphate can help to distinguish SIADH (less than 20%) from CSW (greater than 20%).

To evaluate the amount of solute-free water that the kidney can excrete per unit time, one can determine the *free water clearance (CH$_2$O)*. If urine is hypo-osmotic to plasma, the total urine volume (V in mL/min or L/day) can be viewed as consisting of two components: one that contains all the urinary solute in a concentration isosmotic to plasma (the osmolal clearance or COsm) and one that contains the solute-free water that makes the urine dilute (CH$_2$O). Thus:

Urine flow (V) = osmolar clearance (COsm) + free water clearance (CH$_2$O)

$$CH_2O = V - COsm$$

$$CH_2O = V - [(UOsm / POsm) \times V]$$

A positive CH$_2$O denotes the excretion of excess free water. A negative CH$_2$O indicates reabsorption of excess free water. Positive CH$_2$O in hypertonic conditions or negative CH$_2$O during hypotonicity confirms an abnormal AVP-renal axis response.

## HYPONATREMIA

Hyponatremia is defined as an SNa less than 135 mEq/L. It is one of the most common childhood electrolyte disturbances, affecting up to 25% of hospitalized children.[38–42] Although most cases of hyponatremia are mild and relatively asymptomatic, hyponatremia is clinically important because (1) acute severe hyponatremia can be associated with substantial morbidity and mortality, (2) adverse outcomes are higher in a variety of medical conditions with concomitant hyponatremia, and (3) overly rapid correction of chronic hyponatremia can cause severe neurologic deficits and death.

Hyponatremia occurs when the kidney does not appropriately excrete free water. This occurs with the following mechanisms: (1) diminished generation of free water in the loop of Henle and distal tubule; (2) increased water permeability in the collecting duct, most often from the inappropriate presence of AVP; and (3) excessive fluid intake. A combination of these factors can generate and maintain hyponatremia in any individual patient.

## CLINICAL MANIFESTATIONS

As hyponatremia develops, there is an influx of water from the extracellular to the intracellular compartment, along the osmotic gradient. This fluid shift results in cellular swelling, which can lead to encephalopathy and cerebral edema. Hyponatremia is associated with a broad spectrum

of clinical signs and symptoms, ranging from subtle and nonspecific findings (e.g., headache, nausea, vomiting) to behavioral alterations, weakness, decreased response to tactile and verbal stimuli, seizures, and cerebral herniation. The symptoms do not progress along a predictable course, and children are at particularly high risk of severe complications because of their high brain-to-skull ratio as compared with adults. Although adult brain size is achieved by approximately 6 years of age, adult skull size is not attained until approximately 16 years of age.[43] Thus, less severe cerebral edema may be associated with more severe complications in children. Hypoxia impairs brain cell volume regulation, decreases cerebral perfusion, and thereby increases the probability of developing neuronal lesions in the setting of hyponatremic cerebral edema.[44]

## CLINICAL APPROACH TO HYPONATREMIA

The approach to hyponatremia involves:

1. Confirm hypo-osmolality. As described earlier, exclusion of dilutional hyponatremia and pseudohyponatremia at this stage avoids unnecessary evaluation and intervention.
2. Obtain a detailed history. The history should include a detailed account of fluid balance, sources of sodium and water loss, free water ingestion or administration, change in weight, medications including diuretics, and underlying medical illnesses or conditions that could stimulate nonosmotic release of AVP (e.g., nausea, pain, postoperative state).
3. Determine the patient's volume status. Clinical assessment of the effective circulating volume provides important clues to the cause of hypo-osmolality (Figure 15.5). However, diminished effective circulating volume may have been restored with hypotonic fluids, and a detailed history is therefore critical in such cases.
4. Evaluate urine sodium excretion and osmolality. In the setting of significant hyponatremia, UOsm should be low, usually less than 100 mOsm/kg H$_2$O. If UOsm exceeds 100 mOsm/kg H$_2$O, then the kidney is not excreting free water appropriately. The UNa may then provide additional clues to the cause of the hyponatremia. In the presence of diminished effective circulating volume, the kidneys should be retaining sodium; hence the UNa is generally low (less than 25 mEq/L). In contrast, renal tubular dysfunction, diuretic use, SIADH, and other conditions with renal salt wasting are associated with UNa greater than 25 mEq/L. As noted previously, there

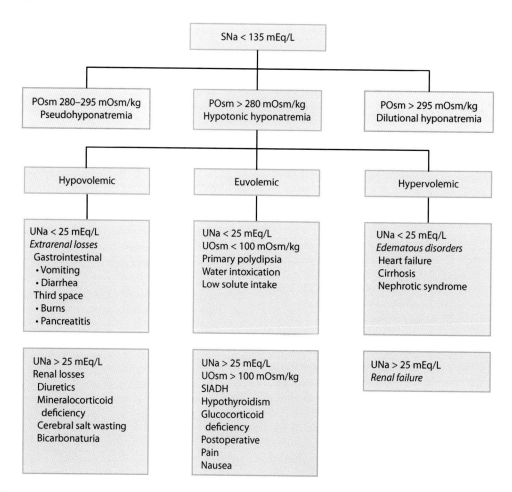

**Figure 15.5** Clinical approach to hyponatremia. POsm, plasma osmolality; SIADH, syndrome of inappropriate antidiuretic hormone secretion; SNa, serum sodium concentration; UNa, urine sodium concentration; UOsm, urine osmolality.

are potential difficulties associated with the use of UNa alone. In particular in the hospital setting, timing of intravenous saline boluses, diuretic administration, and fluid or sodium restriction should be considered. FENa may be helpful in certain cases.

## HYPOVOLEMIC HYPONATREMIA

With hypovolemic hyponatremia, diminished intravascular volume or effective circulating volume leads to baroreceptor-mediated release of AVP with associated AQP2-mediated free water retention. In some cases, diminished GFR is also

---

**KEY POINT**

If UOsm exceeds 100 mOsm/kg $H_2O$ in the setting of hyponatremia, then the kidney is not excreting free water appropriately.

---

present and impairs urinary dilution by decreasing fluid delivery to the distal nephron for excretion. Hyponatremia is often exacerbated when the fluid deficit is replenished with hypotonic fluids. UNa is helpful to determine the source of solute losses (i.e., renal vs. extrarenal) that induced the hypovolemic state.

## Extrarenal losses

Gastric contents and stool are hypotonic. Prolonged vomiting or diarrhea without fluid replacement would therefore be anticipated to cause hypernatremia. However, with low-solute fluid replacement (e.g., free water, tea, diluted juice, hypotonic parenteral fluids), hyponatremia ensues. Third space fluid loss (e.g., sepsis, burns, capillary leak, pancreatitis) with diminished effective circulating volume induces hyponatremia by a similar mechanism. The history and physical examination are critical to appropriate diagnosis in these settings. UNa is typically low, consistent with appropriate renal salt conservation in response to hypovolemia. An exception is ongoing vomiting, which can be associated with bicarbonaturia that causes obligatory urinary cation (sodium) loss; in this case, the UNa may be elevated, but the urine chloride should be low.

## Renal losses

Renal loss of sodium is associated with elevated UNa and may be seen in the following clinical conditions.

**Diuretics:** Diuretic-induced hyponatremia is more common with thiazide diuretics than with loop diuretics. This can be explained by the differences in the tubular site of action of these medications.[45] Loop diuretics inhibit NaCl reabsorption in the thick ascending limb of the loop of Henle. As noted previously, the reabsorption of NaCl without water in the medullary portion of this segment is the first step in the generation of the hyperosmotic gradient in the medullary interstitium. When a loop diuretic is administered, it impairs the accumulation of NaCl in the medulla. Thus, although the associated diuresis stimulates AVP secretion by intravascular volume depletion, the collecting tubule responsiveness to AVP is also reduced because of impairment in the medullary gradient.[45] Therefore, hyponatremia rarely occurs unless there is either diminished distal delivery of fluid as with decreased GFR or high water intake. In contrast, thiazide diuretics impair NaCl reabsorption in the distal convoluted tubule and leave the medullary concentration gradient intact. This means that thiazide-treated patients have limited ability to dilute the urine while still being able to concentrate the urine in the presence of AVP. Thiazides may also directly upregulate AQP2 abundance.[46] These factors contribute to a high risk of hyponatremia. Thiazide-induced hyponatremia typically develops within the first 1 to 2 weeks of therapy if diuretic dose and dietary intake remain constant. However, alterations in free water intake, as with intercurrent illness, may be associated with new-onset hyponatremia after several months of stable therapy. Patients who are susceptible to hyponatremia with thiazide diuretics often demonstrate recurrent hyponatremia when the thiazide is reintroduced.

**Mineralocorticoid deficiency:** In patients with primary mineralocorticoid deficiency, renal sodium wasting leads to intravascular hypovolemia with baroreceptor-mediated AVP secretion, AQP2-mediated water retention, and hyponatremia. Ingestion of water or administration of hypotonic intravenous fluids exacerbates the hyponatremia. Many patients in this setting demonstrate hyperkalemia in association with decreased urine potassium excretion. However, hyperkalemia is not a constant feature of primary mineralocorticoid deficiency in children.[47]

**CSW:** CSW has been described in the setting of subarachnoid hemorrhage, brain injury, meningoencephalitis (most frequently tuberculous), and neurosurgical procedures.[48–50] Although it has been proposed that the initial inciting factor is an increase in brain or atrial natriuretic peptide, studies have not shown consistent elevation of these hormones in CSW.[51,52] In addition, the condition occurs primarily, but not exclusively, with central nervous system disease, a finding leading some authors to propose that the condition be termed "renal salt wasting" because the kidney is the end organ for salt excretion.[53–55] The hallmark of this condition is primary renal natriuresis, which leads to intravascular volume depletion with secondary neurohormonal responses including baroreceptor-mediated AVP secretion. AQP2-mediated water retention and activation of the renin-angiotensin-aldosterone system and sympathetic nervous system are also present in these patients. It can be clinically difficult to distinguish CSW from SIADH.[49] However, several features may be helpful. The key distinguishing feature of CSW is the history of intravascular volume depletion, whereas SIADH is associated with euvolemia. Although both conditions are associated with hypouricemia and elevated fractional excretion of uric acid, these abnormalities resolve with correction of hyponatremia in SIADH but persist in CSW.[56] However, the reliability of this finding to differentiate between CSW and SIADH requires further study, particularly in children.[49] It has been further proposed that the fractional excretion of phosphate can distinguish SIADH (less than 20%) from CSW (greater than 20%). Finally, fluid restriction should induce hypovolemia in the setting of ongoing renal salt loss in CSW, whereas this maneuver is a mainstay of treatment in SIADH.

## EUVOLEMIC HYPONATREMIA

Euvolemic hyponatremia is caused by a relative or absolute excess of body water. Because otherwise healthy kidneys have great capacity to excrete free water, it is uncommon for excessive water ingestion to be the sole cause of hyponatremia, and most cases of euvolemic hyponatremia arise from a relative excess of AVP secretion.

### KEY POINT

Because otherwise healthy kidneys have great capacity to excrete free water, it is uncommon for excessive water ingestion to be the sole cause of hyponatremia, and most cases of euvolemic hyponatremia arise from a relative excess of AVP secretion.

## Syndrome of inappropriate antidiuretic hormone secretion

SIADH is a common cause of severe hyponatremia in hospitalized patients. It is caused by increased AVP secretion in the absence of an osmotic or hypovolemic stimulus and is most commonly seen in disorders of the central nervous or pulmonary systems or with medications (Table 15.1). The criteria were proposed in 1967,[57] and they have remained largely unchanged since that time (Table 15.2). It is not necessary for UOsm to exceed POsm to make the diagnosis of SIADH. In the setting of hypo-osmolality, AVP secretion should be suppressed, resulting in maximally dilute urine.

Table 15.1 Causes of syndrome of inappropriate antidiuretic hormone

**Neurologic and Psychiatric Disorders**
- Infections: meningitis, encephalitis, brain abscess
- Vascular: thrombosis, subarachnoid or subdural hemorrhage, temporal arteritis, cavernous sinus thrombosis, stroke
- Neoplasm
- Skull fracture/traumatic brain injury
- Psychosis
- Other: Guillain-Barré syndrome, acute intermittent porphyria, autonomic neuropathy, postpituitary surgery, multiple sclerosis, seizure disorder, hydrocephalus, lupus cerebritis

**Drugs**
- Intravenous cyclophosphamide
- Carbamazepine
- Vincristine, vinblastine
- Thiothixene
- Thioridazine, other phenothiazines
- Haloperidol
- Tricyclic antidepressants
- Serotonin reuptake inhibitors
- Monoamine oxidase inhibitors
- Bromocriptine
- Clofibrate
- Lorcainide
- General anesthesia
- Opiates
- Nicotine
- Desmopressin

**Pulmonary Disease**
- Pneumonia
- Tuberculosis
- Acute respiratory failure
- Positive pressure ventilation

Table 15.1 Causes of syndrome of inappropriate antidiuretic hormone (Continued)

**Ectopic Production of AVP**
- Carcinoma of lung, duodenum, pancreas, thymus, olfactory, neuroblastoma, bladder, prostate, uterus
- Lymphoma
- Sarcoma
- Leukemia

**Miscellaneous Conditions**
- Acquired immunodeficiency syndrome (AIDS)
- Idiopathic conditions

AVP, arginine vasopressin.

Therefore, UOsm greater than 100 mOsm/kg $H_2O$ reflects inappropriate antidiuresis and is compatible with the diagnosis of SIADH. As noted in Table 15.2, SIADH is a diagnosis of exclusion. Measurement of plasma AVP is not required for the diagnosis of SIADH, for the following reasons: (1) AVP levels are inconsistently elevated in SIADH; (2) the plasma AVP assay suffers from variability related to sample processing and storage; (3) there is often a significant delay in obtaining results that limits clinical utility; and (4) plasma AVP should be relatively elevated in all forms of true hyponatremia, whether hypovolemic, hypervolemic, or euvolemic. It has been suggested that the ratio of copeptin to UNa can reliably distinguish hypovolemic hyponatremia from SIADH,[58] but this assay is not readily available at many centers and so is of limited clinical value currently. In SIADH, plasma uric acid concentration is typically decreased with increased fractional excretion of uric acid. UNa is greater than 20 mEq/L. The difficulties associated with differentiation of SIADH and CSW are described earlier.

## Nephrogenic syndrome of inappropriate antidiuresis

Recent studies in children with hyponatremia have identified genetic mutations of the $V_2$ receptor associated with

Table 15.2 Criteria for diagnosis of syndrome of inappropriate antidiuretic hormone

- Decreased plasma osmolality (<275 mOsm/kg $H_2O$)
- Inappropriate urinary concentration (UOsm > 100 mOsm/kg $H_2O$ with normal renal function) in the setting of plasma hypo-osmolality
- Clinical euvolemia
- Elevated urine sodium excretion (>20 mEq/L) with normal salt and water intake
- Absence of other causes of euvolemic hypo-osmolality (e.g., severe hypothyroidism, hypocortisolism)
- Normal renal function and absence of diuretic use

constitutive activation with increased AQP2 abundance in the absence of AVP binding.[59–62] These patients meet the clinical criteria for SIADH but have undetectable plasma AVP levels. The spectrum of symptoms of nephrogenic syndrome of inappropriate antidiuresis (NSIAD) has been shown to vary markedly within families, ranging from infrequent voiding to incidentally noted hyponatremia to recurrent hyponatremic seizures[63]; some affected patients may not manifest hyponatremia until adulthood.[64] *V2R* mutation analysis is indicated for diagnosis. Children with this condition have been successfully managed with fluid restriction and urea therapy.

## Endocrinopathies

Endocrinopathies including glucocorticoid deficiency and hypothyroidism are associated with failure to suppress AVP, which leads to AQP2-mediated free water retention.[65,66] Although symptoms of these conditions are often nonspecific, usually these endocrinopathies can be quickly excluded as a cause of euvolemic hyponatremia through routine laboratory testing. Thyroid function tests are readily available in most laboratories, and a morning serum cortisol concentration lower than 10 µg/dL in an acutely ill patient suggests glucocorticoid deficiency. In some cases, a formal cosyntropin stimulation test may be needed. Hyponatremia caused solely by hypothyroidism appears to be uncommon,[67] particularly in children, but if present it relates at least in part to diminished GFR and cardiac output in the setting of severe myxedema.

## Primary polydipsia

Patients with primary or psychogenic polydipsia have a primary increase in water intake and often present with complaints of polyuria or excessive thirst. Primary polydipsia is rare in childhood, but it does occur in otherwise healthy children including infants, in children with psychiatric disorders such as schizophrenia,[68,69] in response to anticholinergic or antipsychotic medications that cause dry mouth, and in hypothalamic disease in which thirst regulation is disordered. Because the kidneys' ability to excrete free water is intact, affected patients usually demonstrate normal or slightly reduced SNa with UOsm lower than 100 mOsm/kg $H_2O$. It is only with extreme water intake (e.g., 10 to 15 L/day in adults) or high-volume water ingestion over short periods of time that significant hyponatremia occurs. Other alterations that limit free water excretion, such as concomitant diuretic use or increased AVP secretion (e.g., nausea, postoperative state), may exacerbate the otherwise mild hyponatremia in primary polydipsia. As anticipated, animal models of chronic primary polydipsia are associated with suppressed AVP concentrations and diminished collecting duct AQP2 abundance, with decreased ability to upregulate AQP2 and concentrate the urine in response to acute water deprivation.[70]

## Water intoxication

Water intoxication is a common cause of hyponatremia in children. Infants are at particular risk, not only because of a relatively diminished GFR that limits delivery of the free water load to the distal nephron for excretion, but also because they depend on others to provide a daily free water volume that can be appropriately managed by the infant kidney. Oral free water supplementation or excessive dilution of formula can quickly lead to hypo-osmolar hyponatremia in children dependent on a liquid diet. Because the infant's caloric intake depends primarily on the liquid diet, hunger drives the infant to accept the low-solute formula to the point of water intoxication. Such excessive oral free water supplementation is seen when the caregiver has not been properly educated regarding appropriate infant feeding, as well as in low-income settings where formula may be diluted intentionally to make the available supply last longer.[71,72] Cases of water intoxication have also been reported in infants and children with abusive or psychologically unstable caregivers.[72–74] Older children who depend on tube feedings can develop water intoxication when excess free water is administered through the feeding tube, either erroneously or intentionally. In otherwise healthy adolescents and young adults, significant acute hyponatremia with neurologic complications has been observed with ingestion of large volumes of free water over short periods of time, as in water-drinking contests or following 3,4-methylenedioxy-methamphetamine (Ecstasy) use.[75] Ecstasy has also been demonstrated in experimental models and in case reports to stimulate AVP secretion, an effect that is more pronounced in women than in men.[76–79] In water intoxication, the urine should be maximally dilute in the setting of intact kidney function with suppression of plasma AVP concentration.

## Reset osmostat

In this condition, the kidney retains its ability to concentrate and dilute urine appropriately. However, the threshold for AVP secretion is reset downward to a value less than 275 to 280 mOsm/kg $H_2O$, resulting in a stable but low SNa, usually approximately 125 to 130 mEq/L. This condition is quite rare in the pediatric age group but has been reported in the setting of congenital midline central nervous system defects[80] and quadriplegia.[81]

## Miscellaneous conditions

Other nonosmotic stimuli for AVP release can result in euvolemic hyponatremia, particularly in the setting of free water ingestion or administration of hypotonic parenteral fluids. Pain and nausea are powerful stimuli for AVP secretion.[82,83] The postoperative state is also associated with nonosmotic AVP secretion that usually resolves by the third postoperative day, but it occasionally can persist to the fifth postoperative day.[40,43,84] Such patients are at particular risk of hyponatremia when they receive hypotonic parenteral fluid support; therefore, frequent electrolyte monitoring is indicated.

## HYPERVOLEMIC HYPONATREMIA

Hypervolemic hyponatremia is associated with edema formation secondary to renal sodium and water retention. Diminished effective circulating volume is common in edematous states, including congestive heart failure (by a primary reduction in cardiac output), nephrotic syndrome (by decreased oncotic pressure associated with hypoalbuminemia), and cirrhosis (by decreased peripheral vascular resistance associated with splanchnic vasodilation[85]). In such settings, hyponatremia has several mechanisms, including the following: (1) diminished effective circulating volume stimulates baroreceptor-mediated AVP secretion; (2) decreased GFR and increased proximal tubular NaCl and water reabsorption both limit the amount of fluid delivered to the distal nephron for excretion; (3) stimulation of thirst with hyponatremia is further exacerbated by intake of hypotonic fluids. Of these mechanisms, baroreceptor-mediated AVP secretion appears to be the most significant contributor to hyponatremia because administration of a vasopressin $V_2$ receptor antagonist (vaptan) largely reverses defective water excretion in heart failure and cirrhosis without improving tissue perfusion.[86–88] These effects are less clear in nephrotic syndrome.

Advanced renal failure can be associated with hyponatremia. As the urine becomes isosthenuric (approximately 300 mOsm/kg $H_2O$) with advancing renal failure, the ability to excrete a free water load is impaired despite appropriate suppression of AVP. Retention of ingested water results in hyponatremia. Although this condition lowers the effective serum osmolality and is thus clinically significant, the measured serum osmolality may remain in the normal or even high range because of the contribution of elevated BUN.

## TREATMENT OF HYPONATREMIA

### General considerations

Acute hyponatremia is associated with shift of water intracellularly to maintain osmotic equilibrium. When hyponatremia develops quickly (e.g., over several hours), cerebral edema and associated symptoms can result. In contrast, when hyponatremia develops over a more prolonged time period, brain cells extrude organic solutes ("idiogenic osmoles") from their cytoplasm, thus allowing intracellular osmolality to equal POsm without a marked increase in cell water.[89] This process minimizes brain edema and explains how only mild symptoms can be observed despite severe hyponatremia. This same phenomenon makes the brain susceptible to injury when the chronic hyponatremia is rapidly corrected or overcorrected. Rapid reversal of chronic hyponatremia can exceed the brain's ability to regain the lost idiogenic osmoles and can lead to osmotic demyelination.[90] A biphasic pattern occurs in osmotic demyelination

syndrome (ODS), with initial neurologic improvement on correction of hyponatremia, followed 1 to several days later by new, progressive, and in some cases, permanent neurologic damage. Findings may include confusion, pseudobulbar palsy, or pseudocoma, but many patients are asymptomatic. Magnetic resonance imaging (MRI) is the preferred modality to demonstrate the cerebral demyelinating lesions, which are best seen more than 2 weeks following correction of hyponatremia.

### Management of acute hyponatremia

Brain herniation is typically observed with acute hyponatremia of less than 24 h duration or in the setting of underlying intracranial disorders. Hypoxia from hypoventilation or noncardiogenic pulmonary edema exacerbates hyponatremia-associated brain edema.[44] It has been suggested that a 4 to 6 mEq/L rise in SNa will reverse most serious neurologic manifestations of acute hyponatremia.[90] In the setting of acute *symptomatic* hyponatremia, hypertonic (3%) saline (514 mEq/L) is indicated. Assuming that total body water comprises approximately 50% of total body weight, 1 mL/kg of 3% saline will increase PNa by approximately 1 mEq/L. The goal of hypertonic saline therapy in acute symptomatic hyponatremia is to raise the SNa by approximately 1 mEq/L/h until: (1) the patient becomes alert and seizure-free; (2) PNa increases by 20 to 25 mEq/L; or (3) SNa of 125 to 130 mEq/L is achieved, whichever occurs first. If the child is having seizures or showing other evidence of increased intracranial pressure, the hypertonic saline infusion rate should target a rise in SNa of 4 to 8 mEq/L in the first hour or until seizure activity ceases. Following initial correction, acute hyponatremia can typically be rapidly normalized in forms of water intoxication. This often occurs spontaneously once AVP secretion is suppressed and excess free water ingestion is discontinued. Table 15.3 provides recommendations for management of acute symptomatic hyponatremia.

> ### KEY POINT
>
> In the setting of acute *symptomatic* hyponatremia, hypertonic (3%) saline (514 mEq/L) is indicated.

### Management of chronic hyponatremia

It is clear from numerous animal and human studies that overly rapid correction of chronic hyponatremia can lead to iatrogenic brain damage.[91–93] However, the most appropriate rate and duration of correction of chronic hyponatremia remain a matter of debate. A consensus committee in adults recommended a correction rate of 4 to 8 mEq/L/day in patients with clinical factors suggesting a low risk of ODS and 4 to 6 mEq/L/day in patients with a high risk of ODS.[93] Risk factors for ODS in adults include hypokalemia, severe

Table 15.3 Management of acute symptomatic hyponatremia*

| Indications | Acute water intoxication<br>Known duration of hyponatremia less than 24–48 h<br>Intracranial disorder or increased intracranial pressure<br>Seizures or coma regardless of known chronicity |
| --- | --- |
| Therapy goals | Urgent correction by 4–6 mEq/L to prevent brain herniation and neurologic damage from cerebral ischemia |
| Treatment | Severe symptoms<br>3% saline, 1–2 mL/kg IV over 10 min; may repeat × 2<br>Adults: 3% saline, 100 mL IV over 10 min; may repeat × 2<br>Mild to moderate symptoms<br>3% saline, 0.5–2 mL/kg/h |

*Source:* Verbalis JG, Goldsmith SR, Greenberg A, et al. Diagnosis, evaluation and treatment of hyponatremia: expert panel recommendations. Am J Med. 2013;126 (Suppl 1):S1–42.

* The rate of correction need not be restricted in patients with true acute hyponatremia, nor is relowering of excessive correction indicated. However, if there is any uncertainty about whether the hyponatremia is chronic versus acute, then the limits for correction of chronic hyponatremia should be followed.

Table 15.4 Measures to minimize risk of osmotic demyelination syndrome in correction of chronic hyponatremia

- Highest-risk population: serum sodium concentration <120 mEq/L for >48-h duration
- Increased vigilance indicated for specific risk factors:
  - Hypokalemia
  - Hypoxia
  - Malnutrition
  - Advanced liver disease
- Minimum correction of SNa by 4–8 mEq/L/day, with lower goal of 4–6 mEq/L/day if risk of ODS is high
- Maximum correction of SNa by 10–12 mEq/L/24 h or 18 mEq/L/48 h, with lower goal (8 mEq/L/24 h) if risk of ODS is high

*Source:* Verbalis JG, Goldsmith SR, Greenberg A, et al. Diagnosis, evaluation and treatment of hyponatremia: expert panel recommendations. Am J Med. 2013;126 (Suppl 1):S1–42.
*Abbreviations:* ODS, osmotic demyelination syndrome, SNa, serum sodium.

malnutrition, alcoholism, hypoxia, and advanced liver disease. However, the serum potassium concentration and the degree of the aforementioned medical conditions that increase the risk of ODS have not been defined, nor have the relevant risk factors in adults been correlated with risk of ODS in children. Guidelines for minimization of ODS are noted in Table 15.4. Sterns et al.[94] proposed a "rule of sixes" for management of severe hyponatremic symptoms ("sx"): "six a day makes sense for safety so six in 6 hours for severe sx then stop."

An unexpectedly rapid rate of correction of chronic hyponatremia can occur despite cautious management. This is particularly common in settings in which the pathogenic stimulus for excess AVP secretion is "turned off," such as fluid resuscitation in volume depletion, hydrocortisone treatment of cortisol deficiency, and discontinuation of thiazides. Excretion of maximally dilute urine can raise SNa by more than 2 mEq/L/h. It has therefore been suggested that goal correction rates fall short of rates associated with iatrogenic complications and that frequent monitoring of SNa (e.g., every 2 to 4 hours) and urine volume be instituted.

The longer the duration of hyponatremia and the lower the SNa, the higher is the risk of iatrogenic complications with overcorrection of SNa. Consideration should be given to reversing overcorrection of chronic hyponatremia when initial SNa was less than 120 mEq/L, particularly when known risk factors for ODS are present. In this setting, it is appropriate

to withhold ongoing measures designed to increase SNa (e.g., hypertonic saline) and to prevent further correction induced by urinary free water loss (e.g., replace urinary losses with 5% dextrose in water [D5W] or oral water).

The approach to treatment of hyponatremia should therefore consider (1) the underlying condition that precipitated the hyponatremia, (2) the presence of hyponatremia-associated neurologic symptoms, and (3) the duration of hyponatremia. With these considerations in mind, the discussion focuses on management of specific causes of hyponatremia.

## Management of hypovolemic hyponatremia

With correction of volume depletion, the nonosmotic stimulus for AVP secretion is abolished, and the relative water excess corrects itself by water diuresis. Thus, appropriate monitoring of SNa and urine volume is indicated to avoid overcorrection of hyponatremia, which is frequently chronic. When intravascular volume depletion is evident, isotonic fluid resuscitation is indicated until euvolemia is restored. Such therapy is frequently initiated even before laboratory results are available. Hyponatremia secondary to gastrointestinal fluid loss is rarely of sufficient severity or acuity to require hypertonic saline. Once fluid resuscitation is completed, intravenous or enteral fluid support can be provided as needed, taking into account any ongoing gastrointestinal losses. Appropriate potassium supplementation is indicated in the setting of hypokalemia, which is commonly seen with emesis or stool losses. Potassium is exchangeable with intracellular sodium, so supplementation to correct hypokalemia raises SNa to the same degree as sodium repletion. Patients with acidosis (e.g., ongoing stool bicarbonate loss) may require bicarbonate or acetate support to prevent expansion acidosis. Therapy specific to the underlying disorder should be pursued as appropriate.

Diuretic-induced hyponatremia is chronic. Discontinuation of the offending diuretic and repletion of sodium and potassium deficits reverse the associated hyponatremia. Caution should be exercised to ensure that overly rapid correction does not occur. Administration of potassium raises the SNa to a degree equivalent to that of administering sodium, so potassium dosage should be taken into account in the hyponatremia treatment plan. Enteral water or D5W can be used to slow the rate of correction if necessary.

Fluid resuscitation with isotonic saline is indicated in hypovolemic patients with CSW. Hypertonic saline can be used if altered mental status is present and is believed to relate to the hyponatremia, with correction rates as outlined earlier. Sodium supplementation, either intravenous or oral, may be needed because of ongoing natriuresis.

Mineralocorticoid deficiency is typically chronic. Volume repletion with isotonic saline is indicated. Fludrocortisone is used on a long-term basis for mineralocorticoid replacement and should minimize recurrent hypovolemic hyponatremia. Spontaneous aquaresis with rapid correction of hyponatremia can occur once volume status is restored; therefore, frequent monitoring of SNa is indicated.

## Treatment of euvolemic hyponatremia

Treatment of SIADH should be directed to elimination of the source (e.g., discontinuation of offending medications, appropriate management of tumor, antibiotic treatment of pneumonia). Acute symptomatic hyponatremia in SIADH is most appropriately treated with hypertonic saline. It is critical to recall that patients with euvolemic hyponatremia secondary to SIADH may not respond to isotonic saline, and in some cases, such therapy causes the hyponatremia to worsen because urine sodium excretion increases while free water is retained. For most cases of mild to moderate hyponatremia related to SIADH, fluid restriction is the appropriate initial intervention. General recommendations in this regard include the following: (1) all fluid intake, including parenteral and enteral nutrition and fluid from medications, must be included in the fluid restriction; (2) the degree of restriction required depends on urine output (which may be decreased) and insensible fluid loss; (3) several days of restriction may be required before a significant increase in POsm is observed; and (4) sodium intake should not be restricted in these patients, who may have mild total body sodium depletion resulting from ongoing natriuresis. Predictors of poor response to fluid restriction alone include high UOsm (greater than 500 mOsm/kg $H_2O$) and low urine volume, findings that support the presence of significantly elevated plasma AVP concentration. Urea has been proposed as an alternative oral treatment for SIADH. Urea acts by inducing osmotic water elimination and by promoting passive sodium reabsorption in the ascending limb of the loop of Henle.[95] PNa and tonicity increase progressively, without associated hypertonicity. Reported adverse effects include gastrointestinal upset, poor compliance because of the undesirable taste of the medication, and development of azotemia at high doses. The administration of urea in SIADH can allow for a less strict regimen of fluid restriction. Low dietary solute intake limits free water excretion and should be avoided in patients with SIADH.

Vaptans, specific antagonists of the $V_2$ receptor, have been shown to increase renal free water excretion in adults with euvolemic and hypervolemic hyponatremia. Conivaptan is a $V_1a/V_2$ receptor antagonist available in intravenous form, whereas tolvaptan is a selective $V_2$ receptor antagonist available as an oral agent. In the SALT-1 and SALT-2 randomized placebo-controlled trials (Study of Ascending Levels of Tolvaptan in Hyponatremia) of tolvaptan versus placebo in adults with hyponatremia resulting from cardiac failure, liver failure or SIADH,[96,97] treatment with tolvaptan was associated with a progressive increase in SNa without requirement for water restriction. The largest increase in SNa occurred in patients with the lowest baseline SNa. Vaptans should not be used in conjunction with or immediately after other treatments for hyponatremia such as hypertonic saline because of the potential for excessively rapid correction of hyponatremia. The efficacy of vaptans in severe hyponatremia (SNa less than 120 mEq/L) has not been systematically studied, and current recommendations support hypertonic saline treatment in such cases. Vaptans have not been studied in children, but it is likely that clinical trials will be implemented in pediatric hyponatremia in the near future.

Patients with suspected NSIAD should undergo mutation analysis of the *AVPR2* gene to confirm the diagnosis. Fluid restriction and urea therapy are effective in the management of affected children.[61] Vaptans have not been shown to be effective in the few adult patients with NSIAD in whom they have been attempted.

If glucocorticoid deficiency is suspected, blood should be drawn for baseline plasma cortisol, and glucocorticoid replacement should be provided. Rapid water diuresis following administration of hydrocortisone is consistent with underlying glucocorticoid deficiency, and hyponatremia typically resolves without additional intervention. The associated aquaresis can be associated with rapid or overcorrection of chronic hyponatremia, so close laboratory monitoring is indicated.

The most appropriate treatment for hyponatremia secondary to hypothyroidism is thyroid hormone replacement. Because such hyponatremia is typically mild, fluid restriction can be helpful. Hyponatremic encephalopathy from myxedema is rare in general but particularly in childhood.

Management of primary polydipsia should target normal fluid intake. This can be difficult to accomplish, particularly in the setting of psychiatric disease or altered thirst regulation. Measures to decrease the sensation of thirst (e.g., sour candies to stimulate saliva flow or ice chips to moisten the mouth) may be helpful. Although there are anecdotal reports of clozapine to reduce polydipsia and recurrent hyponatremia in adults with psychiatric disease,[98] similar findings have not been systematically described in childhood, in which clozapine use is rare. Chronic primary polydipsia is associated with impaired urinary concentration and diminished upregulation of AQP2 in rats in response to water deprivation,[70] so a progressive decrease toward normal fluid intake may be preferable in affected patients.

Water intoxication typically rapidly resolves once excess free water ingestion is discontinued. Because the urinary diluting mechanism is intact, SNa can rise rapidly in this situation. Given that most cases of water intoxication are acute, the risk of ODS is low. However, if there is concern for possible chronicity of the water intoxication, overly rapid correction should be avoided.

## Treatment of hypervolemic hyponatremia

Diuretics and fluid and sodium restriction remain the primary treatments for edematous disorders. From a practical standpoint, however, compliance with fluid and sodium restriction is variable, and diuretics can induce electrolyte abnormalities and diminish effective circulating volume. Hyponatremia attributable to nonosmotic AVP secretion in these conditions is chronic and should be managed accordingly. Severely symptomatic patients with heart failure and rapidly falling or very low SNa can be managed with combined hypertonic saline and loop diuretics to prevent fluid overload. However, this treatment must be attempted cautiously. Typical therapies for management of cirrhosis with ascites include fluid and sodium restriction, diuretic therapy, and large-volume paracentesis. Management of nephrotic syndrome includes fluid and sodium restriction, diuretics, and 25% albumin support as clinically indicated.

Vaptans have perhaps their most ideal application in hypervolemic hyponatremia which has been unsuccessfully managed with fluid restriction. In contrast to loop diuretics, vaptans do not cause significant direct intravascular volume depletion and therefore do not stimulate neurohormonal responses of the renin-angiotensin-aldosterone and sympathetic nervous systems, and they do not deplete electrolytes. As noted previously, vaptans effectively induce renal free water excretion in adults with hypervolemic hyponatremia secondary to heart failure and cirrhosis. However, more recent studies in adults with autosomal dominant polycystic kidney disease who used oral tolvaptan at up to twice the maximum dose approved for hyponatremia raised concern for possible irreversible and potentially fatal liver injury,[99] a finding prompting the FDA to recommend limited duration of use in hypervolemic and euvolemic hyponatremia and avoidance of use with underlying liver disease. Conivaptan is not recommended in patients with cirrhosis and portal hypertension because blockade of the $V_1a$ receptor in the splanchnic circulation can increase portal blood flow and precipitate variceal bleeding. Vaptans have not been systematically studied in nephrotic syndrome. As noted previously, these medications have not been studied or approved for use in children.

## HYPERNATREMIA

Hypernatremia is defined as SNa greater than 145 mEq/L. It is less common than hyponatremia but has a broad reported prevalence of 1% to 14%, depending on the population studied.[100-102] Hypernatremia is frequently acquired in the hospital,[38] and it is seen most commonly in children with restricted access to free water and those with chronic disease, critical illness, or underlying neurologic disease. Gastroenteritis is reported to account for only approximately 20% of cases of hypernatremia in hospitalized children.[38] Similar to hyponatremia, many cases of hypernatremia are mild and relatively asymptomatic. However, hypernatremia is clinically important because (1) acute severe hypernatremia can be associated with substantial morbidity and mortality, (2) adverse outcomes are higher in a variety of medical conditions with concomitant hypernatremia, and (3) overly rapid correction of chronic hypernatremia can cause significant neurologic complications and death.

Hypernatremia occurs by the following mechanisms: (1) diminished urinary concentrating capacity with renal free water loss, (2) excess sodium ingestion, and (3) impaired thirst. One or a combination of these factors results in a relative free water deficit in an individual patient.

The body has two primary defense mechanisms against hypernatremia: AVP secretion and thirst. AVP is typically secreted when POsm exceeds 280 mOsm/kg $H_2O$, with maximal secretion greater than 290 to 295 mOsm/kg $H_2O$. The thirst mechanism provides a critical defense against hypernatremia because with intact thirst and free access to water, hypernatremia can be prevented in most cases even with concomitant impairment in urinary concentrating capacity or excess sodium ingestion.

Hypernatremia is always associated with elevated POsm.

### KEY POINT

The thirst mechanism provides a critical defense against hypernatremia because, with intact thirst and free access to water, hypernatremia can be prevented in most cases even with concomitant impairment in urinary concentrating capacity or excess sodium ingestion.

## CLINICAL MANIFESTATIONS

As hypernatremia develops, there is movement of water from the intracellular to the extracellular compartment along the osmotic gradient. This results in transient cerebral dehydration and cell shrinkage. Brain cell volume can decrease by as much as 10% to 15% acutely, with subsequent rapid adaptation. Within 1 hour, the brain increases the intracellular content of sodium, potassium, amino acids, and idiogenic osmoles. Within 1 week, the brain regains approximately 98% of its water content.

Hypernatremia is associated with a broad spectrum of neurologic signs and symptoms, ranging from subtle and nonspecific findings including agitation, irritability, lethargy, hypertonicity, and hyperreflexia to myoclonus, asterixis, chorea, seizures, and rhabdomyolysis. As in hyponatremia, the symptoms do not progress along a predictable time course. Physical findings of intravascular volume depletion may not be as striking in the setting of hypernatremic dehydration because extracellular volume is maintained at the expense of intracellular volume. Mortality is reported to be up to 15%, which is 15 times higher than age-matched mortality rates in children without hypernatremia.[38,43]

However, many deaths are not directly related to the hypernatremia, and this may instead reflect the overall severity of the underlying disease state.

## CLINICAL APPROACH TO HYPERNATREMIA

The approach to hypernatremia involves the following (Figure 15.6):

1. **Obtain a detailed history.** The history should include a detailed account of fluid balance, including recent intake and output. Assessment of intake should include consideration of both enteral and parenteral fluids and the associated free water and sodium content. Sodium supplementation should be reviewed. Consideration should be given to whether the patient's thirst mechanism is intact, whether full access to fluids was provided, and whether fluid ingestion is regulated by the patient or a caregiver. Assessment of output should include the nature and magnitude of both renal and extrarenal losses. Review of recent weights is often valuable. The medication history should be reviewed,

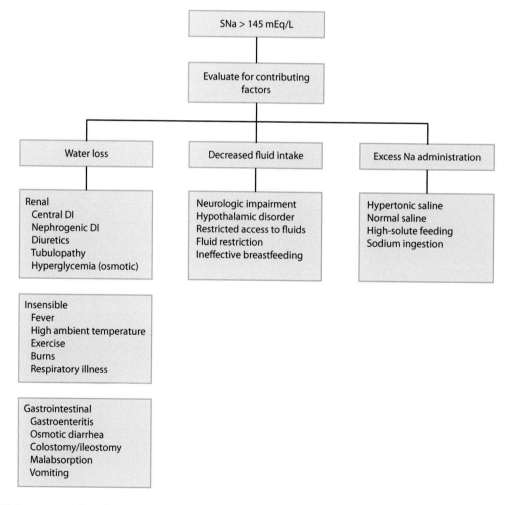

Figure 15.6 Clinical approach to hypernatremia. SNa, serum sodium concentration. DI, diabetes insipidus.

including diuretics. A family history of DI or tubulopathies should be obtained.

2. **Evaluate UOsm.** In the setting of significant hypernatremia, UOsm should be increased to greater than 800 mOsm/kg $H_2O$. If lower UOsm is present, then a renal concentrating defect is present.

The pathogenesis of hypernatremia is typically multifactorial and may involve free water loss, excess sodium administration, and impaired thirst.

---

## KEY POINT

If UOsm is lower than 800 mOsm/kg $H_2O$ in the setting of hypernatremia, then the kidney is not concentrating appropriately.

---

## RENAL WATER LOSS

DI results from the inability to reabsorb free water. This can occur in patients with deficient AVP secretion (central DI or CDI) or when the collecting duct is unresponsive to AVP (NDI). Affected patients experience polyuria with subsequent polydipsia, increased thirst, and potentially hypernatremia.

**CDI** is most often acquired but can also be congenital. Congenital CDI occurs in patients with structural brain malformations that affect hypothalamic or pituitary function. Less commonly observed are autosomal dominant or recessive mutations of the gene encoding AVP-neurophysin II (NPII). Autosomal dominant mutations result from heterozygous AVP gene mutations that are believed to alter processing of the AVP precursor.[103] Accumulation of the misfolded AVP protein in the hypothalamic magnocellular neurons leads to eventual neuronal destruction. Affected patients demonstrate gradual development of DI over several months to years after birth. Autosomal recessive CDI is much less common but is associated with biologically inactive AVP.[103] Acquired forms of CDI are observed in several conditions associated with destruction or degeneration of vasopressinergic neurons. These include primary tumors (e.g., craniopharyngioma, germinoma) or metastases, infection (meningitis, encephalitis), histiocytosis, granulomatous disease, autoimmune disorders (lymphocytic infundibuloneurohypophysitis), and central nervous system trauma or surgical procedures.[104]

**NDI** can be congenital or acquired. Congenital NDI is caused by mutations in the *AVPR2* gene, which is located on chromosome Xq28 or by autosomal dominant or recessive mutations in the *AQP2* gene, which is located on chromosome 12q13 (less than 10%).[105] X-linked NDI is rare, affecting approximately 4 in 1,000,000 boys and men worldwide, but it accounts for 90% of congenital NDI. As anticipated with X-linked disease, males are affected, whereas females are carriers. Most *AVPR2* missense mutations result in a translated but misfolded V2R protein that remains trapped in the endoplasmic reticulum.[105] A few of the mutant receptors reach the cell surface but cannot bind AVP or trigger an intracellular cAMP signal. AQP2 mutant proteins are similarly trapped intracellularly.

Several forms of acquired NDI can affect children. Several of these conditions are known to be associated with impaired function of AQP2 water channels, including hypokalemia,[106] hypercalcemia,[107,108] obstructive uropathy,[109,110] and lithium administration.[111] Additional causes of acquired NDI include sickle cell disease and some primary renal diseases. There are also a variety of tubulopathies that have been associated with vasopressin resistance, including cystinosis and other causes of Fanconi syndrome, nephronophthisis, Bartter syndrome, and syndrome of apparent mineralocorticoid excess[112]; a small case series of affected patients has shown no associated mutations in *AVPR2* or *AQP2*.[113]

Patients with DI experience polyuria, which can be extreme (10 to 15 L/day in adults) and leads to increased thirst and polydipsia. When water access is unlimited, affected patients usually drink enough water to prevent significant hypernatremia. However, restricted water access (including a caregiver's lack of recognition of increased fluid needs), inability to keep fluids down (e.g., vomiting), a coexistent impaired thirst mechanism, or increased extrarenal losses may lead to severe hypernatremia over a matter of hours. Affected children often complain incessantly with attempts to limit their free water intake. Infants with congenital X-linked NDI often present within the first weeks of life with nonspecific symptoms including fever, vomiting, fussiness, and failure to thrive. First-time mothers may not recognize that urine volume is abnormally high. Mental retardation and intracranial calcifications were historically reported in affected male patients with X-linked NDI and are thought to relate to delayed diagnosis with recurrent episodes of dehydration.[114,115] Older children may experience enuresis or nocturia. Ongoing marked polyuria can lead to hydroureteronephrosis and megabladder, as well as functional obstructive uropathy, which in extreme cases can cause end-stage renal disease.

DI is diagnosed by demonstration of hyperosmolality with urine that is inappropriately dilute. With healthy kidneys, urine should be maximally concentrated in response to significant hypernatremia and hyperosmolality. UOsm lower than 800 mOsm/kg $H_2O$ in the setting of hypernatremia or POsm greater than 290 to 295 mOsm/kg $H_2O$ is consistent with DI. Male patients with X-linked NDI frequently manifest baseline UOsm of approximately 50 to 80 mOsm/kg $H_2O$. The discrepancy between UOsm and POsm is more prominent during fluid deprivation. However, if CDI or congenital NDI is suspected, it is dangerous to advise overnight fluid deprivation at home; instead, evaluation is most appropriately conducted in the hospital or clinic setting, where serial laboratory and urine output monitoring is readily available. A standardized fluid deprivation test includes serial measurement of weight, SNa, serum osmolality, urine volume, and UOsm while the patient is fasted and deprived of fluids for up to 8 to 10 hours. The diagnosis of complete DI is confirmed when SOsm rises to more than 300 mOsm/kg $H_2O$ with UOsm lower than 300 mOsm/kg $H_2O$. UOsm in the 300 to 750 mOsm/kg $H_2O$ range suggests partial DI, whereas UOsm greater than 750 mOsm/kg $H_2O$ excludes the diagnosis of DI. If DI is confirmed during the water deprivation test, a plasma sample should be obtained for AVP. The patient is then given vasopressin, often as desmopressin, to distinguish AVP deficiency from AVP unresponsiveness.

When CDI is confirmed, MRI of the brain with focus on the hypothalamic-pituitary region is indicated. CDI is often but not always associated with loss of the posterior pituitary "bright spot" on T1-weighted images. However, the bright spot can also be absent in normal persons.[116] DI may not be immediately apparent in patients with concomitant anterior pituitary–mediated adrenal glucocorticoid deficiency, which is often associated with free water retention. Glucocorticoid replacement may unmask CDI in such patients. It has been suggested that normal findings on brain MRI in CDI warrant ongoing surveillance for tumor, especially hypothalamic stalk lesions.[117] Treatment of CDI includes appropriate management of the primary disease, correction of any fluid deficit, and normalization of urine output with desmopressin. Desmopressin is an AVP analogue with significantly reduced pressor activity and longer half-life as compared with AVP; it can be administered intranasally or by subcutaneous injection. Because of the risk of hyponatremia with limited control of intranasal desmopressin dose, CDI can be managed in infancy with high-dose fluids either orally or by gastrostomy tube placed specifically for high-dose fluid support.

Treatment for congenital NDI has not changed for some decades, although a better understanding of the underlying mechanisms has evolved. Affected patients should be allowed constant access to fluids with high threshold for hypotonic parenteral fluid support when *ad libitum* oral fluid intake is not possible. It is critical to address the high free water need in such patients during parenteral fluid support. Low solute intake decreases the osmotic load for excretion, so dietary sodium restriction of 1 mmol/kg/day has been advocated. In this regard, families benefit from ongoing dietitian support as the child ages. Thiazide diuretics effectively decrease urine volume in congenital NDI. An initial thiazide-induced reduction in sodium reabsorption in the distal tubule increases sodium excretion, with extracellular fluid volume contraction. The associated decrease in GFR results in less fluid delivery to the distal nephron, thus limiting free water excretion. It has also been suggested that thiazides directly affect the AVP-AQP2 cascade, but further studies are needed to elucidate the mechanism.[118] Because hypokalemia is known to impair AQP2-mediated urinary concentration,[106] co-treatment with potassium-sparing diuretics such as amiloride or spironolactone is usually necessary.

Nonsteroidal anti-inflammatory drugs (NSAIDs) also decrease urine volume in congenital NDI by decreasing GFR. Prostaglandin $E_2$ is known to induce trafficking and phosphorylation of AQP2, and prostaglandin inhibition with NSAIDs inhibits endocytic retrieval of AQP2 from the apical membrane.[119] The individual contribution of these effects of NSAIDs to decreased urine volume in NDI is unclear. Indomethacin quite effectively decreases urine volume in congenital NDI, but some practitioners defer NSAIDs in very young children because of the risk of gastritis. Other NSAIDs such as ibuprofen and tolmetin are also effective in congenital NDI. Even with current optimal control of congenital NDI, urine volume is not normal. However, a reduction in urine volume of 50% can often be achieved. From a quality of life standpoint, the reduction in urine volume from 10 to 5 L/day is significant, although the patient remains markedly polyuric. $V_2$ receptor antagonists have been used in vitro as pharmacologic chaperones to rescue the cell-surface expression and functional activity of misfolded mutant $V_2$ receptors associated with specific mutations, but further studies are needed to assess the clinical relevance of these findings.[120,121] A similar approach with thiazides and NSAIDs can be used for management of polyuria caused by impaired urinary concentration associated with specific tubulopathies.

Lithium is the most common cause of acquired NDI in adults. A urinary concentrating defect occurs in approximately 55% of adults receiving long-term therapy, with 20% of patients producing more than 3 L urine per day. Lithium causes NDI by inhibition of adenylyl cyclase in principal cells in the collecting duct, with associated downregulation of AQP2 water channels.[111,122–124] Lithium also reduces UT-A1 protein abundance and interferes with the ability of AVP to phosphorylate UT-A1, thus reducing accumulation of inner medullary interstitial urea with diminished urinary concentrating ability.[125,126] Lithium-induced reduction of UT-B in the inner medulla decreases urea recycling and the efficiency of countercurrent exchange, further limiting urinary concentrating ability. Lithium-induced NDI can be irreversible if it is not quickly diagnosed and lithium is not subsequently discontinued. Amiloride can reduce lithium uptake into principal cells in the collecting duct, and this may lessen the inhibitor effect of intracellular lithium on water reabsorption.[127] Thus, co-treatment with lithium and amiloride is becoming widespread. Other medications known to induce a urinary concentrating defect include amphotericin B, cidofovir, demeclocycline, didanosine, foscarnet, ofloxacin, and orlistat.

Hypercalcemia, hypokalemia, low-protein diets, and obstructive uropathy are known to cause acquired NDI. These acquired forms are rarely as severe as congenital NDI but can result in significant polyuria. These conditions are associated with downregulation of AQP2 expression in the medulla of rat kidneys.[106–109,128,129] Hypokalemia and release of ureteral obstruction are also associated with reduced abundance of UT-A1, UT-A3, and UT-B protein in the kidney medulla in rats.[130,131] These alterations all diminish urinary concentrating ability.

Hypernatremia from free water loss through the kidneys is also observed with excessive osmotic diuretic use and with severe hyperglycemia secondary to osmotic water loss.

## EXTRARENAL WATER LOSS

Excess free water loss occurs with increased insensible losses, including fever, high ambient temperature, prolonged exercise, burns, and respiratory illnesses. Gastrointestinal water loss occurs in association with gastroenteritis, osmotic diarrhea, stool losses through ostomies, malabsorption, or vomiting. The history is critical in the evaluation of such losses. Primary treatment should be directed toward the precipitating factor.

## DECREASED FLUID INTAKE

The thirst mechanism is perhaps the most powerful defense against hypernatremia. Children with structural brain defects with associated hypothalamic disease can have diminished or absent thirst leading to insufficient water intake. More commonly, however, decreased fluid intake is related to an imposed limitation on water. This is particularly common in infants, neurologically impaired children, and others who are unable to communicate the experience of thirst effectively and who therefore rely on attentive caregivers to provide appropriate free water support. Exclusively breast fed newborns of primiparous mothers are at particular risk for hypernatremic dehydration and may suffer from vascular complications, including renal vein thrombosis.[132,133] Prolonged fluid restriction has also been observed as a form of child abuse.[134]

## EXCESS SODIUM ADMINISTRATION

Excess sodium administration is a less common cause of hypernatremia in childhood, but it can be observed both with parenteral administration of fluids with high sodium content and with enteral sodium ingestion. Repeated sodium bicarbonate administration for management of acidosis in the intensive care setting, particularly during prolonged code resuscitation, can result in hypernatremia. Infants and children who receive sodium supplementation for salt-losing disorders (e.g., salt-losing nephropathy) should undergo careful laboratory monitoring to ensure that the SNa remains within the normal range. Table salt is particularly concentrated (1 tsp salt = 104 mEq sodium). When table salt supplementation is prescribed for home administration for children, it is critical that parents measure rather than estimate each dose because salt poisoning can easily occur. Salt poisoning has also been described as a form of child abuse.[134]

## TREATMENT OF HYPERNATREMIA

Treatment of hypernatremia requires provision of adequate free water to normalize the SNa. Hypernatremia is frequently accompanied by volume depletion; therefore, fluid resuscitation with isotonic crystalloid or colloid should be implemented before attempts to correct the free water deficit. Any offending agent (e.g., medication or salt supplementation) that is contributing to hypernatremia should be discontinued. As always, therapy directed toward the primary disease is indicated.

Following volume resuscitation, the composition of parenteral fluid therapy depends on the cause of the hypernatremia. For example, patients with sodium overload or a renal concentrating defect require more hypotonic fluid support than do patients with volume depletion and intact renal concentrating ability. Oral hydration should be instituted as soon as it is safely tolerated. Despite the best efforts of trained medical personnel, children with DI are often much better at self-correcting hypernatremia in response to thirst. Patients with acute hypernatremia that is corrected by oral free water supplementation appear to tolerate a more rapid rate of correction with less frequency of seizures than do patients receiving only parenteral fluid management. Serum electrolytes should be assessed every 2 hours until the patient is neurologically stable.

The free water deficit should always be calculated to devise an appropriate initial fluid management plan. Many pediatricians erroneously assume that simply providing a less hypotonic parenteral fluid than the SNa will correct the hypernatremia. The following formula is useful to determine the minimum amount of fluid necessary to correct hypernatremia:

$$\text{Free water deficit} = 4 \text{ mL} \times \text{Current body weight (kg)} \times [\text{Desired change in SNa in mEq/L}]$$

This formula assumes that total body water is approximately 50% of total body weight. The fluid composition then dictates the amount of fluid required to correct the fluid deficit. For example, to correct a free water deficit of 3 L, 4 L of 0.2% NaCl in water or 6 L of 0.45% NaCl in water would be required because these solutions contain approximately 75% and 50% free water, respectively.[43] It is important to consider the patient's ability to tolerate the proposed quantity of fluid (e.g., in oliguric acute kidney injury). The calculated free water deficit does not account for ongoing losses or maintenance needs. Calculations for free water deficit and maintenance needs should be combined with estimation or quantification of ongoing losses to determine the best fluid management plan to correct hypernatremia in an individual child.

The rate of correction of hypernatremia depends on the severity and the cause of the hypernatremia. As noted earlier, the brain rapidly responds to hypernatremia with generation of idiogenic osmoles to maintain brain volume. Given the relative inability of the brain to extrude idiogenic osmoles, rapid correction of hypernatremia can lead to cerebral edema. Although there are no clinical studies defining the optimal rate of correction of hypernatremia to avoid cerebral edema, empiric data suggest that a rate less than 1 mEq/L/h or 15 mEq/L/24 h is appropriate in the absence of hypernatremic encephalopathy.[43] If severe hypernatremia is present (SNa greater than 170 mEq/L), the target SNa should be higher than 150 mEq/L for the first 48 to 72 hours of therapy.[135] Laboratory studies should be monitored frequently (e.g., every 2 hours), with adjustments to the treatment plan as needed. Seizures occurring during correction of hypernatremia may indicate cerebral edema. Appropriate management includes slowing the rate of correction or consideration of hypertonic saline to increase SNa by a few milliequivalents per liter.[40] Such seizures are typically self-limited and do not necessarily portend adverse long-term neurologic outcome.[135]

## SUMMARY

Hyponatremia and hypernatremia are commonly encountered in pediatric nephrology practice, particularly in hospitalized children. A thorough understanding of the physiologic processes that contribute to urinary concentration and dilution allows for recognition of the specific derangements that generate abnormalities of water metabolism in the individual patient. Appropriate therapy can then be tailored to the patient's needs, with minimization of the risk of potentially severe neurologic complications.

## REFERENCES

1. Darwin C. On the Origin of Species by Means of Natural Selection. London: John Murray; 1859.
2. Smith HW. From Fish to Philosopher. Boston: Little, Brown and Company; 1953.
3. Bernard C. Leçons sur lex phénomènes de la vie communs aux animaux et auz végétaux. Paris: JB Baillerre et Fils; 1885.
4. Kuhn W, Ryffel K. Herstellung konzentrierter Losungen aus verdunnten durch blosse Membranwirking: ein Modellversuch zur der Niere. Z Physiol Chem. 1942;276:145–80.
5. Kokko JP, Rector FCJ. Countercurrent multiplication system without active transport in inner medulla. Kidney Int. 1972;2:214–23.
6. Sands JM, Kokko JP. Countercurrent system. Kidney Int 1990;38:695–9.
7. Stephenson JL. Concentration of urine in a central core model of the renal counterflow system. Kidney Int. 1972;2:85–94.
8. Molony DA, Reeves WB, Andreoli TE. Na$^+$:K$^+$:2Cl$^-$ cotransport and the thick ascending limb. Kidney Int. 1989;36:418–26.
9. Dunn FL, Brennan TJ, Nelson AE, Robertson GL. The role of blood osmolality and volume in regulating vasopressin secretion in the rat. J Clin Invest. 1973;52:3212–9.
10. Robertson GL, Berl T. Pathophysiology of water metabolism. In: Brenner BM, editor. The Kidney. 6th ed. Philadelphia: WB Saunders; 2000. p. 866–924.
11. Morgenthaler NG, Struck J, Alonso C, Bergmann A. Assay for the measurement of copeptin, a stable peptide derived from the precursor of vasopressin. Clin Chem. 2006;52:112–9.
12. Robertson GL. Abnormalities of thirst regulation. Kidney Int. 1984;25:460–9.
13. Schrier RW. Pathogenesis of sodium and water retention in high-output and low-output cardiac failure, nephrotic syndrome, cirrhosis, and pregnancy (1). N Engl J Med. 1988;319:1065–72.
14. Schrier RW. Pathogenesis of sodium and water retention in high-output and low-output cardiac failure, nephrotic syndrome, cirrhosis, and pregnancy (2). N Engl J Med. 1988;319:1127–34.
15. Saito T, Ishikawa SE, Sasaki S, et al. Alteration in water channel AQP-2 by removal of AVP stimulation in collecting duct cells of dehydrated rats. Am J Physiol. 1997;272:F183–91.
16. Hozawa S, Holtzman EJ, Ausiello DA. cAMP motifs regulating transcription in the aquaporin 2 gene. Am J Physiol. 1996;270:C1695–702.
17. Yasui M, Zelenin SM, Celsi G, Aperia A. Adenylate cyclase–coupled vasopressin receptor activates AQP2 promoter via a dual effect on CRE and AP1 elements. Am J Physiol. 1997;272:F443–50.
18. Matsumura Y, Uchida S, Rai T, et al. Transcriptional regulation of aquaporin-2 water channel gene by cAMP. J Am Soc Nephrol. 1997;8:861–7.
19. McGowan AR. The fat and water content of the dead infant's skinfold. Pediatr Res 1979;13:1304–6.
20. Hartnoll G, Betremieux P, Modi N. Body water content of extremely preterm infants at birth. Arch Dis Child Fetal Neonatal Ed. 2000;83:F56–9.
21. Rodriguez G, Ventura P, Samper MP, et al. Changes in body composition during the initial hours of life in breast-fed healthy term newborns. Biol Neonate 2000;77:12–6.
22. Day GM, Radde IC, Balfe JW, Chance GW. Electrolyte abnormalities in very low birthweight infants. Pediatr Res. 1976;10:522–6.
23. Bonilla-Felix M. Development of water transport in the collecting duct. Am J Physiol Renal Physiol. 2004;287:F1093–101.
24. Dobrovic-Jenik D, Milkovic S. Regulation of fetal Na$^+$/K$^+$-ATPase in rat kidney by corticosteroids. Biochim Biophys Acta. 1988;942:227–35.
25. Rane S, Aperia A. Ontogeny of Na-K-ATPase activity in thick ascending limb and of concentrating capacity. Am J Physiol. 1985;249:F723–8.

26. Osathanondh V, Potter EL. Development of human kidney as shown by microdissection. III. Formation and interrelationship of collecting tubules and nephrons. Arch Pathol. 1963;76:290–302.

27. Liu W, Morimoto T, Kondo Y, et al. "Avian-type" renal medullary tubule organization causes immaturity of urine-concentrating ability in neonates. Kidney Int. 2001;60:680–93.

28. Quigley R, Lisec A, Baum M. Ontogeny of rabbit proximal tubule urea permeability. Am J Physiol Regul Integr Comp Physiol. 2001;280:R1713–8.

29. Forrest JN, Jr, Stanier MW. Kidney composition and renal concentration ability in young rabbits. J Physiol. 1966;187:1–4.

30. Edelmann CM, Barnett HL, Troupkou V. Renal concentrating mechanisms in newborn infants: Effect of dietary protein and water content, role of urea, and responsiveness to antidiuretic hormone. J Clin Invest. 1960;39:1062–9.

31. Edelmann CM, Jr, Barnett HL, Stark H. Effect of urea on concentration of urinary nonurea solute in premature infants. J Appl Physiol. 1966;21:1021–5.

32. Imran S, Eva G, Christopher S, Flynn E, Henner D. Is specific gravity a good estimate of urine osmolality? J Clin Lab Anal. 2010;24:426–30.

33. Leech S, Penney MD. Correlation of specific gravity and osmolality of urine in neonates and adults. Arch Dis Child. 1987;62:671–3.

34. Lord RC. Osmosis, osmometry, and osmoregulation. Postgrad Med. J 1999;75:67–73.

35. Aw TC, Kiechle FL. Pseudohyponatremia. Am J Emerg Med. 1985;3:236–9.

36. Katz MA. Hyperglycemia-induced hyponatremia: Calculation of expected serum sodium depression. N Engl J Med. 1973;289:843–4.

37. Hillier TA, Abbott RD, Barrett EJ. Hyponatremia: Evaluating the correction factor for hyperglycemia. Am J Med. 1999;106:399–403.

38. Moritz ML, Ayus JC. The changing pattern of hypernatremia in hospitalized children. Pediatrics. 1999;104:435–9.

39. Moritz ML, Ayus JC. Prevention of hospital-acquired hyponatremia: A case for using isotonic saline. Pediatrics. 2003;111:227–30.

40. Moritz ML, Ayus JC. Preventing neurological complications from dysnatremias in children. Pediatr Nephrol. 2005;20:1687–700.

41. Armon K, Riordan A, Playfor S, et al. Hyponatraemia and hypokalaemia during intravenous fluid administration. Arch Dis Child. 2008;93:285–7.

42. Hasegawa H, Okubo S, Ikezumi Y, et al. Hyponatremia due to an excess of arginine vasopressin is common in children with febrile disease. Pediatr Nephrol. 2009;24:507–11.

43. Moritz ML, Ayus JC. Disorders of water metabolism in children: Hyponatremia and hypernatremia. Pediatr Rev. 2002;23:371–80.

44. Ayus JC, Achinger SG, Arieff A. Brain cell volume regulation in hyponatremia: Role of sex, age, vasopressin, and hypoxia. Am J Physiol Renal Physiol. 2008;295:F619–24.

45. Szatalowicz VL, Miller PD, Lacher JW, et al. Comparative effect of diuretics on renal water excretion in hyponatraemic oedematous disorders. Clin Sci (Lond). 1982;62:235–8.

46. Kim GH, Lee JW, Oh YK, et al. Antidiuretic effect of hydrochlorothiazide in lithium-induced nephrogenic diabetes insipidus is associated with upregulation of aquaporin-2, Na-Cl co-transporter, and epithelial sodium channel. J Am Soc Nephrol. 2004;15:2836–43.

47. Hsieh S, White PC. Presentation of primary adrenal insufficiency in childhood. J Clin Endocrinol Metab. 2011;96:E925–8.

48. Bettinelli A, Longoni L, Tammaro F, et al. Renal salt-wasting syndrome in children with intracranial disorders. Pediatr Nephrol. 2012;27:733–9.

49. Moritz ML. Syndrome of inappropriate antidiuresis and cerebral salt wasting syndrome: Are they different and does it matter? Pediatr Nephrol. 2012;27:689–93.

50. Hardesty DA, Kilbaugh TJ, Storm PB. Cerebral salt wasting syndrome in post-operative pediatric brain tumor patients. Neurocrit Care. 2012;17:382–7.

51. von BP, Ankermann T, Eggert P, et al. Diagnosis and management of cerebral salt wasting (CSW) in children: The role of atrial natriuretic peptide (ANP) and brain natriuretic peptide (BNP). Childs Nerv Syst. 2006;22:1275–81.

52. Costa KN, Nakamura HM, Cruz LR, et al. Hyponatremia and brain injury: Absence of alterations of serum brain natriuretic peptide and vasopressin. Arq Neuropsiquiatr. 2009;67:1037–44.

53. Bitew S, Imbriano L, Miyawaki N et al. More on renal salt wasting without cerebral disease: Response to saline infusion. Clin J Am Soc Nephrol. 2009;4:309–15.

54. Maesaka JK, Imbriano LJ, Ali NM, Ilamathi E. Is it cerebral or renal salt wasting? Kidney Int. 2009;76:934–8.

55. Maesaka JK, Miyawaki N, Palaia T, et al. Renal salt wasting without cerebral disease: Diagnostic value of urate determinations in hyponatremia. Kidney Int. 2007;71:822–6.

56. Maesaka JK, Gupta S, Fishbane S. Cerebral salt-wasting syndrome: Does it exist? Nephron. 1999;82:100–9.

57. Bartter FC, Schwartz WB. The syndrome of inappropriate secretion of antidiuretic hormone. Am J Med. 1967;42:790–806.

58. Fenske W, Stork S, Blechschmidt A, et al. Copeptin in the differential diagnosis of hyponatremia. J Clin Endocrinol Metab. 2009;94:123–9.

59. Carpentier E, Greenbaum LA, Rochdi D, et al. Identification and characterization of an activating F229V substitution in the V2 vasopressin receptor in an infant with NSIAD. J Am Soc Nephrol. 2012;23:1635–40.

60. Cheung CC, Cadnapaphornchai MA, Ranadive SA, et al. Persistent elevation of urine aquaporin-2 during water loading in a child with nephrogenic syndrome of inappropriate antidiuresis (NSIAD) caused by a R137L mutation in the V2 vasopressin receptor. Int J Pediatr Endocrinol. 2012;2012:3.

61. Rosenthal SM, Feldman BJ, Vargas GA, Gitelman SE. Nephrogenic syndrome of inappropriate antidiuresis (NSIAD): A paradigm for activating mutations causing endocrine dysfunction. Pediatr Endocrinol Rev. 2006;4(Suppl 1):66–70.

62. Tenenbaum J, Ayoub MA, Perkovska S, et al. The constitutively active V2 receptor mutants conferring NSIAD are weakly sensitive to agonist and antagonist regulation. PLoS One. 2009;4:e8383.

63. Bockenhauer D, Penney MD, Hampton D, et al. A family with hyponatremia and the nephrogenic syndrome of inappropriate antidiuresis. Am J Kidney Dis. 2012;59:566–8.

64. Decaux G, Vandergheynst F, Bouko Y, et al. Nephrogenic syndrome of inappropriate antidiuresis in adults: High phenotypic variability in men and women from a large pedigree. J Am Soc Nephrol. 2007;18:606–2.

65. Wang W, Li C, Summer SN, et al. Molecular analysis of impaired urinary diluting capacity in glucocorticoid deficiency. Am J Physiol Renal Physiol. 2006;290:F1135–42.

66. Chen YC, Cadnapaphornchai MA, Yang J, et al. Nonosmotic release of vasopressin and renal aquaporins in impaired urinary dilution in hypothyroidism. Am J Physiol Renal Physiol. 2005;289:F672–8.

67. Hanna FW, Scanlon MF. Hyponatraemia, hypothyroidism, and role of arginine-vasopressin. Lancet. 1997;350:755–6.

68. Matsumoto T, Takeya M, Takuwa S, et al. Suppressed urinary excretion of aquaporin-2 in an infant with primary polydipsia. Pediatr Nephrol. 2000;14:48–52.

69. Dogangun B, Herguner S, Atar M, et al. The treatment of psychogenic polydipsia with risperidone in two children diagnosed with schizophrenia. J Child Adolesc Psychopharmacol. 2006;16:492–5.

70. Cadnapaphornchai MA, Summer SN, Falk S, et al. Effect of primary polydipsia on aquaporin and sodium transporter abundance. Am J Physiol Renal Physiol. 2003;285:F965–71.

71. Bruce RC, Kliegman RM. Hyponatremic seizures secondary to oral water intoxication in infancy: Association with commercial bottled drinking water. Pediatrics. 1997;100:E4.

72. Keating JP, Schears GJ, Dodge PR. Oral water intoxication in infants: An American epidemic. Am J Dis Child. 1991;145:985–90.

73. Partridge JC, Payne ML, Leisgang JJ, et al. Water intoxication secondary to feeding mismanagement: A preventable form of familial seizure disorder in infants. Am J Dis Child. 1981;135:38–41.

74. Crumpacker RW, Kriel RL. Voluntary water intoxication in normal infants. Neurology. 1973;23:1251–5.

75. Moritz ML, Kalantar-Zadeh K, Ayus JC. Ecstasy-associated hyponatremia: Why are women at risk? Nephrol Dial Transplant. 2013;28:2206–9.

76. Fallon JK, Shah D, Kicman AT, et al. Action of MDMA (ecstasy) and its metabolites on arginine vasopressin release. Ann N Y Acad Sci. 2002;965:399–409.

77. Forsling ML, Fallon JK, Shah D, et al. The effect of 3,4-methylenedioxymethamphetamine (MDMA, 'ecstasy') and its metabolites on neurohypophysial hormone release from the isolated rat hypothalamus. Br J Pharmacol. 2002;135:649–56.

78. van Dijken GD, Blom RE, Hene RJ, et al. High incidence of mild hyponatraemia in females using ecstasy at a rave party. Nephrol Dial Transplant. 2013;28:2277–83.

79. Wolff K, Tsapakis EM, Winstock AR, et al. Vasopressin and oxytocin secretion in response to the consumption of ecstasy in a clubbing population. J Psychopharmacol. 2006;20:400–10.

80. Gupta P, Mick G, Fong CT, et al. Hyponatremia secondary to reset osmostat in a child with a central nervous system midline defect and a chromosomal abnormality. J Pediatr Endocrinol Metab. 2000;13:1637–41.

81. Gibbs CJ, Lee HA. Severe hyponatraemia in a quadriplegic. Br J Clin Pract. 1994;48:53–4.

82. Kendler KS, Weitzman RE, Fisher DA. The effect of pain on plasma arginine vasopressin concentrations in man. Clin Endocrinol (Oxf). 1978;8:89–94.

83. Rowe JW, Shelton RL, Helderman JH, et al. Influence of the emetic reflex on vasopressin release in man. Kidney Int. 1979;16:729–35.

84. Chung HM, Kluge R, Schrier RW, Anderson RJ. Postoperative hyponatremia: A prospective study. Arch Intern Med. 1986;146:333–6.

85. Martin PY, Ohara M, Gines P, et al. Nitric oxide synthase (NOS) inhibition for one week improves renal sodium and water excretion in cirrhotic rats with ascites. J Clin Invest. 1998;101:235–42.

86. Anderson RJ, Cadnapaphornchai P, Harbottle JA, et al. Mechanism of effect of thoracic inferior vena-cava constriction on renal water excretion. J Clin Invest. 1974;54:1473–9.

87. Ishikawa S, Saito T, Okada K, et al. Effect of vasopressin antagonist on water excretion in inferior vena cava constriction. Kidney Int. 1986;30:49–55.

88. Claria J, Jimenez W, Arroyo V, et al. Blockade of the hydroosmotic effect of vasopressin normalizes water excretion in cirrhotic rats. Gastroenterology. 1989;97:1294–9.

89. Verbalis JG. Brain volume regulation in response to changes in osmolality. Neuroscience 2010;168:862–70.

90. Sterns RH, Riggs JE, Schochet SS, Jr. Osmotic demyelination syndrome following correction of hyponatremia. N Engl J Med. 1986;314:1535–42.

91. Adrogue HJ, Madias NE. The challenge of hyponatremia. J Am Soc Nephrol. 2012;23:1140–8.

92. Moritz ML, Ayus JC. The pathophysiology and treatment of hyponatraemic encephalopathy: An update. Nephrol Dial Transplant. 2003;18:2486–91.

93. Verbalis JG, Goldsmith SR, Greenberg A, et al. Diagnosis, evaluation, and treatment of hyponatremia: Expert panel recommendations. Am J Med. 2013;126(Suppl 1):S1–42.

94. Sterns RH, Hix JK, Silver S. Treating profound hyponatremia: A strategy for controlled correction. Am J Kidney Dis. 2010;56:774–9.

95. Decaux G, Unger J, Brimioulle S, Mockel J. Hyponatremia in the syndrome of inappropriate secretion of antidiuretic hormone: Rapid correction with urea, sodium chloride, and water restriction therapy. JAMA. 1982;247:471–4.

96. Schrier RW, Gross P, Gheorghiade M, et al. Tolvaptan, a selective oral vasopressin V2-receptor antagonist, for hyponatremia. N Engl J Med. 2006;355:2099–112.

97. Verbalis JG, Adler S, Schrier RW, et al. Efficacy and safety of oral tolvaptan therapy in patients with the syndrome of inappropriate antidiuretic hormone secretion. Eur J Endocrinol. 2011;164:725–32.

98. Goldman MB. The assessment and treatment of water imbalance in patients with psychosis. Clin Schizophr Relat Psychoses. 2010;4:115–23.

99. Torres VE, Chapman AB, Devuyst O, et al. Tolvaptan in patients with autosomal dominant polycystic kidney disease. N Engl J Med. 2012;367:2407–18.

100. Eke F, Nte A. A prospective clinical study of patients with hypernatraemic dehydration. Afr J Med Med Sci. 1996;25:209–12.

101. Guarner J, Hochman J, Kurbatova E, Mullins R. Study of outcomes associated with hyponatremia and hypernatremia in children. Pediatr Dev Pathol. 2011;14:117–23.

102. Forman S, Crofton P, Huang H, et al. The epidemiology of hypernatraemia in hospitalised children in Lothian: A 10-year study showing differences between dehydration, osmoregulatory dysfunction and salt poisoning. Arch Dis Child. 2012;97:502–7.

103. Bichet DG. Genetics and diagnosis of central diabetes insipidus. Ann Endocrinol (Paris). 2012;73:117–27.

104. Ghirardello S, Garre ML, Rossi A, Maghnie M. The diagnosis of children with central diabetes insipidus. J Pediatr Endocrinol Metab. 2007;20:359–75.

105. Bichet DG. V2R mutations and nephrogenic diabetes insipidus. Prog Mol Biol Transl Sci. 2009;89:15–29.

106. Marples D, Frokiaer J, Dorup J, et al. Hypokalemia-induced downregulation of aquaporin-2 water channel expression in rat kidney medulla and cortex. J Clin Invest. 1996;97:1960–8.

107. Earm JH, Christensen BM, Frokiaer J, et al. Decreased aquaporin-2 expression and apical plasma membrane delivery in kidney collecting ducts of polyuric hypercalcemic rats. J Am Soc Nephrol. 1998;9:2181–93.

108. Wang W, Li C, Kwon TH, et al. AQP3, p-AQP2, and AQP2 expression is reduced in polyuric rats with hypercalcemia: Prevention by cAMP-PDE inhibitors. Am J Physiol Renal Physiol. 2002;283:F1313–25.

109. Frokiaer J, Christensen BM, Marples D, et al. Downregulation of aquaporin-2 parallels changes in renal water excretion in unilateral ureteral obstruction. Am J Physiol. 1997;273:F213–23.

110. Shi Y, Li C, Thomsen K, et al. Neonatal ureteral obstruction alters expression of renal sodium transporters and aquaporin water channels. Kidney Int. 2004;66:203–15.

111. Marples D, Christensen S, Christensen EI, et al. Lithium-induced downregulation of aquaporin-2 water channel expression in rat kidney medulla. J Clin Invest. 1995;95:1838–45.

112. Bockenhauer D, Bichet DG. Inherited secondary nephrogenic diabetes insipidus: Concentrating on humans. Am J Physiol Renal Physiol. 2013;304:F1037–42.

113. Bockenhauer D, van't HW, Dattani M, et al. Secondary nephrogenic diabetes insipidus as a complication of inherited renal diseases. Nephron Physiol. 2010;116:23–9.

114. Linnanvuo-Laitinen M, Pirttiaho H, Simila S, Lautala P. [Familial nephrogenic diabetes insipidus and mental retardation]. Duodecim. 1985;101:778–82.

115. Schofer O, Beetz R, Bohl J, et al. Mental retardation syndrome with renal concentration deficiency and intracerebral calcification. Eur J Pediatr. 1990;149:470–4.

116. Brooks BS, el GT, Allison JD, Hoffman WH. Frequency and variation of the posterior pituitary bright signal on MR images. AJNR Am J Neuroradiol. 1989;10:943–8.

117. Mootha SL, Barkovich AJ, Grumbach MM, et al. Idiopathic hypothalamic diabetes insipidus, pituitary stalk thickening, and the occult intracranial germinoma in children and adolescents. J Clin Endocrinol Metab. 1997;82:1362–7.

118. Cesar KR, Magaldi AJ. Thiazide induces water absorption in the inner medullary collecting duct of normal and Brattleboro rats. Am J Physiol. 1999;277:F756–60.

119. Pedersen RS, Bentzen H, Bech JN, Pedersen EB. Effect of an acute oral ibuprofen intake on urinary aquaporin-2 excretion in healthy humans. Scand J Clin Lab Invest. 2001;61:631–40.

120. Bernier V, Lagace M, Lonergan M, et al. Functional rescue of the constitutively internalized V2 vasopressin receptor mutant R137H by the pharmacological chaperone action of SR49059. Mol Endocrinol. 2004;18:2074–84.

121. Morello JP, Salahpour A, Laperriere A, et al. Pharmacological chaperones rescue cell-surface expression and function of misfolded V2 vasopressin receptor mutants. J Clin Invest. 2000;105:887–95.

122. Christensen BM, Marples D, Kim YH, et al. Changes in cellular composition of kidney collecting duct cells in rats with lithium-induced NDI. Am J Physiol Cell Physiol. 2004;286:C952–64.

123. Christensen BM, Kim YH, Kwon TH, Nielsen S. Lithium treatment induces a marked proliferation of primarily principal cells in rat kidney inner medullary collecting duct. Am J Physiol Renal Physiol. 2006;291:F39–48.

124. Kwon TH, Laursen UH, Marples D, et al. Altered expression of renal AQPs and Na(+) transporters in rats with lithium-induced NDI. Am J Physiol Renal Physiol. 2000;279:F552–64.

125. Frohlich O, Aggarwal D, Klein JD, et al. Stimulation of UT-A1-mediated transepithelial urea flux in MDCK cells by lithium. Am J Physiol Renal Physiol. 2008;294:F518–24.

126. Klein JD, Gunn RB, Roberts BR, Sands JM. Down-regulation of urea transporters in the renal inner medulla of lithium-fed rats. Kidney Int. 2002;61:995–1002.

127. Batlle DC, von Riotte AB, Gaviria M, Grupp M. Amelioration of polyuria by amiloride in patients receiving long-term lithium therapy. N Engl J Med. 1985;312:408–14.

128. Sands JM, Naruse M, Jacobs JD, et al. Changes in aquaporin-2 protein contribute to the urine concentrating defect in rats fed a low-protein diet. J Clin Invest. 1996;97:2807–14.

129. Frokiaer J, Marples D, Knepper MA, Nielsen S. Bilateral ureteral obstruction downregulates expression of vasopressin-sensitive AQP-2 water channel in rat kidney. Am J Physiol. 1996;270:F657–68.

130. Li C, Klein JD, Wang W, et al. Altered expression of urea transporters in response to ureteral obstruction. Am J Physiol Renal Physiol. 2004;286:F1154–62.

131. Klein JD. Expression of urea transporters and their regulation. Subcell Biochem. 2014;73:79–107.

132. Oddie SJ, Craven V, Deakin K, et al. Severe neonatal hypernatraemia: A population based study. Arch Dis Child Fetal Neonatal Ed. 2013;98:F384–7.

133. Moritz ML, Manole MD, Bogen DL, Ayus JC. Breastfeeding-associated hypernatremia: Are we missing the diagnosis? Pediatrics. 2005;116:e343–7.

134. Dine MS, McGovern ME. Intentional poisoning of children—an overlooked category of child abuse: Report of seven cases and review of the literature. Pediatrics. 1982;70:32–5.

135. Rosenfeld W, deRomana GL, Kleinman R, Finberg L. Improving the clinical management of hypernatremic dehydration: Observations from a study of 67 infants with this disorder. Clin Pediatr (Phila). 1977;16:411–7.

## REVIEW QUESTIONS

1. A 3-month-old male infant presents with seizures. He is euvolemic on examination. Initial laboratory studies include serum sodium of 118 mEq/L with serum osmolality 240 mOsm/kg $H_2O$ and urine osmolality 85 mOsm/kg $H_2O$. Further investigation should be directed toward:
   a. Family history of diabetes insipidus
   b. Home preparation of infant formula
   c. Central nervous system infection as a cause of SIADH
   d. History of sustained fever with increased insensible losses

2. A teenage male patient presents with altered mental status and is found to have a cerebrospinal fluid specimen positive for herpes simplex virus by polymerase chain reaction. He is mildly volume depleted and hypernatremic on admission. What is the most likely cause of his hypernatremia?
   a. Table salt ingestion
   b. Poor fluid intake related to altered mental status
   c. Nephrogenic diabetes insipidus
   d. Surreptitious diuretic use

3. After a few days the patient described in question 2 returns to his usual diet. He then develops hyponatremia with serum sodium of 125 mEq/L, SOsm 258 mOsm/kg $H_2O$, and UOsm 300 mOsm/kg $H_2O$. He is clinically euvolemic. He most likely has:
   a. Primary polydipsia related to increased thirst from hypothalamic dysfunction
   b. Pseudohyponatremia
   c. Central diabetes insipidus
   d. SIADH

4. A 4-week old male infant is admitted with hypovolemia, failure to thrive, and chronic irritability. He is hypernatremic (serum sodium of 159 mEq/L) with UOsm 50 mOsm/kg $H_2O$. The most likely cause of his hypernatremia is:
   a. Child abuse with chronic fluid deprivation
   b. Chronic diarrhea
   c. Nephrogenic diabetes insipidus
   d. Chronic vomiting

5. A 6-month-old male infant with known congenital X-linked nephrogenic diabetes insipidus has been vomiting everything he eats or drinks for the past 36 hours. On presentation, his weight is decreased 1 kg from baseline. His is afebrile with heart rate 165 bpm and capillary refill 4 seconds. Which of the following parenteral fluid therapies is most appropriate at this time?
   a. Fluid bolus with normal saline
   b. Fluid bolus with D5W
   c. D5 0.5 NS at maintenance rate
   d. D5 0.2 NS at maintenance rate

6. A 16-year-old female patient presents to the adolescent medicine clinic with fatigue and recent-onset headache. She is mildly volume depleted with weight stable from 1 month ago at 37 kg. Laboratory tests reveal serum sodium of 122 mEq/L, SOsm 250 mOsm/kg $H_2O$, urine chloride 47 mEq/L, and UNa 55 mEq/L. The most likely cause of her hyponatremia is:
   a. Surreptitious diuretic use
   b. Chronic laxative abuse
   c. Bulimia with chronic vomiting
   d. Primary polydipsia as a means to reduce hunger

7. A 3-year-old girl undergoes a water deprivation test for polyuria and polydipsia. Over the course of a 6-hour test, serum sodium increases from 139 to 142 mEq/L, and UOsm changes from 250 mOsm/kg $H_2O$ to 850 mOsm/kg $H_2O$. The most likely cause of the polyuria is:
   a. Primary polydipsia
   b. Nephrogenic diabetes insipidus
   c. Partial nephrogenic diabetes insipidus
   d. Central diabetes insipidus

8. A 3-year-old boy undergoes a water deprivation test for polyuria and polydipsia. Over the course of a 6-hour test, serum sodium increases from 142 to 148 mEq/L, whereas UOsm remains lower than 100 mOsm/kg $H_2O$. dDAVP is administered and UOsm increases to 850 mOsm/kg $H_2O$. The most likely cause of the polyuria is:
   a. Primary polydipsia
   b. Nephrogenic diabetes insipidus
   c. Partial nephrogenic diabetes insipidus
   d. Central diabetes insipidus

9. A 12-month-old boy presents with hyponatremic seizures. He is euvolemic. The following treatment should be provided now:
   a. Hypertonic saline
   b. Fluid restriction
   c. Conivaptan
   d. Normal saline bolus

10. A 12-month-old boy presents with hypernatremic dehydration with associated seizures. Serum sodium is 162 mEq/L. Following fluid resuscitation, his fluid management plan should include:
   a. Administer normal saline because this has a lower concentration than the current serum sodium.
   b. Provide maintenance parenteral fluid support.
   c. Calculate and correct the free water deficit while providing additional support for maintenance and ongoing losses.
   d. Administer D5 0.2 NS at maintenance.

## ANSWER KEY

1. b
2. b
3. d
4. c
5. a
6. a
7. a
8. d
9. a
10. c

# Nephrotic syndrome

MICHELLE N. RHEAULT

Nephrotic syndrome (NS) is one of the most common glomerular disorders of childhood. It is characterized by proteinuria that is severe enough to cause hypoalbuminemia and edema. The first description of a nephrotic child was published in 1484, when Cornelius Roelans of Belgium described "swelling of the whole body of the child" as one of 52 common diseases of children.[1] Almost 250 years later, the kidney tubules were implicated in the pathogenesis of NS by Theodore Zwinger, who also described deterioration of renal function in some patients.[1,2] Richard Bright described NS in more detail in his classic text from 1827: however, the term "nephrotic syndrome" was not coined until 1929, in the writings of Henry Christian from Boston.[3,4] Outcomes for children with NS were uniformly poor before the introduction of antibiotics in the 1930s, with mortality rates of approximately 67%.[5] With widespread use of sulfonamides and penicillin to treat NS-associated infections, mortality dropped to 35% by 1950.[5] The watershed moment in the history of NS was the introduction of steroids for the treatment of this disorder in the 1950s, which led to clinical remission in a majority of treated patients and a drop in mortality to 9% by 1960.[5]

## DEFINITIONS AND CLASSIFICATION

NS is a clinical description of a constellation of findings that can be caused by a large number of underlying primary and secondary disorders. The International Study of Kidney Disease in Children (ISKDC) defined NS as massive proteinuria (greater than 40 mg/m$^2$/h, or 1000 mg/m$^2$/24 h) leading to hypoalbuminemia (less than 2.5 g/dL), edema, and hyperlipidemia.[6] The urine protein-to-creatinine ratio greater than 2 also correlates well with nephrotic range or massive proteinuria. There are many ways to categorize patients with NS, including by age at presentation, by kidney pathologic features, and by clinical response to corticosteroid therapy. Presentation of NS at less than 3 months of age is termed congenital NS and is often caused by congenital infections or mutations in various podocyte proteins such as nephrin.[7,8] Infantile NS is defined as clinical presentation between 3 months and 1 year of age and often has a genetic basis as well (see Chapter 18). Childhood NS accounts for the majority of patients with NS and is defined as presentation between 1 and 18 years of age.

Children with NS can also be categorized by underlying renal pathologic features. Minimal change NS (MCNS) is the most common histopathologic finding in children with NS (Figure 16.1).[6] Kidney biopsy specimens from patients with MCNS have a normal appearance by light microscopy.[9] By electron microscopy, broadening and retraction of podocyte foot processes ("effacement") are evident. Foot process effacement is the hallmark pathologic finding in NS and is present in most, but not all, affected patients.[10,11] In addition to podocyte effacement by electron microscopy, biopsy samples from children with focal segmental glomerulosclerosis (FSGS) demonstrate light microscopic findings of segmental hyalinosis and sclerosis within some glomeruli or segmental glomerular collapse.[12] Other pathologic

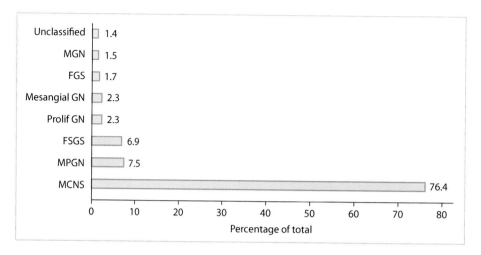

**Figure 16.1** Distribution of renal disorders in 521 children undergoing renal biopsy for diagnosis of nephrotic syndrome. FGS, focal global sclerosis; FSGS, focal segmental glomerulosclerosis; MCNS, minimal change nephrotic syndrome; mesangial GN, mesangial proliferative glomerulonephritis; MGN, membranous glomerulonephritis; MPGN, membrano-proliferative glomerulonephritis; prolif GN, proliferative glomerulonephritis. (Data from International Study of Kidney Disease in Children. Nephrotic syndrome in children: prediction of histopathology from clinical and laboratory characteristics at time of diagnosis. Kidney Int. 1978;13:159–65.)

findings in children with NS can include membranous nephropathy, diffuse mesangial sclerosis, World Health Organization class V lupus nephritis, immunoglobulin A (IgA) nephropathy, Henoch-Schönlein purpura nephritis, membranoproliferative glomerulonephritis, or mesangial proliferative glomerulonephritis (see individual chapters on these disorders).[13] Clinical response to corticosteroids has long been used as a means to classify children with NS because it predicts pathologic findings and long-term renal outcome.[6,14] Achievement of remission in response to corticosteroid therapy requires a marked reduction in urine protein to less than 4 mg/m²/h or urine dipstick of 0 to trace protein for 3 consecutive days with resolution of edema. Terms used for clinical subclassification of NS are as follows:

***Relapse:*** Relapse of NS is defined as recurrence of severe proteinuria (greater than 40 mg/m²/h or urine protein dipstick 2+ or more for 3 consecutive days), often with recurrence of edema.[6]

***Steroid-sensitive NS (SSNS):*** SSNS is defined as complete remission in response to corticosteroid therapy alone. SSNS suggests MCNS on histopathologic examination; 93.7% of steroid-sensitive children up to 6 years of age and 85.7% of steroid-sensitive children between 7 and 16 years of age demonstrate this lesion on kidney biopsy.[6] MCNS generally predicts excellent long-term renal outcome.

***Steroid-dependent NS (SDNS):*** Some children who initially respond to steroids experience a relapse while still receiving steroids or within 2 weeks of discontinuation of treatment and are classified as having SDNS.

***Frequently relapsing NS (FRNS):*** Finally, children who develop more than four relapses in 12 months are classified as having FRNS. Children with SDNS and FRNS may have significant complications from prolonged corticosteroid therapy and may require treatment with other immunosuppressive agents.

***Steroid-resistant NS (SRNS):*** Children with SRNS do not achieve remission despite 4 to 8 weeks of high-dose corticosteroid therapy.[15,16] Approximately 75% of children with SRNS have FSGS lesions on renal biopsy.[17] Failure to achieve remission with steroid therapy is a poor prognostic sign, and alternate therapies such as cyclosporine, mycophenolate, rituximab, and renin-angiotensin system blockade are often tried. No remission in response to any therapy in children with FSGS is associated with only a 47% renal survival at 3 years after presentation, whereas a partial remission (defined as a more than 50% reduction in proteinuria) is a favorable prognostic sign and is associated with 92% renal survival at 3 years.[18]

---

**KEY POINT**

---

SSNS is suggestive of MCNS on histopathologic examination and carries a good prognosis. Children younger than 6 years of age are more likely to have SSNS and MCNS than are older children.

## EPIDEMIOLOGY

The prevalence of NS is estimated at approximately 16 cases per 100,000 children.[19,20] The annual incidence of NS has been estimated to range from 2 to 7 new cases per 100,000 children.[20–23] Whereas the overall incidence of NS appears to be stable, there is some evidence that the histopathologic pattern may be evolving, with more children demonstrating FSGS and fewer demonstrating MCNS, although the underlying reason for this shift is unclear.[21,24–27] In younger children with NS, boys outnumber girls by 2:1, but this gender disparity is not present in adolescents and adults, in whom the incidence among male and female patients is equal.[28]

## Ethnic distribution

Ethnic, geographic, and racial differences in the incidence and histologic patterns in children with NS have been well characterized. In the United Kingdom, South Asian children have a more than fivefold higher incidence of NS than do white children.[22,29] NS appears to be less common among children in Africa; however, when it is present, FSGS lesions are more likely to be found on kidney biopsy.[30–32] NS in children in Sub-Saharan Africa may be more often caused by infections such as human immunodeficiency virus (HIV) infection, hepatitis B, and malaria, and NS is less likely to be steroid responsive than childhood NS in the United States or Europe.[33–35] In the United States, the distribution of NS tends to follow the racial and ethnic distribution of the surrounding community, although some population studies suggest a higher incidence of NS in African Americans.[21,24,36] African-American children presenting with NS are more likely to have SRNS and more rapid progression to end-stage kidney disease.[21,36,37] Biopsy studies have shown increased risk of FSGS in African Americans, with 44% to 47% of children presenting with NS demonstrating FSGS on kidney biopsy compared with 17% to 18% of white children.[21,24] African Americans with SRNS or FSGS are also less like to have an underlying genetic cause for their disease.[38] Sequence variants within the *APOL1* gene encoding apolipoprotein L1 were demonstrated to account for a large fraction of observed increased FSGS risk in African Americans.[39,40] The mechanism by which variants in *APOL1* contribute to increased risk of FSGS is unknown; *APOL1* is expressed in podocytes, and alterations in intrinsic podocyte function may be responsible.[41,42]

## Age at presentation

The peak age of presentation of NS is 2 years, with approximately 60% to 70% of cases occurring in children less than 6 years old.[6,21] The age of initial presentation of NS is also an important predictor of histopathologic features and steroid responsiveness. In seminal reports from the ISKDC, MCNS was diagnosed in 87% of children presenting with NS at less than 6 years of age.[6] In the same study, the median age of diagnosis in patients with MCNS was 3 years, compared with 6 years for FSGS and 10 years for MPGN.[6] Thus, younger children with NS are more likely to have MCNS on biopsy, whereas older children are more

likely to have a less favorable diagnosis of FSGS. Younger children are also more likely to respond to steroids, with 86% of children younger than 6 years of age going into remission compared with 60% of children older than 6 years of age.[6]

## PATHOPHYSIOLOGY OF EDEMA FORMATION

Edema, a state of total body sodium and water excess, is the most common presenting sign of NS and is the result of fluid accumulation in the interstitial space. The pathophysiology of edema formation in nephrotic patients has been studied and debated for almost 100 years.[43] There are two conflicting hypotheses to account for sodium and water retention in nephrotic patients: the "underfill" hypothesis and the "overfill" hypothesis. Both hypotheses are supported by clinical and experimental evidence, and in fact, it is likely that both mechanisms contribute to edema formation in individual patients at varying times in their disease course.[44]

## UNDERFILL HYPOTHESIS

The underfill hypothesis suggests that hypoalbuminemia and the resultant decreased plasma oncotic pressure lead to leakage of fluid from the intravascular to the interstitial space and cause hypovolemia, renal hypoperfusion, activation of the renin-angiotensin-aldosterone system and vasopressin release, and secondary renal sodium and fluid retention. Hypoalbuminemia leads to edema by altering the Starling forces that govern the movement of fluid in the peripheral capillaries.[45]. Briefly, the net movement of fluid between the capillary and the interstitial space compartments represents the algebraic sum of net outward hydrostatic pressure minus net inward oncotic pressure. Tissue oncotic pressure, although a smaller component in the Starling forces, provides an additional mechanism that promotes capillary fluid movement into the interstitial space. As shown in Figure 16.2, net hydrostatic pressure in healthy persons exceeds the oncotic pressure at the arterial end of the capillary and favors movement of capillary fluid into the interstitial space. This constant, slow leak of plasma water into the interstitial space is appropriate and necessary to provide substrate for cells not adjacent to the blood vessel. By the time blood flow reaches the venous end of the capillary bed, hydrostatic pressure decreases to venous pressure levels. Additionally, because of the fluid extravasation, capillary oncotic pressure increases slightly. The net pressure at the venous end of the capillary relationship favors movement of fluid back into the vascular space. However, not all the excess interstitial fluid is removed back into the capillary space, but is eventually removed by lymphatic drainage and returned back into the circulation.

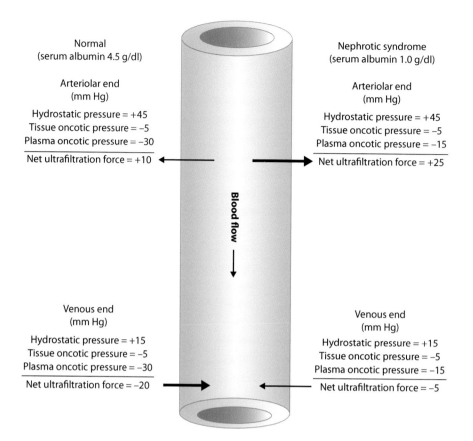

Figure 16.2 Starling forces in the peripheral capillaries that determine the development of edema. The left side depicts normal oncotic and hydrostatic pressure dynamics, and the right side depicts the hypoalbuminemic state, such as nephrotic syndrome. Decreased capillary oncotic pressure resulting from hypoalbuminemia creates a greater net force (+25 mm Hg) across the arterial end of the capillary wall that allows transudation of fluid from the capillary. The net force generated at the venous end of the capillary that favors passage of fluid back into the capillary from the interstitial space is also lower in the nephrotic state, as compared with the normal condition (−5 mm Hg versus −20 mm Hg).

In NS, hypoalbuminemia results in a decrease in the capillary oncotic pressure, whereas capillary hydrostatic pressure remains unchanged, increasing the net driving force for fluid to move out of the capillary into the interstitial space. Furthermore, the net driving force that facilitates flow of fluid from the interstitial space into the venous end of the capillary is also diminished; consequently, less of the interstitial fluid returns to the capillary (see Figure 16.2), and edema formation results. Additionally, low circulating intravascular volume stimulates neurohumoral compensatory mechanisms in an attempt to replenish intravascular volume, including the sympathetic nervous system, the renin-angiotensin-aldosterone system, and vasopressin. In summary, hypoalbuminemia induces movement of fluid from the capillary space into the interstitial space and resultant edema formation.

Clinical evidence to support the underfill hypothesis includes high renin and aldosterone levels and low fractional excretion of sodium in NS, particularly in patients with severe hypoalbuminemia and MCNS.[46–48] Further support comes from studies demonstrating high basal vasopressin levels in patients with NS that can be suppressed by albumin loading, a finding suggesting that hypovolemia is a stimulus for vasopressin release and free water retention in this setting.[49,50] However, these findings are not consistent among all patients with NS, and some studies demonstrate normal or expanded blood volumes with suppressed renin values in these patients.[51,52] In addition, the initial oncotic pressure gradient that develops in response to acute hypoalbuminemia is lost over time because of a parallel decrease in interstitial oncotic pressure.[53,54] Incongruously, some patients and animal models with analbuminemia do not typically develop severe edema, a finding suggesting that hypoalbuminemia alone does not account for edema in nephrotic patients.[55,56] Evidence against a primary role of the renin-angiotensin-aldosterone system in driving sodium and fluid retention comes from studies showing minimal effect on edema and sodium excretion in nephrotic patients treated with angiotensin-converting enzyme (ACE) inhibition or aldosterone blockade.[57–59] Further evidence against the underfill hypothesis was generated in an elegant rat model whereby NS was induced in one kidney while normal contralateral kidney function was maintained.[60] These experiments demonstrated sodium retention in only the nephrotic kidney and pointed to an intrinsic renal mechanism for sodium retention, rather than systemic effects.[60]

## OVERFILL HYPOTHESIS

The alternate overfill hypothesis suggests that patients with NS have primary increased sodium reabsorption with resultant expanded circulatory blood volume and suppression of the renin-angiotensin-aldosterone system.[44] Some studies demonstrate increased expression and apical targeting of the epithelial sodium channel, ENaC, with increased sodium-potassium–adenosine triphosphatase (Na-K-ATPase) activity in the cortical collecting duct in nephrotic animals.[61–64] Modification of extracellular loops of ENaC by urine proteinases such as plasmin that are filtered by the nephrotic kidney activates ENaC and leads to sodium reabsorption.[65] This finding implies that proteinuria itself contributes to sodium retention by ENaC activation. In support of this hypothesis, urine from nephrotic patients, including children, demonstrates elevated plasmin levels that can activate ENaC in vitro.[66,67] Blockade of ENaC with amiloride, a competitive inhibitor, leads to increased sodium excretion.[66,68] Critics of the overfill hypothesis point to studies demonstrating low plasma volume, elevated plasma renin, and a natriuretic response to spironolactone in patients with NS and propose that overfill is more common in animal models of NS than in humans.[69] In addition, the clinical use of amiloride in nephrotic patients demonstrates only a mild diuretic effect.[70]

Clinically, it is important to distinguish whether an individual nephrotic patient is "underfilled" or "overfilled" because this influences management of the edema. Physical examination with particular emphasis on perfusion, pulse, and orthostatic blood pressures may help clarify volume status. Chest x-ray studies may also be useful to evaluate pulmonary vasculature for evidence of intravascular volume overload. It has also been suggested that patients with a fractional excretion of sodium that is lower than 1% and high relative urinary potassium excretion $[U_K/(U_K + U_{Na})]$ of higher than 60% are more likely to have low intravascular volume and that these tests correlate with elevated renin, aldosterone, norepinephrine, and vasopressin levels.[47,71] A fractional excretion of sodium of 0.2% or more identifies volume expanded nephrotic patients.[72]

## CLINICAL APPROACH

In a child with periorbital or generalized edema, a dipstick urinalysis demonstrating 3 to 4+ protein is sufficient to make a preliminary diagnosis of NS. Edema is generally seen in dependent parts of the body, such as ankles, but it can also be seen in the areas with low tissue resistance, such as the eyelids, scrotum, and labia. Periorbital swelling in the morning on awakening and ankle swelling later in the day for ambulating children are common. Scrotal, labial, and penile edema can result in significant discomfort and excoriation of skin in these areas (Figure 16.3). NS should be confirmed by a urine protein-to-creatinine ratio greater than 2 (mg/mg), a serum albumin concentration less than 2.5 g/dL, and the presence of hypercholesterolemia. Once the diagnosis of NS has been established, a thorough investigation for a possible cause must then be undertaken.

## CLINICAL HISTORY AND PHYSICAL EXAMINATION

The clinical history and physical examination should focus on determining whether secondary causes of NS are likely to be present (Table 16.1). A thorough medication exposure

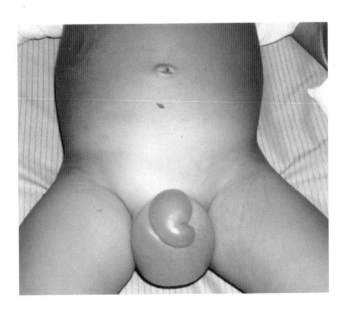

Figure 16.3 Severe scrotal and penile edema in a child with minimal change nephrotic syndrome.

Table 16.1 Causes of Nephrotic Syndrome in Children

| Age at presentation | Causes |
|---|---|
| **Congenital nephrotic syndrome (age <3 mo)** | **Primary**<br>Genetic: *NPHS1, NPHS2, WT1, LAMB2* (Laminin β2, Pierson syndrome), *PLCE1, COQ6, ARHGDIA*<br><br>**Secondary**<br>Infections: syphilis, toxoplasmosis, CMV, HIV, malaria, rubella, hepatitis B<br>Maternal lupus<br>Antenatal membranous nephropathy secondary to anti–neutral endopeptidase antibodies |
| **Infantile nephrotic syndrome (age 3–12 mo)** | **Primary**<br>Genetic: *NPHS1, NPHS2, WT1, LAMB2, PLCE1, COQ6, LMX1B* (nail-patella syndrome)<br>MCNS<br>Galloway-Mowat syndrome<br>Idiopathic conditions |
| **Childhood nephrotic syndrome (age >1 yr)** | **Primary**<br>MCNS<br>FSGS<br>Idiopathic conditions<br>Mutations in *NPHS2, INF2, ACTN4, TRPC6, LMX1B, CD2AP, MYO1E, PTPRO, WT1, COQ6, MYH9*<br>Mesangial proliferative glomerulonephritis (IgM nephropathy, C1q nephropathy)<br>MPGN<br>Membranous nephropathy<br><br>**Secondary**<br>Systemic disease<br>  Henoch-Schönlein purpura<br>  IgA nephropathy<br>  Systemic lupus erythematosus<br>  LCAT deficiency<br>Infections<br>  Hepatitis B and C<br>  HIV<br>  Parvovirus B19<br>Malignancy<br>  Leukemia<br>  Lymphoma (particularly Hodgkin disease)<br>Medications/toxins<br>  Nonsteroidal anti-inflammatory drugs<br>  Penicillamine<br>  Captopril<br>  Tiopronin<br>  Mercury<br>  Pregnancy |

*Abbreviations:* CMV, cytomegalovirus; FSGS, focal segmental glomerulosclerosis; HIV, human immunodeficiency virus; IgA, immunoglobulin A; IgM, immunoglobulin M; LCAT, lecithin cholesterol acyltransferase; MCNS, minimal change nephrotic syndrome; MPGN, membranoproliferative glomerulonephritis.

history is necessary because medications such as nonsteroidal anti-inflammatory drugs, captopril, and penicillamine have been shown to cause NS.[73-75] Risk factors and exposure to hepatitis B, hepatitis C, and HIV should be explored. Joint pain and swelling may be signs of systemic lupus erythematosus or Henoch-Schönlein purpura if a lower extremity purpuric rash is present. A history of gross hematuria may be associated with glomerulonephritis (membranoproliferative glomerulonephritis, IgA nephropathy, mesangial proliferative glomerulonephritis). Easy bruising, fatigue, weight loss, or night sweats may suggest a malignant disease. Cough or difficulty breathing may be a symptom of pleural effusion or pulmonary edema resulting from fluid overload. Menstrual history should be obtained in adolescent girls because Frasier syndrome, *WT1* mutations with 46XY gonadal dysgenesis, can be associated with FSGS and primary amenorrhea. Finally, the possibility of pregnancy should be entertained in postpubertal female patients. A careful family history should be obtained to determine whether any family members are known to have proteinuria or have required kidney dialysis or kidney transplantation to suggest familial NS.

Vital signs including blood pressure and weight should be obtained in all patients with NS. Hypertension is less common in children with MCNS than in those with other diagnoses.[13] Children should be carefully examined to determine the extent of edema, including an abdominal examination for ascites, the presence of periorbital and peripheral edema, and a genitourinary examination to evaluate for scrotal edema.

## INVESTIGATIONS

Recommendations for laboratory studies at initial presentation are listed in Table 16.2.[76] A urinalysis is recommended to confirm proteinuria and for identification of significant hematuria or casts that may represent nephritis rather than primary NS. Hematuria is not always associated with nephritis, however, because microscopic hematuria can be demonstrated in 23% of children with MCNS and in 48% of children with FSGS.[13] Hypocomplementemia should prompt a kidney biopsy for evaluation for membranoproliferative glomerulonephritis or systemic lupus erythematosus. Additional screening studies for viral causes of NS such as parvovirus infection, hepatitis B, hepatitis C, and HIV infection should be considered in at-risk populations. Cytopenias on a complete blood count may suggest systemic lupus erythematosus, parvovirus B19 infection, or malignant disease. In anticipation of immunosuppressive treatment, placement of a PPD (purified protein derivative) or blood testing for tuberculosis with a quantiFERON-TB Gold test (Quest Diagnostics, Madison, NJ) should be considered for high-risk populations.[76,77] Finally, testing for immunity to varicella with varicella immunoglobulin G (IgG) titer is

Table 16.2 Initial evaluation of a child with nephrotic syndrome

**General Tests**

Urinalysis

First morning urine protein to creatinineratio

Serum electrolytes

BUN, creatinine

Serum albumin

Serum complement 3 (C3)

Complete blood count

Cholesterol level

PPD or serum screening for tuberculosis

Varicella titer

**Tests for Selected Populations**

ANA: if any systemic signs of lupus, if C3 is low, if age 10 yr or older

Hepatitis B, hepatitis C, HIV: if high risk or history of exposure

Parvovirus B19: if characteristic rash present, patient is anemic, or history of exposure

Kidney biopsy: if age 12 yr or older

Genetic testing: if family history of nephrotic syndrome or FSGS

*Abbreviations:* ANA, antinuclear antibody; BUN, blood urea nitrogen; FSGS, focal segmental glomerulosclerosis; HIV, human immunodeficiency virus; PPD, purified protein derivative.

recommended. Varicella exposure in a previously varicella-naïve patient should prompt treatment with varicella-zoster immunoglobulin within 96 h of exposure because varicella can be life-threatening in this population.[78] A renal ultrasound examination is not necessary in patients with an initial presentation of NS. However, gross hematuria in a nephrotic patient should prompt renal ultrasound with Doppler studies to evaluate for renal vein thrombosis.

### KEY POINT

Children with NS should have a thorough history and physical examination performed, as well as limited laboratory screening to evaluate for secondary causes of NS.

## KIDNEY BIOPSY

Most young children with NS are steroid responsive and do not require a kidney biopsy because it is overwhelmingly likely that they will have MCNS on histopathologic examination.[13] An initial trial of steroids at 2 mg/kg/day for 6 weeks is recommended, with biopsy reserved for steroid-resistant patients. Kidney biopsy is also recommended for children older than 12 years of age because it is more likely that they will demonstrate pathologic features other than MCNS.[76] Finally, kidney biopsy should be considered in patients with atypical features, including age less than 1 year, gross hematuria, hypocomplementemia, or a suspected viral or malignant cause.

---

## KEY POINTS

Clinical characteristics of MCNS are:

- Usual age of presentation: 2 to 6 years
- Absence of hypertension
- Normal renal function
- No gross hematuria, possible mild microscopic hematuria
- Normal complement profile
- Good response to corticosteroids, usually in 2 weeks

---

## COMPLICATIONS

## THROMBOEMBOLISM

Thromboembolism is a rare, but potentially life-threatening complication of NS that occurs in approximately 3% of affected patients.[79] Most thrombotic episodes are venous in origin; however, arterial thrombosis has been reported rarely (Figure 16.4).[80] The incidence of subclinical disease

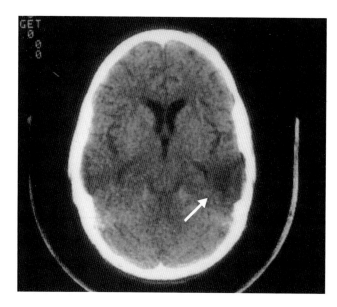

Figure 16.4 A noncontrast computed tomography scan of a 12-year-old girl with nephrotic syndrome that shows a triangular area of infarction affecting the blood flow distribution area of the middle cerebral artery (arrow).

may be higher than previously recognized, with one study demonstrating pulmonary embolism (PE) in 28% of asymptomatic nephrotic children by computed tomography (CT) pulmonary angiography.[81] Symptomatic venous thromboembolism (VTE) most often occurs within the first 3 months after diagnosis of NS and can manifest as clots in the deep leg veins, ileofemoral veins, inferior vena cava, pulmonary veins, renal veins, and sagittal sinus.[80,82] The risk of VTE in nephrotic patients appears to be higher for children with congenital NS, adolescents, and children with membranous nephropathy.[80,83,84] Evaluation of a child with suspected thrombosis should be performed in an urgent manner and include imaging with Doppler or CT angiography to confirm the diagnosis. Clinical Vignette 16.1 describes a patient with PE in FSGS.

The pathophysiology of VTE in NS is likely multifactorial and includes both disease-specific and treatment-related factors (Table 16.3). Nephrotic-range proteinuria leads to loss of anticoagulation factors in the urine such as antithrombin III (ATIII) and protein S, thus shifting the nephrotic patient toward a prothrombotic state.[85,86] In addition, the liver increases synthesis of numerous procoagulant proteins such as factors I, II, V, VII, VIII, X, and XIII and fibrinogen.[85] Diminished fibrinolytic activity has also been reported in NS, with decreased plasminogen and tissue-type plasminogen activator and increased concentrations of inhibitors of fibrinolysis such as lipoprotein (a) and $\alpha_2$-antiplasmin.[85,87] Thrombocytosis is common in children with NS, although the prothrombotic consequences of this abnormality alone are unclear.[88] Regardless of number, platelets from nephrotic patients have been shown to be hyperaggregable.[89,90] Hyperlipidemia and abnormal endothelial cell function have also been implicated in increased thrombosis risk in this population.[91,92] Children with inherited causes of thrombophilia such as factor V Leiden coincident with NS may be at increased risk of thrombosis,

Table 16.3 Risk factors for thromboembolism in nephrotic syndrome

**Disease-Specific Risk Factors**

Platelet hyperaggregability
Increased procoagulation factors I, II, V, VII, VIII, X, and XIII
Decreased anticoagulation factors ATIII and protein S
Diminished fibrinolytic activity: decreased plasminogen, increased lipoprotein (a) and $\alpha_2$-antiplasmin
Hyperlipidemia
Endothelial cell dysfunction

**General Risk Factors**

Intravascular volume depletion
Presence of inherited thrombophilia (e.g., factor V Leiden, prothrombin G20210A)
Indwelling catheters
Presence of antiphospholipid antibodies

*Abbreviations:* ATIII, antithrombin III.

although the incidence of inherited thrombophilia in this population has not been studied.

Iatrogenic factors may also be responsible for an increased risk of thrombosis in nephrotic patients. Indwelling catheters increase the risk of VTE and should be used cautiously in children with NS. A large study showed that nearly 45% of VTE cases in children with NS were associated with indwelling catheters.[80] Diuretic use can cause intravascular volume depletion and increased blood viscosity, which predispose to thrombosis.[93]

Treatment of NS-associated thrombosis is generally initiated with heparin or low-molecular-weight heparin with transition to warfarin in some patients.[79] Because heparin requires ATIII for its mechanism of action, some children require supplementation with recombinant ATIII to maintain optimal anticoagulation effect.[94] There is no generally accepted pharmacologic prevention strategy for thrombosis in children with NS.[95] Prophylactic anticoagulation therapy should be considered for children who suffer relapses after earlier episodes of thrombosis while nephrotic.

---

### KEY POINTS

Children with NS are at increased risk for VTE because of:

- Loss of anticoagulation factors in the urine
- Increased production of prothrombotic factors
- Diminished fibrinolytic activity
- Hemoconcentration due to diuretic therapy
- Iatrogenic factors, such as indwelling venous catheter use

---

## INFECTIONS

Infection is the most common complication of NS, affecting approximately 17% of all NS hospitalizations.[96] It is also the most common cause of mortality in pediatric NS.[97] Parents and primary care providers should be counseled about the increased risk of infection in nephrotic children. Any fever or abdominal pain in a child with NS should prompt urgent evaluation in the clinic or emergency department.

Patients with NS are prone to develop bacterial infections for both disease-specific reasons and as a result of immunosuppressive therapies. Children with lower serum albumin levels appear to be at highest risk of infection.[98] In addition to loss of albumin in the urine, nephrotic patients lose components of the alternative complement pathway, including factors B and D.[99-102] This loss of opsonizing factors increases susceptibility to encapsulated organisms such as *Streptococcus pneumoniae, Haemophilus influenzae,* and *Escherichia coli.* Children with NS also demonstrate low serum IgG levels related to urinary losses as well as T-cell dysfunction that may contribute to risk of infection.[103-105]

The causative organisms for bacterial infections in children with NS may be shifting after the introduction of routine infant immunization with pneumococcal vaccine in 2000.[96,106]

The most common types of infection in nephrotic children are pneumonia, bacteremia, urinary tract infections, peritonitis, cellulitis, and meningitis. Pneumonia is an underrecognized cause of infection in patients with NS. Although early studies suggested that it was rare, more recent reports from the United States and Taiwan both found a high incidence of pneumonia in children hospitalized with NS.[96,107] The presence of severe edema in children with NS predisposes to the development of cellulitis, particularly in areas of skin breakdown. Spontaneous bacterial peritonitis is another common infection in nephrotic children, with an incidence of 2.6% to 5%.[103,108] Spontaneous bacterial peritonitis often manifests with fever, abdominal pain, and leukocytosis in the setting of abdominal ascites, which acts as an excellent culture medium.[103] The most common organisms are *S. pneumoniae* and *E. coli,* but others have been reported.[108,109] If peritonitis is suspected, then paracentesis should be performed to allow peritoneal fluid to be sent for white blood cell count and culture. Peritoneal fluid white blood cell count greater than 250/mm$^3$ in the setting of clinical signs of peritonitis is considered diagnostic.[98] Broad-spectrum antibiotics should be initiated until culture results are available.

The use of prophylactic antibiotics in children with NS remains controversial. Prophylactic penicillin has been recommended by some physicians to prevent infection, particularly in high-risk populations such as those children younger than 2 years old, those with SDNS or FRNS, or those with an earlier episode of pneumococcal infection.[110] Prophylactic antibiotics should be used with caution in children with NS because these drugs have been associated with resistant pneumococcal infections.[111,112] A Cochrane database review found no evidence of benefit for any prophylactic strategy to prevent infection in children or adults with NS.[113]

---

### KEY POINT

Children with NS are prone to developing life-threatening infections including pneumonia, sepsis, peritonitis, and cellulitis from losses of components of the alternative complement pathway in the urine.

---

## ACUTE KIDNEY INJURY

Acute kidney injury (AKI) is common in hospitalized adults with NS (34%) and somewhat less common in the pediatric population (8.5%).[96,114] The etiology of AKI is variable and includes prerenal AKI, acute tubular necrosis, interstitial nephritis, and medication nephrotoxicity, especially resulting from calcineurin inhibitors. Children with NS may have intravascular volume depletion yet receive diuretics for total body fluid overload, thereby precipitating AKI. One randomized controlled trial found that the reversible nephrotoxicity rate for children with SRNS treated with cyclosporine was up to 50% and for tacrolimus was up to 33%.[115] Similarly, ACE inhibitors (ACEIs) and angiotensin receptor blockers (ARBs) have been identified as potential causes of AKI in pediatric NS.[116,117] Antibiotics, particularly aminoglycosides, may have direct nephrotoxic effects or may cause interstitial nephritis.

Renal vein thrombosis may manifest as AKI, typically along with acute hypertension and gross hematuria. Finally, there appears to be an intrinsic decrease in glomerular filtration rate observed in patients with NS that is incompletely understood, but it is hypothesized that severe interstitial edema in the kidney may cause vascular or tubular obstruction.[118,119] Alternately, reduced glomerular permeability may also play a role.[120]

## ENDOCRINE ABNORMALITIES

Hypothyroidism is a frequent complication in children with congenital NS as a result of losses of thyroid-binding protein in the urine, and levothyroxine supplementation is recommended for this population.[121] In older children, free thyroxine and thyroid-stimulating hormone levels are typically normal, although hypothyroidism has been documented in some patients with SRNS.[122]

Children with NS demonstrate decreased 25-hydroxyvitamin D levels in response to urinary excretion of vitamin D–binding protein.[123,124] Suboptimal vitamin D stores may lead to decreased 1,25-dihydroxyvitamin D levels or even secondary hyperparathyroidism and metabolic bone disease.[125,126] Children with SSNS have low vitamin D levels even when they are in remission, although the clinical significance is unclear.[127] Vitamin D supplementation for children with NS has been recommended by some groups, but it is typically reserved for patients with chronic kidney disease or secondary hyperparathyroidism.[128] Treatment with corticosteroids may exacerbate metabolic bone disease in this population.[129]

## HYPERLIPIDEMIA AND ATHEROGENESIS

Hyperlipidemia is a universal finding in NS, including in MCNS. The characteristics of hyperlipidemia in NS are elevated total cholesterol (TC), low-density lipoprotein (LDL), very-low-density lipoprotein (VLDL), and intermediate-density lipoprotein cholesterol fractions. High-density lipoprotein (HDL) cholesterol fraction is usually unchanged, and the LDL/HDL cholesterol ratio is elevated. Serum triglyceride levels are usually normal or only slightly elevated.[130]

Hypoalbuminemia is believed to be the trigger for development of hypercholesterolemia in NS. An inverse relationship between plasma protein level and serum cholesterol level in patients with NS is well known. An even stronger inverse relationship was noted between oncotic pressure and TC level.[131] Indeed, infusion of albumin and other osmotically active molecules was shown to, at least transiently, reduce hepatic VLDL synthesis in patients with NS.[132] Although the precise sequence of events is unclear, the current view holds that hyperlipidemia in NS results from multiple abnormalities in lipid metabolism[130,133–137]:

- LDL receptor deficiency in peripheral tissues leads to diminished catabolism of LDL cholesterol.
- Increased hepatic 3-hydroxy-3-methyl glutaryl-CoA (HMG-CoA) activity causes enhanced hepatic cholesterol synthesis.
- Lecithin cholesterol acyltransferase (LCAT) deficiency from urinary losses reduces extrahepatic uptake of cholesterol and synthesis of HDL cholesterol.

An atherogenic lipid profile in adults with active NS is associated with an increased risk of cardiovascular events, such as myocardial infarction and coronary death.[138] A few reports of myocardial infarction have also been documented in children.[139] Although Zilleruelo et al.[140] found persistent lipid abnormalities in patients with NS, even in remission, long-term cardiovascular risk for children with SSNS is, however, unclear. One retrospective study did not demonstrate any increase in cardiovascular mortality or morbidity in adults with a history of SSNS.[141] Conversely, children with SRNS have a variety of abnormalities suggesting an increased risk for cardiovascular morbidity and mortality, including increased aortic pulse wave velocity, increased carotid intima media thickness, increased left ventricular mass, and hypertension.[142]

Treatment of hyperlipidemia in NS should include dietary counseling to limit dietary fat to less than 30% of total calories and cholesterol to less than 300 mg/day.[76] Most children with SSNS are not treated for their hypercholesterolemia because it is usually transient. Simvastatin and lovastatin are effective and well tolerated in children with persistent nephrotic range proteinuria, and these drugs cause an approximately 40% decrease in TC and LDL cholesterol, as well as a 30% to 40% decrease in triglycerides.[143,144] Because of a risk of rhabdomyolysis in children treated with statins, creatine kinase enzyme activity should be closely monitored.

## OTHER COMPLICATIONS

Respiratory distress in children with NS may result from pleural effusions or decreased effective lung volume caused by ascites. Acute onset of respiratory distress and hypoxia should lead to investigation for pulmonary embolism. Although pulmonary edema is uncommon, it can occur during aggressive treatment of NS with albumin infusions. Patients at high risk for albumin infusion–related respiratory distress include those with decreased glomerular filtration rate, those not receiving adequate diuretics, and those receiving multiple albumin infusions per day.

Intussusception has been reported in children with NS who present with abdominal pain.[145] It is hypothesized that edema of the bowel wall may contribute to development of intussusception.[146] Alternately, peritonitis may induce intramural lymphoid hyperplasia with creation of a lead point for intussusception.[147] A high index of suspicion should be maintained for intussusception in nephrotic children with abdominal pain who do not appear to have peritonitis.

## PRINCIPLES OF MANAGEMENT

Specific immunosuppressive treatments for MCNS and FSGS are discussed in Chapter 17. Principles of treatment of children with NS include management of edema, use of antiproteinuric agents, effective control of hypertension, and prevention of infections through appropriate immunizations.

## EDEMA

Edema is one of the cardinal signs of NS and can sometimes be severe. The goal of edema management in NS is to prevent complications of severe edema such as respiratory distress and skin breakdown, and it can be achieved in most nephrotic children with fluid restriction and sodium restriction to less than 1500 to 2000 mg/day.[76] For children with anasarca or symptomatic edema, pharmacologic management may be necessary with diuretics and 25% albumin infusions. Diuretics should be initiated only in patients for whom significant intravascular volume depletion has been excluded or corrected. If necessary, 25% albumin is given intravenously over 1 to 4 h followed immediately by intravenous diuretics. Slowly increasing the serum albumin to the range of 2.5 to 2.8 g/dL is adequate to restore intravascular oncotic pressure with little clinical benefit from raising the serum albumin to normal levels. The 25% albumin infusions are generally restricted to once daily. Risks of aggressive albumin infusion or concomitant inadequate diuretic therapy include pulmonary edema, respiratory distress, acute hypertension, and congestive heart failure.[148]

### KEY POINTS

- Therapy with 25% albumin infusions should be used only in patients with severe, symptomatic edema.
- Risks of 25% albumin infusions include pulmonary edema, hypertension, respiratory distress, and congestive heart failure.

Furosemide is the most commonly used diuretic for treatment of edema in NS. Furosemide, which is a loop diuretic, acts by inhibiting the sodium potassium-2 chloride (NKCC2) transporter in the thick ascending limb of the loop of Henle. Furosemide is highly protein bound (greater than 95%), with minimal glomerular filtration.[149] It is actively secreted through the organic acid pathway in proximal tubule cells to the tubular lumen, where it reaches the NKCC2 transporter.

Several factors can impair the ability of loop diuretics to function optimally in NS. First, hypoalbuminemia increases the volume of distribution of furosemide by allowing diffusion of free drug into the extravascular space. This, along with a decrease in furosemide that can be bound to albumin because of hypoalbuminemia, reduces the amount of albumin-bound drug that can be delivered to proximal tubule secretory sites.[150] Another factor that limits furosemide activity is binding of filtered albumin in the tubular lumen to secreted furosemide, which limits the free drug that is available to act on the NKCC2 transporter.[151] Several strategies are used to improve the diuretic effect in patients with NS, including more frequent dosing (every 6 to 8 h), higher doses, or even continuous dosing. Doses of up to 200% to 300% of normal are often required to achieve clinical effects, but this may increase the risk of ototoxicity, which correlates with peak levels.[151] Alternately, coadministration of furosemide with 25% albumin can improve efficacy by increasing renal perfusion and increasing delivery of furosemide. Another approach is to add a diuretic with a different mechanism of action for synergistic effects.[152] Metolazone, a thiazide diuretic, acts primarily in the distal tubule but also has some secondary effects on the proximal tubule, and it is often helpful in overcoming diuretic resistance in NS. Blockade of sodium reabsorption at several sites along the nephron can improve the overall diuretic effect.[153,154]

Diuretics should be used with caution in children with NS because of their potential for complications. Diuretic use is an iatrogenic risk factor for development of thrombosis.[93] AKI is increasingly common in nephrotic patients and can be precipitated by further volume depletion induced by diuretics.[96] Electrolyte disturbances induced by diuretics can range from mild to severe hypokalemia and metabolic alkalosis. Finally, hypercalciuria related to use of loop diuretics can cause nephrocalcinosis or kidney stones, particularly in patients who are receiving long-term therapy.[155]

## ANTIPROTEINURIC AGENTS

ACEIs have been shown to slow the progression of proteinuric kidney disease in general and are currently recommended for use in all children with SRNS.[16,76] ACEIs and ARBs decrease proteinuria by decreasing intraglomerular pressure and through a direct alteration of glomerular permselectivity.[156,157] In addition, ACEI and ARBs have antifibrotic effects through inhibition of proinflammatory cytokines.[158] Several studies have demonstrated significant reduction in proteinuria in response to ACEI treatment in children with NS.[157,159,160] The reduction in proteinuria appears to be dose related. One prospective study demonstrated that nephrotic children treated with high-dose enalapril (0.6 mg/kg/day) had greater reductions in proteinuria than did children treated with low-dose enalapril (0.2 mg/kg/day).[160] In most studies, ARBs or the combination of ACEIs and ARBs had similar effects on reduction of proteinuria.[161,162] Rebound proteinuria can be observed in children treated with ACEIs or ARBs. The ESCAPE trial (Effect of Strict Blood Pressure Control and ACE-Inhibition on Progression of Chronic Renal Failure in Pediatric Patients) demonstrated a 50% reduction in proteinuria for children with chronic kidney disease who were treated with ramipril, but proteinuria rebounded to baseline levels after 3 years of therapy.[163] The effect of rebound proteinuria on long-term renal outcomes is unclear.

ACEIs and ARBs are generally well tolerated in children. Adverse effects include hyperkalemia, hypotension, AKI, cough, and angioedema. Children treated with ACEIs or ARBs should have electrolytes and creatinine monitored routinely during therapy. Combination therapy with ACEIs and ARBs may increase the risk of adverse events.[164,165] Women of childbearing age should be counseled about risks of major congenital malformations in pregnancies exposed to ACEIs and ARBs.[166]

## MANAGING HYPERTENSION

Systolic hypertension (defined as greater than the 98th percentile) on first presentation was documented in 21% of children with MCNS and in 49% of children with FSGS in the ISKDC study in the 1970s, but a higher frequency of hypertension has been reported more recently.[13,167,168] Hypertension may be exacerbated by therapies such as corticosteroids or calcineurin inhibitors. Posterior reversible encephalopathy syndrome can be observed in nephrotic children presenting with acute hypertension, headache, or seizures.[169] Children with chronic kidney disease should have blood pressures controlled to the 50th percentile for age and gender in an attempt to slow the progression of renal disease.[163] Children without chronic kidney disease, such as SSNS, should aim for blood pressures lower than the 90th percentile.[170] Nephrotic children and their families should receive low-salt diet education (less than 1500 to 2000 mg) and assistance with body weight management, if necessary. ACEIs or ARBs should be used as first-line pharmacologic therapy for hypertension because of their added antiproteinuric and antifibrotic effects.

## IMMUNIZATIONS

Careful attention should be paid to immunization status in children with NS because they are susceptible to vaccine preventable diseases related to disease-specific effects as well as effects of immunosuppression. Live vaccines should be deferred for 3 months after therapy with cytotoxic agents such as cyclophosphamide. Children receiving at least 2 mg/kg/day of corticosteroids for more than 14 days should not receive live vaccines until 1 month after discontinuation of therapy.[78] Children receiving less than 2 mg/kg/day of corticosteroid may receive live vaccines. Children documented to be nonimmune to varicella based on titers or history should

be vaccinated as soon as appropriate. If exposed to varicella, nonimmune immunocompromised children should receive varicella zoster immune globulin prophylaxis.[78] Children with NS may develop severe, life-threatening varicella infection, and treatment with intravenous acyclovir should be considered at the onset of skin lesions.[76,171]

All children should complete their routine 13-valent pneumococcal vaccine series and also receive the 23-valent pneumococcal vaccine at age 2 years or older. There is evidence that invasive pneumococcal disease decreased in the United States after introduction of the 7-valent pneumococcal vaccine in 2000.[106,172] In children hospitalized with NS, the frequency of peritonitis decreased by 50% from 2000 to 2009, possibly because of vaccine effects, although further study is required.[96] Children with NS, even those in remission, and their families should receive inactivated influenza vaccine yearly.

---

### SUMMARY

Advances in NS and podocyte research are happening at a rapid pace, with new FSGS-causative genes identified on a regular basis. The cause of MCNS remains elusive, but this subject is a large research focus. With the advent of next-generation sequencing, the initial evaluation of new patients with NS will probably soon include large gene panels to determine whether a child's disorder is likely to be steroid resistant.[173] The next 10 to 20 years will also likely see changes in the treatment of NS, with the development of podocyte-specific and nonimmunosuppressive therapies.[174]

---

### Clinical Vignette 16.1

A 14-year-old boy presented to the emergency department with acute shortness of breath and hypoxia. Evaluation demonstrated a pulmonary embolism, and he was started on low-molecular-weight heparin with gradual improvement in his clinical status. Further investigation was notable for the classic features of NS, including proteinuria, hypoalbuminemia, and hyperlipidemia. There was mild leg edema on physical examination. A kidney biopsy demonstrated focal segmental glomerulosclerosis.

### TEACHING POINTS

Most patients with NS present as a result of edema, but some patients may present initially with signs and symptoms of a complication such as infection or thrombosis. This may reflect a delay in diagnosis because the edema may be misdiagnosed (e.g., "allergies") or may not be appreciated. In other cases, the patient may have biochemical evidence of NS, but either mild or no discernible edema.

# REFERENCES

1. Cameron JS. Five hundred years of the nephrotic syndrome: 1484–1984. Ulster Med J. 1985;54(Suppl):S5–19.

2. Zwinger T. Paedojatreja practica, curationem plerum que morborum puerilium per meras observationes, in praxi quotidiana factas, clare et distincte exponens. Basil, Switzerland: Apus E. & J.R. Thurnosios Fratres; 1722.

3. Bright R. Reports of Medical Cases: Selected With a View of Illustrating the Symptoms and Cure of Diseases by a Reference to Morbid Anatomy. London: Longman, Rees, Orme, Browne, and Green; 1827.

4. Cameron JS, Glassock RJ. The Nephrotic Syndrome. New York: Dekker; 1988.

5. Arneil GC, Lam CN. Long-term assessment of steroid therapy in childhood nephrosis. Lancet. 1966;2:819–21.

6. The primary nephrotic syndrome in children: Identification of patients with minimal change nephrotic syndrome from initial response to prednisone. A report of the International Study of Kidney Disease in Children. J Pediatr. 1981;98:561–4.

7. Kestila M, Lenkkeri U, Mannikko M, et al. Positionally cloned gene for a novel glomerular protein—nephrin—is mutated in congenital nephrotic syndrome. Mol Cell. 1998;1:575–82.

8. Jalanko H. Congenital nephrotic syndrome. Pediatr Nephrol. 2009;24:2121–8.

9. Vernier RL, Farquhar MG, Brunson JG, Good RA. Chronic renal disease in children: Correlation of clinical findings with morphologic characteristics seen by light and electron microscopy. AMA J Dis Child. 1958;96:306–43.

10. Kalluri R. Proteinuria with and without renal glomerular podocyte effacement. J Am Soc Nephrol. 2006;17:2383–9.

11. Good KS, O'Brien K, Schulman G, et al. Unexplained nephrotic-range proteinuria in a 38-year-old man: A case of "no change disease." Am J Kidney Dis. 2004;43:933–8.

12. D'Agati VD, Fogo AB, Bruijn JA, Jennette JC. Pathologic classification of focal segmental glomerulosclerosis: A working proposal. Am J Kidney Dis. 2004;43:368–82.

13. Nephrotic syndrome in children: Prediction of histopathology from clinical and laboratory characteristics at time of diagnosis. A report of the International Study of Kidney Disease in Children. Kidney Int. 1978;13:159–65.

14. Buscher AK, Kranz B, Buscher R, et al. Immunosuppression and renal outcome in congenital and pediatric steroid-resistant nephrotic syndrome. Clin J Am Soc Nephrol. 2010;5:2075–84.

15. Niaudet P, Gagnadoux MF, Broyer M. Treatment of childhood steroid-resistant idiopathic nephrotic syndrome. Adv Nephrol Necker Hosp. 1998;28:43–61.

16. Lombel RM, Hodson EM, Gipson DS. Treatment of steroid-resistant nephrotic syndrome in children: New guidelines from KDIGO. Pediatr Nephrol. 2013;28:409–14.

17. McBryde KD, Kershaw DB, Smoyer WE. Pediatric steroid-resistant nephrotic syndrome. Curr Probl Pediatr Adolesc Health Care. 2001;31:280–307.

18. Gipson DS, Chin H, Presler TP, et al. Differential risk of remission and ESRD in childhood FSGS. Pediatr Nephrol. 2006;21:344–9.

19. Eddy AA, Symons JM. Nephrotic syndrome in childhood. Lancet. 2003;362:629–39.

20. Schlesinger ER, Sultz HA, Mosher WE, Feldman JG. The nephrotic syndrome. Its incidence and implications for the community. Am J Dis Child. 1968;116:623–32.

21. Srivastava T, Simon SD, Alon US. High incidence of focal segmental glomerulosclerosis in nephrotic syndrome of childhood. Pediatr Nephrol. 1999;13:13–8.

22. McKinney PA, Feltbower RG, Brocklebank JT, Fitzpatrick MM. Time trends and ethnic patterns of childhood nephrotic syndrome in Yorkshire, UK. Pediatr Nephrol. 2001;16:1040–4.

23. Wyatt RJ, Marx MB, Kazee M, Holland NH. Current estimates of the incidence of steroid responsive idiopathic nephrosis in Kentucky children 1–9 years of age. Int J Pediatr Nephrol. 1982;3:63–5.

24. Bonilla-Felix M, Parra C, Dajani T, et al. Changing patterns in the histopathology of idiopathic nephrotic syndrome in children. Kidney Int. 1999;55:1885–90.

25. Kari JA. Changing trends of histopathology in childhood nephrotic syndrome in western Saudi Arabia. Saudi Med J. 2002;23:317–21.

26. Banaszak B, Banaszak P. The increasing incidence of initial steroid resistance in childhood nephrotic syndrome. Pediatr Nephrol. 2012;27:927–32.

27. Borges FF, Shiraichi L, da Silva MP, et al. Is focal segmental glomerulosclerosis increasing in patients with nephrotic syndrome? Pediatr Nephrol. 2007;22:1309–13.

28. Heymann W, Makker SP, Post RS. The preponderance of males in the idiopathic nephrotic syndrome of childhood. Pediatrics. 1972;50:814–7.

29. Sharples PM, Poulton J, White RH. Steroid responsive nephrotic syndrome is more common in Asians. Arch Dis Child. 1985;60:1014–7.

30. Doe JY, Funk M, Mengel M, et al. Nephrotic syndrome in African children: Lack of evidence for "tropical nephrotic syndrome"? Nephrol Dial Transplant. 2006;21:672–6.

31. Coovadia HM, Adhikari M, Morel-Maroger L. Clinico-pathological features of the nephrotic syndrome in South African children. Q J Med. 1979;48:77–91.

32. Adhikari M, Coovadia HM, Chrystal V, Morel-Maroger L. Absence of 'true' minimal change nephrotic syndrome in African children in South Africa. J Trop Med Hyg. 1983;86:223–8.

33. Abdurrahman MB, Aikhionbare HA, Babaoye FA, et al. Clinicopathological features of childhood nephrotic syndrome in northern Nigeria. Q J Med. 1990;75:563–76.

34. Hendrickse RG, Adeniyi A, Edington GM, et al. Quartan malarial nephrotic syndrome: Collaborative clinicopathological study in Nigerian children. Lancet. 1972;1:1143–9.

35. Ramsuran D, Bhimma R, Ramdial PK, et al. The spectrum of HIV-related nephropathy in children. Pediatr Nephrol. 2012;27:821–7.

36. Sorof JM, Hawkins EP, Brewer ED, et al. Age and ethnicity affect the risk and outcome of focal segmental glomerulosclerosis. Pediatr Nephrol. 1998;12:764–8.

37. Ingulli E, Tejani A. Racial differences in the incidence and renal outcome of idiopathic focal segmental glomerulosclerosis in children. Pediatr Nephrol. 1991;5:393–7.

38. Chernin G, Heeringa SF, Gbadegesin R, et al. Low prevalence of NPHS2 mutations in African American children with steroid-resistant nephrotic syndrome. Pediatr Nephrol. 2008;23:1455–60.

39. Papeta N, Kiryluk K, Patel A, et al. APOL1 variants increase risk for FSGS and HIVAN but not IgA nephropathy. J Am Soc Nephrol. 2011;22:1991–6.

40. Kopp JB, Nelson GW, Sampath K, et al. APOL1 genetic variants in focal segmental glomerulosclerosis and HIV-associated nephropathy. J Am Soc Nephrol. 2011;22:2129–37.

41. Madhavan SM, O'Toole JF, Konieczkowski M, et al. APOL1 localization in normal kidney and nondiabetic kidney disease. J Am Soc Nephrol. 2011;22:2119–28.

42. Reeves-Daniel AM, DePalma JA, Bleyer AJ, et al. The APOL1 gene and allograft survival after kidney transplantation. Am J Transplant. 2011;11:1025–30.

43. Epstein A. Concerning the causation of edema in chronic parenchymatous nephritis. Am J Med Sci. 1917;154:638.

44. Siddall EC, Radhakrishnan J. The pathophysiology of edema formation in the nephrotic syndrome. Kidney Int. 2012;82:635–42.

45. Starling EH. On the Fluids of the Body. Chicago: W. T. Keener & Co.; 1909.

46. Meltzer JI, Keim HJ, Laragh JH, et al. Nephrotic syndrome: Vasoconstriction and hypervolemic types indicated by renin-sodium profiling. Ann Intern Med. 1979;91:688–96.

47. Vande Walle JG, Donckerwolcke RA, Koomans HA. Pathophysiology of edema formation in children with nephrotic syndrome not due to minimal change disease. J Am Soc Nephrol. 1999;10:323–31.

48. Manning RD, Jr. Effects of hypoproteinemia on renal hemodynamics, arterial pressure, and fluid volume. Am J Physiol. 1987;252:F91–8.

49. Rascher W, Tulassay T. Hormonal regulation of water metabolism in children with nephrotic syndrome. Kidney Int Suppl. 1987;21:S83–9.

50. Usberti M, Federico S, Meccariello S, et al. Role of plasma vasopressin in the impairment of water excretion in nephrotic syndrome. Kidney Int. 1984;25:422–9.

51. Geers AB, Koomans HA, Boer P, Dorhout Mees EJ. Plasma and blood volumes in patients with the nephrotic syndrome. Nephron. 1984;38:170–3.

52. Vande Walle J, Donckerwolcke R, Boer P, et al. Blood volume, colloid osmotic pressure and F-cell ratio in children with the nephrotic syndrome. Kidney Int. 1996;49:1471–7.

53. Koomans HA, Geers AB, Dorhout Mees EJ, Kortlandt W. Lowered tissue-fluid oncotic pressure protects the blood volume in the nephrotic syndrome. Nephron. 1986;42:317–22.

54. Fauchald P, Noddeland H, Norseth J. Interstitial fluid volume, plasma volume and colloid osmotic pressure in patients with nephrotic syndrome. Scand J Clin Lab Invest. 1984;44:661–7.

55. Russi E, Weigand K. Analbuminemia. Klin Wochenschr. 1983;61:541–5.

56. Toye JM, Lemire EG, Baerg KL. Perinatal and childhood morbidity and mortality in congenital analbuminemia. Paediatr Child Health. 2012;17:e20–3.

57. Shapiro MD, Hasbargen J, Hensen J, Schrier RW. Role of aldosterone in the sodium retention of patients with nephrotic syndrome. Am J Nephrol. 1990;10:44–8.

58. Brown EA, Markandu ND, Sagnella GA, et al. Evidence that some mechanism other than the renin system causes sodium retention in nephrotic syndrome. Lancet. 1982;2:1237–40.

59. Brown EA, Markandu ND, Sagnella GA, et al. Lack of effect of captopril on the sodium retention of the nephrotic syndrome. Nephron. 1984;37:43–8.

60. Ichikawa I, Rennke HG, Hoyer JR, et al. Role for intrarenal mechanisms in the impaired salt excretion of experimental nephrotic syndrome. J Clin Invest. 1983;71:91–103.

61. Kim SW, Wang W, Nielsen J, et al. Increased expression and apical targeting of renal ENaC subunits in puromycin aminonucleoside-induced nephrotic syndrome in rats. Am J Physiol Renal Physiol. 2004;286:F922–35.

62. Kim SW, de Seigneux S, Sassen MC, et al. Increased apical targeting of renal ENaC subunits and decreased expression of 11betaHSD2 in HgCl2-induced nephrotic syndrome in rats. Am J Physiol Renal Physiol. 2006;290:F674–87.

63. Deschenes G, Doucet A. Collecting duct (Na⁺/K⁺)-ATPase activity is correlated with urinary sodium excretion in rat nephrotic syndromes. J Am Soc Nephrol. 2000;11:604–15.

64. Deschenes G, Gonin S, Zolty E, et al. Increased synthesis and AVP unresponsiveness of Na,K-ATPase in collecting duct from nephrotic rats. J Am Soc Nephrol. 2001;12:2241–52.

65. Carattino MD, Hughey RP, Kleyman TR. Proteolytic processing of the epithelial sodium channel gamma subunit has a dominant role in channel activation. J Biol Chem. 2008;283:25290–5.

66. Svenningsen P, Bistrup C, Friis UG, et al. Plasmin in nephrotic urine activates the epithelial sodium channel. J Am Soc Nephrol. 2009;20:299–310.

67. Andersen RF, Buhl KB, Jensen BL, et al. Remission of nephrotic syndrome diminishes urinary plasmin content and abolishes activation of ENaC. Pediatr Nephrol. 2013;28:1227–34.

68. Deschenes G, Wittner M, Stefano A, et al. Collecting duct is a site of sodium retention in PAN nephrosis: A rationale for amiloride therapy. J Am Soc Nephrol. 2001;12:598–601.

69. Schrier RW, Fassett RG. A critique of the overfill hypothesis of sodium and water retention in the nephrotic syndrome. Kidney Int. 1998;53:1111–7.

70. Bockenhauer D. Over- or underfill: Not all nephrotic states are created equal. Pediatr Nephrol. 2013;28:1153–6.

71. Vande Walle JG, Donckerwolcke RA. Pathogenesis of edema formation in the nephrotic syndrome. Pediatr Nephrol. 2001;16:283–93.

72. Kapur G, Valentini RP, Imam AA, Mattoo TK. Treatment of severe edema in children with nephrotic syndrome with diuretics alone: A prospective study. Clin J Am Soc Nephrol. 2009;4:907–13.

73. Sturgill BC, Shearlock KT. Membranous glomerulopathy and nephrotic syndrome after captopril therapy. JAMA. 1983;250:2343–5.

74. Radford MG, Jr, Holley KE, Grande JP, et al. Reversible membranous nephropathy associated with the use of nonsteroidal anti-inflammatory drugs. JAMA. 1996;276:466–9.

75. Habib GS, Saliba W, Nashashibi M, Armali Z. Penicillamine and nephrotic syndrome. Eur J Intern Med. 2006;17:343–8.

76. Gipson DS, Massengill SF, Yao L, et al. Management of childhood onset nephrotic syndrome. Pediatrics. 2009;124:747–57.

77. Laskin BL, Goebel J, Starke JR, et al. Cost-effectiveness of latent tuberculosis screening before steroid therapy for idiopathic nephrotic syndrome in children. Am J Kidney Dis. 2013;61:22–32.

78. Pickering L, editor. Red Book: 2012 Report of the Committee on Infections Diseases, 29th ed. Elk Grove Village, IL: American Academy of Pediatrics Committee on Infectious Diseases; 2012.

79. Kerlin BA, Haworth K, Smoyer WE. Venous thromboembolism in pediatric nephrotic syndrome. Pediatr Nephrol. 2014;29:989–97.

80. Kerlin BA, Blatt NB, Fuh B, et al. Epidemiology and risk factors for thromboembolic complications of childhood nephrotic syndrome: A Midwest Pediatric Nephrology Consortium (MWPNC) study. J Pediatr. 2009;155:105–10, 10 e1.

81. Zhang LJ, Wang ZJ, Zhou CS, et al. Evaluation of pulmonary embolism in pediatric patients with nephrotic syndrome with dual energy CT pulmonary angiography. Acad Radiol. 2012;19:341–8.

82. Andrew M, Brooker LA. Hemostatic complications in renal disorders of the young. Pediatr Nephrol. 1996;10:88–99.

83. Hamed RM, Shomaf M. Congenital nephrotic syndrome: A clinico-pathologic study of thirty children. J Nephrol. 2001;14:104–9.

84. Mahan JD, Mauer SM, Sibley RK, Vernier RL. Congenital nephrotic syndrome: Evolution of medical management and results of renal transplantation. J Pediatr. 1984;105:549–57.

85. Schlegel N. Thromboembolic risks and complications in nephrotic children. Semin Thromb Hemost. 1997;23:271–80.

86. Hanevold CD, Lazarchick J, Constantin MA, et al. Acquired free protein S deficiency in children with steroid resistant nephrosis. Ann Clin Lab Sci. 1996;26:279–82.

87. Kerlin BA, Ayoob R, Smoyer WE. Epidemiology and pathophysiology of nephrotic syndrome–associated thromboembolic disease. Clin J Am Soc Nephrol. 2012;7:513–20.

88. Dame C, Sutor AH. Primary and secondary thrombocytosis in childhood. Br J Haematol. 2005;129:165–77.

89. Remuzzi G, Mecca G, Marchesi D, et al. Platelet hyperaggregability and the nephrotic syndrome. Thromb Res. 1979;16:345–54.

90. Walter E, Deppermann D, Andrassy K, Koderisch J. Platelet hyperaggregability as a consequence of the nephrotic syndrome. Thromb Res. 1981;23:473–9.

91. Dogra GK, Watts GF, Herrmann S, et al. Statin therapy improves brachial artery endothelial function in nephrotic syndrome. Kidney Int. 2002;62:550–7.

92. Dogra GK, Herrmann S, Irish AB, et al. Insulin resistance, dyslipidaemia, inflammation and endothelial function in nephrotic syndrome. Nephrol Dial Transplant. 2002;17:2220–5.

93. Lilova MI, Velkovski IG, Topalov IB. Thromboembolic complications in children with nephrotic syndrome in Bulgaria (1974–1996). Pediatr Nephrol. 2000;15:74–8.

94. Zaffanello M, Franchini M. Thromboembolism in childhood nephrotic syndrome: A rare but serious complication. Hematology. 2007;12:69–73.

95. Glassock RJ. Prophylactic anticoagulation in nephrotic syndrome: A clinical conundrum. J Am Soc Nephrol. 2007;18:2221–5.

96. Rheault MN, Wei CC, Hains DS, et al. Increasing frequency of acute kidney injury amongst children hospitalized with nephrotic syndrome. Pediatr Nephrol. 2014;29:139–47.

97. Minimal change nephrotic syndrome in children: Deaths during the first 5 to 15 years' observation. Report of the International Study of Kidney Disease in Children. Pediatrics. 1984;73:497–501.

98. Hingorani SR, Weiss NS, Watkins SL. Predictors of peritonitis in children with nephrotic syndrome. Pediatr Nephrol. 2002;17:678–82.

99. Matsell DG, Wyatt RJ. The role of I and B in peritonitis associated with the nephrotic syndrome of childhood. Pediatr Res. 1993;34:84–8.

100. McLean RH, Forsgren A, Bjorksten B, et al. Decreased serum factor B concentration associated with decreased opsonization of Escherichia coli in the idiopathic nephrotic syndrome. Pediatr Res. 1977;11:910–6.

101. Anderson DC, York TL, Rose G, Smith CW. Assessment of serum factor B, serum opsonins, granulocyte chemotaxis, and infection in nephrotic syndrome of children. J Infect Dis. 1979;140:1–11.

102. Ballow M, Kennedy TL, 3rd, Gaudio KM, et al. Serum hemolytic factor D values in children with steroid-responsive idiopathic nephrotic syndrome. J Pediatr. 1982;100:192–6.

103. Krensky AM, Ingelfinger JR, Grupe WE. Peritonitis in childhood nephrotic syndrome: 1970–1980. Am J Dis Child. 1982;136:732–6.

104. Giangiacomo J, Cleary TG, Cole BR, et al. Serum immunoglobulins in the nephrotic syndrome: A possible cause of minimal-change nephrotic syndrome. N Engl J Med .1975;293:8–12.

105. Fodor P, Saitua MT, Rodriguez E, et al. T-cell dysfunction in minimal-change nephrotic syndrome of childhood. Am J Dis Child. 1982;136:713–7.

106. Haddy RI, Perry K, Chacko CE, et al. Comparison of incidence of invasive Streptococcus pneumoniae disease among children before and after introduction of conjugated pneumococcal vaccine. Pediatr Infect Dis J. 2005;24:320–3.

107. Wei CC, Yu IW, Lin HW, Tsai AC. Occurrence of infection among children with nephrotic syndrome during hospitalizations. Nephrology (Carlton). 2012;17:681–8.

108. Uncu N, Bulbul M, Yildiz N, et al. Primary peritonitis in children with nephrotic syndrome: Results of a 5-year multicenter study. Eur J Pediatr. 2012;169:73–6.

109. Tain YL, Lin G, Cher TW. Microbiological spectrum of septicemia and peritonitis in nephrotic children. Pediatr Nephrol. 1999;13:835–7.

110. McIntyre P, Craig JC. Prevention of serious bacterial infection in children with nephrotic syndrome. J Paediatr Child Health. 1998;34:314–7.

111. Milner LS, Berkowitz FE, Ngwenya E, et al. Penicillin resistant pneumococcal peritonitis in nephrotic syndrome. Arch Dis Child. 1987;62:964–5.

112. Ilyas M, Roy S, 3rd, Abbasi S, et al. Serious infections due to penicillin-resistant Streptococcus pneumoniae in two children with nephrotic syndrome. Pediatr Nephrol. 1996;10:639–41.

113. Wu HM, Tang JL, Cao L, et al. Interventions for preventing infection in nephrotic syndrome. Cochrane Database Syst Rev. 2012;4:CD003964.

114. Chen T, Lv Y, Lin F, Zhu J. Acute kidney injury in adult idiopathic nephrotic syndrome. Ren Fail. 2011;33:144–9.

115. Choudhry S, Bagga A, Hari P, et al. Efficacy and safety of tacrolimus versus cyclosporine in children with steroid-resistant nephrotic syndrome: A randomized controlled trial. Am J Kidney Dis. 2009;53:760–9.

116. Olowu WA, Adenowo OA, Elusiyan JB. Reversible renal failure in hypertensive idiopathic nephrotics treated with captopril. Saudi J Kidney Dis Transpl. 2006;17:216–21.

117. Milliner DS, Morgenstern BZ. Angiotensin converting enzyme inhibitors for reduction of proteinuria in children with steroid-resistant nephrotic syndrome. Pediatr Nephrol. 1991;5:587–90.

118. Lowenstein J, Schacht RG, Baldwin DS. Renal failure in minimal change nephrotic syndrome. Am J Med. 1981;70:227–33.

119. Koomans HA. Pathophysiology of edema and acute renal failure in idiopathic nephrotic syndrome. Adv Nephrol Necker Hosp. 2000;30:41–55.

120. Vande Walle J, Mauel R, Raes A, et al. ARF in children with minimal change nephrotic syndrome may be related to functional changes of the glomerular basal membrane. Am J Kidney Dis. 2004;43:399–404.

121. Holmberg C, Antikainen M, Ronnholm K, et al. Management of congenital nephrotic syndrome of the Finnish type. Pediatr Nephrol. 1995;9:87–93.

122. Dagan A, Cleper R, Krause I, et al. Hypothyroidism in children with steroid-resistant nephrotic syndrome. Nephrol Dial Transplant. 2012;27:2171–5.

123. Freundlich M, Bourgoignie JJ, Zilleruelo G, et al. Calcium and vitamin D metabolism in children with nephrotic syndrome. J Pediatr. 1986;108:383–7.

124. Barragry JM, France MW, Carter ND, et al. Vitamin-D metabolism in nephrotic syndrome. Lancet. 1977;2:629–32.

125. Goldstein DA, Haldimann B, Sherman D, et al. Vitamin D metabolites and calcium metabolism in patients with nephrotic syndrome and normal renal function. J Clin Endocrinol Metab. 1981;52:116–21.

126. Malluche HH, Goldstein DA, Massry SG. Osteomalacia and hyperparathyroid bone disease in patients with nephrotic syndrome. J Clin Invest. 1979;63:494–500.

127. Weng FL, Shults J, Herskovitz RM, et al. Vitamin D insufficiency in steroid-sensitive nephrotic syndrome in remission. Pediatr Nephrol. 2005;20:56–63.

128. Gulati S, Sharma RK, Gulati K, et al. Longitudinal follow-up of bone mineral density in children with nephrotic syndrome and the role of calcium and vitamin D supplements. Nephrol Dial Transplant. 2005;20:1598–603.

129. Leonard MB, Feldman HI, Shults J, et al. Long-term, high-dose glucocorticoids and bone mineral content in childhood glucocorticoid-sensitive nephrotic syndrome. N Engl J Med. 2004;351:868–75.

130. Vaziri ND: Molecular mechanisms of lipid disorders in nephrotic syndrome. Kidney Int. 2003;63:1964–76.

131. Appel GB, Blum CB, Chien S, et al. The hyperlipidemia of the nephrotic syndrome: Relation to plasma albumin concentration, oncotic pressure, and viscosity. N Engl J Med. 1985;312:1544–8.

132. Baxter JH, Goodman HC, Allen JC. Effects of infusions of serum albumin on serum lipids and lipoproteins in nephrosis. J Clin Invest. 1961;40:490–8.

133. Chan MK, Persaud JW, Ramdial L, et al. Hyperlipidaemia in untreated nephrotic syndrome, increased production or decreased removal? Clin Chim Acta. 1981;117:317–23.

134. Warwick GL, Caslake MJ, Boulton-Jones JM, et al. Low-density lipoprotein metabolism in the nephrotic syndrome. Metabolism. 1990;39:187–92.

135. Nakahara C, Kobayashi K, Hamaguchi H, et al. Plasma lipoprotein (a) levels in children with minimal lesion nephrotic syndrome. Pediatr Nephrol. 1999;13:657–61.

136. Garnotel R, Roussel B, Pennaforte F, et al. Changes in serum lipoprotein(a) levels in children with corticosensitive nephrotic syndrome. Pediatr Nephrol. 1996;10:699–701.

137. Liu S, Vaziri ND. Role of PCSK9 and IDOL in the pathogenesis of acquired LDL receptor deficiency and hypercholesterolemia in nephrotic syndrome. Nephrol Dial Transplant. 2014;29:538–43.

138. Ordonez JD, Hiatt RA, Killebrew EJ, Fireman BH. The increased risk of coronary heart disease associated with nephrotic syndrome. Kidney Int. 1993;44:638–42.

139. Hopp L, Gilboa N, Kurland G, et al. Acute myocardial infarction in a young boy with nephrotic syndrome: A case report and review of the literature. Pediatr Nephrol. 1994;8: 290–4.

140. Zilleruelo G, Hsia SL, Freundlich M, et al. Persistence of serum lipid abnormalities in children with idiopathic nephrotic syndrome. J Pediatr. 1984;104:61–4.

141. Lechner BL, Bockenhauer D, Iragorri S, et al. The risk of cardiovascular disease in adults who have had childhood nephrotic syndrome. Pediatr Nephrol. 2004;19:744–8.

142. Candan C, Canpolat N, Gökalp S, et al. Subclinical cardiovascular disease and its association with risk factors in children with steroid-resistant nephrotic syndrome. Pediatr Nephrol. 2014;29:95–102.

143. Coleman JE, Watson AR. Hyperlipidaemia, diet and simvastatin therapy in steroid-resistant nephrotic syndrome of childhood. Pediatr Nephrol. 1996;10:171–4.

144. Sanjad SA, al-Abbad A, al-Shorafa S. Management of hyperlipidemia in children with refractory nephrotic syndrome: The effect of statin therapy. J Pediatr. 1997;130:470–4.

145. Cho MH, Hwang HH, Choe BH, et al. The reversal of intussusception associated with nephrotic syndrome by infusion of albumin. Pediatr Nephrol. 2009;24:421–2.

146. Asai K, Tanaka S, Tanaka N, et al. Intussusception of the small bowel associated with nephrotic syndrome. Pediatr Nephrol. 2005;20:1818–20.

147. Kietkajornkul C, Vithayasai N, Ratanaprakarn W, et al. Intussusception associated with a relapsing nephrotic patient: A case report. J Med Assoc Thai. 2003;86(Suppl 3):S596–9.

148. Haws RM, Baum M. Efficacy of albumin and diuretic therapy in children with nephrotic syndrome. Pediatrics. 1993;91:1142–6.

149. Brater DC. Diuretic therapy. N Engl J Med. 1998;339:387–95.

150. Inoue M, Okajima K, Itoh K, et al. Mechanism of furosemide resistance in analbuminemic rats and hypoalbuminemic patients. Kidney Int. 1987;32:198–203.

151. Rybak LP. Furosemide ototoxicity: Clinical and experimental aspects. Laryngoscope. 1985;95:1–14.

152. Sica DA, Gehr TW. Diuretic combinations in refractory oedema states: Pharmacokinetic-pharmacodynamic relationships. Clin Pharmacokinet. 1996;30:229–49.

153. Arnold WC. Efficacy of metolazone and furosemide in children with furosemide-resistant edema. Pediatrics. 1984;74:872–5.

154. Garin EH. A comparison of combinations of diuretics in nephrotic edema. Am J Dis Child. 1987;141:769–71.

155. Mocan H, Yildiran A, Camlibel T, Kuzey GM. Microscopic nephrocalcinosis and hypercalciuria in nephrotic syndrome. Hum Pathol. 2000;31:1363–7.

156. Remuzzi A, Puntorieri S, Battaglia C, et al. Angiotensin converting enzyme inhibition ameliorates glomerular filtration of macromolecules and water and lessens glomerular injury in the rat. J Clin Invest. 1990;85:541–9.

157. Delucchi A, Cano F, Rodriguez E, et al. Enalapril and prednisone in children with nephrotic-range proteinuria. Pediatr Nephrol. 2000;14:1088–91.

158. Remuzzi A, Gagliardini E, Sangalli F, et al. ACE inhibition reduces glomerulosclerosis and regenerates glomerular tissue in a model of progressive renal disease. Kidney Int. 2006;69:1124–30.

159. Yi Z, Li Z, Wu XC, et al. Effect of fosinopril in children with steroid-resistant idiopathic nephrotic syndrome. Pediatr Nephrol. 2006;21:967–72.

160. Bagga A, Mudigoudar BD, Hari P, et al. Enalapril dosage in steroid-resistant nephrotic syndrome. Pediatr Nephrol. 2004;19:45–50.

161. Ellis D, Vats A, Moritz ML, et al. Long-term anti-proteinuric and renoprotective efficacy and safety of losartan in children with proteinuria. J Pediatr. 2003;143:89–97.

162. Supavekin S, Surapaitoolkorn W, Tancharoen W, et al. Combined renin angiotensin blockade in childhood steroid-resistant nephrotic syndrome. Pediatr Int. 2012;54:793–7.

163. Wuhl E, Trivelli A, Picca S, et al. Strict blood-pressure control and progression of renal failure in children. N Engl J Med. 2009;361:1639–50.

164. Mann JF, Schmieder RE, McQueen M, et al. Renal outcomes with telmisartan, ramipril, or both, in people at high vascular risk (the ONTARGET study): A multicentre, randomised, double-blind, controlled trial. Lancet. 2008;372:547–53.

165. Hanevold CD. Acute renal failure during lisinopril and losartan therapy for proteinuria. Pharmacotherapy. 2006;26:1348–51.

166. Cooper WO, Hernandez-Diaz S, Arbogast PG, et al. Major congenital malformations after first-trimester exposure to ACE inhibitors. N Engl J Med. 2006;354:2443–51.

167. Kuster S, Mehls O, Seidel C, Ritz E. Blood pressure in minimal change and other types of nephrotic syndrome. Am J Nephrol. 1990;10(Suppl 1):76–80.

168. Kontchou LM, Liccioli G, Pela I. Blood pressure in children with minimal change nephrotic syndrome during oedema and after steroid therapy: The influence of familial essential hypertension. Kidney Blood Press Res. 2009;32:258–62.

169. Ishikura K, Ikeda M, Hamasaki Y, et al. Nephrotic state as a risk factor for developing posterior reversible encephalopathy syndrome in paediatric patients with nephrotic syndrome. Nephrol Dial Transplant. 2008;23:2531–6.

170. The fourth report on the diagnosis, evaluation, and treatment of high blood pressure in children and adolescents. Pediatrics. 2004;114:555–76.

171. Wiegering V, Schick J, Beer M, et al. Varicella-zoster virus infections in immunocompromised patients: A single centre 6-years analysis. BMC Pediatr. 2011;11:31.

172. Mufson MA, Stanek RJ. Epidemiology of invasive Streptococcus pneumoniae infections and vaccine implications among children in a West Virginia community, 1978–2003. Pediatr Infect Dis J 2004;23:779–81.

173. McCarthy HJ, Bierzynska A, Wherlock M, et al. Simultaneous sequencing of 24 genes associated with steroid-resistant nephrotic syndrome. Clin J Am Soc Nephrol. 2013;8:637–48.

174. Reiser J, Gupta V, Kistler AD. Toward the development of podocyte-specific drugs. Kidney Int. 2010;77:662–8.

## REVIEW QUESTIONS

1. The most likely finding on kidney histopathologic examination for a 2-year-old child with steroid-sensitive nephrotic syndrome is:
   a. Minimal change nephrotic syndrome
   b. Focal segmental glomerulosclerosis
   c. Membranous nephropathy
   d. Membranoproliferative glomerulonephritis
   e. Mesangial proliferative glomerulonephritis

2. Sequence variants in the following gene account for a large fraction of observed FSGS risk in African Americans:
   a. NPHS2
   b. WT1
   c. MYH9
   d. APOL1
   e. COQ6

3. Which of the following is not a component of the "underfill hypothesis" of edema formation in nephrotic syndrome?
   a. Decreased plasma oncotic pressure with leakage of fluid into the interstitial space
   b. Hypovolemia with renal hypoperfusion
   c. Activation of the renin-angiotensin-aldosterone system
   d. Vasopressin release
   e. Increased sodium reabsorption through ENaC

4. Children with an initial presentation of nephrotic syndrome should have all of the following performed, except:
   a. Complement C3 level
   b. Genetic testing for NPHS2 mutations
   c. Serum albumin
   d. PPD
   e. Cholesterol level

5. The following factors cause increased risk for thrombosis in nephrotic syndrome, except:
   a. Increased production of protein S by the liver
   b. Loss of ATIII in the urine
   c. Platelet hyperaggregability
   d. Diminished fibrinolytic activity
   e. Hyperlipidemia

6. Complications of furosemide therapy for treatment of edema in nephrotic syndrome can include all of the following except:
   a. Hypokalemia
   b. Acute kidney injury
   c. Nephrocalcinosis
   d. Metabolic acidosis
   e. Thrombosis

7. Live vaccines (varicella, MMR) can be given to which population of children with nephrotic syndrome?
   a. Children receiving cyclophosphamide
   b. Children receiving 2 mg/kg/day of prednisone

c. Children who have been off high-dose steroids for 1 month

d. Children who have been off high-dose steroids for 1 week

e. Children receiving 2 mg/kg/day of prednisone and exposed to varicella

8. Complications of 25% albumin infusions in nephrotic patients can include all of the following, **except:**

a. Pseudotumor cerebri

b. Respiratory distress

c. Congestive heart failure

d. Acute hypertension

e. Pulmonary edema

9. Which of the following is most suggestive of a cause of nephrotic syndrome other than MCNS?

a. Age 2 years

b. No hematuria

c. Anasarca

d. Stage II hypertension

e. Normal complement 3

10. After receiving intravenous furosemide, a 2-year-old girl with SSNS develops gross hematuria and hypertension. What study should be performed first to evaluate for the cause of the hematuria?

a. Urine calcium-to-creatinine ratio

b. Urine protein-to-creatinine ratio

c. Lasix renogram

d. Renal ultrasound with Doppler

e. Voiding cystourethrogram

## ANSWER KEY

1. a
2. d
3. e
4. b
5. a
6. d
7. c
8. a
9. d
10. d

# 17

# Primary podocytopathies

RAED BOU MATAR, RUDOLPH P. VALENTINI AND WILLIAM E. SMOYER

Nephrotic syndrome is defined by the presence of high-grade proteinuria, hypoalbuminemia, and edema. Hyperlipidemia and hypercoagulability are common associated findings. Increased permeability of the glomerular filtration barrier (GFB) results in massive loss of protein in the urine that leads to the constellation of renal and extrarenal findings characteristic of the disease. Children with nephrotic syndrome commonly present with periorbital swelling, peripheral pitting edema, or ascites. If left untreated, these children are at risk for various complications, including systemic infections, thromboembolism, and pulmonary edema. As discussed in Chapters 10 and 16, a major contributor to the GFB is the *podocyte*, and disruption of podocyte physiology is an important cause of nephrotic syndrome. Nephrotic syndrome in the majority of children results from an abnormality in podocyte structure or function. In such cases, we refer to the disease as a *primary podocytopathy*, which is the subject of this chapter (Table 17.1). In children, the most common primary podocytopathies are minimal change disease (MCD) and focal segmental glomerulosclerosis (FSGS). Secondary podocytopathies are less common and include autoimmune diseases, drug effects, and infections.

## KEY POINT

Nephrotic syndrome is caused by an injury to the podocyte that results in disruption of the GFB.

## THE PODOCYTE

The podocyte, also known as the glomerular visceral epithelial cell, is a terminally differentiated, highly specialized cell located at the urinary side of the glomerular capillary tuft. It plays a central role in: maintenance of the GFB through preservation of a molecular filtration sieve, synthesis of the glomerular basement membrane (GBM), and regulation of other glomerular cell types. In many proteinuric diseases, the podocytes become the target of immunologic or nonimmunologic injury.[1] This leads to a disruption of the podocyte cytoskeleton and widespread foot process effacement. In FSGS, for example, podocyte depletion and detachment from the underlying basement membrane are prominent features.[2]

The kidney maintains homeostasis by facilitating the excretion of body fluids and waste products while retaining physiologically important macromolecules, such as albumin and other plasma proteins. This regulation is possible only in the presence of an intact complex functional structure, the GFB. An intact GFB prevents the passage of molecules larger than 42 Å in diameter or with a molecular

Table 17.1 Classification of the podocytopathies

| Condition | Definition | Examples |
|---|---|---|
| Podocytopathy | Any proteinuric disease resulting from disruption of normal podocyte physiology | |
| Primary glomerulopathy | A glomerular disease with no systemic extrarenal involvement | Minimal change disease, focal segmental glomerulosclerosis, membranoproliferative glomerulonephritis, IgA nephropathy |
| Idiopathic podocytopathy | A primary glomerulopathy characterized by minimal glomerular inflammatory infiltration and a bland urinary sediment | Minimal change disease, focal segmental glomerulosclerosis, membranous nephropathy, mesangial proliferative glomerulonephritis |
| Secondary podocytopathy | A podocytopathy caused by an immune, inflammatory, or mechanical injury to the podocyte resulting from a systemic disorder or a decreased number of nephrons (hyperfiltration injury) | Podocytopathies secondary to hepatitis B, hepatitis C, HIV infection, drugs (heavy metals, penicillamine, gold), autoimmune diseases (systemic lupus erythematosus, Henoch-Schönlein's purpura, Sjögren's syndrome), and morbid obesity |
| Genetic podocytopathy | A glomerular disorder caused by a genetic defect that interferes with normal podocyte structure or function | NPHS2, NPHS1, ACTN4, TRPC6 and Myo1E gene mutations |

Abbreviations: HIV, human immunodeficiency virus; IgA, immunoglobulin A.

weight exceeding approximately 200 kDa.[3] The GFB has three components: the capillary endothelial cell, the GBM, and the glomerular epithelial cells (podocytes). First, the capillary endothelial cells contains pores, known as fenestrations, that are large enough to permit non–size-selective passage of macromolecules. However, these fenestrations contain glycoprotein assemblies that hinder the free filtration of macromolecules.[4] Second, the GBM is mainly composed of type IV collagen, laminin, and glycoproteins. It plays an important role in the restriction of fluid flux.[5] Third, the podocytes are terminally differentiated epithelial cells consisting of a cell body, major processes, and minor processes, also known as foot processes. Podocyte foot processes interdigitate with those of neighboring podocytes. Between the foot processes are highly specialized cell-cell junctions, known as slit diaphragms.[6] Many of the proteins forming or associated with the slit diaphragm have been implicated in the pathogenesis of genetic forms of nephrotic syndrome. These include nephrin,[7] podocin,[8] and TRPC6.[9,10] The slit diaphragm interacts with the actin cytoskeleton of the podocyte foot processes.[11] In view of the central role the podocyte plays in the pathogenesis of proteinuria, the term podocytopathies has become increasingly used to describe various glomerular disorders.

The charge selectivity of the GFB has been the topic of ongoing debate among the scientific community (further discussed in Chapter 10). Charge selectivity was initially supported by experimentally observing significant differences in the sieving coefficients between neutral and anionic proteins (particularly albumin),[12,13] This concept was challenged, however, when newer measurements of the albumin

concentration in the Bowman space that used intravital two-photon microscopy were higher than previously thought. This finding suggested that a proportion of albumin is filtered and then reclaimed by the proximal tubular cells.[14] Studies of charge selectivity in animals with nephrotic syndrome have yielded conflicting results. Some experiments demonstrated a loss of charge selectivity,[15–17] whereas others failed to detect alterations in charge selectivity in patients with MCD or FSGS.[18] Dysregulation of anionic charge has also been detected in other cell membranes in patients with nephrotic syndrome, such as the membranes of red blood cells and platelets, thereby leading to a controversial belief that MCD may be a systemic disorder of cell membrane function.[19]

Glomerular diseases associated with podocyte injury (podocytopathies) have been traditionally classified based on the presence or absence of systemic disease or glomerular inflammation. *Primary glomerulopathies* involve glomerular lesions with no systemic extrarenal (systemic) involvement. Primary glomerulopathies include conditions associated with inflammatory glomerular lesions and an active urinary sediment (red blood cell or white blood cell casts), such as membranoproliferative glomerulonephritis (MPGN) and immunoglobulin A (IgA) nephropathy. In addition, primary glomerulopathies also include *idiopathic podocytopathies*, such as MCD, FSGS, and mesangial proliferative glomerulonephritis (MesProlif GN). Idiopathic podocytopathies are often characterized by minimal glomerular inflammatory infiltration and a bland urinary sediment (MCD and FSGS), with

MesProlif GN often showing some signs of glomerular inflammation. Despite the prevalent nomenclature, a significant proportion of the "idiopathic" podocytopathies have been attributed to underlying genetic mutations, hence the term *genetic podocytopathies*. *Secondary glomerulopathies*, conversely, are associated with systemic diseases such as viral infections (hepatitis B, hepatitis C, human immunodeficiency virus [HIV] infection), drugs (heavy metals, penicillamine, gold), and autoimmune diseases (systemic lupus erythematosus, Henoch-Schönlein purpura, Sjögren's syndrome).

## EPIDEMIOLOGY

Nephrotic syndrome is the most prevalent pediatric glomerular disease. It affects 2 to 7 per 100,000 children annually worldwide and has a cumulative prevalence of 16 per 100,000 children.[20-24] The incidence of nephrotic syndrome in children peaks at the age of 2 years.[20,21] In 1978, a prospective study by the International Study of Kidney Diseases in Childhood (ISKDC) included 521 children between the age of 3 months and 16 years with newly diagnosed with nephrotic syndrome. This study provided invaluable insight into the clinicopathologic features of idiopathic nephrotic syndrome. As a result, the association between certain histopathologic features and steroid responsiveness was gradually established.[25]

An important observation is that the likelihood of having a specific underlying histopathologic lesion varies by age. For example, MCD is the underlying histopathologic feature in more than 90% of children with nephrotic syndrome who are less than 10 years of age. After the age of 10 years, minimal change histology is seen in only approximately 50% of cases. With the exception of the first year of life, the likelihood of MCD generally decreases as the age of disease onset increases. In contrast, the likelihood of FSGS, or resistance to steroid therapy, increases with age at presentation. This was illustrated by a classic ISKDC study of children with nephrotic syndrome who had undergone renal biopsy.[25] In that cohort, the median age at presentation for MCD was 3 years. In contrast, children with FSGS presented at an older age (median, 6 years).[25] None of the patients with MPGN presented before the age of 6 years.[25]

There is a male preponderance of approximately 2:1 among young children with idiopathic nephrotic syndrome. However, this difference disappears in adolescent children, who tend to have equal incidence in boys and girls.[20,21] Whereas MCNS and FSGS are more common in boys, MPGN has a female predominance.[25]

In addition to age and sex differences, ethnicity may also predict the underlying histopathologic features and response to therapy. In a case series of 42 children living in the United Kingdom, Asian children appeared to have a six times higher incidence of steroid-sensitive nephrotic syndrome (SSNS) compared to Europeans.[26] This difference was attributed to the higher incidence of atopy among Asian children. In a report from South Africa, conversely, steroid-sensitive nephrotic syndrome (SSNS) was relatively uncommon among African children (14.4%), even among those with underlying minimal change histologic features, only 44% of whom were responsive to steroids. In this cohort of African children, membranous nephropathy associated with hepatitis B virus was detected in 40% of the cases.[27] Genetic variation at the *MYH9* gene locus may also help explain the high rate of FSGS in African children.[28] In another study from Texas, a relatively high proportion (47%) of African-American children who presented with nephrotic syndrome had FSGS on histopathologic examination. This is in clear contrast to Hispanic and white children with nephrotic syndrome, of whom only 11% and 18% had FSGS on histopathologic examination, respectively.[29] Although Hispanics had the highest incidence of MCD, FSGS was the most common cause of nephrotic syndrome in African-American children.[29] Despite these differences in the underlying histopathologic characteristics, the overall incidence of nephrotic syndrome was found to be equally distributed across various ethnicities in the same report.[29] Similar findings were reported in another study from Kansas City.[22] However, in this study, African-American children appeared to have double the annual incidence of nephrotic syndrome as compared with white children.[22]

Familial forms of idiopathic nephrotic syndrome were first described in the literature in the early 1970s.[30-35] In a European survey of 1877 children with nephrotic syndrome, 3.3% had a family member affected by the disease.[32] Identical twins and other affected siblings tend to have a similar disease presentation, age at onset, underlying histologic features, and response to therapy.[34,35] More recently, various genes have been implicated in the pathogenesis of familial forms of the disease. These are discussed in more detail later.

## PATHOGENESIS

## MINIMAL CHANGE DISEASE

The exact etiology that underlies MCD remains unknown. Anecdotal evidence points to the presence of an unspecified systemic factor that disrupts the GFB, with resulting massive proteinuria and diffuse effacement of the podocyte foot processes. Classically, MCD has been considered primarily a disorder of cell-mediated (T-cell) immune regulation.[36]

However, more recent observations proposed an important contributory role for humoral (B-cell) immunity in the pathogenesis of the disease.[37]

At least two studies support the presence of an unidentified systemic factor in MCD. In the first study, serum collected from a patient with Hodgkin's lymphoma and MCD increased the in vitro permeability of cultured podocytes. The ability of the serum to increase podocyte permeability was abolished by treatment of the underlying Hodgkin's lymphoma.[38] In another report, kidneys transplanted from a patient with MCD into two recipients (with no proteinuria at baseline) resulted in transient proteinuria shortly after the transplant procedure that subsequently resolved spontaneously over a 6-week period.[39]

In 1974, Shalhoub et al.[36] suggested that abnormal T-cell monoclonal proliferation in nephrotic syndrome may produce a lymphokine that is toxic to the GBM. The central role of cell-mediated immunity in the pathogenesis of MCD has been supported by several observations. First, children with atopy appear to have a higher incidence of the disease.[40] Second, severe viral infections, known to suppress cell-mediated immunity, may sometimes induce remission of nephrotic syndrome.[36] Third, MCD appears to be more common among children with malignant diseases, particularly Hodgkin's lymphoma.[41] Fourth, medications known to suppress T-cell function, such as corticosteroids, dramatically induce remission in most children with MCD.[25]

In agreement with Shalhoub's hypothesis, T-cell function appears to be altered during active relapses of MCD.[42] Active MCD is associated with increased numbers of CD4[+] and CD8[+] memory T-cell subsets,[43] as well as with delayed cutaneous hypersensitivity reactions.[44] It also appears that the undifferentiated (CD34[+]) T-cells are involved in the pathogenesis of MCD, rather than the more mature (CD34[−]) cells.[45]

Clinical observations further support a role for T-cell–mediated autoimmunity in MCD. For example, viral upper respiratory infections commonly induce relapses in children with this disease. In addition, case reports indicated that SSNS may rarely be induced by a bee sting or a fire ant bite.[46,47] Bee stings may also precipitate a relapse in children with a known history of nephrotic syndrome.[48] Interestingly, a possible association between food allergies and the development of nephrotic syndrome has also been suggested in small case series. In a series of 42 patients with steroid resistant or steroid-dependent nephrotic syndrome (SDNS), 38% had positive skin testing and 29% had elevated serum IgE levels. Limiting certain antigens in the diet allowed for discontinuation of steroids for a period of 1 to 5 years in 7 of 27 patients with steroid-dependent disease. However, the benefit was not sustained because the majority of patients eventually had one or more relapses.[49]

Several studies attempted to identify cellular-immunity associated genes from peripheral blood mononuclear cells (PBMCs) that may be involved in the pathogenesis of MCD. Using a subtractive cDNA library, genes encoding cytoskeletal proteins and T-cell receptor components, such as Fyb/Slap, L-plastin, and grancalcin, were found to be upregulated during relapsing MCD.[50] Two additional reports yielded similar results using serial analyses of gene expression.[51,52] Collectively, these studies reflect a significantly altered transcriptome of PBMCs in patients with MCD. A subsequent proteomic analysis of PBMCs identified four proteins that were increased in relapsing MCD as compared with controls, three of which (L-plastin, α-tropomyosin, and annexin III) are known to be involved in cytoskeletal rearrangement.[53] Given the cross-sectional design of these studies, it is not possible to conclude that the aforementioned alterations in gene or protein expression are causally associated with MCD.

Cytokine release from T-cells has also been implicated in the pathogenesis of MCD.[54,55] Interleukin 13 (IL-13) gene expression appears to be enhanced in children with SRNS.[56] Moreover, overexpression of IL-13 in transfected rats induced albuminuria, hypoalbuminemia, and podocyte effacement with no structural glomerular lesion seen on light microscopy, thus closely resembling human MCD on histologic examination.[57] IL-13 in concert with other cytokines or microbial agents may trigger upregulation of CD80, a T-cell co-stimulation protein on the podocyte cell surface, and lead to the disruption of its cytoskeletal organization.[51] Further studies are needed before these mechanisms can be generalized to all children with MCD.

Humoral immunity, once considered irrelevant, may also play a role in the pathophysiology of MCD. This role is inferred from the observation that rituximab, an anti-CD20 (B-cell) monoclonal antibody, appears to alter the clinical course of some children with MCD.[37] Alternatively, the depletion of B cells by rituximab may favorably affect nephrosis by its disruption of the role of B cells in antigen presentation and subsequent cytokine production from T cells. Moreover, it has been known for decades that children with MCD have decreased serum IgG levels and increased serum IgM levels compared with the general population, a finding also suggesting humoral dysfunction.[58]

## FOCAL SEGMENTAL GLOMERULOSCLEROSIS

Despite similarities in the presentation, histopathologic features, and response to therapy between FSGS and MCD,[59] they are, in fact, two distinct pathologic entities. Podocyte injury is most probably the initial triggering event in both disorders. However, the underlying molecular mechanisms of injury or response to injury are vastly different between the two diseases. Some children who are initially diagnosed with MCD on a kidney biopsy may occasionally turn out to have FSGS on subsequent biopsies. This can be simply attributed to the focal nature of FSGS, and it raises the possibility of sampling error on an initial biopsy specimen. However, children with focal global sclerosis, with no segmental lesions seen on biopsy, tend to be more responsive to steroids and may follow a course that more closely resembles that of MCD.[60] FSGS may be idiopathic (formerly known as primary), genetic (familial or sporadic), or secondary. Because testing for many of the known genetic mutations is not currently widely available, many patients with sporadic FSGS who are clinically categorized as having "idiopathic" FSGS may actually have underlying undetected genetic mutations.

## Idiopathic focal segmental glomerulosclerosis

Injury to the podocyte (visceral epithelial cell) is thought to be the primary event leading to the development of idiopathic FSGS.[61,62] The initial injury results in effacement of the podocyte foot processes that, if severe, may progress to podocyte apoptosis. Because podocytes are generally unable to replicate, the resulting reduction in the number of podocytes leads to uncovered areas of the GBM. This is followed by formation of adhesions (synechiae) between the GBM and the parietal epithelial cells. Subsequently, filtered plasma proteins begin to accumulate in the area underlying the parietal epithelial cells (periglomerular space) and the subendothelial space, thus triggering interstitial inflammation, hyalinosis, and segmental sclerosis. Finally, advanced disease is characterized by the development of progressive global sclerosis and interstitial fibrosis.

The precise mechanisms underlying podocyte injury in FSGS are poorly understood. Immunologic, inflammatory, genetic, and toxic factors may all play a role. In many patients with FSGS, the injury appears to be mediated by a circulating factor. This notion was supported by several clinical observations. First, there is a relatively high rate of recurrence of FSGS following renal transplantation,[63] and plasmapheresis often improves proteinuria in transplant recipients with recurrence of disease.[64] Second, injection of serum from patients with collapsing glomerulopathy, a severe form of FSGS, into rats may result in transient proteinuria.[65] Third, transient proteinuria was reported in an infant born to a mother with active FSGS.[66]

The soluble urokinase plasminogen activator receptor (suPAR) has been identified as a candidate circulating factor in patients with FSGS.[67] In mouse models, overexpression of suPAR was associated with massive proteinuria, effacement of podocyte foot processes, and segmental glomerular lesions, similar to those seen in human FSGS.[68] In animal studies, suPAR-induced podocyte injury appears to be mediated by activation of $\beta_3$ integrin.[68] However, human studies correlating serum suPAR with clinical activity in idiopathic FSGS have yielded conflicting results. In one report, serum suPAR levels were elevated in 55% of children and in 84% of adults with active FSGS and were suppressed with successful immunosuppressive therapy.[68,69] In another

report, suPAR was specifically elevated in patients with FSGS, but not in other glomerular diseases such as MCD or membranous nephropathy.[68] However, the latter study was heavily criticized for failing to account for differences in glomerular filtration rate (GFR), a key confounding variable among participants in the study.[70] In contrast, a small single center study showed no difference in plasma suPAR levels between children with FSGS and those with other glomerular diseases, or even healthy controls.[71] Notably, high pretransplant serum levels of suPAR were found in a retrospective review of patients who developed post-transplant FSGS recurrence [67] However, because serum suPAR accumulates in advanced renal failure, it did not appear to have prognostic utility when obtained in adult renal transplant candidates. Urine suPAR has also been proposed as an alternate option for use in the pretransplant evaluation of patients with FSGS.[72]

## Genetic variants of focal segmental glomerulosclerosis

Since the discovery of the nephrin gene in 1998,[7] growing numbers of patients with FSGS have been found to have gene mutations inherited in a mendelian fashion.[7,8,73,74] Such mutations may be detected in the majority of infants with congenital or infantile nephrotic syndrome, in children with familial FSGS, and even in a significant number of children with sporadic steroid-resistant FSGS. These genes are mainly involved in the formation or regulation of the slit diaphragm (nephrin, podocin, alpha-actinin-4, TRPC6, CD2AP) or regulation of podocyte differentiation and cytoskeletal stability.

NPHS2 encodes for podocin, a protein exclusively expressed in podocytes that constitutes an integral component of the glomerular slit diaphragm. NPHS2 has been implicated in early-onset autosomal recessive familial FSGS.[8] In addition, NPHS2 mutations have been described in children with sporadic SRNS and adults with autosomal recessive FSGS.[75] In a French multicenter study, NPHS2 mutations were detected in 42% of patients with autosomal recessive SRNS and in 10.5% of patients with sporadic SRNS. Patients with a single mutation of NPHS2 tend to present at an older age than do patients with multiple mutations.[76]

NPHS1 gene mutations are known to cause congenital nephrotic syndrome of the Finnish type.[7] However, NPHS1 mutations have also been reported in older children and young adults with SRNS.[77,78]

Mutations in the inverted formin 2 (INF2) gene have emerged as important causes of autosomal dominant familial FSGS.[73] INF2 encodes for a member of the formin family of actin-regulating proteins, an essential factor that promotes the stability of the podocyte's cytoskeletal structure. INF2 mutations have been detected in 9% to 17% of families with late-onset familial FSGS,[79-81] but these mutations are relatively rare in sporadic FSGS.[79] In one study, mutations in INF2 and WT1 were identified as causative in 20% and 10%

of autosomal dominant SRNS, respectively.[82] *INF2* mutations have also been implicated in the pathogenesis of the neuropathy and glomerulopathy associated with Charcot-Marie-Tooth disease.[83]

*ACTN4* encodes for α-actinin-4, a cytoskeletal protein that appears to be essential for podocyte structural integrity. *ACTN4* mutations were identified in 3.5% of children and adults with familial autosomal dominant FSGS and in less than 1% of those with sporadic FSGS.[84] Mutations in *ACTN4* are often reflected by distinct histologic features on electron microscopy, primarily in the form of electron-dense collections in the podocyte cytoplasm.[85]

The *TRPC6* gene encodes for a calcium-permeable receptor, known as the canonical transient receptor potential six-ion channel. This channel appears to play an important role in the proper function of podocytes and slit diaphragms.[9] Mutations have been classically associated with late-onset familial autosomal dominant FSGS,[86] but they have also been reported in children with sporadic SRNS.[87,88]

Finally, two mutations in the *Myo1E* gene, encoding myosin 1E, were identified in two independent families from Italy and Turkey. Both families had multiple children with autosomal recessive steroid resistant FSGS.[74]

## Secondary focal segmental glomerulosclerosis

### HYPERFILTRATION INJURY

Podocytes are terminally differentiated cells that are generally unable to replicate. In response to nephron loss, such as in chronic kidney disease, renal dysplasia, or nephrectomy, compensatory changes develop in the remaining nephrons, which are manifested as glomerular hypertrophy and intraglomerular hypertension. The increase in the single nephron GFR initially serves to compensate for the reduced total number of nephrons. However, hyperfiltration often exacerbates podocyte shear stress and eventually leads to podocyte detachment from the GBM. The subsequent events that lead to segmental sclerosis are comparable to those described earlier in idiopathic FSGS. Histologically, the presence of glomerular hypertrophy and a patchy distribution of foot process effacement (less than 50% of the total glomerular capillary surface area) may help differentiate secondary forms of FSGS from idiopathic FSGS.[89]

### OBESITY

Similarly, severe obesity may also lead to glomerulomegaly, hyperfiltration, and increased GFR, which infrequently progresses to secondary FSGS.[90] Hemodynamic factors, related to hyperfiltration and intraglomerular hypertension, may also account for the development of FSGS in patients with severe preeclampsia, anabolic steroid abuse,[91] pamidronate,[92] and interferon therapy.[93] Interestingly, prematurity and very low birth weight have been associated

with reduced nephron number and an increased risk for the subsequent development of secondary FSGS.[94,95]

### OTHER RENAL DISEASES

Secondary FSGS may also develop as a consequence of healed inflammatory glomerular lesions, such as those resulting from vasculitis, lupus nephritis, IgA nephropathy or postinfectious nephritis. In the healing phase of glomerular inflammation, extracellular matrix deposition and fibrosis appear to be mediated primarily by overexpression of transforming growth factor-β (TGF-β) in an animal model.[96]

## EVALUATION OF PATIENTS WITH PRIMARY PODOCYTOPATHY

Most children with nephrotic syndrome present with generalized pitting edema. Initial evaluation should be aimed at confirming the diagnosis, screening for complications, assessing the indications for a renal biopsy, and excluding secondary and familial forms of the disease.

## CLINICAL HISTORY

Generalized swelling is usually first noticed in soft tissue regions with weak subcutaneous fasciae, such as the periorbital area, scrotum, or labia. Edema tends to accumulate in gravity-dependent areas, such as the lower extremities in ambulatory patients. The symptoms are frequently preceded by a triggering illness, such as a viral upper respiratory infection. A primary podocytopathy should be suspected in any child who develops progressive swelling with no systemic symptoms (e.g., arthralgias or skin rash) and no known triggers (medications or toxins). Clinical Study 17.1 describes the typical clinical presentation in a young child.

## PHYSICAL EXAMINATION

Systemic hypertension is more common in children with FSGS and secondary podocytopathies when compared with children with MCD. Joint swelling, joint erythema, skin rash, and mouth ulcers are uncommon in primary podocytopathies and warrant evaluation for secondary causes, such as systemic lupus erythematosus.

## LABORATORY STUDIES

The diagnosis of nephrotic syndrome is confirmed by detecting massive proteinuria (300 mg/dL or more) on urine dipstick, low serum albumin (less than 2.5 g/dL), and commonly elevated serum cholesterol or triglycerides on blood chemistry studies. The proteinuria may be quantified by using a spot urine protein-to-creatinine ratio (normal, less than 0.2 mg/mg; nephrotic range, greater than 2.0 mg/mg). Microscopic hematuria is not uncommon in children with primary podocytopathies. Approximately 20% of children with MCD and 50% of those with FSGS manifest microscopic hematuria at initial presentation.[25] In contrast, gross hematuria is relatively rare in children with primary podocytopathies. Elevated blood urea nitrogen (BUN) or creatinine signals concurrent acute kidney injury, often related to intravascular fluid volume depletion, but it can also suggest an alternative diagnosis such as chronic glomerulonephritis or IgA nephropathy.[97]

---

**KEY POINT**

Gross hematuria, elevated blood pressure, elevated BUN or creatinine, and hypocomplementemia are uncommon in MCD and should raise the suspicion of an alternate cause.

---

Additional testing should include complement components (C3 and C4), antinuclear antibodies (ANA), and anti-double stranded (ds) DNA to evaluate for MPGN and lupus. Liver function tests along with serologic testing for hepatitis B virus (HBV), hepatitis C virus (HCV), and HIV may be indicated in sexually active adolescents or other at-risk children.

## INDICATIONS FOR RENAL BIOPSY

A renal biopsy is often unnecessary at the initial presentation of children with nephrotic syndrome. Accumulating evidence has revealed that a thorough initial clinical evaluation of children presenting with nephrotic syndrome predicts, with satisfactory accuracy, the likelihood of subsequent clinical response to corticosteroid therapy.[25] The following criteria have been established that are consistent with a diagnosis of MCD and therefore predict a high probability (greater than 90%) of steroid-responsive disease: (1) children between the age of 1 and 10 years; (2) absence of hypertension, gross hematuria, or elevated serum creatinine; and (3) normocomplementemia. It is recommended that children who satisfy all the aforementioned criteria empirically receive an initial treatment course of daily corticosteroids without the need to obtain a kidney biopsy.[98]

---

**KEY POINT**

Children with the typical clinical and laboratory features of MCD may be treated empirically with steroids, without the need for a renal biopsy.

---

A kidney biopsy should be considered in children who do not fulfill the foregoing criteria or who do not respond to the initial or subsequent courses of corticosteroids. A renal biopsy has also been recommended for all children who are older than 12 years of age on presentation.[99] Older children also are at a greater risk for non-minimal change causes, such as FSGS or lupus nephritis.[99] Although some clinicians recommend a renal biopsy based on age, one could argue that an empiric trial of corticosteroids could be considered in a teenage child who does not fulfill any of the aforementioned criteria of hypertension, gross hematuria, azotemia, or hypocomplementemia. Because the best predictor of long-term prognosis is steroid responsiveness, it would be reasonable to postpone the biopsy and reassess the need for a potential biopsy after the initial 3 to 4 weeks of treatment with corticosteroids. A biopsy will also be required if the initial evaluation uncovers findings that point to a cause other than MCD. Such findings may include systemic hypertension, skin rash, pruritus, weight loss, arthralgias, positive viral serologic test results, or a positive serum ANA or anti ds DNA.

## HISTOLOGIC CLASSIFICATION

## MINIMAL CHANGE DISEASE

Histologically, MCD is defined by the absence of glomerular or tubulointerstitial abnormalities on light microscopy (Figure 17.1) and by the absence of immune deposits on immunofluorescence staining. However, the finding of mild mesangial hypercellularity or occasional globally sclerotic glomeruli does not exclude the diagnosis.[100] On electron microscopy, diffuse podocyte foot process effacement is usually prominent. In some cases of early FSGS, if none of the glomeruli examined on the initial kidney biopsy demonstrate segmental sclerosis, the histologic diagnosis may be labeled as MCD. Subsequently, segmental sclerotic lesions may be seen on a repeat biopsy specimen obtained months to years later. Such situations have led to the controversial belief by some investigators that MCD and FSGS may represent different stages of the same pathologic entity, as discussed earlier.

In children who present with nephrotic syndrome but no systemic symptoms, MCD is the most likely underlying histopathologic process.[25] This was illustrated by the original ISKDC cohort, which included 521 children who presented with symptoms of nephrotic syndrome. In this group, 77% were found to have MCD histologic features on the initial

---

**KEY POINTS**

Histologic variants of MCD disease include:

- C1q nephropathy
- MesProlif GN
- IgM nephropathy

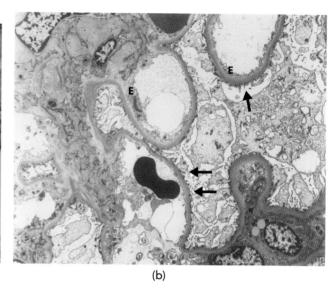

(a)              (b)

Figure 17.1 **(a)** Light microscopy displaying the histologic appearance for minimal change disease. The glomerulus (periodic acid–Schiff stain ×40) shows normal size and cellularity. The capillary loops are thin and uniform. The mesangium is not expanded. **(b)** Electron microscopy showing diffuse effacement of the podocyte foot processes over the urinary aspect of the glomerular basement membrane (arrows). The endothelial cells (E) are unremarkable, and there are no mesangial, subendothelial or subepithelial deposits.

renal biopsy. In the same cohort, 80% of children eventually diagnosed with MCD on renal biopsy presented with nephrosis before the age of 6 years. In contrast, only 50% of children with a histologic diagnosis of FSGS presented at such a young age.[25] In a more recent report, 88% of children who presented with nephrotic syndrome had MCD on renal biopsy.[101]

## MINIMAL CHANGE DISEASE VARIANTS

Histologic variants have been proposed that resemble MCD on light microscopy but are distinguished by ultrastructural characteristics on electron microscopy or immunofluorescence. In view of the limited knowledge of the underlying pathophysiology, it remains unclear whether these disorders represent primary podocyte disorders, similar to MCD or FSGS, or separate pathologic entities with secondary involvement of the podocytes. The clinical significance of these variants lies in their lower response rate to corticosteroid therapy and their less favorable prognosis compared with classic histologic features of MCD.[102–104]

### Mesangial proliferative glomerulonephritis

The MesProlif GN variant *of* MCD is characterized by variable degrees of mesangial proliferation.[105,106] In a series of 29 children with diffuse mesangial hypercellularity, the majority had associated microscopic or gross hematuria, and close to 50% had concurrent systemic hypertension. In the same cohort, 40% of children were steroid resistant, a proportion that far exceeds the 10% rate of steroid resistance that has been previously described in children with classic MCD.[106]

## Immunoglobulin M nephropathy

IgM nephropathy is differentiated from classic MCD by the presence of electron-dense mesangial immune deposits that correspond to granular IgM staining on immunofluorescence staining.[103] These deposits must be differentiated from nonspecific mesangial IgM deposits, a relatively common finding in MCD that, in contrast to those seen in IgM nephropathy, do not correspond to electron-dense deposits on electron microscopy. The prognostic significance of a histopathologic diagnosis of IgM nephropathy remains uncertain. In a study that included 23 children with steroid-resistant or steroid-dependent IgM nephropathy, 88% of those treated with cyclosporine (7 of 8) achieved a partial or complete remission as compared with only 18% of those treated with cyclophosphamide (2 of 11).[107] In another large series of 110 children and adults with IgM nephropathy who were followed for a mean duration of 8 years, 29% were steroid resistant and 57% were steroid dependent. In the same cohort, 36% developed chronic renal insufficiency, and 23% reached end-stage kidney disease (ESKD) over the follow-up period, percentages that far exceed what would be expected in children with classic MCD.[104]

## C1q nephropathy

In the absence of serologic evidence for systemic lupus erythematosus, diffuse mesangial electron-dense deposits associated with predominant C1q staining on immunofluorescence define *C1q nephropathy*. This histologic entity may be associated with MCD,[108] FSGS,[102] or mesangial proliferative lesions on light microscopy. Studies evaluating the prognostic significance of C1q nephropathy have yielded conflicting results. In a report of

12 children with C1q nephropathy, 8 of whom presented with nephrotic syndrome, most had steroid-dependent or steroid-resistant disease. The likelihood of progression to ESKD was very high, particularly in patients with steroid-resistant cases.[109] In contrast, only 3 of 61 children and adults with C1q nephropathy in another report developed renal insufficiency 8 to 15 years following the initial diagnosis.[110] In another review of 72 children and adults with C1q nephropathy, most (77%) of those with MCD histologic features, but only one-third of those with FSGS histologic features, were in complete remission at a mean follow-up of 5.5 years (range, 4 months to 21 years).[108]

# FOCAL SEGMENTAL GLOMERULOSCLEROSIS

As the nomenclature implies, FSGS is histologically characterized by glomerular fibrosis or mesangial collapse (glomerulosclerosis) that affects part of (segmental) the glomerular tuft (Figure 17.2). The lesions typically involve some but not all glomeruli (focal). In the initial stages of disease, most affected glomeruli are juxtamedullary and therefore may be missed on a renal biopsy that samples only cortical tissue.[111] Nonspecific mesangial IgM and C3 deposits are frequently seen in the glomerular sclerotic lesions on immunofluorescence staining. In contrast, staining for IgG is usually negative.[112] Electron microscopy often reveals diffuse podocyte foot process effacement, which is particularly prominent in children with idiopathic FSGS.[113]

Several mutually exclusive histologic variants of FSGS have been described (Columbia classification), the prognostic significance of which is not entirely clear.[114]

## Classic focal segmental glomerulosclerosis

The diagnosis of classic FSGS (FSGS not otherwise specified), the most common form of FSGS, is generally made on exclusion of all other histologic variants. In classic FSGS, segmental glomerulosclerosis is seen in one or more capillary loops and is associated with variable degrees of mesangial matrix expansion and hypercellularity.[89,115]

## Collapsing variant

Collapsing variant FSGS is characterized by the global or segmental collapse of the glomerular capillary tuft (Figure 17.3). Collapsing FSGS has been associated with HIV infection[116] and parvovirus B19 infection.[117,118] It appears to be more common in children of African descent. Clinically, it is correlated with severe nephrotic syndrome that is generally resistant to immunosuppressive therapy and often carries a poor prognosis, almost invariably progressing to ESKD.[119] Because of differences in podocyte number between collapsing FSGS and the other variants, with apparent proliferation in the collapsing lesion versus podocytopenia in the others, it has been suggested that the collapsing variant is a distinct disease.[120] However, no differences in treatment regimen have been proposed.

## Tip variant

Tip variant FSGS is defined by the presence of segmental involvement of the glomerular tuft at the origin of the proximal tubule, at which there is prominent tissue expansion by foam cells or hyaline material.[121] The remainder of the glomerular tuft appears normal by light microscopy, but diffuse podocyte foot process effacement is seen on electron microscopy. Clinically, tip variant has been correlated with an abrupt onset of steroid-sensitive nephrotic syndrome, resembling MCD.[121] Notably, in a small report in adults, as many as 55% of patients with tip variant FSGS on initial biopsy actually underwent spontaneous complete remission without the need for immunosuppressive therapy.[122]

## Perihilar variant

Perihilar variant FSGS is distinguished by segmental sclerosis and hyalinosis in a perihilar pattern. Perihilar variant is seen predominantly in children with secondary FSGS.

---

### KEY POINTS

Histologic variants of FSGS include:

- Classic FSGS (FSGS not otherwise specified)
- Collapsing variant
- Tip variant
- Perihilar variant
- Cellular variant

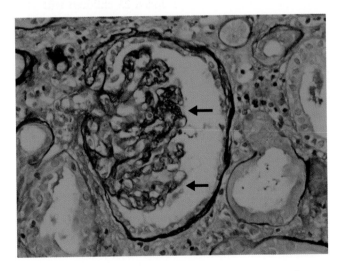

Figure 17.2 Renal biopsy findings in a child with nephrotic syndrome resulting from classic focal segmental glomerulosclerosis. A photomicrograph of a glomerulus (periodic acid–Schiff stain ×40) shows a normal segment of the glomerulus (lower arrow) and the sclerotic (upper arrow) glomerular segment.

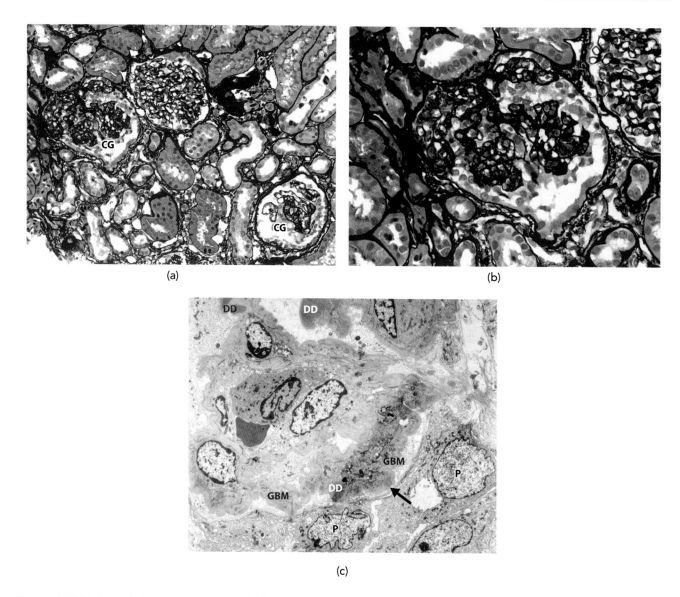

Figure 17.3 Light and electron microscopy findings in a patient with collapsing focal segmental glomerulosclerosis. **(a)** Low-power photomicrograph (Jones stain ×20) shows two glomeruli with retracted and collapsed capillary tufts (CG). The capillary lumina are not preserved. **(b)** Higher-power photomicrograph (Jones stain ×40) of the same patient shows a glomerulus with collapsed capillary tuft, hyperplastic and hypertrophied epithelial cells, and thickened glomerular basement membrane (GBM). **(c)** An electron micrograph shows collapsed capillary loops with obliteration of the capillary lumina. Diffuse effacement of the podocyte (P) foot processes over the urinary aspect of the GBM is also noted. Abundant entrapped electron dense deposits (DD) are seen in the mesangium and on the inner sides of the collapsed glomerular capillary loops (arrow). No subepithelial deposits are present.

## Cellular variant

Finally, cellular variant FSGS is diagnosed when at least one glomerulus shows segmental cellular proliferation. This lesion has been correlated clinically with a poor prognosis, similar to collapsing FSGS.[89]

## Increasing incidence

Several studies have reported an increase in the incidence of FSGS in both children and adults over the last several decades.[22,29,123] It has been frequently debated, however, whether this trend can be simply explained by the more

selective approach to obtaining renal biopsies in modern medicine. In the classic ISKDC cohort, renal biopsies were obtained on all patients who presented with nephrotic syndrome before or shortly after initiating therapy. In the current era, renal biopsies are generally performed only for children who to fail to respond to the initial 4- to 8-week course of steroids and therefore carry a far higher likelihood of having structural glomerular lesions, including FSGS. To minimize this bias, a study compared the incidence of FSGS in a well-defined geographic area between two periods of 8½ years extending from 1985 to 2002. Consistent with previous reports, the annual incidence of FSGS increased from 0.37 to 0.94 cases per 100,000-child population/year between the two eras studied.[123] The basis behind this increase in the incidence of FSGS over time remains unknown.

In older children and adults, detecting occasional glomeruli with global sclerosis on renal biopsy is not uncommon. Focal global glomerulosclerosis (FGGS) is distinguished from FSGS by complete, rather than segmental, scarring of one or more sampled glomeruli. In the absence of significant associated interstitial changes, global sclerosis is considered a nonspecific finding and correlates with a more favorable long-term outcome when compared with FSGS histologic features.[60,124]

Secondary FSGS, a condition attributed to nephron loss, is associated with similar light microscopic findings as those seen in idiopathic FSGS, except for the prominent finding of glomerulomegaly. However, electron microscopy typically reveals focal podocyte foot process effacement in secondary FSGS, mainly confined to the sclerotic lesions, as opposed to the diffuse pattern seen in idiopathic FSGS.[89] Secondary FSGS may be seen in children with reflux nephropathy, renal dysplasia, sickle cell disease, glycogen storage diseases, and congenital heart disease.[125–127] In contrast to idiopathic FSGS, secondary FSGS typically manifests with a more gradual onset of proteinuria, which is usually in the subnephrotic range. Children with secondary FSGS are also less likely to have features of active nephrotic syndrome, such as edema, ascites, and hypoalbuminemia. The disorder is unlikely to respond to immunosuppressive therapy, but it is usually treated with angiotensin blockade and often has a more favorable outcome.[90,128]

# SECONDARY PODOCYTOPATHIES

Podocyte injury may be the result of a systemic illness affecting multiple organs, the mechanism of which varies depending on the underlying origin. Secondary causes of childhood nephrotic syndrome include infectious agents, drugs, metabolic derangements, malignant diseases, and autoimmune diseases (Table 17.2).

## Minimal change disease

### LYMPHOMA

Nephrotic syndrome is infrequently reported in children and adults with Hodgkin's lymphoma. The timing of renal involvement is highly variable. The nephrotic symptoms may precede the diagnosis of Hodgkin's disease by up to several years,[129,130] may occur simultaneously,[131] or may even occur later during remission.[132] MCD appears to be the most common underlying histopathologic lesion in this setting. The nephrotic syndrome commonly remits with successful treatment of the underlying lymphoma.[133,134]

### NONSTEROIDAL ANTI-INFLAMMATORY DRUGS

Nephrotic syndrome, in the form of MCD or membranous nephropathy, with or without concomitant tubulointerstitial nephritis, is a rare side effect of nonsteroidal anti-inflammatory drugs (NSAIDs).[135–137] Glomerular disease has also been reported with the use of the newer selective NSAIDs,

**Table 17.2** Primary and secondary podocytopathies in children

**Primary Causes**
- Minimal change disease (MCD)
- Focal segmental glomerulosclerosis (FSGS)
- MCD variants
  - Mesangial proliferative glomerulonephritis
  - Immunoglobulin M nephropathy
  - C1q nephropathy
- Membranoproliferative glomerulonephritis (MPGN)
  - MPGN type I
  - MPGN type II (dense deposit disease)
  - MPGN type III
- Membranous nephropathy

**Genetic Causes***
- Nonsyndromic
  - *NPHS2* (podocin)
  - *NPHS1* (nephrin)
  - *IFN2* (formin)
  - *ACTN4* (α-actinin-4)
  - TRPC6 (TRPC6)
  - *Myo1E* (nonmuscle myosin-1E)
  - *PLCE1* (phospholipase Cε1)
  - *CD2AP* (CD2-associated protein)
- Syndromic
  - *WT1* (Denysh-Drash syndrome)
  - Mitochondrially encoded tRNA leucine 1 (mitochondrial myopathy, encephalopathy, lactic acidosis, and stroke-like episodes).
  - *ITGB4* (epidermolysis bullosa)
  - *CD151* (epidermolysis bullosa, sensorineural deafness, nail dystrophy)
  - *SCARB* (action myoclonus–renal failure syndrome)
  - *LMX1b* (nail-patella syndrome)
  - Nonmuscle myosin IIA (*MYH9*; Epstein and Fechtner syndrome)
- *LAMB2* (Pierson syndrome)

**Causes of Secondary Minimal Change Disease**
- Lymphoma
- Nonsteroidal anti-Inflammatory drugs (NSAIDs)
- Gold salts
- Penicillamine, bucillamine
- Anti–tumor necrosis factor agents, such as infliximab and etanercept

**Causes of Secondary Focal Segmental Glomerulosclerosis**
- Human immunodeficiency virus (HIV) infection
- Leukemia and lymphoma

*(continued)*

- Anabolic steroids
- Mitochondrial disorders
- Sickle cell disease
- Glycogen storage diseases
- Obesity

**Causes of Secondary Collapsing Glomerulopathy**
- HIV infection
- Parvovirus B19 infection
- Hepatitis C
- Human T-lymphocyte virus type I (HTLV-I) infection
- Cytomegalovirus infection

*  This is a limited list of the more common genetic causes of nephrotic syndrome. The reader is referred to www.omim. org for a more comprehensive and current list of genetic mutations that may cause nephrotic syndrome.

such as the cyclooxygenase 2 (COX-2) inhibitor, celecoxib.[138] However, in another report, celecoxib was successfully used as an alternative in an adult with NSAID-associated nephrotic syndrome without recurrence of the renal symptoms. This finding may suggest that a selective NSAID can sometimes be safely substituted with close monitoring for patients who require continued NSAID therapy.[139]

OTHER MEDICATIONS

In addition to NSAIDs, multiple other anti-inflammatory medications have been linked to the development of nephrotic syndrome. These include gold salts (especially parenteral formulations),[140] penicillamine,[141] bucillamine,[142] and anti–tumor necrosis factor agents, such as infliximab and etanercept.[143] Histologically, the glomerular toxicity of these agents may manifest as MCD, membranous nephropathy,[144] or immune complex glomerulonephritis, among others. In a case series of 33 patients with penicillamine-induced glomerulopathy, proteinuria did not clearly correlate with the dose or duration of therapy. However, 80% of the affected patients presented in the first year of therapy and most patients (close to 90%) had membranous nephropathy on renal biopsy.[141] Tiopronin, a thiol drug with marked structural similarity to penicillamine that is used to treat cystinuria, has also been associated with the development of membranous nephropathy.[145]

# Focal segmental glomerulosclerosis

HUMAN IMMUNODEFICIENCY VIRUS INFECTION

Nephrotic syndrome is the most common presentation of HIV-related nephropathy.[146] In a large series of 71 children with HIV-1–related nephropathy from Africa, 39% had classic FSGS, and 26% had collapsing FSGS. The children with collapsing glomerulopathy had a worse outcome.[147] On electron microscopy, tubuloreticular inclusions may be seen, but they are not considered specific for HIV infection.[116] Fortunately, most children who receive antiretroviral therapy are expected to achieve partial or complete remission.[116] Persistent sterile pyuria has been correlated with declining renal function in HIV-infected children treated with indinavir.[148] In addition to FSGS, other forms of glomerular involvement have been reported with HIV, including immune complex kidney disease (HIVICK) and thrombotic microangiopathies.[149]

LEUKEMIA

A few case reports have identified acute lymphoblastic leukemia that developed in children treated for nephrotic syndrome.[150,151] The relative contribution, if any, of the immunosuppressive therapy to the risk of malignancy in these patients remains uncertain. Moreover, multiple case reports have been described of steroid-sensitive nephrotic syndrome, particularly FSGS or MCD, associated with chronic lymphocytic leukemia.[152-154] Case reports of membranous nephropathy have also been described in patients with acute myeloid leukemia.[155] Hematopoietic stem cell transplantation, with or without graft-versus-host disease, has also been linked to the development of nephrotic syndrome in several pediatric[156] and adult cases.[157-160]

DRUGS

Anabolic steroids, frequently abused to enhance athletic performance, have been associated with the development of secondary FSGS. In a retrospective review of 10 patients, prolonged use of anabolic steroids (8 to 20 years) was associated with significant proteinuria, which progressed to nephrotic syndrome in 3 patients. Renal biopsies revealed FSGS in the majority of cases. In the same report, glomerulomegaly and collapsing glomerulopathy were seen in 4 and 3 patients, respectively. Glomerulopathy improved after discontinuation of the offending agents.[91]

MITOCHONDRIAL DISORDERS

Minor renal tubular abnormalities are the most common renal manifestations of mitochondrial disorders, and these abnormalities affect up to 50% of children with known mitochondrial disease.[91] However, case reports have described glomerular disease in children with mitochondrial disorders, primarily in the form of steroid-resistant FSGS,[161,162] collapsing glomerulopathy, or crescentic glomerulonephritis.[163] Rarely, mutations in the COQ2 gene leading to coenzyme Q10 deficiency, have been detected in patients with collapsing glomerulopathy associated with mitochondrial disease.[163] Characteristic features are detected on electron microscopy in children with COQ2 gene mutations. These features include numerous structurally abnormal mitochondria located in the glomerular and tubular cells. These mitochondria appear enlarged, lack cristae, and have an electron-lucent central core.[163,164] Other closely linked mutations in the coenzyme Q10 pathway have also been described, including mutations in the PDSS2[165] and COQ6 genes.[166] Mutations in the COQ6 gene are also associated with a syndrome of SRNS and sensorineural hearing loss.[166] Treatment with coenzyme Q10 supplements, also known as ubidecarenone, may help alleviate many of the manifestations of coenzyme Q10 deficiency.[161,167]

## SICKLE CELL DISEASE

Renal manifestations of sickle cell disease include hematuria, tubular dysfunction, vascular compromise, and glomerular disease. Proteinuria develops in 25% of patients with SS disease.[168] Histologic patterns suggestive of secondary FSGS are often seen on renal biopsy, in concert with glomerular enlargement and hyperfiltration injury to podocytes.[168] Angiotensin-converting enzyme inhibitors (ACEIs) appear to be beneficial in this setting, by improving glomerular capillary hemodynamics and reducing proteinuria by more than 50% as illustrated in one study.[168] As would be expected with hemodynamic podocyte injury, the onset of proteinuria in sickle cell disease is gradual and not associated with significant swelling. Therefore, a child with sickle cell disease who presents with an acute onset of nephrotic syndrome should be evaluated for alternate causes.[169] In addition to FSGS, collapsing glomerulopathy and MPGN have also been described in patients with sickle cell disease.[170,171]

## OBESITY

Nephrotic syndrome has been associated with severe obesity since the early 1970s.[172] With the emerging epidemic of obesity, the prevalence of obesity-associated glomerulopathy has increased by 10-fold over a 10-year period from 1986 to 1996.[90] *Obesity-induced glomerulopathy* has been attributed to an increase in GFR, hyperfiltration and intraglomerular hypertension.[90,173] In one report, for instance, the average GFR in severely obese adults was 145 mL/min compared with 90 mL/min in their nonobese counterparts.[173] More recently, lack of adiponectin, an adipose tissue–secreted hormone, has also been implicated in the underlying pathogenesis of glomerular injury in obese patients.[174] Glomerulomegaly and variable degrees of segmental or global sclerosis are the most common histologic lesions seen in obesity-related glomerulopathy.[90] By electron microscopy, increased width of individual foot processes, decreased density of podocytes, and decreased numbers of podocytes are prominent features of the disease.[175] Both weight loss and the use of ACEIs are effective treatment options.[176]

## Secondary collapsing glomerulopathy

As previously detailed, HIV is by far the most common viral infection associated with collapsing glomerulopathy. Small case series and case reports have also implicated other viruses, such as parvovirus B19,[118] hepatitis C virus, and human T-lymphocyte virus type I (HTLV-I),[116] and cytomegalovirus (CMV).[119] although a causal relationship has not been established between these viruses and the associated collapsing glomerulopathy. Because

immunosuppressive therapy may be detrimental in patients with such viral infections, a thorough viral workup is warranted before labeling a child as having "idiopathic" collapsing glomerulopathy.[119]

## TREATMENT OF PRIMARY PODOCYTOPATHIES

Since the introduction of corticosteroids in the early 1950s, the outcome for children with nephrotic syndrome has been dramatically altered. Over the following several decades, classic reports from the ISKDC and the Arbeitsgemeinschaft fur Padiatrische Nephrologie (APN) have served to improve the treatment of nephrotic syndrome further.[177-179] In one report, glucocorticoid therapy induced complete remission in 89% of children with nephrotic syndrome.[101] However, steroid responsiveness varied substantially according to the underlying histopathologic features. For instance, 95% to 98% of children with MCD responded to corticosteroid therapy as compared with only 20% of those with FSGS.[98,180] Several presenting features have been identified that may help predict the underlying histopathologic features and, therefore, the response to corticosteroids. Specifically, children between the age of 1 and 10 years, with normal renal function, no gross hematuria, no systemic hypertension, and no hypocomplementemia, are most likely to be steroid sensitive. As discussed earlier, it has been generally recommended that children who fulfill most or all of these features receive empiric treatment with glucocorticoids without resorting to a kidney biopsy.[99] Guidelines have been established for the initial and subsequent treatment regimens for children with nephrotic syndrome. Following the initial course of corticosteroids, the subsequent therapeutic approach varies considerably based on steroid responsiveness, frequency of relapses, and biopsy results, if a biopsy is deemed necessary. A widely used classification based on the response to steroids and frequency of relapses is detailed in Table 17.3.

## STEROID-SENSITIVE NEPHROTIC SYNDROME

Guidelines for the treatment of childhood nephrotic syndrome were published in 2009 by the Children's Nephrotic Syndrome Consensus Conference, an expert panel of pediatric nephrologists (Table 17.4). These recommendations were developed for children 1 to 18 years of age with nephrotic syndrome. The panel recommended that the initial episode of nephrotic syndrome be treated with prednisone 2 mg/kg/day for 6 weeks (maximum, 60 mg per day), followed by 1.5 mg/kg/dose (maximum, 40 mg per dose) given every other day for 6 additional weeks. Prednisone should then be discontinued at the conclusion of the initial treatment course without the need for a tapering regimen.[99] Following this initial regimen, it is estimated that approximately 50%

Table 17.3 Clinical terminology based on response to corticosteroids and the frequency of relapses

| Term | Definition |
|---|---|
| Nephrotic syndrome | The presence of edema, high-grade proteinuria (>40 mg/m²/h or a urine protein-to-creatinine ratio >2.0) and hypoalbuminemia (<2.5 g/dL)* |
| Remission of nephrotic syndrome | Reduction in the spot urine protein-to-creatinine ratio to <0.2 mg/mg, or urine albumin dipstick readings that are negative or trace for 3 consecutive days |
| Relapse of nephrotic syndrome | Following remission, relapse is defined by an increase in the spot urine protein to creatinine (preferably obtained on a first-morning urine sample) to >2.0, or urine albumin dipstick readings exceeding 100 mg/dL (2+ or more) on 3 out of 5 consecutive days |
| Steroid-sensitive nephrotic syndrome (SSNS) | Remission in response to an initial 4–8-wk course of daily corticosteroid therapy |
| Steroid-resistant nephrotic syndrome (SRNS) | Persistent high-grade proteinuria following 4 wk of daily corticosteroids |
| Steroid-dependent nephrotic syndrome (SDNS) | Patients with SSNS who develop a relapse during gradual weaning of the dose of steroids, or within 2 wk of discontinuing steroid therapy |
| Frequent-relapsing nephrotic syndrome (FRNS) | Two or more relapses of nephrotic syndrome within a 6-mo period following initial therapy or four or more relapses within any 12-mo period |

* Hyperlipidemia and hypercoagulability are often associated findings, but they are not considered defining features of nephrotic syndrome.

of children will remain relapse free at 24-month follow-up. However, close to 30% are expected to develop a frequently relapsing course subsequently.[99]

Similar recommendations for the treatment of childhood nephrotic syndrome were published in 2012 by the Kidney Disease: Improving Global Outcomes (KDIGO) working group (see Table 17.4). The group

recommended that oral prednisone be given initially for 4 to 6 weeks as a single daily dose of 60 mg/m²/day or 2 mg/kg/day (maximum, 60 mg/day). This should be followed by alternate-day therapy of 40 mg/m²/per dose or 1.5 mg/kg/dose (maximum, 40 mg on alternate days) to be continued for 2 to 5 months.[181] Unlike the Children's Nephrotic Syndrome Consensus

Table 17.4 Corticosteroid treatment protocols for nephrotic syndrome

| Reference | Initial episode | Infrequent relapses | Frequent relapses |
|---|---|---|---|
| 2009 Children's Nephrotic Syndrome Consensus Conference[99] | Prednisone, 2 mg/kg/day orally for 6 wk (maximum 60 mg/day) to be followed by 1.5 mg/kg/dose (maximum 40 mg/dose) given every other day for 6 additional wk (no taper) | Prednisone, 2 mg/kg/day until the urine dipstick for protein is trace or negative for 3 consecutive days; prednisone dose is then decreased to 1.5 mg/kg administered every other day for at least 4 wk | Prednisone, 2 mg/kg/day until the urine dipstick is trace or negative for 3 days; this is followed by 1.5 mg/kg on alternate days for an additional 4 wk; prednisone is then tapered over a period of 2 mo by 0.5 mg/kg |
| 2012 Kidney Disease Improving Global Outcomes[181] | Prednisone, 60 mg/m²/day or 2 mg/kg per day (maximum 60 mg/day) orally for 4–6 wk as a single daily dose; this is followed by alternate-day therapy of 40 mg/m²/dose or 1.5 mg/kg/dose (maximum 40 mg on alternate days) to be continued for 2–5 mo, then tapered over 2–5 mo | | Prednisone, 60 mg/m²/day or 2 mg/kg/day (maximum 60 mg/day) orally until the child has been in remission for at least 3 days; this followed by alternate-day prednisone for at least 3 mo; prednisone is to be given on alternate days in the lowest dose possible to maintain remission without major side effects |

Conference, the KDIGO group recommended tapering the alternate-day steroid dose over the course of 2 to 5 months. This recommendation was based on a systematic review revealing that prolonged duration of alternate-day therapy, up to 6 months, may reduce the risk of subsequent relapses of the disease.[182]

In patients with newly diagnosed disease, corticosteroids should be given for at least 12 weeks. This is because shorter courses of therapy have been associated with an increased risk of future relapses.[182] In a multicenter controlled trial, 61 children were randomized to receive either standard therapy, in the form of 4 weeks of daily steroids followed by alternate-day therapy, or a short course of daily steroids until they achieved full remission followed by alternate-day therapy. Only 19% of children who received the shorter course were in sustained remission at 2 years as compared with 41% with standard therapy. Moreover, the mean duration of remission in children receiving the shorter course was half of that of the children receiving a longer course.[177] Subsequent studies have further validated the beneficial effect of routinely using a relatively prolonged steroid regimen in the initial treatment of the disease because of its favorable impact on future relapses.[183–185]

Once-daily corticosteroid dosing appears to be as efficacious as twice-daily dosing.[182] A few studies have also inferred that calculating the steroid dose based on body weight, rather than surface area, may result in underdosing of young children who weigh less than 30 kg.[186] This potential underdosing does not appear to alter initial response to therapy, but it may increase the risk of future frequent relapses.[187]

Variations of the foregoing recommended regimens for the initial treatment of childhood nephrotic syndrome have been reported, with limited benefit. In a randomized controlled trial of 104 children, the use of the standard prednisone regimen was compared with standard glucocorticoids in addition to 8 weeks of cyclosporine A. Despite reduced rates of relapse in children treated with cyclosporine during the first year, there was no difference in sustained remission rates between the 2 groups at a follow-up period of 2 years.[188]

The majority of children with nephrotic syndrome will achieve complete remission within 4 weeks of therapy. In the original ISKDC cohort, 92% of children responded to steroid treatment. Of the initial responders approximately 75%, 94%, and 99% did so within the first 2 weeks, 4 weeks, and 8 weeks of therapy, respectively.[98] In a retrospective review of 103 children with idiopathic nephrotic syndrome, a shorter time to a response (less than 7 days) predicted a lower likelihood for an early relapse (within 3 months of discontinuing steroids). A shorter time to response was also associated with a lower risk for either a frequently relapsing or steroid-dependent course. In the same study, the median time to remission on steroids was 7 days.[189]

## INITIAL RELAPSE OR INFREQUENTLY RELAPSING NEPHROTIC SYNDROME

More than 50% of children with nephrotic syndrome who respond to the initial course of steroids will develop at least one relapse of the disease.[99] Relapses are usually spontaneous, but they may sometimes be triggered by an upper respiratory infection. Relapses may occur during tapering of the prednisone dose or at some point following discontinuation of the medication. Some relapses (10% to 23%) may remit spontaneously.[190] The Children's Nephrotic Syndrome Consensus and the KDIGO groups define infrequent relapses as one relapse within 6 months of initial response, or one to three relapses in any 12-month period. Both groups recommended that patients with initial or infrequent relapses be treated with prednisone 2 mg/kg/day until the urine dipstick for protein is trace or negative for 3 consecutive days. The prednisone dose should then be decreased to 1.5 mg/kg administered every other day for at least 4 weeks.[99,181] These recommendations are based on a randomized controlled trial by the ISKDC that compared an 8-week regimen of steroids with another regimen of shorter duration (mean, 12 days). The 8-week regimen was associated with a markedly lower risk of relapse during treatment (8% vs. 40%) and a more prolonged relapse-free period after treatment.[179]

## FREQUENTLY RELAPSING OR STEROID-DEPENDENT NEPHROTIC SYNDROME

In the ISKDC cohort, 30% of children with SSNS eventually developed a frequently relapsing course, defined as four or more relapses per year.[191] Moreover, relapses that occur while tapering steroids or within 2 weeks after discontinuing treatment indicate steroid dependence. Children with steroid dependence or frequent relapses often require prolonged courses of glucocorticoids. The goals of therapy for such children are focused on reducing the incidence of relapses, promoting a sustained remission, and limiting cumulative exposure to corticosteroids. To minimize toxicity, the lowest effective dose of glucocorticoids or steroid-sparing medications should be used to maintain remission. In the absence of significant glucocorticoid-associated adverse effects, extended treatment with low-dose alternate-day prednisone is generally the preferred option. Treatment with steroid-sparing medications, such as cytotoxic agents, calcineurin inhibitors, mycophenolate mofetil (MMF), or rituximab, is also frequently considered when these children manifest significant signs of corticosteroid toxicity.[99]

In the absence of signs of corticosteroid toxicity, the 2009 Children's Nephrotic Syndrome Consensus Conference recommended treatment of frequent relapses with prednisone 2 mg/kg/day until the urine dipstick is trace or negative for 3 days. This should be followed by 1.5 mg/kg on alternate days for an additional 4 weeks. Prednisone should then be tapered in 0.5 mg/kg increments over a period of 2 months.

Alternatively, children with frequently relapsing nephrotic syndrome (FRNS) or SDNS may be treated with oral cyclophosphamide, MMF, or cyclosporine A. Oral cyclophosphamide is prescribed at a dose of 2 mg/kg/day in addition to oral prednisone for a total of 12 weeks (cumulative dose, 168 mg/kg). The cyclophosphamide dose should be based on ideal body weight. MMF is prescribed at a dose of 400 to 600 mg/m$^2$/dose twice daily (maximum, 2 g/day) for 1 to 2 years along with a tapering dose of prednisone. A third option is cyclosporine A at a dose of 3 to 5 mg/kg/day divided twice daily for an average of 2 to 5 years.[99] Although a renal biopsy is not typically performed in FRNS or SDNS, it is recommended that it be performed before starting cyclosporine and periodically (approximately every 2 years) thereafter to document baseline renal histologic features, and monitor for cyclosporine-induced nephrotoxicity, respectively. There is currently insufficient evidence to support recommending one steroid-sparing medication over another. However, cyclophosphamide and MMF are probably the best options because of the side effect profile of cyclosporine (including nephrotoxicity) and the finding that relapse rates are high on tapering. Accordingly, the use of a specific agent depends on the tolerability and the potential for associated side effects.

Guidelines published by KDIGO are consistent with the previously discussed regimen, with only minor differences. The KDIGO group similarly suggested that children with FRNS or SDNS be treated with daily prednisone until the child has been in remission for at least 3 days. This treatment should be followed by alternate-day prednisone for at least 3 months. Prednisone is to be given on alternate days in the lowest dose possible to maintain remission without major side effects. Low-dose daily prednisone may also be given to maintain remission in children with SDNS, particularly when alternate-day therapy fails. In addition, the KDIGO group also suggested using daily prednisone during episodes of upper respiratory infections or other infections to reduce the risk of relapses in children with FRNS or SDNS who are already receiving alternate-day prednisone.[192] The recommendations for using low-dose alternate-day prednisone or daily prednisone for SDNS are based on small observational studies.[193,194]

## Steroid-related side effects

Children with FRNS and SDNS often require prolonged courses of glucocorticoids and are at the highest risk of associated adverse effects. In addition, some patients with SRNS also require long courses of corticosteroids given on alternate days, thus putting them at significant risk for toxicity. Steroid-associated side effects are among the most common causes of iatrogenic morbidity in medicine. Accordingly, management of children with nephrotic syndrome requires in-depth knowledge of the impact, scope, and clinical implication of these adverse effects. A brief discussion of some of the more common toxicities is presented here.

### GROWTH IMPAIRMENT

Glucocorticoids may induce suppression of growth hormone release, insulin-like growth factor I (IGF-I) activity, bone formation, and collagen synthesis.[195,196] However, studies that investigated the impact of prolonged corticosteroids therapy on linear growth in children with nephrotic syndrome have yielded conflicting results.

In a study of 85 children with SRNS with a minimum follow-up of 3 years, 38 children (45%) showed significant linear growth retardation. Higher doses of prednisone, a more prolonged duration of therapy, and older age were identified as risk factors for impaired growth.[197] In another report of 42 children with FRNS or SDNS with a mean follow-up of approximately 12 years, growth impairment correlated with the mean duration and cumulative dose of prednisone. Pubertal growth spurt was delayed in boys in this study, but not in girls. Children who continued to receive prednisone after puberty were at the highest risk for growth impairment. In contrast, early discontinuation of prednisone was associated with partial "catch-up" growth.[198]

Another report of 41 children with nephrotic syndrome also showed reduced final height in girls and boys. Similar to the previous study, delayed puberty was noted in boys, but not girls. Moreover, an abnormal pattern of growth hormone and gonadotropin release was observed in 6 of 8 children with growth impairment.[199] A third study by Leroy et al.[200] investigated the impact of corticosteroids and cyclosporine on the growth parameters of 64 boys with SDNS over a 10-year follow-up period. In concert with other reports, growth impairment was more pronounced in the children who received prednisone beyond 12 years of age. Catch-up growth in late puberty was common among study participants.[200] Conversely, in a small study of 41 children with SDNS followed for a mean of 4.2 years, prednisolone doses up to 0.75 mg/kg/day did not seem to adversely affect linear growth velocity.[201]

Steroid-sparing medications, such as alkylating agents, were associated with improved linear growth in one report.[202] The evidence for use of alternate-day corticosteroid therapy to minimize growth impairment is not conclusive. In one report, linear growth impairment did not occur with alternate-day steroid regimens,[203] whereas another study documented significant growth impairment in children who received alternate-day steroids.[198] Pending further evidence, we suggest using alternate-day steroid regimens when feasible to diminish the likelihood of growth impairment and other long-term adverse effects.

### OSTEONECROSIS

Long-term use of corticosteroids has been associated with an increased risk of osteonecrosis of the femoral head. The underlying mechanism behind this association is not well understood. Fat microemboli involving the terminal bone arterioles have been implicated in the pathogenesis of osteonecrosis. Glucocorticoids may predispose patients to fat microembolization by altering the structure of circulating lipoproteins, inducing fatty liver, or disrupting bone marrow fat cells.[204,205] An alternate theory, based on observations in animal models, suggests that corticosteroids may induce endothelial cell injury of the venules draining the bone, thereby leading to local stasis and subsequent bone necrosis.[206]

Osteonecrosis of the femoral head should be suspected in any child receiving corticosteroids who presents with hip pain, knee pain, or limping. In view of the insidious onset and the often low specificity of presenting symptoms, a high index of suspicion for osteonecrosis in children receiving long-term steroid therapy is crucial. The initial evaluation should include anteroposterior and frog-leg hip x-ray views. However, magnetic resonance imaging of the hip is far more sensitive and is often required for proper staging of the disease.[207]

## CATARACTS

Posterior subcapsular cataracts have been reported in 10% to 56% of children receiving long-term corticosteroid therapy for nephrotic syndrome.[208-212] The development of this complication was associated with a higher total dose and longer duration of corticosteroids therapy in one study.[209] However, other studies found no such correlations.[208,210] Notably, cataracts have been reported even in children receiving alternate-day corticosteroid therapy.[210] Younger children who are exposed to prolonged courses of corticosteroids may be at the highest risk.[212] Cataracts associated with corticosteroids are often bilateral and progress slowly. In children receiving prolonged courses of corticosteroids, routine examination of the lens using an ophthalmoscope is recommended at each clinic visit. Cataracts may be detected as dark gray or black spots located in the posterior aspect of the lens. Even though most children with posterior subcapsular cataracts retain excellent visual acuity,[210,211] amblyopia has been infrequently reported.[212] Accordingly, children suspected to have cataracts should be promptly referred to an ophthalmologist for further evaluation and management.

## Steroid-sparing medications

Prolonged courses of corticosteroids are often prescribed in children with FRNS or SDNS. In the absence of significant side effects, corticosteroids are usually prescribed at the lowest dose possible to maintain a prolonged remission. However, the development of steroid-related adverse effects

> ### KEY POINT
>
> Alkylating agents and MMF are effective steroid-sparing medications used in children with FRNS or SDNS to minimize steroid-induced toxicity.

often necessitates the addition of other immunomodulatory therapies, known as steroid-sparing medications. This strategy aims to maintain remission while further reducing the cumulative dose and duration of corticosteroid therapy. Treatment options in this situation include alkylating agents, MMF, and, less commonly calcineurin, inhibitors.[99] Steroid-sparing medications have been shown to be effective in maintaining remission while minimizing long-term steroid-related toxicities.[99]

## ALKYLATING AGENTS

The effectiveness of cyclophosphamide and chlorambucil as steroid-sparing medications in the treatment of children with FRNS was verified in a meta-analysis of randomized controlled trials. In these trials, cyclophosphamide was given orally at a dose of 2 mg/kg/day for 8 to 12 weeks or chlorambucil was administered at a dose of 0.2 mg/kg/day for 8 to 12 weeks. Both medications were effective in maintaining a prolonged remission in 72% and 36% of the patients at 2 and 5 years, respectively.[213] However, cyclophosphamide appears to be less effective in children with SDNS compared with children with FRNS.[214-216] Moreover, children who are dependent on higher doses of steroids are less likely to respond to treatment with cyclophosphamide compared with children dependent on lower doses.[217]

In addition to oral use, intravenous regimens of cyclophosphamide have also been described in SRNS or SDNS. Two prospective studies compared the efficacy and safety of using monthly intravenous infusions of cyclophosphamide (pulse cyclophosphamide) at a dose of 500 mg/m²/dose for 6 months in SDNS or FRNS with the conventional oral regimens described earlier. Intravenous pulse cyclophosphamide was equally effective and safe in both studies.[218,219] The efficacy of cyclophosphamide may be determined in some patients by certain genetic factors. For instance, the detection of specific polymorphisms in enzymes involved in the metabolism of cyclophosphamide, particularly glutathione-S-transferases, has been associated with increased efficacy of the drug.[220,221]

## Side effects and outcome

The use of alkylating agents in the treatment of nephrotic syndrome has been associated with a significant risk of bone marrow suppression and infections. Other adverse effects, such as hemorrhagic cystitis, alopecia, or infertility, are more commonly seen in children who receive higher doses of cyclophosphamide (cumulative doses in excess of 200 mg/kg/treatment course), such as those used in oncologic protocols. Because such high doses are not recommended for children with nephrotic syndrome, these adverse effects are relatively uncommon in this setting.

In a meta-analysis of 38 studies (1504 children) evaluating the use of alkylating agents in FRNS, leukopenia developed in approximately one-third of children treated with cyclophosphamide or chlorambucil.[213] In view of these results, complete blood counts should be monitored periodically in children receiving either drug, and therapy with alkylating agents should be temporarily held if the white blood cell count drops to less than 3000/mm³. In children who receive pulse (intravenous) treatment, the nadir blood counts often occurs 1 to 2 weeks following cyclophosphamide infusion. Accordingly, most nephrologists monitor complete blood counts at least once every 2 weeks in children receiving monthly pulse cyclophosphamide therapy.

In the same meta-analysis described earlier, serious bacterial infections were observed in 1.5% of children treated with cyclophosphamide and in 6.8% of those treated with chlorambucil.[213] Bacterial infections may occur in the presence or absence of concurrent leukopenia. Other infections, such as pneumocystis, fungal, or viral infections, may also occur. Severe cases of disseminated varicella infection have also been reported in nonimmune children with nephrotic syndrome who were treated with cyclophosphamide.[222,223]

The risk of infertility in patients treated with cyclophosphamide correlates with the total cumulative dose. At the currently recommended doses for children with nephrotic syndrome, the risk is considered trivial in adolescent girls and is relatively low in adolescent boys. In the same meta-analysis, long-term ovarian dysfunction was rare in treated girls and women. However, oligospermia and azoospermia were occasionally seen in adolescent boys and appeared to correlate with the total cumulative dose of cyclophosphamide.[213] In one study, for instance, 13 of 30 young men with nephrotic syndrome developed oligospermia or azoospermia, all of whom received oral cyclophosphamide for more than 16 weeks or received a total cumulative dose exceeding 300 mg/kg body weight, or both.[224]

The risk of malignant disease also appears to be very low. Only 14 cases of malignant disease were detected in the cohort of 1504 children included in the meta-analysis; all these cases occurred in patients receiving doses of alkylating agents that exceeded the currently recommended regimens. Chlorambucil appears to have a less favorable side effect profile, particularly in terms of a higher risk of infection and a potential for inducing seizures. Therefore, cyclophosphamide is considered the preferred alkylating agent for the treatment of FRNS or SDNS.[213]

## CALCINEURIN INHIBITORS

The exact mechanism of action of calcineurin inhibitors (cyclosporine A and tacrolimus) in nephrotic syndrome is unknown. Calcineurin inhibitors suppress IL-2 production by blocking calcineurin, a calcium-dependent serine-threonine phosphatase, thereby inhibiting T-cell activation.[225] However, cyclosporine may also have a direct stabilizing effect on the podocyte cytoskeleton, thus further contributing to its antiproteinuric effect.[226] The effectiveness of cyclosporine in the treatment of SDNS and FRNS has been well established in several trials.[227–231] However, in view of the significant associated risk of irreversible nephrotoxicity, calcineurin inhibitors continue to be considered a third-line choice for FRNS and SDNS, after prednisone and alkylating agents.

Cyclosporine is used as a steroid-sparing medication at a starting dose of 4 to 5 mg/kg/day divided twice daily. The dose should then be adjusted to maintain serum trough levels of 100 to 200 ng/mL by high-performance liquid chromatography (HPLC) assay. Concurrent use of alternate-day prednisone is frequently needed to maintain a stable remission.[181] Two randomized controlled trials showed that cyclosporine was as effective as cyclophosphamide and chlorambucil in inducing remission and in reducing the need for prednisone in SDNS and FRNS. Unlike with alkylating agents, however, the effect of cyclosporine was not sustained once the treatment was stopped.[232,233] In a prospective clinical trial, 49 children with FRNS were successfully treated with cyclosporine for 2 years and were monitored for an additional 2 years after completion of treatment. Two years after stopping cyclosporine, 85% of the children had a relapse at least once, and 61% regressed back to a frequently relapsing course.[234] Hence, the majority of children who respond to calcineurin inhibitors can be expected to have a relapse after discontinuing the medication. Therefore, the treatment should generally be continued for at least 12 to 24 months.

In light of the previous results, prolonged courses of cyclosporine are commonly prescribed in children with FRNS or SDNS. However, the duration of therapy is often limited by the development of adverse effects, particularly chronic nephrotoxicity. Histologically, calcineurin-inhibitor–related renal toxicity manifests as tubulointerstitial fibrosis, classically in a "striped" pattern reflecting the blood supply. The risk of renal toxicity increases with the duration of therapy. In one report, interstitial fibrosis was found in 11% (2 of 18) of children who received cyclosporine for less than 2 years, but in 58% of children who received the drug for more than 2 years.[235] Other common side effects related to cyclosporine therapy include hypertension, tremor, hyperkalemia, gingival hyperplasia, and hypertrichosis.

The optimal duration of calcineurin inhibitor use in children with nephrotic syndrome remains a subject of significant controversy. Some experts recommended limiting treatment to a 2-year duration to reduce the risk of long-term nephrotoxicity.[235] Serial annual or biannual renal biopsies in children who receive the medication for a period in excess of 2 years have also been suggested.[228,236] If histologic evidence for progressive interstitial fibrosis is detected on biopsy, serious consideration should be given for tapering the calcineurin inhibitor and transitioning to an alternative steroid-sparing medication. It has been suggested that in some cases toxicity is not apparent clinically and is observed only on biopsy. Because of a lack of sufficient evidence, however, the 2012 KDIGO group did not support the practice of performing serial renal biopsies in children receiving long-term calcineurin inhibitors for nephrotic syndrome with no laboratory evidence of progressive renal dysfunction.[181] Further studies are needed to clarify the role, if any, of serial biopsies in this setting. Nevertheless, frequent monitoring of renal function, proteinuria, and cyclosporine levels is still considered crucial to screen for early signs of potential nephrotoxicity.

Tacrolimus, also known as FK 506, is a calcineurin inhibitor with a mechanism of action similar to that of cyclosporine. It has been frequently used as an alternative to the older cyclosporine A to avoid cyclosporine-associated cosmetic side effects (gingival hyperplasia and hypertrichosis). Support for its efficacy in the treatment of FRNS and SDNS comes from small retrospective case series.[237] Tacrolimus is usually started at a dose of 0.1 mg/kg/day, divided twice daily. The dose is adjusted to target serum trough levels of 5 to 10 mg/L. Once remission is achieved, the dose is titrated to the lowest possible amount to sustain remission. Although tacrolimus has a generally similar side effect profile compared with cyclosporine, gum hypertrophy and hypertrichosis do not occur with tacrolimus use.

Unfortunately, tacrolimus has been associated with a higher risk of neurotoxicity compared to cyclosporine.[238,239] Tacrolimus has also been associated with a higher risk of insulin-dependent diabetes mellitus compared with cyclosporine. Even though tacrolimus-associated insulin dependency is most often transient and resolves with discontinuation, it may occasionally become permanent.[240,241]

Levamisole is an antihelminthic and is the only immunostimulatory medication with known efficacy in the treatment of FRNS and SDNS. The efficacy and safety of levamisole have been validated in a randomized placebo controlled trial of 61 children with FRNS. After tapering and discontinuing corticosteroids, only 4 children developed a relapse in the treatment group as compared with 14 children in the placebo group when patients monitored for a period of 112 days.[242] Retrospective case series have yielded similar results confirming the efficacy of levamisole use in SDNS.[243-246] In a retrospective study of 51 children with FRNS or SDNS, the efficacy of a 6-month course of levamisole was equivalent to an 8- to 12-week regimen of cyclophosphamide. Both medications reduced the relapse frequency and the total exposure to corticosteroids.[247] Levamisole is usually prescribed at a dose of 2.5 mg/kg on alternate days for 4 to 12 months. Levamisole appears to be generally safe in children at the conventionally prescribed doses. Reported adverse effects include neutropenia, agranulocytosis, flu-like symptoms, seizures, and, rarely, disseminated vasculitis.[248,249] Levamisole was withdrawn from the United States market in 2000 because of the risk of agranulocytosis,[250] but it is still available in many countries worldwide.

## MYCOPHENOLATE MOFETIL AND MIZORIBINE

MMF and mizoribine have been frequently used in the management of children with FRNS and SDNS. The exact mechanism of action of MMF and mizoribine in the treatment of glomerular diseases remains unknown. MMF inhibits T- and B-lymphocyte proliferation through noncompetitive inhibition of inosine monophosphate dehydrogenase (IMPDH), thereby leading to depletion of guanosine triphosphate and deoxyguanosine triphosphate.[251] Clinically, this effect is specific to T and B lymphocytes because all other cells in the body are capable of regenerating purines by a separate scavenger pathway and therefore are generally unaffected. In addition, MMF preferentially suppresses Th2 cytokines in the kidney, particularly IL-4.[252] MMF also inhibits mesangial cell proliferation,[253] and it interferes with the adhesion of activated lymphocytes to endothelial cells.[254]

In comparison with calcineurin inhibitors and alkylating agents, MMF has a generally favorable side effect profile. Most importantly, MMF is not nephrotoxic, and this property renders MMF a very attractive choice for patients with FRNS and SDNS. Evidence to support the effectiveness and safety of MMF and mizoribine in the treatment of FRNS and SDNS comes from small observational case series and retrospective studies.[255-260] In these studies, MMF reduced the need for corticosteroids and the relapse rate by 40% to 70%. Mizoribine appears to be more effective in children less than 10 years of age.[261] In a study of 46 children treated with MMF after remaining steroid dependent despite previous regimens of levamisole and cyclophosphamide, 43% were able to discontinue corticosteroids, and an additional 27% required lower doses of steroids to maintain remission. At a mean follow-up of 3.5 years, 54% of these children required no further alternative immunosuppression.[255]

As is the case with calcineurin inhibitors, relapses are common after MMF is discontinued. In a multicenter study of 33 children with FRNS by the Southwest Pediatric Nephrology Study Group, the relapse rate was decreased in patients receiving MMF from 1 episode every 2 months to 1 episode every 14.7 months. However, in the same series, remission was maintained in only 25% of children with FRNS after stopping MMF.[258]

MMF appears to be less effective in inducing remission when compared with cyclosporine.[262,263] In a multicenter, open-label, crossover trial of 60 children with FRNS, 85% of patients remained relapse free while receiving cyclosporine (1-year duration) as compared with only 64% of patients receiving MMF. In this trial, low serum levels of mycophenolic acid (MPA), an active metabolite of MMF, were correlated with a higher risk for relapse.[264] When considering the choice of MMF versus other immunosuppressive agents, these differences in efficacy should be carefully weighed against the potential for renal (calcineurin inhibitors), hematologic, and gonadal toxicities (alkylating agents).

MMF is usually prescribed at a dose of 400 to 600 mg/m$^2$/dose twice daily (25 to 36 mg/kg/day; maximum dose 1 g twice daily). Adverse reactions associated with MMF include diarrhea, vomiting, leukopenia, anemia, and sepsis. In addition, mizoribine is also known to be associated with hyperuricemia. Most adverse effects are dose dependent and are more common among children less than 6 years of age and transplant recipients.[265] In one study, for example, adverse effects led to stopping MMF in 54% of renal transplant recipients.[266] Enteric-coated mycophenolic acid is an alternative to MMF that is associated with fewer gastrointestinal side effects.[267,268] Because most children require the use of a liquid suspension, enteric-coated mycophenolic acid has limited use in the pediatric population. In light of the significant risk for leukopenia or anemia, periodic monitoring of blood counts in children receiving MMF or mizoribine has been suggested.

In children receiving MMF for the treatment of nephrotic syndrome, gastrointestinal and hematologic side effects appear to be less common. This feature was illustrated in 4 studies evaluating the use of MMF in childhood nephrotic syndrome that included a combined total of 110 children. None of the study participants reported dose-limiting gastrointestinal symptoms, none developed leukopenia, and only 3 children developed mild anemia that required reducing the MMF dose.[256,260,269,270]

### RITUXIMAB

Rituximab is a monoclonal antibody that targets CD20, a B-cell surface marker, thus leading to the depletion of B cells.[271] The rationale for the use of rituximab in glomerular diseases came from evidence that proposed a crucial role for B cells in the regulation of cell-mediated immune response.[272] The efficacy of rituximab in SDNS was evaluated in a single randomized trial and in multiple small observational case series. In a randomized, open-label, controlled trial of 54 children with steroid-dependent and calcineurin-dependent idiopathic nephrotic syndrome, rituximab allowed the temporary withdrawal of prednisone and calcineurin inhibitors in 63% at 3 months and in 50% at 9 months while maintaining a stable remission.[273] Other smaller observational studies yielded similar results, providing further support for its role in the treatment of refractory SDNS.[274-277] Most studies used 1 to 4 infusions of rituximab (375 mg/m² per infusion) given 2 weeks apart during a period of disease remission. Relapses are common, particularly during recovery of B-lymphocyte counts.[278]

The use of MMF as a preferred maintenance medication following rituximab therapy has been suggested. In a prospective nonrandomized controlled pilot study, 9 children with SDNS were treated with rituximab followed by MMF and were compared with 7 children treated only with rituximab. At 1 year of follow-up, 3 of the 9 children in the MMF group had relapses, as compared with 6 of 7 in the control group.[279] In summary, evidence from a single randomized trial and multiple observational studies supports the use of rituximab in the management of refractory SDNS. However, given the current paucity of evidence on the long-term safety of this agent in nephrotic syndrome, rituximab use should be reserved for children with significant steroid-related toxicity who fail to respond to conventional steroid-sparing drugs.

Short-term adverse effects associated with rituximab include infusion-related reactions in the form of myalgias, fever, chills, pruritus, respiratory distress, hypotension, or anaphylaxis. Long-term but rarer adverse effects include infections, fatal pulmonary fibrosis,[280] and progressive multifocal leukoencephalopathy (PML).[281] PML is a rare demyelinating disorder that results from reactivation of latent JC polyoma virus. This delayed complication of rituximab (mean, 5.5 months) carries a 90% mortality rate, based on adult studies.[282]

## STEROID-RESISTANT NEPHROTIC SYNDROME

As previously discussed, most children (80% to 90%) with nephrotic syndrome respond well to an initial 8 weeks of corticosteroid therapy. The lack of a response to an adequate initial course of steroid therapy defines SRNS. Various underlying genetic mutations have been identified in 25% to 52% of children with SRNS.[283-285] Other important causes of steroid resistance include nonadherence to the prescribed medications, inappropriate dosing, inadequate gastrointestinal absorption, concurrent infections, or underlying malignant diseases.

A response to corticosteroids beyond 8 weeks of therapy is uncommon but not impossible. Moreover, such a delayed response has been occasionally reported with intravenous pulse glucocorticoids.[286] Conversely, delayed resistance to steroids is not uncommon in children who are initially steroid responsive.[287] Whether early or delayed, resistance to steroid therapy universally represents an ominous prognostic sign, predicting a 5-year risk of progression to ESKD of more than 50% in some studies.[288-290]

The treatment of children with SRNS is often very challenging. It requires carefully weighing the risk of comorbidities and progressive renal insufficiency in children with unremitting nephrotic syndrome against the potential for nephrotoxicity and serious adverse effects related to immunosuppressive medications. Various therapeutic options has been developed for the treatment of SRNS and may be classified into three major categories (Tables 17.5 and 17.6):

- Supportive therapy
- Immunomodulatory therapy
- Nonimmunosuppressive therapy

## Supportive and adjunctive therapies for steroid-resistant nephrotic syndrome

Children with SRNS require close monitoring and supportive medical care. This includes careful monitoring for infectious and thrombotic complications, electrolyte abnormalities, and volume status. In addition, supportive measures include antihypertensive medications, immunizations, and treatment of edema and dyslipidemia. An overview of the general medical care of children with nephrotic syndrome is presented next, followed by a review of the recommended immunizations. Please refer to Chapter 16 for a detailed discussion of the management of edema and dyslipidemia in these children.

Table 17.5 Components of supportive therapy for children with steroid-resistant nephrotic syndrome

| General medical care | Management of edema | Management of hyperlipidemia |
|---|---|---|
| Identification and treatment of suspected thrombosis:<br>Asymmetric swelling in extremity | Moderate restriction of dietary salt intake | Limit dietary saturated and trans fat |
| | | Increase intake of complex carbohydrates and fiber, including whole grains, fruits, and vegetables |
| Respiratory distress<br>Acute oliguria<br>Gross hematuria<br>Neurologic symptoms | | |
| Identification and treatment of suspected infection: | Avoidance of excessive fluid intake | Regular exercise regimen (30–45 minutes of moderately intense exercise daily) |
| Cellulitis<br>Peritonitis<br>Sepsis | | |
| Maintenance or restoration of intravascular volume | Elevation of extremities | HMG Co-A reductase inhibitors (statins)* |
| Maintenance of adequate protein intake (130%–140% of RDA) | Judicious use of albumin and diuretics (only for severe edema) | |
| Immunizations | Head-out water immersion | |

*Abbreviations:* HMG-CoA, 3-hydroxy-3-methylglutaryl–coenzyme A; RDA, recommended dietary allowance.
*Patients more than 8 years of age.

## GENERAL MEDICAL CARE

Children with SRNS are at a high risk for infectious and thrombotic complications. Common infections in children with active nephrotic syndrome include pneumonia, bacteremia or sepsis, peritonitis, urinary tract infection, and cellulitis.[291] Frequent, careful evaluation for skin infections and skin breakdown is crucial in patients with refractory edema. Prophylactic antibiotics are generally not recommended, but signs of cellulitis such as skin erythema, tenderness, or induration should be promptly evaluated and treated with systemic antibiotics. Skin breakdown can be prevented by frequent repositioning of bedridden patients.

Skin breakdown is of particular concern in boys with severe scrotal edema. Asymmetric swelling of the lower extremity should raise a suspicion for deep vein thrombosis. Thrombotic complications may also manifest with an acute onset of respiratory distress, suggesting pulmonary embolism. The development of acute neurologic deficits may suggest a thrombotic stroke. Careful monitoring of volume status is essential, particularly in children who are maintained on diuretics. Despite generalized salt and water retention, children with SRNS commonly show signs of intravascular fluid depletion and hemoconcentration, both of which generally respond well to intravenous albumin

Table 17.6 Treatment options for children with steroid-resistant nephrotic syndrome

| Immunosuppressive | Immunostimulatory | Nonimmunosuppressive |
|---|---|---|
| Cyclosporine | Levamisole* | ACE inhibitors/angiotensin receptor blockers |
| Tacrolimus | — | Vitamin E* |
| Mycophenolate mofetil | — | Galactose* |
| Pulse IV methylprednisolone | — | — |
| Rituximab | — | — |
| Plasma exchange and immunoadsorption* | — | — |
| Azathioprine* | — | — |

*Abbreviations:* ACE, angiotensin-converting enzyme.
* Less commonly used or controversial.

infusions.[292] In contrast, most children with refractory FSGS develop systemic hypertension. ACEIs are frequently used to control hypertension in view of their antiproteinuric and long-term renoprotective properties.[293-295] Intravenous albumin infusions should be avoided in children with uncontrolled hypertension because of the risk of exacerbating the blood pressure elevation and inducing congestive heart failure (see Chapter 16).

## INFECTIONS AND IMMUNIZATIONS

Before the initiation of steroid therapy, a purified protein derivative (PPD) test should be requested in children with newly diagnosed nephrotic syndrome, to exclude tuberculosis. In children who receive daily or alternate-day corticosteroids at a dose that exceeds 2 mg/kg/day *or* exceeds 20 mg/day for more than 14 days, the American Academy of Pediatrics recommends that all live vaccines should be delayed for at least 1 month after discontinuing corticosteroids. If the dose of corticosteroids exceeds the aforementioned threshold but the duration of treatment is less than 14 days, live vaccines may be administered immediately after discontinuing corticosteroids.[296] Conversely, live vaccines are effective and may be administered safely to children who are receiving lower doses of steroids (less than 2 mg/kg/day *and* less than 20 mg/day). Varicella immunization is particularly important in children with newly diagnosed nephrotic syndrome, given the high risk of morbidity and mortality associated with this infection.[222,223,297-299] To ensure an adequate response, varicella immunization is preferably postponed until the patient is in remission or receiving alternate-day corticosteroids. In children who are in a stable remission, including those receiving alternate-day corticosteroids, varicella vaccine has been shown to be safe and effective, and it has a relatively low risk of inducing a relapse of the disease.[300-302] Immunosuppressed children who are exposed to varicella should receive passive immunoprophylaxis in the form of the varicella-zoster immunoglobulin (VZIG) within 4 days of the exposure. VZIG may prevent or minimize the morbidity associated with varicella infection in this setting. VZIG has not been shown to be effective if it is given more than 96 hours after exposure to varicella.[303] Passive immunoprophylaxis is not recommended in children who have previously completed the two-dose regimen of the varicella vaccine.

Rare cases of vaccination-induced relapses of nephrotic syndrome have been reported.[304] This has led to significant anxiety among parents and health professionals regarding administration of immunizations to children with nephrotic syndrome who are in a stable remission. Based on the available evidence, these concerns do not seem justified because the risk of future infections will likely far outweigh the remote possibility of triggering a relapse. Indeed, in a multicenter study, 29 children with nephrotic syndrome, half of whom were receiving alternate-day prednisone treatment, were immunized with 2 doses of varicella. Of these children, 91% showed serologic evidence of a protective immune response for at least 2 years. None of administered vaccination doses were linked to relapses or other adverse events in this study (also see Chapter 6).[300]

The 2009 Children's Nephrotic Syndrome Consensus recommended that all children with nephrotic syndrome receive the 23-valent polysaccharide pneumococcal vaccine (PPSV23) and the heptavalent conjugated pneumococcal vaccine (PCV7).[99] However, PCV13, a polysaccharide-protein conjugate vaccine that immunizes against 13 pneumococcal serotypes, was introduced in 2010 and has since replaced the PCV7. Accordingly, we suggest that children with nephrotic syndrome receive the PCV13 vaccine in addition to the PPSV23 at the time of initial diagnosis. Children, who are actively nephrotic or receiving immunosuppressive medications, and their household contacts should also receive the annual inactivated influenza vaccine. The group also recommended delaying live vaccines until the dose of prednisone dose has been reduced to less than 2 mg/kg/day (and less than 20 mg total/day). Live vaccines should also be postponed for 3 months following the conclusion of cytotoxic therapy and for 1 month after the conclusion of treatment with other immunosuppressive agents.[99]

## Immunomodulatory therapies for steroid-resistant nephrotic syndrome

As previously discussed, children with refractory nephrotic syndrome are at a markedly increased risk of progression to ESKD. Aside from supportive therapy and treatment of the associated comorbidities, the management of children with SRNS is directed toward two main objectives: (1) complete or partial resolution of proteinuria and (2) halting the progression of renal insufficiency. Therapeutic options are categorized into: immunosuppressive, immunostimulatory, and nonimmune mediated treatments (see Table 17.6).

> ### KEY POINT
>
> Children with SRNS and identified causative genetic mutations are unlikely to respond to immunomodulatory therapy.

Children with SRNS and identified genetic mutations are unlikely to respond to immunomodulatory therapies. This was demonstrated in a study of 91 patients with SRNS or congenital nephrotic syndrome. Genotyping revealed various mutations in 43 of these patients, none of whom attained complete remission with immunosuppressive therapy and only 2 of whom achieved a partial response.[283] In another report of 29 patients with SRNS and identified homozygous or compound heterozygous mutations in *NPHS2,* none achieved complete remission following treatment with cyclosporine A or cyclophosphamide.[305] A third study reported disease-causing mutations in 37 of 110 patients with SRNS. None of the 37 patients achieved a complete remission with immunosuppressive therapy.[285]

## CYCLOSPORINE A

Cyclosporine A is widely used in the treatment of SRNS and is one of the most effective therapies available for this disease. Cyclosporine is generally started at a dose of 150 mg/m$^2$/per day or 4 to 5 mg/kg/day divided twice daily. The dose is titrated to maintain a trough drug level in the range of 100 to 200 ng/mL by HPLC assay. The efficacy of cyclosporine has been demonstrated in several randomized controlled trials,[306–308] as well as observational series.[227,309,310]

In a meta-analysis of 3 randomized trials that included a total of 49 children with SRNS, cyclosporine was more effective in inducing partial or complete remission compared with placebo or no treatment, regardless of the underlying histopathologic features (relative risk [RR], 5.5). Analysis of the subset of patients with FSGS on renal biopsy yielded similar results (RR, 5.8), but the beneficial effect in this subset did not reach statistical significance.[311] In the same meta-analysis, the rate of complete and partial remission in response to cyclosporine therapy was 36% (8 of 22) and 45% (10 of 22), respectively. Furthermore, these data are also consistent with multiple observational studies that showed rates of complete remission with the use of cyclosporine in the range of 46% to 84%.[227,309] In a case series of 65 children with SRNS, the rate of remission varied with the underlying histopathologic features, from 30% in FSGS to 46% in MCD.[227]

---

## KEY POINT

Calcineurin inhibitors are frequently effective in the treatment of SRNS. However, long-term therapy is limited by concerns of irreversible nephrotoxicity.

---

The addition of pulse intravenous methylprednisolone to cyclosporine may increase the cumulative rate of children achieving remission. In a retrospective study of 52 children with biopsy-confirmed FSGS, the combined use of pulse intravenous methylprednisolone and cyclosporine was associated with an 84% cumulative rate of sustained complete remission, compared with only 64% in those who received alternate-day oral prednisone therapy and cyclosporine.[309] In the same report, all 14 children who were diagnosed with MCD by renal biopsy achieved complete remission in response to cyclosporine therapy, regardless of whether it was combined with oral or intravenous corticosteroids.[309]

Cyclosporine appears to be more effective in SRNS compared with either cyclophosphamide or MMF. A multicenter randomized controlled open-label trial compared treatment with cyclosporine with intravenous cyclophosphamide in 32 children with SRNS. At 12 weeks of follow-up, 3 of 17 children (18%) had complete or partial remission in the cyclophosphamide treatment group compared with

9 of 15 children (60%) in the cyclosporine group, thus significantly favoring cyclosporine over cyclophosphamide. The incidence of adverse events was similar between the 2 groups, with the most common complications being infections, systemic hypertension, and Cushing syndrome.[312] In another randomized controlled trial of 138 children and adults with SRNS, a 12-month course of cyclosporine was compared with a combination of intravenous dexamethasone and MMF. Forty-six percent (33 of 72) of patients were in partial or complete remission after 12 months in the cyclosporine group as compared with 33% (22 of 66) in the dexamethasone/MMF group. However, this difference did not reach statistical significance.[313] In the same report, no significant difference was found in the rate of sustained remission between the 2 groups at 26 weeks of follow-up after discontinuing immunosuppression.[313]

Adverse reactions that have been attributed to cyclosporine therapy include nephrotoxicity, systemic hypertension, hyperkalemia, metabolic acidosis, elevated serum creatinine, infections, tremor, seizures, gingival hypertrophy, and hypertrichosis. Nephrotoxicity is of particular concern because it is irreversible and frequently limits the long-term use of cyclosporine. It manifests in the form of progressive interstitial fibrosis on renal biopsy, classically in a striped pattern. In one study, interstitial fibrosis was found on renal biopsy in 11% of children who received the medication for less than 2 years and in 58% of children who received it for more than 2 years.[235] Other factors that were associated with an increased risk of nephrotoxicity included the presence of renal insufficiency at baseline, FSGS histopathologic features, dosage exceeding 5.5 mg/kg/day, and high-grade proteinuria for more than 30 days.[235,314]

Limiting the duration of cyclosporine therapy to reduce the potential for nephrotoxicity has been suggested. However, the optimal duration of therapy remains a subject of considerable debate. In children with SRNS who respond to cyclosporine therapy, an attempt to wean the medication or switch to an alternative non-nephrotoxic option (e.g., MMF) may be reasonable after 1 to 2 years.[235] However, performing serial renal biopsies to monitor for nephrotoxicity in children who receive long-term cyclosporine therapy was not supported by the 2012 KDIGO group, and it remains controversial.[181]

Systemic hypertension may also be linked to calcineurin inhibitors and has been attributed to overactivity of the sodium chloride cotransporter in the distal convoluted tubule.[315] In addition, features of type IV renal tubular acidosis, including hyperkalemia and metabolic acidosis, may be seen in children receiving cyclosporine. Cyclosporine-induced neurotoxicity ranges from a mild tremor that resolves with continued therapy to an acute confusional state, psychosis, or seizures.[316] Seizures related to cyclosporine toxicity have been seen concomitantly with systemic hypertension and imaging findings suggestive of posterior reversible encephalopathy syndrome (PRES).[317,318] Finally, children who develop significant cosmetic adverse effects related to cyclosporine, such gingival hyperplasia or hypertrichosis, may benefit from transitioning to tacrolimus as an alternative agent.

In summary, cyclosporine is currently one of the most effective immunosuppressive agents used in the treatment of SRNS. It is generally well tolerated in the short term, but the risk of progressive irreversible nephrotoxicity limits its long-term use. Accordingly, children who initially respond to cyclosporine therapy should be transitioned to an alternative immunosuppressive agent within 2 years, if feasible.

## TACROLIMUS

Tacrolimus, also known as FK 506, is a calcineurin inhibitor with a mechanism of action similar to that of cyclosporine. Toxicities associated with tacrolimus are similar to those seen with cyclosporine. However, unlike cyclosporine, tacrolimus has not been associated with gum hypertrophy or hypertrichosis, thus rendering it an attractive alternative for children with intolerable cosmetic side effects linked to cyclosporine. However, tacrolimus has been associated with a higher incidence of neurotoxicity and glucose intolerance when compared with cyclosporine.[238,239] In transplant recipients, tacrolimus has also been associated with a higher risk of insulin-dependent diabetes mellitus compared with cyclosporine. Tacrolimus-associated insulin dependency is often transient, resolving with discontinued use, but it may rarely become permanent.[240,241] Tacrolimus is usually started at a dose of 0.1 mg/kg/day divided twice daily. The dose is adjusted to maintain target serum trough levels of 5 to 10 mg/L.

The efficacy of tacrolimus in the treatment of SRNS was demonstrated in a small randomized trial and in several observational reports. A randomized controlled open-label trial compared tacrolimus with cyclosporine for the treatment of SRNS. After 6 months of treatment, complete remission was achieved in 86% (18 of 21) of children who received tacrolimus as compared with 80% (16 of 20) of children who received cyclosporine. The rates of complete remission were also similar between the 2 groups at 12 months of therapy. However, more children developed relapses with cyclosporine as compared with tacrolimus (RR, 4.5).[319] Several other observational studies in children with SRNS, most with relatively short-term follow-up (less than 1 year), reported complete remission rates ranging between 40% and 94% with tacrolimus therapy.[320–325] In a single-center report of 19 children with SRNS treated with tacrolimus followed for an average duration of 55 months, complete remission was observed in 11 patients and partial remission in 6 patients. The mean time to induction of remission with tacrolimus was 8 weeks in this study.[323] Tacrolimus was generally well tolerated in the foregoing studies, with no reports of diabetes mellitus or severe neurotoxicity. However, given the paucity of long-term follow-up data, the long-term safety of tacrolimus in the treatment of SRNS remains uncertain.

In conclusion, limited evidence from a single randomized controlled trial and several observational reports have illustrated the effectiveness and short-term safety of tacrolimus use in SRNS. Tacrolimus appears to have similar efficacy in the treatment of SRNS compared with cyclosporine. However, cyclosporine continues to be the preferred calcineurin inhibitor by many nephrologists, primarily because of the longer-term experience with its use in SRNS. However, tacrolimus is an attractive alternative in children who develop intolerable cosmetic side effects related to cyclosporine use.

## MYCOPHENOLATE MOFETIL

MMF is known to suppress lymphocyte proliferation through inhibition of purine synthesis.[251] However, the specific mechanism of action of MMF in glomerular diseases remains unknown. Evidence for the benefit of MMF in childhood SRNS comes from a single randomized controlled trial and several observational case series. In a multicenter trial, 138 children and young adults were randomized to receive a 12-month course of either cyclosporine or a combination of MMF and intravenous dexamethasone. Partial or complete remission was attained in 33% (22 of 66), compared to 46% (33 of 72) in the cyclosporine-treated group, a difference that did not reach statistical significance.[313] Because the study did not include a group that received dexamethasone monotherapy, it was not possible to attribute the beneficial effect solely to MMF. In a retrospective study of 52 children, 34 of whom were previously resistant to cyclosporine, MMF treatment for at least 6 months induced complete or partial remission in approximately 60% of the cases.[326] In another report of 24 Chinese infants (less than 2 years of age) with SRNS, MMF was used for 6 to 12 months along with a stepwise tapering regimen of daily prednisone therapy; complete remission was achieved in 15 patients and partial remission in 6.[327] In a third study, 9 children and young adults with SRNS were pretreated with weekly intravenous pulse methylprednisolone therapy (15 mg/kg) for 4 to 8 weeks. This was followed by a regimen of MMF and ACEIs or angiotensin receptor blockers (ARBs). Proteinuria, assessed using spot urine protein-to-creatinine ratios, decreased by 43% when compared with baseline in treated patients, a reduction that was sustained after 24 months of observation.[295] An open-label, 6-month trial of MMF in 18 adults with steroid-resistant FSGS showed a marked improvement in proteinuria in 44% (8 of 18), which was sustained in 50% (4 of 8) of the patients for up to 1 year after discontinuing therapy.[328] Considering the observational design of these studies, it was not possible to account for multiple confounding variables. Hence, a causal association between MMF treatment and the observed benefits cannot be ascertained.

MMF may also be helpful in sustaining remission in children who were previously treated successfully with cyclosporine A. This concept was illustrated by an observational study that included 18 children with SRNS in complete remission on cyclosporine. The addition of MMF allowed for successful discontinuation of cyclosporine in 16 children. Of these children, only 21% developed relapses at a mean follow-up of 7 years.[270] In contrast, children who did not respond to cyclosporine monotherapy are unlikely to respond to a combination of MMF and cyclosporine.

This was illustrated by an observational study of 27 adults with cyclosporine-resistant SRNS. At 5 years of follow-up, MMF therapy did not induce complete remission in any of the cyclosporine-resistant patients and was associated with partial remission in only 4 patients (14%). MMF also failed to delay the progression of renal insufficiency in these patients.[329]

In summary, based on several observational studies, MMF appears to be less effective than cyclosporine in children with SRNS. MMF may be more suitable as an adjunct to pulse methylprednisolone or to help sustain remission in children who were previously successfully treated with a calcineurin inhibitor. Randomized controlled trials are needed to define the role of MMF in the treatment of SRNS further.

## RITUXIMAB

Rituximab is a monoclonal antibody against CD 20, a B-cell surface marker. It causes rapid depletion of B cells and suppresses immunoglobulin production. Traditionally, nephrotic syndrome has been considered a disorder of T-cell dysregulation. However, more recent evidence suggested a role for B-cell dysfunction in the pathogenesis of the disease.[330] This led to a growing interest in rituximab as a potential treatment option for SRNS refractory to other therapies. The exact mechanism by which rituximab may be effective in nephrotic syndrome is uncertain. Proposed mechanisms include late induction of regulatory T cells,[331,332] podocyte cytoskeletal stabilization,[333,334] and reduction of suPAR levels.[335] The effect of rituximab may be monitored by enumerating cells that express CD 19, another B-cell surface marker.[336]

Multiple observational studies and case reports have suggested a beneficial role for rituximab in the treatment of children and adults with SRNS.[279,337-345] More recently, an open-label, randomized controlled trial investigated the efficacy of rituximab in 31 children with SRNS who were resistant to calcineurin inhibitors.[346] The control group continued to receive calcineurin inhibitors and prednisone, whereas the intervention group received the same standard therapy in addition to 2 infusions of rituximab 375 mg/m² administered 2 weeks apart. If feasible, prednisone and tacrolimus were gradually tapered and sequentially discontinued within 6 to 8 weeks. At 3 months of follow-up, the rate of proteinuria was not significantly different between the 2 groups. Three patients in each group achieved remission (defined as a protein excretion less than 1 g/m²/day) and were successfully weaned off all medications. All 6 children who showed a response to therapy had a history of delayed resistance to corticosteroids. In this study, severe allergic reactions to rituximab were reported in only 2 patients, but minor reactions were common.[346] This study was powered to detect a 70% difference in proteinuria between the 2 groups and was evaluated for treatment-related effects for only a relatively short duration of 3 months. Therefore, a delayed or more modest effect related to rituximab could have been missed. Similarly, late adverse effects may have

also been missed. In conclusion, the current evidence is not sufficient to recommend for or against the use of rituximab in SRNS. Randomized controlled trials are needed to outline its role in this regard more definitively.

## PULSE INTRAVENOUS METHYLPREDNISOLONE

Pulse intravenous methylprednisolone, in isolation or combined with other immunosuppressive therapy, has been used for decades to induce remission in children with SRNS. In the early 1990s, Mendoza et al.[347] described an 18-month protocol of intravenous high-dose methylprednisolone (30 mg/kg) given three times/week for the first 2 weeks, then weekly for the next 8 weeks, then every other week for the following 8 weeks, then every 4 weeks for 8 doses, followed by every other month for an additional 4 doses.[347] Cyclophosphamide or chlorambucil was added for children who have not responded by 10 weeks of therapy or who had experienced relapse when reducing the frequency of pulse steroids. In the initial cohort, 52% (12 of 23) of children achieved full remission at a mean follow-up of 46 months.[347] Prolonged follow-up of children treated with this protocol (mean, 6.3 years) revealed sustained complete remission in 66% (21 of 32).[348] Multiple variations of this protocol have been subsequently reported with varying success, reporting rates of complete remission in the range of 38% to 82%.[349-353] Moreover, based on a retrospective review, intravenous methylprednisolone therapy, when added to oral cyclosporine, may improve the rate of remission in children with SRNS.[309]

However, despite the generally satisfactory response to the use of intravenous pulse methylprednisolone, the original Mendoza protocol is not commonly used in current practice because of its high cumulative dose of corticosteroids, which has been linked to serious short-term and long-term adverse effects including cataracts (22%), growth retardation (17%), impaired glucose tolerance, and systemic hypertension.[347] The introduction of newer relatively safe and effective alternatives, such as calcineurin inhibitors and MMF, has further reduced the need for intravenous pulse corticosteroids in the treatment of children with SRNS.

## ALKYLATING AGENTS

In view of the availability of safer and more effective alternatives, alkylating agents, including cyclophosphamide and chlorambucil, are no longer recommended for the treatment of SRNS. A meta-analysis of five randomized studies evaluated the efficacy of alkylating agents in the treatment of SRNS. The meta-analysis concluded that there was no significant benefit associated with the use of oral or IV cyclophosphamide in children with SRNS over prednisone alone.[311] Two ISKDC studies reported in 1974 and 1996, compared treatment with oral cyclophosphamide plus prednisone with prednisone alone. The studies included a total of 84 patients and found no significant differences in the number of patients who achieved a complete or partial remission between the two groups.[286,354] Children who received cyclophosphamide, however, responded in a shorter period of time (mean, 38.4 days as compared with 95.5 days with prednisone).

In another report, 30 patients with SRNS received treatment with either chlorambucil or indomethacin. No significant differences were found in the number of patients who achieved complete remission or those who developed ESKD with either treatment.[355] As previously detailed, the efficacy of cyclosporine was superior to that of intravenous cyclophosphamide in a randomized controlled trial of 32 children with SRNS.[312]

## PLASMAPHERESIS AND IMMUNOADSORPTION

Plasma exchange or plasmapheresis is frequently used in children who develop recurrences of FSGS after renal transplant. The benefit observed in transplant recipients has been attributed to the removal of circulating permeability factors, such as suPAR. In children with refractory idiopathic FSGS in native kidneys, treatment with plasma exchange has been reported in small case series and case reports to have varying success. In a report of eight children with steroid-resistant idiopathic FSGS, six sessions of plasma exchange were completed over a 2-week period. Proteinuria decreased significantly in only two of these patients and was sustained in only one of these.[356] In another report of 9 children with cyclosporine-resistant FSGS, two of whom had recurrent disease after renal transplantation, five patients achieved complete remission, and one patient achieved partial remission. However, three of these patients had relapses within 2 years.[357] Multiple other case reports in children and adults with FSGS have also suggested benefit with the use of plasma exchange, although often combined with other immunosuppressive therapies.[358–363]

Despite the widespread use of plasma exchange in recurrent FSGS after kidney transplantation, the evidence for its use in native kidney FSGS remains relatively limited. In one controlled trial, 14 patients with native kidney FSGS were randomized to receive tacrolimus only or tacrolimus with 15 sessions of plasmapheresis. No significant differences were found in proteinuria between the 2 groups at 6 months and 12 months of follow-up (unpublished data).[364]

## AZATHIOPRINE

The current evidence does not justify the use of azathioprine in the treatment of SRNS. A prospective randomized double-blind placebo-controlled trial that included 31 children with SRNS compared the use of a combination of azathioprine and steroids with steroids alone. The study did not detect any benefit from the addition of azathioprine.[365] Azathioprine also did not offer any advantage when it was used in two subsequent small case series of patients with SRNS.[366,367]

## LEVAMISOLE

Levamisole has been frequently used in the treatment of both FRNS and SDNS worldwide. Its use has also been infrequently reported in children with SRNS. This was illustrated in two small observational studies. The first included five children with SRNS who were treated with levamisole 2.5 mg/kg on alternate days. Two of these children also received cyclosporine A. None of the five children with SRNS experienced a remission. Serious adverse reactions were reported in two patients, in the form of agranulocytosis and a severe psoriasis-like cutaneous reaction.[368] The second study included six children with SRNS who were treated with levamisole at 2 mg/kg/day. Levamisole treatment was associated with a marked improvement in proteinuria (from 1.53 g to 0.11 g/day) and decreased need for corticosteroids (from 9086 to 1505 mg).[245] In the latter report, neutropenia developed in 15% of children treated with levamisole. In the absence of randomized controlled trials, there is thus little evidence to support the use of levamisole in children with SRNS.

# Nonimmunosuppressive therapy for steroid-resistant nephrotic syndrome

## ANGIOTENSIN-CONVERTING ENZYME INHIBITORS

ACEIs and ARBs are recommended in children with refractory nephrotic syndrome for their antiproteinuric, antihypertensive, lipid-lowering, and long-term renoprotective effects. Several mechanisms have been proposed for the antiproteinuric effect associated with the use of ACEIs and ARBs. Reduction in the intraglomerular filtration pressure, alteration in glomerular permselectivity, and antifibrotic and lipid-lowering effects all may contribute to reducing proteinuria. First, ACEIs and ARBs acutely reduce the glomerular capillary hydraulic pressure and filtration pressure across the GFB by blocking the vasoconstrictor effect of angiotensin II on both the afferent and efferent glomerular arterioles.[369,370] Second, ACEIs and ARBs alter the permselectivity of the GFB independently of hemodynamic changes,[371,372] thereby providing an explanation for the continued improvement in proteinuria up to several months following the initiation of ACEIs and ARBs.[373] Third, angiotensin II appears to promote the release of profibrotic factors, such as transforming growth factor-β (TGF-β) and epidermal growth factor (EGF), an effect that is mediated by the angiotensin I receptor (AT1 receptor). Hence, ACEIs and ARBs block the release of profibrotic factors and can slow the progression of glomerular and tubulointerstitial fibrosis in chronic kidney disease.[374] Fourth, the use of ACEIs and ARBs is associated with a prominent lipid-lowering effect that exceeds what would be expected in response to decreased proteinuria.[375–377] Angiotensin blockade–induced correction of dyslipidemia may also

> ## KEY POINT
>
> ACEIs and ARBs are recommended in children with refractory nephrotic syndrome for their antiproteinuric, antihypertensive, lipid-lowering, and long-term renoprotective effects.

contribute to the delayed progression of chronic kidney disease in proteinuric diseases.[378]

The beneficial effects of ACEIs and ARBs in proteinuric kidney diseases are well established in large controlled adult studies.[379-381] The benefits appear to be enhanced by concurrent dietary sodium restriction.[382] In children, multiple observational studies have illustrated the antiproteinuric effects of ACEIs and ARBs in SRNS.[294,295,377,383] In a randomized uncontrolled prospective crossover trial of 25 children with SRNS, high-dose (0.6 mg/kg/day) and low-dose enalapril (0.2 mg/kg/day) reduced proteinuria by 52% and 33%, respectively.[293] Moreover, a prospective observational study investigated the use of losartan in 52 children with proteinuria, 22 of whom had associated hypertension. Proteinuria decreased by 34% at a 6-week follow-up visit. Further reductions in proteinuria in the range of 64% to 67% from baseline were noted at 3 subsequent visits between 4.5 months and 2.5 years later.[294]

In a case series, 13 children with SRNS received enalapril at a dose of 0.2 to 0.6 mg/kg/day combined with low-dose prednisone given on alternate days. Total urinary protein and albumin excretion were reduced by 80% and 70%, respectively. In the same study, urine protein electrophoresis showed a shift to a more albumin-selective proteinuria in children treated with enalapril.[383] In another case series of 9 children with SRNS, the combined use of MMF and angiotensin blockade resulted in a 72% reduction in proteinuria at 6 months of follow-up compared with baseline, a benefit that was maintained for at least 24 months. Both total cholesterol and triglycerides also markedly improved.[295]

Adverse effects associated with ACEIs and ARBs include decreased GFR, hyperkalemia, cough, and, rarely, angioedema. The decrease in GFR is most pronounced in children with decreased renal perfusion, such as those with bilateral renal artery stenosis. In conditions with decreased renal perfusion, angiotensin II maintains the filtration pressure through efferent vasoconstriction. ACEIs and ARBs block this defense mechanism and may result in a precipitous drop in the GFR. ACEIs and ARBs may also induce or exacerbate hyperkalemia, most likely through blockade of angiotensin II–induced release of aldosterone. Monitoring of renal function and electrolytes is suggested 5 to 7 days after initiating ACEIs and ARBs and after increases (usually of 50% or more) in the prescribed dose. ACEIs and ARBs should be discontinued in the event of a significant elevation in serum creatinine (greater than 30%) from baseline value or significant hyperkalemia.

## ANTIOXIDANTS

Induction of reactive oxygen species (ROS)[384] and reduced antioxidant enzyme activity[385] have been implicated in the pathogenesis of nephrotic syndrome in animal models. In addition, accumulation of lipid peroxides, a product of oxidative damage, were documented in the renal cortex,[386] glomeruli,[387,388] and urine of animals with glomerular injury.[386-388] The use of ROS scavengers partially ameliorates glomerular injury in some animal models of nephrotic syndrome.[386,389-391]

Total serum antioxidant activity is reduced in children with nephrotic syndrome.[392-394] Total serum antioxidant activity was also significantly lower in children with SSNS who developed subsequent relapses of the disease compared with those with sustained remission.[394] In addition, malondialdehyde, a marker of oxidative stress, is significantly elevated during active disease.[392-394] Antioxidants, such as ascorbic acid and vitamin E, were elevated in some reports,[395] but unchanged in others.[392,393] It remains unclear whether these findings are related to an increase in oxygen free radical generation or suppressed antioxidant defense mechanisms.

The use of vitamin E as an ROS scavenger in the treatment of childhood FSGS was investigated in a small open-label controlled trial. Eleven children with biopsy-proven FSGS, 8 of whom were steroid resistant, were treated with vitamin E 200 IU twice daily. Nine children with other glomerular diseases and high-grade proteinuria were used as controls. After approximately 3 months of therapy, vitamin E was associated with a significant quantitative reduction in proteinuria (from a mean protein to creatinine ratio of 9.7 to 4.1) in the FSGS group, but not in the controls.[396] A subsequent randomized placebo-controlled trial of vitamin E in children with IgA nephropathy yielded similar results, a finding suggesting that the beneficial effect may be generalized to other glomerular diseases, rather than being specific to idiopathic FSGS.[397] Despite these findings, reproduction of these results in long-term randomized controlled studies will be required before vitamin E may be recommended for the treatment of children with SRNS.

## GALACTOSE

In vitro and in vivo evidence suggests that galactose binds avidly to a circulating permeability factor in some patients with FSGS. Binding to galactose may induce rapid inactivation and clearance of the permeability factor. Intravenous and oral administration of galactose in a patient with posttransplant FSGS recurrence resulted in sustained suppression of permeability activity.[285] This study was followed by a case report of an adult with refractory SRNS who was successfully treated with oral galactose, which resulted in remission of the disease and reduced permeability factor activity.[398] Partial remission of nephrotic syndrome was also reported with oral galactose therapy in a toddler with IgM nephropathy and an adolescent girl with mesangioproliferative glomerulonephritis, both of whom were previously refractory to multiple immunosuppressive medications.[399] A prospective study is under way to investigate the role of galactose in SRNS further.

# OTHER TREATMENT-RELATED ADVERSE EFFECTS

## Drug-induced hypertension

Systemic hypertension is common in children with nephrotic syndrome who are maintained on immunosuppressive medications. In this setting, the elevated blood pressure is more likely to be related to the use of corticosteroids or calcineurin inhibitors than to the underlying glomerular disease. The hypertensive effect of corticosteroids is thought to be mediated by an increase in the vasoconstrictor response to endogenous catecholamines[400–402] and to angiotensin II.[401,402] Renal salt retention, mediated through corticosteroid-induced direct activation of mineralocorticoid receptors, may also play a contributory role.[403] Tacrolimus, in contrast, may induce systemic hypertension through activation of sodium chloride cotransporters (NCCs) in the distal convoluted tubules. Tacrolimus-induced hypertension is often associated with hyperkalemia, hypercalciuria, and metabolic acidosis, a syndrome that resembles familial hyperkalemic hypertension (Gordon syndrome), a genetic disease characterized by overactivity of NCC.[315] Similarly, cyclosporine A has been associated with systemic hypertension. However, the underlying mechanisms behind the hypertensive effect of cyclosporine remain undetermined.

In children with persistent proteinuria, ACEIs and ARBs are the preferred antihypertensive medications in view of their antiproteinuric and long-term renoprotective effects. Careful monitoring of electrolytes and renal function is imperative in children with nephrotic syndrome who are treated with ACEIs and ARBs, particularly children with severe anasarca and intravascular volume depletion who are at high risk for acute kidney injury or hyperkalemia.

Based on more recent studies, up to 50% of children with nephrotic syndrome who are treated with calcineurin inhibitors may develop systemic hypertension.[231,237] Classically, calcium channel blockers have been considered the first-line choice in children with calcineurin inhibitor-induced hypertension. However, since uncovering the underlying tubular mechanisms behind the hypertensive effect of tacrolimus, selective blockade of NCC by using thiazide diuretics has been proposed as an alternative.[315] Clinical trials are needed to determine the efficacy of thiazide diuretics in the treatment of calcineurin inhibitor–induced hypertension.

## Drug-induced dyslipidemia

The effect of glucocorticoids on lipid metabolism has been debated in multiple adult studies. After controlling for autoimmune disease activity, diet, physical activity, and other confounding factors, low to moderate doses of glucocorticoids do not appear to adversely affect lipid profiles in adults[404,405] or in children with systemic lupus erythematosus.[406,407] In children with SSNS, glucocorticoids are likely to improve the lipid profiles paradoxically by reducing proteinuria.

Cyclosporine has been associated with elevated triglyceride and lipoprotein A levels, along with an undesirable fall in high-density lipoprotein cholesterol independent of prednisone in renal transplant recipients.[408] However, this effect is more difficult to isolate in children with nephrotic syndrome who are treated with calcineurin inhibitors. Moreover, the antiproteinuric benefit of calcineurin inhibitors in children with nephrotic syndrome will likely outweigh any risk of drug-related dyslipidemia.

## COMPLICATIONS OF THE PODOCYTOPATHIES

The development of acute kidney injury, as well as common infectious, thromboembolic, cardiovascular, and pulmonary complications of nephrotic syndrome, is discussed in detail in Chapter 16. The following sections discuss some of the less common complications that include anemia, endocrine abnormalities, and trace element deficiencies.

## ANEMIA

Anemia related to erythropoietin deficiency or iron deficiency has been described in children with refractory nephrotic syndrome. The anemia has been attributed to urinary losses and increased catabolism of both erythropoietin and transferrin.[409,410] The anemia improves following induction of remission of the disease, but it may also be responsive to exogenous erythropoietin therapy.[411]

## ENDOCRINE ABNORMALITIES AND DEFICIENCY OF TRACE ELEMENTS

Many circulating hormones, vitamins, and trace elements are bound to serum albumin or other binding proteins. In children with active nephrotic syndrome, massive losses of these binding proteins can result in endocrine abnormalities or deficiency symptoms. For example, substantial losses of vitamin D–binding proteins in nephrotic syndrome can result in signs and symptoms of vitamin D deficiency. Secondary hyperparathyroidism with low levels of 25-hydroxy-vitamin D and 1,25-hydroxy-vitamin D have also been detected in children with nephrotic syndrome.[412,413] However, the free and physiologically active fraction of 1,25-hydroxy-vitamin D usually remains normal.[414] This may explain why only a subset of children with nephrotic syndrome develops symptomatic vitamin D abnormalities that require supplementation.[415]

Studies evaluating bone mineral density in children with nephrotic syndrome produced variable results. In an uncontrolled prospective evaluation of 100 children with nephrotic syndrome using dual-energy x-ray absorptiometry (DEXA), osteoporosis was detected in 22%.[416] The low bone mineral density in these children was partially reversed following calcium and vitamin D supplementation.[417] Conversely, Leonard et al.[418] reported similar bone mineral content of the spine in 60 children with nephrotic syndrome and 195 healthy controls. In the same study, the whole body mineral content was increased in children with nephrotic syndrome. These differences were attributed to steroid-induced weight gain, an undesirable adverse effect of corticosteroids that is also associated with increased bone density.[418]

Urinary losses of binding proteins for cortisol and thyroxine may lead to reduced total blood levels of these hormones in children with nephrotic syndrome.[419,420] However, the unbound hormonal fractions remain normal, and symptomatic hypothyroidism or adrenal insufficiency seldom occurs.[413,420] One exception to this rule involves infants with congenital nephrotic syndrome. Unlike other children with nephrotic syndrome, these infants develop massive urinary losses of binding proteins that commonly lead to clinical hypothyroidism and often require supplementation.[421–423] Clinically important hypocortisolism has also been reported in an infant with congenital nephrotic syndrome.[423]

In addition to endocrine abnormalities, deficiencies of zinc and copper have been described in patients with nephrotic syndrome. Zinc and copper are lost into the urine through urinary losses of their associated binding proteins—albumin and ceruloplasmin, respectively[413,424,425] (see Chapter 6).

## PROGNOSIS

## LIKELIHOOD OF ACHIEVING REMISSION

The initial response to steroid therapy is considered the most important long-term prognostic indicator in childhood nephrotic syndrome. This was illustrated in a multicenter study of 389 children with idiopathic nephrotic syndrome who were treated with prednisone and were followed for up to 17 years. Most (76%) children who responded to the initial course of glucocorticoids and were in remission for at least 6 months remained in remission for the entire follow-up period or had relapses rarely. In contrast, children who failed to respond to the initial 8-week course of corticosteroids developed ESKD in 21% of the cases. Moreover, children who failed to respond to both the initial steroid course and subsequent therapies over a period of 6 months developed ESKD in 35% of the cases. Children who responded to the initial course of glucocorticoids but who later developed frequent relapses within the subsequent 6-months period had a more favorable outcome, with 63% eventually becoming relapse free after an average follow-up of 3 years.[191]

In the initial ISKDC cohort, 78% of children who were treated with corticosteroids achieved complete remission.[98] However, the likelihood of responding to corticosteroids differed by the underlying histopathologic features. The steroid-response rate was 93%, 30%, 56%, and 7% in children with MCD, FSGS, MesProlif GN, and MPGN, respectively. None of the children with membranous nephropathy responded to corticosteroids in the ISKDC cohort.[98] Furthermore, the

likelihood of response to steroids varied by age at presentation, with lower response rates seen in older children. This finding is not surprising because a higher age at presentation has been correlated with histopathologic features with poor steroid responsiveness, such as FSGS, MPGN, or membranous nephropathy.[25]

In our current era, a range of effective options may be offered to children who fail to respond to the initial course of corticosteroids. However, many of these children, particularly those with familial disease, may have an identifiable underlying genetic defect that profoundly reduces their probability of responding to immunosuppression. It appears that children with SRNS attributable to the identified genetic mutations to date are unlikely to achieve remission in response to immunosuppressive therapy. This was illustrated in a study of 91 children with SRNS, of whom 43 had identified disease-causing mutations. None of the 43 patients with identified disease-causing mutations achieved complete remission in response to cyclosporine, and only 2 achieved partial remission.[283] Similarly, immunosuppressive therapy failed to induce complete remission in any of 66 patients with SRNS and detected genetic mutations who were included in two other reports.[285,305]

The long-term prognosis of children who are responsive to cyclosporine has not been extensively studied. In a multicenter prospective report, 71% (22 of 31) of children with SRNS who initially attained complete remission in response to cyclosporine continued to require immunosuppressive therapy at 5 years of follow-up. Of these 22 patients, 19 remained on cyclosporine, and 7 developed frequent relapses.[426] Unfortunately, relapses are common during tapering or after discontinuing cyclosporine therapy. By the end of 12 months of cyclosporine treatment, 3 of 6 children who initially responded developed a relapse in one study.[307] The substitution of MMF may reduce the rate of relapse during cyclosporine tapering. In a study of pediatric SRNS, MMF was added sequentially to 18 children who achieved complete remission on cyclosporine A. This was followed by the successful discontinuation of cyclosporine in 16 children. At a mean follow-up of 7 years, only 21% of these children eventually developed relapses. In this study, renal function parameters improved significantly following discontinuation of cyclosporine.[270]

Most studies that have investigated the efficacy of immunosuppressive medications did not include genetic testing. As a result, it is not possible to estimate the response rate of children with nongenetic forms of SRNS to various immunosuppressive medications. When genetic and nongenetic forms of the disease are taken into account, the rates of achieving complete remission in children with SRNS have been reported at 52% for pulse steroids (Mendoza protocol),[347] in the range of 36% to 84% with cyclosporine,[227,306–310] and 40% to 94% with tacrolimus.[319–325] In light of these statistics, it appears highly likely that children with SRNS, particularly those with nongenetic forms of the disease, will achieve remission in response to at least one of the foregoing immunosuppressive options.

---

**KEY POINT**

Clinical response to steroids with entry into complete remission predicts a favorable long-term outcome in children and adults with primary podocytopathies.

## RELAPSE RATE

The majority of children with SSNS (70%) will experience at least one relapse of their disease. However, the probability of developing relapses declines over time. By 8 years following the initial diagnosis, 80% (311 of 389) of children from the original ISKDC cohort with steroid-sensitive MCD had no further relapses.[191] In the same study, the best outcome was seen in children who responded to initial therapy with prednisone and subsequently remained in remission for at least 6 months. Of those, 75% remained in remission or developed rare relapses throughout the follow-up period (mean, 9.4 years).[191]

## END-STAGE KIDNEY DISEASE AND TRANSPLANT RECURRENCE RISK

Persistent high-grade proteinuria that is unresponsive to corticosteroids or other immunosuppressive medications predicts a high risk for progressive renal insufficiency. In the ISKDC cohort of 389 children with MCD, 21% of those who did not respond to the initial course of prednisone progressed to ESKD at a mean follow-up of 9.4 years.[191] Moreover, 35% of those who had unremitting proteinuria for 6 months following the initial prednisone course progressed to ESKD. Overall, 4% to 5% of the ISKDC cohort of children died or progressed to ESKD.[191]

Similar to the foregoing observations in children with MCD, steroid responsiveness also predicted a more favorable outcome in children[289,427] and adults[290] with FSGS. In a report of 60 children with FSGS, 58% of whom were African American, the risk of ESKD was reduced by 90% in those who achieved complete remission at a median follow-up of 33 months.[289] In another retrospective review of 92 children with steroid-resistant FSGS, including 33 patients with late steroid resistance, the lack of an initial response to corticosteroids was also identified as an important risk factor for progression to chronic kidney disease. Other risk factors identified in this study included asymptomatic proteinuria at presentation, baseline renal insufficiency, higher percentage of segmentally sclerotic glomeruli on biopsy, and a high degree of tubulointerstitial fibrosis.[427]

Renal transplantation is considered the treatment of choice in most children with nephrotic syndrome who progress to ESKD. In children with FSGS, however, recurrence of the disease has been reported in 20% to 56% of pediatric allograft recipients.[428–430] In a report by the North American Pediatric Renal Transplant Cooperative Study database (NAPRTCS), recurrent FSGS resulted in the loss of the allograft in 6.1% of children by 5 years after transplantation.[431] Risk factors for FSGS recurrence include a younger age at onset (less than 15 years), rapid progression to ESKD (within 3 years), mesangial proliferative histopathologic features, and a previous history of recurrence.[60,432–434] FSGS recurrence after renal transplantation has also been infrequently reported in children with identified genetic mutations in *NPHS2*[435,436] or *TRPC6*.[437] Effective treatment options include corticosteroids, plasma exchange,[63] and cyclosporine.[438]

## MORTALITY RISK

A dramatic reduction in the mortality rate of children with nephrotic syndrome followed the introduction of antibiotics in the 1940s and corticosteroids in the 1950s. Despite these enormous advances, children with nephrotic syndrome, particularly those who are refractory to conventional therapies, remain at a considerable risk of mortality. Death is often related to disease complications. In the ISKDC study that included 389 children with biopsy-proven MCD, 10 children died (2.6%) over a follow-up period of 5 to 15 years. The deaths were attributed to infection in 6 of these 10 children,[439] a finding highlighting the importance of early recognition and treatment of the infectious complications of nephrotic syndrome.

## ADULTS WITH A HISTORY OF CHILDHOOD NEPHROTIC SYNDROME

Three studies described the clinical course of adults who had a history of childhood SSNS. In the first study, which described adults at a mean duration of 22 years after their initial diagnosis, 33% (14 of 42) reported at least 1 relapse during adulthood, but all had normal renal function. As would be expected, a complicated course and the need for steroid-sparing medications during childhood predicted adult relapses.[440] The second study included 15 adults with persistent biopsy-proven childhood MCD with a frequently relapsing or steroid-dependent course. These patients were evaluated at a median duration of 24 years since initial diagnosis. Similar to the previous report, all patients had normal renal function, but 80% were still being treated with an immunosuppressive medication. The prevalence of treatment-related complications was relatively high. The most common complications were hypertension (47%), osteoporosis (33%), and cataracts (20%).[441] In a third study, which investigated the adult outcome of 117 patients with a history of childhood SSNS, 42% reported at least one relapse during adulthood. A younger age at disease onset (less than 6 years) and a higher number of relapses during childhood were identified as risk factors for continued relapses into adulthood. Steroid-related side effects, particularly in the form of obesity or osteoporosis, were detected in 44% of adults who continued to experience relapses.[442] In summary, these studies clearly demonstrate that the burden of nephrotic syndrome, as well as treatment-related complications, carries over into adulthood in many patients. This finding highlights the importance of appropriate transitioning of patients with nephrotic syndrome to an adult nephrologist for continued follow-up and monitoring.

## SUMMARY

Nephrotic syndrome is one of the most commonly encountered kidney diseases in children. Advances in genetic testing and molecular diagnostics have allowed for better classification of the disease. Moreover, animal and human research studies have contributed to an improved understanding of the underlying pathophysiology. However, many questions remain unanswered in terms of the pathogenesis behind the primary glomerular injury, as well as the mechanisms of edema and dyslipidemia. Furthermore, the pathways by which the most commonly used medications, such as corticosteroids, exert their effect have not been fully elucidated. Despite the monumental improvements in the mortality and morbidity of children with this disease, many children with refractory SRNS, particularly those with underlying genetic mutations, may not fully respond to the currently available therapeutic options. Unfortunately, such children continue to face significant challenges in regard to their quality of life, and they remain at increased risk for treatment-related toxicities as well as infectious, thrombotic, and cardiovascular complications. Additional research is needed to promote a deeper understanding of the underlying pathogenesis and to provide a wider spectrum of safe and effective treatments.

## ACKNOWLEDGMENTS

Special thanks are extended to Dr. Chung-Ho Chang, Renal Pathologist from Children's Hospital of Michigan, for his assistance with the attainment of the histologic photographs and their interpretation.

### Clinical Vignette 17.1

Anthony is a 2-year-old boy with a known history of seasonal allergies who presents to his primary physician with bilateral periorbital swelling of 5 days' duration. His mother initially "self-treated" his facial swelling with over-the-counter diphenhydramine, with minimal response. He does not appear to be in any discomfort and maintains normal activity. His appetite is slightly decreased. His mother has not noticed any changes in his voiding pattern or urine color. His facial swelling appears to be worse in the morning and improves as the day progresses. No apparent triggers are reported, but the mother recalls a transient brief episode of runny nose and dry cough that resolved spontaneously approximately 1 week before the current presentation.

In the office, he appears well and in no acute distress. His blood pressure is 102/56 mm Hg, and his heart rate is 77 beats/min. His physical examination is notable for bilateral periorbital swelling, abdominal fullness with a positive fluid wave but no tenderness, and significant pitting pretibial edema bilaterally. No skin rash or joint abnormalities are noted on examination. A urine dipstick was obtained in the office that shows 4+ protein (greater than 2000 mg/dL). Chemistry panel shows hypoalbuminemia (albumin, 2.1 g/dL) and hypercholesterolemia (total cholesterol, 340 mg/dL). Serum complement levels, blood urea nitrogen, creatinine, and electrolytes are normal.

Anthony is referred to a pediatric nephrologist, who discusses with the family the most likely diagnosis, MCD, as well as the recommended initial empiric therapy (corticosteroids), expected adverse effects, and alternatives to therapy. He is started on oral prednisolone, 2 mg/kg/day, of which he completes 6 weeks, followed by 1.5 mg/kg/dose given on alternate days for an additional 6 weeks. His urine dipstick turns negative for protein approximately 6 days after starting prednisolone therapy, and his generalized swelling completely resolves 3 days later.

## REFERENCES

1. Shankland SJ. The podocyte's response to injury: Role in proteinuria and glomerulosclerosis. Kidney Int. 2006;69:2131–47.
2. Kriz W. The pathogenesis of 'classic' focal segmental glomerulosclerosis: Lessons from rat models. Nephrol Dial Transplant. 2003;18(Suppl 6):vi39–44.
3. Brenner BM, Hostetter TH, Humes HD. Glomerular permselectivity: Barrier function based on discrimination of molecular size and charge. Am J Physiol. 1978;234:F455–60.
4. Rostgaard J, Qvortrup K. Sieve plugs in fenestrae of glomerular capillaries: Site of the filtration barrier? Cells Tissues Organs. 2002;170:132–8.
5. Haraldsson B, Nystrom J, Deen WM. Properties of the glomerular barrier and mechanisms of proteinuria. Physiol Rev. 2008;88:451–87.
6. Karnovsky MJ, Ainsworth SK. The structural basis of glomerular filtration. Adv Nephrol Necker Hosp. 1972;2:35–60.
7. Kestila M, Lenkkeri U, Mannikko M, et al. Positionally cloned gene for a novel glomerular protein—nephrin—is mutated in congenital nephrotic syndrome. Mol Cell. 1998;1:575–82.
8. Boute N, Gribouval O, Roselli S, et al. NPHS2, encoding the glomerular protein podocin, is mutated in autosomal recessive steroid-resistant nephrotic syndrome. Nat Genet. 2000;24:349–54.

9. Reiser J, Polu KR, Moller CC, et al. TRPC6 is a glomerular slit diaphragm–associated channel required for normal renal function. Nat Genet. 2005;37:739–44.

10. Winn MP, Conlon PJ, Lynn KL, et al. A mutation in the TRPC6 cation channel causes familial focal segmental glomerulosclerosis. Science. 2005;308:1801–4.

11. Schwarz K, Simons M, Reiser J, et al. Podocin, a raft-associated component of the glomerular slit diaphragm, interacts with CD2AP and nephrin. J Clin Invest. 2001;108:1621–9.

12. Sorensson J, Ohlson M, Lindstrom K, Haraldsson B. Glomerular charge selectivity for horseradish peroxidase and albumin at low and normal ionic strengths. Acta Physiol Scand. 1998;163:83–91.

13. Ciarimboli G, Schurek HJ, Zeh M, et al. Role of albumin and glomerular capillary wall charge distribution on glomerular permselectivity: Studies on the perfused-fixed rat kidney model. Pflugers Arch. 1999;438:883–91.

14. Russo LM, Sandoval RM, McKee M, et al. The normal kidney filters nephrotic levels of albumin retrieved by proximal tubule cells: Retrieval is disrupted in nephrotic states. Kidney Int. 2007;71:504–13.

15. Kitano Y, Yoshikawa N, Nakamura H. Glomerular anionic sites in minimal change nephrotic syndrome and focal segmental glomerulosclerosis. Clin Nephrol. 1993;40:199–204.

16. Carrie BJ, Salyer WR, Myers BD. Minimal change nephropathy: An electrochemical disorder of the glomerular membrane. Am J Med. 1981;70:262–8.

17. van den Born J, van den Heuvel LP, Bakker MA, et al. A monoclonal antibody against GBM heparan sulfate induces an acute selective proteinuria in rats. Kidney Int. 1992;41:115–23.

18. Taylor GM, Neuhaus TJ, Shah V, et al. Charge and size selectivity of proteinuria in children with idiopathic nephrotic syndrome. Pediatr Nephrol. 1997;11:404–10.

19. Levin M, Smith C, Walters MD, Gascoine P, Barratt TM. Steroid-responsive nephrotic syndrome: A generalised disorder of membrane negative charge. Lancet. 1985;2:239–42.

20. Clark A, Barrat T. Steroid-responsive nephrotic syndrome. In: Barrat T, Avner E, Harmon W, editors. Pediatric Nephrology. Baltimore: Lippincott Williams & Wilkins; 1998. p. 731.

21. Nash M, Edelman C, Bernstein J. The nephrotic syndrome. In: Edelman C, editor. Pediatric Kidney Disease. Boston: Little, Brown and Company; 1992. p. 1247.

22. Srivastava T, Simon SD, Alon US. High incidence of focal segmental glomerulosclerosis in nephrotic syndrome of childhood. Pediatr Nephrol. 1999;13:13–8.

23. Hogg RJ, Portman RJ, Milliner D, et al. Evaluation and management of proteinuria and nephrotic syndrome in children: Recommendations from a pediatric nephrology panel established at the National Kidney Foundation conference on proteinuria, albuminuria, risk, assessment, detection, and elimination (PARADE). Pediatrics. 2000;105:1242–9.

24. McEnery PT, Strife CF. Nephrotic syndrome in childhood: management and treatment in patients with minimal change disease, mesangial proliferation, or focal glomerulosclerosis. Pediatr Clin North Am. 1982;29:875–94.

25. Anonymous. Nephrotic syndrome in children: Prediction of histopathology from clinical and laboratory characteristics at time of diagnosis. A report of the International Study of Kidney Disease in Children. Kidney Int. 1978;13:159–65.

26. Sharples PM, Poulton J, White RH. Steroid responsive nephrotic syndrome is more common in Asians. Arch Dis Child. 1985;60:1014–7.

27. Bhimma R, Coovadia HM, Adhikari M. Nephrotic syndrome in South African children: Changing perspectives over 20 years. Pediatr Nephrol. 1997;11:429–34.

28. Kopp JB, Smith MW, Nelson GW, et al. MYH9 is a major-effect risk gene for focal segmental glomerulosclerosis. Nat Genet. 2008;40:1175–84.

29. Bonilla-Felix M, Parra C, Dajani T, et al. Changing patterns in the histopathology of idiopathic nephrotic syndrome in children. Kidney Int. 1999;55:1885–90.

30. McCurdy FA, Butera PJ, Wilson R. The familial occurrence of focal segmental glomerular sclerosis. Am J Kidney Dis. 1987;10:467–9.

31. Naruse T, Hirokawa N, Maekawa T, et al. Familial nephrotic syndrome with focal glomerular sclerosis. Am J Med Sci. 1980;280:109–13.

32. White RH. The familial nephrotic syndrome. I. A European survey. Clin Nephrol. 1973;1:215–9.

33. Chandra M, Mouradian J, Hoyer JR, Lewy JE. Familial nephrotic syndrome and focal segmental glomerulosclerosis. J Pediatr. 1981;98:556–60.

34. Moncrieff MW, White RH, Glasgow EF, et al. The familial nephrotic syndrome. II. A clinicopathological study. Clin Nephrol. 1973;1:220–9.

35. Roy S, 3rd, Pitcock JA. Idiopathic nephrosis in identical twins. Am J Dis Child. 1971;121:428–30.

36. Shalhoub RJ. Pathogenesis of lipoid nephrosis: A disorder of T-cell function. Lancet. 1974;2:556–60.

37. Yang T, Nast CC, Vo A, Jordan SC. Rapid remission of steroid and mycophenolate mofetil (MMF)–resistant minimal change nephrotic syndrome after rituximab therapy. Nephrol Dial Transplant. 2008;23:377–80.

38. Aggarwal N, Batwara R, McCarthy ET, et al. Serum permeability activity in steroid-resistant minimal change nephrotic syndrome is abolished by treatment of Hodgkin disease. Am J Kidney Dis. 2007;50:826–9.

39. Ali AA, Wilson E, Moorhead JF, et al. Minimal-change glomerular nephritis: Normal kidneys in an abnormal environment? Transplantation. 1994;58:849–52.

40. Abdel-Hafez M, Shimada M, Lee PY, et al. Idiopathic nephrotic syndrome and atopy: Is there a common link? Am J Kidney Dis. 2009;54:945–53.

41. Audard V, Larousserie F, Grimbert P, et al. Minimal change nephrotic syndrome and classical Hodgkin's lymphoma: Report of 21 cases and review of the literature. Kidney Int. 2006;69:2251–60.

42. Sasdelli M, Cagnoli L, Candi P, et al. Cell mediated immunity in idiopathic glomerulonephritis. Clin Exp Immunol. 1981;46:27–34.

43. Yan K, Nakahara K, Awa S, et al. The increase of memory T cell subsets in children with idiopathic nephrotic syndrome. Nephron. 1998;79:274–8.

44. Fodor P, Saitua MT, Rodriguez E, et al. T-cell dysfunction in minimal-change nephrotic syndrome of childhood. Am J Dis Child. 1982;136:713–7.

45. Sellier-Leclerc AL, Duval A, Riveron S, et al. A humanized mouse model of idiopathic nephrotic syndrome suggests a pathogenic role for immature cells. J Am Soc Nephrol. 2007;18:2732–9.

46. Tasic V. Nephrotic syndrome in a child after a bee sting. Pediatr Nephrol. 2000;15:245–7.

47. Swanson GP, Leveque JA. Nephrotic syndrome associated with ant bite. Tex Med. 1990;86:39–41.

48. Cuoghi D, Venturi P, Cheli E. Bee sting and relapse of nephrotic syndrome. Child Nephrol Urol. 1988;9:82–3.

49. Lagrue G, Laurent J, Rostoker G. Food allergy and idiopathic nephrotic syndrome. Kidney Int Suppl. 1989;27:S147–51.

50. Sahali D, Pawlak A, Valanciute A, et al. A novel approach to investigation of the pathogenesis of active minimal-change nephrotic syndrome using subtracted cDNA library screening. J Am Soc Nephrol. 2002;13:1238–47.

51. Ishimoto T, Shimada M, Araya CE, et al. Minimal change disease: A CD80 podocytopathy? Semin Nephrol. 2011;31:320–5.

52. Okuyama S, Komatsuda A, Wakui H, et al. Up-regulation of TRAIL mRNA expression in peripheral blood mononuclear cells from patients with minimal-change nephrotic syndrome. Nephrol Dial Transplant. 2005;20:539–44.

53. Gonzalez E, Neuhaus T, Kemper MJ, Girardin E. Proteomic analysis of mononuclear cells of patients with minimal-change nephrotic syndrome of childhood. Nephrol Dial Transplant. 2009;24:149–55.

54. Garin EH. A comparison of combinations of diuretics in nephrotic edema. Am J Dis Child. 1987;141:769–71.

55. van den Berg JG, Weening JJ. Role of the immune system in the pathogenesis of idiopathic nephrotic syndrome. Clin Sci (Lond). 2004;107:125–36.

56. Cheung W, Wei CL, Seah CC, et al. Atopy, serum IgE, and interleukin-13 in steroid-responsive nephrotic syndrome. Pediatr Nephrol. 2004;19:627–32.

57. Lai KW, Wei CL, Tan LK, et al. Overexpression of interleukin-13 induces minimal-change–like nephropathy in rats. J Am Soc Nephrol. 2007;18:1476–85.

58. Yokoyama H, Kida H, Abe T, et al. Impaired immunoglobulin G production in minimal change nephrotic syndrome in adults. Clin Exp Immunol. 1987;70:110–5.

59. McAdams AJ, Valentini RP, Welch TR. The nonspecificity of focal segmental glomerulosclerosis: The defining characteristics of primary focal glomerulosclerosis, mesangial proliferation, and minimal change. Medicine (Baltimore). 1997;76:42–52.

60. Ellis D, Kapur S, Antonovych TT, et al. Focal glomerulosclerosis in children: Correlation of histology with prognosis. J Pediatr. 1978;93:762–8.

61. Hara M, Yanagihara T, Takada T, et al. Urinary excretion of podocytes reflects disease activity in children with glomerulonephritis. Am J Nephrol. 1998;18:35–41.

62. Hara M, Yanagihara T, Kihara I. Urinary podocytes in primary focal segmental glomerulosclerosis. Nephron. 2001;89:342–7.

63. Dantal J, Bigot E, Bogers W, et al. Effect of plasma protein adsorption on protein excretion in kidney-transplant recipients with recurrent nephrotic syndrome. N Engl J Med. 1994;330:7–14.

64. Cravedi P, Kopp JB, Remuzzi G. Recent progress in the pathophysiology and treatment of FSGS recurrence. Am J Transplant. 2013;13:266–74.

65. Avila-Casado M del C, Perez-Torres I, Auron A, et al. Proteinuria in rats induced by serum from patients with collapsing glomerulopathy. Kidney Int. 2004;66:133–43.

66. Kemper MJ, Wolf G, Muller-Wiefel DE. Transmission of glomerular permeability factor from a mother to her child. N Engl J Med. 2001;344:386–7.

67. Wei C, Trachtman H, Li J, et al. Circulating suPAR in two cohorts of primary FSGS. J Am Soc Nephrol. 2012;23:2051–9.

68. Wei C, El Hindi S, Li J, et al. Circulating urokinase receptor as a cause of focal segmental glomerulosclerosis. Nat Med. 2011;17:952–60.

69. Huang J, Liu G, Zhang YM, et al. Plasma soluble urokinase receptor levels are increased but do not distinguish primary from secondary focal segmental glomerulosclerosis. Kidney Int. 2013;84:366–72.

70. Maas RJ, Deegens JK, Wetzels JF. Serum suPAR in patients with FSGS: Trash or treasure? Pediatr Nephrol. 2013;28:1041–8.

71. Bock ME, Price HE, Gallon L, Langman CB. Serum soluble urokinase-type plasminogen activator receptor levels and idiopathic FSGS in children: A single-center report. Clin J Am Soc Nephrol. 2013;8:1304–11.

72. Franco Palacios CR, Lieske JC, Wadei HM, et al. Urine but not serum soluble urokinase receptor (suPAR) may identify cases of recurrent FSGS in kidney transplant candidates. Transplantation. 2013;96:394–9.

73. Brown EJ, Schlondorff JS, Becker DJ, et al. Mutations in the formin gene INF2 cause focal segmental glomerulosclerosis. Nat Genet. 2010;42:72–6.

74. Mele C, Iatropoulos P, Donadelli R, et al. MYO1E mutations and childhood familial focal segmental glomerulosclerosis. N Engl J Med. 2011;365:295–306.

75. He N, Zahirieh A, Mei Y, et al. Recessive NPHS2 (podocin) mutations are rare in adult-onset idiopathic focal segmental glomerulosclerosis. Clin J Am Soc Nephrol. 2007;2:31–7.

76. Weber S, Gribouval O, Esquivel EL, et al. NPHS2 mutation analysis shows genetic heterogeneity of steroid-resistant nephrotic syndrome and low post-transplant recurrence. Kidney Int. 2004;66:571–9.

77. Philippe A, Nevo F, Esquivel EL, et al. Nephrin mutations can cause childhood-onset steroid-resistant nephrotic syndrome. J Am Soc Nephrol. 2008;19:1871–8.

78. Santin S, Garcia-Maset R, Ruiz P, et al. Nephrin mutations cause childhood- and adult-onset focal segmental glomerulosclerosis. Kidney Int. 2009;76:1268–76.

79. Barua M, Brown EJ, Charoonratana VT, et al. Mutations in the INF2 gene account for a significant proportion of familial but not sporadic focal and segmental glomerulosclerosis. Kidney Int. 2013;83:316–22.

80. Boyer O, Benoit G, Gribouval O, et al. Mutations in INF2 are a major cause of autosomal dominant focal segmental glomerulosclerosis. J Am Soc Nephrol. 2011;22:239–45.

81. Gbadegesin RA, Lavin PJ, Hall G, et al. Inverted formin 2 mutations with variable expression in patients with sporadic and hereditary focal and segmental glomerulosclerosis. Kidney Int. 2012;81:94–9.

82. Lipska BS, Iatropoulos P, Maranta R, et al. Genetic screening in adolescents with steroid-resistant nephrotic syndrome. Kidney Int. 2013;84:206–13.

83. Boyer O, Nevo F, Plaisier E, et al. INF2 mutations in Charcot-Marie-Tooth disease with glomerulopathy. N Engl J Med. 2011;365:2377–88.

84. Kaplan JM, Kim SH, North KN, et al. Mutations in ACTN4, encoding alpha-actinin-4, cause familial focal segmental glomerulosclerosis. Nat Genet. 2000;24:251–6.

85. Henderson JM, Alexander MP, Pollak MR. Patients with ACTN4 mutations demonstrate distinctive features of glomerular injury. J Am Soc Nephrol. 2009;20:961–8.

86. Santin S, Ars E, Rossetti S, et al. TRPC6 mutational analysis in a large cohort of patients with focal segmental glomerulosclerosis. Nephrol Dial Transplant. 2009;24:3089–96.

87. Mir S, Yavascan O, Berdeli A, Sozeri B. TRPC6 gene variants in Turkish children with steroid-resistant nephrotic syndrome. Nephrol Dial Transplant. 2012;27:205–9.

88. Gigante M, Caridi G, Montemurno E, et al. TRPC6 mutations in children with steroid-resistant nephrotic syndrome and atypical phenotype. Clin J Am Soc Nephrol. 2011;6:1626–34.

89. D'Agati V. Pathologic classification of focal segmental glomerulosclerosis. Semin Nephrol. 2003;23:117–34.

90. Kambham N, Markowitz GS, Valeri AM, et al. Obesity-related glomerulopathy: An emerging epidemic. Kidney Int. 2001;59:1498–509.

91. Herlitz LC, Markowitz GS, Farris AB, et al. Development of focal segmental glomerulosclerosis after anabolic steroid abuse. J Am Soc Nephrol. 2010;21:163–72.

92. Dijkman HB, Weening JJ, Smeets B, et al. Proliferating cells in HIV and pamidronate-associated collapsing focal segmental glomerulosclerosis are parietal epithelial cells. Kidney Int. 2006;70:338–44.

93. Markowitz GS, Nasr SH, Stokes MB, D'Agati VD. Treatment with IFN-{alpha}, -{beta}, or -{gamma} is associated with collapsing focal segmental glomerulosclerosis. Clin J Am Soc Nephrol. 2010;5:607–15.

94. Hodgin JB, Rasoulpour M, Markowitz GS, D'Agati VD. Very low birth weight is a risk factor for secondary focal segmental glomerulosclerosis. Clin J Am Soc Nephrol. 2009;4:71–6.

95. Ikezumi Y, Suzuki T, Karasawa T, et al. Low birth-weight and premature birth are risk factors for podocytopenia and focal segmental glomerulosclerosis. Am J Nephrol. 2013;38:149–57.

96. Sharma K, Ziyadeh FN. The emerging role of transforming growth factor-beta in kidney diseases. Am J Physiol. 1994;266:F829–42.

97. Branten AJ, Vervoort G, Wetzels JF. Serum creatinine is a poor marker of GFR in nephrotic syndrome. Nephrol Dial Transplant. 2005;20:707–11.

98. Anonymous. The primary nephrotic syndrome in children: Identification of patients with minimal change nephrotic syndrome from initial response to prednisone. A report of the International Study of Kidney Disease in Children. J Pediatr. 1981;98:561–4.

99. Gipson DS, Massengill SF, Yao L, et al. Management of childhood onset nephrotic syndrome. Pediatrics. 2009;124:747–57.

100. Churg J, Habib R, White RH. Pathology of the nephrotic syndrome in children: A report for the International Study of Kidney Disease in Children. Lancet. 1970;760:1299–302.

101. White RH, Glasgow EF, Mills RJ. Clinicopathological study of nephrotic syndrome in childhood. Lancet. 1970;1:1353–9.

102. Markowitz GS, Schwimmer JA, Stokes MB, et al. C1q nephropathy: A variant of focal segmental glomerulosclerosis. Kidney Int. 2003;64:1232–40.

103. Border WA. Distinguishing minimal-change disease from mesangial disorders. Kidney Int. 1988;34:419–34.

104. Myllymaki J, Saha H, Mustonen J, et al. IgM nephropathy: Clinical picture and long-term prognosis. Am J Kidney Dis. 2003;41:343–50.

105. Waldherr R, Gubler MC, Levy M, et al. The significance of pure diffuse mesangial proliferation in idiopathic nephrotic syndrome. Clin Nephrol. 1978;10:171–9.

106. Anonymous. Childhood nephrotic syndrome associated with diffuse mesangial hypercellularity: A report of the Southwest Pediatric Nephrology Study Group. Kidney Int. 1983;24:87–94.

107. Swartz SJ, Eldin KW, Hicks MJ, Feig DI. Minimal change disease with IgM+ immunofluorescence: A subtype of nephrotic syndrome. Pediatr Nephrol. 2009;24:1187–92.

108. Vizjak A, Ferluga D, Rozic M, et al. Pathology, clinical presentations, and outcomes of C1q nephropathy. J Am Soc Nephrol. 2008;19:2237–44.

109. Kersnik Levart T, Kenda RB, Avgustin Cavic M, et al. C1Q nephropathy in children. Pediatr Nephrol. 2005;20:1756–61.

110. Hisano S, Fukuma Y, Segawa Y, et al. Clinicopathologic correlation and outcome of C1q nephropathy. Clin J Am Soc Nephrol. 2008;3:1637–43.

111. Fogo A, Glick AD, Horn SL, Horn RG. Is focal segmental glomerulosclerosis really focal? Distribution of lesions in adults and children. Kidney Int. 1995;47:1690–6.

112. Morel-Maroger L, Leathem A, Richet G. Glomerular abnormalities in nonsystemic diseases: Relationship between findings by light microscopy and immunofluorescence in 433 renal biopsy specimens. Am J Med. 1972;53:170–84.

113. Fogo A, Hawkins EP, Berry PL, et al. Glomerular hypertrophy in minimal change disease predicts subsequent progression to focal glomerular sclerosis. Kidney Int. 1990;38:115–23.

114. D'Agati VD, Kaskel FJ, Falk RJ. Focal segmental glomerulosclerosis. N Engl J Med. 2011;365:2398–411.

115. D'Agati VD, Fogo AB, Bruijn JA, Jennette JC. Pathologic classification of focal segmental glomerulosclerosis: A working proposal. Am J Kidney Dis. 2004;43:368–82.

116. Laurinavicius A, Hurwitz S, Rennke HG. Collapsing glomerulopathy in HIV and non-HIV patients: A clinicopathological and follow-up study. Kidney Int. 1999;56:2203–13.

117. Tanawattanacharoen S, Falk RJ, Jennette JC, Kopp JB. Parvovirus B19 DNA in kidney tissue of patients with focal segmental glomerulosclerosis. Am J Kidney Dis. 2000;35:1166–74.

118. Moudgil A, Nast CC, Bagga A, et al. Association of parvovirus B19 infection with idiopathic collapsing glomerulopathy. Kidney Int. 2001;59:2126–33.

119. Albaqumi M, Barisoni L. Current views on collapsing glomerulopathy. J Am Soc Nephrol. 2008;19:1276–81.

120. Barisoni L, Schnaper HW, Kopp JB. A proposed taxonomy for the podocytopathies: A reassessment of the primary nephrotic diseases. Clin J Am Soc Nephrol. 2007;2:529–42.

121. Stokes MB, Markowitz GS, Lin J, et al. Glomerular tip lesion: A distinct entity within the minimal change disease/focal segmental glomerulosclerosis spectrum. Kidney Int. 2004;65:1690–702.

122. Deegens JK, Assmann KJ, Steenbergen EJ, et al. Idiopathic focal segmental glomerulosclerosis: A favourable prognosis in untreated patients? Neth J Med. 2005;63:393–8.

123. Filler G, Young E, Geier P, et al. Is there really an increase in non-minimal change nephrotic syndrome in children? Am J Kidney Dis. 2003;42:1107–13.

124. Mongeau JG, Corneille L, Robitaille P, et al. Primary nephrosis in childhood associated with focal glomerular sclerosis: Is long-term prognosis that severe? Kidney Int. 1981;20:743–6.

125. Bhathena DB, Weiss JH, Holland NH, et al. Focal and segmental glomerular sclerosis in reflux nephropathy. Am J Med. 1980;68:886–92.

126. Baker L, Dahlem S, Goldfarb S, et al. Hyperfiltration and renal disease in glycogen storage disease, type I. Kidney Int. 1989;35:1345–50.

127. Tejani A, Phadke K, Adamson O, et al. Renal lesions in sickle cell nephropathy in children. Nephron. 1985;39:352–5.

128. Cameron JS, Turner DR, Ogg CS, et al. The long-term prognosis of patients with focal segmental glomerulosclerosis. Clin Nephrol. 1978;10:213–8.

129. Fouque D, Laville M, Colon S, et al. Cyclosporin A–sensitive nephrotic syndrome preceding Hodgkin's disease by 32 months. Clin Nephrol. 1990;34:1–4.

130. Bhatt N. Nephrotic syndrome preceding Hodgkin's lymphoma by 13 months. Clin Nephrol. 2005;64:228–30.

131. Stephan JL, Deschenes G, Perel Y, et al. Nephrotic syndrome and Hodgkin disease in children: A report of five cases. Eur J Pediatr. 1997;156:239–42.

132. Mori T, Yabuhara A, Nakayama J, et al. Frequently relapsing minimal change nephrotic syndrome with natural killer cell deficiency prior to the overt relapse of Hodgkin's disease. Pediatr Nephrol. 1995;9:619–20.

133. Moorthy AV, Zimmerman SW, Burkholder PM. Nephrotic syndrome in Hodgkin's disease: Evidence for pathogenesis alternative to immune complex deposition. Am J Med. 1976;61:471–7.

134. Cale WF, Ullrich IH, Jenkins JJ. Nodular sclerosing Hodgkin's disease presenting as nephrotic syndrome. South Med J. 1982;75:604–6.

135. Huang JB, Yang WC, Yang AH, et al. Arterial thrombosis due to minimal change glomerulopathy secondary to nonsteroidal anti-inflammatory drugs. Am J Med Sci. 2004;327:358–61.

136. Radford MG, Jr, Holley KE, Grande JP, et al. Reversible membranous nephropathy associated with the use of nonsteroidal anti-inflammatory drugs. JAMA. 1996;276:466–9.

137. Robinson J, Malleson P, Lirenman D, Carter J. Nephrotic syndrome associated with nonsteroidal anti-inflammatory drug use in two children. Pediatrics. 1990;85:844–7.

138. Alper AB, Jr, Meleg-Smith S, Krane NK. Nephrotic syndrome and interstitial nephritis associated with celecoxib. Am J Kidney Dis. 2002;40:1086–90.

139. Mihovilovic K, Ljubanovic D, Knotek M. Safe administration of celecoxib to a patient with repeated episodes of nephrotic syndrome induced by NSAIDs. Clin Drug Investig. 2011;31:351–5.

140. Husserl FE, Shuler SE. Gold nephropathy in juvenile rheumatoid arthritis. Am J Dis Child. 1979;133:50–2.

141. Hall CL, Jawad S, Harrison PR, et al. Natural course of penicillamine nephropathy: A long term study of 33 patients. Br Med J (Clin Res Ed). 1988;296:1083–6.

142. Nagahama K, Matsushita H, Hara M, et al. Bucillamine induces membranous glomerulonephritis. Am J Kidney Dis. 2002;39:706–12.

143. Stokes MB, Foster K, Markowitz GS, et al. Development of glomerulonephritis during anti–TNF-alpha therapy for rheumatoid arthritis. Nephrol Dial Transplant. 2005;20:1400–6.

144. Katz WA, Blodgett RC, Jr, Pietrusko RG. Proteinuria in gold-treated rheumatoid arthritis. Ann Intern Med. 1984;101:176–9.

145. Lindell A, Denneberg T, Enestrom S, et al. Membranous glomerulonephritis induced by 2-mercaptopropionylglycine (2-MPG). Clin Nephrol. 1990;34:108–15.

146. Ramsuran D, Bhimma R, Ramdial PK, et al. The spectrum of HIV-related nephropathy in children. Pediatr Nephrol. 2012;27:821–7.

147. Pardo V, Aldana M, Colton RM, et al. Glomerular lesions in the acquired immunodeficiency syndrome. Ann Intern Med. 1984;101:429–34.

148. van Rossum AM, Dieleman JP, Fraaij PL, et al. Persistent sterile leukocyturia is associated with impaired renal function in human immunodeficiency virus type 1–infected children treated with indinavir. Pediatrics. 2002;110:e19.

149. Bhimma R, Purswani MU, Kala U. Kidney disease in children and adolescents with perinatal HIV-1 infection. J Int AIDS Soc. 2013;16:18596.

150. Bhatia M, Kher K, Minniti CP. Acute lymphoblastic leukemia in a child with nephrotic syndrome. Pediatr Nephrol. 2004;19:1290–3.

151. Mackie FE, Roy LP, Stevens M. Onset of leukaemia after levamisole treatment for nephrotic syndrome. Pediatr Nephrol. 1994;8:527–8.

152. Al-Jehani F, Alsousou J, Gover P. Nephrotic syndrome associated with chronic lymphocytic leukaemia. Hematology. 2004;9:401–3.

153. Rosado MF, Morgensztern D, Abdullah S, et al. Chronic lymphocytic leukemia–associated nephrotic syndrome caused by focal segmental glomerulosclerosis. Am J Hematol. 2004;77:205–6.

154. Aslam N, Nseir NI, Viverett JF, et al. Nephrotic syndrome in chronic lymphocytic leukemia: A paraneoplastic syndrome? Clin Nephrol. 2000;54:492–7.

155. Sahiner S, Ayli MD, Yuksel C, et al. Membranous nephropathy associated with acute myeloid leukemia. Transplant Proc. 2004;36:2618–9.

156. Miura K, Sekine T, Takamizawa M, et al. Early occurrence of nephrotic syndrome associated with cord blood stem cell transplantation. Clin Exp Nephrol. 2012;16:180–2.

157. Wang HH, Yang AH, Yang LY, et al. Chronic graft-versus-host disease complicated by nephrotic syndrome. J Chin Med Assoc. 2011;74:419–22.

158. Heras M, Saiz A, Sanchez R, et al. Nephrotic syndrome resulting from focal segmental glomerulosclerosis in a peripheral blood stem cell transplant patient. J Nephrol. 2007;20:495–8.

159. Kalayoglu-Besisik S, Yurci A, Yazici H, et al. Long-term outcome of nephrotic syndrome in an allogeneic hematopoietic stem cell recipient without typical features of graft versus host disease. Transplantation. 2007;83:1407–8.

160. Ikee R, Yamamoto K, Kushiyama T, et al. Recurrent nephrotic syndrome associated with graft-versus-host disease. Bone Marrow Transplant. 2004;34:1005–6.

161. Rotig A, Appelkvist EL, Geromel V, et al. Quinone-responsive multiple respiratory-chain dysfunction due to widespread coenzyme Q10 deficiency. Lancet. 2000;356:391–5.

162. Doleris LM, Hill GS, Chedin P, et al. Focal segmental glomerulosclerosis associated with mitochondrial cytopathy. Kidney Int. 2000;58:1851–8.

163. Diomedi-Camassei F, Di Giandomenico S, Santorelli FM, et al. COQ2 nephropathy: A newly described inherited mitochondriopathy with primary renal involvement. J Am Soc Nephrol. 2007;18:2773–80.

164. Barisoni L, Diomedi-Camassei F, Santorelli FM, et al. Collapsing glomerulopathy associated with inherited mitochondrial injury. Kidney Int. 2008;74:237–43.

165. Lopez LC, Schuelke M, Quinzii CM, et al. Leigh syndrome with nephropathy and CoQ10 deficiency due to decaprenyl diphosphate synthase subunit 2 (PDSS2) mutations. Am J Hum Genet. 2006;79:1125–9.

166. Heeringa SF, Chernin G, Chaki M, et al. COQ6 mutations in human patients produce nephrotic syndrome with sensorineural deafness. J Clin Invest. 2011;121:2013–24.

167. Montini G, Malaventura C, Salviati L. Early coenzyme Q10 supplementation in primary coenzyme Q10 deficiency. N Engl J Med. 2008;358:2849–50.

168. Falk RJ, Scheinman J, Phillips G, et al. Prevalence and pathologic features of sickle cell nephropathy and response to inhibition of angiotensin-converting enzyme. N Engl J Med. 1992;326:910–5.

169. Nasr SH, Markowitz GS, Sentman RL, D'Agati VD. Sickle cell disease, nephrotic syndrome, and renal failure. Kidney Int. 2006;69:1276–80.

170. Bhathena DB, Sondheimer JH. The glomerulopathy of homozygous sickle hemoglobin (SS) disease: Morphology and pathogenesis. J Am Soc Nephrol. 1991;1:1241–52.

171. Serjeant GR. Sickle-cell disease. Lancet. 1997;350:725–30.

172. Weisinger JR, Kempson RL, Eldridge FL, Swenson RS. The nephrotic syndrome: A complication of massive obesity. Ann Intern Med. 1974;81:440–7.

173. Chagnac A, Weinstein T, Herman M, et al. The effects of weight loss on renal function in patients with severe obesity. J Am Soc Nephrol. 2003;14:1480–6.

174. Sharma K, Ramachandrarao S, Qiu G, et al. Adiponectin regulates albuminuria and podocyte function in mice. J Clin Invest. 2008;118:1645–56.

175. Chen HM, Liu ZH, Zeng CH, et al. Podocyte lesions in patients with obesity-related glomerulopathy. Am J Kidney Dis. 2006;48:772–9.

176. Shen WW, Chen HM, Chen H, et al. Obesity-related glomerulopathy: Body mass index and proteinuria. Clin J Am Soc Nephrol. 2010;5:1401–9.

177. Anonymous. Short versus standard prednisone therapy for initial treatment of idiopathic nephrotic syndrome in children. Arbeitsgemeinschaft fur Padiatrische Nephrologie. Lancet. 1988;1:380–3.

178. Ehrich JH, Brodehl J. Long versus standard prednisone therapy for initial treatment of idiopathic nephrotic syndrome in children. Arbeitsgemeinschaft fur Padiatrische Nephrologie. Eur J Pediatr. 1993;152:357–61.

179. Anonymous. Alternate-day versus intermittent prednisone in frequently relapsing nephrotic syndrome: A report of "Arbeitsgemeinschaft fur Padiatrische Nephrologie." Lancet. 1979;1:401–3.

180. Arneil GC. The nephrotic syndrome. Pediatr Clin North Am. 1971;18:547–59.

181. Lombel RM, Gipson DS, Hodson EM, Kidney Disease: Improving Global Outcomes. Treatment of steroid-sensitive nephrotic syndrome: New guidelines from KDIGO. Pediatr Nephrol. 2013;28:415–26.

182. Hodson EM, Willis NS, Craig JC. Corticosteroid therapy for nephrotic syndrome in children. Cochrane Database Syst Rev. 2007;(4):CD001533.

183. Brodehl J. The treatment of minimal change nephrotic syndrome: Lessons learned from multicentre co-operative studies. Eur J Pediatr. 1991;150:380–7.

184. Hodson EM, Knight JF, Willis NS, Craig JC. Corticosteroid therapy in nephrotic syndrome: A meta-analysis of randomised controlled trials. Arch Dis Child. 2000;83:45–51.

185. Bagga A, Hari P, Srivastava RN. Prolonged versus standard prednisolone therapy for initial episode of nephrotic syndrome. Pediatr Nephrol. 1999;13:824–7.

186. Feber J, Al-Matrafi J, Farhadi E, et al. Prednisone dosing per body weight or body surface area in children with nephrotic syndrome: Is it equivalent? Pediatr Nephrol. 2009;24:1027–31.

187. Saadeh SA, Baracco R, Jain A, et al. Weight or body surface area dosing of steroids in nephrotic syndrome: Is there an outcome difference? Pediatr Nephrol. 2011;26:2167–71.

188. Hoyer PF, Brodeh J. Initial treatment of idiopathic nephrotic syndrome in children: Prednisone versus prednisone plus cyclosporine A. A prospective, randomized trial. J Am Soc Nephrol. 2006;17:1151–7.

189. Vivarelli M, Moscaritolo E, Tsalkidis A, et al. Time for initial response to steroids is a major prognostic factor in idiopathic nephrotic syndrome. J Pediatr. 2010;156:965–71.

190. Wingen AM, Muller-Wiefel DE, Scharer K. Spontaneous remissions in frequently relapsing and steroid dependent idiopathic nephrotic syndrome. Clin Nephrol. 1985;23:35–40.

191. Tarshish P, Tobin JN, Bernstein J, Edelmann CM, Jr. Prognostic significance of the early course of minimal change nephrotic syndrome: Report of the International Study of Kidney Disease in Children. J Am Soc Nephrol. 1997;8:769–76.

192. Mattoo TK, Mahmoud MA. Increased maintenance corticosteroids during upper respiratory infection decrease the risk of relapse in nephrotic syndrome. Nephron. 2000;85:343–5.

193. Elzouki AY, Jaiswal OP. Long-term, small dose prednisone therapy in frequently relapsing nephrotic syndrome of childhood: Effect on remission, statural growth, obesity, and infection rate. Clin Pediatr (Phila). 1988;27:387–92.

194. Srivastava RN, Vasudev AS, Bagga A, Sunderam KR. Long-term, low-dose prednisolone therapy in frequently relapsing nephrotic syndrome. Pediatr Nephrol. 1992;6:247–50.

195. Allen DB. Growth suppression by glucocorticoid therapy. Endocrinol Metab Clin North Am. 1996;25:699–717.

196. Allen DB, Julius JR, Breen TJ, Attie KM. Treatment of glucocorticoid-induced growth suppression with growth hormone: National Cooperative Growth Study. J Clin Endocrinol Metab. 1998;83:2824–9.

197. Donatti TL, Koch VH, Fujimura MD, Okay Y. Growth in steroid-responsive nephrotic syndrome: A study of 85 pediatric patients. Pediatr Nephrol. 2003;18:789–95.

198. Emma F, Sesto A, Rizzoni G. Long-term linear growth of children with severe steroid-responsive nephrotic syndrome. Pediatr Nephrol. 2003;18:783–8.

199. Rees L, Greene SA, Adlard P, et al. Growth and endocrine function in steroid sensitive nephrotic syndrome. Arch Dis Child. 1988;63:484–90.

200. Leroy V, Baudouin V, Alberti C, et al. Growth in boys with idiopathic nephrotic syndrome on long-term cyclosporin and steroid treatment. Pediatr Nephrol. 2009;24:2393–400.

201. Simmonds J, Grundy N, Trompeter R, Tullus K. Long-term steroid treatment and growth: A study in steroid-dependent nephrotic syndrome. Arch Dis Child. 2010;95:146–9.

202. Padilla R, Brem AS. Linear growth of children with nephrotic syndrome: Effect of alkylating agents. Pediatrics. 1989;84:495–9.

203. Polito C, Oporto MR, Totino SF, et al. Normal growth of nephrotic children during long-term alternate-day prednisone therapy. Acta Paediatr Scand. 1986;75:245–50.

204. Jones JP, Jr. Fat embolism and osteonecrosis. Orthop Clin North Am. 1985;16:595–633.

205. Solomon L. Idiopathic necrosis of the femoral head: Pathogenesis and treatment. Can J Surg. 1981;24:573–8.

206. Nishimura T, Matsumoto T, Nishino M, Tomita K. Histopathologic study of veins in steroid treated rabbits. Clin Orthop Relat Res. 1997;334:37–42.

207. Malizos KN, Karantanas AH, Varitimidis SE, et al. Osteonecrosis of the femoral head: Etiology, imaging and treatment. Eur J Radiol. 2007;63:16–28.

208. Limaye SR, Pillai S, Tina LU. Relationship of steroid dose to degree of posterior subcapsular cataracts in nephrotic syndrome. Ann Ophthalmol. 1988;20:225–7.

209. Hayasaka Y, Hayasaka S, Matsukura H. Ocular findings in Japanese children with nephrotic syndrome receiving prolonged corticosteroid therapy. Ophthalmologica. 2006;220:181–5.

210. Brocklebank JT, Harcourt RB, Meadow SR. Corticosteroid-induced cataracts in idiopathic nephrotic syndrome. Arch Dis Child. 1982;57:30–4.

211. Bachmann HJ, Schildberg P, Olbing H, et al. Cortisone cataract in children with nephrotic syndrome. Eur J Pediatr. 1977;124:277–83.

212. Ng JS, Wong W, Law RW, et al. Ocular complications of paediatric patients with nephrotic syndrome. Clin Experiment Ophthalmol. 2001;29:239–43.

213. Latta K, von Schnakenburg C, Ehrich JH. A meta-analysis of cytotoxic treatment for frequently relapsing nephrotic syndrome in children. Pediatr Nephrol. 2001;16:271–82.

214. Anonymous. Effect of cytotoxic drugs in frequently relapsing nephrotic syndrome with and without steroid dependence. N Engl J Med. 1982;306:451–4.

215. Azib S, Macher MA, Kwon T, et al. Cyclophosphamide in steroid-dependent nephrotic syndrome. Pediatr Nephrol. 2011;26:927–32.

216. Kyrieleis HA, Levtchenko EN, Wetzels JF. Long-term outcome after cyclophosphamide treatment in children with steroid-dependent and frequently relapsing minimal change nephrotic syndrome. Am J Kidney Dis. 2007;49:592–7.

217. Zagury A, de Oliveira AL, de Moraes CA, et al. Long-term follow-up after cyclophosphamide therapy in steroid-dependent nephrotic syndrome. Pediatr Nephrol. 2011;26:915–20.

218. Prasad N, Gulati S, Sharma RK, et al. Pulse cyclophosphamide therapy in steroid-dependent nephrotic syndrome. Pediatr Nephrol. 2004;19:494–8.

219. Gulati S, Pokhariyal S, Sharma RK, et al. Pulse cyclophosphamide therapy in frequently relapsing nephrotic syndrome. Nephrol Dial Transplant. 2001;16:2013–7.

220. Vester U, Kranz B, Zimmermann S, et al. The response to cyclophosphamide in steroid-sensitive nephrotic syndrome is influenced by polymorphic expression of glutathione-S-transferases-M1 and -P1. Pediatr Nephrol. 2005;20:478–81.

221. Sharda SV, Gulati S, Tripathi G, et al. Do glutathione-S-transferase polymorphisms influence response to intravenous cyclophosphamide therapy in idiopathic nephrotic syndrome? Pediatr Nephrol. 2008;23:2001–6.

222. Scheinman JI, Stamler FW. Cyclophosphamide and fatal varicella. J Pediatr. 1969;74:117–9.

223. Resnick J, Schanberger JE. Varicella reactivation in nephrotic syndrome treated with cyclophosphamide and adrenal corticosteroids. J Pediatr. 1973;83:451–4.

224. Watson AR, Rance CP, Bain J. Long term effects of cyclophosphamide on testicular function. Br Med J (Clin Res Ed). 1985;291:1457–60.

225. Borel JF. Mechanism of action of cyclosporin A and rationale for use in nephrotic syndrome. Clin Nephrol. 1991;35(Suppl 1):S23–30.

226. Faul C, Donnelly M, Merscher-Gomez S, et al. The actin cytoskeleton of kidney podocytes is a direct target of the antiproteinuric effect of cyclosporine A. Nat Med. 2008;14:931–8.

227. Niaudet P, Habib R. Cyclosporine in the treatment of idiopathic nephrosis. J Am Soc Nephrol. 1994;5:1049–56.

228. Niaudet P, Broyer M, Habib R. Treatment of idiopathic nephrotic syndrome with cyclosporin A in children. Clin Nephrol. 1991;35(Suppl 1):S31-6.

229. Kano K, Kyo K, Yamada Y, et al. Comparison between pre- and posttreatment clinical and renal biopsies in children receiving low dose ciclosporine-A for 2 years for steroid-dependent nephrotic syndrome. Clin Nephrol. 1999;52:19–24.

230. Habib R, Niaudet P. Comparison between pre- and posttreatment renal biopsies in children receiving ciclosporine for idiopathic nephrosis. Clin Nephrol. 1994;42:141–6.

231. Mahmoud I, Basuni F, Sabry A, et al. Single-centre experience with cyclosporin in 106 children with idiopathic focal segmental glomerulosclerosis. Nephrol Dial Transplant. 2005;20:735–42.

232. Niaudet P. Comparison of cyclosporin and chlorambucil in the treatment of steroid-dependent idiopathic nephrotic syndrome: A multicentre randomized controlled trial. The French Society of Paediatric Nephrology. Pediatr Nephrol. 1992;6:1–3.

233. Ponticelli C, Edefonti A, Ghio L, et al. Cyclosporin versus cyclophosphamide for patients with steroid-dependent and frequently relapsing idiopathic nephrotic syndrome: A multicentre randomized controlled trial. Nephrol Dial Transplant. 1993;8:1326–32.

234. Ishikura K, Yoshikawa N, Nakazato H, et al. Two-year follow-up of a prospective clinical trial of cyclosporine for frequently relapsing nephrotic syndrome in children. Clin J Am Soc Nephrol. 2012;7:1576–83.

235. Iijima K, Hamahira K, Tanaka R, et al. Risk factors for cyclosporine-induced tubulointerstitial lesions in children with minimal change nephrotic syndrome. Kidney Int. 2002;61:1801–5.

236. Anonymous. Safety and tolerability of cyclosporin A (Sandimmun) in idiopathic nephrotic syndrome. Collaborative Study Group of Sandimmun in Nephrotic Syndrome. Clin Nephrol. 1991;35(Suppl 1):S48–60.

237. Sinha MD, MacLeod R, Rigby E, Clark AG. Treatment of severe steroid-dependent nephrotic syndrome (SDNS) in children with tacrolimus. Nephrol Dial Transplant. 2006;21:1848–54.

238. Anonymous. A comparison of tacrolimus (FK 506) and cyclosporine for immunosuppression in liver transplantation: The U.S. Multicenter FK506 Liver Study Group. N Engl J Med. 1994;331:1110–5.

239. Anonymous. Randomised trial comparing tacrolimus (FK506) and cyclosporin in prevention of liver allograft rejection. European FK506 Multicentre Liver Study Group. Lancet. 1994;344:423–8.

240. Dittrich K, Knerr I, Rascher W, Dotsch J. Transient insulin-dependent diabetes mellitus in children with steroid-dependent idiopathic nephrotic syndrome during tacrolimus treatment. Pediatr Nephrol. 2006;21:958–61.

241. Trompeter R, Filler G, Webb NJ, et al. Randomized trial of tacrolimus versus cyclosporin microemulsion in renal transplantation. Pediatr Nephrol. 2002;17:141–9.

242. Anonymous. Levamisole for corticosteroid-dependent nephrotic syndrome in childhood: British Association for Paediatric Nephrology. Lancet. 1991;337:1555–7.

243. Mongeau JG, Robitaille PO, Roy F. Clinical efficacy of levamisole in the treatment of primary nephrosis in children. Pediatr Nephrol. 1988;2:398–401.

244. Boyer O, Moulder JK, Grandin L, Somers MJ. Short- and long-term efficacy of levamisole as adjunctive therapy in childhood nephrotic syndrome. Pediatr Nephrol. 2008;23:575–80.

245. Sumegi V, Haszon I, Ivanyi B, et al. Long-term effects of levamisole treatment in childhood nephrotic syndrome. Pediatr Nephrol. 2004;19:1354–60.

246. Elmas AT, Tabel Y, Elmas ON. Short- and long-term efficacy of levamisole in children with steroid-sensitive nephrotic syndrome. Int Urol Nephrol. 2013;45:1047–55.

247. Alsaran K, Grisaru S, Stephens D, Arbus G. Levamisole vs. cyclophosphamide for frequently-relapsing steroid-dependent nephrotic syndrome. Clin Nephrol. 2001;56:289–94.

248. Barbano G, Ginevri F, Ghiggeri GM, Gusmano R. Disseminated autoimmune disease during levamisole treatment of nephrotic syndrome. Pediatr Nephrol. 1999;13:602–3.

249. Menni S, Pistritto G, Gianotti R, et al. Ear lobe bilateral necrosis by levamisole-induced occlusive vasculitis in a pediatric patient. Pediatr Dermatol. 1997;14:477–9.

250. Chang A, Osterloh J, Thomas J. Levamisole: A dangerous new cocaine adulterant. Clin Pharmacol Ther. 2010;88:408–11.

251. Eugui EM, Almquist SJ, Muller CD, Allison AC. Lymphocyte-selective cytostatic and immunosuppressive effects of mycophenolic acid in vitro: Role of deoxyguanosine nucleotide depletion. Scand J Immunol. 1991;33:161–73.

252. Penny MJ, Boyd RA, Hall BM. Mycophenolate mofetil prevents the induction of active Heymann nephritis: Association with Th2 cytokine inhibition. J Am Soc Nephrol. 1998;9:2272–82.

253. Hauser IA, Renders L, Radeke HH, et al. Mycophenolate mofetil inhibits rat and human mesangial cell proliferation by guanosine depletion. Nephrol Dial Transplant. 1999;14:58–63.

254. Allison AC, Kowalski WJ, Muller CJ, et al. Mycophenolic acid and brequinar, inhibitors of purine and pyrimidine synthesis, block the glycosylation of adhesion molecules. Transplant Proc. 1993;25:67–70.

255. Banerjee S, Pahari A, Sengupta J, Patnaik SK. Outcome of severe steroid-dependent nephrotic syndrome treated with mycophenolate mofetil. Pediatr Nephrol. 2013;28:93–7.

256. Afzal K, Bagga A, Menon S, et al. Treatment with mycophenolate mofetil and prednisolone for steroid-dependent nephrotic syndrome. Pediatr Nephrol. 2007;22:2059–65.

257. Fujinaga S, Ohtomo Y, Umino D, et al. A prospective study on the use of mycophenolate mofetil in children with cyclosporine-dependent nephrotic syndrome. Pediatr Nephrol. 2007;22:71–6.

258. Hogg RJ, Fitzgibbons L, Bruick J, et al. Mycophenolate mofetil in children with frequently relapsing nephrotic syndrome: A report from the Southwest Pediatric Nephrology Study Group. Clin J Am Soc Nephrol. 2006;1:1173–8.

259. Novak I, Frank R, Vento S, et al. Efficacy of mycophenolate mofetil in pediatric patients with steroid-dependent nephrotic syndrome. Pediatr Nephrol. 2005;20:1265–8.

260. Bagga A, Hari P, Moudgil A, Jordan SC. Mycophenolate mofetil and prednisolone therapy in children with steroid-dependent nephrotic syndrome. Am J Kidney Dis. 2003;42:1114–20.

261. Yoshioka K, Ohashi Y, Sakai T, et al. A multicenter trial of mizoribine compared with placebo in children with frequently relapsing nephrotic syndrome. Kidney Int. 2000;58:317–24.

262. Gellermann J, Querfeld U. Frequently relapsing nephrotic syndrome: Treatment with mycophenolate mofetil. Pediatr Nephrol. 2004;19:101–4.

263. Dorresteijn EM, Kist-van Holthe JE, Levtchenko EN, et al. Mycophenolate mofetil versus cyclosporine for remission maintenance in nephrotic syndrome. Pediatr Nephrol. 2008;23:2013–20.

264. Gellermann J, Weber L, Pape L, et al. Mycophenolate mofetil versus cyclosporin A in children with frequently relapsing nephrotic syndrome. J Am Soc Nephrol. 2013;24.1689–97.

265. Bunchman T, Navarro M, Broyer M, et al. The use of mycophenolate mofetil suspension in pediatric renal allograft recipients. Pediatr Nephrol. 2001;16:978–84.

266. Butani L, Palmer J, Baluarte HJ, Polinsky MS. Adverse effects of mycophenolate mofetil in pediatric renal transplant recipients with presumed chronic rejection. Transplantation. 1999;68:83–6.

267. Pape L, Ahlenstiel T, Kreuzer M, Ehrich JH. Improved gastrointestinal symptom burden after conversion from mycophenolate mofetil to enteric-coated mycophenolate sodium in kidney transplanted children. Pediatr Transplant. 2008;12:640–2.

268. Vilalta Casas R, Vila Lopez A, Nieto Rey JL, et al. Mycophenolic acid reaches therapeutic levels whereas mycophenolate mofetil does not. Transplant Proc. 2006;38:2400–1.

269. Fujinaga S, Ohtomo Y, Hirano D, et al. Mycophenolate mofetil therapy for childhood-onset steroid dependent nephrotic syndrome after long-term cyclosporine: Extended experience in a single center. Clin Nephrol. 2009;72:268–73.

270. Gellermann J, Ehrich JH, Querfeld U. Sequential maintenance therapy with cyclosporin A and mycophenolate mofetil for sustained remission of childhood steroid-resistant nephrotic syndrome. Nephrol Dial Transplant. 2012;27:1970–8.

271. Maloney DG, Grillo-Lopez AJ, White CA, et al. IDEC-C2B8 (rituximab) anti-CD20 monoclonal antibody therapy in patients with relapsed low-grade non-Hodgkin's lymphoma. Blood. 1997;90:2188–95.

272. Sanz I, Anolik JH, Looney RJ. B cell depletion therapy in autoimmune diseases. Front Biosci. 2007;12:2546–67.

273. Ravani P, Magnasco A, Edefonti A, et al. Short-term effects of rituximab in children with steroid- and calcineurin-dependent nephrotic syndrome: A randomized controlled trial. Clin J Am Soc Nephrol. 2011;6:1308–15.

274. Sellier-Leclerc AL, Macher MA, Loirat C, et al. Rituximab efficiency in children with steroid-dependent nephrotic syndrome. Pediatr Nephrol. 2010;25:1109–15.

275. Sellier-Leclerc AL, Baudouin V, Kwon T, et al. Rituximab in steroid-dependent idiopathic nephrotic syndrome in childhood: Follow-up after CD19 recovery. Nephrol Dial Transplant. 2012;27:1083–9.

276. Fujinaga S, Hirano D, Nishizaki N, et al. Single infusion of rituximab for persistent steroid-dependent minimal-change nephrotic syndrome after long-term cyclosporine. Pediatr Nephrol. 2010;25:539–44.

277. Guigonis V, Dallocchio A, Baudouin V, et al. Rituximab treatment for severe steroid- or cyclosporine-dependent nephrotic syndrome: A multicentric series of 22 cases. Pediatr Nephrol. 2008;23:1269–79.

278. Kamei K, Ito S, Nozu K, et al. Single dose of rituximab for refractory steroid-dependent nephrotic syndrome in children. Pediatr Nephrol. 2009;24:1321–8.

279. Ito S, Kamei K, Ogura M, et al. Maintenance therapy with mycophenolate mofetil after rituximab in pediatric patients with steroid-dependent nephrotic syndrome. Pediatr Nephrol. 2011;26:1823–8.

280. Chaumais MC, Garnier A, Chalard F, et al. Fatal pulmonary fibrosis after rituximab administration. Pediatr Nephrol. 2009;24:1753–5.

281. Pradhan M, Furth S. Rituximab in steroid-resistant nephrotic syndrome in children: A (false) glimmer of hope? J Am Soc Nephrol. 2012;23:975–8.

282. Carson KR, Evens AM, Richey EA, et al. Progressive multifocal leukoencephalopathy after rituximab therapy in HIV-negative patients: A report of 57 cases from the Research on Adverse Drug Events and Reports project. Blood. 2009;113:4834–40.

283. Buscher AK, Kranz B, Buscher R, et al. Immunosuppression and renal outcome in congenital and pediatric steroid-resistant nephrotic syndrome. Clin J Am Soc Nephrol. 2010;5:2075–84.

284. Hildebrandt F. Genetic kidney diseases. Lancet. 2010;375:1287–95.

285. Santin S, Bullich G, Tazon-Vega B, et al. Clinical utility of genetic testing in children and adults with steroid-resistant nephrotic syndrome. Clin J Am Soc Nephrol. 2011;6:1139–48.

286. Tarshish P, Tobin JN, Bernstein J, Edelmann CM, Jr. Cyclophosphamide does not benefit patients with focal segmental glomerulosclerosis: A report of the International Study of Kidney Disease in Children. Pediatr Nephrol. 1996;10:590–3.

287. Straatmann C, Ayoob R, Gbadegesin R, et al. Treatment outcome of late steroid-resistant nephrotic syndrome: A study by the Midwest Pediatric Nephrology Consortium. Pediatr Nephrol. 2013;28:1235–41.

288. Abrantes MM, Cardoso LS, Lima EM, et al. Predictive factors of chronic kidney disease in primary focal segmental glomerulosclerosis. Pediatr Nephrol. 2006;21:1003–12.

289. Gipson DS, Chin H, Presler TP, et al. Differential risk of remission and ESRD in childhood FSGS. Pediatr Nephrol. 2006;21:344–9.

290. Troyanov S, Wall CA, Miller JA, et al. Focal and segmental glomerulosclerosis: Definition and relevance of a partial remission. J Am Soc Nephrol. 2005;16:1061–8.

291. Rheault MN, Wei CC, Hains DS, et al. Increasing frequency of acute kidney injury amongst children hospitalized with nephrotic syndrome. Pediatr Nephrol. 2014;29:139–47.

292. Haws RM, Baum M. Efficacy of albumin and diuretic therapy in children with nephrotic syndrome. Pediatrics. 1993;91:1142–6.

293. Bagga A, Mudigoudar BD, Hari P, Vasudev V. Enalapril dosage in steroid-resistant nephrotic syndrome. Pediatr Nephrol. 2004;19:45–50.

294. Ellis D, Vats A, Moritz ML, et al. Long-term antiproteinuric and renoprotective efficacy and safety of losartan in children with proteinuria. J Pediatr. 2003;143:89–97.

295. Montane B, Abitbol C, Chandar J, et al. Novel therapy of focal glomerulosclerosis with mycophenolate and angiotensin blockade. Pediatr Nephrol. 2003;18:772–7.

296. American Academy of Pediatrics. Immunocompromised children. In: Pickering LK, Baker CJ, Kimberlin DW, editors. Red Book: Report of the Committee on Infectious Diseases, 29th ed. Elk Grove Village, IL: American Academy of Pediatrics; 2012. p. 74–90.

297. Close GC, Houston IB. Fatal haemorrhagic chickenpox in a child on long-term steroids. Lancet. 1981;2:480.

298. Mate ES, Fisher BK. Fatal chickenpox in a patient with nephrotic syndrome. Int J Dermatol. 1993;32:794–7.

299. Gangaram HB, Cheong IK. Fatal haemorrhagic chickenpox complicating nephrotic syndrome. Med J Malaysia. 1993;48:446–8.

300. Furth SL, Arbus GS, Hogg R, et al. Varicella vaccination in children with nephrotic syndrome: A report of the Southwest Pediatric Nephrology Study Group. J Pediatr. 2003;142:145–8.

301. Alpay H, Yildiz N, Onar A, et al. Varicella vaccination in children with steroid-sensitive nephrotic syndrome. Pediatr Nephrol. 2002;17:181–3.

302. Quien RM, Kaiser BA, Deforest A, et al. Response to the varicella vaccine in children with nephrotic syndrome. J Pediatr. 1997;131:688–90.

303. Marin M, Guris D, Chaves SS, Schmid S, et al. Prevention of varicella: Recommendations of the Advisory Committee on Immunization Practices (ACIP). MMWR Recomm Rep. 2007;56:1–40.

304. Abeyagunawardena AS, Goldblatt D, Andrews N, Trompeter RS. Risk of relapse after meningococcal C conjugate vaccine in nephrotic syndrome. Lancet. 2003;362:449–50.

305. Ruf RG, Lichtenberger A, Karle SM, et al. Patients with mutations in NPHS2 (podocin) do not respond to standard steroid treatment of nephrotic syndrome. J Am Soc Nephrol. 2004;15:722–32.

306. Garin EH, Orak JK, Hiott KL, Sutherland SE. Cyclosporine therapy for steroid-resistant nephrotic syndrome: A controlled study. Am J Dis Child. 1988;142:985–8.

307. Ponticelli C, Rizzoni G, Edefonti A, et al. A randomized trial of cyclosporine in steroid-resistant idiopathic nephrotic syndrome. Kidney Int. 1993;43:1377–84.

308. Lieberman KV, Tejani A. A randomized double-blind placebo-controlled trial of cyclosporine in steroid-resistant idiopathic focal segmental glomerulosclerosis in children. J Am Soc Nephrol. 1996;7:56–63.

309. Ehrich JH, Geerlings C, Zivicnjak M, et al. Steroid-resistant idiopathic childhood nephrosis: Overdiagnosed and undertreated. Nephrol Dial Transplant. 2007;22:2183–93.

310. Hamasaki Y, Yoshikawa N, Hattori S, et al. Cyclosporine and steroid therapy in children with steroid-resistant nephrotic syndrome. Pediatr Nephrol. 2009;24:2177–85.

311. Hodson EM, Willis NS, Craig JC. Interventions for idiopathic steroid-resistant nephrotic syndrome in children. Cochrane Database Syst Rev. 2010;11:CD003594.

312. Plank C, Kalb V, Hinkes B, et al. Cyclosporin A is superior to cyclophosphamide in children with steroid-resistant nephrotic syndrome-a randomized controlled multicentre trial by the Arbeitsgemeinschaft fur Padiatrische Nephrologie. Pediatr Nephrol. 2008;23:1483–93.

313. Gipson DS, Trachtman H, Kaskel FJ, et al. Clinical trial of focal segmental glomerulosclerosis in children and young adults. Kidney Int. 2011;80:868–78.

314. Meyrier A. Treatment of idiopathic nephrosis by immunophillin modulation. Nephrol Dial Transplant. 2003;18(Suppl 6):vi79–86.

315. Hoorn EJ, Walsh SB, McCormick JA, et al. The calcineurin inhibitor tacrolimus activates the renal sodium chloride cotransporter to cause hypertension. Nat Med. 2011;17:1304–9.

316. Wijdicks EF, Wiesner RH, Krom RA. Neurotoxicity in liver transplant recipients with cyclosporine immunosuppression. Neurology. 1995;45:1962–4.

317. Schwartz RB, Bravo SM, Klufas RA, et al. Cyclosporine neurotoxicity and its relationship to hypertensive encephalopathy: CT and MR findings in 16 cases. AJR Am J Roentgenol. 1995;165:627–31.

318. Trullemans F, Grignard F, Van Camp B, Schots R. Clinical findings and magnetic resonance imaging in severe cyclosporine-related neurotoxicity after allogeneic bone marrow transplantation. Eur J Haematol. 2001;67:94–9.

319. Choudhry S, Bagga A, Hari P, et al. Efficacy and safety of tacrolimus versus cyclosporine in children with steroid-resistant nephrotic syndrome: A randomized controlled trial. Am J Kidney Dis. 2009;53:760–9.

320. Bhimma R, Adhikari M, Asharam K, Connolly C. Management of steroid-resistant focal segmental glomerulosclerosis in children using tacrolimus. Am J Nephrol. 2006;26:544–51.

321. Gulati S, Prasad N, Sharma RK, et al. Tacrolimus: A new therapy for steroid-resistant nephrotic syndrome in children. Nephrol Dial Transplant. 2008;23:910–3.

322. Loeffler K, Gowrishankar M, Yiu V. Tacrolimus therapy in pediatric patients with treatment-resistant nephrotic syndrome. Pediatr Nephrol. 2004;19:281–7.

323. Roberti I, Vyas S. Long-term outcome of children with steroid-resistant nephrotic syndrome treated with tacrolimus. Pediatr Nephrol. 2010;25:1117–24.

324. Wang W, Xia Y, Mao J, et al. Treatment of tacrolimus or cyclosporine A in children with idiopathic nephrotic syndrome. Pediatr Nephrol. 2012;27:2073–9.

325. Butani L, Ramsamooj R. Experience with tacrolimus in children with steroid-resistant nephrotic syndrome. Pediatr Nephrol. 2009;24:1517–23.

326. de Mello VR, Rodrigues MT, Mastrocinque TH, et al. Mycophenolate mofetil in children with steroid/cyclophosphamide-resistant nephrotic syndrome. Pediatr Nephrol. 2010;25:453–60.

327. Li Z, Duan C, He J, et al. Mycophenolate mofetil therapy for children with steroid-resistant nephrotic syndrome. Pediatr Nephrol. 2010;25:883–8.

328. Cattran DC, Wang MM, Appel G, et al. Mycophenolate mofetil in the treatment of focal segmental glomerulosclerosis. Clin Nephrol. 2004;62:405–11.

329. Segarra Medrano A, Vila Presas J, Pou Clave L, et al. Efficacy and safety of combined cyclosporin A and mycophenolate mofetil therapy in patients with cyclosporin-resistant focal segmental glomerulosclerosis. Nefrologia. 2011;31:286–91.

330. Kemper MJ, Altrogge H, Ganschow R, Muller-Wiefel DE. Serum levels of immunoglobulins and IgG subclasses in steroid sensitive nephrotic syndrome. Pediatr Nephrol. 2002;17:413–7.

331. Vallerskog T, Gunnarsson I, Widhe M, et al. Treatment with rituximab affects both the cellular and the humoral arm of the immune system in patients with SLE. Clin Immunol. 2007;122:62–74.

332. Bruneau S, Dantal J. New insights into the pathophysiology of idiopathic nephrotic syndrome. Clin Immunol. 2009;133:13–21.

333. Fornoni A, Sageshima J, Wei C, et al. Rituximab targets podocytes in recurrent focal segmental glomerulosclerosis. Sci Transl Med. 2011;3:85ra46.

334. Chan AC. Rituximab's new therapeutic target: The podocyte actin cytoskeleton. Sci Transl Med. 2011;3:85ps21.

335. Alachkar N, Wei C, Arend LJ, et al. Podocyte effacement closely links to suPAR levels at time of posttransplantation focal segmental glomerulosclerosis occurrence and improves with therapy. Transplantation. 2013;96:649–56.

336. Vancsa A, Szabo Z, Szamosi S, et al. Long-term effects of rituximab on B cell counts and autoantibody production in rheumatoid arthritis: Use of high-sensitivity flow cytometry for more sensitive assessment of B cell depletion. J Rheumatol. 2013;40:565–71.

337. Fernandez-Fresnedo G, Segarra A, Gonzalez E, et al. Rituximab treatment of adult patients with steroid-resistant focal segmental glomerulosclerosis. Clin J Am Soc Nephrol. 2009;4:1317–23.

338. Peters HP, van de Kar NC, Wetzels JF. Rituximab in minimal change nephropathy and focal segmental glomerulosclerosis: Report of four cases and review of the literature. Neth J Med. 2008;66:408–15.

339. Gulati A, Sinha A, Jordan SC, et al. Efficacy and safety of treatment with rituximab for difficult steroid-resistant and -dependent nephrotic syndrome: Multicentric report. Clin J Am Soc Nephrol. 2010;5:2207–12.

340. Prytula A, Iijima K, Kamei K, et al. Rituximab in refractory nephrotic syndrome. Pediatr Nephrol. 2010;25:461–8.

341. Sugiura H, Takei T, Itabashi M, et al. Effect of single-dose rituximab on primary glomerular diseases. Nephron Clin Pract. 2011;117:c98–105.

342. Kari JA, El-Morshedy SM, El-Desoky S, et al. Rituximab for refractory cases of childhood nephrotic syndrome. Pediatr Nephrol. 2011;26:733–7.

343. Kisner T, Burst V, Teschner S, et al. Rituximab treatment for adults with refractory nephrotic syndrome: A single-center experience and review of the literature. Nephron Clin Pract. 2012;120:c79–85.

344. Kong WY, Swaminathan R, Irish A. Our experience with rituximab therapy for adult-onset primary glomerulonephritis and review of literature. Int Urol Nephrol. 2013;45:795–802.

345. Ochi A, Takei T, Nakayama K, et al. Rituximab treatment for adult patients with focal segmental glomerulosclerosis. Intern Med. 2012;51:759–62.

346. Magnasco A, Ravani P, Edefonti A, et al. Rituximab in children with resistant idiopathic nephrotic syndrome. J Am Soc Nephrol. 2012;23:1117–24.

347. Mendoza SA, Reznik VM, Griswold WR, et al. Treatment of steroid-resistant focal segmental glomerulosclerosis with pulse methylprednisolone and alkylating agents. Pediatr Nephrol. 1990;4:303–7.

348. Tune BM, Kirpekar R, Sibley RK, et al. Intravenous methylprednisolone and oral alkylating agent therapy of prednisone-resistant pediatric focal segmental glomerulosclerosis: A long-term follow-up. Clin Nephrol. 1995;43:84–8.

349. Chang JW, Yang LY, Wang HH. Low-dose methylprednisolone pulse therapy in Chinese children with steroid resistant focal segmental glomerulosclerosis. Pediatr Int. 2007;49:349–54.

350. Hari P, Bagga A, Jindal N, Srivastava RN. Treatment of focal glomerulosclerosis with pulse steroids and oral cyclophosphamide. Pediatr Nephrol. 2001;16:901–5.

351. Pena A, Bravo J, Melgosa M, et al. Steroid-resistant nephrotic syndrome: Long-term evolution after sequential therapy. Pediatr Nephrol. 2007;22:1875–80.

352. Waldo FB, Benfield MR, Kohaut EC. Therapy of focal and segmental glomerulosclerosis with methylprednisolone, cyclosporine A, and prednisone. Pediatr Nephrol. 1998;12:397–400.

353. Adhikari M, Bhimma R, Coovadia HM. Intensive pulse therapies for focal glomerulosclerosis in South African children. Pediatr Nephrol. 1997;11:423–8.

354. Anonymous. Prospective, controlled trial of cyclophosphamide therapy in children with nephrotic syndrome. Report of the International study of Kidney Disease in Children. Lancet. 1974;2:423–7.

355. Kleinknecht C, Broyer M, Gubler MC, Palcoux JB. Irreversible renal failure after indomethacin in steroid-resistant nephrosis. N Engl J Med. 1980;302:691.

356. Feld SM, Figueroa P, Savin V, et al. Plasmapheresis in the treatment of steroid-resistant focal segmental glomerulosclerosis in native kidneys. Am J Kidney Dis. 1998;32:230–7.

357. Franke D, Zimmering M, Wolfish N, et al. Treatment of FSGS with plasma exchange and immunadsorption. Pediatr Nephrol. 2000;14:965–9.

358. Vecsei AK, Muller T, Schratzberger EC, et al. Plasmapheresis-induced remission in otherwise therapy-resistant FSGS. Pediatr Nephrol. 2001;16:898–900.

359. Ginsburg DS, Dau P. Plasmapheresis in the treatment of steroid-resistant focal segmental glomerulosclerosis. Clin Nephrol. 1997;48:282–7.

360. Oliveira L, Wang D, McCormick BB. A case report of plasmapheresis and cyclophosphamide for steroid-resistant focal segmental glomerulosclerosis: Recovery of renal function after five months on dialysis. Ther Apher Dial. 2007;11:227–31.

361. Ghiggeri GM, Musante L, Candiano G, et al. Protracted remission of proteinuria after combined therapy with plasmapheresis and anti-CD20 antibodies/cyclophosphamide in a child with oligoclonal IgM and glomerulosclerosis. Pediatr Nephrol. 2007;22:1953–6.

362. Kuhn C, Kuhn A, Markau S, et al. Effect of immunoadsorption on refractory idiopathic focal and segmental glomerulosclerosis. J Clin Apher. 2006;21:266–70.

363. Kanai T, Shiraishi H, Ito T, et al. Plasma exchange and tacrolimus therapy for focal segmental glomerulosclerosis collapsing variant and the cytokine dynamics: A case report. Ther Apher Dial. 2010;14:603–5.

364. Mattoo TK, Mentser M, Kaskel FJ, et al. Plasmapheresis in steroid-resistant FSGS. Poster session presented at: Kidney Week. Annual Conference of the American Society of Nephrology, 2012, San Diego, CA.

365. Abramowicz M, Barnett HL, Edelmann CM, Jr, et al. Controlled trial of azathioprine in children with nephrotic syndrome: A report for the international study of kidney disease in children. Lancet. 1970;1:959–61.

366. McIntosh RM, Griswold W, Smith FG, Jr, et al. Azathioprine in glomerulonephritis: A long-term study. Lancet. 1972;1:1085–9.

367. Cade R, Mars D, Privette M, et al. Effect of long-term azathioprine administration in adults with minimal-change glomerulonephritis and nephrotic syndrome resistant to corticosteroids. Arch Intern Med. 1986;146:737–41.

368. Tenbrock K, Muller-Berghaus J, Fuchshuber A, et al. Levamisole treatment in steroid-sensitive and steroid-resistant nephrotic syndrome. Pediatr Nephrol. 1998;12:459–62.

369. Anderson S, Rennke HG, Garcia DL, Brenner BM. Short and long term effects of antihypertensive therapy in the diabetic rat. Kidney Int. 1989;36:526–36.

370. Brunner HR. ACE inhibitors in renal disease. Kidney Int. 1992;42:463–79.

371. Remuzzi A, Puntorieri S, Battaglia C, et al. Angiotensin converting enzyme inhibition ameliorates glomerular filtration of macromolecules and water and lessens glomerular injury in the rat. J Clin Invest. 1990;85:541–9.

372. Remuzzi A, Perticucci E, Ruggenenti P, et al. Angiotensin converting enzyme inhibition improves glomerular size-selectivity in IgA nephropathy. Kidney Int. 1991;39:1267–73.

373. Gansevoort RT, de Zeeuw D, de Jong PE. Dissociation between the course of the hemodynamic and antiproteinuric effects of angiotensin I converting enzyme inhibition. Kidney Int. 1993;44:579–84.

374. Ruiz-Ortega M, Ruperez M, Esteban V, et al. Angiotensin II: A key factor in the inflammatory and fibrotic response in kidney diseases. Nephrol Dial Transplant. 2006;21:16–20.

375. Trachtman H, Gauthier B. Effect of angiotensin-converting enzyme inhibitor therapy on proteinuria in children with renal disease. J Pediatr. 1988;112:295–8.

376. Milliner DS, Morgenstern BZ. Angiotensin converting enzyme inhibitors for reduction of proteinuria in children with steroid-resistant nephrotic syndrome. Pediatr Nephrol. 1991;5:587–90.

377. Lama G, Luongo I, Piscitelli A, Salsano ME. Enalapril: Antiproteinuric effect in children with nephrotic syndrome. Clin Nephrol. 2000;53:432–6.

378. Grone EF, Grone HJ. Does hyperlipidemia injure the kidney? Nat Clin Pract Nephrol. 2008;4:424–5.

379. Apperloo AJ, de Zeeuw D, Sluiter HE, de Jong PE. Differential effects of enalapril and atenolol on proteinuria and renal haemodynamics in non-diabetic renal disease. BMJ. 1991;303:821–4.

380. Kunz R, Friedrich C, Wolbers M, Mann JF. Meta-analysis: Effect of monotherapy and combination therapy with inhibitors of the renin angiotensin system on proteinuria in renal disease. Ann Intern Med. 2008;148:30–48.

381. Gansevoort RT, Sluiter WJ, Hemmelder MH, et al. Antiproteinuric effect of blood-pressure-lowering agents: A meta-analysis of comparative trials. Nephrol Dial Transplant. 1995;10:1963–74.

382. Heeg JE, de Jong PE, van der Hem GK, de Zeeuw D. Efficacy and variability of the antiproteinuric effect of ACE inhibition by lisinopril. Kidney Int. 1989;36:272–9.

383. Delucchi A, Cano F, Rodriguez E, et al. Enalapril and prednisone in children with nephrotic-range proteinuria. Pediatr Nephrol. 2000;14:1088–91.

384. Gwinner W, Landmesser U, Brandes RP, et al. Reactive oxygen species and antioxidant defense in puromycin aminonucleoside glomerulopathy. J Am Soc Nephrol. 1997;8:1722–31.

385. Wang JS, Yang AH, Chen SM, et al. Amelioration of antioxidant enzyme suppression and proteinuria in cyclosporin-treated puromycin nephrosis. Nephron. 1993;65:418–25.

386. Trachtman H, Schwob N, Maesaka J, Valderrama E. Dietary vitamin E supplementation ameliorates renal injury in chronic puromycin aminonucleoside nephropathy. J Am Soc Nephrol. 1995;5:1811–9.

387. Kawamura T, Yoshioka T, Bills T, et al. Glucocorticoid activates glomerular antioxidant enzymes and protects glomeruli from oxidant injuries. Kidney Int. 1991;40:291–301.

388. Srivastava RN, Diven S, Kalia A, et al. Increased glomerular and urinary malondialdehyde in puromycin aminonucleoside-induced proteinuria in rats. Pediatr Nephrol. 1995;9:48–51.

389. Diamond JR, Bonventre JV, Karnovsky MJ. A role for oxygen free radicals in aminonucleoside nephrosis. Kidney Int. 1986;29:478–83.

390. Milner LS, Wei SH, Houser MT. Amelioration of glomerular injury in doxorubicin hydrochloride nephrosis by dimethylthiourea. J Lab Clin Med. 1991;118:427–34.

391. Thakur V, Walker PD, Shah SV. Evidence suggesting a role for hydroxyl radical in puromycin aminonucleoside-induced proteinuria. Kidney Int. 1988;34:494–9.

392. Mishra OP, Gupta AK, Prasad R, et al. Antioxidant status of children with idiopathic nephrotic syndrome. Pediatr Nephrol. 2011;26:251–6.

393. Ghodake SR, Suryakar AN, Ankush RD, et al. Role of free radicals and antioxidant status in childhood nephrotic syndrome. Indian J Nephrol. 2011;21:37–40.

394. Bakr A, Abul Hassan S, Shoker M, et al. Oxidant stress in primary nephrotic syndrome: Does it modulate the response to corticosteroids? Pediatr Nephrol. 2009;24:2375–80.

395. Mathew JL, Kabi BC, Rath B. Anti-oxidant vitamins and steroid responsive nephrotic syndrome in Indian children. J Paediatr Child Health. 2002;38:450–37.

396. Tahzib M, Frank R, Gauthier B, et al. Vitamin E treatment of focal segmental glomerulosclerosis: Results of an open-label study. Pediatr Nephrol. 1999;13:649–52.

397. Chan JC, Mahan JD, Trachtman H, et al. Vitamin E therapy in IgA nephropathy: A double-blind, placebo-controlled study. Pediatr Nephrol. 2003;18:1015–9.

398. De Smet E, Rioux JP, Ammann H, et al. FSGS permeability factor–associated nephrotic syndrome: Remission after oral galactose therapy. Nephrol Dial Transplant. 2009;24:2938–40.

399. Kopac M, Meglic A, Rus RR. Partial remission of resistant nephrotic syndrome after oral galactose therapy. Ther Apher Dial. 2011;15:269–72.

400. Whitworth JA. Adrenocorticotrophin and steroid-induced hypertension in humans. Kidney Int Suppl. 1992;37:S34–7.

401. Saruta T, Suzuki H, Handa M, et al. Multiple factors contribute to the pathogenesis of hypertension in Cushing's syndrome. J Clin Endocrinol Metab. 1986;62:275–9.

402. Pirpiris M, Sudhir K, Yeung S, et al. Pressor responsiveness in corticosteroid-induced hypertension in humans. Hypertension. 1992;19:567–74.

403. Ulick S, Wang JZ, Blumenfeld JD, Pickering TG. Cortisol inactivation overload: A mechanism of mineralocorticoid hypertension in the ectopic adrenocorticotropin syndrome. J Clin Endocrinol Metab. 1992;74:963–7.

404. Choi HK, Seeger JD. Glucocorticoid use and serum lipid levels in US adults: The Third National Health and Nutrition Examination Survey. Arthritis Rheum. 2005;53:528–35.

405. Leong KH, Koh ET, Feng PH, Boey ML. Lipid profiles in patients with systemic lupus erythematosus. J Rheumatol. 1994;21:1264–7.

406. Sarkissian T, Beyene J, Feldman B, et al. Longitudinal examination of lipid profiles in pediatric systemic lupus erythematosus. Arthritis Rheum. 2007;56:631–8.

407. Sarkissian T, Beyenne J, Feldman B, et al. The complex nature of the interaction between disease activity and therapy on the lipid profile in patients with pediatric systemic lupus erythematosus. Arthritis Rheum. 2006;54:1283–90.

408. Hilbrands LB, Demacker PN, Hoitsma AJ, et al. The effects of cyclosporine and prednisone on serum lipid and (apo)lipoprotein levels in renal transplant recipients. J Am Soc Nephrol. 1995;5:2073–81.

409. Vaziri ND. Erythropoietin and transferrin metabolism in nephrotic syndrome. Am J Kidney Dis. 2001;38:1–8.

410. Feinstein S, Becker-Cohen R, Algur N, et al. Erythropoietin deficiency causes anemia in nephrotic children with normal kidney function. Am J Kidney Dis. 2001;37:736–42.

411. Bayes B, Serra A, Junca J, Lauzurica R. Successful treatment of anaemia of nephrotic syndrome with recombinant human erythropoietin. Nephrol Dial Transplant. 1998;13:1894–5.

412. Freundlich M, Bourgoignie JJ, Zilleruelo G, et al. Calcium and vitamin D metabolism in children with nephrotic syndrome. J Pediatr. 1986;108:383–7.

413. Harris RC, Ismail N. Extrarenal complications of the nephrotic syndrome. Am J Kidney Dis. 1994;23:477–97.

414. Koenig KG, Lindberg JS, Zerwekh JE, et al. Free and total 1,25-dihydroxyvitamin D levels in subjects with renal disease. Kidney Int. 1992;41:161–5.

415. Auwerx J, De Keyser L, Bouillon R, De Moor P. Decreased free 1,25-dihydroxycholecalciferol index in patients with the nephrotic syndrome. Nephron. 1986;42:231–5.

416. Gulati S, Godbole M, Singh U, et al. Are children with idiopathic nephrotic syndrome at risk for metabolic bone disease? Am J Kidney Dis. 2003;41:1163–9.

417. Gulati S, Sharma RK, Gulati K, et al. Longitudinal follow-up of bone mineral density in children with nephrotic syndrome and the role of calcium and vitamin D supplements. Nephrol Dial Transplant. 2005;20:1598–603.

418. Leonard MB, Feldman HI, Shults J, et al. Long-term, high-dose glucocorticoids and bone mineral content in childhood glucocorticoid-sensitive nephrotic syndrome. N Engl J Med. 2004;351:868–75.

419. Afrasiabi MA, Vaziri ND, Gwinup G, et al. Thyroid function studies in the nephrotic syndrome. Ann Intern Med. 1979;90:335–8.

420. Feinstein EI, Kaptein EM, Nicoloff JT, Massry SG. Thyroid function in patients with nephrotic syndrome and normal renal function. Am J Nephrol. 1982;2:70–6.

421. Muranjan MN, Kher AS, Nadkarni UB, Kamat JR. Congenital nephrotic syndrome with clinical hypothyroidism. Indian J Pediatr. 1995;62:233–5.

422. Chadha V, Alon US. Bilateral nephrectomy reverses hypothyroidism in congenital nephrotic syndrome. Pediatr Nephrol. 1999;13:209–11.

423. Warady BA, Howard CP, Hellerstein S, et al. Congenital nephrosis in association with hypothyroidism and hypoadrenocorticism. Pediatr Nephrol. 1993;7:79–80.

424. Niel O, Thouret MC, Berard E. Anemia in congenital nephrotic syndrome: Role of urinary copper and ceruloplasmin loss. Blood. 2011;117:6054–5.

425. Stec J, Podracka L, Pavkovcekova O, Kollar J. Zinc and copper metabolism in nephrotic syndrome. Nephron. 1990;56:186–7.

426. Hamasaki Y, Yoshikawa N, Nakazato H, et al. Prospective 5-year follow-up of cyclosporine treatment in children with steroid-resistant nephrosis. Pediatr Nephrol. 2013;28:765–71.

427. Paik KH, Lee BH, Cho HY, et al. Primary focal segmental glomerular sclerosis in children: Clinical course and prognosis. Pediatr Nephrol. 2007;22:389–95.

428. Jungraithmayr TC, Bulla M, Dippell J, et al. Primary focal segmental glomerulosclerosis: Long-term outcome after pediatric renal transplantation. Pediatr Transplant. 2005;9:226–31.

429. Fuentes GM, Meseguer CG, Carrion AP, et al. Long-term outcome of focal segmental glomerulosclerosis after pediatric renal transplantation. Pediatr Nephrol. 2010;25:529–34.

430. Tejani A, Stablein DH. Recurrence of focal segmental glomerulosclerosis posttransplantation: A special report of the North American Pediatric Renal Transplant Cooperative Study. J Am Soc Nephrol. 1992;2:S258–63.

431. Baum MA, Stablein DM, Panzarino VM, et al. Loss of living donor renal allograft survival advantage in children with focal segmental glomerulosclerosis. Kidney Int. 2001;59:328–33.

432. Pinto J, Lacerda G, Cameron JS, et al. Recurrence of focal segmental glomerulosclerosis in renal allografts. Transplantation. 1981;32:83–9.

433. Striegel JE, Sibley RK, Fryd DS, Mauer SM. Recurrence of focal segmental sclerosis in children following renal transplantation. Kidney Int Suppl. 1986;19:S44–50.

434. Baum MA. Outcomes after renal transplantation for FSGS in children. Pediatr Transplant. 2004;8:329–33.

435. Srivastava T, Garola RE, Kestila M, et al. Recurrence of proteinuria following renal transplantation in congenital nephrotic syndrome of the Finnish type. Pediatr Nephrol. 2006;21:711–8.

436. Becker-Cohen R, Bruschi M, Rinat C, et al. Recurrent nephrotic syndrome in homozygous truncating NPHS2 mutation is not due to anti-podocin antibodies. Am J Transplant. 2007;7:256–60.

437. Schachter ME, Monahan M, Radhakrishnan J, et al. Recurrent focal segmental glomerulosclerosis in the renal allograft: Single center experience in the era of modern immunosuppression. Clin Nephrol. 2010;74:173–81.

438. Canaud G, Zuber J, Sberro R, et al. Intensive and prolonged treatment of focal and segmental glomerulosclerosis recurrence in adult kidney transplant recipients: A pilot study. Am J Transplant. 2009;9:1081–6.

439. Anonymous. Minimal change nephrotic syndrome in children: Deaths during the first 5 to 15 years' observation. Report of the International Study of Kidney Disease in Children. Pediatrics. 1984;73:497–501.

440. Ruth EM, Kemper MJ, Leumann EP, et al. Children with steroid-sensitive nephrotic syndrome come of age: Long-term outcome. J Pediatr. 2005;147:202–7.

441. Kyrieleis HA, Lowik MM, Pronk I, et al. Long-term outcome of biopsy-proven, frequently relapsing minimal-change nephrotic syndrome in children. Clin J Am Soc Nephrol. 2009;4:1593–600.

442. Fakhouri F, Bocquet N, Taupin P, et al. Steroid-sensitive nephrotic syndrome: From childhood to adulthood. Am J Kidney Dis 2003;41:550–7.

## REVIEW QUESTIONS

1. A 3-year-old boy presents with bilateral periorbital swelling and abdominal distention. Blood pressure is 104/66 mm Hg. Urine dipstick revealed 4+ proteinuria and moderate blood. You discuss the likelihood of response to steroid therapy with the family. Children who are *least* likely to respond to corticosteroids include:
   a. Asians
   b. African Americans
   c. Hispanics
   d. Native Americans
   e. Whites

2. A 16-year-old female patient with morbid obesity is being referred by her primary physician for evaluation of persistent proteinuria. Physical examination is significant for morbid obesity and acanthosis nigricans. Urinalysis showed 2+ proteinuria but no other abnormalities. She is normotensive. A spot urine protein-to-creatinine ratio on a first morning urine specimen was 1.6 mg/mg. You anticipate that her renal biopsy will *most likely* show:
   a. Glomeruli of large diameter
   b. Subepithelial and subendothelial dense deposits
   c. Diffuse foot process effacement
   d. Splitting and proliferation of the glomerular basement membrane
   e. Increased number and density of podocytes

3. Acceptable options for the treatment of children with steroid-resistant nephrotic syndrome include all of the following *except*:
   a. Oral cyclophosphamide
   b. Mycophenolate mofetil
   c. Tacrolimus
   d. Cyclosporine
   e. Use of angiotensin-converting enzyme inhibitors for refractory proteinuria

4. A 6-year-old girl presents with progressive generalized swelling of 2 weeks' duration. She has no reported changes in her urine color. Blood pressure measurements in the office are normal. Laboratory workup reveals high-grade proteinuria and severe hypoalbuminemia. Serum complement levels are normal. You suspect minimal change disease, and you inform parents that her prognosis is *most closely* linked to the following parameter:
   a. Presence or absence of systemic hypertension on presentation
   b. Age at onset less than 10 years
   c. Grade of peripheral edema on initial presentation
   d. Clinical response to oral prednisolone
   e. Detection and degree of microscopic hematuria on initial urine dipstick

5. A 12-year-old boy with history of steroid-resistant nephrotic syndrome presents for follow-up. He has been treated with cyclosporine, prednisone, lisinopril, and amlodipine for the last 5 months. His cyclosporine levels have been monitored periodically and have been consistently in the therapeutic range. Laboratory workup obtained this morning again showed therapeutic cyclosporine level, persistent high-grade proteinuria, and hypoalbuminemia. His serum creatinine is elevated at 1.5 mg/dL. You also note that his most recent previous creatinine level obtained 8 weeks ago was 0.8 mg/dL. The *most appropriate* next step in the management of this patient is to:

a. Admit to the hospital for albumin and Lasix infusions.
b. Discontinue lisinopril.
c. Stop cyclosporine therapy and replace with tacrolimus.
d. Encourage oral hydration and repeat kidney function tests in 1 week.
e. Arrange for a repeat renal biopsy.

6. A 17-year-old African-American male patient is recently diagnosed with primary focal segmental glomerulosclerosis (FSGS). A *high likelihood* of steroid response has been associated with the following histologic variant:

a. Tip lesion
b. Collapsing glomerulopathy
c. Perihilar variant
d. Cellular variant
e. Classic variant

## ANSWER KEY

1. b
2. a
3. a
4. d
5. b
6. a

# 18

# Nephrotic syndrome in the first year of life

## CHRISTER HOLMBERG AND HANNU JALANKO

Nephrotic syndrome (NS) in the first year of life manifests unique clinical and causal challenges. NS occurring in the first 3 months of life is defined as the congenital nephrotic syndrome (CNS); NS with onset between 4 and 12 months is known as infantile NS (INS), and NS appearing after the first year is recognized as childhood NS. In the youngest patients, mutations in the podocyte-associated genes or the syndromic disorders are the most common causes of NS. In contrast, minimal change nephrotic syndrome (MCNS) is the most prevalent form of NS later in childhood.

MCNS and some secondary forms of NS are often treatable, unlike NS resulting from gene mutations or syndromes. Overall, NS during the first year of life is an uncommon but severe disease. The affected children usually develop end-stage renal disease (ESRD) and require treatment with dialysis and renal transplantation (RTx). Classification of NS in the first year of life, based on primary and secondary causes is given in Table 18.1.

---

### KEY POINT

NS during the first year of life is an uncommon but severe disease. Affected children develop ESRD and require treatment with dialysis and RTx.

---

## PODOCYTE FUNCTION AND PROTEINURIA

Each of our kidneys contains approximately one million nephrons that filter 100 to 200 L of plasma from the glomerular capillaries daily into the urinary space. Most of the ultrafiltrate is reabsorbed by the renal tubules and collecting ducts. Normally, blood cells and plasma proteins are not lost into the urine. The glomerular capillary wall forms an efficient filtration barrier, which consists of three layers: fenestrated endothelium, the glomerular basement membrane (GBM), and the epithelium or podocyte layer.[1]

Podocytes are specialized neuron-like cells that possess a cell body, major and minor processes, and foot processes that attach to the GBM (Figures 18.1 and 18.2). The foot processes are linked by a specialized structure, the slit diaphragm (SD). Although all these components contribute to the regulation of renal filtration, the SD plays the most important role in preventing urinary protein losses. The main component of the SD is nephrin, a 1241-residue cell adhesion protein of the immunoglobulin family. Nephrin consists of an extracellular part with eight immunoglobulin-like modules and one type-III fibronectin domain.[2] The

---

### KEY POINTS

- Podocytes are now being recognized as an important cell structure in the glomerular filtration barrier.
- SD is the most important structure involved in preventing loss of protein from the glomerular capillaries into the urinary space.
- SD is chiefly composed of nephrin, which forms a zipper-like barrier across the foot processes.

---

Table 18.1 Classification of nephrotic syndrome in the first years of life

**Primary causes**

1. Podocytopathies (restricted to the kidney)
   - Nephrin gene defect *(NPHS1)*
   - Podocin gene defect *(NPHS2)*
   - Phospholipase Cα1 gene defect *(PLCε1)*
2. Syndromes
   - Wilms tumor gene 1 defect *(WT1)*
   - Laminin β2 gene defect *(LAMβ2)*
   - Cation channel defect *(TRPC6)*
   - Coenzyme Q synthetase disturbances *(PDSS2)*
   - PHB-propenyl transferase defect *(COQ2)*
   - RhoGDIβ defect *(ARGHDIA)*
   - Nail-patella *(LMX1B* gene defect)
   - Lowe *(OCRL* gene defect)
   - Herlitz junctional epidermolysis bullosa *(LAMβ3* gene defect)
   - Galloway-Mowat (gene defect unknown)

**Secondary causes**

- Infections (syphilis, cytomegalovirus, human immunodeficiency virus)
- Immunologic (infantile lupus erythematosus/maternal)
- Idiopathic nephrotic syndrome

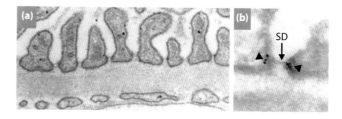

Figure 18.2 Electron microscopy of the glomerular capillary wall. **(a)** Capillary wall with normal podocyte foot processes and the slit diaphragms. **(b)** Normal slit diaphragm (SD) between podocyte foot processes.

extracellular part of one nephrin molecule binds to nephrin from an adjacent foot process (homophilic binding), as well as to other SD proteins, such as Neph1. These components form a zipper-like structure of the SD that is visible with electron microscopy (Figure 18.3). The intracellular part of nephrin contains nine tyrosine residues, which may be phosphorylated and are important in signal transduction from the SD into the podocyte.[3]

Besides nephrin, the proper function of the SD involves additional components, such as Neph1, Neph2, Neph3, and FAT.[4-6] These SD proteins, especially nephrin and Neph1, interact with adapter proteins podocin, CD2AP, and ZO-1 located in the cytosolic part of the foot processes.[7,8] These adapter proteins link the SD proteins to the actin cytoskeleton, which is vital to podocyte morphology (see Figure 18.3). Podocin belongs to the stomatin family and binds nephrin to lipid rafts, thus contributing to signal transduction.[8] Mutations in the podocin gene, *NPHS2*, and in the nephrin gene, *NPHS1*, are the two most common causes of primary CNS.[9]

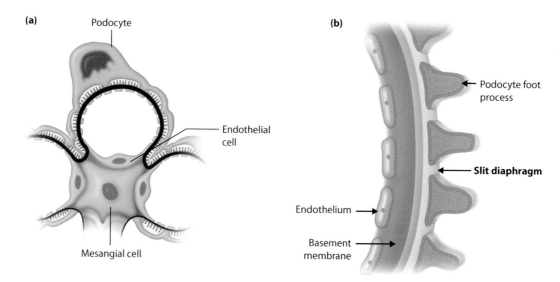

Figure 18.1 **(a)** Illustration of cross section of a glomerular capillary showing the three glomerular cells: podocyte (epithelial cell), endothelial cell, and mesangial cell. **(b)** Illustration of cross section of a capillary wall showing the three layers of the glomerular filtration barrier: fenestrated endothelium, basement membrane, and epithelial layers comprising the podocyte foot processes and the slit diaphragm.

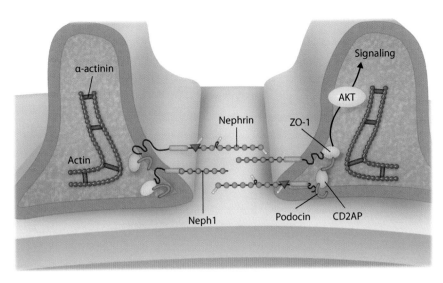

Figure 18.3 Illustration depicting a simplified model of the slit diaphragm and podocyte foot process. Anchoring of nephrin, Neph1, and podocin to the podocytes and formation of the slit diaphragm are shown.

## GENETIC MUTATIONS IN NEPHROTIC SYNDROME

### *NPHS1* (NEPHRIN)

In 1956, Hallman's group described the first patients with NS whose clinical features are compatible with *NPHS1* gene mutation.[10] Norio[11] showed that this autosomal recessive disease occurs in 1 in 8200 newborns in Finland. In the late 1990s, Kestilä et al.[2] located the gene responsible for CNF on chromosome 19q13.1 and named it nephrotic syndrome gene 1 *(NPHS1)*; its gene product was named nephrin.

Two main mutations are present in the Finnish children: Fin-major and Fin-minor.[2,3] Approximately 60% of Finnish patients are homozygous for the Fin-major mutation, 20% are compound heterozygotes for the Fin-major and Fin-minor mutations, and 10% are homozygous for the Fin-minor mutation.[12] The Fin-major mutation is a two-base pair deletion in exon 2, which causes a frameshift and an early translational stop. The Fin-minor is a nonsense mutation in exon 26. Both of these mutations lead to a total absence of nephrin in the SD filaments by electron microscopy. Today, more than 200 different *NPHS1* mutations have been described worldwide (www.biobase-international.com), including nonsense and missense mutations, frameshifts, small insertions or deletions, and splice-site changes. Most are individual mutations located quite evenly along the gene and often lead to a severe form of CNS. However, studies have also described "mild" mutations leading to an unusual phenotype.[13] Although Fin-major and Fin-minor mutations are rare outside Finland, the 1481delC mutation is common in Mennonites and leads to a truncated protein of 547 residues, and homozygous nonsense mutation R1160X in exon 27 frequently occurs in Maltese children.[14,15]

### Clinical features

Pregnancy with an affected fetus is usually uneventful. A high concentration of α-fetoprotein (AFP) in the amniotic fluid during the second trimester is often a sign of fetal proteinuria.[16] However, this finding is not diagnostic for homozygous *NPHS1* mutation, because fetal carriers of the Fin-major or Fin-minor mutation also may have a temporarily high concentration of AFP.[17] Amniotic fluid AFP may be elevated in other disorders, such as the presence of neural tube defects. Thus, only genetic testing is diagnostic. At birth, the amniotic fluid is often stained with meconium and the placenta is usually more than 25% of the newborn's weight; the child may be born prematurely.[18]

---

**KEY POINTS**

- The gene product of NPHS1 is nephrin and is present in SDs.
- Fin-major and Fin-minor were the two earliest described mutations in *NPHS1* in Finland. These are rare mutations in non-Finnish populations.
- More than 200 mutations have been recorded in the *NPHS1*, worldwide.

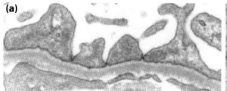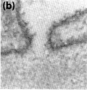

Figure 18.4 **(a)** Electron microscopy showing capillary wall of a patient with congenital nephrotic syndrome secondary to *NPHS1* mutation, demonstrating aberrant podocyte foot processes, with effacement. **(b)** "Empty" podocyte slit, without the (SD) filament is seen in a higher resolution.

Severe proteinuria is often evident right after birth, and NS develops within the first days or weeks. Children with *NPHS1* mutations have no extrarenal malformations, but growth and development may progress slowly. Protein deficiency may cause affected children to exhibit muscular hypotonia and mild atrophic brain changes. Some patients with *NPHS1* mutation have exhibited athetoid cerebral palsy, the cause of which is unknown.[19] Renal function is initially normal, unless the patient is severely dehydrated, and an ultrasound reveals oversize kidneys (as much as twice their normal size). Left untreated, a patient with *NPHS1* mutation grows insufficiently, is prone to thrombotic and infectious complications, and usually dies during the first year of life.

## Renal pathology

By light microscopy, the glomeruli show mesangial expansion and degenerative changes. Dilated proximal tubules, interstitial fibrosis, and glomerular sclerosis develop over time. Electron microscopy reveals effacement of foot processes, as is common in all proteinuric disorders (Figure 18.4).[20] A total absence of the SD filaments by electron microscopy due to absence of nephrin also may be seen (Figure 18.4B). Scanning electron microscopy may show loss of normal podocyte architecture and an aberrant podocyte structure (Figure 18.5).

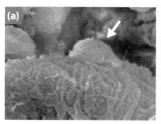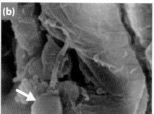

Figure 18.5. **(a)** Scanning electron microscopy (SEM) of a normal glomerular capillary wall showing podocyte soma and filaments. **(b)** SEM of a patient with congenital nephrotic syndrome resulting from *NPHS1* mutation showing aberrant podocyte structure and a lack of primary and secondary epithelial branching that normally covers the glomerular basement membrane.

## *PODOCIN*

In 2000, Boute et al.[7] reported a new podocyte gene, *NPHS2*, in autosomal recessive steroid-resistant nephrotic syndrome (SRNS) and its gene product was named podocin.[7] Podocin is an intracellular linker protein that interacts with nephrin and serves as a scaffold for the SD. Mutations in the *NPHS2* can lead to typical CNS, but also may manifest later in life as steroid-resistant NS.[21] Researchers have described more than 100 pathogenic mutations. In one report on 80 European families, *NPHS2* mutations accounted for 39% of the CNS cases and 35% of the INS cases. Hinkes et al.[22] found *NPHS2* mutations in 18% of more than 400 patients in a worldwide cohort of SRNS ranging in age from birth to 21 years. Severe truncating mutations resulted in early onset of NS (from birth to 9.1 years; mean 1.75 years). Overall, *NPHS2* mutations account for approximately 20% of sporadic and 40% of familial cases of SRNS.[21] The *R138Q* mutation is common in Europe, and patients with homozygous mutations develop NS early in life. Nephrin expression may be distorted in CNS resulting from *NPHS2* mutations.[15,21]

---

### KEY POINT

Mutations in the podocin gene, *NPHS2*, and in the nephrin gene, *NPHS1*, are the two most common causes of primary CNS.

---

### KEY POINTS

- NS caused by *NPHS2* mutations is more variable with less severe proteinuria than NS caused by *NPHS1* mutations.
- FSGS is the most common renal pathology seen in *NPHS2* mutation (podocin).

---

## Clinical features

NS resulting from *NPHS2* mutations may exhibit less severe proteinuria than NS caused by *NPHS1* gene mutation.[23] Renal failure develops at a mean age of 6.6 years, significantly later than in *NPHS1* mutations.[22] Only podocytes express podocin, and affected children show no extrarenal malformations, although some patients with cardiac anomalies have been reported.[24] With regard to renal histology, focal segmental glomerulosclerosis (FSGS) is the most common pathologic process noted, but MCNS and mesangial proliferative glomerulopathy have also been reported.[21,24]

# *WT1* GENE MUTATION

The Wilms tumor suppressor gene *(WT1)*, located on chromosome 11p13, encodes for transcription factor WT1 of the zinc finger family, which is located in the podocytes. WT1 regulates numerous target genes that are important for renal morphogenesis and also development of genitalia in fetal life.[26] These include some of the podocyte proteins, such as nephrin. Researchers have described a variety of *WT1* mutations that affect renal development or predispose to tumor formation.[27] These disorders include the Denys-Drash syndrome (DDS), Frasier syndrome, and WAGR syndrome (Wilms tumor, aniridia, genitourinary anomalies, and mental retardation).[27–31]

DDS is characterized by male pseudohermaphroditism, 46,XY karyotype, and diffuse mesangial sclerosis (DMS) noted in renal biopsy. Patients with DDS have a high risk for Wilms tumor. DDS results from heterozygous mutations in exons 8 and 9 of *WT1*, of which over 60 germline mutations have so far been described. The most prevalent of these mutations is *R394W*, located at zinc finger 3.[32] In most patients with DDS, *WT1* expression in podocytes is either absent or reduced.[27]

Clinically, DDS can be categorized into (1) genotypic males with all three abnormalities; (2) genotypic males with nephropathy and ambiguous external, internal, or both genitalia only; and (3) genotypic females with glomerulopathy and Wilms tumor only. Proteinuria and NS develop usually during the first few months of life, ESRD occurs within a year, and DMS is histologically evident.[28]

*WT1* analysis in young patients with NS is important for early detection and tumor prophylaxis. Nephropathy is usually discovered at the age of a few months, sometimes at birth. To avoid the development of Wilms tumor, bilateral nephrectomy is recommended in all patients with DDS nephropathy resulting from *WT1* mutations at the time of developing ESRD.[33] RTx is usually the treatment of choice. *WT1* mutations also may cause isolated DMS.[32,34]

Frasier syndrome is also an autosomal dominantly inherited condition in which females present with amenorrhea, streaked gonads, 46,XY karyotype, and progressive nephropathy leading to ESRD. Proteinuria is usually detected between 2 and 6 years of age, and kidney biopsy reveals FSGS. Frasier syndrome results from point mutations in intron 9 of *WT1* and is characterized by male pseudohermaphroditism and glomerulopathy.[35] Indeed, patients with 46,XY exhibit complete male-to-female gender reversal. Frasier syndrome is associated with gonadoblastomas but not with Wilms tumor.

Mutations in *WT1* also can cause an isolated kidney disease with NS. The histopathologic diagnosis in these cases may be DMS or FSGS.[36] In a recent study, *WT1* mutations were observed in 5 of 110 (4.5%) of patients with SRNS. All patients were less than 5 years of age at onset of NS.[37] In a worldwide cohort of 164 cases of sporadic SRNS, 15 patients exhibited seven different mutations exclusively in exons 8 and 9 of *WT1*, suggesting that screening for *WT1* exons 8 and 9 in patients with sporadic SRNS is sufficient to detect pathogenic mutations.[38]

# PHOSPHOLIPASE Cε1 GENE (*PLCε1*) MUTATIONS

*PLCε1* belongs to the phospholipase family of proteins that catalyse the hydrolysis of phosphoinositides, which are involved in a broad range of intracellular functions.[39] *PLCε1* was found to associate with IQGAP1, a protein that interacts with nephrin. The precise function of *PLCε1* in podocytes, however, remains unclear.

In 2006, Hinkes et al.[40] identified mutations in *PLCε1* as a cause of early-onset NS. The age at onset in the 12 patients varied from 2 months to 4 years, and the age at ESRD was from 5 to over 13 years. No extrarenal manifestations were observed, and kidney histologic examination showed DMS in most patients. Two siblings with a missense mutation exhibited characteristics of FSGS. Interestingly, two other affected individuals responded to immunosuppressive therapy, making this the first report of a molecular cause of NS that may have resolved after therapy. In a subsequent study, Gbadegesin et al.[41] identified 40 children from 35 families with idiopathic DMS from a worldwide cohort of 1368 children with NS. The age of onset varied from 1 month to 6 years. Truncating mutations in *PLCε1* were detected in 10 of 35 (29%) of the families, and, interestingly, *WT1* mutations were seen in only 3 of 35 (8.5%) of the families. Except in one family, all the mutations detected were homozygous loss-of-function mutations. One child had two compound heterozygous mutations. Fourteen children were placed on corticosteroid or cyclosporine (CsA) therapy, but none responded. Age at ESRD varied from 8 months to 5 years.

Thus far, the results show that *PLCε1* mutations are a major genetic cause of isolated DMS, and subjects with this type of histologic lesion should be screened for *PLCε1* mutations. Such mutations also may lead to FSGS with a relatively

---

## KEY POINTS

- Bilateral nephrectomy is highly recommended in patients with DDS because of the high risk for Wilms tumor.
- Patients with Frasier syndrome have a high risk for gonadoblastoma but not Wilms tumor. Therefore, bilateral nephrectomy is generally not necessary.

---

## KEY POINT

*PLCε1* mutations usually have DMS pathology, but FSGS also can be seen.

late onset of proteinuria. *PLCε1* mutations, however, remain an infrequent cause of FSGS. A Dutch study found no *PLCε1* mutations in 19 cases of childhood-onset FSGS.[42] Similarly, no *PLCε1* mutations were found in 125 Spanish patients with SRNS ranging from congenital to adult onset.[43] Interestingly, some individuals with *PLCε1* mutations may remain asymptomatic, implying that modifier genes may interact with *PLCε1* to cause DMS or FSGS.

## *LAMβ2* GENE MUTATIONS (PIERSON SYNDROME)

The *LAMβ2* gene encodes for the laminin β2-chain expressed in the GBM, eye, and central nervous system.[44] Pierson syndrome (OMIM 609049) consists of CNS (with DMS histology), ocular changes (microcoria, lens cornea, and retina abnormalities and possibly blindness), and in surviving children, neurologic deficits (hypotonia and psychomotor retardation). Pierson syndrome usually results from biallelic truncated mutations in the *LAMβ2*, but variants also exist, as do milder forms of cases involving *LAMβ2* mutations. Matejas et al.[45] reviewed the findings of 51 patients from 39 families with *LAMβ2* mutations. The age of most of the patients at diagnosis was younger than 3 months, and only four patients were older than 1 year; their age at ESRD onset was mainly under 1 year (from 1 week to 16 years). Renal biopsy showed DMS histology in 73%, FSGS in 14%, and minimal changes in 8% of the patients. Neurodevelopmental deficits were observed in 82% of the patients, and all but two patients had some ocular abnormalities. Among patients with isolated NS, *LAMβ2* mutations are rare. However, in patients with CNS without *NPHS1* or *NPHS2* mutations, and especially in those with eye abnormalities, this syndrome should be considered.

---

### KEY POINTS

- Pierson syndrome manifests as CNS, eye abnormalities, neurologic manifestations, DMS, or, sometimes FSGS.
- Pierson syndrome is caused by *LAMβ2* mutations that encodes for the lamininβ2-chain of the GBM.

---

## RARE MUTATIONS CAUSING CONGENITAL NEPHROTIC SYNDROME

A few other gene defects associated with podocytopathies may cause NS during the first months of life, although these presentations are much less common than those described previously.[9] Mutations in the cation channel gene *TRPC6*, *PDSS2* coding for coenzyme Q synthetase, *COQ2* for PHB-propenyl transferase, and *ARHGDIA* regulating RHO GTPase activity in podocytes all can cause NS.[46-50] *PDSS2*

and *COQ2* defects lead to mitochondrial disorders with several extrarenal symptoms, and *ARHGDIA* mutations have been associated with early NS accompanied by the rapid development of ESRD and DMS.

The Galloway-Mowat syndrome, first described in 1968, consists of congenital microcephaly, CNS, and hiatal hernia.[51,52] Subsequently, additional anomalies have been described, including dysmorphic clinical features, as well as ocular, limb, cardiac, and diaphragmatic anomalies.[53] The gene responsible for Galloway-Mowat syndrome has not yet been isolated. CNS has been described in single patients with nail-patella syndrome, Lowe syndrome, Herlitz junctional epidermolysis bullosa, and sialic acid storage disease.[54-58]

## NONGENETIC FORMS OF CONGENITAL AND INFANTILE NEPHROTIC SYNDROME

NS in newborn infants has been described in association with a multitude of neonatal infections, such as cytomegalovirus infection, toxoplasmosis, congenital rubella, and human immunodeficiency virus infection.[59-62] Congenital syphilis can cause membranous nephropathy that is curable by penicillin therapy.[63] These reversible or treatable diseases need to be ruled out in all patients with CNS. Lupus erythematosus with nuclear antibodies, hypocomplementemia, and glomerulonephritis, but with poor response to therapy has been described in infants.[64] Membranous nephropathy resulting from fetomaternal alloimmunization with neutral endopeptidase antibodies and CNS also has been reported.[65] It is important to remember that idiopathic NS with minimal change histology, which is by far the most common form of childhood NS, usually occurs in toddlers and school-age children but can sometimes present during the first year of life.

---

### DIAGNOSTIC EVALUATION

## EVALUATION OF RENAL DISEASE

NS is sometimes difficult to detect in infants, but edema, hypoproteinemia, hypoalbuminuria, hyperlipidemia, and heavy proteinuria are the cardinal signs. The serum albumin level is typically less than 15 g/L (<1.5 g/dL), and proteinuria

---

### KEY POINTS

- NS is sometimes difficult to detect in infants, but edema, hypoproteinemia, hyperlipidemia, and heavy proteinuria are the cardinal signs.
- Heavy and constant proteinuria (5 to 100 g/L) inevitably leads to life-threatening edema, and protein substitution by parenteral albumin infusions is mandatory.

Table 18.2 Diagnostic points in a child with nephrotic syndrome during the first year of life

| Clinical manifestation | Possible disorder |
| --- | --- |
| Large placenta | NPHS1, intrauterine proteinuria |
| Nephrotic syndrome during the first month | NPHS1, infections |
| Ocular malformations | LAMβ2, syndromic disorders |
| Genital malformations | WT1 |
| Neurologic problems | LAMβ2, PDSS2, COQ2, ARGHDIA syndromes |
| High creatinine during first months | NPHS2, WT1 |
| Renal ultrasound-large kidneys | NPHS1 |
| Ultrasound—small kidneys | DMS/WT1 |

is in nephrotic range. Other serum proteins can be lost into the urine, thus lowering immunoglobulin G, transferrin, apoproteins, LPL, antithrombin III, ceruloplasmin, vitamin D–binding protein, and thyroid-binding globulin. The severity of proteinuria, however, varies and can be modest initially. Serum creatinine and cystatin C can be normal during the first weeks or months, and ultrasound can show the nonspecific finding of large hyperechoic kidneys (Table 18.2).[19]

## ROLE OF RENAL BIOPSY

The indications for renal biopsy remain unclear. Histologic lesions such as FSGS, MCNS, and DMS, as well as glomerular mesangial expansion, are not specific to the gene defect involved. On the other hand, clinical findings and histologic examination together can suggest the cause. The severity of the histologic lesions also helps in developing treatment strategies.

## ESTABLISHING GENETIC DIAGNOSIS

The etiologic diagnosis is helpful in choosing therapy and assessing prognosis, following associated symptoms, and genetic counseling for the family. Examination should include possible renal and nonrenal malformations, genital abnormalities (karyotype), and neurologic and ocular defects, because these may compel the search for a mutation in the most likely gene. In newborns, a placental weight greater than 25% of birth weight is typical of classic NPHS1 mutation, but may occur in other entities with congenital NS.

Patients with CNS or INS should first be screened for mutations in NPHS1 and NPHS2. In a large study of early-onset NS, 74% of all patients presenting during the first week of life carried an NPHS1 mutation and 11% had an NPHS2 defect.[23] Conversely, NPHS2 mutations accounted for 37%

of those seen after the first month, and only 16% carried an NPHS1 mutation. In this study, 5.6% had a WT1, LAMε2, or PLCε1 mutation, and 18.7% had no known mutations. If a kidney biopsy shows FSGS histologic findings, the patient shows signs of renal failure, or both, screening for NPHS2 mutations is always the first option. On the other hand, all cases with DMS histology require WT1 and PLCε1 analyses. Individually sequencing several genes can be time-consuming and costly. However, next-generation genetic analysis of several genes simultaneously is now available at a reasonable price.

## TREATMENT

## MAINTAINING HOMEOSTASIS AND GROWTH

The magnitude of the protein losses into the urine is crucial for therapeutic decisions in infants with NS. Heavy and constant proteinuria inevitably leads to life-threatening edema, and protein substitution by parenteral albumin infusions is mandatory (Table 18.3). On the other hand, patients with moderate proteinuria (2 to 5 g/L) may be managed without parenteral albumin substitution, especially if proteinuria is associated with renal failure and reduced urinary output. Daily albumin infusions are necessary in severe NS and can be administered in one to three infusions per day together with 0.5 mg/kg furosemide, initially in three 2-hour infusions and later as one 6-hour infusion at night. Normally, 20% to 25% albumin, depending on which is available, is infused (3 to 4 g/kg/day) through a permanently placed

Table 18.3 Treatment strategies in children with nephrotic syndrome in the first year of life

- Exclude and treat infectious/immunologic causes
- Maintain the patient without severe edema (IV albumin)
- Provide sufficient calories (nasogastric tube/gastrostomy)
- Administer ACE inhibitors (and indomethacin) especially in cases with moderate proteinuria
- Begin anticoagulation to avoid thrombotic complications
- Treat consequences of other protein losses (thyroxine, balanced fat diet, active treatment of infections)
- Early nephrectomy and dialysis in children with uremia, delayed growth and development, frequent infections, or reduced quality of life
- Renal transplantation when the patient has attained a sufficient weight (>10 kg for extraperitoneal placement)

deep-vein catheter. One should aim for normal growth and a nonedematous state. If protein loss is less severe, only a few infusions per week may be needed to maintain the fluid balance and albumin concentration at approximately 1.5 g/dL (15 g/L).[19,66]

Infants with severe NS have traditionally been treated with a high-energy (130 kcal/kg/day) and high-protein (3 to 4 g/kg/day) diet, although neonates with CNS can manage for some time with breast milk or cows' milk formulas. Glucose polymers are administered to increase energy intake, and a mixture of rapeseed and sunflower oil serves to balance lipid levels. The children also receive vitamin $D_3$ (10 to 30 μg/day), multivitamin preparations, magnesium, and calcium. Most infants need a nasogastric tube or gastrostomy to ensure their energy intake.[67,68]

---

### KEY POINT

Most infants with CNS need a nasogastric tube or gastrostomy to provide adequate caloric intake.

---

Patients with constant proteinuria often have low levels of serum thyroid-binding globulin; for such patients, thyroxine substitution is recommended. An imbalance of plasma coagulation factor levels contributes to hypercoagulability and raises the risk for thrombosis; in such cases, warfarin, (and aspirin) therapy are recommended. Antithrombin III (50 U/kg) may be administered before surgical procedures. Prophylactic use of immunoglobulins has been recommended to prevent the consequences of urinary immunoglobulin loss, but in our hands this has proved to be ineffective. Similarly, the use of prophylactic antibiotics may increase the likelihood of infection with resistant organisms.[69] Immunization programs should be performed after nephrectomy and before RTx. Patients with NS warrant a high degree of vigilance for septic infections.

---

### KEY POINTS

- Thyroxine replacement is required for most patients with CNS.
- Hypercoagulability needs to be addressed.

---

## MEDICAL MANAGEMENT OF PROTEINURIA

In the great majority of infants with genetic NS, proteinuria fails to respond to medication. However, a few patients with NPHS1 with "mild" mutations have reportedly responded to antiproteinuric medication with angiotensin-converting enzyme (ACE) inhibitors and indomethacin.[12,66] Thus, in non-Finnish patients with less severe mutations, a 3- to 4-month course of ACE inhibitor or angiotensin II (ATII)

blocker with indomethacin may be worth trying. In patients with SRNS resulting from NPHS2 mutations, antiproteinuric therapy has proved ineffective. In general, patients with NS often receive ACE inhibitors or ATII blockers, especially if the clinical findings support the diagnosis of idiopathic NS.

---

### KEY POINTS

- For children with heavy proteinuria, early bilateral nephrectomy, dialysis, and subsequent renal transplantation is often the therapy of choice.
- A few patients with NPHS1 with "mild" mutations have reportedly responded to antiproteinuric medication with ACE inhibitors and indomethacin.
- Antiproteinuric therapy in SRNS resulting from NPHS2 mutations has proved to be ineffective.

---

Prednisone is the drug of choice in patients with nongenetic forms of NS. In practice, because the genetic analysis of patients with NS takes time, prednisone is often administered on admission, except in neonates with severe CNS. Some studies have reported success with single patients, but most of these had no known gene mutation.[9,24]

Recent data suggest that CsA might improve proteinuria, mainly in patients with WT1 mutations.[40,70–73] CsA directly stabilizes the podocyte actin cytoskeleton by inhibiting the degradation of synaptopodin.[74] Some patients with FSGS and NPHS2 mutations as well as patients with DMS and PCLε1 mutations have also responded to CsA.[40,71,72] In addition, one report indicates that a patient with a coenzyme Q10 deficiency responded to coenzyme Q10 supplementation.[75] However, the long-term results of these medications and the magnitude of their side effects remain unclear.

## DIALYSIS

As long as the child grows and develops normally and the quality of life is acceptable for the patient and family, conservative therapy for NS and for progressive uremia can continue.[19,66] However, thrombotic events and infections may occur, and the risk for permanent neurologic complications is greatest during this period. In infants with moderate proteinuria, unilateral nephrectomy may be indicated to reduce proteinuria and the need for IV albumin replacement. On the other hand, for children with heavy proteinuria, early bilateral nephrectomy, dialysis, and subsequent RTx is often the therapy of choice.[68] In patients with NPHS1 with Fin-major or Fin-minor mutations, and in those who fail to respond to ACE inhibitors, we usually perform bilateral nephrectomy and begin peritoneal dialysis (PD) when the patient has attained a weight of about 7 kg. The PD catheter is inserted before initiation of PD.[67] The diet and medication administered to the proteinuric child are optimized following nephrectomy, some centers providing additional

IV albumin for the first 2 to 3 days after nephrectomy to normalize serum albumin.[19]

With aggressive therapy, growth and development can be normalized during PD in infants with minimal comorbidities.[68] However, long-term PD therapy is suboptimal for the child and the child's family and early RTx is recommended.[76]

# RENAL TRANSPLANTATION

In most centers, RTx is performed after an infant with NS has reached the weight of approximately 10 kg. The donor kidney usually comes from a living (parental) or deceased adult donor. The graft can be placed intraperitoneally or extraperitoneally depending on the preferred technique. Transplanting an adult kidney into an infant requires large amounts of fluids (2500 mL/m$^2$/day) to provide adequate perfusion of the graft.[77] Extra fluids are continued for several months after the surgery. RTx and the postoperative therapy in infants is otherwise quite similar to that in older recipients.

## KEY POINT

Transplanting an adult kidney into an infant requires excessive fluids (2500 mL/m$^2$/day) to provide adequate perfusion of the graft.

Today, the long-term results of RTx in infants, when performed in experienced centers, are comparable to those in older children.[78,79] Long-term patient and graft survival rates are over 90%. The likelihood that NS will recur in the allografts of patients with a genetic form of NS is minimal. However, recurrences have occurred in patients with *NPHS1* (Fin-major homozygotes) and *NPHS2* mutations. One-third of the Fin-major homozygotes develop anti-nephrin antibodies to this previously absent protein after RTx. The cause of recurrence in *NPHS2* is elusive. Most of these patients responded to plasma exchange, cyclophosphamide, anti-CD20 monoclonal antibodies (Rituximab), or a combination of these.[80]

## LONG-TERM OUTCOME

With the first CNS children having reached adulthood, we know that with aggressive therapy from birth, children without comorbidities can enjoy normal growth and development.[68,81,82] Final height in 105 Finnish children transplanted at a mean age of 4.5 years was –1.2 standard deviation (SD) in boys and –1.7 SD in girls (45% of patients CNS of the Finnish type), puberty was normal, and psychomotor development was acceptable.[83-88] Moreover, families with an infant with CNS living in developed societies with adequate social support seemed to cope well.[76]

## SUMMARY

NS in the first year of life is a rare, usually severe disease that in most cases can be treated only with RTx after nephrectomy of the diseased native kidneys. However, the long-term outcome for these children critically depends on early diagnosis and early institution of supportive treatment with subsequent PD and RTx.

## REFERENCES

1. Jalanko H, Patrakka J, Tryggvason K, Holmberg C. Genetic kidney diseases disclose the pathogenesis of proteinuria. Ann Med. 2001;33:526–33.
2. Kestilä M, Lenkkeri M, Männikkö M, et al. Positionally cloned gene for a novel glomerular protein-nephrin is mutated in congenital nephrotic syndrome. Mol Cell. 1998;1:575–82.
3. Ruotsalainen V, Ljungberg P, Wartiovaara J, et al. Nephrin is specifically located at the slit diaphragm of glomerular podocytes. Proc Natl Acad Sci U S A. 1996:7962–7.
4. Donoviel DB, Freed DD, Vogel H, et al. Proteinuria and perinatal lethality in mice lacking NEPH1, a novel protein with homology to nephrin. Mol Cell Biol. 2001;21:4829–36.
5. Inoue T, Yaoita E, Kurihara H, et al. FAT is a component of glomerular slit diaphragms. Kidney Int. 2001;59:1003–12.
6. Gerke P, Huber TB, Sellin L, et al. Homodimerisation and heterodimerisation of the glomerular podocyte proteins nephrin and NEPH1. J Am Soc Nephrol. 2003;14:918–26.
7. Boute N, Gribouval O, Roselli S, et al. NPHS2, encoding the glomerular protein podocin, is mutated in autosomal recessive steroid-resistant nephrotic syndrome. Nat Genet. 2000;24:349–54.
8. Schwarz K, Simons M, Reiser J, et al. Podocin, a raft-associated component of the glomerular slit diaphragm, interacts with CD2AP and nephrin. J Clin Invest. 2001;108:1621–9.
9. Hinkes BG, Mucha B, Vlangos CN, et al. Nephrotic syndrome in the first year of life: Two thirds of cases are caused by mutations in 4 genes (NPHS1, NPHS2, WT1 and LAMB2). Pediatrics. 2007;119:e907–19.
10. Ahvenainen EK, Hallman N, Hjelt L. Nephrotic syndrome in newborn and young infants. Ann Paediatr Fenn. 1956;2:227–41.
11. Norio R. Heredity in congenital nephrotic syndrome: A genetic study of 57 Finnish families with a review of reported cases. Ann Paediatr Fenn. 1966;12(Suppl 27):1–94.

12. Patrakka J, Kestilä M, Wartiovaara J, et al. Congenital nephrotic syndrome (NPHS1): Features resulting from different mutations in Finnish patients. Kidney Int. 2000;58:972–80.

13. Philippe A, Nevo F, Esquivel EL, et al. Nephrin mutations can cause childhood-onset steroid resistant nephrotic syndrome. J Am Soc Nephrol. 2008;19:1871–8.

14. Bolk S, Puffenberg EG, Hudson J, et al. Elevated frequency and allelic heterogeneity of congenital nephrotic syndrome, Finnish type, in the old order Mennonites. Am J Hum Genet. 1999;65:1785–90.

15. Koziell A, Grech V, Hussain S, et al. Genotype/phenotype correlations of NPHS1 and NPHS2 mutations in nephrotic syndrome advocate a functional interrelationship in glomerular filtration. Hum Mol Genet. 2002;11:379–88.

16. Seppälä M, Rapola J, Huttunen NP, et al. Congenital nephrotic syndrome: Prenatal diagnosis and genetic counselling by estimation of amniotic-fluid and maternal serum alpha-fetoprotein. Lancet. 1976;2:123–5.

17. Patrakka J, Martin P, Salonen R, et al. Proteinuria and prenatal diagnosis of congenital nephrosis in fetal carriers of nephrin gene mutations. Lancet. 2002;359:1575–7.

18. Laakkonen H, Lönnqvist T, Uusimaa J, et al. Muscular dystonia and athetosis in six patients with congenital nephrotic syndrome of the Finnish type (NPHS1). Pediatri Nephrol. 2006;21:182–9.

19. Jalanko H, Holmberg C. Congenital nephrotic syndrome. In: Avner E, Harmon WE, Niaudet P, Yoshikawa N, editors. Pediatric Nephrology. New York: Springer, 2009. pp. 601–19.

20. Roselli S, Moutkine I, Gribouval O, et al. Plasma membrane targeting of podocin through the classical exocytic pathway: Effect of NPHS2 mutations. Traffic. 2004;5:37–44.

21. Weber S, Gribouval O, Esquivel EL, et al. NPHS2 mutation analysis shows genetic heterogeneity of steroid-resistant nephrotic syndrome and low post-transplant recurrence. Kidney Int. 2004;66:571–9.

22. Hinkes B, Vlangos C, Heeringa S, et al. Specific podocin mutations correlate with age of onset in steroid-resistant nephrotic syndrome. J Am Soc Nephrol. 2008;19:365–71.

23. Machua E, Benoit G, Nevo F, et al. Genotype-phenotype correlations in non-Finnish congenital nephrotic syndrome. J Am Soc Nephrol. 2010;21:1209–17.

24. Ruf RG, Lichtenberger A, Karle SM, et al. Patients with mutations in NPHS2 (podocin) do not respond to standard steroid treatment of nephrotic syndrome. J Am Soc Nephrol. 2004;15:722–32.

25. Frischberg Y, Feinstein S, Rinat C, et al. The heart of children with steroid-resistant nephrotic syndrome: Is it all podocin? J Am Soc Nephrol. 2006;17:227–31.

26. Call KM, Glaser T, Ito CY, et al. Isolation and characterization of a zinc finger polypeptide gene at the human chromosome 11 Wilms' tumor locus. Cell. 1990;60:509–20.

27. Niaudet P, Gubler MC. WT1 and glomerular disease. Pediatr Nephrol. 2006;21:1653–60.

28. Denys P, Malvaux P, Van Den Berghe H, et al. Association of an anatomo-pathological syndrome of male pseudohermaphroditism, Wilms' tumor, parenchymatous nephropathy and XX/XY mosaicism. Arch Fr Pediatr. 1967;24:729–39.

29. Drash A, Sherman F, Hartmann WH, et al. A syndrome of pseudohermaphroditism, Wilms' tumor, hypertension, and degenerative renal disease. J Pediatr. 1970;76:585–93.

30. Barbaux S, Niaudet P, Gubler MC, et al. Donor splice-site mutations in WT1 are responsible for Frasier syndrome. Nat Genet. 1997;17:467–70.

31. Klamt B, Koziell A, Poulat F, et al. Frasier syndrome is caused by defective alternative splicing of WT1 leading to an altered ratio of WT1+/-KTS splice isoforms. Hum Mol Genet. 1998;7:709–14.

32. Habib R, Gubler MC, Antignac C, Gagnadoux MF. Diffuse mesangial sclerosis: A congenital glomerulopathy with nephrotic syndrome. Adv Nephrol. 1993;22:43–56.

33. Hu M, Zhang GY, Arbuckle S, et al. Prophylactic bilateral nephrectomies in two paediatric patients with missense mutations in the WT1 gene. Nephrol Dial Transplant. 2004;19:223–6.

34. Hahn H, Cho YM, Park YS, et al. Two cases of isolated diffuse mesangial sclerosis with WT1 mutations. J Korean Med Sci. 2006;21:160–4.

35. Hildebrandt F. Genetic kidney diseases. Lancet. 2010;375:1287–95.

36. Ito S, Takata A, Hataya H, et al. Isolated diffuse mesangial sclerosis and Wilm's tumor suppressor gene. J Pediatr. 2001;138:425–8.

37. Ruf R, Schultheiss M, Lichtenberger A, et al. Prevalence of WT1 mutations in a large cohort of patients with steroid-resistant and steroid-sensitive nephrotic syndrome. Kidney Int. 2004;66:564–70.

38. Mucha B, Ozaltin F, Hinkes B, et al. Mutations in the Wilms' tumor 1 gene cause isolated steroid resistant nephrotic syndrome and occurs in exons 8 and 9. Pediatr Res. 2006;59:325–31.

39. Chaib H, Hoskins BE, Ashraf S, et al. Identification of BRAF as a new interactor of PLCε1, the protein mutated in nephrotic syndrome type 3. Am J Physiol Ren Physiol 2008;294:F93-99.

40. Hinkes B, Wiggins RC, Gbadegesin R, et al. Positional cloning uncovers mutations in PLCE1 responsible for a nephrotic syndrome variant that may be reversible. Nat Genet. 2006;38:1397–405.

41. Gbadegesin R, Hinkes B, Hoskins B, et al. Mutations in PLCE1 are a major cause of isolated diffuse

mesangial sclerosis (IDMS). Nephrol Dial Transplant. 2008;23:1291–7.

42. Löwik M, Levtchenko E, Westra D, et al. Bigenetic heterozygosity and development of steroid-resistant focal segmental glomerulosclerosis. Nephrol Dial Transplant. 2008;23:3146–51.

43. Santin S, Bullich G, Tazon-Vega B, et al. Clinical utility of genetic testing in children and adults with steroid-resistant nephrotic syndrome. Clin J Am Soc Nephrol. 2011;6:1139–48.

44. Zenker M, Aigner T, Wendler O, et al. Human laminin beta2 deficiency causes congenital nephrosis with mesangial sclerosis and distinct eye abnormalities. Hum Mol Genet. 2004;13:2625–32.

45. Matejas V, Hinkes B, Alkandari F, et al. Mutations in the human laminin beta2 (LAMB2) gene and the associated phenotypic spectrum. Hum Mutat. 2010;31:992–1002.

46. Gigante M, Caridi G, Montemurno E, et al. TRPC6 mutations in children with steroid-resistant nephrotic syndrome and atypical phenotype. Clin J Am Soc Nephrol. 2011; 6:1626–34.

47. Diomedi-Camassei F, Di Giandomenico S, Santorelli FM, et al. COO2 nephropathy: A newly described inherited mitochondriopathy with primary renal involvement. J Am Soc Nephrol. 2007;18:2773–80.

48. Heeringa S, Chernin G, Chaki M, et al. COQ6 mutations in human patients produce nephrotic syndrome with sensorineural deafness. J Clin Invest. 2011;121:2013–24.

49. Gupta IR, Baldwin C, Auguste D, et al. ARGHDIA: A novel gene implicated in nephrotic syndrome. J Med Genet. 2013;50:330–8.

50. Gee HY, Saisawat P, Ashraf S, et al. ARGHDIA mutations cause nephrotic syndrome via defective RHO GTPase signaling. J Clin Invest. 2013;123:3243–53.

51. Galloway WH, Mowat AP. Congenital microcephaly with hiatus hernia and nephrotic syndrome in two sibs. J Med Genet. 1968;5:319–21.

52. Srivastava T, Whiting JM, Garola RE, et al. Podocyte proteins in Galloway-Mowat syndrome. Pediatr Nephrol. 2001;16:1022-1029.

53. Meyers KE, Kaplan P, Kaplan BS. Nephrotic syndrome, microcephaly, and developmental delay: Three separate syndromes. Am J Med Genet. 1999;82:257-–60.

54. Bongers EM, Gubler MC, Knoers NV, et al. Nail-patella syndrome: Overview on clinical and molecular findings. Pediatr Nephrol. 2002;17:703–12.

55. Heidet L, Bongers EM, Sich M, et al. in vivo expression of putative LMX1B targets in nail-patella syndrome kidneys. Am J Pathol. 2003;163:145–55.

56. Nielsen KF, Steffensen GK. Congenital nephrotic syndrome associated with Lowe's syndrome. Clin Nephrol Urol. 1990;10:92–5.

57. Hata D, Miyazaki M, Seto S, et al. Nephrotic syndrome and aberrant expression of laminin isoforms in glomerular basement membranes for an infant with Herlitz junctional epidermolysis bullosa. Pediatrics. 2005;116:e601–7.

58. Sperl W, Grober W, Quatacker J, et al. Nephrosis in two siblings with infantile sialic acid storage disease. Eur J Pediatr. 1990;149:477–82.

59. Besbas N, Bayrakci US, Kale G, et al. Cytomegalovirus-related congenital nephrotic syndrome with diffuse mesangial sclerosis. Pediatr Nephrol. 2006;21:740–2.

60. Shahin B, Papadopoulou ZL, Jenis EH. Congenital nephrotic syndrome associated with congenital toxo-plasmosis. J Pediatr. 1974;85:366–70.

61. Esterley JR, Oppenheimer EH. Pathological lesions due to congenital rubella. Arch Pathol. 1969;87:380–88.

62. Ross MJ, Klotman PE. Recent progress in HIV-associated nephropathy. J Am Soc Nephrol. 2002;13:2997–3004.

63. Basker M, Agrawal I, Bendon KS. Congenital nephrotic syndrome: A treatable cause. Ann Trop Paediatr. 2007;27:87–90.

64. Dudley J, Fenton T, Unsworth J, et al. Systemic lupus erythematosus presenting as congenital nephrotic syndrome. Pediatr Nephrol. 1996;10:752–5.

65. Debiec H, Guigonis V, Mougenot B, et al. Antenatal membranous glomerulonephritis due to anti-neutral endopeptidase antibodies. N Engl J Med. 2002;346:2053–60.

66. Holmberg C, Antikainen M, Rönnholm K, et al. Management of congenital nephrotic syndrome of the Finnish type. Pediatr Nephrol. 1995;9:87–93.

67. Laakkonen H, Hölttä T, Lönnqvist T, et al. Peritoneal dialysis in children under two years of age. Nephrol Dial Transplant. 2008;23:1747–53.

68. Laakkonen H, Happonen JM, Marttinen E, et al. Normal growth and intravascular volume status with good metabolic control during peritoneal dialysis in infancy. Pediatr Nephrol. 2010;25:1529–38.

69. Ljungberg P, Holmberg C, Jalanko H. Infections in infants with congenital nephrosis of the Finnish type. Pediatr Nephrol. 1997;11:148–52.

70. Gellerman J, Ehrich JH, Querfeld U. Sequential maintenance therapy with cyclosporine A and mycophe-nolate mofetil for sustained remission of childhood steroid-resistant nephrotic syndrome. Nephrol Dial Transplant. 2012;27:1970–8.

71. Stefanidis C, Querfeld U. The podocyte as a target: Cyclosporin A in the management of the nephrotic syndrome caused by WT1 mutations. Eur J Pediatr. 2011;170:1377–82.

72. Buescher A, Weber S. The podocytopathies. Eur J Pediatr. 2012;171:1151–60.

73. Boyer O, Benoit G, Gribouval O, et al. Mutational analysis of the PLCE1 gene in steroid resistant nephrotic syndrome. J Med Genet. 2010;47:445–52.

74. Faul C, Donnelly M, Merscher-Gomez, et al. The actin cytoskeleton of kidney podocytes is a direct target of the antiproteinuric effect of cyclosporine A. Nat Med. 2008;14:931–8.

75. Montini G, Malaventura C, Salviati L. Early coenzyme Q10 supplementation in primary coenzyme Q10 deficiency. New Engl J Med. 2008;358:2849–50.

76. Laakkonen H, Taskinen S, Rönnholm K, et al. Parent-child and spousal relationships in families with a young child with end-stage renal disease. Pediatr Nephrol. 2014;29:289–95.

77. Salvatierra O Jr, Singh T, Shiffrin R, et al. Successful transplantation of adult-size kidneys into infants requires maintenance of high aortic blood flow. Transplantation. 1998;66:819–23.

78. Foster BJ, Dahhou M, Zhang X, et al. Association between age and graft failure rates in young kidney transplant recipients. Transplantation. 2011;92:1237–3.

79. Hertelius M, Celsi G, Edstrom Halling S, et al. Renal transplantation in infants and small children. Pediatr Nephrol. 2012;27:145–50.

80. Holmberg C, Jalanko H. Congenital nephrotic syndrome and recurrence of proteinuria after renal transplantation. Pediatr Nephrol. 2014;29:2309-17.

81. Quist E, Laine J, Rönnholm K, et al. Graft function 5-7 years after renal transplantation in early childhood. Transplantation. 1999;67:1043–9.

82. Quist E, Marttinen E, Rönnholm K, et al. Growth after renal transplantation in infancy or early childhood. Pediatr Nephrol. 2002;17:438–43.

83. Tainio J, Qvist E, Vehmas R, et al. Pubertal development is normal in adolescents after renal transplantation in childhood. Transplantation. 2011;92:404–9.

84. Laakkonen H, Lönnquist T, Valanne L, et al. Neurological development in 21 children on peritoneal dialysis in infancy. Pediatr Nephrol. 2011;26:1863–71.

85. Haavisto A, Jalanko H, Sintonen H, et al. Quality of life in adult survivors of pediatric kidney transplantation. Transplantation. 2011;92:1322–26.

86. Haavisto A, Korkman M, Holmberg C, et al. Neuropsychological profile of children with kidney transplants. Nephrol Dial Transplant. 2012;27:2594–601.

87. Johnson RJ, Warady BA. Long-term neurocognitive outcomes of patients with end-stage renal disease during infancy. Pediatr Nephrol. 2013;28:1283–91.

88. van Strahlen KJ, Borzych-Duzalka D, Hataya H, et al. Survival and clinical outcomes of children starting renal replacement therapy in the neonatal period. Kidney Int. 2014;86:168–74.

## REVIEW QUESTIONS

1. Congenital nephrotic syndrome is *best defined* as:
   a. Nephrotic syndrome during the first year of life
   b. Nephrotic syndrome during the first 6 years of life
   c. Nephrotic syndrome during the first 3 months of life
   d. End-stage renal disease and proteinuria in infancy
   e. Proteinuria and hematuria with uremia at birth

2. The *most common* causes of congenital nephrotic syndrome are:
   a. *WT1* mutations
   b. *WT1* and *PLCε1* mutations
   c. Neonatal infections
   d. Galloway-Mowat syndrome
   e. *NPHS1* and *NPHS2* mutations

3. Which of the following is *most important* in regulating glomerular protein filtration?
   a. The capillary endothelium
   b. Mesangial cell function
   c. The basement membrane
   d. The slit diaphragm
   e. The podocyte cell bodies

4. Congenital nephrotic syndrome secondary to *NPHS1* mutation:
   a. Is most commonly seen in Turkish children
   b. Is caused by a mutation in the podocin gene
   c. Usually manifests after the first 3 months of life
   d. Is caused by a nephrin gene mutation
   e. Reacts to cyclosporin A medication

5. Congenital nephrotic syndrome secondary to *NPHS2* mutation:
   a. Presents during the first month of life
   b. Is characterized by severe NS and ocular malformations
   c. Is caused by a mutation in the podocin gene
   d. Shows DMS in renal biopsy
   e. Reacts to ACE inhibitors and indomethacin

6. The *most typical* symptoms of congenital nephrotic syndrome is (are):
   a. Severe nephrosis during the first 3 months of life
   b. Malformations and end-stage renal failure
   c. Hematuria, high fever, and a typical rash
   d. Proteinuria and gastrointestinal malformations
   e. Edema, high creatinine level, and high blood pressure during the first months of life

7. Congenital nephrotic syndrome is *most effectively* treated by:
   a. Dialysis and early renal transplantation
   b. ACE inhibitors and indomethacin with cyclosporin A
   c. The patients recover spontaneously
   d. Penicillin
   e. High-dose immunosuppression

8. Which of the following *best represents* the long-term outcome of congenital nephrotic syndrome?
   a. Remains poor, with death during the first years of life
   b. Has improved, because most patients respond to the medication
   c. Is poor regardless of intervention, because the disease mostly reappears in the graft
   d. Is good with early support, dialysis, and renal transplantation
   e. Is poor because graft survival is still only 50% at 5 years

## ANSWER KEY

1. c
2. e
3. d
4. d
5. c
6. a
7. a
8. d

# 19

# Membranoproliferative glomerulonephritis

CARLA M. NESTER AND DANNIELE G. HOLANDA

As advances are made in our understanding of the mechanistic underpinnings of membranoproliferative glomerulonephritis (MGPN), the classification and nomenclature of MPGN as a clinicopathologic entity is being revisited. Children with MPGN may present with nephritic syndrome, nephrotic syndrome, asymptomatic proteinuria, or a nephritic-nephrotic clinical picture. Despite an increased understanding of its pathogenesis, optimal treatment of MPGN remains uncertain.

## HISTORICAL PERSPECTIVE AND NOMENCLATURE

MPGN is the pathologic term used to describe a pattern of glomerular injury noted on kidney biopsy. When the ultrastructural abnormalities that characterize MPGN are present on the kidney biopsy in the absence of immune deposits, the term membranoproliferative *pattern* is often preferred, instead of membranoproliferative *glomerulonephritis*. MPGN pattern is commonly seen in the late phase of thrombotic microangiopathy, chronic allograft rejection, and radiation-induced glomerulonephritis.

The term *secondary* MPGN applies when the characteristic pathologic findings are seen in renal biopsy in association with a defined disease process (e.g., systemic lupus erythematosus, hepatitis B or hepatitis C). The list of secondary causes of MPGN is extensive (Table 19.1). MPGN is designated *idiopathic* (or simply MPGN) when there is no evidence for an underlying disease. The secondary forms of MPGN are more common in adults, and the idiopathic forms of MPGN are more common in children. This chapter will focus on the idiopathic forms of MPGN in children.

Historically, MPGN has been classified into three morphologic types based on the location of the immune deposits noted on electron microscopy of the kidney biopsy sample (Figure 19.1): types I, II, and III. Type I, often referred to as *MPGN* (without the Roman numeral designation), is the most common variant and is characterized predominantly by the presence of subendothelial immune complex deposits. The immune complexes identified by immunofluorescence may include immunoglobulin, complement, or a combination of the two. The presence of immune deposits has led to the presumption that an important aspect of the pathogenesis of MPGN I is immune complex–mediated inflammation, with subsequent complement activation from chronic antigen stimulation.

The pathologic feature characteristic of MPGN II is the presence of distinct, dense, osmiophilic, sausage-shaped intramembranous deposits on electron microscopy. The historical term *MPGN II* as a disease entity is a misnomer because only 25% of patients with this disorder demonstrate any glomerular proliferative changes that are characteristic of MPGN.[1-6] In keeping with this distinctive pathologic picture, the dense deposit disease (DDD) is considered the

**KEY POINTS**

- MPGN classification is based on the location of immune deposits seen on electron microscopy of the kidney biopsy sample.
- The nomenclature of MPGN is in flux and is likely to be reconsidered.
- The term *C3 glomerulopathy* (C3G) is being proposed to capture a subgroup of patients with renal morphologies that manifest within the spectrum of MPGN.

preferred term. Additional criteria for the disease definition of DDD include the presence of predominant complement component 3 (C3) deposits on immunofluorescence staining of the kidney biopsy.[5,7–12]

Type III MPGN, considered by some to be a morphologic variant of type I and by others to represent a distinct category, has a more complex distribution of immune deposits. The electron microscopy of MPGN III not only demonstrates subendothelial and occasional intramembranous deposits but also includes subepithelial deposits.

The MPGN nomenclature, mainly types I and III, is in flux. In 2007, Servais et al. suggested that it may be important mechanistically, therapeutically, and prognostically to differentiate MPGN based on the predominant immunostaining, as opposed to the location of the deposits.[14] As noted previously, the diagnostic immunostaining requirement for DDD was a predominant C3 pattern on renal biopsy. Servais et al. hypothesized that the important pathologic distinction for all of the MPGNs was not the *location* of the deposits, but the *specificity*. The authors supported their theory by demonstrating that a significant proportion of the patients with C3 only on the kidney biopsy

Table 19.1 Secondary causes of membranoproliferative glomerulonephritis

| | |
|---|---|
| Rheumatologic disorders | Genetic disorders |
|   Systemic lupus erythematosus |   Alpha-1–antitrypsin deficiency |
|   Sjögren's syndrome |   Hereditary complement deficiencies |
|   Henoch Schönlein purpura |   Down syndrome |
|   Rheumatoid arthritis |   Gaucher disease |
|   Sarcoidosis |   Kartagener syndrome |
|   Psoriasis |   Sickle cell disease |
|   Takayasu arteritis |   Partial lipodystrophy |
|   Polyarteritis |   Wiskott-Aldrich syndrome |
|   Hypocomplementemic urticarial vasculitis |   Prader-Willi syndrome |
| Infection |   Turner syndrome |
|   Infected ventricular shunt |   Hereditary angioedema |
|   Endocarditis |   Familial Mediterranean fever |
|   Visceral abscess |   Addison disease |
|   Tuberculosis | Gastrointestinal disease |
|   Lyme disease |   Chronic active hepatitis |
|   Mycoplasma |   Cirrhosis |
|   Hepatitis B or C |   Celiac disease and sprue |
|   Human immunodeficiency virus |   Diabetes mellitus |
|   Hantavirus |   Ulcerative colitis |
|   Filariasis | Renal disease |
|   Malaria |   Alport syndrome |
|   Schistosomiasis |   C1q nephropathy |
|   *Candida* endocrinopathy |   PCKD |
| Malignancy |   POEMS syndrome |
|   Amyloidosis |   Cushing's disease |
|   Plasma cell dyscrasia |   Immunoglobulin deposition disease |
|   Leukemia or lymphoma |   Radiation nephritis |
|   Epithelial tumors | Other |
|   Malignant melanoma |   Bone marrow transplantation |
|   Desmoplastic tumors |   Immunoglobulin deficiency |
|   Ovarian tumors |   Drug abuse |
|   Castleman disease |   Organizing pneumonia |

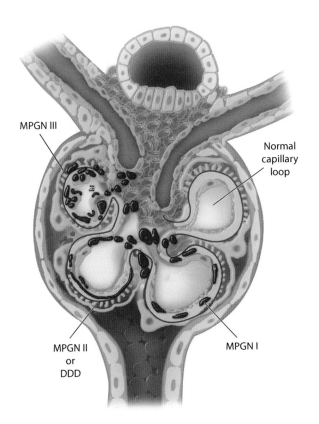

Figure 19.1 Classification of membranoproliferative glomerulonephritis (MPGN) by location of electron-dense deposits. MPGN I deposits are classically subendothelial and occasionally intramembranous. The defining deposits of MPGN II (dense deposit disease [DDD]) are the elongated, sausage-shaped intramembranous deposits. MPGN III has the most complex array of deposits, including subendothelial, intramembranous and subepithelial. Podocyte pathology is not depicted in this cartoon; however, it may be present in each of the MPGNs.

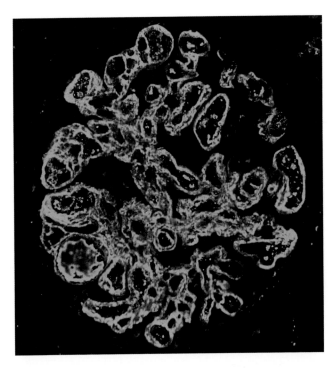

Figure 19.2 Immunofluorescence pattern in dense deposit disease. There is a strong capillary wall staining of C3 as well as mesangial C3 staining.

immunostaining had genetic mutations in complement genes, an acquired complement abnormality, or both.[14–22] Servais et al. further proposed that distinguishing a group of MPGN patients with a primary complement abnormality facilitates a more directed treatment approach.

The term *C3 glomerulopathy* (C3G) has been proposed as a new categorization of the diseases that would include entities formerly classified as MPGN I or MPGN III and MPGN II, all with C3 predominance on immunofluorescence (Figure 19.3). This recategorization of MPGN pathologic subtypes, based on the presence of *isolated* or *predominant* C3 deposits on kidney biopsy, has been embraced by several other authors.[13,23–26] The updated nomenclature includes two major categories: MPGN (alternatively called *immune complex MPGN* or simply *MPGN*), types I or III and C3G. C3G is currently separated into two subcategories: DDD and C3 glomerulonephritis (C3GN). Those who do not have the characteristic dense deposits noted in DDD are designated as C3GN (regardless of whether the MPGN pattern is type I or II). Gale

et al.[15] suggested CFHR5 nephropathy as another subcategory of C3G. CFHR5 nephropathy meets the histologic criteria of C3G yet has a well-described, unique, genetic, complement-based etiology.[15] A consensus statement on the definition of these terms, recapping our current understanding of the underlying pathologic processes, and identifying knowledge gaps was recently issued.[13]

Undoubtedly, the published literature is based on a heterogeneous description of patients who may or may not share the degree of disease characteristics previously presumed. When discussing epidemiology, treatment, and prognosis in this chapter, we use the older nomenclature for our primary discussion. However, to facilitate understanding of the disease process, newer terminology will also be included.

## EPIDEMIOLOGY

Although MPGN was originally reported in children, it is seen less frequently in children than in adults.[27–29] The true incidence of MPGN remains unknown. Estimates of prevalence have been extrapolated from data in patients who underwent kidney biopsy for indications of abnormal kidney function, proteinuria, hematuria, or a combination of these. The diagnosis of MPGN is reported in 5% to 10% of U.S. patients and 9.6% of U.K. patients undergoing a kidney biopsy for the evaluation of glomerular diseases.[28,30–34]

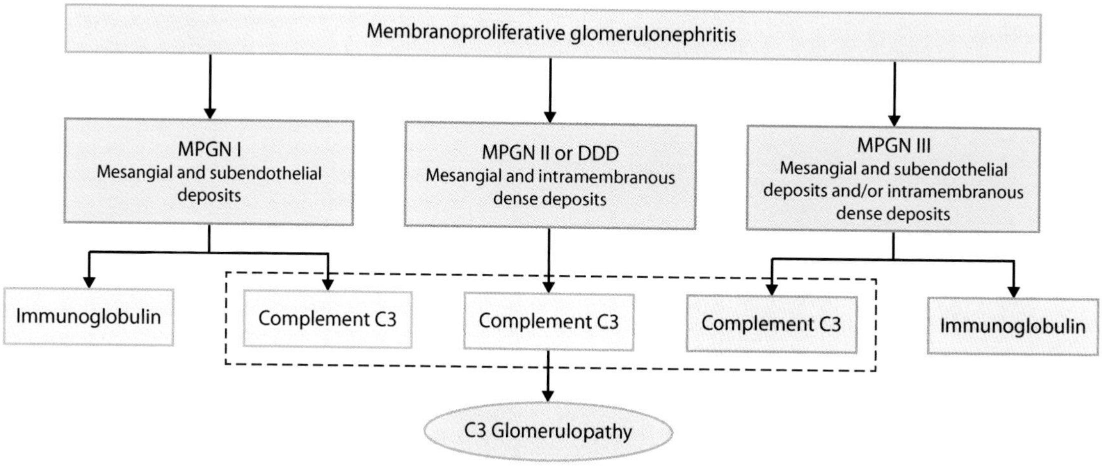

Figure 19.3 Renal pathology in membranoproliferative glomerulonephritis (MPGN). Three types of MPGN have historically been recognized: MPGN I, dense deposit disease [DDD], and MPGN III. MPGN I is often referred to as immune complex MPGN when immunoglobulin is the primary immunostaining. When C3 is the predominant immunostaining, regardless of the electron microscopy findings, C3 glomerulopathy is the preferred term.

Whereas MPGN is the most common primary glomerulonephritis in developing countries, it appears to be on the decline in some industrialized countries.[29] Hygienic, environmental, and socioeconomic factors are presumed to play a role in this disparity, but no firm relationships have been established. Local practice pattern, including indications for performing a kidney biopsy, may affect the reported incidence estimates.

MPGN is one of the least common types of glomerulonephritides in children. Three single-center reviews support the adult predominance and demonstrate ethnic differences. Nawaz et al.[28] presented a 5-year review of biopsies performed in their center. Of 348 biopsy samples, 13% were designated as MPGN, with an adult-to-pediatric ratio of 4:1.[28] Golay et al.[27] reported from their center that 5.25% of 666 biopsies were classified as MPGN, with 25% in children. In contrast, Kawamura et al.[29] reported that only 1.2% of 6369 biopsies were MPGN, 30% of which were in children.

Many reports suggest that the global incidence of MPGN in adults has not changed substantially over time. However, a declining incidence of MPGN in children from industrialized countries has been reported.[29,35–37] The reasons for this decline of MPGN in children have not been identified.

The incidence of C3G as a subset of MPGN is unknown. Undoubtedly, a number of C3G cases were previously designated as MPGN I, II, or III. Disease-specific data are impossible to tease out from previously published literature. The initial study of Servais et al.[22] described 19 cases over a 33-year period, 5 of which were in patients under the age of 18. In a follow-up study, they reported an additional 134 cases, 39% occurring in children.[14]

In the United States, idiopathic MPGN predominantly affects whites. Type I disease affects women more often than men, but a nearly equal sex distribution is seen in MPGN type II. On the other hand, in a multicenter French report, both type I and type II/DDD were more common in male patients.[14] As in the United States, the French group reported that MPGN I was more common in adults and DDD was more common in children. DDD tends to affect children between 5 and 15 years of age. As noted previously, secondary forms of MPGN lesions are also more common in adults and the epidemiology parallels that of the underlying disease.

## KEY POINTS

- The incidence of MPGN may be declining in the industrialized countries.
- Light microscopy of MPGN demonstrates intense cellularity of the glomeruli, with increase in mesangial cell and cytoplasm.
- Silver stain may demonstrate a "double-contoured" glomerular basement membrane.
- Immunofluorescence shows capillary loop and mesangial deposition of C3 and immunoglobulin G (IgG).
- Electron microscopy findings are variable, depending of the type of MPGN.

## PATHOLOGY

A combination of light microscopy, immunofluorescence, and electron microscopy is necessary to define and stratify MPGN into the generally accepted variants. The characteristic light microscopy renal biopsy findings are as follows:

1. Light microscopy shows cellular (proliferative) glomeruli, with a lobular appearance. This morphologic picture results from an extensive mesangial cell and endothelial cell proliferation. These findings in older literature were also referred to as mesangiocapillary glomerulonephritis (see Figure 19.1 and 19.4A to C).
2. Glomerular basement membranes are thickened and double contoured because of interposition of the mesangial cytoplasmic extensions into the basement membranes and new basement membrane formation in response to immune complex deposition (see Figure 19.1 and Figure 19.4D). This morphologic finding

in light microscopy is sometimes referred to as "tram-tracking". These findings are better demonstrated with stains that highlight the basement membrane, such as Jones methenamine silver stain.

Immunofluorescence microscopy demonstrates a granular to thick semilinear (or pseudolinear) pattern of immune deposits consisting of either IgG and C3 or isolated C3 deposits (see Figure 19.2). Lesser degrees of IgA, IgM, and C1q may be present. Electron microscopy has a variable pattern of electron-dense deposits, depending on the subtype of MPGN.

Based on location, quality, and specificity of immune deposits on immunofluorescence and electron microscopy findings, MPGN is further classified by the by these methods into three distinct subtypes (Table 19.2). MPGN I is

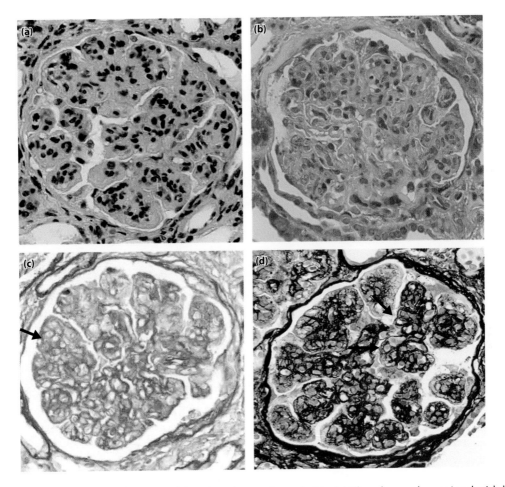

Figure 19.4 Light microscopy in membranoproliferative glomerulonephritis. **(a)** The glomerulus stained with hematoxylin and eosin (H&E) stain shows increased glomerular cellularity. The lobulated appearance of the capillary tuft results from an increase in mesangial cell numbers and increased endocapillary hypercellularity. Several neutrophils are seen infiltrating the glomerular tuft. **(b)** The glomerulus stained with periodic acid–Schiff (PAS) stain demonstrates glomerular tuft lobulation and mesangial cell proliferation. Capillary wall thickening is also noted. **(c)**. A glomerulus stained with trichrome stain showing mesangial proliferative changes. Arrow points to the lobulated glomerular tuft with very few open capillaries. Close inspection of the glomerular basement membranes shows numerous areas of double-contoured appearance. **(d)**. The Jones methenamine silver stain is ideal for outlining glomerular basement membrane (black, or argyrophilic). This figure shows thickened glomerular basement membranes and double contours or tram-rack of the basement membrane (arrows). This appearance results from proliferation and interposition of the mesangial cytoplasm, almost splitting the basement membrane, or to the presence of immune deposits along the contour of the basement membrane, as is seen in the dense deposit disease.

Table 19.2 Classification of membranoproliferative glomerulonephritis based on immunofluorescence microscopy and electron microscopy findings

| | Electron microscopy microscopy | Immunofluorescence |
|---|---|---|
| MPGN type I | Granular and/or thick linear interrupted pattern of deposits with either IgG and C3 or isolated C3 deposits. Lesser degrees of IgA, IgM, and C1q may be present. | Subendothelial deposits |
| MPGN type II | Granular and/or band ("ribbon")–like C3 deposits. | Long, dense, band ("ribbon")-- like or "sausage"-shaped deposits in the lamina densa of the glomerular capillary basement membrane and subendothelial space |
| MPGN type III | Granular to the semilinear pattern of deposits with either IgG and C3 or isolated C3 deposits. Lesser degrees of IgA, IgM and C1q may be present. | Subendothelial, intramembranous and subepithelial deposits |

characterized by presence of subendothelial electron-dense deposits (see Figures 19.1 and 19.5), MPGN II has ribbon-like or sausage-like electron-dense deposits in the lamina densa (see Figures 19.1 and 19.6), and MPGN III has electron-dense deposits in the subendothelial, intramembranous, and subepithelial areas (see Figures 19.1 and 19.7)

## PATHOGENESIS

A detailed understanding of the pathogenesis of MPGN I, II, and III is not yet established. It is likely that a diverse set of pathogenic pathways lead to the pathologic findings seen in MPGN. In some cases, MPGN is a manifestation of an underlying disorder, such as chronic antigen exposure and subsequent kidney injury from immune complex deposition and complement activation. This is designated as the

Table 19.3 Clinical features at membranoproliferative glomerulonephritis presentation

| | Children* (%) | Children and adults† (%) |
|---|---|---|
| Hematuria | 33 (100%) | 83 (58.8%) |
| Macroscopic hematuria | 13 (39.4%) | |
| Nephrotic syndrome | 23 (69.7%) | 58 (41/1% |
| Non-nephrotic proteinuria | 10 (30.3%) | |
| Hypertension | 18 (54.5%) | 43 (30.5%) |
| Renal failure | 9(27.2%) | |
| Hypocomplementemia | 19 (57.5%) | |
| Low C3 | 14 (42%) | 53 (46.1%) |
| Low C3 and C4 | 5 | 2 (1.7%) |

*Sources:* Ren Fail. 2014 Sep;36(8):1221-5; Clin Exp Nephrol. 2013 Apr;17(2):248-54.
* 33 children with idiopathic membranoproliferative glomerulo-nephritis (MPGN).
† 52 children and 82 adults with idiopathic MPGN.

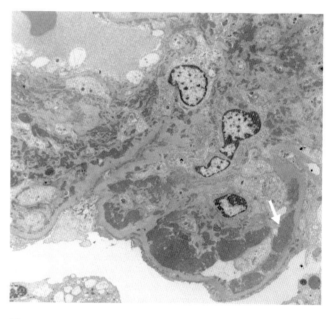

Figure 19.5 Electron microscopy pathologic finding of membranoproliferative glomerulonephritis I. Arrow indicates subendothelial deposits.

secondary form of MPGN (see Table 19.1). The idiopathic MPGN is not associated with any apparent underlying disorder. It remains unclear whether abnormalities in the complement cascade will eventually be identified in some of these patients.

Two primary mechanisms have been proposed for the pathogenesis of idiopathic MPGN. In both of them, involvement of complement cascade plays a central role. In the first proposed mechanism, immune complex deposition in the glomeruli activates the classic pathway of complement. Immune activation of component C1 (active form: C1qC1rC1s) leads to the cleavage of C4 and C2. Cleavage of C4 and C2 leads to the generation of C4b and C2a and the subsequent formation of C4b2a, the classic pathway C3 convertase (Figure 19.8). The C3 convertase cleaves C3

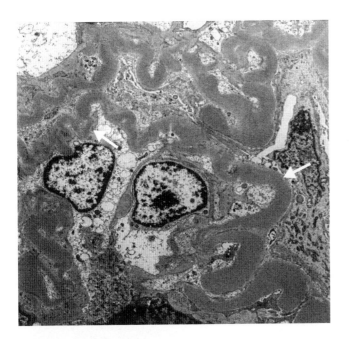

Figure 19.6 Electron microscopic pathology of dense deposit disease, or membranoproliferative glomerulonephritis II. Arrows points to intramembranous bandlike or "sausage-like" electron-dense deposits.

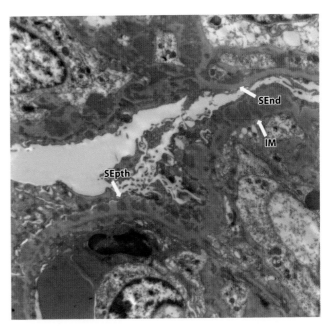

Figure 19.7 Electron microscopy pathologic image of membranoproliferative glomerulonephritis III. Arrows shows electron-dense deposits in subepithelial (SEpth) space, subendothelial (SEnd) space, and intramembranous (IM) region.

into C3a, an anaphylatoxin, and C3b, which joins the C3 convertase to form the C5 convertase (C4b2aC3b). The C5 convertase cleaves C5 into C5a (another anaphylatoxin) and C5b. The cleavage product C5b is the first protein of the terminal complement complex. The joining of C5b to C6, C7, C8, and C9 generates the membrane attack complex (MAC). Production of MAC causes cell activation or damage to the glomerular capillary wall.

## KEY POINTS

- MPGN is mediated by an activated complement system.
- Some patients have circulating C3-nephritic factor(s), which is an antibody that combines with the C3 convertase and prevents its catabolism. This results in an "always on" alternative complement pathway and downstream activation.
- Rare patients with MPGN may have inherited complement gene abnormalities.

In addition to MAC-induced tissue damage, the cleavage products C3a and C5a are potent anaphylatoxins. Anaphylatoxin generation triggers the accumulation of white blood cells capable of releasing oxidants and proteases that facilitate glomerular damage. In addition, anaphylatoxin activity plays a role in precipitating mesangial proliferation. Mesangial proliferation leads to the classic clinical

findings of MPGN: hematuria, proteinuria, and a reduction in glomerular filtration.

To understand the second mechanism of MPGN, it is necessary to understand normal function of the alternative pathway (AP) of complement (see Figure 19.8). Through this pathway, complement is activated as part of innate immunity, in the absence of immune complexes. C3b (produced by spontaneous hydrolysis of C3) is the first protein of the AP. It reacts with factor B and properdin to form the AP C3 convertase (C3bBb). As in the classic pathway, the C3 convertase cleaves C3 to C3a and C3b. This step is known as the amplification loop of the AP. This amplification loop facilitates accelerated cleavage of additional C3. Additional C3b molecules combine with the AP C3 convertase to form the AP C5 convertase (C3bBbC3b). The end-result of AP activation is also MAC and anaphylatoxin production.

The second pathologic mechanism for MPGN involves an underlying primary complement abnormality. In this instance, injury is not associated with activation of the classic pathway of complement but results from dysregulation of the AP. The final steps are the same: formation of complement breakdown products, anaphylatoxin, and the terminal complement complex (C5b-9). However, the underlying initiating event of disease is the loss of normal control of the AP leading to uncontrolled AP activity. Dysregulation of the AP may be primarily at the C3 convertase (presence of circulating C3 nephritic factors), at the C5 convertase or terminal complement pathway (denoted by elevated C5b-9), or both. Because the AP has an amplification loop,

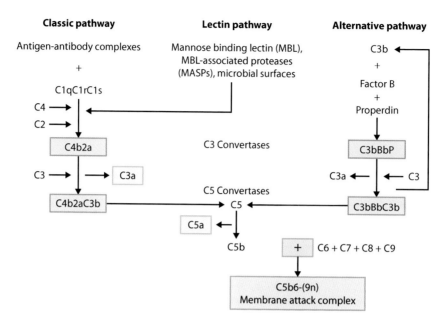

Figure 19.8 The complement cascade. The classical pathway, lectin pathway and the alternative pathway generate C3 convertase. Downstream complement activation eventually leads to the formation of the membrane attack complex (MAC).

uncontrolled activity can result in marked complement activity.

Two important discoveries have helped define the underlying disease mechanism in the second scenario. The first was the discovery of the C3 nephritic factors.[38] C3 nephritic factors are antibodies that bind to and prevent the normal breakdown of the AP C3 convertase, leading to AP dysregulation (Figure 19.9). The interaction of C3 nephritic factors with the AP C3 convertase leads to a constantly activated state of the AP.[38–41] A more active AP leads to an amplified production of C3 breakdown products. C3 breakdown products are deposited on the glomerular basement membrane, triggering a cascade of complement inflammatory responses. Why some patients develop circulating C3 nephritic factor remains unknown. C3 nephritic factors are present in up to 50% of MPGN I patients and in as many as 85% of patients with DDD.[25,42–44] C3 nephritic factors have been reported in 45% of C3GN patients.[14]

Genetic complement abnormalities also play an important role in the pathogenesis of MPGN, although these occur with less frequency than C3 nephritic factors. Both familial and sporadic forms of genetic complement abnormalities are well-documented in MPGN.[17–19,21,25,45,46] One large cohort found that genetic mutations in the complement regulatory proteins factor H (CFH), factor I (CFI), or membrane cofactor protein (MCP) were present in 16.8%, 17.2%, and 19.6% of idiopathic MPGN I, DDD, and C3GN patients, respectively. The association of gene mutations of complement regulatory proteins and MPGN has been substantiated in multiple ethnic groups.[24,47–51] Mutations in the complement factor H–related proteins CFHR1, CFHR3, and CFHR5 have been implicated in C3GN.[15,16,18,52] These mutations are primarily present in proteins that normally regulate the AP, and their impact is likely via dysregulation of

the AP. Consistent with the relative low frequency of genetic abnormalities in this disease population, there are very few reports of multiple family members being affected.

## CLINICAL MANIFESTATIONS

Clinical manifestations of MPGN vary, depending on the severity of the disease (see Table 19.3). Idiopathic MPGN often presents with high-grade proteinuria, nephrotic syndrome, hypertension, and glomerular hematuria (see Table 19.2).[1,7,9,35,42,53–56] MPGN accounts for more than 7% of children and 12% of adults with idiopathic nephrotic syndrome. Gross hematuria can simulate clinical features of poststreptococcal glomerulonephritis in some at initial presentation. Hypocomplementemia, with low C3 is common, but C4 also may be low in an occasional patient. Respiratory illness may precede onset in some patients with MPGN. Children tend to have a more acute presentation and a slower decline in renal function than adults. Rapidly progressive disease is also well described in children. In contrast to adults, children are more likely to have hematuria at onset and less likely to have renal insufficiency.[42] Hypertension is present in half of children at presentation, and renal dysfunction occurs in 25% to 50% of patients.

Clinical manifestations of the different types of MPGN are indistinguishable on presentation. Patients with DDD may have unique chronic clinical complications. These patients may have ophthalmologic findings of drusen, which are electron-dense deposits in the retina between the collagenous layer of the Bruch membrane and the retinal pigmented epithelial cells.[57] Presence of drusen carries an approximately 10% risk for long-term visual problems.[58]

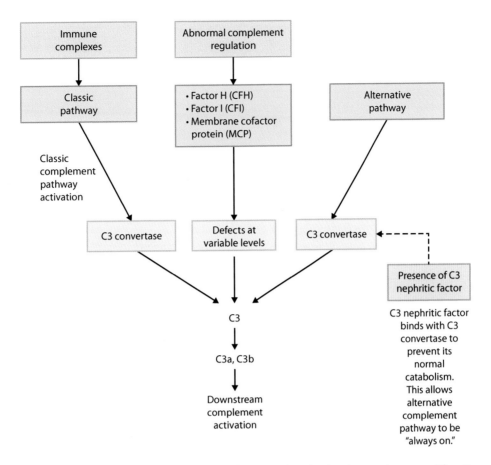

Figure 19.9 Pathogenesis of complement pathway dysregulation and activation in membranoproliferative glomerulone-phritis (MPGN). Inherited defects of complement pathways that are associated with MPGN are listed but are not shown in relation to the site of their dysregulation.

Occasionally, patients with DDD also develop acquired partial lipodystrophy, a disease characterized by the loss of fat from the face, neck, shoulders, arms, forearms and thorax.[58] Lower extremities are generally spared.

---

## KEY POINTS

- Despite morphologic subtypes, clinical manifestations of MPGN are indistinguishable.
- MPGN can manifest with gross hematuria, proteinuria, and low serum complement C3 level features that can be mistaken for poststreptococcal glomerulonephritis.
- Nephrotic syndrome, hypertension, and renal dysfunction are common findings of MPGN.

## EVALUATION

Renal biopsy with light microscopy, immunofluorescence, and electron microscopy studies establishes the diagnosis of MPGN and allows its classification into the subtypes of MPGN I, MPGN II, or MPGN III. Further investigations are generally guided by the patient's exposure history, potential comorbid conditions, and clinical examination. The goal of the workup is to determine if there is an underlying or treatable disease process. For instance, identifying systemic lupus erythromatosus or a monoclonal gammopathy in a patient with MPGN offers a specific treatment target.[59] Although diseases that are associated with MPGN (see Table 19.1) may be considered, a practical approach includes a much more limited laboratory evaluation (Table 19.4, top). If no associated disease is identified, the patient's disease is labeled idiopathic MPGN and treatment will be based on current knowledge about its treatment and response to therapy. Care must be taken to rule out a postinfectious glomerulonephritis (PIGN) process as the cause of MPGN. Postinfectious MPGN is most often a self-limited glomerular disease that requires only supportive care. Whereas extreme presentations of PIGN may require immunosuppression and renal replacement, this presentation is unusual enough that it should trigger close follow-up to ensure that the diagnosis is not actually idiopathic MPGN that was triggered by an infection.

As a result of our better understanding of the role of complement in the pathogenesis of MPGN and related diseases, and with the publication of the C3G consensus statement,

Table 19.4 Evaluation of patients with membranoproliferative glomerulonephritis*

| Immunoglobulin dominant immunostaining | | |
|---|---|---|
| **Infection** | **Organ dysfunction** | **Immune abnormality** |
| HCV, HBV, HIV | Liver function studies | ANA, ANCA, ENA |
| ASO | Chest x-ray | Rheumatoid factor |
| Tick-borne viral studies | Renal ultrasound | Cryoglobulins |
| Blood cultures | Protein electrophoresis | C3, C4, CH50 |
| | | C3 nephritic factor |
| **Evaluating MPGN with C3 Dominant† Immunostaining** | | |
| Autoantibodies and protein deficiencies | Serum complement activity assays | Screen for genetic variants and/or copy number variation |
| C3 nephritic factors | Alternative pathway function | CFH |
| FHAA | | CFI |
| FBAA | C3 breakdown products | MCP |
| FH level | C5 breakdown products | C3 |
| FB level | | CFB |
| Properdin level | Terminal complement cascade activity | CFHR1-5 |
| CD46 expression on leukocytes | Hemolytic assay | Copy number variation in the CFH-CFHR region |
| Western blot for FHR proteins | | |

* The investigations for immunoglobulin dominant forms are designed to identify secondary associations (see Table 19.1) that may influence a treatment plan. The workup of C3 dominant glomerulonephritis remains the most controversial and is likely to change as the pathologic mechanisms behind disease become better defined.
† Dominant refers to 2 orders of magnitude over other positive stains.
ANA, antinuclear antibody; ANCA, anticytoplasmic autoantibody; ENA, extractible nuclear antigens; C4, complement C4; CH50, classical pathway 50% activity; FHAA, factor H autoantibody; FBAA, factor B autoantibody; CFH, factor H, CFI, factor I; MCP, membrane cofactor protein; CFI, factor I; CFHR1-5, complement factor H related 1, 3, 3, 4 and 5.

recommendations are to evaluate the patient according to the specificity of immune staining on immunofluorescence.[13] Accordingly, if the patient has a predominant C3 deposition pattern on immunofluorescence, the assumption is that the patient's disease is driven by an abnormal complement system. In this case, it is appropriate to assess complement proteins and genes to define the disease pathogenesis. Table 19.4 (bottom) outlines a comprehensive complement system evaluation. Although this workup serves to further define a given patient's pathologic process and complement abnormality, the absence of approved, directed therapeutics (unapproved anticomplement therapy to be discussed later) limits the clinical usefulness of this workup at this time. It is anticipated, however, that understanding the underlying pathologic condition will allow directed therapy in the near future.

It is worth noting that C3 predominance is often present by immunofluorescence in a patient with PIGN who requires a kidney biopsy (as is low peripheral C3 at presentation). Most often, knowledge of the clinical course will facilitate separation from C3G. If there is confusion, per consensus, PIGN is ruled out by a steady improvement of glomerular signs and normalization of the peripheral C3

over the subsequent 12 weeks. If either is still abnormal after 12 weeks, it is appropriate to reassign the patient's diagnosis to C3G and continue to follow the patient for chronic glomerulonephritis.

## TREATMENT

The treatment of the secondary MPGNs is dictated by the cause. In some cases, the focus is treating the primary disease while monitoring the kidney response to this primary therapy. In cases of MPGN associated with lupus nephritis, treatment is guided by trial data and based on the histologic class of lupus. Finally, in other cases, a standard approach to a proliferative glomerulonephritis (e.g., high-dose steroids) may be used. Treatment of idiopathic MPGN has not been uniformly satisfying, and available options are based primarily on retrospective reviews and case reports. No up-to-date randomized controlled trials are available to guide care. The small number of patients studied and the relatively short follow-up time further compromise the usefulness of available data. Finally, because most trials, to date, included patients with all three types of MPGN (and patients with C3G), analysis of treatment results are likely to be confounded.

Treatment strategies for idiopathic MPGN have included corticosteroids, immunosuppressive agents, antiplatelet regimens, plasma exchange, and biologic agents. As with all glomerular diseases, patients should receive therapy to maintain a normal blood pressure and minimize proteinuria using angiotensin-converting enzyme inhibitors or angiotensin receptor blockers. In addition, growth and development should be monitored closely, with a focus on appropriate chronic kidney disease markers and nutrition.

> ## KEY POINTS
>
> - There is no clear consensus on the treatment of MPGN.
> - The International Study of Kidney Diseases (ISKD) protocol for alternate-day steroids for 2 years or more is often used in children.
> - The value of steroid-sparing therapies has yet to be confirmed in randomized controlled trials.

## CORTICOSTEROIDS

Retrospective and prospective studies have demonstrated a beneficial effect of steroid therapy on renal survival in pediatric patients with MPGN.[60,61] Steroid use was tested in the International Study of Kidney Disease in Children trial (ISKDC), a prospective, multicenter, randomized trial of 80 children, with predominantly type I MPGN (before the new classification), heavy proteinuria, and glomerular filtration rates of 70 mL/min/1.73 m² or greater.[62] The patients were randomized to receive either 40 mg/m² of prednisone every other day or placebo for a mean duration of treatment of 41 months. Treatment failure (30% increase in serum creatinine) occurred less frequently (40%) in patients treated with prednisone than in those who received placebo (55%). Of the treatment group, 61% versus 12% of the placebo group had stable renal function at the end of the study. Similar results have been reported in the combined adult and pediatric cohorts.[63] It is unclear what impact a presumed heterogeneous population of patients may have had on treatment outcome. It is important to note that the reported success of steroid use in MPGN involves alternate-day therapy, used for 24 to 40 months.[60,62] Nonetheless, steroids remain the mainstay of therapy for MPGN. Because treatment failures were as high as 40%, and because a protracted course of steroid therapy is not without adverse effects, other treatment options have been evaluated. Particularly, it appears that non-nephrotic children may forego steroid treatment without compromising long-term kidney function.[26]

## ANTICOAGULANTS

Anticoagulants (heparin, warfarin, aspirin, dipyridamole), combined with or without steroids have been inconsistently successful, and long-term benefit has not been established.[53]

## CYCLOPHOSPHAMIDE

In one study, 19 pediatric and adult patients with MPGN were treated with a prolonged regimen of pulse methylprednisolone, oral prednisone, and cyclophosphamide.[27] Of these, 15 achieved complete remission and 3 achieved a partial remission. Despite this success, the side effects of cyclophosphamide limit its usefulness as a primary treatment agent. In practice, cyclophosphamide is generally reserved for patients with rapidly progressive renal failure or a recent deterioration in renal function, especially those with crescentic histopathology.

## MYCOPHENOLATE MOFETIL

Mycophenolate mofetil (MMF) is an inosine monophosphate dehydrogenase inhibitor, which inhibits the proliferation of T and B cells. Such an inhibitory action is expected to limit inflammatory reaction in the kidney, particularly as it applies to anaphylatoxin response. MMF was proposed for the treatment of MPGN as a steroid-sparing option. Few data exist to determine MMF's efficacy as a primary agent, but MMF is being increasingly used for treating patients with other forms of immune-mediated renal disease, particularly those resistant to steroids.[64] In idiopathic MPGN, preliminary studies suggest that the combination of MMF and corticosteroids can, in the short term, reduce proteinuria and may preserve renal function.[28,29]

## CYCLOSPORINE

The role of calcineurin inhibitors for treating idiopathic MPGN is unclear. Two studies have suggested there may be some benefit from cyclosporine, particularly if high-grade proteinuria is present.[65,66] Bagheri et al.[67] used cyclosporine to treat 18 patients with MPGN who were resistant to steroids, aspirin, and dipyridamole. Long-term reductions in proteinuria with preservation of renal function were observed in 17 of the patients, suggesting that cyclosporine can be considered in corticosteroid-resistant primary MPGN.

## PLASMA EXCHANGE

The data for plasma therapy in MPGN I are limited. Plasma therapy for C3GN is supported by data derived from experimental animal models.[68,69] Support for effectiveness in humans comes from a handful of case reports.[21,70,71] As a treatment strategy in humans, plasma therapy has appeal either as a mechanism for removing abnormal disease-causing proteins (i.e., C3 nephritic factors), or replacing deficient proteins (e.g., genetic complement factor H deficiency). A number of issues make this a less palatable option. Among the deterrents to the routine use of this therapy are (1) the fact that the vast majority of patients with MPGN do not have genetic mutations causing protein deficiencies, (2) we lack scientific proof that reducing the C3 nephritic titer is protective of renal health, and (3) the risks of placing a catheter, especially given the lack of evidence for effectiveness. Currently, plasma therapy remains a fourth- or fifth-line consideration for the treatment of MPGN.

## RITUXIMAB

Rituximab, a chimeric IgG1 monoclonal antibody that specifically targets the CD20 surface antigen expressed on B lymphocytes, has been considered for the treatment of MPGN. Similar to plasma therapy, the purported mechanism relates to the reduction of an abnormal complement-related circulating protein.[72] Few convincing examples of its success, however, are reported in the literature.[73]

## ECULIZUMAB

Over the last decade, great advances have been made in our understanding of the complement-mediated renal diseases such as C3G and, to a lesser extent, MPGN. Given the role of complement dysregulation in the pathogenesis of these diseases, anticomplement treatment makes theoretical sense. A therapeutic role for eculizumab, an anti-C5 therapy (i.e., anti-C5a and anti-C5b) is supported by a number of case reports, especially in C3G.[50,74-76] The larger of these reports was a prospective, uncontrolled trial in six adults with native or recurrent post-transplant DDD or C3GN.[50] At the conclusion of a 1-year course of eculizumab, a clinical improvement was observed in three of the patients. Alternatively, a handful of reports have cataloged the failure of eculizumab in C3G.[76] Eculizumab is currently not approved by the U.S. Food and Drug Administration for MPGN or C3G, and the expense of this agent limits its availability off label. Trial data to support its efficacy are required to determine the role of eculizumab in the treatment of MPGN

## OUTCOME

The natural history of MPGN is variable. Some patients appear to have a single nephritic-nephrotic episode followed by relative preservation of their kidney function and minimal, if any, residual signs of glomerular disease, such

> ### KEY POINTS
>
> - MPGN has a high recurrence rate in kidney transplants.
> - Histologic recurrence of DDD (MPGN II), without significant clinical manifestations, is common.

as hematuria, proteinuria, and hypertension.[77-79] More frequently, patients have a chronic relapsing and remitting course of nephritis and nephrotic syndrome. Progression to end-stage renal disease (ESRD) is common, regardless of MPGN subtype.[1,7,42,43,80,81] Unfortunately, it is not possible to predict who will progress to ESRD. Habib et al. suggested that crescents or significant kidney dysfunction at presentation increases the risk for progression to ESRD.[1,14,82] In a small cohort of children, severe tubulointerstitial damage was the best predictor of outcome.[83] Others have failed to document a relationship with presentation and disease progression.[84] Reports have been variable regarding outcomes in relation to treatment regimens employed.[14]

## TRANSPLANT

Given the presumed heterogeneity of the historical MPGN populations, it is not surprising that the post-transplant recurrence estimate is difficult to establish. Historical estimates have ranged from 2% to 20% for MPGN. Higher estimates are reported for DDD.[85] The North American Pediatric Renal Transplant Cooperative Study performed a retrospective cohort study of 8000 pediatric transplant recipients (including 75 children with DDD); 11 of 29 grafts lost in patients with DDD patients were due to DDD recurrence. Histologic recurrence of DDD is reported to be as high as in 90% patients. Higher estimates of recurrence have been reported in more contemporary cohorts of MPGN, making MPGN one of the more common glomerular diseases to recur in kidney transplants.[42,86-92]

## COMPLICATIONS

The complications that result from MPGN disease are primarily related to the features of chronic glomerular disease and include chronic kidney disease, effects on growth, hypertension, bone health, and cardiac status. In patients treated with immunosuppression, each of the immune suppressants comes with its own set of cautions and side effects (e.g., infertility, cystitis, bone changes, gum and renal abnormalities, risk for cancer). The use of these agents in this setting is not unique to their use in other settings, with the exception that patients with significant renal dysfunction may have accentuated side effects of agents that are classically renally excreted.

## SUMMARY

MPGN comprises a heterogeneous group of diseases that share distinct kidney biopsy pathologic findings. MPGN is an important renal disease in children. Progressive renal disease is common, with approximately 50% renal survival at 10 years in some affected children. Idiopathic MPGN is more common in children and young adults, whereas MPGN lesions are more commonly secondary to chronic infections in adults. New insights into the role of complement regulation in renal injury are adding to our understanding of the cause of injury in the C3G subcategory of MPGN. Randomized control trials for the treatment of MPGN are limited, and the mainstay of therapy includes standard renal protective agents (antihypertensive and antiproteinuric treatments). Small cohort studies guide adding anticellular immunosuppression. More data are required for the use of anticomplement therapy in patients with C3G. Transplant recurrence is frequent. Genetic studies currently do not have a clinical role, but in the future may help define targeted therapies.

### Clinical Vignette 19.1

An 8-year-old boy presented with a 2-week history of fatigue and poor appetite and 5-day history of intermittent painless gross hematuria. He had no history of rash or joint pains. The review of systems was otherwise negative, with no history of recent infections. His medical history was negative for any illness.

Physical examination was significant for a moderately ill–appearing boy who was afebrile, with a blood pressure of 124/88 mm Hg. Lung, abdomen, skin, and joint examinations were normal. The patient had 1+ edema of ankles bilaterally. The urine was tea colored, and was positive for blood and protein. The urine protein-to-creatinine ratio was 2.0 His serum creatinine was 1.8 mg/dL, and serum albumin was 1.8 g/dL (normal 3.8 to 5.4 g/dL). Complement C3 was 14 mg/dL (normal greater than 90 mg/dL), and C4 was normal. Antinuclear antibody, antineutrophil cytoplasmic antibodies, and antistreptolysin were negative. Epstein-Barr virus and cytomegalovirus polymerase chain reaction results were negative. Because of rising serum creatinine and evolving oliguria, a renal biopsy was done and revealed diffuse proliferative changes and a lobulated appearance of the glomerular capillary loops. Silver staining revealed "tram-track" appearance of the glomerular basement membrane. There was no evidence of chronic tubulointerstitial damage. Immunofluorescence staining showed an isolated C3 deposition along the capillary loops, and electron microscopy demonstrated findings of diffuse foot process effacement, subepithelial deposits, with an occasional "hump," and subendothelial electron-dense deposits. Tuboreticular inclusions were absent. The biopsy was consistent with MPGN .

The patient was treated with three daily doses of pulse intravenous methylprednisolone (10 mg/kg/doses) and then continued on high-dose steroids for 1 month. Over the subsequent 6 weeks, his C3 values increased, at 63 mg/dL at 2 weeks and 74 mg/dL at 3 weeks; the levels remained at low normal for the next 6 months. After 1 month of high-dose steroids, he was placed on a weaning dose of oral steroids to complete his course of immune suppression by 12 weeks after presentation. The patient was followed in clinic for 2 years with no recurrence of gross hematuria, proteinuria, or hypertension. His serum creatinine returned to normal by 3 months after presentation (0.4 mg/dL), and his ratio of urine protein to creatinine returned to normal by 12 months. Microscopic hematuria persisted for 12 months.

### TEACHING POINTS

- This clinical case makes several important points relevant to the diagnosis and management of patients with MPGN.
- This patient simulated the clinical manifestations of poststreptococcal glomerulonephritis, which is the most common cause of hypocomplementemic acute glomerulonephritis in children. Although this patient did not have history of preceding infectious event before onset of gross hematuria, many patients with MPGN have history or laboratory evidence of recent viral or even streptococcal infection.
- Advancing acute kidney injury and progressive proteinuria, as was the case in this patient, should suggest the possible diagnosis of MPGN in a hypocomplementemic patient with glomerulonephritis. Indeed, these clinical findings led to his renal biopsy and eventual diagnosis of MPGN. The renal biopsy showed a proliferative glomerulonephritis with subepithelial and subendothelial C3 immune deposits.
- Interestingly, the biopsy also showed subepithelial "humps," indicating that a postinfectious onset could not be completely ruled out.
- A normal serum C4 and ANA points away from the diagnosis of systemic lupus erythematosus, in which a diffuse proliferative picture can also be seen in the renal biopsy. Often, patients with MPGN may continue to demonstrate low to low-normal levels of complement level for an extended time, as was the case in this patient.
- Given the acute oliguric presentation and renal dysfunction, intravenous steroids were used to treat this patient. Those with persistent hypocomplementemia and proteinuria can be considered for alternate-day, long-term steroid therapy, per the ISKDC protocol.

# REFERENCES

1. Habib R, Gubler MC, Loirat C, et al. Dense deposit disease: A variant of membranoproliferative glomerulonephritis. Kidney Int. 1975;7:204–15.

2. Walker PD, Ferrario F, Joh K, et al. Dense deposit disease is not a membranoproliferative glomerulonephritis. Mod Pathol. 2007;20:605–16.

3. Sibley RK, Kim Y. Dense intramembranous deposit disease: New pathologic features. Kidney Int. 1984;25:660–70.

4. Razzaque MS, Yamaguchi K, Taguchi T. An unusual case of dense deposit disease with nodular sclerotic lesions of the glomeruli. Clin Nephrol. 1999;51:326–8.

5. Joh K, Aizawa S, Matsuyama N, et al. Morphologic variations of dense deposit disease: Light and electron microscopic, immunohistochemical and clinical findings in 10 patients. Acta Pathol Jpn. 1993;43:552–65.

6. The Southwest Pediatric Nephrology Study Group. Dense deposit disease in children: Prognostic value of clinical and pathologic indicators. Am J Kidney Dis. 1985;6:161–9.

7. Davis AE, Schneeberger EE, Grupe WE, et al. Membranoproliferative glomerulonephritis (MPGN type I) and dense deposit disease (DDD) in children. Clin Nephrol. 1978;9:184–93.

8. Belgiojoso GB, Tarantino A, Bazzi C, et al. Immunofluorescence patterns in chronic membranoproliferative glomerulonephritis (MPGN). Clin Nephrol. 1976;6:303–10.

9. Burkholder PM, Bradford WD. Proliferative glomerulonephritis in children: A correlation of varied clinical and pathologic patterns utilizing light, immunofluorescence, and electron microscopy. Am J Pathol. 1969;56:423–67.

10. Jenis EH, Sandler P, Hill GS, et al. Glomerulonephritis with basement membrane dense deposits. Arch Pathol. 1974;97:84–91.

11. Kim Y, Vernier RL, Fish AJ, et al. Immunofluorescence studies of dense deposit disease: The presence of railroad tracks and mesangial rings. Lab Invest. 1979;40:474–80.

12. West CD, Witte DP, McAdams AJ. Composition of nephritic factor-generated glomerular deposits in membranoproliferative glomerulonephritis type 2. Am J Kidney Dis. 2001;37:1120–30.

13. Pickering MC, D'Agati VD, Nester CM, et al. C3 glomerulopathy: Consensus report. Kidney Int. 2013;84:1079–89.

14. Servais A, Noel LH, Roumenina LT, et al. Acquired and genetic complement abnormalities play a critical role in dense deposit disease and other C3 glomerulopathies. Kidney Int. 2012;82:454–64.

15. Gale DP, de Jorge EG, Cook HT, et al. Identification of a mutation in complement factor H-related protein 5 in patients of Cypriot origin with glomerulonephritis. Lancet 2010;376:794–801.

16. Athanasiou Y, Voskarides K, Gale DP, et al. Familial C3 glomerulopathy associated with CFHR5 mutations: Clinical characteristics of 91 patients in 16 pedigrees. Clin J Am Soc Nephrol. 2011;6:1436–46.

17. Martinez-Barricarte R, Heurich M, Valdes-Canedo F, et al. Human C3 mutation reveals a mechanism of dense deposit disease pathogenesis and provides insights into complement activation and regulation. J Clin Invest. 2010;120:3702–12.

18. Malik TH, Lavin PJ, Goicoechea de Jorge E, et al. A hybrid CFHR3-1 gene causes familial C3 glomerulopathy. J Am Soc Nephrol. 2012;23:1155–60.

19. Tortajada A, Yebenes H, Abarrategui-Garrido C, et al. C3 glomerulopathy-associated CFHR1 mutation alters FHR oligomerization and complement regulation. J Clin Invest. 2013;123:2434–46.

20. Medjeral-Thomas N, Malik TH, Patel MP, et al. A novel CFHR5 fusion protein causes C3 glomerulopathy in a family without Cypriot ancestry. Kidney Int. 2014;85:933–7.

21. Licht C, Heinen S, Jozsi M, et al. Deletion of Lys224 in regulatory domain 4 of factor H reveals a novel pathomechanism for dense deposit disease (MPGN II). Kidney Int. 2006;70:42–50.

22. Servais A, Fremeaux-Bacchi V, Lequintrec M, et al. Primary glomerulonephritis with isolated C3 deposits: A new entity which shares common genetic risk factors with haemolytic uraemic syndrome. J Med Genet. 2007;44:193–9.

23. Sethi S, Nester CM, Smith RJ. Membranoproliferative glomerulonephritis and C3 glomerulopathy: Resolving the confusion. Kidney Int. 2012;81:434–41.

24. Sethi S, Fervenza FC, Zhang Y, et al. C3 glomerulonephritis: Clinicopathological findings, complement abnormalities, glomerular proteomic profile, treatment, and follow-up. Kidney Int. 2012;82:465–73.

25. Servais A, Noel LH, Fremeaux-Bacchi V, et al. C3 glomerulopathy. Contrib Nephrol. 2013;181:185–93.

26. Pickering M, Cook HT. Complement and glomerular disease: New insights. Curr Opin Nephrol Hypertens. 2011;20:271–7.

27. Golay V, Trivedi M, Abraham A, et al. The spectrum of glomerular diseases in a single center: A clinicopathological correlation. Indian J Nephrol. 2013;23:168–75.

28. Nawaz Z, Mushtaq F, Mousa D, et al. Pattern of glomerular disease in the Saudi population: A single-center, five-year retrospective study. Saudi J Kidney Dis Transpl. 2013;24:1265–70.

29. Kawamura T, Usui J, Kaseda K, et al. Primary membranoproliferative glomerulonephritis on the decline: Decreased rate from the 1970s to the 2000s in Japan. Clin Exp Nephrol. 2013;17:248–54.

30. Swaminathan S, Leung N, Lager DJ, et al. Changing incidence of glomerular disease in Olmsted County,

Minnesota: A 30-year renal biopsy study. Clin J Am Soc Nephrol. 2006;1:483–7.

31. Braden GL, Mulhern JG, O'Shea MH, et al. Changing incidence of glomerular diseases in adults. Am J Kidney Dis. 2000;35:878–83.

32. Maisonneuve P, Agodoa L, Gellert R, et al. Distribution of primary renal diseases leading to end-stage renal failure in the United States, Europe, and Australia/New Zealand: Results from an international comparative study. Am J Kidney Dis. 2000;35:157–65.

33. Hanko JB, Mullan RN, O'Rourke DM, et al. The changing pattern of adult primary glomerular disease. Nephrol Dial Transplant. 2009;24:3050–4.

34. Briganti EM, Dowling J, Finlay M, et al. The incidence of biopsy-proven glomerulonephritis in Australia. Nephrol Dial Transplant. 2001;16:1364–7.

35. Study Group of the Spanish Society of Nephrology. Decreasing incidence of membranoproliferative glomerulonephritis in Spanish children. Pediatr Nephrol. 1990;4:266–7.

36. Iitaka K, Saka T, Yagisawa K, et al. Decreasing hypocomplementemia and membranoproliferative glomerulonephritis in Japan. Pediatr Nephrol 2000;14:794–6.

37. West CD. Idiopathic membranoproliferative glomerulonephritis in childhood. Pediatr Nephrol. 1992;6:96–103.

38. Daha MR, Fearon DT, Austen KF. C3 nephritic factor (C3NeF): Stabilization of fluid phase and cell-bound alternative pathway convertase. J Immunol. 1976;116:1–7.

39. Scott DM, Amos N, Sissons JG, et al. The immunogloblin nature of nephritic factor (NeF). Clin Exp Immunol. 1978;32:12–24.

40. Thompson RA. C3 inactivating factor in the serum of a patient with chronic hypocomplementaemic proliferative glomerulo-nephritis. Immunology. 1972;22:147–58.

41. Spitzer RE, Vallota EH, Forristal J, et al. Serum C3 lytic system in patients with glomerulonephritis. Science. 1969;164:436–7.

42. Cameron JS, Turner DR, Heaton J, et al. Idiopathic mesangiocapillary glomerulonephritis: Comparison of types I and II in children and adults and long-term prognosis. Am J Med. 1983;74:175–92.

43. Swainson CP, Robson JS, Thomson D, MacDonald MK. Mesangiocapillary glomerulonephritis: A long-term study of 40 cases. J Pathol. 1983;141:449–68.

44. Schwertz R, Rother U, Anders D, et al. Complement analysis in children with idiopathic membranoproliferative glomerulonephritis: A long-term follow-up. Pediatr Allergy Immunol. 2001;12:166–72.

45. Pickering MC, Cook HT. Translational mini-review series on complement factor H: Renal diseases associated with complement factor H—Novel insights from humans and animals. Clin Exp Immunol. 2008;151:210–30.

46. Wong EK, Anderson HE, Herbert AP, et al. Characterization of a factor H mutation that perturbs the alternative pathway of complement in a family with membranoproliferative GN. J Am Soc Nephrol. 2014;25:2425–33.

47. Xiao X, Pickering MC, Smith RJ. C3 glomerulopathy: The genetic and clinical findings in dense deposit disease and C3 glomerulonephritis. Semin Thromb Hemost. 2014;40:465–71.

48. Servais A, Noel LH, Dragon-Durey MA, et al. Heterogeneous pattern of renal disease associated with homozygous factor H deficiency. Hum Pathol. 2011;42:1305–11.

49. Vaziri-Sani F, Holmberg L, Sjoholm AG, et al. Phenotypic expression of factor H mutations in patients with atypical hemolytic uremic syndrome. Kidney Int. 2006;69:981–8.

50. Bomback AS, Smith RJ, Barile GR, et al. Eculizumab for dense deposit disease and C3 glomerulonephritis. Clin J Am Soc Nephrol. 2012;7:748–56.

51. Alper CA, Abramson N, Johnston RB, Jr, et al. Increased susceptibility to infection associated with abnormalities of complement-mediated functions and of the third component of complement (C3). N Engl J Med. 1970;282:350–4.

52. Neary J, Dorman A, Campbell E, et al. Familial membranoproliferative glomerulonephritis type III. Am J Kidney Dis. 2002;40:E1.

53. Donadio JV, Jr, Slack TK, Holley KE, et al. DM. Idiopathic membranoproliferative (mesangiocapillary) glomerulonephritis: A clinicopathologic study. Mayo Clin Proc. 1979;54:141–50.

54. Bohle A, Gartner HV, Fischbach H, et al. The morphological and clinical features of membranoproliferative glomerulonephritis in adults. Virchows Arch A Pathol Anat Histol. 1974;363:213–24.

55. Lu DF, Moon M, Lanning LD, et al. Clinical features and outcomes of 98 children and adults with dense deposit disease. Pediatr Nephrol. 2012;27:773–81.

56. Park SJ, Kim YJ, Ha TS, et al. Dense deposit disease in Korean children: A multicenter clinicopathologic study. J Korean Med Sci. 2012;27:1215–21.

57. Duvall-Young J, MacDonald MK, McKechnie NM. Fundus changes in (type II) mesangiocapillary glomerulonephritis simulating drusen: A histopathological report. Br J Ophthalmol. 1989;73:297–302.

58. Appel GB, Cook HT, Hageman G, et al. Membranoproliferative glomerulonephritis type II (dense deposit disease): An update. J Am Soc Nephrol. 2005;16:1392–403.

59. Sethi S, Fervenza FC. Membranoproliferative glomerulonephritis: A new look at an old entity. N Engl J Med. 2012;366:1119–31.

60. McEnery PT. Membranoproliferative glomerulo-nephritis: The Cincinnati experience—Cumulative renal survival from 1957 to 1989. J Pediatr. 1990;116:S109–14.

61. Ford DM, Briscoe DM, Shanley PF, et al. Childhood membranoproliferative glomerulonephritis type I: Limited steroid therapy. Kidney Int. 1992;41:1606–12.

62. Tarshish P, Bernstein J, Tobin JN, et al. Treatment of mesangiocapillary glomerulonephritis with alternate-day prednisone: A report of the International Study of Kidney Disease in Children. Pediatr Nephrol. 1992;6:123–30.

63. Nasr SH, Valeri AM, Appel GB, et al. Dense deposit disease: Clinicopathologic study of 32 pediatric and adult patients. Clin J Am Soc Nephrol. 2009;4:22–32.

64. De S, Al-Nabhani D, Thorner P, et al. Remission of resistant MPGN type I with mycophenolate mofetil and steroids. Pediatr Nephrol. 2009;24:597–600.

65. Singh A, Tejani C, Tejani A. One-center experience with cyclosporine in refractory nephrotic syndrome in children. Pediatr Nephrol. 1999;13:26–32.

66. Erbay B, Karatan O, Duman N, et al. The effect of cyclosporine in idiopathic nephrotic syndrome resistant to immunosuppressive therapy. Transplant Proc. 1988;20:289–92.

67. Bagheri N, Nemati E, Rahbar K, et al. Cyclosporine in the treatment of membranoproliferative glomerulonephritis. Arch Iran Med. 2008;11:26–9.

68. Jansen JH, Hogasen K, Harboe M, Hovig T. In situ complement activation in porcine membranoproliferative glomerulonephritis type II. Kidney Int. 1998;53:331–49.

69. Pickering MC, Cook HT, Warren J, et al. Uncontrolled C3 activation causes membranoproliferative glomerulonephritis in mice deficient in complement factor H. Nat Genet. 2002;31:424–8.

70. McGinley E, Watkins R, McLay A, et al. Plasma exchange in the treatment of mesangiocapillary glomerulonephritis. Nephron. 1985;40:385–90.

71. Oberkircher OR, Enama M, West JC, et al. Regression of recurrent membranoproliferative glomerulonephritis type II in a transplanted kidney after plasmapheresis therapy. Transplant Proc. 1988;20:418–23.

72. Guiard E, Karras A, Plaisier E, et al. Patterns of non-cryoglobulinemic glomerulonephritis with monoclonal Ig deposits: Correlation with IgG subclass and response to rituximab. Clin J Am Soc Nephrol. 2011;6:1609–16.

73. Kattah AG, Fervenza FC, Roccatello D. Rituximab-based novel strategies for the treatment of immune-mediated glomerular diseases. Autoimmun Rev. 2013;12:854–9.

74. Radhakrishnan S, Lunn A, Kirschfink M, et al. Eculizumab and refractory membranoproliferative glomerulonephritis. N Engl J Med. 2012;366:1165–6.

75. Vivarelli M, Pasini A, Emma F. Eculizumab for the treatment of dense-deposit disease. N Engl J Med. 2012;366:1163–5.

76. Daina E, Noris M, Remuzzi G. Eculizumab in a patient with dense-deposit disease. N Engl J Med. 2012;366:1161-3.

77. Marks SD, Rees L. Spontaneous clinical improvement in dense deposit disease. Pediatr Nephrol. 2000;14:322–4.

78. Ikeda M, Honda M, Hasegawa O. Another example of spontaneous improvement in a case of dense deposit disease. Pediatr Nephrol. 2001;16:609–10.

79. West CD, McAdams AJ, Witte DP. Acute non-proliferative glomerulitis: A cause of renal failure unique to children. Pediatr Nephrol. 2000;14:786–93.

80. di Belgiojoso B, Tarantino A, Colasanti G, et al. The prognostic value of some clinical and histological parameters in membranoproliferative glomerulonephritis (MPGN): Report of 112 cases. Nephron. 1977;19:250–8.

81. Somers M, Kertesz S, Rosen S, et al. Non-nephrotic children with membranoproliferative glomerulonephritis: Are steroids indicated? Pediatr Nephrol. 1995;9:140–4.

82. Little MA, Dupont P, Campbell E, et al. Severity of primary MPGN, rather than MPGN type, determines renal survival and post-transplantation recurrence risk. Kidney Int. 2006;69:504–11.

83. Çaltik Yilmaz A, Aydog Ö, Ayküz SG, et al. The relation between treatment and prognosis of childhood membranoproliferative glomerulonephritis. Ren Fail. 2014;36:1221–5.

84. Nasr SH, Valeri AM, Appel GB, et al. Dense deposit disease: Clinicopathologic study of 32 pediatric and adult patients. Clin J Am Soc Nephrol. 2009;4:22–32.

85. Braun MC, Stablein DM, Hamiwka LA, et al. Recurrence of membranoproliferative glomerulonephritis type II in renal allografts: The North American Pediatric Renal Transplant Cooperative Study experience. J Am Soc Nephrol. 2005;16:2225–33.

86. Kotanko P, Pusey CD, Levy JB. Recurrent glomerulonephritis following renal transplantation. Transplantation. 1997;63:1045–52.

87. Mathew TH. Recurrence of disease following renal transplantation. Am J Kidney Dis. 1988;12:85–96.

88. Cameron JS. Recurrent disease in renal allografts. Kidney Int. (Suppl) 1993;43:S91–4.

89. Cameron JS. Recurrent renal disease after renal transplantation. Curr Opin Nephrol Hypertens. 1994;3:602–7.

90. Ramos EL, Tisher CC. Recurrent diseases in the kidney transplant. Am J Kidney Dis. 1994;24:142–54.
91. Hariharan S, Adams MB, Brennan DC, et al. Recurrent and de novo glomerular disease after renal transplantation: A report from Renal Allograft Disease Registry (RADR). Transplant 1999;68:635–41.
92. Lorenz EC, Sethi S, Leung N, et al. Recurrent membranoproliferative glomerulonephritis after kidney transplantation. Kidney Int. 2010;77:721–8.

## REVIEW QUESTIONS

1. What is the *major* distinguishing pathologic feature of the MPGN kidney biopsy?
   a. Immunoglobulin deposition on immunofluorescence
   b. Mesangial interposition into the glomerular basement membrane
   c. Mesangial cell proliferation
   d. Podocyte effacement
2. Why was the name MPGN II changed to dense deposit disease?
   a. Only 25% of patients actually had MPGN.
   b. MPGN II is the only MPGN with intramembranous deposits.
   c. Dense deposits were the sole disease-defining characteristic.
3. Which is the classic laboratory finding in MPGN patients?
   a. Low platelet count
   b. Hypocomplementemia
   c. Genetic abnormality
   d. Positive bacterial cultures
4. Which of the following is *not* a known cause of secondary MPGN?
   a. Systemic lupus erythematosus
   b. Viral infection
   c. Licorice intoxication
   d. Immunoglobulin deficiency
5. Name the required immune deposit location for dense deposit disease.
   a. Subendothelial deposits
   b. Intramembranous deposits
   c. Subepithelial deposits
   d. Mesangial deposits.
6. What is the ratio of MPGN presentation in children compared to that in adults?
   a. ¼:1
   b. ½:1
   c. ¾:1
   d. 1:1

7. The *most* likely pathologic cause of dense deposit disease is:
   a. A genetic mutation
   b. An autoantibody
   c. A protein inhibitor
   d. An exposure
8. What is the risk for end-stage renal disease for a patient with MPGN?
   a. 25%
   b. 50%
   c. 75%
   d. 100%
9. Of the MPGN diseases, which is the *most* likely to result in end-stage renal disease?
   a. DDD
   b. MPGN I
   c. MPGN III
   d. C3GN
10. What is the risk for recurrence after transplant for MPGN?
    a. 25%
    b. 50%
    c. 75%
    d. 100%
11. Which treatment for MPGN is supported by a randomized controlled trial?
    a. Steroid therapy
    b. None
    c. Mycophenolate mofetil
    d. Rituximab
12. What is the presentation biomarker that is associated with the *greatest* likelihood of advancing to end-stage renal disease?
    a. Proteinuria greater than 2 g
    b. Degree of interstitial fibrosis on presentation biopsy
    c. Degree of creatinine elevation at time of kidney biopsy
    d. Unknown

## ANSWER KEY

1. b
2. a
3. b
4. c
5. b
6. a
7. b
8. b
9. a
10. b
11. a
12. d

# 20

# Membranous nephropathy

GEORGES DESCHÊNES

Membranous nephropathy (MN) is an uncommon disorder in children. It is an immune complex glomerulonephritis characterized by thickened glomerular basement membrane (GBM), presence of subepithelial immune deposits, and lack of cellular proliferation or infiltration within glomeruli.[1] The subepithelial immune deposits always contain immunoglobulin G (IgG) and frequently complement C3.[2] Proteinuria and nephrotic syndrome are the common manifestation of the disease at onset.[3] Although the idiopathic form of the disease is much more common in adults, secondary disorders, such as systemic lupus erythematosus (SLE) and infectious diseases, are common causes of MN in children.[4] This chapter discusses the clinical manifestations, renal biopsy characteristics, etiologies and therapy of children with MN.

was noted to be 22% in children 13 to 19 years of age in whom biopsy was performed for the diagnosis of nephrotic syndrome, suggesting that it might be more common in older children.[10] MN is an uncommon cause of end-stage renal disease (ESRD) in children. The 2013 U.S. Renal Data System data indicate that MN accounted for only 0.6% of pediatric ESRD patients in the United States.[11] There is no gender or racial predilection for childhood MN.[6]

A higher incidence of MN has been formerly reported from endemic geographic regions with a high prevalence of hepatitis B or malarial infection.[9,12] However, with control of hepatitis B with immunization and effective treatment and prevention of malaria, the incidence of MN resulting from these infectious causes appears to be significantly declining.[13,14]

## EPIDEMIOLOGY

MN is an uncommon cause of proteinuria in childhood, while it remains a leading cause of nephrotic syndrome in adults.[5,6] In the International Study of Kidney Disease in Children (ISKDC) MN was seen in only 1.5% of the 521 children with nephrotic syndrome (12 weeks to 16 years).[7] In a Japanese study, 163 children (3 to 15 years) had kidney biopsies to investigate hematuria or proteinuria; the incidence of MN was 6.7%.[8] The incidence of MN among 463 Taiwanese children (younger than 17 years) who underwent biopsy for primary glomerular disease, was 11.7%.[9] In one study from the United States, the incidence of MN

## RENAL PATHOLOGY

### LIGHT AND IMMUNOFLUORESCENCE MICROSCOPY

Thickening of the glomerular wall is the main feature of MN on light microscopy, using trichrome or hematoxylin-eosin staining (Figure 20.1A). Staining with basement membrane stains, such as Jones silver stain or periodic acid–Schiff stain, shows that the GBM is thickened and exhibits argyrophilic projections, known as "spikes" that extend toward the epithelial aspect (see Figure 20.1B). This picture results from the fact that the subepithelial immune deposits sit in

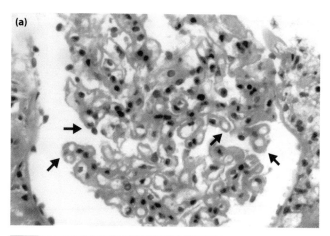

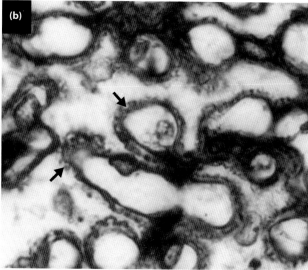

Figure 20.1 (a) Light microscopy (hematoxylin and eosin stain) showing thickened glomerular capillary wall (arrows) in a patient with membranous nephropathy. Absence of cellular or mesangial matrix proliferation is the hallmark of membranous nephropathy. (b) Jones silver–stained renal biopsy showing typical spikes of membranous nephropathy. Arrows point to the site of immune deposits (which do not stain) with proliferation of surrounding glomerular basement membrane giving rise to the morphologic picture of spikes.

between the projections of GBM and are not stained by the GBM stain (Figure 20.2). Glomeruli may be affected in a segmental fashion.

Immunofluorescence shows IgG and C3 deposits along the periphery of the glomerular capillary wall. Primary or idiopathic MN is characterized by deposition of IgG4 and IgG1.[15] In contrast, secondary forms of MN primarily demonstrate IgG1, IgG2, and IgG3 in the immunofluorescence staining.[15,16] Tubular atrophy and interstitial fibrosis can be seen in long-standing and severe disease and correlate with the progression to chronic kidney disease (CKD) and ESRD.[17] Long-standing and progressive MN eventually leads to sclerosis of glomeruli. Immune deposits may be seen in mesangial location, and occasionally crescents may be associated with MN.[18]

## ELECTRON MICROSCOPY

Depending on the duration of the disease, electron microscopy may demonstrate a variable pattern in MN (Figure 20.3).[19] Early MN (stage I) is characterized by finely granular, discontinuous electron-dense deposits that are located along the epithelial aspect of the GBM, under the epithelial cell foot processes. Over time, the GBM proliferates and surrounds the electron-dense deposits (stage II). Basement membrane stains (silver stain) at this stage result in the typical picture of spikes noted in light microscopy. Eventually, GBM proliferation envelopes the electron-dense deposits and incorporates them into the GBM (stage III). Finally, the electron-dense deposits in the GBM demonstrate resorption or dissolution and GBM repair ensues (stage IV). The site of electron-dense deposits in the GBM at this stage is often represented by a scalloped appearance. These stages of evolution of immune deposits in MN are depicted in Figure 20.3 and described in Table 20.1.

---

### KEY POINTS

- The definition of MN relies on the characteristic renal histologic findings.
- Electron microscopy provides histologic staging of the disease.

---

## CLINICAL FEATURES AND DIAGNOSIS

The diagnosis of MN should be suspected in patients with steroid-resistant nephrotic syndrome, especially in those in whom the onset of nephrotic syndrome occurs after 10 years of age. Proteinuria, which can be nephrotic or subnephrotic range, is the clinical hallmark of MN and is associated with low serum albumin in almost all patients.[3,6] Although microscopic hematuria is commonly observed in children with MN, gross hematuria has been described in up to 40% of children with idiopathic MN.[4,6,20] Hypertension at presentation is uncommon in children with MN. Renal function is usually normal at onset in children with MN, but renal dysfunction and development of CKD may be noted during disease progression.[20] Serum complement C3 and C4 are normal in the primary or idiopathic form of MN, but can be low in MN as a result of SLE. Differences between MN in children and adults are summarized in Table 20.2. A secondary cause of MN should be diligently sought in children.

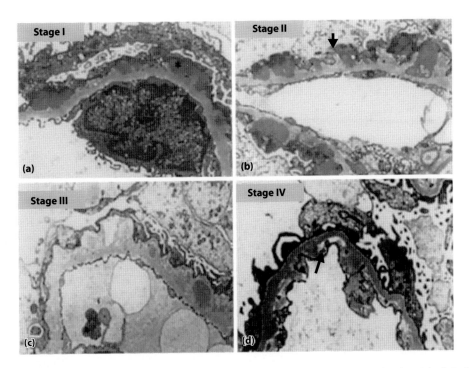

Figure 20.2 Electron microscopy staging of membranous nephropathy. **(a)** Stage 1: Initial subepithelial electron dense-deposits. **(b)** Stage 2: Basement membrane enveloping electron-dense deposits (arrow head). The projection of basement membrane between the deposits gives rise to the characteristic spikes in the silver-stained sections in light microscopy. **(c)** Stage 3: Electron-dense deposits incorporated into the basement membrane. **(d)** Stage 4: Repair of the basement membrane and resolution of the dense deposits, giving rise to scalloped electron-lucent appearance (arrow) along the endothelial aspect of the glomerular basement membrane. (Reproduced with permission from: Yokoyama H, Yoshimoto K, Wada T, et al. Electron-dense deposition patterns and the outcomes of idiopathic membranous nephropathy in Japanese. Med Electron Microsc. 2002;35:81–6.)

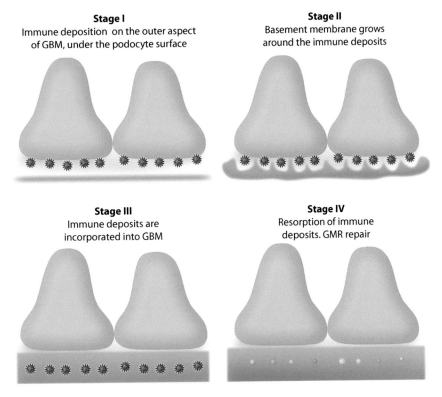

Figure 20.3 A diagrammatic representation of the four stages of membranous nephropathy, demonstrating the life cycle of the subepithelial immune deposits.

Table 20.1 Electron microscopy classification of membranous nephropathy

| Stage | Definition |
|---|---|
| I | Scattered subepithelial deposits without significant thickening of the GBM. Foot process effacement seen. |
| II | Widely distributed subepithelial deposits. Spikes are seen between the electron-dense deposits. The GBM is thickened. |
| III | GBM fuses over the deposits and envelopes them. Deposits become intramembranous in location. |
| IV | Resorption of deposits, leaving behind irregularly thickened lamina densa of the GBM. |

*Source:* Churg J, Sobin LH. Renal disease: classification and atlas of glomerular diseases. Tokyo: Igaku-shoin, 1982, p. 52.
*Abbreviation:* GBM, glomerular basement membrane.

---

## KEY POINTS

- Nephrotic syndrome and proteinuria are hallmarks of MN.
- Gross hematuria is common in children and raises the possibility of associated renal vein thrombosis.

## CAUSES OF MEMBRANOUS NEPHROPATHY

MN is an immune complex glomerulonephritis that exhibits characteristics of an autoimmune disease in adults, as well as in many children. Although most cases are characterized as being idiopathic, discovery of numerous glomerular antigens and circulating antibodies to these antigens has redefined the notion of idiopathic MN. MN in children is often secondary to an underlying disorder. Table 20.3 lists the causes of MN and brief descriptions of some of the common causes of MN are provided in the following section.

## PRIMARY OR IDIOPATHIC

Except in areas where the hepatitis B virus infection is endemic, the primary or idiopathic form of the disease is the most frequently observed etiology in adults.[4] Many patients with the primary or idiopathic MN have an autoimmune disease in which the kidneys are the specific target organ of the autoantibodies (see discussion of pathogenesis).[21] One such target podocyte antigen is phospholipase A2 receptor (PLA2R). Most adult

Table 20.2 Demographic, clinical, and morphologic differences between pediatric and adult forms of membranous nephropathy

| Disease features | Pediatric membranous nephropathy (%) | Adult membranous nephropathy (%) |
|---|---|---|
| **Disease type or subtype** | | |
| Proportion of primary nephrotic syndrome cases that have MN | <5 in younger children and 5–20 in adolescents. | 15–30 |
| MN cases that have primary ("idiopathic") disease | Minority | Majority |
| Proportion of primary MN that is PLA$_2$R-associated | 45 (more common in adolescents) | 70–80 |
| **Demographic and clinical features** | | |
| • Male predominance | Variable | Yes |
| • Nephrotic syndrome | 40–75 | 75 |
| • Hypertension | <10 | 30 |
| • Thromboembolic events | <5 | 10–20 |
| • Spontaneous remission | Common | 30 |
| • Progressive renal impairment | <25 | 30–40 |
| **Pathologic features** | | |
| • Mesangial deposits | Up to 50 | 30 |
| • Segmental distribution of deposits | Occasional | Very rare |

*Source:* Ayalon R, Beck LH Jr. Membranous nephropathy: not just a disease for adults. Pediatr Nephrol. 2015;30:31–9. Reproduced with permission

Table 20.3 Causes of membranous nephropathy

**Primary Membranous glomerular nephritis**
- Autoantibodies to phospholipase A2 Receptor1 (PLA2R1)
- Autoantibodies to thrombospondin type-1 domain-containing 7A (THSD7A)
- Antibodies to cationic bovine serum albumin (cBSA) in children
- Idiopathic (antigen origin unknown at this point)

**Secondary membranous glomerular nephritis**
- Autoimmune diseases
  - Systemic lupus erythematosus
  - Antithyroid antibody mediated
  - Mixed connective tissue disorders
  - Rheumatoid arthritis
  - Sjögren syndrome
- Infectious diseases
  - Hepatitis B infection
  - Malaria
  - Schistosomiasis
  - Syphilis
- Drugs
  - Captopril
  - Nonsteroidal anti-inflammatory drugs (NSAIDs)
  - Gold
  - Probenecid
  - Penicillamine
  - Lithium
  - Mercury
- Malignancy
  - Leukemias
  - Lymphomas
  - Solid organ malignancies
- Miscellaneous disorders
  - Renal transplantation (de novo)
  - Bone marrow transplantation
  - Sickle cell disease

## KEY POINTS

- The most common cause of MN in adults is primary.
- Primary is now characterized as an autoimmune disorder.
- Approximately 70% of patients with primary MN have circulating antibodies against PLA2R, a podocyte antigen.
- cBSA, as a planted antigen, may cause MN in young children.

## SYSTEMIC LUPUS ERYTHEMATOSUS

MN occurs in 20% of the children with SLE nephropathy and may be indistinguishable from the idiopathic MN by light microscopy in the renal biopsy.[24] Mixed proliferative and MN pathology also can be seen in patients with SLE, and clinical manifestations consist of proteinuria and nephrotic syndrome.

## RENAL AND ALLOGENEIC BONE MARROW TRANSPLANTATION

In children, recurrence of MN in a renal allograft has not been reported. By contrast, de novo membranous nephropathy leads to graft loss in 60% of patients.[87] In adults, recurrence of MN in renal transplants has been reported in approximately 30% cases, whereas de novo disease is noted much more commonly in protocol transplant biopsies.[25] The recurrent form of transplant MN occurs early in the course of transplantation and can be associated with graft loss in 50% cases. De novo disease, conversely, occurs later in the transplant course, and may be asymptomatic or associated with mild proteinuria. Hepatitis C infection may be seen in patients with de novo transplant MN.[25] Rarely, MN also has been reported in allogeneic bone marrow transplantation and is usually associated with graft-versus-host disease.[26]

## MEMBRANOUS NEPHROPATHY IN THE NEONATE

MN has been well described in neonates as a result of maternal syphilitic infection.[27] Prematurity, hepatitis and splenomegaly, respiratory distress, skin lesions, especially over the soles and palms, cerebrospinal fluid abnormalities, jaundice, and periostitis are possible findings of neonatal syphilis. When associated with MN, these neonates exhibit massive proteinuria and nephrotic syndrome.[27]

Rarely, neonatal MN also may occur as a result of the placental transfer of anti-neutral endopeptidase (NEP) IgG antibodies from the mother to the fetus. These mothers lack NEP because of gene deletion and have undergone previous alloimmunization because of blood transfusion, prior pregnancy or miscarriage.[28] Patients present early in the neonatal course with severe proteinuria and nephrotic syndrome.

patients (70%) with idiopathic MN have autoantibodies against PLA2R.[22] Whether this antibody test can serve to definitively differentiate primary from secondary forms of MN in adults and children is being investigated.

In children below 5 years of age, cationic bovine serum albumin (cBSA) originating from the trypsin digestion of cow's milk or beef protein in the gut has been linked to the development of MN.[23] It is possible that many of the idiopathic forms of MN will eventually be recognized as autoimmune disorders with glomerular or exogenous antigens serving as the causal triggers for the immune response.

NEP was the first podocyte antigen discovered to be associated MN.

## VIRAL INFECTIONS

Hepatitis B virus (HBV) infection in children is a common cause of MN in some geographic regions of the world where HBV infection is endemic.[9,13] This results from glomerular co-deposition of viral antigens and their cognate antibodies.[9] Universal HBV vaccination of children has led to a decreased incidence of HBV-related MN.[13]

Another viral cause of MN in children is the human immunodeficiency virus (HIV) infection. HIV-associated MN is far less frequent than HIV-associated nephropathy or collapsing glomerulopathy.[29] Epstein-Barr virus (EBV) infection also, rarely, has been reported to be responsible for MN in children.[30]

## DRUGS AND TOXINS

Drugs and toxins can lead to MN. Of the drugs in clinical use, captopril and nonsteroidal anti-inflammatory drugs (NSAIDs) have been well described to cause MN.[31,32] Treatment of adults with rheumatoid arthritis with gold salts has been reported to cause MN.[33] Isolated pediatric cases of MN have been reported after use of D-penicillamine and bucillamine.[33–35]

## PATHOGENESIS OF MEMBRANOUS NEPHROPATHY

Heymann nephritis is an experimental model of MN that has been studied extensively since the 1950s.[36]. In experimental models, as well as in human disease, subepithelial deposition of immune complex formation is the histologic hallmark of MN. The presence of immune complexes in this location sets the stage for complement activation and subsequent podocyte injury. The pathogenesis of subepithelial immune complex formation in experimental and human MN can involve one of the three possible mechanisms discussed in the following section.

### Podocyte antigen–induced in situ immune complex formation

Studies done in the 1970s and1980s demonstrated that circulating antibodies can bind in situ to glomerular antigens in Heymann nephritis and lead to the development of subepithelial immune deposits.[37] These antibodies are thought to traverse the GBM and bind to antigens present on the basal surface of podocytes. In Heyman nephritis, the antibodies bind toGp330, also known as megalin.[38]

Megalin is not the target antigen in human MN since it is not present on the surface of human podocytes. In a seminal discovery in 2002, fetomaternal alloimmunization to NEP, a podocyte antigen, caused MN in a newborn.[28] The mother of the patient did not possess the NEP antigen and had been alloimmunized during a previous pregnancy. Passive transfer of antibodies in this fetus resulted in severe neonatal MN that was confirmed by renal biopsy. Subsequently, Beck et al.[39] demonstrated that antibodies directed against a podocyte antigen, M-type PLA2R, were present in 70% of idiopathic MN in adults, but not in secondary MN. More recently, antibodies to another podocyte antigen, thrombospondin type-1 domain-containing 7A (THSD7A), were detected in a subset of adult idiopathic MN patients who are negative for anti-PLA2R antibodies.[40]

It is possible that additional autoantibodies to podocyte antigens will be discovered. The role of testing for these autoantibodies in diagnosis, prognosis and management is not defined.

### Planted antigen-antibody immune complex formations

cBSA, when injected into rabbits, leads to nephrotic syndrome with pathologic findings of MN.[41] cBSA is believed to navigate across the GBM along an electrostatic charge gradient (since it is positively charged). It is then trapped (or "planted") in the subepithelial region, and interacts later with antibodies generated by the host to form immune complex.

The demonstration of MN in children who develop antibodies to cBSA has substantiated the existence of planted antigens as a pathogenic mechanism of MN in patients.[23] Planted cBSA in these children with MN has been suggested to orignitate from trypsin digestion of cow's milk or beef protein in the gut. The cBSA is readily absorbed via the more permeable gastrointestinal tract of the infant and is

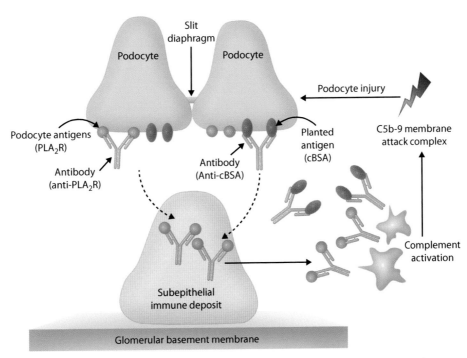

Figure 20.4 Pathogenesis of podocyte injury in membranous nephropathy. Autoantibodies to inherent podocyte antigens (PLA2R) or the planted (cBSA) antigens attach to the appropriate antigen site on the podocytes. The immune complexes detach from the podocytes and form the subepithelial deposits. Local complement activation results in formation of the membrane attack complex (MAC), which leads to sublethal podocyte injury. (Based on: Beck LH Jr, Salant DJ. Membranous nephropathy: from models to man. J Clin Invest. 2014;124:2307–14.)

subsequently trapped in the subepithelial space of the glomerular capillary wall. The development of antibodies to cBSA results binding to the planted antigen (cBSA) in the glomerular capillary wall and the development of MN.

## Circulating immune complex formation

Evidence for circulating immune complexes (CICs) as the pathogenic mechanism of subepithelial immune complex formation in MN is scant. An experimental model using ferritin-antiferritin antibody–induced MN has provided some evidence that immune complexes may be formed along the endothelial side of the glomerular capillary wall and then translocate into the subepithelial space.[42] The presence of CICs in HBV-associated MN has been suggested as a human equivalent of circulating immune complex–induced MN.[43]

## PODOCYTES INJURY AND COMPLEMENT ACTIVATION

After formation of in situ immune complexes on the basal aspect of podocytes, these immune complexes dislodge from podocyte surfaces and migrate onto the epithelial aspect of the GBM to form the subepithelial immune deposits.[44] Eventually, these antigen-antibody immune complexes lead to complement activation and formation of the terminal complement (C5b-9) membrane attack complex

(MAC). MAC in sublytic concentration is instrumental in inducing podocyte injury via mechanisms that involve cellular calcium influx, oxidative injury, and disruption of the actin cytoskeleton (Figure 20.4).[44,45] The consequences of these cellular events within the podocytes are simplification of the podocyte cell structure, loss or displacement of slit diaphragms, podocyte detachment, and development of proteinuria.[44–46] Indeed, MAC excretion has been well documented in the urine of patients with idiopathic MN that improves or disappears on treatment with immunosuppressive agents.[47] It has been suggested that MAC also may be involved in the tubulointerstitial damage observed in patients with MN.[48]

> ### KEY POINT
>
> Podocyte injury in MN results from local complement activation and formation of MAC.

## MANAGEMENT

There is no clear consensus on the treatment of children with MN. Immunosuppressive therapies have been recommended on the belief that MN is an autoimmune disorder.

All of the immunosuppressive regimens are associated with significant side effects, including renal toxicity associated with calcineurin inhibitor therapy, and need to be chosen carefully. Evidence-based data with the use of immunosuppressive treatments in children are lacking, and therapy decisions are often based on the safety and efficacy data obtained in in adults. Supportive therapies for treatment of edema, use of antiproteinuric agents, prevention of infections, and treatment of hypertension need to be considered in all patients with MN. These therapies are briefly discussed in the following section and are described in detail in Chapters 16 and 17.

## IMMUNOSUPPRESSIVE REGIMENS

There are no definitive guidelines for the treatment of idiopathic MN in children; the approach is largely based on trials in adults. Prolonged corticosteroid therapy, alkylating agents, calcineurin inhibitors, and rituximab have been used in treating MN. However, the most appropriate strategy for treatment has yet to emerge. This is further complicated by the fact that spontaneous improvement of nephrotic syndrome and proteinuria is common (approximately 30%) in MN. A brief review of the immunosuppressive agents used for treatment of MN is given later, which relies heavily on the experience in adult patients.

---

### KEY POINTS

- Immunosuppressive regimens are the primary form of therapy in MN.
- Corticosteroid therapy as a monotherapy is not recommended.

---

## Corticosteroids

Corticosteroids as a monotherapy are ineffective in the treatment of adult patients with MN. An early study compared using 8 weeks of alternate-day corticosteroids with placebo. Corticosteroids produced a significantly slower decline in glomerular filtration rate (GFR), with doubling of creatinine at 3 years in 24% in the treatment arm and 36% in the placebo arm.[48] The Medical Research Council Trial in the United Kingdom, using short-term prednisone therapy did not find any difference in renal function or proteinuria at 36 months between the treatment and placebo arms.[49] Another randomized controlled 6-month trial of alternate-day corticosteroids also failed to demonstrate any beneficial effects of the therapy.[50] Based on the lack of definitive evidence of benefit, the Kidney Disease Improving Global Outcomes (KDOQI) guidelines do not recommend corticosteroids as a monotherapy for treatment of MN.[51]

## Corticosteroids and alkylating agents in cyclical therapy

Alkylating agents (chlorambucil and cyclophosphamide), used cyclically with steroids for 6 months, were shown to be effective in inducing remission of nephrotic syndrome by Ponticelli et al.[53] Being a cyclical therapy, the Ponticelli regimen uses monthly cycles of intravenous steroids and alkylating agent. In the first month, intravenous pulse prednisolone is administered daily for three doses and then oral methylprednisolone (0.5 mg/kg/day) is used for 27 days. In month 2, oral chlorambucil is administered in a dose of (0.15 to 0.2 mg/kg/day). Alternatively, oral cyclophosphamide (2 mg/kg/day) can be used for 30 days. These cycles are repeated for a total of 6 months. In a recently reported randomized controlled trial of adults with MN with declining function, immunosuppression consisting of 6 months of therapy with prednisolone and chlorambucil in a format similar to that in the Ponticelli regimen was found to slow the decline of renal function compared to the control group.[53] Although effective, alkylating agents can be associated with significant side effects and infectious complications.

## Calcineurin inhibitor therapy

Cyclosporine, a calcineurin inhibitor, is effective in reducing proteinuria in patients with MN. In some randomized controlled trials, cyclosporine was superior to placebo in preserving renal function.[54,55] In the controlled study by Alexopoulos et al.,[56] complete remission of nephrotic syndrome after 6 months of therapy was higher when cyclosporine was combined with corticosteroids (19% vs. 5%).[56] However, the partial remission rate was similar in the two groups. Failure to respond to cyclosporine after 6 months of treatment was noted in 17% of the combination group (cyclosporine and corticosteroids) and in 15% of patients in the cyclosporine monotherapy group. The dose of cyclosporine used in this study was 2 to 4 mg/kg/day in two divided doses, and the dose was adjusted to keep the plasma cyclosporine level at approximately 100 ng/mL.

Cyclosporine should be used cautiously in patients with decreased renal function. Comparing the Ponticelli regimen, cyclosporine, and supportive care, the U.K. randomized controlled trial demonstrated a higher risk for decline in renal function in patients receiving cyclosporine.

The appropriate duration of cyclosporine therapy in MN is unclear. KDIGO guidelines recommend at least 6-months of therapy in those who respond and possible extension of therapy to 1 year.[52] Relapses of proteinuria and nephrotic syndrome occur in 40% to 50% of patients after discontinuation of cyclosporine.

The mechanism by which cyclosporine reduces proteinuria in nephrotic states, including MN, is poorly understood. Possible mechanisms include suppressing the immune system, selective vasoconstrictive action on the afferent arteriole, and enhancing the selectivity of the glomerular capillary barrier.[57] More recently, cyclosporine has been shown to have a stabilizing effect on the actin cytoskeleton of podocytes.[58,59]

Tacrolimus is also effective in controlling proteinuria in MN. The dose of tacrolimus in the randomized controlled trial by Praga et al.[60] was 0.05 mg/kg, given twice daily for 12 months and then tapered over 6 months. Remission of proteinuria occurred in 58%, 82%, and 94% after 6, 12, and 18 months of treatment, respectively. This compared with the remission rate of 10%, 24%, and 35% in the control group at 6, 12, and 18 months, respectively.

In a head-to-head comparison of tacrolimus and cyclophosphamide, Xu et al.[61] reported a remission rate of 65.1% in the tacrolimus group compared to a 44.2% remission rate in the cyclophosphamide group after 2 months of treatment. Both groups also received low-dose steroids. Mean time to partial or complete remission of proteinuria was 2.2 months in the tacrolimus group and 3.9 months in the cyclophosphamide group. However, the response was similar after 6 months of treatment, but there were fewer side effects in the tacrolimus arm of the study. Similarly, Chen et al.[62] noted that compared to the group receiving cyclophosphamide plus prednisone, tacrolimus plus prednisone provided a higher remission rate at 6 months (85% vs. 65%), but the remission rate was similar at 12 months of treatment. In the Cochrane meta-analysis of 39 studies in adults, there was no clear superiority of cyclosporine over alkylating agents (cyclophosphamide).[63] The number of studies using tacrolimus in this meta-analysis was too small to make any specific recommendations.

As is the case with cyclosporine, the relapse rate after discontinuation of tacrolimus is high. Patients on either of the two calcineurin inhibitor therapies become "dependent" on such treatments and therefore at risk of long-term nephrotoxicity.

## Mycophenolate mofetil

Mycophenolate mofetil (MMF) is a potential therapeutic choice for some patients with MN.[64] However, the type of patients with MN who may benefit from MMF therapy remains unclear at this time. Using historical controls of MN patients who had been treated with daily cyclophosphamide (1.5 mg/kg/day), Branten et al.[65] treated a group of 32 adult MN patients with MMF (1 g twice daily). MMF reduced proteinuria comparable to the response with cyclophosphamide, but 38% of patients treated with MMF had relapse of nephrotic syndrome on cessation of treatment compared to 13% in the cyclophosphamide group. Of the patients treated with MMF, 16% failed to respond to the therapy. Dussol et al.[66] evaluated MMF monotherapy in adults for 12 months (randomized controlled) and compared it to symptomatic treatment along with angiotensin-converting enzyme inhibitor (ACEI) therapy. Although proteinuria improved in both groups, none of the MMF patients developed complete remission of proteinuria at 6 months.

Being an immunosuppressive agent, MMF may be considered in patients with idiopathic or primary MN with circulating anti-PLA2R antibodies. However, given the paucity of available data and a high relapse rate after discontinuation of therapy, the therapeutic role of MMF in the treatment of MN is unclear.

## Rituximab

Rituximab is a monoclonal antibody that binds to the CD20 antigen on B cells, resulting in their deletion. Rituximab was approved by the U.S. Food and Drug Administration (FDA) in 1997 for treatment of non-Hodgkin's lymphoma and later for chronic lymphocytic leukemia, rheumatoid arthritis, granulomatosis with polyangiitis (Wegener granulomatosis), and microscopic polyangiitis.[67]

In an open-label clinical trial of rituximab, Fervenza et al.[68] treated 15 patients with MN using two doses intravenously 2 weeks apart (1 g/dose). They noted a mean of 48% reduction in proteinuria in 66% of patients, which occurred gradually over 12 months. However, 33% patients failed to respond. Disappearance of anti-PLA2R circulating antibodies has been noted after treatment with rituximab.[69] Ruggenenti et al.[70] extended their previously reported study on safety and efficacy of rituximab in 100 MN patients. Follow-up of rituximab (375 mg/m$^2$) therapy over 29 months resulted in a complete remission of proteinuria in 27% patients, and another 38% achieved partial remission. In this study, 35% patients did not fulfill the criteria for a partial or complete remission, but were noted to have a reduction in the degree of proteinuria. Remission with rituximab therapy was gradual and was attained over a median of 7.1 months. An important finding was that complete remission was associated with a significant improvement of GFR of approximately 13 mL/min/1.73 m$^2$. Interestingly, of those who achieved partial or complete remission, 27% had recurrence of proteinuria that ranged from 7 through 116 months (median 42 months) after rituximab treatment.

Interestingly, Fervenza et al.[68] found no relationship between the response rate and the number of B cells in the blood or CD20 cells in the kidney biopsy. Randomized controlled trials of rituximab use in MN are lacking, and recommendations related to its use in children cannot be made with confidence.

## Adrenocorticotropin hormone gel therapy

Adrenocorticotrophin hormone (ACTH) was approved by the FDA for clinical use in 1952. A new formulation of ACTH in gel was approved by the FDA for treatment of edematous states (nephrotic syndrome) in 2010.[71] HP Acthar Gel (ACTH; Mallinckrodt, St. Louis, MO) is obtained from porcine pituitary gland and is currently the only approved product available in the United States. It has been shown to reduce proteinuria in a variety of kidney disorders, including MN.[72-74] There is some optimism about the use of ACTH gel therapy in the treatment of MN, but recommendations in children are currently inappropriate in view of a complete lack of substantial data.

## SUPPORTIVE THERAPY

Supportive treatment of MN should be considered in all nephrotic patients for relief of edema, curtailing proteinuria, and preventing complications. These measures are also discussed in Chapters 16 and 17.

---

### KEY POINT

Supportive therapy should be considered as an adjunct to immunosuppressive treatment in all patients with MN.

---

### Antiproteinuric and renoprotective therapy

ACEIs and angiotensin receptor–blocking agents (ARBs) are well accepted as adjuncts in nephrotic patients to curb proteinuria. Apart from their antiproteinuric impact, ACEIs and ARBs are also renoprotective. Treatment with ACEIs, ARBs, or both is effective in achieving complete or partial remission in patients with MN and should be considered in all patients with MN.[75]

### Managing hypertension and cardiovascular risks

Hypertension should be effectively controlled to lower cardiovascular risk and to slow progression of renal disease. Because of their antiproteinuric as well as antihypertensive effects, ACEIs and ARBs are the preferred initial therapy for hypertension in MN patients. Intensified blood pressure control, with a target between the 50th and 95th percentiles has been recommended in patients with CKD for optimal renoprotection, and should be the goal in patients with MN.[76] Hypercholesterolemia is common in MN and is routinely treated with statins in adults. The role of statins in children with nephrotic syndrome is not clearly defined.[77]

### Managing edema

Diuretics are important in the management of edema in most nephrotic patients, including those with MN. Although not studied specifically in MN, a combination of furosemide, thiazides, and potassium-sparing diuretics can be considered for relief of edema. These therapies are also discussed in Chapters 16 and 17.

### Prevention of thromboembolism

The prolonged nephrotic syndrome that occurs in some patients with membranous nephropathy increases the risk of thromboembolic complications. Renal vein thrombosis has been reported to be especially common in patients with MN.[78] Zhang et al.[79] studied renal computed tomography (CT) venography and pulmonary CT angiography in 512 patients (9 to 81 years of age) with nephrotic syndrome of all causes, 80 of whom were children. Pulmonary embolism or renal vein thrombosis was diagnosed in 35% patients. MN as the cause of nephrotic syndrome was the leading cause of these two thromboembolic complications (48%) in this study. Thrombotic complications involving other large vessels have also been reported in patients with MN.[80] The annual incidence of venous thrombosis (mostly pulmonary embolism and deep vein thrombosis) in adult patients with nephrotic syndrome has been estimated to be 1.02%, and the risk for arterial thrombosis (mostly myocardial infarction) has been estimated to be 1.45%.[81] These observations point to the importance of preventing thromboembolism in patients with MN.

Nephrotic children who may be at high risk for thromboembolic complications are difficult to identify. But the severity of proteinuria has been identified as a risk factor for thromboembolism in children.[82] There are no definitive guidelines for employing anticoagulants or antiplatelet agents in nephrotic syndrome, including in MN. For established thromboembolism, intravenous heparin therapy is the traditional approach, but low-molecular-weight heparin (enoxaparin [Lovenox]) may offer an alternative in some patients. If indicated, heparin may be necessary as long as the nephrotic state persists in these patients or at least for 3 to 6 months. Thrombolysis may be needed in patients with arterial thromboembolic events.[83]

### Prevention of infections

Infections such as spontaneous bacterial peritonitis or sepsis may occur in children with MN. Strategies for preventing these infectious complications in nephrotic patients are discussed in Chapters 16 and 17 and should be employed in these MN patients. These include pneumococcal vaccinations and intravenous immunoglobulin in select patients.

## NATURAL HISTORY OF MEMBRANOUS NEPHROPATHY

The natural history of MN is unique in that spontaneous remission of proteinuria and nephrotic syndrome in untreated patients is relatively common. The second clinically relevant aspect of the natural history of MN in adults is that progression of renal dysfunction occurs slowly and over many years. Noel et al.[78] followed 116 patients with MN for a mean of 4.5 years (2 months to 21 years) without any treatment. Of these, 23.5% developed clinical remission of nephrotic syndrome, some with residual mild-to-moderate proteinuria. Remission was noted more commonly in patients with stage I electron microscopy renal biopsy findings.

## KEY POINTS

- Spontaneous remission of primary or idiopathic MN is common in adult studies (approximately 30%).
- Spontaneous remission is more common with stage I renal pathology and lower baseline proteinuria.

In a cohort of 116 patients with idiopathic MN from the Mayo Clinic, 72 patients did not receive any treatment and 42 patients received various immunosuppressive therapies.[84] Of the untreated patients, 57% had remission of proteinuria, 10% had persistent proteinuria, and 33% continued to have nephrotic syndrome. In contrast, in the treated group, 40% developed remission, 12% had persistent proteinuria, and 48% had persistent nephrotic syndrome. In an Italian study of 107 patients who received only diuretics or antihypertensive medications and were followed for a mean duration of 52 months, 65% of patients followed for at least 5 years developed clinical remission of proteinuria.[85] Serum creatinine in the entire group increased from a mean of 1.1 ± 0.5 mg to 1.4 ± 1.2 mg during the observational period. Polanco et al.[86] observed a multicenter cohort of 328 patients with nephrotic syndrome secondary to MN. Spontaneous remission of nephrotic syndrome occurred in 32% over a mean interval of 14.7 ± 11.4 months. Remission was more likely in patients with lower baseline proteinuria. Relapse of nephrotic syndrome occurred in only 5.7% of patients, and reduction of proteinuria by 50% in the first year was associated with remission of nephrotic syndrome.

Given the possibility of spontaneous remission in adult patients with MN, conservative therapy, such as with ACEIs, ARBs, and diuretics, has been recommended by some.[75] However, clinical, renal biopsy, or laboratory characteristics of patients who might respond to such a therapeutic approach remain unclear.

## SUMMARY

MN is a relatively unusual cause of nephrotic syndrome in children. The underlying etiology varies in different regions of the world because of differences in the prevalence of infections such as hepatitis B and HIV infection and autoimmune disorders, especially lupus. The majority of adult idiopathic MN is due to autoantibodies to PLA2R. Children may develop MN as a result of autoantibodies to cBSA or alloantibodies to NEP. Treatment, determined by the underlying cause, includes antiviral agents and immunosuppressive medications.

## Clinical Vignette 20.1

An 8-year-old girl was noted by her parents to have facial swelling. She was diagnosed with nephrotic syndrome. Daily oral prednisone for 4 weeks at a dose of 60 mg/m²/day and three additional intravenous pulses of methylprednisolone did not produce remission of proteinuria, and she was considered to have steroid-resistant nephrotic syndrome. Renal biopsy was performed, which showed typical findings of MN with thickening of the GBM and presence of spikes in the basement membrane on silver staining. Immunofluorescence showed IgG and C3 deposits. Electron microscopy demonstrated subepithelial electron-dense deposits characteristic of stage II classification. Estimated GFR was in the normal range. Viral serologic findings and polymerase chain reaction results were negative, and no drug or toxic exposure was detected. Serum complement levels were normal, anti-DNA autoantibodies were negative, and anti-PLA2R and anti-BSA antibodies were negative.

Treatment of MN was begun with tacrolimus and alternate-day prednisone. She was also started on anticoagulation with low-molecular-weight heparin. Complete remission of proteinuria and nephrotic syndrome was achieved in 4 weeks. Anticoagulation was stopped after the recovery of serum albumin to a normal level. Enalapril was started for renoprotection. Prednisone was stopped in 9 months, and tacrolimus was discontinued 26 months after initiation.

The patient relapsed with nephrotic-range proteinuria 4 months after discontinuing tacrolimus, while she was still taking enalapril. Tacrolimus was restarted, and full remission was again noted in 8 weeks. The trough level of tacrolimus was maintained less than 8 ng/L. Because of a decrease in GFR, despite complete remission of proteinuria, enalapril had to be discontinued. Prednisone was not restarted in this relapse.

A second renal biopsy was performed in year 3 after onset of the disease because of the decline in GFR and suspected nonadherence to therapy. Tubular atrophy and interstitial fibrosis were observed in 20% of the biopsy field, possibly as a result of tacrolimus therapy. The patient was started on rituximab therapy, to minimize the tacrolimus dose. B-cell depletion lasted 6 months. Unfortunately, her proteinuria reappeared following B-cell repletion.

### TEACHING POINTS

- In children, MN is classically discovered following the investigation of steroid-resistant nephrotic syndrome. The diagnosis relies on the renal biopsy findings, especially the findings of immunofluorescence staining and electron microscopy.
- This patient was investigated thoroughly for a secondary cause of MN, as well as autoantibodies, and was eventually diagnosed to have idiopathic MN.

- Addition of tacrolimus to prednisone achieved a clinical and biochemical remission of proteinuria. Enalapril was used as a renoprotective and antiproteinuric agent, but it did not result in significant improvement in proteinuria.
- Unfortunately, MN in this patient continued to have a relentless chronic clinical course and she became "dependent" on tacrolimus therapy.
- Development of CKD, characterized by chronic interstitial disease in this patient could be attributed to persistent proteinuria and tacrolimus therapy. It is possible that she will develop ESRD.
- The choice of rituximab instead of cyclophosphamide as a B cell–depleting agent was based on the report of Beck et al.[69] despite the absence of anti-PLA2R autoantibodies. This therapy choice over cyclophosphamide was favoured in view of the lack of gonadal toxicity in females with rituximab.

# REFERENCES

1. Wasserstein AG. Membranous glomerulonephritis. J Am Soc Nephrol. 1997;8:664–74.
2. Glassock RJ. Attending rounds: An older patient with nephrotic syndrome. Clin J Am Soc Nephrol. 2012;7:665–70.
3. Hladunewich MA, Troyanov S, Calafati J, et al. The natural history of the non-nephrotic membranous nephropathy patient. Clin J Am Soc Nephrol. 2009;4:1417–22.
4. Lee BH, Cho HY, Kang HG, et al. Idiopathic membranous nephropathy in children. Pediatr Nephrol. 2006;21:1707–15.
5. Chen A, Frank R, Vento S, et al. Idiopathic membranous nephropathy in pediatric patients: Presentation, response to therapy, and long-term outcome. BMC Nephrol. 2007;8:11.
6. Menon S, Valentini RP. Membranous nephropathy in children: Clinical presentation and therapeutic approach. Pediatr Nephrol. 2010;25:1419–28.
7. International Study of Kidney Disease in Children. Nephrotic syndrome in children: Prediction of histopathology from clinical and laboratory characteristics at time of diagnosis: A report of the International Study of Kidney Disease in Children. Kidney Int. 1978;13:159–65.
8. Takekoshi Y, Tanaka M, Shida N, et al. Strong association between membranous nephropathy and hepatitis-B surface antigenaemia in Japanese children. Lancet. 1978;18;2:1065–8.
9. Hsu HC, Wu CY, Lin CY, et al. Membranous nephropathy in 52 hepatitis B surface antigen (HBsAg) carrier children in Taiwan. Kidney Int. 1989;36:1103–7.
10. Moxey-Mims MM, Stapleton FB, Feld LG. Applying decision analysis to management of adolescent idiopathic nephrotic syndrome. Pediatr Nephrol. 1994;8:660–4.
11. 2013 U.S. Renal Data System annual data, report. Pediatric ESRD. Available at: http://www.usrds.org/2013/pdf/v2_ch8_13.pdf. Accessed on January 2, 2015.
12. Hendrickse RG, Adeniyi A, Edington GM, et al. Quartan malarial nephrotic syndrome: Collaborative clinicopathological study in Nigerian school children. Lancet. 1972;1:1143–9.
13. Liao MT, Chang MH, Lin FG, et al. Universal hepatitis B vaccination reduces childhood hepatitis B virus-associated membranous nephropathy. Pediatrics. 2011;128:e600–4.
14. Olowu WA, Adelusola KA, Adefehinti O, et al. Quartan malaria-associated childhood nephrotic syndrome: Now a rare clinical entity in malaria endemic Nigeria. Nephrol Dial Transplant. 2010;25:794–801.
15. Doi T, Mayumi M, Kanatsu K, et al. Distribution of IgG subclasses in membranous nephropathy. Clin Exp Immunol. 1984;58:57–62.
16. Noël LH, Aucouturier P, Monteiro RC, et al. Glomerular and serum immunoglobulin G subclasses in membranous nephropathy and anti-glomerular basement membrane nephritis. Clin Immunol Immunopathol. 1988;46:186–94.
17. Troyanov S, Roasio L, Pandes M, et al. Renal pathology in idiopathic membranous nephropathy: A new perspective. Kidney Int. 2006;69:1641–8.
18. Rodriguez EF, Nasr SH, Larsen CP, et al. Membranous nephropathy with crescents: A series of 19 cases. Am J Kidney Dis. 2014;64:66–73.
19. Churg J, Sobin LH. Renal disease: Classification and atlas of glomerular diseases. Tokyo: Igaku-shoin, 1982, p. 52.
20. Tsukahara H, Takahashi Y, Yoshimoto M, et al. Clinical course and outcome of idiopathic membranous nephropathy in Japanese children. Pediatr Nephrol. 1993;7:387–91.
21. Ardalan M. Triggers, bullets and targets, puzzle of membranous nephropathy. Nephrourol Mon. 2012;4:599–602.
22. Ronco P, Debiec H, Imai H. Circulating antipodocyte antibodies in membranous nephropathy: Pathophysiologic and clinical relevance. Am J Kidney Dis. 2013;62:16–9
23. Debiec H, Lefeu F, Kemper MJ, et al. Early-childhood membranous nephropathy due to cationic bovine serum albumin. N Engl J Med. 2011;364:2101–10.
24. Wong SN, Chan WK, Hui J, et al. Membranous lupus nephritis in Chinese children: A case series and review of the literature. Pediatr Nephrol. 2009;24:1989–96.

25. Aline-Fardin A, Rifle G, Martin L, et al. Recurrent and de novo membranous glomerulopathy after kidney transplantation. Transplant Proc 2009; 41: 669–671.

26. Wang HH, Yang AH, Yang LY, et al. Chronic graft-versus-host disease complicated by nephrotic syndrome. J Chin Med Assoc. 2011;74:419-22.

27. Palcoux JB, Gaulme J, Demeocq F, et al. Extramembranous glomerulonephritis during congenital syphilis. Arch Fr Pediatr. 1979;36:691–5.

28. Debiec H, Guigonis V, Mougenot B, et al. Antenatal membranous glomerulonephritis due to anti-neutral endopeptidase antibodies. N Engl J Med. 2002;346:2053–60.

29. Purswani MU, Chernoff MC, Mitchell CD, et al. Chronic kidney disease associated with perinatal HIV infection in children and adolescents. Pediatr Nephrol. 2012;27:981–9.

30. Araya CE, Gonzalez-Peralta RP, Skoda-Smith S, et al. Systemic Epstein-Barr virus infection associated with membranous nephropathy in children. Clin Nephrol. 2006;65:160–4.

31. Sturgill BC, Shearlock KT. Membranous glomerulopathy and nephrotic syndrome after captopril therapy. JAMA. 1983;250:234–5.

32. Nawaz FA, Larsen CP, Troxell ML. Membranous nephropathy and nonsteroidal anti-inflammatory agents. Am J Kidney Dis. 2013;62:1012–7.

33. Hall CL. The natural course of gold and penicillamine nephropathy: A long-term study of 54 patients. Adv Exp Med Biol. 1989;252:247–56.

34. Kawasaki Y, Suzuki J, Sike T, et al. Bucillamine-induced nephropathy in a child with juvenile rheumatoid arthritis and Kartagener's syndrome. Pediatr Int. 2000;42:316–8.

35. Theodoni G, Printza N, Karyda S, et al. D-penicillamine induced membranous glomerulonephritis in a child with Wilson's disease. Hippokratia. 2012;16:94.

36. Heymann W, Hackel DB, Harwod S. et al. Production of the nephrotic syndrome in rats by Freund's adjuvants and rat kidney suspensions. Proc Soc Exp Biol Med. 1959;10:60–4.

37. Couser WG, Steinmuller DR, Stilmant MM, et al. Experimental glomerulonephritis in the isolated perfused rat kidney. J Clin Invest. 1978; 62:1275–87.

38. Farquhar MG, Saito A, Kerjaschki D, et al. The Heymann nephritis antigenic complex: Megalin (gp330) and RAP. J Am Soc Nephrol. 1995;6:35–47.

39. Beck LH Jr, Bonegio RG, Lambeau G, et al. M-type phospholipase A2 receptor as target antigen in idiopathic membranous nephropathy. N Engl J Med. 2009;361:11–21.

40. Tomas NM, Beck LH Jr, Meyer-Schwesinger C, et al. Thrombospondin type-1 domain-containing 7A in idiopathic membranous nephropathy. N Engl J Med. 2014;371:2277–87

41. Border WA, Ward HJ, Kamil ES, et al. Induction of membranous nephropathy in rabbits by administration of an exogenous cationic antigen. J Clin Invest. 1982;69:451–61.

42. Fujigaki Y, Nagase M, Honda N. Intraglomerular basement membrane translocation of immune complex (IC) in the development of passive in situ IC nephritis of rats. Am J Pathol. 1993;142:831–842.

43. Takekoshi Y, Tanaka M, Miyakawa Y, et al. Free "small" and IgG associated "large" hepatitis B e antigen in the serum and glomerular capillary walls of two patients with membranous glomerulonephritis. N Engl J Med. 1979;300:814–9.

44. Beck LH Jr, Salant DJ. Membranous nephropathy: From models to man. J Clin Invest. 2014;124:2307–14.

45. Cybulsky AV, Quigg RJ, Salant DJ. Experimental membranous nephropathy redux. Am J Physiol Renal Physiol. 2005;289:F660–71.

46. Nangaku M, Shankland SJ, William G. Couser WG. Cellular response to injury in membranous nephropathy. J Am Soc Nephrol. 2005;16:1195–204.

47. Kon SP, Coupes B, Short CD, et al. Urinary C5b-9 excretion and clinical course in idiopathic human membranous nephropathy. Kidney Int. 1995;48:1953–8.

48. Papagianni AA, Alexopoulos E, Leontsini M, et al. C5b-9 and adhesion molecules in human idiopathic membranous nephropathy. Nephrol Dial Transplant. 2002;17:57–63.

49. Anonymous. Collaborative study of the adult idiopathic nephritic syndrome: A controlled study of short-term prednisone treatment in adults with membranous nephropathy. N Engl J Med. 1979;301:1301–6.

50. Cameron JS, Healy MJ, Adu D. The Medical Research Council Trial of short-term high-dose alternate day prednisone in idiopathic membranous nephropathy with nephritic syndrome in adults. Q J Med. 1990;274:133–56.

51. Cattran DC, Delmore T, Roscoe J, et al. A randomized controlled trial of prednisone in patients with idiopathic membranous nephropathy. N Engl J Med. 1989;320:210–5.

52. International Society of Nephrology. Kidney disease: Improving global outcomes (KDIGO) clinical practice guideline for glomerulonephritis. Idiopathic membranous nephropathy. Kidney Int Suppl. 2012;2:186–97.

53. Ponticelli C, Zucchelli P, Passerini P, et al. A randomized trial of methylprednisolone and chlorambucil in idiopathic membranous nephropathy. N Engl J Med. 1989;320:8–13.

54. Howman A, Chapman TL, Langdon MM, et al. Immunosuppression for progressive membranous nephropathy: A UK randomised controlled trial. Lancet. 2013;381:744–51.

55. Cattran DC, Greenwood C, Ritchie S, et al. A controlled trial of cyclosporine in patients with progressive membranous nephropathy. Canadian Glomerulonephritis Study Group. Kidney Int. 1995;47:1130–5.

56. Alexopoulos E, Papagianni A, Tsamelashvili M, et al. Induction and long-term treatment with cyclosporine in membranous nephropathy with the nephrotic syndrome. Nephrol Dial Transplant. 2006;21:3127–32.

57. Ambalavanan S, Fauvel JP, Sibley RK, et al. Mechanism of the antiproteinuric effect of cyclosporine in membranous nephropathy. J Am Soc Nephrol. 1996;7:290–8.

58. Schönenberger E, Ehrich JH, Haller H, et al. The podocyte as a direct target of immunosuppressive agents. Nephrol Dial Transplant. 2011;26:18–24.

59. Faul C, Donnelly M, Merscher-Gomez S, et al. The actin cytoskeleton of kidney podocytes is a direct target of the antiproteinuric effect of cyclosporine A. Nat Med. 2008;14:931–8.

60. Praga M, Barrio V, Juárez GF, et al. Tacrolimus monotherapy in membranous nephropathy: A randomized controlled trial. Kidney Int. 2007;71:924–30.

61. Xu J, Zhang W, Xu Y, et al. Tacrolimus combined with corticosteroids in idiopathic membranous nephropathy: A randomized, prospective, controlled trial. Contrib Nephrol. 2013;181:152–62.

62. Chen M, Li H, Li XY, Lu FM, et al. Tacrolimus combined with corticosteroids in treatment of nephrotic idiopathic membranous nephropathy: A multi-center randomized controlled trial. Am J Med Sci. 2010;339:233–8.

63. Chen Y, Schieppati A, Chen X, et al. Immunosuppressive treatment for idiopathic membranous nephropathy in adults with nephrotic syndrome. Cochrane Database Syst Rev. 2014;(10):004293.

64. Miller G, Zimmerman R 3rd, Radhakrishnan J, et al. Use of mycophenolate mofetil in resistant membranous nephropathy. Am J Kidney Dis. 2000;36:250–6.

65. Branten AJ, du Buf-Vereijken PW, Vervloet M, et al. Mycophenolate mofetil in idiopathic membranous nephropathy: A clinical trial with comparison to a historic control group treated with cyclophosphamide. Am J Kidney Dis. 2007;50:248–56.

66. Dussol B, Morange S, Burtey S, et al. Mycophenolate mofetil monotherapy in membranous nephropathy: A 1-year randomized controlled trial. Am J Kidney Dis. 2008;52:699–705.

67. Annonymus. Package insert of Rituxan. Available at: http://www.gene.com/download/pdf/rituxan_prescribing.pdf. Accessed January 5, 2015.

68. Fervenza FC, Cosio FG, Erickson SB, et al. Rituximab treatment of idiopathic membranous nephropathy. Kidney Int. 2008;73:117–25.

69. Beck LH Jr, Fervenza FC, Beck DM, et al. Rituximab-induced depletion of anti-PLA2R autoantibodies predicts response in membranous nephropathy. J Am Soc Nephrol. 2011;22:1543–50.

70. Ruggenenti P, Cravedi P, Chianca A, et al. Rituximab in idiopathic membranous nephropathy. J Am Soc Nephrol. 2012; 23:1416–25.

71. Approval package for H.P. Acthar Gel. Available at http://www.accessdata.fda.gov/drugsatfda_docs/nda/2010/022432Orig1s000Approv.pdf. Accessed August 8, 2015.

72. Ponticelli C, Passerini P, Salvadori M, et al. A randomized pilot trial comparing methylprednisolone plus a cytotoxic agent versus synthetic adrenocorticotropic hormone in idiopathic membranous nephropathy. Am J Kidney Dis. 2006;47:233-40.

73. Rauen T, Michaelis A, Floege J, et al. Case series of idiopathic membranous nephropathy with long-term beneficial effects of ACTH peptide 1-24. Clin Nephrol. 2009 ;71:637-42.

74. Hladunewich MA, Cattran D, Beck LH, et al. A pilot study to determine the dose and effectiveness of adrenocorticotrophic hormone (H.P. Acthar® Gel) in nephrotic syndrome due to idiopathic membranous nephropathy. Nephrol Dial Transplant. 2014;29:1570-7.

75. van den Brand JA, van Dijk PR, Hofstra JM, Wetzels JF. Long-term outcomes in idiopathic membranous nephropathy using a restrictive treatment strategy. J Am Soc Nephrol. 2014;25:150–8.

76. Wuhl E, Trivelli A, Picca S, et al. Strict blood-pressure control and progression of renal failure in children. N Engl J Med. 2009;361:1639–50.

77. Daniels SR, Greer FR; Committee on Nutrition. Lipid screening and cardiovascular health in childhood. Pediatrics. 2008;122:198–208.

78. Noel LH, Zanetti M, Droz D, Barbanel C: Long-term prognosis of idiopathic membranous glomerulonephritis: Study of 116 untreated patients. Am J Med. 1079;66:82–90.

79. Zhang LJ, Zhang Z, Li SJ, et al. Pulmonary embolism and renal vein thrombosis in patients with nephrotic syndrome: Prospective evaluation of prevalence and risk factors with CT. Radiology. 2014;273:897–906.

80. Hsu HF, Huang SY. Carotid artery thrombosis in a child with membranous nephropathy associated with factor V Leiden mutation. Pediatr Int. 2012;54:573–4.

81. Mahmoodi BK, ten Kate MK, Waanders F, et al. High absolute risks and predictors of venous and arterial thromboembolic events in patients with nephrotic syndrome: Results from a large retrospective cohort study. Circulation. 2008;117:224–30.

82. Kerlin BA, Blatt NB, Fuh B, et al. Epidemiology and risk factors for thromboembolic complications of childhood nephrotic syndrome: A Midwest Pediatric Nephrology Consortium (MWPNC) study. J Pediatr. 2009;155:105–110.

83. Kerlin BA, Ayoob R, Smoyer WE. Epidemiology and pathophysiology of nephrotic syndrome-associated thromboembolic disease. Clin J Am Soc Nephrol. 2012;7:513–20.

84. Donadio JV Jr, Torres VE, Velosa JA, et al. Idiopathic membranous nephropathy: The natural history of untreated patients. Kidney Int. 1988;33:708–15.

85. Schieppati A, Mosconi L, Perna A, et al. Prognosis of untreated patients with idiopathic membranous nephropathy. N Engl J Med. 1993;229:85–89, 1993.

86. Polanco N, Gutiérrez E, Covarsí A, et al. Spontaneous remission of nephrotic syndrome in idiopathic membranous nephropathy. J Am Soc Nephrol. 2010;21:697–704.

87. Heidet L, Gagnadoux ME, Beziau A, et al. Recurrence of de novo membranous glomerulonephritis on renal grafts. *Clin Nephrol* 1994;41:31

## REVIEW QUESTIONS

1. Membranous nephropathy is:
   a. The leading cause of nephrotic syndrome in adults
   b. The leading cause of nephrotic syndrome in children
   c. Idiopathic in most cases, whatever the patient age
   d. Mainly associated with lupus nephropathy

2. The diagnosis of membranous nephropathy relies on:
   a. Nephrotic-range proteinuria
   b. The age at onset of nephrotic syndrome
   c. Renal biopsy findings of thickened glomerular capillary wall, immunopathology, and electron microscopy showing subepithelial deposits
   d. Low circulating C3 and C4 in the plasma

3. The treatment of idiopathic membranous nephropathy includes all *except*:
   a. Prednisone + calcineurin antagonists
   b. Prednisone + alkylating agents
   c. Immunosuppression and ACE inhibitors
   d. Immunosuppression and ARBs
   e. Complement blockade by eculizumab

4. Circulating anti-PLA2R antibodies are seen in patients with:
   a. Membranous nephropathy associated with systemic lupus erythematosus
   b. Membranous nephropathy associated with drugs and toxins
   c. Primary or idiopathic membranous nephropathy
   d. Membranous nephropathy associated with hepatitis B

5. Corticosteroids, as a monotherapy, can produce long-lasting remission in patients with membranous nephropathy.
   a. True
   b. False

## ANSWER KEY

1. a
2. c
3. e
4. c
5. b

# 21

# Acute glomerulonephritis

## DIEGO H. AVILES AND V. MATTI VEHASKARI

Acute glomerulonephritis is a well-described complication of streptococcal and other infections in children. The narrative of hematuria and edema (dropsy) following scarlet fever provided a clinical description of acute glomerulonephritis, and for over a century this condition was known as the Bright disease.[1] It is likely, however, that many of the patients with Bright disease actually had some form of chronic glomerulonephritis. The term *acute postinfectious glomerulonephritis* (APIGN) refers to the broad group of acute nephritis that follows a variety of infectious events. APIGN may result from a variety of other bacterial and viral infectious agents, such as staphylococci, pneumococci, *Yersinia*, *Mycoplasma pneumoniae*, influenza virus, adenovirus, coxsackie virus, Epstein-Barr virus, varicella virus, mumps virus, measles virus, and parvovirus B19 (Table 21.1). APIGN can also occur in states of chronic bacterial infections, such as acute endocarditis, ventriculoatrial shunt infections, and deep-seated abscesses.

The term *acute poststreptococcal glomerulonephritis* (APSGN) is reserved for acute glomerulonephritis that develops after infection with group A β-hemolytic streptococci (GAS). Although generally a self-limited disease, APSGN may lead to life-threatening complications such as severe hypertension and encephalopathy, acute kidney injury (AKI), need for dialysis, and pulmonary edema. This chapter will primarily focus on the clinical aspects of APSGN. Viral infections resulting in glomerulonephritis are discussed separately in Chapter 29.

## EPIDEMIOLOGY

APSGN may occur at any age, but it is more commonly encountered between the ages of 2 and 15 years.[2–5] Peak incidence in a recent study from New Zealand was noted to be between 5 and 9 years of age.[4] Occurrence of APSGN below 2 years of age has been reported, but is rare.[6] Most studies report a slight male preponderance.[3–5] Global prevalence of severe GAS-associated systemic disease (rheumatic fever and APSGN) remains a public health concern. Estimated prevalence of severe GAS associated systemic illnesses is at least 18.1 million cases (mostly rheumatic fever), with 1.78 million new cases occurring annually.[7] With improvement in living standards, the incidence of APSGN has significantly declined in the Western world. This declining trend in APSGN was well documented in the United States from 1961 to 1988 in a regional study from Memphis, Tennessee by Roy and Stapleton.[5] In a comparative analysis of APSGN in Florida, Ilyas and Tolaymat[6] noted that the prevalence of the disease had decreased from 2.18 in 100,000 population in the 1959 to 1973 cohort, to 0.64 in 100,000 population in the 1999 to 2006 cohort. ASPGN, however, remains a public health concern in some global regions.[3,5,7–9] For example, the endemic incidence of APSGN reported from Santiago, Chile in the decade of the 1980s was 37.5 in 100,000, which decreased to 15.3 in the decade of 1990s.[3] During GAS epidemics, the prevalence of APSGN was recorded to be 103.8 in 100,000 population in this study. In another recent study

Table 21.1 Microorganisms associated with acute postinfectious glomerulonephritis

**Bacterial infections**
- Group A β-hemolytic streptococcus
- Staphylococci
- *Streptococcus pneumoniae*
- *Yersinia*
- *Mycoplasma pneumoniae*
- *Mycobacterium tuberculosis*
- Syphilis
- Brucellosis
- *Rickettsia rickettsii*
- *Granulicatella adiacens*

**Viral infections**
- Hepatitis B
- Hepatitis C
- HIV-1 infection
- Cytomegalovirus (especially in immunocompromised and kidney transplant patients)
- Parvovirus B19
- Influenza virus
- Adenovirus
- Coxsackie virus
- Epstein-Barr virus
- Varicella virus
- Mumps virus

**Parasitic infections**
- Malaria
- Schistosomiasis

**Fungal infections**
- Histoplasmosis
- Cryptococcosis
- Coccidioidomycosis

from Auckland Metropolitan area in New Zealand, annual incidence of APSGN was estimated to be 9.7 in 100,000.[4] This study also established an inverse relationship between incidence of APSGN and socioeconomic status. Association with overcrowding and low socioeconomic status has been established in other studies.[3]

**KEY POINTS**

- APSGN is the most common form of acute glomerulonephritis encountered in children, worldwide.
- APSGN is uncommon in children younger than 2 years of age.
- The peak incidence of APSGN is 5 to 9 years.

APSGN follows upper respiratory or skin infection with GAS. A bimodal distribution of APSGN is well described. Pharyngotonsillitis is a more common antecedent to APSGN in temperate climates and occurs during winter and spring months. Impetigo-associated APSGN, on the other hand, is more common during summer and autumn months and occurs more frequently in the tropical regions with warm and humid climate.[3,6] Interestingly, a trend of decreasing impetigo-associated APSGN has been observed since the 1960s in the United States in several studies.[4,5] A recent study from Florida noted that antecedent pharyngitis has replaced skin infection as the main source of streptococcal infection in APSGN.[4] Pharyngitis-associated APSGN was noted in 64% of the recently observed cases (1999 to 2006 cohort), whereas impetigo-associated APSGN formed the bulk (66%) of APSGN cases in the earlier era (1957 to 1973) in this study.[4] Epidemic outbreaks of APSGN may occur, especially in overcrowded and poor sanitation conditions.[3,9]

**KEY POINTS**

- Tonsillopharyngitis as a source of GAS infection is more common in the United States and developed countries.
- Pyoderma as a source of GAS is more common in Australia and less developed countries.

Studies of epidemic and nonepidemic APSGN have well documented that subclinical disease is common.[10-17] Siblings of affected patients are more at risk for asymptomatic APSGN, but parents also can be affected.[12,13] Screening of family members of index cases within 7 days revealed abnormal urinalysis in 22.3% of siblings, and definitive diagnosis of APSGN was made in 9.4% of the siblings. Prospective screening of family contacts by Rodríguez-Iturbe et al.[12] demonstrated that asymptomatic cases of APSGN are four times more common than symptomatic cases and that the attack rate in siblings was 37.8%.

## CLINICAL MANIFESTATIONS

The onset of clinical APSGN usually has a dramatic clinical presentation that occurs 7 to 14 days after pharyngotonsillitis and as long as 6 weeks following impetigo.[14] Scabies is often present in those manifesting pyoderma. Scarlet fever may be a manifesting feature of some cases.[11] The primary infection may remain undetected in some cases. Typical initial

Table 21.2 Clinical manifestations and laboratory findings of acute poststreptococcal glomerulonephritis in children

| Clinical and laboratory findings | Berrios et al.[3] (%) | Ilyas and Tolaymat[6] (%) | Roy and Tapleton[5] (%) |
|---|---|---|---|
| Edema | 100 | 78 (data derived) | 83 (S) 82.6 (P) |
| Arterial hypertension | 97 | 75 (data derived) | 42.3 (S), 80.6 (P) |
| Oliguria | 92 | Not reported | Not reported |
| Hematuria | 90 | 82 | 59.5 (S), 47.2 (P) |
| Moderate proteinuria | 73 | Not reported | 27.1 (S) |
| Nephrotic proteinuria | 3 | Not reported | Not reported |
| Decreased C3 | 95 | 88 | 72.9 (S), 94.5 (P) |
| Increased ASO titer | | 84 | 83.3 (S), 70.8 (P) |
| Increased serum creatinine | | | |
| Mild/moderate | 52 | 40 | 88.1 (S), 91.7 (P) |
| Severe | 0.5 | Not reported | Not reported |
| Chest x-ray: Pulmonary edema | Not reported | 50 | Not reported |

*Abbreviations:* P, pyoderma-associated acute poststreptococcal glomerulonephritis (APSGN); S, sore throat–associated APSGN; ASO, anti-streptolysin O.

manifestations of APSGN consist of a combination of gross hematuria, oliguria, hypertension, mild lower extremity, periorbital edema, and a modest impairment in the renal function (Table 21.2). Dull abdominal pain or flank pain and malaise may be present. Mild fever can be seen in approximately half of the patients, often attributed to an underlying tonsillopharyngitis, and hepatomegaly may be noted in some.[6] As shown in Figure 21.1, gross hematuria may last for a few weeks, but microscopic hematuria in APSGN can persist for several months to a year in some patients. Proteinuria in APSGN is short-lived and disappears in 4 to 6 weeks. Persistence of proteinuria should raise suspicion about the diagnosis and may be an indication for a renal biopsy in these patients.

Painless gross hematuria with brownish (the color of cola or tea) discoloration of urine is present in up to 50% to 90% of the patients and may be the only manifestation at presentation.[2,3,5,6,15] Significant leukocyturia may be seen in some patients with APSGN. Proteinuria is common (25% to 75%), and frank nephrotic syndrome is seen in 3% to 27%.[3,5,15] Oliguria and edema are observed in 80% to 100%, and pulmonary edema secondary to fluid overload may be seen on chest radiographs (Figure 21.2) in approximately half of patients.[3,6,10] Azotemia with modest elevation of serum creatinine is noted in 40% to 80% of patients on presentation, and severe azotemia requiring dialysis occurs in fewer than 1% cases.[3,5,6,15] Occasionally, a quickly rising serum creatinine level may represent transition to a crescentic form of glomerulonephritis.[16] Characteristically, serum C3 level is very low, often 20% of normal, in patients with APSGN.

## KEY POINTS

- Edema, hematuria (cola-colored urine), and hypertension are the characteristic manifestations of APSGN.
- Pulmonary edema may be seen in up to 50% cases on chest radiograph.
- Leukocyturia, with a positive test for leukocyte esterase, may be present.
- Azotemia, proteinuria, and severely low complement C3 level are characteristic of APSGN.

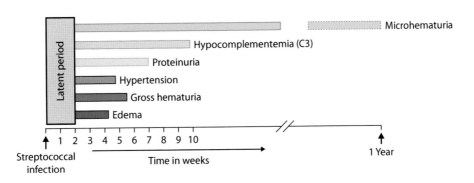

Figure 21.1 Time course of clinical manifestations of acute poststreptococcal glomerulonephritis.

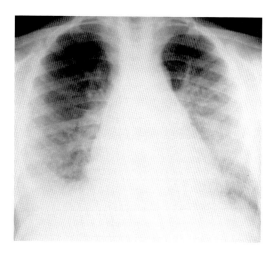

Figure 21.2 Chest radiograph of a patient with poststreptococcal glomerulonephritis showing pulmonary edema.

Hypertension is an almost a universal finding in patients with clinical APSGN, being present in 80% to 90% cases.[3,5,6,15] Occasionally, patients may present with severe hypertension and hypertensive encephalopathy as the only manifestation of APSGN.[17] Radiographically defined posterior reversible encephalopathy syndrome (PRES) has been reported as a presenting manifestation in patients with APSGN.[18] Magnetic resonance imaging findings of multiple abnormal foci of increased density in white and gray matter suggestive of a vasculitic lesion have also been reported in some patients with APSGN.[19] Whether these patients had PRES rather than true vasculitis is unclear.

## PATHOLOGY

A diagnostic renal biopsy is generally not necessary in children suspected to have APSGN. Adults, on the other hand, may have APIGN as a result of infective agents other than GBS and renal biopsies are generally recommended.[20] Light microscopy in the acute phase of APSGN shows diffuse endocapillary cell proliferation and narrowing of the glomerular capillary lumens (Figure 21.3A).[15,20,21] Infiltration of the glomeruli with neutrophils and monocytes is a characteristic finding in early biopsies, but monocytes may be more abundant in later stages of APSGN.[15] Glomerular crescents and a clinical presentation of rapidly progressive glomerulonephritis (RPGN) can be seen rarely in patients with APSGN.[22]

Immunofluorescence microscopy reveals coarsely granular staining of the capillary loops with IgG and complement C3. The presence of IgM and IgA is variable.[14] Three distinct immunofluorescence patterns, symbolizing the nature of immune deposits visualized in the glomeruli, described by Sorger et al.[23] are starry sky (generalized distribution), tree stalk (mesangial), and garland (capillary wall). The starry sky pattern denotes IgG, IgM, and IgA, combined with C3 deposition in the endocapillary-mesangial distribution.

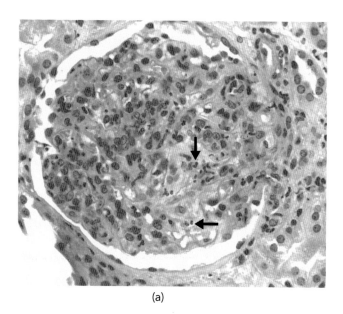

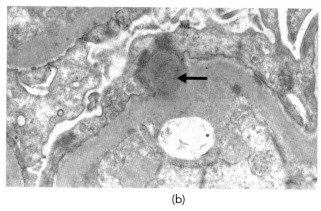

(a)                                        (b)

Figure 21.3 Acute poststreptococcal glomerulonephritis. (a) Light micrograph showing a glomerulus with endocapillary proliferation in a patient with acute poststreptococcal glomerulonephritis. Glomerular capillaries are obliterated in many areas as a result of endothelial cell swelling. Numerous neutrophils (arrows) are noted in the glomerulus. (b) Electron micrograph showing a characteristic large subepithelial deposit or "hump" (arrow) in a patient with poststreptococcal glomerulonephritis. (Photomicrographs courtesy of Dr. Randall Craver, Louisiana State University.)

This pattern is usually seen in the early phase of the disease—within the first few weeks. The tree stalk, or mesangial pattern, consists mainly of C3 deposition along the mesangium. The garland type of immune deposits may be more characteristic of patients with heavy subepithelial immune deposits, often associated with severe proteinuria.[23] After the acute phase, mesangial hypercellularity with positive immunofluorescence may persist for months to years, despite clinical recovery.[21]

---

### KEY POINTS

- Renal biopsy is not necessary in the diagnosis of APSGN in children.
- Severe endocapillary proliferation and narrowing of glomerular capillary lumens are characteristic.
- Distinct immunofluorescence patterns with IgG and C3 deposition are seen along the glomerular capillary wall.
- "Humps" of electron-dense deposits in subepithelial location are characteristic of APSGN.

---

The hallmark of APSGN is electron microscopy finding of large subepithelial deposits (humps), believed to be immune complexes (see Figure 21.3B). Electron-dense deposits can sometimes be noted in the subendothelial or even intramembranous regions.[24] Subepithelial electron-dense deposits are also seen in membranous glomerulopathy, which is distinguished from APSGN by lack of any glomerular endocapillary proliferation and inflammatory infiltrate.

## PATHOGENESIS

Infection by GAS elicits an antibody response in most patients, and in some it leads to the development of non-suppurative complication, such as acute rheumatic fever or APSGN. Epidemiologic data suggest that the clinically affected patients of APSGN are outnumbered by those who are asymptomatic, by a ratio of 1:4. Therefore, not all infected patients develop clinical disease, suggesting that apart from the bacterial virulence and nephritogenicity, host factors may be equally important in the pathogenesis of APSGN. The last two decades have produced some of the groundbreaking information about our understanding of the nephritogenicity of GBS and pathogenesis of APSGN.

## NEPHRITOGENICITY OF STREPTOCOCCI

Most cases of APSGN are associated with group A streptococcal infections, although epidemics with group C streptococci have been reported.[25] Zoonotic infection involving an equine source of streptococcus also has been reported, less commonly.[26] The glomerular inflammatory lesions in APSGN, are believed to result from the host immune response to the preceding streptococcal infection. Not all strains of streptococci result in APSGN, and the causative organisms are referred to as nephritogenic strains. Lancefield M serotypes 1, 2, 3, 4, 12, 18, and 25 are most commonly seen with pharyngitis-associated APSGN, whereas serotypes 2, 49, 55, 57, and 60 are commonly encountered with skin infection–associated APSGN.[27] GAS that cause pharyngotonsillitis and pyoderma can also be typed using characteristics of the *emm* gene subfamily in their chromosomes.[28]

---

### KEY POINTS

- Not all strains of GAS cause nephritis.
- Strains causing APSGN are referred to as *nephritogenic strains*.
- Nephritogenic GAS strains do not cause rheumatic fever.

---

## NEPHRITOGENIC ANTIGENS

In the past, the streptococcal M antigen has been considered as the primary nephritogenic antigen involved in the glomerular inflammatory response in APSGN.[29] Newer evidence, however, does not support the relevance of M antigen as a nephritogenic antigen.[30] Elegant studies done in the last two decades have focused on two separate antigens that may be associated with the nephritogenic potential of the streptococci. Evolving consensus suggests that both antigens may be involved in the pathogenesis of APSGN. These two streptococcal antigens are nephritis-associated plasmin receptor (NAPlr) and streptococcal pyrogenic exotoxin B (SpeB). Once deposited in the glomerular structures, both of these antigens induce complement activation, promote glomerular tissue injury, and induce chemoattractants and inflammatory response in the mesangial and endocapillary sites.[31]

---

### KEY POINTS

- Streptococcal M antigen is not considered to be the nephritogenic antigen.
- NAPlr and SpeB streptococcal antigens are involved in the pathogenesis of APSGN.

---

## Nephritis-associated plasmin receptor

Yoshizawa et al. isolated a 43-kDa protein from GSA, which they designated as NAPlr.[32-34] NAPlr is highly similar to previously reported streptococcus plasmin(ogen) receptor Plr, or glyceraldehyde-3-phosphate dehydrogenase (GAPDH). NAPlr induces an antibody response in the infected host, which has been well documented in patients with APSGN. NAPlr has been shown to be localized to the endothelial aspect of the GBM and the mesangium in the glomeruli.[33] This localization has been noted in 100% of APSGN patients within 2 weeks of onset of the disease and disappears beyond 90 days. Also, the anti-NAPlr antibodies persist in the host for a prolonged period and can be detected at lower levels for as long as 10 years after the onset of APSGN. The NAPlr antigen is restricted by the GBM because of its anionic charge.

In APSGN, NAPlr binds to the plasmin and prevents its breakdown in the glomerular tissues, which results in local tissue injury. Plasmin is known to have multiple physiologic roles, which include fibrinolysis, extracellular matrix turnover, cell migration, wound healing, angiogenesis, and activation of metalloproteins.[34] Plasmin-induced glomerular tissue damage may be mediated by degrading extracellular matrix proteins, such as fibronectin or laminin. The proposed net effect of these interactions is damage to the GBM.[32-34] Yoshizawa's investigative group proposed that NAPlr bound to plasmin also encourages endocapillary and mesangial proliferation and inflammatory response in APSGN (Figure 21.4).[34] Additionally, impaired GBM permeability might allow the NAPlr to transgress from the endothelial aspect of the GBM into the subepithelial space, where it may bind with the anti-NAPlr antibody to give rise to *in situ* immune complex formation. Alternatively, immune complexes of NAPlr and anti-NAPlr antibody could be preformed on the endothelial side and then migrate to the subepithelial area, where they form the humps seen in the renal biopsy of patients with APSGN.

## Pyrogenic exotoxin B

SpeB is a cationic extracellular cysteine proteinase generated by proteolysis of a zymogen precursor (zSpeB) and is produced by the nephritogenic GAS.[35-37] As with NAPlr, SpeB has been demonstrated to be present in the biopsy samples of patients with APSGN, and high titers of antibodies to SpeB are seen in sera of APSGN patients during convalescence. Another feature that SpeB shares with NAPlr is that it also acts as a plasmin-binding receptor, can activate metalloproteinases, and can degrade human fibronectin.[38] In contrast to NAPlr, SpeB is a cationic antigen and has the potential to move across the intact anionically charged GBM. Indeed, SpeB is the only streptococcal antigen that has been documented to be co-deposited with IgG and complement C3 in the subepithelial humps that are the hallmark of APSGN.[38]

## CIRCULATING IMMUNE COMPLEX FORMATION

The role of circulating immune complexes in the pathogenesis of APSGN is controversial. In the 1960s and 1970s, the presence of glomerular immune complexes was considered to be the evidence for "trapped" circulating antigen-antibody complexes in APSGN. The experimental correlate cited for this pathogenetic mechanism was the serum sickness model of acute glomerulonephritis induced in rabbits by a single injection of bovine serum albumin.[39,40] This experimental model is also characterized

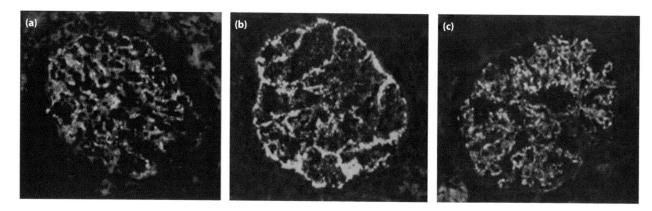

Figure 21.4 Illustrative patterns of complement C3 immunofluorescence observed in renal biopsy samples from patients with postinfectious glomerulonephritis. (a) Mesangial pattern: Mesangial C3 deposits are present, particularly toward the axial region of the glomerulus. (b) Garland or capillary wall pattern: Heavy C3 deposits are present along the glomerular basement membrane (GBM). (c) Starry sky or diffuse pattern: Many small deposits of C3 are present along the GBM and in the mesangium. (Reproduced with permission from: Kanjanabuch T, Kittikowit W, Eiam-Ong S. An update on acute postinfectious glomerulonephritis worldwide. Nat Rev Nephrol. 2009;5:259–69.)

by self-limited acute proliferative glomerulonephritis characterized by complement and IgG deposition, and hypocomplementemia.

Presence of circulating immune complexes in APSGN has been documented in several older reports.[41-43] In a year-long study of 30 children with APSGN from Taiwan, Lin[43] reported a high level of circulating immune complexes, using Raji cell radioimmune assay.[43] Circulating immune complexes were noted to be highest in the first 3 days after the onset of gross hematuria, and the levels gradually returned to baseline normal by 9 months. Some evidence to suggest that these circulating immune complexes contain streptococcal antigens has been presented, but these findings have not been verified or explored further with more direct techniques, or any of the more modern investigative techniques.[44] Evidence supporting the involvement of circulating immune complexes in APSGN with the newly discovered nephritogenic streptococcal antigens (NAPlr and SpeB) has yet to be presented convincingly.

## COMPLEMENT ACTIVATION

Hypocomplementemia and profoundly low levels of complement C3 are common findings in APSGN.[45] Complement C4 level, on the other hand, is generally normal. The immune complexes in renal biopsy samples of patients with APSGN also demonstrate complement C3, along with C5b-9 membrane attack complex and IgG in them.[46] Deposition of early classic complement pathway components (C4 and C1q) is generally lacking.[47] These findings largely suggest that alternative complement activation pathway is likely to be involved in APSGN. However, Wyatt et al.[45] presented some evidence of classic pathway involvement in patients with APSGN, despite normal serum C4 level. Hisano et al.[47] provided evidence for activation of both the alternative pathway and lectin pathway in the biopsies of patients with APSGN.

---

**KEY POINTS**

- Complement activation is the hallmark of APSGN.
- Alternative complement pathway is the predominant pathway for complement activation in APSGN.
- Lectin pathway may be involved in some.

---

## Host susceptibility factors

Host susceptibility and disease-modifying factors for APSGN are not fully understood. Increased frequency of HLA-DRW4 and HLA-DRB1*3011 has been reported in APSGN patients,[48,49] Whether this represents a true susceptibility to APSGN in these patients remains unclear. Similarly, a higher prevalence of eNOS4a (eNOS4a/a and eNOS4a/b) genotype has been noted in patients with APSGN, compared to healthy controls.[50] These findings suggest that "aa" and "ab" genotypes or "a" allele of eNOS4 have a greater likelihood of developing APSGN.

---

**KEY POINT**

Host susceptibility factors remain unclear but may be important in the pathogenesis of APSGN.

---

## Final pathways of glomerular inflammation and injury

Irrespective of initiating streptococcal antigen, the final common pathway of setting up glomerular inflammation and injury in APSGN is likely to be multifaceted (Figure 21.5).[20] These pathogenetic complement-activating mechanisms include a combination of (1) glomerular in situ immune complex formation by antibodies directed against planted cationic bacterial antigens, such as SpeB, (2) entrapment of circulating bacterial antigen-antibody immune complexes; (3) deposition of bacterial antigens, such as NAPlr, that bind to plasminogen, inducing local tissue injury, (Figure 21.6). Once the complement activation and plasmin-induced local tissue injury are initiated, multiple chemoattractants in the glomerular space promote inflammation and injury.[20,34] Host response and susceptibility characteristics may modify the inflammatory response, injury, and clinical manifestation of APSGN.

## EDEMA AND HYPERTENSION

Fluid overload is frequently present in APSGN, even in a mild disease. It is mostly the consequence of inappropriate tubular sodium (Na) reabsorption, not the result of reduced GFR. Proximal tubular avidity for Na during the acute phase of APSGN has been well described.[51] Fractional excretion of Na (FeNa) of 0.5 or less is common in APSGN, especially in patients developing hypertension.[52,53] These observations indicate that enhanced tubular Na absorption underlies the development of fluid overload and hypertension in these patients.[52] Plasma renin activity has been reported to be low or normal in the early phase of APSGN, perhaps reflecting a state of plasma volume expansion in these patients.[53,54]

---

**KEY POINTS**

- ASPGN is characterized by increased tubular Na reabsorption, fluid retention, and a low FeNa.
- Plasma renin activity is low to normal.

---

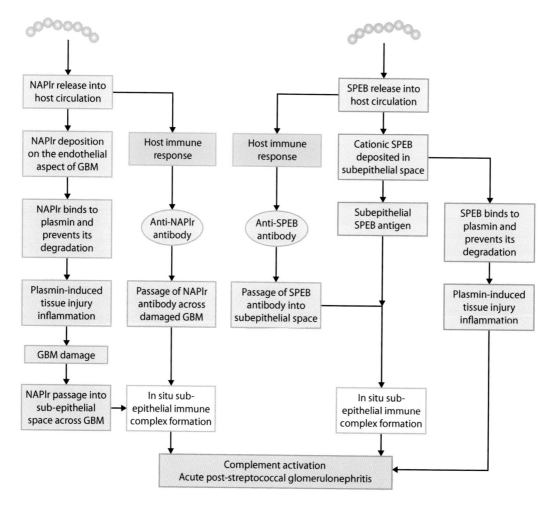

Figure 21.5 Mechanisms through which streptococcal antigens, nephritis-associated plasmin receptor (NAPlr) and strepto-coccal pyrogenic exotoxin B (SpeB), induce glomerular injury in acute poststreptococcal glomerulonephritis. Both antigens induce a host antibody response, which leads to in situ immune complex deposition. NAPlr also induces endocapillary inflammation and injury by binding to plasmin. SpeB being cationic in charge can also directly move into the subepithe-lial location to form in situ immune complexes. In contrast, because NAPlr is anionic in charge, it requires glomerular basement membrane (GBM) permeability to change via plasmin-induced injury to transgress into the subepithelial sites. Concepts based on data in references 33, 34, 37, and 48.

## DIFFERENTIAL DIAGNOSIS

Several renal diseases may mimic clinical manifestations of of ASPGN. These include other immune complex glomer-ulonephritides such as IgA nephritis, nephritis associated with systemic lupus nephritis (SLE), membranoprolifera-tive glomerulonephritis (MPGN), and Henoch-Schönlein nephritis. IgA nephritis, in particular, is easy to misdiag-nose as APSGN because of the presentation of gross hema-turia with respiratory infection. However, gross hematuria in IgA nephropathy occurs within 24 to 48 hours of onset of upper respiratory tract infection (usually viral) and is often referred to as *synpharyngitic* hematuria. Clinical and labo-ratory features distinguishing APSGN and IgA nephropa-thy are listed in Table 21.3.

Nephritis may be the first sign of SLE, sometimes even before extrarenal manifestations appear. Presence of hypo-complementemia in SLE nephritis can further complicate the clinical distinction between the two clinical disor-ders. However, presence of antinuclear antibody and anti-double-stranded DNA antibody in SLE can be a diagnostic differentiation of SLE from APSGN. MPGN can manifest with clinical features similar to those of APSGN, includ-ing gross hematuria, edema, increased serum creatinine, hypertension, and presence of hypocomplementemia. However, the clinical course of APSGN is one of progres-sive improvement in contrast to that of MPGN, which is characterized by progressive worsening of proteinuria, nephrotic syndrome, edema, and presence of severe hyper-tension. A renal biopsy is eventually necessary to clinch the diagnosis.

Table 21.3 Clinical and laboratory features distinguishing acute nephritic syndromes of immunoglobulin A nephropathy and acute poststreptococcal glomerulonephritis

| Clinical and laboratory findings | APSGN | IgA nephropathy |
|---|---|---|
| Latent period from URI to onset of gross hematuria | 10-14 days. Longer with pyoderma | Synpharyngitic association: Within 48 hours of onset of URI |
| Oliguria | Common | Not common |
| Increased serum creatinine | Common | Not common |
| Edema | Present | Absent |
| Hypertension | Present | Usually absent |
| Group A streptococcal infection | Positive bacteriologic evidence | Usually negative, often viral |
| Serologic evidence for streptococcal infection | Positive | Negative |
| Serum complement C3 | Low, recovers by 6-8 wk | Normal |

# DIAGNOSIS OF ACUTE POSTSTREPTOCOCCAL GLOMERULONEPHRITIS

## Patient history

Streptococcal pharyngitis typically precedes the development of gross hematuria and other symptoms of APSGN by 7 to 14 days. In temperate climates, a history of recent skin infection should be ascertained; this may have occurred several weeks before the onset of nephritis. In addition, any infectious disease during the preceding month should be recorded (see Table 21.1), as well as infections in family members and other daily contacts.

## Throat culture

Throat culture for GAS should be obtained, even though positive findings may not be always present by the time of the patient's presentation. It should also be recognized that up to 20% of healthy individuals are streptococcal carriers.[55,56]

## Streptococcal antibody titers

Streptolysin O is a toxin secreted by the streptococcus, which is present in all streptococci, but its gene expression varies.[57] Anti–streptolysin O (ASO) antibody titer is elevated in patients with recent streptococcal infection, but a preferred method is to demonstrate a rising titer of the serum ASO antibody at an interval of 2 weeks. Other antigens against which host antibody titer can be measured as evidence of recent streptococcal infection include anti-DNase B and antihyaluronidase antibodies.

The streptozyme panel, which includes antibodies against five streptococcal antigens, is a more sensitive test than the commonly used ASO titer. ASO antibody titer tends to be higher in APSGN associated with tonsillitis or pharyngitis, whereas in impetigo-associated disease the anti-DNase B antibody or antihyaluronidase antibody (included in the streptozyme panel) is more consistently positive, even in the absence of elevated ASO titer.[57–59] In acute glomerular nephritis secondary to nonstreptococcal infections, specific antibody titers should be obtained, when possible.

## Complement studies

Low complement C3 is central in the diagnosis of APSGN. Typically, it is markedly decreased (less than 40 mg/dL) from the very onset of the disease and normalizes in 2 to 8 weeks.[45,60,61] Persistence of low complement C3 beyond 8 weeks likely indicates a diagnosis other than APSGN. Approximately 15% of patients with APSGN do not demonstrate a low C3 level, perhaps reflecting a transient complement utilization and rapid recovery in these patients.[61] Complement C4 levels, in contrast, are normal in most patients with APSGN, but can be transiently low in some patients, especially in the first 1 to 2 weeks.[61] Apart from APSGN, low complement C3 is also seen in SLE and MPGN (Table 21.4). Some

Table 21.4 Acute glomerulonephritis associated with C3 hypocomplementemia

- Acute poststreptococcal glomerulonephritis
- Membranoproliferative glomerulonephritis
- Nephritis associated with systemic lupus erythematosus
- Glomerulonephritis associated with subacute bacterial endocarditis
- Glomerulonephritis associated with ventriculoatrial shunt infection

patients with atypical APSGN may exhibit persistent urinary abnormalities, along with abnormalities of complement C3 and C4. Some of these patients may have inherited abnormalities of complement-regulating proteins and persistent activation of alternative complement pathway.[62]

## RENAL BIOPSY

A diagnostic renal biopsy is not necessary in most typical cases of APSGN. An exception is a rapid deterioration of renal function, raising a suspicion of MPGN, SLE-associated nephritis, rapidly progressive glomerulonephritis, and IgA nephropathy. Persistently low complement C3 beyond 8 weeks, or prolonged proteinuria also indicate a need for tissue diagnosis in order to rule out chronic glomerulonephritis, such as MPGN or C3-associated nephropathy.

Table 21.4 presents a two-step approach to the diagnosis of acute glomerulonephritis. If the clinical presentation is strongly suggestive of APSGN, the first step may confirm the diagnosis and render the second step unnecessary. If APSGN appears unlikely, or is ruled out by the initial laboratory result, a more extended evaluation, possibly including renal biopsy, will be necessary.

Table 21.5 Evaluation of acute nephritic syndrome

**Initial evaluation when APSGN is strongly suspected**
- Urinalysis and urine microscopy
- Blood count (rule out hemolytic-uremic syndrome)
- Blood urea nitrogen, creatinine, electrolytes, serum albumin
- Quantify proteinuria (urine protein:creatinine ratio)
- Throat culture
- Culture of skin infections
- Streptococcal antibody titers (ASO, antihyaluronidase, antistreptokinase, anti-NAD, anti-DNase B)
- Complement C3, C4
- Chest radiograph to rule out pulmonary edema

**Further evaluation of acute nephritis if APSGN not present or is unlikely**
- Hepatitis B panel, hepatitis C titer
- HIV-1 antibody
- ANA (full lupus panel if ANA is positive)
- ANCA
- Anti-GBM antibody titer
- Renal biopsy as indicated

*Abbreviations:* ANA, anti-nuclear antibody; ANCA, anti-neutrophil cytoplasmic antibody; ASO, anti–streptolysin O; GBM, glomerular basement membrane; HIV, human immunodeficiency virus,

## MANAGEMENT

## SUPPORTIVE THERAPY

The mainstay of treatment of APIGN consists of supportive therapy. Children without volume expansion, hypertension, electrolyte problems, or decreased kidney function need only close follow-up. Patients who develop moderate-to-severe hypertension, renal impairment, or hyperkalemia generally require hospitalization for monitoring fluid and electrolyte balance as well as for managing hypertension.

## ANTIBIOTICS

Antibiotic treatment after the onset of APSGN does not alter the course of the disease. In epidemics, antibiotic prophylaxis given to family members may reduce the risk for spread of APSGN.[3,5,63] During epidemics of GAS infection, universal penicillin prophylaxis to all children has been shown to prevent transmission of nephritogenic strains of GAS and protect against glomerulonephritis.[64–66] Routine prophylaxis of general population and outside the household contacts, however, is not recommended.

In a large-scale prospective study, treatment of 4782 patients with culture-proved GAS tonsillopharyngitis, treatment with oral penicillin V resulted in GSA eradication rate of 84%.[67] APSGN sequelae occurred in only five (0.1%) of the treated patients in this study, reaffirming that appropriate and timely treatment of GAS infection prevents development of APSGN.

## FLUID OVERLOAD AND HYPERTENSION

When present, hypertension is the result of sodium retention and volume expansion. Therefore, treatment is directed at sodium restriction and diuretic therapy, in addition to antihypertensive medication, if necessary. The combination of a loop or thiazide diuretic with a calcium channel blocker is usually effective. Caution should be exercised with the use of angiotensin-converting enzyme inhibitors or angiotensin receptor blockers because of the risk for hyperkalemia or acute kidney injury. Interestingly, in two studies the use of captopril was noted to be therapeutically efficient in reducing blood pressure without any significant change in renal function.[68,79] Serum potassium was, unfortunately, not monitored in these studies.

## HYPERKALEMIA

Hyperkalemia is commonly seen in patients with APSGN, especially if renal function is compromised and daily intake of potassium remains unchecked. Hyporeninemic hypoaldosteronism seen in patients with APSGN has

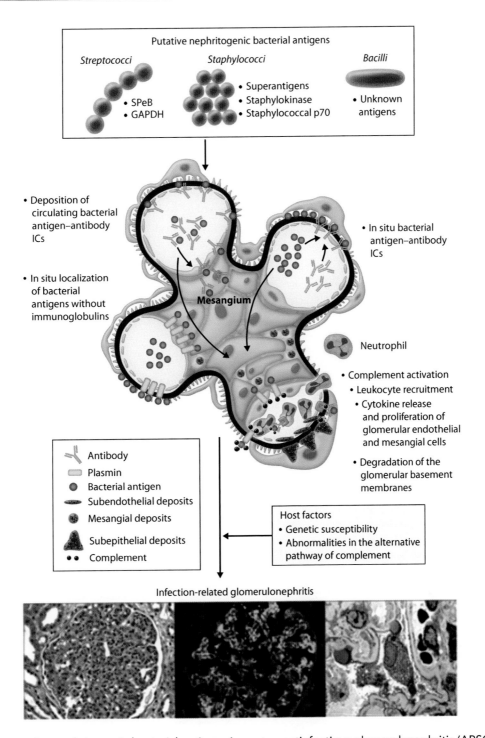

Figure 21.6 The putative nephritogenic bacterial antigens in acute postinfectious glomerulonephritis (APSGN) cause glomerular injury through multiple potential mechanisms that include the following: **(1)** passive glomerular entrapment of circulating bacterial antigen-antibody immune complexes; **(2)** glomerular in situ immune complex (IC) formation by antibodies directed against planted cationic bacterial antigens or intrinsic glomerular antigens via molecular mimicry; and **(3)** glomerular in situ localization of circulating cationic bacterial antigens without immunoglobulin, potentially promoting plasmin activation in the mesangium and glomerular basement. Any combination of these mechanisms may act in concert and initiate complement cascade activation via the alternative and lectin pathways. The resultant complement activation in glomeruli leads to the generation of chemotactins C3a and C5a, recruitment of neutrophils and monocytes, and leukocyte-mediated injury. In addition, locally activated plasmin degrades the glomerular basement membrane directly or through the activation of metalloproteinases and may promote inflammation. Predisposing host factors such as genetic susceptibility and dysregulation of the alternative complement pathway may contribute to pathogenesis. *GAPDH*, glyceraldehyde-3-phosphate dehydrogenase; *NAPlr*, nephritis-associated plasmin receptor; *SpeB*, streptococcal pyrogenic exotoxin B. (Reproduced with permission from: Nasr SH, Radhakrishnan J, D'Agati VD. Bacterial infection-related glomerulonephritis in adults. Kidney Int. 2013;83:792–803.

been suggested to be the cause of hyperkalemia in these patients.[70] Mildly elevated serum potassium level can be treated with restriction of potassium intake in the diet, and use of potassium exchange resin sodium polystyrene sulfonate (Kayexalate®) orally. Severe hyperkalemia should be treated as an emergency using an inhaled $\beta_2$-adrenergic stimulant salbutamol, intravenous bicarbonate, intravenous glucose and insulin, or calcium carbonate, as appropriate. Salbutamol inhalation can provide a quick response (30 minutes) and lower serum potassium to a more manageable level, and its effect can last up to 2 hours.[71] Rare cases of life-threatening or symptomatic hyperkalemia require treatment with dialysis, in conjunction with pharmacologic therapy.

## Dialysis

In addition to treating hyperkalemia, hemodialysis or continuous venovenous hemofiltration may be necessary to treat severe cases of uremia or volume overload, especially if diuretic-unresponsive anuria or oliguria is present. Most patients requiring dialysis support for management of fluid overload, hyperkalemia, and uremia in APSGN have severe renal disease with crescentic renal pathology.[72]

## TREATMENT OF CRESCENTIC ACUTE POSTSTREPTOCOCCAL GLOMERULONEPHRITIS

A rapidly progressive clinical course with crescents in the renal biopsy represents therapeutic challenges, such as fluid overload, hypertension, hyperkalemia, and potential for long-term renal damage. Apart from supportive management, there are no clear, evidence-based, and well-accepted guidelines for treatment of such patients. Treatment with quadruple therapy consisting of prednisone, azathioprine, cyclophosphamide, dipyridamole, and heparin was not shown to be superior to supportive therapy alone in a study by Roy et al.[73] In another nonrandomized study of crescentic APSGN, steroids, with or without cyclophosphamide, did not provide any convincing therapeutic advantage.[23]

## CLINICAL COURSE AND PROGNOSIS

The acute morbidity of ASPGN is well known and clinically challenging in some patients.[77] However, several long-term studies in children have documented an excellent long-term outcome in a majority of patients with this disease.[74-76] Potter et al.[74] followed 760 patients, of whom 41 were adults, for 2 to 6 years after onset of APSGN. Of these, only 1.8% patients had persistent urinary abnormalities and only one patient had developed chronic kidney disease (CKD). In half of the patients, urinary abnormalities disappeared on their own in the following 2 years of observation. Hypertension was present in only 1.4% patients.

Clark et al.[75] prospectively followed a cohort of 36 children with biopsy-proven APSGN between 1962 and 1970. After a mean follow-up of 9.5 years (range, 5.4 to 12.4 years), although minor urinary abnormalities were noted in 20% cases, no one developed CKD and hypertension was noted in only one patient, who also had history of recurrent pyelonephritis. Similarly, Popović-Rolović et al.[76] found hypertension in 3.4%, proteinuria in 2.3%, and microhematuria in 2.3% of APSGN patients after follow-up of 10 to 17 years.

Prognosis of APSGN in adults has been reported to be less optimistic compared to that in children. Lien et al.[77] followed 57 adult patients with APSGN for a period of 1 to 14 years (mean, 7 years). Of these, 5 patients died, 2 with CKD. Glomerular obsolescence was noted on repeat renal biopsy in 3 of the 11 patients who underwent biopsy for evidence of ongoing proteinuria, hematuria, or abnormal renal function. Chugh et al.[78] reported that of the 192 patients (142 adults and 51 children) followed in India up to 10 years (mean, 4.8 years), 10 patients developed CKD or end-stage renal disease (ESRD). Hypertension was noted in 15% of patients during follow-up. Similarly, Srisawat et al.[79] noted that 14% of their patients with APIGN developed ESRD, none had APSGN, and all had other infective causes for acute glomerulonephritis. In summary, adults with APSGN need to be followed more closely and for a longer time than children.

## SUMMARY

Despite a decrease in the incidence, APSGN is still one of the most common kidney diseases in children. The disease is relatively benign in most children, but it can have considerable early morbidity in some, such as hypertensive encephalopathy and hyperkalemia. In most cases, the diagnosis is easily made and treatment consists of supportive measures. Full recovery is expected in most children. Atypical cases may present diagnostic challenges and severe cases require a renal biopsy. Improving overcrowding and poor living conditions can reduce the burden of the disease worldwide.

### Clinical Vignette 21.1

A 10-year-old African-American boy presented to the emergency department with the complaints of passing dark brown urine and swelling around his eyes since waking up the same morning. On further questioning, the patient reported having a slight sore throat within the previous month but a throat culture was not obtained. He denied any such previous illness.

His physical examination revealed moderate periorbital and pretibial edema and a few bilateral basal pulmonary crackles. His blood pressure was 150/102 mm Hg. Laboratory evaluation demonstrated normal CBC; serum sodium, 138 mmol/L; potassium, 5.2 mmol/L; chloride, 106 mmol/L; bicarbonate, 18 mmol/L; blood urea nitrogen (BUN), 20 mg/dL, creatinine, 1.7 mg/dL; and urine with 3+ and 2+ protein. The patient was admitted to hospital for treatment of his hypertension and further diagnostic evaluation.

The patient's hypertension responded to intravenous furosemide and oral calcium channel blocker (amlodipine) therapy. The day after admission his blood pressure was 128/80 mm Hg; serum creatinine, 1.5 mg/dL; BUN, 35 mg/dL; and electrolytes within normal limits. The ASO titer was positive at 1:400 (international units/mL), and his complement C3 level was low at 30 mg/dL (normal is greater than 90 mg/dL). The antinuclear antibody (ANA) test was negative and throat culture was negative for GAS. Based on the clinical presentation and laboratory results, the diagnosis of APSGN was made. On the third day, his serum creatinine was 1 mg/dL. He was discharged from the hospital the following day on oral amlodipine therapy. Antibiotics were not prescribed in view of negative throat culture results.

At a follow-up appointment 1 week after discharge, a serum creatinine was 0.7 mg/dL. Four weeks later the patient's basic metabolic panel and serum C3 level were normal, and urinalysis shows microscopic hematuria only. His blood pressure in the outpatient clinic was 96/66 mm Hg, and his amlodipine therapy was discontinued.

## TEACHING POINTS

- The apparent short duration of illness and decreased renal function point toward acute disease such as APSGN, rapidly progressive glomerulitis, or an exacerbation of a previously undiagnosed chronic glomerulonephritis, such as IgA nephropathy and MPGN. Absence of signs of systemic disease makes generalized vasculitis unlikely.
- The presence of proteinuria, hematuria, hypertension, azotemia, and low C3 points to three possibilities: APSGN, MPGN, and nephritis of SLE. A negative ANA suggests that the patient is unlikely to have SLE nephritis. A declining serum creatinine was shown on day 2; although this is a positive development, the possibility of MPGN could not be ruled out in that time frame. However, further decline of serum creatinine on day 3 made the diagnosis of APSGN more likely.
- Had the serum creatinine continued to rise, MPGN would have been the more likely diagnosis at that time and he would have needed a diagnostic renal biopsy.
- Treatment of this patient was mainly directed at control of his blood pressure, and a combination of diuretics and calcium channel blockers was sufficient to normalize it.

- Antibiotics were not prescribed for this patient because throat culture was negative for GAS. If the throat culture would have been positive, oral antibiotics would have been appropriate from a public health perspective to eradicate the infection in this patient and prevent its transmission to others in his circle of contacts.
- The parents of this child should be informed that he may continue to have microscopic hematuria for a number of months, even though he has no active renal disease. His overall prognosis should be excellent.

## REFERENCES

1. Bright R. Cases and observations illustrative of renal disease accompanied with the secretion of albuminous urine. Guy Hosp Rep. 1836;1:338–341.
2. Eison TM, Ault BH, Jones DP, et al. Post-streptococcal acute glomerulonephritis in children: Clinical features and pathogenesis. Pediatr Nephrol. 2011;26:165–80
3. Berrios X, Lagomarsino D, Solar E, et al. Post-streptococcal acute glomerulonephritis in Chile: 20 years of experience. Pediatr Nephrol. 2004;19:306–312.
4. Wong W, Lennon DR, Crone S, et al. Prospective population-based study on the burden of disease from post-streptococcal glomerulonephritis of hospitalised children in New Zealand: Epidemiology, clinical features and complications. J Paediatr Child Health. 2013;49:850–5.
5. Roy S, Stapleton FB. Changing perspectives in children hospitalized with poststreptococcal acute glomerulonephritis. Pediatr Nephrol. 1990;4:585–8.
6. Ilyas M, Tolaymat A. Changing epidemiology of acute post-streptococcal glomerulonephritis in Northeast Florida: A comparative study. Pediatr Nephrol. 2008;23:1101–6.
7. Bingler MA, Ellis D, Moritz ML. Acute post-streptococcal glomerulonephritis in a 14-month-old boy: Why is this uncommon? Pediatr Nephrol. 2007;22:448–50.
8. Carapetis JR, Steer AC, Mulholland EK, et al. The global burden of group A streptococcal diseases. Lancet Infect Dis. 2005;5:685–94.
9. Jackson SJ, Steer AC, Campbell H. Systematic review: Estimation of global burden of non-suppurative sequelae of upper respiratory tract infection—Rheumatic fever and post-streptococcal glomerulonephritis. Trop Med Int Health. 2011;16:2–11.
10. Anthony BF, Kaplan EL, Chapman SS, et al. Epidemic acute nephritis with reappearance of type 49 streptococcus. Lancet. 1967;2:787–90.
11. Reinstein CR. Epidemic of nephritis at Red Lake, Minnesota. J Pediatr. 1955;47:25–34.

12. Rodríguez-Iturbe B, Rubio L, García R. Attack rate of poststreptococcal nephritis in families: A prospective study. Lancet. 1981;1:401–3.

13. Tasic V, Polenakovic M. Occurrence of subclinical post-streptococcal glomerulonephritis in family contacts. J Paediatr Child Health. 2003;39:177–9.

14. Sagel I, Treser G, Ty A, et al. Occurrence and nature of glomerular lesions after group A streptococcal infections in children. Ann Intern Med. 1973;79:492–9.

15. Lewy JE, Salinas-Madrigal L, Herdson PB, et al. Clinico-pathologic correlations in acute poststreptococcal glomerulonephritis: A correlation between renal functions, morphologic damage and clinical course of 46 children with acute poststreptococcal glomerulonephritis. Medicine (Baltimore) 1971;50:453–501.

16. Modai D, Pik A, Behar M, et al. Biopsy proven evolution of post streptococcal glomerulonephritis to rapidly progressive glomerulonephritis of a post infectious type. Clin Nephrol. 1985;23:198–202.

17. Batson BN, Baliga R. Post-streptococcal hypertensive encephalopathy with normal urinalysis. Pediatr Nephrol. 2003;18:73.

18. Zaki SA, Shanbag P. Unusual presentation of poststreptococcal glomerulonephritis as posterior reversible encephalopathy syndrome. J Pediatr Neurosci. 2014;9:42–4.

19. Rovang RD, Zawada ET Jr, Santella RN, et al. Cerebral vasculitis associated with acute poststreptococcal glomerulonephritis. Am J Nephrol. 1997;17:89–92.

20. Nasr SH, Radhakrishnan J, D'Agati VD. Bacterial infection-related glomerulonephritis in adults. Kidney Int. 2013;83:792–803.

21. Jennings RB, Earle DP. Post-streptococcal glomerulonephritis: Histopathologic and clinical studies of the acute, subsiding acute and early chronic latent phase's. J Clin Invest. 1961;40:1525–95.

22. Wong W, Morris MC, Zwi J. Outcome of severe acute post-streptococcal glomerulonephritis in New Zealand children. Pediatr Nephrol. 2009;24:1021–6.

23. Sorger K, Gessler U, Hubner FK, et al. Subtypes of acute postinfectious glomerulonephritis: Synopsis of clinical and pathological features. Clin Nephrol. 1982;17:114–128.

24. Michael AF Jr, Drummond KN, Good RA, et al. Acute poststreptococcal glomerulonephritis: Immune deposit disease. J Clin Invest. 1966;45:237–48.

25. Mori Y, Yamashita H, Umeda Y, et al. Association of parvovirus 19 infection with acute glomerulonephritis in healthy adults: Case report and review of the literature. Clin Nephrol 2002;57:69–73

26. Thorley AM, Campbell D, Moghal NE, et al. Post streptococcal acute glomerulonephritis secondary to sporadic Streptococcus equi infection. Pediatr Nephrol. 2007;22:597–9.

27. Dillon HC. Pyoderma and nephritis. Ann Rev Med 1967;18:207–18.

28. Bessen DE, Sotir CM, Readdy TL, et al. Genetic correlates of throat and skin isolates of group A streptococci. J Infect Dis. 1996;173:896–900.

29. Zabriskie JB, Utermohlen V, Read SE, et al. Streptococcus-related glomerulonephritis. Kidney Int. 1973;3:100–4.

30. Rodríguez-Iturbe B, Batsford S. Pathogenesis of poststreptococcal glomerulonephritis a century after Clemens von Pirquet. Kidney Int. 2007;71:1094–104.

31. Rodríguez-Iturbe B, Musser JM. The current state of poststreptococcal glomerulonephritis. J Am Soc Nephrol. 2008;19:1855–64.

32. Yoshizawa N, Oshima S, Sagel I, et al. Role of a streptococcal antigen in the pathogenesis of acute poststreptococcal glomerulonephritis: Characterization of the antigen and a proposed mechanism for the disease. J Immunol 1992;148:3110–3116.

33. Yoshizawa N, Yamakami K, Fujino M, et al. Nephritis-associated plasmin receptor and acute poststreptococcal glomerulonephritis: Characterization of the antigen and associated immune response. J Am Soc Nephrol. 2004;15:1785–93.

34. Oda T, Yoshizawa N, Yamakami K, et al. The role of nephritis-associated plasmin receptor (NAPlr) in glomerulonephritis associated with streptococcal infection. J Biomed Biotechnol. 2012;2012:417675. Article ID 4176759. doi 10.1155/2012/417675.

35. Poon-King R, Bannan J, Viteri A, et al. Identification of an extracellular plasmin binding protein from nephritogenic streptococci. J Exp Med. 1993;178:759–63.

36. Cu GA, Mezzano S, Bannan JD, et al. Immunohistochemical and serological evidence for the role of streptococcal proteinase in acute post-streptococcal glomerulonephritis. Kidney Int. 1998;54:819–26.

37. Batsford SR, Mezzano S, Mihatsch M, et al. Is the nephritogenic antigen in post-streptococcal glomerulonephritis pyrogenic exotoxin B (SPE B) or GAPDH? Kidney Int. 2005;68:1120–9.

38. Vogt A, Batsford S, Rodríguez-Iturbe B, et al. Cationic antigens in poststreptococcal glomerulonephritis. Clin Nephrol. 1983;20:271–9.

39. Dixon FJ, Feldman JD, Vazquez JJ. Experimental glomerulonephritis: The pathogenesis of a laboratory model resembling the spectrum of human glomerulonephritis. J Exp Med. 1961;113:899–920

40. Fish AJ, Michael AF, Vernier RL, et al. Acute serum sickness nephritis in the rabbit: An immune deposit disease. Am J Pathol. 1966;49:997–1022.

41. Mohammed I, Ansell BM, Holborow EJ, et al. Circulating immune complexes in subacute infective endocarditis and post-streptococcal glomerulonephritis. J Clin Pathol. 1977;30:308–11.

42. van de Rijn I, Fillit H, Brandeis WE, et al. Serial studies on circulating immune complexes in post-streptococcal sequelae. Clin Exp Immunol. 1978;34:318–25.

43. Lin CY. Serial studies of circulating immune complexes in poststreptococcal glomerulonephritis. Pediatrics. 1982;70:725–7.

44. Friedman J, van de Rijn I, Ohkuni H, et al. Immunological studies of post-streptococcal sequelae: Evidence for presence of streptococcal antigens in circulating immune complexes. J Clin Invest. 1984;74:1027–34.

45. Wyatt RJ, Forristal J, West CD, et al. Complement profiles in acute post-streptococcal glomerulonephritis. Pediatr Nephrol. 1988;2:219–23.

46. Matsell DG, Wyatt RJ, Gaber LW. Terminal complement complexes in acute poststreptococcal glomerulonephritis. Pediatr Nephrol. 1994; 8:671–76

47. Hisano S, Matsushita M, Fujita T, et al. Activation of the lectin complement pathway in post-streptococcal acute glomerulonephritis. Pathol Int 2007;57:351–7.

48. Layrisse Z, Rodríguez-Iturbe B, Garcia-Ramirez R, et al. Family studies of the HLA system in acute post-streptococcal glomerulonephritis. Hum Immunol. 1983;7:177–85.

49. Bakr A, Mahmoud LA, Al-Chenawi F, Salah A. HLA-DRB1 alleles in Egyptian children with poststreptococcal acute glomerulonephritis. Pediatr Nephrol. 2007;22:376–9.

50. Dursun H, Noyan A, Matyar S, et al. Endothelial nitric oxide synthase gene intron 4 a/b VNTR polymorphism in children with APSGN. Pediatr Nephrol. 2006; 21:1661–5.

51. Leme CE, Ribeiro CA Jr, Silva HB. Renal tubular sodium reabsorption during the recovery from the oliguric phase of acute nephritis. Biomedicine. 1975;23:92–6.

52. Mota-Hernandez F, Feiman R, Gordillo-Paniagua G. Predictive value of fractional excretion of filtered sodium for hypertension in acute post-streptococcal glomerulonephritis. J Pediatr. 1984;104:560–3.

53. Ozdemir S, Saatçi U, Beşbaş N, et al. Plasma atrial natriuretic peptide and endothelin levels in acute poststreptococcal glomerulonephritis. Pediatr Nephrol. 1992;6:519–22.

54. Powell HR, Rotenberg E, Williams AL, Credie MC. Plasma renin activity in acute post-streptococcal glomerulo-nephritis and the haemolytic-uraemic syndrome. Arch Dis Child. 1974;49:802–7.

55. Maekawa S, Fukuda K, Yamauchi T, et al. Follow-up study of pharyngeal carriers of beta-hemolytic streptococci among s3chool children in Sapporo City during a period of 2 years and 5 months. J Clin Microbiol. 1981;13:101–22.

56. Strömberg A, Schwan A, Cars O. Throat carrier rates of beta-hemolytic streptococci among healthy adults and children. Scand J Infect Dis. 1988;20:411–7.

57. Parks T, Smeesters PR, Curtis N, et al. ASO titer or not? When to use streptococcal serology: A guide for clinicians. Eur J Clin Microbiol Infect Dis. 2015;34:945–9.

58. Dodge WF, Spargo BH, Travis LB, et al. Poststreptococcal glomerulonephritis: A prospective study in children. N Engl J Med. 1972; 286: 273–8.

59. Meekin GE, Martin DR, Dawson KP. Probable association of M type 57 streptococcal skin infection with acute glomerulonephritis in the Tauranga area. N Z Med J. 1980;91:456–60.

60. West CD, Northway JD, Davis NC. Serum levels of beta-1C globulin, a complement component, in the nephritidies, lipoid nephrosis and other conditions. J Clin Invest. 1964; 43:1507-17.

61. Cameron JS, Vick RM, Ogg SC, et al. Plasma C3 and C4 concentrations in management of glomerulonephritis. Br Med J. 1973;3:668–72.

62. Sethi S1, Fervenza FC, Zhang Y, et al. Atypical postinfectious glomerulonephritis is associated with abnormalities in the alternative pathway of complement. Kidney Int. 2013;83:293–9.

63. Rodríguez-Iturbe B. Epidemic poststreptococcal glomerulonephritis. Kidney Int. 1984;25:129–36.

64. Johnston F, Carapetis J, Patel MS, et al. Evaluating the use of penicillin to control outbreaks of acute poststreptococcal glomerulonephritis. Pediatr Infect Dis J. 1999;18:327–32.

65. Atkins, R. C. How bright is their future? Poststreptococcal glomerulonephritis in indigenous communities in Australia. Med J Aust. 2001;174:489–90.

66. Streeton CL, Hanna JN, Messer RD, Merianos A. An epidemic of acute poststreptococcal glomerulonephritis among aboriginal children. J Paediatr Child Health. 1995;31:245–8.

67. Adam D, Scholz H, Helmerking M. Short-course antibiotic treatment of 4782 culture-proven cases of group A streptococcal tonsillopharyngitis and incidence of poststreptococcal sequelae. J Infect Dis. 2000;182:509–16.

68. Morsi MR, Madina EH, Anglo AA, et al. Evaluation of captopril versus reserpine and furosemide in treating hypertensive children with acute post-streptococcal glomerulonephritis. Acta Paediatr. 1992;81:145–9.

69. Parra G, Rodríguez-Iturbe B, Colina-Chourio J. Short-term treatment with captopril in hypertension due to acute glomerulonephritis. Clin Nephrol. 1988;29:58–62.

70. Don BR, Schambelan M. Hyperkalemia in acute glomerulonephritis due to transient hyporeninemic hypoaldosteronism. Kidney Int. 1990;38:1159–63.

71. Allon M, Smeesters PR, Curtis N, Steer AC. Nebulized albuterol for acute hyperkalemia in patients on hemodialysis. Ann Intern Med. 1989;110:426–9.

72. Blyth CC, Robertson PW, Rosenberg AR. Post-streptococcal glomerulonephritis in Sydney: A 16-year retrospective review. J Paediatr Child Health. 2007;43:446–50.

73. Roy S 3rd, Murphy WM, Arant BS Jr. Poststreptococcal crescentic glomerulonephritis in children: Comparison of quintuple therapy versus supportive care. J Pediatr. 1981;98:403–10.

74. Potter EV, Abidh S, Sharrett AR, et al. Clinical healing two to six years after poststreptococcal glomerulonephritis in Trinidad. N Engl J Med. 1978;298:767–72.

75. Clark G, White RH, Glasgow EF, et al. Poststreptococcal glomerulonephritis in children: Clinicopathological correlations and long-term prognosis. Pediatr Nephrol. 1988;2:381–8.

76. Popović-Rolović M, Kostić M, Antić-Peco A, et al. Medium- and long-term prognosis of patients with acute poststreptococcal glomerulonephritis. Nephron. 1991;58:393–9.

77. Lien JW, Mathew TH, Meadows R. Acute post-streptococcal glomerulonephritis in adults: A long-term study. Q J Med. 1979;48:99–111.

78. Chugh KS, Malhotra HS, Sakhuja V, et al. Progression to end stage renal disease in post-streptococcal glomerulonephritis (PSGN)—Chandigarh Study. Int J Artif Organs. 1987;10:189–94.

79. Srisawat N, Aroonpoonsub L, Lewsuwan S, et al. The clinicopathology and outcome of post-infectious glomerulonephritis: Experience in 36 adults. J Med Assoc Thai. 2006;89(Suppl 2):S157–62.

## REVIEW QUESTIONS

1. The typical "deposits" in acute poststreptococcal glomerulonephritis seen by electron microscopy are in which of the following locations?
   a. Mesangial
   b. Subendothelial
   c. Subepithelial
   d. Intramembranous

2. Typical glomerular anti-IgG immunofluorescence in acute poststreptococcal glomerulonephritis shows which of the following patterns?
   a. Linear along capillary loops
   b. Granular along capillary loops
   c. Granular in mesangium
   d. No immunofluorescence

3. Acute postinfectious glomerulonephritis most commonly follows infection by which of the following organisms?
   a. Group A β-hemolytic streptococcus
   b. Group B β-hemolytic streptococcus
   c. Group C β-hemolytic streptococcus
   d. Group C streptococcus

4. Which of the following is true regarding scabies-associated acute postinfectious glomerulonephritis?
   a. The latent period is longer than in tonsillitis-associated disease.
   b. It is usually not caused by group A β-hemolytic streptococcus.
   c. Complement C3 is typically not decreased.
   d. An antigen from *Sarcoptes scabiei* is present in the glomeruli.

5. Which of the following statements is true regarding the epidemiology of acute poststreptococcal glomerulonephritis?
   a. It is more common in affluent societies.
   b. During epidemics, subclinical disease is more common than symptomatic disease.
   c. Epidemics are usually caused by non–group A streptococci.
   d. Antibiotic prophylaxis is not effective.

6. A 9-year-old boy presents with symptomless gross hematuria. He has had a sore throat for 2 days. His basic metabolic panel is normal. Which of the following is the *most* helpful diagnostic test?
   a. Complement C3 level
   b. Complement C4 level
   c. Throat culture
   d. ASO titer

7. A 6-year-old girl has painless gross hematuria and puffy eyes. She denies any recent illness. Her BP is 139/76; BUN, 34 mg/dL; creatinine, 1.3 mg/dL; serum albumin, 2.9 g/dL; and complement, C3 23 mg/dL. Urine is positive for blood and protein. Which of the following is the *most* appropriate treatment?
   a. Amoxicillin
   b. Intravenous steroids
   c. Chlorothiazide or furosemide
   d. Observation only

8. A 9-year-old boy presents with puffy eyes and headache. He remembers having a recent sore throat. His BP is 150/90 mm Hg, and he has mild periorbital and pretibial edema. Blood urea nitrogen (BUN) is 30 mg/dL; creatinine, 1.3 mg/dL; and complement C3, 20 mg/dL. Intravenous nicardipine and furosemide are started to control his hypertension. The next day his metabolic panel shows sodium, 132 mmol/L; potassium, 4.8 mmol/L; chloride, 100 mmol/L; carbon dioxide, 20

mmol/L; BUN, 60 mg/dL; and creatinine, 3.2 mg/dL. Which of the following is the *most* appropriate next step?

a. Hemodialysis
b. Continuous venovenous hemofiltration
c. Renal biopsy
d. Intravenous steroid treatment

9. Hypertension in acute postinfectious glomerulonephritis is mainly due to which of the following?

a. Activated sympathomimetic nervous system
b. Decreased glomerular filtration rate
c. Elevated plasma renin level secondary to nephritis
d. Increased fluid volume expansion resulting from increased tubular sodium absorption

## ANSWER KEY

1. c
2. b
3. a
4. a
5. b
6. a
7. c
8. c
9. d

# 22

# Rapidly progressive glomerulonephritis and vasculitis

FRANCA IOREMBER AND V. MATTI VEHASKARI

Rapidly progressive glomerulonephritis (RPGN) is a rare clinical disorder characterized by sudden and rapid deterioration of kidney function over days or weeks and by histologic findings of glomerular injury associated with extensive "crescent" formation. Glomerular crescents are cellular or fibrotic, crescent-shaped formations outside the glomerular capillary tuft in the Bowman space that ultimately result in global glomerular sclerosis. Some crescents may occasionally be seen in severe forms of glomerulonephritis, but in a stricter sense the term *crescentic glomerulonephritis* is used only when crescents affect more than 50% of the glomeruli in an adequate kidney biopsy.[1,2] This definition is arbitrary, however, and patients with a lesser degree of crescent formation may progress to full-blown RPGN. The diagnosis of RPGN must be made promptly because a delay in the initiation of therapy can lead to irreversible renal injury and loss of kidney function. The best predictors of outcome for all types of crescentic glomerulonephritis are the severity of kidney dysfunction at presentation and the initiation of therapy.[3,4] Another poor prognostic indicator is the severity of crescents present in the renal biopsy.[3–6]

## CLASSIFICATION

RPGN is classified into three broad categories (Table 22.1) based on pathologic and immunopathologic features: (1) immune complex–mediated crescentic glomerulonephritis, (2) pauci-immune crescentic glomerulonephritis, and (3) anti–glomerular basement membrane (anti-GBM) antibody disease. As noted in Table 22.1, several specific diseases can result in RPGN and are classifiable into one of the three distinct categories.

Childhood RPGN is frequently caused by vasculitis, which includes immune complex–mediated disorders, such as Henoch-Schönlein purpura (HSP) nephritis and lupus nephritis, and all of the conditions included under the classification of pauci-immune RPGN.

### KEY POINTS

Three types of RPGN are:

- Immune complex–mediated disease
- Pauci-immune disease
- Anti-GBM antibody disease

Consensus criteria for classification of vasculitides for the pediatric population were developed by the European League Against Rheumatism (EULAR) and the Pediatric Rheumatology European Society (PReS) in 2006.[7,8] This classification uses vessel size to categorize vasculitis into large-, medium-, and small-vessel

Table 22.1 Causes of rapidly progressive glomerulonephritis*

**Immune Complex RPGN (45% of Pediatric Cases)**
- Systemic vasculitis
  - HSP
  - SLE
- Isolated renal disease
  - IgA nephropathy
  - MPGN type 1 and 3
  - Dense deposit disease (DDD)
  - APIGN

**Pauci-immune RPGN (42% of Pediatric Cases)**
- ANCA-associated vasculitis (AAV)
  - Microscopic polyangiitis
  - Granulomatosis with polyangiitis (formerly Wegener granulomatosis)
  - Eosinophilic granulomatosis with polyangiitis (formerly Churg-Strauss syndrome)
  - Renal limited disease
  - Drug-induced disease
  - ANCA-negative vasculitis

**Anti-GBM Antibody–Associated RPGN (12% of Pediatric Cases)**
- Idiopathic (autoimmune anti-GBM antibodies)
- After renal transplantation in Alport syndrome
- Combined anti-GBM and ANCA

*Abbreviations:* AAV, ANCA-associated vasculitis; ANCA, anti–neutrophil cytoplasmic antibodies; APIGN, acute postinfectious glomerulonephritis; GBM, glomerular basement membrane; HSP, Henoch-Schönlein purpura; IgA, immunoglobulin A; MPGN, membranoproliferative glomerulonephritis; RPGN, rapidly progressive glomerulonephritis; SLE, systemic lupus erythematosus.
* Vasculitides not associated with RPGN are not included.

Table 22.2 Classification of pediatric vasculitis

**Predominantly large-vessel disease**
- Takayasu arteritis

**Predominantly medium-vessel vasculitis**
- Childhood polyarteritis nodosa
- Cutaneous polyarteritis
- Kawasaki disease

**Predominantly small-vessel vasculitis**
a. Granulomatous
  - Granulomatosis with polyangiitis
  - Eosinophilic granulomatosis with polyangiitis
b. Nongranulomatous
  - Microscopic polyangiitis
  - Henoch-Schönlein purpura
  - Isolated cutaneous leukocytoclastic vasculitis
  - Hypocomplementemic urticarial vasculitis

**Other vasculitides**
- Behçet disease
- Vasculitis secondary to infection (including hepatitis B associated–polyarteritis nodosa), malignant diseases, and drugs including hypersensitivity vasculitis)
- Vasculitis associated with connective tissue diseases
- Isolated vasculitis of the central nervous system
- Cogan syndrome
- Unclassified

diseases (Table 22.2). In general, RPGN largely results from small-vessel vasculitides. Most other forms of vasculitis are rarely, if ever, a cause of acute renal disease, with the exception of polyarteritis nodosa (PAN) and Kawasaki disease, both of which may manifest with renal disease that is histologically distinct from RPGN. PAN predominantly affects medium-sized blood vessels, causes necrotizing vasculitis, and often spares the glomeruli.[9,10] The major renal manifestation of Kawasaki disease is tubulointerstitial nephritis. This chapter discusses the clinical, pathologic, and management aspects of diseases that cause RPGN.

## EPIDEMIOLOGY

RPGN is a rare disease in all populations, especially in children. Most incidence estimates come from biopsy materials. In a large study of 632 renal biopsies with crescentic glomerulonephritis, only 11.6% were pediatric cases.[3] Overall, pauci-immune crescentic glomerulonephritis was the predominant subtype in adults and made up 60% of the total number of cases. In children, the number of immune-complex mediated and pauci-immune RPGN were similar, each accounting for 45% and 42% of cases respectively. Anti-GBM disease comprised 12% of the total number of pediatric patients in this study. In another pediatric report of 33 cases of RPGN from India, immune complex–mediated crescentic glomerulonephritis accounted for 45.5%, whereas pauci-immune

---

### KEY POINTS

- Most types of RPGN are caused by small-vessel vasculitides.
- Pauci-immune RPGN is more common in adults.
- In children, distribution of immune-complex mediated and pauci-immune RPGN is almost equal.
- Anti-GBM disease is rare in children.

disease comprised the remaining 54.5% cases.[11] RPGN affects more whites than African Americans in a ratio of 7:1, with no gender predilection.[3,12,13]

Whereas the overall incidence of all RPGN in the general population is unknown, the incidence of pauci-immune glomerulonephritis has been estimated at 4 per million.[14] The annual incidence of RPGN secondary to anti–neutrophil cytoplasmic antibody–associated vasculitis (AAV) in both European and North American populations is approximately 10 to 20/million, with a peak age of onset at 65 to 74 years.[13] In Japan, the annual incidence is reported to be as high as 22.6/million.[15] Available data suggest significant geographic differences among AAV subtypes. Data from Europe, India, and Japan have shown that granulomatosis with polyangiitis (GPA, formerly known as Wegener granulomatosis) is the most common subtype of AAV in Europe and India, whereas microscopic polyangiitis (MPA) predominates in Japan.[13,15–18] These regional differences may be explained by genetic and environmental risk factors.[19]

Available data estimate the annual incidence of anti-GBM disease at 1 case per million in the general population, and this disorder is even less common in children.[20–24] The peak age of incidence is in the third decade in young men, and a second peak, in the sixth and seventh decades, affects both sexes equally.[25]

## PATHOGENESIS AND PATHOLOGY

Glomerular crescents are the hallmark in all forms of RPGN, crescents are the hallmark findings in all forms of RPGN, and they need to be documented for the diagnosis in an adequate renal biopsy. The percentage of glomeruli with crescents on renal biopsy correlates with the severity of renal failure and with long-term prognosis.[3,26,27] Glomerular crescents can be of two types: (1) cellular crescents; and (2) crescents with varying degrees of fibrin organization, including fibrocellular and fibrous crescents.[28] Cellular crescents develop first and eventually organize into fibrous crescents as the disease progresses. Ultimately, the entire glomerular tuft may be replaced by fibrous material, with resultant cessation of filtration and glomerular death (global sclerosis).

### KEY POINTS

- Glomerular crescents crescents are the hallmark of RPGN.
- The initiating event in crescent formation is disruption of the glomerular capillary wall.
- Crescents are derived from proliferating parietal cells and podocytes, as well as from recruitment of circulating monocytes, neutrophils, and macrophages.

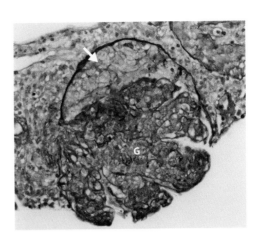

Figure 22.1. Light microscopy showing a glomerulus with cellular crescent (arrow). Compression of the glomerular tuft (G) by the crescent is also evident. (Figure courtesy of Dr. Bhaskar Kallakuri, Department of Pathology, Georgetown University Hospital, Washington DC.)

Cellular crescents are defined by the presence of two or more layers of cells in a crescent-shaped formation in the periphery of the Bowman space (Figure 22.1). These cells are derived from proliferating parietal cells and podocytes and from recruitment of circulating monocytes and macrophages. There is also evidence of local proliferation of macrophages within the Bowman space.[29–31] The initiating event in crescent formation appears to be disruption of the glomerular capillary wall, which is a common pathway for all types of RPGN.[3,32] Lysis of the GBM results from release of serine proteinases and matrix metalloproteinases derived from activated monocytes and neutrophils infiltrating into the glomerular tuft.[3]

Disruption of the glomerular capillary wall allows passage of plasma coagulation factors to leak into the Bowman space. These factors result in the formation of fibrin on contact with a tissue factor, a transmembrane protein expressed in different cell types, including monocytes and macrophages. The tissue factor has been shown to also possess proinflammatory properties, thus facilitating further macrophage and T-cell recruitment from the circulation into the Bowman space.[3,33,34] Other chemotactic factors such as fibrin, monocyte chemoattractant protein-1 (MCP-1), macrophage colony-stimulating factor, and macrophage migration-inhibitory factor also play major roles in cellular recruitment.[28] Macrophage-derived proinflammatory cytokines including interleukin-1 (IL-1) and tumor necrosis factor-α (TNF-α) exacerbate glomerular injury and promote further macrophage infiltration and glomerular cell proliferation (Figure 22.2).[28] The entry of T cells and fibroblasts into the Bowman space, as occurs through tears in the GBM, leads to progressive deposition of collagen and transition from cellular crescents into fibrocellular and eventually fibrous crescents. This transition may be orchestrated by transforming growth factor-β (TGF-β). Within a week or so, a gradual loss of macrophages, T cells,

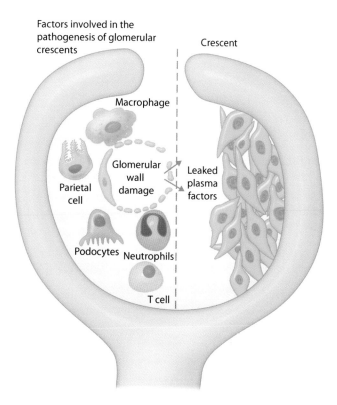

Factors involved in the pathogenesis of glomerular crescents

Crescent

Macrophage

Glomerular wall damage

Parietal cell

Leaked plasma factors

Podocytes  Neutrophils

T cell

Figure 22.2 A diagrammatic representation of pathogenesis of crescents in rapidly progressive glomerulonephritis. The initiating event in crescent formation appears to be disruption of the glomerular capillary wall. Lysis of the glomerular basement membrane results from release of serine proteinases and matrix metalloproteinases derived from activated monocytes and neutrophils infiltrating into the glomerular tuft. Cells forming crescents are derived from proliferating parietal cells and podocytes, as well as from recruitment of circulating monocytes and macrophages.

and fibroblasts from the Bowman space occurs, a process mediated by apoptosis that leads to glomerular scarring (Figure 22.3).[3,28,35,36] In general, crescent formation is less common in immune-complex glomerulonephritides than in other forms of RPGN-causing conditions.

## IMMUNE COMPLEX MEDIATED RAPIDLY PROGRESSIVE GLOMERULONEPHRITIS

Immune complex glomerulonephritides may, in their most severe form, also progress to RPGN. Two of the most common diseases, HSP and systemic lupus erythematosus (SLE), are systemic vasculitides, but the renal disease in both disorders is triggered by immune complex deposition in the glomeruli. Other immune complex diseases that have the potential to develop into RPGN include immunoglobulin A (IgA) nephropathy, acute postinfectious glomerulonephritis (APIGN), and membranoproliferative glomerulonephritis (MPGN) including $C_3$ nephropathy.[3] More than 90% of cases of APIGN result from streptococcal infections. RPGN

is uncommon in all of the foregoing diseases and probably occurs in fewer than 10% of all cases. RPGN may be encountered in any type of MPGN, but it is not clear whether the risk of RPGN is influenced by the type of MPGN.

---

### KEY POINTS

- HSP and SLE are the two most common causes of immune complex–mediated RPGN in childhood.
- Rarely, other glomerulonephritides may also progress to RPGN.

---

The initiating pathogenetic events are the accumulation of immune complexes in glomeruli and the activation of complement coagulation factors and other mediators of glomerular injury. If the disorder is severe enough, crescent formation follows, as described earlier. The immune complexes may be either preformed circulating complexes that are trapped in the glomerular filter or complexes formed in situ.[37,38] In the latter case, a circulating antigen may possess affinity to the glomerular capillary wall, with secondary binding of antibody.

The characteristic finding on renal biopsy in immune complex–induced RPGN, in addition to crescents, is the presence of immune deposits in the glomeruli. The immune complexes are often easier to identify in the better-preserved glomeruli. The location and type of immune material are specific to each primary disease, thus giving rise to mesangial or granular capillary loop immunofluorescence with antibodies against appropriate immunoglobulins. The exception is MPGN type 2, in which only complement C3 is seen by standard immunofluorescence. In advanced disease, the underlying primary disease may no longer be recognizable on renal biopsy because of the extensive glomerulosclerosis.

## PAUCI-IMMUNE CRESCENTIC GLOMERULONEPHRITIS

Pauci-immune crescentic glomerulonephritis is the most common cause of RPGN in adults and also a common cause of RPGN in children.[3] The three commonly described vasculitides in this category are (1) microscopic polyangiitis, (2) GPA (formerly Wegener granulomatosis), and (3) eosinophilic granulomatosis with polyangiitis (EGPA; formerly Churg-Strauss syndrome). Most cases of pauci-immune glomerulonephritis involve inflammation and necrosis of small blood vessel walls. Renal biopsy characteristically shows glomerular crescents and vasculitis of small vessels, with paucity or absence of immunoglobulins by immunofluorescence. Common to most of these small-vessel vasculitides is the presence of circulating anti–neutrophil cytoplasmic

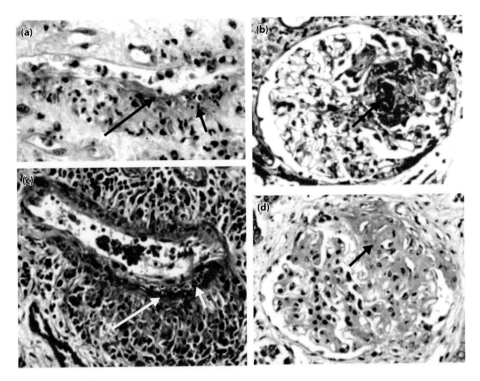

Figure 22.3 Microscopic polyangiitis demonstrating vasculitis lesions. (a) and (c) Fibrinoid necrosis (long arrows) and fragmentation of nuclei or leukocytoclasia (short arrows) affecting small blood vessels (venulitis). The inflammatory infiltrate in the affected areas consists of a mixture of neutrophils and mononuclear leukocytes. (b) Glomerulus with similar fibrinoid necrosis (arrow) and an acute inflammatory reaction. (d) Masson trichrome–stained glomerulus demonstrating residual chronic segmental sclerosis (arrow) after acute inflammatory glomerular disease in rapidly progressive glomerulonephritis. (From Jennette JC, Falk RJ, Hu P, et al. Pathogenesis of antineutrophil cytoplasmic antibody-associated small-vessel vasculitis. Annu Rev Pathol. 2013;8:139–60.)

antibodies (ANCAs) that target specific antigens in cytoplasmic granules.[39–44] The term *ANCA-associated vasculitis* (AAV) is often used to describe these vasculitides. Rarely, AAV may be induced by drugs, such as hydralazine and propylthiouracil. AAV is a frequent cause of pulmonary-renal syndromes.[45,46]

---

### KEY POINTS

- Pauci-immune RPGN usually results from small-vessel vasculitides.
- Three common types are:
  - Microscopic polyangiitis
  - GPA (formerly Wegener granulomatosis)
  - EGPA (formerly Churg-Strauss syndrome)
  - Circulating ANCA is present in more than 70% of cases.

---

ANCA test results are negative in approximately 10% to 30% of patients with pauci-immune RPGN, and anti–endothelial cell antibodies are found in more than 50% of these cases, thus suggesting their pathogenic and clinical significance.[43] These patients tend to exhibit fewer extrarenal

symptoms compared with ANCA-positive patients.[44] Some patients with pauci-immune glomerulonephritis have no evidence of systemic vasculitis or other organ involvement and are referred to as having renal limited vasculitis (RLV). Several cases of RLV have been reported in the pediatric literature.[47]

The pathophysiologic mechanisms in pauci-immune glomerulonephritis are complex and involve both humoral and cellular immune systems. The hallmark of AAV is the formation of ANCA against granular cytoplasmic antigens, including proteinase-3 (PR3) and myeloperoxidase (MPO). Whereas GPA is predominantly associated with cytoplasmic antibodies directed against PR3 (cytoplasmic ANCA or cANCA), MPA and EGPA are more often associated with perinuclear antibodies against MPO (perinuclear ANCA or pANCA).[48–50] Lysosomal membrane protein-2 (LAMP2) has been proposed as another major target for ANCA, but this hypothesis remains controversial.[51–53] Granulomatous inflammation is present in GPA and EGPA but not in MPA.[48–50]

The precise cause of ANCA autoimmunity is unclear, but once in the circulation, ANCA activates neutrophils and monocytes. This process is facilitated by neutrophil priming with cytokines that causes the release and display of antigens on the surface of neutrophils, where they interact with ANCA. Once ANCA binds to antigens, neutrophil activation is induced by Fc receptor engagement.[48,50,53] Activated neutrophils release factors that activate the alternative complement pathway, thereby leading to the generation of C5a, which recruits and activates additional neutrophils.[50,54,55] This inflammatory amplification loop generates the localized necrotizing inflammation in blood vessels, including in renal vessels. T lymphocytes and monocytes are further recruited into the site of severe injury and replace neutrophils that have undergone leukocytoclasia during acute inflammation. Mild vascular injury may resolve with vessel wall remodeling, but with more severe injury fibrosis and sclerosis may result.[50] The formation of extravascular granulomatosis in AAV may occur as a result of intense localized inflammation, caused by activated extravascular neutrophils, that leads to tissue necrosis and fibrin formation.

## ANTI–GLOMERULAR BASEMENT MEMBRANE DISEASE

Anti-GBM disease is rare in all age groups and is characterized by the presence of circulating autoantibodies to the GBM and linear deposition of immunoglobulin G (IgG) along the GBM and alveolar basement membrane.[25,56] Anti-GBM disease is the most aggressive form of RPGN and may involve the kidneys alone (Goodpasture disease), or be accompanied by pulmonary hemorrhage (Goodpasture syndrome). In anti-GBM disease, the primary target of the circulating IgG autoantibodies is the noncollagenous 1 (NC1) domain of the $\alpha_3$-chain of type IV collagen, with specific binding to the $E_A$ and $E_B$ epitopes.[57,58] All IgG subclasses (1 through 4) are known to be present in patients with anti-GBM disease who have moderate to severe renal injury requiring dialysis. In patients who have pathogenic anti-GBM autoantibodies but normal kidney function, IgG1, IgG2, and IgG4 predominate. Natural anti-GBM IgG antibodies are also known to be present in the sera of healthy individuals and are predominantly of the IgG2 and IgG4 subclass.[20,59] The circulating antibody level in anti-GBM disease correlates with the severity of renal disease and serum creatinine concentrations.[20,60] Anti-GBM antibodies

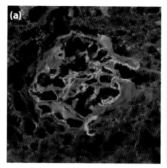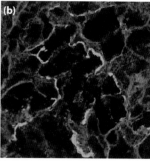

Figure 22.4 Immunofluorescence staining showing immunoglobulin G linear staining of the (a) glomerular and (b) alveolar basement membrane in a patient with Goodpasture syndrome. (Reproduced with permission from Williamson S, Phillips C, Andreoli S, et al. A 25-year experience with pediatric anti–glomerular basement membrane disease. Pediatr Nephrol. 2011;26:85–91.)

have been reported to coexist with ANCA in approximately one-third of cases of crescentic glomerulonephritis in both adults and children.[61–64] Lung and kidney involvement (pulmonary-renal syndrome) may be associated with anti-GBM antibodies alone, with a combination of ANCA and anti-GBM antibodies, or with ANCA alone.

The pathogenesis of vascular tissue injury in anti-GBM disease is similar to that in AAV.[25] Circulating anti-GBM IgG attacks the NCI domain of $\alpha_3$-chain of type IV collagen present in both the kidney and the lungs, and this process leads to crescentic glomerulonephritis and pulmonary hemorrhage. In contrast to AAV, in which immunoglobulin deposits occur only at the sites of vascular injury, anti-GBM disease and immune complex glomerulonephritis are characterized by deposits of immunoglobulin throughout the involved vasculature.[50]

Unless the diagnosis is made early and therapy is instituted promptly, anti-GBM disease rapidly progresses to renal failure and end-stage renal disease (ESRD), with a fatal outcome in approximately one-half of all cases. In almost all patients, circulating IgG autoantibodies can be detected by enzyme-linked immunosorbent assay (ELISA). Renal biopsy typically shows necrotizing crescentic glomerulonephritis and linear deposition of IgG, and less frequently C3, along the GBM (Figure 22.4). Rarely, RPGN due to anti-GBM antibodies occurs in patients with Alport syndrome who receive a kidney transplant. The anti-GBM antibodies develop in these recipients because the type IV collagen present in the transplanted kidney is perceived as a foreign antigen by the recipient, who lacks it in the native kidney.[65,66]

## CLINICAL MANIFESTATIONS

Table 22.3 depicts the clinical and laboratory findings in different types of RPGN. The clinical presentation of RPGN limited to the kidney can vary from asymptomatic

---

### KEY POINTS

- Anti-GBM disease is the least common form of RPGN in both children and adults.
- Anti-GBM disease results from circulating IgG autoantibodies that target the noncollagenous 1 (NC1) domain of the $\alpha_3$-chain of type IV collagen in the GBM and the alveolar basement membrane.

Table 22.3 Differential diagnosis of rapidly progressive glomerulonephritis in children

| | Pauci-immune GN | | | | Immune complex GN | | | | |
| --- | --- | --- | --- | --- | --- | --- | --- | --- | --- |
| | GPA | EGPA | MPA | RLV | MPGN | APIGN | SLE | HSP | aGBM |
| **Symptoms** | | | | | | | | | |
| Constitutional | ++ | ++ | ++ | | | + | ++ | ++ | ++ |
| Pulmonary | ++ | ++ | ++ | | | | | | ++ |
| Arthralgia | ++ | | | | | | ++ | ++ | |
| Sinusitis | + | ++ | | | | | | | |
| Oral ulcers | + | | | | | | + | | |
| Nasal ulcers | + | | | | | | | | |
| Skin | + | ++ | + | | | | ++ | ++ | |
| **Laboratory Findings** | | | | | | | | | |
| Low C3 | | | | | ++ | ++ | ++ | | |
| cANCA | ++ | + | + | | | | | | + |
| pANCA | + | ++ | ++ | ++ | | | | | + |
| ANA | | | | | | | ++ | | |
| aGBM | | | | | | | | | ++ |
| Eosinophilia | + | ++ | | | | | | | |
| Streptozyme | | | | | | ++ | | | |
| **Imaging** | | | | | | | | | |
| Granulomas | ++ | ++ | | | | | | | |

++, More than 50% of patients; +, fewer than 50% of patients; aGBM, anti–glomerular basement membrane antibody disease; ANA, antinuclear antibody; APIGN, acute post-infectious glomerulonephritis; cANCA, cytoplasmic anti–neutrophil cytoplasmic antibody; EGPA, eosinophilic granulomatosis with polyangiitis; GPA, granulomatosis with polyangiitis; HSP, Henoch-Schönlein purpura; MPA, microscopic polyangiitis; MPGN, membranoproliferative glomerulonephritis; pANCA, perinuclear cANCA, cytoplasmic anti–neutrophil cytoplasmic antibody; RLV, renal limited vasculitis; SLE, systemic lupus erythematosus.

proteinuria and hematuria in early stages to life-threatening renal failure requiring dialysis or hypertensive crises. Vague constitutional symptoms, such as malaise and loss of appetite, may be present and may precede other disease manifestations. Gross hematuria is present in many patients, especially in patients with IgA nephropathy, APSGN, or MPGN. Symptoms and signs may evolve over days to weeks.

Extrarenal symptoms may predominate initially in many patients with RPGN. The most common extrarenal symptoms include malaise, fever, weight loss, arthralgias, and upper respiratory tract symptoms.[67–69] Characteristic skin lesions are often present in HSP and SLE. Respiratory tract symptoms and signs in children with GPA include sinusitis, epistaxis, hemoptysis, nasal and oral ulcers, otitis media, hearing loss, and pulmonary nodules or infiltrates. A retrospective analysis of pediatric patients with GPA showed that constitutional symptoms, glomerulonephritis, and upper and lower respiratory tract symptoms predominated at the initial diagnosis.[69,70] Arthritis, eye and skin involvement, and hypertension were less common.

In pediatric EGPA, pulmonary and cardiac involvement is more common than in adults. The most common respiratory findings are asthma and sinusitis, which are present in 91% and 77% of children, respectively.[71] Eosinophilia is frequently present. Additional pulmonary findings in these patients include eosinophilic pleural effusion and eosinophilic microabscesses.[72]

In anti-GBM disease, arthralgia and myalgia are less common symptoms, and hypertension is also uncommon, except in the presence of severe renal failure. Hemoptysis is seen as a result of alveolar hemorrhage in these patients.[25,56,73] The relative involvement of the kidneys and lungs in anti-GBM disease is variable. Although most patients present with both renal and alveolar disease, isolated renal involvement occurs in 30% to 40% of all cases. Occasionally, patients may present with pulmonary hemorrhage alone, without overt renal disease, although they may have urinary abnormalities.[73] The conditions to be considered in the differential diagnosis of RPGN are listed in Table 22.3.

## DIAGNOSTIC EVALUATION

The diagnosis of RPGN must be made rapidly to enable early institution of therapy. Evaluation should start with a thorough history and a physical examination. Laboratory investigations taken into consideration in the investigations

Table 22.4 Evaluation of suspected rapidly progressive glomerulonephritis

**Laboratory Tests**
- Complete blood count
- Comprehensive metabolic panel
- Peripheral blood smear (to rule out HUS)
- Urinalysis, urine protein-to-creatinine ratio
- Complement C3 and C4 and total complement
- ANA (full lupus panel if ANA positive)
- ANCA (cANCA and pANCA)
- Anti-GBM antibody titers
- Streptococcal antibody titers (ASO, anti-DNase B and antihyaluronidase)
- Culture of throat and skin lesions (for suspected APSGN)

**Radiologic Imaging**
- Chest x-ray study
- Renal ultrasound examination
- Computed tomography scan of orbit, sinuses, trachea, and chest

**Tissue Diagnosis**
- Renal biopsy

*Abbreviations:* ANA, antinuclear antibody; ANCA, anti–neutrophil cytoplasmic antibody; APSGN, acute poststreptococcal glomerulonephritis; ASO, anti–streptolysin O; cANCA, cytoplasmic anti–neutrophil cytoplasmic antibody; GBM, glomerular basement membrane; HUS, hemolytic-uremic syndrome, pANCA, perinuclear anti–neutrophil cytoplasmic antibody.

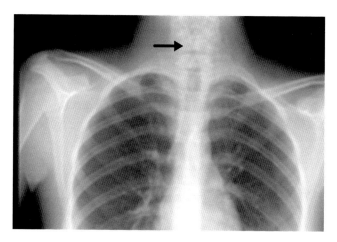

Figure 22.5 Subglottic narrowing (arrow) in a patient with granulomatosis with polyangiitis.

of RPGN are listed in Table 22.4. The goals of evaluation are to identify the underlying immunopathologic mechanisms and determine the activity and severity of renal involvement. Laboratory investigations should include the following: complete blood count; comprehensive metabolic panel; complement C3, complement C4, and total complement; ANA, ANCA, anti-GBM antibodies; urinalysis, and quantitative measurement of urinary protein excretion. Radiologic investigations is indicated in patients with pulmonary manifestations or if the diagnosis of GPA is being actively considered.

ANCA is usually of the IgG class, although IgA and immunoglobulin M (IgM) ANCAs have been described.[74] Although ANCA is strongly associated with pauci-immune crescentic glomerulonephritis, a negative ANCA test result does not exclude the diagnosis. Approximately 90% of patients with GPA have a positive test result for ANCA, mostly for PR3-ANCA (cANCA), whereas 70% of MPA patients have a positive test result for ANCA, mostly to MPO (pANCA). Of EGPA patients, only 50% are ANCA positive, but this varies with stage of renal and lung involvement.[74] ANCA has been reported in other nonvasculitic disorders, including SLE, rheumatoid arthritis, inflammatory bowel disease, autoimmune hepatitis, tuberculosis,

subacute bacterial endocarditis, and malignant diseases.[74,75] The international guidelines for ANCA testing recommend screening for ANCA by immunofluorescence test (IFT). If results are positive, ANCA testing by ELISA is required.[76] IFT is more sensitive for ANCA, and ELISA is more specific for cANCA and pANCA.

In suspected APSGN, streptococcal antibody titers should be obtained. Erythrocyte sedimentation rate (ESR) and C-reactive panel, although nonspecific, may help establish the presence of inflammation. Radiologic studies should include a renal ultrasound examination, which may show enlarged echogenic kidneys. A chest x-ray study and computed tomography (CT) scan of the orbit, sinuses, trachea, and chest may be necessary in suspected GPA. Imaging studies of the upper airway may identify subglottic stenosis (Figure 22.5). Radiography of the chest may also demonstrate infiltrative pulmonary disease (Figure 22.6), pulmonary hemorrhage, pleural effusions, or granulomatous lesions.

A renal biopsy is essential for tissue diagnosis. It provides information necessary for categorization of RPGN and to

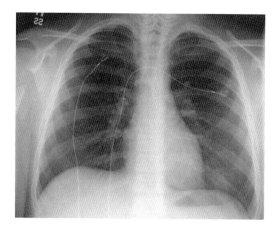

Figure 22.6 Chest x-ray film of a patient with granulomatosis with polyangiitis (Wegener granulomatosis) showing bibasilar pulmonary infiltrates, especially on the left side.

determine the severity of renal involvement. Inability to obtain a renal biopsy because of a patient's instability should not delay the initiation of therapy.[2]

## TREATMENT

Treatment of RPGN must be initiated as soon as the diagnosis is suspected and sometimes even before a renal biopsy is obtained. The aims of early treatment of RPGN are to halt disease progression, reverse renal injury, induce remission, and preserve renal function. In general, the treatment can be arbitrarily divided into two phases: (1) induction of remission and (2) maintenance of disease remission.

## INDUCTION OF REMISSION

Standard treatment strategies involve the use of corticosteroids, immunosuppressive agents, and plasmapheresis. More recent experience with therapeutic agents such as rituximab, mycophenolate mofetil (MMF), leflunomide, antibodies to cytokines, and signal transduction inhibitors is encouraging.

### Glucocorticoids

High-dose corticosteroids form part of the initial therapy for crescentic glomerulonephritis in most regimens.[2,3,77–79] The rationale for the use of high-dose steroids in the form of "pulse methylprednisolone" includes the rapid anti-inflammatory properties of this regimen and the possible effect on reduction of ANCA-producing plasma cells in AAV. Kidney Disease Improving Global Outcomes (KDIGO) recommends the use of pulse methylprednisolone as an initial therapy in RPGN in combination with cyclophosphamide.[79]

An intravenous dose of methylprednisolone 10 mg/kg/day (maximum dose, 500 mg daily) is given for 3 days, followed by oral prednisone at a dose of 2 mg/kg/day (maximum, 60 mg daily), which is tapered over several months. There is no evidence that 1000 mg of methylprednisolone is more effective than 500 mg.[79] A meta-analysis involving 983 patients showed that long-term low-dose glucocorticoid therapy administered for more than 12 months reduced relapse rates.[80]

### Cyclophosphamide

Cyclophosphamide, an alkylating agent, is the most common immunosuppressant used in combination with glucocorticoids for the treatment of patients with RPGN. Cyclophosphamide has been shown to be effective in inducing remission in these patients, and KDIGO recommends its use as part of the initial therapy in patients with crescentic glomerulonephritis.[79] Oral and parenteral routes are equally effective in inducing remission. A randomized trial of more than 140 patients with newly diagnosed AAV compared pulse with oral cyclophosphamide for the induction of remission.[81,82] Pulse intravenous cyclophosphamide was as effective as the oral route in inducing remission, with the advantage of a reduced total cumulative cyclophosphamide dose and fewer cases of leukopenia. The recommended dose of intravenous cyclophosphamide is 0.5 to 0.75 g/m², given every 3 to 4 weeks for 3 to 6 months. The cyclophosphamide dose should be adjusted to keep the leukocyte count between 3 and 5 $10^3/\mu L$ at 2 weeks after treatment. Other regimens for intravenous cyclophosphamide pulse therapy also exist. Oral cyclophosphamide is usually given at a dose of 1.5 to 2mg/kg/day for 3 months and not more than 6 months.[77,79] The oral cyclophosphamide dose should also be adjusted to keep the leukocyte count between 3 and 5 $10^3/\mu L$. Currently, there is no convincing evidence that longer treatment with cyclophosphamide reduces relapse rates. In patients who are dialysis dependent and who have severe renal damage on histologic examination, the mortality rate appears to be increased.[83] Therefore, in patients who are dialysis dependent at 3 months after initiation of therapy and who have no evidence of ongoing extrarenal manifestations of vasculitis, cyclophosphamide should be discontinued.[79,83]

### Plasmapheresis

The use of plasmapheresis as an adjunctive therapy in the management of RPGN has attracted interest since the 1980s. Plasmapheresis aims to remove antibodies in patients with anti-GBM disease or AAV. A randomized trial of high-dose methylprednisolone or plasma exchange as adjunctive therapy for severe renal vasculitis showed that high-dose methylprednisolone was less effective in facilitating renal recovery as compared with plasma exchange.[84] Early plasmapheresis in combination with corticosteroids and cyclophosphamide has been shown to improve renal outcomes in patients with

RPGN associated with severe renal failure.[84-,88] In patients with RPGN associated with pulmonary hemorrhage, the addition of plasmapheresis to induction therapy significantly improved patient survival.[87-90] More recent meta-analyses demonstrated an improvement in the risk of ESRD in patients with renal vasculitis in whom plasmapheresis was added to induction therapy.[81,91] Currently, the EULAR and KDIGO recommend the addition of plasmapheresis to initial induction therapy with corticosteroids and cyclophosphamide in patients with RPGN associated with severe renal disease and pulmonary hemorrhage.[79,92] Duration of plasmapheresis therapy is not clearly defined, but 7 to 14 sessions have been performed in various studies.[84,86,87,89]

## Newer induction therapies

Although current therapies have dramatically reduced the mortality associated with RPGN, induction of remission is often slow, requiring 3 to 6 months of therapy, by which time renal tissue damage and chronic kidney disease commence. Furthermore, approximately 20% to 30% of patients fail to achieve complete remission, and relapse is common, even after full remission.[93] Drug toxicity and infection rates also remain high with current induction agents. Alternative immunosuppressive medications such as rituximab and MMF have attracted attention as potential remission-inducing agents. A head-to-head comparison of rituximab and cyclophosphamide as induction therapy for AAV demonstrated that rituximab was effective in inducing remission in severe AAV and had a better side effect profile.[94] Based on these findings, the Food and Drug Administration (FDA), in April 2011, approved rituximab (in combination with glucocorticoids) as a front-line agent for treating adult patients with GPA and MPA. In patients with refractory cases of AAV, rituximab has also been shown to be effective in inducing remission.[95,96] Data on MMF as an effective remission-inducing agent are weak and insufficient to support its use as induction therapy for crescentic glomerulonephritis. Other emerging agents currently being investigated include TNF-$\alpha$ antagonists, high-dose intravenous immunoglobulin, antithymocyte globulin, and alemtuzumab.

## Maintenance therapy

Maintenance therapy should be initiated in patients who have achieved remission. The toxicity of long-term use of cyclophosphamide makes this drug an unattractive option for use as a maintenance agent for patients with crescentic glomerulonephritis. Current options for maintenance therapy include azathioprine, MMF, leflunomide, and methotrexate.[92] Available evidence supports the use of azathioprine as a first-line agent for maintenance of remission in crescentic glomerulonephritis. A randomized controlled trial in 144 patients with AAV showed that withdrawal of cyclophosphamide and substitution with azathioprine after induction of remission did not increase relapse rates.[97] Another randomized study compared azathioprine and MMF for maintenance of remission in AAV and found that MMF was less effective than azathioprine for maintaining remission in these patients.[98] KDIGO currently recommends azathioprine as first-line maintenance therapy. In patients who do not tolerate azathioprine, MMF can be substituted. If patients are intolerant to both azathioprine and MMF, methotrexate may then be considered. Methotrexate is not safer than azathioprine and should not be used in patients with a glomerular filtration rate of less than 60 mL/min/1.73 m$^2$.[99] Maintenance therapy should be continued for at least 18 months in patients who remain in remission.[79]

---

## KEY POINTS

Maintenance therapies for RPGN include:

- Azathioprine
- MMF
- Methotrexate

---

The foregoing recommendations are largely based on studies in adults with pauci-immune RPGN. Because immune complex RPGN is common in children and has a better prognosis, it is possible that a less intensive treatment regimen may be sufficient in selected pediatric cases.

## CLINICAL COURSE AND PROGNOSIS

RPGN constitutes a medical emergency. In the absence of prompt therapy, morbidity, mortality, and the risk of progression to ESRD are high. With the introduction of immunosuppressive therapy and tools for early diagnosis, the clinical course and prognosis of vasculitis has dramatically improved over the last several decades.[100,101] The current patient survival rate for AAV ranges from 75% to 100% at 5 years.[101] Severe kidney injury at presentation, a higher Birmingham Vasculitis Activity score, a higher white blood cell count, and lower hemoglobin levels are poor prognostic factors in long-term survival.[4,11,102]

The histologic predictors of poor renal survival are a low percentage of normal glomeruli, a high percentage of crescentic glomeruli, extensive tubular atrophy, and interstitial fibrosis at the time of biopsy. The percentage of normal glomeruli at biopsy is the best predictor of dialysis independence over time.[5,6,103,104] Similar findings also have been published in the pediatric population.[11,105-107] Children with immune complex crescentic glomerulonephritis have better renal survival and are more likely to be dialysis free at follow up than are children with pauci-immune glomerulonephritis. A single center study of children with crescentic glomerulonephritis showed a renal survival of 94% at 3 years in those with immune complex glomerulonephritis compared with 63% in those with pauci-immune glomerulonephritis.[105]

## COMPLICATIONS

Crescentic glomerulonephritis is associated with serious adverse events related to the disease itself and to immunosuppressive therapy. Target organ damage resulting from the disease process includes renal failure, as well as respiratory failure secondary to pulmonary hemorrhage and edema. The intensity of immunosuppression during the induction phase of therapy is associated with a high risk of infection with bacterial, fungal, viral, and parasitic organisms.[107,108] Approximately 10% to 20% of patients will die of serious infections in the first 3 months of therapy.[47] Overall, the leading causes of death in the first year of diagnosis are infections and active vasculitis.[101,108] Factors that increase the risk of infection include leukopenia, immune dysfunction induced by therapy, and renal failure. High cumulative doses of cyclophosphamide are associated with irreversible gonadal failure causing infertility and an increased risk of malignant diseases such as nonmelanoma skin cancer and urinary tract cancers.[108] Osteoporosis, hypertension, and weight gain are some of the adverse effects of high dose steroid exposure. These complications must be discussed with patients and their families before therapy is initiated.

## SUMMARY

RPGN is a rare but devastating disease that may result in ESRD or death if it is left untreated or if treatment is significantly delayed. Its highly variable presentation, depending on the specific diagnosis and extent of organ involvement, may cause diagnostic difficulties. The index of suspicion should therefore be high whenever a patient presents with nephritic syndrome, acutely worsening kidney function, or systemic manifestations consistent with vasculitis, pulmonary hemorrhage, or granuloma formation. Although current treatment regimens have greatly improved the outlook, evolving new medications, especially biologic agents, are likely to improve the prognosis further.

### Clinical Vignette 22.1

A 10-year-old girl presented with a 4-week history of worsening malaise, weight loss, and intermittent fevers. She was diagnosed with sinusitis by her pediatrician 6 weeks earlier and received two courses of oral antibiotics, with no improvement. On physical examination, she was not in any distress. Her blood pressure was 130/90 mm Hg. She had paranasal tenderness, and there was no pedal edema. The rest of her physical examination was unremarkable. Laboratory data revealed blood urea nitrogen of 76 mg/dL and creatinine of 4.5 mg/dL, normal electrolytes, and serum albumin of 3.0 g/dL. Hemoglobin and hematocrit was 8.7 g/dL and 28%, respectively. Urinalysis shows hematuria and proteinuria with a urine protein-to-creatinine ratio of 1.8 mg/mg. Renal biopsy was performed urgently, and results show necrotizing glomerulonephritis, with 70% of glomeruli exhibiting fibrocellular crescents (Figure 22.7). Immunofluorescence was negative. Electron microscopy did not reveal any electron-dense deposits. The diagnosis of rapidly progressive glomerulonephritis was established.

### TEACHING POINTS

Based on the biopsy findings, the patient in Clinical Vignette 22.1 has pauci-immune rapidly progressive glomerulonephritis. Further characterization revealed negative serologic results for antinuclear antibodies (ANAs), anti–glomerular basement membrane antibodies, and myeloperoxidase (MPO) antibodies, but the proteinase-3 (PR3) antibody level was high at 701 absorbance units arbitany units/mL (normal, 0 to 19). Chest x-ray was normal. A high-resolution CT scan of the chest, however, revealed multiple bilateral mostly peripheral and vasocentric lung nodules and wedged peripheral

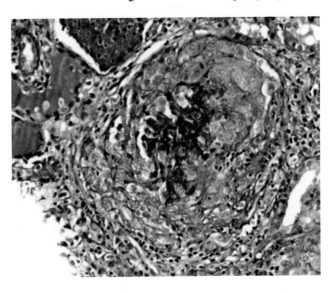

Figure 22.7 Proliferation of parietal epithelial cells forms a nearly circumferential epithelial crescent surrounding a collapsed glomerular tuft. (Courtesy of Dr. Randall Craver, Louisiana State University, Baton Rouge, LA.)

densities. There were areas of early cavitation in both upper and left lower lobes, and subglottic tracheal narrowing (see Figure 22.5) was also noted. Collectively, these findings suggested granulomatosis with polyangiitis, formerly known as Wegener granulomatosis. Renal biopsy confirmed the presence of severe proliferative glomerulonephritis with cellular crescents.

Induction therapy was initiated with high-dose methylprednisolone pulses and cyclophosphamide. The patient received three pulses of methylprednisolone and then was transitioned to oral steroids. Cyclophosphamide was given parenterally every 4 weeks for 6 months. Remission was achieved by 14 weeks of therapy. After cyclophosphamide infusions, azathioprine was initiated as maintenance therapy. The patient remained in remission 16 months after diagnosis. Follow-up CT scan of her chest after 5 months of therapy showed complete resolution of her lung lesions. Her kidney function and hematologic indices remained normal. Her upper respiratory tract symptoms also resolved.

# REFERENCES

1. Markowitz GS, Radhakrishnan J, D'Agati VD. An overlapping etiology of rapidly progressive glomerulonephritis. Am J Kidney Dis. 2004;43: 388–93.
2. Kambham N. Crescentic glomerulonephritis: An update on pauci-immune and anti-GBM disease. Adv Anat Pathol. 2012;19:111–24.
3. Jennette JC. Rapidly progressive crescentic glomerulonephritis. Kidney Int. 2003;63:1164–77.
4. Flossmann O, Berden A, de Groot K, et al. Long-term patient survival in ANCA-associated vasculitis. Ann Rheum Dis. 2011;70:488–94.
5. Li Z, Gou S, Chen M, et al. Predictors for outcomes in patients with severe ANCA-associated glomerulonephritis who were dialysis-dependent at presentation: A study of 89 cases in a single Chinese center. Semin Arthritis Rheum. 2013;42:515–21.
6. de Lindvan Wijngaarden RA, Hauer HA, Wolterbeek R, et al. Clinical and histologic determinants of renal outcome in ANCA-associated vasculitis: A prospective analysis of 100 patients with severe renal involvement. J Am Soc Nephrol. 2006;17:2264–74.
7. Ozen S, Ruperto N, Dillon MJ, et al. EULAR/PReS endorsed consensus criteria for the classification of childhood vasculitides. Am Rheum Dis. 2006;65:936–41.
8. Ruperto N, Ozen S, Pistorio A, et al. EULAR/PRINTO/PRES criteria for Henoch-Schonlein purpura, childhood polyarteritis nodosa, childhood Wegener granulomatosis and childhood Takayasu arteritis: Ankara 2008. Part I. Overall methodology and clinical characterization. Ann Rheum Dis. 2010;69:790–7.
9. Oe Y, Nakaya I, Yahata M, et al. Classic polyarteritis nodosa presenting with rapidly progressive renal insufficiency. Clin Nephrol. 2010;74:315–8.
10. Bakkaloglu SA, Ekim M, Tumer N, et al. Severe renal impairment in the case of classic polyarteritis nodosa. Pediatr Nephrol. 2001;16:148–50.
11. Sinha A, Puri K, Hari P, et al. Etiology and outcome of crescentic glomerulonephritis. Indian Pediatr. 2013;50:283–8.
12. Gardner-Medwin JM, Dolezalova P, Cummins C, et al. Incidence of Henoch-Schonlein purpura, Kawasaki disease, and rare vasculitides in children of different ethnic origins. Lancet. 2002;360:1197–1202.
13. Watts R. What is known about the epidemiology of the vasculitides? Best Pract Res Clin Rheumatol. 2005;19:191–207.
14. Hedger N, Stevens J, Drey N, et al. Incidence and outcome of pauci-immune rapidly progressive glomerulonephritis in Wessex, UK: A 10-year retrospective study. Nephrol Dial Transplant. 2000;15:1593–9.
15. Fujimoto S, Watts R, Kobayashi S, et al. Comparison of the epidemiology of anti–neutrophil cytoplasmic antibody–associated vasculitis between Japan and the UK. Rheumatology. 2001;50:1916–20.
16. Kobayashi S, Fujimoto S. Epidemiology of vasculitides: Differences between Japan, Europe and North America. Clin Exp Nephrol. 2013;17:611–4.
17. Watts R, Scott DG, Jayne DR, et al. Renal vasculitis in Japan and the UK—are there differences in epidemiology and clinical phenotype? Nephrol Dial Transplant. 2008;23:3928–31.
18. Suzuki Y, Takeda Y, Sato D, et al. Clinicoepidemiological manifestations of RPGN and ANCA-associated vasculitides: An 11-year retrospective hospital-based study in Japan. Mod Rheumatol. 2010;20:54–62.
19. Gibelin A, Maldini C, Mahr A. Epidemiology and etiology of Wegener granulomatosis, microscopic polyangiitis, Churg-Strauss syndrome and Goodpasture syndrome: Vasculitides with frequent lung involvement. Semin Respir Crit Care Med. 2011;32:264–73.
20. Cui Z, Zhao M. Advances in human antiglomerular basement membrane disease. Nat Rev Nephrol. 2011;7:697–705.
21. Hirayama K, Yamagata K, Kobayashi M, et al. Anti–glomerular basement membrane antibody disease in Japan: Part of the nationwide rapidly progressive glomerulonephritis survey in Japan. Clin Exp Nephrol. 2008;12:339–47.
22. Lahmer T, Heemann U. Anti–glomerular basement membrane antibody disease: A rare autoimmune disorder affecting the kidney and the lung. Autoimmun Rev. 2012;12:169–73.
23. Williamson S, Phillips C, Andreoli S, et al. A 25-year experience with pediatric anti–glomerular basement membrane disease. Pediatr Nephrol. 2011;26:85–91.

24. Bayat A, Kamperis K, Herlin T. Characteristics and outcome of Goodpasture's disease in children. Clin Rheumatol. 2012;31:1745–51.

25. Hirayama K and Yamagata K. Anti-Glomerular Basement Membrane Disease. In Update on Glomerulopathies - Clinical and Treatment Aspects, Sharma P (Ed.), Intech Publishers, Shanghai, China. 2011; 251-76.

26. Couser WG. Rapidly progressive glomerulonephritis: Classification, pathogenetic mechanisms, and therapy. Am J Kidney Dis. 1988;11:449–64.

27. Hans-Joachim A. Diagnosis and management of crescentic glomerulonephritis: State of the art. Saudi J Kidney Dis Transplant. 2000;11:353–61.

28. Atkins R, Nikolic-Paterson DJ, Song Q, et al. Modulators of crescentic glomerulonephritis. J Am Soc Nephrol. 1996;7:2271–78.

29. Lan HY, Nikolic-Paterson DJ, Mu W, et al. Local macrophage proliferation in the pathogenesis of glomerular crescent formation in rat anti–glomerular basement membrane (GBM) glomerulonephritis. Clin Exp Immunol. 1997;110:233–40.

30. Singh SK, Jeansson M, Quaggin SE. New insights into the pathogenesis of cellular crescents. Curr Opin Nephrol Hypertens. 2011;20:258–62.

31. Bariety J, Bruneval P, Meyrier A, et al. Podocyte involvement in human immune crescentic glomerulonephritis. Kidney Int. 2005;68:1109–19.

32. Bonsib SM. Glomerular basement membrane discontinuities: Scanning electron microscopic study of acellular glomeruli. Am J Pathol. 1985;119:357–60.

33. Grandaliano G, Gesualdo L, Ranieri E, et al. Tissue factor, plasminogen activator inhibitor-1, and thrombin receptor expression in human crescentic glomerulonephritis. Am J Kidney Dis. 2000;35:726–38.

34. Cunningham MA, Kitchin AR, Tipping PG, et al. Fibrin independent proinflammatory effects of tissue factor in experimental crescentic glomerulonephritis. Kidney Int. 2004;66:647–54.

35. Reynolds J, Moss J, Duda MA, et al. The evolution of crescentic nephritis and alveolar haemorrhage following induction of autoimmunity to glomerular basement membrane in an experimental model of Goodpasture's disease. J Pathol. 2003;200:118–29.

36. Lan HY, Nikolic-Paterson DJ, Atkins RC. Involvement of activated periglomerular leukocytes in the rupture of Bowman's capsule and glomerular crescent progression in experimental glomerulonephritis. Lab Invest. 1992;67:743–51.

37. Lin C. Serial studies of circulating immune complexes in poststreptococcal glomerulonephritis. Pediatrics. 1982;70:725–7.

38. Choi J, Yu C, Jung H, et al. A case of progressive IgA nephropathy in a patient with exacerbation of Crohn's disease. BMC Nephrol. 2012;13:84–8.

39. Lane SE, Watts RA, Shepstone L, et al. Primary systemic vasculitis: Clinical features and mortality. Q J Med. 2005;98:97–111.

40. Pallan L, Savage CO, Harper L. ANCA-associated vasculitis: From bench research to novel treatments. Nat Rev Nephrol. 2009;5:278–86.

41. Ozen S, Fuhlbrigge RC. Update in paediatric vasculitis. Best Pract Res Clin Rheumatol. 2009;23:679–88.

42. Chen M, Kallenberg CG, Zhao M. ANCA-negative pauci-immune crescentic glomerulonephritis. Nat Rev Nephrol. 2009;5:313–18.

43. Cong M, Chen M, Zhang J, et al. Anti–endothelial cell antibodies in antineutrophil cytoplasmic antibodies negative pauci-immune crescentic glomerulonephritis. Nephrology 2008;13:228–34.

44. Chen M, Yu F, Wang SX, et al. Antineutrophil cytoplasmic autoantibody–negative pauci-immune crescentic glomerulonephritis. J Am Soc Nephrol. 2007;18:599–605.

45. Lin Y, Zheng W, Tian X, et al. Antineutrophil cytoplasmic antibody–associated vasculitis complicated with diffuse alveolar hemorrhage. J Clin Rheumatol. 2009;15:341–44.

46. Lee RW, D'Cruz DP. Pulmonary renal vasculitis syndromes. Autoimmun Rev. 2010;9:657–60.

47. Krmar RT, Kagebrand M, Hansson ME, et al. Renal-limited vasculitis in children: A single center retrospective long-term follow-up analysis. Clin Nephrol. 2013;80:388–94.

48. Wilde B, Paassen P, Witzke O, et al. New pathophysiological insights and treatment of ANCA-associated vasculitis. Kidney Int. 2011;79:599–612.

49. Gomez-Puerta JA, Bosch X. Anti–neutrophil cytoplasmic antibody pathogenesis in small-vessel vasculitis. Am J Pathol. 2009;175:1790–98.

50. Jennette JC, Falk RJ, Hu P, et al. Pathogenesis of antineutrophil cytoplasmic antibody–associated small-vessel vasculitis. Annu Rev Pathol. 2013;8:139–60.

51. Roth AJ, Brown MC, Smith RN, et al. Anti-LAMP-2 antibodies are not prevalent in patients with antineutrophil cytoplasmic autoantibody glomerulonephritis. J Am Soc Nephrol. 2012;23:545–55.

52. Bosch X, Mirapeix E. LAMP-2 illuminates pathogenesis of ANCA glomerulonephritis. Nat Rev Nephrol. 2009;5:247–9.

53. Kain R, Firmin DA, Rees AJ. Pathogenesis of small vessel vasculitis associated with autoantibodies to neutrophils cytoplasmic antigens: New insights from animal models. Curr Opin Rheumatol. 2010;22:15–20.

54. Xiao H, Schreiber A, Heeringa P. Alternative complement pathway in the pathogenesis of disease mediated by antineutrophil cytoplasmic antibodies. Am J Pathol. 2007;170:52–64.

55. Savage CO. Pathogenesis of anti–neutrophil cytoplasmic autoantibody (ANCA)–associated vasculitis. Clin Exp Immunol. 2011;164(Suppl 1):23–6.

56. Salama AD, Levy JB, Lightstone L, et al. Goodpasture's disease. Lancet. 2001;358:917–20.

57. Pedchenko V, Bondar O, Fogo A, et al. Molecular architecture of the Goodpasture autoantigen in anti-GBM nephritis. N Engl J Med. 2010;363:343–54.

58. Borza D, Hudson B. Molecular characterization of the target antigens of anti–glomerular basement membrane antibody disease. Semin Immunopathol. 2003;24:345–61.

59. Zhao J, Yan Y, Cui Z, et al. The immunoglobulin G subclass distribution of anti-GBM autoantibodies against rHα3 (IV) NC1 is associated with disease activity. Hum Immunol. 2009;70:425–9.

60. Yang R, Hellmark T, Zhao J, et al. Levels of epitope-specific autoantibodies correlate with renal damage in anti-GBM disease. Nephrol Dial Transplant. 2009;24:1838–44.

61. Rutgers A, Slot M, Paassen P, et al. Coexistence of anti–glomerular basement membrane antibodies and myeloperoxidase-ANCAs in crescentic glomerulonephritis. Am J Kidney Dis. 2005;46:253–62.

62. Bogdanovic R, Minic P, Markovic-Lipkovski, et al. Pulmonary renal syndrome in a child with coexistence of anti–neutrophil cytoplasmic antibodies and anti-glomerular basement membrane disease: Case report and literature review. BMC Nephrol. 2013;14:66–73.

63. Hellmark T, Niles JL, Collins AB, et al. Comparison of anti-GBM antibodies in sera with or without ANCA. J Am Soc Nephrol. 1997;8:376–85.

64. Yang R, Hellmark T, Zhao J, et al. Antigen and epitope specificity of anti–glomerular basement membrane antibodies in patients with Goodpasture disease with or without anti-neutrophil cytoplasmic antibodies. J Am Soc Nephrol. 2007;18:1338–43.

65. Hudson B, Tryggvason K, Sundaramoorthy M, et al. Alport's syndrome, Goodpasture's syndrome and type IV collagen. N Engl J Med. 2003;348:2543–56.

66. Charytan D, Torre A, Khurana M, et al. Allograft rejection and glomerular basement membrane antibodies in Alport's syndrome. J Nephrol. 2004;17:431–5.

67. McMahon N, Cooper M, Iorember F, et al. Just chronic sinusitis? Clin Pediatr. 2012;51:1099–1102.

68. Shimizu M, Sekiguchi T, Kishi N, et al. A case of a 6-year-old girl with anti–neutrophil cytoplasmic autoantibody–negative pauci-immune crescentic glomerulonephritis. Clin Exp Nephrol. 2011;15:596–601.

69. Akikusa JD, Schneider R, Harvey EA, et al. Clinical features and outcome of pediatric Wegener's granulomatosis. Arthritis Rheum. 2007;57:837–44.

70. Orlowski JP, Clough JD, Dyment PG. Wegener's granulomatosis in the pediatric age group. Pediatrics. 1978;61:83–90.

71. Zwerina J, Eger G, Englbrecht M, et al. Churg-Strauss syndrome in childhood: A systematic literature review and clinical comparison with adult patients. Semin Arthritis Rheum. 2008;39:108–15.

72. Boyer D, Vargas SO, Slattery D, et al. Churg-Strauss syndrome in childhood: A clinical and pathologic review. Pediatrics. 2006;118:e914–20.

73. Pusey CD. Anti–glomerular basement membrane disease. Kidney Int. 2003;64:1535–50.

74. Sinclair D, Stevens JM. Role of antineutrophil cytoplasmic antibodies and glomerular basement membrane antibodies in the diagnosis and monitoring of systemic vasculitides. Ann Clin Biochem. 2007;44:432–42.

75. Csernok E. ANCA testing: The current stage and perspectives. Clin Exp Nephrol. 2013;17:615–8.

76. Savige J, Gillis D, Benson E, et al. International consensus statement on testing and reporting of antineutrophil cytoplasmic antibodies (ANCA). Am J Clin Pathol. 1999;111:507–13.

77. Li X, Chen N. Management of crescentic glomerulonephritis: What are the recent advances? Contrib Nephrol. 2013;181:229–39.

78. Jindal K. Management of idiopathic crescentic and diffuse proliferative glomerulonephritis: Evidence-based recommendations. Kidney Int. 1999;55(Suppl 70):S33–40.

79. KDIGO Clinical practice guideline for glomerulonephritis. Kidney Int. 2012;2:233–39.

80. Walsh M, Merkel P, Mahr A, et al. Effects of duration of glucocorticoid therapy on relapse rate in antineutrophil cytoplasmic antibody–associated vasculitis: A meta-analysis. Arthritis Care Res. 2010;62:1166–73.

81. Harper L, Morgan MD, Walsh M, et al. Pulse versus daily oral cyclophosphamide for induction of remission in ANCA-associated vasculitis: Long-term follow-up. Ann Rheum Dis. 2012;71:955–60.

82. Groot K, Harper L, Jayne DR, et al. Pulse versus daily oral cyclophosphamide for induction of remission in antineutrophil cytoplasmic antibody–associated vasculitis. Ann Intern Med. 2009;150:670–80.

83. Lind van Wijngaarden RA, Hauer HA, Wolterbreek R, et al. Chances of recovery for dialysis-dependent ANCA–associated glomerulonephritis. J Am Soc Nephrol. 2007;18:2189–97.

84. Jayne DR, Gaskin G, Rasmussen N, et al. Randomized trial of plasma exchange or high-dosage methylprednisolone as adjunctive therapy for severe renal vasculitis. J Am Soc Nephrol. 2007;18:2180–88.

85. Walters GD, Willis NS, Craig JC. Interventions for renal vasculitis in adults: A systematic review. BMC Nephrol. 2010;11:12–34.

86. Gregersen JW, Kristensen T, Krag SR, et al. Early plasma exchange improves outcome in PR3-ANCA–positive renal vasculitis. Clin Exp Rheumatol. 2012;30(Suppl 70):S39–47.

87. Levy JB, Turner AN, Rees AJ, et al. Long-term outcome of anti–glomerular basement membrane antibody disease treated with plasma exchange and immunosuppression. Ann Intern Med. 2001;134:1033–42.

88. Lind van Wijngaarden RA, Hauer HA, Wolterbreek R, et al. Clinical and histologic determinants of renal outcome in ANCA-associated vasculitis: A prospective analysis of 100 patients with severe renal involvement. J Am Soc Nephrol. 2006;17:2264–74.

89. Klemmer PJ, Chalermskulrat W, Reif MS, et al. Plasmapheresis therapy for diffuse alveolar hemorrhage in patients with small-vessel vasculitis. Am J Kidney Dis. 2003;42:1149–53.

90. Cui Z, Zhao J, Jia X, et al. Anti–glomerular basement membrane disease: Outcomes of different therapeutic regimens in a large single-center Chinese cohort study. Medicine (Baltimore). 2011;90:303–11.

91. Walsh M, Catapano F, Szpirt W, et al. Plasma exchange for renal vasculitis and idiopathic rapidly progressive glomerulonephritis: A meta-analysis. Am J Kidney Dis. 2011;57:566–74.

92. Mukhtyar C, Guillevin L, Cid MC, et al. EULAR recommendations for the management of primary small and medium vessel vasculitis. Ann Rheum Dis. 2009;68:310–17.

93. Hiemstra TF, Jayne D. Newer therapies for vasculitis. Best Pract Res Clin Rheumatol. 2009;23:379–89.

94. Stone JH, Merkel PA, Spiera R, et al. Rituximab versus cyclophosphamide for ANCA-associated vasculitis. N Engl J Med. 2010;363:221–32.

95. Jones, RB, Ferraro AJ, Chaudhry AN, et al. A multicenter survey of rituximab therapy for refractory antineutrophil cytoplasmic antibody–associated vasculitis. Arthritis Rheum. 2009;60:2156–68.

96. Walsh M, Jayne D. Rituximab in the treatment of anti–neutrophil cytoplasm antibody associated vasculitis and systemic lupus erythematosus: Past, present and future. Kidney Int. 2007;72:676–82.

97. Jayne D, Rasmussen N, Andrassy K, et al. A randomized trial of maintenance therapy for vasculitis associated with antineutrophil cytoplasmic autoantibodies. N Engl J Med. 2003;349:36–44.

98. Hiemstra TF, Walsh M, Mahr A, et al. Mycophenolate mofetil vs. azathioprine for remission maintenance in antineutrophil cytoplasmic antibody–associated vasculitis: A randomized controlled trial. JAMA. 2010;304:2381–8.

99. Pagnoux C, Mahr A, Hamidou MA, et al. Azathioprine or methotrexate maintenance for ANCA-associated vasculitis. N Engl J Med. 2008;359:2790–803.

100. Stratta P, Marcuccio C, Campo A, et al. Improvement in relative survival of patients with vasculitis: Study of 101 cases compared to the population. Int J Immunopathol Pharmacol. 2008;21:631–42.

101. Phillip R, Luqmani R. Mortality in systemic vasculitis: A systemic review. Clin Exp Rheumatol. 2008;26(Suppl 51):S94–104.

102. Day CJ, Howie AJ, Nightingale P, et al. Prediction of ESRD in pauci-immune necrotizing glomerulonephritis: Quantitative histomorphometric assessment and serum creatinine. Am J Kidney Dis. 2010;55:250–8.

103. Hauer HA, Bajema IM, Houwelingen HC, et al. Determinants of outcome in ANCA-associated glomerulonephritis: A prospective clinic-histopathological analysis of 96 patients. Kidney Int. 2002;62:1732–42.

104. Vergunst CE, Gurp E, Hagen EC, et al. An index for renal outcome in ANCA-associated glomerulonephritis. Am J Kidney Dis. 2003;41:532–8.

105. Alsaad A, Oudah N, Al Ameer A, et al. Glomerulonephritis with crescents in children: Etiology and predictors of renal outcome. ISRN Pediatr. 2011;2011:507298.

106. Siomou E, Tramma D, Bowen C, et al. ANCA-associated glomerulonephritis/systemic vasculitis in childhood: Clinical features—Outcome. Pediatr Nephrol. 2012;27:1911–20.

107. Charlier C, Henegar C, Launay O, et al. Risk factors for major infections in Wegener granulomatosis: Analysis of 113 patients. Ann Rheum Dis. 2009;68:658–63.

108. Wall N, Harper L. Complications of long term therapy for ANCA-associated systemic vasculitis. Nat Rev Nephrol. 2012;8:523–32.

## REVIEW QUESTIONS

1. The diagnosis of RPGN requires which of the following?
   a. Low complement C3 and deteriorating renal function

    b. Glomerular crescents on biopsy and positive ANCA

    c. Glomerular crescents and deteriorating renal function

    d. Glomerular crescents and linear anti-IgG immunofluorescence

2. A 13-year-old girl has hemoptysis and is found to have serum creatinine of 8.5 mg/dL. Which of the following test results is most likely to be abnormal?

    a. ANA

    b. Anti-GBM antibody

    c. Complement C3

    d. ANCA

3. A 15-year-old girl is found to have proteinuria and serum creatinine of 1.8 mg/dL. A week later her s-Cr is 4.8 mg/dL. Her hepatitis C titer is positive. Her renal biopsy shows crescents in 12 of 18 glomeruli. Immunofluorescence is most likely to show which of the following capillary loop patterns?

    a. Linear staining for anti-IgG, negative for C3

    b. Granular staining for IgG and C3

    c. Granular staining for C3, negative for IgG

    d. Granular staining for IgG, negative for C3

4. Which of the following statements is true regarding RPGN in children?

    a. It is less common than in adults.

    b. The most common cause is anti-GBM antibodies.

    c. It is a frequent complication of APSGN.

    d. It is ANCA positive in most cases.

5. A 17-year-old patient has chronic sinusitis, cough, and oral ulcers. Chest x-ray study shows nodular lung densities. Laboratory evaluation reveals positive cANCA. Which of the following is the most likely diagnosis?

    a. Granulomatosis with polyangiitis

    b. Systemic lupus erythematosus

    c. Dense deposit disease

    d. Microscopic polyangiitis

6. Which if the following is true of PAN?

    a. It predominantly involves small vessels.

    b. It predominantly involves medium-size vessels.

    c. It is a common cause of crescentic glomerulonephritis.

    d. Renal histology is indistinguishable from RPGN.

7. Which of the following is the currently recommended regimen for initiation therapy of severe RPGN?

    a. Cyclophosphamide and high-dose steroids only

    b. Cyclophosphamide, high-dose steroids and plasmapheresis

    c. High-dose steroids and plasmapheresis only

    d. Cyclophosphamide and plasmapheresis

8. RPGN caused by which of the following primary diseases is least likely to result in ESRD?

    a. Goodpasture disease

    b. Granulomatosis with polyangiitis

    c. IgA nephropathy

    d. Eosinophilic granulomatosis with polyangiitis

9. Which of the following is true of ANCA?

    a. It is present in all patients with pauci-immune RPGN.

    b. It activates neutrophils by binding to surface antigens.

    c. pANCA is predominantly seen with GPA.

    d. It is produced in response to known antigenic stimuli.

10. An 11-year-old girl has a 6-week history of malaise and weight loss. Serum BUN and creatinine are 75 mg/dL and 6.4 mg/dL, respectively. Electrolytes are unremarkable. She is suspected to have RPGN; additional laboratory evaluation is pending. The most appropriate next step is:

    a. Start intravenous fluids and monitor kidney function.

    b. Arrange an immediate renal biopsy.

    c. Start cyclophosphamide and high-dose steroids.

    d. Start intermittent hemodialysis.

## ANSWER KEY

1. c
2. b
3. b
4. a
5. a
6. b
7. b
8. c
9. b
10. b

# 23

# Immunoglobulin A nephropathy and Henoch-Schönlein purpura nephritis

M. COLLEEN HASTINGS AND ROBERT J. WYATT

Immunoglobulin A (IgA) nephropathy (IgAN) is the most common chronic glomerulonephritis in childhood, and Henoch-Schönlein purpura (HSP) is the most common vasculitis diagnosed in children and has nephritis as its most frequent chronic manifestation.[1,2] Because of shared pathogenic features, IgAN and HSP nephritis (HSPN) are discussed together in this chapter.[3]

In 1969, Jean Berger[4] reported IgA deposition in the mesangial region of glomeruli from children and young adults who were experiencing macroscopic hematuria during viral upper respiratory infections. In that report, Berger also described similar IgA deposits in patients with HSP. Some children diagnosed with HSPN subsequently have one or more episodes of macroscopic hematuria in the absence of rash, joint, or abdominal symptoms.[5] Meadow and Scott[6] reported identical twins with simultaneous adenovirus infections; one of them developed the clinical phenotype of HSP, the other had isolated macroscopic hematuria, and both had mesangial IgA deposits. HSP has occurred in children who previously had one or more episodes of isolated macroscopic hematuria with an interval between the episode and onset of HSP as long as 12 years.[7,8]

## EPIDEMIOLOGY

Few studies have determined population-based incidence for IgAN in children and adolescents. Many have relied on inferences from the percentage of cases in renal biopsy series. In Memphis, Tennessee and Seoul, Korea, the reported biopsy series incidence is approximately 10%,[1,9] whereas in Japan it is considerably higher, ranging from 24% to 30%.[10,11] In an Italian registry, IgAN and HSPN together accounted for approximately 30% of pediatric renal biopsy diagnoses.[12]

In central and eastern Kentucky, from 1985 through 1994, the incidence of IgAN was 5.6 cases per million persons per year for children 1 to 9 years of age and 10.2 cases per million persons per year for those 10 to 19 years of age.[13] The reported incidence of IgAN in Italy for children under the age of 15 years was 3.1 cases per million persons per year from 1992 through 1994. For children under the age of 15 years in Venezuela, the incidence of IgAN was only 0.3 cases per million persons per year in 1998.[14] From 1983 to 1999, the incidence was 45 cases per million persons per year for children under age 15 in Yonaga City, Japan.[15] The increased incidence in Japan compared to other areas of the world may reflect a true racial or ethnic difference in incidence.[16] However, additional explanations include increased detection through school screening programs, better diagnostic acuity of Japanese primary care physicians, and an aggressive approach of Japanese pediatric nephrologists toward biopsies for children with isolated microscopic hematuria or low levels of proteinuria.

Data from adult biopsy series suggested that IgAN is rare in persons of African descent and very few cases of IgAN have been reported from the continent of Africa.[17,18] However, in Shelby county (Memphis), Tennessee, for the period 1985 through 1995, the incidence of IgAN was higher for African-American children than white children (5.7 vs. 3.0 cases per million persons per year).[19] We continue to diagnose a significant number of African-American patients with IgAN.[20]

Population-based incidence for HSP from different regions was more than 100 cases per million persons per year, or at least 20-fold higher than that of IgAN.[1] However, because only 20% to 40% of children with HSP develop nephritis, which is often mild, the incidence of persistent HSPN appears similar to or even lower than that of IgAN.[1]

North American and European pediatric studies of IgAN find a male-to-female predominance of approximately two to one.[21,22] However, Japanese data that include school screening programs found no gender predominance.[15] Males and females are affected equally with HSP, but for HSPN there appears to be a slight male predominance of approximately 1.5 to 1.[1,23-27]

## PATHOLOGIC FEATURES

Renal histologic features in HSPN are strikingly similar to those in IgAN.[28,29] In both IgAN and HSPN, IgA is the dominant or codominant immunoglobulin that deposits mainly in the glomerular mesangium.[23,30] Only the IgA1 subclass is found in the deposits.[31]

The Oxford classification (Table 23.1) was developed to define lesions that may predict outcome of IgAN.[32,33] Figure 23.1A to E show some of the pathologic features examined as prognostic markers in the Oxford cohort that included both adult and pediatric patients. Light microscopic features in IgAN and HSPN are quite variable: glomeruli may have normal histologic findings, mesangial

proliferation and expansion without glomerular sclerosis or other chronic changes, endocapillary proliferation, focal segmental glomerulosclerosis with or without mesangial proliferation, focal necrosis (affecting a minority of glomeruli), adhesion of the glomerular tuft to Bowman's capsule and formation of crescents, or a combination of these. The presence of chronic tubular and interstitial injury is not often seen in the initial biopsy sample for pediatric IgAN and HSPN, but when present indicates progressive disease.[34]

> **KEY POINTS**
>
> - IgAN and HSP are both characterized by dominant deposition of IgA in the glomerular mesangium.
> - Most consider these two disorders as part of the same clinical spectrum.

Figure 23.1F shows this mesangial pattern as demonstrated by direct immunofluorescence. These deposits almost always can be seen by electron microscopy, typically in the paramesangial region where the basement membrane covers the mesangium. The immune deposits also may occur in the capillary loops, particularly during the early phase of aggressive HSPN and IgAN.[35,36] IgG, IgM, and complement C3 deposits are frequently seen on immunofluorescence, but IgA may be the sole immunoglobulin present in approximately 15% of biopsy samples.[37] Electron microscopy usually shows electron-dense material corresponding

Table 23.1 Oxford classification of immunoglobulin A nephropathy (MEST score)

| Biopsy variable | Definition | Score |
|---|---|---|
| Mesangial hypercellularity | <4 mesangial cells/mesangial area = 0<br>4–5 mesangial cells/mesangial area = 1<br>6–7 mesangial cells/mesangial area = 2<br>>8 mesangial cells/mesangial area = 3<br>The mesangial hypercellularity score is the mean score for all glomeruli. If more than half the glomeruli have more than three cells in a mesangial area, this is categorized as M1. | M0 ≤ 0.5<br>M1 > 0.5 |
| Endocapillary hypercellularity | Hypercellularity secondary to increased number of cells within the glomerular capillary lumina causing narrowing of the lumina | E0: Absent<br>E1: Present |
| Segmental glomerulosclerosis | Any amount of the tuft involved in sclerosis, but not involving the whole tuft or the presence of an adhesion | S0: Absent<br>S1: Present |
| Tubular atrophy/interstitial fibrosis | Percentage of cortical area involved by the tubular atrophy or interstitial fibrosis, whichever is greater | T0: 0–25%<br>T1: 26%–50%<br>T2: >50% |

*Source:* Adapted from Cattran DC, Coppo R, Cook HT, et al. The Oxford classification of IgA nephropathy: rationale, clinico-pathological correlations, and classification. Kidney Int. 2009;76,534–45.

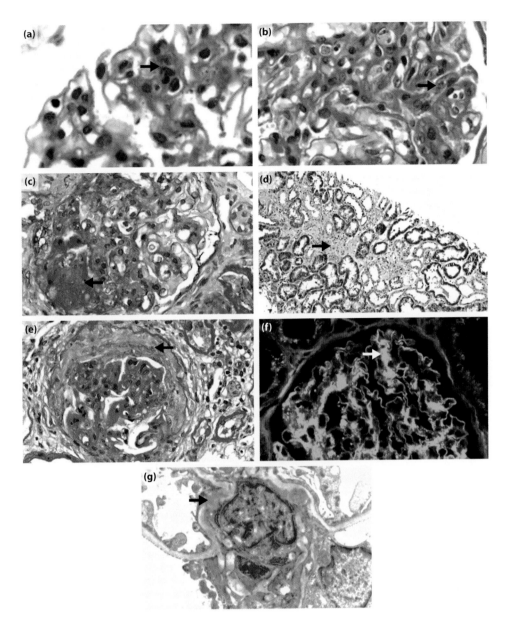

Figure 23.1 Pathologic characteristics of immunoglobulin A nephropathy. **(a)** Periodic acid–Schiff (PAS) stain shows mesangial hypercellularity, with four or more cells per mesangial area (arrow). **(b)** PAS shows segmental endocapillary proliferation with occlusion of the capillary lumen (arrow). **(c)** PAS shows segmental glomerulosclerosis and adhesion, with focal accumulation of hyaline and obliteration of the capillary lumen (arrow). **(d)** Trichrome stain shows tubular atrophy and interstitial fibrosis, with severe interstitial scarring and loss of tubules (arrow). **(e)** PAS shows a glomerular crescent; a circumferential layer of epithelial cells surrounds the glomerular tuft (arrow). **(f)** Immunofluorescence stain with fluorescein-conjugated anti-IgA antibodies) shows diffuse mesangial staining for IgA (arrow). **(g)** Electron micrograph of a glomerular capillary tuft in a specimen fixed in osmium tetroxide shows electron-dense material in the mesangial area (arrow), a finding that is consistent with the accumulation of immune complexes. (Reproduced with permission from: Wyatt RJ, Julian BA. IgA nephropathy. N Engl J Med. 2013;368:2402–14.)

to immunodeposits on immunofluorescence microscopy. These are generally in mesangial and paramesangial areas but are occasionally in subepithelial and subendothelial portions of glomerular basement membranes.[38]

Children seem to have fewer chronic-appearing lesions at the time of biopsy than adults with IgAN. Comparing kidney biopsy samples obtained from Japanese children to those from Japanese adults with IgAN, pediatric patients had increased glomerular hypercellularity although adult patients had more mesangial matrix expansion without hypercellularity; more adhesions, crescents, or both; and more tubulointerstitial damage.[39] Pediatric biopsy samples from the Oxford cohort also had more mesangial and endocapillary hypercellularity but less segmental glomerulosclerosis and tubulointerstitial injury compared to biopsy samples obtained from adult subjects.[40]

## PATHOGENESIS

The multiple hit hypothesis has been proposed to explain the pathogenesis of IgAN as well as HSPN (Figure 23.2).[1,41,42] The initiating or first hit is the presence in the serum of galactose-deficient (or underglycosylated) IgA1 in which in some of the carbohydrate side chains (O-glycans) at the hinge region terminate in N-acetylgalactosamine (GalNAc) or sialylated GalNac, rather than galactose. IgA1 differs from IgA2 and the other immunoglobulins in that it has a hinge region that contains O-linked glycans composed of N-acetylgalactosamine (GalNAc) linked to galactose (Figure 23.3).[43-45] Attachment of the galactose requires β1,3 galactosyltransferase. Galactose-deficient IgA1 can be detected in serum samples from patients with IgAN and HSPN by an increased affinity for binding to various lectins such as *Helix aspersa* that are specific for terminal GalNAc.[45,46]

The second hit involves generation of antiglycan antibodies that recognize the terminal GalNac residue on galactose deficient-IgA1. These antibodies may be either IgG or IgA.[47] This points to IgAN being an autoimmune disorder. The third hit consists of the formation of nephritogenic circulating immune complexes containing galactose-deficient IgA1 and antiglycan antibody.[48] These complexes then deposit in the glomerular mesangium by virtue of decreased clearance from the circulation, increased affinity for binding to mesangial structures, or both.[49-51]

> ### KEY POINTS
>
> - A multi-hit hypothesis has been suggested to explain the pathogenesis of IgAN.
> - The primary abnormality in IgAN is the presence of galactose-deficient (or underglycosylated) IgA1 in the serum of these patients.

The fourth hit incorporates all of the pathways of glomerular injury after deposition of the nephritogenic complexes in the mesangium and activation of the mesangial cells. Some of these mechanisms include the secretion of extracellular matrix components,[52] induction of nitric oxide synthase,[53] and the release various mediators of renal injury such as angiotensin II,[54] proinflammatory and profibrotic cytokines,[52,54] and growth factors.[53] Most, if not all, of these mechanisms of injury are not specific to IgAN.

## GENETICS

In 1985, Julian et al.[55] described a pedigree containing eight patients with IgAN who descended over 200 years from one of the earliest settlers of Pike County, Kentucky. Many similar pedigrees were subsequently described from eastern Kentucky and northern Italy.[56-58] A study of the French Society of Nephrology described 40 families in which two or more first-, second-, or third-degree relatives had IgAN, with five families having a member with HSP.[59] In addition, 18 other families had one member with IgAN and one or two with HSP.

> ### KEY POINTS
>
> - Familial IgAN has been reported from several parts of the world, but most cases of IgAN are sporadic.
> - No gene or gene product has yet been identified as pathognomonic for IgAN.
> - Serum galactose-deficient IgA1 level is elevated in approximately 75% patients with IgAN and is a heritable trait.

Gharavi et al.[60] used members of 30 pedigrees from Italy and Kentucky to demonstrate linkage to a locus on chromosome 6 in 60% of the pedigrees. This locus at 6q22-23 was named *IgAN1*. However, no gene or gene product from that locus of pathogenic importance for IgAN has yet been identified.

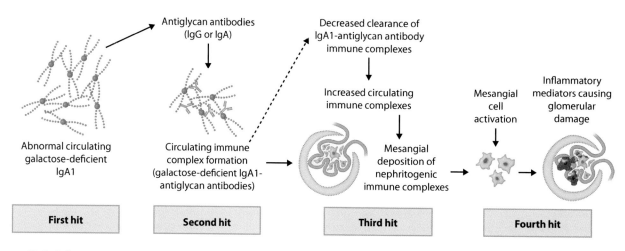

Figure 23.2 Schematic representation of the multi-hit pathogenesis of immunoglobulin A nephropathy.

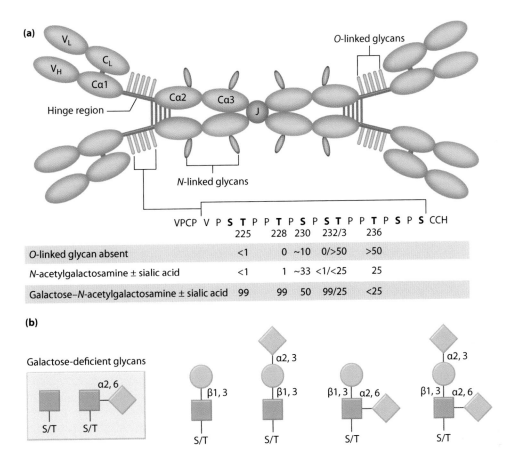

| | 225 | 228 | 230 | 232/3 | 236 |
|---|---|---|---|---|---|
| *O*-linked glycan absent | <1 | 0 | ~10 | 0/>50 | >50 |
| *N*-acetylgalactosamine ± sialic acid | <1 | 1 | ~33 | <1/<25 | 25 |
| Galactose–*N*-acetylgalactosamine ± sialic acid | 99 | 99 | 50 | 99/25 | <25 |

Figure 23.3 Structure of human immunoglobulin A1 (IgA1). IgA exists in several forms in the circulation: monomers, dimers, trimers, larger polymers, and secretory IgA. The IgA1 dimer is composed of two monomers linked by a joining chain. Each heavy chain has two N-linked (attached to a nitrogen molecule) glycan (carbohydrate) side chains and a hinge region between the first and second constant-region domains (Cα1 and Cα2, respectively). This hinge region is longer in IgA1 than in IgA2, and the longer IgA1 segment is rich in proline, threonine, and serine amino acid residues. Within the IgA1 hinge region, three to six glycans are attached to an oxygen molecule of a serine or threonine residue (O-linked). The dimer depicted has five O-linked glycans at each of the four hinge regions. The numbered amino acids indicate the six most common sites of attachment of O-glycans. The composition and number of the O-glycans differ substantially among the IgA1 molecules in a person, constituting microheterogeneity for the structure of the hinge region. The numbers below the position indicators show the frequency (percentage) of the compositional variations of an IgA1 myeloma protein that mimics the structure of poorly glycosylated IgA1 in patients with IgA nephropathy. As compared with healthy persons, patients with IgA nephropathy have more circulating IgA1 molecules with O-linked hinge-region glycans that do not include galactose (galactose-deficient IgA1). Panel B shows O-glycan variants of IgA1. Synthesis of the O-linked glycans proceeds in a stepwise manner, starting with attachment of N-acetylgalactosamine to some of the hinge-region serine or threonine amino acids. The glycan is normally extended by attachment of galactose. Sialic acid can be attached to N-acetylgalactosamine, galactose, or both. If sialic acid is attached to N-acetylgalactosamine before attachment of galactose, subsequent attachment of galactose is not possible. An imbalance in the activities or expression of specific glycosyltransferases in patients with IgA nephropathy accounts for the increased production of galactose-deficient O-linked glycans in the IgA1 hinge region with increased sialic acid residues. Cα denotes constant-region domain on alpha heavy chain, CL constant-region domain on light chain, VH variable region on heavy chain, and VL variable region on light chain. Squares indicate N-acetylgalactosamine, circles galactose, and diamonds sialic acid. (Reproduced with permission from: Wyatt RJ, Julian BA. IgA nephropathy. N Engl J Med. 2013;368:2402–14.)

Serum galactose-deficient IgA1 level is a heritable trait in whites with IgAN and HSPN nephritis and in Asians and African Americans with IgAN.[61–63] Approximately 75% of patients with IgAN have a level above the 90th percentile for healthy controls and approximately 30% to 40% of first-degree relatives of patients with IgAN also have significantly elevated serum galactose-deficient IgA1 level.[61,64] The majority of first-degree relatives with elevated serum

galactose-deficient IgA1 levels do not develop clinical manifestations of IgAN of HSPNs.[61,65] This suggests that additional factors are necessary for the disease to be clinically expressed.

Genome-wide association studies (GWAS) have the capablity to detect common susceptibility for complex traits without *a priori* mechanistic hypotheses.[66] A GWAS comprising a discovery cohort of 1194 IgAN cases and 902 controls of Chinese Han ancestry and follow-up cohorts of Han Chinese (740 cases, 750 controls) and European ancestry (1273 cases, 1201 controls) found five susceptibility loci. Three were on chromosome 6p21 in the major histocompatibility complex, and one was on chromosome 1q32 in the complement factor H (CFH) gene cluster. A single deletion of CFHR1,3 (complement factor H–related proteins 1 and 3) conferred a 30% reduction in the risk for developing IgAN. The fifth locus was on chromosome 22q12 in a region encoding oncostatin and leukemia inhibitory factor, which are cytokines involved in mucosal immunity and inflammation. All five loci were replicated in a meta-analysis comprising 12 cohorts of Asian, European, and African-American ancestry.[67]

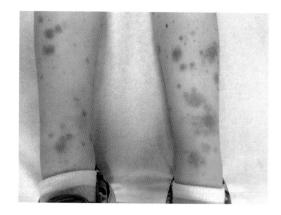

Figure 23.4 Classic distribution of Henoch-Schönlein purpura rash in the lower extremities in a child.

## CLINICAL PRESENTATION

In the United States, 75% of children and adolescents with IgAN present with macroscopic hematuria.[22,34,67.] Such episodes typically occur during an upper respiratory tract infection, with macroscopic hematuria clearing after a period of 2 to 4 days. Children also may present with microscopic hematuria with or without proteinuria or, more rarely, isolated proteinuria. Gross hematuria is not generally seen before the age of 3 years.[68]

Approximately 10% of children presenting with macroscopic hematuria have an acute kidney injury, but fewer than 5% have chronically impaired renal function at diagnosis.[22,34] Before the widespread use of normative blood pressure data based on gender, age, and height percentiles, hypertension at presentation of pediatric IgAN appeared to be unusual. The use of such normative data suggests that approximately 25% of pediatric patients in the United States are hypertensive at presentation.[69] However, severe hypertension in children presenting with normal renal function is rare. As a result of school screening programs, the majority of cases in Japan are detected with asymptomatic microscopic hematuria, proteinuria, or both.[10,15] Some children detected by screening will subsequently have a typical episode of macroscopic hematuria during an upper respiratory tract infection.

Fewer than 10% of children with IgAN present with overt nephrotic syndrome.[22,70] IgAN and steroid-responsive idiopathic nephrotic syndrome have occurred in the same child, and the clinical manifestations of one may appear several years after the other.[71,72] Treatment with corticosteroids should be directed toward the steroid-responsive idiopathic nephrotic syndrome and not withheld because of the presence of IgAN.[72]

The peak incidence of HSP is between 4 and 6 years of age, although individuals may present later in childhood or even as adults.[73] The child initially manifests with a typical rash that spreads from lower extremities up toward the buttocks and can be seen on the trunk and extensor surfaces of upper extremities (Figure 23.4). Scalp edema has been described in some patients. Other manifestations include abdominal pain or arthritis. Joint swelling and pain may be a dominant clinical manifestation in some. Intussusception may be seen in some patients with HSP, which manifests with intermittent abdominal pain and gastrointestinal bleeding. Urinalysis is often normal at the time of presentation, even in some who subsequently develop severe nephritis. HSPN may actually develop after all other manifestations of HSP have resolved.[73] Thus, it is imperative that all patients with

---

### KEY POINTS

- Synpharyngitic macroscopic hematuria is common in children with IgAN.
- Ten percent of children present with acute kidney injury.
- Hypertension is common in children at presentation (approximately 25%).
- Nephrotic syndrome is uncommon (less than 10%).

---

### KEY POINTS

- The peak incidence of HSP is seen in early childhood (4 to 6 years of age).
- Nephritis in HSP can occur after the nonrenal manifestations have subsided.
- Urinalysis may be normal early in the course of HSP.
- Proteinuria and nephrotic syndrome require close monitoring.
- Persistent proteinuria, nephrotic syndrome, and renal dysfunction are indications for a renal biopsy and treatment.

HSP should have a urinalysis performed every other week for at least 2 months from onset. Approximately 25% of children with HSPN will have macroscopic hematuria.[1,74] Approximately 10% to 20% of pediatric patients with HSPN will develop nephrotic syndrome.[75-77]

## EVALUATION AND DIAGNOSIS

Serum galactose-deficient IgA1 and antiglycan antibodies levels show some promise as diagnostic markers, but at the present time assays appropriate for use in the clinical laboratory are not available.[78] With no specific serologic marker for IgAN, diagnosis remains dependent on examination of cortical renal tissue obtained via kidney biopsy. In contrast, the diagnosis of HSPN is based on the presence of typical clinical features of HSP and clinical evidence of nephritis.[79] In HSPN, renal biopsy is usually reserved for patients with significant proteinuria who may require treatment. The renal biopsy findings in HSPN and IgAN are indistinguishable,[80] although patients with HSPN are more likely to have significant crescentic involvement.[1,23]

Initial laboratory tests for evaluation of suspected IgAN should include serum creatinine and albumin, serum complement C3, fluorescent antinuclear antibody (to exclude systemic lupus erythematosus [SLE]), urinalysis, and quantitation of urinary protein excretion by either a timed urine collection or random ratio of urine protein to creatinine. Except in the rare instance of preexisting deficiencies of an individual complement component or regulatory protein, serum concentrations of C3 and C4 are normal in both IgAN and HSPN.[23,81-83] For HSPN, perinuclear antineutrophil cytoplasmic antibodies (p-ANCA) and cytoplasmic ANCA (c-ANCA) and platelet counts may be necessary. Although the serum IgA level is usually above the mean and often significantly elevated in IgAN and HSPN, the sensitivity of the assay is too low for its use as a diagnostic test for either condition.[23,81,84]

The differential diagnosis of IgAN includes C1q nephropathy, IgG nephropathy, and SLE.[85-87] Poststreptococcal acute glomerulonephritis rarely manifests with a rash that appears similar to the HSP rash, and this diagnosis should be entertained when the serum C3 level is depressed.[88] Another unusual presentation is HSPN with typical systemic manifestations but without mesangial immune complex deposition.[81]

## OUTCOME

The outcome for pediatric patients with IgAN ranges from complete resolution of all clinical signs of disease to end-stage renal disease (ESRD).[22,34,36,69,81,89-91] At least one-third of pediatric patients with IgAN eventually have a normal urinalysis result, including some with severe histologic changes such as focal segmental sclerosis and crescents[69] or nephrotic syndrome.[22,34,69,81,89] In 181 Japanese children

with IgAN with a mean follow-up time of 7.3 years, 50.3% had achieved a clinical remission, 13.2% had persistent isolated hematuria, 32.6% had persistent hematuria and proteinuria, and 4% had advanced to ESRD at the time of last clinical examination.[92] The same group retrospectively analyzed 96 Japanese children with minor glomerular abnormalities, focal mesangial proliferation, or both, who did not receive medication for treatment of IgAN and found that 57 achieved spontaneous remission with a mean time from onset to remission of $5.9 \pm 0.4$ years.[93]

---

### KEY POINTS

- IgAN may progress to ESRD in 20% of cases.
- In unselected cases of HSPN, ESRD is seen in 3% of cases.

---

Kidney survival data for pediatric IgAN indicate that about 20% of patients eventually progress to ESRD, as often as adults.[2-5] In 2007, in a Memphis cohort of 67 white patients, predicted renal survival was 91% at 10 years and 80% at 20 years.[94] These findings are similar to predicted renal survival in a Finnish pediatric cohort (n = 55), with 93% renal survival at 10 years and 87% renal survival at 20 years.[95]

In Japan, 5% of pediatric patients with IgAN reached ESRD by 10 years from diagnosis in cohorts analyzed in the late 1980s.[90,91] Yata et al.[96] reported actuarial renal survival from the time of apparent disease onset in children diagnosed from 1976 to 2004 as 96.4% at 10 years, 84.5% at 15 years, and 73.9% at 20 years, with improved renal survival in those children diagnosed between 1990 and 2004 (98.8% at 10 years and 98.8% at 15 years). Studies of renal survival in pediatric patients with IgAN are summarized in Table 23.2.

Precise outcome for HSPN is difficult to determine because of wide differences in severity of cases reported from various tertiary care hospitals.[98-102] Data from "unselected" patients suggest that the risk for ESRD is approximately 1% for all children with HSP and 3% for those with HSPN.[75,77,98] Clearly, some pediatric patients with HSPN will progress to ESRD.[24,25,98] In Germany, 22% of patients with HSPN were predicted to reach ESRD by 10 years from onset.[24]

## PROGNOSIS

The optimal primary endpoint for studies of prognostic markers and treatment of glomerular diseases is progression to ESRD or a surrogate marker that closely associates with this end point. For pediatric patients with IgAN, clinical markers at diagnosis that associate with progressive loss of kidney function, ESRD, or both are magnitude of proteinuria and severe histologic features on kidney biopsy.[2-4]

Table 23.2 Kidney survival rates for pediatric immunoglobulin A nephropathy and Henoch-Schönlein purpura nephritis using the Kaplan-Meier method

| Study | Period | Location | Number | 5-year survival | 10-year survival | 20-year survival |
|---|---|---|---|---|---|---|
| **IgA Nephropathy** | | | | | | |
| Kusomoto et al. [90] | Before 1987 | Japan | 98 | 99 | 95 | 82 |
| Yoshikawa et al.[91] | Before 1989 | Japan (Kobe and Tokyo) | 258 | 95 | 94 | 89 |
| Wyatt et al.[22] | 1973–1994 | Kentucky and Tennessee | 103 | 94 | 87 | 70 |
| Ariceta et al.[89] | Before 2000 | Spain | 58 | 100 | 93 | |
| Nozawa et al.[92] | 1979–2004 | Japan | 181 | | 92 | 89 |
| Ronkainen et al.[95] | Before 2004 | Finland | 55 | 98 | 93 | 87 |
| Hastings et al.[94] | 1974–2006 | Tennessee (white) | 67 | 96 | 91 | 80 |
| Yata et al.[96] | 1976–2004 | Japan | 500 | 96 | 85 | 74 |
| **HSP Nephritis** | | | | | | |
| Scharer et al.[25] | 1969—1996 | Germany | 64 | 82 | 78 | 68 |
| Butani and Morgenstern [97] | 1950–1995 | Mayo Clinic | 52 | 92 | 88 | 80 |
| Coppo et al.[24] | 1980–2004 | Italy | 83 | 95 | 90 | |

*Source:* Adapted from Sanders JT, Wyatt RJ. IgA nephropathy and Henoch-Schönlein purpura nephritis. Curr Opin Pediatr. 2008;20:163–70.
*Abbreviation:* HSP, Henoch-Schönlein purpura.

Numerous studies of adults with IgAN have indicated that hypertension and renal function at time of presentation are important prognostic indicators.[102]

The use of serial measurements of urinary protein excretion averaged over 6-month intervals after renal biopsy has better prognostic value than a single measurement of proteinuria at the time of diagnosis.[103] In an adult population of Chinese patients with IgAN, time-averaged urinary protein excretion greater than 1.0 g/day was associated with a risk for ESRD that was 46 times the risk among patients with values of less than 0.5 g/day.[104]

Hypertension has been significantly related to progression in only one pediatric report.[34] However, blood pressures greater than 140/90 mm Hg are usually associated with loss of renal function in adult cohorts.[106-111] Proteinuria and hypertension were used in an adult study together to accurately predict decline in glomerular filtration rate and risk for dialysis or death.[111,112]

Numerous adult studies that have associated poor renal function at the time of diagnosis with development of ESRD.[115,116] There are not enough large pediatric studies that have evaluated baseline renal function and progression of disease in children. It is reasonable to assume that a child with impaired renal function at the time of diagnosis would be at increased risk for development of ESRD.

Hematuria, whether macroscopic or microscopic, does not correlate with prognosis, and early studies suggesting that gross hematuria was associated with better outcome were likely affected by lead time bias.[116] Two reports that both included the patients from Memphis suggested that African Americans had a significantly worse outcome than whites.[22,34] However, for Memphis patients diagnosed since 1990 there was no difference in outcome based on race.[20] Our most recent kidney survival data for the entire Memphis IgAN cohort also shows no difference in progression to ESRD based on gender.

The Oxford cohort was developed to determine histologic predictors of progression.[32,33] Patients with estimated glomerular filtration rate (eGFR) less than 30 mL/min/1.73 m² (CKD4) were excluded from the study, and progression to ESRD or more than 50% decline from entry eGFR was used as the primary outcome measure during validation for this biopsy classification schema. The Oxford cohort included 206 adult and 59 pediatric patients with IgAN from 17 centers (located in Asia, Europe, and North America) and required urinary protein excretion greater than 500 mg/day and more than 12 months of follow-up time.

Mesangial hypercellularity (M), segmental glomerulosclerosis/adhesion (S), and tubular atrophy and interstitial fibrosis (T) were the histologic features independently associated with loss of renal function (see Figure 23.1). Endocapillary proliferation (E) was associated with progression in patients not treated with corticosteroids or other immunosuppressive drugs. Grading of these four histologic features constitute the MEST score.[33]

Coppo et al.[40] verified the MEST with a subgroup analysis of the data from the pediatric patients in the Oxford cohort. Other groups have applied this classification schema to their cohorts of children with IgAN. In a Swedish study, the mesangial hypercellularity score greater than 0.5, the presence of endocapillary hypercellularity, or tubular atrophy/interstitial fibrosis of greater than 25% was significantly associated with a poor renal outcome, but segmental glomerulosclerosis was not.[117] Shima et al.[118] found in 161 Japanese children with newly diagnosed IgAN from 1977 to 1989 that mesangial hypercellularity score, endocapillary hypercellularity, tubular atrophy, and crescents were significant predictors of renal outcome in a univariate analysis.

Severe histologic findings and nephrotic syndrome are markers of poor prognosis for HSPN.[23,101] Logistic regression analysis in a German cohort found that renal insufficiency at presentation and nephrotic syndrome were significant independent predictors of outcome.[25] Although many clinicians feel that younger children are less likely to have severe or progressive HSPN, age at presentation does not significantly associate with outcome.[24,25,99]

## TREATMENT STRATEGIES

There are no solid, evidence-based guidelines for the treatment of pediatric IgAN and HSPN.[72] This is due to factors such as (1) the small number of patients at single centers; (2) the difficulty, time, and expense in organizing randomized controlled trials (RCTs); and (3) progression from normal function to ESRD may take several decades. In addition, distinct treatment strategies may be applied to acute and chronic phases of disease.

Rapidly progressive or severe crescentic IgAN and HSPN are usually treated with high-dose intravenous methylprednisolone pulses followed by oral corticosteroids and sometimes other immunosuppressive agents, such as cyclophosphamide.[120-123] All published data on this approach are from uncontrolled case series. This treatment may be effective in some instances, but a poor outcome cannot be avoided if the glomerular lesions are too far advanced before therapy is begun.[72]

Treatment with an angiotensin-converting enzyme inhibitor (ACEI) or angiotensin receptor blocker is recommended as initial therapy for with IgAN.[123] A recent RCT in children and young adults showed that ACEI treatment was associated with better prognosis.[124] Our group and others now use this approach for both hypertensive and normotensive pediatric patients.[71,125] In an RCT of mycophenolate mofetil (MMF) for pediatric and adult patients with IgAN, many patients had such significant reduction in proteinuria in response to 3 months of ACEI and fish oil treatment that they were no longer eligible for randomization to MMF or placebo.[126]

### KEY POINTS

- Treatment of rapidly progressive nephritis should be undertaken urgently. Intravenous methylprednisolone is the initial drug of choice.
- Use of ACEIs or angiotensin receptor blockers is the recommended therapy in early IgAN.

Although there are no RCTs supporting the approach, corticosteroid therapy is indicated for pediatric patients with IgAN or HSPN who have the nephrotic syndrome.[72] An RCT for adult and pediatric patients with IgAN compared alternate-day prednisone, fish oil capsules, and placebo and showed no significant advantage with respect to time to ESRD for any arm of the trial.[127] Current Kidney Disease: Improving Global Outcomes (KDIGO) guidelines for glomerular disease suggest that corticosteroids should be initiated in high-risk patients only if proteinuria remains above 1 g/day after supportive care has been optimized for 3 to 6 months and only if GFR remains above 50 mL/min/1.73 m$^2$ (level 2C evidence).[123] The Therapeutic Evaluation of Steroids in IgA Nephropathy Global Study (TESTING Study) is an RCT currently enrolling patients 14 years or older with proteinuria higher than 1 g/day to evaluate the use of methylprednisolone versus placebo in patients with IgAN already on maximal RAS blockade (http://clinicaltrials.gov/show/NCT01560052). Coppo[128] postulated that there may be a legacy effect—that is, benefit to early and aggressive treatment of mild IgAN with low-grade proteinuria at presentation that might prevent sclerosis and interstitial fibrosis leading to loss of GFR later in the course of the disease.

### SUMMARY

As illustrated in the following case report, some patients who originally have HSPN will enter a chronic phase in which the clinical phenotype is that of IgAN. Patients with HSPN and IgAN with persistent proteinuria, flares, or both characterized by macroscopic hematuria during viral illness appear to be at risk for eventual progression to ESRD. In such cases decisions about treatment are difficult and sometimes not supported by evidence from RCTs. Future advances will depend on delineation of the earliest pathogenetic mechanisms in IgAN and HSPN with specific therapy targeted toward such mechanisms.

### ACKNOWLEDGMENTS

This work was supported by a generous gift from Donald and Anna Waite. The authors thank Dr. Patrick Walker for providing renal pathologic images in Figure 23.1.

### Clinical Vignette 23.1

A previously well 5-year-old white male presented with the typical features of HSP: purpuric rash distributed on the lower limbs, swollen ankles, abdominal pain, and microscopic hematuria. Two weeks later he developed macroscopic hematuria. He had transient hypertension with a maximum blood pressure of 120/85 mm Hg that resolved without treatment. Pertinent laboratory tests included hemoglobin, 11.3 g/dL; platelet count, 519 ×

$10^9$/mL; serum creatinine, 0.5 mg/dL; serum albumin, 2.8 g/dL; serum cholesterol, 242 mg/dL; complement C3, 92 mg/dL (normal); and a negative antinuclear antibody test. The urinalysis had a specific gravity of 1.015 with 2+ protein and a sediment that showed too numerous to count (TNTC) red blood cells (RBCs), 5 to 10 white blood cells (WBCs) per high-power field (hpf), and several granular casts/hpf. Random ratio of urine protein to creatinine increased from 0.62 to 4.1 over the next 7 days. Renal biopsy showed diffuse mesangial proliferative glomerulonephritis with focal sclerosis in 9% and cellular crescents in 12% of the glomeruli. Immunofluorescence showed mesangial deposition of IgA (3+), IgG (2+), complement C3 (3+), and properdin (2+). Alternate-day prednisone was begun at a dose of 40 mg/m$^2$ every other day and continued in a tapering dose for 18 months. At this era, an ACEI was not used for treatment of nonhypertensive glomerular disease. One month after treatment was stopped the urine had TNTC RBC/hpf, but the ratio of urine protein to creatinine was normal (0.13).

The child was not seen again until age 10, when he had an episode of macroscopic hematuria associated with exercise. At this time he had no rash or joint or abdominal symptoms. His serum creatinine was 0.5 mg/dL, and the ratio of urine protein to creatinine was 2.8. Alternate-day prednisone was again begun at 40 mg/m$^2$ per dose, and a fish oil supplement (MaxEPA) was added. After 4 months he was lost to follow-up until he returned at age 14 after another episode of macroscopic hematuria during a flulike illness. His serum creatinine level was 0.9 mg/dL and albumin was 3.1 g/dL. Urinalysis showed specific gravity of 1.020 with 2+ protein. Microscopic examination of unspun urine showed TNTC RBCs/hpf, 20% of which were dysmorphic. The ratio of urine protein to creatinine was 4.1. A second renal biopsy showed diffuse mesangial proliferation with 20% obsolescent glomeruli, but minimal focal sclerosis and no crescents. There was minimal interstitial fibrosis. The immunofluorescence pattern was similar to that of the first biopsy sample except for the presence of IgM with 1+ intensity. He was normotensive, with no HSP rash. With no therapeutic intervention, 2 weeks after the biopsy the ratio of urine protein to creatinine fell to 1.07 and 10 mg per day of the ACEI fosinopril was begun.

One year later he had yet another episode of macroscopic hematuria with a viral illness. Over the next 2 months his serum creatinine increased from 0.7 to 2.2 mg/dL and albumin fell to 2.9 g/dL; the ratio of urine protein to creatinine was up to 5.9. A third renal biopsy was performed that showed diffuse mesangial proliferation with 10% of the glomeruli having cellular crescents. Several glomeruli showed segmental sclerosis and fibrous adhesions to Bowman's capsule. Alternate-day prednisone at 40 mg/m$^2$ per dose and MMF (initial dose of 600 mg/m$^2$/day, advanced to 900 mg/m$^2$/day)

were started. The prednisone was discontinued after 10 months and MMF after 14 months when the serum creatinine was 0.7 mg/dL; albumin, 3.2 g/dL; and ratio of urine protein to creatinine, 2.5. Three years later, at age 17, he developed macroscopic hematuria again and nephrotic syndrome shortly after undergoing a tonsillectomy. Serum creatinine was 1.7 mg/dL; albumin, 2.0 g/dL; and ratio of urine protein to creatinine, 4.6. He had severe edema with ascites. He slowly improved after treatment with alternate-day prednisone, MMF, fosinopril, and losartan. At the last follow-up, he continued to have microscopic hematuria with a serum creatinine of 1.1 mg/dL; serum albumin, 3.4 g/dL, and ratio of urine protein to creatinine, 0.75.

## TEACHING POINTS

This patient presented at 5 years of age with classic clinical features of HSPN. Five years later, he developed episodes of recurrent gross hematuria that were preceded by exercise and flu-like illnesses. HSP-like rash was absent in these hematuria events. The clinical course of this patient is reminiscent of a transition from HSPN to IgAN. Interestingly, the first renal biopsy of this patient documented that 9% of glomeruli were affected by chronicity changes indicated by focal glomerular sclerosis, a finding that is less likely to be present during acute phase of HSP nephritis. It can, therefore, be argued that even though this patient presented with classic clinical features of acute HSPN, it is more likely that he had an underlying IgA nephropathy of much longer duration. Although an accurate MEST score for IgAN (Oxford classification) was not developed for this patient, histologic features, presence of renal insufficiency at presentation, and nephrotic syndrome are considered indicators of poor outcome in HSPN-IgAN spectrum of disorders. [23,25,101,117,118]

From a therapeutic perspective, remission of proteinuria after steroid therapy for HSPN provided clinical relief to the patient. Yet the renal disease in this patient progresses, as documented by the second renal biopsy, development of nephrotic syndrome, and onset of CKD. This patient did not receive the benefit of ACE-inhibition as an anti-proteinuric and renoprotective therapy, since such a therapy was not considered to be the standard of care in the era of this patient's clinical presentation. At present, ACE inhibition and ARB therapies should be considered as a part of ongoing management of IgA nephropathy, unless contraindications for their use exist.

## REFERENCES

1. Delos Santos NM, Wyatt RJ. Pediatric IgA nephropathies: Clinical aspects and therapeutic approaches. Semin Nephrol. 2004;24:269–86.
2. Saulsbury FT. Henoch-Schönlein purpura. Curr Opin Rheumatol. 2001;13:35–40.

3. Wyatt RJ, Julian BA. IgA nephropathy. N Engl J Med. 2013;368:2402–14.

4. Berger J. IgA glomerular deposits in renal disease. Transplant Proc. 1969;1:939–44.

5. Waldo FB. Is Henoch-Schönlein purpura the systemic form of IgA nephropathy? Am J Kidney Dis. 1988;12:373–7.

6. Meadow SR, Scott DG. Berger disease: Henoch-Schönlein syndrome without the rash. J Pediatr. 1985;106:27–32.

7. Hughes FJ, Wolfish NM, McLaine PN. Henoch-Schönlein syndrome and IgA nephropathy: A case report suggesting a common pathogenesis. Pediatr Nephrol. 1988;2:389–92.

8. Watanabe T, Takada T, Kihara I, Oda Y. Three cases of Henoch-Schönlein purpura preceded by IgA nephropathy. Pediatr Nephrol. 1995;9:674.

9. Cho BS, Kim SD, Choi YM, Kang HH. School urinalysis screening in Korea: Prevalence of chronic renal disease. Pediatr Nephrol. 2001;16:1126–8.

10. Utsunomiya Y, Kado T, Koda T, et al. Features of IgA nephropathy in preschool children. Clin Nephrol. 2000;54:443–8.

11. Yoshikawa N, Tanaka R, Iijima K. Pathophysiology and treatment of IgA nephropathy in children. Pediatr Nephrol. 2001;16:446–57.

12. Coppo R, Gianoglio B, Porcellini MG, Maringhini S. Frequency of renal diseases and clinical indications for renal biopsy in children (report of the Italian National Registry of Renal Biopsies in Children). Group of Renal Immunopathology of the Italian Society of Pediatric Nephrology and Group of Renal Immunopathology of the Italian Society of Nephrology. Nephrol Dial Transplant. 1998;13:293–7.

13. Wyatt RJ, Julian BA, Baehler RW, et al. Epidemiology of IgA nephropathy in central and eastern Kentucky for the period 1975 through 1994. Central Kentucky Region of the Southeastern United States IgA Nephropathy DATABANK Project. J Am Soc Nephrol. 1998;9:853–8.

14. Coppo R, Camilla R, Alfarano A, et al. Upregulation of the immunoproteasome in peripheral blood mononuclear cells of patients with IgA nephropathy. Kidney Int. 2009;75:536–41.

15. Utsunomiya Y, Koda T, Kado T, et al. Incidence of pediatric IgA nephropathy. Pediatr Nephrol. 2003;18:511–5.

16. Kiryluk K, Li Y, Sanna-Cherchi S, et al. Geographic differences in genetic susceptibility to IgA nephropathy: GWAS replication study and geospatial risk analysis. PLoS Genet. 2012;8:e1002765.

17. Jennette JC, Wall SD, Wilkman AS. Low incidence of IgA nephropathy in blacks. Kidney Int. 1985;28:944–50.

18. Seedat YK, Nathoo BC, Parag KB, et al. IgA nephropathy in blacks and Indians of Natal. Nephron. 1988;50:137–41.

19. Sehic AM, Gaber LW, Roy S, et al. Increased recognition of IgA nephropathy in African-American children. Pediatr Nephrol. 1997;11:435–7.

20. Lau KK, Gaber LW, Delos Santos NM, et al. Pediatric IgA nephropathy: Clinical features at presentation and outcome for African-Americans and Caucasians. Clin Nephrol. 2004;62:167–72.

21. Lévy M, Gonzalez-Burchard G, Broyer M, et al. Berger's disease in children: Natural history and outcome. Medicine (Baltimore). 1985;64:157–80.

22. Wyatt RJ, Kritchevsky SB, Woodford SY, et al. IgA nephropathy: Long-term prognosis for pediatric patients. J Pediatr. 1995;127:913–9.

23. Levy M, Broyer M, Arsan A, Levy-Bentolila D, et al. Anaphylactoid purpura nephritis in childhood: Natural history and immunopathology. Adv Nephrol Necker Hosp. 1976;6:183–228.

24. Coppo R, Mazzucco G, Cagnoli L, et al. Long-term prognosis of Henoch-Schönlein nephritis in adults and children. Italian Group of Renal Immunopathology Collaborative Study on Henoch-Schönlein purpura. Nephrol Dial Transplant. 1997;12:2277–83.

25. Scharer K, Krmar R, Querfeld U, Ruder H, et al. Clinical outcome of Schönlein-Henoch purpura nephritis in children. Pediatr Nephrol. 1999;13:816–23.

26. Ronkainen J, Nuutinen M, Koskimies O. The adult kidney 24 years after childhood Henoch-Schönlein purpura: A retrospective cohort study. Lancet. 2002;360:666–70.

27. Yoshikawa N, Ito H, Yoshiya K, Nakahara C, et al. Henoch-Schöenlein nephritis and IgA nephropathy in children: A comparison of clinical course. Clin Nephrol. 1987;27:233–7.

28. Davin JC. Henoch-Schönlein purpura nephritis: Pathophysiology, treatment, and future strategy. Clin J Am Soc Nephrol. 2011;6:679–89.

29. Evans DJ, Williams DG, Peters DK, et al. Glomerular deposition of properdin in Henoch-Schönlein syndrome and idiopathic focal nephritis. Br Med J. 1973;3:326–8.

30. Wyatt RJ, Julian BA, Bhathena DB, et al. IgA nephropathy: Presentation, clinical course, and prognosis in children and adults. Am J Kidney Dis. 1984;4:192–200.

31. Conley ME, Cooper MD, Michael AF. Selective deposition of immunoglobulin A1 in immunoglobulin A nephropathy, anaphylactoid purpura nephritis, and systemic lupus erythematosus. J Clin Invest. 1980;66:1432–6.

32. Roberts IS, Cook HT, Troyanov S, et al. The Oxford classification of IgA nephropathy: Pathology definitions, correlations, and reproducibility. Kidney Int. 2009;76:546–56.

33. Cattran DC, Coppo R, Cook HT, et al. The Oxford classification of IgA nephropathy: Rationale, clinico-pathological correlations, and classification. Kidney Int. 2009;76:534–45.

34. Hogg RJ, Silva FG, Wyatt RJ, et al. Prognostic indicators in children with IgA nephropathy: Report of the Southwest Pediatric Nephrology Study Group. Pediatr Nephrol. 1994;8:15–20.

35. Andreoli SP, Yum MN, Bergstein JM. IgA nephropathy in children: Significance of glomerular basement membrane deposition of IgA. Am J Nephrol. 1986;6:28–33.

36. Yoshikawa N, Ito H, Nakamura H. Prognostic indicators in childhood IgA nephropathy. Nephron. 1992;60:60–7.

37. Barratt J, Feehally J. IgA nephropathy. J Am Soc Nephrol. 2005;16:2088–97.

38. Haas M. IgA nephropathy and Henoch-Schöenlein purpura nephritis. In: Jennette JC, Olsen JL, Schwartz MM, FG S, editors. Heptinstall's Pathology of the Kidney. vol I. 6th ed. Philadelphia: Lippincott, Williams and Wilkins; 2007. pp. 423–86.

39. Ikezumi Y, Suzuki T, Imai N, et al. Histological differences in new-onset IgA nephropathy between children and adults. Nephrol Dial Transplant. 2006;21:3466–74.

40. Coppo R, Troyanov S, Camilla R, et al. The Oxford IgA nephropathy clinicopathological classification is valid for children as well as adults. Kidney Int. 2010;77:921–7.

41. Suzuki H, Kiryluk K, Novak J, et al. The pathophysiology of IgA nephropathy. J Am Soc Nephrol. 2011;22:1795–803.

42. Lau KK, Suzuki H, Novak J, Wyatt RJ. Pathogenesis of Henoch-Schönlein purpura nephritis. Pediatr Nephrol. 2010;25:19–26.

43. Barratt J, Feehally J, Smith AC. Pathogenesis of IgA nephropathy. Semin Nephrol. 2004;24:197–217.

44. Mestecky J, Tomana M, Crowley-Nowick PA, et al. Defective galactosylation and clearance of IgA1 molecules as a possible etiopathogenic factor in IgA nephropathy. Contrib Nephrol. 1993;104:172–82.

45. Tomana M, Matousovic K, Julian BA, et al. Galactose-deficient IgA1 in sera of IgA nephropathy patients is present in complexes with IgG. Kidney Int. 1997;52:509–16.

46. Allen AC, Willis FR, Beattie TJ, et al. Abnormal IgA glycosylation in Henoch-Schönlein purpura restricted to patients with clinical nephritis. Nephrol Dial Transplant. 1998;13:930–4.

47. Berthoux F, Suzuki H, Thibaudin L, et al. Autoantibodies targeting galactose-deficient IgA1 associate with progression of IgA nephropathy. J Am Soc Nephrol. 2012;23:1579–87.

48. Tomana M, Novak J, Julian BA, et al. Circulating immune complexes in IgA nephropathy consist of IgA1 with galactose-deficient hinge region and antiglycan antibodies. J Clin Invest. 1999;104:73–81.

49. Novak J, Julian BA, Tomana M, et al. Progress in molecular and genetic studies of IgA nephropathy. J Clin Immunol. 2001;21:310–27.

50. Novak J, Vu HL, Novak L, et al. Interactions of human mesangial cells with IgA and IgA-containing immune complexes. Kidney Int. 2002;62:465–75.

51. Novak J, Tomana M, Matousovic K, et al. IgA1-containing immune complexes in IgA nephropathy differentially affect proliferation of mesangial cells. Kidney Int. 2005;67:504–13.

52. Novak J, Julian BA, Mestecky J, et al. Glycosylation of IgA1 and pathogenesis of IgA nephropathy. Semin Immunopathol. 2012;34:365–82.

53. Amore A, Conti G, Cirina P, et al. Aberrantly glycosylated IgA molecules downregulate the synthesis and secretion of vascular endothelial growth factor in human mesangial cells. Am J Kidney Dis. 2000;36:1242–52.

54. Lai KN. Pathogenesis of IgA nephropathy. Nat Rev Nephrol. 2012;8:275–83.

55. Julian BA, Quiggins PA, Thompson JS, et al. Familial IgA nephropathy: Evidence of an inherited mechanism of disease. N Engl J Med. 1985;312:202–8.

56. Wyatt RJ, Rivas ML, Julian BA, et al. Regionalization in hereditary IgA nephropathy. Am J Hum Genet. 1987;41:36–50.

57. Lavigne KA, Woodford SY, Barker CV, et al. Familial IgA nephropathy in southeastern Kentucky. Clin Nephrol. 2010;73:115–21.

58. Scolari F, Amoroso A, Savoldi S, et al. Familial clustering of IgA nephropathy: Further evidence in an Italian population. Am J Kidney Dis. 1999;33:857–65.

59. Levy M. Familial cases of Berger's disease and anaphylactoid purpura: More frequent than previously thought. Am J Med. 1989;87:246–8.

60. Gharavi AG, Yan Y, Scolari F, et al. IgA nephropathy, the most common cause of glomerulonephritis, is linked to 6q22-23. Nat Genet. 2000;26:354–7.

61. Gharavi AG, Moldoveanu Z, Wyatt RJ, et al. Aberrant IgA1 glycosylation is inherited in familial and sporadic IgA nephropathy. J Am Soc Nephrol. 2008;19:1008–14.

62. Kiryluk K, Moldoveanu Z, Sanders JT, et al. Aberrant glycosylation of IgA1 is inherited in both pediatric IgA nephropathy and Henoch-Schönlein purpura nephritis. Kidney Int. 2011;80:79–87.

63. Hastings MC, Moldoveanu Z, Julian BA, et al. Galactose-deficient IgA1 in African Americans with IgA nephropathy: Serum levels and heritability. Clin J Am Soc Nephrol. 2010;5:2069–74.

64. Moldoveanu Z, Wyatt RJ, Lee JY, et al. Patients with IgA nephropathy have increased serum galactose-deficient IgA1 levels. Kidney Int. 2007;71:1148–54.

65. Lin X, Ding J, Zhu L, Shi S, et al. Aberrant galactosylation of IgA1 is involved in the genetic susceptibility of Chinese patients with IgA nephropathy. Nephrol Dial Transplant. 2009;24:3372–5.

66. Wellcome Trust Case Control Consortium. Genome-wide association study of 14,000 cases of seven common diseases and 3,000 shared controls. Nature. 2007;447:661–78.

67. Kher KK, Makker SP, Moorthy B. IgA nephropathy (Berger's disease): A clinicopathologic study in children. Int J Pediatr Nephrol. 1983;4:11–8.

68. Coppo R. Pediatric IgA nephropathy: Clinical and therapeutic perspectives. Semin Nephrol. 2008;28:18–26.

69. Santos NM, Ault BH, Gharavi AG, et al. Angiotensin-converting enzyme genotype and outcome in pediatric IgA nephropathy. Pediatr Nephrol. 2002;17:496–502.

70. Kitajima T, Murakami M, Sakai O. Clinicopathological features in the Japanese patients with IgA nephropathy. Jpn J Med. 1983;22:219–22.

71. Southwest Pediatric Nephrology Study Group. Association of IgA nephropathy with steroid-responsive nephrotic syndrome. Am J Kidney Dis. 1985;5:157–64.

72. Wyatt RJ, Hogg RJ. Evidence-based assessment of treatment options for children with IgA nephropathies. Pediatr Nephrol. 2001;16:156–67.

73. Hurley RM, Drummond KN. Anaphylactoid purpura nephritis: Clinicopathological correlations. J Pediatr. 1972;81:904–11.

74. Calvino MC, Llorca J, Garcia-Porrua C, et al. Henoch-Schönlein purpura in children from northwestern Spain: A 20-year epidemiologic and clinical study. Medicine (Baltimore). 2001;80:279–90.

75. Amoli MM, Thomson W, Hajeer AH, et al. Interleukin 1 receptor antagonist gene polymorphism is associated with severe renal involvement and renal sequelae in Henoch-Schönlein purpura. J Rheumatol. 2002;29:1404–7.

76. Stewart M, Savage JM, Bell B, et al. Long-term renal prognosis of Henoch-Schönlein purpura in an unselected childhood population. Eur J Pediatr. 1988;147:113–5.

77. Saulsbury FT. Henoch-Schönlein purpura in children: Report of 100 patients and review of the literature. Medicine (Baltimore). 1999;78:395–409.

78. Hastings MC, Moldoveanu Z, Suzuki H, et al. Biomarkers in IgA nephropathy: Relationship to pathogenetic hits. Expert Opin Med Diagn. 2013;7:615–27.

79. Mills JA, Michel BA, Bloch DA, et al. The American College of Rheumatology 1990 criteria for the classification of Henoch-Schönlein purpura. Arthritis Rheum. 1990;33:1114–21.

80. Evans DJ, Williams DG, Peters DK, et al. Glomerular deposition of properdin in Henoch-Schönlein syndrome and idiopathic focal nephritis. Br Med J. 1973;3:326–8.

81. Levy M, Gonzalez-Burchard G, Broyer M, et al. Berger's disease in children: Natural history and outcome. Medicine (Baltimore). 1985;64:157–80.

82. Wyatt RJ, Julian BA, Rivas ML. Role for specific complement phenotypes and deficiencies in the clinical expression of IgA nephropathy. Am J Med Sci. 1991;301:115–23.

83. Garcia-Fuentes M, Martin A, Chantler C, et al. Serum complement components in Henoch-Schönlein purpura. Arch Dis Child. 1978;53:417–9.

84. Julian BA, Wyatt RJ, McMorrow RG, et al. Serum complement proteins in IgA nephropathy. Clin Nephrol. 1983;20:251–8.

85. Lau KK, Gaber LW, Delos Santos NM, et al. C1q nephropathy: Features at presentation and outcome. Pediatr Nephrol. 2005;20:744–9.

86. Iskandar SS, Browning MC, Lorentz WB. C1q nephropathy: A pediatric clinicopathologic study. Am J Kidney Dis. 1991;18:459–65.

87. Yoshikawa N, Iijima K, Shimomura M, et al. IgG-associated primary glomerulonephritis in children. Clin Nephrol. 1994;42:281–7.

88. Goodyer PR, de Chadarevian JP, Kaplan BS. Acute poststreptococcal glomerulonephritis mimicking Henoch-Schönlein purpura. J Pediatr. 1978;93:412–5.

89. Ariceta G, Gallego N, Lopez-Fernandez Y, et al. Long-term prognosis of childhood IgA nephropathy in adult life. Med Clin (Barc). 2001;116:361–4.

90. Kusumoto Y, Takebayashi S, Taguchi T, et al. Long-term prognosis and prognostic indices of IgA nephropathy in juvenile and in adult Japanese. Clin Nephrol. 1987;28:118–24.

91. Yoshikawa N, Ito H, Nakamura H. IgA nephropathy in children from Japan: Clinical and pathological features. Child Nephrol Urol. 1988;9:191–9.

92. Nozawa R, Suzuki J, Takahashi A, et al. Clinicopathological features and the prognosis of IgA nephropathy in Japanese children on long-term observation. Clin Nephrol. 2005;64:171–9.

93. Shima Y, Nakanishi K, Hama T, et al. Spontaneous remission in children with IgA nephropathy. Pediatr Nephrol. 2013;28:71–6.

94. Hastings MC, Delos Santos NM, et al. Renal survival in pediatric patients with IgA nephropathy. Pediatr Nephrol. 2007;22:317–8.

95. Ronkainen J, Ala-Houhala M, Autio-Harmainen H, et al. Long-term outcome 19 years after childhood IgA nephritis: A retrospective cohort study. Pediatr Nephrol. 2006;21:1266–73.

96. Yata N, Nakanishi K, Shima Y, Togawa H, et al. Improved renal survival in Japanese children with IgA nephropathy. Pediatr Nephrol. 2008;23:905–12.

97. Koskimies O, Mir S, Rapola J, et al. Henoch-Schönlein nephritis: Long-term prognosis of unselected patients. Arch Dis Child. 1981;56:482–4.

98. Butani L, Morgenstern BZ. Longterm outcome of children with Henoch-Schonlein purpura nephritis. Clin Pediatr (Phila). 2007;46:505-511.

99. Counahan R, Winterborn MH, White RH, et al. Prognosis of Henoch-Schönlein nephritis in children. Br Med J. 1977;2:11–4.

100. Bunchman TE, Mauer SM, Sibley RK, et al. Anaphylactoid purpura: Characteristics of 16 patients who progressed to renal failure. Pediatr Nephrol. 1988;2:393–7.

101. Goldstein AR, White RH, Akuse R, et al. Long-term follow-up of childhood Henoch-Schönlein nephritis. Lancet. 1992;339:280–2.

102. Barbour SJ, Reich HN. Risk stratification of patients with IgA nephropathy. Am J Kidney Dis. 2012;59:865–73.

103. Reich HN, Troyanov S, Scholey JW, et al. Remission of proteinuria improves prognosis in IgA nephropathy. J Am Soc Nephrol. 2007;18:3177–83.

104. Le W, Liang S, Hu Y, Deng K, et al. Long-term renal survival and related risk factors in patients with IgA nephropathy: Results from a cohort of 1155 cases in a Chinese adult population. Nephrol Dial Transplant. 2012;27:1479–85.

105. Beukhof JR, Kardaun O, Schaafsma W, et al. Toward individual prognosis of IgA nephropathy. Kidney Int. 1986;29:549–56.

106. Alamartine E, Sabatier JC, Guerin C, et al. Prognostic factors in mesangial IgA glomerulonephritis: An extensive study with univariate and multivariate analyses. Am J Kidney Dis. 1991;18:12–9.

107. Bartosik LP, Lajoie G, Sugar L, et al. Predicting progression in IgA nephropathy. Am J Kidney Dis. 2001;38:728–35.

108. Li PK, Ho KK, Szeto CC, et al. Prognostic indicators of IgA nephropathy in the Chinese: Clinical and pathological perspectives. Nephrol Dial Transplant. 2002;17:64–9.

109. Lv J, Zhang H, Zhou Y, et al. Natural history of immunoglobulin A nephropathy and predictive factors of prognosis: A long-term follow up of 204 cases in China. Nephrology (Carlton). 2008;13:242–6.

110. Goto M, Kawamura T, Wakai K, et al. Risk stratification for progression of IgA nephropathy using a decision tree induction algorithm. Nephrol Dial Transplant. 2009;24:1242–7.

111. Mackinnon B, Fraser EP, Cattran DC, et al. Validation of the Toronto formula to predict progression in IgA nephropathy. Nephron Clin Pract. 2008;109:c148–53.

112. Berthoux F, Mohey H, Laurent B, et al. Predicting the risk for dialysis or death in IgA nephropathy. J Am Soc Nephrol. 2011;22:752–61.

113. Frimat L, Briançon S, Hestin D, et al. IgA nephropathy: Prognostic classification of end-stage renal failure. L'Association des Néphrologues de l'Est. Nephrol Dial Transplant. 1997;12:2569–75.

114. Radford MG, Donadio JV, Bergstralh EJ, et al. Predicting renal outcome in IgA nephropathy. J Am Soc Nephrol. 1997;8:199–207.

115. Manno C, Strippoli GF, D'Altri C, et al. A novel simpler histological classification for renal survival in IgA nephropathy: A retrospective study. Am J Kidney Dis. 2007;49:763–75.

116. D'Amico G, Minetti L, Ponticelli C, et al. Prognostic indicators in idiopathic IgA mesangial nephropathy. Q J Med. 1986;59:363–78.

117. Edström Halling S, Söderberg MP, Berg UB. Predictors of outcome in paediatric IgA nephropathy with regard to clinical and histopathological variables (Oxford classification). Nephrol Dial Transplant. 2012;27:715-22.

118. Shima Y, Nakanishi K, Hama T, et al. Validity of the Oxford classification of IgA nephropathy in children. Pediatr Nephrol. 2012;27:783–92.

119. Niaudet P, Murcia I, Beaufils H, Broyer M, et al. Primary IgA nephropathies in children: Prognosis and treatment. Adv Nephrol Necker Hosp. 1993;22:121–40.

120. Niaudet P, Habib R. Methylprednisolone pulse therapy in the treatment of severe forms of Schönlein-Henoch purpura nephritis. Pediatr Nephrol. 1998;12:238–43.

121. Oner A, Tinaztepe K, Erdogan O. The effect of triple therapy on rapidly progressive type of Henoch-Schönlein nephritis. Pediatr Nephrol. 1995;9:6–10.

122. Bergstein J, Leiser J, Andreoli SP. Response of crescentic Henoch-Schöenlein purpura nephritis to corticosteroid and azathioprine therapy. Clin Nephrol. 1998;49:9–14.

123. Kidney Disease IGO Clinical practice guidelines for glomerulonephritis. Immunoglobulin A nephropathy. Kidney Int Suppl. 2012;S209–17.

124. Coppo R, Peruzzi L, Amore A, et al. IgACE: A placebo-controlled, randomized trial of angiotensin-converting enzyme inhibitors in children and young people with IgA nephropathy and moderate proteinuria. J Am Soc Nephrol. 2007;18:1880–8.

125. Bhattacharjee R, Filler G. Additive antiproteinuric effect of ACE inhibitor and losartan in IgA nephropathy. Pediatr Nephrol. 2002;17:302–4.

126. Hogg RJ, Wyatt RJ, Scientific Planning Committee of the North American IgA Nephropathy Study. A randomized controlled trial of mycophenolate mofetil in patients with IgA nephropathy ISRCTN62574616. BMC Nephrol. 2004;5:3.

127. Hogg RJ, Lee J, Nardelli N, Julian BA, et al. Clinical trial to evaluate omega-3 fatty acids and alternate day prednisone in patients with IgA nephropathy: Report from the Southwest Pediatric Nephrology Study Group. Clin J Am Soc Nephrol. 2006;1:467–74.

128. Coppo R. Is a legacy effect possible in IgA nephropathy? Nephrol Dial Transplant. 2013;28:1657–62.

# REVIEW QUESTIONS

1. Which of the following histopathologic features is *not* included as a part of the Oxford classification?
   a. Mesangial hypercellularity
   b. Endocapillary hypercellularity
   c. Segmental glomerulosclerosis
   d. Tubular atrophy/interstitial fibrosis
   e. Crescent formation

2. The increased incidence of IgA nephropathy in Asian countries such as Japan may be due to all of the following, *except:*
   a. True racial or ethnic differences in incidence
   b. Increased detection through school screening programs
   c. An aggressive approach by pediatric nephrologists in these countries for performing renal biopsies in children with isolated microscopic hematuria or low levels of proteinuria
   d. Increased serum levels of immunoglobulin A in these populations

3. On renal biopsy, IgA nephropathy is characterized by which of the following:
   a. Dominant or codominant deposition of immunoglobulin A, mainly in the glomerular mesangium
   b. Subepithelial humps
   c. Patchy foot process effacement
   d. Prominent subendothelial deposits
   e. Apple-green birefringence under polarized light

4. A multi-hit hypothesis may explain the pathogenesis of IgA nephropathy. The first hit is thought to be due to:
   a. The presence in the serum of galactose-deficient (or underglycosylated) IgA1 in which in some carbohydrate side chains (*O*-glycans) of the hinge region terminate in *N*-acetylgalactosamine (GalNAc) or sialylated GalNac rather than galactose
   b. The generation of antiglycan antibodies recognizing this terminal GalNac
   c. The formation of nephritogenic circulating immune complexes containing galactose-deficient IgA1 and antiglycan antibody
   d. Secretion of extracellular matrix components, induction of nitric oxide synthase, and the release various mediators of renal injury such as angiotensin II, proinflammatory and profibrotic cytokines, and growth factors

5. Which of the following statements is *false*?
   a. Serum galactose-deficient IgA1 level is elevated in approximately 75% patients with IgA nephropathy; this is a heritable trait.
   b. The majority of first-degree relatives with elevated serum galactose-deficient IgA1 levels do not develop clinical manifestations of IgA nephropathy of HSP nephritis.
   c. A locus at 6q22-23 named IgAN1 is associated with the production of galactose-deficient immunoglobulin A.
   d. Susceptibility loci for IgA nephropathy have been found on chromosome 6p21 in the major histocompatibility complex and on chromosome 1q32 in the complement factor H (CFH) gene cluster.

6. In the United States, the percentage of children who have gross hematuria at the time of presentation with IgA nephropathy is approximately:
   a. 10%
   b. 25%
   c. 50%
   d. 75%
   e. 90%

7. The peak incidence of Henoch-Schönlein purpura is between ages:
   a. 1 to 3 years
   b. 2 to 4 years
   c. 4 to 6 years
   d. 6 to 8 years
   e. 10 to 12 years

8. The percentage of children with IgA nephropathy who present with overt nephrotic syndrome is:
   a. Less than 10%
   b. 10% to 25%
   c. 25% to 50%
   d. 50% to 75%
   e. Greater than 75%

9. The diagnosis of IgA nephropathy is dependent on:
   a. Serum galactose-deficient IgA1 and antiglycan antibody levels
   b. Serum immunoglobulin A levels
   c. Low C3 levels
   d. Genetic testing for IgAN1
   e. Examination of cortical renal tissue obtained via kidney biopsy

10. A normal urinalysis may eventually be seen in what percentage of pediatric patients diagnosed with IgA nephropathy?
    a. 10%
    b. 20%
    c. 33%
    d. 70%
    e. 90%

11. All of the following features may predict loss of renal function in children and adults with IgA nephropathy, *except:*
    a. Serial measurements of urinary protein excretion averaged over 6 month intervals after renal biopsy
    b. Severe histologic features on kidney biopsy
    c. Hypertension
    d. Renal function at time of presentation
    e. Persistent hematuria

12. The mainstay of treatment for persistent proteinuria in the setting of IgA nephropathy is:
    a. High-dose intravenous corticosteroids
    b. Low-dose oral corticosteroids
    c. Angiotensin-converting enzyme inhibitors or angiotensin receptor blockers
    d. Tonsillectomy
    e. Cyclophosphamide

## ANSWER KEY

1. e
2. d
3. a
4. a
5. c
6. d
7. b
8. a
9. e
10. c
11. e
12. c

# 24

# Thrombotic microangiopathies

JOHN D. MAHAN AND STEPHEN CHA

## INTRODUCTION

Thrombotic microangiopathies (TMAs) are diverse clinical conditions characterized by endothelial injury and microvascular thrombotic lesions that often involve the kidneys and can affect a variety of organs, such as the nervous system and the gastrointestinal (GI) tract. The most common forms of TMA encountered during childhood are the hemolytic uremic-syndrome (HUS), and to a significantly lesser extent thrombotic thrombocytopenia (TTP). All TMAs, especially HUS, are characterized by the triad of microangiopathic hemolytic anemia, thrombocytopenia, and microvascular thrombosis in the kidneys and other organs.

## HISTORICAL DEVELOPMENTS

HUS was first described by Gasser in 1955, and the systemic character of HUS was subsequently defined.[1] Kaplan and Drummond[2] identified several distinct entities that can manifest as HUS and emphasized that HUS was a syndrome with a common pathologic outcome. HUS is now considered as a part of the broader group of TMA. TTP, first described by Moschcowitz[3] in 1925, is a distinct clinicopathologic condition that can mimic the clinical characteristics of HUS. Indeed, although these criteria seem distinct, in real life the clinical forms are often incomplete or changing during the course of the disorder, complicating a precise separation of the two entities and their evaluation and treatment.

The TMAs can occur as sporadic disorders, in epidemic outbreaks, or in a genetic or familial pattern.[4–7] Although HUS and TTP are uncommon diseases, they represent common causes of acute kidney injury (AKI) in infants and children, in both the developed and undeveloped countries.[8] Although most children experience complete recovery of renal function after a single TMA disorder, chronic kidney disease (CKD) characterized by hypertension, proteinuria, renal insufficiency, or a combination of these complicates a significant minority of the survivors. Children with severe clinical disease and those with an inherited form of HUS often progress to end-stage renal disease (ESRD).

The discovery that endothelial cell injury underlies this broad spectrum of TMA disorders has come into focus during the last two decades. In the 1980s, Karmali et al.[9] defined the presence of microvascular injury in diarrhea-associated HUS and the critical role of a verotoxin produced by specific strains of Escherichia coli. This verotoxin was subsequently found to be a member of a family of toxins first identified with Shigella and known as Shiga toxin (Stx). This relationship and the eventual link of TTP to abnormally high levels of ultra-large Von Willebrand factor (vWF) multimers caused by congenital or acquired reductions in ADAMTS13 (a disintegrin and metalloproteinase with a thrombospondin type 1 motif, member 13) activity was established at approximately the same time.[10] A decade later, Warwicker et al.[7] confirmed the association of atypical HUS (aHUS) to defects in a region on chromosome 1 that contains the genes for several complement regulatory proteins. Mutations in complement factor H (CFH), complement factor I (CFI), membrane cofactor protein (MCP, CD46), factor B, C3, and thrombomodulin have now been found to cause many of the familial cases of aHUS.[4] These discoveries have allowed a more comprehensive understanding of the pathogenesis, evaluation, and treatment of the entire spectrum of TMA disorders and provide a more rational and effective approach to the care of these children with complicated disease.[4,11]

## NOMENCLATURE

TMA encompasses a number of different clinicopathologic disorders, most prominently HUS and TTP (Table 24.1). The nomenclature of TMA, and particularly of HUS, has evolved over the last decade. HUS caused by Stx-producing E. coli (STEC) and usually preceded by a diarrheal prodrome had been previously designated as D-positive HUS (diarrhea-associated. All other forms of HUS that were not associated with preceding diarrhea were classified as D-negative HUS.

With the development of a better understanding of the pathogenesis of HUS, the classification of HUS into subtypes is also undergoing a redefinition. The D-positive HUS caused by the STEC is now referred to as the STEC-HUS. Nondiarrheal, or D-negative HUS, on the other hand, comprises multiple clinical entities that have varied causes and pathogenesis. The term *atypical HUS* (aHUS) is now beginning to be used in a more restricted manner to indicate the genetic, or familial, form of TMA resulting from a dysfunctional regulation of the complement cascade. With increasing availability of genetic testing, it is likely that more patients with the familial, or genetic, form of aHUS will be detected. HUS from pneumococcal infection is a less common but a well-recognized clinical form of TMA. HIV infection–associated TMA is an important infection-triggered disorder seen in both children and adults. Drugs, malignancies, and pregnancy-associated TMA are sometimes encountered in specific clinical circumstances.

## DIAGNOSTIC CRITERIA FOR THROMBOTIC MICROANGIOPATHIES

TMA is characterized by the triad of hemolytic anemia, thrombocytopenia, and organ dysfunction, especially renal dysfunction. Hemolytic anemia in TMA is microangiopathic, with peripheral smear of blood demonstrating burr cells, helmet cells or schistocytes, and teardrop cells (Figure 24.1). Anemia is thought to be due to direct

**TAble 24.1** Etiopathologic classification of thrombotic microangiopathies

1. Diarrhea-associated HUS
   a. STEC infection
   b. Non-STEC infection
2. Atypical HUS secondary to complement dysregulation
   a. Complement factor H
   b. Complement factor I
   c. Membrane cofactor protein (MCP, CD46)
   d. Factor B
   e. C3
   f. Thrombomodulin
3. *Streptococcus* pneumonia–associated HUS
4. HUS secondary to systemic infections
   a. *Mycoplasma pneumoniae*
   b. Human immunodeficiency virus infection
   c. Cocksackie virus, influenza virus
   d. Epstein-Barr virus
   e. Rubella
   f. Histoplasmosis
5. Thrombotic thrombocytopenia
   a. Congenital (Upshaw-Schulman syndrome)
   b. ADAMTS13 deficiency or antibody related
6. Drug-associated thrombotic microangiopathies
   a. Cyclosporine, tacrolimus
   b. Mithramycin
   c. Ticlodipine, clopidogrel
   d. Bevacizumab
7. Stem cell and bone marrow transplantation related
8. Malignant hypertension
9. Collagen vascular diseases and vasculitides (systemic lupus erythromatosus, Kawasaki disease)
10. Cancers
11. Pregnancy (HELLP syndrome: hemolytic anemia, elevated liver enzymes, low platelets)
12. Ionizing radiation

*Source:* HUS, hemolytic-uremic syndrome; *STEC*, Shiga toxin-producing *Escherichia coli.*

mechanical injury of the red blood cells (RBCs) caused by thrombosis in the microvascular circulation. Because anemia is nonimmune in nature, the direct Coombs test is negative in all cases, except *Streptococcus pneumoniae*-associated HUS (explained later). Hemolysis is further confirmed by an elevated serum lactic dehydrogenase (LDH) level and elevated reticulocyte count. Thrombocytopenia is modest in most at onset, but can rapidly reach below $50,000/mm^3$. Blood urea nitrogen (BUN) and serum creatinine may be elevated at presentation, and BUN may be elevated out of proportion to rise in creatinine (Cr) (BUN/Cr ratio greater than 20) in some patients because of the presence of dehydration caused by the diarrheal disease.

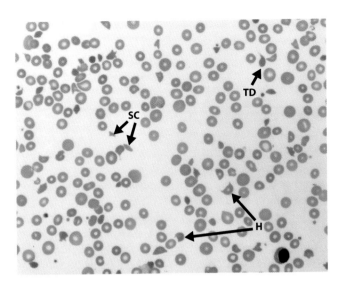

Figure 24.1 Peripheral smear from a child with HUS demonstrating fragmented RBCs and schistocytes.

## SHIGA TOXIN–PRODUCING *ESCHERICHIA COLI*–ASSOCIATED HEMOLYTIC-UREMIC SYNDROME

## EPIDEMIOLOGY

STEC-HUS is the most common form of HUS noted during childhood. Since 2001, *E. coli* O157 and non-O157 STEC infections resulting in human illness have been designated as notifiable illness in the Nationally Notifiable Diseases Surveillance System in the United States, resulting in more complete data acquisition on the disease. Annually, 110,000 cases of diarrhea caused by *E. coli* are identified in the United States. Of this, approximately 3200 (3%) require hospitalization.[12] HUS develops in 5% to 8% of patients affected by STEC in the United States. A meta-analysis of the published reports observed that of the patients with *E. coli* O157:H7 diarrheal disease, 17.2% patients in small studies (fewer than 50 cases) and 4.2% in large studies (more than 1000 cases) developed HUS.[13] Children below 5 years of age infected by STEC are disproportionately susceptible to development of HUS and may have an infection rate of up to 15%.[14,15]

STEC-HUS accounts for 90% of all cases of HUS in childhood.[16] The overall incidence of STEC-HUS in the United States, including in adults, is 1.5 per 100,000 population.[14] However, STEC-HUS is more common in children younger than 5 years of age, wherein its incidence has been reported to be as high as 6.5 cases per 100,000 population.[14]

Median age of STEC-HUS in one study from the United States was 4 years (range, 3 months to 64 years). The disease was dominant in the age group younger than 18 years, and only 12% of total patients in this study were over 18 years of age.[16] A similarly high incidence of STEC-HUS in children younger than 5 years of age also has been reported from other geographic regions.[6,15,17] A recent epidemic of

STEC-HUS in Germany caused by *E. coli* O104:H4, however, was, characterized by an exceptionally high incidence in adults (median age, 42 years) and older children and may reflect a changing epidemiologic trend.[18] In part, this demographic shift has been attributed to the type of vector (salad) involved in the transmission of *E. coli* in this epidemic.

---

### KEY POINTS

- HUS secondary to *E. coli* infection is the most common form of HUS in children (90%).
- STEC-HUS occurs in 1.5 to 2 patients per 100,000 population.
- STEC-HUS is more common in children younger than 5 years of age (6.5 per 100,000 population.)

---

Peak incidence of STEC-HUS occurs in the summer months of May through September, but sporadic cases occur throughout the year.[16] Equal sex distribution of the STEC-HUS has been recognized in most studies.[16] One study reported a significantly low incidence of STEC-HUS in African-Americans.[19] A decreasing trend in STEC-HUS was reported in the United States by the Centers for Disease Control and Prevention (CDC) in 2011, compared to the 2006 to 2008 era, but the trend appears to have halted in 2013.[20]

## MICROBIOLOGY OF *ESCHERICHIA COLI* INFECTION

The most common *E. coli* serotype identified in patients with hemorrhagic colitis and HUS in the United States is O157:H7.[13,16,17,21] *E. coli* serotypes are diverse, and by now over 200 different types of STEC have been characterized.[21] Non-O157:H7 *E. coli*, such as O111 and O104:H4 and even nonserotypable *E. coli*, are an emerging subgroup of *E. coli* that can cause outbreaks of enterocolitis and HUS.[22–24] The important characteristic of *E. coli* that results in HUS is the ability to produce the Shiga toxin. Because Stx-producing *E. coli* frequently causes symptoms of hemorrhagic diarrhea, the term *enterohemorrhagic E. coli* is sometimes used to identify it. Studies have shown that 0.3% to 0.9% of stool samples submitted for routine culture are STEC positive, and approximately 50% of these are the *E. coli* O157:H7 strain.[25] In patients with diarrhea due to *E. coli* O157:H7, it can be recovered in 100% of stool samples if the culture is obtained in the first 2 days and the yield declines to 33% after 7 days.[3,26]

Cattle are the largest reservoir for STEC, in which it may cause bloody diarrhea but usually by a commensal organism.[27] Undercooked hamburgers have been the vector of several epidemics of HUS in the United States and Canada. Other potential vectors of STEC include domestic animals (sheep), wild animals (deer, seagulls), humans, water, other beverages, and other food sources. Transmission of STEC commonly occurs through ingestion of contaminated food products (beef, fruit, and produce washed in contaminated water), visits to dairy farms and petting zoos, and exposure to airborne organisms.[28, 29] Contact with contaminated dirt also has been implicated in the transmission of these bacteria.[29] Person-to-person spread of *E. coli* O157:H7, especially in day care and family groups, is well known.[30]

---

### KEY POINTS

- *E. coli* serotype O157:H7 is the most common pathogen associated with STEC-HUS.
- Other serotypes may be involved in STEC-HUS.

---

## SHIGA TOXIN

STEC was first linked to acute colitis in humans by Riley et al.[31] in 1983 and to epidemic HUS in children by Karmali et al.[9] in 1985. The Stx family of toxins elaborated by *E. coli* are also referred to as *verotoxins* because of their observed toxicity in monkey kidney vero cells.

The Stx produced by STEC is composed of a biologically active subunit A and a receptor unit B. The B subunit is composed of five subunits, through which the toxin binds to specific glycoprotein receptors on susceptible cells.[33] STEC produce two types of Stx, known as Stx1 and Stx2, and each have their subvariants, Stx1c, Stx2c, Stx2d, Stx2e, Stx2f, and Stx2g.[3,32] STEC toxins are structurally similar to the toxins produced by *Shigella dysenteriae* type 1, and are thus named Shiga toxins (or Shiga-like toxins). Some strains of STEC can produce both types of Stx1 and Stx2 toxins. Stx2 has been shown to be a more toxic and virulent form of Shiga toxin in mice. The STEC toxins are potent inhibitors of protein synthesis in endothelial cells.[32]

## PATHOGENESIS OF SHIGA TOXIN–PRODUCING *ESCHERICHIA COLI* HEMOLYTIC-UREMIC SYNDROME

In humans, STEC infection causes both bloody and nonbloody diarrhea. Only approximately 5% to 8% of children with STEC-associated hemorrhagic colitis develop HUS.[14,15,26] Virulence factors such as enterocyte attachment factors affect the ability of these organisms to produce human disease.[32–34] The severity of the colitis usually correlates with the clinical severity of the HUS.[35]

After a person ingests contaminated or poorly cooked food, STEC results in colitis that can be associated with bloody diarrhea. Stx and lipopolysaccharides produced by these organisms are then absorbed from the colonic mucosa into the systemic circulation

(Figure 24.2).[36] In the past, endotoxemia caused by Stx was difficult to demonstrate.[37] Recent findings of circulating Stx in some patients with HUS by Brigotti et al.[38] support the hypothesis of endotoxemia-induced pathogenesis of HUS. The role of leukocytes and RBCs in the carriage of Stx from the gut to kidney and other organs also has been in demonstrated in STEC-HUS.[38,39]

Through its subunit B, Stx binds to the glycoprotein galabiosyl ceramide and globotriosyl ceramide (Gb3) receptors on the surface of GI epithelial and endothelial cells (Figure 24.3). The active fragment of Stx (subunit A) is internalized into the cells and interferes with ribosomal protein synthesis through depurination. This leads to apoptosis of the affected cells and eventual cell death.[9,40–42] Apart from glomerular endothelial cells, Gb3 receptors for Stx are also present on podocytes and mesangial cells.[39] Stx binding to glomerular and renal tubular cells can be quite unpredictable because of variable cellular Gb3 expression on these cells. Stx binding or Gb3 expression has not been shown to be greater in the glomeruli or renal tissue of younger subjects compared to older subjects.[43]

---

### KEY POINTS

- Stx subunit B attaches to GB3 receptor on the GI epithelial cells and other host cells.
- Subunit A is internalized and interferes with cellular protein synthesis.
- Stx endotoxemia has been difficult to demonstrate but may be present.

---

The receptor-mediated internalization of the Stx is essential in cellular injury and inducing a prothrombotic state.[39] Endothelial cells, in response to subunit A demonstrate altered gene expressions, increased prothrombotic protein production, and release of von Willebrand (vW) multimers into the circulation that cause platelets to adhere to these multimers and form microvascular clots.[44] Other cells, such as monocytes and neutrophils, are induced by Stx to release proinflammatory mediators such as interleukin-1 and tumor necrosis factor (TNF) and upregulate adhesion molecules that can augment adherence to endothelial cells, further enhancing the vascular and cellular injury in HUS.[43–46] As endothelial surfaces are injured, platelet and coagulation factor deposition results in microvascular thrombi formation and, ultimately, the TMA that characterizes HUS.[47] Documentation of hypocomplementemia, with low C3 complement, along with increased levels of activated factor B and soluble membrane attack complex (MAC) detected during active HUS in some patients suggest a possible role for alternative complement activation in the pathogenesis of STEC-HUS.[48–50]

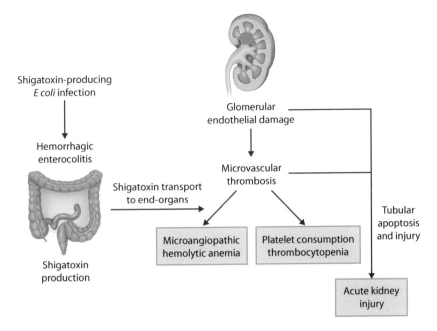

Figure 24.2 Pathogenesis of Shiga toxin–producing *Escherichia coli* hemolytic-uremic syndrome–related acute kidney injury.

Most studies suggest that antibiotic treatment of STEC-mediated gastroenteritis is associated with a higher incidence of HUS, presumably as a result of release of Stx into the circulation.[51,52] Based on in vitro experiments in mice, induction of bacteriophages in *E. coli* by antibiotics (quinolones) has been proposed as a mechanism for this enhanced Stx production.[53] However, in a meta-analysis of clinical reports and studies, treatment with antibiotics failed to demonstrate an increased likelihood of HUS with antibiotic use in STEC diarrhea.[54]

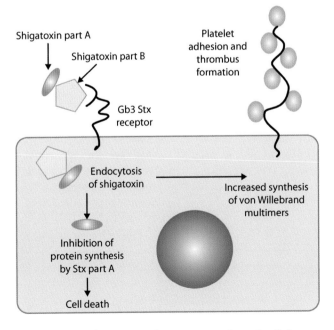

Figure 24.3 A diagrammatic representation of cellular events leading to microvascular thrombosis and organ injury in Shiga toxin (Stx)–producing *Escherichia coli* hemolytic-uremic syndrome.

## CLINICAL MANIFESTATIONS

STEC-HUS primarily affects young children, in whom the disease is also more severe. STEC-HUS is more common in the summer and autumn months and may occur both sporadically and in localized epidemics. Some studies have reported a higher incidence of HUS among rural than urban populations in the United States and in other countries.[3,5,17] Siegler et al.,[55] on the other hand, did not see a significant difference in the incidence of STEC-HUS in urban and rural settings.

Three clinically indistinct phases, diarrheal prodrome, onset of HUS, and recovery phase or progression to ESRD, are noted in the course of STEC- HUS in children.

### Diarrheal prodrome

Signs of GI illness, characterized by abdominal pain, vomiting, and diarrhea, precede the onset of STEC-HUS. A diarrheal prodrome is noted in 85% to 95% of patients with STEC-induced HUS, and usually lasts 3 to 4 days.[6,16,17,55] Although stools are usually bloody, some may have only streaks of blood visible in the diarrheal stool.[55] Severe cases may be associated with intussusception or intestinal perforation.[56,57] GI manifestations may be minimal or transient.

### Acute disease phase

HUS evolves in 5 to 7 days after onset of diarrheal prodrome.[6,16,17,55] Anorexia, weakness, pallor, and jaundice are the presenting manifestations in many children with HUS. These findings represent development of profound anemia as a result of microangiopathic hemolysis. Platelet count of approximately 75,000/mm$^3$ is common at presentation. Normal platelet count has been reported in 13% patients with HUS.[58] As thrombocytopenia becomes more significant, purpura or petechiae may develop

---

### KEY POINTS

- Onset of STEC-HUS can be sudden, 4 to 6 days after diarrhea.
- Oliguria, paleness, and puffiness are early manifestations.
- Neurologic manifestations can occur in 30% patients with STEC-HUS.

---

Oliguria or hematuria may be the initial recognition of HUS by many parents of the affected children. These manifestations may evolve over a few hours to a few days, depending on the severity of the disease. Progressive and severe renal injury is usually associated with anuria. Oligoanuria, as a manifestation of AKI in HUS, has been reported in 50% to 60% patients and eventual need for dialysis arises in 40% to 50% of patients with STEC-HUS.[56,59] Duration of necessary dialysis varies from 1 to 2 weeks in most patients. Hyponatremia secondary to fluid overload (dilutional hyponatremia), high anion gap metabolic acidosis, and hyperkalemia may be seen at presentation.

Central nervous system symptoms, such as lethargy, irritability, seizures, cortical blindness, paresis, and coma, have been reported in 25% to 30% of affected children.[16,60,61] Complications of renal insufficiency, such as hypertension, electrolyte disturbances, and uremia, may contribute to the CNS symptoms, as well. Evidence of other significant organ system damage in HUS may become apparent as the condition progresses. Pancreatic injury in some patients with HUS can lead to hyperglycemia and diabetes mellitus.[62]

## Recovery phase

Once oliguria and AKI set in, dialysis support for treatment of hypervolemia, electrolyte disturbances, and hypertension may be necessary for 1 to 2 weeks. It is uncommon for dialysis to be required beyond 4 weeks in most patients, unless associated complications occur or progression to ESRD is impending. Recovery of platelet count often precedes renal recovery by 3 to 5 days. Urine output can increase rapidly in patients headed toward recovery of renal function. Sometimes a phase of polyuria can be seen while recovering from oligoanuric HUS. Mild proteinuria can be seen in the recovery phase and may persist for several months, but nephrotic-range proteinuria is unusual. Prolonged anuria indicates severe renal disease that may lead to nonrecovery of renal function and development of ESRD. Sequential renal ultrasound evaluations may demonstrate declining renal size in these patients over 6 to 8 weeks of the disease.

## ATYPICAL HEMOLYTIC-UREMIC SYNDROME

HUS without any accompanying diarrheal illness has, in past, been classified as D-negative HUS. One subcategory of D-negative HUS, characterized by severe clinical disease, frequent progression to ESRD, recurrent disease episodes, and sometimes familial occurrence, is now recognized as a separate clinical disorder and is designated the atypical hemolytic uremic syndrome (aHUS). Complement dysfunction resulting from mutations in one or multiple complement regulatory proteins is recognized as the underlying mechanism in these patients.

## INCIDENCE AND DEMOGRAPHICS

The incidence of aHUS is not known precisely. It is estimated that aHUS comprises 5% to 10% of all cases of childhood HUS, and more than 1000 cases have been reported worldwide.[63] The incidence of aHUS in the United States, derived indirectly from the Synsorb Study, has been estimated to be 2 in 1,000,000 population, representing 11% of all cases of HUS in the study.[64] These data may, indeed, be an under-representation of true incidence in the general population.

The initial presentation of aHUS may occur as early as the first day of life to as late as adulthood. In the International Registry of Recurrent and Familial HUS/TTP data, 60% of the reported cases were younger than 18 years of age, whereas in the French national study, 42% patients were younger than 18 years of age.[65,66] The mean age of presentation in the French series was 1.5 years.[66] Early presentation of the disease has been reported to be especially common in patients with the CFH gene mutations.

The male-to-female sex ratio was nearly equal in the International Registry patients (M/F, 125:131).[65] The French series also showed an equal male-to-female ratio (M/F, 47:42) in children younger than 18 years of age, but there was a preponderance of females among the adult patients with aHUS (M/F, 32:93).[66]

---

### KEY POINTS

- aHUS is a rare disorder (1 to 2 per 1,000,000 population) and accounts for fewer than 10% of all cases of HUS in childhood.
- Family history of aHUS may be present in 30% cases.
- Genetic mutations in complement-regulating proteins or complement cause this disorder.

A family history of aHUS may be present in approximately 30% of patients.[65–67] A recognized trigger of an episode of aHUS is recorded in 30% to 50% patients and varies from a trivial viral respiratory infection, otitis media, or sinusitis in the majority of patients to severe systemic infectious diseases in the minority. Precipitation of an episode of aHUS also has been noted after exposure to certain drugs, hypertension, or pregnancy. Diarrheal illnesses can occasionally trigger aHUS, making it difficult at presentation to distinguish aHUS from STEC-induced HUS in such cases.

## ATYPICAL HEMOLYTIC-UREMIC SYNDROME AS A COMPLEMENT DYSFUNCTION DISORDER

Many, but not all, patients presenting with the clinical features of aHUS demonstrate mutations of the alternative complement pathway. Inherited deficiency or dysfunction of factor H or factor I, factors that exert inhibitory control over the alternative complement pathway, are the most commonly described genetic defects of complement regulation associated with aHUS.[65–69] Other less frequent genetic defects in complement regulation associated with an aHUS include factor B and reduced expression of membrane cofactor protein (MCP, CD46).[70–73] Recently, mutations affecting diacylglycerol transferase an enzyme present in endothelial cells, also has been described as a cause of aHUS.[74] Some of these patients do not manifest clinical disease until adulthood, even though the genetic predisposition is present, when a triggering event occurs.

## COMPLEMENT CASCADE AND ITS REGULATION

Complement serves as an important mediator of immune responses. The entire complement pathway is composed of over 30 protein molecules that are synthesized in the liver. The complement pathway participates in tissue inflammation by generation of chemoattractants in areas of inflammation, opsonization of bacteria, and bacterial cell lysis. Three separate mechanisms can initiate the complement cascade: (1) classical pathway, (2) lectin pathway, and (3) alternative pathway. Although all three pathways are initiated by different triggers, they all result in generation of a common effector molecule called C3 convertase (Figure 24.4). C3 convertase is responsible for enzymatic degradation of complement C3. This part of the complement cascade is known as the early complement pathway. After C3 convertase is generated, complements C5 through C9 are activated, leading to the formation of MAC, and C5a. MAC is involved in cell lysis and activation of platelets and is prothrombotic

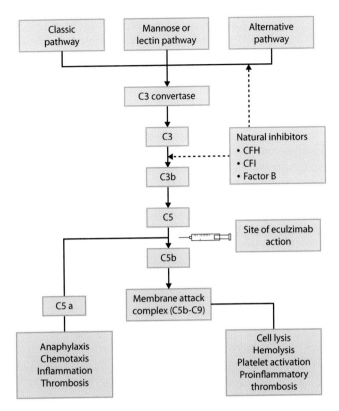

Figure 24.4 Diagrammatic representation of complement pathways showing the inhibitory control sites by complement factor H (CFH) and complement factor I (CFI). Site of action of eculizumab is also shown.

and proinflammatory. C5a, on the other hand, promotes anaphylaxis, chemotaxis, inflammation, and thrombosis. This segment of complement pathway beyond the formation of C3 convertase is also known as the terminal complement pathway.[75]

If not regulated, the complement cascade can result in unregulated generation of proinflammatory molecules detrimental to the host. Several circulating and tissue-bound proteins provide an inhibitory control mechanism on the complement pathway and prevent unwarranted complement activation that can be harmful to the host.

## GENETICS OF ATYPICAL HEMOLYTIC-UREMIC SYNDROME

Genetic mutations in one or more of the complement regulatory proteins have been documented in 40% to 60% of individuals with aHUS.[65–73] These disorders represent an incomplete gene penetrance, and additional triggers, such as an infection, drugs, or bone marrow transplant, are often necessary to precipitate an episode of aHUS in susceptible individuals. Concurrent multiple complement-regulating gene defects also have been described in some individuals with aHUS, and such patients appear to have the greatest risk for progression to ESRD, as well as recurrence after renal transplant.[72]

# COMPLEMENT REGULATION PROTEINS AND ATYPICAL HEMOLYTIC-UREMIC SYNDROME

Without the appropriate inhibitory control in the complement activation process, excessive C3 convertase and eventually C5a and C5b can occur. C5a induces significant changes in endothelial cells to a prothrombotic, inflammatory phenotype capable of chemotactic effects on circulating leukocytes. The C5b fraction leads to generation of the MAC, a molecular assembly that leads to lysis of endothelial and other cells. The end-result of complement activation is vascular injury and development of a prothrombotic state, leading to TMA.[65,72]

Although a number of complement regulatory protein defects have been characterized and the phenotype-genotype correlation well established, understanding of the broad range of mutations and their phenotypic outcome is still evolving. Some of the defined complement regulatory protein defects leading to aHUS include the following:

1. **Complement factor H:** CFH is one of the proteins that bind to C3b and the C3 convertase formed in the alternative pathway at the cell surface and degrades both of them.[76] Diminished CFH allows unchecked C3 convertase formation on endothelial cells. Mutations in CFH are the most common genetic defect noted in aHUS, accounting for 20% to 30% of all cases (Table 24.2).[65-68]
2. **Antibodies to complement factor H:** Autoantibodies to CFH can result in a nonfunctional or poorly functional CFH and lead to aHUS. In large studies, these antibodies have been identified in 3% to 7% of patients with aHUS.[65,66,76]

3. **Complement factor I:** CFI is a serene protease that cleaves C3b and C4b. In its absence there is increased C3 convertase formation and initiation of the both the proximal and terminal parts of the complement cascade. Mutations that result in decreased CFI activity have been reported in 4% to 9% of patients with aHUS.[65,66,76]
4. **Membrane cofactor protein:** Membrane cofactor protein (MCP, also known as CD46) is an important cofactor for CFI in degrading C3b and C4b.[71,75,76] Mutations in MCP have been documented in 7% to 19% of patients with aHUS.[65-68,76]
5. **Complement C3:** Complement C3 plays a central role in the complement cascade as the precursor protein for C3 convertase. A gain in function mutation affecting complement C3 can result in the enhanced formation of C3 convertase and activation of complement cascade.[76] C3 mutations have been reported in 4% to 9% of patients with aHUS.[65-68,76]
6. **Thrombomodulin:** Thrombomodulin (TM), encoded by the *THBD* gene, is involved in the inactivation of C3b by CFI.[75,76] THBD gene mutation is involved in fewer than 5% of patients with aHUS.[65-68]
7. **Factor B:** Factor B is involved in the alternative complement pathway, where it is cleaved by factor D into Ba and Bb. The subfraction Bb results in the formation of C3 convertase of the alternative pathway. This is an uncommon complement dysfunction caused by gain in function mutation of the gene regulating factor B. Factor B mutations account for 0% to 3% of aHUS.[76]
8. **Undefined genetic mutations:** In each of the three large genetic studies, reported so far, 30% to 60% of patients with aHUS did not have any known genetic mutation.[65-68]

Table 24.2 Summary of the frequency distribution, risk for end-stage renal disease death and transplant recurrence in various genetic mutations associated with atypical hemolytic-uremic syndrome

| | Noris et al.[66] (N = 273) (%) | Frémeaux-Bacchi V[67] (N = 214) (%) | Maga TK et al.[68] (N = 144) (%) | Risk for ESRD or death in 3 years[66] (%) | Recurrence risk in kidney transplant[66] (%) |
|---|---|---|---|---|---|
| Participating population | International | France | United States | | |
| Family history of HUS | 29.6 | 19.6 | – | – | – |
| No mutations detected | 53 | 33.6 | 54 | 50–60 | 50–60 |
| CHF | 24 | 27.5 | 27 | 70–90 | 50–60 |
| CHF antibody | 3 | 6.5 | 0 | 60–70 | 35–40 |
| MCP | 7 | 9.3 | 5 | 6–10 | 15–20 |
| CFI | 4 | 8.4 | 8 | 60–70 | 10–15 |
| C3 | 4 | 8.4 | 2 | 60–75 | 10–15 |
| *THBD* | 5 | 0 | 3 | 50–70 | 10–15 |
| CHFB | 1 | 0 | 4 | – | – |
| CHF R5 | 0 | 0 | 5 | – | – |
| Combined | 0 | 4.3 | 0 | – | – |

*Abbreviation:* HUS, hemolytic-uremic syndrome.

## CLINICAL MANIFESTATIONS

Most children have their first episode of aHUS before 2 years of age. Mean age of presentation of children with aHUS in the French series was 1.5 years. Family history of the aHUS may be present in 30% of patients.[65,66]

The episode of aHUS is often preceded by an infective event or exposure to specific drugs or occurs during pregnancy in adult women. Occasionally, viral and other diarrheal illness may trigger aHUS, making the differentiation from STEC-induced HUS difficult at presentation.

Onset of clinical symptoms, such as pallor and decreased urine output, indicative of hemolytic anemia and renal dysfunction, can occur insidiously but may also appear abruptly following an illness. The classic diagnostic triad of hemolytic anemia, thrombocytopenia, and renal failure, evolves in most patients (70% to 80%).[63,65,66] Extrarenal manifestations, particularly neurologic and cardiovascular involvement, are common, especially in aHUS patients with CFH mutations.[65,66] Reduced complement C3 level is present in approximately 30% to 50% of patients, most notably in aHUS secondary to complement C3 mutations and CFH mutations.[65,66]

## CLINICAL OUTCOME OF ATYPICAL HEMOLYTIC-UREMIC SYNDROME

The clinical course of aHUS can be characterized by recurrent episodes of hemolysis and renal dysfunction. A relapsing pattern has been reported in 10% to 60% of cases, depending on the type of genetic mutation.[65,66] Most relapses (80%) occur within the first year of onset of aHUS.[66] Recurrences of aHUS are most commonly observed in patients with CFH gene mutations.[65] The International Registry of Recurrent and Familial HUS/TTP reported that ESRD or death occurred within the first 3 years of the onset of aHUS in 70% of patients.[65] Of all the genetic mutations in complement regulation, aHUS associated with MCP mutations has the most favorable outcome, with ESRD or death reported in fewer than 10% patients.[65,76] Interestingly, the prognosis of aHUS in patients without any identifiable mutation does not appear to be better than that seen in those with well-documented gene mutations.[65,66,77]

Table 24.3 Acute complications of hemolytic-uremic syndrome

| Organ system | Complication |
|---|---|
| • Neurologic | • Irritability |
|  | • Seizures |
|  | • Coma |
|  | • Cerebral infarction |
|  | • Cortical blindness |
|  | • Paresis |
| • Cardiac | • Coronary artery occlusion |
|  | • Cardiomyopathy |
|  | • Myocardial infarction |
| • Gastrointestinal tract | • Ileus |
|  | • Intussusception |
|  | • Infarction |
|  | • Perforation |
|  | • Stricture |
| • Pancreas | • Pancreatitis |
|  | • Pancreatic failure (diabetes mellitus) |
| • Liver | • Hepatocellular injury |
| • Testes | • Infarction |
| • Skeletal muscles | • Myopathy |

## HEMOLYTIC-UREMIC SYNDROME IN PNEUMOCOCCAL DISEASE

An atypical form of HUS (D-HUS) caused by invasive *S. pneumoniae* infection termed SpHUS is an uncommon but well-described clinical disorder. Because many of these patients also suffer from significant *S. pneumoniae* systemic disease and may even have concurrent disseminated intravascular coagulopathy (DIC), recognition of aHUS in these patients may be difficult. A high index of suspicion is an important key to the diagnosis of SpHUS in such sick patients.

## INCIDENCE AND DEMOGRAPHICS

SpHUS is a rare form of HUS. Over a 21-year period, only 14 patients with SpHUS were reported from the Children's Hospital of Philadelphia, suggesting occurrence of 0.63 cases per year.[78] In another study from the United Kingdom, a total of 45 patients were reported nation-wide over a 7-year period.[79] This suggests a yearly incidence of 6.4 new cases of SpHUS per year in the entire United Kingdom. Based on hospital discharge data over a 5-year period, SpHUS comprised 4.6% of all HUS cases admitted to hospitals in the United States.[80]

SpHUS generally occurs in young children. Median age of presentation in the United Kingdom was 13 months (range, 5 to 39 months).[79] In two studies reported from the United States, the mean age of presentation was 22 months (range, 4 to 62 months) and 27 months (range, 4 to 56 months).[78,81] In an analysis of 58 other reported cases, Brandt et al.[82] found the mean age of presentation to be 16.2 months. A slight female dominance has been reported by some.[70,80] Seasonal distribution in cases from the United Kingdom suggests that majority (74%) of cases occurred between October and March.[79]

## SITE OF INFECTION AND BACTERIOLOGY

In more than 75% of patients with SpHUS, the primary source of infection is in the lungs, usually pneumonia. The second most common source of infection is meningitis. Empyema, as a complication of pneumonia, has been noted commonly in these patients and may represent the invasive nature of this organism.[78-83] Specific serotypes of *S. pneumoniae* may be relevant in the etiopathogenesis of SpHUS. Two separate studies of SpHUS have noted a high prevalence of infection by *S. pneumoniae* serotype A19.[78,81]

## PATHOGENESIS

Klein et al.,[84] in 1977, proposed that the neuraminidase produced by *S. pneumoniae* exposes the hidden or cryptic Thomsen-Friedenreich antigen (T-antigen) present normally on RBCs, platelets, endothelial cells, glomeruli, and hepatocytes. This observation was based on the finding that the T-antigen was found exposed on the RBCs and the glomeruli in two children who died of pneumococcal sepsis and pneumonia. Klein et al. proposed that once neuraminidase exposes the T-antigen on the RBCs, platelets, and endothelial cells, these sites react with the naturally occurring circulating serum immunoglobulin M (IgM) antibodies to the T-antigen. This may lead to complement activation, vascular injury, and development of TMA, although there is now evidence that the pathogenesis is more complex than this straight forward explanation.[85,86]

A role for CFH, a potent inhibitor of alternative complement pathway activation, in the pathogenesis of SpHUS has been speculated by some.[87,88] These investigators suggest that desialylation of RBCs and endothelial cells by pneumococcal neuraminidase also may destroy binding sites for CFH on these host cells that could promote complement activation.

---

**KEY POINTS**

- Neuraminidase in *S. pneumonia* exposes the T-antigens on RBCs and other cells.
- Naturally occurring IgM antibodies against T-antigen react with the exposed T-antigen to initiate cellular damage and hemolysis.

---

## CLINICAL FEATURES

In contrast to classic *E. coli*-induced HUS, patients with SpHUS are younger and usually sicker. Acute renal injury, evidenced by oliguria and rise of serum creatinine may lead to the incidental discovery of TMA in some of these patients. A higher proportion of patients with SpHUS (up to 80%) require supportive dialysis, and there is a higher frequency of serious extrarenal complications.[78,79,81,82]

One of the distinguishing features of SpHUS is that these patients have a positive direct Coombs test. This distinguishes SpHUS patients from those with other forms of TMA and can be used as a screening test in suspected cases with *S. pneumoniae*-induced HUS.

---

**KEY POINT**

Renal failure needing dialysis or continuous renal replacement therapy is very frequent (80%) in SpHUS.

---

**THROMBOTIC MICROANGIOPATHIES IN OTHER INFECTIONS**

HUS has been reported in a variety of infectious diseases that may be associated with diarrhea, such as *Salmonella, Shigella, Yersinia,* and *Campylobacter* infections.[89,90] Some viral infections, such as the human immunodeficiency virus (HIV), Coxsackie virus, influenza virus, Epstein-Barr virus, and rubella virus, have been associated with HUS.[91-94]

HIV-associated TMA may manifest abruptly and at any stage of HIV infection. The pathogenesis of TMA in HIV infection remains unclear. Some patients have been reported to have deficiency of ADAMTS13, whereas others have normal plasma levels.[94] Endothelial injury by the virus or antiretroviral drugs remains a possibility. Oliguric renal failure and ESRD can result after a relatively short clinical course.[90,94,95]

## DRUG-INDUCED THROMBOTIC MICROANGIOPATHIES

TMA, in particular the classic HUS phenotype, has been reported in association with some drugs and malignancies. Clinically, these cases mimic patients with aHUS. Calcineurin inhibitors (cyclosporine and tacrolimus), commonly used in renal and other transplants, are well known causes of TMA.[96] Chemotherapeutic agents, such as mitomycin C, cytosine arabinoside, cisplatinum, and gemcitabine, have been associated with drug-induced HUS.[97] Antiplatelet drugs, such as ticlopidine and clopidogrel, can cause HUS.[98] Antiangiogenesis treatment of malignancies also has been associated with a TMA disorder. TMA has been reported after treatment with biologic agents that block the activity of vascular endothelial growth factor (VEGF).[99]

## THROMBOTIC THROMBOCYTOPENIA

TTP is an uncommon but life-threatening form of TMA that rarely occurs in children. The clinical manifestations and some of the laboratory features of TTP can, at times, be indistinguishable from those of HUS. The differentiation may be complicated further by the fact that neurologic and other organ dysfunction also can be encountered in children with HUS.

## KEY POINTS

- SpHUS is an uncommon form of HUS and may be under-recognized.
- The highest incidence is in children younger than 3 years of age.
- Complicated pneumonia is a common association.
- Presence of a positive direct Coombs test, in addition to other features of HUS, is diagnostic for spHUS.

## INCIDENCE AND DEMOGRAPHICS

The true incidence of TTP in childhood remains uncertain. The Oklahoma TTP-HUS Registry recently analyzed their experience over the 17 years (1996 to 2013) during which 79 patients were diagnosed to have TTP.[100] The incidence of TTP in children (younger than 18 years) in this group was 0.09 in 1,000,000 children per year. This compared to the incidence of 2.88 in 1,000,000 per year in adults. These observations suggest that that only 3% of patients with TTP are younger than 18 years of age. Most of the children affected by TTP are older, in contrast with STEC-HUS, in which most patients are younger than 5 years of age.[100,101] The sex distribution of TTP in children is reported to be similar to that seen in adults, with TTP more common in females.

## KEY POINTS

- TTP is mostly a disease of the adult population.
- In TTP, females are affected more than males.

## PATHOGENESIS

The role of von Willibrand factor (vWF) in the pathogenesis of TTP has been well characterized in the last decade. vWF is synthesized by endothelial cells and megakaryocytes and stored as ultra-large vWF multimers in Weibel-Palade bodies in the endothelium and as a granules in platelets. vWF is secreted as multimers into the plasma compartment but remains associated with the endothelial cell surface, providing binding sites for platelets and promoting platelet aggregation. Stress or injury to endothelial cells, and vasopressin, lead to increased vWF release.

The vWF cleaving protease known as ADAMTS13 (a dysintegrin and metalloprotease with thrombospondin-like motifs type 13) is now recognized to be critical in maintaining intravascular clotting homeostasis.[11,102] ADAMTS13 cleaves the vWF multimers by proteolytic degradation.[102] Lacking adequate concentration of ADAMTS13 enzyme in plasma, the plasma multimers of vWF accumulate and promote platelet aggregation and formation of thrombi within the vascular tree (Figure 24.5). These thrombi usually lack fibrin and are composed mostly of platelet aggregates.[102] The platelet-rich microvascular thrombi of TTP are typically found at the arteriolar-capillary junction, a site characterized by high sheer stress. The vascular beds usually affected by microvascular thrombosis in TTP are in the brain, heart, spleen, kidneys, pancreas, adrenals, lungs, and eyes.

Inherited deficiency of ADAMTS13 is now well established as a cause of TTP in children. Several mutations in the gene encoding ADAMTS13 have been described and are associated with development of the inherited variant of TTP.[102-105] The inherited form of TTP seen during childhood is also known as Upshaw-Schulman syndrome, named after the initial discoverers of the defect.[105,106]

TTP in adults usually results from acquired IgG antibodies directed against ADAMTS13.[107,108] Circulating immune complexes containing ADAMTS13 have been documented in about a third of these patients.[109] TTP is considered by some to be an autoimmune disorder.

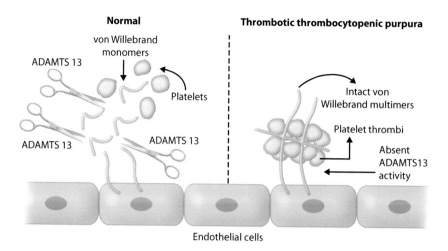

**Normal**

**Thrombotic thrombocytopenic purpura**

von Willebrand monomers

ADAMTS 13

Platelets

ADAMTS 13

ADAMTS 13

Intact von Willebrand multimers

Platelet thrombi

Absent ADAMTS13 activity

Endothelial cells

Figure 24.5 Pathogenesis of thrombotic thrombocytopenia. Left side of the cartoon demonstrates the role of ADAMTS13 in breaking down vWF in normal individuals. Right side of the cartoon shows the generation of platelet thrombi in TTP. Absence or inactivation of ADAMTS 13 leads to accumulation of von Willibrand factor multimers in plasma, promotes adherence of platelets to vWF multimers, and develops microvascular thrombosis.

---

> ## KEY POINTS
>
> - TP is caused by deficiency or absence of vWF factor–cleaving protease known as ADAMTS13.
> - Mutations in *ADAMTS13* gene can result in the congenital form of TTP in children and adults known as Upshaw-Schulman syndrome.

## CLINICAL FEATURES

### Upshaw-Schulman syndrome

Inherited TTP resulting from genetic mutation and absence of ADAMTS13 (Upshaw-Schulman syndrome) often manifests with neonatal hyperbilirubinemia secondary to microangiopathic hemolytic anemia. In a review of 43 patients with the Upshaw-Schulman syndrome from Japan, 43% patients had history of neonatal hyperbilirubinemia that required exchange transfusion.[110] Recurrent episodes of TTP and associated AKI are common in these patients, and ESRD develops in approximately 20%.[111] Even with congenital deficiency of ADAMTS13, more than half of the patients are diagnosed later in life (15 to 45 years).[110,111] TTP in these patients is usually triggered by infection or pregnancy.

### Antibody-mediated thrombotic thrombocytopenia

The clinical and laboratory criteria used by Moschcowitz[3] to describe patients with the TTP pentad are

- Features of systemic illness, such as fever
- Microangiopathic hemolytic anemia
- Thrombocytopenia
- AKI
- Neurologic involvement

Classic (antibody-mediated) TTP is seen in older adolescents and adults and affects females more than males. At presentation, the clinical pentad noted here is not observed universally and may be seen in only 40% to 50% of cases. The triad of microangiopathic hemolytic anemia, thrombocytopenia, and neurologic manifestations, on the other hand, is the most common manifestation and is seen in 80% to 90% of patients.[112] Clinical presentation of patients with TTP can be quite dramatic, with neurologic manifestations such as headache, confusion, seizures, or coma.[111,112] Most patients also have nonspecific clinical complaints, such as fever, malaise, and nausea. Involvement of the GI system can manifest as abdominal pain, pancreatitis, and GI bleeding.[112–114] AKI requiring renal replacement therapy evolves quickly in 40% to 75% of cases.[110,111] Thrombocytopenia-related petechial manifestations or even frank bleeding diatheses also can be seen.

> ## KEY POINTS
>
> - All features of the TTP pentad are seen in only 40% to 50% of cases.
> - Renal disease is seen less commonly in TTP than HUS.
> - Extrarenal manifestations are common.
> - The acute mortality rate of TTP is high.

# DIFFERENTIATING HEMOLYTIC-UREMIC SYNDROME FROM THROMBOTIC THROMBOCYTOPENIA

The majority of children (85% to 95%) with STEC-HUS display a GI prodrome, and neurologic involvement and seizures are less common (15% to 30%). In contrast, fever, feeling of being unwell, and neurologic symptoms dominate in TTP. ADAMTS13 assay allows a clearer distinction between TTP and HUS. Plasma ADAMTS13 levels are very low in TTP patients and are normal (greater than 10%) in patients with HUS. Antibodies to ADAMTS13 are seen in acquired forms of TTP, whereas these are absent in inherited forms of TTP.[114]

# PATHOLOGY OF THROMBOTIC MICROANGIOPATHY

## Vascular pathology

Irrespective of the underlying cause of TMA, the characteristic pathologic lesions consist of endothelial cell injury and small vessel thrombosis, platelet aggregation, vascular injury, and organ dysfunction.[1,115,116] The endothelial cells are swollen, they may be detached from the underlying basement membrane, and the subendothelial space is filled with amorphous material and fibrin. Platelet-fibrin thrombi are present within the vascular lumen and hinder vascular blood flow. Pathologic studies demonstrate that fibrin vascular thrombi tend to predominate in HUS and that platelet thrombi are more prominent in the vascular injury associated with TTP.[11]

## Renal pathology

The morphologic findings of renal injury in HUS and all forms TMAs consist of glomerular, arteriolar and interlobular arterial endothelial cell injury and thrombosis and signs of tubular cell injury and acute tubular necrosis (ATN). Glomerular thrombi and thrombosis affecting the interlobular arteries are classic features of HUS (Figure 24.6).[117-119] The extent of ATN can be variable and may be prominent in some. Earliest electron microscopy findings consist of endothelial cell swelling, vacuolization, and separation of the endothelial cell from the basement membrane with "fluffy" and fibrillar material and platelet fragments appearing under the separated endothelial cells. Later, mesangial matrix and cell expansion, endothelial cell necrosis, and small and larger vessel occlusion with platelet and fibrin thrombi are evident.[119,120] Positive staining for fibrinogen, C3, and IgM in the vascular lesions is characteristic.[118]

As the acute phase of the disease wanes and renal biopsies are obtained during follow-up of patients with CKD secondary to TMA, most patients demonstrate varying degrees of glomerular sclerosis and chronic tubulointerstitial damage and fibrosis.

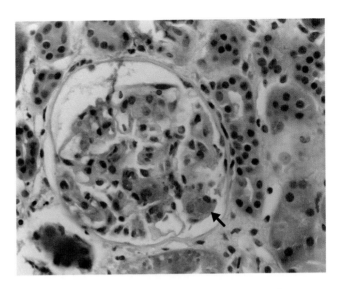

Figure 24.6 Light microscopy showing a glomerulus affected by thrombosis (arrow) in Shiga toxin–producing *Escherichia coli* hemolytic-uremic syndrome.

> ## KEY POINTS
>
> - Endothelial damage is the hallmark of TMA.
> - Microvascular thrombosis affects glomeruli, arterioles, and interlobar arteries of the kidney.

# EVALUATION AND DIAGNOSIS

A general diagnostic evaluation pathway of a patient with suspected TMA is shown in in Figure 24.7. Clinical and laboratory diagnostic techniques are essential in establishing the diagnosis of various types of TMA.

## Urinalysis

The urinalysis typically demonstrates hematuria, proteinuria, and cellular casts, although early in the course hematuria may be the only abnormality. Urine also may be visibly brown or muddy in some cases.

## Hematologic profile

All patients have evidence of microangiopathic hemolytic anemia with low hemoglobin and peripheral smear demonstrating evidence of fragmented RBCs (see Figure 24.1) and schistocytes. Thrombocytopenia with evidence of new large platelets and a high mean platelet volume is generally seen. The reticulocyte count is typically elevated in response to intravascular hemolysis, although eventually, as renal insufficiency develops, the reticulocyte count will be low.

The leukocyte count is often elevated early in the course of HUS.[121] The direct and indirect Coombs tests are negative in STEC-HUS and aHUS, but the direct Coombs test is positive in SpHUS. The plasma

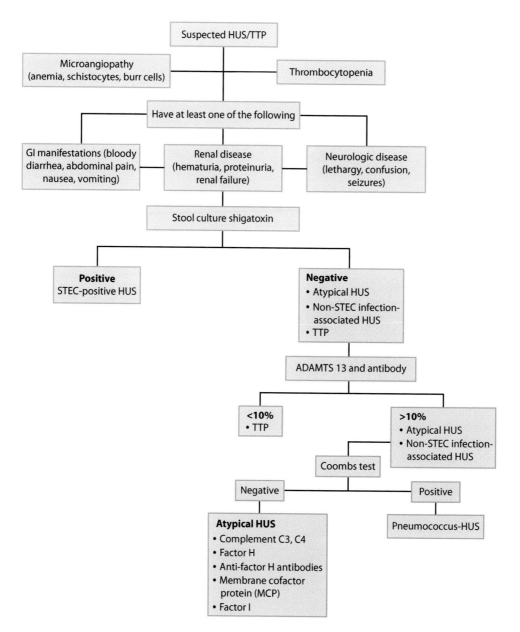

Figure 24.7 Diagnostic evaluation pathway in patients with thrombotic microangiopathy. *GI*, gastrointestinal; *HUS*, hemolytic-uremic syndrome; *STEC*, Shiga toxin–producing *Escherichia coli*; *TTP*, thrombotic thrombocytopenic purpura.

haptoglobin is low and indirect bilirubin high. Plasma LDH is elevated as a result of red cell lysis. The prothrombin and partial thromboplastin times are normal. Evidence of activation of the fibrinolytic system (increased levels of fibrin degradation products) is commonly seen, when assessed.

## STOOL CULTURE AND SHIGA TOXIN ASSAY

Evidence of STEC infection can be determined by stool culture, detection of Stx in stool, and/or polymerase chain reaction (PCR) assays for Stx in the stool. CDC recommendations include collection of stool as early as

possible after onset of diarrhea for detection of STEC and other pathogens.[122] In extenuating circumstances the stool sample may be stored for 24 hours in an unpreserved manner or in transport medium for up to 48 hours. Stx in testing on the bacterial culture obtained in broth provides better diagnostic yield than testing on the stool itself.[122] Immunoassay or PCR testing for Stx is now possible using several commercially available kits. It has been observed that stool culture alone on sorbitol MacConkey agar failed to detect a positive culture in 28% cases of STEC infection, and PCR for detection of the Stx gene missed 11% cases.[123] The CDC as well as other experts recommend using at least two methods for detection of STEC and Stx.[122–124] Newer research studies, including detection of Stx on the surface of circulating neutrophils, offer other promising methods for more rapid detection of Stx-mediated HUS in the future.[125] DNA-based Stx gene detection has not yet been approved by the U.S. Food and Drug Administration.

---

### KEY POINTS

- Stool culture should be inoculated on appropriate media for detection of STEC.
- Assaying Stx on cultured organisms rather than on stool itself gives better results.
- Stx assay and stool culture give better diagnostic yield for STEC than either one alone.

---

## Renal function

The degree of kidney injury may be quite variable but usually manifests over 5 to 7 days after first evidence of renal involvement.[6,16,18,55] Laboratory evidence of acute renal failure injury in more severely affected patients include elevated BUN and creatinine, hyperkalemia, metabolic acidosis, hypocalcemia, hyperphosphatemia, and hyperuricemia.

## Other organ dysfunction

Other less frequent laboratory findings, typically seen in more severely affected patients, include elevations of liver enzymes, creatine kinase, amylase, and lipase. For patients with pregnancy-associated HUS or HUS seen with medications, vasculitides, or other secondary disorders, the diagnosis is usually not difficult to establish.

## Complement assay

The European Pediatric Study Group for HUS has defined the algorithm that should be followed for diagnosis of aHUS and its treatment. After ruling out the possibility of STEC-HUS and SpHUS, complement studies need to be obtained in all cases in which aHUS is being considered. It is important to note that despite being a disorder of dysregulated complement pathways, a normal serum complement C3 level does not always rule out aHUS.[126] Other studies that need to be considered in these patients include CFH and CFI plasma assay; antibody against CFH, MCP (CD46) expression on mononuclear leukocytes; and gene mutation analysis for CFH, CFI, MCP, factor B, and C3.

## ADAMTS-13 AND ANTIBODY ASSAY

In patients considered to have TTP, plasma level of ADAMTS13 and antibody to ADAMTS13 (also known as inhibitor) should be determined before plasmapheresis is undertaken. The congenital or inherited form of TTP should be suspected in newborns with severe jaundice and hemolytic anemia of unclear cause. Severe deficiency of ADAMTS13 (less than 10%), without any antibody detection should be considered as presumptive evidence of this disorder and an indication for plasma infusion therapy. Congenital TTP can manifest at any age and may be considered even in older children. Presence of antibody to ADAMTS13 suggests the diagnosis of acquired (classic) form of TTP.[127]

---

### MANAGEMENT OF SHIGA TOXIN–PRODUCING *ESCHERICHIA COLI* HEMOLYTIC-UREMIC SYNDROME

Most children with STEC-HUS recover with appropriate supportive care and management of acute renal failure. Supportive management of volume deficit or excess, anemia, hypertension, and electrolyte abnormalities is the mainstay of treatment of established HUS.

## ANTIBIOTIC USE

Antibiotic therapy is not indicated for D positive HUS or idiopathic HUS and has been associated with worse outcome in some studies and been shown to be of no benefit or harm in most studies.[51,52] Often, in diarrhea-associated HUS, by the time the child presents with signs of HUS, the diarrheal illness is resolving and stool cultures may actually be negative.

## INTRAVASCULAR VOLUME

Judicious volume expansion early in the course of HUS has been demonstrated to attenuate the degree of renal impairment.[128–130] Serum albumin is often low in these children, and replacement with intravenous albumin may be useful; however, no controlled studies using this intervention have been reported.[131] Most importantly, once acute renal failure and oliguria have set in, fluid balance needs to be maintained with judicious use of intravenous and oral fluid intake to avoid fluid overload and associated complications.

## ANEMIA AND THROMBOCYTOPENIA

Treatment of anemia with judicious RBC transfusions is usually directed to keep the hemoglobin level greater than 8.0 mg/dL. Erythropoietin administration may be useful to maintain the hemoglobin count in case of prolonged renal insufficiency. Platelet transfusions may increase microvascular thrombosis, and are generally not recommended in TMA.[132] Platelet transfusion, however, may be clinically indicated in a minority of patients, especially in those who may require surgery. In one study, platelet transfusions based on clinical needs in STEC-HUS was not associated with adverse outcome.[133]

## ACUTE RENAL INJURY

Management of acute oliguric renal failure requires (1) strict attention to fluid balance, (2) treatment of hypertension, and (3) correction of metabolic disturbances, such as hyperkalemia, metabolic acidosis, hypocalcemia, and hyperphosphatemia.[8,17,84,85] Dialysis support becomes necessary once anuria or significant oliguria develops in a patient with evidence of progressive renal insufficiency. In most young children, peritoneal dialysis (PD) is the modality of choice.[8] The advantage of PD in these patients is that it is technically easy, and placement of the dialysis catheter can be done by the bedside in the intensive care unit. Continuous renal replacement therapy (CRRT) also can be used in the treatment of AKI associated with HUS and may be especially suited in patients with intra-abdominal complications, such as pancreatitis or colitis. Regional citrate anticoagulation is preferred over heparinization in such patients because of the potential risk for bleeding. When dialysis is required, it is generally needed for 5 to 7 days, although some patients have recovered after more than a month of dialysis support, albeit with evidence of some chronic renal insufficiency. Providing adequate nutrition is important in all cases of HUS with significant AKI and may require parenteral nutritional therapy until the GI tract has recovered.

## ECULIZUMAB IN SHIGA TOXIN–PRODUCING *ESCHERICHIA COLI* HEMOLYTIC-UREMIC SYNDROME

There is new interest in the use of eculizumab, a monoclonal antibody to C5, for the treatment of STEC-HUS. The rationale for this therapy is the observation that alternative complement pathway is likely to be involved in the pathogenesis of STEC-HUS.[51] Reports of children with severe STEC-HUS who received this drug have been encouraging, with reversal of hematologic abnormalities and improvement in neurologic symptoms with this therapy.[134] However, a subsequent clinical trial of eculizumab with plasma exchange in the German STEC-HUS epidemic did not establish superiority of eculizumab and plasma exchange over plasma exchange alone.[135,136] At present, the use of eculizumab has not been accepted universally for treatment of STEC-HUS but may be considered for the most severe cases, especially with neurologic manifestations.

---

### KEY POINT

Although eculizumab has been used in STEC-HUS, its efficacy in this disorder is unclear at this time.

---

## OTHER THERAPIES

For STEC-HUS, other therapies such as intravenous streptokinase, intravenous gamma-globulin, Stx-binding antitoxins, and corticosteroids have been shown to have no impact on clinical outcome.[137–140] Recent experience with plasma infusions and plasmapheresis in STEC-HUS in Germany has revived interest in these treatments for resistant or very sick patients with STEC-HUS.[135,136]

## PREVENTING HEMOLYTIC-UREMIC SYNDROME

Prevention strategies are most useful to minimize exposure to STEC and include appropriate meat processing, food handling, and preparation.[141] All parts of food, especially meats, must be cooked to a core temperature of 70° C. Salads and sprouts are a common source of spread of STEC, and their cultivation, washing, and storage need to be carefully supervised in the supply chain. Simple measures, such as hand and food washing as well as avoidance of ingestion of raw and rare beef, remain effective strategies for prevention of acquisition of STEC infections and HUS.

## MANAGEMENT OF ATYPICAL HEMOLYTIC-UREMIC SYNDROME

Patients with aHUS may present with an infection-triggered hemolytic crisis, acute onset of renal dysfunction, or neurologic complications, such as seizures. Supportive care, including dialysis therapy should be individualized. Some of the specific treatment options to be considered in this disorder are outlined in the following section.

### PLASMAPHERESIS

Expert opinion favors providing plasmapheresis as the most effective initial therapy in aHUS.[125] This recommendation stems from the observation that high mortality rate, neurologic complications, and ESRD are common in this group of patients. Plasmapheresis should be begin within 24 hours of the presumptive diagnosis of aHUS. Fresh frozen plasma is used for plasmapheresis, and the treatment is continued until the platelet count normalizes.

### ECULIZUMAB

Eculizumab has now been established as the standard of care for patients with aHUS.[145] This humanized monoclonal IgG2/4 antibody functions as a terminal complement inhibitor by binding to C5, thus blocking the production of C5a and C5b, activated complement proteins that trigger the TMA response (see Figure 24.4). Early initiation of eculizumab therapy is associated with more rapid control of aHUS disease manifestations and has been reported to improve short-term and long-term outcomes.[143] In the prospective phase 2 trial of eculizumab, treatment over 26 weeks resulted in a mean increase in platelet count of $73 \times 10^9$ and a relapse-free clinical course in 80% of patients. Chronic dialysis was discontinued in four of five patients in the trial. A sustained increase in estimated glomerular filtration rate (GFR) and decrease in proteinuria were noted in the treated patients, and earlier start of therapy was associated with a better renal outcome.[142]

Eculizumab is administered weekly until normalization of the platelet count and the microangiopathic anemia improves. The pediatric dose recommendations for eculizumab are 600 mg per dose for children below 40 kg body weight and 900 mg per dose in those weighing above 40 kg body weight. Eculizumab is administered in a solution strength of 5 mg/mL and can be diluted with normal saline from its original strength of 10 mg/mL concentration. Infusion should last over 35 minutes, and patients need to be premedicated to prevent any cytokine-mediated or allergic manifestation. The half-life of eculizumab is 12.1 days.[144] Frequency of follow-up infusions is every 2 to 4 weeks, based on the clinical response. At this point, eculizumab is considered to be a life-long treatment for aHUS. Discontinuation of eculizumab has been associated with recurrence of disease, and most clinicians continue antibody therapy indefinitely.[145] Further studies are needed to determine the appropriate dosage, timing, and frequency of eculizumab infusions to preserve renal function and prevent HUS relapses and establish specific treatment parameters for specific genetic conditions.

## LIVER TRANSPLANTATION

Failure rate in kidney transplantation in patients with aHUS attributable to disease recurrence is as high as 80% to 90%, especially in patients with CFH and CFI mutations.[146] Transplantation of a healthy liver, alone or with a kidney transplant, has been seen as an option for replacing deficient complement CHF or CFI. Early experience with such liver transplantation strategies in these patients was disappointing, but recent clinical successes have generated renewed interest in liver or combined liver and kidney transplantation in patients with aHUS.[147,148] At present, the recommendation of the Consensus Study Group is to consider liver only transplantation in patients in whom the renal function has recovered, and the dual liver and kidney transplantation in those with ESRD.[147] Plasmapheresis, plasma replacement, and eculizumab therapy in the perioperative period may evolve as adjuncts in improving patient and graft survival in aHUS.[149]

---

### KEY POINTS

- Liver transplant may provide definitive therapy for correcting complement dysfunction in some patients with aHUS.
- Role of liver transplantation in aHUS is not clearly defined and needs to be evaluated.

## MANAGEMENT OF THROMBOTIC THROMBOCYTOPENIC PURPURA

General and supportive care of patients with TTP, as outlined earlier, should be considered in all patients. This includes institution of dialysis therapy, if needed. Neurologic, cardiac, and GI manifestations should be addressed appropriately.

## PLASMAPHERESIS AND PLASMA THERAPY

Prompt institution of plasmapheresis is now regarded as the most appropriate initial treatment of TTP in adults and the one that is associated with best outcomes.[150] Plasmapheresis has been able to decrease the mortality in TTP from 94.5% to 13% in the last two decades.[151] The purpose of plasmapheresis is twofold: (1) To remove the anti-ADAMTS13 antibody in the acquired type of TTP and (2) to provide new source of ADAMTS13 via the fresh frozen plasma used in the plasmapheresis. Superiority of plasmapheresis over plasma infusions has been well established in the acquired form of TTP.[152]

Daily 1.5 blood volume plasmapheresis is usually initiated in patients with TTP after the diagnosis is presumptively considered. Fresh frozen plasma is used as the replacement fluid. Rise of platelet count is used as a guide to the success of plasmapheresis and is usually continued for a few days beyond normalization of the platelet count.[153]

In the inherited form of TTP (Upshaw-Schulman syndrome), periodic plasma infusion therapy is able to provide the plasma ADAMTS13 that is lacking.[154] Several case reports of long-term use of this therapy resulting in prolongation of life and preventing ESRD have been reported in the literature.[157] Although many patients require frequent plasma infusions, some may need it only during acute infections that might precipitate these events.[154]

## RITUXIMAB

Rituximab, a monoclonal antibody directed to CD20 on the surface of β cells, has recently been reported to be effective in TTP. In the phase 2 safety trial, rituximab given in a dose of 375 mg/m$^2$ within 3 days of the diagnosis of TTP was compared with the standard therapy consisting of plasmapheresis and steroids.[156] Rituximab was continued weekly for 4 doses. Median time to sustained normalization of platelets was 12 days, and by the second dose, 68% of cases had a platelet count greater than 50,000/mm$^3$. Of the 37 patients in the rituximab group, 4 developed a relapse of TTP at a median duration of 27 months. In comparison, the plasmapheresis group developed a relapse in 21 of the 38 patients at a median duration of 18 months. The relapse rate TTP in this study was reduced from 55.2% to 10.8% with rituximab. In retrospective analysis, Westwood et al.[157] reported on their use of rituximab as an adjunct, in addition to protocol plasmapheresis. They were able to achieve remission in 95% of patients in the rituximab therapy group. Earlier treatment with rituximab (less than 3 days) was shown to be more effective in reducing hospitalization, achieving a faster remission, and decreasing the need for plasmapheresis treatments. Relapse of TTP occurred in 13.4% patients at a median duration of 24 months. ADAMTS13 levels normalized in 3 months after initiation of rituximab in all patients.

The role of rituximab in inducing remission in patients with TTP, alone or in addition to plasmapheresis, is evolving and may become an acceptable modality of treatment in these patients.

## CORTICOSTEROIDS AND OTHER IMMUNOSUPPRESSIVE AGENTS

Corticosteroids have been used as immunosuppressive therapy for TTP since the 1960s.[158] Even after the development of plasmapheresis as a treatment of choice in acute TTP, corticosteroids have continued to be adjunct therapeutic agents to decrease the recurrence of TTP and reduce their clinical severity.[154] Controlled, randomized studies on the efficacy of steroids are lacking, and data from small series do not allow fair evaluation of such a regimen.[159] Similarly, other immunosuppressives, such as cyclosporine and cyclophosphamide, also have been used in clinical studies, but their therapeutic role remains unclear.[159]

## PROGNOSIS OF THROMBOEMBOLIC MICROANGIOPATHIES

## SHIGA TOXIN–PRODUCING *ESCHERICHIA COLI* HEMOLYTIC-UREMIC SYNDROME

The prognosis of STEC-HUS is generally good. Most children recover fully from the acute episode without obvious sequelae and without subsequent relapses.[104] Acute mortality in children with STEC-HUS is reported as 2% to 5%.[55,59] The cause of death in children with STEC-HUS is usually due to neurologic complications, such as a stroke, or GI complications, such as intestinal perforation and ischemic necrosis of the bowel.[55,59] Autopsies performed in children dying early in the course of illness have shown presence of brain edema and infarction in most patients.[160] Although acute renal failure itself is rarely a cause of death in STEC-HUS patients in the present era, this was reported as a leading cause of mortality in children before the 1970s.[58]

Evidence of CKD, such as proteinuria and decreased GFR, may be seen in up to 30% to 50% of children who recover from STEC-HUS. During a median follow-up of 6.5 years (range, 1 to 16 years), Siegler et al.[55] noted the presence of proteinuria or decreased GFR in 31% of cases, and combined proteinuria and decreased GFR in 12.5% of children who recovered from STEC-HUS. ESRD occurred in 3.6% of patients in this series extending over 20 years. In the more recent epidemic, STEC-HUS associated with a contaminated water supply in Canada (Walkerton epidemic), the overall renal outcome was better, with none of the children experiencing abnormal GFR or significant proteinuria.[161] In Argentina, where STEC-HUS is endemic, ESRD has been reported in 3.4% and proteinuria with decreased GFR in 16.1% of children followed over a mean duration of 13 years (range, 10 to 19.6 years).[59] Although long-term studies have yet to be reported, the short-term data from the German epidemic of *E. coli* O104:H4 documented ESRD in 1% of patients and CKD (stage 3 and 4) in 3.3% of cases.[23]

Hypertension may develop after recovery from HUS, sometimes requiring multiple medications for adequate control of blood pressure. In large series, the incidence of residual hypertension has ranged from 6.5% to 17.7%.[55,57] The incidence of hypertension has been noted to be higher in children with more severe disease that is characterized by oliguria exceeding 10 days.[162] Neurologic sequelae, such as seizures, delayed development, and hemiparesis, have been reported in 7% to 9% of cases. Despite a high incidence of seizures at onset, residual seizures in the short-term studies in the German epidemic of *E. coli* O104:H4 was only 3.3%.[23]

In a large cohort of STEC-HUS from Utah, predictors of adverse outcome such as residual neurologic sequelae, hypertension, renal disease, or death have been reported to be age younger than 2 years, leukocyte count greater than 20,000/mm$^3$, and presence of anuria in the diarrheal prodrome.[56] Others have also reported duration of oliguria to be a predictor of CKD with recovery of renal function occurring in 92.8% of those with oliguria lasting fewer than 10 days and in only 69.2% patients with oliguria longer than 10 days.[59]

A significantly lower platelet count was reported to be associated with acute neurologic complications in the German outbreak.[23]

## ATYPICAL HEMOLYTIC-UREMIC SYNDROME

High early mortality and ESRD are the hallmarks of patients with aHUS secondary to dysregulation of complement pathways. Mortality rate during the presenting episode depends on the type of genetic mutation in the patient. It has been reported to be as high as 30% in patients with CFH mutations and the best early survival (100%) has been reported with MCP mutations.[163] Similarly, development of ESRD is also variable and occurs in 60% to 70% patients with CFH, CFI, or C3 gene mutations. Those with MCP gene mutations appear to have a better prognosis for ESRD (6% to 19%).[63,65,72,163] Recurrence of aHUS and graft loss in 3 years is also high in these patients.[72] These findings suggest a heterogeneity in the clinical outcome and the importance of genotype-phenotype correlation in patients with aHUS.

## STREPTOCOCCUS PNEUMONIAE– ASSOCIATED HEMOLYTIC-UREMIC SYNDROME

SpHUS occurs in the background of invasive pneumococcal disease, and most patients are significantly sick. Early mortality rate in these patients has ranged from 3% to 11%.[79,81] Hospital length of stay of patients with SpHUS is generally longer than STEC-HUS. In one comparative study, median hospital stay for SpHUS was 21 days, versus 8 days in STEC-HUS.[80] A greater need for dialysis therapy (70% to 75%) in SpHUS has been well recognized, and ESRD has been reported in 23% to 28% patients.[81,82]

## THROMBOTIC THROMBOCYTOPENIA

High mortality of TTP at onset is well known. Amorosi and Ultmann[164] reviewed 255 previously reported patients and 16 of their own patients in 1966 and noted that 72% of patients died by 90 days of onset. After introduction of plasmapheresis, the immediate mortality rate declined to 29% by the 1990s and currently stands at 10% to 13%.[150-152] Even after a successful treatment of the clinical disease at onset, recurrences of TTP are common and often occur within the first year. With maintenance therapy using rituximab, the relapse rate has been reduced to 13.4%.[157] Early mortality usually results from neurologic or cardiovascular disease associated with TTP.

## SUMMARY

HUS is a clinical syndrome characterized by the triad of microangiopathic hemolytic anemia, thrombocytopenia, and renal injury. Although there are many distinct causes of HUS in children, up to 90% of cases are related to GI infection (diarrhea-associated HUS) with STEC or *Shigella*. Supportive care is essential to good outcome, and the course and outcome are related to the underlying cause. With diarrhea-associated HUS, mortality is now less than 5% but a large number of survivors exhibit signs of proteinuria, hypertension, or renal insufficiency and deserve continued follow-up.

Improved public health prevention strategies remain the best option to decrease the frequency of diarrhea-associated HUS in children. Early detection of STEC infection offers promise to provide opportunities to minimize disease severity. For children with established STEC colitis, supportive care is the mainstay. HUS continues to be a challenge in terms of prevention; even for severely affected children, appropriate supportive management of acute renal insufficiency and nonrenal complications can provide a good outcome.

Children with diarrhea-negative HUS are a more heterogeneous group. aHUS resulting from inherited complement disorders is emerging as a distinct entity. Treatment with eculizumab and liver transplantation provides new hope in such patients. SpHUS caused by *S. pneumonia* infection may be an under-recognized clinical disorder. Management of TTP is also undergoing rethinking with the use of rituximab as a possible maintenance therapy, after prompt plasmapheresis has stabilized the patient's clinical course.

### Clinical Vignette 24.1

A 19-month-old white boy was admitted from the emergency department (ED) with a 5-day history of low-grade fever, anorexia, and watery diarrhea. His parents reported eating at a barbecue 2 days before his GI symptoms started. On the day of admission his stools were streaked with blood. In the ED he was noted to be pale, fatigued, and slightly dehydrated. He had intermittent abdominal colic and vomited once.

Initial laboratory studies showed proteinuria and microhematuria on urinalysis. Hemoglobin was 11.0 mg/dL; white blood cell (WBC) count, 22,400/mm³; platelets, 177,000/mm³; reticulocyte count, 5.6%; and LDH 4980 units/L. Serum creatinine was 1.0 mg/dL; BUN, 34 mg/dL; sodium, 134 mmol/L; potassium, 3.8 mmol/L; bicarbonate, 18 mmol/L; chloride, 98 mmol/L; calcium, 8.8 mg/dL; phosphorus, 4.8 mg/dL; and albumin, 2.8 mg/dL. Liver transaminases, amylase, and lipase were normal. Creatine kinase was elevated, at 448 units/L. Bacterial stool cultures were sent for examination. The stool was positive for fecal WBCs.

Intravenous hydration was initiated on admission. On hospital day 2 his hemoglobin was 8.3 mg/dL and platelets 74,000/mm³. His stool culture was positive for *E. coli* O157:H7. A rectal prolapse needed to be reduced with use of sedation. His serum creatinine increased to 1.8 mg/dL and urine output declined to less than 0.5 mL/kg/h. A PD catheter was inserted on the third hospital day because of anuria and progressive azotemia. Severe hypertension was treated with short-acting and long-acting calcium channel blockers. He was started on intravenous erythropoietin for anemia but required two RBC transfusions to maintain his hemoglobin above 8.0 mg/dL during the first week on PD. Total parenteral nutrition (TPN) was initiated on hospital day 5, and he subsequently required insulin therapy for control of hyperglycemia. At that time his lipase was elevated, at 1266 mg/dL.

On hospital day 6, on the third day after starting PD, hydrothorax was noted and PD was discontinued for 2 days. Hydrothorax did not reoccur on restarting PD. His TPN and insulin therapy were able to be discontinued on hospital day 22 after resumption of oral intake. PD was performed for 29 days before substantial urine output returned, and PD was able to be discontinued.

By hospital day 35 his urine output and oral intake were good and serum creatinine was 1.2 mg/dL. His PD catheter was removed on day 36, and he was discharged to home the following day on enalapril 1.25 mg twice daily. His serum creatinine was 0.9 mg/dL at 6 months after resolution of HUS.

Three years after his recovery, further renal impairment was noted, with no evidence of active HUS. His hypertension worsened, and he developed progressive renal insufficiency. He received a successful renal transplant 14 years after his recovery from acute HUS and is now doing well, with no signs of recurrent HUS.

## TEACHING POINTS

- This boy's clinical presentation was typical for diarrhea-associated HUS. His initial complete blood count had only mild anemia and an elevated WBC count. Thrombocytopenia, anemia, and renal dysfunction became more impressive over the next few days, and dialysis was started once severe oliguria was noted in this setting.

- He did not receive antibiotic therapy. RBC transfusions and erythropoietin were employed. Platelet transfusion was not employed.

- His blood pressure was difficult to manage and required acute management. He continued to require antihypertensive therapy at the time of discharge, and his renal function has not normalized.

- Long-term outcome of this case was characteristic of the subset of children who do not experience complete recovery of HUS and stresses the need for continued follow-up of affected patients.

## REFERENCES

1. Gasser C, Gautier E, Steck A, et al. Hemolytic-uremic syndrome: Bilateral necrosis of the renal cortex in acute acquired hemolytic anemia. Schweiz Med Wochenschr. 1955;85:905–9.
2. Kaplan B S, Drummond K N. Hemolytic uremic syndrome is a syndrome. N Engl J Med. 1978;298:964–66
3. Moschcowitz E. An acute febrile pleiochromic anemia with hyaline thrombosis of the terminal arterioles and capillaries: An undescribed disease. Arch Int Med. 1925;36:89–93.
4. Noris M, Mescia F, Remuzzi G. STEC-HUS, atypical HUS and TTP are all diseases of complement activation. Nat Rev Nephrol. 2012;8:622–33.
5. Tarr PI, Gordon CA, Chandler WL. Shiga-toxin-producing *Escherichia coli* and haemolytic uraemic syndrome. Lancet. 2005;365:1073–86.
6. Lynn RM, O'Brien SJ, Taylor CM, et al. Childhood hemolytic uremic syndrome: United Kingdom and Ireland. Emerg Infect Dis. 2005;1:590–6.
7. Warwicker P, Goodship TH, Donne RL, et al. Genetic studies into inherited and sporadic hemolytic uremic syndrome. Kidney Int. 1998;53:836–44.
8. Mishra OP, Gupta AK, Pooniya V, et al. Peritoneal dialysis in children with acute kidney injury in children with acute kidney injury: A developing country experience. Perit Dial Int. 2012;32:431–6.
9. Karmali MA, Petric M, Lim C, et al. The association between idiopathic hemolytic uremic syndrome and infection by verotoxin-producing *Escherichia coli*. J Infect Dis. 1985;151:775–82.
10. Moake JL, Turner NA, Stathopoulos NA, et al. Involvement of large plasma von Willebrand factor (vWF) multimers and unusually large vWF forms derived from endothelial cells in shear stress-induced platelet aggregation. J Clin Invest. 1986;78:1456–61.
11. Chapman K, Seldon M, Richards R. Thrombotic microangiopathies, thrombotic thrombocytopenic purpura, and ADAMTS-13. Semin Thromb Hemost. 2012;38:47–54.

12. Enterohemorrahagic *Escherichia coli.* Available at: http://www.cdc.gov/ncidod/dbmd/diseaseinfo/enterohemecoli_t.htm. Accessed April 11, 2014.

13. Keithlin J, Sargeant J, Thomas MK, et al. Chronic sequelae of *E. coli* O157: Systematic review and meta-analysis of the proportion of *E. coli* O157 cases that develop chronic sequelae. Foodborne Pathog Dis. 2014;11:79–95.

14. Gould H L, Demma L, Jones TF, et al. Hemolytic uremic syndrome and death in persons with *Escherichia coli* O157:H7 Infection, Foodborne Diseases Active Surveillance Network Sites, 2000–2006. Clin Infect Dis. 2009;49:1480–5

15. López EL, Contrini MM, Glatstein E, et al. An epidemiologic surveillance of Shiga-like toxin-producing *Escherichia coli* infection in Argentinean children: Risk factors and serum Shiga-like toxin 2 values. Pediatr Infect Dis J. 2012;31:20–4.

16. Banatvala N, Griffin PM, Greene KD, et al. The United States National prospective hemolytic uremic syndrome study: Microbiologic, serologic, clinical, and epidemiologic findings. J Infect Dis. 2001;183:1063–70.

17. Elliott EJ, Robins-Browne RM, O'Loughlin EV, et al. Nationwide study of haemolytic uraemic syndrome: Clinical, microbiological, and epidemiological features. Arch Dis Child. 2001;85:125–31.

18. Frank C, Werber D, Cramer JP, et al. Epidemic profile of Shiga-toxin-producing *Escherichia coli* O104:H4 outbreak in Germany. N Engl J Med. 2011;365:1771–80

19. Jernigan SM, Waldo FB. Racial incidence of hemolytic uremic syndrome. Pediatr Nephrol. 1994;8:545–7.

20. Anonymous. Incidence and trends of infection with pathogens transmitted commonly through food. Foodborne Diseases Active Surveillance Network, 10 U.S. Sites, 996–2012. MMWR. 2013;62:283–7.

21. Nataro JP, Kaper JB. Diarrheagenic *Escherichia coli.* Clin Microbiol Rev. 1998;11:142-201.

22. Pollock KGJ, Bhojani S, Beattie TJ, et al. Highly virulent *Escherichia coli* O26 in Scotland. Emerging Infect Dis. 2011;17:1777–9.

23. Loos S, Ahlenstiel T, Kranz B, et al. An outbreak of Shiga-toxin producing *E. coli* O104:H4 hemolytic uremic syndrome in Germany: Presentation and short-term outcome in children. Clin Infect Dis. 2012;55:753–9.

24. Mody RK, Luna-Gierke RE, Jones TF, et al. Infections in pediatric postdiarrheal hemolytic uremic syndrome: Factors associated with identifying Shiga toxin-producing *Escherichia coli.* Arch Pediatr Adolesc Med. 2012;166:902–9.

25. Slutsker L, Ries AA, Greene KD, et al. *Escherichia coli* O157:H7 diarrhea in the United States: Clinical and epidemiologic features. Ann Intern Med. 1997;126:505–13.

26. Tarr PI, Neill MA, Clausen CR, et al. *Escherichia coli* O157:H7 and the hemolytic uremic syndrome: Importance of early cultures in establishing the etiology. J Infect Dis. 1990;162:553–6.

27. Renter DG, Checkley SL, Campbell J, et al. Shiga toxin-producing *Escherichia coli* in the feces of Alberta feedlot cattle. Can J Vet Res. 2004;68:150–3.

28. Strachan NJ, Dunn GM, Locking ME, et al. *Escherichia coli* O157: Burger bug or environmental pathogen? Int J Food Microbiol. 2006;112:129–37.

29. Boyce TG, Swerdlow DL, Griffin PM. *Escherichia coli* O157:H7 and the hemolytic-uremic syndrome. N Engl J Med. 1995;333:364–8.

30. Locking MJ, Pollock KGJ, Allison LJ, et al. *Escherichia coli* O157 infection and secondary spread, Scotland, 1999-2008. Emerg Infect Dis. 2011;17:524–7.

31. Riley LW, Remis RS, Helgerson SD, et al. Hemorrhagic colitis associated with a rare *Escherichia coli* serotype. *N Engl J Med. 1983;308:681–5.*

32. Obrig TG. *Escherichia coli* shiga toxin mechanisms of action in renal disease. Toxins. 2010;2:2769–94.

33. Werber D, Fruth A, Buchholz U, et al. Strong association between shiga toxin-producing *Escherichia coli* O157 and virulence genes *stx2* and *eae* as possible explanation for predominance of serogroup O157 in patients with haemolytic uraemic syndrome. Eur J Clin Microbiol Infect Dis. 2003;22:726–30.

34. Ethelberg S, Olsen KE, Scheutz F, et al. Virulence factors for hemolytic uremic syndrome, Denmark. Emerg Infect Dis. 2004;10:842–7.

35. López EL, Devoto S, Fayad A, et al. Association between severity of gastrointestinal prodrome and long-term prognosis in classic hemolytic-uremic syndrome. J Pediatr. 1992;120:210–5.

36. Cleary TG. The role of Shiga-toxin-producing *Escherichia coli* in hemorrhagic colitis and hemolytic uremic syndrome. Semin Pediatr Infect Dis. 2004;15:260–5.

37. Ochoa TJ, Cleary TG. Epidemiology and spectrum of disease of *Escherichia coli* O157. Curr Opin Infect Dis. 2003;16:259–63.

38. Brigotti M, Tazzari PL, Ravanelli E, et al. Clinical relevance of shiga toxin concentrations in the blood of patients with hemolytic uremic syndrome. Pediatr Infect Dis J. 2011;30:486–90.

39. Obrig TG, Karpman D. Shiga toxin pathogenesis: Kidney complications and renal failure. Curr Top Microbiol Immunol. 2012;357:105–36.

40. Ray PE, Liu XH. Pathogenesis of Shiga toxin-induced hemolytic uremic syndrome. Pediatr Nephrol. 2001;16:823–39.

41. Van Setten PA, van Hinsbergh VW, Van den Heuvel L P et al. Verocytotoxin inhibits mitogenesis and protein synthesis in purified human

glomerular mesangial cells without affecting cell viability: Evidence for two distinct mechanisms. J Am Soc Nephrol.1997;8:1877–88.

42. Schuller S, Frankel G, Phillips AD. Interaction of Shiga toxin from *Escherichia coli* with human intestinal epithelial cell lines and explants: Stx2 induces epithelial damage in organ culture. Cell Microbiol. 2004;6:289–301.

43. Ergonul Z, Clayton F, Fogo AB, et al. Shigatoxin-1 binding and receptor expression in human kidneys do not change with age. Pediatr Nephrol. 2003;18:246–53.

44. Petruzziello TN, Mawji IA, Khan M, Marsden PA. Verotoxin biology: Molecular events in vascular endothelial injury. Kidney Int Suppl. 2009;75:S17–9.

45. Fitzpatrick MM, Shah V, Trompeter RS, et al. Interleukin-8 and polymorphoneutrophil leucocyte activation in hemolytic uremic syndrome of childhood. Kidney Int. 1992;42:951–6.

46. van Setten PA, van Hinsbergh VW, van der Velden TJ, et al. Effects of TNF alpha on verocytotoxin cytotoxicity in purified human glomerular microvascular endothelial cells. Kidney Int. 1997;51:1245–56.

47. Proesmans W. The role of coagulation and fibrinolysis in the pathogenesis of diarrhea-associated hemolytic uremic syndrome. Semin Thromb Hemost. 2001;27:201–5.

48. Thurman JM, Marians R, Emlen W, et al. Alternative pathway of complement in children with diarrhea-associated hemolytic uremic syndrome. Clin J Am Soc Nephrol 2009;4:1920–4.

49. Morigi M, Galbusera M, Gastoldi S, et al. Alternative pathway activation of complement by Shiga toxin promotes exuberant C3a formation that triggers microvascular thrombosis. J Immunol. 2011;187:172–80.

50. Orth D, Khan AB, Naim A, et al. Shiga toxin activates complement and binds factor H: Evidence for an active role of complement in hemolytic uremic syndrome. J Immunol. 2009;182:6394–400

51. Wong CS, Jelacic S, Habeeb RL, et al. The risk of the hemolytic-uremic syndrome after antibiotic treatment of *Escherichia coli* O157:H7 infections. N Engl J Med. 2000;342:1930–6.

52. Proulx F, Turgeon JP, Delage G, et al. Randomized, controlled trial of antibiotic therapy for *Escherichia coli* O157:H7 enteritis. J Pediatr. 1992;121:299–303.

53. Zhang X, McDaniel AD, Wolf LE, et al. Quinolone antibiotics induce Shiga toxin-encoding bacteriophages, toxin production, and death in mice. *J Infect Dis.* 2000;181:664–70.

54. Safdar N, Said A, Gangnon RE, et al. Risk of hemolytic uremic syndrome after antibiotic treatment of *Escherichia coli* O157:H7 enteritis: A meta-analysis. JAMA. 2002;288:996–1001.

55. Siegler RL, Pavia AT, Christofferson RD, et al. A 20-year population-based study of postdiarrheal hemolytic uremic syndrome in Utah. Pediatrics. 1994;94:35–40.

56. Rahman RC, Cobeñas CJ, Drut R, et al. Hemorrhagic colitis in postdiarrheal hemolytic uremic syndrome: Retrospective analysis of 54 children. Pediatr Nephrol. 2012;27:229–33

57. Brandt ML, O'Regan S, Rousseau E, et al. Surgical complications of the hemolytic-uremic syndrome. J Pediatr Surg. 1990;25:1109–12.

58. Sallée M1, Ismail K, Fakhouri F, et al. Thrombocytopenia is not mandatory to diagnose haemolytic and uremic syndrome. BMC Nephrol. 2013;14:3. doi: 10.1186/1471-2369-14-3.

59. Spizzirri FD, Rahman RC, Bibiloni N, et al. Childhood hemolytic uremic syndrome in Argentina: Long-term follow-up and prognostic features. Pediatr Nephrol. 1997;11:156–60.

60. Eriksson KJ, Boyd SG, Tasker RC. Acute neurology and neurophysiology of haemolytic-uraemic syndrome. Arch Dis Child. 2001;84:434–5.

61. Siegler RL. Spectrum of extrarenal involvement in postdiarrheal hemolytic-uremic syndrome. J Pediatr. 1994;125:511–8.

62. Robitaille P, Gonthier M, Grignon A, et al. Pancreatic injury in the hemolytic-uremic syndrome. Pediatr Nephrol. 1997;11:631–32

63. Loirat C, Frémeaux-Bacchi V. Atypical hemolytic uremic syndrome. Orphanet J Rare Dis. 2011, 6:60 doi: 10.1186/1750-1172-6-60.

64. Constantinescu AR, Bitzan M, Weiss LS, et al. **Non-enteropathic hemolytic uremic syndrome: Causes and short-term course.** *Am J Kidney Dis.* 2004;43:976–82.

65. Noris M, Caprioli J, Bresin E, et al. Relative role of genetic complement abnormalities in sporadic and familial aHUS and their impact on clinical phenotype. Clin J Am Soc Nephrol. 2010;5:1844–59.

66. Frémeaux-Bacchi V, Fakhouri F, Garnier A, et al. Genetics and outcome of atypical hemolytic uremic syndrome: A nationwide French series comparing children and adults. Clin J Am Soc Nephrol. 2013;8:554–62.

67. Maga TK, Nishimura CJ, Weaver AE, et al. Mutations in alternative pathway complement proteins in American patients with atypical hemolytic uremic syndrome. Hum Mut. 2010;31:E1445–60.

68. Landau D, Shalev H, Levy-Finer G, et al. Familial hemolytic uremic syndrome associated with complement factor H deficiency. J Pediatr. 2001:138:412–17.

69. Warwicker P, Donne RL, Goodship JA, et al. Familial relapsing haemolytic uraemic syndrome and complement factor H deficiency. Nephrol Dial Transplant. 1999;14:1229–33.

70. Richards A, Kemp EJ, Liszewski MK, et al. Mutations in human complement regulator, membrane cofactor protein (CD46), predispose to development of familial hemolytic uremic syndrome. Proc Natl Acad Sci U S A. 2003;100:12966–71.

71. Noris M, Brioschi S, Caprioli J, et al. Familial haemolytic uraemic syndrome and an MCP mutation. Lancet. 2003;362:1542–7.

72. Bresin E, Rurali E, Caprioli J, et al.; European Working Party on Complement Genetics in Renal Diseases. Combined complement gene mutations in atypical hemolytic uremic syndrome influence clinical phenotype. J Am Soc Nephrol. 2013;24:475–86.

73. Kavanagh D, Richards A, Frémeaux-Bacchi V, et al. Screening for complement system abnormalities in patients with atypical hemolytic uremic syndrome. Clin J Am Soc Nephrol. 2007;2:591–6.

74. Lemaire M, Frémeaux-Bacchi V, Schaefer F, et al. Recessive mutations in DGKE cause atypical hemolytic-uremic syndrome. Nat Genet. 2013;45:53–6.

75. Janeway CA Jr, Travers P, Walport M, et al. Immunobiology: The Immune System in Health and Disease. 5th edition. New York: Garland Science; 2001. The complement system and innate immunity. http://www.ncbi.nlm.nih.gov/books/NBK27100/.

76. Hirt-Minkowski P, Dickenmann M, Schifferli JA. Atypical hemolytic uremic syndrome: Update on the complement system and what is new. Nephron Clin Pract. 2010;114:c219–35.

77. Sellier-Leclerc A-N, Frémeaux-Bacchi V, Dragon-Durey M-A, et al. Differential impact of complement mutations on clinical characteristics in atypical hemolytic uremic syndrome. J Am Soc Nephrol. 2007;18:2392–400.

78. Copelovitch L, Kaplan BS. Streptococcus pneumoniae–associated hemolytic uremic syndrome: Classification and the emergence of serotype 19A. Pediatrics. 2010;125:e174–82.

79. Waters AM, Kerecuk L, Luk D. Hemolytic uremic syndrome associated with invasive pneumococcal disease: The United Kingdom experience. J Pediatr. 2007;151:140–4.

80. Veesenmeyer AF, Edmonson MB. Trends in US hospital stays for Streptococcus pneumoniae-associated hemolytic uremic syndrome. Pediatr Infect Dis J. 2013;32:731–5.

81. Banerjee R, Hersh AL, Newland J, et al. Streptococcus pneumoniae-associated hemolytic uremic syndrome among children in North America. Pediatr Infect Dis J. 2011;30:736–9.

82. Brandt J, Wong C, Mihm S, et al. Invasive pneumococcal disease and hemolytic uremic syndrome. Pediatrics. 2002;110:371–76.

83. Loupiac A, Elayan A, Cailliez M, et al. Diagnosis of Streptococcus pneumoniae–associated hemolytic uremic syndrome. Pediatr Infect Dis J. 2013;32:1045–49.

84. Klein PJ, Bulla M, Newman RA, et al. Thomsen-Friedenreich antigen in haemolytic-uraemic syndrome. Lancet. 1977;2:1024–5.

85. Cochran, JB, Panzarino VM, Maes LY, et al. Pneumococcus-induced T-antigen activation in hemolytic uremic syndrome and anemia. Pediatr Nephrol. 2004;19:317–21.

86. Coats MT, Murphy T, Paton JC, et al. Exposure of Thomsen-Friedenreich antigen in Streptococcus pneumoniae infection is dependent on pneumococcal neuraminidase A. Microb Pathog. 2011;50:343–9.

87. Ault BH. Factor H and the pathogenesis of renal diseases. Pediatr Nephrol. 2000;14:1045–53.

88. Spinale JM, Ruebner RL, Kaplan BS, et al. Update on Streptococcus pneumoniae associated hemolytic uremic syndrome. Curr Opin Pediatr. 2013;25:203–8.

89. Albaqali A, Ghuloom A, Al Arrayed A, et al. Hemolytic uremic syndrome in association with typhoid fever. Am J Kidney Dis. 2003;41:709–13.

90. Delans RJ, Biuso JD, Saba SR, et al. Hemolytic uremic syndrome after Campylobacter-induced diarrhea in an adult. Arch Intern Med. 1984;144:1074–6.

91. Turner ME, Kher K, Rakusan T, et al. Atypical hemolytic uremic syndrome in human immunodeficiency virus-1-infected children. Pediatr Nephrol. 1997;11:161–3.

92. Austin TW, Ray CG. Coxsackie virus group B infections and the hemolytic-uremic syndrome. J Infect Dis. 1973;127:698–701.

93. Lee MH, Cho KS, Kahng KW, et al. A case of hemolytic uremic syndrome associated with Epstein-Barr virus infection. Korean J Intern Med. 1998;13:131–5.

94. Malak S, Wolf M, Millot GA, et al. Human immunodeficiency virus–associated thrombotic microangiopathies: Clinical characteristics and outcome according to ADAMTS13 activity. Scand J Immunol. 2008;68:337–44.

95. Becker S, Fusco G, Fusco J, et al. HIV-associated thrombotic microangiopathy in the era of highly active antiretroviral therapy: An observational study. Clin Infect Dis. 2004;39(Suppl 5):S267–75.

96. Said T, Al-Otaibi T, Al-Wahaib S, et al. Posttransplantation calcineurin inhibitor-induced hemolytic uremic syndrome: Single-center experience. Transplant Proc. 2010; 42:814-6.

97. Blake-Haskins JA, Lechleider RJ, Kreitman RJ. Thrombotic microangiopathy with targeted cancer Agents. Clin Cancer Res 2004;19:317–21.

98. Bennett CL, Jacob S, Dunn BL, et al. Ticlopidine-associated ADAMTS13 activity deficient thrombotic thrombocytopenic purpura in 22 persons in Japan: A report from the Southern Network on Adverse Reactions (SONAR). Br J Haematol. 2013;161:896–8.

99. Bollée G, Patey N, Cazajous G, et al. Thrombotic microangiopathy secondary to VEGF pathway inhibition by sunitinib. Nephrol Dial Transplant. 2009;24:682-5.

100. Reese JA, Muthurajah DS, Kremer Hovinga JA, et al. Children and adults with thrombotic thrombocytopenic purpura associated with severe, acquired ADAMTS13 deficiency: Comparison of incidence, demographic and clinical features. Pediatr Blood Cancer. 2013;60:1676–82.

101. Loirat C, Paul C, Agnès V, et al. Thrombotic thrombocytopenic purpura in children. Curr Opin Pediatr. 2013;25:216–24.

102. De Ceunynck K, De Meyer SF, Vanhoorelbeke K. Unwinding the von Willebrand factor strings puzzle. Blood. 2013;121:270–7.

103. Schneppenheim R, Budde U, Oyen F, et al. von Willebrand factor cleaving protease and ADAMTS13 mutations in childhood TTP. Blood. 2003;101:1845–50.

104. Licht C, Stapenhorst L, Simon T, et al. Two novel ADAMTS13 gene mutations in thrombotic thrombocytopenic purpura/hemolytic-uremic syndrome (TTP/HUS). Kidney Int. 2004;66:955–8.

105. Schulman I, Pierce M, Lukens A, et al. Studies on thrombopoiesis. I. A factor in normal plasma required for platelet production: Chronic thrombocytopenia due to its deficiency. Blood. 1960;16:943–57.

106. Upshaw JD. Congenital deficiency of a factor in normal plasma that reverses microangiopathic hemolysis and thrombocytopenia. N Engl J Med. 1978;298:1350–2.

107. Tsai HM, Lian EC. Antibodies to von Willebrand factor-cleaving protease in acute thrombotic thrombocytopenic purpura. N Engl J Med. 1998;339:1585–94.

108. Ferrari S, Scheiflinger F, Rieger M, et al. Prognostic value of anti-ADAMTS13 antibody features (Ig isotype, titer, and inhibitory effect) in a cohort of 35 adult French patients undergoing a first episode of thrombotic microangiopathy with undetectable ADAMTS13 activity. Blood. 2007;109:2815–22.

109. Lotta LA, Valsecchi C, Pontiggia S, et al. Measurement and prevalence of circulating ADAMTS13-specific immune complexes in autoimmune thrombotic thrombocytopenic purpura. J Thromb Haemost. 2014;12:329–36.

110. Fujimura Y, Matsumoto M, Isonishi A, et al. Natural history of Upshaw-Schulman syndrome based on ADAMTS13 gene analysis in Japan. J Thromb Haemost. 2011;9(Suppl 1):283–301.

111. Loirat C, Veyradier A, Girma JP, et al. Thrombotic thrombocytopenic purpura associated with von Willebrand factor-cleaving protease (ADAMTS13) deficiency in children. Semin Thromb Hemost. 2006;32:90–7.

112. Ridolfi RL, Bell WR. Thrombotic thrombocytopenic purpura: Report of 25 cases and review of the literature. Medicine (Baltimore). 1981;60:413–28.

113. Veyradier A, Meyer D. Thrombotic thrombocytopenic purpura and its diagnosis. J Thromb Haemostasis. 2005;3:2420–7.

114. Barrows BD, Teruya J. Use of the ADAMTS13 activity assay improved the accuracy and efficiency of the diagnosis and treatment of suspected acquired thrombotic thrombocytopenic purpura. Arch Pathol Lab Med. 2014;138:546–9.

115. Ruggenenti P, Noris M, Remuzzi G. Thrombotic microangiopathy, hemolytic uremic syndrome, and thrombotic thrombocytopenic purpura. Kidney Int. 2001;60:831–46.

116. Zoja C, Morigi M, Remuzzi G. The role of the endothelium in hemolytic uremic syndrome. J Nephrol. 2001;4:S58–82.

117. Taylor CM, Chua C, Howie AJ, et al. Clinicopathological findings in diarrhoea-negative haemolytic uraemic syndrome. Pediatr Nephrol. 2004;19:419–25.

118. Inward CD, Howie AJ, Fitzpatrick MM, et al.: Renal histopathology in fatal cases of diarrhoea-associated haemolytic uraemic syndrome. British Association for Paediatric Nephrology. Pediatr Nephrol. 1997;11:556–9.

119. Koster FT, Boonpucknavig V, Sujaho S, et al. Renal histopathology in the hemolytic-uremic syndrome following shigellosis. Clin Nephrol. 1984;21:126–33.

120. Halevy D, Radhakrishnan J, Markowitz G, et al. Thrombotic microangiopathies. Crit Care Clin. 2002;18:309–20.

121. Buteau C, Proulx F, Chaibou M, et al. Leukocytosis in children with Escherichia coli O157:H7 enteritis developing the hemolytic-uremic syndrome. Pediatr Infect Dis J. 2000;9:642–7.

122. Gould LH, Bopp C, Strockbine N, et al. Recommendations for diagnosis of shiga toxin–producing *Escherichia coli* Infections by clinical laboratories. MMWR. 2009;58:12–4.

123. Klein EJ, Stapp JR, Clausen CR, et al. Shiga toxin-producing *Escherichia coli* in children with diarrhea: Prospective point-of-care study. *J Pediatr*. 2002;141:172–7.

124. Cohen MB. Shiga toxin–producing *E. coli*: Two tests are better than one. J Pediatr 2002;141:155–6.

125. Tazzari PL, Ricci F, Carnicelli D, et al.: Flow cytometry detection of Shiga toxins in the blood from children with hemolytic uremic syndrome. Cytometry B Clin Cytom. 2004;61:40–4.

126. Ariceta G, Besbas N, Johnson S, et al. Guideline for the investigation and initial therapy of diarrhea-negative hemolytic uremic syndrome. Pediatr Nephrol. 2009; 24:687–96.

127. Peyvandi F, Palla R, Lotta LA, et al. ADAMTS-13 assays in thrombotic thrombocytopenic purpura. J Thromb Haemost. 2010;8:631–40.

128. Thomas DE, Elliott EJ. Interventions for preventing diarrhea-associated hemolytic uremic syndrome: Systematic review. BMC Public Health. 2013;13:799.

129. Ake JA, Jelacic S, Ciol M A, et al. Relative nephroprotection during *Escherichia coli* O157:H7 infections: Association with intravenous volume expansion. Pediatrics. 2005;115:e673–80.

130. Hickey CA, Beattie TJ, Cowieson J, et al. Early volume expansion during diarrhea and relative nephroprotection during subsequent hemolytic uremic syndrome. Arch Pediatr Adolesc Med. 2011;165:884–9.

131. Serebruany VL, Christenson MJ, Pescetti J, et al. Hypoproteinemia in the hemolytic-uremic syndrome of childhood. Pediatr Nephrol. 1993;7:72–3.

132. Harkness DR, Byrnes JJ, Lian EC. Hazard of platelet transfusion in thrombotic thrombocytopenic purpura. JAMA. 1981;246:1931–3.

133. Balestracci A, Martin SM, Toledo I, et al. Impact of platelet transfusions in children with post-diarrheal hemolytic uremic syndrome. Pediatr Nephrol. 2013;28:919–25.

134. Lapeyraque AL, Malina M, Frémeaux-Bacchi V, et al. Eculizumab in severe Shiga-toxin–associated HUS. N Engl J Med. 2011;364:2561–3.

135. Kielstein JT, Beutel G, Fleig S, et al. Best supportive care and therapeutic plasma exchange with or without eculizumab in Shiga-toxin-producing *E. coli* O104:H4 induced haemolytic-uraemic syndrome: An analysis of the German STEC-HUS registry. Nephrol Dial Transplant. 2012;27:3807–15.

136. Menne J, Nitschke M, Stingele R, et al. Validation of treatment strategies for enterohaemorrhagic *Escherichia coli* O104:H4 induced haemolytic uraemic syndrome: Case-control study. BMJ. 2012;345:e4565

137. Diekmann L. Treatment of the hemolytic-uremic syndrome with streptokinase and heparin. Klin Padiatr. 1980;192:430–5.

138. Robson WL, Fick GH, Jadavji T, et al. The use of intravenous gammaglobulin in the treatment of typical hemolytic uremic syndrome. Pediatr Nephrol. 1991;5:289–92.

139. Trachtman H, Cnaan A, Christen E, et al. Effect of an oral Shiga toxin-binding agent on diarrhea-associated hemolytic uremic syndrome in children: A randomized controlled trial. JAMA. 2003;290:1337–44.

140. Perez N, Spizzirri F, Rahman R, et al. Steroids in the hemolytic uremic syndrome. Pediatr Nephrol. 1998;12:101–4.

141. Reill, A. Prevention and control of enterohaemorrhagic *Escherichia coli* (EHEC) infections: Memorandum from a WHO meeting. World Health Organization consultation on prevention and control of enterohaemorrhagic *Escherichia coli* (EHEC) infections. Bull World Health Organ. 1998;76:245–55.

142. Legendre CM, Licht C, Muus P, et al. Terminal complement inhibitor eculizumab in atypical hemolytic uremic syndrome. N Engl J Med. 2013;368:2169–81.

143. Kavanagh D, Goodship TH, Richards A. Atypical hemolytic uremic syndrome. Semin Nephrol. 2013;33:508–30.

144. U.S. Food and Drug Administration. Highlights of Prescribing Information: Soliris [online], 2011. Available at: http://www.accessdata.fda.gov/drugsatfda_docs/label/2011/125166s172lbl.pdf. Accessed April 14, 2014.

145. Carr R, Cataland SR. Relapse of aHUS after discontinuation of therapy with eculizumab in a patient with aHUS and factor H mutation. Ann Hematol. 2013;92:845–6.

146. Bresin E, Daina E, Noris M, et al. Outcome of renal transplantation in patients with non-Shiga toxin-associated hemolytic uremic syndrome: Prognostic significance of genetic background. Clin J Am Soc Nephrol. 2006;1:88–99.

147. Saland JM, Ruggenenti P, Remuzzi G; Consensus Study Group. Liver-kidney transplantation to cure atypical hemolytic uremic syndrome. J Am Soc Nephrol. 2009;20:940–9.

148. Saland J. Liver-kidney transplantation to cure atypical HUS: Still an option post-eculizumab? Pediatr Nephrol. 2014;29:329–32.

149. Nester C, Stewart Z, Myers D, et al. Pre-emptive eculizumab and plasmapheresis for renal transplant in atypical hemolytic uremic syndrome. Clin J Am Soc Nephrol. 2011;6:1488–94.

150. George JN. Thrombotic thrombocytopenic purpura. N Engl J Med. 2006;354:1927–35.

151. von Baeyer H. Plasmapheresis in thrombotic microangiopathy-associated syndromes: Review of outcome data derived from clinical trials and open studies. Ther Apher. 2002;6:320–8

152. Rock GA, Shumak KH, Buskard NA, et al. Comparison of plasma exchange with plasma infusion in the treatment of thrombotic thrombocytopenic purpura. N Engl J Med. 1991;325:393–7.

153. Forzley BR, Sontrop JM, Macnab JJ, et al.: Treating TTP/HUS with plasma exchange: A single centre's 25-year experience. Br J Haematol. 2008;143:100–6.

154. George JN. Congenital thrombotic thrombocytopenic purpura: Lessons for recognition and management of rare syndromes. Pediatr Blood Cancer. 2008;50:947–8.

155. Mise K, Ubara Y, Matsumoto M, et al. Long term follow up of congenital thrombotic thrombocytopenic purpura (Upshaw-Schulman syndrome) on hemodialysis for 19 years: A case report. BMC Nephrol. 2013;14:156.

156. Scully M1, McDonald V, Cavenagh J, et al. A phase 2 study of the safety and efficacy of rituximab with plasma exchange in acute acquired thrombotic thrombocytopenic purpura. Blood. 2011;118:1746–53

157. Westwood JP, Webster H, McGuckin S, et al. Rituximab for thrombotic thrombocytopenic purpura: Benefit of early administration during acute episodes and use of prophylaxis to prevent relapse. J Thromb Haemost. 2013;11:481–90.

158. Distenfeld A, Oppenheim E. The treatment of acute thrombotic thrombocytopenic purpura with corticosteroids and splenectomy: Report of three cases. Ann Intern Med. 1966;65:245–51.

159. Cataland SR, Jin M, Ferketich AK, et al. An evaluation of cyclosporin and corticosteroids individually as adjuncts to plasma exchange in the treatment of thrombotic thrombocytopenic purpura. Br J Haematol. 2007;136:146–9.

160. Oakes RS, Siegler RL, McReynolds MA, et al. Predictors of fatality in postdiarrheal hemolytic uremic syndrome. Pediatrics. 2006;117:1656–62.

161. Matsell DG, White CT. An outbreak of diarrhea-associated childhood hemolytic uremic syndrome: The Walkerton epidemic. Kidney Int Suppl. 2009;112:S35–7.

162. Oakes RS, Kirkham JK, Nelson RD, et al. Duration of oliguria and anuria as predictors of chronic renal-related sequelae in post-diarrheal hemolytic uremic syndrome. Pediatr Nephrol. 2008;23:1303–8.

163. Caprioli J, Noris M, Brioschi S, et al. Genetics of HUS: The impact of MCP, CFH, and IF mutations on clinical presentation, response to treatment, and outcome. Blood. 2006;108:1267–79.

164. Amorosi EL, Ultmann JE. Thrombotic thrombocytopenic purpura: Report of 16 cases and review of the literature. Medicine (Baltimore). 1966;45:139–59.

## REVIEW QUESTIONS

1. Which of the following molecules is involved in the pathogenesis of pneumococcal HUS?
   a. Factor H
   b. Globotriosyl ceramide (Gb3)
   c. Membrane cofactor protein (CD46)
   d. Neuraminic acid
   e. von Willebrand factor cleaving protease ADAMTS13

2. Which of the following laboratory findings is associated with pneumococcal HUS but not seen in atypical HUS?
   a. Hypocomplementemia
   b. Microangiopathic hemolytic anemia
   c. Normal or slightly elevated prothrombin time
   d. Positive result of a Coombs test
   e. Positive result of a peanut lectin activity test

3. Which of the following is associated with a poor outcome in pneumococcal HUS?
   a. Family history of aHUS
   b. History of recurrent pneumococcal infections
   c. Meningitis
   d. Serotype of *S. pneumoniae*
   e. Severity of thrombocytopenia

4. In the treatment of a patient with pneumococcal HUS, which of the following approaches should be avoided?
   a. Calcium channel blockers
   b. Continuous venovenous hemofiltration
   c. Hemodialysis
   d. Peritoneal dialysis
   e. Transfusion of unwashed packed red blood cells

5. In the comparison of children with pneumococcal HUS and STEC-HUS, which of the following is *true*?
   a. Children with pneumococcal HUS are not more likely to require acute dialysis.
   b. There is no gender predisposition in STEC-HUS.
   c. Children with pneumococcal HUS are more likely to be younger at presentation.
   d. Children with pneumococcal HUS are less likely to develop chronic kidney disease.
   e. Children with STEC-HUS are more likely to require red blood cell and platelet transfusions.

6. In children with STEC-HUS, which of the following *E. coli* serotypes is most commonly identified?
   a. O157
   b. O104
   c. O97
   d. O144
   e. Nontypable
7. What is the *most* accurate statement about the Shiga-like toxin that results in diarrhea-associated HUS?
   a. It binds to ceramide receptors on susceptible cells.
   b. It binds only to endothelial cells.
   c. It binds to the T antigen on RBCs.
   d. It inhibits ADAMTS-13.
   e. It is only toxic in cows.
8. TMA has been associated with which of the following medications?
   a. Calcineurin inhibitors
   b. Cyclophosphamide
   c. Eculizumab
   d. Erythropoietin
   e. Rituximab
9. Which of the following is the *most common* long-term sequela of STEC-HUS?
   a. CKD stage 3 to 5
   b. ESRD
   c. GI malabsorption
   d. Proteinuria
   e. Seizures
10. What is the *most commonly* defined genetic abnormality in individuals with aHUS?
    a. C3
    b. Factor H
    c. Factor I
    d. Factor 2
    e. Thrombomodulin

## ANSWER KEY

1. d
2. d
3. c
4. e
5. c
6. a
7. a
8. a
9. d
10. b

# 25

# Tubulointerstitial nephritis

ROSSANA BARACCO, GAURAV KAPUR, AND TEJ K. MATTOO

Approximately 80% of the renal parenchyma consists of renal tubules and the interstitium. These structures provide support and hold together the nephrons and the renal vasculature. Inflammatory lesions of these structures, or tubulointerstitial nephritis (TIN), constitute a heterogeneous disorder that is commonly involved in renal pathologic findings.[1] Progressive tubulointerstitial damage correlates well with progression of renal disease and deterioration of glomerular and tubular functions.[2–4]

## DEFINITION AND CLASSIFICATION

TIN is characterized by inflammatory infiltrate, edema, and fibrosis affecting renal tubules and the interstitium.[5] Clinicopathologically, TIN may be acute or chronic in onset.

- *Acute tubulointerstitial nephritis (ATIN)* is characterized by an acute inflammatory cell-mediated response that is associated with a rapid decline in renal function.
- *Chronic tubulointerstitial nephritis (CTIN)*, also called *chronic tubulointerstitial nephropathy*, is characterized by a protracted onset and a slow decline in renal function.[6]

These two types of TIN may represent a continuum in the spectrum of initial acute inflammatory cell-mediated response that transforms into interstitial fibrosis over time. This transition to fibrosis can occur quickly, sometimes as early as a week after onset of the disorder.[4] TIN is defined as primary in origin when the inflammation is limited to the tubules and the interstitium and glomeruli and vessels are either not involved or show minor involvement. Secondary TIN results from diseases that initially involve glomerular or vascular structures.[6]

## EPIDEMIOLOGY

The precise incidence of TIN is unclear. It accounts for 8% to 27% of the reported cases of acute kidney injury (AKI) in adults and up to 7% in children.[7–11] A lower reported incidence of primary TIN in children may represent a lack of recognition of the disorder in routine renal biopsies.[12] Among 171 army recruits in Finland who underwent renal biopsy for proteinuria or hematuria, two cases had TIN and the reported incidence was 0.7 per 100,000 population.[13] TIN is estimated to account for 22% to 33% of cases with chronic kidney disease (CKD) in adults.[14,15] CTIN is commonly seen in association with obstructive uropathy and vesicoureteral reflux (VUR), both of which are significant causes of CKD and end-stage renal disease (ESRD) in children.[16–20]

## ACUTE TUBULOINTERSTITIAL NEPHRITIS

### ETIOLOGY

ATIN may occur in four distinct clinical settings (Table 25.1): exposure to drugs, infections, immunologic disorders, and idiopathic. Drugs and infections are the two leading causes of ATIN in children.[26–29]

## KEY POINTS

- TIN is characterized by an inflammatory infiltrate, edema, or fibrosis of renal tubules and the renal interstitium.
- Multiple antigens can cause ATIN by becoming targets of an immune reaction that is characterized by cell-mediated interstitial damage.

## Drug-induced acute tubulointerstitial nephritis

Exposure to drugs is the most common cause of ATIN in adults.[24,25] The list of drugs reported to cause ATIN is ever expanding (Table 25.2). Of these, penicillins, nonsteroidal anti-inflammatory drugs (NSAIDs), rifampin, and sulfonamide derivatives account for the majority of reported cases.[30] Drug-induced ATIN is a rare idiosyncratic reaction and occurs in only a small subset of patients exposed to any specific medication. It is not dose-dependent and typically occurs with repeated exposure to the drug. Structurally similar drugs may induce cross-reactivity, as evidenced by recurrent ATIN after cephalosporin administration in individuals with previous penicillin-induced ATIN.[30] The mechanisms by which drugs can induce ATIN include binding of the drug to the tubular basement membrane (TBM) and forming antigenic heptans, drug mimicking a normally present antigen in the TBM, drug being trapped in the interstitium and acting as a trapped or "planted" antigen, or forming antigen-antibody complexes in circulation that are trapped in the interstitium (Figure 25.1).

## Infection-associated acute tubulointerstitial nephritis

Infection-associated ATIN may complicate the clinical course of many bacterial, viral, fungal, and parasitic infections (see Table 25.1). It may occur as a result of direct invasion of the renal interstitium (pyelonephritis) or as an immune-mediated reaction to a systemic infection. Polyoma BK virus–induced interstitial nephritis has been reported in renal transplant patients and in a child receiving chemotherapy for leukemia.[30,31] Primary infection with this virus or reactivation of the latent virus in immunosuppressed patients in the renal epithelium is believed to induce interstitial nephritis. The presence of typical

Table 25.1 Etiologic classification of acute tubulointerstitial nephritis

A. DRUG EXPOSURE (see Table 25.2 for drug list)
- Immunologic mechanisms: Antibiotics, anti-inflammatory drugs (NSAID), diuretics
- Toxic mechanisms: Aminoglycosides
- Unknown mechanisms

B. INFECTIONS

**Reactive (sterile), infective agent not in renal parenchyma**

- Bacteria: *Yersinia pseudotuberculosis, Mycoplasma, Streptococcus pneumoniae,* β-hemolytic streptococcus, *Salmonella*
- Viruses: Rubeola virus, Epstein-Barr virus, human immunodeficiency virus, hepatitis viruses
- Parasites: *Toxoplasma gondii, Leishmania donovani*

**Infectious interstitial nephritis**

- Bacteria: Acute bacterial pyelonephritis, *Leptospira, Mycobacteria, Treponema pallidum*
- Viruses: Cytomegalovirus, adenovirus, polyoma virus (BK)
- Fungi: *Candida, Histoplasma capsulatum, Aspergillus* sp.
- Rickettsiae: *Rickettsia rickettsii, Rickettsia conorii, Rickettsia prowazekii*
- Parasites: *Plasmodium* spp., *Schistosoma* sp..

C. IMMUNOLOGIC
- Anti-TBM antibodies
  - Primary anti-TBM nephritis
  - Secondary anti-TBM nephritis
    - Membranous GN
    - Anti-GBM disease
    - Miscellaneous GN
- Immune complex deposition
  - Primary immune complex nephritis
  - Secondary Immune complex nephritis
    - SLE
    - Sjögren syndrome
    - Membranous GN
    - MPGN
    - Miscellaneous GN
- T-cell mechanisms
  - Primary T-cell nephritis
    - Allograft rejection
    - TINU
    - Sarcoidosis
  - Secondary T-cell nephritis
    - Associated with nephropathies
    - Tubulointerstitial nephritis

D. IDIOPATHIC

*Abbreviations: GBM*, glomerular basement membrane; *GN*, glomerulonephritis; *MPGN*, membranoproliferative glomerulonephritis; *SLE*, systemic lupus erythematosus; *TBM*, tubular basement membrane; *TINU*, tubulointerstitial nephritis with uveitis.

Table 25.2 Drugs associated with acute tubulointerstitial nephritis

**Antimicrobial Agents**
Acyclovir
AMPICILLIN[*,†]
Amoxicillin
Aztreonam
Carbenicillin
Cefaclor
Cefamandole
Cefazolin
Cephalexin
Cephaloridine
Cephalothin
Cephapirin
Cephradine
Cefixitin
Cefotetan
Cefotaxime
CIPROFLOXACIN
Cloxacillin
Colistin
Cotrimoxazole[†]
Erythromycin
Ethambutol
Foscarnet
Gentamicin
Indinavir
Interferon
Isoniazid
Lincomycin
METHICILLIN[†]
Mezlocillin
Minocycline
Nafcillin
Nitrofurantoin[†]
Norfloxacin
Oxacillin[†]
PENICILLIN G[†]
Piperacillin
Piromidic acid
Polymyxin acid[†]
Quinine
RIFAMPICIN[†]
Spiramycin[†]
SULFONAMIDES
Teicoplanin

**Nonsteroidal Anti-inflammatory Drugs**
Alclofenac
Azapropazone
ASPIRIN
Benoxaprofen
Diclofenac
Diflunisal[†]
Fenclofenac
FENOPROFEN
Flurbiprofen
IBUPROFEN
INDOMETHACIN
Tetracycline
Vancomycin
Ketoprofen
Mefenamic acid
Meloxicam
Mesalazine (5-ASA)
NAPROXEN
Niflumic acid
Phenazone
PHENYLBUTAZONE
PIROXICAM
Pirprofen
Sulfasalazine
Sulindac
Suprofen
TOLEMETIN
ZOMEPIRAC

**ANALGESICS**
Aminopyrine
Antipyrine
Antrafenine
Clometacin[†]
Floctafenine[†]
Glafenine[†]
Metamizole
Noramidopyrine

**ANTICONVULSANTS**
Carbamazepine
Diazepam

**Diuretics**
Chlorthalidone
Ethacrynic acid
FUROSEMIDE[†]
Hydrochlorothiazide[†]
Indapamide
Tienilic acid[†]
Triamterene[†]
**Miscellaneous**
ALLOPURINOL[†]
α-Methyldopa
Azathioprine
Bethanidine[†]
Bismuth salts
Captopril[†]
Carbimazole[†]
Chlorpropamide[†]
Cyclosporine
CIMETIDINE
Clofibrate
Clozapine
Cyamethazine[†]
D-penicillamine
Fenofibrate[†]
Gold salts
Griseofulvin
Interferon
Interleukin-2
OMEPRAZOLE
PHENINDIONE[†]
Phenothiazine
Phenylpropanolamine
Probenecid
Propranolol
Propylthiouracil
Ranitidine
Streptokinase
Sulfinpyrazone
Warfarin

*Source:* Adapted from and reproduced with permission from: Rossert J. Drug-induced acute interstitial nephritis. Kidney Int. 2001;60:804.
[*] Drugs most commonly involved are shown in capital letters.
[†] Drugs that can induce granulomatous acute interstitial nephritis.

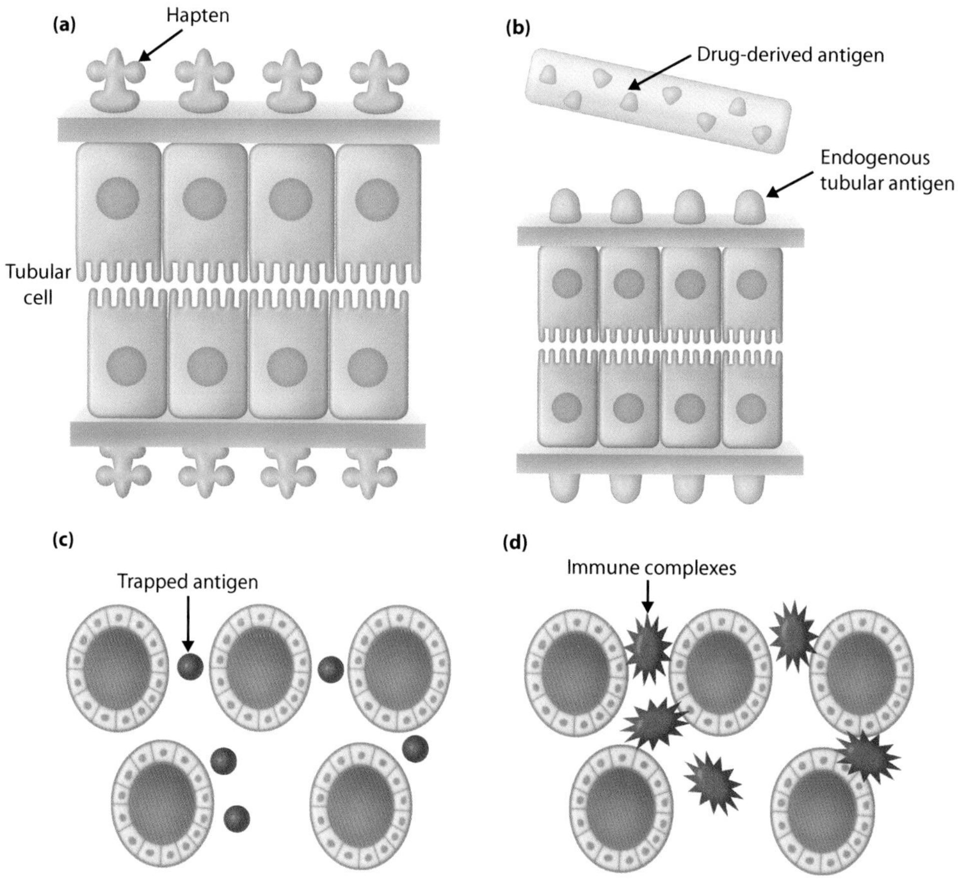

Figure 25.1 Mechanisms whereby a drug (or one of its metabolites) can induce acute interstitial nephritis. (a) The drug can bind to a normal component of the tubular basement membrane (TBM) and act as a hapten. (b) The drug can mimic an antigen normally present within the TBM or the interstitium and induce an immune response that will also be directed against this antigen. (c) The drug can bind to the TBM or deposit within the interstitium and act as a planted ("trapped") antigen. (d) The drug can elicit the production of antibodies and become deposited in the interstitium as circulating immune complexes. (Adapted and reproduced with permission from: Rossert J. Drug-induced acute interstitial nephritis. Kidney Int. 2001;60:804–17.)

basophilic or amphophilic intranuclear inclusions on renal biopsy is diagnostic. Distinguishing polyoma viral infection from allograft rejection is critical in the management of these patients.

## Immunologically mediated acute tubulointerstitial nephritis

Antibodies, immune complexes, or T cells may mediate ATIN by immune mechanisms.[7] Primary TIN resulting from anti-TBM antibody[32,33] and immune complex deposition is rare.[34] Linear deposits of immunoglobulin G (IgG) and complement along the TBM, with relative sparing of glomeruli and vessels, characterize primary anti-TBM nephritis.[7] Systemic lupus erythematosus (SLE) is the most important cause of ATIN seen in association with glomerulonephritis in children,[19] and the degree of tubulointerstitial lesions has been proposed to predict renal outcome in lupus nephritis.[35] Secondary ATIN also may be seen in association with membranous glomerulonephritis, shunt

nephritis, and immunoglobulin A (IgA) nephropathy.[7] Patients with glomerular and tubulointerstitial involvement have worse renal function than those with isolated glomerular involvement.[36] ATIN also has been described as an extraintestinal manifestation of Crohn disease.[37] Allograft rejection, TIN with uveitis (TINU), and sarcoidosis manifest with predominant tubulointerstitial damage mediated by T cells.[7]

## PATHOGENESIS

The immune mechanisms producing tubulointerstitial damage, like any other immune-mediated reaction, have an antigen recognition phase, immune regulatory phase, and effector phase (Figure 25.2).

## ANTIGENS

The antigens causing ATIN may be derived from the interstitial cells or may be planted into the interstitial

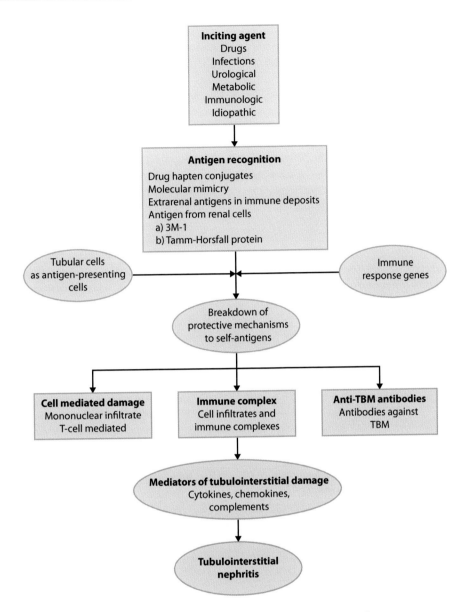

Figure 25.2 Pathogenesis of tubulointerstitial nephritis. *TBM*, tubular basement membrane.

microenvironment from the circulation. The nephritogenic antigens derived from the renal cells and the TBM include 3M-1 antigen,[38] Heymann nephritis protein (gp330, megalin)[39] and Tamm-Horsfall protein.[40-42] 3M-1 (TIN antigen) is the antigen of anti-TBM disease and has been characterized and mapped to chromosome 6 in humans.[38] Immunohistochemical studies have indicated that TIN antigen is defective in kidney tissues of patients with juvenile nephronophthisis.[42] Genetic deletion of the TIN antigen gene has been identified to cause TIN resulting in CKD.[43] Allotypic differences in the expression of the gene may occasionally result in anti-TBM disease in renal transplants of these patients.[44,45] Tamm-Horsfall protein may be an inciting antigen, especially following lower tract obstruction.[46]

Molecular mimicry of infectious agents,[47,48] drugs acting as haptens,[49] and toxic damage to the interstitium exposing cryptic nephritogenic neoantigens,[50] are other mechanisms whereby tubulointerstitial antigens may become targets.

Studies also have shown that induction of TIN could be a consequence of viral proteins, as in renal disease related to the Epstein-Barr virus (EBV)[51] and human immunodeficiency virus (HIV).[52] Experimental evidence suggests that native renal cells can process and present the antigen to T cells[53,54]; upregulate cell surface proteins, including intracellular adhesion molecule 1 (ICAM)[55] and vascular cell adhesion molecule 1 (VCAM)[56]; and enhance production of cytokines and chemokines.[57] Induced class II major histocompatibility complex (MHC) expression by renal tubular cells in response to inflammation or proinflammatory cytokines[49,58] may promote autoimmune injury by facilitating expression of self-antigens.

## IMMUNE RESPONSE

Genetic factors play a role not only in antigen expression[59] but also in immune response to a particular antigen[60] (immune response genes). Successful recognition of antigens leads to activation of nephritogenic T cells, which sequentially activates the nephritogenic immune response. Regulation of autoimmune B-cell and T-cell response may occur either during the maturational phase or by a fully differentiated effector mechanism. Interstitial nephritis is relatively uncommon, because nephritogenic B-cell and T-cell activation is self-limited by downregulatory events.[60,61] These regulatory events include complementary interactions in immune system[61] or regulation of target antigen presentation.[62] The immune response genes carried by specific individuals are important in determining the host immune response. Suppressor T cells are an important component of the immunoregulatory process. Models of autoimmune interstitial nephritis provide evidence for peripheral inactivation of autoreactive clones regulating suppressor T cells.[63] Breakdown of the tolerance to self-parenchymal antigens is needed for spontaneous TIN, and the details of these mechanisms need to be elucidated.

# EFFECTOR MECHANISMS

## Cell-mediated response

The predominant effector mechanism in acute interstitial nephritis is cell-mediated immunity. The majority of the infiltrating cells (>50%) in TIN are T lymphocytes; the CD4/CD8 ratio is at least 1, and the infiltrating T cells and tubular epithelial cell express class II MHC. Studies in animal models of TIN have revealed that nephritogenic helper T cells producing interstitial nephritis are usually CD4 and class II restricted,[64] whereas the effector cells are usually CD8 and class I restricted.[65,66] They induce toxic cellular damage by releasing inflammatory cytokines or by direct cell-mediated cytotoxicity by releasing proteases.[65]

## Antibody-mediated response

Antibody-mediated damage is less common and may occur as anti-TBM nephritis or immune complex–mediated TIN. Human anti-TBM nephritis has been reported in patients who received drugs such as methicillin, those who underwent renal transplantation, or in cases without an underlying abnormality.[31,45,67,68] Immune complex and complement deposition are seen in patients with SLE.[69] Tamm-Horsfall protein[37,38] and Heymann antigen of brush border[36] have been implicated in local immune complex formation in the interstitium. Tamm-Horsfall protein is localized in the interstitium in the setting of urinary tract obstruction or reflux nephropathy, suggesting that it may be a target antigen in previously damaged kidneys.[70]

# Amplification of tubular damage and interstitial fibrosis

Infiltration of T cells or antibody-mediated damage triggers processes that augment and amplify tubulointerstitial injury and inflammation. These include chemoattraction of inflammatory cells such as eosinophils and macrophages, release of soluble factors, and activation of the complement cascade. The soluble factors include chemokines, complement, luminal proteins, cytokines (profibrotic and proinflammatory), and proteinases.[71] Interstitial fibrosis is the final common pathway, especially for diseases associated with glomerular proteinuria or presence of inflammatory cells in the tubulointerstitium.[72,73] Transforming growth factor beta (TGF-$\beta$) is the most important profibrotic cytokine.[74] Specific inhibition of TGF-$\beta$ in ureteral obstruction[75] reduces renal fibrosis. Myofibroblasts play an important role in elaboration of interstitial fibrosis and may evolve from differentiation of tubular epithelial cells into fibroblasts (epithelial to mesenchymal transformation), resident interstitial cells, macrophages, or endothelial cells.[71] Immune-mediated mechanisms of various cytokines may trigger this transformation, as well as result in tubular cell damage. Thus, tubular atrophy and interstitial fibrosis coexist.

# PATHOLOGY

Renal biopsy findings in ATIN demonstrate a mononuclear cell infiltrate within the interstitium, most prominently observed in the cortical interstitium (Figure 25.3A).

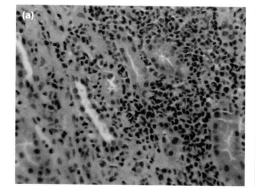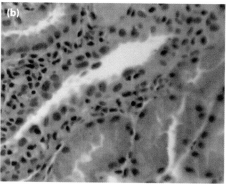

Figure 25.3 (a) Light microscopy showing acute interstitial inflammatory infiltrate consisting of mononuclear cells in a patient with acute interstitial nephritis. The patient presented with acute kidney injury and proteinuria. (b) Inflammatory cell infiltration into the tubules resulting in tubulitis.

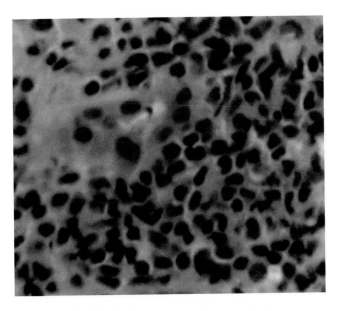

Figure 25.4 Granuloma in the renal interstitium in a patient with sarcoidosis.

The presence of infiltrating lymphocytes between tubular epithelial cells (tubulitis) is common in severe cases (see Figure 25.3B). The interstitial mononuclear infiltrate consists mostly of T lymphocytes, and B cells and plasma cells constitute a minor fraction. Eosinophils may be present, especially in drug-induced ATIN. Interstitial granulomas with giant cells may be seen with medication-associated TIN (methicillin, thiazides) and sarcoidosis (Figure 25.4). Variable degrees of tubular necrosis and regeneration are usually present. The glomeruli are generally normal, but associated nephrotic syndrome with minimal change has been reported in TIN caused by NSAIDS.[21] In ATIN secondary to infections, neutrophils may dominate as the cell type. Interstitial edema may be observed. Based on immunofluorescence findings on renal biopsy, ATIN can be classified into three subtypes:

1. No antibodies or immune deposits (pauci-immune)
2. Immune complex deposits present along the basement membrane (Figure 25.5)
3. Linear immunofluorescence staining for IgG and complement along the TBM, also known as anti–tubular basement disease (Figure 25.6)[22,23]

## CLINICAL MANIFESTATIONS AND DIAGNOSIS

Clinical manifestations of ATIN can range from asymptomatic proteinuria to renal failure (Table 25.4). Many patients have constitutional symptoms such as fever (especially during infection-associated ATIN), fatigue, anorexia, weight loss, nausea, and vomiting.[26–29] Approximately 30% to 40% of patients with ATIN have nonoliguric AKI.[11] ATIN should be suspected in any patient who presents with AKI

of unclear cause. With drug-induced ATIN, the patient may exhibit other features of allergic process such as rash, fever, or eosinophilia. The classic triad of fever, arthralgia, and rash occurs in fewer than 10% of such patients.[24,76] Such signs are even less common in ATIN resulting from NSAIDS.[73]

In drug-induced TIN, renal manifestations develop on average 10 days after starting the medication; however, they can occur as early as one day and as late as months after the inciting medication is started.[78] The urinary abnormalities in ATIN consist of microscopic or macroscopic hematuria, sterile pyuria, and white blood cell casts. Mild proteinuria, usually less than 1 g/day is frequently observed. Nephrotic syndrome has been associated with TIN caused by NSAIDS,[78] and nephrotic-range proteinuria has occasionally been reported with nephropathies induced by lithium, ampicillin, and rifampicin.[79] Eosinophiluria, which is defined as the presence of eosinophils greater than 1% of total urinary leucocytes (by Hansel stain), is seen in only approximately 25% of patients. However, eosinophiluria also can be seen in other forms of renal injury and inflammation and is not, by itself, diagnostic of ATIN.[80] Renal ultrasound reveals normal or enlarged kidneys, depending on the degree of interstitial edema. Clinical manifestations of acute TIN in adults reported in two separate studies are shown in Table 25.3.

Renal tubular epithelial cell damage and abnormalities in tubular function are common; sometimes these abnormalities may be limited to specific tubular segments.[25] Fanconi syndrome and tubular acidosis are seen rarely in ATIN but are relatively more common in CTIN. Urinary $\beta_2$ microglobulin excretion is elevated[81,82] and could reflect renal inflammatory activity. Urinary biomarkers have been studied in ATIN; among them, monocyte chemotactic peptide-1 (MCP-1) has been identified to correlate well with acute lesions, such as interstitial edema and inflammatory infiltration, seen in kidney biopsy samples of patients with drug-induced ATIN.[83] N-acetyl-β-D-glucosaminidase (NAG), has been proposed to correlate with more rapid progression of renal dysfunction in patients with CTIN.[84] In

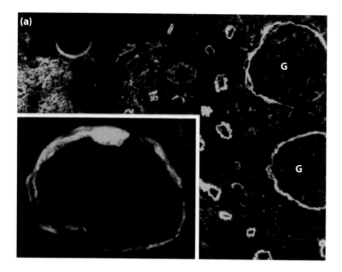

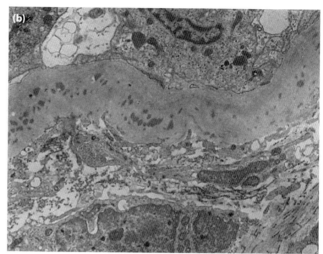

Figure 25.5 **(a)** Immunofluorescence microscopy showing intense staining of the tubular basement membranes (TBMs) and Bowman capsule with IgG in a finely granular pattern. The glomerular tufts (G) are negative for immunofluorescence staining. Inset shows the TBMs with finely granular staining pattern at 400× magnification. **(b)** Electron microscopy showing atrophic tubular epithelium and thickened TBM with scattered electron-dense deposits. (Reproduced with permission from: Vaseemuddin M, Schwartz MM, Dunea G, et al. Idiopathic hypocomplementemic immune-complex mediated tubulointerstitial nephritis. Nat Clin Pract Nephrol. 2007;3:50–8.)

view of the nonspecific nature of the clinical and laboratory features of ATIN, a kidney biopsy is often indicated to confirm the diagnosis.

## TREATMENT

### Eliminating the inciting drug or agent

The therapy of ATIN should begin by eliminating the possible inciting factors, such as drugs or infections. In choosing therapeutic options, potentially cross-reacting drugs (e.g., penicillin by cephalosporin) should be avoided. Many patients with mild ATIN may show recovery of their renal

Table 25.3 Clinical and laboratory features at presentation in adult patients with acute tubulointerstitial nephritis

| Clinical Manifestations | Percentage of patients manifesting (%) |
|---|---|
| Acute renal failure | 100 |
| Acute renal failure requiring dialysis | 40 |
| Arthralgia* | 45 |
| Fever | 36 |
| Skin rash | 22 |
| Eosinophilia (>500 eosinophils/mm³) | 35 |
| Microhematuria† | 67 |
| Gross hematuria† | 5 |
| Leukocyturia† | 82 |
| Non-nephrotic proteinuria | 93 |
| Nephrotic-range proteinuria | 2.5 |
| Complete nephrotic syndrome | 0.8 |

*Solution:* Praga M, González E. Acute interstitial nephritis. Kidney Int. 2010;77:956–61. Reproduced with permission

\* Data from Clarkson MR, Giblin L, O'Connell FP, et al. Acute interstitial nephritis: clinical features and response to corticosteroid therapy. Nephrol Dial Transplant. 2004;19:2778–83.

† Data from González E, Gutiérrez E, Galeano C, et al. Early steroid treatment improves renal function recovery in patients with drug-induced acute interstitial nephritis. Kidney Int. 2008;73: 940–46.

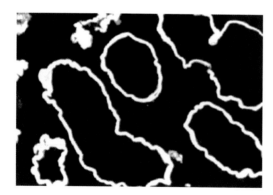

Figure 25.6 Immunofluorescence microscopy showing linear immunoglobulin G deposits in a patient with acute interstitial nephritis. (Reproduced with permission from: Markowitz GS, Seigle RL, D'Agati VD. Three-year-old boy with partial Fanconi syndrome. Am J Kidney Dis.1999;34:184–8.)

disease after discontinuation of the inciting drug, and no further treatment may be necessary. Supportive care involving maintenance of fluid balance, monitoring of blood chemistry, and dialysis may be necessary for patients with renal dysfunction.

## Corticosteroids

The role of corticosteroids in the treatment of ATIN remains unclear[9,24,30] because of conflicting studies, some of which revealed no benefit with corticosteroids[76] and others reported improvement of serum creatinine and decreased need for dialysis.[24,85,86] A study in children observed improvement in renal function within 1 week of initiation of corticosteroid therapy after a period of observation with no spontaneous recovery.[87]

A small prospective study showed that children with ATIN who received prednisone had a faster recovery of renal function.[88] There is a need for prospective randomized controlled trials to address this. We recommend administering corticosteroids when the renal function is not improving after removing the offending agent or if there is significant inflammatory infiltration seen in the biopsy sample. Corticosteroids are generally administered daily as oral prednisone (2 mg/kg/day) for 4 weeks, followed by gradual tapering.[19,22,30]

Methylprednisolone intravenous pulse therapy (5 to 10 mg/kg/dose) for 1 to 3 days, followed by oral prednisone has been used in severe cases of ATIN, especially those with severe AKI.[19,30] There is no available evidence to suggest that cyclosporine or cyclophosphamide is of benefit in patients resistant to steroids.[30]

## Mycophenolate mofetil

Mycophenolate mofetil (MMF) has been used in a limited number of case reports and small studies in patients with ATIN in whom corticosteroids alone were not effective.[89–91] Although encouraging, sufficient data are not available to make recommendations about MMF in patients with ATIN.

## PROGNOSIS

The prognosis for recovery of renal function after ATIN in children is usually excellent.[26,28,29,78] Poor prognosis in ATIN is associated with the presence of tubular atrophy.[24,30,78] However, data on relationship of interstitial fibrosis[19,30,92–94] and degree of cellular involvement and tubulitis[19,30,95] with the outcome of ATIN are unclear. Poor recovery of renal function also has been reported in patients with protracted oliguria lasting over 3 weeks, and in the presence of a preexisting renal disease.[24,95] There is no obvious correlation between peak serum creatinine or clinical severity of the disease at presentation with long-term outcome of ATIN.[19,24]

## CHRONIC TUBULOINTERSTITIAL NEPHRITIS

### ETIOLOGY

Chronic tubulointerstitial nephritis (CTIN) results from numerous infectious, metabolic, structural, toxic, or hereditary factors. CTIN is commonly seen in children in association with obstructive uropathy and VUR. Interstitial damage and progressive fibrosis in these disorders may result from renal immune responses that amplify tubulointerstitial injury, induced by high urinary tract pressures in the setting of infection.[19] Some drugs, such as calcineurin inhibitors (cyclosporine and tacrolimus) are particularly likely to cause CTIN, whereas others can cause both ATIN and CTIN. CTIN secondary to chronic cyclosporine toxicity is characterized by tubular atrophy, interstitial fibrosis, and vascular hyalinosis and sclerosis.[96] With the exception of cisplatinum, none of the drugs that cause AKI commonly results in CKD.[6] Conditions that may be associated with CTIN are listed in Table 25.5. The hyperosmolar, acidic, and hypoxic environment of the renal medulla favors precipitation of many metabolites (e.g., calcium, uric acid, and oxalate), resulting in tubulointerstitial injury and CTIN.[1]

### PATHOLOGY

Unlike ATIN, CTIN is a slowly progressive disorder characterized by renal tubular atrophy and interstitial fibrosis. Interstitial inflammatory cell infiltration may be minimal or even absent. The deposited extracellular matrix consists of a combination of collagen I, III, and V from interstitial fibroblasts and type IV derived from endothelial and tubular cells.[7] Tubular atrophy with thickened and wrinkled TBM is generally present. In contrast to ATIN, glomeruli in CTIN often show ischemic changes with shrinking of the glomerular tuft and wrinkling of the Bowman capsule (Figure 25.7).[7] Periglomerular fibrosis is also commonly seen. The end result of CTIN can be small and shrunken kidneys with prominent parenchymal scarring and pelvicalyceal dilatation.

Table 25.4 Common clinical manifestations of tubulointerstitial nephritis

**Symptoms**
- Fever
- Nausea
- Anorexia
- Abdominal Pain
- Vomiting
- Weight loss
- Growth Failure (CTIN especially)
- Eye pain (TINU)
- Polyuria
- Rash (usually with allergic drug reactions)

**Investigations**
- Urinalysis
  - Hematuria
  - Proteinuria (modest), urine protein excretion is usually less than 1.0 g/day
  - Leukocyturia, eosinophiluria, white cell and tubular cell casts
- Blood chemistry
  - Increased creatinine
  - Predominant segmental tubular defects
    - Proximal tubular defects: Proximal RTA, Fanconi syndrome
    - Distal tubular defects: Hyperkalemia, sodium wasting, distal RTA
    - Medullary defects: Sodium wasting, polyuria
  - Anemia: Normochromic normocytic
  - Eosinophilia
  - Increased erythrocyte sedimentation rate

**Radiology**
- Ultrasonography
  - Enlarged hyperechoic kidneys (ATIN)
  - Small contracted kidneys (CTIN)

**Renal biopsy**
- Diagnostic gold standard

*ACTIN*, acute tubulointerstitial nephritis; *CTIN*, chronic tubulointerstitial nephritis; *RTA*, renal tubular acidosis; *TINU*, tubulointerstitial nephritis with uveitis.

---

## KEY POINTS

- CTIN is often the end result of numerous types of renal injuries and inflammatory processes.
- Urinary obstruction and VUR are commonly associated with CTIN in children.
- Growth failure and inability to concentrate urine may be the only presenting manifestations of CTIN in children.

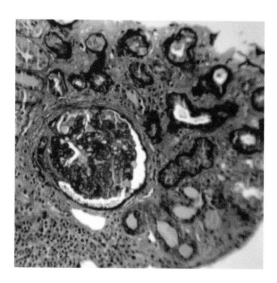

Figure 25.7 Glomerulus in a patient with chronic tubulointerstitial nephritis showing periglomerular fibrosis and ischemic glomeruli with collapsed capillary lumens.

## CLINICAL MANIFESTATIONS AND DIAGNOSIS

The clinical, laboratory, and radiologic manifestations of CTIN are similar to those observed in ATIN (see Table 25.5).[19] However, individuals with CTIN may have no evidence of renal disease, may have asymptomatic proteinuria, or may be first diagnosed as a result of the onset of CKD. Nonspecific symptoms such as weight loss, fatigue, anorexia, and vomiting may be present, and polyuria and polydipsia may be prominent features of the illness. Growth retardation may be a prominent manifestation of CTIN in children.[19] Polyuria resulting from inability to concentrate urine because of chronic tubular dysfunction is a common manifestation and may lead to nocturnal enuresis and urinary frequency.

Renal ultrasound usually reveals small, hyperechogenic kidneys. In association with CKD, skeletal radiographs may reveal changes of renal osteodystrophy. Generally, CTIN tends to progress more slowly than other forms of renal disease.[11] A kidney biopsy is often needed to confirm the diagnosis.

## TREATMENT

There is currently no known effective therapy for CTIN. As in ATIN, when an offending agent is identified it should be discontinued and supportive care initiated. For example, calcineurin inhibitor therapy may be associated with CTIN in renal transplants as well in native kidneys, where this class of drugs may be used as steroid-sparing agents. However, the damage may be irreversible and the disease course self-perpetuating.[19] Management of hypertension and prevention of further renal damage in the form

Table 25.5 Etiologic classification of chronic tubulointerstitial nephritis

**Drug related**
- Analgesic nephropathy
- Cyclosporine
- Cisplatinum
- Lithium
- Phenacetin
- Propylthiouracil
- Nitrosoureas

**Cakut**
- Posterior urethral valves
- Renal dysplasia
- Uretropelvic junction obstruction
- Vesicoureteric reflux
- Prune belly syndrome

**Metabolic**
- Oxalate nephropathy
- Urate nephropathy
- Hypokalemic nephropathy
- Hypercalcemic nephropathy
- Cysteine nephropathy

**Heavy metals**
- Lead
- Mercury
- Cadmium

**Hereditary**
- Alport syndrome
- Nephronophthisis-medullary cystic disease complex
- Sickle cell disease
- Laurence-Moon-Bardet-Biedl syndrome

**Immunologic**
All of the immunologic causes listed in Table 25.1

**Miscellaneous**
- Radiation nephritis
- Balkan nephropathy
- Hypoxic disorders
- Anorexia nervosa
- Hemorrhagic fever

CAKUT, congenital anomalies of the kidney and urinary tract.

of infection or from nephrotoxic agents are the focus of treatment. The beneficial effect of angiotensin-converting enzyme inhibitors (ACEIs) in CTIN-induced proteinuria can be predicted, but these have yet to be confirmed in clinical studies.[9]

## TUBULOINTERSTITIAL NEPHRITIS UVEITIS

Dobrin et al.[97] described the association of tubulointerstitial nephritis with uveitis and granulomas in the bone marrow. This uncommon condition is now recognized as a separate clinicopathologic entity and is known as tubulointerstitial nephritis uveitis (TINU) syndrome.

TINU tends to affect young women, but the disorder has been reported in both sexes, as well as in older patients.[98] Cases of familial TINU have been described,[99,100] suggesting an underlying genetic component. An association between TINU and certain human leukocyte antigens (HLAs) has been reported. Levinson et al.[101] found HLA-DQA1*01, HLA-DQB1*05, and HLADRB1*01. Renal lesions are characterized by acute interstitial nephritis with predominant T-cell infiltration into the interstitium. Ocular disease is commonly bilateral and is characterized by anterior uveitis. Ocular manifestations may occur before, simultaneous with, or up to several months subsequent to the onset of renal disease.[100] Manifestations of uveitis include ocular pain, redness, photophobia, itching, and visual impairment, and can be the presenting manifestation of the disorder. However, recent studies suggest that uveitis is underdiagnosed in patients with TIN, as it is asymptomatic in 50% to 58% of patients.[87,100] A prospective study of children with TIN recommends that patients with TIN be evaluated by an ophthalmologist even if there are no ocular complaints and followed at 3-month intervals for at least 1 year.[97] Fever and other nonspecific symptoms such as fatigue and anorexia also may be present.[88]

Laboratory findings of TINU are notable for markedly elevated ESR, normocytic and normochromic anemia, elevated creatinine, and elevated immunoglobulins. Patients with TINU have been reported to have serologic evidence of autoantibodies, including antinuclear antibody (ANA), rheumatoid factor, and cytoplasmic antineutrophil cytoplasmic antibodies (c-ANCA). TINU has also been reported in association with herpes zoster, EBV infection, toxoplasmosis, and insect bites, as well as systemic diseases such as hyperthyroidism and hypothyroidism, rheumatoid arthritis, and lymphadenopathy. In children and adolescents with this syndrome, TIN spontaneously resolves and its long-term prognosis is good, but uveitis often relapses. Systemic steroids may be required for treatment of both uveitis and TIN.[87]

---

**KEY POINT**

Patients with ATIN should have an ophthalmologic evaluation, because uveitis can be asymptomatic.

## SUMMARY

TIN is an important cause of AKI and should be considered in patients with no obvious cause for renal failure. History of infection, drug ingestion, skin rashes, or other constitutional symptoms may be present. The clinical features are nonspecific, and strong clinical suspicion is needed to make a diagnosis, which, depending on the clinical course of the patient, may need to be confirmed by renal biopsy. Patients with TIN should be evaluated for uveitis even in the absence of ocular symptoms. Studies support the role of systemic corticosteroid therapy in ATIN. Elimination of the causative agent such as medication and instigation of supportive care are recommended. The prognosis for ATIN is usually good, and very few patients progress to CTIN. On the other hand, CTIN indicates chronic progressive renal damage that involves interstitial fibrosis and glomerular and tubular damage. Recent research has focused on various factors involved in the pathogenesis of TIN and, with better understanding of the immunologic process involved, may help in determining the best targets for treatment.

### Clinical Vignette 25.1

A 16-month-old girl with no significant medical history presented to the emergency department (ED) with fever, fussiness, vomiting, and diarrhea. Five days before presentation she had been seen at her pediatrician's office for fever and upper respiratory tract symptoms. She was prescribed oral azithromycin for otitis media. Fevers continued and her mother gave her around-the-clock ibuprofen. She then developed vomiting and nonbloody diarrhea, significantly decreased oral intake, and increased fussiness. The mother noted no wet diapers for 1 day before bringing her to ED. In the ED, she was afebrile, tachycardic with a heart rate of 142 beats/min. Her blood pressure was normal at 106/62 mm Hg, and on examination she looked dehydrated. Relevant laboratory test results revealed serum potassium, 5.2 mEq/L; bicarbonate, 17 mEq/L; blood urea nitrogen, 60 mg/dL; and creatinine, 5.2 mg/dL. Complete blood count showed a white blood cell count of $18.0 \times 10^3/\mu L$; hemoglobin, 11.8 g/dL; and platelets 540,000/$\mu$L. Complement levels were normal, and serology studies, including ANA and ANCA titers, were negative. After three normal saline boluses her hydration status improved; however, she remained anuric. She was admitted, and her blood chemistry on the next day showed further deterioration in blood chemistry values, including renal function.

A kidney biopsy was done, and a peritoneal dialysis catheter was placed at the same time. Kidney biopsy showed severe interstitial nephritis; the interstitium was edematous and markedly expanded with severe inflammatory infiltrate and many eosinophils. Immunofluorescence was negative. Intravenous methylprednisolone was given for 3 days followed by oral prednisone 2 mg/kg/day. After 2 days of methylprednisolone the patient began producing small amounts of urine. She continued to slowly improve and was weaned off dialysis 10 days later. She received prednisone 2 mg/kg/day for 1 month, after which it was slowly weaned over the course of 5 months. Her renal function on follow-up has been normal for 4 years.

### TEACHING POINTS

- Patients with ATIN usually have nonoliguric AKI, but this patient was anuric on presentation, with rapidly deteriorating renal function.
- The diagnostic value of renal biopsy in such patients is demonstrated by this case. The renal biopsy was remarkable for severe interstitial inflammation with significant amount of eosinophils, a picture typically seen in drug-induced ATIN.
- She had a history of taking two different medications (ibuprofen and azithromycin), either of which could have been the responsible for her ATIN.
- Another confounding aspect of her presentation was the symptoms suggestive of a viral infection, which included diarrhea, vomiting, and lethargy.
- Significant dehydration is likely to have added a prerenal component to her AKI.
- Treatment with corticosteroids resulted in clinical improvement. Whether this improvement was because of the removal of the offending agent or a result of corticosteroids that she received is difficult to ascertain.
- The patient has now been labeled as being allergic to both ibuprofen and azithromycin, the two drugs potentially inciting ATIN in this patient.

## REFERENCES

1. Schwartz MM. Prologue to section III. In: Jennette JC, Olson JL, Schwartz MM, Silva FG, editors. Heptinstall's Pathology of the Kidney, 5th ed. Philadelphia: Lippincott-Raven, 1998: 657–65.
2. Nath KA. Tubulointerstitial changes as a major determinant in the progression of renal damage. Am J Kidney Dis. 1992;20:1–17.
3. Bohle A, Wehrmann M, Bogenschutz O, et al. The long-term prognosis of the primary glomerulonephritides. Pathol Res Pract. 1992;188:908–24.
4. Neilson EG. Pathogenesis and therapy of interstitial nephritis. Kidney Int. 1989;35:1257–70.
5. Dillon M. Tubulointerstitial nephropathy. In: Edelmann C, editor. Pediatric Kidney Diseases, 2nd ed. Boston: Little, Brown; 1992.

6. Cavallo T. Tubulointerstitial nephritis. In: Jenette JC, Olson JL, Schwartz MM, Silva FG, editors. Heptinstall's Pathology of the Kidney, 5th ed. Philadelphia: Lippincott-Raven; 1998.

7. Wilson DM, Turner DR, Cameron JS, et al. Value of renal biopsy in acute intrinsic renal failure. Br Med J. 1976;2:459–61.

8. Linton AL, Clark WF, Driedger AA, et al. Acute interstitial nephritis due to drugs: Review of the literature with a report of nine cases. Ann Intern Med. 1980;93:735–41.

9. Farrington K, Levison DA, Greenwood RN, et al. Renal biopsy in patients with unexplained renal impairment and normal kidney size. Q J Med. 1989;70:221–33.

10. Ekonayan G. Tubulointerstitial nephropathies. In: Massry SG, Glasscock RJ, editors. Textbook of Nephrology, 3rd ed. Baltimore: Williams & Wilkins; 1995.

11. Greising J, Trachtman H, Gauthier B, Valderrama E. Acute interstitial nephritis in adolescents and young adults. Child Nephrol Urol. 1990;10:189–95.

12. Jones CL, Eddy AA. Tubulointerstitial nephritis. Pediatr Nephrol. 1992;6:572–86.

13. Pettersson E, von Bonsdorff M, Tornroth T, Lindholm H. Nephritis among young Finnish men. Clin Nephrol. 1984;22:217–22.

14. Murray T, Goldberg M. Chronic interstitial nephritis: Etiologic factors. Ann Intern Med. 1975;82:453–9.

15. Rostand SG, Kirk KA, Rutsky EA, et al. Racial differences in the incidence of treatment for end stage renal disease. N Engl J Med. 1982;306:1276–9.

16. Tejani A, Butt K, Glassberg K, et al. Predictors of eventual end stage renal disease in children with posterior urethral valves. J Urol. 1986;136:857–60.

17. Smith GH, Canning DA, Schulman SL, et al. The long-term outcome of posterior urethral valves treated with primary valve ablation and observation. J Urol. 1996;155:1730–4.

18. Hostetter TH, Nath KA, Hostetter MK. Infection-related chronic interstitial nephropathy. Semin Nephrol. 1988;8:11–6.

19. Alon US. Tubulointerstitial nephritis. In: Avner ED, Harmon WE, Niaudet P, editors. Pediatric Nephrology, 5th ed. Philadelphia: Lippincott Williams & Wilkins; 2004.

20. North American Pediatric Renal Transplant Cooperative Study (NAPRTCS). 2004 annual report. Boston: NAPRTCS; 2004:8-4, 13-4.

21. Alpers CE. The kidney. In: Kumar V, Abbas AK, Faust N, editors. Robbins and Cotran Pathologic Basis of Disease, 7th ed. Philadelphia: WB Saunders; 2004. p. 1483.

22. Kelly CJ, Neilson EG. Tubulointerstitial disease. In: Brenner BM, editor. Brenner & Rector's The Kidney, 7th ed. Philadelphia: WB Saunders; 2004. p. 1483.

23. Bergstein J, Litman N. Interstitial nephritis with anti-tubular-basement-membrane antibody. N Engl J Med. 1975;292:875–8.

24. Baker RJ, Pusey CD. The changing profile of acute tubulointerstitial nephritis. Nephrol Dial Transplant. 2004;19:8–11.

25. Toto RD. Acute tubulointerstitial nephritis. Am J Med Sci. 1990;299:392–410.

26. Hawkins EP, Berry PL, Silva FG. Acute tubulointerstitial nephritis in children: Clinical, morphologic, and lectin studies. A report of the Southwest Pediatric Nephrology Study Group. Am J Kidney Dis. 1989;14:466–71.

27. Koskimies O, Holmberg C. Interstitial nephritis of acute onset. Arch Dis Child. 1985;60:752–5.

28. Ellis D, Fried WA, Yunis EJ, Blau EB. Acute interstitial nephritis in children: A report of 13 cases and review of the literature. Pediatrics. 1981;67:862–72.

29. Kobayashi Y, Honda M, Yoshikawa N, Ito H. Acute tubulointerstitial nephritis in 21 Japanese children. Clin Nephrol. 2000;54:191–7.

30. Meyers C. Acute interstitial nephritis. In: Greenberg A, editor. Primer on Kidney Diseases, 3rd ed. San Diego: Academic Press; 2001.

31. Inaba H, Jones DP, Gaber LW, et al. BK virus-induced tubulointerstitial nephritis in a child with acute lymphoblastic leukemia. J Pediatr. 2007;151:215–7.

32. Brentjens JR, Matsuo S, Fukatsu A, et al. Immunologic studies in two patients with antitubular basement membrane nephritis. Am J Med. 1989;86:603–8.

33. Clayman MD, Michaud L, Brentjens J, et al. Isolation of the target antigen of human anti-tubular basement membrane antibody-associated interstitial nephritis. J Clin Invest. 1986;77:1143–7.

34. Ellis D, Fisher SE, Smith WI, Jr, Jaffe R. Familial occurrence of renal and intestinal disease associated with tissue autoantibodies. Am J Dis Child. 1982;136:323–6.

35. Yu F, Wu LH, Tan Y, et al. Tubulointerstitial lesions of patients with lupus nephritis classified by the 2003 International Society of Nephrology and Renal Pathology Society system. Kidney Int. 2010;77:820–9.

36. Levy M, Guesry P, Loirat C, et al. Immunologically mediated tubulo-interstitial nephritis in children. Contrib Nephrol. 1979;16:132–40.

37. Marcus SB, Brown JB, Melin-Aldana H, Strople JA. Tubulointerstitial nephritis: An extraintestinal manifestation of Crohn disease in children. J Pediatr Gastroenterol Nutr. 2008;46:338–41.

38. Clayman MD, Martinez-Hernandez A, Michaud L, et al. Isolation and characterization of the nephritogenic antigen producing anti-tubular basement membrane disease. J Exp Med. 1985;161:290–305.

39. Noble B, Mendrick DL, Brentjens JR, Andres GA. Antibody-mediated injury to proximal tubules in the rat kidney induced by passive transfer of homologous anti-brush border serum. Clin Immunol Immunopathol. 1981;19:289–301.

40. Hoyer JR. Tubulointerstitial immune complex nephritis in rats immunized with Tamm-Horsfall protein. Kidney Int. 1980;17:284–92.

41. Cavallone D, Malagolini N, Serafini-Cessi F. Binding of human neutrophils to cell-surface anchored Tamm-Horsfall glycoprotein in tubulointerstitial nephritis. Kidney Int. 1999;55:1787–99.

42. Ikeda M, Takemura T, Hino S, Yoshioka K. Molecular cloning, expression, and chromosomal localization of a human tubulointerstitial nephritis antigen. Biochem Biophys Res Commun. 2000;268:225–30.

43. Takemura Y, Koshimichi M, Sugimoto K, et al. A tubulointerstitial nephritis antigen gene defect causes childhood-onset chronic renal failure. Pediatr Nephrol. 2010;25:1349–53.

44. Wilson CB. Individual and strain differences in renal basement membrane antigens. Transplant Proc. 1980; 12(Suppl):69–73.

45. Sugusaki T, Kano K, Andres G, et al. Antibodies to tubular basement membrane elicited by stimulation with allogenic kidney. Kidney Int. 1980;21:557–64.

46. Fasth AL, Hoyer JR, Seiler MW. Extratubular Tamm-Horsfall protein deposits induced by ureteral obstruction in mice. Clin Immunol Immunopathol. 1988;47:47–61.

47. Mayrer AR, Miniter P, Andriole VT. Immunopathogenesis of chronic pyelonephritis. Am J Med. 1983;75:59–70.

48. Sherlock JE. Interstitial nephritis in rats produced by *E. coli* in adjuvant: Immunological findings. Clin Exp Immunol. 1977;30:154–9.

49. Border WA, Lehman DH, Egan JD, et al. Antitubular basement-membrane antibodies in methicillin-associated interstitial nephritis. N Engl J Med. 1974;291:381–4.

50. McCluskey RT, Colvin RB. Immunologic aspects of renal tubular and interstitial diseases. Annu Rev Med. 1978;29:191–203.

51. Becker JL, Miller F, Nuovo GJ, et al. Epstein-Barr virus infection of renal proximal tubule cells: Possible role in chronic interstitial nephritis. J Clin Invest. 1999;104:1673–81.

52. Bruggeman LA, Ross MD, Tanji N, et al. Renal epithelium is a previously unrecognized site of HIV-1 infection. J Am Soc Nephrol. 2000;11:2079–87.

53. Wuthrich RP, Glimcher LH, Yui MA, et al. MHC class II, antigen presentation and tumor necrosis factor in renal tubular epithelial cells. Kidney Int. 1990;37:783–92.

54. Mendrick DL, Kelly DM, Rennke HG. Antigen processing and presentation by glomerular visceral epithelium in vitro. Kidney Int. 1991;39:71–8.

55. Tang WW, Feng L, Mathison JC, Wilson CB. Cytokine expression, upregulation of intercellular adhesion molecule-1, and leukocyte infiltration in experimental tubulointerstitial nephritis. Lab Invest. 1994;70:631–8.

56. Wuthrich RP. Intercellular adhesion molecules and vascular cell adhesion molecule-1 and the kidney. J Am Soc Nephrol. 1992;3:1201–11.

57. Wuthrich RP, Sibalic V. Autoimmune tubulointerstitial nephritis: Insight from experimental models. Exp Nephrol. 1998;6:288–93.

58. Halloran PF, Jephthah-Ochola J, Urmson J, Farkas S. Systemic immunologic stimuli increase class I and II antigen expression in mouse kidney. J Immunol. 1985;135:1053–60.

59. Neilson EG, Phillips SM. Murine interstitial nephritis. I. Analysis of disease susceptibility and its relationship of pleiomorphic gene products defining both immune-response genes and a restrictive requirement for cytotoxic T cells at H-2K. J Exp Med. 1982;155:1075–85.

60. Neilson EG, Clayman MD, Haverty T, et al. Experimental strategies for the study of cellular immunity in renal disease. Kidney Int. 1986;30:264–79.

61. Neilson EG, Zakheim B. T cell regulation, anti-idiotypic immunity, and the nephritogenic immune response. Kidney Int. 1983;24:289–302.

62. Halloran PF, Wadgymar A, Autenried P. The regulation of expression of major histocompatibility complex products. Transplantation. 1986;41:413–20.

63. Kelly CJ, Roth DA, Meyers CM. Immune recognition and response to the renal interstitium. Kidney Int. 1991;39:518–30.

64. Mann R, Zakheim B, Clayman M, et al. Murine interstitial nephritis. IV. Long-term cultured L3T4+ T cell lines transfer delayed expression of disease as I-A-restricted inducers of the effector T cell repertoire. J Immunol. 1985;135:286–93.

65. Mann R, Kelly CJ, Hines WH, et al. Effector T cell differentiation in experimental interstitial nephritis. I. The development and modulation of effector lymphocyte maturation by I-J+ regulatory T cells. J Immunol. 1987;138:4200–8.

66. Meyers CM, Kelly CJ. Effector mechanisms in organ-specific autoimmunity. I. Characterization of a CD8+ T cell line that mediates murine interstitial nephritis. J Clin Invest. 1991;88:408–16.

67. Wilson C. The renal response to immunological injury. In: Brenner BM, Rector FD Jr, editors. The Kidney, 4th ed. Philadelphia: WB Saunders; 1991.

68. Wilson CB, Lehman DH, McCoy RC, et al. Antitubular basement membrane antibodies after renal transplantation. Transplantation. 1974;18:447–52.

69. Lehman DH, Wilson CB, Dixon FJ. Extraglomerular immunoglobulin deposits in human nephritis. Am J Med. 1975;58:765–96.

70. Zager RA, Cotran RS, Hoyer JR. Pathologic localization of Tamm-Horsfall protein in interstitial deposits in renal disease. Lab Invest. 1978;38:52–7.

71. Harris DC. Tubulointerstitial renal disease. Curr Opin Nephrol Hypertens. 2001;10:303–13.

72. Remuzzi G, Bertani T. Pathophysiology of progressive nephropathies. N Engl J Med. 1998;339:1448–56.

73. Strutz F, Neilson EG. The role of lymphocytes in the progression of interstitial disease. Kidney Int Suppl. 1994;45:S106–10.

74. Rerolle JP, Hertig A, Nguyen G, et al. Plasminogen activator inhibitor type 1 is a potential target in renal fibrogenesis. Kidney Int. 2000;58:1841–50.

75. Isaka Y, Tsujie M, Ando Y, et al. Transforming growth factor-beta 1 antisense oligodeoxynucleotides block interstitial fibrosis in unilateral ureteral obstruction. Kidney Int. 2000;58:1885–92.

76. Clarkson MR, Giblin L, O'Connell FP, et al. Acute interstitial nephritis: Clinical features and response to corticosteroid therapy. Nephrol Dial Transplant. 2004;19:2778–83.

77. Murray MD, Brater DC. Renal toxicity of the nonsteroidal anti-inflammatory drugs. Annu Rev Pharmacol Toxicol. 1993;33:435–65.

78. Rossert J. Drug-induced acute interstitial nephritis. Kidney Int. 2001;60:804–17.

79. Brezin JH, Katz SM, Schwartz AB, Chinitz JL. Reversible renal failure and nephrotic syndrome associated with nonsteroidal anti-inflammatory drugs. N Engl J Med. 1979;301:1271–3.

80. Ruffing KA, Hoppes P, Blend D, et al. Eosinophils in urine revisited. Clin Nephrol. 1994;41:163–6.

81. Dehne MG, Boldt J, Heise D, et al. Tamm-Horsfall protein, alpha-1- and beta-2-microglobulin as kidney function markers in heart surgery. Anaesthesist. 1995;44:545–51.

82. Tsai CY, Wu TH, Yu CL, et al. Increased excretions of beta2-microglobulin, IL-6, and IL-8 and decreased excretion of Tamm-Horsfall glycoprotein in urine of patients with active lupus nephritis. Nephron. 2000;85:207–14.

83. Wu Y, Yang L, Su T, et al. Pathological significance of a panel of urinary biomarkers in patients with drug-induced tubulointerstitial nephritis. Clin J Am Soc Nephrol. 2010;5:1954–9.

84. Shi Y, Su T, Qu L, et al. Evaluation of urinary biomarkers for the prognosis of drug-associated chronic tubulointerstitial nephritis. Am J Med Sci. 2013;346:283–8.

85. Gonzalez E, Gutierrez E, Galeano C, et al. Early steroid treatment improves the recovery of renal function in patients with drug-induced acute interstitial nephritis. Kidney Int. 2008;73:940–6.

86. Raza MN, Hadid, Keen CE, et al. Acute tubulointerstitial nephritis, treatment with steroid and impact on renal outcomes. Nephrology. 2012;17:748–53.

87. Jahnukainen T, Ala-Houhala M, Karikoski R, et al. Clinical outcome and occurrence of uveitis in children with idiopathic tubulointerstitial nephritis. Pediatr Nephrol. 2011;26:291–9.

88. Jahnukainen T, Saarela V, Arikoski P, et al. Prednisone in the treatment of tubulointerstitial nephritis in children. Pediatr Nephrol. 2013;28:1253–60.

89. Preddie DC, Markowitz GS, Radhakrishnan J, et al. Mycophenolate mofetil for the treatment of interstitial nephritis. Clin J Am Soc Nephrol. 2006;1:718–22.

90. Moudgil A, Przygodzki RM, Kher KK. Successful steroid-sparing treatment of renal limited sarcoidosis with mycophenolate mofetil. Pediatr Nephrol. 2006;21:281–5.

91. Leeaphorn N, Stokes MB, Ungprasert P, et al. Idiopathic granulomatous interstitial nephritis responsive to mycophenolate mofetil therapy. Am J Kidney Dis. 2014;63:696–9.

92. Laberke HG, Bohle A. Acute interstitial nephritis: Correlations between clinical and morphological findings. Clin Nephrol. 1980;14:263–73.

93. Ivanyi B, Hamilton-Dutoit SJ, Hansen HE, Olsen S. Acute tubulointerstitial nephritis: Phenotype of infiltrating cells and prognostic impact of tubulitis. Virchows Arc. 1996;428:5–12.

94. Bhaumik SK, Kher V, Arora P, et al. Evaluation of clinical and histological prognostic markers in drug-induced acute interstitial nephritis. Ren Fail. 1996;18:97–104.

95. Kida H, Abe T, Tomosugi N, et al. Prediction of the long-term outcome in acute interstitial nephritis. Clin Nephrol. 1984;22:55–60.

96. Myers BD, Ross J, Newton L, et al. Cyclosporine-associated chronic nephropathy. N Engl J Med. 1984;311:699–705.

97. Dobrin R, Vernier R, Fish A. Acute eosinophilic interstitial nephritis and renal failure with bone marrow–lymph node granulomas and anterior uveitis. Am J Med. 1975;59:325–33.

98. Mandeville JT, Levinson RD, Holland GN. The tubulointerstitial nephritis and uveitis syndrome. Surv Ophthalmol 2001;46:195–208.

99. Dusek J, Urbanova I, Stejskal J, et al. Tubulointerstitial nephritis and uveitis syndrome in a mother and her son. Pediatr Nephrol. 2008;23:2091–3.

100. Saarela V, Nuutinen M, Ala-Houala M et al. Tubulointerstitial nephritis and uveitis syndrome in children: A prospective multicenter study. Ophthalmology. 2013;120:1476–81.

101. Levinson RD, Park MS, Rikkers SM, et al. Strong associations among specific HLA-DQ and HLA-DR alleles and the tubulointerstitial nephritis and uveitis syndrome. Invest Ophthalmol Vis Sci. 2003;44:653–7.

## REVIEW QUESTIONS

1. Which of the following is true regarding drug-induced ATIN?
   a. ATIN secondary to NSAIDs can present as nephrotic syndrome.
   b. The triad of fever, rash, and arthralgia is present in the majority of patients with drug-induced ATIN.
   c. Eosinophiluria is pathognomonic for ATIN.
   d. Renal injury always develops soon after starting the offending drug.
   e. Drug-induced ATIN is dose-dependent.

2. The typical features on light microscopy of a kidney biopsy in a patient with ATIN are:
   a. Tubular atrophy and interstitial fibrosis with minimal interstitial inflammatory cell infiltration
   b. Diffuse endocapillary proliferation with crescents and necrosis
   c. Diffuse thickening of the glomerular basement membrane
   d. Diffuse mesangial proliferation
   e. Interstitial mononuclear cell infiltration with variable degrees of tubular necrosis and regeneration

3. A 15-year-old boy with a history of obstructive uropathy who received a kidney transplant 8 years ago has an elevated creatinine level. Renal biopsy shows interstitial stripe fibrosis and tubular atrophy. These findings are characteristic of:
   a. Interstitial nephritis secondary to BK virus
   b. Acute cellular rejection
   c. Calcineurin inhibitor chronic interstitial damage
   d. Interstitial nephritis secondary to NSAIDs use
   e. Chronic transplant nephropathy

4. A 5-year-old girl presents with fever, fatigue, and abdominal pain and is admitted to the hospital because of AKI with a creatinine value of 1.3. According to history obtained, she had been taking amoxicillin for 4 days for strep throat. Her physical examination is normal; her urinalysis reveals a specific gravity of 1.009, negative findings for blood and protein, 10 to 20 white blood cells, and no casts. You suspect ATIN secondary to amoxicillin. Which of the following is the next *best* step in her management?
   a. Schedule her for a renal biopsy.
   b. Discontinue amoxicillin and follow creatinine trend.
   c. Administer pulse corticosteroids followed by oral prednisone.
   d. Check eosinophils in the urine, if negative, continue workup looking for other causes of AKI.
   e. Change amoxicillin to a cephalosporin.

5. Which of the following urinary biomarkers has been associated with the acute changes seen in ATIN?
   a. N-acetyl-$\beta$-D-glucosaminidase (NAG)
   b. Kidney injury molecule-1 (KIM-1)
   c. Neutrophil gelatinase-associated lipocalin (NGAL)
   d. Monocyte chemotactic peptide-1 (MCP-1)
   e. $\beta_2$-Microglobulin

6. A 10-year-old boy presents with nonoliguric AKI. He has a renal biopsy performed that shows severe interstitial inflammation with predominant mononuclear cell infiltrate and no granulomas; immunofluorescence is negative. There is no history of medication use or evidence of any viral or bacterial infection. The patient receives corticosteroids and his renal function returns to normal. Regarding further evaluation and follow-up, which of the following is the *most* accurate statement?
   a. He will need follow-up with a nephrologist for at least 1 year.
   b. He can follow up with his primary care physician for yearly checkups only and does not need specialty care.
   c. He needs an ophthalmology evaluation now and every 3 months for the next year in addition to follow-up with a nephrologist.
   d. He needs follow-up with a rheumatologist because of the possibility of underlying autoimmune disease.

7. A 12-year-old girl, previously healthy, presents with nausea and vomiting. She has been taking ibuprofen for a knee injury for the last 7 days. She has mild pitting edema on both lower extremities. Her laboratory results reveal significant proteinuria with a ratio of urine protein to creatinine of 5.9, elevated serum creatinine of 3.5 mg/dL, normal electrolytes, and a low serum albumin of 2.0 g/dL. You suspect ATIN secondary to NSAIDs and stop the medication. Over the next 2 days her creatinine continues to rise and you decide to perform a renal biopsy. Which of the following would be the *most* appropriate step in her management while you wait for the results of her biopsy?
   a. Administer albumin followed by furosemide
   b. Administer intravenous fluids
   c. Check complements and serologic findings and test for viral and bacterial infections
   d. Start intravenous methylprednisolone 10 mg/kg
   e. Start mycophenolate mofetil

8. Which of the following condition can cause secondary tubulointerstitial nephritis?
   a. Membranous nephropathy
   b. Inflammatory bowel disease
   c. Systemic lupus erythematosus
   d. IgA nephropathy
   e. All of the above

9. Regarding CTIN, which of the following statements is true?
   a. In children, the most common cause of CTIN is lupus nephritis.
   b. NSAIDs are the most common causes of drug-related CTIN in children.
   c. CTIN progresses rapidly to end-stage renal disease.
   d. Polyuria, polydipsia, and nocturnal enuresis may be the only manifesting symptoms in children with CTIN.
   e. Corticosteroids are effective in the treatment of CTIN.

10. Regarding prognosis of ATIN in children, which of the following statements is true?
    a. The recovery of renal function depends on the severity of disease at presentation.
    b. Prognosis is independent from the presence of tubular atrophy.
    c. Prognosis is worse in patients with underlying renal disease and when there is prolonged oliguria (more than 3 weeks).
    d. Most children with ATIN progress slowly to CTIN.
    e. All of the above.

## ANSWER KEY

1. a
2. e
3. c
4. b
5. a
6. c
7. d
8. e
9. d
10. c

# Kidney in systemic diseases

# 26

# Lupus nephritis

CARLA M. NESTER, DAVID B. THOMAS, AND DEBBIE S. GIPSON

Systemic lupus erythematosus (SLE) is a rheumatologic disease associated with significant morbidity and mortality in children.[1–11] It is a chronic autoimmune, inflammatory disease well known for affecting multiple organ systems including the kidney. Presenting symptoms and disease-defining clinical parameters are protean[12,13] (Table 26.1). The pathology of SLE is complex, and disease results from a combination of an inherent susceptibility to the environment and genetically determined abnormalities in the immune system. Although SLE is less common in children than in adults, renal involvement *(lupus nephritis)* in children is more common and more severe than in adults.[14] Lupus nephritis is seen in 60% to 80% of children at presentation, depending on the patient's age and ethnicity.[15,16] When lupus nephritis is not part of the initial constellation, it is likely to evolve and often becomes one of the most significant prognostic factors for long-term morbidity and mortality in a child with this disease.[17–20]

estimated prevalence in the general population of 50 per 100,000 when all ages are included.[24] Variations in the reported prevalence of SLE are likely to be influenced by referral bias, as well as the ethnic makeup of the selected populations studied. The relative risk of SLE in nonwhite pubescent girls compared with white pubescent girls has been estimated to be 7 for Asian girls, 4.5 for African-American girls, and 3 for Hispanic girls.[18] The burden of SLE in the African-American and Hispanic populations is compounded by an increased severity and worse prognosis.[21,25]

## KEY POINTS

- Renal involvement in lupus is both more common and more severe in children than in adults.
- The relative risk of SLE is higher in Asian, African-American, and Hispanic girls and women.

## EPIDEMIOLOGY

SLE is significantly more common in girls and women than in boys and men.[21] The female-to-male ratio rises from 2:1 in prepubertal children, to 4.5:1 in adolescence, and finally to approximately 10:1 in adults.[22,23] The prevalence of SLE in children is estimated to be as high as 10 per 100,000 individuals, compared with an

## PATHOGENESIS

A complete understanding of the pathologic underpinnings of SLE remains to be defined. The production of pathogenic autoantibodies represents the hallmark of SLE and indicates that a major component of the pathology is loss of *immune tolerance*.[26] The acceptance of self-antigens is known as tolerance. Normally, B cells

Table 26.1 Clinical manifestations of systemic lupus erythematosus in children*

| Clinical and laboratory features | Manifestations in patients N = 189 (%) | Manifestations in <8 year olds (%) | Manifestations in 8–12 year olds (%) | Manifestations in >12 year olds (%) | P value |
|---|---|---|---|---|---|
| Malar rash | 67 | 36 | 70 | 69 | 0.05 |
| Discoid rash | 4 | 7 | 2 | 4 | 0.43 |
| Photosensitivity | 28 | 21 | 29 | 28 | 0.93 |
| Oral ulcers | 35 | 29 | 39 | 34 | 0.69 |
| Arthritis | 37 | 29 | 34 | 40 | 0.59 |
| Serositis | | | | | |
|   Pericarditis | 5 | 0 | 9 | 5 | 0.45 |
|   Pleuritis | 13 | 7 | 11 | 17 | 0.50 |
| Nephritis | | | | | |
|   Proteinuria | 51 | 57 | 48 | 52 | 0.79 |
|   Hematuria | 44 | 71 | 39 | 44 | 0.09 |
|   Cellular casts | 11 | 7 | 11 | 11 | 1.00 |
| Neurologic involvement | 11 | 14 | 7 | 12 | 0.56 |
| Hematologic involvement | | | | | |
|   Leukopenia | 32 | 29 | 32 | 32 | 1.00 |
|   Hemolytic anemia | 30 | 36 | 34 | 28 | 0.65 |
|   Lymphopenia | 53 | 36 | 41 | 61 | 0.02 |
|   Thrombocytopenia | 31 | 14 | 36 | 30 | 0.31 |
| Immune abnormalities | | | | | |
|   Anti-dsDNA antibody | 94 | 100 | 93 | 93 | 0.79 |
|   Anti-Smith antibody | 21 | 21 | 11 | 12 | 0.55 |
|   Antinuclear antibody | 99 | 100 | 100 | 98 | 1.00 |

Source: Adapted from Lee PY, Yeh KW, Yao TC, et al. The outcome of patients with renal involvement in pediatric-onset systemic lupus erythematosus-a 20-year experience in Asia. Lupus. 2013;22:1534–40.

* Renal disease is seen in more than 50% patients. Data are representative of an Asian population.

that are able to recognize an individual's own antigens are tightly controlled and eliminated. SLE is characterized by a global loss of self-tolerance and activation of autoreactive T and B cells.[27] The results are the production of pathogenic autoantibodies and tissue injury. Autoantibodies are produced to self-antigens such as DNA, nuclear proteins, and certain cytoplasmic proteins.[28] The stimulus for generation of these autoantibodies is likely fostered by a failure to clear apoptotic debris containing nuclear proteins and chromatin effectively.[29] These self-antigens are then recognized by the abnormal, self-reactive B cells. B-cell and T-cell cooperation leading to B-cell activation results in the creation of both effector and memory B cells. Effector B cells release immunoglobulin G (IgG) autoantibodies into the circulation that form antigen-antibody complexes. These complexes accumulate in the small vessels of organs, where they stimulate local inflammation by activating complement pathways and by binding of Fc receptors, thus leading to mast cell degranulation and local infiltration of macrophages and neutrophils. This aberrant immune regulation provides the backdrop for maladaptive responses to environmental antigens.

As another measure of the complexity of SLE, there are now more than 60 genetic loci associated with this disease (Table 26.2).[30–60] The genetic susceptibility to SLE is supported by familial aggregation, the disease concordance rate in twins, and the increased sibling risk for SLE.[61–66] The genetic contribution appears to involve multiple loci with small to modest individual effect.

## KEY POINT

Lupus nephritis results from aberrant immune regulation and is influenced by both environmental factors and genetic risk.

Because SLE may affect the vascular, glomerular, and tubulointerstitial compartments of the kidney to differing degrees, lupus nephritis can manifest in a variety of histologic patterns. Glomerular involvement results not only from the deposition of immune complexes but also from glomerular response and injury caused by antigen specificity and complement stimulation. The pathologic classification of lupus nephritis is based on the criteria set forth by the International Society of Nephrology (ISN) and the Renal Pathology Society (RPS).[67,68] This

Table 26.2 Genes associated with systemic lupus susceptibility*

| | | | | | |
|---|---|---|---|---|---|
| FCGR2A | HLA-DR3 | C1q | TNIP1 | PTTG1 | ACP5 |
| FCGR3A | IKZF1 | C1s | UBE2L3 | PXK | ELF1 |
| FCGR2B | IL21 | C2 | C1r | TMEM39A | ETS1 |
| FCGR3B | LYN | C4 | ATG5 | TNXB | IFIH1 |
| TREX1 | MSH5 | FAS | DNASE1 | UHRFiBP1 | IRAK1 |
| TYK2 | NCF2 | FASL | DNASE1L3 | WDFY4 | IRF5 |
| AFF1 | PRDM1 | FcR | GSR | XKR6 | IRF7 |
| BANK1 | PTPN22 | UBE2L3 | NDUFS4 | ICAM | IRF8 |
| BLK | STAT4 | PRKCB | NOS1 | IL10 | TLR7 |
| HLA-DR2 | TNFSF4 | SLC15A4 | CLEC16A | IFR8 | |
| ETS1 | UBASH3A | TNFAIP3 | JAZF1 | ITGAM | |

* These genes, which are involved in immune complex processing, T- and B-cell signally, interferon pathways, Toll-like receptor function, and multiple other pathways, have been implicated in the pathogenesis of systemic lupus erythematosus.

classification system is a refinement of the historical World Health Organization (WHO) classification system, with the major advances being (1) elimination of the normal biopsy category, (2) elimination of the subcategories of membranous class V lupus, (3) sharper delineations among all the classes, and (4) the addition of subclasses to the diffuse proliferative (class IV) lupus nephritis category. Although the ISN classification is the preferred system, familiarity with the WHO classification system is essential because most available trial data are based on this older classification.

# PATHOLOGY

The WHO classification of lupus nephritis has been in use in clinical studies since the 1980s (Table 26.3). In 2003, the ISN and RPS provided further refinement of the pathologic classification of lupus nephritis (Table 26.4). An abbreviated version of this classification for clinical use is given in Table 26.5.

Class I lupus nephritis is minimal mesangial lupus nephritis. The glomeruli are normal by light microscopy, but there is evidence of renal involvement by immune

Table 26.3 World health organization classification of systemic lupus erythematosus (modified in 1982)

| | |
|---|---|
| Class I | **Normal glomeruli** |
| | a. Nil (by all techniques) |
| | b. Normal by light microscopy, but deposits by electron or immunofluorescence microscopy |
| Class II | **Pure mesangial alterations (mesangiopathy)** |
| | a. Mesangial widening and/or mild hypercellularity (+) |
| | b. Moderate hypercellularity (++) |
| Class III | **Focal segmental glomerulonephritis (associated with mild or moderate mesangial alterations)** |
| | a. With active necrotizing lesions |
| | b. With active and sclerosing lesions |
| | c. With sclerosing lesions |
| Class IV | **Diffuse glomerulonephritis (severe mesangial, endocapillary, or mesangiocapillary proliferation and/or extensive subendothelial deposits)** |
| | a. Without segmental lesions |
| | b. With active necrotizing lesions |
| | c. With active and sclerosing lesions |
| | d. With sclerosing lesions |
| Class V | **Diffuse membranous glomerulonephritis** |
| | a. Pure membranous glomerulonephritis |
| | b. Associated with lesions of category II (a or b) |
| | c. Associated with lesions of category III (a–c) |
| | d. Associated with lesions of category IV (a–d) |
| Class VI | **Advanced sclerosing glomerulonephritis** |

*Source:* Weening JJ, D'Agati VD, Schwartz MM, et al. The classification of glomerulonephritis in systemic lupus erythematosus revisited. Kidney Int. 2004;65:521–30.

+, ++, an integer scoring system of 0, + = 1, ++ = 2, etc., with increasing number reflecting worsening hypercellularity.

Table 26.4 Detailed International Society Of Nephrology/Renal Pathology Society 2003 classification of lupus nephritis

| | |
|---|---|
| **Class I** | **Minimal mesangial lupus nephritis** |
| | Normal glomeruli by light microscopy, but mesangial immune deposits by immunofluorescence |
| **Class II** | **Mesangial proliferative lupus nephritis** |
| | Purely mesangial hypercellularity of any degree or mesangial matrix expansion by light microscopy, with mesangial immune deposits |
| | A few isolated subepithelial or subendothelial deposits possibly visible by immunofluorescence or electron microscopy, but not by light microscopy |
| **Class III** | **Focal lupus nephritis**[a] |
| | Active or inactive focal, segmental, or global endocapillary or extracapillary glomerulonephritis involving <50% of all glomeruli, typically with focal subendothelial immune deposits, with or without mesangial alterations |
| **Class III (A)** | Active lesions: focal proliferative lupus nephritis |
| **Class III (A/C)** | Active and chronic lesions: focal proliferative and sclerosing lupus nephritis |
| **Class III (C)** | Chronic inactive lesions with glomerular scars: focal sclerosing lupus nephritis |
| **Class IV** | **Diffuse lupus nephritis**[b] |
| | Active or inactive diffuse, segmental, or global endocapillary or extracapillary glomerulonephritis involving ≥50% of all glomeruli, typically with diffuse subendothelial immune deposits, with or without mesangial alterations; this class is divided into diffuse segmental (IV-S) lupus nephritis when ≥50% of the involved glomeruli have segmental lesions, and diffuse global (IV-G) lupus nephritis when ≥50% of the involved glomeruli have global lesions; segmental is defined as a glomerular lesion that involves less than half of the glomerular tuft; this class includes cases with diffuse wire loop deposits but with little or no glomerular proliferation |
| **Class IV-S (A)** | Active lesions: diffuse segmental proliferative lupus nephritis |
| **Class IV-G (A)** | Active lesions: diffuse global proliferative lupus nephritis |
| **Class IV-S (A/C)** | Active and chronic lesions: diffuse segmental proliferative and sclerosing lupus nephritis |
| **Class IV-G (A/C)** | Active and chronic lesions: diffuse global proliferative and sclerosing lupus nephritis |
| **Class IV-S (C)** | Chronic inactive lesions with scars: diffuse segmental sclerosing lupus nephritis |
| **Class IV-G (C)** | Chronic inactive lesions with scars: diffuse global sclerosing lupus nephritis |
| **Class V** | **Membranous lupus nephritis** |
| | Global or segmental subepithelial immune deposits or their morphologic sequelae by light microscopy and by immunofluorescence or electron microscopy, with or without mesangial alterations |
| | Class V lupus nephritis possible in combination with class III or IV, in which case both classes will be diagnosed |
| | Class V lupus nephritis possibly showing advanced sclerosis |
| **Class VI** | **Advanced sclerotic lupus nephritis** |
| | ≥90% of glomeruli globally sclerosed without residual activity |

Source: Weening JJ, D'Agati VD, Schwartz MM, et al. The classification of glomerulonephritis in systemic lupus erythematosus revisited. Kidney Int. 2004;65:521–30.
[a] Indicates the proportion of glomeruli with active and with sclerotic lesions.
[b] Indicates the proportion of glomeruli with fibrinoid necrosis and/or cellular crescents.

complex deposition that is visible on immunofluorescence microscopy or electron microscopy (Figure 26.1). Class II lupus nephritis includes mesangioproliferative lesions visible by light microscopy (Figure 26.2). Class III focal proliferative lupus nephritis is defined as nephritis involving less than 50% of all glomeruli and is divided

Table 26.5 Abbreviated International Society Of Nephrology/Renal Pathology Society 2003 classification of lupus nephritis[*]

| | |
|---|---|
| Class I | Minimal mesangial lupus nephritis |
| Class II | Mesangial proliferative lupus nephritis |
| Class III | Focal lupus nephritis[a] |
| Class IV | Diffuse segmental (IV-S) or global (IV-G) lupus nephritis[b] |
| Class V | Membranous lupus nephritis[c] |
| Class VI | Advanced sclerosing lupus nephritis |

Source: Weening JJ, D'Agati VD, Schwartz MM, et al. The classification of glomerulonephritis in systemic lupus erythematosus revisited. Kidney Int. 2004;65:521–30.
[*] Indications and grading (mild, moderate, severe) tubular atrophy, interstitial inflammation and fibrosis, severity of arteriosclerosis, or other vascular lesions, when seen in the biopsy.
[a] Indicates the proportion of glomeruli with active lesions and with sclerotic lesions.
[b] Indicates the proportion of glomeruli with fibrinoid necrosis and cellular crescents.
[c] Class V may occur in combination with class III or IV, in which case both classes will be diagnosed.

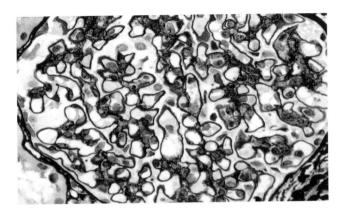

Figure 26.1 Class I (ISN/RPS 2003) minimal mesangial lupus glomerulonephritis. Glomeruli are normal by light microscopy but are positive for immune complex deposition by immunofluorescence microscopy.

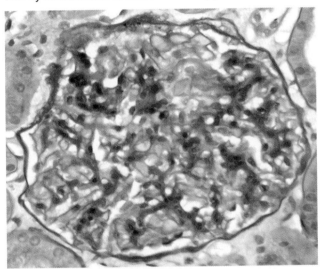

Figure 26.2 Class II (ISN/RPS 2003) mesangial proliferative lupus glomerulonephritis: only mesangial proliferation (more than three mesangial cells per mesangial area in a 3-μm section) with any degree of matrix expansion by light microscopy, positive immunofluorescence microscopy, and electron microscopy for immune complex deposition (original magnification: 200×, periodic acid–Schiff stain).

into active (A) and chronic (C) lesions. The active lesions include endocapillary hypercellularity, leukocyte infiltrates, karyorrhexis, necrosis, cellular crescents, and hyaline thrombi. The chronic lesions are characterized by sclerosis, adhesions, or fibrous crescents. Class IV diffuse proliferative lupus nephritis involves the same lesions as in class III, but with greater than 50% of all glomeruli affected with active, chronic, or both (acute and chronic) findings (Figure 26.3). Additionally, class IV is subdivided into global (G), involving the entire affected glomerulus, or segmental (S), affecting less than half of the affected glomerulus (Figure 26.4). Class V lupus nephritis

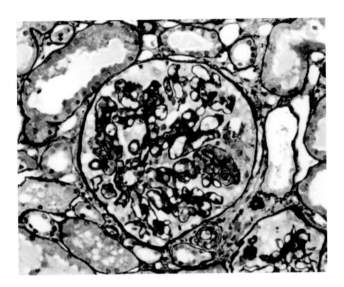

Figure 26.3 Lupus nephritis class III (A). Light micrograph showing a glomerulus with segmental endocapillary hypercellularity, mesangial hypercellularity, capillary wall thickening, and early segmental capillary necrosis (methenamine silver). (From Weening JJ, D'Agati VD, Schwartz MM, et al. The classification of glomerulonephritis in systemic lupus erythematosus revisited. Kidney Int. 2004;65:521–30.)

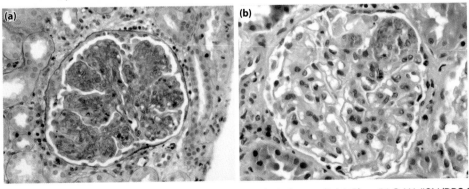

Figure 26.4 Class IV lesions involve greater than 50% of the total sampled glomeruli. (a) Class IV-G (A) (ISN/RPS 2003) diffuse proliferative lupus glomerulonephritis. The endocapillary hypercellularity involves more than half the individual tuft in greater than 50% of glomeruli sampled. The active or chronic tubulointerstitial injury and vascular findings are reported separately. (b) Class IV-S (A) (ISN/RPS 2003) diffuse proliferative glomerulonephritis. Glomeruli have segmental (less than 50% of the individual glomerulus) tuft injury but lesions are present in greater than 50% of the total sampled glomeruli. In this example with necrosis at the 1 o'clock position. Both images (a) and (b) are active lesions ("A") with no chronic glomerular capillary tuft injury (e.g. "C").

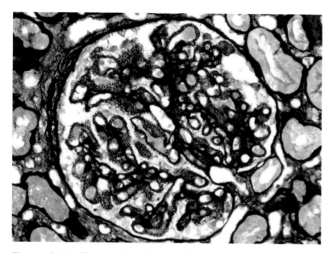

Figure 26.5 Class V (ISN/RPS 2003) membranous lupus glomerulonephritis. Light microscopy, immunofluorescence microscopy, and electron microscopy reveal subepithelial deposits that are global, segmental, or diffusely distributed. Associated mesangial alterations are frequently present. When a class V lesion has additional tuft abnormalities, then a designation of combine class V and III or IV is warranted, depending on the distribution of the additional lesions.

is membranous lupus nephritis and is characterized by subepithelial deposits in the majority of capillary loops (Figure 26.5). Class V lupus nephritis may be coincident with class III and class IV lesions. Class VI sclerosing lupus nephritis is the end result (chronic lesions) of renal lupus involvement, with more than 90% globally sclerotic glomeruli (Figure 26.6). In the Glomerular Disease Collaborative Network patient registry (Table 26.6), the diffuse proliferative lesion (class IV) was the most commonly observed pathologic feature (54%).

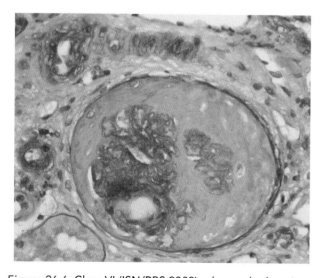

Figure 26.6 Class VI (ISN/RPS 2003) advanced sclerosis lupus glomerulonephritis. Glomerular sclerosis was present in greater than 90% of glomeruli, without any residual acuity of lesions.

Table 26.6 Distribution of classification of lupus nephritis lesions in children and adolescents from the Glomerular Disease Collaborative Network patient registry.

| Classification | Lesion | N = 80 | Percentage (%) |
|---|---|---|---|
| I | Mesangial immune complex | 3 | 4 |
| II | Mesangioproliferative | 12 | 15 |
| III | Focal proliferative | 14 | 17 |
| IV | Diffuse proliferative | 43 | 54 |
| V | Membranous | 8 | 10 |
| VI | Sclerosis | 0 | 0 |

*Solution:* Data from Clinical Coordinating Center, University of North Carolina, Division of Nephrology and Hypertension, Chapel Hill, NC.

Immunofluorescence in SLE nephritis is associated with granular deposition of IgA, IgG, IgM and complements C3, C4, and C1q in the capillary walls and the mesangium. This pattern of extensive glomerular immune deposition is sometimes referred to as a "full house" immune localization and is characteristic of lupus nephritis. Although IgA nephropathy and Henoch-Schönlein purpura (HSP) nephritis also have IgA glomerular deposition, "full house" immune deposition is not characteristically observed in either of these clinical disorders.

## KEY POINTS

- Polyclonal (kappa and lambda) IgG and complement components (C3, C1q) are characteristic of lupus nephritis glomerular deposits.
- When all three immunoglobulin isotypes, IgG, IgM and IgA are present, the pattern is often referred to as "full house" staining.

## CLINICAL MANIFESTATIONS

The initial presentation of SLE is typically recognized by the extrarenal symptoms. SLE is often more acute and more severe with onset in children before the age of 16 years.[69,70] The aggregates of immune complexes in SLE can deposit throughout the body, with resulting multiorgan systemic involvement and a broad spectrum of possible clinical presentations.[13,16,23,71] As the disease progresses, additional organ system involvement can alter the individual patient's clinical manifestations. Generalized symptoms of fever, fatigue, weight loss, and anorexia are common. Abdominal pain caused either by vasculitis or by serositis occurs frequently in children with SLE. Rash occurs in more than 50% of patients with SLE, and alopecia is also frequent.[16,72,73] Musculoskeletal complaints, such as arthralgias, arthritis, myalgias, or myositis, occur in nearly 86% of children; both large and small joints are affected similarly.[72,73]

Pulmonary involvement occurs in more than 75% of children, and it can manifest as pleuritis, dyspnea, and restrictive lung disease. Pericarditis and endocarditis are well-known clinical indicators of cardiac involvement in pediatric SLE. Neuropsychiatric symptoms, typically attributable to central nervous system vasculitis, are frequent in pediatric SLE and include headache, chorea, cranial nerve palsies, seizures, and psychiatric and behavioral problems. Hematologic abnormalities such as normochromic, normocytic anemia, hemolytic anemia, neutropenia, lymphopenia and thrombocytopenia are common. Manifestations of "polyserositis," such synovitis, pleuritis, and pericarditis, should raise the diagnostic concern of SLE in patients with multisystem disease.

Justification for initial and serial evaluation for renal disease in SLE is supported by the observation that up to 80% of children with SLE develop nephritis over the course of their disease.[22] Clinically evident lupus nephritis may produce a combination of hematuria, proteinuria, edema, diminished glomerular filtration rate, or hypertension. Abnormal urinary sediment consisting of cellular casts and sterile pyuria secondary to renal inflammation is frequently present. Renal tubular dysfunction may be present, and this can manifest as metabolic acidosis, normoglycemic glycosuria, and electrolyte imbalance, especially hyperkalemia.

## EVALUATION AND DIAGNOSIS

The diagnosis of lupus nephritis most often is made in a patient with other signs and symptoms of SLE. The clinical history and examination should prompt the screening for serum antinuclear antibodies (ANAs). In patients with SLE, these autoantibodies associate with their complementary antigen and form immune complexes that either are detected in the circulation or are found as immune deposits in tissue biopsy specimens. The immunofluorescent ANA screen allows for the detection of antibodies that bind an array of potential nuclear antigens such as DNA, RNA, and proteins. Although ANAs are present in as many as 95% of patients with SLE, as many as 30% of persons with a positive screening ANA titer of 1:40 are healthy and without lupus.[74] The false-positive rate drops to 3% if the reported titer is 1:320. Because diseases other than SLE are associated with positive ANA test results, the predictive value of a positive test result depends on the test population. In patients with other rheumatic and collagen vascular diseases, a positive ANA test result

may have only a 20% to 35% predictive value for SLE.[75] However, the negative predictive value, the probability of having SLE if the ANA test result is negative, is less than 0.14%. Consequently, if the ANA test result is positive and SLE is suspected, tests for anti–double stranded DNA (anti-dsDNA) and anti-Smith (anti-Sm) antibodies should be ordered. These autoantibodies are the most specific for SLE. Although anti-dsDNA and anti-Sm antibody specificity is much greater than screening ANA, the sensitivity is much lower, 40% to 90% and 5% to 30%, respectively.[22] Antiphospholipid antibodies may occur in 29% to 87% of children with SLE.[76-79] The increased risk of thrombotic events in children with antiphospholipid antibodies is well known.[77,79]

The anti-DNA antibodies are the most highly associated autoantibodies in lupus nephritis. The pathogenicity of anti-DNA antibodies in this setting is suggested by three separate observations: (1) anti-DNA levels tend to correlate with the relative activity of lupus nephritis,[80-82] (2) the anti-DNA antibody can be isolated from the glomeruli of the affected kidneys,[83] and (3) nephritis can be induced in normal mice by administration of monoclonal anti-DNA antibodies.[84] Lupus nephritis can be present in the absence of anti-DNA, a finding suggesting additional or alternative mediators.

Immune complexes of SLE can activate the classic complement pathway. Therefore, the detection of the consumption of complement may also be useful in supporting the diagnosis of lupus nephritis. Hypocomplementemia, both low C3 and C4, is found at presentation in more than three-fourths of patients with SLE and is more common with lupus nephritis.[84,85] Because of the activation of the classic complement pathway in SLE, serum C4 is often used as an index of the inflammatory state and disease activity in lupus nephritis. Successful treatment of SLE typically results in improvement in C4 and C3. However, in patients with a genetic C4 deficiency, complement C4 remains persistently decreased. Along with positive autoimmune serologic findings, patients with lupus nephritis have a varying degree of renal dysfunction. Alternatively, renal dysfunction may be minimal or even absent in lupus nephritis.

The most useful laboratory studies to support the diagnosis of nephritis in a patient with SLE includes the urinary sediment urine protein to creatinine ratio from a first morning specimen, serum creatinine, and renal biopsy. The renal biopsy findings are used to define the class of lupus nephritis and also drive the choice of immunosuppressive therapy in a given patient. Additional laboratory evaluation includes a complete and differential blood cell count to screen for anemia, thrombocytopenia, and leukopenia because pancytopenia or suppression of individual cell lines can be seen on presentation of uncontrolled SLE. Serum albumin is often used to define the impact of proteinuria further. The ratio of serum albumin to globulin is generally reversed in SLE (normal, 2:1) because of the presence of hyperglobulinemia resulting from high serum levels of multispectrum antibodies in these patients.

Diffuse lupus glomerulonephritis (class IV) is seen in 20% to 50% of all children presenting with SLE who undergo renal biopsy,[86] with a higher incidence in African-American and Hispanic children. In the Glomerular Disease Collaborative Network patient registry, with a predominantly African-American patient group, 54% of children and adolescents who underwent biopsy for diagnosis and classification of lupus nephritis had diffuse lupus glomerulonephritis (class IV).

Just as the overall systemic disease may wax and wane, and involve new systems, lupus nephritis may recur, or it may change to a different pathologic class over time. Relapse of renal disease after treatment of lupus nephritis may be identified by the laboratory evaluation of urinalysis, the degree of proteinuria, the presence of hypoalbuminemia, and the rise in serum creatinine (Table 26.7) in these patients.

---

## KEY POINT

Renal pathologic features of lupus nephritis can change over time.

---

## DIFFERENTIAL DIAGNOSIS

The differential diagnosis for a patient suspected of having SLE nephritis can be narrowed based on the presence or absence of other clinical and laboratory findings. HSP can manifest with joint pain, systemic symptoms, nephritis, and a purpuric rash. HSP is, however, characterized by an absence of significant ANAs. Furthermore, the renal biopsy results in HSP demonstrate a dominant IgA staining pattern on immunofluorescence that is not seen in SLE.

Peri-infectious syndromes may also masquerade as SLE, especially if both nephritis and arthritis are clinically present. Unfortunately, the ANA test result may also be positive in this setting, thus complicating the picture. If the kidney biopsy findings are inconclusive, and the history of a preceding infection is convincing, the presumed infection is treated and the patient is observed. Close follow-up is warranted, and the aggressive immunosuppressive regimen required for proliferative lupus nephritis lesions is reserved for patients with a confirmed diagnosis.

ANA positivity can be seen in other rheumatologic diseases that may involve the kidney, particularly in mixed connective tissue disease and rheumatoid arthritis (RA). The diagnosis of RA may be established by radiologic evaluation of the affected joints, which may show erosions and deforming arthritis. Therefore, a presentation with renal disease, a positive ANA test result, and deforming arthritis is suggestive of RA. Finally, thrombotic thrombocytopenia purpura (TTP), which may occur in the setting of SLE, can lead to significant renal disease with symptoms of oligoanuria, acute renal failure, hemolytic anemia, and thrombocytopenia, far exceeding those expected with the classic lupus nephritis lesion. An assessment of the ADAMTS13 (a disintegrin and metalloproteinase with a thrombospondin type 1 motif, member 13) level should be sufficient to differentiate this disease from SLE. Because TTP does not respond to the therapy used to treat lupus nephritis, it is crucial that this disorder is identified and treated appropriately.

## TREATMENT STRATEGIES

To date, there are no randomized controlled trials or comprehensive cohort studies to suggest the optimal treatment for children with lupus nephritis. Therapy for pediatric lupus nephritis is based on the histologic classification of

---

## KEY POINTS

- Treatment for lupus nephritis is based on the renal biopsy pathologic findings.
- Class I and II lupus may respond to corticosteroids and management of extrarenal manifestations of SLE.
- Proliferative lupus nephritis (class III and IV) requires escalation of immunotherapy regimen.

---

Table 26.7 Laboratory parameters used to identify uncontrolled systemic lupus erythematosus nephritis relapse.

| Relapse | | |
| Mild | Moderate | Severe |
| --- | --- | --- |
| Hematuria increasing. RBC casts may be present | Increasing serum creatinine (within 30% of baseline) | Serum creatinine increasing ≥ 30% over baseline |
| Sterile Pyuria. WBC casts may be present | Proteinuria increasing up to 2 fold from baseline and UPC < 5 g/g | Proteinuria increasing and UPC ≥ 5 g/g |

the renal lesion and the results of clinical trials conducted in adults with lupus nephritis. It remains unclear whether a given lesion on a pediatric biopsy equates to that seen on an adult biopsy and whether the findings in adult trials can be generalized to children. However, the standard of care at present involves the use of those drugs that were found to be successful in adult trials. Given this situation, determining the optimal balance between potential benefits and adverse side effects continues to be a priority in the treatment and future research of the pediatric patient with lupus nephritis.

# CLASS I AND II LUPUS NEPHRITIS

Minimizing the inflammatory state with the use of immunosuppressive drugs remains the primary therapeutic modality in the treatment of SLE and lupus nephritis. In addition, patients with all classes of lupus nephritis may benefit from supportive measures such as adequate nutrition, optimal blood pressure control, and diuretics for edema. ISN classes I and II occur less frequently in patients who have undergone biopsy. (see Table 26.4).

In general, treatment for class I is directed at the treatment of the SLE extrarenal manifestations. Treatment of class II lupus nephritis is guided by the degree of proteinuria. Corticosteroid treatment alone may be effective in reducing urine protein to less than 3 g/day. If corticosteroids are ineffective, or if there is a relapse of urine protein with an attempt to reduce or wean from steroid treatment, it is reasonable to consider calcineurin inhibitor therapy for patients with class II lupus. The risk of long-term immune suppression when there is no clear evidence that class I and II lesions have long-term renal health import must be considered. Careful surveillance is required to ensure that if transformation to a more severe kidney lesion occurs, the lesion can be identified and treated in a timely fashion.

# CLASS III AND IV LUPUS NEPHRITIS

Clinical trials data indicate that corticosteroids alone are not effective for inducing remission in patients with actively proliferative lupus nephritis. Corticosteroids are more appropriately combined with at least one other immunosuppressant agent in this setting. Patients with focal proliferative glomerulonephritis (class III) or diffuse proliferative lupus nephritis (class IV) are at the greatest risk of progression to end-stage renal disease (ESRD) if the nephritis is left uncontrolled.[9,11,87] These two clinicopathologic subgroups of lupus nephritis are best treated with another immunosuppressive, in addition to corticosteroids. Additional indicators for aggressive immunotherapy for class III lupus nephritis are (1) elevated creatinine level at the time of renal biopsy, (2) severe nephritic syndrome, (3) the presence of crescent formation in the biopsy specimen, (4) severe tubulointerstitial disease, and (5) evidence of vasculitis.[88]

In general, immunosuppression treatment regimens are separated into two phases: (1) induction, a time of maximal immune suppression exposure; and (2) maintenance, when immune suppression can be reduced, with the goal to limit side effects yet maintain renal remission. The ideal second agent and the length of treatment with additional immunosuppressants continue to evolve.

## Cyclophosphamide

The initial National Institutes of Health (NIH) regimen, which included 2 years of cyclophosphamide exposure combined with corticosteroids, improved renal survival and set the stage for future regimens.[89–97] Unfortunately, this regimen is also associated with significantly higher morbidity in patients. The NIH lupus nephritis treatment regimen (2001 version) involved induction with intravenous methylprednisolone, 1 g/$m^2$ of body surface area, administered as a monthly bolus for at least 12 months, and it could be extended to 36 months.[9] Intravenous cyclophosphamide was given in a dose of 1000 mg/$m^2$ of body surface area, as a monthly bolus for 6 consecutive months, and then once every 3 months for at least 24 additional months. Patients failing to respond after 1 year could be considered for recycling of therapy. Recycling was limited to no more than twice.

Because of side effects associated with high-dose cyclophosphamide use in the NIH regimen, the Euro-Lupus Nephritis Trials (ELNT) compared the efficacy of low-dose intravenous cyclophosphamide with the standard high-dose NIH regimen.[96,97] All adult patients received three daily 750-mg intravenous methylprednisolone pulses, followed by oral glucocorticoid therapy at an initial dose of 0.5 mg equivalent prednisolone/kg/day for 4 weeks. After 4 weeks, glucocorticoids were tapered by 2.5 mg prednisolone every 2 weeks. The high-dose cyclophosphamide group received eight intravenous cyclophosphamide (Cytoxan) pulses within a year, given as six monthly pulses followed by two quarterly pulses. The initial cyclophosphamide dose was 0.5 g/$m^2$ of body surface area, and the subsequent doses were increased by 250 mg, according to the white blood cell count nadir measured on day 14, with a maximum of 1500 mg per pulse. Patients assigned to the low-dose group received six fortnightly intravenous cyclophosphamide pulses at a fixed dose of 500 mg. In both arms of the trial, azathioprine (2 mg/kg/day) was started 2 weeks after the last Cytoxan dose. Mean serum creatinine in the low-dose group was 1.0 ± 0.6 mg/dL, and it was 1.0 ± 0.4 mg/dL in the high-dose group, at 10-year follow-up. Similarly, 10-year follow-up proteinuria was 0.5 ± 1.0 g/day in the low-dose group and $0.6 \pm 1.3$ in the high-dose group. The investigators concluded that low-dose intravenous cyclophosphamide followed by azathioprine (now known as "Euro-Lupus regimen") achieved remission rates as favorable as those of the high-dose cyclophosphamide therapy. Because this trial was conducted in white patients of European ancestry, its application to wider ethnic groups remains to be validated.

## Mycophenolate mofetil

Although cyclophosphamide continues to be one of the cornerstones of therapy (both oral and intravenous regimens have trial support), efforts are under way to achieve remission with the fewest side effects. A mycophenolate mofetil (MMF) induction regimen has received considerable attention. MMF induction in patients with active lupus nephritis (class III, IV, or V) as compared with intravenous cyclophosphamide was shown to result in a greater number of complete and partial remissions of lupus nephritis.[98] The youngest patient enrolled in this trial was 19 years old. In this induction phase study, the most severe infections were noted in the cyclophosphamide-treated group. Follow-up data continue to support the usefulness of MMF induction; MMF-induced patients had similar plasma creatinine concentrations, urinary protein, and activity of urine sediment as patients who underwent induction with cyclophosphamide therapy. Although there was a trend toward a greater relapse rate in the MMF-induction patients (15%) compared with cyclophosphamide (11%), this study opened the door to using MMF as induction therapy, particularly in those patients with the greatest risk for the infertility side effects of cyclophosphamide.[98] Additional small studies in children have also shown a modest benefit of MMF in active or progressive lupus nephritis.[99-101] Long-term follow-up of MMF induction in lupus nephritis, compared with the data on efficacy of cyclophosphamide, is limited at present.

---

### KEY POINT

MMF can be an effective induction agent in a selected population with proliferative lupus nephritis.

---

A major advantage of the use of MMF, especially in children, is its ease of administration (as an oral medication). However, treatment regimens need to limit MMF use in female patients at risk for pregnancy, given the risk of fetal malformation and miscarriage during the first trimester with the use of this agent.

## Rituximab

Rituximab (Rituxan) is a humanized monoclonal antibody initially approved for treatment of B-cell malignant diseases. Rituximab has been considered in uncontrolled retrospective studies as an induction agent for patients with proliferative lupus nephritis. Its therapeutic mechanism is that of destruction of a specific population of B cells. Because B cells are the progenitors of the antibody-producing plasma cells, their modulation, in theory, could modulate SLE, an antigen-antibody driven disease. The efficacy and safety of a regimen of rituximab as compared with placebo were tested in the adult Lupus Nephritis Assessment with Rituximab (LUNAR) study).[102] Although rituximab therapy led to a greater response profile (greater reduction in anti-dsDNA and C3/C4 levels), it did not improve the clinical outcomes of the treated patient population (72 patients) at 1 year.

Failure of the LUNAR study dampened the expectation of the usefulness of rituximab as an induction agent, but its role in "resistant" proliferative glomerulonephritis is still being considered. Three separate uncontrolled studies have suggested the effectiveness of rituximab in this setting.[103-105] In a retrospective review of 19 patients who had rituximab added to their regimen after standard therapy (cyclophosphamide and prednisolone) failed, all patients responded with improved renal function, serologic findings, and hematologic profiles.[104] In another trial, the addition of rituximab allowed shortening of the cyclophosphamide regimen.[106] Sufficient follow-up to draw formal conclusions about long-term remission rates remains unclear.

## Other biologic agents

Belimumab (Benlysta) is the newest anti–B-cell drug to be used in the setting of SLE. Belimumab is a human monoclonal antibody that inhibits the soluble form of the B-cell survival factor, B-lymphocyte stimulator (BLyS). It is approved by the Food and Drug Administration for patients with SLE who continue to have active antibody-positive lupus despite standard therapy (including glucocorticoids, antimalarial drugs, and immunosuppressive agents). Although belimumab was found to improve the SLE responder index (SRI)

---

### KEY POINT

Rituximab and other biologic agents have not succeeded as induction agents in proliferative lupus nephritis.

---

in patients in randomized, controlled trials, there is no evidence for its efficacy in lupus nephritis.[107] Some more recent case reports, however, support its use as a maintenance agent in lupus nephritis.[108] Abatacept (Orencia), another monoclonal antibody that inhibits T-cell responsiveness by blocking the second signal from the antigen-presenting cell, has been approved for use in juvenile arthritis. In one trial, the addition of abatacept to a regimen of cyclophosphamide followed by azathioprine did not improve the outcome of lupus nephritis at either 24 weeks or 52 weeks.[109]

## Plasmapheresis

Plasmapheresis has not been formally studied in lupus nephritis in children. In adult patients, a randomized controlled trial of plasmapheresis, with a standardized treatment protocol consisting of prednisone and cyclophosphamide, failed to improve the outcome of severe lupus nephritis.[110] Although plasmapheresis as a treatment modality for lupus nephritis has been abandoned, case reports support its use in the setting of antiphospholipid or TTP overlap with lupus syndromes.[111]

### KEY POINT

Plasmapheresis, as a supportive therapy, has not been effective in the treatment of lupus nephritis.

## CLASS V OR MEMBRANOUS LUPUS NEPHRITIS

Membranous lupus nephritis has the potential for morbidity secondary to uncontrolled nephrotic syndrome and, less commonly, chronic kidney disease or ESRD. Treatment of this disorder is not as clearly defined as that for the proliferative lesions, and no randomized trials have been published. Treatment regimens have included supportive therapy with angiotensin-converting enzyme inhibition in combination with systemic SLE-targeted immunosuppressive regimens or angiotensin-converting enzyme inhibition in combination with additional immunosuppressive agents including cyclosporine, azathioprine, MMF, or cyclophosphamide, with or without corticosteroids.[112] A retrospective review

### KEY POINT

Treatment of class V lupus nephritis consists of supportive management of nephrotic syndrome and modest immunosuppressive therapy.

found no significant difference in achievement of response in either hematuria or proteinuria for membranous lupus nephritis as opposed to proliferative lupus nephritis.[113]

The low risk of ESRD from membranous lupus nephritis (approximately 5% to 15% at 10 years) has encouraged a less aggressive approach to management compared with proliferative lupus nephritis lesions.[114] However, the significant morbidity associated with uncontrolled nephrotic syndrome, including the potential for accelerated atherosclerosis, thrombosis, and infections, supports intervention. In addition, a retrospective review documented that the coexistence of membranous and proliferative lupus nephritis portends a worse renal prognosis than does the presence of a proliferative lesion alone (16.1% vs. 6%) and therefore justifies a more aggressive treatment plan.[113]

## DILEMMA OF TREATMENT SELECTION IN CHILDREN

Limited randomized data exist for the application of each of the foregoing treatment modes in children. In general, pediatric nephrologists extrapolate from the adult patient literature to build treatment plans that reflect the best randomized controlled data combined with experience. Toward that end, proliferative lupus nephritis lesions are approached with combination regimens. A combination of corticosteroids and cyclophosphamide is the most frequently used regimen, although the length of therapy is variable. Reported steroid regimens have varied considerably; consistently, however, once remission has been established, steroids are tapered to the lowest clinically effective dose to limit side effects. Alternative induction regimens with agents such as MMF and corticosteroids are used because they offer fewer side effects, but long-term renal survival data are lacking. Similar to azathioprine, MMF has also gained a place in the maintenance phase of therapy for lupus nephritis lesions in children. Although not specifically structured for pediatric care, the American College of Rheumatology has suggested treatment guidelines which could provide a road map when considering the treatment options for pediatric patients with lupus nephritis (Figures 26.7 and 26.8).[115]

## PATIENT OUTCOME

Although the 5-year survival for children with lupus nephritis is 83% to 97%, the 5-year renal survival can be variable and depends on the renal pathologic features.[21] Overall improvement in the prognosis of SLE, as well as lupus nephritis, has been demonstrated since the 1980s. In a retrospective analysis of children with WHO class III and IV lupus nephritis who were seen in the 1965 to

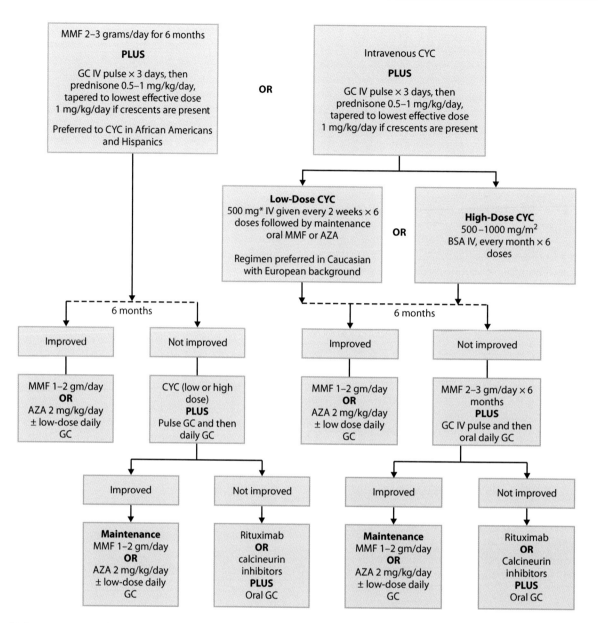

Figure 26.7 American College of Rheumatology guidelines for induction therapy in adult patients with biopsy-proven class III/IV lupus nephritis. Dosing of drugs in pediatric patients should be appropriately adjusted. AZA, azathioprine; BSA, body surface area; CYC, cyclophosphamide; GC, glucocorticoids; IV, intravenous; MMF, mycophenolate mofetil; *dose may require adjustment in children less than 1 year of age. (From Hahn BH, McMahon MA, Wilkinson A, et al. American College of Rheumatology guidelines for screening, treatment, and management of lupus nephritis. Arthritis Care Res [Hoboken]. 2012;64:797–808.)

1992 era, survival was reported to be 82.8% at 5 years and 67.7% at 10 years, and renal survival was 44.4% at 5 years and 29% at 10 years.[116] In a retrospective study of 66 Canadian children with biopsy-proven class IV lupus nephritis (1984 to 1991), the renal survival rate at 5, 10, and 15 years was 87%, 72%, and 65%, respectively.[117] During a mean follow-up of 11 years, the overall mortality rate was 6%, with sepsis the most common cause of death. Pereira et al.[21] reported renal survival in childhood-onset lupus nephritis over a 30-year period (1980 to 2010). This retrospective study suggested that modern treatment protocols seem to offer a survival advantage, with 5-year renal survival rates as high at 91%. Indicators

of poor overall renal prognosis included nephrotic-range proteinuria, renal function lower than normal at presentation, and proliferative nephritis. In addition, escalating urine protein concentrations despite treatment portend a poorer renal prognosis.

## KEY POINT

Indicators of poor renal prognosis include nephrotic range proteinuria, poor renal function at presentation, and a proliferative lesion on biopsy examination.

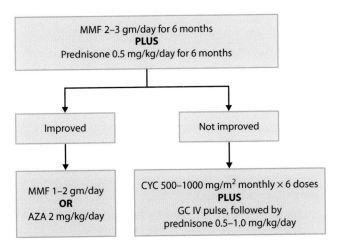

**Figure 26.8** American College of Rheumatology guidelines for induction therapy in adult patients with biopsy-proven class V (membranous) lupus nephritis. Dosing of drugs in pediatric patients should be appropriately adjusted. AZA, azathioprine; CYC, cyclophosphamide; GC, glucocorticoids; IV, intravenous; MMF, mycophenolate mofetil. (From Hahn BH, McMahon MA, Wilkinson A, et al. American College of Rheumatology guidelines for screening, treatment, and management of lupus nephritis. Arthritis Care Res [Hoboken]. 2012;64:797–808.)

## COMPLICATIONS

Complications resulting from lupus nephritis can be divided into two main categories: (1) those that result from the chronic disease itself and (2) those that are related to the toxicity of therapeutic regimens. Infection is a major cause of morbidity in pediatric patients with SLE, presumably resulting from hypocomplementemia and decreased number and function of neutrophils.[21,116,117] This problem is further complicated by the therapeutic use of immunosuppressive agents. Long-term follow-up of one NIH trial documented that 26% of patients taking cyclophosphamide developed a serious bacterial infection.[92] This number increased to 32% when steroids were added to the treatment regimen. These data are among the primary driving forces behind defining newer, less immunosuppressive, yet effective therapies.

Infertility is a significant concern associated with therapy for lupus nephritis. Boumpas et al.[118] reported that 51% of women who are more than 30 years old are at risk of ovarian failure after treatment with cyclophosphamide. The concomitant use of a gonadotropin-releasing hormone agonist, such as leuprolide acetate, has been suggested to induce a state of ovarian protection from the cyclophosphamide effect,[119] although general agreement on its efficacy and protocols describing how it is to be used are lacking. Bladder cancer and lymphoproliferative disorders have been documented following cyclophosphamide. In children and adolescents, the incidence of these side effects from the currently low-dose cyclophosphamide regimens is unknown but presumably low.

Steroid therapy alone or in conjunction with other immunosuppressives is associated with further complications. Avascular necrosis has been reported in as many as 30% of patients treated with significant methylprednisolone exposure. Cataracts without visual impairment are a well-documented morbidity associated with significant steroid use. Hyperglycemia, short stature, and osteopenia may also be caused by intense or prolonged courses of corticosteroids.

## SUMMARY

SLE is a multisystem, autoimmune disorder that occurs in children, adolescents, and adults. Although SLE is more common in girls and women, in general, it affects African-American children more severely (Clinical Vignette 26.1). Renal disease associated with SLE can be quite diverse in pathologic features, as well as in long-term outcome. Whereas membranous nephropathy has a better clinical outlook, diffuse proliferative lesions are associated with risk of progressive chronic kidney disease and ESRD. Treatment with steroids and cyclophosphamide has been the "gold standard" for treatment of severe lupus nephritis, but MMF and lower-dose cyclophosphamide are being shown to be equally effective in controlling lupus-associated nephritis. Failure of some of the monoclonal biologic agents in recent years has been disappointing, and their role in treatment of lupus nephritis remains unclear at this point. Management of these patients requires care by a team of specialists, to optimize therapy and minimize the side effects of immunosuppressive therapies. Clearly, randomized, controlled trials of treatments found to be effective in adult populations also need to be conducted in children and adolescents, to develop the most effective treatment protocols for this age group.

### Clinical Vignette 26.1

A 15-year-old African-American girl presents with a history of fatigue, joint swelling, and anorexia. She denied having had fever, but had an unintended 6-pound weight loss in the last 2 months. She reported a new symptom of shortness of breath while in dance class and denied facial or extremity edema. She has had bilateral wrist and knee pain and swelling for approximately 2 months. She reported visual sensitivity to light and appearance of a faint pink rash on her cheeks several times over the last 2 months. She denied mouth ulcers but has had increased hair loss over the previous 3 months. Past medical history is significant for gastroesophageal reflux. Family history is significant for systemic lupus erythematosus (SLE) in an aunt.

Urinalysis revealed the following: specific gravity, 1.022; 3+ protein; 3+ blood; 25 to 30 red blood cells (RBCs)/hpf; 5 to 10 white blood cells (WBCs)/hpf; 5 to 10 RBC casts; urine protein-to-creatinine ratio, 5.2; blood urea nitrogen (BUN), 31 mg/dL; creatinine, 2.8 mg/dL; albumin, 3.0 g/dL; WBC count, 4200/mm³; hematocrit, 28%; platelet count, 100,000/mm³; antinuclear antibodies (ANAs), 1:1280; Anti-dsDNA, 1:32; complement C3, 48 mg/dL (normal, 83 to 177 mg/dL); complement C4, 9 mg/dL (normal, 15 to 45 mg/dL); erythrocyte sedimentation rate (ESR), 32 mm/h; and C-reactive protein (CRP), 4 mg/dL (normal, less than 1.0 mg/dL).

Renal biopsy showed that more than 50% of glomeruli had evidence of endocapillary hypercellularity (Figure 26.9). Almost half of the affected glomeruli had cellular crescent formation, with distortion of the Bowman capsule. Moderate interstitial edema and some tubules contained prominent RBC casts. Scattered interstitial mononuclear leukocytes were also noted. The arteries and arterioles had no sclerotic or inflammatory changes. On immunofluorescence microscopy, findings were predominantly mesangial and some glomerular capillary wall granular staining with antisera specific for immunoglobulin G (IgG) 2+, IgA 1+, IgM 1+, C3 3+, C1Q 1+, kappa light chains 2+, and lambda light chains 1+. There was no extraglomerular staining. Electron microscopy revealed numerous mesangial and subendothelial immune complex–type electron-dense deposits. Rare subepithelial and intramembranous deposits were also identified. Endothelial tubuloreticular inclusions were present. There was effacement of the visceral epithelial cell foot processes with focal microvillous

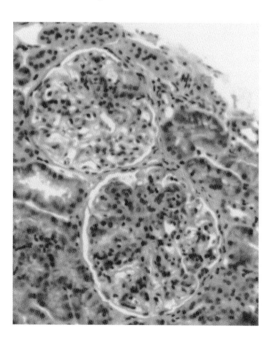

Figure 26.9 Renal biopsy findings in the patient. The glomerulus on the right has endocapillary hypercellularity in the 5 to 10 o'clock position. In contrast, other capillary loops are open, with luminal red blood cells present.

transformation. Pathologic findings were consistent with class IV diffuse proliferative glomerulonephritis.

The patient was treated with a combination of corticosteroids and mycophenolate mofetil (MMF). The hematuria and proteinuria improved by 2.5 months, with a urine protein-to-creatinine ratio of 2.0, urinary microscopy showing 5 to 10 RBC/hpf, and serum creatinine decreasing to 1.5 mg/dL. Angiotensin-converting enzyme therapy was added. By 6 months the urine protein-to-creatinine ratio was 0.5, urinalysis showed 2 to 5 RBC/hpf of urine, and serum creatinine was 0.8 mg/dL. Based on this response, her steroid regimen was progressively weaned, she was begun on maintenance therapy with MMF, and she was continued on an angiotensin-converting enzyme inhibitor.

## TEACHING POINTS

The patient in Clinical Vignette 26.1 presented with symptoms that are highly suggestive of systemic lupus erythematosus (SLE). The presence of hematuria, proteinuria, and red blood cell (RBC) casts in the urinary sediment, along with elevated blood urea nitrogen (BUN) and creatinine, is indicative of SLE nephritis, possibly with a diffuse proliferative pathologic process. Renal biopsy demonstrated a crescentic form of acute proliferative glomerular lesion, compatible with class IV lesions (ISN/RPS 2003). This patient received induction therapy with steroids and mycophenolate mofetil (MMF) and then maintenance therapy with MMF alone. Normalization of proteinuria and renal function occurred over the next 6 months.

Although induction with intravenous steroids and cyclophosphamide is the "gold standard" for treatment of the proliferative form of lupus nephritis, MMF and steroids were chosen for induction. The rationale for picking this regimen was that cyclophosphamide has greater potential for side effects, and, more importantly, investigators have demonstrated equipotency by MMF in lupus nephritis in some of the more recent clinical trials. This patient will need to be followed by the rheumatology and nephrology teams to monitor overall care of her SLE, with modulation of immunosuppression and monitoring of proteinuria and renal functions.

## REFERENCES

1. Levy DM, Kamphuis S. Systemic lupus erythematosus in children and adolescents. Pediatr Clin North Am. 2012;59:345–64.
2. Pineles D, Valente A, Warren B, et al. Worldwide incidence and prevalence of pediatric onset systemic lupus erythematosus. Lupus. 2011;20:1187–92.
3. Gottlieb BS, Ilowite NT. Systemic lupus erythematosus in children and adolescents. Pediatr Rev. 2006;27:323–30.

4. Benseler SM, Silverman ED. Systemic lupus erythematosus. Rheum Dis Clin North Am. 2007;33:471–98, vi.

5. Mok CC, Mak A, Chu WP, et al. Long-term survival of southern Chinese patients with systemic lupus erythematosus: A prospective study of all age-groups. Medicine (Baltimore). 2005;84:218–24.

6. Lilleby V, Flato B, Forre O. Disease duration, hypertension and medication requirements are associated with organ damage in childhood-onset systemic lupus erythematosus. Clin Exp Rheumatol. 2005;23:261–9.

7. Gutierrez-Suarez R, Ruperto N, Gastaldi R, et al. A proposal for a pediatric version of the Systemic Lupus International Collaborating Clinics/American College of Rheumatology Damage Index based on the analysis of 1,015 patients with juvenile-onset systemic lupus erythematosus. Arthritis Rheum. 2006;54:2989–96.

8. Ramirez Gomez LA, Uribe Uribe O, Osio Uribe O, et al. Childhood systemic lupus erythematosus in Latin America: The GLADEL experience in 230 children. Lupus. 2008;17:596–604.

9. Tucker LB, Uribe AG, Fernandez M, et al. Adolescent onset of lupus results in more aggressive disease and worse outcomes: Results of a nested matched case-control study within LUMINA, a multiethnic US cohort (LUMINA LVII). Lupus. 2008;17:314–22.

10. Hiraki LT, Benseler SM, Tyrrell PN, et al. Ethnic differences in pediatric systemic lupus erythematosus. J Rheumatol. 2009;36:2539–46.

11. Hersh AO, Trupin L, Yazdany J, et al. Childhood-onset disease as a predictor of mortality in an adult cohort of patients with systemic lupus erythematosus. Arthritis Care Res (Hoboken). 2010;62:1152–9.

12. Barsalou J, Levy DM, Silverman ED. An update on childhood-onset systemic lupus erythematosus. Curr Opin Rheumatol. 2013;25:616–22.

13. Lee PY, Yeh KW, Yao TC, et al. The outcome of patients with renal involvement in pediatric-onset systemic lupus erythematosus: A 20-year experience in Asia. Lupus. 2013;22:1534–40.

14. Mak A, Mok CC, Chu WP, et al. Renal damage in systemic lupus erythematosus: A comparative analysis of different age groups. Lupus. 2007;16:28–34.

15. Cameron JS. Lupus nephritis in childhood and adolescence. Pediatr Nephrol. 1994;8:230-49.

16. Platt JL, Burke BA, Fish AJ, et al. Systemic lupus erythematosus in the first two decades of life. Am J Kidney Dis. 1982;2:212–22.

17. Bartosh SM, Fine RN, Sullivan EK. Outcome after transplantation of young patients with systemic lupus erythematosus: A report of the North American pediatric renal transplant cooperative study. Transplantation. 2001;72:973–8.

18. Hiraki LT, Feldman CH, Liu J, et al. Prevalence, incidence, and demographics of systemic lupus erythematosus and lupus nephritis from 2000 to 2004 among children in the US Medicaid beneficiary population. Arthritis Rheum. 2012;64:2669–76.

19. Emre S, Bilge I, Sirin A, et al. Lupus nephritis in children: Prognostic significance of clinicopathological findings. Nephron. 2001;87:118–26.

20. Baqi N, Moazami S, Singh A, et al. Lupus nephritis in children: A longitudinal study of prognostic factors and therapy. J Am Soc Nephrol. 1996;7:924–9.

21. Pereira T, Abitbol CL, Seeherunvong W, et al. Three decades of progress in treating childhood-onset lupus nephritis. Clin J Am Soc Nephrol. 2011;6:2192–9.

22. Cameron JS. Lupus nephritis. J Am Soc Nephrol. 1999;10:413–24.

23. Lehman TJ, McCurdy DK, Bernstein BH, et al. Systemic lupus erythematosus in the first decade of life. Pediatrics. 1989;83:235–9.

24. Rosenberg AM. Systemic lupus erythematosus in children. Springer Semin Immunopathol. 1994;16:261–79.

25. Alarcon GS, McGwin G, Jr., Petri M, et al. Baseline characteristics of a multiethnic lupus cohort: PROFILE. Lupus. 2002;11:95–101.

26. Shlomchik MJ, Craft JE, Mamula MJ. From T to B and back again: Positive feedback in systemic autoimmune disease. Nat Rev Immunol. 2001;1:147–53.

27. Shlomchik MJ. Sites and stages of autoreactive B cell activation and regulation. Immunity. 2008;28:18–28.

28. Carroll MC. A protective role for innate immunity in systemic lupus erythematosus. Nat Rev Immunol. 2004;4:825–31.

29. Casciola-Rosen LA, Anhalt G, Rosen A. Autoantigens targeted in systemic lupus erythematosus are clustered in two populations of surface structures on apoptotic keratinocytes. J Exp Med. 1994;179:1317–30.

30. Cui Y, Sheng Y, Zhang X. Genetic susceptibility to SLE: Recent progress from GWAS. J Autoimmun. 2013;41:25–33.

31. Forton AC, Petri MA, Goldman D, Sullivan KE. An osteopontin (SPP1) polymorphism is associated with systemic lupus erythematosus. Hum Mutat. 2002;19:459.

32. Graham RR, Cotsapas C, Davies L, et al. Genetic variants near TNFAIP3 on 6q23 are associated with systemic lupus erythematosus. Nat Genet. 2008;40:1059–61.

33. Karassa FB, Trikalinos TA, Ioannidis JP, FcgammaRIIa-SLE Meta-Analysis Investigators. Role of the Fcgamma receptor IIa polymorphism in susceptibility to systemic lupus erythematosus and lupus nephritis: A meta-analysis. Arthritis Rheum. 2002;46:1563–71.

34. Koene HR, Kleijer M, Swaak AJ, et al. The Fc gam-maRIIIA-158F allele is a risk factor for systemic lupus erythematosus. Arthritis Rheum. 1998;41:1813–8.

35. Kyogoku C, Dijstelbloem HM, Tsuchiya N, et al. Fcgamma receptor gene polymorphisms in Japanese patients with systemic lupus erythematosus: Contribution of FCGR2B to genetic susceptibility. Arthritis Rheum. 2002;46:1242–54.

36. Lee-Kirsch MA, Gong M, Chowdhury D, et al. Mutations in the gene encoding the 3'-5' DNA exonuclease TREX1 are associated with systemic lupus erythematosus. Nat Genet. 2007;39:1065–7.

37. Bronson PG, Chaivorapol C, Ortmann W, et al. The genetics of type I interferon in systemic lupus erythematosus. Curr Opin Immunol. 2012;24:530–7.

38. Cunninghame Graham DS, Morris DL, Bhangale TR, et al. Association of NCF2, IKZF1, IRF8, IFIH1, and TYK2 with systemic lupus erythematosus. PLoS Genet. 2011;7:e1002341.

39. Fu Q, Zhao J, Qian X, et al. Association of a functional IRF7 variant with systemic lupus erythematosus. Arthritis Rheum. 2011;63:749–54.

40. Gateva V, Sandling JK, Hom G, et al. A large-scale replication study identifies TNIP1, PRDM1, JAZF1, UHRF1BP1 and IL10 as risk loci for systemic lupus erythematosus. Nat Genet. 2009;41:1228–33.

41. Jacob CO, Zhu J, Armstrong DL, et al. Identification of IRAK1 as a risk gene with critical role in the pathogenesis of systemic lupus erythematosus. Proc Natl Acad Sci U S A. 2009;106:6256–61.

42. Kaufman KM, Zhao J, Kelly JA, et al. Fine mapping of Xq28: Both MECP2 and IRAK1 contribute to risk for systemic lupus erythematosus in multiple ancestral groups. Ann Rheum Dis. 2013;72:437–44.

43. Krausgruber T, Blazek K, Smallie T, et al. IRF5 promotes inflammatory macrophage polarization and TH1-TH17 responses. Nat Immunol. 2011;12:231–8.

44. Salloum R, Franek BS, Kariuki SN, et al. Genetic variation at the IRF7/PHRF1 locus is associated with autoantibody profile and serum interferon-alpha activity in lupus patients. Arthritis Rheum. 2010;62:553–61.

45. Shen N, Fu Q, Deng Y, et al. Sex-specific association of X-linked Toll-like receptor 7 (TLR7) with male systemic lupus erythematosus. Proc Natl Acad Sci U S A. 2010;107:15838–43.

46. Sullivan KE, Piliero LM, Dharia T, et al. 3' polymorphisms of ETS1 are associated with different clinical phenotypes in SLE. Hum Mutat. 2000;16:49–53.

47. Wang D, John SA, Clements JL, et al. Ets-1 deficiency leads to altered B cell differentiation, hyper-responsiveness to TLR9 and autoimmune disease. Int Immunol. 2005;17:1179–91.

48. Wang S, Adrianto I, Wiley GB, et al. A functional haplotype of UBE2L3 confers risk for systemic lupus erythematosus. Genes Immun. 2012;13:380–7.

49. Yang W, Shen N, Ye DQ, et al. Genome-wide association study in Asian populations identifies variants in ETS1 and WDFY4 associated with systemic lupus erythematosus. PLoS Genet. 2010;6:e1000841.

50. Adrianto I, Wen F, Templeton A, et al. Association of a functional variant downstream of TNFAIP3 with systemic lupus erythematosus. Nat Genet. 2011;43:253–8.

51. Musone SL, Taylor KE, Lu TT, et al. Multiple polymorphisms in the TNFAIP3 region are independently associated with systemic lupus erythematosus. Nat Genet. 2008;40:1062–4.

52. Sheng YJ, Gao JP, Li J, et al. Follow-up study identifies two novel susceptibility loci PRKCB and 8p11.21 for systemic lupus erythematosus. Rheumatology (Oxford). 2011;50:682–8.

53. Criswell LA, Pfeiffer KA, Lum RF, et al. Analysis of families in the multiple autoimmune disease genetics consortium (MADGC) collection: The PTPN22 620W allele associates with multiple autoimmune phenotypes. Am J Hum Genet. 2005;76:561–71.

54. Kozyrev SV, Abelson AK, Wojcik J, et al. Functional variants in the B-cell gene BANK1 are associated with systemic lupus erythematosus. Nat Genet. 2008;40:211–6.

55. Lee YH, Song GG. Associations between TNFSF4 and TRAF1-C5 gene polymorphisms and systemic lupus erythematosus: A meta-analysis. Hum Immunol. 2012;73:1050–4.

56. Lu R, Vidal GS, Kelly JA, et al. Genetic associations of LYN with systemic lupus erythematosus. Genes Immun. 2009;10:397–403.

57. Namjou B, Sestak AL, Armstrong DL, et al. High-density genotyping of STAT4 reveals multiple haplotypic associations with systemic lupus erythematosus in different racial groups. Arthritis Rheum. 2009;60:1085–95.

58. Nath SK, Han S, Kim-Howard X, et al. A nonsynonymous functional variant in integrin-alpha(M) (encoded by ITGAM) is associated with systemic lupus erythematosus. Nat Genet. 2008;40:152–4.

59. Wang B, Zhu JM, Fan YG, et al. Association of the −1082G/A polymorphism in the interleukin-10 gene with systemic lupus erythematosus: A meta-analysis. Gene. 2013;519:209–16.

60. Takeuchi T, Suzuki K. CD247 variants and single-nucleotide polymorphisms observed in systemic lupus erythematosus patients. Rheumatology (Oxford). 2013;52:1551–5.

61. Block SR, Winfield JB, Lockshin MD, et al. Studies of twins with systemic lupus erythematosus: A review of the literature and presentation of 12 additional sets. Am J Med. 1975;59:533–52.

62. Deapen D, Escalante A, Weinrib L, et al. A revised estimate of twin concordance in systemic lupus erythematosus. Arthritis Rheum. 1992;35:311–8.

63. Arnett FC, Reveille JD, Wilson RW, et al. Systemic lupus erythematosus: Current state of the genetic hypothesis. Semin Arthritis Rheum. 1984;14:24–35.

64. Hunnangkul S, Nitsch D, Rhodes B, et al. Familial clustering of non-nuclear autoantibodies and C3 and C4 complement components in systemic lupus erythematosus. Arthritis Rheum. 2008;58:1116–24.

65. Murashima A, Fukazawa T, Hirashima M, et al. Long term prognosis of children born to lupus patients. Ann Rheum Dis. 2004;63:50–3.

66. Tsao BP. The genetics of human systemic lupus erythematosus. Trends Immunol. 2003;24:595–602.

67. Weening JJ, D'Agati VD, Schwartz MM, et al. The classification of glomerulonephritis in systemic lupus erythematosus revisited. J Am Soc Nephrol. 2004;15:241–50.

68. Weening JJ, D'Agati VD, Schwartz MM, et al. The classification of glomerulonephritis in systemic lupus erythematosus revisited. Kidney Int. 2004;65:521–30.

69. Tucker LB, Menon S, Schaller JG, Isenberg DA. Adult- and childhood-onset systemic lupus erythematosus: A comparison of onset, clinical features, serology, and outcome. Br J Rheumatol. 1995;34:866–72.

70. Meislin AG, Rothfield N. Systemic lupus erythematosus in childhood: Analysis of 42 cases, with comparative data on 200 adult cases followed concurrently. Pediatrics. 1968;42:37–49.

71. Hochberg MC. Updating the American College of Rheumatology revised criteria for the classification of systemic lupus erythematosus. Arthritis Rheum. 1997;40:1725.

72. Carreno L, Lopez-Longo FJ, Monteagudo I, et al. Immunological and clinical differences between juvenile and adult onset of systemic lupus erythematosus. Lupus. 1999;8:287–92.

73. Rood MJ, ten Cate R, van Suijlekom-Smit LW, et al. Childhood-onset systemic lupus erythematosus: Clinical presentation and prognosis in 31 patients. Scand J Rheumatol. 1999;28:222–6.

74. Tan EM, Feltkamp TE, Smolen JS, et al. Range of antinuclear antibodies in "healthy" individuals. Arthritis Rheum. 1997;40:1601–11.

75. Shiel WC, Jr., Jason M. The diagnostic associations of patients with antinuclear antibodies referred to a community rheumatologist. J Rheumatol. 1989;16:782–5.

76. Massengill SF, Hedrick C, Ayoub EM, et al. Antiphospholipid antibodies in pediatric lupus nephritis. Am J Kidney Dis. 1997;29:355–61.

77. Molta C, Meyer O, Dosquet C, et al. Childhood-onset systemic lupus erythematosus: Antiphospholipid antibodies in 37 patients and their first-degree relatives. Pediatrics. 1993;92:849–53.

78. Ravelli A, Caporali R, Di Fuccia G, et al. Anticardiolipin antibodies in pediatric systemic lupus erythematosus. Arch Pediatr Adolesc Med. 1994;148:398–402.

79. Seaman DE, Londino AV, Jr., Kwoh CK, et al. Antiphospholipid antibodies in pediatric systemic lupus erythematosus. Pediatrics. 1995;96:1040–5.

80. Bootsma H, Spronk P, Derksen R, et al. Prevention of relapses in systemic lupus erythematosus. Lancet. 1995;345:1595–9.

81. Smeenk RJ, van den Brink HG, Brinkman K, et al. Anti-dsDNA: Choice of assay in relation to clinical value. Rheumatol Int. 1991;11:101–7.

82. ter Borg EJ, Horst G, Hummel EJ, et al. Measurement of increases in anti–double-stranded DNA antibody levels as a predictor of disease exacerbation in systemic lupus erythematosus: A long-term, prospective study. Arthritis Rheum. 1990;33:634–43.

83. Winfield JB, Faiferman I, Koffler D. Avidity of anti-DNA antibodies in serum and IgG glomerular eluates from patients with systemic lupus erythematosus: Association of high avidity antinative DNA antibody with glomerulonephritis. J Clin Invest. 1977;59:90–6.

84. Singsen BH, Bernstein BH, King KK, Hanson V. Systemic lupus erythematosus in childhood correlations between changes in disease activity and serum complement levels. J Pediatr. 1976;89:358–69.

85. Klein MH, Thorner PS, Yoon SJ, et al. Determination of circulating immune complexes, C3 and C4 complement components and anti-DNA antibody in different classes of lupus nephritis. Int J Pediatr Nephrol. 1984;5:75–82.

86. Malleson PN. The role of the renal biopsy in childhood onset systemic lupus erythematosus: A viewpoint. Clin Exp Rheumatol. 1989;7:563–6.

87. Austin HA, Balow JE. Natural history and treatment of lupus nephritis. Semin Nephrol. 1999;19:2–11.

88. Austin HA, 3rd, Boumpas DT, Vaughan EM, Balow JE. High-risk features of lupus nephritis: Importance of race and clinical and histological factors in 166 patients. Nephrol Dial Transplant. 1995;10:1620–8.

89. Austin HA, 3rd, Klippel JH, Balow JE, et al. Therapy of lupus nephritis: Controlled trial of prednisone and cytotoxic drugs. N Engl J Med. 1986;314:614–9.

90. Boumpas DT, Austin HA, 3rd, Vaughn EM, et al. Controlled trial of pulse methylprednisolone versus two regimens of pulse cyclophosphamide in severe lupus nephritis. Lancet. 1992;340:741–5.

91. Gourley MF, Austin HA, 3rd, Scott D, et al. Methylprednisolone and cyclophosphamide, alone or in combination, in patients with lupus nephritis: A randomized, controlled trial. Ann Intern Med. 1996;125:549–57.

92. Illei GG, Austin HA, Crane M, et al. Combination therapy with pulse cyclophosphamide plus pulse methylprednisolone improves long-term renal outcome without adding toxicity in patients with lupus nephritis. Ann Intern Med. 2001;135:248–57.

93. Lehman TJ, Onel K. Intermittent intravenous cyclophosphamide arrests progression of the renal chronicity index in childhood systemic lupus erythematosus. J Pediatr. 2000;136:243–7.

94. Lehman TJ, Sherry DD, Wagner-Weiner L, et al. Intermittent intravenous cyclophosphamide therapy for lupus nephritis. J Pediatr. 1989;114:1055–60.

95. Valeri A, Radhakrishnan J, Estes D, et al. Intravenous pulse cyclophosphamide treatment of severe lupus nephritis: A prospective five-year study. Clin Nephrol. 1994;42:71–8.

96. Houssiau FA, Vasconcelos C, D'Cruz D, et al. Immunosuppressive therapy in lupus nephritis: The Euro-Lupus Nephritis Trial, a randomized trial of low-dose versus high-dose intravenous cyclophosphamide. Arthritis Rheum. 2002;46:2121–31.

97. Houssiau FA, Vasconcelos C, D'Cruz D, et al. The 10-year follow-up data of the Euro-Lupus Nephritis Trial comparing low-dose and high-dose intravenous cyclophosphamide. Ann Rheum Dis. 2010;69:61–4.

98. Chan TM, Li FK, Tang CS, et al. Efficacy of mycophenolate mofetil in patients with diffuse proliferative lupus nephritis. Hong Kong-Guangzhou Nephrology Study Group. N Engl J Med. 2000;343:1156–62.

99. Aragon E, Chan YH, Ng KH, et al. Good outcomes with mycophenolate-cyclosporine–based induction protocol in children with severe proliferative lupus nephritis. Lupus. 2010;19:965–73.

100. Buratti S, Szer IS, Spencer CH, et al. Mycophenolate mofetil treatment of severe renal disease in pediatric onset systemic lupus erythematosus. J Rheumatol. 2001;28:2103–8.

101. Kazyra I, Pilkington C, Marks SD, Tullus K. Mycophenolate mofetil treatment in children and adolescents with lupus. Arch Dis Child. 2010;95:1059–61.

102. Rovin BH, Furie R, Latinis K, et al. Efficacy and safety of rituximab in patients with active proliferative lupus nephritis: The Lupus Nephritis Assessment with Rituximab study. Arthritis Rheum. 2012;64:1215–26.

103. Marks SD, Patey S, Brogan PA, et al. B lymphocyte depletion therapy in children with refractory systemic lupus erythematosus. Arthritis Rheum. 2005;52:3168–74.

104. Podolskaya A, Stadermann M, Pilkington C, et al. B cell depletion therapy for 19 patients with refractory systemic lupus erythematosus. Arch Dis Child. 2008;93:401–6.

105. Willems M, Haddad E, Niaudet P, et al. Rituximab therapy for childhood-onset systemic lupus erythematosus. J Pediatr. 2006;148:623–7.

106. MacDermott EJ, Lehman TJ. Prospective, open-label trial of rituximab in childhood systemic lupus erythematosus. Curr Rheumatol Rep. 2006;8:439–41.

107. Furie R, Petri M, Zamani O, et al. A phase III, randomized, placebo-controlled study of belimumab, a monoclonal antibody that inhibits B lymphocyte stimulator, in patients with systemic lupus erythematosus. Arthritis Rheum. 2011;63:3918–30.

108. Kraaij T, Huizinga TW, Rabelink TJ, et al. Belimumab after rituximab as maintenance therapy in lupus nephritis. Rheumatology (Oxford). 2014;53:2122–4.

109. ACCESS Trial Group. Treatment of lupus nephritis with abatacept: The abatacept and cyclophosphamide combination efficacy and safety study. Arthritis Rheumatol. 2014;66:3096–104.

110. Lewis EJ, Hunsicker LG, Lan SP, et al. A controlled trial of plasmapheresis therapy in severe lupus nephritis. N Engl J Med. 1992 ;326:1373–9.

111. Sendzischew MA, Vieregge GB, Green DF, et al. Plasma exchange for concurrent lupus nephritis and antiphospholipid syndrome. Clin Kidney J. 2014;7:86–9.

112. Kolasinski SL, Chung JB, Albert DA. What do we know about lupus membranous nephropathy? An analytic review. Arthritis Rheum. 2002;47:450–5.

113. Boneparth A, Ilowite N, for the CARRA Registry Investigators. Comparison of renal response parameters for juvenile membranous plus proliferative lupus nephritis versus isolated proliferative lupus nephritis: A cross-sectional analysis of the CARRA Registry. Lupus. 2014;11;23:898–904.

114. Mok CC. Membranous nephropathy in systemic lupus erythematosus: A therapeutic enigma. Nat Rev Nephrol. 2009;5:212–20.

115. Hahn BH, McMahon MA, Wilkinson A, et al. American College of Rheumatology guidelines for screening, treatment, and management of lupus nephritis. Arthritis Care Res (Hoboken). 2012;64:797–808.

116. Baqi N, Moazami S, Singh A, et al. Lupus nephritis in children: A longitudinal study of prognostic factors and therapy. J Am Soc Nephrol. 1996;7:924–9.

117. Hagelberg S, Lee Y, Bargman J, et al. Long-term followup of childhood lupus nephritis. J Rheumatol. 2002;29:2635–42.

118. Boumpas DT, Austin HA, 3rd, Vaughan EM, et al. Risk for sustained amenorrhea in patients with systemic lupus erythematosus receiving intermittent pulse cyclophosphamide therapy. Ann Intern Med. 1993;119:366–9.

119. Slater CA, Liang MH, McCune JW, et al. Preserving ovarian function in patients receiving cyclophosphamide. Lupus. 1999;8:3–10.

## REVIEW QUESTIONS

1. Renal biopsy was performed in a 15-year-old African-American girl with known SLE for 3 months and a recently noted abnormal serum creatinine of 1.5 mg/dL for 2 weeks. The light microscopy findings of the renal biopsy were compatible with class IV (ISN/RPS 2003) changes. Recommendation for treatment of SLE nephritis in this case should be:
   a. Intravenous steroids and intravenous cyclophosphamide
   b. Intravenous steroids and rituximab
   c. Intravenous steroids and mycophenolate mofetil
   d. Option a or option c
   e. Option b or option c
2. SLE is more severe and more common in African Americans.
   a. True
   b. False
3. Indicator(s) of poor renal prognosis in lupus nephritis is (are):
   a. Nephrotic range proteinuria
   b. Increased serum creatinine at presentation
   c. Class III or IV renal pathologic features in renal biopsy
   d. All of the above
   e. None of the above
4. Glomerular mesangial and capillary wall immune deposits of IgA can be seen in:
   a. SLE nephritis
   b. IgA nephritis
   c. HSP nephritis
   d. All of the above
   e. Only b and c
5. Renal prognosis of class V lupus nephritis at 10 years is:
   a. ESRD in more than 50% patients
   b. ESRD in 10% to 25% patients
   c. ESRD in fewer than 5% patients
6. SLE is associated with:
   a. No genetic predisposition
   b. Familial aggregation
   c. Autosomal recessive inheritance
   d. Autosomal dominant inheritance
7. Steroids alone are effective in treatment of class III and class IV lupus nephritis.
   a. True
   b. False
8. The most common cause of death in lupus nephritis is:
   a. End-stage renal disease
   b. Associated cerebritis
   c. Overwhelming sepsis
   d. Thromboembolic complications
9. Morbidity associated with class V (membranous) lupus nephritis is caused by:
   a. Proteinuria and edema
   b. Thromboembolic events
   c. Infective events
   d. All of the above
10. Patients with class V (membranous) lupus nephritis should receive induction therapy with pulse IV steroids and IV Cytoxan protocol.
    a. True
    b. False
11. In treatment of proliferative lupus nephritis (class III and IV), mycophenolate mofetil (MMF) induction therapy is:
    a. Less effective than NIH regimen of IV Cytoxan
    b. More effective than NIH regimen of IV Cytoxan
    c. At least as effective as NIH regimen of IV Cytoxan
    d. There are no convincing comparative data available.

## ANSWER KEY

1. d
2. a
3. d
4. d
5. b
6. b
7. b
8. c
9. d
10. b
11. c

# 27

# Kidney disease in sickle cell anemia

IBRAHIM F. SHATAT AND SHERRON M. JACKSON

Sickle cell disease (SCD) affects more than 100,000 or 1 In 500 African Americans (AAs) in the United States. In SCD, a single gene mutation results in the substitution of valine for glutamate on the β chain of hemoglobin. This causes the abnormal sickle hemoglobin (HbS) to polymerize and form strands or fiber-like structures in hypoxic (or deoxygenated) state. Moreover, these strands of HbS bunch up together to form bundles that distort red blood cells (RBCs) into elongated sickled shapes. Such RBCs are prone to hemolysis and also to blocking tissue capillaries, thereby resulting in impaired oxygen delivery to every organ system in the body and tissue damage. Within the kidney, the entire nephron is affected by vaso-occlusion, ischemia, and infarction associated with SCD, ultimately leading to nephron loss. Evidence of renal disease in SCD or sickle cell nephropathy (SCN) begins early in childhood, and it can progress to chronic kidney disease (CKD) in adults. A schematic representation of renal manifestations of SCD by age is presented in Figure 27.1. This chapter discusses the epidemiology, pathogenesis, clinical manifestations, evaluation, and treatment of SCN in children and young adults.

## EPIDEMIOLOGY

The spectrum of renal disease in SCD begins in early childhood, and it often manifests as hyposthenuria and polyuria. The age of onset of other renal disorders is variable. Although nephron injury in SCD starts in infancy, SCN manifests more prominently in the second decade of life. Studies in children have clearly characterized some of the common manifestations of SCN, including microalbuminuria, hyperfiltration, nephrotic syndrome, and CKD. Polyuria, enuresis, hematuria, renal papillary necrosis (RPN), and renal medullary carcinoma (RMC) are other well-described renal manifestations of SCD. In general, patients with homozygous SS disease (HbSS) demonstrate more significant renal injury than do patients with hemoglobin S-C disease (HbSC) or hemoglobin Sβ thalassemia. The prevalence of renal manifestations in patients with SCD and trait increases with age. Frequently, the renal manifestations correlate with the severity of SCD, as measured by the degree of hemolysis, hemoglobin levels, and the presence of other sickle cell morbidities.[1]

In a study of more than 2000 medical records of children with SCD, the prevalence of gross hematuria was 6.3%. Preexisting hematuria was significantly associated with the risk of early development of acute kidney injury (AKI) and CKD. Hematuria may originate from either kidney, although a preponderance of left-sided renal bleeding has been observed.[2,3]

### KEY POINT

The spectrum of kidney complications begins in childhood as hyposthenuria.

Proteinuria is the hallmark of glomerular injury. Early studies reported the prevalence of proteinuria

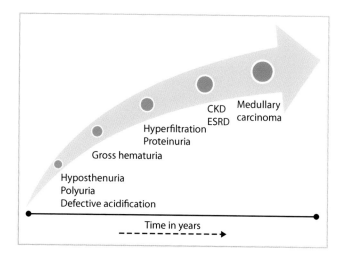

Figure 27.1 Kidney disease manifestations of sickle cell disease from childhood through young adulthood. CKD, chronic kidney disease; ESRD, end-stage renal disease.

in young children with SCD to be 5% to 6%.[4,5] In more recent studies, the prevalence of microalbuminuria and proteinuria in teens and young adults with SCD was 16% to 40%.[6–11] McPherson et al.[6] examined the prevalence and clinical correlates of albuminuria and CKD in 410 pediatric patients. Of these patients, 20.7% had microalbuminuria, 26.5% met the Kidney Disease Improving Global Outcomes study (KDIGO) definition for CKD, with CKD I in 14.8% and CKD II in 11.6%.[6] The prevalence of CKD in adults with SCD ranges from 5% to 30%.[12,13] Adults with SCD develop CKD at a much younger age than do patients with HbSC. Hypertension, proteinuria, nephrotic syndrome, hematuria, and anemia generally predict progressive and severe renal disease. Patients with CKD have a significantly higher mortality rate compared with patients with SCD patients who do

not have CDK, and this is true for both HbSS and HbSC.[12] Guasch et al.[14] studied 300 adult patients with HbSS and noticed that sickle glomerulopathy affected the majority of older adults, and its prevalence was much higher than previously reported on the basis of dipstick protein. Sixty-eight percent of patients had increased albumin excretion rates. Approximately 26% of those patients demonstrated macroalbuminuria and evidence of CKD.[14]

## PATHOGENESIS

An outline of the pathogenesis of renal disease in SCD, primarily based on the principles of microvascular obstruction and tissue damage, is shown in Figure 27.2. However, the clinical spectrum of SCN cannot be fully explained by vaso-occlusive pathophysiologic processes alone. Genetic factors undoubtedly influence renal and other complications in SCD. Platt et al.[15] and Lebensburger et al.[16] identified low fetal hemoglobin levels as a risk factor in adults with early death. It has long been noted that the presence of β globin Central African Republic haplotype is associated with renal involvement.[17] Some studies suggest that microdeletions of α globin genes in α thalassemia are protective and are associated with lower prevalence of proteinuria.[18] Genetic polymorphisms may explain the variation for risk of developing CKD.

## HEMATURIA

Microscopic or painless visible hematuria is a common manifestation of injury to different parts of the nephron or the collecting system in SCD. Hematuria is especially common in patients with sickle cell trait.

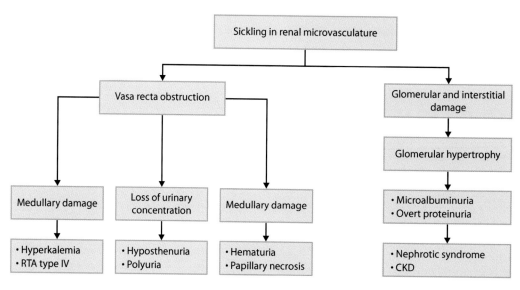

Figure 27.2 Pathogenesis of nephropathy in sickle cell disease. CKD, chronic kidney disease; RTA, renal tubular acidosis.

Sickling in the renal microcirculation, especially In the vasa recta, is promoted by the hypoxemic, acidic, and high osmotic renal medullary environment. This leads to microvascular obstruction, vascular congestion, ischemia, papillary injury, and hematuria.

## URINARY CONCENTRATING DEFECT

The earliest evidence of kidney injury in SCD consists of a defective urinary concentrating ability and hyposthenuria. The clinical consequences are the development of enuresis and polyuria and the potential for dehydration and worsening vaso-occlusive symptoms.[19] Cumulative damage to the renal medulla, vasa recta, and collecting ducts occurs after repeated vaso-occlusive events, and infarctions lead to the loss of the medullary concentration gradient needed for water reabsorption.[20] Blood transfusions have transiently reversed the concentrating defect, but the defect ultimately becomes an irreversible feature of SCN in children and young adults.[21]

## TUBULAR DYSFUNCTION

Defects in urinary acidification and potassium excretion (type IV renal tubular acidosis [RTA]) in the distal tubule have been well described in SCD. However, these defects are not universal, and some patients seldom experience hyperkalemia or metabolic acidosis. The underlying mechanism is unclear but may be related to repeat sickling events, abnormal medullary blood flow, and chronic ischemia reperfusion injury. The hyperkalemia is not related to aldosterone deficiency but is believed to result from target organ damage resulting from medullary fibrosis and distal tubular damage. Aldosterone and renin levels may indeed be elevated in these patients, possibly in response to the relative hypovolemia and hyperkalemia.[19]

Patients with SCD demonstrate an enhanced proximal tubular activity with increased reabsorption of sodium, phosphorus, and $\beta_2$-microglobulin.[3] Increased tubular secretion of creatinine and uric acid is also well known and may reflect a functional adaptation to high uric acid generation.[22] Enhanced tubular secretion of creatinine may result in a lower than expected serum creatinine level in patients with SCD. Proximal tubular dysfunction is seen in young

### KEY POINT

Patients with SCD have an increased proximal tubule activity with increased reabsorption of sodium and phosphorus, whereas tubular secretion of creatinine and uric acid is enhanced.

children and is independent of glomerular damage. Marsenic et al.[23] reported increased excretion of urinary retinol-binding protein (marker of proximal tubular dysfunction) in 15% of their study population.

## HYPERFILTRATION

Localized prostaglandin release and increased nitrous oxide synthase contribute to increased renal blood flow in SCD.[13] Renal plasma flow is elevated in excess of glomerular filtration rate (GFR), and the result is a lower than normal filtration fraction, which can be reversed with prostaglandin inhibition.[24] Hyperfiltration peaks in childhood and declines in adulthood.[25]

## IRON OVERLOAD

Early studies confirmed hemosiderin deposition in tubular epithelium, but it is unclear whether the iron deposits cause renal damage.[26,27] Schein et al.[28] detected kidney iron on magnetic resonance imaging and determined that the renal iron is the result of chronic hemolysis (evidenced by increased lactate dehydrogenase levels) and does not correlate with hepatic iron stores.

## TUMORIGENESIS

RMC is an epithelial malignant tumor arising from the collecting duct epithelium. This tumor occurs almost exclusive in young black patients with sickle cell hemoglobinopathies, mainly sickle cell trait.[29] Chronic medullary hypoxia may be involved in the pathogenesis of RMC. A role of genetic abnormalities in the pathogenesis of RMC has been proposed, but no consistent genotype has been observed in these patients.[30,31]

### KEY POINT

RMC occurs almost exclusively in young black patients with sickle trait (HbAS).

## RENAL PAPILLARY NECROSIS

The exact mechanism of RPN is not entirely understood, but several factors contributing to this process have been described. It is well established that dehydration, acidosis, decreased oxygen tension, and high osmolality present in the renal medulla are the main triggers of RBC sickling in this anatomic region of the kidney. Additionally, blood

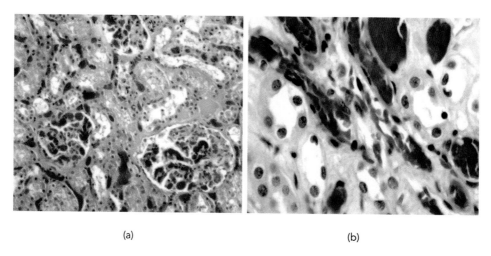

(a)                                                      (b)

Figure 27.3 **(a)** Light microscopy of renal biopsy in a patient who died in sickle crisis. Red blood cell sickling is seen within the glomerular capillaries. There are also extensive congestion and sickling in the peritubular capillaries. **(b)** Marked red blood cell sickling is evident within the vasa recta. (From Fogo A. Sickle cell nephropathy. Am J Kidney Dis. 2001;37:E34–5.1.)

flow in the vasa recta is much slower than in the cortical vessels, thus leading to more time for the hyperosmolar interstitium to induce RBC sickling. This process, in turn, increases the viscosity of blood, which causes even further slowing of the medullary blood flow. The sluggish flow ultimately leads to the formation of microthrombi and local microinfarctions, as well as a reduction in the number of functional vasa recta in the medulla. Loss of the vasa recta disrupts the concentration gradient in the medulla and results in isosthenuria.[32]

## SICKLE GLOMERULOPATHY

The presence of sickle cells in the glomeruli and congestion of the peritubular capillaries can be demonstrated in the renal biopsy specimens of patients with SCD, especially during sickle crises (Figure 27.3). Glomerular enlargement, increased intraglomerular pressure, and hyperfiltration are the hallmarks of established SCN and are thought to contribute to the development of focal segmental glomerulosclerosis (FSGS) seen in these patients (Figure 27.4). FSGS is the most common glomerular disorder seen in SCN.[33,34] In a review of 18 renal biopsy specimens from patients with SCD and glomerular involvement, Maigne et al.[27] described 4 histopathologic variants in SCD: FSGS in 39%, membranoproliferative glomerulonephritis (MPGN) in 28%, thrombotic microangiopathy glomerulopathy in 17%, and specific SCD

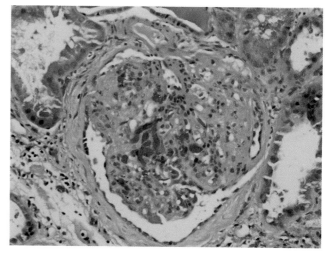

Figure 27.4 Sickle glomerulopathy. Light microscopy of a 16-year-old patient with HbSS disease and proteinuria showing focal segmental glomerulosclerosis. Red blood cell sickling in the glomerular capillaries is also seen. (Courtesy of Dr. Sally Self.)

glomerulopathy characterized by glomerular hypertrophy and congested peritubular capillaries in 17%. Long-term follow-up analysis revealed that 50% of patients exhibited CKD.[27] Apart from glomerular lesions, focal areas of tubulointerstitial fibrosis adjacent to sclerotic glomeruli are commonly seen. Immunofluorescence staining is nonspecific and may be positive for immunoglobulin M (IgM), C3, and C1q in the sclerotic segments. Results of electron microscopy are generally negative for immune electron-dense deposits.[33]

## KEY POINT

FSGS is the most common glomerular disorder observed in SCD associated with proteinuria or nephrotic syndrome.

## BLOOD PRESSURE

Children with SCD have lower clinic or office blood pressure (BP) readings than their healthy counterparts. This observation has been attributed to poor urinary concentrating ability, volume depletion, lower body weight, anemia, reduced left ventricular afterload, and decreased blood viscosity secondary to anemia. Altered vascular responsiveness to angiotensin II and nitric oxide resistance are also believed to contribute to altered vascular reactivity and relatively low BP.[35,36] Available evidence suggests that children with SCD have increased prevalence of blunted BP dipping and nighttime hypertension.[37] The concept of "relative hypertension" (BP that is within normal limits but elevated to peer SCD population) has been considered in patients with SCD and has been implicated in silent cerebral infarcts in these patients.[38]

## CLINICAL MANIFESTATIONS

*Sickle cell nephropathy* (SCN) is the term used for the plethora of clinical, biochemical, and pathologic renal abnormalities seen in patients with SCD. These manifestations often begin during early childhood, but their full clinical impact may not be evident until later in adolescence or young adulthood. The current model of SCN suggests that destruction of renal medulla induces production of renal vasodilating substances that feed back to the glomerulus and cause hyperfiltration. In turn, hyperfiltration leads to glomerulosclerosis and proteinuria, with impacts on kidney function and CKD.

## HEMATURIA

Hematuria is, by far, the most common complication of sickle cell trait (HbAS). It can occur at any age and is more often reported with HbAS.[3] In a large study of SCD (HbSS), the prevalence of hematuria was 6.3%.[2] Hematuria was significantly associated with earlier development of CKD in patients in this study.[2] In a cohort of SCD-affected children from Saudi Arabia, hematuria and hemoglobinuria were present in 8.5% and 14.5%, respectively.[39] Gross hematuria associated with passage of clots or development of "clot colic" should alert the clinician to the possibility of papillary necrosis, either secondary to SCD or from excessive use of nonsteroidal anti-inflammatory agents (NSAIDs) by these patients for relief of pain.

Alternative causes of hematuria, such as stones, neoplasms, and urinary tract infection, should always be considered in patients with SCD, and the diagnostic workup should be similar to what may be indicated in other patients.

## RENAL PAPILLARY NECROSIS

RPN is due to ischemic injury to the renal medulla seen in SCD and other disorders, such as analgesic abuse and urinary tract infections, particularly in the setting of diabetes mellitus (Figure 27.5). Although RPN is much more

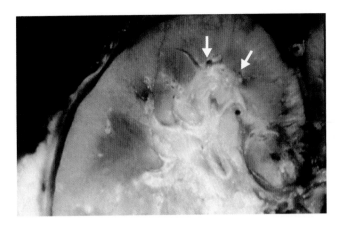

Figure 27.5 Papillary necrosis. Cut section of the kidney showing loss of the papillary tips in upper pole pyramids (arrows). (Figure is in public domain, reproduced from Lonergan GJ, Cline DB, Abbondanzo SL. Sickle cell anemia: from the archives of the AFIP. RadioGraphics 2001;21:971–94.)

common in SCD (HbSS), it can also be seen in patients with sickle cell trait (HbAS).[40]

RPN commonly manifests with painless gross hematuria, and bleeding is typically mild and unilateral when visualized by cystoscopy. Left kidney involvement is more frequent, presumably because of its larger size and unique blood supply. Apart from gross hematuria, other symptoms of RPN include flank pain, abdominal pain, nausea, and vomiting. Fever, if present, is typically the result of superimposed infection. Papillary sloughing and passage of the tissue down the ureter can cause intense colicky flank or abdominal pain, in addition to hematuria. Confirmation of papillary sloughing can be sought by preserving the tissue passed in urine (often embedded in a clot) in formalin and by tissue microscopy in pathologic examination.

## BLOOD PRESSURE

Clinic BP in patients with SCD is generally lower than that of the general population.[41] Systemic hypertension occurs in 2% to 6% of adults with SCD, compared with the published prevalence of 28% in the adult African-American population of the United States.[42,43] Transient hypertension in SCD is common during pain crises and in patients with CKD.

In a natural history study of 3317 patients with SCD who were 2 years old and older, significantly lower BP was correlated with body mass index, hemoglobin, renal function, and age, but the strength of the correlation varied among age and sex subgroups.[41] The risk for occlusive stroke increased with systolic BP (SBP) but not diastolic BP (DBP) in this study. Mortality was also related to elevated BP in male patients and to a lesser extent in female patients. In subjects with HbSC disease, BP also deviated from normal but to a lesser degree.[41] In another study examining factors associated with silent cerebral infarcts in SCD, the authors identified relatively high SBP as an independent determinant of such infarcts in these children.[37]

Adult and pediatric studies have also demonstrated a correlation between higher BP and microalbuminuria, an independent cardiorenal mortality risk factor.[9,13,43] In a study of 90 children with SCD, Becton et al.[9] found that clinic BP classification (prehypertensive and hypertensive) was independently associated with the presence of microalbuminuria. Stallworth et al.[2] reported that preexisting hypertension was significantly associated with the risk of developing AKI in children with SCD.

The prevalence of ambulatory hypertension and abnormal BP patterns on 24-h ambulatory BP (ABP) monitoring has not been well reported in children with SCD. One study, of 24-h ABP in 38 asymptomatic children with SCD, demonstrated that 17 (43.6%) subjects had ambulatory hypertension, whereas 4 (10.3%) were hypertensive based on their clinic BP.[38] Mean SBP dip and DBP dip were 8.3 ± 5.9% and 14.7 ± 7.6%, respectively. Twenty-three (59%) subjects had impaired SBP dipping, 7 (18%) had impaired DBP dipping, and 5 (13%) had reversed dipping. Clinic BP and ABP correlated modestly. These findings emphasize the need for close monitoring of patients with SCD to prevent long-term cardiac mortality risks.

## RENAL MEDULLARY CARCINOMA

RMC is a rare and highly aggressive tumor that is seen almost exclusively in young black patients with sickle cell trait (Figure 27.6). Dimashkieh et al.[44] reviewed 55 cases of RMC reported in the literature, and the average age at tumor presentation was 21 years, with a male-to-female ratio of 2:1. The right kidney was involved three times more commonly.

Of the 55 patients, 50 patients had HbAS, 2 patients had HbSC, and 1 patient had HbSS disease, thus highlighting its occurrence in patients with sickle trait. The most common symptoms at the time of presentation of RMC are flank pain, hematuria, weight loss, and abdominal pain, but some patients present with cough secondary to metastatic involvement of the lungs.[32,44]

## PROTEINURIA AND CHRONIC KIDNEY DISEASE

The reported prevalence of microalbuminuria and proteinuria in patients with SCD HbSS and HbSC genotypes ranges from 16% to 40%.[9,11] The prevalence of proteinuria in other genotypes is not well described. The prevalence of microalbuminuria increases with age, and this finding is uncommon before 7 years of age.[11] Microalbuminuria and proteinuria in SCD correlate with the number of vaso-occlusive crises, the severity of hemolysis, hemoglobin level, increasing age, BP, and pulmonary hypertension in children.[9] Many of these patients eventually develop overt proteinuria, which suggests an established sickle glomerulopathy. Although overt proteinuria may be seen up to 25% of patients with SCD, clinically evident nephrotic syndrome occurs in only 4% of cases.[33,45] FSGS is the dominant pathologic finding in 80% of such cases on renal biopsy. As many as 70% of patients with SCD and SCN may go on to develop end-stage renal disease (ESRD) in 2 years after diagnosis.[45] Hypertension and severe anemia are the other predictors of development of ESRD in patients with SCD.[12,46]

CKD can result from SCD and progression of SCN in children. In a cross-sectional observational study in 410 patients with SCD, 11.6% of these patients were noted to have CKD II.[9] The incidence of CKD I and CKD II combined was 26.5%. HbSC and HbSβ+ genotypes were associated with a higher risk for CKD in this study. In a smaller study of 48 children with SCD, Bodas et al.[47] found CKD II in 8.3% cases.

Although traditional thinking has been that sickle cell trait (HbAS), which affects 1 in 12 African Americans in the

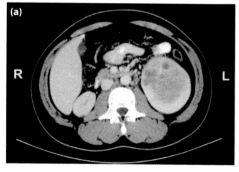
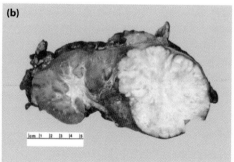

Figure 27.6 Renal medullary carcinoma. (a) Computed tomography scan of the abdomen showing a left kidney mass in a patient with renal medullary carcinoma. (b) Gross photograph of a well-circumscribed tumor involving the lower pole of the kidney. (From Dimashkieh H, Choe J, Mutema G. Renal medullary carcinoma: a report of 2 cases and review of the literature. Arch Pathol Lab Med. 2003;127:e135–8.)

United States, does not lead to CKD, more recent reevaluations have demonstrated HbAS is also associated with a higher risk for CKD and ESRD.[48,49] Based on the US Renal Data System (USRDS) database, SCD as a cause of ESRD accounts for 0.1% of all patients started on hemodialysis in the United States.[50]

---

## KEY POINT

Microalbuminuria or proteinuria affects 16% to 40% of patients with SCD and is the hallmark of glomerular injury.

---

## ACUTE KIDNEY INJURY

AKI occurs frequently in patients with SCD, and it can manifest as an isolated organ injury or as part of acute multiorgan failure syndrome.[51] Sklar et al.[52] reported a twofold or greater increase in serum creatinine in 12 of 116 (10.3%) hospitalized patients with SCD. AKI was seen most often in association with infections and in patients with lower hemoglobin (mean, 6.4 vs. 8.7 g/dL). Volume depletion was the most common precipitating factor of AKI. The incidence of AKI in hospitalized adult patients has been shown to vary with the severity of vaso-occlusive complication (VOC). AKI in one study was reported in 2.3% with pain crisis, 6.9% for moderate acute chest syndrome, and 13.6% for severe acute chest syndrome.[53] The use of NSAIDs may also be a causative factor in the precipitation of AKI in some patients with SCD.[54] Rhabdomyolysis leading to AKI during severe exercise has also been reported in patients with sickle cell trait.[55]

## TUBULAR DYSFUNCTION AND ENURESIS

The most common clinically manifest tubular abnormality in SCD is a urinary concentrating defect. The urine concentrating defect is unique to sickling hemoglobinopathies and is not seen in other anemias. In contrast, urinary dilution is normal.[21]

Most patients with HbSS are unable to achieve a urine maximal concentration of approximately 500 mOsm/kg after 14 to 17 hours of thirst and exogenously administered pitressin, compared with mean osmolality of 1055 ± 188 mOsm/kg in controls.[56] The defective urine concentrating ability appears to be age dependent, being less pronounced in infants and in children up to age 7 years.[56,57] Even patients with sickle trait have a diminished urinary concentrating capacity.[58] The urine concentrating defect in SCD is resistant to exogenous pitressin therapy, a finding indicating that the diabetes insipidus in SCD is of "nephrogenic" origin.[56] The nephrogenic diabetes insipidus associated with SCD is likely the result of hemodynamic changes in the renal medulla and vasa recta induced by ongoing sickling and tubulointerstitial damage.

An inability to concentrate urine in SCD results in an increased frequency of urination and enuresis in children with SCD and makes them susceptible to dehydration. Improvement in the concentrating defect in response to pharmacologic doses of intranasal desmopressin acetate (DDAVP) is variable and seems to be related to the percentage of sickle hemoglobin present in erythrocytes; vasopressin generation is normal.[58] Early indications are that treatment with hydroxyurea improves urine concentrating ability in children.[59]

Incomplete distal RTA may complicate SCD, but it is not usually a clinical problem.[19] The minimum urine pH achieved in response to ammonium chloride loading is not as low as in controls (5.8 vs. 5.1), but total ammonium excretion is normal. Consequently, titratable acidity is reduced.[60] Distal RTA with hyperkalemia (type IV) has also been described in SCD, with a reduced ability to lower urine pH in response to acid load and inadequate urinary potassium secretion, especially in patients with decreased renal function.[61] Metabolic acidosis and hyperkalemia in SCD are believed to result from aldosterone-independent end-organ failure secondary to medullary fibrosis and tubulointerstitial damage. β Blockers, potassium-sparing diuretics, or angiotensin-converting enzyme inhibitors (ACEIs) should be used with caution in patients with SCD because these drugs may cause hyperkalemia.

Because of the enhanced proximal tubular sodium reabsorption in patients with SCD, diuretic response may be poor. Similarly, because of enhanced proximal tubular phosphate reabsorption, which usually parallels sodium reabsorption, hyperphosphatemia may be seen in in some patients with SCD, especially in the presence of an increased phosphate load generated by hemolysis.[19]

In summary, the tubular dysfunction of SCD manifests a defect in urine concentration, whereas dilution is maintained. Hydrogen ion and potassium secretion functions are only mildly affected, and proximal tubular mechanisms are exaggerated.

---

## KEY POINTS

- SCD is associated with a defect in urine concentration, whereas urine dilution capability is well maintained.
- SCD is characterized by supranormal proximal tubular function.

---

## CLINICAL MANAGEMENT

## HEMATURIA

Patients with SCD (HbSS) and sickle cell trait (HbAS) who develop gross hematuria need a thorough evaluation for all the usual diagnostic entities, such as urinary tract infection or renal stones. However, conditions that are unique to these patients, such as RPN and the distinctive RMC, must also be considered in the diagnostic evaluation. Initial investigations should include urine analysis, culture, and renal ultrasound. Renal ultrasound findings can be nondescript and nonspecific, except in patients with RPN. A review of ultrasound studies in young patients with SCD (10 to 20 years old) found diffusely increased echogenicity in 9% and increased medullary echodensity in 3%.[62] Surprisingly, echodensity was greater in the clinically milder genotypes: 37% and 79% in patients with SC and S-Thal, respectively. These findings may indicate subclinical nephrocalcinosis or iron deposition.

Because of the radiation-associated risk, renal computed tomography (CT) scan should be considered only if it is diagnostically essential. If sustained gross hematuria is present, cystoscopy with ureteroscopy may be required. More recently, magnetic resonance urography (MRU) has been used to define the renal anatomy and function (Figure 27.7).

Continued gross hematuria should be considered a form of renal sickle crisis in patients known to have HbSS or HbAS. The treatment of hematuria in SCD involves bed rest, analgesics, and adequate fluid intake to ensure a high urinary flow. Blood transfusion to reduce the burden of circulating RBCs with sickle hemoglobin should be considered.

Vasopressin and ε-amino caproic acid (EACA or Amicar) have both been used with variable success in controlling severe urologic hemorrhage associated with HbSS or HbAS.[63,64] However, caution must be exercised when using EACA because this antifibrinolytic agent may predispose to the formation of clots that can obstruct the urinary collecting system. If prolonged and life-threatening bleeding is localized to one side, a limited surgical approach may be considered. Unilateral nephrectomy is generally not recommended because bleeding may recur in the contralateral kidney.

RPN can be a diagnostic and management challenge in patients with HbSS and HbAS. These patients present with persistent hematuria and may have abdominal pain resulting from clot-induced colic. Renal ultrasound evaluation may be sufficient to demonstrate a roughened, sloughed papillary tip with a preserved base of the calyx or formation of a sinus that communicates between the renal pelvis and the calyx (Figure 27.8). An intravenous pyelogram (IVP) may show the classic "ring shadow" (Figure 27.9) in the area of necrotic papilla, but this procedure carries the risk for AKI in these patients. Eventually, a calcified papilla may be evident in a renal ultrasound scan or an abdominal x-ray study. The presence of sloughed papillae in the urine is diagnostic, but It has low sensitivity. In some cases, direct visualization of renal calyces with ureteroscopy is required to reach the diagnosis.[32]

Apart from the principles of therapy described previously for managing renal hemorrhage, low-dose, oral EACA may be considered in patients with RPN who have severe hemorrhagic manifestations.[64,65] ACEIs have been shown to induce a 50% increase in papillary blood flow in experimental studies, and these drugs may be considered as preventive therapy in these patients.[20] However, during an episode of active bleeding, ACEI therapy may aggravate hematuria by increasing blood flow to the tissues affected by hemorrhage. Ureteroscopy and the use of a balloon ureteral dilator to tamponade the bleeding site has also successfully stopped bleeding in some patients with RPN.[66]

## PROTEINURIA AND NEPHROTIC SYNDROME

Evaluation of proteinuria in patients with SCD should begin with quantification of the degree of proteinuria. First morning urine sample should be used to quantify urinary protein excretion (urine protein-to-creatinine ratio). A 24-h urine collection is generally not necessary in children. Serum total protein and albumin, along with renal function and serum cholesterol, should also be measured. Tubular proteinuria can also occur in patients with SCD as a result of tubulointerstitial damage, and it needs to be evaluated by urine protein electrophoresis. Eventually, patients with progressively increasing proteinuria or nephrotic syndrome should undergo a renal biopsy to confirm the presence and type of sickle glomerulopathy. As indicated earlier, glomerular hypertrophy and FSGS are the dominant pathologic lesions in such cases.

Treatment of microalbuminuria, as well as of overt proteinuria, by ACEIs has been found to useful in small and short-duration studies.[8,33,45,46] A Cochrane review of

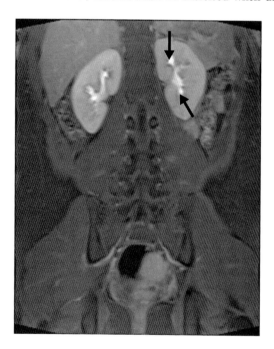

Figure 27.7 Coronal postcontrast fat-saturated T1-weighted three-dimensional magnetic resonance volumetric interpolated breath-hold examination (VIBE) demonstrates partially sloughed material within the medial left upper pole minor calyx (upper arrow) giving a subtle golf ball-on-a-tee calyceal contour. The left lower pole minor calyx is clubbed from resorption of the papilla (lower arrow). (Courtesy of Dr. Paul G. Thacker, Jr.)

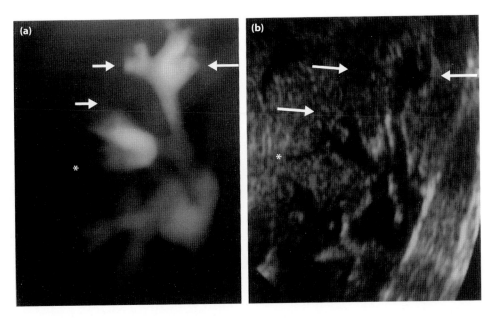

Figure 27.8 Renal papillary necrosis. **(a)** Tomographic intravenous pyelography of an 18-year-old patient with abdominal pain and hematuria. Papillary necrosis is evident from blunted medullary cavities, especially the upper pole (arrows). The bases of the calyces are preserved. The middle pole calyx has a possible sinus tract (*). **(b)** Ultrasonographic visualization of the same kidney. The middle pole exhibits deep extensions into the papilla, likely to be sinus tracts. (Courtesy of Dr. JI Scheinman. From Scheinman JI. Sickle cell disease and the kidney. Nat Clin Pract Nephrol. 2009;5:78–88.)

the literature, however, was unable to find evidence that administration of ACEIs is associated with improvement in microalbuminuria and proteinuria in SCD.[67] There is also no well-documented evidence to suggest that corticosteroids or other immunosuppressive therapies are helpful in inducing remission of nephrotic syndrome in such patients. Moreover, corticosteroids are tolerated poorly by patients

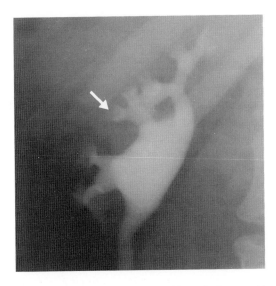

Figure 27.9 Papillary necrosis in sickle cell disease. Frontal view of the right kidney obtained during excretory urography showing a small, round collection of contrast material in an area of missing papillary tip (arrow). (Figure is in public domain, reproduced from Lonergan GJ, Cline DB, Abbondanzo SL. Sickle cell anemia: from the archives of the AFIP. RadioGraphics 2001;21:971–94.)

with SCD and may also precipitate veno-occlusive crises in these patients.[68]

## CHRONIC KIDNEY DISEASE

Hyperfiltration is the hallmark of SCD in early infancy, which continues throughout childhood and in young adults in most patients.[6,69,70] A gradual decline in estimated GFR (eGFR) is noted in patients with SCD throughout childhood, adolescence, and adulthood. CKD in patients with SCD is uncommon before the teen years, and CKD stage II has been reported in approximately 11% patients.[6]

In part, because of supernormal proximal tubular secretion of creatinine in SCD, creatinine clearance often overestimates the GFR. The Pediatric Hydroxyurea Phase III Trial (BABY HUG) study evaluated GFR in infants by using 99m-technetium ($^{99m}$Tc)–diethylene triamine penta-acetic acid (DTPA) and creatinine clearance estimates using Schwartz formulas.[69,70]. The mean DTPA GFR in this study was 125.2 ± 34.4 mL/min/m$^2$, whereas the Schwartz classic formula estimates were higher, at 184.4 ± 55.5 mL/min/1.73 m$^2$.[69] eGFR based on the CKid-Schwartz (k = 0.413) formula, however, correlated better with DTPA-derived GFR in infants.[70] A disparity of up to 30% may be noted between creatinine clearance and inulin clearance in patients with SCD.[19,71] Additionally, many children with SCD are underweight, with low muscle mass, and this feature adds to the complexity of interpreting GFR estimates based on serum creatinine. Whether serum cystatin-C is better indicator of renal function than serum creatinine in SCD is unclear.[10,72]

Although serum creatinine has its drawbacks as a marker for estimating GFR, mostly leading to its overestimation, formulas based on serum creatinine remain the most practiced bedside and practical standards. National Heart, Lung and Blood Institute (NHLBI) guidelines for the management of SCD recommend checking renal function (creatinine, blood urea nitrogen, urinalysis) annually for children 12 months old and older as part of the suggested routine clinical laboratory evaluations.[73]

As CKD advances in patients with SCD, they need to be followed and cared for in a manner similar to other patient groups with a similar stage of renal dysfunction. A unique aspect in the management of SCD-related CKD and ESRD is the treatment of associated anemia. Whereas erythropoietin (EPO) use in anemia of CKD and ESRD is an accepted therapy, its safety and effectiveness in SCD-related CKD and ESRD have not been well established. In general, EPO response in SCD-related CKD and ESRD has been noted to be unpredictable. The dose of EPO for adequate erythropoiesis in these patients is significantly higher than the standard dose (less than 200 units/kg/dose), sometimes as high as 1500 units/kg/dose.[74,75] Past concerns with use of EPO in patients with SCD-related CKD and ESRD have been increased veno-occlusive sickle cell crises and increased thrombotic events.[74] However, more recent experience in the treatment of these patients with EPO found the therapy to be safe and effective, although some patients have experienced increased veno-occlusive sickle cell crises.[75]

## BLOOD PRESSURE

Because BP in patients with SCD is generally lower than in the general population, "normal" BP readings in these patients may indeed reflect elevated BP. However, optimum target BP in SCD has not been established. It is also unclear whether treatment is needed for such patients with "normal" BP and whether there would be any beneficial effects of such therapy. In general, there should be a lower threshold for treating these patients for hypertension. It is also important to consider the class of antihypertensive agents prescribed for these patients. Because an increased risk of hyperkalemia in SCD can be seen with the use of β blockers and ACEIs, caution should be exercised in the use of these drugs. Diuretic agents in patients with SCD, who have obligate hyposthenuria, can cause dehydration and also can precipitate vaso-occlusive events.

## RENAL TUBULAR DISORDERS

Treatment of tubular disorders in SCD is usually unnecessary in patients with normal renal function. The risk of dehydration caused by decreased urinary concentrating ability requires prompt treatment of underlying conditions, as well as appropriate intravenous fluid therapy. The BABY HUG trial data suggest that urinary concentrating ability in SCD can be improved with the use of hydroxyurea, and this option can be considered in such patients.[70,76] Metabolic

acidosis should also be avoided because it may facilitate the onset of veno-occlusive crisis.

### KEY POINT

Hydroxyurea is associated with better urine concentrating ability and less renal enlargement.

Hyperuricemia, resulting from increased urate production, may be aggravated by diuretics (especially thiazides) that inhibit urate secretion. Severe hemolysis, ACEIs, or β blockers can aggravate hyperkalemia, especially in the presence of renal insufficiency. The use of these drugs, as noted previously, should be considered cautiously.

## DIALYSIS AND KIDNEY TRANSPLANTATION

The prolonged survival of patients with SCD has led to an increase in the prevalence of SCN and ESRD.[12,77] The average age of renal failure is 40 years, but early signs, such as microalbuminuria, may be apparent at an earlier age.[78] Adequate predialysis care reduces mortality among patients with SCD and ESRD. Using data provided by the Centers for Medicare and Medicaid Services (CMS), McClellan et al.[79] examined the relationship between mortality and pre-ESRD care in incident patients with SCD and ESRD. These investigators found that patients with SCD and ESRD who received predialysis nephrology care had a lower death rate than did patients with SCD and ESRD who did not receive predialysis nephrology care.[79] Patients with SCD and ESRD also had inferior survival rates compared with patients with ESRD from other causes at 1 year after starting dialysis.

### KEY POINT

Adequate predialysis care reduces mortality among patients with ESRD who have SCD.

In the years 1989 to 1995, ESRD from SCD accounted for only 0.5% and 0.2% of the pediatric patients registered in the dialysis and transplant arms, respectively, of the North American Pediatric Renal Transplant Cooperative Study (NAPRTCS) database. Mean graft survival at 12 and 24 months after transplant was 89% and 71%, respectively. Patient survival was 89%.[80] Huang et al.[81] reported improved survival among kidney transplant recipients with SCD from 2000 to 2011, compared with the 1988 to 1999 era. Multivariate Cox proportional hazard models, however, revealed an increased mortality risk with SCD in both eras. Despite a less satisfactory outcome, available evidence strongly indicates that transplantation is a better option for the patient with SCD and ESRD. Increased vaso-occlusive crises and allograft sickling events, however, remain challenges in these patients. SCN has been reported to recur in the transplanted kidney after as short a time as 3.5 years.[82]

## SUMMARY

SCD is a multiorgan disorder that can affect the kidney and lead to CKD and ESRD. Renal injury or SCN starts early in childhood. Efforts to prevent sickling, examine potential renoprotective agents, and develop biomarkers to identify early kidney injury and patients at risk of disease progression are among the most important avenues in understanding and preventing the renal consequences of SCD.

Kidney transplantation offers better survival option for patients with ESRD. With advances in the transplant field, bone marrow coupled with kidney transplantation is becoming a more promising option for patients with SCD and ESRD.

More emphasis is needed on well-structured transition care programs from childhood to adulthood. Children with SCD have lower clinic or office BP than their healthy counterparts. The significance of having normal BP for age, sex, and height (relative hypertension) in children with SCD is unknown. Abnormalities in ABP measurements and patterns in children with SCD are prevalent and require more attention from health care providers. ABP monitoring is a valuable tool in identifying masked hypertension and abnormalities in circadian BP.

# REFERENCES

1. Lonsdorfer A, Comoe L, Yapo AE, et al. Proteinuria in sickle cell trait and disease: An electrophoretic analysis. Clin Chim Acta. 1989;181:239–47.
2. Stallworth JR, Tripathi A, Jerrell JM. Prevalence, treatment, and outcomes of renal conditions in pediatric sickle cell disease. South Med J. 2011;104:752–6.
3. Pham PT, Pham PC, Wilkinson AH, et al. Renal abnormalities in sickle cell disease. Kidney Int. 2000;57:1–8.
4. Sklar AH, Campbell H, Caruana RJ, et al. A population study of renal function in sickle cell anemia. Int J Artif Organs. 1990;13:231–6.
5. Wigfall DR, Ware RE, Burchinal MR, et al. Prevalence and clinical correlates of glomerulopathy in children with sickle cell disease. J Pediatr. 2000;136:749–53.
6. McPherson Yee M, Jabbar SF, et al. Chronic kidney disease and albuminuria in children with sickle cell disease. Clin J Am Soc Nephrol. 2011;6:2628–33.
7. McKie KT, Hanevold CD, Hernandez C, et al. Prevalence, prevention, and treatment of microalbuminuria and proteinuria in children with sickle cell disease. J.Pediatr Hematol Oncol. 2007;29:140–4.
8. Alvarez O, Lopez-Mitnik G, Zilleruelo G. Short-term follow-up of patients with sickle cell disease and albuminuria. Pediatr Blood Cancer. 2008;50:1236–9.
9. Becton LJ, Kalpatthi RV, Rackoff E, et al. Prevalence and clinical correlates of microalbuminuria in children with sickle cell disease. Pediatr Nephrol. 2010;25:1505–11.
10. Aygun B, Mortier NA, Smeltzer MP, et al. Glomerular hyperfiltration and albuminuria in children with sickle cell anemia. Pediatr Nephrol. 2011;26:1285–90.
11. Dharnidharka VR, Dabbagh S, Atiyeh B, et al. Prevalence of microalbuminuria in children with sickle cell disease. Pediatr Nephrol. 1998;12:475–8.
12. Powars DR, Elliott-Mills DD, Chan L, et al. Chronic renal failure in sickle cell disease: Risk factors, clinical course, and mortality. Ann Intern Med. 1991;115:614–20.
13. Thompson J, Reid M, Hambleton I, et al. Albuminuria and renal function in homozygous sickle cell disease: Observations from a cohort study. Arch Intern Med. 2007;167:701–8.
14. Guasch A, Navarrete J, Nass K, et al. Glomerular involvement in adults with sickle cell hemoglobinopathies: Prevalence and clinical correlates of progressive renal failure. J Am Soc Nephrol. 2006;17:2228–35.
15. Platt OS, Brambilla DJ, Rosse WF, et al. Mortality in sickle cell disease: Life expectancy and risk factors for early death. N Engl J Med. 1994 9;330:1639–44.
16. Lebensburger J, Johnson SM, Askenazi DJ, et al. Protective role of hemoglobin and fetal hemoglobin in early kidney disease for children with sickle cell anemia. Am J Hematol. 2011;86:430–2.
17. Powars DR, Meiselman HJ, Fisher TC, et al. Beta-S gene cluster haplotypes modulate hematologic and hemorheologic expression in sickle cell anemia: Use in predicting clinical severity. Am J Pediatr Hematol Oncol. 1994;16:55–61.
18. Guasch A, Zayas CF, Eckman JR, et al. Evidence that microdeletions in the alpha globin gene protect against the development of sickle cell glomerulopathy in humans. J Am Soc Nephrol. 1999;10:1014–9.
19. Allon M. Renal abnormalities in sickle cell disease. Arch Intern Med. 1990;150:501–4.
20. Sabatini S. Pathophysiologic mechanisms of abnormal collecting duct function. Semin Nephrol. 1989;9:179–202.
21. Statius van Eps LW, Schouten H, La Porte-Wijsman LW, et al. The influence of red blood cell transfusions on the hyposthenuria and renal hemodynamics of sickle cell anemia. Clin Chim Acta. 1967;17:449–61.
22. Davies SC, Hewitt PE. Sickle cell disease. Br J Hosp Med. 1984;31:440–4.

23. Marsenic O, Couloures KG, Wiley JM. Proteinuria in children with sickle cell disease. Nephrol Dial Transplant. 2008;23:715–20.

24. Allon M, Lawson L, Eckman JR, et al. Effects of non-steroidal antiinflammatory drugs on renal function in sickle cell anemia. Kidney Int. 1988;34:500–6.

25. Ataga KI, Orringer EP. Renal abnormalities in sickle cell disease. Am J Hematol. 2000;63:205–11.

26. Chauhan PM, Kondlapoodi P, Natta CL. Pathology of sickle cell disorders. Pathol Annu. 1983;18:253–76.

27. Maigne G, Ferlicot S, Galacteros F, et al. Glomerular lesions in patients with sickle cell disease. Medicine (Baltimore). 2010;89:18–27.

28. Schein A, Enriquez C, Coates TD, et al. Magnetic resonance detection of kidney iron deposition in sickle cell disease: A marker of chronic hemolysis. J Magn Reson Imaging. 2008;28:698–704.

29. Baig MA, Lin YS, Rasheed J, et al. Renal medullary carcinoma. J Natl Med Assoc. 2006;98:1171–4.

30. Swartz MA, Karth J, Schneider DT, et al. Renal medullary carcinoma: Clinical, pathologic, immunohistochemical, and genetic analysis with pathogenetic implications. Urology. 2002;60:1083–9.

31. Walsh A, Kelly DR, Vaid YN, et al. Complete response to carboplatin, gemcitabine, and paclitaxel in a patient with advanced metastatic renal medullary carcinoma. Pediatr Blood Cancer. 2010;55:1217–20.

32. Kiryluk K, Jadoon A, Gupta M, et al. Sickle cell trait and gross hematuria. Kidney Int. 2007;71:706–10.

33. Falk RJ, Scheinman J, Phillips G, et al. Prevalence and pathologic features of sickle cell nephropathy and response to inhibition of angiotensin-converting enzyme. N Engl J Med. 1992;326:910–5.

34. Bhathena DB, Sondheimer JH. The glomerulopathy of homozygous sickle hemoglobin (SS) disease: Morphology and pathogenesis. J Am Soc Nephrol. 1991;1:1241–52.

35. Hatch FE, Crowe LR, Miles DE, et al. Altered vascular reactivity in sickle hemoglobinopathy: A possible protective factor from hypertension. Am J Hypertens. 1989;2:2–8.

36. Wood KC, Hsu LL, Gladwin MT. Sickle cell disease vasculopathy: A state of nitric oxide resistance. Free Radic Biol Med. 2008;44:1506–28.

37. Shatat IF, Jakson SM, Blue AE, et al. Masked hypertension is prevalent in children with sickle cell disease: A Midwest Pediatric Nephrology Consortium study. Pediatr Nephrol. 2013;28:115–20.

38. DeBaun MR, Armstrong FD, McKinstry RC, et al. Silent cerebral infarcts: A review on a prevalent and progressive cause of neurologic injury in sickle cell anemia. Blood. 2012;119:4587–96.

39. Aleem A. Renal abnormalities in patients with sickle cell disease: A single center report from Saudi Arabia. Saudi J Kidney Dis Transpl. 2008;19:194–9.

40. Osegbe DN. Haematuria and sickle cell disease: A report of 12 cases and review of the literature. Trop Geogr Med. 1990;42:22–7.

41. Pegelow CH, Colangelo L, Steinberg M, et al. Natural history of blood pressure in sickle cell disease: Risks for stroke and death associated with relative hypertension in sickle cell anemia. Am J Med. 1997;102:171–7.

42. Guasch A, Cua M, You W, et al. Sickle cell anemia causes a distinct pattern of glomerular dysfunction. Kidney Int. 1997;51:826–33.

43. Johnson CS, Giorgio AJ. Arterial blood pressure in adults with sickle cell disease. Arch Intern Med. 1981;141:891–3.

44. Dimashkieh H, Choe J, Mutema G. Renal medullary carcinoma: A report of 2 cases and review of the literature. Arch Pathol Lab Med. 2003;127:e135–8.

45. Bakir AA, Hathiwala SC, Ainis H, et al. Prognosis of the nephrotic syndrome in sickle glomerulopathy: A retrospective study. Am J Nephrol. 1987;7:110–5.

46. Foucan L, Bourhis V, Bangou J, et al. A randomized trial of captopril for microalbuminuria in normotensive adults with sickle cell anemia. Am J Med. 1998;104:339–42.

47. Bodas P, Huang A, O'Riordan MA, et al. The prevalence of hypertension and abnormal kidney function in children with sickle cell disease: A cross sectional review. BMC Nephrol. 2013;14:237.

48. Derebail VK, Nachman PH, Key NS, et al. High prevalence of sickle cell trait in African Americans with ESRD. J Am Soc Nephrol. 2010;21:413–7.

49. Naik RP, Derebail VK, Grams ME, et al. Association of sickle cell trait with chronic kidney disease and albuminuria in African Americans. JAMA. 2014;312:2115–25.

50. Abbott KC, Hypolite IO, Agodoa LY. Sickle cell nephropathy at end-stage renal disease in the United States: Patient characteristics and survival. Clin Nephrol. 2002;58:9–15.

51. Hassell KL, Eckman JR, Lane PA. Acute multiorgan failure syndrome: A potentially catastrophic complication of severe sickle cell pain episodes. Am J Med. 1994;96:155–62.

52. Sklar AH, Perez JC, Harp RJ, et al. Acute renal failure in sickle cell anemia. Int J Artif Organs. 1990;13:347–51.

53. Audard V, Homs S, Habibi A, et al. Acute kidney injury in sickle patients with painful crisis or acute chest syndrome and its relation to pulmonary hypertension. Nephrol Dial Transplant. 2010;25:2524–9.

54. Simckes AM, Chen SS, Osorio AV, et al. Ketorolac-induced irreversible renal failure in sickle cell disease: A case report. Pediatr Nephrol. 1999;13:63–7.

55. Koppes GM, Daly JJ, Coltman CA, Jr., et al. Exertion-induced rhabdomyolysis with acute renal failure and disseminated intravascular coagulation in sickle cell trait. Am J Med. 1977;63:313–7.

56. Keitel HG, Thompson D, Itano HA. Hyposthenuria in sickle cell anemia: A reversible renal defect. J Clin Invest. 1956;35:998–1007.

57. Miller ST, Wang WC, Iyer R, et al. Urine concentrating ability in infants with sickle cell disease: Baseline data from the phase III trial of hydroxyurea (BABY HUG). Pediatr Blood Cancer. 2010;54:265–8.

58. Gupta AK, Kirchner KA, Nicholson R, et al. Effects of alpha-thalassemia and sickle polymerization tendency on the urine-concentrating defect of individuals with sickle cell trait. J Clin Invest. 1991;88:1963–8.

59. Alvarez O, Miller ST, Wang WC, et al. Effect of hydroxyurea treatment on renal function parameters: Results from the multi-center placebo-controlled BABY HUG clinical trial for infants with sickle cell anemia. Pediatr Blood Cancer. 2012;59:668–74.

60. de Jong PE, de Jong-van den Berg LT, Schouten H, et al. The influence of indomethacin on renal acidification in normal subjects and in patients with sickle cell anemia. Clin Nephrol. 1983;19:259–64.

61. Kurtzman NA. Acquired distal renal tubular acidosis. Kidney Int. 1983;24:807–19.

62. Walker TM, Serjeant GR. Increased renal reflectivity in sickle cell disease: Prevalence and characteristics. Clin Radiol. 1995;50:566–9.

63. John EG, Schade SG, Spigos DG, et al. Effectiveness of triglycyl vasopressin in persistent hematuria associated with sickle cell hemoglobin. Arch Intern Med. 1980;140:1589–93.

64. Immergut MA, Stevenson T. The use of epsilon amino caproic acid in the control of hematuria associated with hemoglobinopathies. J Urol. 1965;93:110–1.

65. Gabrovsky A, Aderinto A, Spevak M, et al. Low dose, oral epsilon aminocaproic acid for renal papillary necrosis and massive hemorrhage in hemoglobin SC disease. Pediatr Blood Cancer. 2010;54:148–50.

66. Herard A, Colin J, Youinou Y, et al. Massive gross hematuria in a sickle cell trait patient with renal papillary necrosis: Conservative approach using a balloon ureteral catheter to tamponade the papilla bleeding. Eur Urol. 1998;34:161–2.

67. Sasongko TH, Nagalla S, Ballas SK. Angiotensin-converting enzyme (ACE) inhibitors for proteinuria and microalbuminuria in people with sickle cell disease. Cochrane Database Syst Rev. 2013;3:CD009191..

68. Darbari DS, Castro O, Taylor JG, 6th, et al. Severe vaso-occlusive episodes associated with use of systemic corticosteroids in patients with sickle cell disease. J Natl Med Assoc. 2008;100:948–51.

69. Ware RE, Rees RC, Sarnaik SA, et al. Renal function in infants with sickle cell anemia: Baseline data from the BABY HUG trial. J Pediatr. 2010;156:66–70.e1.

70. Alvarez O, Miller ST, Wang WC, et al. Effect of hydroxyurea treatment on renal function parameters: Results from the multi-center placebo-controlled BABY HUG clinical trial for infants with sickle cell anemia. Pediatr Blood Cancer. 2012;59:668–74.

71. Herrera J, Avila E, Marín C,et al. Impaired creatinine secretion after an intravenous creatinine load is an early characteristic of the nephropathy of sickle cell anaemia. Nephrol Dial Transplant. 2002;17:602–7.

72. Alvarez O, Zilleruelo G, Wright D, et al. Serum cystatin C levels in children with sickle cell disease. Pediatr Nephrol. 2006;21:533–7.

73. Annonymous. The Management of Sickle Cell Disease, 4th ed. National Heart Lung and Blood Institute. Division of Blood Diseases and Resources. NIH Publication: 02-2117. Bethesda, MD: National Institutes of Health; 2002.

74. Tomson CRV, Edmunds ME, Chambers K, et al. Effect of human recombinant erythropoietin on erythropoiesis in homozygous sickle cell anaemia and renal failure. Nephrol Dial Transplant. 1992;7:817–21.

75. Little JA, McGowan VR, Kato GJ, et al. Combination erythropoietin-hydroxyurea therapy in sickle cell disease: Experience from the National Institutes of Health and a literature review. Haematologica. 2006;91:1076–83.

76. Miller ST, Wang WC, Iyer R, et al. Urine concentrating ability in infants with sickle cell disease: Baseline data from phase III trial of hydroxyurea (BABY HUG). Pediatr Blood Cancer. 210;54:256–8.

77. Powars DR, Chan LS, Hiti A, et al. Outcome of sickle cell anemia: A 4-decade observational study of 1056 patients. Medicine (Baltimore). 2005;84:363–76.

78. Wesson DE. The initiation and progression of sickle cell nephropathy. Kidney Int. 2002;61:2277–86.

79. McClellan AC, Luthi JC, Lynch JR, et al. High one year mortality in adults with sickle cell disease and end-stage renal disease. Br J Haematol. 2012;159:360–7.

80. Warady BA, Sullivan EK. Renal transplantation in children with sickle cell disease: A report of the North American Pediatric Renal Transplant Cooperative Study (NAPRTCS). Pediatr Transplant. 1998;2:130–3.

81. Huang E, Parke C, Mehrnia A, et al. Improved survival among sickle cell kidney transplant recipients in the recent era. Nephrol Dial Transplant. 2013;28:1039–46.

82. Miner DJ, Jorkasky DK, Perloff LJ, et al. Recurrent sickle cell nephropathy in a transplanted kidney. Am J Kidney Dis. 1987;10:306–13.

## REVIEW QUESTIONS

1. Hematuria is *more often* reported with:
   a. HbSS
   b. HbSC
   c. HbS/β thal
   d. Hb AS
   e. Hb AA
2. The *most common* manifestation of tubular abnormality in SCD is:
   a. Urine concentration defect
   b. Urine acidification defect
   c. Edema
   d. Urine dilution defect
   e. a and d
3. In patients with sickle cell disease, the *most common* glomerular pathologic finding on renal biopsy is:
   a. Minimal change disease
   b. FSGS
   c. MPGN
   d. IgA nephropathy
   e. Membranous nephropathy
4. All the following statements about sickle cell nephropathy are correct *except:*
   a. Treatment of hematuria in SCD involves bed rest and maintenance of a high urinary flow.
   b. Patients with sickle cell disease are at a lower risk of developing hyperkalemia when treated with ACEIs and β blockers.
   c. The reported prevalence of microalbuminuria and proteinuria in patients with sickle cell disease ranges from 16% to 40%.
   d. Renal medullary carcinoma is present almost exclusively in young black patients with sickle cell trait.
   e. Children with sickle cell disease have lower clinic BP measurements than their age-, sex-, height-matched counterparts.
5. All of the following statements regarding tubular function in patients with sickle cell disease are correct *except:*
   a. Sodium reabsorption is increased.
   b. Phosphate reabsorption is increased.
   c. Potassium reabsorption is increased.
   d. Urate secretion is increased.
   e. Creatinine secretion is increased.
6. The *earliest* manifestation of kidney injury in childhood is:
   a. Acidosis
   b. Enuresis
   c. Hyposthenuria
   d. Hypertension
   e. Proteinuria
7. Mechanisms of renal injury include all of the following *except:*
   a. Immune complex deposits in the basement membrane
   b. Hypoxia in the vasa recta
   c. Polymerization of sickle hemoglobin
   d. Hyperfiltration in the glomerulus
   e. Medullary fibrosis
8. All of the following factors are strong predictors of chronic kidney disease *except:*
   a. Proteinuria
   b. Hematuria
   c. CAR haplotype
   d. Nephrotoxic medications
   e. Nephrotic syndrome
9. All of the following are known correlates of microalbuminuria and proteinuria *except:*
   a. Degree of hemolysis
   b. Increasing age
   c. Elevated blood pressure
   d. Pulmonary hypertension
   e. Higher hemoglobin levels

## ANSWER KEY

1. d
2. a
3. b
4. b
5. c
6. c
7. a
8. d
9. e

# 28

# Kidney disease associated with diabetes mellitus and metabolic syndrome

## KANWAL KHER AND MICHELE MIETUS-SNYDER

Diabetes mellitus is the most common metabolic disorder affecting humans. The hallmark of this condition is hyperglycemia, which can develop from a lack of insulin production, peripheral resistance to the metabolic actions of insulin, or both. In adults, diabetes mellitus is the leading cause of chronic kidney disease (CKD), loss of vision, and nontraumatic amputations. This chapter will discuss the clinical spectrum of renal disease seen in diabetes mellitus and obesity-metabolic syndrome. Both of these disorders, although well recognized in adults, are increasingly being encountered in children and adolescents.

## CLASSIFICATION OF DIABETES

From a clinical point of view, diabetes mellitus is classified into distinct types. Type 1 diabetes mellitus (DM1) is more common in childhood and adolescence and results from insulin deficiency, usually secondary to immune destruction of pancreatic β cells in the islets of Langerhans. On the other hand, type 2 diabetes mellitus (DM2) is more common in adults and results from resistance to insulin in peripheral tissues. The incidence of DM2 in children and adolescents has, however, been rising globally in the last decade.[1] A combination of relative insulin deficiency

and peripheral resistance to insulin action can be seen in some patients, especially in young adults.

## EPIDEMIOLOGY OF DIABETES MELLITUS

The SEARCH for Diabetes in Youth Study estimates that 191,986 children and adults younger than 20 years of age have diabetes mellitus in the United States. Of this, 166,984 have DM1 and 20,262 have DM2. The remaining 4740 patients have other forms of diabetes.[2] Overall prevalence of diabetes mellitus in children and adolescents is estimated to be 2.22 per 1000 children, with the majority of this (1.93 of 1000 children) accounted for by DM1 and 0.24 of 1000 by DM2.[3]

## DIABETIC NEPHROPATHY

Diabetic renal disease or nephropathy (DN) is an insidious and a common complication of diabetes mellitus. At its onset, DN is clinically silent and the only detectable abnormality may be presence of microalbuminuria (or also known as albuminuria). Overt proteinuria, nephrotic syndrome, hypertension, and a decline in renal function eventually evolve in these patients.

## EPIDEMIOLOGY

DN is the single largest cause of end-stage renal disease (ESRD) in adults in the United States, accounting for 44.1% cases.[4] In contrast, diabetes mellitus is a lesser known cause of ESRD in children and adolescents. The number of patients with the diagnosis of ESRD secondary to diabetes, between 0 and 19 years of age in the United States Renal Data System (USRDS) in the 2008 to 2012 era was only 57 of 6204 patients, representing only 0.9% of the pediatric ESRD population. Of the 57 patients, 34 had DM2 and 23 had DM1.[4] It is important to recognize that many children with diabetes mellitus are likely to grow into adulthood and will remain at risk for development of DN and ESRD later in their lives.

---

### KEY POINTS

- Diabetes mellitus is the most common cause of ESRD in adults.
- Diabetes mellitus is an uncommon cause of ESRD in children.
- Risk for DN rises with duration of diabetes mellitus.

---

In general, the risk for developing DN increases with the increasing duration of diabetes mellitus. Using microalbuminuria as evidence for DN, the German Diabetes Documentation System in children and young adults with DM1 demonstrated that 4.3% had abnormal urinary microalbumin excretion. Extending the follow-up data to age 40 years in these children showed that 25% patients eventually developed microalbuminuria.[5] Swedish data in childhood-onset DM1 with a mean disease duration of 29 years demonstrated microalbuminuria in 20% cases, and frank proteinuria was noted in another 12% of cases.[6] In Brazilian children with DM1, Salgado et al.[7] reported the incidence of microalbuminuria to be 11.2% after a mean disease duration of 11.32 ± 4.02 years. ESRD in this population was reported to be 2.9%. The cumulative incidence of ESRD in Finnish children with DM1 was 2.2% at 20 years and 7.8% at 30 years following the diagnosis of disease.[8] Several

---

### KEY POINTS

- Of children with DM1, 25% to 40% eventually develop DN in their lifetime.
- Risk for DN may be decreased by good glycemic control.

---

studies have observed that microalbuminuria occurs earlier in DM2 in children and young adults compared to DM1.[9,10]

## PATHOGENESIS OF DIABETIC NEPHROPATHY

DN in both DM1 and DM2 is believed to be the consequence of poorly controlled hyperglycemia. An integrated view of the mechanisms leading to renal injury in diabetes mellitus is evolving. Available evidence points to accumulation of injurious metabolic by-products, such as glycosylated compounds, involvement of the renin-angiotensin system, and endothelial and podocyte injury being involved in the pathogenesis of DN (Figure 28.1).

### Formation of advanced glycation end products

Glucose in diabetic patients reacts nonenzymatically with proteins, lipids, and nucleic acids to form Schiff bases characterized by carbon-nitrogen double bonds. Rearrangement of Schiff bases leads to the formation of intermediate Amadori products, eventually forming advanced glycation end products (AGEs), such as carboxymethyl lysine, pentosidine, imidazolone, and pyrraline. AGEs bind to lysozymes and specific cellular receptors, such as receptor for AGE (RAGE).[11] Consequences of this interaction are diverse alterations of cellular functions, such as decreased production of nitric oxide (NO) and increased production of oxidative radicals, cytokines, and growth factors. This shift in the internal milieu of the tissues promotes damage of cellular structures and is believed to play a leading role in the pathogenesis of DN.

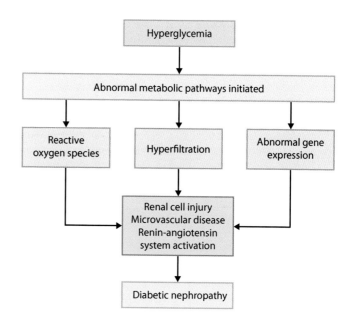

Figure 28.1 An over view of the pathogenic pathways and mediators in the development of diabetic nephropathy.

## Increased oxidative stress

Due to the persistent hyperglycemic state in diabetes mellitus, as much as 30% of glucose may be metabolized via the polyol pathway, depleting intracellular nicotinamide adenine dinucleotide phosphate (NADPH). These intracellular events lead to enhanced intracellular oxidative stresses, generated by decreased NO synthesis.[11]

## Vascular injury and profibrotic events

Hyperglycemia induces intracellular protein kinase (PKC) with profound downstream impact on the expression of genes that modulate effects on vascular tone, vascular permeability, and angiogenesis. Specifically, PKC activation is associated with downregulation of nitric oxide synthase (eNOS) and upregulation of endothelin 1 and vascular endothelial growth factor (VEGF).[12] All of these lead to vascular injury, increased vascular permeability, increased production of profibrotic cytokine transforming growth factor β-1 (TGB β-1), and mesangial matrix expansion.[12] An imbalance in the factors that promote vascular injury and those that prevent vascular injury is believed to be involved in the pathogenesis of diabetic microvascular disease and DN.[11–13]

## Podocyte injury

Hyperglycemia induces podocyte injury and apoptosis via a variety of mechanisms and may be a mediator of glomerular injury in DN.[14] Moreover, insulin also plays a profound role in maintaining the actin cytoskeletal and structural integrity of podocytes. The action of insulin is mediated via insulin receptors present on the podocyte cell surface.[15] Morphometric studies of renal biopsies in diabetic patients have demonstrated a decreased podocyte number, even before the onset of microalbuminuria, suggesting podocyte injury to be an early pathogenic event of DN.[16–18]

## Renin-angiotensin system

Experimental work by Brenner and colleagues laid the foundation for our understanding of the role played by renin-angiotensin system in the pathogenesis of DN.[19] Diabetic rats have been shown to have increased intraglomerular pressure, hyperfiltration, relative vasoconstriction at the efferent end of the glomerular capillary, and resultant albuminuria.[20] Renin was proposed as the possible agent for these intraglomerular vascular changes. Using the angiotensin-converting enzyme (ACE) inhibitor enalapril, Zatz et al.[21] further demonstrated an improvement in intraglomerular pressure, hyperfiltration, and improvement in albuminuria in this experimental diabetes model. Brenner et al.[22] eventually proposed a central role for the renin-angiotensin system in the evolution of hyperfiltration and DN. At a clinical level, however, the plasma renin level in DN is variable and can be either normal or suppressed.[23,24] These findings and other experimental evidence suggests the possible role of intrarenal renin-angiotensin activation in these patients.[25–27]

## Glomerular hyperfiltration

Increased glomerular filtration rate (GFR) or hyperfiltration has been well documented in early DN.[19,28] As noted earlier, Brenner et al. demonstrated hyperfiltration in experimental diabetes mellitus model and proposed its central role in the pathogenesis of DN.[20–22] Hyperfiltration has been demonstrated to result in progressive injury to the surviving nephrons, resulting in ongoing renal injury and eventual nephron loss. Hyper-reninemia was proposed by Brenner et al.[22] to cause selective efferent arteriolar constriction, leading to intraglomerular hypertension and resultant hyperfiltration.

---

### KEY POINTS

- The renin-angiotensin system has been implicated in the pathogenesis of glomerular hyperfiltration and ongoing renal injury.
- Use of ACE and angiotensin-receptor blockers (ARBs) has improved the prognosis of DN.

---

Leading away from glomerulocentric pathogenesis of hyperfiltration in patients with DN, some investigators have suggested a possible role of tubuloglomerular feedback (TGF) in its pathogenesis.[29] TGF refers to a protective mechanism in which increased tubular sodium concentration resulting from hyperfiltration stimulates a proportionate feedback to the corresponding afferent arterioles of the glomeruli, causing them to constrict and reduce glomerular blood flow and GFR. TGF is mediated by release of adenosine triphosphate (ATP) from the macula densa in response to increased tubular sodium concentration as a result of increased GFR. ATP is converted to adenosine, which binds to the adenosine A1 receptor (A1AR) in the afferent arteriole, causing vasoconstriction. In contrast, decreased distal sodium delivery to macula densa results in vasodilatation of the afferent arteriole and an increase in the superficial nephron GFR.[29,30] A clear understanding of the role played by TGF in the pathogenesis of DN has not emerged yet.

## Genetic predisposition

DN develops in only approximately 30% to 40% of patients with DM. Some epidemiologic observations suggest the possibility of familial clustering of DN.[31] So far, no definitive susceptibility genes for DN have been identified. Recent genome-wide association scan for susceptibility to DN, using single nucleotide polymorphisms (SNPs) genotyping, has revealed possible associations with two candidate loci near FRMD3 and CARS genes.[32] In a Japanese study SNP-rs1411766 in chromosome 13q was found to be highly associated with DN.[3]

Table 28.1 Clinical stages in the evolution of diabetic nephropathy

| Clinical stage | Disease duration (Yr) | Glomerular filtration rate | Microalbuminuria | Hyperfiltration |
|---|---|---|---|---|
| Latent disease stage | Begins early <10 | Elevated | No | Yes |
| Microalbuminuria stage | 10–15 | Normal or elevated | Yes | Yes |
| Overt proteinuria stage | >15 | Normal or decreased | Overt albuminuria | No |
| End-stage renal disease | 30-40 | Severely decreased | Overt albuminuria | No |

## CLINICAL MANIFESTATIONS

Although a few cases of early onset of DN have been reported in childhood, it is unusual to see overt DN before a decade of established disease state.[34] Kimmelstiel and Wilson[35] described the autopsy findings of DN in patients who manifested proteinuria, nephrotic syndrome, and hypertension. Although advanced DN is well known to be associated with severe proteinuria and CKD, early observable manifestations of DN are subtle and characterized by increased GFR (hyperfiltration) and microalbuminuria.

Clinical course of DN is a continuum of clinical manifestations that can be arbitrarily divided into following four stages (Table 28.1).

### Latent disease

Hyperglycemia-induced hyperfiltration is an early observable abnormality in DM.[28] At this stage, patients are asymptomatic, blood pressure is normal, and there is no detectable microalbuminuria. Renal size is normal or slightly increased on ultrasound examination. In DM1, this phase can last for 10 to 15 years of the disease during childhood.

### Microalbuminuria stage

Presence of microalbuminuria (also known as albuminuria) in patients with DM1 or DM2 is now recognized as an early marker of DN.[36–38] Most studies indicate that it takes 10 to 15 years for microalbuminuria to be noticed in patients with childhood onset of DM1.[39] In a Danish study, none of the patients younger than 15 years of age had an elevated albumin excretion rate.[40] In the Oxford Regional Prospective Study, the cumulative prevalence of microalbuminuria was 25.7% (95% confidence interval [CI] 21.3% to 30.1%) after 10

years of DM and in 50.7% (CI 40.5% to 60.9%) after 19 years of diabetes.[41]

Patients continue to have hyperfiltration in the microalbuminuria stage, but as the disease progresses, GFR declines and may appear to be "normal."[36,37] Presence of a normal GFR and microalbuminuria in a patient with DM1 or DM2 of long-standing duration should be viewed as an indicator of disease progression. Blood pressure is usually normal in this stage of DN but nephromegaly may be noted by ultrasound evaluation.[42] With effective therapy, regression of microalbuminuria has been reported in some patients with DM1.[43,44]

## ALBUMINURIA DETECTION

Available urine protein detecting dipsticks (Albustix or Multistix) are only able to detect proteinuria greater than 30 mg/dL. Low-level proteinuria, below 30 mg/dL, is defined as microalbuminuria (also known as albuminuria), which can be detected by immunodiffusion or other laboratory techniques. Although a 24-hour urine collection is the most accurate method for quantifying microalbuminuria, timed urine collections are often difficult or inaccurate in children. Consequently, a spot sample of ratio of urine microalbumin (or albumin) to creatinine (ACR) is a practical alternative. Using this technique, microalbuminuria is defined as urinary albumin to creatinine ratio (ACR) of greater than 30 mg/g of creatinine. Diagnostic reliability of spot urine albumin to creatinine ratio and its linear correlation with microalbuminuria in a 24 hour urine sample is well established.[45,46] To avoid erroneous results because of orthostatic proteinuria seen in older children and adolescents, it is recommended that ACR be obtained in the first morning sample of urine.[46] Guidelines for diagnosis of albuminuria are presented in Table 28.2.

---

### KEY POINTS

- DN has a long latent period, which manifests with hyperfiltration (increased GFR) only.
- Microalbuminuria is a marker of DN.
- Microalbuminuria should be assayed in the first morning urine sample to avoid overestimation because of orthostatic proteinuria.

---

Table 28.2 Definition of normal and abnormal urinary albumin excretion

| | 24-Hour urinary albumin (mg/24 hr) | Spot urine albumin/creatinine (mg/g creatinine) |
|---|---|---|
| Normal | 15–50 | <10–15 |
| Microalbuminuria | 30–299 | <30 |
| Overt proteinuria | >300 | >200 |

## Overt proteinuria stage

Overt proteinuria develops in an advanced stage of DN in a patient with progressive disease. The degree of proteinuria in DN can range from moderate (approximately 500 mg/day) to severe (greater than 3 g/day) and can be associated with nephrotic syndrome. Decline of renal function and hypertension is common at this clinical stage.[35,37,39] Transitioning from (micro)albuminuria to overt proteinuria takes 10 to 15 years.[39–42] Rapid progression from microalbuminuria to CKD, without an identifiable overt proteinuria stage, has been reported occasionally.[47]

## End-stage renal disease

With declining renal function in DN, proteinuria usually decreases and nephrotic syndrome may seem to improve. In general, the time course of ESRD in most studies involving children with DM1 has been noted to be 25 to 30 years (Figure 28.2), but early onset of ESRD also has been reported.[5,48,49] In the cohort of patients with DM1 from 1970 to 1980, the unadjusted cumulative incidence of ESRD at 25 years was 9.3%.[48] The unadjusted hazard of ESRD in this study was noted to be reduced by 70% compared to the cohort from 1922 to 1969. The authors credit better glycemic control to be an important factor in reducing the incidence of ESRD in the 1970 to 1980 cohort. Similarly, in another study of DM1 children, ESRD at 40 years of the disease duration was noted to be 9.4%.[5] Hypertension, if uncontrolled, may further accentuate progression of renal injury, accelerating the onset of ESRD. In addition to ESRD, patients demonstrate evidence of microvascular disease in other organs, such as retinopathy, loss of vision, coronary artery disease (CAD), and stroke. Joslin Clinic data suggest that despite significant (85%) use of ACE inhibitors (ACEIs) in patients, cumulative risk for ESRD in white patients with DM1 (1991 and 2004 cohort) remains high (52%).[49]

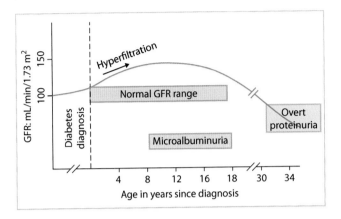

Figure 28.2 Time course of clinical events in the progression of nephropathy in type 1 diabetes mellitus.

## RENAL PATHOLOGY

The hallmark of DN in its advanced state is the lesion known as diabetic glomerulosclerosis, which was first described by Kimmelstiel and Wilson[35] in 1936. These patients had diabetes mellitus, advanced proteinuria, and hypertension, and renal pathologic findings on autopsy demonstrated glomerulosclerosis. Early renal lesions of DN, however, can be subtle and may be difficult to differentiate from other nondiabetic nephropathies. A consensus report of the Renal Pathology Society proposed four classes of morphologic changes in DN (Table 28.3). These classes are reflective of progression of the renal disease in these patients (Figure 28.3).[50] Although DN

Table 28.3 Renal pathology in diabetic nephropathy*

| Class | Pathologic description | Basement membrane | Mesangial lesion | Nodular sclerosis |
|---|---|---|---|---|
| I | Glomerular basement membrane thickening | Thickening on electron microscopy | Normal | No |
| II | Mesangial expansion | | | No |
| | IIa (mild) | Thickened | Mesangial expansion affecting < 25% | |
| | IIb (severe) | Thickened | Mesangial expansion affecting > 25% | |
| III | Nodular sclerosis (Kimmelstiel-Wilson lesions) | Wrinkled and thickened | Mesangial expansion, mesangiolysis | Yes — Lesions affect < 50% glomeruli; at least one convincing Kimmelstiel-Wilson lesion |
| IV | Advanced diabetic glomerulosclerosis | Wrinkled and thickened | | Yes — Lesions affect > 50% of glomeruli |

* Based on the classification proposed by: Cohen-Tervaert TW, Mooyaart AL, Amann K, et al.; Renal Pathology Society. Pathologic classification of diabetic nephropathy. J Am Soc Nephrol. 2010;21:556–63.

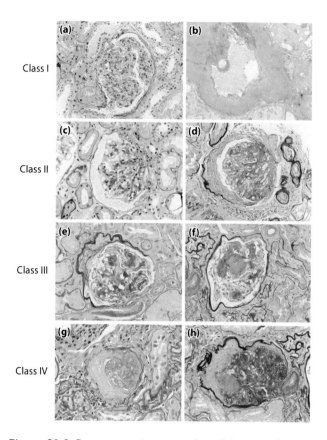

Class I

Class II

Class III

Class IV

Figure 28.3 Representative examples of the morphologic lesions in diabetic nephropathy (DN). Class I glomerular changes in panels (a) and (b). **(a)** Glomerulus showing only mild ischemic changes, with splitting of Bowman's capsule. No clear mesangial alteration. **(b)** Electron microscopy of this glomerulus showing the thickened glomerular basement membrane with a mean width of 671 nm, enabling the lesion to be categorized as class I. Class II glomerular change in panels (c) and (d). **(c)** The mesangial expansion does not exceed the mean area of a capillary lumen (IIa), whereas in panel **(d)** it does (IIb). Class III glomerular changes in panels (e) and (f). **(e)** The lesion in panel (e) is not as convincing for Kimmelstiel-Wilson lesion; therefore (on the basis of the findings in this glomerulus) the finding is consistent with class IIb. **(f)** Class III Kimmelstiel-Wilson lesion. For the purpose of the classification, at least one convincing Kimmelstiel-Wilson lesion (as in panel [f]) needs to be present. Class IV glomerular lesion in panels (g) and (h). **(g)** This is an example of glomerulosclerosis (glomerulus from the same biopsy as panel [h]). **(h)** Signs of class IV DN consist of hyalinosis of the glomerular vascular pole and a remnant of a Kimmelstiel-Wilson lesion on the opposite site of the pole. For the purpose of the classification, signs of DN should be histopathologically or clinically present to classify a biopsy with global glomerulosclerosis in more than 50% of glomeruli as class IV. (Reproduced with permission from: Cohen-Tervaert TW, Mooyaart AL, Amann K, et al.; Renal Pathology Society. Pathologic classification of diabetic nephropathy. J Am Soc Nephrol. 2010;21:556–63.)

---

### KEY POINT

The Renal Pathology Society has proposed four morphologic classes of DN.

---

classification is primarily based on changes noted in glomeruli, concomitant tubulointerstitial changes often accompany the glomerular lesions and must be considered in the prognostication of the clinical disease. In general, the histopathology of DN in DM1 is indistinguishable from that of DM2.

It is important to recognize that diabetic patients also can have nondiabetic renal disease, such as glomerulonephritis and tubulointerstitial nephritis.[51] These also need to be carefully distinguished from DN.

## MANAGING DIABETIC NEPHROPATHY

Pediatric nephrologists are increasingly asked to participate in the care of diabetic children, adolescents, and young adults. Care of these patients is best considered as a team of clinical providers, educators, nurses, and nutritionists. Such a team management approach can prevent and reduce the incidence of complications such as DN, retinopathy, cardiovascular disease, and neuropathy associated with DM.

### Glycemic control

In general, there has been a decline in the prevalence of DN in DM1 since the 1950s. This has been largely attributed to a better glycemic control in diabetic patients. The American Diabetic Association (ADA) recommends a hemoglobin (Hb) A1c goal of 7% in adults with DM1 and DM2.[52] Target HbA1c in children and adolescents recommended by the International Society for Pediatric and Adolescent Diabetes (ISPAD) consensus guidelines of 2009 is less than 7.5%.[53] Unfortunately, available pediatric data suggest that targets for glycemic control are rarely met in children and adolescents. Amed et al.[54] reported that only 7.4% of patients with diabetes mellitus in the pediatric age group achieved target HbA1c and the needed compliance for follow-up (missed clinic visits).

---

### KEY POINTS

- Good glycemic control is $HbA_{1c}$ goal of 7.
- Good glycemic control is the best strategy for prevention of DN.
- Target glycemic control is difficult in children.

---

A tighter control of diabetes and lowering the target of HbA1c to 6.5% has been suggested by some studies in adults.[55,56] These studies point to a substantial decline in microvascular disease, including DN in patients treated with a tighter HbA1c target. In the Diabetes Control and Complications Trial (DCCT) that evaluated intensive treatment protocol to achieve near normal glucose control in patients with DM1 in a randomized controlled study demonstrated a 50% reduction in the risk for impaired renal function compared to conventional therapy.[55] Similarly, the international consortium of investigators in the ADVANCE collaborative reported a 65% reduction in the risk for ESRD in patients with DM2 in whom a tight glycemic control target HbA1c of 6.5% or less was maintained over a median duration of 5 years.[56] A meta-analysis of tight glycemic control of DM2 has also suggested a lower incidence of microalbuminuria, but the evidence for reduction in the renal end points of doubling of serum creatinine and ESRD was less convincing.[57] Concern has, however, been expressed by some that despite a positive impact of tight glycemic control on microvascular disease and nephropathy, such an approach may not be advocated at this time because of adverse cardiovascular outcome noted in the Action to Control Cardiovascular Risk in Diabetes (ACCORD) study.[58,59]

## Early detection of nephropathy

Microalbuminuria (or albuminuria) is the hallmark of early DN, which can progress to overt proteinuria. Microalbuminuria is also an independent risk factor for cardiovascular disease and ESRD in diabetic patients.[60,61] Except in a rare patient, microalbuminuria in DM1 usually appears in those with the disease duration of more than a decade after onset. On the other hand, microalbuminuria is an early feature of DM2. This difference has been attributed to possible endothelial injury and hypertension that often accompanies DM2.[62] Another interesting feature of pediatric DM1 is that microalbuminuria has been reported to be reversible with effective treatment.[44]

The Kidney Disease Outcomes Quality Initiative (KDOQI) guidelines of the National Kidney Foundation recommend that screening for microalbuminuria be initiated after 5 years of onset of DM1, and at the time of diagnosis of DM2.[63] This screening should consist of measuring urinary ACR in a spot urine sample obtained in the clinic and checking serum creatinine to estimate GFR. An elevated ACR should be reconfirmed in a first morning sample in an adolescent diabetic patient, preferably within 3 months.

## Angiotensin-converting enzyme inhibitors

The therapeutic role of ACEIs in reducing the rate of progression of DM is well established.[64–66] The effectiveness of ACEIs was initially demonstrated in the murine models of diabetes and the five-sixth renal ablation models established by Brenner et al.[19–22] More recently, therapeutic effectiveness of ARBs, alone or in concert with an ACEI, to reduce

microalbuminuria and progression of DN also has been established.[67–69]

### KEY POINTS

- ACEIs and ARBs have helped slow the progression of DN at the microalbuminuria stage.
- Risk for hyperkalemia with ACEI and ARBs requires close monitoring.
- Early use of ACEI and ARBs to prevent development of microalbuminuria is unclear.

The timing of ACEI and ARB therapies in DM1 and DM2, however, has been a subject of considerable debate. Although it is tempting to consider that early start of ACEIs and ARBs might prevent the onset of microalbuminuria in diabetic patients, clinical trials have provided mixed results. Mauer et al. suggested that ACEI may not help in preventing onset of microalbuminuria in those without it, but others have demonstrated benefits of ACEIs and ARBs therapy in patients with DM2 without evidence of microalbuminuria.[66,70,71] KDOQI guidelines (2012) recommend against early use of ACEI and ARBs in DM1 and DM2 as a strategy to prevent DN in patients with normal blood pressure (nonhypertensive patients).[72]

Combined use of ACEIs and ARBs in treatment of DN has been suggested by some to be beneficial in preventing the progression of DN, since this drug combination blocks the entire cascade of the renin-angiotensin system. This combination has been shown to have an additive effect in reducing proteinuria in some studies.[73] Others have not been able to demonstrate a significant clinical benefit of combining ACEIs and ARBs in the treatment of adult patients with diabetes.[74] Some recent studies have, indeed, suggested that there is an increased risk for side effects, such as hyperkalemia and acute kidney injury in patients treated with a combination of ACEI and ARBs. These studies discourage the use of combination therapy in the treatment of DN.[75,76]

The antirenin drug aliskiren has been approved as a therapeutic agent for treatment of hypertension, and its use in treatment of early DN has been considered in clinical trials.[77] However, despite improved microalbuminuria, the incidence of hyperkalemia, hypotension, worsening of renal function, and death has been reported in a significant number of patients in these studies.[77,78] In 2012, the U.S. Food and Drug Administration issued a safety alert against the use of the combination of aliskiren, ACEIs, and ARBs for treatment of DN.[79]

## Cardiovascular disease and hypertension

The Joslin Clinic study in juvenile-onset DM1 demonstrated that most of the CAD-related deaths occurred beyond the third decade of life.[80] The cumulative mortality in the Framingham Heart Study from CAD was 35% ± 5%, compared to 8% in males and 4% in females in the nondiabetic population.[81] The risk factors associated with CAD in diabetes are hypertension, lipid profile abnormalities, atherosclerosis, and endothelial injury.[82]

Onset of hypertension in DM1 often coincides with the development of overt DN and proteinuria.[83] As a part of the metabolic syndrome or obesity-associated DM2, hypertension may be present at the time of initial detection of the disease. For pediatric patients, the ADA recommends that blood pressure readings higher than the 95th percentile for age and gender be considered thresholds for pharmacotherapy for hypertension.[84] Interestingly, an intensive effort to reduce systolic BP to 120 mm Hg in adults in the ACCORD study did not reduce the rate of a composite outcome of fatal and nonfatal major cardiovascular events in adults with DM2.[85] Cochrane meta-analysis also concluded that there is no clear evidence to suggest that blood pressure lower than accepted standard targets need to be achieved in hypertensive patients with diabetes.[86]

Apart from being an effective antihypertensive treatment, ACEIs and ARBs also have a beneficial effect on DN and remain the drugs of choice for treatment of hypertension in this population. Calcium channel blockers are also effective therapies in treating hypertension in diabetic patients and are neutral in their impact on glycemic control.[87] These are usually used as adjuncts to ACEIs and ARBs in the management of hypertension in diabetic patients. A recent report about calcium channel blockers helping β cell loss in the pancreas is interesting and may change the utility of calcium channel blockers in the management of hypertension in diabetes.[88] Thiazide diuretics and β blockers should be avoided in patients with prediabetes and diabetes, because this class of drugs is known to worsen the glycemic control in patients with diabetes and even accelerate the development of diabetes in those with impaired glucose metabolism.

In addition to pharmacotherapy, usual hypertension management strategies, such as lower salt intake, exercise, and caffeine avoidance should also be instituted in the management of hypertension in diabetics patients. Weight reduction strategies in metabolic syndrome and DM2 associated with obesity should be an important element in the management of hypertension in these patients.

Dyslipidemia is a common finding in diabetic children with poor glycemic control, magnifying their risk for CAD. Lipid abnormalities consisting of elevated total cholesterol and low-density lipoprotein (LDL) cholesterol, low high-density lipoprotein (HDL) cholesterol, elevated apolipoprotein B, and a relatively normal to elevated serum triglyceride level.[89-92] Dyslipidemia is more common in DM2 versus DM1. In a large study of young adults and adolescents, DM2 dyslipidemia was demonstrated in 33% of patients compared to 19% of patients with DM1.[91] Although duration of the disease does not appear to influence dyslipidemia in diabetic patients, poor glycemic control over time is associated with a worse lipid profile.[92] It is prudent to address the dyslipidemia in these patients by appropriate dietary advice and use of statins. Indeed, in adults with DM2, the use of statins has significantly increased to 52.2% of subjects during the years 2007 to 2010.[93] In a recent pediatric study, however, only 1% of pediatric patients with diabetes-associated dyslipidemia were recorded to be receiving any pharmacotherapy.[91]

## METABOLIC SYNDROME

The term *syndrome X* was coined in 1988 to denote an association of cardiovascular mortality with hypertension, dyslipidemia, and insulin resistance, resulting from of obesity.[94,95] Other expressions have been proposed over the past several decades to describe this clinical constellation, but most have adopted the term *metabolic syndrome* (MetS). The criteria proposed for defining MetS by the third report of the National Cholesterol Education Program Expert Panel on Detection, Evaluation, and Treatment of High Blood Cholesterol in Adults (Adult Treatment Panel III) (ATPIII) and those from the World Health Organization (WHO) are most widely used and are listed in Tables 28.4 and Table 28.5.[96-98]

## CLINICAL CONSTELLATION

Although obesity is easily definable by body mass index (BMI) or weight criteria (Table 28.6), MetS is a constellation of clinical findings and its definition is still somewhat loose.

Table 28.4 Adult treatment panel III clinical criteria for metabolic syndrome in adults

| Risk factor | Defining level |
| --- | --- |
| Abdominal obesity, given as waist circumference | |
| Men | >102 cm (>40 inches) |
| Women | >88 cm (>35 inches) |
| Triglycerides | ≥150 mg/dL |
| High-density lipoprotein cholesterol | |
| Men | <40 mg/dL |
| Women | <50 mg/dL |
| Blood pressure | ≥130/≥85 mm Hg |
| Fasting glucose | ≥110 mg/dL |

*Source:* Reproduced from: Anonymous. Third report of the National Cholesterol Education Program Expert Panel on Detection, Evaluation, and Treatment of High Blood Cholesterol in Adults (Adult Treatment Panel III). NIH Publication No. 02-5215, September 2002. Bethesda, MD: National Institutes of Health.

Table 28.5 World health organization clinical criteria for metabolic syndrome

Insulin resistance, identified by one of the following:

- Type 2 diabetes
- Impaired fasting glucose
- Impaired glucose tolerance
- For those with normal fasting glucose levels (<110 mg/dL), glucose uptake below the lowest quartile for background population under investigation under hyperinsulinemic, euglycemic conditions

Plus any two of the following:

- Antihypertensive medication and/or high blood pressure (≥140 mm Hg systolic or ≥ 90 mm Hg diastolic)
- Plasma triglycerides ≥ 150 mg/dL (≥1.7 mmol/L)
- High-density lipoprotein < 35 mg/dL (<0.9 mmol/L) in men or < 39 mg/dL (1.0 mmol/L) in women
- Body mass index > 30 kg/m² and/or waist-to-hip ratio > 0.9 in men, > 0.85 in women
- Urinary albumin excretion rate ≥ 20 μg/min or albumin-to-creatinine ratio ≥ 30 mg/g

Table 28.6 Characteristics of obesity-associated focal segmental glomerulosclerosis

Identifying features of obesity-associated and metabolic syndrome–associated FSGS

**Clinical features**
- Patients may not manifest edema
- Modest and subnephrotic-range proteinuria is usual
- Higher albumin than idiopathic FSGS
- Lower cholesterol than idiopathic FSGS
- More indolent course with slower progression

**Biopsy features**
- Large glomeruli
- Modest foot-process effacement on electron microscopy
- Increased foot-process width
- Segmental sclerosis is less common compared to idiopathic FSGS
- Global sclerosis is comparable to idiopathic FSGS
- Hyperplasia of juxtaglomerular apparatus is common

**Gene expressions**
Glomerular gene expression heightened for:
- Lipid metabolism
- Inflammatory cytokines
- Insulin resistance

FSGS, focal segmental glomerulosclerosis.

Table 28.7 Classification of obesity by body mass index

| Obesity classification | Body mass index (kg/m²) |
|---|---|
| Ideal | 18.5–24.9 |
| Overweight | 25.0–29.9 |
| Obesity | ≥30 |
| Class I | 30–34.9 |
| Class II | 35.0–39.9 |
| Class III | ≥40 |

Source: World Health Organization. Obesity: preventing and managing the global epidemic. Report of a WHO Consultation. WHO Technical Report Series 894. Geneva: World Health Organization; 2000. Document is in public domain.

A common approach is to require existence of at least three of the following clinical and biochemical findings:

- Increased waist circumference
- Hyperglycemia
- Elevated systolic and/or diastolic blood pressure
- Elevated fasting triglycerides
- Low HDL cholesterol
- Microalbuminuria

There are no universally accepted criteria for definition of MetS in children and adolescents.[99] Consensus, however, exists in that the common constellation of clinical and biochemical findings associated with the insulin resistance experienced in children and adolescents are often precipitated by excess weight, notably ectopic adiposity.[100] As with BMI, changing percentile norms must be considered when evaluating waist measures in children and adolescents. A more meaningful alternative is to consider the waist-to-height ratio, which is normally at or just below 50%, but reaches between 50% and 60% and above with severe visceral adiposity.[101] Ethnic and racial factors affect the MetS diagnostic parameters in adults, and adjusted ethnic and racial specific cutoffs have been proposed.[102]

## KEY POINT

Pediatric criteria for MetS have yet to be established.

## EPIDEMIOLOGY

As with adults, the pediatric prevalence of MetS varies considerably and is a function of the criteria chosen, as well as the population demographics. In the 2430 children reported in the Third National Health and Nutrition Examination Survey (1988 to 1994), overall MetS prevalence was 4%, but its prevalence in overweight children was 30%.[103] As the degree of obesity increases, the prevalence of MetS increases, occurring in 38.7% of moderately obese (mean BMI 33.4 kg/m$^2$) and 49.7% of severely obese (mean BMI 40.6 kg/m$^2$) children and adolescents.[104]

---

**KEY POINT**

The prevalence of MetS in obese children may be as high as 30%.

---

## ETIOPATHOGENESIS

### Genetics

The MetS clusters in families and its prevalence varies across ethnic groups.[105,106] Heritability has been estimated to be as high as 24% to 61%, but no short list of candidate genes has emerged from study in this area.[107] Both candidate gene analyses and genome-wide association scans have hinted at complex gene networks with pleiotropic effects.[108,109] Multiple candidate genes have been identified, each making a small contribution to the pathologic processes of MetS. Many of these genes contribute to insulin regulation and energy metabolism.[110] Environmental triggers, such as a sedentary lifestyle and an energy-rich diet, may be equally important in in the causation of obesity and activation of these genetic influences.[111]

### Intestinal microbiome

Some of the most provocative theories on the origins of the MetS relate to the possible interactions between human superorganism cells and resident gut flora. Intestinal bacteria have been causally implicated in the inflammatory processes associated with obesity and insulin resistance by increasing gut permeability, permitting excessive microbial translocation.[112]

### Adipocyte-triggered systemic inflammation

It is increasingly apparent that obesity triggers systemic inflammatory response and insulin resistance, both of which are present in MetS. Preadipocytes are phagocytic cells that resemble macrophages in both morphology and patterns of gene expression.[113] In obesity, as in an infection, adipose tissue and infiltrated monocytes and macrophages release proinflammatory adipokines (Figure 28.4), notably TNF-α, interleukin-6 (IL-6), retinol binding protein-4 (RBP-4),

---

**KEY POINT**

Obesity leads to a state of inflammation and insulin resistance.

---

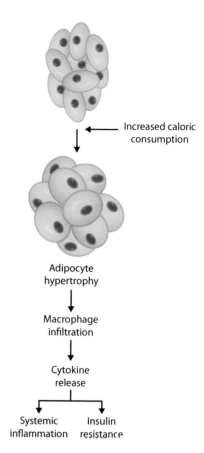

Figure 28.4 Obesity as an inflammatory state. Obesity is characterized by hyperplasia of the adipose cells. Excess calories are shunted into ectopic and hypertrophied adipocytes. Adipocyte dysfunction leads to monocyte and macrophage infiltration in the location of ectopic hypertrophied adipocytes. Release of cytokines from these tissue sites leads to a state of ongoing inflammation and insulin resistance.

and leptin, together with macrophage chemoattractant protein-1 (MCP-1). The mechanism for insulin resistance during inflammation induced by obesity is believed to be a physiologic response to make glucose available for the metabolic needs of an activated immune system.[114] Aging and a sedentary lifestyle also may influence this proinflammatory state in obesity and has been proposed as a possible mechanism for the development of MetS.[115]

### Nutrient metabolic quality

Not all calories are created equal. Qualitative and quantitative nutrient features are important in microbial translocation of endotoxin across the intestinal barrier—the putative inflammatory root cause of insulin resistance and the MetS. Diets high in calorie content, such as refined starches, sugar, saturated and trans fats, and low in long-chain polyunsaturated omega fatty acids, natural antioxidants, and fiber from fruits and vegetables have been shown to promote inflammation and insulin resistance, and contribute to the development of the MetS.[116] Low consumption of fish, fruit, and vegetables, combined with a sedentary lifestyle, has been considered an important factor in the development of MetS and preventable cardiovascular deaths.[117,118] Additionally, excess intake of branched-chain amino acids (protein), ethanol, and fructose can overwhelm hepatic clearance mechanisms and their metabolic accumulation may be associated with the MetS.[119] Fortunately, a fourth injurious dietary additive, trans-fatty acids, is being eased out of the food supply. These four substrates that are not regulated by insulin deliver metabolic intermediates to hepatic mitochondria and promote lipogenesis and the ectopic adipose storage—a feature characteristic of MetS.

## Defective adipose tissue storage of calories

Obesity is characterized by a diminished differentiation and proliferation (hyperplasia) of the adipose cells to meet the storage demands of excess calories. Without sufficient adipose cells for fat storage, excess calories are shunted into ectopic and hypertrophied adipocytes. These hypertrophied adipocytes become dysfunctional, have inadequate vascular supply, and are at a heightened risk for apoptosis. As shown in Figure 28.4, the outcome of adipocyte dysfunction is monocyte and macrophage infiltration and initiation of an inflammatory cycle in these tissue sites.[120]

## RENAL PATHOLOGIC FINDINGS IN OBESITY-RELATED GLOMERULOPATHY

The impact of obesity on renal glomerular structure has been well known since the early 1970s and has been further characterized recently.[121,122] Obesity and increased BMI are, indeed, independent risk factors for development of CKD, ESRD, and hypertension.[123,124]

Obesity and MetS lead to similar renal injury and are often grouped together under the heading of obesity-related glomerulopathy (ORG). Two pathologic lesions pathognomonic of ORG are glomerulomegaly and focal segmental glomerulosclerosis (FSGS). Glomerular hypertrophy is the most widely described abnormality in ORG (Figure 28.5). In age-matched patients (3.6 to 30 years), Cohen[122] noted a significant increase in the glomerular area in obese patients. Others have also demonstrated glomerulomegaly in the renal biopsies of obese children and adults.[125–127] In a study of 6818 renal biopsies, Kambham et al.[121] noted that the mean glomerular diameter in patients with ORG was 226 ± 246 mm (range, 172 to 300 μm), compared to 168 ± 12 μm (range, 138 to 186 μm) in age- and sex-matched controls.[121] Animal models of obesity (Zucker obese rats) also demonstrate glomerulomegaly as a part of their systemic organ dysfunction profile.[128]

The second type of renal lesions seen in association with obesity is FSGS (O-FSGS). Prevalence of O-FSGS in the renal biopsies of obese patients is unclear and variable (Table 28.6). Whereas erra et al. reported O-FSGS in only 5.3% of white patients from Spain, two studies from China noted O-FSGS to be present in 55.6% to 70% of obese patients with proteinuria.[124,126-129] All of these studies were conducted in adult patients. Although similar to classic FSGS, the following findings distinguish O-FSGS from classic FSGS (Figure 28.6)[121,127–130]:

- Glomerulomegaly as a prominent feature
- A lesser degree of global sclerosis and segmental sclerosis in the affected glomeruli
- A lesser degree of the foot process effacement (fusion)
- Tubulointerstitial disease less prominent
- Mesangial matrix expansion and sclerosis, along with basement membrane thickening—changes suggestive of "diabetes-like" morphology

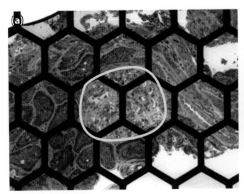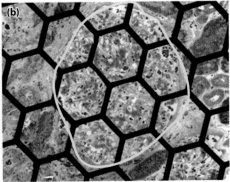

Figure 28.5 Glomerular hypertrophy seen in light microscopy. **(a)** A normal-sized glomerulus (area < 30,000 μm²) and **(b)** an excessively enlarged one (area > 40 000 μm²). (Reproduced with permission from: Goumenos DS, Kawar B, El Nahas M, et al. Early histological changes in the kidney of people with morbid obesity. Nephrol Dial Transplant. 2009;24:3732–8.)

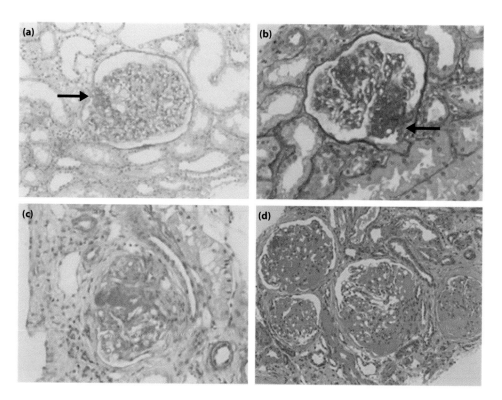

Figure 28.6 Representative light microscopy, immunohistology, and electron microscopy of obesity associated–focal segmental glomerulosclerosis (O-FSGS). (a) Mild or early FSGS with segmental increase in mesangial cellularity and matrix (arrow). (b) In advanced stages of FSGS, segmental sclerosis enlarges and the capillary tuft begins to adhere to Bowman's capsule (arrow). (c) When segmental adhesion and sclerosis proceed, more of the capillary lumen is obliterated and global sclerosis is about to develop. (d) In addition to focal glomerulosclerosis in the four adjacent glomeruli, glomerular size is increased, indicative of glomerular hypertrophy. (Reproduced with permission from: Amann K, Benz K. Structural renal changes in obesity and diabetes. Semin Nephrol. 2013;33:23–33.)

## RENAL MANIFESTATIONS OF OBESITY-RELATED GLOMERULOPATHY AND METABOLIC SYNDROME

Patients with ORG and MetS may be clinically asymptomatic but may have elevated urinary microalbumin excretion. Proteinuria, when present, is usually subnephrotic in range, but nephrotic-range proteinuria has been reported in a minority of cases. Serum albumin is usually better preserved, despite significant proteinuria, and a clinical nephrotic state is uncommon.[125] For example, Kambham et al.[121] noted a nephrotic-range proteinuria in 48%, but clinical nephrotic syndrome was present in only 5.6% cases of ORG. Hypertension is common in these patients. Hyperfiltration, resulting in increased GFR, is noted in the early stages of ORG-MetS.[121,124] This is followed by gradually increasing serum creatinine, which has been seen in 35% to 50% patients in some studies, eventually leading to ESRD in

some.[123] The annual ESRD rate in white patients with ORG-MetS has been estimated to be approximately 7%.[131]

## MANAGEMENT

Management of renal consequences of obesity and metabolic syndrome is directly linked to effective of metabolic syndrome. Management of these patients is best offered by a multidisciplinary team consisting of a nutritionist, exercise trainer, nephrologist, and a specialist in lipid disorder. The strategy includes weight reduction, identification and treatment of risk factors for coronary heart disease, and treatment of hyperfiltration.

### Weight reduction

Weight reduction is part of the composite management of MetS, referred to as *therapeutic lifestyle changes* (TLCs).[96] TLC alone has been shown to decrease the incidence of MetS in at-risk adults by 41%.[132] TLC also reduces the incidence of diabetes mellitus in patients with prediabetes.[133] Additionally, modest weight loss is also associated with a decrease in fasting insulin and leptin and an increase in adiponectin levels.[134] The positive impact of weight reduction on the degree of proteinuria also has been documented

---

**KEY POINT**

Obesity- and MetS-induced FSGS is usually associated with modest subnephrotic-range proteinuria.

in some studies.[125] Reduction of saturated fat, trans fats, and cholesterol in the diet has the added benefit of lowering serum LDL cholesterol profile, a risk factor for coronary heart disease (CHD).

## Insulin-sensitizing agents

Metformin, a drug originally derived from the plant *Galega officinalis,* which had been used for treatment of diabetes mellitus, is also useful in the treatment of MetS.[132,135] Metformin also has been noted to reduce the incidence of diabetes mellitus in patients with prediabetes.[133] Metformin provides a dual impact by decreasing hepatic glucose synthesis as well as by increasing glucose uptake in peripheral tissues. In effect, metformin increases tissue sensitivity to insulin and is also referred to as an insulin sensitizer. Thiazolidinediones, also known as glitazones (rosiglitazone and pioglitazone), are other types of clinically useful insulin sensitizers in MetS prediabetes management.[136,137]

## Hypertension and glomerular hyperfiltration

ACEIs and ARBs are recommended to be the primary therapeutic choice in treatment of hypertension in patients with MetS. Apart from managing hypertension, the advantage of ACEIs and ARBs in MetS patients is their ability to diminish glomerular hyperfiltration.[138] Use of ACEIs and ARBs also helps reduce microalbuminuria and overt proteinuria in these patients.[125]

## Dyslipidemia

To reduce CHD risk, use of statins has been highly recommended in adults with MetS.[96] However, this benefit has to be balanced with the reported diabetogenic potential of statins in adults.[139] Although useful in children with dyslipidemia, the Expert Panel on Integrated Guidelines for Cardiovascular Health and Risk Reduction in Children and Adolescents does not recommended statin use below 10 years of age.[140,141]

## SUMMARY

Metabolic syndrome and obesity-related diabetes (type 2) is being increasingly encountered in children and adolescents. Good glycemic control is essential in preventing nephropathy and other microvascular complications of diabetes. Use of ACEIs in early treatment of nephropathy associated with diabetes is recommended to prevent onset of proteinuria, CKD, and ESRD. Unfortunately, these drugs have not been shown to forestall onset of nephropathy, when used as preventive agents in the early course of the disease. Macrovascular complications, such as CAD, atherosclerosis, and stroke continue to be the leading causes of mortality, in addition to CKD and need for dialysis and transplantation.

## Clinical Vignette 28.1

A 17-year-old Hispanic female with known obesity presented to the renal clinic for management of hypertension. She was the product of 37 weeks of gestation born via cesarean section, with a birth weight 9 lb. Pregnancy was complicated by maternal obesity, a 50-lb weight gain during pregnancy, and eclampsia, but there was no history of gestational diabetes in the mother. The patient was not breast fed and was advanced on formula and progressed by 4 months to rice cereal and onto solid foods in response to a "robust appetite." The patient had always been husky for age and had accelerated weight gain with menarche at 8.5 years.

The patient was initially referred to multidisciplinary care at an obesity clinic at 12 years of age, when her BMI was above the 95th percentile, with central adipose distribution (waist-to-height ratio, 68%). Review of systems was positive for gastrointestinal reflux disease and heavy snoring during sleep. She had no history of sleep apnea, but she reported daytime sleepiness. She has been on oral contraceptives and has had regular menstrual cycle. Weight management strategies were discussed at the initial visit, but she was lost to follow-up until this referral for new onset of hypertension

The patient's family history was positive for DM2 on the maternal side of the family with associated hypertension and dyslipidemia. Her maternal great-grandmother also had DM2 and was on dialysis by 60 years of age. Her paternal grandfather had a stroke in his 50s.

The patient is in grade 11 and has been struggling academically. She reports long-standing difficulty in keeping up with her peers in physical education. She does not seek after-school activities and watches TV for an average of 4 to 6 hours per day.

Physical examination showed height, 60 inches (5th percentile); weight, 180 lb (97th percentile); BMI, 37.2 kg/m$^2$ (99th percentile); and blood pressure, 128/78 mm Hg (systolic SBP 97th percentile, diastolic 88th percentile). Moderate acanthosis nigricans was seen around the back of her neck. Ambulatory blood pressure monitoring (ABPM) showed more than 75% of daytime readings and more than 90% of nighttime readings exceeding limits for age, gender, and height. Blunted nocturnal dipping was noted.

A fasting metabolic screen showed total cholesterol, 180 mg/dL (high); triglycerides, 185 mg/dL (high); HDL cholesterol, 38 mg/dL (low); non-HDL cholesterol, 182 mg/dL (high); lipoprotein a, 95 nmol/L (high); LDL cholesterol, 105 mg/dL (high); glucose, 95 mg/dL (normal); 2-hour oral glucose tolerance test, 148 mg/dL (abnormal); fasting insulin, 35 mU/L(high); HbA1c 6.2% (high); alanine transaminase, 34 international units/L (high); normal electrolytes, blood urea nitrogen (BUN), 16 mg/dL; and creatinine, 1.1 mg/dL. Urinalysis was negative for protein; the urine (micro) albumin-to-creatinine ratio (ACR) was 3.0 mg/mmol and 25-OH vitamin D was 12 (low).

## TEACHING POINTS

- This 17-year-old adolescent female of Hispanic ancestry with a lifelong history of obesity presented with clinical and biochemical evidence of insulin resistance and cardiometabolic sequelae consistent with MetS. These include central adiposity, hypertriglyceridemia, low HDL level, and systolic hypertension. Hyperglycemia is masked by hyperinsulinism, but her 2-hour oral glucose tolerance test result is abnormal and the elevated HbA1c reflects suboptimal glucose regulation. Elevated ALT is consistent with nonalcoholic fatty liver disease. Disordered sleep history is suggestive of obstructive sleep apnea that can aggravate insulin resistance. BUN and creatinine levels are both at upper limits of normal. Evidence of prediabetes, as well as the lack of nocturnal dipping on ABPM and upper range of normal ACR heightens the potential for CKD.[123,134]
- She is at an increased risk for insulin resistance on the basis of her Latino ancestry, positive family history of DM2 and early cardiovascular disease, large size for gestational age birth weight, maternal obesity, and excessive maternal weight gain during gestation.
- Her risk is further accentuated by a sedentary lifestyle and poor dietary habits. Although there is ample room for lifestyle improvements, this patient will need adjunct insulin-sensitizing and antihypertensive medications with intensive reinforcement of nutritional and activity changes.
- She is also at high risk for developing CKD later in life.[142] Measures need to be implemented to stem this momentum toward a diagnosis of DM2 and CKD.

## REFERENCES

1. Pinhas-Hamiel O, Zeitler P. The global spread of type 2 diabetes mellitus in children and adolescents. J Pediatr. 2005;146:693–700.
2. Pettit DJ, Talton J, Dabelea D, et al.; SEARCH for Diabetes in Youth Study Group. Prevalence of diabetes mellitus in U.S. youth in 2009. The SEARCH for Diabetes in Youth Study. Diabetes Care. 2014;37:402–8.
3. Fagot-Campagna A, Pettitt DJ, Engelgau M, et al. Type 2 diabetes among North American children and adolescents: An epidemiologic health perspective. J Pediatr. 2000;136:664–72.
4. United States Renal Data System. US Renal Data System 2012 Annual Data Report: Atlas of End-Stage Renal Disease in the United States. Bethesda, MD: National Institutes of Health, National Institute of Diabetes and Digestive and Kidney Diseases. Available at: http://www.usrds.org. Accessed September 9, 2013.
5. Raile K, Galler A, Hofer S, et al. Diabetic nephropathy in 27,805 children, adolescents, and adults with type 1 diabetes: Effect of diabetes duration, A1C, hypertension, dyslipidemia, diabetes onset, and sex. Diabetes Care. 2007;30:2523–28.
6. Dahlquist G, Stattin E-L, Rudberg S. Urinary albumin excretion rate and glomerular filtration rate in the prediction of diabetic nephropathy: A long-term follow-up study of childhood onset type-1 diabetic patients. Nephrol Dial Transplant. 2001;16:1382–86.
7. Salgado PP, Silva IN, Vieira EC, et al. Risk factors for early onset of diabetic nephropathy in pediatric type 1 diabetes. J Pediatr Endocrinol Metab. 2010;23:1311–20.
8. Finne P, Reunanen A, Stenman S, et al. Incidence of end-stage renal disease in patients with type 1 diabetes. JAMA. 2005;294:1782–7.
9. Maahs DM, Snively BM, Bell RA, et al. Higher prevalence of elevated albumin excretion in youth with type 2 than type 1 diabetes. The SEARCH for Diabetes in Youth Study. Diabetes Care. 2007;30:2593–8.
10. Eppens M, Craig ME, Cusumano J, et al. Prevalence of diabetes complications in adolescents with type 2 compared with type 1 diabetes. Diabetes Care. 2006;29:1300–6.
11. Vallon V, Komers R. Pathophysiology of the diabetic kidney. Compr Physiol. 2011;1:1175–232.
12. Noh H, King GL. The role of protein kinase C activation in diabetic nephropathy. Kidney Int. 2007;106(Suppl):S49–53.
13. Kanwar YS, Sun L, Xie P, et al. A glimpse of various pathogenetic mechanisms of diabetic nephropathy. Annu Rev Pathol Mech Dis. 2011;6:395–423.
14. Susztak K, Raff A, Schiffer M, et al. Glucose-induced reactive oxygen species cause apoptosis of podocytes. Diabetes. 2006;55:225–33.
15. Welsh GI, Hale LJ, Eremina V, et al. Insulin signaling to the glomerular podocyte is critical for normal kidney function. Cell Metab. 2010;12:329–40.
16. Li JJ, Kwak SJ, Jung DS J, et al. Podocyte biology in diabetic nephropathy. Kidney Int. 2007;72:S36–42.
17. Weil EJ, Lemley KV, Yee B, Lovato T, et al. Podocyte detachment in type 2 diabetic nephropathy. Am J Nephrol. 2011;33(Suppl 1):21–4
18. Weil E J, Lemley KV, Mason CC, et al. Podocyte detachment and reduced glomerular capillary endothelial fenestration promote kidney disease in type 2 diabetic nephropathy. Kidney Int. 2012;82:1010–7.
19. Hostetter TH, Troy JL, Brenner BM. Glomerular hemodynamics in experimental diabetes mellitus. Kidney Int. 1981;19:410–15.

20. Hostetter TH, Rennke HG, Brenner BM. The case for intrarenal hypertension in the initiation and progression of diabetic and other glomerulopathies. Am J Med. 1982;72:375–80.

21. Zatz RB, Dunn RB, Meyer TW, et al. Prevention of diabetic glomerulopathy by pharmacological amelioration of glomerular capillary hypertension. J Clin Invest. 1986;77:1925–30.

22. Brenner BM, Lawler EV, Mackenzie HS. The hyperfiltration theory: A paradigm shift in nephrology. Kidney Int. 1996;49:1774–7.

23. Price DA, Porte LE, Gordon M, et al. The paradox of the low-renin state in diabetic nephropathy. J Am Soc Nephrol 1999;10:2382–91.

24. Perez GO, Lespier L, Jacobi J. Hyporeninemia and hypoaldosteronism in diabetes mellitus. Arch Intern Med. 1977;137:852–55.

25. Toma I, Kang JJ, Sipos A, et al. Succinate receptor GPR91 provides a direct link between high glucose levels and renin release in murine and rabbit kidney. J Clin Invest. 2008;118:2526–34.

26. Peti-Peterdi J. High glucose and renin release: The role of succinate and GPR91. Kidney Int. 2010;78:1214–7.

27. Peti-Peterdi J, Gevorgyan H, Lam L, Riquier-Brison A. Metabolic control of renin secretion. Pflugers Archiv 2013;465:53–8.

28. Mogensen CE, Andersen MJ. Increased kidney size and glomerular filtration rate in early juvenile diabetes. Diabetes. 1973;22:706–12.

29. Thomson SC, Vallon V, Blantz RC. Kidney function in early diabetes: The tubular hypothesis of glomerular filtration. Am J Physiol Renal Physiol. 2004;28.F8–15.

30. Persson P, Hansell P, Palm F. Tubular reabsorption and diabetes-induced glomerular hyperfiltration. Acta Physiol (Oxf). 2010;200:3–10.

31. Seaquist ER, Goetz FC, Rich S, et al. Familial clustering of diabetic kidney disease. N Engl J Med. 1989;320:1161–65.

32. Pezzolesi MG, Poznik GD, Mychaleckyj JC, et al. Genome-wide association scan for diabetic nephropathy susceptibility genes in type 1 diabetes. Diabetes. 2009;58:1403–10.

33. Maeda S, Araki S, Babazono T, et al. Replication study for the association between four loci identified by a genome-wide association study on European American subjects with type 1 diabetes and susceptibility to diabetic nephropathy in Japanese subjects with type 2 diabetes. Diabetes. 2010;59:2075–79.

34. Chobanian MC, Chevalier RL, Sturgill BC, et al. Early onset of clinical diabetic nephropathy in children: A new subgroup? Int J Pediatr Nephrol. 1984;5:23–9.

35. Kimmelstiel P, Wilson C. Intercapillary lesions of the glomeruli of the kidney. Am J Pathol. 1936;12:83–96.

36. Mogensen CE, Christensen CK. Predicting diabetic nephropathy in insulin-dependent patients. N Engl J Med. 1984;311:89–93.

37. Mogensen CE. Microalbuminuria predicts clinical proteinuria and early mortality in maturity-onset diabetes. N Engl J Med. 1984;310:356–60.

38. National Kidney Foundation. Clinical practice guidelines and clinical practice recommendations for diabetes and chronic kidney disease. Am J Kidney Dis. 2007;49(Suppl 2):S12–154.

39. Krolewski AS, Warram JH, Christlieb AR, et al. The changing natural history of nephropathy in type I diabetes. Am J Med. 1985;78:785–94.

40. Olsen BS, Sjølie AK, Hougaard P, et al. The significance of the prepubertal diabetes duration for the development of retinopathy and nephropathy in patients with type 1 diabetes. J Diabetes Complications. 2004;18:160–4.

41. Amin R, Widme B, Prevost AT, et al. Risk of microalbuminuria and progression to macroalbuminuria in a cohort with childhood onset type 1 diabetes: Prospective observational study. BMJ. 2008;336:697–701.

42. Raile K, Galler A, Hofer S, et al. Diabetic nephropathy in 27,805 children, adolescents, and adults with type 1 diabetes: Effect of diabetes duration, A1C, hypertension, dyslipidemia, diabetes onset, and sex. Diabetes Care. 2007;30:2523–28.

43. Frazer FL, Palmer LJ, Clarey A, et al. Relationship between renal volume and increased albumin excretion rates in children and adolescents with type 1 diabetes mellitus. J Pediatr Endocrinol Metab. 2001;14:875–81.

44. Perkins BA, Ficociello LH, Silva KH, et al. Regression of microalbuminuria in type 1 diabetes. N Engl J Med. 2003;348:2285–93.

45. Assadi FK. Quantitation of microalbuminuria using random urine samples. Pediatr Nephrol. 2002;17:107–110.

46. Witte EC, Heerspink HJL, de Zeeuw D, et al. First morning voids are more reliable than spot urine samples to assess microalbuminuria. J. Am Soc Nephrol 2009;20:436–443.

47. Perkins BA, Ficociello LH, Roshan B, et al. In patients with type 1 diabetes and new-onset microalbuminuria the development of advanced chronic kidney disease may not require progression to proteinuria. Kidney Int. 2010;77:57–64.

48. LeCaire TJ, Klein BEK, Howard KP, et al. Risk for end-stage renal disease over 25 years in the population-based WESDR cohort. Diabetes Care. 2014;37:381–8.

49. Rosolowsky ET, Skupien J, Smiles AM, et al. Risk for ESRD in type 1 diabetes remains high despite renoprotection. J Am Soc Nephrol. 2011;22:545–53.

50. Cohen-Tervaert TW, Mooyaart AL, Amann K, et al.; Renal Pathology Society. Pathologic classification of diabetic nephropathy. J Am Soc Nephrol. 2010;21:556–63.

51. Kasinath BS, Mujais SK, Spargo BS, et al. Nondiabetic renal disease in patients with diabetes mellitus. Am J Med. 1983;75:613–17.

52. American Diabetes Association. Standards of medical care in diabetes: 2013. Diabetes Care. 2013;36(Suppl 1): S11–66.

53. ISPAD clinical practice consensus guidelines 2009: Compendium. Pediatr Diabetes. 2009;10(Suppl 12):71–81.

54. Amed S, Nuernberger K, McCrea P, et al. Adherence to clinical practice guidelines in the management of children, youth, and young adults with type 1 diabetes: A prospective population cohort study. J Pediatr. 2013;163:543–8.

55. The DCCT/EDIC Research Group: Intensive diabetes therapy and glomerular filtration rate in type 1 diabetes. N Engl J Med. 2011;365:2366–76.

56. Perkovic V, Heerspink HL, Chalmers J, et al.; ADVANCE Collaborative Group. Intensive glucose control improves kidney outcomes in patients with type 2 diabetes. Kidney Int. 2013;83:517–23.

57. Coca SG, Ismail-Beigi F, Haq N, et al. Role of intensive glucose control in development of renal endpoints in type 2 diabetes: Systematic review and meta-analysis. Arch Intern Med. 2012;172:761–9.

58. Skyler JS, Bergenstal R, Bonow RO. Glycemic control and the prevention of cardiovascular events: Implications of the ACCORD, ADVANCE, and VA Diabetes Trials—Position statement of the American Diabetes Association and a scientific statement of the American College of Cardiology Foundation and the American Heart Association. J Am Coll Cardiol. 2009;53:298–304.

59. Shurraw S, Tonelli M. Intensive glycemic control in type 2 diabetics at high cardiovascular risk: Do the benefits justify the risks? Kidney Int. 2013;83:346–8.

60. Stehouwerb CDA, Smulders YM. Microalbuminuria and risk for cardiovascular disease: Analysis of potential mechanisms. J Am Soc Nephrol. 2006;17:2106–11.

61. Weir MR. Microalbuminuria and cardiovascular disease. Clin J Am Soc Nephrol. 2007;2:581–90.

62. Yokoyama H, Okudaira M, Otani T, et al.: Higher incidence of diabetic nephropathy in type 2 than in type 1 diabetes in early-onset diabetes in Japan. Kidney Int. 2000;58:302–11.

63. National Kidney Foundation. KDOQI clinical practice guidelines and clinical practice recommendations for diabetes and chronic kidney disease. Am J Kidney Dis. 2007;49(2 Suppl 2):S1-180.

64. Cook J, Daneman D, Perlman K, et al. Angiotensin converting enzyme inhibitor therapy to decrease microalbuminuria in normotensive children with insulin-dependent diabetes mellitus. J Pediatr. 1990;117:39–45.

65. EUCLID Study Group. Randomised placebo-controlled trial of lisinopril in normotensive patients with insulin dependent diabetes and normoalbuminuria or microalbuminuria. Lancet. 1997;349:1787–92.

66. ACE Inhibitors in Diabetic Nephropathy Trialist Group. Should all patients with type 1 diabetes mellitus and microalbuminuria receive angiotensin-converting enzyme inhibitors? A meta-analysis of individual patient data. Ann Intern Med. 2001;134:370–9.

67. Parving H-H, Hommel E, Jensen BR, et al. Long-term beneficial effect of ACE inhibition on diabetic nephropathy in normotensive type 1 diabetic patients. Kidney Int. 2001;60:228–34.

68. Brenner BM, Cooper ME, de Zeeuw D, et al. Effects of losartan on renal and cardiovascular outcomes in patients with type 2 diabetes and nephropathy. N Engl J Med. 2001;345:861–9.

69. Bilous R, Chaturvedi N, Sjolie AK, et al. Effect of candesartan on microalbuminuria and albumin excretion rate in diabetes: Three randomized trials. Ann Intern Med. 2009;151:11–20.

70. Mauer M, Zinman B, Gardiner R, et al. Renal and retinal effects of enalapril and losartan in type 1 diabetes. N Engl J Med. Jul 2 2009;361:40-51

71. Hirst JA, Taylor KS, Stevens RJ, et al. The impact of renin–angiotensin–aldosterone system inhibitors on type 1 and type 2 diabetic patients with and without early diabetic nephropathy. Kidney Int. 2012;81:674–83.

72. National Kidney Foundation. KDOQI clinical practice guidelines for diabetes and CKD: 2012 Update. Am J Kidney Dis. 2012;60:850–86.

73. Jennings DL, Kalus JS, Coleman CI, et al. Combination therapy with an ACE inhibitor and an angiotensin receptor blocker for diabetic nephropathy: A meta-analysis. Diabet Med. 2007;24:486–93.

74. Juarez GF, Luño J, Barrio V, et al. Effect of dual blockade of the renin-angiotensin system on the progression of type 2 diabetic nephropathy: A randomized trial. Am J Kidney Dis. 2013;61:211–8.

75. Mann JF, Schmieder RE, McQueen M, et al. Renal outcomes with telmisartan, ramipril, or both, in people at high vascular risk (the ONTARGET study): A multicentre, randomised, double-blind, controlled trial. Lancet. 2009;372:547–53.

76. Fried LF, Emanuele N, Zhang JH, et al. Combined angiotensin inhibition for the treatment of diabetic nephropathy. N Engl J Med. 2013;369:1892–903.

77. Parving H-H, Persson F, Lewis JB, et al.; AVOID Study Investigators. Aliskiren combined with losartan in type 2 diabetes and nephropathy. N Engl J Med. 2008;358:2433–46.

78. Parving H-H, Brenner BM, McMurray JJV, et al. Cardiorenal end points in a trial of aliskiren for type 2 diabetes. N Engl J Med. 2012;367:2204–13.

79. U.S. Food and Drug Administration. FDA drug safety communication: New warning and contraindication for blood pressure medicines containing aliskiren (Tekturna): 4-20-2012. http://www.fda.gov/drugs/drugsafety/ucm300889.htm. Accessed on November 10, 2013.

80. Krolewski AS, Kosinski EJ, Warram JH, et al. Magnitude and determinants of coronary artery disease in juvenile-onset, insulin-dependent diabetes mellitus. Am J Cardiol. 1987;59:750–5.

81. Preis SR, Hwang SJ, Coady S, et al. Trends in all-cause and cardiovascular disease mortality among women and men with and without diabetes mellitus in the Framingham Heart Study, 1950 to 2005. Circulation. 2009;119:1728–35.

82. Rodriguez BL, Fujimoto WY, Mayer-Davis EJ, et al. Prevalence of cardiovascular disease risk factors in U.S. children and adolescents with diabetes: The SEARCH for diabetes in youth study. Diabetes Care. 2006;29:1891–6.

83. Christlieb AR, Warram JH, Krolewski AS, et al. Hypertension: The major risk factor in juvenile-onset insulin-dependent diabetics. Diabetes. 1981;30(Suppl 2):90–6.

84. American Diabetes Association. Standards of medical care in diabetes: 2013. Diabetes Care. 2013;36(Suppl 1):S11–66.

85. The ACCORD Study Group: Effects of intensive blood-pressure control in type 2 diabetes mellitus. N Engl J Med. 2010;362:1575–85.

86. Arguedas JA, Leiva V, Wright JM. Blood pressure targets for hypertension in people with diabetes mellitus. Cochrane Database Syst Rev. 2013;(10)008277.

87. Nosadini R, Tonolo G. Cardiovascular and renal protection in type 2 diabetes mellitus: The role of calcium channel blockers. J Am Soc Nephrol. 2002;13(Suppl 3):S216–23.

88. Xu G, Chen J, Jing G, et al. Preventing β-cell loss and diabetes with calcium channel blockers. Diabetes. 2012;61:848–56.

89. Guy J, Ogden L, Wadwa RP, et al.: Lipid and lipoprotein profiles in youth with and without type 1 diabetes: The SEARCH for Diabetes in Youth Case-Control Study. Diabetes Care. 2009;32:416–20.

90. Vergès B. Lipid disorders in type 1 diabetes. Diabetes Metab. 35: 353–60, 2009.

91. Kershnar AK, Daniels SR, Imperatore G, et al. Lipid abnormalities are prevalent in youth with type 1 and type 2 diabetes: The SEARCH for Diabetes in Youth Study. J Pediatr. 2006;149:314–9.

92. Reh CM, Mittelman SD, Wee C-P, et al. A longitudinal assessment of lipids in youth with type 1 diabetes. Pediatr Diabetes. 2011:12:365–71.

93. Wong HK, Ong KL, Cheung CL, Utilization of glucose, blood pressure, and lipid lowering medications among people with type II diabetes in the United States, 1999-2010. Ann Epidemiol. 2014;24:516–21.

94. Reaven GM. Banting lecture 1988: Role of insulin resistance in human disease. Diabetes. 1988;37:1595–607.

95. Reaven GM. Role of insulin resistance in human disease (syndrome X): An expanded definition. Annu Rev Med. 1993;44:121-31.

96. Anonymous. Third report of the National Cholesterol Education Program Expert Panel on Detection, Evaluation, and Treatment of High Blood Cholesterol in Adults (Adult Treatment Panel III). NIH Publication No. 02-5215, September 2002. Bethesda, MD: National Institutes of Health; 2002.

97. Alberti KG, Zimmet PZ. Definition, diagnosis and classification of diabetes mellitus and its complications. I. Diagnosis and classification of diabetes mellitus provisional report of a WHO consultation. Diabet Med. 1998;15:539–53.

98. World Health Organization. Report of a WHO consultation: Definition of metabolic syndrome in definition, diagnosis, and classification of diabetes mellitus and its complications. I. Diagnosis and classification of diabetes mellitus. Geneva: World Health Organization, Department of Noncommunicable Disease Surveillance; 1999.

99. Steinberger J, Daniels SR, Eckel RH, et al. Progress and challenges in metabolic syndrome in children and adolescents. Circulation. 2009;119:628–47.

100. Fox CS, Massaro JM, Hoffmann U, et al. Abdominal visceral and subcutaneous adipose tissue compartments. association with metabolic risk factors in the Framingham Heart Study. Circulation. 2007;116:39–48.

101. Kuba VM, Leone C, Damiani D. Is waist-to-height ratio a useful indicator of cardio-metabolic risk in 6-10-year-old children? BMC Pediatr. 2013,13:91.

102. Alberti KG, Eckel RH, Grundy SM, et al. Harmonizing the metabolic syndrome: A joint interim statement of the International Diabetes Federation Task Force on Epidemiology and Prevention; National Heart, Lung, and Blood Institute; American Heart Association; World Heart Federation; International Atherosclerosis Society; and International Association for the Study of Obesity. Circulation. 2009;120:1640–5.

103. Cook S, Weitzman M, Auinger P, et al. Prevalence of a metabolic syndrome phenotype in adolescents: Findings from the third National Health and Nutrition Examination Survey, 1988-1994. Arch Pediatr Adolesc Med. 2003;157:821–7.

104. Weiss R, Dziura J, Burgert TS, et al. Obesity and the metabolic syndrome in children and adolescents. N Engl J Med. 2004;350:2362–74.

105. Bosy-Westphal A, Onur S, Geisler C, et al. Common familial influences on clustering of metabolic syndrome traits with central obesity and insulin resistance: The Kiel obesity prevention study. Int J Obes (Lond). 2007;31:784–90.

106. Cameron AJ, Shaw JE, Zimmet PZ. The metabolic syndrome: Prevalence in worldwide populations. Endocrinol Metab Clin North Am. 2004;33:351–75.

107. van Dongen J, Willemsen G, Chen WM, et al. Heritability of metabolic syndrome traits in a large population-based sample. J Lipid Res. 2013;54:2914–23.

108. Povel CM, Boer JM, Reiling E, Feskens EJ. Genetic variants and the metabolic syndrome: A systematic review. Obes Rev. 2011;12:952–67.

109. Monda KL, North KE, Hunt SC, et al. The genetics of obesity and the metabolic syndrome. Endocr Metab Immune Disord Drug Targets. 2010;10:86–108.

110. Sjögren M, Lyssenko V, Jonsson A, et al. The search for putative unifying genetic factors for components of the metabolic syndrome. Diabetologia. 2008;51:2242–51.

111. Parker VE, Semple RK. Genetics in endocrinology: Genetic forms of severe insulin resistance: What endocrinologists should know. Eur J Endocrinol. 20131;169:R71–80.

112. Everard A, Cani PD. Diabetes, obesity and gut microbiota. Best Pract Res Clin Gastroenterol. 2013;27:73–83.

113. Wisse BE. The inflammatory syndrome: The role of adipose tissue cytokines in metabolic disorders linked to obesity. J Am Soc Nephrol. 2004;15:2792–800.

114. Stumvoll M, Goldstein BJ, van Haeften TW. Type 2 diabetes: Principles of pathogenesis and therapy. Lancet. 2005;365:1333–46.

115. Mietus-Snyder M, Krauss RM. Lipid metabolism in children and adolescents: Impact on vascular biology. J Clin Lipidol. 2008;2:127–37.

116. Riccardi G. Dietary treatment of the metabolic syndrome: The optimal diet. Br J Nutr. 2000;83(Suppl 1):S143–8.

117. Huth PJ, Fulgoni VL 3rd, Keast DR, et al. Major food sources of calories, added sugars, and saturated fat and their contribution to essential nutrient intakes in the U.S. diet: Data from the National Health and Nutrition Examination Survey (2003-2006). Nutr J. 2013;12:116. doi 10.1186/1475-2891-12-116.

118. Huffman MD, Capewell S, Ning H, et al. Cardiovascular health behavior and health factor changes (1988-2008) and projections to 2020: Results from the National Health and Nutrition Examination Surveys. Circulation. 2012;125:2595–602.

119. Bremer AA, Mietus-Snyder M, Lustig RH. Toward a unifying hypothesis of metabolic syndrome. Pediatrics. 2012;129:557–70.

120. Bays HE. Is "sick fat" a cardiovascular disease? State-of-the-art paper. J Am Coll Cardiol. 2011;57:2461–73.

121. Kambham N, Markowitz G, Valeri A, et al. Obesity-related glomerulopathy: An emerging epidemic. Kidney Int. 59:1498–509, 200.

122. Cohen AH. Massive obesity and the kidney: A morphologic and statistical study. Am J Pathol. 1975;81:117–30.

123. Hsu CY, McCulloch CE, Iribarren C, et al.: Body mass index and risk for end-stage renal disease. Ann Intern Med. 2006;144:21–8.

124. Serra A, Romero R, Lopez D, et al. Renal injury in the extremely obese patients with normal renal function. Kidney Int. 2008;73:947–55.

125. Adelman RD, Restaino IG, Alon US, Blowey DL. Proteinuria and focal segmental glomerulosclerosis in severely obese adolescents. J Pediatr. 2001;138:481–5.

126. Shen WW, Chen HM, Chen H, et al. Obesity-related glomerulopathy: Body mass index and proteinuria. Clin J Am Soc Nephrol. 2010;5:1401–9.

127. Goumenos DS, Kawar B, El Nahas M, et al. Early histological changes in the kidney of people with morbid obesity. Nephrol Dial Transplant. 2009;24:3732–8.

128. Hayden MR, Sowers JR. Childhood-adolescent obesity in the cardiorenal syndrome: Lessons from animal models. Cardiorenal Med. 2011;1:75–86.

129. Chen HM, Li SJ, Chen HP, et al. Obesity-related glomerulopathy in China: A case series of 90 patients. Am J Kidney Dis. 2008;52:58–65.

130. Danilewicz M, Wagrowska-Danielwicz M. Morphometric and immunohistochemical insight into focal segmental glomerulosclerosis in obese and non-obese patients. Nefrologia 2009;29:35–41.

131. Darouich S, Goucha R, Jaafoura MH, et al. Clinicopathological characteristics of obesity-associated focal segmental glomerulosclerosis. Ultrastruct Pathol. 2011;35:176–2.

132. Orchard TJ, Temprosa M, Goldberg R, et al. The effect of metformin and intensive lifestyle intervention on the metabolic syndrome: The Diabetes Prevention Program randomized trial. Ann Intern Med. 2005;142:611–9.

133. Knowler WC, Barrett-Connor E, Fowler SE, et al. Reduction in the incidence of type 2 diabetes with lifestyle intervention or metformin. N Engl J Med. 2002;346:393–403.

134. Jensen DE, Nguo K, Baxter KA, et al. Fasting gut hormone levels change with modest weight loss in obese adolescents. Pediatr Obes. 2015, doi: 10.1111/ijpo.275.

135. Rojas LBA, Gomes MB. Metformin: An old but still the best treatment for type 2 diabetes. Diabetol Metab Syndr. 2013;5:6.

136. Godarzi MO, Brier-Ash M. Metformin revisited: Re-evaluation of its properties and role in the pharmacopoeia of modern antidiabetic agents. Diabetes Obes Metab. 2005;6:654–65.

137. Mogul HR, Freeman R, Nguyen K, et al. Carbohydrate modified diet & insulin sensitizers reduce body weight & modulate metabolic syndrome measures in EMPOWIR (enhance the

metabolic profile of women with insulin resistance): A randomized trial of normoglycemic women with midlife weight gain. PLoS One. 2014;9:e108264. doi 10.1371/journal.pone.0108264.

138. Sharma AM. Is there a rationale for angiotensin blockade in the management of obesity hypertension? Hypertension. 2004;44:12–9.
139. Sattar N, Preiss D, Murray HM, et al. Statins and risk of incident diabetes: A collaborative meta-analysis of randomized statin trials. Lancet. 2010; 375:735–42.
140. Eiland LS, Luttrell PK. Use of statins for dyslipidemia in the pediatric population. J Pediatr Pharmacol Ther. 2010;15:160–72.
141. Expert Panel on Integrated Guidelines for Cardiovascular Health and Risk Reduction in Children and Adolescents. Summary report. Pediatrics. 2011;128(Suppl 5):S213–56.
142. Ejerblad E, Fored CM, Lindblad P, et al. Obesity and risk for chronic renal failure. J Am Soc Nephrol. 2006;17:1695–702.

## REVIEW QUESTIONS

1. In the pediatric age group (up to 19 years), diabetes mellitus accounts for ESRD in:
   a. 10% to 15%
   b. 20% to 50%
   c. >1%
   d. >10%
2. Advanced glycation products result from nonenzymatic reaction of glucose with proteins, lipids, and nucleic acids.
   a. True
   b. False
3. Podocyes lack insulin receptors.
   a. True
   b. False
4. Renin-angiotensin induces glomerular injury in diabetic nephropathy by:
   a. Systemic hypertension
   b. Glomerular hypertension
   c. Increasing podocyte apoptosis
   d. Increasing tubular sodium concentration and inducing tubuloglomerular feedback
5. The classic pathologic lesion in diabetic nephropathy is:
   a. Kimmelstiel-Wilson lesion
   b. Large glomeruli (glomerulomegaly)
   c. Focal segmental glomerulosclerosis
   d. Wire loop lesion
6. The latent phase of diabetic nephropathy in diabetes mellitus type 1 lasts:
   a. <5 years
   b. 5 to 10 years
   c. 10 to 15 years
   d. 30 to 40 years
7. Microalbuminuria in a diabetic 17-year-old girl is best tested in a:
   a. Random sample obtained in any time
   b. Random sample obtained late in the afternoon
   c. First morning urine sample
   d. Random sample obtained after ambulating for 4 hours
8. Microalbuminuria in a patient with diabetes mellitus type 1 indicates:
   a. Early diabetic nephropathy
   b. No clinical significance
   c. Onset of ESRD
   d. Development of Kimmelstiel-Wilson lesion
9. A 25-year-old man with onset of diabetes mellitus at 3 years of age had been lost to follow-up in nephrology for 3 years. He had sporadic visits with his internist and endocrinologist. Upon his return to the nephrology clinic, his estimated GFR was 100 mL/min/1.73 m$^2$, and he now has well-documented microalbuminuria and his hemoglobin A1c was 11.5%. His previous known GFR, obtained 3 years ago, was 135 mL/min/1.73 m$^2$. Which of the following best reflects diabetic nephropathy in this patient?
   a. His disease has not progressed, because he has a normal GFR.
   b. He is now cured of diabetic nephropathy, because he does not have hyperfiltration
   c. Microalbuminuria in presence of normal GFR has no clinical significance.
   d. His renal disease has progressed, because he now has albuminuria and his GFR has should be considered to have declined from a state of hyperfiltration to "normal."
10. Which of the following statements *best* characterizes the use of angiotensin-converting enzyme inhibitors in diabetic nephropathy?
    a. ACEIs are ideally started at the time of the diagnosis of diabetes mellitus to prevent development of microalbuminuria.
    b. Evidence to suggest that ACEIs prevent development of microalbuminuria is lacking.
    c. ACEIs improve diabetes control.
    d. ACEIs prevent progression of microalbuminuria.
11. The central findings of metabolic syndrome are:
    a. Insulin resistance and hyperglycemia
    b. Hypertension
    c. Obesity with increased waist circumference
    d. Dyslipidemia
    e. Microalbuminuria
    f. All of the above
    g. Only a, b, and e
12. Obesity and metabolic syndrome are characterized by molecular markers of systemic inflammation.
    a. True.
    b. False.

13. Renal pathologic findings in obesity and metabolic syndrome characteristically demonstrate:
    a. Glomerulomegaly (large glomeruli)
    b. FSGS with less pronounced morphologic changes
    c. Basement membrane thickening
    d. Lesser degree of foot-process fusion
    e. All of the above
    f. Only a, b, and d

## ANSWER KEY

1. d
2. a
3. b
4. b
5. a
6. c
7. c
8. a
9. d
10. d
11. f
12. a
13. e

# 29

# Kidney in viral infections

JEFFREY B. KOPP

Viral infections can cause a variety of renal diseases, which can lead to significant morbidity. Renal injury by human immunodeficiency virus (HIV-1), hepatitis B virus (HBV), and hepatitis C virus (HCV) has been well described. The clinical manifestations of these viral infections can range from subtle abnormalities, such as sodium wasting, microscopic hematuria, or proteinuria, to severe nephritic syndrome, nephrotic syndrome, acute kidney injury (AKI), and thrombotic microangiopathy (TMA). Diagnostic evaluation of viral infections has significantly improved in the last decade with availability of viral load detection by quantitative polymerase chain reaction (PCR) testing for many agents in both urine and blood. Therapeutic approaches to treatment of viral infections also have been advanced, especially in the case of HIV-1 infection. This chapter will review the three important viral pathogens noted here and also include a brief description of nephropathies related to cytomegalovirus (CMV), parvovirus B19 (PVB19), and Epstein-Barr virus (EBV).

## HUMAN IMMUNODEFICIENCY-1 VIRUS

## EPIDEMIOLOGY

In 1983, reports of the first cases of pediatric acquired immunodeficiency syndrome (AIDS) occurred in the United States.[1,2] AIDS was initially described in two age groups of the pediatric population:

1. Infants infected through vertical transmission
2. Children who acquired infection through blood transfusions

Subsequently, pediatric AIDS became a major public health concern worldwide, particularly in sub-Saharan Africa, where approximately 600,000 children are born with HIV-1 infection per year.[3] By the end of 2001 in the United States, pediatric AIDS cases represented approximately 1.2% of the total cases of AIDS, predominantly affecting minority populations. African Americans make up approximately 65% of all children with HIV-1 infection or AIDS, and more than 40% of these children are at risk for renal complications.[3-5]

### KEY POINTS

- Approximately 40% of children with HIV infection are at risk for renal complications.
- The morphologic type of renal disease is variable.

## CLINICOPATHOLOGIC VARIANTS

HIV-1 infection is associated with a variety of glomerular diseases (Table 29.1): (1) HIV-associated collapsing glomerulopathy (frequently referred to as HIV-associated nephropathy [HIVAN], (2) HIV-associated glomerulonephritis (HIV-associated GN), and (3) HIV-associated thrombotic microangiopathy (HIV-associated TMA).[6-10]

Table 29.1 Renal diseases associated with viral infections

| | |
|---|---|
| HIV-1 | • Collapsing glomerulopathy |
| | • Glomerulonephritis |
| |   • Lupus-like glomerulonephritis |
| |   • Membranoproliferative glomerulonephritis |
| |   • IgA nephropathy |
| | • Others |
| |   • Membranous nephropathy |
| |   • Fibrillary and immunotactoid nephropathy |
| |   • Thrombotic microangiopathy |
| HBV | • Membranous nephropathy—most common in children |
| | • Membranoproliferative glomerulonephritis |
| | • IgA nephropathy |
| | • Polyarteritis nodosa |
| HCV | • Membranoproliferative glomerulonephropathy (with or without cryoglobulinemia) |

*Abbreviations:* HBV/HCV, hepatitis B/C virus; HIV, human immunodeficiency virus; IgA, immunoglobulin A.

Among African-American patients, collapsing glomerulopathy is the most common clinicopathologic disorder, whereas HIV-associated GN is most prevalent among white, Hispanic, and Asian patients. During early years of the AIDS epidemic in children, Strauss et al.[4] estimated the prevalence of childhood HIVAN to be approximately 10% to 15%. These data were based on clinical criteria, histology from studies of predominantly African American pediatric patients, or both.

# Human immunodeficiency virus collapsing glomerulopathy

## CLINICAL MANIFESTATIONS AND BACKGROUND

Patients with HIVAN often present with asymptomatic proteinuria and are usually normotensive. Renal ultrasound classically shows enlarged, echogenic kidneys. Although HIVAN can occur at any stage of the disease, including the time of seroconversion, it is most commonly seen in patients with advanced HIV disease.[11] In the initial years of the HIV epidemic, this syndrome was characterized by a rapid progression to end-stage renal disease (ESRD). Further, these patients also had increased mortality on dialysis.

Abbott et al.,[12] using the data from the U.S. Renal Data System (USRDS), showed that 2-year survival was 36% for patients with HIVAN on dialysis, compared to 64% for those with ESRD of other causes between 1992 and 1997. In recent years, with the widespread use of combined antiretroviral therapy (cART), the incidence of HIVAN has plummeted.

Patients of African descent have striking susceptibility to developing HIVAN, with nearly 90% of the cases occurring in black individuals. Of patients with HIVAN, 25% have first-degree or second-degree family members with ESRD, suggesting a genetic predisposition to glomerular injury.[13] HIVAN is the third leading cause of ESRD in blacks 20 to 64 years of age, after diabetes mellitus and hypertension.[7] Based on the USRDS, the relative risk for ESRD from HIV-associated nephropathy is approximately 18-fold increased among African Americans compared to white patients.[14] The basis for this striking predilection is a pair of variants in *APOL1*, encoding apolipoprotein L1, that are exclusively present in individuals of African descent and make up 35% of alleles in African Americans.[15] The presence of two *APOL1* risk alleles is associated with an odds ratio of 29 for HIVAN.[16]

## PATHOLOGIC FINDINGS

The renal histologic findings are characterized by segmental or global collapse and sclerosis of the glomerular tuft (Figure 29.1). Podocytes, which are normally postmitotic

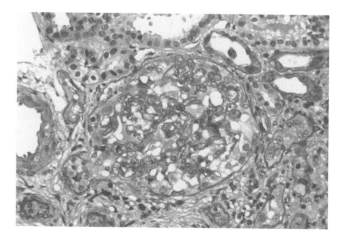

Figure 29.1 HIV-associated collapsing glomerulopathy in a 33-year-old patient. The light microscopy shows collapse of the glomerular tuft. Vacuolization and crowding of the glomerular epithelial cells are commonly seen and reflect the primary epithelial cell injury in this disease.

cells, reenter the cell cycle and proliferate, in some cases forming pseudocrescents, and lose differentiation markers. There is tubular injury with atrophy and microcyst formation (Figure 29.2).

## PATHOGENESIS

The HIV-1 genome contains nine genes (*gag, pol, vif, vpr, vpu, rev, tat, env,* and *nef*), which encode 15 proteins. These viral accessory proteins have pleiotropic effects on cell function and are implicated in renal injury. *vpr* induces G2 cell cycle arrest, perturbs mitochondrial functions, induces (and in some cells prevents) apoptosis, and alters gene transcription by acting as a coactivator. Roles of other accessory proteins in inducing renal injury have not been excluded. *tat* and *nef* each induce proliferation of podocytes, a distinctive feature of HIVAN.[17,18] A series of studies using transgenic mice bearing various portions of this genome have suggested which genes may be responsible for renal injury. HIV-1 transgenic mice carrying a replication defective HIV-1 provirus that lacks *gag* and *pol* develop renal disease characterized by podocyte dysplasia and proliferation, glomerular capillary tuft collapse, focal segmental glomerulosclerosis (FSGS), and tubular injury and do so even in the absence of immunosuppression and viral replication.[19,20] Deletion of *nef* from the transgene reduced the severity of interstitial nephritis, but it did not prevent the development of glomerular disease in one transgenic line.[21] More recently, mice bearing *tat* and *vpr* or *vpr* alone developed FSGS.[22] These data from transgenic mice indicate that *vpr* induces FSGS and *nef* contributes to interstitial nephritis.[22-24]

Because expression of HIV-1 gene products within podocytes and tubular epithelial cells can induce all the features of HIV-associated FSGS, the next question has been to understand how those gene products enter renal parenchymal cells. The data regarding direct infection of renal epithelium by HIV-1 have long been controversial. Bruggeman et al.[25] provided supportive evidence to suggest that HIV-1 viruses can directly infect the renal tissue. They detected HIV-1 in the renal tissue by RNA in situ hybridization and DNA in situ PCR. HIV-1 RNA was detected in renal tubular epithelial cells, glomerular visceral and parietal epithelial cells, and interstitial leukocytes. In addition, the distribution of HIV-1 infection of renal tubules is similar to the pattern of microcystic tubular disease, a prominent histologic feature of the nephropathy. These findings support the direct infection of renal parenchyma by the HIV-1 virus.[26]

---

### KEY POINTS

- The kidney may serve as a reservoir for HIV-1.
- Evidence suggests direct infection of the kidney cells by HIV-1 virus.

---

Infection of renal epithelial cells by HIV-1 has another important implication. The kidney may serve as a reservoir for HIV-1. Marras et al.[27] detected variation in the HIV-1 envelope sequences in the renal tubular epithelium of HIV-infected patients, indicating that renal epithelium can support viral replication. Furthermore, the envelope sequences of HIV-1 found in renal epithelium were distinct from the sequences derived from the same patient's peripheral blood samples, suggesting that the renal epithelium is a distinct reservoir for viral replication from the blood.

## TREATMENT

Although HIVAN is an important cause of renal failure in the United States, no randomized controlled trials have been carried out to assess various therapies. Thus, recommendations are based on retrospective or uncontrolled studies. It is likely that cART prevents the onset or slows progression of HIVAN (based on the epidemiologic evidence of fewer patients reaching ESRD in recent years) and may reverse clinical manifestations (based on anecdotal reports).[11,28] Angiotensin-converting enzyme inhibitors (ACEIs) also have been shown to reduce proteinuria and progression of renal disease in HIV-infected patients.[29,30]

The role of immunosuppressive therapy has been explored but it is no longer considered appropriate. Studies using prednisone in patients with renal dysfunction and HIV-1 infection show some efficacy in preserving renal function and reducing proteinuria.[31,32] However, these studies are not well controlled and not all reported patients underwent renal biopsy. Another retrospective study suggested the efficacy of combination therapy with cART and glucocorticoids.[33] The mean renal survival to

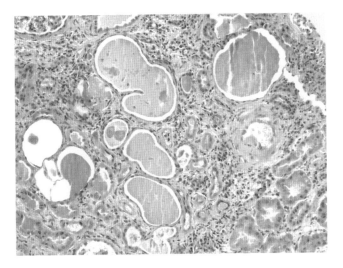

Figure 29.2 HIV-associated tubulointerstitial changes in a 20-year-old patient. The pathologic findings include asymmetric, occasionally massive, tubular epithelial cell cytoplasmic protein resorption droplets, acute tubular epithelial injury with focal simplification, and variable microcystic change.

ESRD was 26 months for those treated with the combination therapy, 6 months for those given cART alone, and 3 months for those given neither cART nor glucocorticoids. Although no studies have suggested the efficacy of glucocorticoids in children with HIVAN, a very small study reported remission of proteinuria with cyclosporine therapy in three children who had steroid-resistant renal disease.[34] Again, the study was not a controlled trial and was done before the era of cART, making it difficult to draw any conclusion.

Several novel therapies have been tested in animal models of HIVAN and offer some prospect for translation to clinical care. Cyclin-dependent kinase inhibitors were found to inhibit podocyte proliferation and induce re-expression of normal podocyte differentiation markers in vitro.[35] Gherardi et al.[36] reported reversal of collapsing glomerulopathy in HIV-transgenic mice with cyclin-dependent kinase inhibitors. He and colleagues demonstrated that retinoid acts in a similar fashion.[37] Sharma et al.[38] showed that Notch pathway inhibition attenuates glomerular injury in HIV-transgenic mice.

## Human immunodeficiency virus–associated immune complex kidney disease

In the absence of a national registry of renal biopsy findings, the true prevalence of HIV-associated immune complex kidney disease is unknown. Several different histologic descriptions have been reported for HIV-associated GN, including a lupus-like pattern, membranoproliferative glomerulonephritis (MPGN), membranous nephropathy (MN), fibrillary and immunotactoid GN, postinfectious GN, and immunoglobulin A (IgA) nephropathy. It is not always possible to discern if the renal disease is a consequence of the HIV-1 infection or if it is a coincidental occurrence. For example, patients with HIV disease are often coinfected with HBV or HCV, each of which can be associated with glomerular diseases, such as membranous glomerulopathy and MPGN.

The pathogenesis of these forms of HIV-associated immune complex kidney disease is not clear. In IgA nephropathy, immune complexes containing HIV proteins have been found in the mesangium, possibly delivered from plasma, or forming in situ, leading to renal parenchymal inflammation.[39] Guidelines for treatment are limited by the lack of prospective, randomized, and controlled trials, but therapies have included antiretroviral therapy, ACE inhibitors, and prednisone.[40,41]

## Human immunodeficiency virus and thrombotic microangiopathy

Since the first report of HIV-associated TMA in 1984, it has been increasingly recognized as a common microvascular injury in this infection.[42] A retrospective study demonstrated that 15 of 224 AIDS patients (7%) had evidence of TMA at the time of death.[43] The pathologic findings include occlusive thrombi in small arteries and arterioles, and detachment of glomerular endothelial cells from the basement membrane (Figure 29.3). Affected patients typically present with hemolytic-uremic syndrome characterized by renal insufficiency, microangiopathic hemolytic anemia, and thrombocytopenia. The pathogenesis of TMA involves endothelial injury caused by toxins, vasoactive peptides, or immune factors. Infection of microvascular endothelial cells by HIV-1 has not been confirmed, and the mechanisms that induce microvascular damage in HIV-1 infection are poorly understood. There are no data to suggest that HIV-associated TMA should be treated differently from idiopathic or autoimmune forms of TMA. Therapies have included plasmapheresis, prednisone, or both, with limited success in HIV-associated TMA.

## Drug-induced nephrotoxicity in human immunodeficiency virus infection

Drug-induced acute renal failure, with or without chronic progression, is a common cause for renal insufficiency in the HIV population. Examples include AKI kidney injury resulting from pentamidine, foscarnet, cidofovir, amphotericin B, and aminoglycosides.[44–46] Acute renal failure also may result from crystal precipitation following the use of sulfadiazine or intravenous acyclovir.[47,48] Indinavir may cause renal calculi and obstruction.[49]

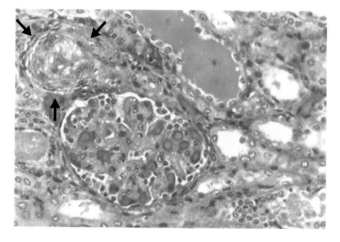

Figure 29.3 Light microscopy of renal biopsy in a child with HIV-associated thrombotic microangiopathy. The glomerular capillaries are collapsed, and red cell fragments are present in several capillary loops. Arrows outline an arteriole with endothelial swelling and luminal narrowing secondary to thrombosis. (Reproduced with permission from Turner ME, Kher K, Rakusan T, et al. Atypical hemolytic uremic syndrome in human immunodeficiency virus-1-infected children. Pediatr Nephrol. 1997;11:161.)

## KEY POINT

Tenofovir toxicity increases with duration of use and, if not discontinued after toxicity occurs, may lead to chronic kidney disease.

In recent years, tenofovir, a nucleoside analogue reverse transcriptase inhibitor (NtRTI) has emerged as the most common cause of drug-associated renal dysfunction (Table 29.2). Its renal toxicity is predominantly characterized by proximal tubular dysfunction, demonstrated by normoglycemic glucosuria, proteinuria, hematuria, and hypophosphatemia.[50,51] The proteinuria associated with tenofovir is usually mild, but nephrotic-range proteinuria also has been described.[52] Some patients also developed signs of distal tubular toxicity, presenting with diabetes insipidus.[53] The frequency of tenofovir renal toxicity in prospective cohort studies rises with increased therapy duration.[54-56] Prompt recognition of the syndrome and discontinuation of tenofovir therapy offers the best chance for improvement in renal function, although complete reversal may not occur. Continued administration of tenofovir may lead to chronic kidney disease in some patients. Renal function improves in most patients on discontinuation of the drug, but persistent glucosuria and proteinuria with elevated creatinine, suggesting irreversible damage, have been documented in some cases.[55,56] Renal biopsies in these patients have shown acute tubular necrosis, particularly involving proximal tubules.[51]

Tenofovir, an acyclic nucleoside phosphonate, belongs to a unique class of nucleoside analogues, which also include cidofovir and adefovir. Many of the adverse effects associated with these agents have been attributed to mitochondrial toxicity, because phosphorylated forms of some nucleoside reverse transcription inhibitors are potent inhibitors of mitochondrial DNA polymerase.[57] Drug-related deficiencies in the mitochondrial oxidative phosphorylation system lead to disruption in pyruvate oxidation and increased lactic acid production.[58] Thus, organs rich in mitochondria, such as muscle, liver, and kidney (particularly the proximal tubules), are at increased risk for the clinical toxicities, which can manifest as myopathy, liver

### Table 29.2  Features of tenofovir renal toxicity

| | |
|---|---|
| Presentation | Fanconi syndrome |
| | Hypokalemia |
| | Proteinuria (usually < 3 g/day) |
| | Diabetes insipidus (rare) |
| | Nephritic syndrome (rare) |
| Onset | At any time during therapy |
| Renal biopsy | Acute tubular necrosis involving mostly proximal tubules |
| Risk factor | Concurrent use of lopinavir/ritonavir |

steatosis, lactic acidosis, and Fanconi syndrome. These nucleoside analogues undergo renal tubular secretion through proximal tubules (via human renal organic anion transporter-1). Therefore, the accumulation of the drug in the proximal tubules likely plays an important role in nephrotoxicity. Given the possible nephrotoxicity, patients taking tenofovir (especially those also on lopinavir or atazanavir, which can increase the serum concentration level of tenofovir) need to be monitored regularly. The decision regarding when the drug should be stopped needs to be individualized.

## The new face of human immunodeficiency virus kidney disease

The widespread and chronic use of cART has led to a new set of renal diseases, similar to those seen in the general population, including particularly diabetic nephropathy and arterionephrosclerosis.[59] In many cases, these appear after a decade or more of cART therapy and thus may affect HIV-positive individuals at substantially younger ages compared to the general population, who tend to manifest renal dysfunction resulting from these diseases after the age of 50 or 60. The mechanisms are likely complex but include a chronic inflammatory state associated with low-level viral replication and immune activation and the effects of cART that promote disorders of glucose and lipid metabolism, including diabetes mellitus and metabolic syndrome.[60]

## HEPATITIS B VIRUS

Chronic HBV infection is a global public health problem affecting approximately 350 million people, or 5% of the world's population. The prevalence of HBV carriers varies from less than 1% in nonendemic areas (North America, Western Europe, Australia, and New Zealand) to 3% to 5% in intermediate areas (Mediterranean countries, Japan, Central Asia, Middle East, and Latin and South America) and to 10% to 20% in endemic areas (Southeast Asia, China, and sub-Saharan Africa).[61]

In nonendemic areas, HBV infection is predominantly a disease of adults, being transmitted largely through intravenous drug use or sexual contact. In the endemic countries, however, HBV is a common disease of childhood, with either vertical or horizontal transmission. This difference in the age at initial infection is likely to be responsible for the wide variability in prevalence of chronic HBV infection in different parts of the world.

The risk for chronicity in HBV infection is inversely related to the age at infection.[62] The risk for chronic infection in infants younger than 1 year of age is thus as high as 90% compared to 10% to 40% at 4 to 6 years and 1% to 5% in adults. Given that the majority of HBV infection cases occur during the first year of life in many endemic areas, it is not surprising that the burden related to the complications of chronic HBV infection is also highest in these areas.

> ## KEY POINT
>
> Chronic HBV is most commonly associated with MN in children, but may cause other glomerular lesions as well.

## CLINICOPATHOLOGIC VARIANTS

Various clinicopathologic forms of renal diseases have been described in patients with chronic HBV infection. These include MN, MPGN, mesangial proliferative GN, IgA nephropathy, and polyarteritis nodosa (see Table 29.1).[62,63] Although there also have been reports of lupus nephritis, FSGS, and minimal-change nephrotic syndrome, it is unclear if these were incidental findings. The most widely accepted pathogenesis for HBV-associated renal disease is the deposition of immune complexes of viral antigen and host antibody.

### Membranous nephropathy

MN is the most common form of HBV-associated nephritis in children, accounting for more than 85% of HBV-associated renal disease undergoing renal biopsy. HBV envelope antigen (HBeAg) is believed to be the primary antigen present in the subepithelial deposits.[64] Approximately 30% to 60% of children with HBV-associated membranous nephropathy (HBV-associated MN) undergo spontaneous remission, usually in association with development of anti-HBeAg seroconversion, over 6 to 24 months.[65] In a study of 71 children with HBV-associated MN from Cape Town, South Africa, the average time of clearance of HBeAg to remission was 5 months.[63] This is in contrast to adults, who tend to develop progressive nephropathy in approximately 25% of affected individuals. The presentation of HBV-associated MN also differs between pediatric and adult patients. Whereas adults tend to present with nephrotic syndrome, children can remain asymptomatic and the proteinuria may be incidentally discovered during a routine urine and serologic screening. In addition, there is a stronger male predominance in children affected by HBV-associated MN and children are also less likely to experience acute hepatitis compared to adults.[62]

### Mesangioproliferative glomerulonephritis (immunoglobulin A nephropathy)

Chronic HBV infection has been associated with mesangial proliferative GN with deposition of IgA and HBV surface antigen in the mesangium.[66] Bhimma et al.[67] reported that 6 of 23 children with HBV-associated nephropathy other than membranous disease had mesangial proliferative GN. It is unclear if the deposited IgA has anti-HBV surface antibody activity.

## Membranoproliferative glomerulonephritis

HBV-associated membranoproliferative glomerulonephritis (MPGN) is characterized by the deposition of antigen-antibody complexes in the mesangium and subendothelial space. These glomerular deposits are mainly composed of IgG and complement C3, and both HBV surface and envelope antigens have been implicated in this GN.[68] MPGN typically occurs in association with mixed cryoglobulinemia, particularly in the setting of coinfection with HCV.

## Polyarteritis nodosa

Polyarteritis nodosa, a large-vessel vasculitis caused by antigen-antibody complex deposition in the vessels can be associated with infection with HBV.[69] The clinical presentation is comparable to that of polyarteritis that is not associated with HBV and typically occurs within 4 months after the onset of HBV infection.

## TREATMENT

Therapy for HBV renal diseases has focused on antiviral therapies, although the data from controlled studies are limited. In general, immunosuppression for HBV-associated renal disease is of no proved benefit, particularly in children with MN in whom spontaneous recovery over 6 to 24 months is common.

### Antiviral therapies

Currently, the three medications approved for treatment of chronic HBV infection in adults are interferon-$\alpha$ (IFN-$\alpha$), lamivudine, and adefovir dipivoxil. Of these, IFN-$\alpha$ and lamivudine are approved for use in children in the United States. Several controlled trials in children with HBV infection have evaluated the efficacy of IFN-$\alpha$ in different parts of the world. Response rate, defined as HBeAg seroconversion or disappearance of plasma HBV DNA, tends to be highest in Western countries at 20% to 58% and lower in Asian countries at approximately 17%.[70-74] The difference in response rates may not be due to ethnicity but rather to the fact that a higher proportion of patients from endemic areas are infected at birth and are in the immune-tolerant phase of infection. It is unclear why such patients are less likely to respond to antiviral therapy. Based on current data, IFN-$\alpha$ may be effective therapy for HBV-associated MN, particularly in young children in nonendemic areas.

Experience with lamivudine in children with chronic HBV infection is limited. Although the available data suggest its efficacy and safety in children, the benefit of lamivudine must be balanced against the risk for selecting resistant mutants. Children with higher baseline alanine aminotransferase and histologic activity index scores on liver biopsy are more likely to respond to lamivudine.[75] The optimal duration of therapy is unclear. Lamivudine should be used for at least 1 year and continued for at least 6 months after HBeAg seroconversion. Adefovir has been evaluated as monotherapy for adults with chronic HBV infection and those who have developed resistance to lamivudine.[76] Other potential antiviral agents that require further studies in children include pegylated IFN, famciclovir, and lobucavir.

## Immunosuppression

Glucocorticoids or cytotoxic agents, which are used in primary MN, have no proved benefit in patients with HBV-associated MN.[77] Indeed, immunosuppression may lead to greater viral replication and exacerbation of chronic hepatitis. One exception may be in patients with active vasculitis who may require a short course of steroid treatment to control the inflammatory response.[78]

## Immunoprophylaxis

The most important strategy to improve morbidity and mortality associated with chronic HBV infection is immunoprophylaxis. HBV vaccination given as part of routine immunization in endemic areas is highly effective in reducing the incidence of HBV-associated MN.

## HEPATITIS C VIRUS

HCV infection, the leading indication for liver transplantation, remains a significant cause for morbidity and mortality in adults. It is, however, a less common cause of liver disease in children. In the United States, 60,000 to 100,000 children (0.2% to 0.4% of all children) are estimated to have chronic infection with HCV, although the specific incidence in children is unknown.[79] The prevalence is much higher in children (50% to 95%) who received multiple transfusions of blood and blood products before 1992.[80]

The predominant route of HCV infection in children is perinatal transmission. The incidence of vertical transmission of HCV is approximately 2% to 5% in HCV RNA–positive mothers, but coinfection with HIV-1 can more than quadruple the risk to approximately 20%.[81] Among adolescents, risk factors also include intravenous or intranasal drug use and use of contaminated tattoo instruments.

The natural history of HCV in the pediatric population is now better defined. In general, infections acquired early in infancy (either by transfusion or vertical transmission) can undergo spontaneous clearance more frequently than infections acquired later in life, and the reported cure rates

vary from 9% to 45%.[82–85] Another general observation is that HCV is often mild and less progressive during childhood, although hepatic cirrhosis generally occurs in the third decade of life.[85]

---

**KEY POINT**

MPGN is the predominant glomerular disease associated with HCV, most often related to cryoglobulinemia.

---

## HEPATIC C NEPHROPATHY

The predominant glomerular disease associated with HCV is MPGN, usually in the setting of cryoglobulinemia.[86] Other forms of glomerular disease associated with HCV in adults include MN and fibrillary and immunotactoid glomerulonephropathy.[87–89] To date, no studies have examined whether treatment of children with HCV infection reduces their subsequent risk for cirrhosis, hepatocellular carcinoma, or renal complications. There are no systemic studies of HCV-associated nephropathy in children. Interestingly, 19% of children with ESRD tested for HCV infection in one study in the 1990s were found to have a positive result, suggesting that HCV may be an important association in progressive renal disease in children.[90] On the other hand, HCV appears to be less commonly associated with MPGN in children.[91]

## CLINICAL MANIFESTATIONS

Unlike with HBV, in children with HCV renal disease is rare, usually occurring in those with long-standing infection and the available clinical data is scant. In adults, HCV-associated renal disease is characterized by proteinuria, nephrotic syndrome, microscopic hematuria, elevated serum creatinine, hypocomplementemia (low C3 and C4), falsely positive antinuclear antibodies, and positive rheumatoid factor.[89] Cryoglobulins are detected in 50% to 70% of patients. Despite a mild clinical course of HCV infection in children, it is unknown if these patients will continue to have a benign course in the future. Those with cryoglobulinemia also may present with palpable purpura, arthralgia, and neuropathy.

## PATHOLOGIC FINDINGS

The predominant glomerular disease associated with HCV is MPGN (Figure 29.4), usually in the setting of cryoglobulinemia. Histopathologic examination shows typical changes associated with MPGN, including lobular glomeruli, increased mesangial cellularity, and intracapillary accumulations of eosinophilic material representing precipitated

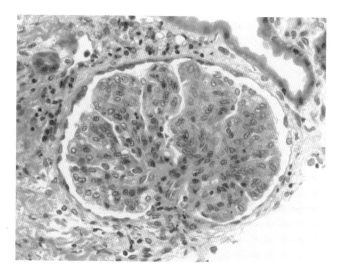

Figure 29.4 Light microscopy of hepatitis C virus–associated membranoproliferative glomerulonephritis in a 15-year-old patient. The glomerular tuft has a lobular appearance with focal areas of increased glomerular cellularity and mesangial expansion.

immune complexes or cryoglobulins.[87–89] Electron microscopy shows subendothelial immune complex deposits (Figure 29.5) and may have a finely fibrillary or tactoid pattern characteristic of cryoglobulin deposition. Although the pathogenesis of glomerular injury in HCV is unclear, it is believed to result from deposition of circulating immune complexes of HCV, anti-HCV, and rheumatoid factor at the site of injury. Apart from MPGN and immunotactoid nephropathy, IgA nephropathy and MN have also reported in patients with HCV infection.[92]

## TREATMENT

The therapy for renal diseases associated with HCV, particularly MPGN, focuses on treatment with antiviral agents. A few small and nonrandomized studies have evaluated the efficacy of the combination therapy in HCV-associated MPGN with IFN-α and ribavirin.[93–101] In general, these studies have suggested efficacy in lowering or clearing viral titers, improving clinical symptoms (related to cryoglobulinemia) and decreasing proteinuria, with variable impact on renal function.

HCV therapy has been revolutionized recently by the introduction of new direct acting anti-viral agents, replacing ribavirin and interferon alpha for some viral genotypes. The current list of these new agents, generally used in particular combinations, includes ledispasvir, sofosubvir, paritaprevir, ombitasvir, dasabuvir, daclatasvir, simeprevir and telaprevir. Case reports suggest that these agents can be safely used in renal transplant patients (1) and in hemodialysis patients (2). Results of the use of these agents in HCV glomerular disease are likely to appear soon.

For more severe or acute cryoglobulinemic renal disease or systemic vasculitis, antiviral therapy does not seem to prevent progression of renal injury.[102] In such cases, combination therapy with anti-inflammatory and cytotoxic drugs may be necessary to prevent new antibody formation. Plasmapheresis is also frequently used in conjunction to remove the circulating cryoglobulins. Although there are no controlled trials, observations suggest that this regimen may lead to improvement in renal function in over 50% of patients.[102,103]

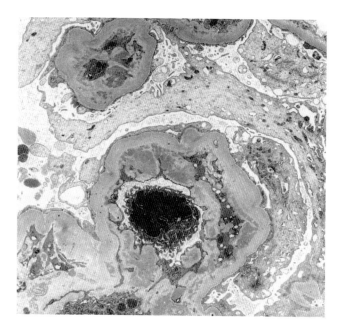

Figure 29.5 Electron micrograph of HCV-associated type I membranoproliferative glomerulonephritis. The glomerular capillary wall is markedly thickened with immune deposits and by interposition of mesangial cell processes.

## CYTOMEGALOVIRUS

Primary infection with human CMV occurs most often in childhood or in industrialized countries, in the teenage and young adult years. The evidence linking CMV infection to glomerulopathy is moderately strong; although still limited to isolated case reports of the syndromes listed later, many have shown convincing localization of viral DNA or protein to glomeruli. Renal manifestations include MPGN, MN,

### KEY POINT

PVB19 is the only parvovirus clearly linked to human glomerulopathy.

TMA, collapsing glomerulopathy, and interstitial nephritis.[104-107] Some but not all cases have involved immunocompromised patients, including renal transplant.

## HUMAN PARVOVIRUS B19

PVB19, a single-stranded DNA virus discovered by an Australian virologist, Yvonne Cossart, in 1975, is the only parvovirus clearly linked to human disease.[108] In 1993, Brown et al.[109] discovered that the receptor for PVB19 is blood-group P antigen or globoside (Gb4). This explains the primary tropism of PVB19 for erythroid precursors. Gb4 is also expressed in other cell types, such as lung, heart, liver, kidneys, synovium, endothelium, and vascular smooth muscle.[110] PVB19 is the etiologic agent of erythema infectiosum, or fifth disease, a highly contagious childhood exanthem. PVB19 also has been implicated in a wide spectrum of diseases, including polyarthropathy, acute aplastic crisis (particularly in patients with increased erythropoiesis), chronic anemia (in immunocompromised hosts), and hydrops fetalis.[111] In addition, PVB19 has been increasingly reported in association with various renal diseases (Table 29.3).

## ACUTE GLOMERULONEPHRITIS AND THROMBOTIC MICROANGIOPATHY

The most frequently reported renal disease in PVB19 infection is acute postinfectious glomerulonephritis (AGN). Nineteen cases of PVB19-associated AGN have been reported to date in children and adults without any underlying diseases.[108-120] PVB19-induced AGN typically occurs within 2 weeks (range, 3 to 45 days) of the viral infection. Usual presentation is with acute nephritic syndrome and hypocomplementemia.

The histopathologic description of PVB19-induced AGN includes endocapillary, mesangial proliferative GN or both. Immunofluorescence typically shows granular deposition of C3, IgG, IgM, or a combination of these along capillary walls and in the mesangium. Electron microscopy may demonstrate subendothelial electron-dense

deposits; subepithelial deposits are generally absent. Immunohistochemical analysis using monoclonal antibody against PVB19 antigen has shown positive staining along capillary walls and in the mesangium, suggesting that the immune complexes with PVB19 may be implicated in the development of AGN.[112,115,116] The diagnosis of acute PVB19-associated GN is suggested by immunostaining of kidney tissue and specific IgM antibody and plasma PCR detection of the viral genome.

Renal biopsies of some patients with B19-induced AGN also had features consistent with TMA, including subendothelial widening, mesangiolytic changes, and thrombotic lesions (Figure 29.6).[112,115] Although the exact pathogenesis is unknown, PVB19 may cause endothelial injury by an immune complex–mediated mechanism and by direct cytotoxicity of the endothelial cells. The observation that the vascular endothelial cells express PVB19 receptor suggests that the virus may directly infect and injure endothelial cells.[111] PVB19 infection has been associated with TMA in four renal allograft recipients and in a healthy adult.[121,122] Given that PVB19 may cause renal injury through various pathways, AGN and TMA may represent phenotypic variants of the same disease, rather than two distinct pathologic entities.

## TREATMENT

Most of the patients with PVB19-induced AGN recovered spontaneously without any specific treatment. Clearance of PVB19 and fall of IgM titers usually take approximately 8 weeks following the initial infection. Low titers, however, may persist up to 6 months, and some patients may not show full recovery for 6 months. The therapy for patients with no underlying medical conditions thus remains supportive. For immunocompromised hosts or those with persistent symptoms, intravenous immunoglobulin may be considered. Successful treatment of chronic PVB19 infection with intravenous immunoglobulin therapy has been reported in patients with lymphoma, acute PVB19-induced

Table 29.3 Renal manifestation of parvovirus B19 infection

| Presentation | Acute nephritic syndrome |
| --- | --- |
| | Hypocomplementemia |
| | Proteinuria |
| Onset | 2 weeks (3–45 days) after infection |
| Renal biopsy | Mesangial proliferative glomerulopathy |
| | Thrombotic microangiopathy |
| | Focal segmental glomerulosclerosis |
| | Collapsing glomerulopathy |

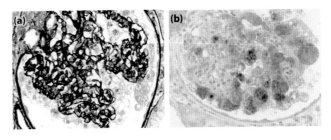

Figure 29.6 Photomicrograph of a glomerulus from a patient with early parvovirus B19–associated collapsing glomerulopathy. (a) Podocytes are enlarged with cytoplasmic vacuoles and protein reabsorption droplets. Capillaries are obliterated as a result of collapse of the walls, and mononuclear leukocytes are spread in the capillary lumens. (b) Parvovirus B19 immunostaining reveals viral protein within the enlarged podocytes.

myocarditis, PVB19-induced chronic fatigue syndrome, and recurrent PVB19 infection with collapsing glomerulopathy in a renal transplant patient.[123-126]

# FOCAL SEGMENTAL GLOMERULOSCLEROSIS AND COLLAPSING GLOMERULOPATHY

The initial cases of FSGS in patients with PVB19 infection were observed in patients with sickle cell disease. Markenson et al.[127] first described the link between renal disease and PVB19 in two siblings with sickle cell disease who developed nephrotic syndrome following PVB19-induced aplastic crises. Wierenga et al.[128] also described a similar report in seven patients with sickle cell disease presenting with nephrotic syndrome following PVB19 infection. The renal biopsy performed during the acute phase in four patients revealed segmental proliferative GN without significant immune complex deposition. In the fifth patient who underwent renal biopsy 4 months following the onset of symptoms, the diagnosis of FSGS was made. Tolaymat et al.[129] reported a similar pediatric case of FSGS and established the first direct association between glomerular disease and PVB19 by demonstrating the viral DNA in renal specimens by PCR. Tanawattanacharoen et al.[130] examined PVB19 DNA in renal biopsy specimens and found that the prevalence of the viral DNA was greater among patients with idiopathic FSGS and collapsing FSGS (85%) than other glomerular diseases (54%). Similarly, Moudgil et al.[131] also reported 78% prevalence of PVB19 DNA in renal biopsies of patients with collapsing glomerulopathy compared to the prevalence of 26% in controls. Despite these studies, the link between PVB19 and collapsing glomerulopathy remains to be fully demonstrated, with more studies needed of localization of viral protein or DNA to glomeruli at the time of initial presentation.

The renal prognosis of patients developing FSGS in the setting of sickle cell disease remains guarded. Among the seven patients reported by Wierenga et al.,[128] only one recovered completely, one reached ESRD within 3 months and died, and the rest had persistently impaired creatinine clearance, four with proteinuria. Because sickle cell disease itself is associated with adaptive FSGS, it is unclear how much of the progression of the renal disease in these patients is directly attributable to PVB19 infection. The benefit of immunosuppressive therapy in these patients also remains unclear, and management needs to be individualized with frequent monitoring and aggressive control of other renal risk factors such as hypertension and avoidance of nephrotoxins.

## EPSTEIN-BARR VIRUS

Although the most common clinical presentation with EBV infection is infectious mononucleosis in adolescents and adults, most EBV infections are asymptomatic

or nonspecific in infants and children.[132] The diagnosis of EBV infection in children is challenging, not only because of its atypical presentation but also because EBV serology in children differs from that in adults or adolescents. First, heterophil antibodies are rarely seen in young children. Second, although IgM antibodies to EBV capsid antigen are considered to be a reliable marker of the infection, it is detected by the conventional indirect immunofluorescence method in a limited number of children.[133] Third, antibody to EBV nuclear antigen (anti-EBV NA IgG), a late-onset antibody, tends to develop earlier in children than in adults.[134] Therefore, detection of anti-EBV NA IgG does not rule out the possibility of acute EBV infection in children.

## CLINICAL MANIFESTATIONS

Mild renal involvement in EBV infection may be present in approximately 16% of patients with infectious mononucleosis.[135] Acute renal failure in patients with EBV infection is rare, and its incidence has been reported to be 1.6% in one study, although this rate may be higher in more severely affected individuals.[135] In a recent retrospective study of 165 Taiwanese children hospitalized with serologically proved primary EBV infection, Tsai et al.[136] reported that 8 had acute renal failure (4.8%). Fever was the most common presentation in these 8 children, with the classic triad of fever, pharyngitis, and lymphadenopathy being present in only 1 patient. Specific renal manifestation included bilateral flank pain and evidence of tubular damage, such as microscopic hematuria, mild proteinuria, glucosuria, or poor concentrating ability on urinalysis (Table 29.4). The creatinine levels typically peaked within 3 weeks following the clinical onset (range, 3 to 17 days) in this study. Except for 1 patient who died of gastrointestinal bleeding, the remaining 7 children recovered their renal function within 1 week to 1 month.

## PATHOLOGIC FINDINGS

The most common pathologic abnormality in renal failure associated with EBV infection is acute tubulointerstitial nephritis. Other reported forms of EBV-associated renal disease are distinctively rare and include immune complex GN, minimal-change disease, and hemolytic uremic syndrome.[137-139] Although the pathogenesis of EBV-associated

Table 29.4 Renal manifestation of Epstein-Barr virus–associated nephropathy

| | |
|---|---|
| Presentation | Bilateral flank pain |
| | Microscopic hematuria |
| | Mild proteinuria |
| | Tubular dysfunctions: Fanconi syndrome, urinary frequency resulting from impaired urine concentrating ability |
| Onset | 3-17 days following clinical onset |
| Renal biopsy | Tubulointerstitial nephropathy |

interstitial nephritis remains enigmatic, Becker et al.[140] postulated that EBV infection of renal proximal tubular cells may evoke a cellular immune response that leads to interstitial damage. Using in situ hybridization and PCR, these authors detected EBV DNA exclusively in the renal tissue of patients with idiopathic chronic interstitial nephritis. The EBV genome was detected primarily in renal proximal tubular cells. Moreover, the authors detected the CD21 antigen, the receptor for EBV in B lymphocytes, also on proximal tubular cells and this was significantly upregulated with EBV infection. The authors speculate that induction of interstitial nephritis by EBV may be the consequence of cellular immune response by infected proximal tubular epithelial cells.

# TREATMENT

The role of glucocorticoid therapy remains unclear in treatment of patients with complications of EBV infection. Therapy with glucocorticoids has led to variable results. In the absence of data derived from controlled studies, specific guidelines regarding indications for glucocorticoid use in EBV-associated interstitial nephritis are difficult to formulate. Likewise, there is no conclusive evidence regarding efficacy of acyclovir to improve outcome or prevent complications in EBV infection.

## SUMMARY

A number of viruses have been associated with human renal disease. They may cause disease by infecting the cells, such as is the case with HIV, but frequently they cause disease through the formation of immune complexes, as is the case with hepatitis viruses. Recognition of viruses as possible agents of renal disease is emerging as a new field in nephrology, especially as it relates to kidney transplantation. Lessons learned from the 2014 Ebola infection epidemic reinforce our need to understand pathogenesis of kidney disease in viral infections and develop effective measures to prevent and treat such infection disorders.[141,142] Quick and early diagnostic tools and containment strategies will be the primary key in effective management of globally transmissible viral diseases. Because specific antiviral treatments do not exist for all viral infections, therapeutic needs in this area should spur growth in the pharmaceutical advances in the years to come.

## ACKNOWLEDGMENT

The authors would like to thank Dr. Cynthia Nast for providing the images of parvovirus-associated collapsing glomerulopathy and Dr. David Thomas for providing the images of HIVAN and MPGN.

### Clinical Vignette 29.1

A 9-year-old girl presents with bilateral leg edema and thirst. She has been well until these symptoms appeared recently. Three months ago she visited her parents' relatives in the Philippines for an extended visit. While there she had a brief febrile illness characterized by anorexia and mild abdominal pain. Parasite workup was unremarkable, and she recovered after several days.

On physical examination she was not ill appearing. Findings were confined to 2+ pitting edema extending half-way between the ankles and the knees on the tibia. Urinalysis showed 3+ protein and trace blood. Serum chemistry findings included normal electrolytes; blood urea nitrogen and creatinine of 15 mg/dL and 0.62 mg/dL, respectively; and albumin of 2.1 g/dL and cholesterol of 217 mg/dL. Serum complement levels were normal. A percutaneous renal biopsy was performed and revealed thickened glomerular basement membranes. Electron microscopy showed dense epimembranous deposits with thickened glomerular basement membrane that in some places suggested a spikelike appearance. A diagnosis of MN was made. A blood test for HBeAg was positive, and the patient was started on pegylated IFN-α therapy.

### TEACHING POINTS

- This vignette presents a typical case of a child with MN secondary to hepatitis B. The diagnosis of MN was suggested by the normal complement levels in the face of a nephritic-nephrotic clinical presentation.
- MN is sufficiently uncommon in children that an infectious cause must be ruled out before presuming that it is idiopathic.
- The fact that this patient was in a country where hepatitis B is more endemic than in the United States and that she had a gastrointestinal illness further suggested the possibility of hepatitis B.
- Importantly, the appropriate treatment is to address the presence of the viral infection.

## REFERENCES

1. Oleske J, Minnefor A, Cooper R, Jr, et al. Immune deficiency syndrome in children. JAMA. 1983;249:2345–49.
2. Rubinstein A, Sicklick M, Gupta A, et al. Acquired immunodeficiency with reversed T4/T8 ratios in infants born to promiscuous and drug-addicted mothers. JAMA.1983; 249:2350–6.
3. Ray PE, Xu L, Rakusan T, et al. A 20-year history of childhood HIV-associated nephropathy. Pediatr Nephrol. 2004;19:1075–92.

4. Strauss J, Abitbol C, Zilleruelo G, et al. Renal disease in children with the acquired immunodeficiency syndrome. N Engl J Med. 1989;321:625–30.

5. Connor E, Gupta S, Joshi V, et al. Acquired immunodeficiency syndrome-associated renal disease in children. J Pediatr. 1988;113:39–44.

6. Kopp JB. Renal dysfunction in HIV-1-infected patients. Curr Infect Dis Rep. 2002;4:449–60.

7. Ross MJ, Klotman PE. Recent progress in HIV-associated nephropathy. J Am Soc Nephrol. 2002;13:2997–3004.

8. Herman ES, Klotman PE. HIV-associated nephropathy: Epidemiology, pathogenesis, and treatment. Semin Nephrol. 2003;23:200–8.

9. Kimmel PL, Barisoni L, Kopp JB. Pathogenesis and treatment of HIV-associated renal diseases: Lessons from clinical and animal studies, molecular pathologic correlations, and genetic investigations. Ann Intern Med. 2003;139:214–26.

10. Weiner NJ, Goodman JW, Kimmel PL. The HIV-associated renal diseases: Current insight into pathogenesis and treatment. Kidney Int. 2003;63:1618–31.

11. Winston JA, Bruggeman LA, Ross MD, et al. Nephropathy and establishment of a renal reservoir of HIV type 1 during primary infection. N Engl J Med. 2001;344:1979–84.

12. Abbott KC, Hypolite I, Welch PG, et al. Human immunodeficiency virus/acquired immunodeficiency syndrome-associated nephropathy at end-stage renal disease in the United States: Patient characteristics and survival in the pre highly active antiretroviral therapy era. J Nephrol. 2001;14:377–83.

13. Freedman BI, Soucie JM, Stone SM, et al. Familial clustering of end-stage renal disease in blacks with HIV-associated nephropathy. Am J Kidney Dis. 1999;34:254–8.

14. Kopp JB, Winkler C. HIV-associated nephropathy in African Americans. Kidney Int Suppl. 2003;63(Suppl 83):S43–9.

15. Genovese G, Friedman DJ, Ross MD, et al. Association of trypanolytic ApoL1 variants with kidney disease in African Americans. Science. 2010;29:841–5.

16. Kopp JB, Nelson GW, Sampath K, et al. APOL1 genetic variants in focal segmental glomerulosclerosis and HIV-associated nephropathy. J Am Soc Nephrol. 2011;22:2129–37.

17. Conaldi PG, Bottelli A, Baj A, et al. Human immunodeficiency virus-1 tat induces hyperproliferation and dysregulation of renal glomerular epithelial cells. Am J Pathol. 2002;161:53–61.

18. Husain M, Gusella GL, Klotman ME, et al. HIV-1 Nef induces proliferation and anchorage-independent growth in podocytes. J Am Soc Nephrol. 2002;13:1806–15.

19. Dickie P, Felser J, Eckhaus M, et al. HIV-associated nephropathy in transgenic mice expressing HIV-1 genes. Virology. 1991;185:109–19.

20. Kopp JB, Klotman ME, Adler SH, et al. Progressive glomerulosclerosis and enhanced renal accumulation of basement membrane components in mice transgenic for human immunodeficiency virus type 1 genes. Proc Natl Acad Sci U S A. 1992;89:1577–8.

21. Kajiyama W, Kopp JB, Marinos NJ, et al. Glomerulosclerosis and viral gene expression in HIV-transgenic mice: Role of nef. Kidney Int. 2000;58:1148–59.

22. Dickie P, Roberts A, Uwiera R, et al. Focal glomerulosclerosis in proviral and c-fms transgenic mice links Vpr expression to HIV-associated nephropathy. Virology. 2004;322:69–81.

23. Kajiyama W, Kopp JB, Marinos NJ, et al. Glomerulosclerosis and viral gene expression in HIV-transgenic mice: Role of nef. Kidney Int. 2000;58:1148–59.

24. Hanna Z, Kay DG, Cool M, et al. Transgenic mice expressing human immunodeficiency virus type 1 in immune cells develop a severe AIDS-like disease. J Virol. 1998;72:121–32.

25. Bruggeman LA, Ross MD, Tanji N, et al. Renal epithelium is a previously unrecognized site of HIV-1 infection. J Am Soc Nephrol. 2000;11:2079–87.

26. Ross MJ, Bruggeman LA, Wilson PD, et al. Microcyst formation and HIV-1 gene expression occur in multiple nephron segments in HIV-associated nephropathy. J Am Soc Nephrol. 2001;12:2645–51.

27. Marras D, Bruggeman LA, Gao F, et al. Replication and compartmentalization of HIV-1 in kidney epithelium of patients with HIV-associated nephropathy. Nat Med. 2002;8:522–26.

28. Wali RK, Drachenberg CI, Papadimitriou JC, et al. HIV-1-associated nephropathy and response to highly-active antiretroviral therapy. Lancet. 1998;352:783–4.

29. Kimmel PL, Mishkin GJ, Umana WO. Captopril and renal survival in patients with human immunodeficiency virus nephropathy. Am J Kidney Dis. 1996;28:202–08.

30. Burns GC, Paul SK, Toth IR, et al. Effect of angiotensin-converting enzyme inhibition in HIV-associated nephropathy. J Am Soc Nephrol. 1997;8:1140–6.

31. Smith MC, Austen JL, Carey JT, et al. Prednisone improves renal function and proteinuria in human immunodeficiency virus-associated nephropathy. Am J Med. 1996;101:41–8.

32. Eustace JA, Nuermberger E, Choi M, et al. Cohort study of the treatment of severe HIV-associated nephropathy with corticosteroids. Kidney Int. 2000;58:1253–60.

33. Navarrete JE, Pastan S. Effect of highly active antiretroviral treatment and prednisone in biopsy-proven HIV-associated nephropathy (abstract). J Am Soc Nephrol. 2000;11:93A.

34. Ingulli E, Tejani A, Fikrig S, et al. Nephrotic syndrome associated with acquired immunodeficiency syndrome in children. J Pediatr. 1991;119:710–16.

35. Nelson PJ, Gelman IH, Klotman PE. Suppression of HIV-1 expression by inhibitors of cyclin-dependent kinases promotes differentiation of infected podocytes. J Am Soc Nephrol. 2001;12:2827–31.

36. Gherardi D, D'Agati V, Chu TH, et al. Reversal of collapsing glomerulopathy in mice with the cyclin-dependent kinase inhibitor CYC202. J Am Soc Nephrol. 2004;15:1212–22.

37. Ratnam KK, Feng X, Chuang PY, et al. Role of the retinoic acid receptor-α in HIV-associated nephropathy. Kidney Int. 2011;79:624–34.

38. Sharma M, Magenheimer LK, Home T, et al. Inhibition of Notch pathway attenuates the progression of human immunodeficiency virus-associated nephropathy. Am J Physiol Renal Physiol. 2013;304:F1127–36.

39. Kimmel PL, Phillips TM, Ferreira-Centeno A, et al. Brief report: Idiotypic IgA nephropathy in patients with human immunodeficiency virus infection. N Engl J Med. 1992;327:702–6.

40. Mattana J, Siegal FP, Schwarzwald E, et al. AIDS-associated membranous nephropathy with advanced renal failure: Response to prednisone. Am J Kidney Dis. 1997;30:116–9.

41. Alarcon-Zurita A, Salas A, Anton E, et al. Membranous glomerulonephritis with nephrotic syndrome in a HIV positive patient: Remarkable remission with triple therapy. Nephrol Dial Transplant. 2000;15:1097–98.

42. Alpers CE. Light at the end of the TUNEL: HIV-associated thrombotic microangiopathy. Kidney Int. 2003;63:385–96.

43. Gadallah MF, el-Shahawy MA, Campese VM, et al. Disparate prognosis of thrombotic microangiopathy in HIV-infected patients with and without AIDS. Am J Nephrol. 1996;16:446–50.

44. Lachaal M, Venuto RC. Nephrotoxicity and hyperkalemia in patients with acquired immunodeficiency syndrome treated with pentamidine. Am J Med. 1989;87:260–3.

45. Deray G, Martinez F, Katlama C, et al. Foscarnet nephrotoxicity: Mechanism, incidence and prevention. Am J Nephrol. 1989;9:316–21.

46. Ortiz A, Justo P, Sanz A, et al. Tubular cell apoptosis and cidofovir-induced acute renal failure. Antivir Ther. 2005;10:185–90.

47. Becker K, Jablonowski H, Häussinger D. Sulfadiazine-associated nephrotoxicity in patients with the acquired immunodeficiency syndrome. Medicine (Baltimore). 1996;75:185–94.

48. Gunness P, Aleksa K, Bend J, et al. Acyclovir-induced nephrotoxicity: The role of the acyclovir aldehyde metabolite. Transl Res. 2011;158:290–301.

49. Gagnon RF, Alli AI, Watters AK, et al. Indinavir crystalluria. Kidney Int. 2006; 70:2047.

50. Hall AM. Update on tenofovir toxicity in the kidney. Pediatr Nephrol. 2013;28:1011–23.

51. Herlitz LC, Mohan S, Stokes MB, et al. Tenofovir nephrotoxicity: Acute tubular necrosis with distinctive clinical, pathological, and mitochondrial abnormalities. Kidney Int. 2010;78:1171–7.

52. Kelly MD, Gibson A, Bartlett H, et al. Tenofovir-associated proteinuria. AIDS. 2013;27:479–81.

53. Irizarry-Alvarado JM, Dwyer JP, Brumble LM, et al. Proximal tubular dysfunction associated with tenofovir and didanosine causing Fanconi syndrome and diabetes insipidus: A report of 3 cases. AIDS Read. 2009;19:114–21.

54. Horberg M, Tang B, Towner W, et al. Impact of tenofovir on renal function in HIV-infected, antiretroviral-naive patients. J Acquir Immune Defic Syndr. 2010;53:62–9.

55. Young J, Schäfer J, Fux CA, Furrer H, et al.; The Swiss HIV Cohort Study. Renal function in patients with HIV starting therapy with tenofovir and either efavirenz, lopinavir or atazanavir. J Acquir Immune Defic Synd. 2012;26:567–75.

56. Wever K, van Agtmael MA, Carr A. Incomplete reversibility of tenofovir-related renal toxicity in HIV-infected men. J Acquir Immune Defic Syndr. 2010;55:78–81.

57. Martin JL, Brown CE, Matthews-Davis N, et al. Effects of antiviral nucleoside analogs on human DNA polymerases and mitochondrial DNA synthesis. Antimicrob Agents Chemother. 1994;38:2743–9.

58. Perazella MA. Tenofovir-induced kidney disease: An acquired renal tubular mitochondriopathy. Kidney Int. 2010;78:1060–3.

59. Mallipattu SK, Salem F, Wyatt CM. The changing epidemiology of HIV-related chronic kidney disease in the era of antiretroviral therapy. Kidney Int. 2014;86:259–65.

60. Paula AA, Falcão MC, Pacheco AG. Metabolic syndrome in HIV-infected individuals: Underlying mechanisms and epidemiological aspects. AIDS Res Ther. 2013;10:32–9.

61. Maynard JE. Hepatitis B: Global importance and need for control. Vaccine. 1990;8(Suppl):S18–20.

62. Bhimma R, Coovadia HM. Hepatitis B virus-associated nephropathy. Am J Nephrol. 2004;24:198–211.

63. Gilbert RD, Wiggelinkhuizen J. The clinical course of hepatitis B virus-associated nephropathy. Pediatr Nephrol. 1994;8:11–14.

64. Hirose H, Udo K, Kojima M, et al. Deposition of hepatitis Be antigen in membranous glomerulonephritis: Identification by F(ab¢)2 fragments of monoclonal antibody. Kidney Int. 1984;26:338–41.

65. Takekoshi Y, Tochimaru H, Nagata Y, et al. Immunopathogenetic mechanisms of hepatitis B virus-related glomerulopathy. Kidney Int Suppl. 1991;35:S3–39.

66. Lai KN, Lai FM, Lo S, et al. IgA nephropathy associated with hepatitis B virus antigenemia. Nephron. 1987;47:141–3.

67. Bhimma R, Coovadia HM, Adhikari M. Hepatitis B virus-associated nephropathy in black South African children. Pediatr Nephrol. 1998;12:479–84.

68. Lee HS, Choi Y, Yu SH, et al. A renal biopsy study of hepatitis B virus-associated nephropathy in Korea. Kidney Int. 1988;34:537–43.

69. Pagnoux C, Seror R, Henegar C, et al. Clinical features and outcomes in 348 patients with polyarteritis nodosa: A systematic retrospective study of patients diagnosed between 1963 and 2005 and entered into the French Vasculitis Study Group Database. Arthritis Rheum. 2010;62:616–26.

70. Ruiz-Moreno M, Rua MJ, Molina J, et al. Prospective, randomized controlled trial of interferon-alpha in children with chronic hepatitis B. Hepatology. 1991;13:1035–9.

71. Barbera C, Bortolotti F, Crivellaro C, et al. Recombinant interferon-alpha 2a hastens the rate of HBeAg clearance in children with chronic hepatitis B. Hepatology. 1994;20:287–90.

72. Sokal EM, Conjeevaram HS, Roberts EA, et al. Interferon alfa therapy for chronic hepatitis B in children: A multinational randomized controlled trial. Gastroenterology. 1998;114:988–95.

73. Lai CL, Lok AS, Lin HJ, et al. Placebo-controlled trial of recombinant alpha 2-interferon in Chinese HBsAg-carrier children. Lancet.1987;2:877–80.

74. Lai CL, Lin HJ, Lau JN, et al. Effect of recombinant alpha 2 interferon with or without prednisone in Chinese HBsAg carrier children. Q J Med. 1991;78:155–63.

75. Jonas MM, Mizerski J, Badia IB, et al. Clinical trial of lamivudine in children with chronic hepatitis B. N Engl J Med. 2002;346:1706–13.

76. Marcellin P, Chang TT, Lim SG, et al. Adefovir dipivoxil for the treatment of hepatitis B e antigen-positive chronic hepatitis B. N Engl J Med. 2003;348:808–16.

77. Lai FM, Tam JS, Li PK, et al. Replication of hepatitis B virus with corticosteroid therapy in hepatitis B virus related membranous nephropathy. Virchows Arch A Pathol Anat Histopathol. 1989;414:279–84.

78. Guillevin L, Lhote F. Treatment of polyarteritis nodosa and microscopic polyangiitis. Arthritis Rheum. 1988;41:2100–5.

79. Alter MJ, Kruszon-Moran D, Nainan OV, et al. The prevalence of hepatitis C virus infection in the United States, 1988 through 1994. N Engl J Med. 1999;341:556–62.

80. Jonas MM. Children with hepatitis C. Hepatology. 2002;36(5 Suppl 1):S173–8.

81. Yeung LT, King SM, Roberts EA. Mother-to-infant transmission of hepatitis C virus. Hepatology. 2001:34:223–9.

82. Tovo PA, Pembrey LJ, Newell ML. Persistence rate and progression of vertically acquired hepatitis C infection: European paediatric hepatitis C virus infection. J Infect Dis. 2000;181:419–24.

83. Minola E, Prati D, Suter F, et al. Age at infection affects the long-term outcome of transfusion-associated chronic hepatitis C. Blood. 2002;99:4588–91.

84. Zuccotti GV, Torcoletti M, Salvini F, et al. Infants vertically infected with hepatitis C: A long term longitudinal follow-up. Pediatr Med Chir. 2004;26:50–2.

85. Bortolotti F, Verucchi G, Cammà C, et al. Long-term course of chronic hepatitis C in children: From viral clearance to end-stage liver disease. Gastroenterology. 2008;134:1900–1907.

86. Uchiyama-Tanaka Y, Mori Y, Kishimoto N, et al. Membranous glomerulonephritis associated with hepatitis C virus infection: Case report and literature review. Clin Nephrol. 2004;61:144–50.

87. Markowitz GS, Cheng JT, Colvin RB, et al. Hepatitis C viral infection is associated with fibrillary glomerulonephritis and immunotactoid glomerulopathy. J Am Soc Nephrol.1998;9:2244–52.

88. El-Serag H, Hampel H, Yeh C, et al. Extrahepatic manifestations of hepatitis C among United States male veterans. Hepatology. 2002;36:1439–45.

89. Johnson RJ, Gretch DR, Yamabe H, et al. Membranoproliferative glomerulonephritis associated with hepatitis C virus infection. N Engl J Med. 1993;328:465–70.

90. Molle ZL, Baqi N, Gretch D, et al. Hepatitis C infection in children and adolescents with end-stage renal disease. Pediatr Nephrol. 2002;17:444–9.

91. Nowicki MJ, Welch TR, Ahmad N, et al. Absence of hepatitis B and C viruses in pediatric idiopathic membranoproliferative glomerulonephritis. Pediatr Nephrol. 1995;9:16–8.

92. Sumida K, Ubara Y, Hoshino J, et al. Hepatitis C virus-related kidney disease: Various histological patterns. Clin Nephrol. 2010;74:446–56.

93. Alric L, Plaisier E, Thebault S, et al. Influence of antiviral therapy in hepatitis C virus-associated cryoglobulinemic MPGN. Am J Kidney Dis. 2004;43:617–23.

94. Meyers CM, Seeff LB, Stehman-Breen CO, et al. Hepatitis C and renal disease: An update. Am J Kidney Dis. 2003;42:631–57.

95. Loustaud-Ratti V, Liozon E, Karaaslan H, et al. Interferon alpha and ribavirin for membranoproliferative glomerulonephritis and hepatitis C infection. Am J Med. 2002;113:516–9.

96. Sabry AA, Sobh MA, Sheaashaa HA, et al. Effect of combination therapy (ribavirin and interferon) in HCV-related glomerulopathy. Nephrol Dial Transplant. 2002;17:1924–30.

97. Lopes EP, Valente LM, Silva AE, et al. Therapy with interferon-alpha plus ribavirin for membranoproliferative glomerulonephritis induced by hepatitis C virus. Braz J Infect Dis. 2003;7:353–7.

98. Zuckerman E, Keren D, Slobodin G, et al. Treatment of refractory, symptomatic, hepatitis C virus related mixed cryoglobulinemia with ribavirin and interferon-alpha. J Rheumatol. 2000;27:2172–8.

99. Wirth S, Pieper-Boustani H, Lang T, et al. Peginterferon alfa-2b plus ribavirin treatment in children and adolescents with chronic hepatitis C. Hepatology, 2005;41:1013–8.

100. Sawinsksi D, Kaur N, Ajeti A, Trofe-Clark J, Lim M, Bleicher M, Goral S, Forde KA, Bloom RD. Successful treatment of hepatitis C in renal transplant recipient with direct acting- antiviral agents. Am J Transplant, in press.

101. Dumortier J, Guillaud O, Gagnieu, M-C, Janbon B, Juillard L, Morelon M, Leroy V.  Anti-triple therapy with telaprevir in haemodialysed HCV patients. J Clin Virol, 56:146–149, 2015.

102. D'Amico G. Renal involvement in hepatitis C infection: Cryoglobulinemic glomerulonephritis. Kidney Int. 1998;54:650–71.

103. Madore F, Lazarus JM, Brady HR. Therapeutic plasma exchange in renal diseases. J Am Soc Nephrol. 1996;7:367–86.

104. Andresdottir MB, Assmann KJ, Hilbrands LB, et al. Type I membranoproliferative glomerulonephritis in a renal allograft: A recurrence induced by a cytomegalovirus infection? Am J Kidney Dis. 2000;35:E6.

105. Georgaki-Angelaki H, Lycopoulou L, Stergiou N, et al. Membranous nephritis associated with acquired cytomegalovirus infection in a 19-month-old baby. Pediatr Nephrol. 2009;24:203–6.

106. Shiraishi N, Kitamura K, Hayata M, Ogata T, et al. Case of anti-glomerular basement membrane antibody-induced glomerulonephritis with cytomegalovirus-induced thrombotic microangiopathy. Intern Med J. 2012;42:e7–11.

107. Chandra P, Kopp JB. Viruses and collapsing glomerulopathy: A brief critical review. Clin Kidney J. 2013;6:1–5.

108. Cossart YE, Field AM, Cant B, et al. Parvovirus-like particles in human sera. Lancet. 1975;1:72–3.

109. Brown KE, Anderson SM, Young NS. Erythrocyte P antigen: Cellular receptor for B19 parvovirus. Science. 1993;262:114–7.

110. Cooling LL, Koerner TA, Naides SJ. Multiple glycosphingolipids determine the tissue tropism of parvovirus B19. J Infect Dis. 1995;172:1198–205.

111. Young NS, Brown KE. Parvovirus B19. N Engl J Med. 2004;350:586–97, 2004.

112. Ohtomo Y, Kawamura R, Kaneko K, et al. Nephrotic syndrome associated with human parvovirus B19 infection. Pediatr Nephrol. 2003;18:280–2.

113. Iwafuchi Y, Morita T, Kamimura A, et al. Acute endocapillary proliferative glomerulonephritis associated with human parvovirus B19 infection. Clin Nephrol. 2002;57:246–50.

114. Schmid ML, McWhinney PH, Will EJ. Parvovirus B19 and glomerulonephritis in a healthy adult. Ann Intern Med. 2000;132:682.

115. Komatsuda A, Ohtani H, Nimura T, et al. Endocapillary proliferative glomerulonephritis in a patient with parvovirus B19 infection. Am J Kidney Dis. 2000;36:851–4.

116. Nakazawa T, Tomosugi N, Sakamoto K, et al. Acute glomerulonephritis after human parvovirus B19 infection. Am J Kidney Dis. 2000;35:E31.

117. Taylor G, Drachenberg C, Faris-Young S. Renal involvement of human parvovirus B19 in an immunocompetent host. Clin Infect Dis. 2001;32:1671–9.

118. Takeda S, Takaeda C, Takazakura E, et al. Renal involvement induced by human parvovirus B19 infection. Nephron. 2001;89:280–5.

119. Mori Y, Yamashita H, Umeda Y, et al. Association of parvovirus B19 infection with acute glomerulonephritis in healthy adults: Case report and review of the literature. Clin Nephrol. 2002;57:69–73.

120. Bleumink GS, Halma C, van Vliet AC, et al. Human parvovirus B19 and renal disease? Neth J Med. 2000;56:163–5.

121. Seward EW, Rustom R, Nye FJ, et al. Haemolytic-uraemic syndrome following human parvovirus infection in a previously fit adult. Nephrol Dial Transplant. 1999;14:2472–3.

122. Iwafuchi Y, Morita T, Kamimura A, et al. Human parvovirus B19 infection associated with hemolytic uremic syndrome. Clin Exp Nephrol. 2000;4:156.

123. Isobe Y, Sugimoto K, Shiraki Y, et al. Successful high-titer immunoglobulin therapy for persistent parvovirus B19 infection in a lymphoma patient treated with rituximab-combined chemotherapy. Am J Hematol. 2004;77:370–3.

124. Stouffer GA, Sheahan RG, Lenihan DJ, et al. The current status of immune modulating therapy for myocarditis: A case of acute parvovirus myocarditis treated with intravenous immunoglobulin. Am J Med Sci. 2003;326:369–74.

125. Kerr JR, Cunniffe VS, Kelleher P, et al. Successful intravenous immunoglobulin therapy in 3 cases of parvovirus B19-associated chronic fatigue syndrome. Clin Infect Dis. 2003;36:e100–6.

126. Barsoum NR, Bunnapradist S, Mougil A, et al. Treatment of parvovirus B-19 (PV B-19) infection allows for successful kidney transplantation without disease recurrence. Am J Transplant. 2002;2:425–8.

127. Markenson AL, Chandra M, Lewy JG, et al. Sickle cell anemia: The nephrotic syndrome and hypoplastic crises in a sibship. Am J Med. 1978;64:719–23.

128. Wierenga KJ, Pattison JR, Brink N, et al. Glomerulonephritis after human parvovirus infection in homozygous sickle-cell disease. Lancet. 1995;346:475–6.

129. Tolaymat A, Al Mousily F, MacWilliam K, et al. Parvovirus glomerulonephritis in a patient with sickle cell disease. Pediatr Nephrol. 1999;13:340–2.

130. Tanawattanacharoen S, Falk RJ, Jennette JC, et al. Parvovirus B19 DNA in kidney tissue of patients with focal segmental glomerulosclerosis. Am J Kidney Dis. 2000;35:1166–74.

131. Moudgil A, Nast CC, Bagga A, et al. Association of parvovirus B19 infection with idiopathic collapsing glomerulopathy. Kidney Int. 2001;59:2126–33.

132. Cohen JI. Epstein-Barr virus infection. N Engl J Med. 2000;343:481–92.

133. Wakiguchi H, Hisakawa H, Kubota H, et al. Serodiagnosis of infectious mononucleosis in children. Acta Paediatr Jpn. 1998;40:328–32.

134. Sumaya CV, Ench Y. Epstein-Barr virus infectious mononucleosis in children. I. Clinical and general laboratory findings. Pediatrics. 1985;75:1003–10.

135. Lee S, Kjellstrand CM. Renal disease in infectious mononucleosis. Clin Nephrol. 19789:236–40.

136. Tsai JD, Lee HC, Lin CC, et al. Epstein-Barr virus-associated acute renal failure: Diagnosis, treatment, and follow-up. Pediatr Nephrol. 2003;18:667–74.

137. Wallace M, Leet G, Rothwell P. Immune complex-mediated glomerulonephritis with infectious mononucleosis. Aust N Z J Med. 1974;4:192–5.

138. Greenspan G. The nephrotic syndrome complicating infectious mononucleosis: Report of a case. Calif Med. 1963;98:162.

139. Shashaty GG, Atamer MA. Hemolytic uremic syndrome associated with infectious mononucleosis. Am J Dis Child. 1974;127:720–2.

140. Becker JL, Miller F, Nuovo GJ, et al. Epstein-Barr virus infection of renal proximal tubule cells: Possible role in chronic interstitial nephritis. J Clin Invest. 1999;104:1673–81.

141. Chertow DS, Kleine C, Edwards JK, et al. Ebola virus disease in West Africa: Clinical manifestations and management. N Engl J Med. 2014;371:2054–7.

142. West TE, von Saint André-von Arnim A. Clinical presentation and management of severe Ebola virus disease. Ann Am Thorac Soc. 2014;11:1341–50.

## REVIEW QUESTIONS

1. HIVAN may manifest with which of the following?
   a. Immune complex glomerulonephritis
   b. Collapsing glomerulopathy
   c. Drug-induced nephrotoxicity
   d. None of the above
   e. All of the above

2. The incidence of HIVAN is:
   a. Increasing
   b. Decreasing
   c. Holding steady

3. The *most* common form of kidney disease associated with hepatitis B infection is:
   a. Membranoproliferative glomerulonephritis
   b. Postinfectious glomerulonephritis
   c. Minimal-change disease
   d. Membranous nephropathy
   e. Focal segmental glomerulosclerosis

4. A 9-year-old child presents with fever, rash, enlarged spleen, and swollen gums. Urinalysis shows 2+ protein and 3+ blood. A kidney biopsy shows a proliferative lesion with epimembranous immune complex deposits. This child is likely to have infection with which of the following viruses?
   a. Hepatitis C
   b. Hepatitis B
   c. Human immunodeficiency virus-1
   d. Epstein-Barr
   e. Parvovirus B19

## ANSWER KEY

1. e
2. b
3. d
4. d

# PART F

# Kidney failure

---

# 30

# Acute kidney injury

PRASAD DEVARAJAN AND STUART L. GOLDSTEIN

Acute kidney injury (AKI) is defined functionally as a rapid decline in glomerular filtration rate (GFR) that leads to accumulation of waste products such as blood urea nitrogen (BUN) and creatinine. The term *acute kidney injury* has largely replaced acute renal failure (ARF) because ARF overemphasizes the discrete event of failed kidney function, whereas AKI accounts for a continuum of renal dysfunction that better characterizes the clinical spectrum of AKI. AKI is a common problem affecting all ages, the leading reason to seek nephrology consultation, and associated with serious consequences and unsatisfactory therapeutic options.[1-5] The etiology of AKI varies widely according to age, geographic region, and clinical setting. Functional AKI induced by dehydration (or prerenal azotemia) is usually reversible with early fluid therapy. However, despite decades of research and technical advances in clinical care, the prognosis for patients with intrinsic AKI in the intensive care setting remains poor, and clinicians now recognize that patients are dying "of," and not just "with," AKI.[6,7] Moreover, a significant proportion of children with severe AKI will have long-term sequelae including chronic kidney disease (CKD). Fortunately, the cellular and molecular tools of modern science are providing critical new insights into the pathogenetic mechanisms of AKI. These newly discovered pathways are yielding novel early biomarkers for the prediction of AKI and its consequences, as well as innovative strategies for the proactive treatment and prevention of AKI.

## DEFINITIONS

The most important advances in the AKI field would not have been possible without a standardized AKI definition, which took initial form as the empirically proposed RIFLE criteria (Risk, Injury, Failure, Loss, and End-Stage Kidney Disease) in 2004, with pediatric modifications (pRIFLE) in 2007 (Table 30.1).[8,9] The RIFLE criteria have been subjected to multiple validation studies in adults and children, and almost all these studies uniformly demonstrated an independent association with increasing AKI severity, morbidity, and mortality.[10,11] Further refinement of the RIFLE criteria (the Acute Kidney Injury Network or AKIN criteria) included the addition of another criterion point of a 0.3 mg/dL serum creatinine rise

Table 30.1 pRIFLE classification of acute kidney injury

| Stage | Estimated creatinine clearance* | Urine output |
|---|---|---|
| R = Risk | eCCl decrease by 25% | <0.5 mL/kg/h for 8 h |
| I = Injury | eCCl decrease by 50% | <0.5 mL/kg/h for 16 h |
| F = Failure | eCCl decrease by 75% or eCCl <35 mL/min/1.73 m² | <0.3 mL/kg/h for 24 h or anuric for 12 h |
| L = Loss | Persistent failure >4 wk | — |
| E = End stage | End-stage renal disease (persistent failure >3 mo) | — |

*Solution:* Akcan-Arikan A, Zappitelli M, Loftis LL, et al. Modified RIFLE criteria in critically ill children with acute kidney injury. Kidney Int. 2007;71:1028–35.

*Abbreviations:* eCCl, estimated creatinine clearance; pRIFLE, pediatric risk, injury, failure, loss, and end-stage renal disease.

* The estimated creatinine clearance is calculated using the modified Schwartz formula.

in less than 48 h, given that both adult and pediatric studies have shown independent associations with poor outcomes at this creatinine threshold.[12–14] Finally, in 2012, RIFLE, AKIN, and pRIFLE were harmonized into a single definition by the Kidney

---

## KEY POINTS

- Despite limitations of serum creatinine, the KDIGO AKI definition and staging should be used to guide clinical care.
- The KDIGO AKI can also be used as a standardized criterion and outcome measure in AKI studies.
- Advances in critical care have increasingly rendered pediatric AKI a hospital-acquired disease, especially in developed countries.

---

Table 30.2 Kidney disease improving global outcomes (KDIGO) acute kidney injury criteria

| Stage | Serum creatinine | Urine output |
|---|---|---|
| 1 | 1.5–1.9 times baseline OR ≥0.3 mg/dL rise increase | <0.5 mL/kg/h for 6–12 h |
| 2 | 2.0–2.9 times baseline | <0.5 mL/kg/h for ≥12 h |
| 3 | 3.0 times baseline OR Increase to ≥4.0 mg/dL (>18 yr of age) OR Decrease in eGFR <35 mL/min/1.73m² (<18 yr of age) OR Initiation of renal replacement therapy | ≤0.3 mL/kg/h for ≥24 h OR Anuria for ≥12 h |

*Solution:* Kidney Disease: Improving Global Outcomes (KDIGO) Acute Kidney Injury Work Group—KDIGO clinical practice guideline for acute kidney injury. Kidney Int Suppl. 2012;2:1–138.

*Abbreviations:* eGFR, estimated glomerular filtration rate.

Disease Improving Global Outcomes (KDIGO) AKI Consensus Conference (Table 30.2).[15] It is recommended that the KDIGO AKI definition and staging be used to guide clinical care and as a standardized criterion and outcome measure in AKI studies until supplemented or supplanted by validation, acceptance, and widespread clinical integration of the novel AKI biomarkers discussed later in this chapter. One limitation of the KDIGO AKI definition is the use of serum creatinine to estimate GFR because changes in serum creatinine concentrations often lag behind changes in GFR until a steady state has been reached.

## CLINICAL CLASSIFICATION

Traditionally, AKI has been classified as prerenal (functional response of structurally normal kidneys to hypoperfusion, usually associated with dehydration, sepsis, or other diseases leading to hypotension), intrinsic renal (involving structural damage to the renal parenchyma usually from nephrotoxic medications, prolonged hypoperfusion, or glomerulonephritis), or postrenal (urinary tract obstruction). This classification remains convenient for understanding mechanisms, as well as the clinical approach to AKI. With the discovery and validation of novel AKI functional and structural biomarkers (discussed later), the terminology is changing to functional, structural, and combined AKI, to depict the clinical situation and therapeutic response more appropriately.[16]

---

## KEY POINTS

A clinically useful classification categorizes AKI into:

- Prerenal
- Intrinsic renal
- Postrenal

## EPIDEMIOLOGIC CLASSIFICATION

AKI may also be classified according to the epidemiologic circumstances in which it occurs. Community-acquired AKI is more likely to be associated with a single predominant insult, most commonly volume depletion, and it is frequently reversible. The medical approach is often conservative and expectant, including discontinuing the insult, providing supportive fluid and electrolyte management, and awaiting spontaneous recovery of renal function. In contrast, hospital-acquired AKI, especially in the critical care setting, is frequently multifactorial and is often part of more extensive multiorgan failure. This form of AKI often accompanies other organ disease processes and markedly complicates their management and outcomes. Management is more aggressive, with early initiation of renal replacement therapies to optimize the overall care of the severely compromised patient. Recovery may be partial, and there are significant short-term and long-term consequences.

### KEY POINTS

AKI may be classified by epidemiologic association:

- Community-acquired AKI, often reversible and associated with a common source of renal insult
- Hospital-acquired AKI, often multifactorial, severe, and frequently associated with multiorgan failure

## OLIGURIC AND NONOLIGURIC ACUTE KIDNEY INJURY

AKI may also be classified according to the urine output as being nonoliguric, oliguric (urine output less than 1 mL/kg/h in infants, less than 0.5 mL/kg/h in children, or less than 400 mL/day in adults), or anuric. Measurement of urine output is especially useful in the critical care setting because the degree of oliguria reflects the severity of the kidney injury, has important implications for volume and electrolyte imbalances, and provides prognostic information. However, even moderately severe forms of AKI secondary to

### KEY POINTS

Based on urine output, AKI can be classified into:

- Oliguric AKI
- Nonoliguric AKI

nephrotoxins, and the majority of AKI seen in neonatal intensive care, are typically nonoliguric.

## EPIDEMIOLOGY

Advances in the care for critically ill neonates, infants with congenital heart disease, and children with bone marrow and solid organ transplantation, sepsis, and hypotension have led to a dramatic broadening of the epidemiology of pediatric AKI. Older pediatric epidemiologic data were mostly generated from single centers and reported hemolytic-uremic syndrome and other primary renal diseases as the most prevalent causes. More recent single-center data have detailed the underlying causes of pediatric AKI in large cohorts of children and have demonstrated nephrotoxic medication exposure or nonrenal primary illnesses as the most common causes of AKI. In fact, primary kidney diseases encompass only 7% to 10% of cases of AKI in hospitalized children.[1,17]

Although the precise incidence of pediatric AKI is not known, it appears to be rising, especially in hospitalized children.[18] AKI rates based on hospital coding data from a large US multicenter dataset revealed a rate of 3.9 per 1000 at-risk pediatric hospitalizations.[19] In addition, the specific clinical setting and patient's clinical condition often determine AKI development rates. For instance, 40% of all children undergoing cardiac surgical procedures develop AKI.[20–22] AKI rates of 20% have been reported in very low birth weight infants.[23] Whereas 10% of all patients in a pediatric intensive care unit (ICU) develop AKI,[24] the rate increases to 60% to 80% in children receiving invasive mechanical ventilation and one vasoactive medication.[9,25] Outside the ICU, 25% of all noncritically ill children receiving an aminoglycoside or three or more nephrotoxic medications will develop AKI.[26–28] Thus, advances in critical care have increasingly rendered pediatric AKI a hospital-acquired disease, especially in developed countries. Such data are important to understand because they can allow clinicians to stratify risk in patients for more active surveillance and potentially decrease or mitigate AKI rates and severity.

## PRERENAL AZOTEMIA AND FUNCTIONAL ACUTE KIDNEY INJURY

Prerenal AKI should be considered an appropriate functional response of intrinsically normal kidneys to hypoperfusion. It is the most common form of AKI encountered globally, accounting for 40% to 55% of all cases. Oliguria in this clinical circumstance represents an appropriate renal response to preserve intravascular volume. Prerenal azotemia is often associated with dehydration, sepsis, or other causes leading to transient hypoperfusion, and it is usually rapidly reversed by restoration of renal perfusion. However, it is critical to understand that functional AKI or prerenal azotemia does not automatically imply fluid responsiveness, and in some situations, such as liver failure, heart failure, and nephrotic syndrome, fluid restriction is the mainstay of treatment.[29] The common causes of prerenal azotemia are listed in Table 30.3.

## PATHOPHYSIOLOGY

The kidneys are endowed with 25% of the cardiac output at rest, to perform critical homeostatic functions, and any decrease in circulatory volume evokes a primeval systemic response leading to the release of potent vasoactive agents (Figure 30.1). These responses help maintain perfusion to other organs by normalizing circulatory volume and blood pressure, but at the potential expense of GFR. There is an intense baroreceptor-mediated activation of the sympathetic nervous system and renin-angiotensin axis, with resultant renal vasoconstriction mediated by angiotensin II and norepinephrine. In addition, angiotensin II promotes avid sodium and water reabsorption by the uninjured tubule cells, thus often resulting in the oliguria and decreased fractional excretion of sodium (FENa) that are the hallmarks of prerenal AKI. Furthermore, the release of antidiuretic hormone in response to hypovolemia and a rise in extracellular osmolality result in

Table 30.3 Common causes of prerenal azotemia or functional acute kidney injury

| Mechanism | Etiology |
| --- | --- |
| Volume depletion | Dehydration |
| | Hemorrhage |
| | Diuretic overuse |
| | Burns |
| | Shock |
| | Nephrotic syndrome |
| | Diabetes mellitus |
| | Diabetes insipidus |
| Decreased cardiac output | Cardiac failure |
| | Arrhythmias |
| Peripheral vasodilatation | Sepsis |
| | Anaphylaxis |
| | Antihypertensive agents (e.g., nifedipine) |
| Renal vasoconstriction | Sepsis |
| | Nonsteroidal anti-inflammatory drugs |
| | ACE inhibitors |
| | Hepatorenal syndrome |

*Abbreviation:* ACE, angiotensin-converting enzyme.

enhanced water reabsorption by the intact collecting duct, which further contributes to the oliguria.

Concomitantly, at least three distinct intrarenal compensatory mechanisms are brought into play that help maintain GFR in the prerenal states (Figure 30.2). Myogenic autoregulation refers to the rapid dilatation of the afferent arterioles in physiologic response to a reduction in lateral stretch following hypoperfusion.

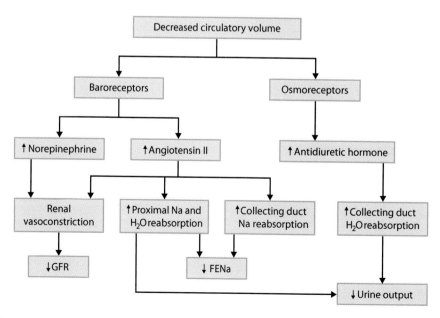

Figure 30.1 Pathophysiology of prerenal and functional acute kidney injury. FENa, fractional excretion of sodium; GFR, glomerular filtration rate; Na, sodium.

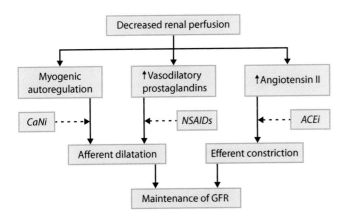

Figure 30.2 Mechanisms that maintain glomerular filtration rate (GFR) in prerenal and functional acute kidney injury. Iatrogenic interference can precipitate a reduction in GFR. These include the use of calcineurin inhibitors (CaNi), nonsteroidal anti-inflammatory drugs (NSAIDs), and angiotensin-converting enzyme inhibitors (ACEi). Broken lines represent inhibitory effects.

Calcineurin inhibitors such as tacrolimus and cyclosporine are known to impair the myogenic response and render the transplanted kidney more susceptible to prerenal azotemia. The role of this response in hypoperfusion states has been challenged, and some investigators have suggested a more important role for autoregulation in maintaining intraglomerular pressure during systemic hypertension.[30] A more effective compensatory mechanism mediating afferent arteriolar dilatation involves the intrarenal production of vasodilatory prostaglandins.[31] Under normal physiologic conditions, the cyclooxygenase (constitutional COX-1 and inducible COX-2) enzyme systems catalyze the intrarenal production of prostaglandins that mediate afferent arteriolar dilatation. This system is dramatically upregulated by volume depletion. Nonsteroidal anti-inflammatory drugs inhibit this response and can precipitate AKI, especially in the presence of decreased circulatory volume.[32,33] For example, the use of indomethacin for patent ductus arteriosus closure in neonates results in AKI in as many as 40% of cases.

Another common pediatric situation in which AKI may occur is the use of ibuprofen in febrile children with a dehydrating illness. A third mechanism for maintaining GFR involves the differential effect of angiotensin II on the efferent arteriole. Whereas angiotensin II tends to constrict both the afferent and efferent arterioles, this effect is more marked in the efferent arteriole, and it leads to increased hydrostatic pressure across the glomerulus.[34] Obvious interference with this compensation occurs following angiotensin-converting enzyme (ACE) inhibitor therapy. In clinical practice, the use of ACE inhibitors markedly increases the incidence of AKI in patients at risk (e.g., undergoing cardiac surgery) preoperatively and postoperatively.[35,36]

Compensatory mechanisms that maintain GFR in prerenal azotemia can be overwhelmed during states of prolonged reduction in renal perfusion pressure, and intrinsic AKI can then ensue. Thus, prerenal and intrinsic AKI can, therefore, be considered along a continuum of renal hypoperfusion states and can evolve from former to the latter in appropriate clinical situations. Substantial evidence for this concept derives from clinical studies demonstrating increased concentrations of biomarkers of tubule damage in patients with prerenal AKI.[37]

> **KEY POINT**
>
> Prostaglandins maintain GFR by mediating afferent arteriolar dilatation. Nonsteroidal anti-inflammatory drugs (NSAIDs) inhibit this response and can precipitate intrinsic AKI in prerenal states.

> **KEY POINTS**
>
> - Prerenal azotemia is usually rapidly reversed by restoration of renal perfusion.
> - Some forms of prerenal AKI (liver failure, heart failure, and nephrotic syndrome) require fluid restriction.

## INTRINSIC ACUTE KIDNEY INJURY

Intrinsic AKI is most frequently caused by prolonged ischemia or nephrotoxins (Tables 30.4 and 30.5), and it

Table 30.4 Common causes of intrinsic or structural acute kidney injury

| Mechanism | Etiology |
| --- | --- |
| Acute tubular necrosis | Prolonged renal ischemia |
| | Nephrotoxic drugs and toxins |
| | Myoglobinuria |
| | Hemoglobinuria |
| | Multiorgan failure |
| | Sepsis |
| Renal vascular diseases | Thrombotic microangiopathies |
| | Vasculitides |
| Interstitial diseases | Interstitial nephritis |
| | Infections |
| | Infiltrative disorders |
| Glomerulonephritides | Acute postinfectious glomerulonephritis |
| | Crescentic glomerulonephritis |

Table 30.5 Drugs and nephrotoxins toxins commonly associated with intrinsic acute kidney injury

| Mechanism of AKI | Drugs, toxins, and clinical states |
|---|---|
| Hemodynamic alterations leading to reduced GFR | ACEIs |
| | ARBs |
| | Calcineurin inhibitors (cyclosporine, tacrolimus) |
| | Interleukin-2 |
| | NSAIDs |
| | Radiocontrast drugs |
| Tubular cell toxins | Acyclovir |
| | Adefovir |
| | Aminoglycosides |
| | Amphotericin B |
| | Calcineurin inhibitors |
| | Carboplatin |
| | Cephalosporins |
| | Cidofovir, adefovir, tenofovir |
| | Cisplatin |
| | Ganciclovir |
| | Iphosphamide |
| | Pentamidine |
| | Radiocontrast drugs |
| | Vancomycin |
| | Zoledronate |
| Intratubular crystal precipitation | Acyclovir |
| | Foscarnet |
| | Indinavir |
| | Methotrexate |
| | Sulfonamides |
| | Triamterene |
| Osmotic renal tubular injury | Dextran |
| | IVIG |
| | Mannitol |
| Myoglobinuria-induced tubular cell injury and obstruction | Cocaine |
| | Ethyl alcohol |
| | Hyperosmolar states |
| | Hypokalemia |
| | Polymyositis |
| | Snake bite |
| | Statins |
| | Viral infection |
| | Wild mushroom poisoning |
| Hemoglobinuria-induced tubular cell injury and obstruction | Carboplatin |
| | Cephalosporins (cefotetan and cephalothin) |
| | Cisplatin |
| | Clavulanate (in Augmentin) |
| | ECMO therapy induced hemolysis |
| | G-6-PD–associated drug induced hemolysis |
| | Nitrofurantoin |
| | Piperacillin |

*Abbreviations:* ACEIs, angiotensin converting enzyme inhibitors; AKI, acute kidney injury; ARBs, angiotensin receptor blockers; ECMO, extracorporeal membrane oxygenator; G-6-PD, glucose-6-phosphate dehydrogenase; GFR, glomerular filtration rate; IVIG, intravenous immunoglobulin; NSAIDs, nonsteroidal anti-inflammatory drugs.

is associated pathologically with acute tubular necrosis (ATN). Consequently, it is common clinical practice to use the terms intrinsic AKI and ATN interchangeably. In the clinical setting, intrinsic AKI is frequently multifactorial, with concomitant ischemic, nephrotoxic, and septic components and with overlapping pathogenic mechanisms.

## MORPHOLOGY OF HUMAN ACUTE TUBULAR NECROSIS

ATN is a misnomer because frank tubular cell necrosis is rarely found in human AKI. Instead, one sees effacement and loss of proximal tubule apical brush border, disruption of microvilli, patchy loss of tubule cells with exposure of denuded basement membrane, focal proximal tubular dilatation and distal tubular casts, and areas of cellular regeneration (Figure 30.3). Necrotic cell death is restricted to the outer medullary regions (S3 segment of the proximal tubule and medullary thick ascending limb of Henle's loop). Conversely, apoptotic cell death has been reported in both distal and proximal tubules, in both ischemic and nephrotoxic forms of human AKI.[38,39] An intense inflammatory response, with peritubular accumulation of leukocytes, is typical in experimental models of AKI but appears to be less prominent in human AKI. In addition, peritubular capillaries in the outer medulla display a striking vascular congestion.[40–44] The molecular, biochemical, and cellular mechanisms underlying these morphologic changes are identifying several novel pathways.[45–48] Only selected mechanisms that are currently providing promising therapeutic approaches are outlined in this chapter.

## HEMODYNAMIC ALTERATIONS

Intrinsic AKI is characterized by persistent hemodynamic abnormalities (Figure 30.4). Total renal blood flow is reduced to approximately 50% of normal in response to persistent renal vasoconstriction in established AKI.[49] Furthermore, there are regional alterations in renal blood flow, with marked congestion of the outer medullary region. Oxygen tension is normally low in this region, which ironically contains tubular segments with high energy requirements, namely the S3 segment of the proximal tubule and medullary thick ascending limb. The postischemic congestion worsens the relative hypoxia, thereby leading to prolonged injury and necrotic cell death in these segments. Mechanisms underlying these hemodynamic alterations relate primarily to endothelial damage.[42–44] This damage

### KEY POINT

Intrinsic AKI is frequently multifactorial, with concomitant ischemic, nephrotoxic, and septic components and with overlapping pathogenic mechanisms.

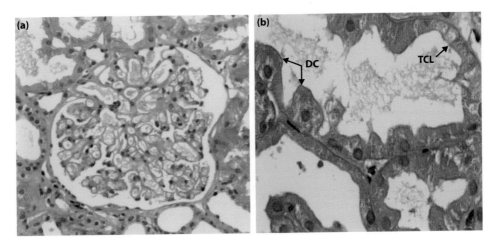

Figure 30.3 Renal biopsy in acute kidney injury. **(a)** Light microscopy showing normal glomerular structure, tubular cell loss, proteinaceous material, and cellular debris in the tubular lumen. **(b)** Higher-power view of the renal tubules demonstrating focal tubular cells loss (TCL) and dedifferentiation or "simplification" of tubular cells (DC). Immunofluorescence (not shown) was negative. (Reproduced under the terms of the Creative Commons Attribution License from Silva S, Maximino J, Henrique R, et al. J Med Case Rep. 2007;1:121.)

leads to a local imbalance of vasoactive substances, including enhanced release of the vasoconstrictor endothelin and reduced release of vasodilatory endothelium-derived nitric oxide.[49] Indeed, plasma endothelin levels are increased in human patients with septic AKI. However, although endothelin receptor antagonists ameliorate ischemic AKI in animals, human data are lacking.[50] A human trial of endothelin receptor antagonist for prevention of contrast-induced AKI resulted in a paradoxical exacerbation of nephrotoxicity.[51] It is now apparent that these hemodynamic abnormalities cannot fully account for the profound loss of renal function, and several human trials of vasodilators such as dopamine have failed to demonstrate improvement in GFR in established AKI despite augmentation of renal blood flow.[52]

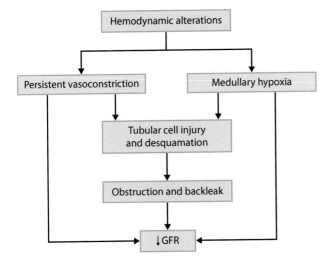

Figure 30.4 Pathophysiology of intrinsic and structural acute kidney injury: hemodynamic alterations and their consequences. GFR, glomerular filtration rate.

## TUBULAR DYNAMICS

Three well-known alterations in tubular dynamics in intrinsic AKI are obstruction, backleak, and activation of tubuloglomerular feedback.[49] The consistent findings of proximal tubular dilatation and distal tubular casts in human AKI are indicative of obstruction to tubular fluid flow. The intraluminal casts stain strongly for Tamm-Horsfall protein, which is normally secreted by the thick ascending limb as a monomer. Conversion into a gel-like polymer is enhanced by the increased luminal sodium concentration typically encountered in the distal tubule in AKI as a result of impaired proximal tubule sodium reabsorption.[53] This provides an ideal environment for cast formation along with desquamated tubule cells and brush-border membranes. However, it is unlikely that obstruction alone can account for the profound dysfunction in clinical AKI because human studies using forced diuresis with furosemide or mannitol did not improve the renal recovery rate of patients with established AKI.[54–56] Similarly, although movement of the glomerular filtrate back into the circulation has been shown to occur, this accounts for only a very minor component of the decrease in GFR in human AKI.[49] Finally, a role for activation of tubuloglomerular feedback has been proposed.[57] By physiologic considerations, the increased delivery of sodium chloride to the macula densa caused by abnormalities in the injured proximal tubule would be expected to induce afferent arteriolar constriction, mediated by adenosine through A1 adenosine receptor (A1AR) activation, and thereby decrease GFR.[58] Thus, research efforts have focused on specific adenosine receptor antagonists as potential therapeutic agents. Initial animal studies using the nonselective adenosine receptor antagonist theophylline yielded encouraging results in terms of preserving renal blood flow when the drug was administered before ischemic injury and in improving blood flow in established ischemic AKI. However, in more recent studies, genetic deletion of the A1AR resulted in paradoxical worsening of ischemic renal injury, and exogenous activation of A1AR was renoprotective.[59] Thus, tubuloglomerular feedback activation following ischemic injury may represent a beneficial phenomenon that limits wasteful delivery of ions and solutes to the damaged tubules. The protective effects of adenosine inhibition on renal blood flow preservation may be mediated by distinct A2 adenosine receptor activation and are currently under investigation.[60]

## ALTERATIONS IN TUBULAR CELL METABOLISM

A profound reduction in intracellular adenosine triphosphate (ATP) content is a hallmark of AKI that occurs early after injury, and it triggers a number of metabolic consequences in tubule cells.[61] These events are detailed later, and their interrelationship is illustrated in Figure 30.5.

Alterations in tubule cell adenine nucleotide metabolism have been well documented. Oxygen deprivation leads to a rapid degradation of ATP to adenosine monophosphate (AMP) and to hypoxanthine. These metabolites are freely diffusible, and their depletion precludes resynthesis of ATP during reperfusion. In addition, ATP depletion results in mitochondrial damage with cessation of oxidative phosphorylation, thus leading to further depletion of energy stores. Although provision of exogenous adenine nucleotides or thyroxine (which stimulates mitochondrial ATP regeneration) can ameliorate the cellular injury in animal models of ischemic AKI, these substances have proven

ineffective in established human AKI.[62] An increase in free intracellular calcium has also been documented following AKI, but its role has remained controversial. Increased intracellular calcium could potentially lead to activation of proteases and phospholipases. A meta-analysis suggested that calcium channel blockers may provide some protection from renal injury in the transplant setting, but evidence for their efficacy in other forms of AKI is currently lacking.[63]

There is now substantial evidence for the role of reactive oxygen species in the pathogenesis of intrinsic AKI. During reperfusion, the conversion of accumulated hypoxanthine to xanthine generates hydrogen peroxide and superoxide. In the presence of iron, hydrogen peroxide forms the highly reactive hydroxyl radical. Concomitantly, ischemia induces nitric oxide synthase in tubule cells, and the nitric oxide generated interacts with superoxide to form peroxynitrate, which results in cell damage through oxidant injury, as well as protein nitrosylation.[61] Furthermore, at the subcellular level, mitochondrial swelling and damage are early and well-documented consequences of hypoxic, ischemic, and nephrotoxic tubule cell injury. The resultant alterations in the mitochondrial electron transport chain lead to a significant increase in superoxide production and release. Indeed, human studies have documented a dramatic increase in oxidative stress with AKI.[64] Several scavengers of reactive oxygen molecules protect against ischemic AKI in animal models, but human studies have been inconclusive. As an alternative approach, the iron scavenger deferoxamine ameliorates ischemia-reperfusion injury in animal models, but the associated toxicity precludes its clinical use in human AKI. Three advances have emerged in the area of iron chelation. The first is the

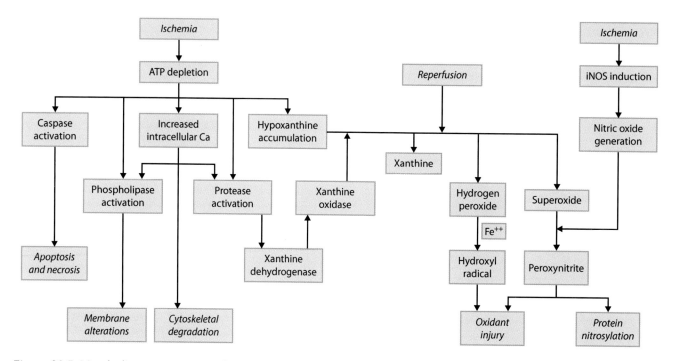

Figure 30.5 Metabolic consequences of acute ischemia and reperfusion injury to kidney tubule cells. Inhibition of these pathways may provide novel therapeutic approaches to acute kidney injury. ATP, adenosine triphosphate; Ca, calcium; Fe++, iron, iNOS, inducible nitric oxide synthase.

availability of human apotransferrin, an iron-binding protein that protects against renal ischemia-reperfusion injury in animals by abrogating renal superoxide formation.[65] The second is the discovery of neutrophil gelatinase–associated lipocalin (NGAL), an endogenous iron-transporting protein, as one of the most highly induced genes and proteins in the kidney following early AKI.[66] Administration of NGAL provided significant functional protection in an animal model of AKI.[67] The third is the availability of deferiprone, an iron chelator that is approved by the Food and Drug Administration to treat patients with thalassemia and iron overload resulting from blood transfusions. The potential therapeutic use of NGAL and deferiprone in human AKI is currently under investigation.

## ALTERATIONS IN TUBULAR CELL STRUCTURE

The cell biologic response of the tubule cell to ischemic or nephrotoxic AKI is multifaceted and includes loss of cell polarity and brush borders, cell death, dedifferentiation of viable cells, proliferation, and restitution of a normal epithelium, as illustrated in Figure 30.6. The major mechanisms underlying this morphologic sequence of events are summarized here.

AKI results in an early, rapid disruption of the apical actin cytoskeleton and redistribution of actin from the apical domain and microvilli into the cytoplasm.[68] This results in loss of brush-border membranes, which contribute to cast formation and obstruction. Disruption of the apical cytoskeleton also results in loss of tight junctions and occludens junctions that accounts for the backleak of glomerular filtrate. Ischemic and nephrotoxic insults also result in the early disruption of at least two normally basolaterally

polarized proteins, namely sodium, potassium-ATPase (Na,K-ATPase) and integrins. The Na,K-ATPase is normally tethered to the spectrin-based cytoskeleton at the basolateral domain by the adapter protein ankyrin. This provides the driving force for the normal reabsorption of salt and water by the proximal tubule. Tubule cell injury leads to a reversible cytoplasmic accumulation of Na,K-ATPase, ankyrin, and spectrin in viable cells.[69] Postulated mechanisms leading to loss of Na,K-ATPase polarity include disruption of the cortical actin cytoskeleton and cleavage of spectrin by ischemia-induced activation of proteases such as calpain.[49] The consequence is impaired proximal tubular sodium reabsorption leading to the high FENa that is characteristic of intrinsic AKI. The $\beta_1$-integrins are normally polarized to the basal domain, where they mediate cell-substratum adhesions. Tubule cell injury leads to a redistribution of integrins to the apical membrane, with consequential detachment of viable cells from the basement membrane. There is good evidence for abnormal adhesion between these exfoliated cells within the tubular lumen, mediated by an interaction between apical integrin and the Arg-Gly-Asp (RGD) motif of integrin receptors.[70] Administration of synthetic RGD compounds attenuated tubular obstruction and renal impairment in animal models of ischemic AKI, but human studies are lacking.

AKI leads to tubule cell death by at least two pathophysiologic mechanisms.[71] Necrosis is characterized by loss of membrane integrity, cytoplasmic swelling, nuclear pyknosis, cellular fragmentation, and an inflammatory response. Apoptosis is characterized by cytoplasmic and nuclear shrinkage, DNA fragmentation, and breakdown of the cell into apoptotic bodies that are rapidly removed by phagocytosis. These two forms of cell death frequently coexist and are two extremes of a continuum. Following

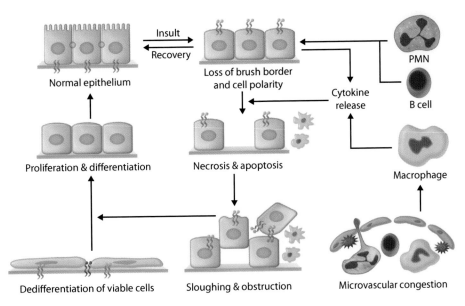

Figure 30.6 Structural consequences of acute ischemia and reperfusion injury to kidney tubule cells. Novel therapeutic approaches in acute kidney injury have targeted prevention of cell death, inhibition of inflammation, and acceleration of the endogenous recovery process. PMN, polymorphonuclear leukocyte.

AKI, the mode of cell death depends primarily on the severity of the insult and the resistance of the cell type. Necrosis occurs following more severe injury and in the more susceptible proximal tubules that normally have to operate at high levels of energy consumption. Apoptosis predominates during physiologic cell death, after less severe injury, and especially in the injury-resistant distal nephron segments. Mounting evidence now indicates that apoptosis is a major mechanism of early tubule cell death in both animal and human models of AKI.[71-80] Considerable attention has therefore been directed toward unraveling the molecular pathways involved in renal tubule cell apoptosis. Multiple intracellular signaling pathways, including the intrinsic (Bcl-2 family, cytochrome c, caspase 9), extrinsic (Fas, Fas-associated death domain protein [FADD], caspase 8), and regulatory (p53) factors, appear to be activated during AKI, as illustrated in Figure 30.7. In addition, the mitochondrial damage that occurs early in AKI results in direct release

of cytochrome c, with activation of downstream apoptotic pathways. Inhibition of apoptosis holds promise in AKI, and certain pharmacologic agents that inhibit p53 or the caspases are currently under investigation.[81] One promising example is the use of small interfering RNA molecules (siRNA) that inhibit p53, which have been shown in animal studies to provide structural and functional protection against ischemic and nephrotoxic AKI.[82] Human trials of p53 siRNA are currently under way.

Renal tubule cells possess a remarkable ability to regenerate and proliferate after ischemic injury.[83] Morphologically, repair is heralded by the appearance of dedifferentiated tubule cells. In the next phase, the cells upregulate genes encoding for a variety of growth factors such as insulin-like growth factor I (IGF-I), hepatocyte growth factor (HGF), fibroblast growth factor (FGF), and bone morphogenetic protein 7 (BMP-7), and undergo marked proliferation. In the final phase, cells undergo redifferentiation until the normal fully polarized epithelium is restored. Thus, during recovery from ischemia, renal tubule cells recapitulate processes similar to those during normal kidney development.[80,83,84] Understanding the molecular mechanisms of repair may provide clues to accelerating recovery from AKI. The potential use of growth factors, progenitor cells, and mesenchymal stem cells (MSCs) as therapeutic strategies in AKI is currently under active investigation.[85,86] Most notable among these are MSCs that promote kidney repair by secreting growth factors (vascular endothelial growth factor [VEGF], HGF, IGF-I) with potent antiapoptotic, mitogenic, anti-inflammatory, and angiogenic properties. Modified MSCs that have been expanded from normal bone marrow cells and rendered immune privileged and genetically stable are currently being investigated for safety and efficacy in human AKI.

## INFLAMMATORY RESPONSE AND COMPLEMENT

There is now increasing evidence in animal and human studies for a prominent role of inflammation in the pathogenesis of AKI.[40,41] The major components of this response include endothelial injury, leukocyte recruitment, and production of inflammatory mediators by tubule cells. Endothelial injury plays a critical role in the pathophysiology of AKI. It is manifested by endothelial swelling, endothelial apoptosis, narrowing of the blood vessels, abnormal retrograde blood flow on reperfusion, and the induction of adhesion molecules such as intercellular adhesion molecule 1 (ICAM-1) and P-selectin that promote endothelial-leukocyte interactions. Although ablation of the ICAM-1 gene and pretreatment with ICAM-1 antibody rendered mice resistant to ischemic AKI, human trials with anti–ICAM-1 antibody did not prevent AKI in deceased donor kidney transplant recipients.[87] Morphologically, neutrophils, macrophages, dendritic cells, B cells, and T cells have all been shown to aggregate in peritubular capillaries following ischemic AKI in humans, and the relative roles of these leukocyte

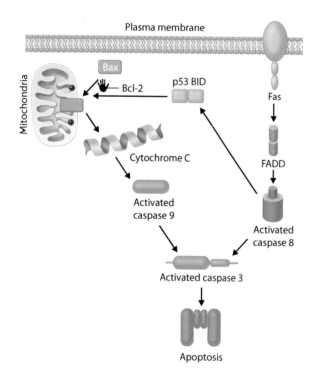

Figure 30.7 Major tubule cell apoptotic pathways in human acute kidney injury (AKI). The extrinsic pathway requires activation of plasma membrane receptors such as Fas and the tumor necrosis factor receptor TNF-R1, with subsequent signal transduction and activation of caspase 8. The intrinsic pathway requires translocation of Bax to the mitochondria, thereby forming pores for the release of cytochrome c and activation of caspase 9. Cross-talk between these pathways is provided largely by the regulatory molecule p53. Bax translocation is prevented by Bcl-2 and Bcl-xL. Both caspases 8 and 9 activate caspase 3, which initiates the final morphologic cascades of apoptosis. Inhibition of the central regulatory molecule p53 and the terminal executor caspases hold promise in human AKI. BID, BH3 interacting death domain; FADD, Fas-associated death domain protein.

subtypes remain under investigation.[48] Neutrophils are the first inflammatory cells to attach to the activated endothelium and accumulate in the peritubular capillary network in both animal and human AKI. They produce reactive oxygen species and cytokines that aggravate the kidney injury. However, blockade of neutrophil function or neutrophil depletion provides only partial protection from AKI in animal models. Similarly, experimental models depleting macrophages or dendritic cells have resulted in partial amelioration of AKI. Translation of these immune cell depletion approaches to human AKI is likely to be challenging.

The injured proximal tubule epithelium is an active participant in the inflammatory response and can generate some mediators that potentiate the process. These include cytokines such as tumor necrosis factor-α (TNF-α) and interleukin-6 (IL-6), and the chemotactic cytokines (monocyte chemoattractant protein-1 [MCP-1], IL-8, RANTES [regulated on activation, normal T cell expressed and secreted]). Human studies have shown that the plasma levels of the proinflammatory cytokines IL-6 and IL-8 predict death in adults with AKI.[88] Strategies that modulate the inflammatory response may provide significant beneficial effects in human AKI. One promising example is α-melanocyte-stimulating hormone (α-MSH), a potent anti-inflammatory and antiapoptotic cytokine that inhibits several proinflammatory cytokines (TNF-α, IL-10), and neutrophil adhesion molecules. In animal studies, α-MSH and its synthetic analogues protect from AKI that was caused by ischemia-reperfusion, nephrotoxins, and sepsis.[89] Human clinical trials using synthetic α-MSH analogues are currently ongoing.

The complement system is an important contributor to inflammation after ischemic AKI. The primary mechanism is by activation of the alternative complement pathway, leading to marked upregulation of the C5a component on proximal tubule cells and macrophages.[90] Pharmacologic inhibition of this pathway by using synthetic C5a receptor blockers resulted in dramatic protection from ischemic AKI in animal models.[91] Human trials should be highly feasible, given the selective nature, stability, and excellent bioavailability of synthetic C5a receptor antagonists.

## SEPSIS

Although sepsis is one of the most common causes of AKI, the pathogenesis of septic AKI remains incompletely understood, in part because of the limitations of rodent models. Small studies have revealed the surprising finding that unlike in ischemic or nephrotoxic AKI, human patients with early septic AKI demonstrate a paradoxical increase in renal blood flow despite a reduction in GFR. Large animal models of septic AKI have confirmed this finding of GFR deterioration despite renal vasodilation and increased renal blood flow.[92] Thus, septic AKI is a hyperemic injury that contrasts with the persistent vasoconstriction characteristic of ischemic AKI. It is likely that the same mechanisms that lead to systemic arterial vasodilation in sepsis

are also operative at the level of the glomerular arterioles. Dilation of both afferent and efferent arterioles, but with a greater efferent than afferent dilation, may account for the decreased GFR despite the increased renal blood flow. Other unique aspects of septic AKI could include an exacerbated endothelial dysfunction and more pronounced complement activation.[93] C5a receptor blockers are especially efficacious in animal models of septic AKI.

## POSTRENAL ACUTE KIDNEY INJURY

Postrenal AKI is a result of obstruction to the outflow tract on both sides and is uncommon beyond the neonatal period. Postrenal AKI is usually reversed by relief of the obstruction, but it is accompanied by very significant postobstructive diuresis. The common causes of postrenal AKI are listed in Table 30.6. The pathophysiology and management of the obstructive nephropathy syndrome that can result from congenital obstruction are detailed in Chapter 47.

## CLINICAL MANIFESTATIONS OF ACUTE KIDNEY INJURY

Until it becomes severe, AKI is largely asymptomatic, and its detection must begin with having a high index of suspicion and an awareness of the risk factors. AKI most commonly manifests with a progressive accumulation of fluid or nitrogenous wastes in a predisposed patient who has been exposed to one or more of the etiologic factors outlined in Tables 30.3 to 30.6. Less frequently, one encounters an increase in BUN and creatinine that is not readily explained. In all cases, the evaluation requires a complete history, physical examination, laboratory evaluation, renal imaging, and, rarely, a kidney biopsy. A diligent search for all drugs and medications ingested is especially important,

Table 30.6 Common causes of postrenal acute kidney injury

| Mechanism | Etiology |
| --- | --- |
| Congenital | Posterior urethral valves |
| | Ureteropelvic junction obstruction in a solitary kidney |
| | Bilateral ureterovesicular obstruction |
| Acquired | Calculi |
| | Clots |
| | Neurogenic bladder |
| | Drugs that cause urinary retention |
| | External compression by pelvic and abdominal tumors |
| | Bladder tumors |

even when another obvious cause for AKI is evident. The initial approach to a patient with known or suspected AKI should be directed toward (1) identifying the underlying cause, (2) distinguishing between prerenal and intrinsic AKI, (3) discriminating between AKI and CKD, (4) determining the severity of AKI, and (5) considering a diagnostic fluid challenge.

## IDENTIFYING THE UNDERLYING CAUSE

The initial history should be directed toward uncovering an obvious risk factor for AKI, such as those listed in Tables 30.3 to 30.5. Additional relevant aspects of the AKI history and physical examination are shown in Table 30.7 and Table 30.8, respectively. These aspects, in combination with a careful urinalysis with microscopy, yield the cause of AKI in the majority of cases. A short duration of vomiting, diarrhea, or decreased oral intake associated with decreased urine output and typical physical findings of dehydration suggests prerenal volume-responsive functional AKI. Bloody diarrhea with oliguria is consistent with the hemolytic-uremic syndrome. A history of pharyngitis or impetigo a few weeks before the onset of gross hematuria

---

**KEY POINT**

Assessing the degree of fluid overload is critical for management and prognosis of patients with AKI.

---

Table 30.7 Relevant history in patients with suspected acute kidney injury

- Fluid loss
  - Diarrhea
  - Vomiting
  - Burns
  - Surgery
  - Shock
- Nephrotoxic agents
  - Nonsteroidal anti-inflammatory drugs
  - Antibiotics and other nephrotoxins
  - Contrast agents
- Glomerular disease
  - Streptococcal infection (poststreptococcal glomerulonephritis)
  - Bloody diarrhea (hemolytic-uremic syndrome)
  - Fever, joint complaints, rash (systemic lupus erythematosus)
- Obstruction
  - Anuria
  - Poor urinary stream

Table 30.8 Relevant clinical examination in acute kidney injury

| Clinical sign | Diagnostic interpretation |
| --- | --- |
| Signs of intravascular volume depletion | Prerenal azotemia |
| Signs of fluid retention: edema, hypertension | Fluid overload, intrinsic renal disease |
| Signs of underlying systemic diseases associated with renal involvement: butterfly rash, joint swelling, purpuric rash, fever, macular rash, palpably enlarged kidneys | Systemic lupus erythematosus Henoch-Schönlein purpura Interstitial nephritis Polycystic or multicystic kidney disease Renal vein thrombosis |
| Signs of urinary obstruction: poor urinary stream, urinary dribbling, palpably enlarged urinary bladder, history of urinary catheterization | Bladder outlet obstruction |

or edema suggests poststreptococcal glomerulonephritis. Edema should also prompt a search for nephrotic syndrome, cardiac failure, or liver failure, which would suggest prerenal or functional AKI that should not be treated with fluid resuscitation. Fever, joint complaints, and a malar rash are indicative of systemic lupus erythematosus. In hospitalized patients, nephrotoxic medications or periods of hypotension are commonly associated with intrinsic AKI, and they should be diligently sought.

The urinalysis is the most important noninvasive test in the diagnostic evaluation. Typically, the urine in conditions that result in prerenal AKI contains little protein or blood. In contrast, proteinuria and hematuria are prominent in causes leading to intrinsic AKI. A heme-positive urine by dipstick in the absence of red blood cells in the sediment suggests hemolysis or rhabdomyolysis. Characteristic findings on microscopic examination of the urine sediment can suggest certain diagnoses. Muddy brown granular casts and epithelial cell casts are highly suggestive of intrinsic AKI

---

**KEY POINTS**

- The initial approach to a patient with suspected AKI should be directed toward the following:
  - Identifying the underlying cause
  - Distinguishing among prerenal (functional), intrinsic (structural), and postrenal AKI
  - Determining the severity of AKI
- The urinalysis and determination of fractional sodium excretion are the most important bedside tools in the diagnostic evaluation of AKI.

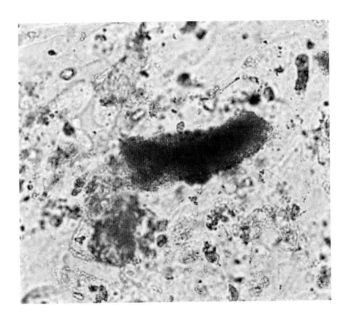

Figure 30.8 Urine microscopy of a patient with acute kidney injury after a cardiac surgical procedure shows a "muddy brown" cast.

or ATN (Figure 30.8). The finding of red blood cell casts is diagnostic of glomerulonephritis. The concurrent findings of red blood cell casts, dysmorphic red blood cells, heavy proteinuria, or lipiduria indicate a "nephritic" urinary sediment. This is commonly associated with AKI caused by glomerulonephritides. Pyuria with white cell and granular or waxy casts are suggestive of tubular or interstitial disease or urinary tract infection. White blood cells and white blood cell casts may also be seen in acute glomerulonephritis.

## DISTINGUISHING BETWEEN PRERENAL AND INTRINSIC ACUTE KIDNEY INJURY

This determination is important because (1) the treatment and prognosis are different, and (2) prompt identification and management of prerenal AKI can prevent the progression to intrinsic AKI. As noted earlier, urinalysis with microscopy often provides an initial differentiation between prerenal and intrinsic AKI. The further distinction is based on the principle that prerenal or functional AKI is associated with maximal reabsorption of solutes and water by the intact proximal tubule, whereas the proximal tubule cell damage typical of intrinsic or structural AKI results in impaired reabsorptive capacity. Urinary indices based on this principle are shown in Table 30.9.

The FENa is a convenient bedside screening test for making this distinction. It is calculated from measured concentrations of sodium (Na) and creatinine (Cr) in the urine (U) and plasma (P), as follows:

$$FENa = ([U / P]Na) / ([U / P]Cr) \times 100$$

An FENa of less than 1% suggests prerenal AKI, in which the reabsorption of almost all the filtered sodium

Table 30.9 Urinary indices in prerenal and intrinsic acute kidney injury

| Test | Prerenal AKI | Intrinsic AKI |
|---|---|---|
| Urine specific gravity | >1,020 | <1,012 |
| Urine/plasma creatinine | >40 | <20 |
| Urine Na (mEq/L) | <20 | >40 |
| FENa | <1% | >2% |

AKI, acute kidney injury; FENa, fractional excretion of sodium.

represents an appropriate response to decreased perfusion. An FENa greater than 2% suggests intrinsic AKI with proximal tubule injury. An FENa between 1% and 2% is nondiagnostic. In neonates, the FENa is generally higher because of their decreased ability to reabsorb sodium that results from immaturity of proximal tubule function. Further, FENa determinations should be interpreted in the context of such considerations as hydration status and sodium intake. The FENa can be low (less than 1%) in conditions such as congestive heart failure, nephrotic syndrome, contrast nephropathy, or pigment nephropathy. The FENa can be high following administration of loop or distal tubule diuretics or administration of a sodium load, which increases urinary sodium excretion. The fractional excretion of urea (FEUrea) has been proposed as a more accurate determinant of prerenal AKI in children, especially in patients receiving diuretics.[94]

By the same principle of increased proximal tubule solute reabsorption, the BUN-to-creatinine ratio in the serum is markedly elevated (to more than 20) in prerenal AKI. This is because the proximal tubule can avidly reabsorb urea but is impermeable to creatinine. However, increases in BUN without AKI can be encountered in patients receiving steroids or total parenteral nutrition, in catabolic states, and in those with gastrointestinal bleeding.

## DISTINGUISHING BETWEEN ACUTE KIDNEY INJURY AND CHRONIC KIDNEY DISEASE

A kidney and bladder ultrasound scan is a sensitive, noninvasive modality that not only can differentiate between AKI and CKD, but also can rule out a postrenal cause. Typically, the kidneys in AKI are normal or enlarged, with increased echogenicity, whereas those in CKD are frequently small and shrunken. Other distinguishing features are shown in Table 30.10.

## DETERMINING THE SEVERITY OF ACUTE KIDNEY INJURY

Estimating the baseline pre-illness serum creatinine can determine the severity of AKI and allow for classification based on the pRIFLE and KDIGO criteria. This estimation is best achieved when a previously drawn serum creatinine

Table 30.10 Features distinguishing acute kidney injury from chronic kidney disease

| Clinical and laboratory parameter | Acute kidney injury | Chronic kidney disease |
|---|---|---|
| Onset of kidney disease | Sudden | Long-standing kidney disease |
| Hypertension | Onset with AKI | Long-standing hypertension |
| Linear growth | Normal | Linear growth retardation |
| Urinalysis | "Muddy brown" casts | No "muddy brown" casts |
| | No broad urinary casts | Broad waxy urinary casts |
| BUN and creatinine | Progressively increasing | Stable, but elevated BUN and creatinine |
| Bone x-ray studies for osteodystrophy | Normal bone x-ray study | Renal osteodystrophy |
| Parathyroid hormone | Normal | Elevated |
| Anemia | Usually mild and explainable by acute onset of disease | Anemia usually severe, normocytic and normochromic |
| Renal ultrasound | Normal or enlarged kidneys; may be echogenic | Small shrunken and echogenic kidneys |

Abbreviations: AKI, acute kidney injury; BUN, blood urea nitrogen.

level is available. If not, the baseline kidney function in children can be estimated using the Schwartz formula:

$$\text{Estimated creatinine clearance in mL/min} = kL / Pcr$$

where L = height (cm), Pcr = plasma creatinine in mg/dL, and k = proportionality constant.

The value of the proportionality constant was previously reported to be age dependent and was quoted to be 0.45 in the first year of life, 0.55 in children and adolescent girls, and 0.70 in adolescent boys. More recent investigations allowed for a simplification of this formula and indicated that a single uniform k value of 0.413 provides a good approximation of GFR in children between 1 and 16 years of age and both genders.[95] However, this simplification was derived in patients with CKD and has not been validated for use in AKI.

Another important index of AKI severity is the degree of fluid overload, which is especially useful in the assessment of the critically ill patient. Several pediatric AKI studies have demonstrated that increasing degrees of fluid overload are independently associated with mortality.[96-98] The extent of fluid overload during a hospitalization period can be estimated by the following formula:

$$\text{Fluid overload (\%)} = [\text{Total fluid in (liters)} - \text{Total fluid out (liters)}] / \text{Admission weight in kg}] \times 100$$

The importance of assessing fluid overload was demonstrated by the Prospective Pediatric Continuous Renal Replacement Therapy (ppCRRT) Registry Group, through the analysis of its 340-patient cohort by using a tripartite classification for percentage of fluid overload at CRRT initiation.[98] Patients who developed a greater than 20% fluid overload at CRRT initiation had a significantly higher mortality rate (66%) than did patients who had a 10% to 20% fluid overload (43%) and those with a less than 10% fluid overload (29%). The association between degree of fluid overload and mortality remained after adjusting for intergroup differences and severity of illness. When fluid overload was dichotomized to greater than 20% and less than 20%, patients with a greater than 20% fluid overload had an adjusted mortality odds ratio (OR) of 8.5 (95% confidence interval [CI], 2.8 to 25.7).

Routine laboratory evaluation for the presence of metabolic complications can also assist in establishing AKI severity. AKI is associated with several life-threatening complications, about which the clinician must constantly be diligent. Fortunately, these complications are uncommon in patients who receive dialytic therapies. Common complications are listed in Table 30.11. Hyponatremia is usually dilutional (secondary to fluid retention and administration of hypotonic fluids). Less common causes of hyponatremia include sodium depletion (hyponatremic dehydration) and hyperglycemia (serum sodium concentration decreases by 1.6 mEq/L for every 100 mg/dL increase in serum glucose higher than 100 mg/dL). Hypernatremia in AKI is usually a result of excessive sodium administration (inappropriate fluid therapy or overzealous sodium bicarbonate administration).

Hyperkalemia in AKI results from reduction in GFR, reduction in tubular secretion of potassium, increased catabolism, and metabolic acidosis (each 0.1-unit reduction in arterial pH raises serum potassium by 0.3 mEq/L). Hyperkalemia is most pronounced in patients with excessive endogenous production (rhabdomyolysis, hemolysis, and tumor lysis syndrome). High–anion gap metabolic acidosis is secondary to the impaired renal excretion of acid

---

**KEY POINT**

Fluid overload greater than 20% at CRRT initiation is associated with higher patient mortality.

Table 30.11 Complications of acute kidney injury

| Metabolic | Cardiovascular | Gastrointestinal | Neurologic | Hematologic | Infectious |
|---|---|---|---|---|---|
| Hyperkalemia | Pulmonary edema | Nausea, vomiting, anorexia | Altered mental status | Anemia | Pneumonia |
| Metabolic acidosis | Arrhythmias | Malnutrition | Irritability | Bleeding | Sepsis |
| Hyponatremia | Pericarditis | Gastritis | Seizures | — | Infected IV sites |
| Hypocalcemia | Myocardial Infarction | GI bleeding | Somnolence | — | — |
| Hyperphosphatemia | Hypertension | GI ulcers | Coma | — | — |

*Abbreviations:* GI, gastrointestinal; IV, intravenous.

and the impaired reabsorption and regeneration of bicarbonate. Acidosis is most severe in shock, sepsis, or impaired respiratory compensation. Hypocalcemia results from increased serum phosphate and impaired renal conversion of vitamin D to the active form. Hypocalcemia is most pronounced in patients with rhabdomyolysis. Metabolic acidosis increases the fraction of ionized calcium (the active form). Therefore, overzealous bicarbonate therapy can decrease the concentration of ionized calcium and precipitate symptoms of hypocalcemia, including tetany, seizures, and cardiac arrhythmias. Hyperphosphatemia in AKI is primarily caused by impaired renal excretion, and it can aggravate hypocalcemia. During recovery from AKI, the vigorous diuretic phase may be accompanied by significant volume depletion, hypernatremia, hypokalemia, and hypophosphatemia.

## ROLE OF DIAGNOSTIC FLUID CHALLENGE

A common clinical situation is one in which patients present with an increase in BUN and serum creatinine and with a history and physical findings consistent with a prerenal cause, but the duration of the prerenal insult is unknown. Another common diagnostic dilemma occurs when a patient presents with an increase in serum creatinine, but the cause is unclear. In both these cases, a fluid challenge may be diagnostic as well as therapeutic. Typically, fluid challenges in children consist of crystalloid at a dose of 10 to 20 mL/kg, repeated once or twice until urine output improves. A reduction in BUN and serum creatinine would indicate a prerenal cause, whereas an absence of improvement in these parameters (or the development of fluid overload, or both) would confirm the diagnosis of intrinsic AKI. Fluid challenges should be avoided in children with prerenal AKI because of non–volume-responsive states such as liver failure, heart failure, and nephrotic syndrome.

## ROLE OF KIDNEY BIOPSY

A renal biopsy is rarely indicated in AKI, but it should be considered when noninvasive evaluation fails to establish a diagnosis. Renal biopsy in children with AKI is most commonly indicated in patients with suspected rapidly progressive or crescentic glomerulonephritis, in suspected lupus nephritis to classify the renal disease, and in kidney transplant recipients with suspected acute allograft rejection. Pathologic findings of AKI in the renal biopsy include normal appearing glomeruli, renal tubules demonstrating tubular cell loss, the presence of denuded tubular epithelial cells in the tubular lumen, and a lack of an inflammatory interstitial infiltrate (see Figure 30.8). Acute renal transplant allograft rejection, conversely, has distinct pathologic findings.

## CONCERNS WITH USING SERUM CREATININE MEASUREMENTS

A progressive increase in serum creatinine (typically 1 to 2 mg/dL/day) is the hallmark of intrinsic AKI, and it has served as a biomarker of AKI for several decades. However, serum creatinine concentration is a flawed AKI biomarker, for several reasons: Serum creatinine does not differentiate the nature, type, and timing of the renal insult.[99] Changes in serum creatinine concentrations often lag behind changes in GFR until a steady state has been reached, which can take several days. Dialysis readily clears serum creatinine, thereby rendering this marker useless in the assessment for improving renal function once dialysis has begun. Even normal serum creatinine concentrations can vary widely with age, gender, diet, muscle mass, nutrition status, medications, and hydration status. In the acute setting, it is estimated that more than 50% of kidney function must be lost before the serum creatinine even begins to rise. However, animal studies have shown that although AKI can be prevented or treated by several maneuvers, these measures must be instituted very early after the

---

### KEY POINT

Using serum creatinine for the diagnosis of AKI is fraught with imprecisions, but it is currently the most widely available tool.

insult, well before the serum creatinine rises. The lack of early biomarkers of AKI in humans has hitherto impaired our ability to launch potentially effective therapies in a timely manner.

## NOVEL BIOMARKERS

The genomic and proteomic tools of modern science have identified novel markers for the early stress response of the kidney that serendipitously appear in the urine or plasma well before a change in serum creatinine is detected.[99] Many of these markers are being developed and validated as early noninvasive biomarkers for the prediction of AKI and its clinical outcomes in humans. This is a rapidly evolving field, and the current status of the most promising examples is summarized in Table 30.12.

The most widely studied and validated early biomarker of AKI in children is NGAL.[100] In a prospective study of 71 children undergoing cardiopulmonary bypass (CPB), levels of NGAL in the urine and plasma were significantly elevated within 2 h of bypass in those children who subsequently developed AKI (defined as a 50% increase in serum creatinine) 1 to 3 days postoperatively.[101] A subsequent prospective study of 374 infants and children undergoing CPB confirmed these findings and additionally established cutoff thresholds, as well as a strong association between early NGAL measurements and hard clinical outcomes, including length of hospital stay and the duration and severity of AKI.[102] A prospective multicenter study of 311 children undergoing cardiac surgical procedures confirmed the early rise of plasma and urine NGAL concentrations (within 6 h postoperatively) in subjects who developed an increase in serum creatinine 2 days later. Early NGAL concentrations were also shown to be associated with longer hospital and ICU stays and with longer duration of mechanical ventilation. Furthermore, the additional of NGAL significantly improved the risk prediction for AKI over clinical models alone.[103] A multicenter pooled analysis of existing NGAL studies in children and adults has been published, confirming the utility of this marker for the early diagnosis of AKI and its clinical outcomes in several clinical situations.[104] One study examined a combination of biomarkers in 220 children undergoing cardiac surgical procedures.[21] Urinary NGAL was increased in AKI patients within 2 h of bypass initiation, urine IL-18 and liver-type fatty acid binding protein (L-FABP) were increased within 6 h, and urine kidney injury molecule 1 (KIM-1) increased at the 12-h time point. All markers correlated with AKI severity and clinical outcomes, and improved the risk prediction for AKI over clinical models. Thus, they represent temporally sequential markers, and a panel of such biomarkers may therefore help establish the timing of injury and plan appropriate therapies. Standardized clinical laboratory platforms for the measurement of urine and plasma NGAL are now available in most countries globally.

Table 30.12 Novel urinary biomarkers for the prediction of acute kidney injury and its outcomes*

| Biomarker | Source | Function | Cardiac surgery | Kidney transplant | ICU/ED |
|---|---|---|---|---|---|
| NGAL | Distal tubule and collecting duct | Regulates iron trafficking, promotes tubule cell survival | 2 h post-CPB 2 days pre-AKI Predicts AKI severity, dialysis, and death | 6 h post-transplant 2–3 days pre-DGF Predicts long-term graft loss | On admission 1–2 days pre-AKI Predicts AKI severity, dialysis, and death |
| IL-18 | Proximal tubule | Promotes tubule cell apoptosis and necrosis | 6 h post-CPB 2 days pre-AKI Predicts AKI severity, dialysis, and death | 6 h post-transplant 2–3 days pre-DGF predicts long-term graft loss | On admission 1–2 days pre-AKI Predicts AKI severity, dialysis, and death |
| L-FABP | Proximal tubule | Antioxidant, suppresses tubulointerstitial damage | 6 h post-CPB 2 days pre-AKI Not tested for outcomes | Not tested | On admission 1–2 days pre-AKI Predicts AKI severity, dialysis, and death |
| KIM-1 | Proximal tubule | Promotes epithelial regeneration, regulates apoptosis | 12 h post-CPB 1 day pre-AKI Not tested for outcomes | Not tested | On admission 1–2 days pre-AKI Predicts AKI severity, dialysis, and death |

*Abbreviations:* AKI, acute kidney injury, typically defined as AKIN stage I or greater; CPB, cardiopulmonary bypass; DGF, delayed graft function; ICU, intensive care unit; ED, emergency department; IL-18, interleukin-18; KIM-1, kidney injury molecule 1; L-FABP, liver-type fatty acid binding protein; NGAL, neutrophil gelatinase–associated lipocalin.

* Times shown (in hours or days) are the earliest time points when the biomarker becomes significantly increased from baseline.

## PREVENTION

Preventive measures include vigorous fluid administration in patients at high risk for developing AKI, adequate fluid repletion in those patients with hypovolemia, avoidance of hypotension in critically ill children by providing inotropic support as needed, and close monitoring of renal function and drug levels in children receiving nephrotoxic medications.

## HYDRATION

Vigorous fluid administration has been successfully employed to prevent AKI in patients at high risk, including those with hemoglobinuria, myoglobinuria, early tumor lysis syndrome, renal transplantation, other major surgical procedures, and use of nephrotoxic agents such as radiocontrast, cisplatin, and amphotericin. The efficacy of preoperative hydration strategies was demonstrated by a meta-analysis of 20 randomized controlled trials that investigated the renoprotective effects of perioperative hemodynamic optimization among 4220 adult surgical patients who were undergoing elective or emergency procedures.[105] Postoperative AKI was significantly reduced by perioperative hemodynamic optimization when compared with the control group of patients who did not receive similar goal-directed therapy (OR, 0.64; 95% CI, 0.50 to 0.83).

---

### KEY POINTS

- The only proven measures to prevent AKI are vigorous, goal-directed fluid administration, avoidance of hypotension, and minimizing of exposure to nephrotoxic medications.
- Management of AKI includes treatment of the underlying cause, fluid and electrolyte management, nutritional support, adjustment of drug dosing, and renal replacement therapy.

---

## FLUID RESUSCITATION

A child with a clinical history and physical examination findings consistent with hypovolemia and impending or established prerenal AKI requires immediate vigorous intravenous fluid therapy with normal saline (10 to 20 mL/kg over 30 min, repeated twice if necessary, until urine output is reestablished). Careful observation should be employed to avoid excessive hydration. If urine output does not improve after restoration of intravascular volume, more invasive monitoring may be required to guide further therapy. In children not responsive to volume repletion alone, preservation of blood pressure and renal perfusion with appropriate inotropic agents is essential to prevent AKI.[106–109]

## MINIMIZING NEPHROTOXIC IMPACTS

The importance of monitoring serum creatinine levels as a measure of kidney function in children receiving nephrotoxic drugs has been brought into focus in a retrospective single-center study of 1660 noncritically ill hospitalized children.[27] Children who developed AKI as defined by the serum creatinine–based pRIFLE criteria had significantly greater odds of exposure to one or more nephrotoxic medications than did patients without AKI (OR, 1.7; 95% CI, 1.04 to 2.9). Both increasing dose and duration of nephrotoxin use were associated with increased development of AKI. It is crucial that clinicians caring for patients requiring potentially nephrotoxic drugs use appropriate drug dosing based on the knowledge of altered pharmacokinetics in early AKI and be vigilant in monitoring for drug efficacy and toxicity. One study demonstrated decreasing AKI duration when systematic daily serum creatinine monitoring policy was put into practice for children who received multiple nephrotoxic medications.[28]

## INTERVENTIONS OF UNCLEAR BENEFIT

These include mannitol, loop diuretics, low-dose dopamine, fenoldopam, atrial natriuretic peptide, and N-acetylcysteine. The potential use of these agents in AKI prevention is discussed here.

### Mannitol

Experimental studies suggest that mannitol may be protective by causing diuresis (which minimizes intratubular cast formation) and by acting as a free radical scavenger (thereby minimizing cell injury). In the clinical setting, the efficacy of mannitol for prevention of AKI is inconclusive, and its use can result in significant side effects including volume expansion, hyperosmolality, and pulmonary edema. Its use for prevention of AKI is not recommended.

### Loop diuretics

Furosemide induces forced diuresis, and it also reduces active sodium chloride (NaCl) transport in the thick ascending limb of the loop of Henle; the ensuing decrease in energy requirement may protect the tubule cells in the presence of a decrease in energy delivery. However, the available evidence from clinical studies in adults does not support the routine use of diuretics as prophylaxis for AKI.[55] Although controlled studies have demonstrated that the administration of furosemide to patients in the early stages of AKI does not significantly alter the natural history of the disease, furosemide can potentially convert the syndrome from an oliguric form to a nonoliguric form and therefore simplify fluid, electrolyte, and nutritional management. In addition, a prospective assessment of a furosemide challenge, or furosemide "stress" test, was able to predict which adult patients would have worsening AKI based on a lack of response to the furosemide within 2 h.[110]

## Dopamine

The use of a low "renal dose" of the inotropic agent dopamine (0.5 to 3 mg/kg/min) had been common in the critical care setting because of its renal vasodilatory and natriuretic effects. However, prospective randomized studies of adult patients at risk for AKI have not shown a beneficial renoprotective effect of "low-dose" dopamine.[111,112] There are risks associated with even low-dose dopamine, including tachycardia, arrhythmias, myocardial ischemia, and intestinal ischemia. Therefore, the routine use of dopamine for prevention of AKI is not recommended.

## Fenoldopam

This is a potent, short-acting, selective dopamine A-1 receptor agonist that increases renal blood flow and decreases systemic vascular resistance. A meta-analysis of 16 randomized studies with a total of 622 adult patients administered fenoldopam and 668 given placebo or other therapy (principally low-dose dopamine) for the prevention or treatment of AKI concluded that fenoldopam significantly reduced the risk for AKI, the need for dialysis, and mortality rates.[113] Experience with fenoldopam in the pediatric age group is limited. A small prospective single-center randomized double-blind controlled trial of children undergoing CPB revealed a significant reduction in the urinary AKI biomarker NGAL at the end of the surgical procedure and 12 hours after ICU admission in the group receiving fenoldopam.[114] Confirmation of the benefits of fenoldopam in a large multicenter randomized controlled trial is required before routinely recommending this agent for the prevention of AKI.

## Natriuretic peptides

Atrial natriuretic peptide (ANP) and B-type natriuretic peptide (BNP) block tubular reabsorption of sodium and vasodilate the afferent arteriole. The renoprotective effects of these agents have been evaluated primarily in trials of adults undergoing cardiac surgical procedures and with congestive heart failure. Although initial data seemed promising, more recent evidence from large randomized trials failed to show a clinic benefit from these agents.[115,116] Pediatric data for the renoprotective effects of natriuretic peptides are limited. In a small retrospective study of 20 children with decompensated heart failure, recombinant human BNP (nesiritide) resulted in increased urine output and decreased serum creatinine concentrations.[117] Pending further randomized controlled trial data, the routine use of natriuretic peptides for prophylaxis against AKI is not recommended.

## N-acetylcysteine

N-acetylcysteine (NAC) is a free radical scavenger antioxidant agent that counteracts the deleterious effects of reactive oxygen species in the generation of tubule cell injury and also has vasodilatory properties. Several meta-analyses examined the efficacy of NAC in the prevention of AKI following cardiac and other major surgical procedures, as well as the prevention of contrast-induced nephropathy in adults. Given that the overall direction of the data is toward benefit and the agent is well tolerated and relatively inexpensive, the use of NAC in high-risk patients is generally recommended.[15] Although NAC is commonly used in children for treatment of acetaminophen toxicity and other forms of acute liver failure, data for its renoprotective effects in the pediatric population are limited. The routine use of NAC for AKI prophylaxis in children is therefore not recommended, with the exception of judicious use in children with CKD who are at high risk for contrast-induced nephropathy.

## MANAGEMENT

The basic principles of the general management of the child with AKI include treatment of the underlying cause, fluid and electrolyte management, nutritional support, adjustment of drug dosing, and renal replacement therapy. In general, prompt consultation and referral to a pediatric nephrologist are recommended for the management of intrinsic AKI, especially in the critically ill child.

## FLUID VOLUME BALANCE

Appropriate immediate fluid management is crucial in children with AKI. Based on the underlying cause, comorbid conditions, and possible previous therapy, the child may be hypovolemic, euvolemic, or hypervolemic. Accurate initial assessment, and careful follow-up with accurate records of fluid input and output as well as body weights, physical examinations, and additional invasive monitoring as needed, will guide the appropriate fluid therapy. A child with a clinical history and physical examination consistent with hypovolemia requires immediate intravenous fluid therapy in an attempt to restore renal function and prevent the progression of prerenal AKI to intrinsic AKI. Commonly used fluids are crystalloid solutions, such as normal saline (10 to 20 mL/kg given over 30 min, repeated twice as needed, monitoring vital signs for appropriate responses). If urine output does not increase and renal function fails to improve with the restoration of intravascular volume, bladder catheterization is recommended to confirm the anuria, and other forms of invasive monitoring may be required to assess the child's fluid status adequately and help guide further therapy. Conversely, a child with signs of fluid overload may require immediate fluid removal or fluid restriction. In such a child who is fluid replete and oliguric for less than 24 h, a trial of furosemide may be attempted to convert the AKI from an oliguric type to a nonoliguric type. Furosemide-induced diuresis can simplify fluid, electrolyte, and nutritional management. Furosemide should be promptly discontinued if the bolus doses do not result in a diuretic response, as would be expected in patients with established AKI. Care should be taken to avoid hypotension from overzealous diuretic therapy because that can increase the risk of nonrecovery of kidney function or death. The risk of ototoxicity from furosemide use in this setting remains significant. In addition, there is evidence in adults with established AKI that the use of diuretics may be associated with adverse clinical outcomes. Diuretics should not be used to postpone initiation of dialysis. Early consideration for renal replacement therapy is essential in a child with AKI and fluid overload, especially if the required fluid restriction is a hindrance to adequate nutrition.

Once euvolemia has been established, the clinician must pay careful attention to ongoing fluid losses (insensible water loss of approximately 300 to 500 mL/m$^2$/day in addition to replacement of urine and gastrointestinal losses) and gains (fluids, medications, and nutrition administered). Insensible water losses are higher in febrile children and lower in ventilated children with decreased respiratory losses. In patients with fluid overload, the achievement of negative balance may require replacement of less than the total urine output. Renal replacement therapy should be considered for children in intensive care with AKI and a greater than 10% fluid overload who are not expected to recover kidney function expeditiously.

## ELECTROLYTE AND ACID-BASE BALANCE

Appropriate electrolyte management is crucial in children with AKI and is also based on the underlying cause, comorbid conditions, and expected complications. In general, electrolyte disturbances are asymptomatic and require a high index of suspicion and routine monitoring for early detection. Patients with oligoanuric AKI should not receive potassium or phosphorus unless they exhibit significant hypokalemia or hypophosphatemia. Sodium intake should be restricted to 2 to 3 mEq/kg/day, to prevent sodium and fluid retention with resultant hypertension. Children with polyuric AKI are at risk for electrolyte losses, which may need to be replaced. Ongoing therapy in such patients can be guided by monitoring of plasma and urinary electrolytes.

Hyperkalemia in children with AKI is usually asymptomatic, but it can constitute a medical emergency. Symptoms are nonspecific and may include malaise, nausea, and muscle weakness. Electrocardiographic changes should be looked for in all patients suspected to have hyperkalemia, including (in sequence according to the severity of hyperkalemia) tall peaked T waves, prolonged PR interval, flattened P waves, widened QRS complex, and ventricular tachycardia and fibrillation. The management of hyperkalemia depends on the onset and severity and is outlined in Table 30.13. Mild to moderate hyperkalemia (serum potassium of 5.5 to 6.5 mEq/L) is treated by eliminating all sources of potassium from the diet or intravenous fluids and administration of an ion exchange resin such as sodium polystyrene sulfonate. This therapy requires several hours of contact with the colonic mucosa to be effective. In addition, patients with hyperkalemia who continue to have some urine output may benefit from the kaliuresis induced by intravenous administration of loop diuretics such as furosemide, but care should be exercised to avoid fluid depletion and hypotension. Emergency treatment is indicated when the serum potassium exceeds 6.5 mEq/L or if any electrocardiographic changes are present. In addition to ion exchange resin, such patients should receive calcium gluconate on an emergency basis to counteract the effects of hyperkalemia on the myocardium. Uptake of potassium by cells can be stimulated by infusion of glucose and insulin (in the absence of significant fluid overload), the β-agonist albuterol by nebulizer, or intravenous sodium bicarbonate. In practice, the definitive therapy for significant hyperkalemia in oliguric AKI often includes dialysis, and the nondialytic therapy outlined earlier serves mostly to tide over the crisis.

High–anion gap metabolic acidosis is common in AKI. Administration of sodium bicarbonate should be initiated only in life-threatening situations in which respiratory compensation is inadequate, or the acidosis is contributing to worsening hyperkalemia. In cases of severe or progressive acidosis following shock, serious infections, or other hypercatabolic states, supplemental bicarbonate may be required to correct and maintain arterial pH to more than 7.2 until the underlying disease is controlled. In general, children with serum bicarbonate levels that are greater

Table 30.13 Nondialytic pharmacotherapy of hyperkalemia

| Agent | Mechanism | Dose | Onset of action |
|---|---|---|---|
| Sodium polystyrene sulfonate (Kayexalate) | Exchanges Na$^+$ for K$^+$ across colonic mucosa | 1 g/kg PO or PR with sorbitol | 1–2 h |
| Calcium gluconate | Stabilizes the myocardial membrane potential | 50 mg/kg IV (max. dose 2 grams) over 5–15 min | Immediate |
| Glucose and insulin | Stimulate cellular uptake of K$^+$ | Glucose 0.5 g/kg, insulin 0.1 unit/kg over 30 min | 30 min |
| β Agonists (albuterol) | Stimulate cellular uptake of K$^+$ | 5–10 mg dose by nebulizer | 30 min |
| Sodium bicarbonate | Shifts K$^+$ into cells | 1 mEq/kg IV over 10 min | 15 min |

Abbreviations: IV, intravenously; K$^+$, potassium; Na$^+$, sodium, PO, orally; PR, rectally.

than 14 mEq/L or with an arterial pH greater than 7.2 do not require bicarbonate administration. Overzealous use of bicarbonate therapy in AKI can precipitate hypocalcemia and hypernatremia.

## NUTRITIONAL SUPPORT

AKI is associated with marked catabolism, and aggressive nutritional support is crucial to enhance the recovery process. Adequate calories to account for maintenance requirements and supplemental calories to combat excessive catabolism should be administered. Infants should receive at least 120 Kcal/kg/day, and older children should be administered at least 150% of maintenance caloric intake. In addition, AKI in critically ill children results in abnormal amino acid synthesis, as well as increased protein catabolism. Furthermore, all forms of renal replacement therapy (including continuous venovenous hemofiltration [CVVH], continuous venovenous hemodialysis [CVVHD], and continuous venovenous hemodialfiltration [CVVHDF]) result in amino acid losses of up to 20% of the amount normally provided by parenteral nutrition.[118] Therefore, children with AKI should be provided with at least 3 g/kg/day of daily protein intake, and those undergoing renal replacement therapy should receive replacement for the additional 20% of amino acid losses. Some recommendations aim to maintain the BUN at the 40 to 80 mg/dL range as a guide to determine whether adequate protein intake is being provided for children undergoing replacement therapy. Hyperalimentation should be considered early because the majority of children with AKI will encounter nausea and anorexia and will not be able to tolerate the oral or other enteral routes. If adequate protein and calorie nutrition cannot be achieved because of fluid restriction, renal replacement therapy should be instituted early in the course of the illness.

## DRUG DOSING

Nephrotoxic agents should be avoided in AKI because they may worsen the injury and delay recovery of function. Critically ill children with AKI are at risk for adverse outcomes of drug therapy. It has been reported that approximately half of patients with reduced renal clearance receive drug doses that are 2.5 times higher than the recommended maximum dose. Drug dosing in the setting of AKI is complicated by several factors. Pharmacokinetic changes include decreases in protein binding and drug metabolism. The volume of distribution of hydrophilic agents can increase as a result of fluid overload and decreased binding of the drug to serum proteins, and drug doses must be adjusted to account for these changes. Serum creatinine–based renal function estimations most often overestimate renal clearance in AKI. Many drugs are significantly cleared by renal replacement therapies. To ensure efficacy and prevent toxicity, therapeutic drug monitoring is highly recommended. However, in the absence of drug monitoring (as is the case for most

medications), adequate concentrations can be inferred only from the clinical response.

Pharmacologic management of children with AKI is best accomplished by close collaboration and consultation with trained pharmacology and pharmacy teams. In general, the dose of all medications should be adjusted based on residual renal function, to avoid toxic accumulation of drugs and their metabolites that are normally excreted by the kidney, as well as to avoid worsening the AKI. When the GFR falls to less than 50% of normal, most drugs excreted by the kidney require modifications in dose or scheduling. However, patients with documented AKI in the early phase with a rising creatinine should be assumed to have a GFR of less than 10 mL/min, and medications should be dosed accordingly, irrespective of the absolute value of the serum creatinine, because of the known delay in serum creatinine to rise to steady-state levels. Where possible, treatment should be modified empirically according to systemic drug-level targets.

## RENAL REPLACEMENT THERAPY

The common indications for acute dialytic therapy in AKI include the following: (1) fluid overload that is unresponsive to diuretics or is a hindrance to adequate nutrition; (2) hyperkalemia that is unresponsive to nondialytic therapy; (3) refractory hypertension; and (4) symptomatic uremia, including pericarditis, pleuritis, and neurologic symptoms. The choices available include hemodialysis (HD), peritoneal dialysis (PD), and CRRT. These modalities are described in detail in other chapters, and only general comments pertaining to AKI are included here. The choice of dialysis modality depends on the clinical status of the patient, the expertise of the physician, and the availability of appropriate resources. HD requires central vascular access, specialized equipment and technical personnel, anticoagulation (except in patients with coagulopathy), and the ability to tolerate a large extracorporeal volume. Critically ill patients frequently require pressor support for effective HD. The advantage of HD in the setting of AKI lies in its ability to correct imbalances in fluid, electrolyte, and acid-base status rapidly. The advantages of PD include ease of performance and no requirement for specialized equipment, personnel, or systemic anticoagulation. PD is frequently the therapy of choice in neonates and small infants.

The transition from the use of adaptive CRRT equipment to production of hemofiltration machines with volumetric control allowing for accurate ultrafiltration flows has led to a change in pediatric renal replacement therapy modality prevalence patterns.[119,120] Accurate ultrafiltration and blood flow rates are crucial for pediatric CRRT because the extracorporeal circuit volume can comprise more than 15% of a small pediatric patients' total blood volume, and small inaccuracies in ultrafiltration may represent a large percentage of the patient's total body water. Polls of US pediatric nephrologists demonstrate increased CRRT use over PD as the preferred modality for treating pediatric AKI. CRRT is especially useful in the presence of hemodynamic instability and multiorgan dysfunction because it allows for gentle, continuous management of fluid overload.

## CRITICALLY ILL PEDIATRIC PATIENTS

As opposed to adults, children tend to develop severe and life-threatening multiorgan dysfunction syndrome very early in their ICU course. Methods to identify patients at risk and aggressive initiation of supportive measures such as CRRT could conceivably improve the outcome. For example, children who receive CRRT and have a requirement for pressor support display a higher mortality than those who do not need pressors in the course of their AKI treatment.[121] As noted earlier, more recent data demonstrate that worsening fluid overload is an independent risk factor for mortality in critically ill children who receive CRRT, irrespective of the severity of illness.[98] These results suggest that early initiation of CRRT at lesser degrees of fluid overload may allow for more optimal nutrition and blood product provision without the further accumulation of fluid or catabolic waste products, thereby improving the outcome.

## INFANTS

Infants and neonates with AKI present unique problems for renal replacement therapy provision. Delivery of HD or CRRT entails a significant portion of their blood volume to be pumped through the extracorporeal circuit. Therefore, extracorporeal circuit volumes that comprise more than 10% to 15% of patient blood volume should be primed with whole blood to prevent hypotension and anemia. Because the prime volume is not discarded, it is important to not reinfuse the blood into the patient at the end of the treatment, to prevent volume overload and hypertension. Short-term PD requires much less technical expertise, expense, and equipment compared with intermittent HD and CRRT. PD catheters can be placed quickly and easily. Initial dwell volumes should be limited to 10 mL/kg of the patient's body weight, to minimize intra-abdominal pressure and the potential for fluid leakage along the catheter tunnel. Although PD may deliver less efficient solute removal than HD or CRRT, its relative simplicity and minimal associated side effects allow for renal replacement therapy provision in settings lacking pediatric dialysis–specific support and personnel. CRRT has been prescribed since the mid-1980s for treatment of AKI in critically ill infants. A more recent evaluation of the CVVH course for 90 infants weighing less than 10 kg demonstrated very few technical complications using newer CVVH machinery.[122,123] Survival for infants receiving CRRT has been noted to be at 35% to 38%, which is similar to survival rates for older children. A newer neonatal CRRT device, the Cardio-Renal, Pediatric Dialysis Emergency Machine (CARPEDIEM), with a low extracorporeal volume of 42 mL and fluid balance errors of only 1 mL/h, is undergoing evaluation in Europe currently.[124]

## CONGENITAL HEART DISEASE

Using recent definitions, the incidence of infant AKI after CPB ranges from 40% to 60%, with survival rates ranging up to 90%.[20,21,103,125] Risk factors for death include increasing underlying complexity of the congenital heart disease and poor cardiac function. A trend toward providing PD therapy earlier in the post-CPB course has been reported, and a study of 20 patients demonstrated 80% patient survival.[126] Improved survival with early PD initiation may result from prevention of fluid overload and from increased clearance of CPB-induced proinflammatory cytokines. Some institutions have advocated the prophylactic use of PD immediately postoperatively to prevent fluid accumulation in patients with high-risk underlying diagnoses such as hypoplastic left heart syndrome, transposition of the great arteries, or anomalous pulmonary venous return.

## PROGNOSIS AND OUTCOME

In general, pediatric AKI has serious short-term and long-term consequences. The outcome depends on the cause, the age of the child, and comorbidities. In terms of mortality, severe AKI requiring renal replacement therapy in children is still associated with a mortality rate of approximately 30% to 50%, and this has not changed appreciably since the 1980s. Infants less than 1 year of age have the highest mortality rate. In the largest study reported to date, 3396 admissions to a single pediatric ICU in the United States were retrospectively analyzed using RIFLE criteria to define AKI.[24] Those patients who presented with AKI on admission to the ICU had a 32% mortality rate, and those who developed AKI at any time during the ICU stay had a 30% mortality rate. AKI on admission to the ICU was associated with an increased risk of mortality (adjusted OR, 5.4; 95% CI, 3.5 to 8.4). Development of AKI during the ICU stay was associated with an even greater risk of mortality (adjusted OR, 8.7; 95% CI, 6.0 to 12.6) and a fourfold increase in length of hospital stay.

Despite important technical advances in renal replacement therapies and critical care, children with severe AKI have a concomitant increasing severity of illness, so that an improvement in survival rates is not readily apparent. In a

---

## KEY POINTS

- Severe AKI requiring renal replacement therapy in children is still associated with a mortality rate of 30% to 50%.
- Long-term follow-up for development of CKD is warranted for children who survive an episode of AKI.

retrospective analysis of 344 patients from the Prospective Pediatric Continuous Renal Replacement Therapy (ppCRRT) Registry, the overall mortality rate was 42%.[17] There was better survival in patients with principal diagnoses of drug intoxication (100%), primary renal disease (84%), tumor lysis syndrome (83%), and inborn errors of metabolism (73%). Survival was lowest in patients with liver disease or transplant (31%), pulmonary disease or transplant (45%), and bone marrow transplant (45%).

Information regarding the long-term outcome of children after an episode of AKI is beginning to accumulate. In a multicenter pooled analysis of 3476 children with hemolytic-uremic syndrome who were followed up for a mean of 4.4 years, the combined average death and end-stage renal disease rate was 12% (95% CI, 10% to 15%), and the combined average renal sequelae rate (CKD, proteinuria, hypertension) was 25% (95% CI, 20% to 30%).[127] Thus, long-term follow-up appears to be warranted after an acute episode of hemolytic-uremic syndrome. Long-term follow-up of premature infants with neonatal AKI has shown a 45% rate of renal insufficiency.[128] Prominent risk factors for progression include an increased random urine protein-to-creatinine ratio and a serum creatinine level greater than 0.6 mg/dL at 1 year of age. More recent long-term follow-up studies demonstrate that 40% to 60% of patients surviving an AKI episode have a sign of CKD, including proteinuria, hyperfiltration, low estimated GFR, or hypertension.[129,130] Collectively, these data strongly suggest that long-term follow-up is warranted for children who survive an episode of AKI.

## SUMMARY

Acute kidney injury represents a very significant and potentially devastating problem in pediatric medicine. The precise incidence of pediatric AKI is not known, but it appears to be rising. Outstanding advances in basic research have illuminated the pathogenesis of AKI and have paved the way for successful therapeutic approaches in animal models. However, translational research efforts in humans have yielded disappointing results. A major reason for this is the lack of early markers for AKI, akin to troponins in acute myocardial disease, and hence an unacceptable delay in initiating therapy. In current clinical practice, AKI is typically diagnosed by measuring serum creatinine, which is an unreliable indicator during acute changes in kidney function. However, animal studies have shown that although AKI can be prevented or treated by several maneuvers, these measures must be instituted very early after the insult. The lack of early AKI biomarkers in humans has hitherto crippled our ability to launch potentially effective therapies in a timely manner. Fortunately, several potential candidates are currently being developed and tested as sequential noninvasive early biomarkers for the prediction

of AKI and its severity. It is likely that not any one biomarker but a collection of strategically selected proteins may provide the hitherto elusive "AKI panel" for the early and rapid diagnosis of AKI. Such a tool would be indispensable for the timely institution of potentially effective therapies in human intrinsic AKI, a common clinical condition still associated with a dismal prognosis and in which early intervention is desperately needed. Clinical Vignette 30.1 illustrates the course of AKI in a young boy.

## ACKNOWLEDGMENT

Studies completed by the authors and reported herein were funded by a grant from the National Institutes of Health (P50 DK096418).

### Clinical Vignette 30.1

A previously healthy 5-year-old 20-kg boy was brought to the emergency department 2 days ago, with complaints of fever, vomiting, and ankle pain. On arrival, he had a temperature of 103° F, heart rate of 150/min, blood pressure of 76/42 mm Hg, and a tender erythematous rash over his left ankle. Laboratory test results showed a blood urea nitrogen (BUN) of 45 mg/dL and serum creatinine 0.8 mg/dL. He received two fluid boluses of 0.9% NaCl (40 mL/kg in total), as well as intravenous ceftriaxone. With no improvement in blood pressure, he was transferred to the intensive care unit. He remained hypotensive and required multiple additional fluid boluses and vasopressors. By the next morning, the initial blood culture results returned positive for Gram-positive cocci in clusters. Intravenous vancomycin was added to his regimen. The BUN was 80 mg/dL and serum creatinine was 2.0 mg/dL.

By the second day, the patient developed oliguria and peripheral and pulmonary edema, and he needed mechanical ventilation. His weight was now 25 kg, and the total fluid intake and output were very imbalanced (6 L in and 1 L out). The BUN was 120 mg/dL and the serum creatinine was 4.5 mg/dL. Multiple doses of intravenous furosemide failed to result in a diuretic response. A kidney ultrasound scan done at the bedside showed bilaterally enlarged and echogenic kidneys, with no hydronephrosis. The blood culture returned positive for methicillin-resistant *Staphylococcus aureus*. A nephrology consultation was requested.

### TEACHING POINTS

1. At the time of renal consultation, it was quite obvious that the child in Clinical Vignette 30.1 had acute kidney injury (AKI). However, even at

the time of initial presentation to the emergency department, there was evidence of AKI. A healthy 5-year-old child should have a serum creatinine in the 0.5 mg/dL range. At presentation, the history of fever and vomiting and the physical findings of tachycardia and hypotension would be compatible with community-acquired prerenal AKI secondary to dehydration. The initial elevated blood urea nitrogen (BUN)–to-creatinine ratio (45/0.8 = 56) also supports this assessment. If measured before fluid therapy, the fractional excretion of sodium (FENa) would have been less than 0.1%.

2. Sometime during the early course of his illness, there was clearly a deleterious shift from prerenal to intrinsic AKI. This is evidenced by several findings. First, both the BUN and serum creatinine continued to rise despite aggressive fluid resuscitation. Second, he was nonresponsive to loop diuretics. Third, the absence of shrunken kidneys on ultrasound makes chronic kidney disease less likely, and the absence of hydronephrosis eliminates obstruction. Fourth, many potential causes of intrinsic AKI are apparent, including prolonged hypotension, sepsis, and nephrotoxins.

3. This child already satisfies the indications for initiation of renal replacement therapy. First, he has severe fluid overload (25%). Second, his high fluid requirements (for nutrition, vasopressor drips, antibiotics, crystalloids and colloids, and blood products) are likely to continue. Third, he requires clearance of accumulating uremic toxins. Given his tenuous clinical condition, the treatment of choice would be continuous renal replacement therapy. In addition, adequate nutrition should be provided (by total parenteral nutrition), potassium intake should be restricted, and additional nephrotoxin use should be avoided. Antibiotics should be continued to treat the underlying cause. His short-term prognosis remains guarded and depends on the efficacy of renal and other supportive care. He will require long-term follow-up because he is at risk for developing chronic kidney disease in the future.

# REFERENCES

1. Hui-Stickle S, Brewer ED, Goldstein SL. Pediatric ARF epidemiology at a tertiary care center from 1999 to 2001. Am J Kidney Dis. 2005;45:96–101.

2. Devarajan P. Update on mechanisms of ischemic acute kidney injury. J Am Soc Nephrol. 2006;17:1503–20.

3. Goldstein SL. Advances in pediatric renal replacement therapy for acute kidney injury. Semin Dialy. 2011;24:187–91.

4. Uchino S, Kellum JA, Bellomo R, et al. Acute renal failure in critically ill patients: A multinational, multicenter study. JAMA. 2005;294:813–8.

5. Askenazi DJ, Ambalavanan N, Goldstein SL. Acute kidney injury in critically ill newborns: What do we know? What do we need to learn? Pediatr Nephrol. 2009;24:265–74.

6. Singbartl K, Kellum JA. AKI in the ICU: Definition, epidemiology, risk stratification, and outcomes. Kidney Int. 2012;81:819–25.

7. Kellum JA, Angus DC. Patients are dying of acute renal failure. Crit Care Med. 2002;30:2156–7.

8. Bellomo R, Ronco C, Kellum JA, et al. Acute renal failure—Definition, outcome measures, animal models, fluid therapy and information technology needs: The Second International Consensus Conference of the Acute Dialysis Quality Initiative (ADQI) Group. Crit Care. 2004;8:R204–12.

9. Akcan-Arikan A, Zappitelli M, Loftis LL, et al. Modified RIFLE criteria in critically ill children with acute kidney injury. Kidney Int. 2007;71:1028–35.

10. Srisawat N, Hoste EE, Kellum JA. Modern classification of acute kidney injury. Blood Purif. 2010;29:300–7.

11. Slater MB, Anand V, Uleryk EM, Parshuram CS. A systematic review of RIFLE criteria in children, and its application and association with measures of mortality and morbidity. Kidney Int. 2012;81:791–8.

12. Mehta RL, Kellum JA, Shah SV, et al. Acute Kidney Injury Network: Report of an initiative to improve outcomes in acute kidney injury. Crit Care. 2007;11.

13. Chertow GM, Burdick E, Honour M, et al. Acute kidney injury, mortality, length of stay, and costs in hospitalized patients. J Am Soc Nephrol. 2005;16:3365–70.

14. Price JF, Mott AR, Dickerson HA, et al. Worsening renal function in children hospitalized with decompensated heart failure: Evidence for a pediatric cardiorenal syndrome? Pediatr Crit Care Med. 2008;9:279–84.

15. Kidney Disease: Improving Global Outcomes (KDIGO) Acute Kidney Injury Work Group—KDIGO clinical practice guideline for acute kidney injury. Kidney Int Suppl. 2012;2:1–138.

16. McCullough PA, Bouchard J, Waikar SS, et al. Implementation of novel biomarkers in the diagnosis, prognosis, and management of acute kidney injury: Executive summary from the tenth consensus conference of the Acute Dialysis Quality Initiative (ADQI). Contrib Nephrol. 2013;182:5–12.

17. Symons JM, Chua AN, Somers MJ, et al. Demographic characteristics of pediatric continuous renal replacement therapy: A report of the prospective pediatric continuous renal replacement therapy registry. Clin J Am Soc Nephrol. 2007;2:732–8.

18. Vachvanichsanong P, Dissaneewate P, Lim A, McNeil E. Childhood acute renal failure: 22-year experience in a university hospital in southern Thailand. Pediatrics. 2006;118:e786–91.

19. Sutherland SM, Ji J, Sheikhi FH, et al. AKI in hospitalized children: Epidemiology and clinical associations in a national cohort. Clin J Am Soc Nephrol. 2013;8:1661–9.

20. Blinder JJ, Goldstein SL, Lee VV, et al. Congenital heart surgery in infants: Effects of acute kidney injury on outcomes. J Thorac Cardiovasc Surg. 2012;143:368–74.

21. Krawczeski CD, Goldstein SL, Woo JG, et al. Temporal relationship and predictive value of urinary acute kidney injury biomarkers after pediatric cardiopulmonary bypass. J Am Coll Cardiol. 2011;58:2301–9.

22. Zappitelli M, Bernier PL, Saczkowski RS, et al. A small post-operative rise in serum creatinine predicts acute kidney injury in children undergoing cardiac surgery. Kidney Int. 2009;76:885–92.

23. Koralkar R, Ambalavanan N, Levitan EB, et al. Acute kidney injury reduces survival in very low birth weight infants. Pediatr Res. 2011;69:354–8.

24. Schneider J, Khemani R, Grushkin C, Bart R. Serum creatinine as stratified in the RIFLE score for acute kidney injury is associated with mortality and length of stay for children in the pediatric intensive care unit. Crit Care Med. 2010;38:933–9.

25. Plotz FB, Bouma AB, van Wijk JA, et al. Pediatric acute kidney injury in the ICU: An independent evaluation of pRIFLE criteria. Intensive Care Med. 2008;34:1713–7.

26. Zappitelli M, Parikh CR, Akcan-Arikan A, et al. Ascertainment and epidemiology of acute kidney injury varies with definition interpretation. Clin J Am Soc Nephrol. 2008;3:948–54.

27. Moffett BS, Goldstein SL. Acute kidney injury and increasing nephrotoxic-medication exposure in noncritically-ill children. Clin J Am Soc Nephrol. 2011;6:856–63.

28. Goldstein SL, Kirkendall E, Nguyen H, et al. Electronic health record identification of nephrotoxin exposure and associated acute kidney injury. Pediatrics. 2013;132:e756–67.

29. Endre ZH, Kellum JA, Di Somma S, et al. Differential diagnosis of AKI in clinical practice by functional and damage biomarkers: Workgroup statements from the tenth Acute Dialysis Quality Initiative Consensus Conference. Contrib Nephrol. 2013;182:30–44.

30. Loutzenhiser R, Bidani AK, Wang X. Systolic pressure and the myogenic response of the renal afferent arteriole. Acta Physiol Scand. 2004;181:407–13.

31. Breyer MD, Hao C, Qi Z. Cyclooxygenase-2 selective inhibitors and the kidney. Curr Opin Crit Care. 2001;7:393–400.

32. Perazella MA. Renal vulnerability to drug toxicity. Clin J Am Soc Nephrol. 2009;4:1275–83.

33. Perazella MA. Drug-induced renal failure: Update on new medications and unique mechanisms of nephrotoxicity. Am J Med Sci. 2003;325:349–62.

34. Ichihara A, Kobori H, Nishiyama A, Navar LG. Renal renin-angiotensin system. Contrib Nephrol. 2004;143:117–30.

35. Arora P, Rajagopalam S, Ranjan R, et al. Preoperative use of angiotensin-converting enzyme inhibitors/angiotensin receptor blockers is associated with increased risk for acute kidney injury after cardiovascular surgery. Clin J Am Soc Nephrol. 2008;3:1266–73.

36. Moffett BS, Goldstein SL, Adusei M, et al. Risk factors for postoperative acute kidney injury in pediatric cardiac surgery patients receiving angiotensin-converting enzyme inhibitors. Pediatr Crit Care Med. 2011;12:555–9.

37. Nejat M, Pickering JW, Devarajan P, et al. Some biomarkers of acute kidney injury are increased in pre-renal acute injury. Kidney Int. 2012;81:1254–62.

38. Safirstein RL. Acute renal failure: From renal physiology to the renal transcriptome. Kidney Int Suppl. 2004;S62–6.

39. Castaneda MP, Swiatecka-Urban A, Mitsnefes MM, et al. Activation of mitochondrial apoptotic pathways in human renal allografts after ischemia reperfusion injury. Transplantation. 2003;76:50–4.

40. Bonventre JV, Zuk A. Ischemic acute renal failure: An inflammatory disease? Kidney Int. 2004;66:480–5.

41. Friedewald JJ, Rabb H. Inflammatory cells in ischemic acute renal failure. Kidney Int. 2004;66:486–91.

42. Molitoris BA, Sutton TA. Endothelial injury and dysfunction: Role in the extension phase of acute renal failure. Kidney Int. 2004;66:496–9.

43. Sutton TA, Fisher CJ, Molitoris BA. Microvascular endothelial injury and dysfunction during ischemic acute renal failure. Kidney Int. 2002;62:1539–49.

44. Sutton TA, Mang HE, Campos SB, et al. Injury of the renal microvascular endothelium alters barrier function after ischemia. Am J Physiol Renal Physiol. 2003;285:F191–8.

45. Sharfuddin AA, Molitoris BA. Pathophysiology of ischemic acute kidney injury. Nat Rev Nephrol. 2011;7:189–200.

46. Bonventre JV, Yang L. Cellular pathophysiology of ischemic acute kidney injury. J Clin Invest. 2011;121:4210–21.

47. Heyman SN, Evans RG, Rosen S, Rosenberger C. Cellular adaptive changes in AKI: Mitigating renal hypoxic injury. Nephrol Dial Transplant. 2012;27:1721–8.

48. Kinsey GR, Sharma R, Okusa MD. Regulatory T cells in AKI. J Am Soc Nephrol. 2013;24:1720–6.

49. Schrier RW, Wang W, Poole B, Mitra A. Acute renal failure: Definitions, diagnosis, pathogenesis, and therapy. J Clin Invest. 2004;114:5–14.

50. Jerkic M, Miloradovic Z, Jovovic D, et al. Relative roles of endothelin-1 and angiotensin II in experimental post-ischaemic acute renal failure. Nephrol Dial Transplant. 2004;19:83–94.

51. Wang A, Holcslaw T, Bashore TM, et al. Exacerbation of radiocontrast nephrotoxicity by endothelin receptor antagonism. Kidney Int. 2000;57:1675–80.

52. Lameire NH, De Vriese AS, Vanholder R. Prevention and nondialytic treatment of acute renal failure. Curr Opin Crit Care. 2003;9:481–90.

53. Wangsiripaisan A, Gengaro PE, Edelstein CL, Schrier RW. Role of polymeric Tamm-Horsfall protein in cast formation: Oligosaccharide and tubular fluid ions. Kidney Int. 2001;59:932–40.

54. Cantarovich F, Rangoonwala B, Lorenz H, et al. High-dose furosemide for established ARF: A prospective, randomized, double-blind, placebo-controlled, multicenter trial. Am J Kidney Dis. 2004;44:402–9.

55. Bagshaw SM, Bellomo R, Kellum JA. Oliguria, volume overload, and loop diuretics. Crit Care Med. 2008;36:S172–8.

56. Gambaro G, Bertaglia G, Puma G, D'Angelo A. Diuretics and dopamine for the prevention and treatment of acute renal failure: A critical reappraisal. J Nephrol. 2002;15:213–9.

57. Kwon O, Corrigan G, Myers BD, et al. Sodium reabsorption and distribution of Na⁺/K⁺-ATPase during postischemic injury to the renal allograft. Kidney Int. 1999;55:963–75.

58. Schnermann J. Homer W. Smith Award lecture. The juxtaglomerular apparatus: From anatomical peculiarity to physiological relevance. J Am Soc Nephrol. 2003;14:1681–94.

59. Lee HT, Xu H, Nasr SH, et al. A1 adenosine receptor knockout mice exhibit increased renal injury following ischemia and reperfusion. Am J Physiol Renal Physiol. 2004;286:F298–306.

60. Laubach VE, French BA, Okusa MD. Targeting of adenosine receptors in ischemia-reperfusion injury. Expert Opin Ther Targets. 2011;15:103–18.

61. Siegel NJ, Van Why SK, Devarajan P. Pathogenesis of acute renal failure. In: Avner ED, Harmon WE, Niaudet P, editors. Pediatric Nephrology. 5th ed. Philadelphia: Lippincott Williams & Wilkins; 2004. p. 1223–32.

62. Acker CG, Flick R, Shapiro R, et al. Thyroid hormone in the treatment of post-transplant acute tubular necrosis (ATN). Am J Transplant. 2002;2:57–61.

63. Shilliday IR, Sherif M. Calcium channel blockers for preventing acute tubular necrosis in kidney transplant recipients. Cochrane Database Syst Rev. 2004;1:CD003421.

64. Himmelfarb J, McMonagle E, Freedman S, et al. Oxidative stress is increased in critically ill patients with acute renal failure. J Am Soc Nephrol. 2004;15:2449–56.

65. de Vries B, Walter SJ, von Bonsdorff L, et al. Reduction of circulating redox-active iron by apo-transferrin protects against renal ischemia-reperfusion injury. Transplantation. 2004;77:669–75.

66. Mishra J, Ma Q, Prada A, et al. Identification of neutrophil gelatinase-associated lipocalin as a novel early urinary biomarker for ischemic renal injury. J Am Soc Nephrol. 2003;14:2534–43.

67. Mishra J, Mori K, Ma Q, et al. Amelioration of ischemic acute renal injury by neutrophil gelatinase–associated lipocalin. J Am Soc Nephrol. 2004;15:3073–82.

68. Molitoris BA. Actin cytoskeleton in ischemic acute renal failure. Kidney Int. 2004;66:871–83.

69. Woroniecki R, Ferdinand JR, Morrow JS, Devarajan P. Dissociation of spectrin-ankyrin complex as a basis for loss of Na-K-ATPase polarity after ischemia. Am J Physiol Renal Physiol. 2003;284:F358–64.

70. Horton MA. Arg-gly-Asp (RGD) peptides and peptidomimetics as therapeutics: Relevance for renal diseases. Exp Nephrol. 1999;7:178–84.

71. Kaushal GP, Basnakian AG, Shah SV. Apoptotic pathways in ischemic acute renal failure. Kidney Int. 2004;66:500–6.

72. Supavekin S, Zhang W, Kucherlapati R, et al. Differential gene expression following early renal ischemia/reperfusion. Kidney Int. 2003;63:1714–24.

73. Kelly KJ, Plotkin Z, Vulgamott SL, Dagher PC. P53 mediates the apoptotic response to GTP depletion after renal ischemia-reperfusion: Protective role of a p53 inhibitor. J Am Soc Nephrol. 2003;14:128–38.

74. Del Rio M, Imam A, DeLeon M, et al. The death domain of kidney ankyrin interacts with Fas and promotes Fas-mediated cell death in renal epithelia. J Am Soc Nephrol. 2004;15:41–51.

75. Burns AT, Davies DR, McLaren AJ, et al. Apoptosis in ischemia/reperfusion injury of human renal allografts. Transplantation. 1998;66:872–6.

76. Oberbauer R, Rohrmoser M, Regele H, et al. Apoptosis of tubular epithelial cells in donor kidney biopsies predicts early renal allograft function. J Am Soc Nephrol. 1999;10:2006–13.

77. Schwarz C, Hauser P, Steininger R, et al. Failure of BCL-2 up-regulation in proximal tubular epithelial cells of donor kidney biopsy specimens is associated with apoptosis and delayed graft function. Lab Invest. 2002;82:941–8.

78. Hoffmann SC, Kampen RL, Amur S, et al. Molecular and immunohistochemical characterization of the onset and resolution of human renal allograft ischemia-reperfusion injury. Transplantation. 2002;74:916–23.

79. Hauser P, Schwarz C, Mitterbauer C, et al. Genome-wide gene-expression patterns of donor kidney biopsies distinguish primary allograft function. Lab Invest. 2004;84:353–61.

80. Devarajan P, Mishra J, Supavekin S, et al. Gene expression in early ischemic renal injury: Clues towards pathogenesis, biomarker discovery, and novel therapeutics. Mol Genet Metab. 2003;80:365–76.

81. Devarajan P. Apoptosis and necrosis. In: Ronco C, Bellomo R, Kellum JA, eds. Critical Care Nephrology, 2nd ed. Philadelphia: Saunders Elsevier; 2009.

82. Molitoris BA, Dagher PC, Sandoval RM, et al. siRNA targeted to p53 attenuates ischemic and cisplatin-induced acute kidney injury. J Am Soc Nephrol. 2009;20:1754–64.

83. Bonventre JV. Dedifferentiation and proliferation of surviving epithelial cells in acute renal failure. J Am Soc Nephrol. 2003;14(Suppl 1):S55–61.

84. Hammerman MR. Recapitulation of phylogeny by ontogeny in nephrology. Kidney Int. 2000;57:742–55.

85. Rookmaaker MB, Verhaar MC, van Zonneveld AJ, Rabelink TJ. Progenitor cells in the kidney: Biology and therapeutic perspectives. Kidney Int. 2004;66:518–22.

86. Morigi M, Imberti B, Zoja C, et al. Mesenchymal stem cells are renotropic, helping to repair the kidney and improve function in acute renal failure. J Am Soc Nephrol. 2004;15:1794–804.

87. Salmela K, Wramner L, Ekberg H, et al. A randomized multicenter trial of the anti–ICAM-1 monoclonal antibody (enlimomab) for the prevention of acute rejection and delayed onset of graft function in cadaveric renal transplantation: A report of the European Anti–ICAM-1 Renal Transplant Study Group. Transplantation. 1999;67:729–36.

88. Simmons EM, Himmelfarb J, Sezer MT, et al. Plasma cytokine levels predict mortality in patients with acute renal failure. Kidney Int. 2004;65:1357–65.

89. Doi K, Hu X, Yuen PS, et al. AP214, an analogue of alpha-melanocyte–stimulating hormone, ameliorates sepsis-induced acute kidney injury and mortality. Kidney Int. 2008;73:1266–74.

90. Peng Q, Li K, Smyth LA, et al. C3a and C5a promote renal ischemia-reperfusion injury. J Am Soc Nephrol. 2012;23:1474–85.

91. Lewis AG, Kohl G, Ma Q, et al. Pharmacological targeting of C5a receptors during organ preservation improves kidney graft survival. Clin Exp Immunol. 2008;153:117–26.

92. Zarjou A, Agarwal A. Sepsis and acute kidney injury. J Am Soc Nephrol. 2011;22:999–1006.

93. Wan L, Bagshaw SM, Langenberg C, et al. Pathophysiology of septic acute kidney injury: What do we really know? Crit Care Med. 2008;36:S198–203.

94. Fahimi D, Mohajeri S, Hajizadeh N, et al. Comparison between fractional excretions of urea and sodium in children with acute kidney injury. Pediatr Nephrol. 2009;24:2409–12.

95. Schwartz GJ, Munoz A, Schneider MF, et al. New equations to estimate GFR in children with CKD. J Am Soc Nephrol. 2009;20:629–37.

96. Foland JA, Fortenberry JD, Warshaw BL, et al. Fluid overload before continuous hemofiltration and survival in critically ill children: A retrospective analysis. Crit Care Med. 2004;32:1771–6.

97. Goldstein SL, Somers MJ, Baum MA, et al. Pediatric patients with multi-organ dysfunction syndrome receiving continuous renal replacement therapy. Kidney Int. 2005;67:653–8.

98. Sutherland SM, Zappitelli M, Alexander SR, et al. Fluid overload and mortality in children receiving continuous renal replacement therapy: The Prospective Pediatric Continuous Renal Replacement Therapy Registry. Am J Kidney Dis. 2010;55:316–25.

99. Devarajan P. Biomarkers for the early detection of acute kidney injury. Curr Opin Pediatr. 2011;23:194–200.

100. Devarajan P. Neutrophil gelatinase–associated lipocalin: A promising biomarker for human acute kidney injury. Biomark Med. 2010;4:265–80.

101. Mishra J, Dent C, Tarabishi R, et al. Neutrophil gelatinase–associated lipocalin (NGAL) as a biomarker for acute renal injury after cardiac surgery. Lancet. 2005;365:1231–8.

102. Krawczeski CD, Woo JG, Wang Y, et al. Neutrophil gelatinase–associated lipocalin concentrations predict development of acute kidney injury in neonates and children after cardiopulmonary bypass. J Pediatr. 2011;158:1009–15e1.

103. Parikh CR, Devarajan P, Zappitelli M, et al. Postoperative biomarkers predict acute kidney injury and poor outcomes after pediatric cardiac surgery. J Am Soc Nephrol. 2011;22:1737–47.

104. Haase M, Devarajan P, Haase-Fielitz A, et al. The outcome of neutrophil gelatinase–associated lipocalin-positive subclinical acute kidney injury: A multicenter pooled analysis of prospective studies. J Am Coll Cardiol. 2011;57:1752–61.

105. Brienza N, Giglio MT, Marucci M, Fiore T. Does perioperative hemodynamic optimization protect renal function in surgical patients? A meta-analytic study. Crit Care Med. 2009;37:2079–90.

106. Filler G. Acute renal failure in children: Aetiology and management. Paediatr Drugs. 2001;3:783–92.

107. Michael M, Kuehnle I, Goldstein SL. Fluid overload and acute renal failure in pediatric stem cell transplant patients. Pediatr Nephrol. 2004;19:91–5.

108. Goldstein SL. Fluid management in acute kidney injury. J Intensive Care Med. 2014;29:183–9.

109. Brierley J, Carcillo JA, Choong K, et al. Clinical practice parameters for hemodynamic support of pediatric and neonatal septic shock: 2007 update from the American College of Critical Care Medicine. Crit Care Med. 2009;37:666–88.

110. Chawla LS, Davison DL, Brasha-Mitchell E, et al. Development and standardization of a furosemide stress test to predict the severity of acute kidney injury. Crit Care. 2013;17:R207.

111. Lassnigg A, Donner E, Grubhofer G, et al. Lack of renoprotective effects of dopamine and furosemide during cardiac surgery. J Am Soc Nephrol. 2000;11:97–104.

112. Lauschke A, Teichgraber UK, Frei U, Eckardt KU. "Low-dose" dopamine worsens renal perfusion in patients with acute renal failure. Kidney Int. 2006;69:1669–74.

113. Landoni G, Biondi-Zoccai GG, Tumlin JA, et al. Beneficial impact of fenoldopam in critically ill patients with or at risk for acute renal failure: A meta-analysis of randomized clinical trials. Am J Kidney Dis. 2007;49:56–68.

114. Ricci Z, Luciano R, Favia I, et al. High-dose fenoldopam reduces postoperative neutrophil gelatinase–associated lipocaline and cystatin C levels in pediatric cardiac surgery. Crit Care. 2011;15:R160.

115. Gottlieb SS, Stebbins A, Voors AA, et al. Effects of nesiritide and predictors of urine output in acute decompensated heart failure: Results from ASCEND-HF (Acute Study of Clinical Effectiveness of Nesiritide and Decompensated Heart Failure). J Am Coll Cardiol. 2013;62:1177–83.

116. Yancy CW, Krum H, Massie BM, et al. Safety and efficacy of outpatient nesiritide in patients with advanced heart failure: Results of the Second Follow-Up Serial Infusions of Nesiritide (FUSION II) trial. Circ Heart Fail. 2008;1:9–16.

117. Jefferies JL, Price JF, Denfield SW, et al. Safety and efficacy of nesiritide in pediatric heart failure. J Card Fail. 2007;13:541–8.

118. Zappitelli M, Juarez M, Castillo L, et al. Continuous renal replacement therapy amino acid, trace metal and folate clearance in critically ill children. Intensive Care Med. 2009;35:698–706.

119. Flynn JT. Choice of dialysis modality for management of pediatric acute renal failure. Pediatr Nephrol. 2002;17:61–9.

120. Warady BA, Bunchman T. Dialysis therapy for children with acute renal failure: Survey results. Pediatr Nephrol. 2000;15:11–3.

121. Bunchman TE, McBryde KD, Mottes TE, et al. Pediatric acute renal failure: Outcome by modality and disease. Pediatr Nephrol. 2001;16:1067–71.

122. Symons JM, Brophy PD, Gregory MJ, et al. Continuous renal replacement therapy in children up to 10 kg. Am J Kidney Dis. 2003;41:984–9.

123. Askenazi DJ, Goldstein SL, Koralkar R, et al. Continuous renal replacement therapy for children ≤10 kg: A report from the prospective pediatric continuous renal replacement therapy registry. J Pediatr. 2013;162:587–92e3.

124. Ronco C, Garzotto F, Ricci Z. CA.R.PE.DI.E.M. (Cardio-Renal Pediatric Dialysis Emergency Machine): Evolution of continuous renal replacement therapies in infants. A personal journey. Pediatr Nephrol. 2012;27:1203–11.

125. Morgan CJ, Zappitelli M, Robertson CM, et al. Risk factors for and outcomes of acute kidney injury in neonates undergoing complex cardiac surgery. J Pediatr. 2013;162:120–7e1.

126. Sorof JM, Stromberg D, Brewer ED, et al. Early initiation of peritoneal dialysis after surgical repair of congenital heart disease. Pediatr Nephrol. 1999;13:641–5.

127. Garg AX, Suri RS, Barrowman N, et al. Long-term renal prognosis of diarrhea-associated hemolytic uremic syndrome: A systematic review, meta-analysis, and meta-regression. JAMA. 2003;290:1360–70.

128. Abitbol CL, Bauer CR, Montane B, et al. Long-term follow-up of extremely low birth weight infants with neonatal renal failure. Pediatr Nephrol. 2003;18:887–93.

129. Askenazi DJ, Feig DI, Graham NM, et al. 3–5 year longitudinal follow-up of pediatric patients after acute renal failure. Kidney Int. 2006;69:184–9.

130. Mammen C, Al Abbas A, Skippen P, et al. Long-term risk of CKD in children surviving episodes of acute kidney injury in the intensive care unit: A prospective cohort study. Am J Kidney Dis. 2012;59:523–30.

## REVIEW QUESTIONS

1. You have just initiated peritoneal dialysis for a 5-year-old boy with acute kidney injury (AKI) resulting from hemolytic-uremic syndrome following infection with Shiga toxin–producing *E. coli*. The family is inquiring about the chances of renal function recovery. Of the following, the *most* appropriate statement regarding the natural history of AKI is:
   a. Complete renal recovery is the rule.
   b. Kidney transplantation is the only hope for renal recovery.
   c. Progression to chronic kidney disease occurs in 25% of children with dialysis requiring HUS.
   d. Renal recovery is aided by the use of diuretics.
   e. Renal recovery is unusual in children with dialysis-requiring AKI.

2. A 4-week-old infant with cyanotic heart disease, renal dysplasia, and a baseline serum creatinine of 1.2 mg/dL undergoes a diagnostic cardiac catheterization with contrast. Five days later, in preparation for cardiac surgery, the anesthesiologist checks a renal panel and notes that the serum creatinine is now 2.2 mg/dL. The urine output is normal, and the urinalysis shows a trace amount of protein. Of the following options, the most likely explanation for the increase in serum creatinine is:
   a. Contrast nephropathy
   b. Laboratory error
   c. Prerenal azotemia
   d. Worsening cardiac function
   e. Worsening chronic kidney disease

3. A 3-day-old infant was born at 36 weeks of gestation by emergency cesarean section for fetal distress and placental abruption. Apgar scores were 2 and 3 at 1 and 5 minutes, respectively. He was placed on mechanical ventilation and given intravenous hydration. He also received a single dose of ampicillin and gentamicin,

which was not continued because the result of admission blood culture was negative. Today, the serum creatinine is 2.5 mg/dL. Of the following, the most likely cause of the acute kidney injury is:

a. Nephrotoxicity
b. Perinatal asphyxia
c. Prematurity
d. Respiratory distress syndrome
e. Sepsis

4. You have initiated therapy with enalapril for essential hypertension in a 14-year-old boy. At follow-up 2 weeks later, his blood pressure has normalized. However, the serum potassium level is 5.5 mEq/L in a nonhemolyzed sample (increased from a baseline of 4.2 mEq/L). Of the following, the most likely explanation for the hyperkalemia is:

a. Decreased glomerular filtration rate
b. Decreased renal blood flow
c. Excessive dietary intake of potassium
d. Increased distal tubular reabsorption of potassium
e. Increased proximal tubular reabsorption of potassium

5. You are seeing a 10-day-old male infant born at 38 weeks of gestation. The delivery was complicated by placental abruption and a tight nuchal cord, with Apgar scores of 2 and 3 at 1 and 5 minutes, respectively, requiring initiation of mechanical ventilation. For the past 2 days, his serum creatinine concentration has been 1.6 mg/dL, increased from 1.2 mg/dL at 1 day of age. The serum electrolytes are normal, and the infant does not have oliguria, edema, or hypertension. Of the following, the most appropriate statement regarding the current serum creatinine measurement is that it:

A. Is normal for his age
B. Is not reflective of kidney dysfunction because the urine output is normal
C. Reflects acute kidney injury
D. Reflects maternal renal function
E. Reflects physiologic maturation

6. You are seeing a 3-year-old girl who was admitted 5 days ago with oliguric acute kidney injury secondary to fever, vomiting, and dehydration. Her oral intake has remained poor, and she has been on an intravenous regimen of D5 0.25% NaCl to replace insensible water losses. Today, the serum sodium is 148 mEq/L, her weight is down by 5%, and her parents report many wet diapers last night. Of the following, the most likely cause of the hypernatremia in this patient is:

a. Excessive glucose intake
b. Excessive sodium administration
c. Laboratory error
d. Recovering acute kidney injury
e. Worsening acute kidney injury

7. You are consulted on a 2-year-old boy with tetralogy of Fallot who is scheduled to undergo a definitive intracardiac repair procedure. During infancy, he underwent a palliative Blalock-Taussig shunt placement and developed moderate postoperative acute kidney injury that resolved spontaneously. Of the following, the most appropriate intervention to reduce the risk of developing acute kidney injury following his upcoming intracardiac repair is the preoperative administration of:

a. Fluids to optimize perioperative hemodynamics
b. Furosemide to induce diuresis
c. Mannitol to scavenge free radicals
d. N-acetylcysteine to provide an antioxidant
e. Renal-dose dopamine to induce renal vasodilation

8. You are consulting on a 5-year-old girl who was admitted to the ICU 2 days ago for the management of sepsis. Laboratory testing today shows a bicarbonate level of 14 mmol/L, BUN 50 mg/dL, and serum creatinine 2.0 mg/dL. The ICU team is contemplating bicarbonate therapy for the metabolic acidosis. Of the following, the most likely consequence of bicarbonate therapy in this situation is:

a. Hyperchloremia
b. Hyperkalemia
c. Hyperphosphatemia
d. Hypocalcemia
e. Hyponatremia

9. You are seeing a 6-yearold boy who was admitted to the critical care unit 3 days ago with septic shock. He has required multiple boluses of crystalloids and colloids for hypotension and multiple blood products for disseminated intravascular coagulation. His urine output has been decreasing for the past 24 h, and he has been anuric for the past 12 h. He has developed generalized edema, and his weight is now 26 kg (up from an admission weight of 20 kg). He has received two doses of intravenous furosemide (3 mg/kg) during the past 12 h, with no diuretic response. Of the following, the most appropriate next step in his management is:

a. Continue furosemide every 6 h.
b. Initiate mannitol diuresis.
c. Start fenoldopam.
d. Initiate a trial of IV normal saline bolus.
e. Prepare for renal replacement therapy.

10. You are seeing a 5-year-old boy who initially presented to the emergency department about 24 h ago with a 3-day history of fever, vomiting, poor oral intake, and 1 day of no urine output. Initial assessment in the emergency department found tachycardia, hypotension, lethargy, and diffuse abdominal tenderness. He was given fluid resuscitation, started on intravenous vancomycin (10 mg/kg/dose every 6 h) and gentamicin (2.5 mg/kg/dose every 8 h), and admitted for close observation. He continues to have anuria. The serum creatinine concentration today is 1.6 mg/dL (increased from 0.8 mg/dL at

initial presentation). Of the following, the *most* appropriate next step in the management of this patient's intravenous antibiotic regimen is:

a. Adjust the antibiotics for a glomerular filtration rate (GFR) of 75 mL/min.
b. Adjust the antibiotics for a GFR of 50 mL/min.
c. Adjust the antibiotics for a GFR of 10 mL/min.
d. Continue the current regimen of antibiotics.
e. Stop all antibiotics.

## ANSWER KEY

1. c
2. a
3. b
4. a
5. c
6. d
7. a
8. d
9. e
10. c

# Chronic kidney disease

KIRTIDA MISTRY

Chronic kidney disease (CKD), which includes end-stage renal disease (ESRD), is a major public health concern in the United States and worldwide. Once ESRD develops, lifesaving renal replacement therapy (RRT), either dialysis or renal transplant, is required to ameliorate the complications of advanced kidney failure. Despite advances in the delivery of RRT, outcomes in adults and children remain disappointing, with significant morbidity and mortality and decreased quality of life.

In the United States, the prevalent ESRD population in all age groups increased over 10-fold from 60,000 in 1980 to 615,899 in 2011, and medical management costs totaled $49.3 billion in 2011.[1] The last three decades have seen a steady increase in the incidence of pediatric ESRD in the United States. Since 2000, the adjusted incident rate of ESRD for patients 0 to 19 years of age has increased 10.1%.[1] This chapter will provide a general overview of pediatric CKD, including epidemiology, causes, classification, pathophysiology, clinical manifestations, and management, including strategies to slow progression.

## DEFINITION AND CLASSIFICATION IN CHILDREN

CKD refers to irreversible anatomic or functional kidney damage. The National Kidney Foundation Kidney Disease Outcomes Quality Initiative (KDOQI) guidelines defined and classified CKD in 2002 (Table 31.1).[2] There are two pediatric exceptions: (1) the criteria for duration longer than 3 months does not apply to infants younger than 3 months, and (2) the glomerular filtration rate (GFR) criteria of less than 60 mL/min/1.73 m$^2$ cannot be used in children under 2 years of age since developmental immaturity in this age group is associated with mean GFR of less than this value. Thus, the diagnostic criteria for reduced GFR in this particular population must be compared to age-matched normative values (Table 31.2).[2,3] The KDOQI classification has been modified and adopted by the Kidney Disease Improving Global Outcomes (KDIGO) work group in 2004 and revised in 2012 (Table 31.3).[3,4]

Table 31.1 Kidney Disease Outcomes Quality Initiative (KDOQI) criteria for the definition of chronic kidney disease

1. Kidney damage for 3 months or longer, as defined by structural or functional abnormalities of the kidney, with or without decreased glomerular filtration rate, manifest by either:
   a. Pathologic abnormalities
   b. Markers of kidney damage, including abnormalities in the composition of the blood or urine, or abnormalities in imaging tests
2. Glomerular filtration rate less than 60 mL/min/1.73 m² for 3 months or longer, with or without kidney damage

Source: KDOQI clinical practice guidelines for chronic kidney disease: evaluation, classification, and stratification. Am J Kidney Dis. 2002;39:S1–266.

GFR in children may be estimated (eGFR), using serum creatinine and length (Table 31.4) by numerous mathematical formulas.[5-7] The original Schwartz and Counahan-Barratt formulas were derived using the Jaffe method of serum creatinine measurement,

Table 31.2 Normative glomerular filtration rate values using inulin clearance in healthy children younger than 2 years

| Age | Mean GFR ± SD (mL/min/1.73 m²) |
|---|---|
| **Preterm babies** | |
| 1–3 days | 14.0 ± 5 |
| 1–7 days | 18.7 ± 5.5 |
| 4–8 days | 44.3 ± 9.3 |
| 3–13 days | 47.8 ± 10.7 |
| 8–14 days | 35.4 ± 13.4 |
| 1.5–4 mo | 67.4 ± 16.6 |
| **Term Babies** | |
| 1–3 days | 20.8 ± 5.0 |
| 3–4 days | 39.0 ± 15.1 |
| 4–14 days | 36.8 ± 7.2 |
| 6–14 days | 54.6 ± 7.6 |
| 15–19 days | 46.9 ± 12.5 |
| 1–3 mo | 85.3 ± 35.1 |
| **Infants** | |
| 4–6 mo | 87.4 ± 22.3 |
| 7–12 mo | 96.2 ± 12.2 |
| 1–2 yr | 105.2 ± 17.3 |

Source: Schwartz GJ, Furth SL. Glomerular filtration rate measurement and estimation in chronic kidney disease. Pediatr Nephrol. 2007;22:1839–48. Reproduced with permission.

Table 31.3 Chronic kidney disease stages according to glomerular filtration rate

| | KDOQI | | KDIGO | |
|---|---|---|---|---|
| Stage | GFR in mL/min/1.73 m² | Category | GFR in mL/min/1.73 m² | |
| 1 | ≥90 | G1 | ≥90 | |
| 2 | 60–89 | G2 | 60–89 | |
| 3 | 30–59 | G3a | 45–59 | |
| 4 | 15–29 | G3b | 30–44 | |
| 5 | <15 or dialysis | G4 | 15–29 | |
| | | G5 | <15 | |

Abbreviations: GFR, glomerular filtration rate; KDOQI, Kidney Disease Outcomes Quality Initiative; KDIGO, Kidney Disease Improving Global Outcomes.

## KEY POINTS

- CKD is characterized by irreversible anatomic or functional kidney damage, even though GFR may be normal.
- Because GFR is normally low in the first 2 years of life, comparison to age-matched norms of GFR should be considered in defining CKD in such patients.

in which serum creatinine is determined by a colorimetric reaction with alkaline picrate. The modified Schwartz formula is based on the enzymatic method for measuring serum creatinine, a methodology adopted by most laboratories. The modified Schwartz equation is the currently preferred method for calculating eGFR in children, but should be used only if serum creatinine is measured by the enzymatic method. An equation using serum creatinine, blood urea nitrogen (BUN), cystatin C, and height has been proposed to enhance accuracy in of eGFR (see Table 31.4).

The serum creatinine values are lower by 0.3 to 0.4 mg/dL when measured by the enzymatic method compared to the Jaffe reaction. Hence, the estimated GFR is higher if the enzymatic method is used.[8] In patients

## KEY POINTS

- Original Schwartz GFR estimation formula is used when serum creatinine is measured by Jaffe method.
- Modified Schwartz formula is applicable only if serum creatinine is measured by enzymatic method.
- MDRD equation should be used only in individuals 18 years of age and older.

Table 31.4 Estimation of the glomerular filtration rate

| Equation for eGFR in mL/min/1.73 m² | Method of serum creatinine measurement |
|---|---|
| **Original Schwartz** | Jaffe reaction |

$$\frac{k \times \text{length in cm}}{\text{Serum creatinine in mg/dL}}$$

| Age | Value of k |
|---|---|
| Preterm infants | 0.33 |
| Full term infants | 0.45 |
| Children ≤ 13 years and adolescent girls | 0.55 |
| Adolescent boys up to age 18 years | 0.7 |

| **Counahan-Barratt** | Jaffe reaction |
|---|---|

$$\frac{0.43 \times \text{length in cm}}{\text{Serum creatinine in mg/dL}}$$

| **Modified Schwartz** | Enzymatic |
|---|---|

$$\frac{0.413 \times \text{length in cm}}{\text{Serum creatinine in mg/dL}}$$

| **Schwartz using creatinine and cystatin C** | Enzymatic |
|---|---|

$39.1 \times (\text{Height/serum creatinine in mg/dL})^{0.516} \times (1.8/\text{cystatin C})^{0.294} \times (30/\text{BUN})^{0.169} \times (1.099) \text{ if male} \times (\text{Height}/1.4)^{0.188}$

| **Modification of Diet in Renal Disease** | Enzymatic |
|---|---|

$175 \times (\text{Serum creatinine in mg/dL})^{-1.154} \times (\text{Age})^{-0.203} \times (0.742 \text{ if female}) \times (1.212 \text{ if African American})$

*Abbreviation:* eGFR, estimated glomerular filtration rate.

18 years and older, the most frequently used equation for estimating GFR is the Modification of Diet in Renal Disease (MDRD) study equation (see Table 31.3).[9] This equation is not applicable in children, but has been validated in white and African-American populations between the ages of 18 and 70 years with GFR less than 60 mL/min/1.73 m².[9]

# EPIDEMIOLOGY

The National Health and Nutrition Examination Survey (NHANES) data demonstrated that 10.8% of the population, or approximately 19.2 million people, in the United States have CKD.[10] It is important to note that clinical CKD, especially ESRD or stage 5 CKD, represents the tip of the iceberg of the CKD spectrum in the community (Figure 31.1). Most pediatric epidemiologic studies have focused on patients with more advanced CKD or ESRD, excluding patients with milder forms of CKD, who may advance to ESRD in adulthood. Consequently, there is limited information about the epidemiology of the early stages of CKD in the pediatric population.

The most complete published pediatric epidemiologic data come from the ItalKid Project, a prospective, population-based Italian registry of children and young adults younger than 20 years old with an eGFR less than

75 mL/min/1.73 m².[11] The mean incidence of CKD in this study was 12.1 cases and point prevalence 74.7 per million. The male-to-female ratio in the study was 2.03, a finding also seen in other registries, including the North American Pediatric Renal Trials and Collaborative Studies (NAPRTCS).[12] In the ItalKid study, 57.6% of all cases were

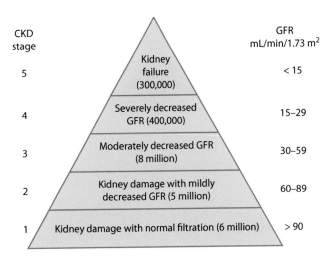

Figure 31.1 National Kidney Foundation and Kidney Disease Outcomes Quality Initiatives stages of chronic kidney disease (CKD). GFR, glomerular filtration rate. (Prevalence data in the triangle from: Coresh J, Selvin E, Stevens LA, et al. Prevalence of chronic kidney disease in the United States. JAMA. 2007;298:2038–47.)

due to hypoplasia and dysplasia, with or without urologic malformations.[11] This contrasts with adults, in whom type 2 diabetes and hypertension account for the majority of patients with CKD.[1]

Not surprisingly, studies evaluating more severe stages of CKD reveal lower incidences and prevalence. In Sweden, the incidence and prevalence rate of KDOQI stage 4 and 5 (KDIGO category G4 and G5) CKD in children 6 months to 16 years was estimated to be 7.7 and 21 per million, respectively.[13] Similarly, the annual incidence of CKD in Lorraine, France was reported to be 7.5 per million children under 16 years of age.[14] In Japan, a national study revealed prevalence of CKD stages 3 to 5 to be only 2.98 In 100,000 children.[15]

In the United States, epidemiologic data outlining the incidence of the early stages of CKD are lacking. In the United States Renal Data System (USRDS), the incidence rate of ESRD between 2007 and 2011 in children up to 19 years, was 15.2 per million population.[1] The incidence increases with age in children, and children under 4 years have the lowest incidence of ESRD.[12]

Worldwide comparative data published by the USRDS in 2005 revealed the highest unadjusted incidence of pediatric ESRD to be in the United States (Figure 31.2).[16] The prevalence in this analysis (Figure 31.3) is highest in Italy, although a wider age range of 0 to 24 years is reported in the Italian data.

There are striking racial and ethnic variations in the incidence and prevalence of ESRD in the United States, with the highest rates reported in African Americans and the lowest in whites.[1] Outcomes also vary by race. In the NAPRTCS 2008 Annual Report, whites with CKD are more likely to receive a transplant and African Americans are more likely to initiate dialysis.[17]

## ETIOLOGY

In the vast majority of children with CKD, it is secondary to congenital anomalies of the kidney and urinary tract (CAKUT). This contrasts with disease in adults, who most commonly have CKD secondary to glomerular disease, most commonly diabetic nephropathy, followed by hypertensive glomerulosclerosis and other chronic glomerulonephritides.

CAKUT and congenital nephropathies account for roughly two-thirds of cases of pediatric CKD in the more economically developed countries, whereas acquired causes prevail in less developed countries.[18] Table 31.5 shows the causes of CKD in children in the United States, as reported in the NAPRTCS database. CAKUT progresses more slowly to ESRD than

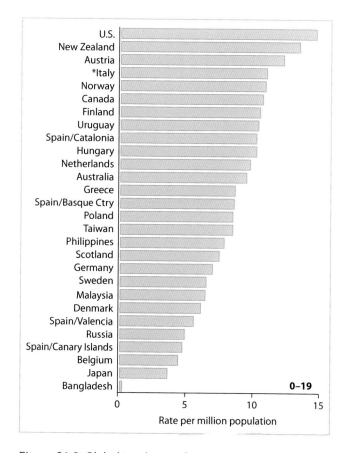

Figure 31.2 Global incidence of end-stage renal disease in 2003, ages 0 to 19 years. For Italy, the age group is 0 to 24 years. (Reproduced from: U.S. Renal Data System. 2005 Annual Data Report: Atlas Of End-Stage Renal Disease in the United States. Bethesda, MD: National Institutes of Health, National Institute of Diabetes and Digestive and Kidney Diseases; 2005.

glomerulonephritis; therefore, registries determining the causes of CKD primarily using data from ESRD patients, like USRDS, report lower incidence of CAKUT. The causes of CKD from various global registries and studies are compiled in Table 31.6.[1,11,17,19–22]

## KEY POINTS

- CAKUT is the most common cause of CKD in children, worldwide.
- Racial differences are seen in the prevalence of CKD in children.
- FSGS is the most common acquired cause of CKD in African-American children.

Although CAKUT predominates as the cause of CKD in children in the NAPRTCS registry, a racial difference in the cause of CKD and ESRD is evident.[17] Whereas patients with focal segmental glomerulosclerosis (FSGS) comprise 14.4% of all dialysis patients, patients with FSGS account for 23.7%

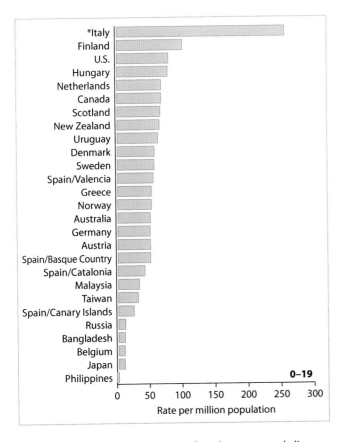

Figure 31.3 Global prevalence of end-stage renal disease in 2003, ages 0 to 19 years. For Italy, the age group is 0 to 24 years. (Reproduced from: U.S. Renal Data System. 2005 Annual Data Report: Atlas Of End-Stage Renal Disease in the United States. Bethesda, MD: National Institutes of Health, National Institute of Diabetes and Digestive and Kidney Diseases; 2005.

of African-American dialysis patients and 30% of African-American dialysis patients 13 years of age or older. The next most prevalent diagnoses among African-American children younger than 13 years of age are obstructive uropathy and renal dysplasia (both 11.5%) and in patients 13 years of age and older the diagnosis is lupus nephritis (10.1%).[17] FSGS accounts for 11.7% of all white dialysis patients. Renal dysplasia (15.7%) remains most common for white children, and obstructive uropathy (13.8%) is also most prevalent among whites 13 years of age and older.[23]

## PROGRESSION

Most patients with CKD progress to ESRD slowly over a period of many years, sometimes over decades. Disease-independent pathways play a decisive role in the progression of renal injury in established CKD. Several mechanisms are postulated to play a role in the progressive loss of kidney function and include perturbations in filtration or hemodynamics, hypertension, proteinuria, podocyte injury, proinflammatory cytokines, and profibrotic growth factors (Figure 31.4).

Table 31.5 2008 North American Pediatric Renal Trials and Collaborative Studies (NAPRTCS) showing details of cause of chronic kidney disease in 7037 participants in the U.S. Voluntary Registry

| Primary diagnosis | N = 7037* | Percentage |
|---|---|---|
| Obstructive uropathy | 1454 | 20.66 |
| Aplasia/hypoplasia/dysplasia | 1220 | 17.33 |
| Reflux nephropathy | 613 | 8.71 |
| Focal segmental glomerulosclerosis | 594 | 8.44 |
| Polycystic kidney disease | 278 | 3.95 |
| Prune belly | 193 | 2.74 |
| Renal infarct | 158 | 2.24 |
| Hemolytic uremic syndrome | 141 | 2.00 |
| SLE nephritis | 114 | 1.63 |
| Familial nephritis | 111 | 1.57 |
| Cystinosis | 104 | 1.47 |
| Pyelo/interstitial nephritis | 99 | 1.40 |
| Medullary cystic disease | 90 | 1.27 |
| Chronic glomerulonephritis | 82 | 1.16 |
| Membranoproliferative glomerulonephritis type 1 | 75 | 1.0 |
| Congenital nephrotic syndrome | 75 | 1.0 |
| Berger's (IgA) nephritis | 66 | 0.93 |
| Idiopathic crescentic glomerulonephritis | 47 | 0.65 |
| Henoch-Schönlein nephritis | 43 | 0.60 |
| Membranoproliferative glomerulonephritis type II | 30 | 0.42 |
| Sickle cell nephropathy | 14 | 0.19 |
| Diabetic glomerulonephritis | 11 | 0.15 |
| Oxalosis | 7 | 0.1 |
| Drash syndrome | 6 | 0.1 |
| Other | 1110 | 182 |
| Unknown | 15.77 | 2.58 |

Source: North American Pediatric Renal Trials and Collaborative Studies. NAPRTCS 2008 annual report. Reproduced with permission.
IgA, immunoglobulin A; SLE, systemic lupus erythematosus.

### KEY POINT

Progression of CKD to ESRD is multifactorial.

## HYPERFILTRATION

Reduced nephron mass (number), whether congenital or acquired, is associated with hyperfiltration in the surviving nephrons. Elegant experiments conducted by Brenner and colleagues established that nephron loss leads to compensatory hypertrophy, intraglomerular hypertension, increased

Table 31.6 Global comparative data showing causes of chronic kidney disease in different geographic regions of the world

| Study | NAPRTCS | ItalKid | ANZDATA | The UK renal registry | USRDS | ESPN/ERA-EDTA (Europe) | Japanese |
|---|---|---|---|---|---|---|---|
| Reference | 16 | 11 | 19 | 20 | 1 | 21 | 22 |
| Time frame (year) | 1994–2007 | 1990–2000 | 1963–2006 | 2008 Point prevalent | 2007–2011 Incident | 2011 incident | 1998 Prevalent |
| eGFR (mL/min/1.73 m$^2$) | <75 | <75 | ESRD | ESRD | ESRD | ESRD | ESRD |
| Age (yr) | 0–20 | 0–20 | 0–18 | 0–16 | 0–19 | 0–15 | 0–19 |
| Number of patients | 7037 | 1197 | 1485 | 905 | 6821 | 594 | 582 |
| CAKUT (%) | 2867 (40.7) | 689 (57.6) | 252 (16.9) | 378 (41.8) | 1642 (24) | 234 (39.4) | 178 (30.6) |
| Reflux nephropathy (%) | 594 (8.4) | | 280 (18.9) | 86 (9.5) | 684 (10) | | 30 (5.2) |
| Congenital/hereditary nephropathy (%) | 671 (9.5) | 199 (16.6) | 192 (12.9) | | | 115 (19.4) | 109 (18.7) |
| Primary and secondary glomerulonephritis (%) | 1183 (16.8) | 68 (5.7) | 444 (29.9) | 150 (16.6) | 2061 (30.2) | 101 (17) | 174 (29.9) |
| Renal infarct/ischemia (%) | 158 (2.2) | 49 (4.1) | 18 (1.2) | | | 6 (1) | 11 (1.9) |
| Hemolytic uremic syndrome (%) | 141 (2) | 43 (3.6) | 48 (3.2) | | 124 (1.8) | 18 (3) | 13 (2.2) |
| Pyelo/interstitial nephritis (%) | 99 (1.4) | 24 (2) | 18 (1.2) | 60 (6.6) | 329 (4.8) | 13 (2.2) | 41 (7) |
| Wilms tumor/malignancy (%) | 32 (0.5) | 4 (0.3) | | 7 (0.8) | 126 (1.8) | | 2 (0.3) |
| Other (%) | 1110 (15.8) | 81 (6.8) | 233 (15.7) | 70 (7.7) | | 60 (10.1) | 24 (4.1) |
| Unknown/missing (%) | 182 (2.6) | 40 (3.3) | | 154 (17) | 314 (4.6) | 47 (7.9) | 34 (5.8) |

ANZDATA, Australia and New Zealand Dialysis and Transplant Registry; CAKUT, congenital anomalies of the kidneys and urinary tract; ESPN/ERA-EDTA, Registry of the European Society for Paediatric Nephrology and the European Renal Association and European Dialysis and Transplantation Association; eGFR, estimated glomerular filtration rate; ESRD, end-stage renal disease; NAPRTCS, North American Pediatric Renal Trials and Collaborative Studies; USRDS, United States Renal Data System.

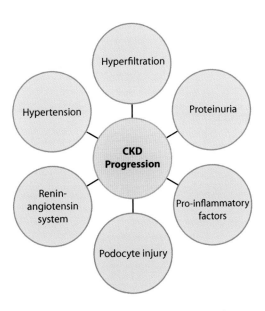

Figure 31.4 Schematic diagram representing factors involved in the progression of chronic kidney disease (CKD).

single-nephron GFR (hyperfiltration), and eventual glomerular injury and glomerulosclerosis in the remnant nephron population.[24–29] These adaptive changes, although an attempt to maintain GFR in the face of nephron loss, result in ongoing glomerular injury and eventual glomerulosclerosis in the surviving nephrons, perpetuating nephron loss. The mechanisms by which hyperfiltration leads to glomerulosclerosis are not entirely clear, but possibilities include glomerular vasodilatation, glomerular hypertension, and stretch-induced cellular injury.[29–31] It is likely that many of these pathogenic mechanisms are interrelated.

The subject of glomerular hyperfiltration and glomerular injury has been studied well in renal disease associated with diabetes mellitus.[32–34] Hyperfiltration in these patients precedes any overt manifestation of renal disease, including microalbuminuria. Amelioration of hyperfiltration by angiotensin-converting enzyme inhibitors (ACEIs) and preventing progression of renal disease in diabetes mellitus have been substantiated in several clinical studies.[35,36] Indeed, ACEIs are now recommended for prevention of hyperfiltration-induced glomerular injury and microalbuminuria in diabetes mellitus. KDOQI, however, does not recommend starting ACEIs in normotensive patients with diabetes with normal urinary microalbulinuria.[37]

Other children at risk for hyperfiltration injury and increased likelihood for CKD are those born with decreased nephron mass as a result of low birth weight, presence of a solitary kidney, those who have undergone therapeutic uninephrectomy, and those with sickle cell disease.[38–41] The clinical implications of hyperfiltration in the congenital and acquired disorders in children are beginning to be understood. The impact of solitary kidney on development of renal injury was studied in the KIMONO study in the Netherlands.[42] Of the 407 children with a solitary kidney,

37% met the criteria for evidence of renal injury, such as presence of hypertension, proteinuria, an impaired GFR, or the need to use renoprotective agents. CKD developed in 6% of these children during follow-up (mean of 9 years). Sanna-Cherchi[43] et al. also cautioned about a poor renal outcome of patients with solitary kidney in the spectrum of CAKUT. In contrast, Wikstad et al.[44] did not report any patients with CKD among 36 patients with single kidney (congenital and uninephrectomy) who were followed for 7 to 40 years. These investigators, however, demonstrated hyperfiltration in all of their patients, and microalbuminuria was present in 47%. Use of ACEIs in patients with a solitary kidney to reduce glomerular hypertension and ameliorate injury in CAKUT, although intuitive, has not been examined in well-controlled clinical studies. At least one study from Italy reports no clear benefit of ACEI in children with CAKUT.[45]

Definition of hyperfiltration in published studies is variable and not clearly delineated in either adults or children.[46] In children, there is an added requirement to consider age-related and gender-related normal values for accurate representation of hyperfiltration. GFR above two standard deviations (SDs) from the mean for age is a suggested definition of hyperfiltration.[47] Lacking any clinical markers of hyperfiltration, microalbuminuria is used as a surrogate of hyperfiltration-induced renal injury, especially in diabetic patients. It is important to recognize that hyperfiltration is an important physiologic response to metabolic challenges, such as following a protein meal and during pregnancy.[48,49]

## SYSTEMIC HYPERTENSION

Systemic hypertension is a well-known hemodynamic risk-factor for progression of CKD.[50,51] Conversely, CKD is also a recognizable risk factor for all-cause cardiovascular mortality.[52] In an observational study of 23 patients with CKD secondary to chronic glomerulonephritis, a significant correlation was demonstrated between blood pressure and the rate of decline of renal function.[53] The impact of blood pressure control on progression of CKD was studied in the MDRD study in adults. Improved blood pressure control in this study was shown to lower rate of decline of GFR in patients who had nondiabetic renal disease with proteinuria exceeding 1 g/day.[54] In the NAPRTCS study of 3834 patients aged 2 to 17 years, hypertension was determined to be an independent predictor of progression of CKD to ESRD.[55]

The degree to which systemic blood pressure needs to be lowered to achieve a positive impact on progression of CKD has been a matter of debate. Intensive blood pressure control, using drugs to inhibit the renin-angiotensin-aldosterone system (RAAS) in patients with CKD and significant proteinuria (>1 g/day) was studied by Bianchi et al.[56] These investigators demonstrated that the rate of decline of eGFR was lower in patients on an intensive blood pressure control regimen. However, the study also pointed out that such a therapy did not reverse the progression of CKD and the side effects associated with such intensive therapy were likely to be severe and unacceptable. The Effect of Strict Blood Pressure

Control and ACE Inhibition on the Progression of CRF in Pediatric Patients (ESCAPE) trial in children recommended that for a protective effect on progression of CKD, 24-hour mean blood pressure targets need to be set below the 50th percentile for age and gender.[57] Sarafidis et al.[58] reviewed this subject and suggested that the degree of blood pressure decline should be tailored in patients with CKD to the cause of the CKD, and whether significant proteinuria is present.

The pathophysiologic mechanisms by which systemic hypertension induces progressive renal damage are complex and include presence of preglomerular vasodilatation and efferent arteriolar constriction induced by RAAS, allowing transmission of elevated systemic blood pressure to the glomeruli, intraglomerular hypertension, and intraglomerular endothelial injury.[59,60]

# RENIN-ANGIOTENSIN-ALDOSTERONE SYSTEM

The RAAS is an important regulator of blood pressure, extracellular volume, and tissue perfusion. Renal diseases are often characterized by an increased renin production (hyper-reninemia) and have an activated RAAS. Renin produced in the juxtaglomerular apparatus of the kidney converts angiotensinogen to angiotensin I (ATI), which transforms to angiotensin II (ATII) by the action of ACE in the pulmonary vascular bed. ATII, a potent vasoconstrictor, mediates its action by binding to angiotensin type 1 and 2 receptors in the heart, blood vessels, and kidneys. ATII action, mediated via the type 1 receptor on the cardiovascular system, results in vasoconstriction and cardiac hypertrophy.[61] Another aspect of ACE is that it also hydrolyzes and inactivates bradykinin, a vasodilator.[62,63] It is postulated that the vasodilatory effect of ACEIs on the kidney (efferent arteriole) is mediated via bradykinin, apart from inhibiting RAAS.[64]

The RAAS promotes progression of CKD by hemodynamic and nonhemodynamic mechanisms. ATII, acting on the glomerular capillaries leads to predominant efferent arteriolar vasoconstriction, increasing intraglomerular hydrostatic pressure, promoting intraglomerular hypertension, and increasing single-nephron GFR (hyperfiltration). Evidence from experimental studies in animals indicates that the abnormally high transcapillary hydrostatic pressure

results in impairment in the size selectivity of the glomerular filtration barrier, leading to proteinuria.[65]

ATII also acts as a nonhemodynamic promoter of glomerular injury. ATII is a growth-promoting factor that regulates cell proliferation, apoptosis, and fibrosis.[66,67] It also enhances production of proinflammatory cytokine response, such as tumor necrosis factor alpha (TNF-α), interleukin-1 (IL-1), interleukin-6 (IL-6), and chemokines (e.g., monocyte chemoattractant protein-1 [MCP-1]), all of which promote inflammation and are likely to worsen glomerular injury.[66] ATII enhances production of cell adhesion molecules, reactive oxygen species, and profibrotic growth factors, all of which induce and perpetuate glomerular injury.[61] Other glomerulosclerosis-promoting actions of AT II consist of inducing hyperplasia and hypertrophy in the vascular smooth muscle cells and glomerular mesangial cells.[68]

Finally, ATII stimulates aldosterone production in the adrenal cortex. In turn, aldosterone mediates distal nephron sodium and water retention and potassium excretion. Adverse effects of aldosterone on the kidney and in the pathogenesis of fibrosis are summarized in the report by Remuzzi et al.[69] Aldosterone promotes endothelial remodeling, making these cells larger and stiffer, contributing to protein leak through intercellular gaps, and the endothelial dysfunction observed in hyperaldosteronism.[70] Other mechanisms whereby aldosterone can induce kidney injury includes induction of reactive $O_2$ species; increased expression of proinflammatory cytokines and growth factors such as osteopontin, MCP-1, IL-6, and IL-1; and inhibition of extracellular matrix degradation.[71-73]

The protective impact of blocking RAAS on progression of CKD has been well documented in clinical studies.[74] Some early studies have demonstrated regression of glomerulosclerosis by inhibition of aldosterone pathways, opening the door for potentially new therapeutic approaches in the prevention and progression of CKD.[75,76]

# PODOCYTE AND GLOMERULAR CELL INJURY

Injury to various cell lines within the glomeruli is relevant to progression of CKD. The terminally differentiated glomerular visceral epithelial cells or podocytes are capable of hypertrophy but not hyperplasia. Thus, when these cells are injured or lost, they cannot be replaced by new cells. Podocytes are pivotal in maintaining the permselectivity of the filtration barrier and are the source of vascular

---

## KEY POINTS

- ATII mediates progression of CKD via hemodynamic and nonhemodynamic mechanisms.
- Use of ACEIs in preventing progression of CKD has been well studied in diabetic nephropathy, and this therapy is used in most other forms of CKD, as well.
- Controlled trials of ACEIs in preventing progression of CKD in CAKUT are scant.

---

## KEY POINTS

- Podocytes are a biologically active and essential part of filtration barrier.
- Podocyte loss or injury leads to progressive glomerulosclerosis.

endothelial growth factor (VEGF) and angiopoeitin, which maintain capillary endothelial growth and permeability.[77,78] Podocyte injury or loss leads to progressive glomerulosclerosis in many glomerular diseases, including idiopathic and inherited forms of FSGS.[79,80]

Endothelial injury also generates growth factors that lead to cell proliferation; metabolic derangements, especially lipid accumulation; and increased extracellular matrix deposition.[81] Mesangial cells, when injured and under the influence of ATII and cytokines, hypertrophy, with increased extracellular matrix production, a major source of scar tissue in glomerulosclerosis.[82]

## GROWTH FACTORS AND CYTOKINES

Many cytokines and growth factors are proinflammatory and profibrotic and play a role in progression of CKD. ATII increases the expression of transforming growth factor-1, TNF, osteopontin, vascular cell adhesion molecule-1, nuclear factor-B, platelet-derived growth factor, basic fibroblast growth factor, plasminogen activator inhibitor-1, and insulin-like growth factor (IGF).[61,69]

## PROTEINURIA AND HYPERLIPIDEMIA

Proteinuria is a manifestation of many renal diseases, and it also can mediate ongoing inflammation and fibrosis in the kidney. Significance of proteinuria as a prognostic indicator in progression of CKD has been demonstrated in numerous clinical studies.[54,83] Inflammatory response induced by proteinuria promotes ongoing tubulointerstitial and renal injury and fibrosis by (1) direct tubular toxicity of protein, (2) via complement activation in the tubular lumens.[84–87] Reducing proteinuria in CKD is accompanied by an improvement in the rate of decline of GFR.[88]

Lipid metabolism is altered in CKD and contributes to atherosclerosis and glomerulosclerosis. Small, dense low-density lipoprotein (LDL) particles are increased in concentration and cause antioxidant renal and vascular damage.[89] The role of dyslipidemia in progression is not fully established. Although the MDRD study was not able to establish dyslipidemia as an independent risk factor for progression of CKD, other clinical and experimental evidence has linked dyslipidemia to progression of CKD.[90–94] Moreover, dyslipidemia of CKD is a risk factor for cardiovascular disease and has been linked to abnormalities in the carotid intima media in children with CKD.[95,96] Statins, although advocated for use in adults with dyslipidemia of CKD, are not recommended in children younger than 18 years of age.[97]

## CLINICAL MANIFESTATIONS

Clinical manifestations of CKD in children depend on the cause. Children with glomerular disease may have gross hematuria and/or edema. Many congenital abnormalities are detected prenatally by ultrasound. Approximately 0.5% of pregnancies are found to have a fetal abnormality of the kidney or urinary tract.[98] These anomalies may be causative of CKD and ESRD in infants and children. Other children with CKD may present with more subtle symptoms such as polydipsia, polyuria, nocturia, and enuresis secondary to the urine concentrating defect associated with CKD, especially in diseases such as renal dysplasia or nephronophthisis. Other children with CKD may manifest poor linear growth, abnormal urinalysis, or the presence of hypertension.

In some cases, children present for the first time because of symptoms of uremia resulting from advanced CKD and ESRD (Table 31.7). Normocytic, normochromic anemia is sometimes the first manifestation of CKD in children, which may have been discovered during hematology consultation for evaluation of anemia. Others may be evaluated in endocrinology for growth retardation before being discovered to have CKD. Although it occurs less frequently now, some patients with CKD may be discovered because of renal osteodystrophy and associated skeletal deformities.

Table 31.7 Clinical manifestations of uremia

| System | Clinical manifestation |
| --- | --- |
| Metabolic | Electrolyte abnormalities: Hyperkalemia, metabolic acidosis, hyponatremia |
| | Hypocalcemia |
| | Hyperphosphatemia |
| | Hyperuricemia |
| Musculoskeletal | Bone pain |
| | Renal osteodystrophy |
| | Muscle cramps and/or weakness |
| Hematologic | Iron deficiency |
| | Anemia |
| | Platelet dysfunction |
| Neurologic | Cognitive impairment |
| | Headache |
| | Seizures |
| | Encephalopathy |
| Cardiovascular | Hypertension |
| | Pericarditis |
| | Pulmonary edema |
| Gastrointestinal | Anorexia |
| | Weight loss |
| | Nausea, emesis |
| Endocrine | Poor growth |
| | Amenorrhea |
| | Dyslipidemia |
| | Insulin resistance |
| | Delayed puberty |
| Integumentary | Pruritus |
| | Hyperpigmentation or hypopigmentation |
| Other | Fatigue, edema, insomnia, pica |

Screening to identify children at risk for developing CKD may improve the rate of early detection and provide opportunities for early intervention (Table 31.8). American Academy of Pediatrics guidelines recommend monitoring growth from birth and blood pressure during annual visits with primary care physicians, beginning at age 3 years. Blood pressure should be monitored from the newborn period if there are risk factors, as delineated in the Fourth Report on the Diagnosis, Evaluation, and Treatment of High Blood Pressure in Children and Adolescents.[99]

The most common complications of CKD and associated prevalence rates are: hypertension 60% to 70%, anemia 37% to 38%, metabolic bone disease 17%, growth failure 12% to 16%, and fluid and electrolyte disturbances 12%.[100,101] The prevalence of all complications increase with advancing CKD.[101]

## HYPERTENSION AND CARDIOVASCULAR DISEASE

Children on dialysis have the same risk factors for development of cardiovascular disease as adults. These include hypertension, dyslipidemia, physical inactivity, hyperhomocysteinemia, hyperparathyroidism, inflammation, and left ventricular hypertrophy (LVH).[102] Hypertension is most commonly the result of fluid overload or activation of the RAAS. It also may be, at times, attributed to medications used to treat glomerular diseases, such as corticosteroids and calcineurin inhibitors.

Table 31.8 Risk factors for the development of chronic kidney disease in children

Preterm birth
Small for gestational age
Family history of genetic kidney disease
History of acute kidney injury
Congenital anomalies of the kidneys and urinary tract (CAKUT)
Vesicoureteral reflux, especially high-grade and associated with recurrent urinary tract infection and scarring
History of acute nephritis
History of nephrotic syndrome
History of hemolytic-uremic syndrome
History of Henoch-Schönlein purpura
Hypertension
Diabetes
Obesity
Systemic and autoimmune conditions that affect the kidneys (e.g., systemic lupus erythematosus)
Sickle cell trait or sickle cell disease
Spina bifida and neurogenic bladder

---

### KEY POINT

Cardiovascular disease is the leading cause of death and morbidity in children with ESRD.

---

Children with CKD and ESRD have increased mortality rate and adjusted all-cause mortality is 6.5 to 7.9 times greater than in the general population.[1] Cardiovascular disease is the leading cause of death in adults and children with ESRD.[23,103,104] In fact, cardiovascular mortality surpasses that from infection in children with ESRD.[1] In a study of children and young adults 0 to 30 years of age in the USRDS database, cardiac deaths were approximately 1000 times more frequent in those who developed ESRD during childhood than in the general pediatric population.[105] The most common cardiovascular events in children on dialysis are arrhythmias (19.6%), valvular heart disease (11.7%), cardiomyopathy (9.6%), and cardiac arrest (3%).[106]

LVH, left ventricular dilation, and systolic and diastolic dysfunction are known complications in pediatric chronic dialysis patients.[107] The prevalence of LVH in pediatric dialysis patients is high and may be more prevalent in hemodialysis versus peritoneal dialysis patients.[107] LVH usually results from hypertension, but other factors such as anemia, fluid overload, hyperparathyroidism, and uremia also contribute.[108,109]

Data about the prevalence and consequences of atherosclerosis in children with CKD is emerging. Carotid intimal-medial thickness abnormalities, coronary artery calcification, and decreased arterial wall compliance are indicators of atherosclerosis and predict cardiovascular disease. Whereas the incidence of coronary artery calcifications may be low in pediatric patients, young adults who present with ESRD in childhood have evidence of calcification.[110] Risk factors for vascular calcifications include duration of dialysis, severity and duration of hyperphosphatemia, high calcium intake, and severity of hyperparathyroidism.[110,111]

## ANEMIA

Parameters for the diagnosis of anemia are gender-dependent and age-dependent. The KDOQI guidelines define anemia as a hemoglobin concentration less than the 5th percentile for children older than 1 year and more than 2 SD below the mean for infants (Table 31.9).[112] Anemia adversely affects patient quality of life, and studies show an improvement following its correction.[113-115]

As kidney function declines, anemia worsens.[116] In the Chronic Kidney Disease in Children (CKiD) study, patients with a GFR less than 30 mL/min/1.73 m$^2$ had a fourfold to fivefold higher risk for anemia compared to those with a GFR of 50 mL/min/1.73 m$^2$ or greater.[100] In adults with

Table 31.9 Hemoglobin values in different age groups for diagnosis of anemia

| Age | Hemoglobin (g/dL) level 2 standard deviations below the mean |
|---|---|
| 1–3 days | 14.5 |
| 1 wk | 13.5 |
| 2 wk | 12.5 |
| 1 mo | 10 |
| 2 mo | 9 |
| 3–6 mo | 9.5 |
| 6–12 mo | 10.5 |

| Age (years) | 5th percentile hemoglobin (g/dL) | |
|---|---|---|
| | Male | Female |
| 1–2 | 10.7 | 10.8 |
| 3–5 | 11.2 | 11.1 |
| 6–8 | 11.5 | 11.5 |
| 9–11 | 12 | 11.9 |
| 12–14 | 12.4 | 11.7 |
| 15–19 | 13.5 | 11.5 |

Source: Kidney Disease Outcomes Quality Initiative. Clinical practice guidelines and clinical practice recommendations for anemia in chronic kidney disease. Am J Kidney Dis. 2006;47:S11–145.

CKD, hemoglobin begins to decline when eGFR is below 60 mL/min/1.73 m$^2$.[117] In the CKiD study, there was a linear decrease in hemoglobin below a threshold iohexol measured GFR of 43 mL/min/1.73 m$^2$, independent of age, race, gender, and underlying diagnosis.[116]

The pathophysiology of anemia in CKD is primarily due to erythropoietin deficiency, although iron and vitamin deficiencies, reduced red blood cell life span, bone marrow suppression secondary to retained inhibitors in uremia, blood loss, and chronic inflammation play a role. Erythropoietin is produced by interstitial peritubular fibroblasts in the renal cortex in response to hypoxia.[118]

Patients with CKD are at increased risk for iron deficiency secondary to chronic blood loss because of platelet dysfunction and hemodialysis. However, they also have altered iron homeostasis. Dietary iron is absorbed in the duodenum and recycled from senescent red blood cells. Circulating transferrin transports iron to maturing red blood cells for incorporation into hemoglobin. Most of the body's iron is bound to hemoglobin. A smaller proportion is stored in hepatocytes and macrophages in the reticuloendothelial system.

Transferrin deficiency of unclear cause leads to reduced iron transport in CKD. This contributes to increased accumulation of stored iron as ferritin, leading to functional iron deficiency. Additionally, there is an inherent inability to mobilize stored iron from macrophages and hepatocytes. This may be partially mediated by hepcidin, a small peptide secreted by the liver that inhibits intestinal iron absorption

and iron release from the reticuloendothelial system.[119] Hepcidin is inhibited by iron deficiency and upregulated in inflammation and CKD.[120] Reduced renal clearance of hepcidin may also lead to higher levels in CKD. Hepcidin levels correlate with ferritin levels and markers of inflammation and increase with deteriorating renal function, being highest in dialysis patients.[121,122]

# CHRONIC KIDNEY DISEASE AND MINERAL AND BONE DISORDER

The mineral and endocrine functions of the kidney are critically important in the regulation of bone formation and remodeling during growth. Aberrations or disruption of these functions begin during early stage 3 CKD and progress as severity of renal failure advances. Bone abnormalities are almost universal in dialysis patients.

Normal kidney function maintains mineral homeostasis. In healthy children, calcium balance is positive to sustain growth and bone mineral accumulation. The process of optimizing peak bone mass by young adulthood is critical to maintaining life-long bone health and protecting against osteoporosis in adulthood.[123,124] Thus, bone disease resulting from CKD in childhood has long-term consequences.

Along with its effect on the skeletal system, disordered mineral and bone metabolism in children with CKD also affects the cardiovascular system. Therefore, the KDIGO guidelines recommend using the term *CKD-MBD* for describing the full spectrum of this disorder. *Renal osteodystrophy* is the term used to described the impact on the skeletal system.[125] Although biochemical abnormalities of mild hyperparathyroidism and 1,25-dihydroxyvitamin D (1,25-D) deficiency may occur before stage 3 CKD, most children are asymptomatic.[126] With advancing CKD, renal osteodystrophy also progresses with manifestations of skeletal deformities, fractures, muscle and bone pain, avascular necrosis, and growth failure.

As CKD progresses, normal serum and tissue concentrations of phosphorus and calcium are disrupted and perturbations occur in the regulation of parathyroid hormone (PTH), 25-hydroxyvitamin D (25-D), 1,25-D, fibroblast growth factor-23 (FGF-23), and growth hormone. In children, monitoring of serum levels of calcium, phosphorus, PTH, and alkaline phosphatase should begin at CKD stage 2.[127]

Hyperphosphatemia usually begins in stage 3 CKD as a result of reduced glomerular clearance of phosphate. This leads to a lower ionized calcium and secondary hyperparathyroidism. The kidney fails to respond adequately to PTH, which normally promotes phosphaturia and calcium reabsorption. Hyperphosphatemia also inhibits the 1α-hydroxylase enzyme in proximal tubular cells, decreasing 1,25-D levels, which in turn, worsens hypocalcemia secondary to reduced gastrointestinal absorption.

FGF-23 is a hormone secreted by osteocytes, and its primary target of action is the kidney. It promotes phosphaturia and decreases production of calcitriol.[128] Stimuli for FGF-23 secretion include increased dietary phosphorus intake and increased 1,25-D levels.[129] Compared to serum PTH and phosphorus, FGF-23 level rises more dramatically and earlier in CKD, presumably as a physiologic adaptation to maintain normal serum phosphate levels.[130] Studies in adults have shown that increased FGF-23 is more strongly associated with mortality than elevated phosphorus.[131,132] It has been shown to be associated with LVH, endothelial dysfunction, and progression of CKD.[133] Other CKD-MBD abnormalities include vitamin D receptor downregulation and skeletal resistance to the calcemic effect of PTH.[134]

## KEY POINTS

- FGF 23 regulates phosphorus and vitamin D metabolism.
- FGF-23 level rises earlier than that of phosphorus in CKD and tracks more closely with mortality than hyperphosphatemia.
- FGF-23 is associated with findings of LVH.

## GROWTH FAILURE

Impaired growth is a complication of CKD, and it increases with progression of CKD. Along with short stature, poor growth is associated with increased morbidity and mortality in children with CKD.[135,136] The risk for death increases by 14% for each 1 SD score (SDS) decrease in height.[135] Short children with CKD have higher rates of hospitalization and poorer school attendance.

Quality of life is also adversely affected by short stature. Adults with childhood onset of ESRD are significantly more likely to have a positive perception of quality of life if they are satisfied with their adult height.[137] In the CKiD population, parents reported an increase in physical and social functioning in children who exhibited catch-up growth as measured by increase in height SDS.[138]

## KEY POINTS

- Poor growth is associated with increased morbidity and mortality in children with CKD.
- Malnutrition is one of the most important contributors to growth impairment in children with CKD.
- Growth hormone level is normal in CKD.
- IGF-1 levels are low to normal.
- Target resistance to IGF-1 is common.

Regular assessment of nutrition and growth is recommended for children with stage 2 or higher CKD.[139] In the general population, short stature is defined as height more than 2 SD below the mean height of other children the same age and gender. This correlates to height less than the 2.5th percentile. A single measurement of height is much less important in assessing growth than is the pattern of growth over a period of time. A slowed growth velocity that progressively deviates from a previously defined percentile is concerning.

Normal growth velocity in children fluctuates with age. Although there are variations around this, growth velocity is roughly 25 cm/yr in the first year of life, 10 cm/yr from age 1 to 4 years, and 5 cm/yr from age 4 years to puberty. There are three phases of growth: infantile, childhood, and pubertal, each under the influence of different predominant environmental or hormonal factors.[140] The infantile phase refers to the first 2 years, when growth velocity is at its most rapid. Although nutritional status is the primary determinant of growth during this time, growth hormone begins to play an increasingly important role after the first 12 months. The childhood phase has a slower, more constant rate of growth under the primary influence of growth hormone and thyroid hormone. Finally, the pubertal phase is characterized by the more rapid growth velocity of 8 to 14 cm/yr, with gonadal sex steroids and growth hormone providing the stimulus.[116]

Calculation of mid-parental height provides insight to the expected adult height of the child. The calculation is as follows:

Female: {[Father's height (cm) − 13 cm] + Mother's height (cm)} ÷ 2.

Male: {[Mother's height (cm) + 13 cm] + Father's height (cm)} ÷ 2.

The value obtained in the above calculation, ±8.5 cm provides the 3rd and the 95th percentile values of expected mid-parental height in the child.

KDOQI guidelines define short stature as height SDS less than −1.88 or height for age less than the 3rd percentile.[139] In the general population, the prevalence of short stature is approximately 3% to 5%. In the NAPRTCS registry, almost 37% of children with CKD had growth impairment at the time of enrollment.[16] Factors associated with more severe height deficits were young age, lower GFR, and anemia.[16] The NAPRTCS 2011 annual dialysis report shows that at dialysis initiation, patients have a mean SDS of −1.60. Height deficits are worse for males and younger patients.[23]

The pathogenesis of short stature in children with CKD is multifactorial. Contributing factors include comorbid conditions, malnutrition, CKD-MBD (renal osteodystrophy, hyperparathyroidism or hypoparathyroidism), abnormalities in the growth hormone insulin like growth factor-1 (IGF-1) IGF-1 axis, fluid and electrolyte disturbances, metabolic acidosis, inadequate dialysis, and medications (e.g., corticosteroids).

## KEY POINT

Short stature is defined as height SDS less than −1.88 or height-for-age below the 3rd percentile.

Malnutrition is one of the primary contributors to growth impairment in children with CKD. The impact of nutrition is especially important in infants, who may never achieve catch-up growth because of the dramatic growth that occurs during infancy. Reduced caloric intake because of anorexia, nausea, and vomiting is common in CKD, and almost all children with these symptoms have some form of disordered gut motility, ranging from gastroesophageal reflux and delayed gastric emptying to gastric dysrhythmias.[142] Furthermore, altered taste sensation, excessive and preferred water intake over food in polyuric children, the increased intra-abdominal pressure associated with peritoneal dialysis, and elevated levels of inflammatory cytokines such as leptin, TNF-α, IL-1, and IL-6 are additional factors contributing to reduced intake.[143]

Metabolic demands and nutritional losses also may be higher in patients with CKD. Metabolic demands increase during times of acute illness and infection, and inflammation is associated with increased energy expenditure. Amino acid and protein losses during peritoneal dialysis demand increased intake to maintain adequate nutrition in children with already compromised ability to maintain sufficient intake.[144] Sodium deficiency has been associated with poor growth, and adequate replenishment is important for their continued growth. Children with polyuric, salt-wasting CKD can maintain or improve growth when repleted with sodium and water.[145]

Growth hormone is an anabolic peptide that stimulates growth. Perturbation in the growth hormone axis is an important contributor to short stature in children with CKD. Growth hormone is secreted in a pulsatile manner by the anterior pituitary gland in response to the balance between two hypothalamic hormones: the stimulatory influence of growth hormone–releasing hormone (GHRH) and inhibitory effect of somatostatin. The largest and most predictable growth hormone peak occurs soon after onset of sleep.

Once produced by the anterior pituitary, growth hormone acts in the liver and the local tissue sites to stimulate production of IGF-1. Although liver is the dominant source of circulating IGF-1, tissue level and local production of IGF-1 under the influence of growth hormone are believed to be a significant determinants of growth.[146] In animal studies, circulating levels of IGF-1 must be reduced by more than 85% before growth is affected.[147]

Growth hormone levels are increased in children with CKD, likely as a result of increased secretion and reduced renal clearance, whereas IGF-1 levels are usually normal (Figure 31.5).[146,148] These findings are suggestive of

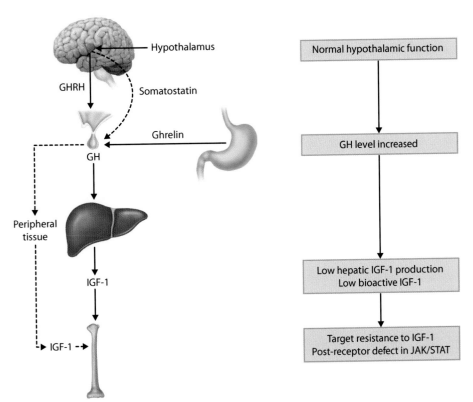

Figure 31.5 The growth hormone (GH)–insulin-like growth factor 1 (IGF-1) axis involved in linear growth in children. Abnormalities in the growth hormone axis seen in chronic kidney disease (CKD) are represented in the right side boxes. Somatostatin inhibits and GHRH stimulated growth hormone secretion. GHRH, growth hormone–releasing hormone; JAK, Janus kinase; STAT, signal transducer and activator of transcription.

peripheral resistance to growth hormone and IGF-1.[149,150] The mechanism of growth hormone resistance appears to be the result of altered postreceptor signaling, rather than reduced number of growth hormone receptors in target organs.[149] Growth hormone binds to its target cell membrane growth hormone receptor, stimulating phosphorylation of Janus kinase 2 (JAK2), a tyrosine kinase. This sequentially stimulates phosphorylation of the growth hormone receptor and cytoplasmic STAT signaling proteins 1, 3, and 5, which translocate to the cell nucleus and activate genes regulated by growth hormone, including the *IGF-1* gene. Suppressor of cytokine signaling *(SOCS)* genes are also activated by this process, and they serve as a negative feedback mechanism, suppressing JAK2. In animal models, impaired phosphorylation of JAK2 and STAT proteins, possibly because of upregulation of SOCS2 and 3, contribute to growth hormone resistance and growth retardation in CKD.[151] Chronic inflammation is believed to be the stimulus for SOCS upregulation in CKD.[152]

Bioavailability of IGF-1 is also significantly altered in CKD. Almost all of the IGF-1 in the bloodstream is bound to six IGF binding proteins (IGFBP 1 to 6) and is inactive, with only 1% being free and bioactive.[153] In CKD, clearance of the IGFBP is reduced, increasing their circulating level and making even less free IGF-1 available for its biologic activity.[154]

Another GHRH, ghrelin, is synthesized in the stomach and to a lesser extent in the hypothalamus and pancreatic islet cells.[147] It has been shown to cause hyperphagia and obesity in rats, increases appetite and food intake in humans, and may stimulate growth hormone secretion.[155] However, its exact role in growth hormone axis regulation and impact on growth is still being investigated.[156]

## FLUID AND ELECTROLYTE ABNORMALITIES

Hyperkalemia is common in CKD and worsens as GFR declines. The principal cause of hyperkalemia in CKD is decreased renal excretion of potassium. Hypoaldosteronism, which may be due to decreased renin production by the kidney or to medications that either inhibit aldosterone production or block its action, may be the additional cause of hyperkalemia in some. Hyperkalemia also may be secondary to movement of potassium from the intracellular into the extracellular space, as is seen in metabolic acidosis or use of medications such as β-adrenergic blockers.

The kidney has an important role in the excretion of acid produced by normal metabolism. A normal Western diet results in the production of 1 to 3 mEq/kg/day hydrogen ions in children, which must be buffered and subsequently excreted by the kidney. Impaired acid excretion is common in CKD, especially as GFR decreases to less than 30 mL/min/1.73 m². Adverse consequences associated with metabolic acidosis include muscle wasting, bone disease, impaired growth, insulin insensitivity, abnormalities in growth hormone and thyroid hormone secretion, and increased β₂-microglobulin accumulation.

## NEUROCOGNITIVE FUNCTION

Before the 1980s, CKD in children, especially if it developed during infancy, was associated with developmental delay of gross motor and language skills, microcephaly, hypotonia, seizures, and dyskinesia.[157] These complications have decreased because of a variety of interventions, including improved nutrition of infants with tube feedings, discontinuation of the use aluminum-based binders, and improved dialysis technology.[158]

Approximately 12% to 23% of children with ESRD have cerebral atrophy on neuroimaging.[159,160] Electroencephalogram (EEG) abnormalities are found in about 25% to 50% of children with CKD. EEG slowing worsens as CKD progresses, and children with CKD have slower peripheral nerve conduction velocities.[161] Potential clinical risk factors for development of neurocognitive deficits include increased disease severity, longer duration of disease, and younger age of onset of kidney disease.[162] Studies evaluating intelligence quotient (IQ) scores in older children are limited. Most children with CKD have normal IQs.[163] However, when compared with siblings, children with CKD, even following transplant, have significantly lower IQs.[164]

Speech and language are adversely affected in children with CKD.[165] Memory, especially short-term visual and verbal memory, is reduced, deficiencies in executive functioning required for problem solving are present, and attention span is diminished.[164,165] The central nervous system adverse effects of CKD have long-term consequences. Verbal performance and full-scale IQ scores and educational attainment are reduced in adults with childhood-onset ESRD.[166] Lower rates of employment and low occupational level are associated with dialysis longer than 8 years.[167]

## QUALITY OF LIFE

A Dutch study evaluated quality of life of adults with childhood-onset ESRD, adult-onset ESRD, and the general population.[168] Compared with the general population, dialysis patients had a higher prevalence of impaired quality of life in physical functioning, role limitations because of physical health, social functioning, and general health perception. Quality of life is substantially impaired in adults with new-onset ESRD.[169] A higher number of comorbid conditions, a lower hemoglobin level, and lower residual renal function were independently related to poorer quality of life.[169]

## ENDOCRINE DYSFUNCTION

### THYROID HORMONE AXIS

CKD affects both the hypothalamus-pituitary-thyroid axis and peripheral thyroid hormone metabolism. Adult uremic patients have higher rates of thyromegaly, goiter, nodules, and carcinoma.[170] The most common thyroid abnormality is sick euthyroid syndrome, a condition characterized by abnormal thyroid function tests in the setting of nonthyroid illness. The prominent alterations are low serum triiodothyronine ($T_3$) and elevated reverse $T_3$ ($rT_3$), also termed low $T_3$ syndrome. Unlike in other conditions with sick euthyroid syndrome, CKD does not cause elevated total $rT_3$ because of redistribution to the extravascular space and increased cellular uptake. However, free $rT_3$ is elevated as a result of reduced renal clearance.[170]

Serum thyroid-stimulating hormone (TSH) concentrations are usually normal or elevated in CKD, but its response to thyroid-releasing hormone (TRH) is reduced. TSH bioavailability may be reduced.[170] Total and free $T_4$ and $T_3$ levels are usually decreased, and patients can have clinical or subclinical hypothyroidism. In hemodialysis patients receiving heparin anticoagulation, free $T_4$ may be elevated secondary to heparin-induced inhibition of $T_4$ binding to its binding proteins.[170]

### GONADAL HORMONES

Delayed pubertal progression occurs in children with CKD, and this further increases the risk for growth retardation. These children exhibit a state of compensated hypergonadotrophic hypogonadism with elevated gonadotropins and decreased or low-normal gonadal hormones.[171] They also have evidence of hypothalamic-pituitary-gonadal dysregulation with blunted response of luteinizing hormone to gonadotropins and decreased luteinizing hormone pulsatility and bioactivity, leading to anovulation in females.[171] Finally, estradiol and testosterone levels are reduced secondary to uremia, either through direct toxic effects or hyporesponsiveness of the gland.[171]

## MANAGEMENT

The goals of therapy in children with CKD are:

1. Treat reversible kidney disease
2. Slow progression to ESRD
3. Manage complications
4. Prepare for RRT

The complexity of care, economic demands, and emotional burden to the patients and their families tend to increase as CKD advances. Compared to adults, children with CKD require more resources, specialized care, and care coordination to achieve optimum outcomes.[172] Support from a multidisciplinary team that includes the nephrologist, primary care physician, pharmacist, nurse, social worker, dietitian, and psychologist is crucial to success. Other members of the team may include other subspecialists such as surgeons and urologists, child life specialists, educators and school counselors, and speech, occupational, and physical therapists.

## TREATMENT OF REVERSIBLE KIDNEY DISEASE

There are many causes of an acute decline of GFR in the setting of CKD. Every attempt should be made to prevent acute or chronic renal injury, ameliorate its effect, and treat the underlying cause promptly to prevent irreversible and accelerated progression of CKD. Common causes of acute kidney injury include volume depletion, use of nonsteroidal anti-inflammatory agents, administration of nephrotoxic medications, contrast nephropathy, RAAS blockade, and urinary outflow obstruction. Early referral to a nephrologist and appropriate management may lessen the burden and severity of complications and, in fact, reduces mortality.[173]

## SLOWING PROGRESSION

Therapeutic interventions at earlier stages of CKD to prevent additional nephron loss and kidney function decline are effective in adults. These strategies include RAAS blockade, blood pressure control, proteinuria reduction, strict glycemic control in diabetics, and dietary protein restriction. Many of these strategies to slow progression in adults have been adopted in the care of pediatric patients with CKD, and data to support their use is increasing.

Inhibition of the RAAS, using either ACEIs or angiotensin receptor blockers (ARBs), is effective in preventing and slowing the rate of GFR decline in CKD. This benefit is likely tightly correlated to the antiproteinuric effect of these agents, but exceeds their antihypertensive effect. In the Ramipril Efficacy in Nephropathy (REIN) study of chronic nondiabetic nephropathies, ACEIs were superior in reducing the rate of GFR decline, despite equivalent blood pressure control, compared to placebo.[174] There may be an additional benefit of combining an ACEI and an ARB, especially in diabetic patients, which results in greater reduction of proteinuria and blood pressure; however, long-term studies are lacking on their effect on CKD progression.[175] In addition, there is an increased incidence of adverse events.

Because aldosterone appears to play a role in renal fibrosis, independent of ATII, the aldosterone receptor antagonists spironolactone and eplerenone have been studied in adults with CKD. In a randomized study, the addition of spironolactone to an ACEI or ARB led to a smaller decline in GFR than occurred in the control group but was associated with significantly more hyperkalemia.[176]

Hypertension is common in patients with CKD and is a modifiable risk factor for reducing cardiovascular disease and slowing progression of CKD. All patients with CKD should have their blood pressure monitored regularly. Unfortunately, data suggest that hypertension is underdiagnosed and undertreated in children with CKD.[177,178]

Effective blood pressure control delays the progression of CKD in adults, and antihypertensive agents that inhibit the RAAS provide superior protection because of their added antiproteinuric, anti-inflammatory and antifibrotic properties. The ESCAPE trial showed that aggressive blood pressure control in children with stage 2 to 4 CKD (eGFR 15 to 80 mL/min/1.73 m²), targeting a 24-hour mean arterial blood pressure less than the 50th percentile, was superior in delaying rate of deterioration of GFR compared to a target between the 50th and 90th percentiles.[57] All patients received the maximum dose of ramipril, an ACEI, and thus the benefit was due to improved blood pressure control not to an ACEI effect.

Current KDOQI guidelines for children with CKD and recommendations from the National High Blood Pressure Education Program Working Group (NHBPEP) for all children are for target blood pressure below the 90th percentile, or less than 120/80 mm Hg, whichever is lower.[179] The KDIGO guideline recommends initiating antihypertensive therapy in children with CKD when blood pressure is consistently greater than the 90th percentile for age, gender, and height.[3] Based on the findings in the ESCAPE trial, KDIGO recommendations are to achieve target blood pressure (particularly if proteinuria is present) below the 50th percentile for age, gender, and height, unless limited by symptoms or signs of hypotension. Because of the proved benefits of these agents, it is recommended that an ARB or ACEI be used in children with CKD in whom treatment with blood pressure–lowering drugs is indicated, irrespective of the level of proteinuria.[3]

Other factors that may slow progression to ESRD include protein restriction in experimental models and clinical adult studies.[180,181] The mechanism involves reduced cytokine expression, reduced intraglomerular pressure, and increased matrix synthesis.[182] In general, the effect on slowing progression is small and there is a concern of malnutrition. In children, there is no evidence that protein restriction delays progression of CKD.[183] The adverse effects on nutrition and growth remain of significant concern, and thus the current recommendations are to provide children with their recommended daily allowance of protein.

Cholesterol-lowering therapy with statins and correction of anemia have been studied in adults; however, little evidence exists that these interventions slow progression of CKD. Although no association was found between hyperuricemia and progression, there may be some evidence that

allopurinol slows progression of renal disease in patients with CKD and reduces cardiovascular and hospitalization risk.[59,160,184,185]

## MANAGEMENT OF COMPLICATIONS

KDOQI and KDIGO guidelines are available for the management of anemia, CKD-MBD, and nutrition in CKD.[3,112,124,125,139,186,187] These topics are reviewed in detail in other chapters (Chapters 32, 33, and 34). The focus in this chapter will be on growth hormone therapy in children with CKD.

## GROWTH HORMONE THERAPY

Growth impairment, defined by KDOQI as height SDS less than –1.88 or height-for-age below the 3rd percentile, is common in children with CKD.[139] Regular assessment of nutrition and growth is recommended for all children with CKD stage 2 or higher. Weight for age, length or height for age, length or height velocity for age, and body mass index for age should all be plotted and monitored. Mid-parental height should be calculated and plotted to gauge genetic potential.

The pathogenesis of short stature in children with CKD is multifactorial and includes comorbid conditions, malnutrition, CKD-associated bone disease, abnormalities in the growth hormone–IGF-1 axis, fluid and electrolyte disturbances, metabolic acidosis, inadequate dialysis, and medications (e.g., corticosteroids). Improving growth therefore requires corrective management of malnutrition, electrolyte abnormalities, metabolic acidosis, hyperparathyroidism, and optimization of dialysis adequacy before the initiation of recombinant human growth hormone (rhGH).

rhGH is effective and safe in treating short stature in children with CKD, yet in the NAPRTCS registry there appears to be significant undertreatment of this condition. Whereas almost 37% of children with CKD had growth impairment at the time of enrollment, only 6.3% of patients were on growth hormone therapy at entry.[16,188]

Unfortunately, children with CKD and short stature very often do not attain normal adult height. Even following renal transplant, final adult height remains significantly reduced.[189,190] In a retrospective study, median height SDS was below the 3rd percentile for age at initiation of dialysis, decreased during dialysis, and did not improve following kidney transplant; approximately 74% of patients had a final height below the 3rd percentile.[190]

The effect of growth hormone treatment on the final adult height of children with CKD was studied by Haffner et al.[191] The adult height of 38 children with CKD who were treated with growth hormone for up to 8.8 years was compared with that of 50 children with CKD who did not receive growth hormone. Height SDS improved significantly in the group treated with growth hormone from a mean of –2.85 to –1.5, compared to deterioration from a mean of –1.5 to

-2.1 in the control group. Thus, the children treated with rhGH had catch-up growth and the untreated children had persistent growth failure. Even though the mean final adult height was below the genetic target height, 65% of the treated children reached an adult height within the normal range (within 2 SD of normal height). The mean final adult height was approximately 11.1 cm and 16 cm below the genetic target height in rhGH-treated and untreated children, respectively.[191]

Following renal transplantation, growth is adversely affected by glucocorticoid therapy, allograft dysfunction, and abnormalities in the growth hormone–IGF-1 axis.[192] Treatment with rhGH improves growth in children following transplant without increasing the rate of allograft rejection or loss.[193] Children with CKD before reaching ESRD requiring RRT with either dialysis or renal transplant have a better response to growth hormone therapy.[194] Thus, rhGH should be initiated early in CKD when indicated, to maximize growth potential.

The recommended rhGH dose for the treatment of growth failure in CKD is 0.35 mg/kg/wk (28 international units/m$^2$/wk), divided into once-daily subcutaneous injections administered in the evening. This dose is higher than that used in patients with growth hormone deficiency. Based on the pathophysiology and results of clinical studies, to be effective, rhGH needs to be prescribed in pharmacologic doses. The dose should be adjusted periodically for weight gain. Emerging data suggest that much higher doses of rhGH (0.7 mg/kg/wk) during puberty improve growth potential even further without significant adverse effects.[195] Further study is required before extending this to the CKD population.

Active malignancy is a contraindication to rhGH use, and caution should be exercised in patients at risk for developing malignancies. Once nutritional and metabolic factors have been corrected and a decision made to initiate rhGH, eligibility should be confirmed by obtaining bone age radiograph, thyroid studies, and hemoglobin A1c. Pubertal stage should be assessed.

Once treatment is initiated, patients should be monitored for adverse effects such as benign intracranial hypertension, glucose intolerance, and slipped capital femoral epiphysis. Patients should have an annual bone age x-ray. If response to therapy is poor despite adequate adherence, referral to an endocrinologist may be required for further evaluation.[196]

Growth hormone therapy should be discontinued when the epiphyses close, and once the patient's height goal has been achieved (based on mid-parental height or 50th percentile for age). It should also be discontinued if the patient develops malignancy, slipped capital femoral epiphyses, benign intracranial hypertension, severe hyperparathyroidism (PTH greater than 900 pg/mL for stage 5 CKD, lower values for earlier CKD stages), nonadherence, and at the time of renal transplant.[196] Growth should be monitored following discontinuation and, if there are no contraindications, can be restarted if growth failure recurs.

## PREPARING FOR RENAL REPLACEMENT THERAPY

Patients and families should be prepared for the progression of CKD to ESRD. Planning for RRT, whether dialysis or renal transplant, should begin during stage 4 CKD or when the GFR is less than 30 mL/min/1.73 m$^2$.[2] As renal function declines, patients should be followed more closely for development of uremic symptoms.

Determination should be made about the timing of the initiation of RRT and type and placement of dialysis access. Veins for dialysis access should be preserved. Generally, it is recommended that RRT be initiated when eGFR declines to less than 15 mL/min/1.73 m$^2$. Earlier RRT may be required if symptoms or signs of uremia develop or if CKD-BMD, malnutrition, growth impairment, or neurocognitive dysfunction is difficult to manage.

Patients and families should receive counseling for choices of RRT, and psychosocial and economic preparation. It is advisable for them to meet with the dialysis and transplant teams before initiating RRT. Social work, psychological, and child life support become increasingly important to provide support to the child and family and help them cope with the medical, psychosocial, and economic implications of impending RRT.

Children are more likely to undergo preemptive transplantation than adults, especially when there are available living donors.[172] Race, economic factors, and educational background are factors that determine rates of preemptive renal transplantation using deceased donors.[197]

The rate of preemptive transplant in children in the NAPRTCS registry is approximately 25%.[16] The rate of preemptive transplantation differs significantly between recipients of living (34%) and deceased donor (13%) allografts; between males (28%) and females (20%); and across races, with preemptive transplantation rates of 31% in whites, 14% in blacks, and 16% in Hispanics.[16] The 6- to 12-year-old age group is most likely to be preemptively transplanted, with a rate of 28%.

There is some evidence that preemptive transplant is beneficial and associated with improved long-term outcomes of graft survival than transplantation following dialysis.[197,198] However, it is uncertain whether patient survival is improved. Unless contraindications exist, preemptive transplant should be pursued in all children, irrespective of whether a living donor is available.

In addition to close clinical monitoring of progression of CKD, reciprocal plot of serum creatinine over time (usually years) may provide an approximate time range when a target serum creatinine necessary to initiate RRT would be reached (Figure 31.6).[199] Such a plot facilitates planning for placement of an arteriovenous fistula or peritoneal dialysis catheter or planning for transplant surgery. The caveat in this approach is that decline of renal function and rise of serum creatinine seldom bear a linear relationship over time and a rapid decline of renal function and a steep slope in the plot are possible and may not be predictable.

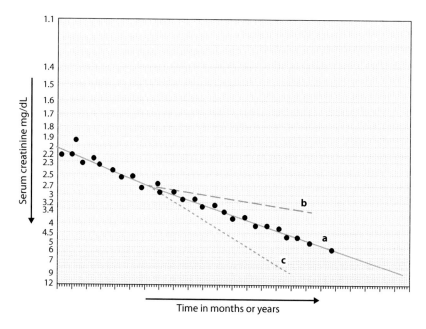

**Figure 31.6** Reciprocal relationship of serum creatinine and time. *Plot a* represents a linear and a predictable plot for reaching a target serum creatinine (e.g., 10 mg/dL in an adult) for starting dialysis therapy. *Plot b* represents an improvement in the rate of decline of renal function. *Plot c* represents an accelerated decline of renal function.

## OUTCOME IN CHILDREN

Children with CKD have a higher mortality rate than age-related and gender-related cohorts. The mortality rate in children 1 to 19 years of age in the United States in 2011 was 0.256 per 1000 population.[200] This compares to an overall mortality rate of 41 per 1000 patient-years at risk for children receiving renal replacement therapies. The risk is highest in patients undergoing hemodialysis (64 in 1000 patient-years), followed by peritoneal dialysis (45 in 1000 patient-years) and kidney transplant (10.4 in 1000 patient-years).[1]

Similarly high mortality rate (3.6%) of children with CKD was also reported in the NAPRTCS registry.[16] One-year outcomes of pediatric ESRD patients on dialysis in the USRDS database is unchanged since 2002, with 38% receiving a kidney transplant and 4% dying.[1] Mortality rate adjusted for age, gender, race, Hispanic ethnicity, and diagnosis is highest in the youngest children, possibly reflecting an increased survival of neonates with significant comorbidities.[1]

For children beginning ESRD therapy in 2002 to 2006, the 5-year survival was 89%, with the lowest survival in children younger than 4 years (80%). By modality, the highest 5-year survival probability was in children with a transplant (96%), compared to 75% and 80% in those treated with hemodialysis or peritoneal dialysis, respectively.[1]

In Australia and New Zealand, 10- and 20-year survival of pediatric patients with ESRD was 79% and 66%, respectively.[201] Mortality in children was 30 times higher than children without ESRD. Overall, a trend toward improved survival was observed over the four decades of the study. Risk factors for death included young age when RRT is initiated (four times higher in children under 1 year of age vs. those 15 to 19 years of age) and treatment with dialysis (more than four times higher risk than those with a renal transplant).

## SUMMARY

CKD is a complex disorder that presents numerous management challenges, especially in the very young. Because almost half of the patients have abnormalities of the urinary tract, a close collaboration between urologists and nephrologist is essential for a successful outcome. Impact of CKD on the families and caregivers at home can be substantial, and providing support through teams of appropriate ancillary staff is an essential aspect of the care of these patients. Preparation of children and families for dialysis and kidney transplantation also requires specialized care. Although hemodialysis is possible even in neonates, vascular access remains challenging in children. Many children require dialysis through a central catheter, adding to the lack of eventual vascular resources in these patients. Transplantation is the goal for all children with CKD, but the life span of even a successful kidney transplant is finite. Despite these challenges, significant progress has been made in the care of children with CKD in the last 20 years. This includes availability of treatments, such as erythropoietin and growth hormone therapy. With technology galloping toward the development of replacement organs from patient's own cells, let us hope that the next 20 years will remain full of promise for children with CKD.

# REFERENCES

1. U.S. Renal Data System. USRDS 2013 Annual Data Report: Atlas of Chronic Kidney Disease and End-Stage Renal Disease in the United States. Bethesda, MD: National Institutes of Health, National Institute of Diabetes and Digestive and Kidney Diseases; 2013.

2. Kidney Disease Outcomes Quality Initiative. Clinical practice guidelines for chronic kidney disease: Evaluation, classification, and stratification. Am J Kidney Dis. 2002;39:S1–266.

3. Kidney Disease: Improving Global Outcomes CKD Work Group. KDIGO 2012 clinical practice guideline for the evaluation and management of chronic kidney disease. Kidney Int Suppl. 2013;3:1–150.

4. Levey AS, Eckardt KU, Tsukamoto Y, et al. Definition and classification of chronic kidney disease: A position statement from Kidney Disease: Improving Global Outcomes (KDIGO). Kidney Int. 2005;67:2089–100.

5. Schwartz GJ, Brion LP, Spitzer A. The use of plasma creatinine concentration for estimating glomerular filtration rate in infants, children, and adolescents. Pediatr Clin North Am. 1987;34:571–90.

6. Schwartz GJ, Furth SL. Glomerular filtration rate measurement and estimation in chronic kidney disease. Pediatr Nephrol. 2007;22:1839–48.

7. Counahan R, Chantler C, Ghazali S, et al. Estimation of glomerular filtration rate from plasma creatinine concentration in children. Arch Dis Child. 1976;51:875–8.

8. Apple F, Bandt C, Prosch A, et al. Creatinine clearance: Enzymatic vs Jaffe determinations of creatinine in plasma and urine. Clin Chem. 1986;32:388–90.

9. Levey AS, Stevens LA, Schmid CH, et al. A new equation to estimate glomerular filtration rate. Ann Intern Med. 2009;150:604–12.

10. Coresh J, Selvin E, Stevens LA, et al. Prevalence of chronic kidney disease in the United States. JAMA. 2007;298:2038–47.

11. Ardissino G, Dacco V, Testa S, et al. Epidemiology of chronic renal failure in children: Data from the ItalKid project. Pediatrics. 2003;111:e382–7.

12. Warady BA, Chadha V. Chronic kidney disease in children: The global perspective. Pediatr Nephrol. 2007;22:1999–2009.

13. Esbjorner E, Berg U, Hansson S. Epidemiology of chronic renal failure in children: A report from Sweden 1986-1994. Swedish Pediatric Nephrology Association. Pediatr Nephrol. 1997;11:438–42.

14. Deleau J, Andre JL, Briancon S, Musse JP. Chronic renal failure in children: An epidemiological survey in Lorraine (France) 1975-1990. Pediatr Nephrol. 1994;8:472–6.

15. Ishikura K, Uemura O, Ito S, et al. Pre-dialysis chronic kidney disease in children: Results of a nationwide survey in Japan. Nephrol Dial Transplant. 2013;28:2345–55.

16. U.S. Renal Data System. USRDS 2005 Annual Data Report: Atlas of End-Stage Renal Disease in the United States, Bethesda, MD: National Institutes of Health, National Institute of Diabetes and Digestive and Kidney Diseases; 2005.

17. North American Pediatric Renal Trials and Collaborative Studies. 2008 Annual Report: Renal Transplantation, Dialysis, Chronic Renal Insufficiency. 2008. Available at https://web.emmes.com/study/ped/annlrept/Annual%20Report%20-2008.pdf. Accessed December 25, 2015.

18. Harambat J, van Stralen KJ, Kim JJ, Tizard EJ. Epidemiology of chronic kidney disease in children. Pediatr Nephrol. 2012;27:363–73.

19. Orr NI, McDonald SP, McTaggart S, et al. Frequency, etiology and treatment of childhood end-stage kidney disease in Australia and New Zealand. Pediatr Nephrol. 2009;24:1719–26.

20. Lewis MA, Shaw J, Sinha MD, et al. Demography of the UK paediatric renal replacement therapy population in 2008. Nephron Clin Pract. 2008;115(Suppl 1):c278–88.

21. European Renal Association and European Dialysis and Transplant Association. Registry 2011. Available at http://www.espn-reg.org/files/ESPN%20 ERAEDTA%20AR2011.pdf. Accessed March 16, 2015.

22. Hattori S, Yosioka K, Honda M, Ito H. The 1998 report of the Japanese National Registry data on pediatric end-stage renal disease patients. Pediatr Nephrol. 2002:17:456–61.

23. North American Pediatric Renal Trials and Collaborative Studies. 2011 annual report: Dialysis. 2011.

24. Hostetter TH, Olson JL, Rennke HG, et al. Hyperfiltration in remnant nephrons: A potentially adverse response to renal ablation. Am J Physiol. 1981;241:F85–93.

25. Hostetter TH, Troy JL, Brenner BM. Glomerular hemodynamics in experimental diabetes mellitus. Kidney Int. 1981;19:410–15.

26. Hostetter TH. Progression of renal disease and renal hypertrophy. Annu Rev Physiol. 1995;57:263–78.

27. Anderson S, Meyer TW, Rennke HG, et al. Control of glomerular hypertension limits glomerular injury in rats with reduced renal mass. J Clin Invest. 1985;76:612–9.

28. Shimamura T, Morrison AB. A progressive glomerulosclerosis occurring in partial five-sixths nephrectomized rats. Am J Pathol. 1975;79:95–106.

29. Hostetter TH. Hyperfiltration and glomerulosclerosis. Semin Nephrol. 2003;23:194–9.

30. Srivastava T, Celsi GE, Sharma M, et al. Fluid flow shear stress over podocytes is increased in the solitary kidney. Nephrol Dial Transplant. 2014;29:65–72.

31. Huang C, Bruggeman LA, Hydo LM, et al. Shear stress induces cell apoptosis via a c-Src-phospholipase D-mTOR signaling pathway in cultured podocytes. Exp Cell Res. 2012;318:1075–85.

32. Chatzikyrkou C, Haller H. Diabetes: Hyperfiltration-a risk factor for nephropathy in T1DM? Nat Rev Endocrinol. 2012;8:385–6.

33. Ruggenenti P, Porrini EL, Gaspari F, et al. Glomerular hyperfiltration and renal disease progression in type 2 diabetes. Diabetes Care. 2012;35:2061–8.

34. Hostetter TH, Troy JL, Brenner BM. Glomerular hemodynamics in experimental diabetes mellitus. Kidney Int. 1981;19:410–15.

35. Lewis EJ, Hunsicker LG, Bain RP, Rohde RD. The effect of angiotensin-converting–enzyme inhibition on diabetic nephropathy. N Engl J Med. 1993;329:1456–62.

36. Brenner BM, Cooper ME, de Zueew, et al.; RENAAL Study Investigators. Effects of losartan on renal and cardiovascular outcomes in patients with type 2 diabetes and nephropathy. N Engl J Med. 2001;345:861–9.

37. National Kidney Foundation. KDOQI clinical practice guideline for diabetes and CKD: 2012 update. Am J Kidney Dis. 2012;60:850–86.

38. Brenner BM, Garcia DL, Anderson S. Glomeruli and blood pressure: Less of one, more the other? Am J Hypertens. 1988;1(4 Part 1):335–47.

39. Luyckx VA, Brenner BM. Low birth weight, nephron number, and kidney disease. Kidney Int Suppl. 2005;97:S68–77.

40. Benz K, Amann K. Maternal nutrition, low nephron number and arterial hypertension in later life. Biochim Biophys Acta. 2010;1802:1309–17.

41. Westland R, Kurvers RA, van Wijk JA, et al. Risk factors for renal injury in children with a solitary functioning kidney. Pediatrics. 2013;131:e478–85.

42. Haymann JP, Stankovic K, Levy P, et al. Glomerular hyperfiltration in adult sickle cell anemia: A frequent hemolysis associated feature. Clin J Am Soc Nephrol. 2010;5:756–61.

43. Sanna-Cherchi S, Ravani P, Corbani V, et al. Renal outcome in patients with congenital anomalies of the kidney and urinary tract. Kidney Int. 2009;76:528–33.

44. Wikstad I, Celsi G, Larsson L, et al. Kidney function in adults born with unilateral renal agenesis or nephrectomized in childhood. Pediatr Nephrol. 1988;2:177–82.

45. Ardissino G, Vigano S, Testa S, et al. No clear evidence of ACEi efficacy on the progression of chronic kidney disease in children with hypodysplastic nephropathy: Report from the ItalKid Project database. Nephrol Dial Transplant. 2007;22:2525–30.

46. Cachat F, Combescure C, Cauderay M, et al. A systematic review of glomerular hyperfiltration assessment and definition in the medical literature. Clin J Am Soc Nephrol. 2015;10:382–9.

47. Helal I, Fick-Brosnahan GM, Reed-Gitomer B, et al. Glomerular hyperfiltration: Definitions, mechanisms and clinical implications. Nat Rev Nephrol. 2012;8:293–300.

48. Simon AH, Lima PR, Almerinda M, et al. Renal haemodynamic responses to a chicken or beef meal in normal individuals. Nephrol Dial Transplant. 1998;13:2261–4.

49. Odutayo A, Hladunewich M. Obstetric nephrology: Renal hemodynamic and metabolic physiology in normal pregnancy. Clin J Am Soc Nephrol. 2012;7:2073–80.

50. Klag MJ, Whelton PK, Randall BL, et al. Blood pressure and end-stage renal disease in men. N Engl J Med. 1996;334:13–8.

51. Tozawa M, Iseki K, Iseki C, et al. Blood pressure predicts risk of developing end-stage renal disease in men and women. Hypertension. 2003;41:1341–1345.

52. Sarafidis PA, Bakris GL. Microalbuminuria and chronic kidney disease as risk factors for cardiovascular disease. Nephrol Dial Transplant. 2006;21:2366–74.

53. Shimamatsu K, Onoyama K, Harada A, et al. Effect of blood pressure on the progression rate of renal impairment in chronic glomerulonephritis. J Clin Hypertens. 1985;1:239–44.

54. Klahr S, Levey AS, Beck GJ, et al. The effects of dietary protein restriction and blood-pressure control on the progression of chronic renal disease. Modification of Diet in Renal Disease Study Group. N Engl J Med. 1994;330:877–84.

55. Mitsnefes M, Ho PL, McEnery PT. Hypertension and progression of chronic renal insufficiency in children: A report of the North American Pediatric Renal Transplant Cooperative Study (NAPRTCS). J Am Soc Nephrol. 2003;14:2618–22.

56. Bianchi S, Bigazzi R, Campese VM. Intensive versus conventional therapy to slow the progression of idiopathic glomerular diseases. Am J Kidney Dis. 2010;55:671–81.

57. Wühl E, Trivelli A, Picca S, et al. ; ESCAPE Trial Group. Strict blood-pressure control and progression of renal failure in children. N Engl J Med. 2009;361:1639–50.

58. Sarafidis PA, Ruilope LM. Aggressive blood pressure reduction and renin-angiotensin system blockade in chronic kidney disease: Time for re-evaluation? Kidney Int. 2014;85:536–46.

59. Bidani AK, Griffin KA. Pathophysiology of hypertensive renal damage: Implications for therapy. Hypertension. 2004;44:595–601.

60. Ravera M, Re M, Deferrari L, et al. Importance of blood pressure control in chronic kidney disease. J Am Soc Nephrol. 2006;17(4 Suppl 2):S98–103.

61. Remuzzi G, Perico N, Macia M, Ruggenenti P. The role of renin-angiotensin-aldosterone system in the progression of chronic kidney disease. Kidney Int Suppl. 2005;99:S57–65.

62. Dorer FE, Kahn JR, Lentz KE, et al. Hydrolysis of bradykinin by angiotensin-converting enzyme. Circ Res. 1974;34:824–7.

63. Linz W, Wiemer G, Gohlke P, et al. Contribution of kinins to the cardiovascular actions of angiotensin-converting enzyme inhibitors. Pharmacol Rev. 1995;47:25–49.

64. Kon V, Fogo A, Ichikawa I. Bradykinin causes selective efferent arteriolar dilation during angiotensin I converting enzyme inhibition. Kidney Int. 1993;44:545–50.

65. Yoshioka T, Rennke HG, Salant DJ, et al. Role of abnormally high transmural pressure in the permselectivity defect of glomerular capillary wall: A study in early passive Heymann nephritis. Circ Res. 1987;61:531–8.

66. Ruiz-Ortega M, Ruperez M, Lorenzo O, et al. Angiotensin II regulates the synthesis of proinflammatory cytokines and chemokines in the kidney. Kidney Int Suppl. 2002;62:S12–22.

67. Wolf G, Neilson EG. Angiotensin II as a renal growth factor. J Am Soc Nephrol. 1993;3:1531–40.

68. Fogo AB. Mechanisms of progression of chronic kidney disease. Pediatr Nephrol. 2007;22:2011–22.

69. Remuzzi G, Cattaneo D, Perico N. The aggravating mechanisms of aldosterone on kidney fibrosis. J Am Soc Nephrol. 2008;19:1459–62.

70. Oberleithner H. Aldosterone makes human endothelium stiff and vulnerable. Kidney Int. 2005;67:1680–2

71. Blasi ER, Rocha R, Rudolph AE, et al. Aldosterone/salt induces renal inflammation and fibrosis in hypertensive rats. Kidney Int. 2003;63:1791–800.

72. Brown NJ. Aldosterone and end-organ damage. Curr Opin Nephrol Hypertens. 2005;14:235–41.

73. Farquharson CA, Struthers AD. Spironolactone increases nitric oxide bioactivity, improves endothelial vasodilator dysfunction, and suppresses vascular angiotensin I/angiotensin II conversion in patients with chronic heart failure. Circulation 2000;101:594–7.

74. Hsu TW, Liu JS, Hung SC, et al. Renoprotective effect of renin-angiotensin-aldosterone system blockade in patients with predialysis advanced chronic kidney disease, hypertension, and anemia. JAMA Intern Med. 2014;174:347–54.

75. Aldigier JC, Kanjanbuch T, Ma LJ, et al. Regression of existing glomerulosclerosis by inhibition of aldosterone. J Am Soc Nephrol. 2005;16:3306–14.

76. Ma LJ, Nakamura S, Aldigier JC, et al. Regression of glomerulosclerosis with high-dose angiotensin inhibition is linked to decreased plasminogen activator inhibitor-1. J Am Soc Nephrol. 2005;16:966–76.

77. Eremina V, Cui S, Gerber H, et al. Vascular endothelial growth factor a signaling in the podocyte-endothelial compartment is required for mesangial cell migration and survival. J Am Soc Nephrol. 2006;17:724–35.

78. Clement LC, Avila-Casado C, Macé C, et al. Podocyte-secreted angiopoietin-like-4 mediates proteinuria in glucocorticoid-sensitive nephrotic syndrome. Nat Med. 2011;17:117–22.

79. Wharram BL, Goyal M, Wiggins JE, et al. Podocyte depletion causes glomerulosclerosis: Diphtheria toxin-induced podocyte depletion in rats expressing human diphtheria toxin receptor transgene. J Am Soc Nephrol. 2005;16:2941–52.

80. Fukuda A, Chowdhury MA, Venkatareddy MP, et al. Growth-dependent podocyte failure causes glomerulosclerosis. J Am Soc Nephrol. 2012;23:1351–63.

81. Gerritsen ME, Bloor CM. Endothelial cell gene expression in response to injury. FASEB J. 1993;7:523–32.

82. Liu Y. Renal fibrosis: New insights into the pathogenesis and therapeutics. Kidney Int. 2006;69:213–7.

83. Fathallah-Shaykh SA, Flynn JT, Pierce CB, et al. Progression of Pediatric CKD of nonglomerular origin in the CKiD cohort. Clin J Am Soc Nephrol. 2015;10:571–7.

84. Sanchez-Niño MD, Fernandez-Fernandez B, Perez-Gomez MV, et al. Albumin-induced apoptosis of tubular cells is modulated by BASP1. Cell Death Dis. 2015;6:e1644.

85. Sheerin NS, Sacks SH. Leaked protein and interstitial damage in the kidney: Is complement the missing link? Clin Exp Immunol. 2002;130:1–3.

86. Boor P, Konieczny A, Villa L, et al. Complement C5 mediates experimental tubulointerstitial fibrosis. J Am Soc Nephrol. 2007;18:1508–15.

87. Gorriz JL, Martinez-Castelao A. Proteinuria: Detection and role in native renal disease progression. Transplant Rev (Orlando). 2012;26:3–13.

88. de Goeij MC, Liem M, de Jager DJ, et al. Proteinuria as a risk marker for the progression of chronic kidney disease in patients on predialysis care and the role of angiotensin-converting enzyme inhibitor/angiotensin II receptor blocker treatment. Nephron Clin Pract. 2012;121:c73–82.

89. Ruan XZ, Varghese Z, Moorhead JF. An update on the lipid nephrotoxicity hypothesis. Nat Rev Nephrol. 2009;5:713–21.

90. Chawla V, Greene T, Beck GJ, et al. Hyperlipidemia and long-term outcomes in nondiabetic chronic kidney disease. Clin J Am Soc Nephrol. 2010;5:1582–7.

91. Kasiske BL, O'Donnell MP, Schmitz PG, Kim Y, Keane WF. Renal injury of diet-induced hypercholesterolemia in rats. Kidney Int. 1990;37:880–91.

92. Chen SC, Hung CC, Kuo MC, et al. Association of dyslipidemia with renal outcomes in chronic kidney disease. PLoS One. 2013;8:e55643.

93. Cases A, Coll E. Dyslipidemia and the progression of renal disease in chronic renal failure patients. Kidney Int Suppl. 2005;99:S87–93.

94. Abrass CK. Cellular lipid metabolism and the role of lipids in progressive renal disease. Am J Nephrol. 2004;24:46–53.

95. Kotur-Stevuljević J, Peco-Antić A, Spasić S, et al. Hyperlipidemia, oxidative stress, and intima media thickness in children with chronic kidney disease. Pediatr Nephrol. 2013;28:295–303.

96. Brady TM, Schneider MF, Flynn JT, et al. Carotid intima-media thickness in children with CKD: Results from the CKiD study. Clin J Am Soc Nephrol. 2012;7:1930–7.

97. Sarnak MJ, Bloom R, Muntner P, et al. KDOQI US Commentary on the 2013 KDIGO clinical practice guideline for lipid management in CKD. Am J Kidney Dis. 2015;65:354–66.

98. Scott JE, Renwick M. Antenatal diagnosis of congenital abnormalities in the urinary tract: Results from the Northern Region Fetal Abnormality Survey. Br J Urol. 1988;62:295–300.

99. National High Blood Pressure Education Program Working Group on High Blood Pressure in Children and Adolescents. The fourth report on the diagnosis, evaluation, and treatment of high blood pressure in children and adolescents. Pediatrics. 2004;114:555–76.

100. Furth SL, Abraham AG, Jerry-Fluker J, et al. Metabolic abnormalities, cardiovascular disease risk factors, and GFR decline in children with chronic kidney disease. Clin J Am Soc Nephrol. 2011;6:2132–40.

101. Wong H, Mylrea K, Feber J, et al. Prevalence of complications in children with chronic kidney disease according to KDOQI. Kidney Int. 2006;70:585–90.

102. Kidney Disease Outcomes Quality Initiative. Clinical practice guidelines for cardiovascular disease in dialysis patients. Am J Kidney Dis. 2005;45:S1–153.

103. Mitsnefes MM. Cardiovascular morbidity and mortality in children with chronic kidney disease in North America: Lessons from the USRDS and NAPRTCS databases. Perit Dial Int. 2005;25(Suppl 3):S120–2.

104. Mitsnefes MM. Cardiovascular disease in children with chronic kidney disease. J Am Soc Nephrol. 2012;23:578–85.

105. Parekh RS, Carroll CE, Wolfe RA, Port FK. Cardiovascular mortality in children and young adults with end-stage kidney disease. J Pediatr. 2002;141:191–7.

106. Chavers BM, Li S, Collins AJ, Herzog CA. Cardiovascular disease in pediatric chronic dialysis patients. Kidney Int. 2002;62:648–53.

107. Mitsnefes MM, Daniels SR, Schwartz SM, et al. Severe left ventricular hypertrophy in pediatric dialysis: Prevalence and predictors. Pediatr Nephrol. 2000;14:898–902.

108. Matteucci MC, Wuhl E, Picca S, et al. Left ventricular geometry in children with mild to moderate chronic renal insufficiency. J Am Soc Nephrol. 2006;17:218–26.

109. Mitsnefes MM, Daniels SR, Schwartz SM, et al. Changes in left ventricular mass in children and adolescents during chronic dialysis. Pediatr Nephrol. 2001;16:318–23.

110. Goodman WG, Goldin J, Kuizon BD, et al. Coronary-artery calcification in young adults with end-stage renal disease who are undergoing dialysis. N Engl J Med. 2000;342:1478–83.

111. Civilibal M, Caliskan S, Adaletli I, et al. Coronary artery calcifications in children with end-stage renal disease. Pediatr Nephrol. 2006;21:1426–33.

112. Kidney Disease Outcomes Quality Initiative. Clinical practice guidelines and clinical practice recommendations for anemia in chronic kidney disease. Am J Kidney Dis. 2006;47:S11–145.

113. Levin NW. Quality of life and hematocrit level. Am J Kidney Dis. 1992;20:16–20.

114. Wolcott DL, Marsh JT, La Rue A, et al. Recombinant human erythropoietin treatment may improve quality of life and cognitive function in chronic hemodialysis patients. Am J Kidney Dis. 1989;14:478–85.

115. Moreno F, Sanz-Guajardo D, Lopez-Gomez JM, et al. Increasing the hematocrit has a beneficial effect on quality of life and is safe in selected hemodialysis patients. J Am Soc Nephrol. 2000;11:335–42.

116. Fadrowski JJ, Pierce CB, Cole SR, et al. Hemoglobin decline in children with chronic kidney disease: Baseline results from the chronic kidney disease in children prospective cohort study. Clin J Am Soc Nephrol. 2008;3:457–62.

117. Astor BC, Muntner P, Levin A, et al. Association of kidney function with anemia: The Third National Health and Nutrition Examination Survey (1988-1994). Arch Intern Med. 2002;162:1401–8.

118. Donnelly S. Why is erythropoietin made in the kidney? The kidney functions as a critmeter. Am J Kidney Dis. 2001;38:415–25.

119. Ganz T. Hepcidin, a key regulator of iron metabolism and mediator of anemia of inflammation. Blood 2003;102:783–8.

120. Coyne DW. Hepcidin: Clinical utility as a diagnostic tool and therapeutic target. Kidney Int. 2011;80:240–4.

121. Zaritsky J, Young B, Wang HJ, et al. Hepcidin: A potential novel biomarker for iron status in chronic kidney disease. Clin J Am Soc Nephrol. 2009;4:1051–6.

122. Ashby DR, Gale DP, Busbridge M, et al. Plasma hepcidin levels are elevated but responsive to erythropoietin therapy in renal disease. Kidney Int. 2009;75:976–81.

123. Bachrach LK. Acquisition of optimal bone mass in childhood and adolescence. Trends Endocrinol Metab. 2001;12:22–8.

124. Kidney Disease Outcomes Quality Initiative. Clinical practice guidelines for bone metabolism and disease in children with chronic kidney disease. Am J Kidney Dis. 2005;46:700–811.

125. Kidney Disease: Improving Global Outcomes. Clinical practice guideline for the diagnosis, evaluation, prevention, and treatment of Chronic Kidney Disease-Mineral and Bone Disorder (CKD-MBD). Kidney Int Suppl. 2009;76:S1–130.

126. Martinez I, Saracho R, Montenegro J, Llach F. The importance of dietary calcium and phosphorus in the secondary hyperparathyroidism of patients with early renal failure. Am J Kidney Dis. 1997;29:496–502.

127. Uhlig K, Berns JS, Kestenbaum B, et al. KDOQI US commentary on the 2009 KDIGO clinical practice guideline for the diagnosis, evaluation, and treatment of CKD-mineral and bone disorder (CKD-MBD). Am J Kidney Dis. 2010;55:773–99.

128. Wahl P, Wolf M. FGF23 in chronic kidney disease. Adv Exp Med Biol. 2012;728:107–25.

129. Liu S, Quarles LD. How fibroblast growth factor 23 works. J Am Soc Nephrol. 2007;18:1637–47.

130. Isakova T, Wahl P, Vargas GS, et al. Fibroblast growth factor 23 is elevated before parathyroid hormone and phosphate in chronic kidney disease. Kidney Int. 2012;79:1370–8.

131. Gutierrez OM, Mannstadt M, Isakova T, et al. Fibroblast growth factor 23 and mortality among patients undergoing hemodialysis. N Engl J Med. 2008;359:584–92.

132. Isakova T, Xie H, Yang W, et al. Fibroblast growth factor 23 and risks of mortality and end-stage renal disease in patients with chronic kidney disease. JAMA. 2011;305:2432–9.

133. Faul C, Amaral AP, Oskouei B, et al. FGF23 induces left ventricular hypertrophy. J Clin Invest. 2011;121:4393–408.

134. Malluche HH, Mawad HW, Monier-Faugere MC. Renal osteodystrophy in the first decade of the new millennium: Analysis of 630 bone biopsies in black and white patients. J Bone Miner Res. 2011;26:1368–76.

135. Wong CS, Gipson DS, Gillen DL, et al. Anthropometric measures and risk of death in children with end-stage renal disease. Am J Kidney Dis. 2000;36:811–9.

136. Furth SL, Hwang W, Yang C, et al. Growth failure, risk of hospitalization and death for children with end-stage renal disease. Pediatr Nephrol. 2002;17:450–5.

137. Rosenkranz J, Reichwald-Klugger E, Oh J, et al. Psychosocial rehabilitation and satisfaction with life in adults with childhood-onset of end-stage renal disease. Pediatr Nephrol. 2005;20:1288–94.

138. Al-Uzri A, Matheson M, Gipson DS, et al. The impact of short stature on health-related quality of life in children with chronic kidney disease. J Pediatr. 2013;163:736–41.

139. Kidney Disease Outcomes Quality Initiative. Clinical practice guideline for nutrition in children with CKD: 2008 update—Executive summary. Am J Kidney Dis. 2009;53:S11–104.

140. Karlberg J. A biologically-oriented mathematical model (ICP) for human growth. Acta Paediatr Scand Suppl. 1989;350:70–94.

141. Clark PA, Rogol AD. Growth hormones and sex steroid interactions at puberty. Endocrinol Metab Clin North Am. 1996;25:665–81.

142. Ravelli AM, Ledermann SE, Bisset WM, et al. Foregut motor function in chronic renal failure. Arch Dis Child. 1992;67:1343–7.

143. Mak RH, Cheung W, Cone RD, Marks DL. Leptin and inflammation-associated cachexia in chronic kidney disease. Kidney Int. 2006;69:794–7.

144. Utaka S, Avesani CM, Draibe SA, et al. Inflammation is associated with increased energy expenditure in patients with chronic kidney disease. Am J Clin Nutr. 2005;82:801–5.

145. Parekh RS, Flynn JT, Smoyer WE, et al. Improved growth in young children with severe chronic renal insufficiency who use specified nutritional therapy. J Am Soc Nephrol. 2001;12:2418–26.

146. Roelfsema V, Clark RG. The growth hormone and insulin-like growth factor axis: Its manipulation for the benefit of growth disorders in renal failure. J Am Soc Nephrol. 2001;12:1297–306.

147. Yakar S, Rosen CJ, Beamer WG, et al. Circulating levels of IGF-1 directly regulate bone growth and density. J Clin Invest. 2002;110:771–81.

148. Haffner D, Schaefer F, Girard J, et al. Metabolic clearance of recombinant human growth hormone in health and chronic renal failure. J Clin Invest. 1994;93:1163–71.

149. Schaefer F, Chen Y, Tsao T, et al. Impaired JAK-STAT signal transduction contributes to growth hormone resistance in chronic uremia. J Clin Invest. 2001;108:467–75.

150. Sun DF, Zheng Z, Tummala P, et al. Chronic uremia attenuates growth hormone-induced signal transduction in skeletal muscle. J Am Soc Nephrol. 2004;15:2630–6.

151. Rabkin R, Sun DF, Chen Y, et al. Growth hormone resistance in uremia, a role for impaired JAK/STAT signaling. Pediatr Nephrol. 2005;20:313–8.

152. Kaysen GA. The microinflammatory state in uremia: Causes and potential consequences. J Am Soc Nephrol. 2001;12:1549–57.

153. Juul A, Flyvbjerg A, Frystyk J, et al. Serum concentrations of free and total insulin-like growth factor-I, IGF binding proteins -1 and -3 and IGFBP-3 protease activity in boys with normal or precocious puberty. Clin Endocrinol (Oxf). 1996;44:515–23.

154. Tonshoff B, Blum WF, Wingen AM, Mehls O. Serum insulin-like growth factors (IGFs) and IGF binding proteins 1, 2, and 3 in children with chronic renal failure: Relationship to height and glomerular filtration rate. The European Study Group for Nutritional Treatment of Chronic Renal Failure in Childhood. J Clin Endocrinol Metab. 1995;80:2684–91.

155. Wren AM, Seal LJ, Cohen MA, et al. Ghrelin enhances appetite and increases food intake in humans. J Clin Endocrinol Metab. 2001;86:5992.

156. Kojima M, Hosoda H, Date Y, et al. Ghrelin is a growth-hormone-releasing acylated peptide from stomach. Nature. 1999;402:656–60.

157. Bock GH, Conners CK, Ruley J, et al. Disturbances of brain maturation and neurodevelopment during chronic renal failure in infancy. J Pediatr. 1989;114:231–8.

158. Greenbaum LA, Warady BA, Furth SL. Current advances in chronic kidney disease in children: Growth, cardiovascular, and neurocognitive risk factors. Semin Nephrol. 2009;29:425–34.

159. Schnaper HW, Cole BR, Hodges FJ, Robson AM. Cerebral cortical atrophy in pediatric patients with end-stage renal disease. Am J Kidney Dis. 1983;2:645–50.

160. Steinberg A, Efrat R, Pomeranz A, Drukker A. Computerized tomography of the brain in children with chronic renal failure. Int J Pediatr Nephrol. 1985;6:121–6.

161. Gipson DS, Duquette PJ, Icard PF, Hooper SR. The central nervous system in childhood chronic kidney disease. Pediatr Nephrol. 2007;22:1703–10.

162. Slickers J, Duquette P, Hooper S, Gipson D. Clinical predictors of neurocognitive deficits in children with chronic kidney disease. Pediatr Nephrol. 2007;22:565–72.

163. Brouhard BH, Donaldson LA, Lawry KW, et al. Cognitive functioning in children on dialysis and post-transplantation. Pediatr Transplant. 2000;4:261–7.

164. Fennell RS, Fennell EB, Carter RL, et al. A longitudinal study of the cognitive function of children with renal failure. Pediatr Nephrol. 1990;4:11–5.

165. Gipson DS, Hooper SR, Duquette PJ, et al. Memory and executive functions in pediatric chronic kidney disease. Child Neuropsychol. 2006;12:391–405.

166. Groothoff JW, Grootenhuis M, Dommerholt A, et al. Impaired cognition and schooling in adults with end stage renal disease since childhood. Arch Dis Child. 2002;87:380–5.

167. Groothoff JW, Grootenhuis MA, Offringa M, et al. Social consequences in adult life of end-stage renal disease in childhood. J Pediatr. 2005;146:512–7.

168. Groothoff JW, Grootenhuis MA, Offringa M, et al. Quality of life in adults with end-stage renal disease since childhood is only partially impaired. Nephrol Dial Transplant 2003;18:310–7.

169. Merkus MP, Jager KJ, Dekker FW, et al. Quality of life in patients on chronic dialysis: Self-assessment 3 months after the start of treatment. The Necosad Study Group. Am J Kidney Dis. 1997;29:584–92.

170. Iglesias P, Díez JJ. Thyroid dysfunction and kidney disease. Eur J Endocrinol. 2009;160:503–15.

171. Rashid R, Neill E, Maxwell H, Ahmed SF. Growth and body composition in children with chronic kidney disease. Br J Nutr. 2007;97:232–8.

172. Stapleton FB, Andreoli S, Ettenger R, et al. Future workforce needs for pediatric nephrology: An analysis of the nephrology workforce and training requirements by the Workforce Committee of the American Society of Pediatric Nephrology. J Am Soc Nephrol. 1997;8:S5–8.

173. Khan SS, Xue JL, Kazmi WH, et al. Does predialysis nephrology care influence patient survival after initiation of dialysis? Kidney Int. 2005;67:1038–46.

174. The GISEN Group (Gruppo Italiano di Studi Epidemiologici in Nefrologia). Randomised placebo-controlled trial of effect of ramipril on decline in glomerular filtration rate and risk of terminal renal failure in proteinuric, non-diabetic nephropathy. Lancet. 1997;349:1857–63.

175. Jacobsen P, Andersen S, Rossing K, Jensen BR, Parving H-H. Dual blockade of the renin-angiotensin system versus maximal recommended dose of ACE inhibition in diabetic nephropathy. Kidney Int. 2003;63:1874–80.

176. Bianchi S, Bigazzi R, Campese VM. Long-term effects of spironolactone on proteinuria and kidney function in patients with chronic kidney disease. Kidney Int. 2006;70:2116–23.

177. Flynn JT, Mitsnefes M, Pierce C, et al. Blood pressure in children with chronic kidney disease: A report from the Chronic Kidney Disease in Children study. Hypertension. 2008;52:631–7.

178. Mitsnefes M, Flynn J, Cohn S, et al. Masked hypertension associates with left ventricular hypertrophy in children with CKD. J Am Soc Nephrol. 2010;21:137–44.

179. Kidney Disease Outcomes Quality Initiative. Clinical practice guidelines on hypertension and antihypertensive agents in chronic kidney disease. Am J Kidney Dis. 2004;43:S1–290.

180. Mitch WE. Dietary protein restriction in chronic renal failure: Nutritional efficacy, compliance, and progression of renal insufficiency. J Am Soc Nephrol. 1991;2:823–31.

181. Bernhard J, Beaufrere B, Laville M, Fouque D. Adaptive response to a low-protein diet in predialysis chronic renal failure patients. J Am Soc Nephrol. 2001;12:1249–54.

182. Fukui M, Nakamura T, Ebihara I, et al. Low-protein diet attenuates increased gene expression of platelet-derived growth factor and transforming growth factor-beta in experimental glomerular sclerosis. J Lab Clin Med. 1993;121:224–34.

183. Chaturvedi S, Jones C. Protein restriction for children with chronic renal failure. Cochrane Database Syst Rev. 2007;(4)006863.

184. Madero M, Sarnak MJ, Wang X, et al. Uric acid and long-term outcomes in CKD. Am J Kidney Dis. 2009;53:796–803.

185. Goicoechea M, de Vinuesa SG, Verdalles U, et al. Effect of allopurinol in chronic kidney disease progression and cardiovascular risk. Clin J Am Soc Nephrol. 2010;5:1388–93.

186. Kidney Disease Outcomes Quality Initiative. Clinical practice guideline and clinical practice recommendations for anemia in chronic kidney disease: 2007 update of hemoglobin target. Am J Kidney Dis. 2007;50:471–530.

187. Kidney Disease: Improving Global Outcomes Anemia Work Group. KDIGO clinical practice guideline for anemia in chronic kidney disease. Kidney Int Suppl. 2012;2:279–335.

188. Seikaly MG, Salhab N, Warady BA, Stablein D. Use of rhGH in children with chronic kidney disease: Lessons from NAPRTCS. Pediatr Nephrol. 2007;22:1195–204.

189. Nissel R, Brazda I, Feneberg R, et al. Effect of renal transplantation in childhood on longitudinal growth and adult height. Kidney Int. 2004;66:792–800.

190. Hokken-Koelega AC, van Zaal MA, van Bergen W, et al. Final height and its predictive factors after renal transplantation in childhood. Pediatr Res. 1994;36:323–8.

191. Haffner D, Wühl E, Schaefer F, et al. Effect of growth hormone treatment on the adult height of children with chronic renal failure. N Engl J Med. 2000;343:923–30.

192. Jabs K, Van Dop C, Harmon WE. Growth hormone treatment of growth failure among children with renal transplants. Kidney Int Suppl. 1993;43:S71–5.

193. Fine RN, Stablein D. Long-term use of recombinant human growth hormone in pediatric allograft recipients: A report of the NAPRTCS Transplant Registry. Pediatr Nephrol. 2005;20:404–8.

194. Wühl E, Haffner D, Nissel R, et al. Short dialyzed children respond less to growth hormone than patients prior to dialysis. German Study Group for Growth Hormone Treatment in Chronic Renal Failure. Pediatr Nephrol. 1996;10:294–8.

195. Mauras N, Attie KM, Reiter EO, et al. High dose recombinant human growth hormone (GH) treatment of GH-deficient patients in puberty increases near-final height: A randomized, multicenter trial. Genentech, Inc., Cooperative Study Group. J Clin Endocrinol Metab. 2000;85:3653–60.

196. Mahan JD, Warady BA. Assessment and treatment of short stature in pediatric patients with chronic kidney disease: A consensus statement. Pediatr Nephrol. 2006;21:917–30.

197. Kasiske BL, Snyder JJ, Matas AJ, et al. Preemptive kidney transplantation: The advantage and the advantaged. J Am Soc Nephrol. 2002;13:1358–64.

198. Vats AN, Donaldson L, Fine RN, Chavers BM. Pretransplant dialysis status and outcome of renal transplantation in North American children: A NAPRTCS Study. North American Pediatric Renal Transplant Cooperative Study. Transplantation. 2000;69:1414–9.

199. Mitch WE, Walser M, Buffington GA, et al. A simple method of estimating progression of chronic renal failure. Lancet. 1976;2:1326–8.

200. Hamilton BE, Hoyert DL, Martin JA, et al. Annual summary of vital statistics: 2010-2011. Pediatrics. 2013;131:548–58.

201. McDonald SP, Craig JC. Long-term survival of children with end-stage renal disease. N Engl J Med. 2004;350:2654–62.

## REVIEW QUESTIONS

1. The *most* common cause of CKD in children is:
   a. Focal segmental glomerulosclerosis
   b. Polycystic kidney disease
   c. Congenital anomalies of the kidneys and urinary tract (CAKUT)
   d. Immune-mediated glomerulonephritis
   e. Hemolytic-uremic syndrome
2. The incidence of ESRD in children:
   a. Decreases with increasing age
   b. Remains the same throughout childhood and adolescence
   c. Is highest in children younger than 4 years
   d. Increases with advancing age
3. In the United States, FSGS is the predominant cause of CKD in:
   a. African Americans
   b. Hispanics
   c. Whites
   d. Native Americans
   e. Asian Americans
4. Mortality of children with ESRD is highest in which age group?
   a. 0 to 4 years
   b. 5 to 14 years
   c. 15 to 19 years
5. Angiotensin II plays a role in progression of CKD by:
   a. Causing predominant afferent over efferent arteriolar vasoconstriction
   b. Decreasing single-nephron GFR
   c. Increasing proinflammatory cytokines, chemokines, and cell adhesion molecules
   d. Stimulating aldosterone, which itself is injurious to the kidney
   e. a, b, and d
   f. c and d
6. What is the *most* common complication of CKD in children?
   a. Anemia
   b. Hypertension
   c. Fluid and electrolyte abnormalities
   d. Growth failure
   e. Mineral and bone disorder

7. The prevalence of LVH in pediatric dialysis patients is:
    a. 10%
    b. 20%
    c. 30%
    d. Up to 50%
    e. Up to 75%
8. In children the fastest rate of growth occurs:
    a. During infancy
    b. Age 1 to 4 years
    c. Age 4 to 10 years
    d. During puberty
9. All of the following contribute to growth impairment in children with CKD, *except:*
    a. Malnutrition
    b. Anemia
    c. GH deficiency
    d. Altered post–receptor signaling of JAK2 and STAT proteins
    e. Reduced bioavailability of IGF-1
10. All of the following central and neurocognitive deficits occur in children with CKD *except:*
    a. Cerebral atrophy
    b. Speech and language delay
    c. Lower educational attainment
    d. Lower IQ scores
    e. Macrocephaly and hydrocephalus

11. In children with CKD, all but one of the following therapeutic interventions slow progression.
    a. ACE-inhibitors or angiotensin receptor blockers
    b. Blood pressure control
    c. Minimizing proteinuria
    d. Cholesterol-lowering therapy

## ANSWER KEY

1. c
2. d
3. a
4. a
5. f
6. b
7. e
8. a
9. c
10. e
11. d

# 32

# Anemia in chronic kidney disease

## MEREDITH ATKINSON

Anemia is a common complication in children with chronic kidney disease (CKD), and it increases in prevalence with advancing disease stage. In addition to being costly to treat, anemia is associated with a variety of adverse clinical consequences including death, hospitalizations, and the development and progression of cardiovascular risk factors such as left ventricular hypertrophy (LVH).[1-3] The introduction of recombinant human erythropoietin (rHuEPO) in the late 1980s revolutionized anemia management by decreasing the need for red blood cell transfusions in patients with CKD. However, there is increasing concern about potential adverse effects of treatment with erythropoiesis-stimulating agents (ESAs). Anemia management in children continues to focus on avoiding transfusions by correction of iron deficiency and the use of ESAs. This chapter reviews the definition, risk factors, and pathophysiology of anemia in children with CKD, with specific attention to current therapeutic strategies and ongoing challenges in its management. The Kidney Disease: Improving Global Outcomes (KDIGO) workgroup published an evidence-based clinical practice guideline for anemia in chronic kidney disease.[4]

## DEFINITION, MONITORING, AND INITIAL EVALUATION

Normal hemoglobin (Hb) levels vary among individual persons based on age and sex.[5-7] The application of adult normative Hb thresholds has been shown to underestimate the prevalence of anemia substantially in patients with CKD who are less than 18 years old.[8] Consequently, the KDGIO clinical practice guideline for anemia uses World Health Organization (WHO) age-specific Hb values to define the level at which an evaluation for the cause of anemia should be initiated (Table 32.1).[4] An alternative source for specific Hb thresholds to define anemia in children 1 to 19 years old is the National Health and Nutrition Examination Survey (NHANES) III data from 1988 to 1994, which reports age- and sex-specific fifth percentile values (Table 32.2).[5] In children without an established diagnosis of anemia, Hb should be measured at least annually in those with stage 3 CKD, at least twice annually in those with stage 4 to 5 CKD, and at least every 3 months in those undergoing dialysis. Hb should be measured more frequently for clinical indications and in children with known anemia.[4]

Because anemia in children with CKD may not be associated solely with EPO deficiency (particularly in patients with only mildly impaired renal function), the initial laboratory evaluation should include a complete blood count to assess red blood cell indices (mean corpuscular hemoglobin, mean corpuscular volume, and mean corpuscular hemoglobin concentration), the absolute reticulocyte count, and serum ferritin and transferrin saturation (TSAT) to assess the adequacy of iron for erythropoiesis.[4] Vitamin $B_{12}$ and folate deficiency are uncommon but easily correctable causes of anemia and should be included in an initial laboratory evaluation, particularly in the setting of macrocytosis.[4] Anemia with concurrent lymphopenia or thrombocytopenia should prompt an evaluation for malignancy, autoimmune disease, or drug toxicity. Microcytosis is most commonly secondary to iron deficiency, but it may be caused by a hereditary hemoglobinopathy, which should be screened for if indicated. Reticulocytosis may result from chronic blood loss or hemolysis, and it should prompt testing for blood in the stool and

Table 32.1 World Health Organization age-specific hemoglobin thresholds for the definition of anemia in children

| Age (yr) | Hemoglobin (g/dL) |
|----------|-------------------|
| 0.5–5 | <11.0 |
| 5–12 | <11.5 |
| 12–15 | <12.0 |
| >15: male | <13.0 |
| >–15: female | <12.0 |

Source: Kidney Disease: Improving Global Outcomes (KDIGO) Anemia Work Group. KDIGO clinical practice guideline for anemia in chronic kidney disease. Kidney Int. Suppl. 2012;2:279–335.

Table 32.2 Age- and sex-specific fifth percentile hemoglobin values for children 1 to 19 years of age based on population-based data from the National Health and Nutrition Examination Survey (NHANES) 1988 to 1994

| Age (yr) | Hemoglobin (g/dL) | |
|----------|------|--------|
| | Male | Female |
| 1–2 | 10.7 | 10.8 |
| 3–5 | 11.2 | 11.1 |
| 6–8 | 11.5 | 11.5 |
| 9–11 | 12.0 | 11.9 |
| 12–14 | 12.4 | 11.7 |
| 15–19 | 13.5 | 11.5 |

Source: Hollowell JG, van Assendelft OW, Gunter EW, et al. Hematological and iron-related analytes—reference data for persons aged 1 year and over: United States, 1988–94. Data from the Third National Health Examination Survey. Vital Health Stat 11. 2005;(247):1–156.

serum markers of hemolysis. The use of aluminum-containing phosphate binders has historically been linked to aluminum toxicity and anemia, but the rare use of these binders has virtually eliminated this complication.[9] Other correctable causes of anemia that are not CKD should be ruled out in patients before initiation of treatment with an ESA.

---

## KEY POINT

The initial anemia evaluation in children with CKD should include a complete blood count with red blood cell indices and reticulocyte count, assessment for iron and other nutritional deficiency, and screening for occult blood loss if indicated.

---

## EPIDEMIOLOGY AND RISK FACTORS

The level of kidney function is the key risk factor for the development of anemia in CKD. Data from the North American Pediatric Renal Trials and Collaborative Studies

(NAPRTCS) cohort has consistently shown that the risk for anemia increases as CKD stage advances, with a prevalence of 73% at stage 3, 87% at stage 5, and more than 93% at stage 5.[10,11] Within the Chronic Kidney Disease in Children (CKiD) cohort study, Hb declined as iohexol-determined glomerular filtration rate decreased to less than 43 mL/min/1.73 m$^2$, although anemia can also be observed at higher rates.[12] Furthermore, among children prescribed an ESA, more than 20% of those at stage 4 and more than 40% at stage 5 demonstrate persistently low Hb levels.[10]

Other independent risk factors for the anemia of CKD include treatment with antihypertensive agents[10,11]; hypertension may be a marker of disease severity, but ACE inhibitors may also contribute to anemia by inhibition of erythropoiesis.[13] In the International Pediatric Peritoneal Dialysis Network (IPPN) registry, low residual renal function, low serum albumin, increased parathyroid hormone levels, high serum ferritin, and the use of bioincompatible dialysate were associated with low Hb levels.[14] Race is also a recognized risk factor for anemia. Among children enrolled in the CKiD study, African Americans have consistently lower Hb levels than white children, even after adjusting for level of kidney function.[7] Although normal Hb levels in healthy children differ by race and ethnicity, current anemia management guidelines do not recommend varying Hb targets or approach to treatment by race.[15]

## ADVERSE ASSOCIATIONS

The anemia of CKD is associated with substantial morbidity in children. Among children on dialysis, low Hb is a strong and independent predictor of death and is associated with increased frequency of hospitalization.[1,14,16,17] Even in the predialysis population, anemia has been associated with an almost 40% increased risk for all-cause hospitalization in children with stage 2 to 5 CKD.[11] Anemia is an important cardiovascular risk factor in children, and it increases the risk for development of LVH independently of elevation in blood pressure, even in mild to moderate CKD.[2,18,19] In children receiving peritoneal dialysis, both hypertension and LVH increase with increasing degree of anemia.[14] Anemia also adversely affects quality of life, including neurocognitive development and exercise capacity.[20] Anemic adolescents with CKD report greater limitations in physical functioning, schoolwork, and activities with friends and family, independent of level of kidney function.[21] Correction of anemia with ESAs has been associated with increased catch-up growth in children with CKD.[22] Finally, there is some evidence in adults that early treatment of mild anemia delays the initiation of renal replacement therapy, and anemia in adolescents with CKD is associated with an accelerated decline in glomerular filtration rate.[23,24] Data from the NAPRTCS registry has also shown anemia to be a risk factor for CKD progression.[25] One proposed mechanism for this is increased production of profibrotic cytokines secondary to renal tissue hypoxia.

Although these and other comorbidities are multifactorial in origin, anemia likely contributes to their development, and its treatment may mitigate some of the risk.

An additional potential adverse effect of anemia is an increase in human leukocyte antigen (HLA) antibodies in patients requiring red blood cell transfusions. Leukoreduction of blood products has been shown to be ineffective for decreasing HLA sensitization, and red blood cell transfusions lead to clinically significant increases in HLA antibody strength and breadth, thus adversely affecting the viability of future transplants.[26,27]

---

### KEY POINT

The adverse associations of anemia in children with CKD include increased risk for hospitalization and death, decreased quality of life, and increased risk for LVH.

---

## PATHOGENESIS

A complex interaction of factors is responsible for decreasing Hb values as kidney disease progresses (Table 32.3 and Figure 32.1), but impaired EPO production by failing kidneys is a central cause. EPO is a 30.4-kDa glycoprotein encoded by a gene on the seventh chromosome that was first identified and cloned in 1985.[28-30] Although human EPO is produced by hepatocytes prenatally, the primary production site shifts to the peritubular fibroblasts in the renal cortex at

Table 32.3 Pathogenic factors in the development of the anemia of chronic kidney disease in children

- Impaired or dysregulated erythropoietin production
- Iron-restricted erythropoiesis
  - Absolute iron deficiency
  - Functional iron deficiency
  - Impaired iron trafficking
- Inflammation (chronic or acute)
- Nutritional deficiencies
  - Folic acid, vitamin $B_{12}$, carnitine
  - Uremia or inadequate dialysis
  - Hyperparathyroidism or bone mineral metabolism disorder
- Chronic blood loss, hemolysis
- Medications (ACEi, nonadherence)
- Pure red cell aplasia
- Hemoglobinopathies

ACEi, angiotensin converting enzyme inhibitor.

birth.[31] Circulating EPO regulates erythroid proliferation and survival, primarily by an antiapoptotic mechanism, by binding to cell surface receptors of erythroid progenitor cells in the bone marrow.[28,29] EPO also acts as a growth factor to enhance red blood cell maturation.[29] The primary stimulus for EPO expression is hypoxia; EPO production is increased by a hypoxia-inducible transcription factor that controls the EPO gene.[28,31] Although EPO production can be decreased in CKD by destruction of peritubular fibroblasts, dysregulation of the renal oxygen-sensing mechanism has also been shown to contribute to inappropriately low EPO production in patients, independent of damage to EPO-producing cells.[32] EPO production in CKD may also be downregulated by the decreased distal tubular sodium reabsorption caused by decreased GFR, which then signals a decrease in EPO production.[28,33] Although measurement of EPO in patients with CKD has revealed levels in the normal to slightly increased range, the levels are inappropriately low for the degree of anemia; EPO levels are 10 to 100 times higher in anemic patients with normal kidney function.[9,28]

Iron-restricted erythropoiesis is also an important cause of the anemia of CKD. Iron restriction may be secondary to absolute iron deficiency, to functional iron deficiency in which accessible iron stores are depleted by an ESA-stimulated bone marrow, or to impaired iron trafficking in the setting of inflammation.[34] The markers of iron status most often used clinically are serum ferritin, a marker of stored iron, and TSAT, which measures circulating iron available for delivery to the bone marrow. Children with CKD are at risk for absolute iron deficiency because of a variety of factors, including decreased nutritional intake and poor enteral absorption, as well as blood loss through the gastrointestinal tract, menstruation, frequent phlebotomy, and hemodialysis.[9,33] Patients with absolute iron deficiency have low serum ferritin and TSAT levels. In patients with functional iron deficiency who are receiving ESAs, the rate of enteral iron absorption or release from reticuloendothelial cells is inadequate to meet the demands for erythropoiesis.[34] These patients often have low TSAT values with normal or high levels of ferritin, and selected patients may benefit from treatment with intravenous (IV) iron.[35] Inflammation also results in impaired iron trafficking through the actions of the iron-regulatory protein hepcidin, production of which is directly upregulated by inflammatory cytokines and which is cleared from the circulation by glomerular filtration.[34,36] Hepcidin causes internalization and degradation of the primary cellular iron exporter, ferroportin, that result in trapping of stored iron within enterocytes and reticuloendothelial cells.[36,37]

---

### KEY POINT

Impaired EPO production and iron-restricted erythropoiesis are primary causes of the anemia of CKD.

---

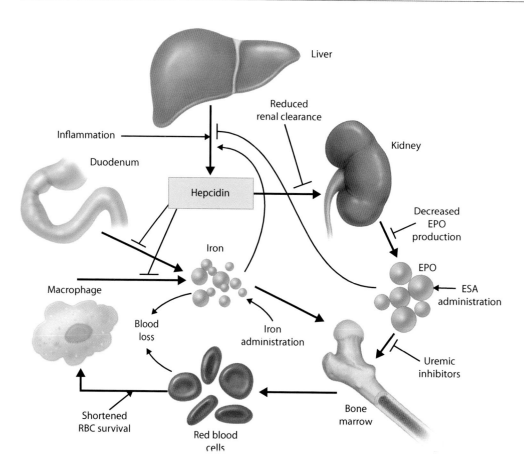

Figure 32.1 Schematic representation of the mechanisms underlying anemia of chronic kidney disease (CKD). Iron and erythropoietin (EPO) are crucial for red blood cell (RBC) production in the bone marrow. Iron availability is controlled by the liver hormone hepcidin, which regulates dietary iron absorption and macrophage iron recycling from senescent RBCs. Several feedback loops control hepcidin levels, including iron and EPO. In patients with CKD (particularly in patients with end-stage kidney disease who are undergoing hemodialysis), hepcidin levels have been found to be highly elevated, presumably from reduced renal clearance and induction by inflammation, leading to iron-restricted erythropoiesis. CKD also inhibits EPO production by the kidney and may also lead to circulating uremic-induced inhibitors of erythropoiesis, shortened RBC life span, and increased blood loss. The black and gray arrows represent normal physiology (black for iron and hormonal fluxes and gray for regulatory processes). The blue arrows represent the additional effects of CKD (blue for activation and red for inhibition). ESA, erythropoiesis-stimulating agent. (Adapted from Babitt JL, Lin HY. Mechanisms of anemia in CKD. J Am Soc Nephrol.. 2012;23:1631–4.)

Beyond iron deficiency, nutritional deficiencies of vitamin $B_{12}$, folate, carnitine, and vitamin C may also contribute to anemia in CKD. Deficiency of folate, which is required for DNA synthesis during erythropoiesis, has been observed in children undergoing dialysis, and when it was corrected in a small pediatric hemodialysis cohort, Hb increased and ESA dose requirement decreased.[38] CKD, and especially long-term hemodialysis, is a leading cause of secondary carnitine deficiency because of its ready dialyzability, among other contributing factors, including decreased dietary intake.[39] Some studies have suggested that L-carnitine supplementation can prolong red cell life span and stimulate erythropoiesis by inhibiting apoptosis, but there have been no large-scale randomized clinical trials conducted to evaluate whether supplementation is effective as an adjunctive treatment for anemia in patients undergoing dialysis.[39] Vitamin C enhances absorption of dietary iron, contributes to the mobilization of intracellular

stored iron, and increases carnitine synthesis. Vitamin C deficiency is common in patients undergoing dialysis as a result of restricted nutritional intake, increased vitamin C catabolism in the setting of inflammation, and perhaps dialytic clearance.[40] However, as with carnitine, there have been no clinical trials to assess the effects of vitamin C supplementation on anemia in patients undergoing dialysis.[40]

Chronic uremia also contributes to anemia through hemolysis; exposure to uremic serum shortens the life span of erythrocytes from healthy subjects, with cell survival time decreased by as much as 50%.[30] The mechanisms seem to be premature changes in the cell membrane and cytoskeleton of red blood cells resulting from uremic toxins and increased oxidative stress.[41] Initially, increased red blood cell production compensates for anemia, but this mechanism is no longer effective once EPO production decreases.[30] Hyperparathyroidism has also been associated with ESA hyporesponsiveness, likely because of decreased bone marrow production of red blood cells in the setting of myelofibrosis.[28,42,43] Finally, ESA-induced pure red cell aplasia (PRCA) is an increasingly rare hematologic disorder that was first described in the late 1990s. PRCA is characterized by a severe and progressive normocytic anemia, reticulocytopenia, and the almost complete absence of erythroid precursors in the bone marrow; affected patients become transfusion dependent.[44] ESA-induced PRCA is secondary to the development of neutralizing antibodies that block the interaction between an ESA (including epoetin alfa or beta, darbepoetin alfa, or endogenous EPO) and its receptor.[44] Most initial cases of ESA-induced PRCA were seen in countries where epoetin alfa formulated with a polysorbate 80 stabilizer was administered subcutaneously to patients with CKD, and regulatory advisories have subsequently discouraged this practice.[45] The evaluation of suspected PRCA includes bone marrow examination and measurement of anti-EPO antibodies.[44]

## TREATMENT

## IRON SUPPLEMENTATION

Both absolute iron deficiency and defects in iron handling make substantial contributions to the development of anemia because red blood cells cannot be produced in the absence of iron. The goal of iron supplementation is to prevent iron deficiency in ESA-treated patients, to raise Hb in iron-deficient patients not yet treated with ESAs, and to reduce the ESA dose required to maintain Hb levels. Iron supplementation is indicated in patients with depleted iron stores and in patients who are likely to have a clinically significant increase in red blood cell production.[4] However, the challenge is to avoid the use of iron in patients who are unlikely to benefit. Patients with hepcidin-mediated iron sequestration are unlikely to absorb enteral iron supplements or to mobilize iron stored as ferritin for the purposes of erythropoiesis. It is clear that administration of iron, and in particular IV iron, increases oxidative stress; hence iron should not be given to patients who cannot use it effectively to increase red blood cell production.[34,46,47]

### Assessment of iron stores

The gold standard test for quantification of body iron stores is bone marrow iron staining, but for practical considerations this is rarely performed clinically.[48] The most widely available and clinically utilized tests are serum ferritin, considered to be a reflection of stored iron, and TSAT, an indicator of the amount of iron available for transport to the bone marrow for erythropoiesis.[48–50] Ferritin and transferrin provide the safe storage and transport, respectively, of the highly reactive iron element. There are various other potentially useful markers of iron status in patients with CKD including reticulocyte Hb content, percentage of hypochromic red blood cells, soluble transferrin receptor, and

erythrocyte zinc protoporphyrin, but none have yet achieved widespread clinical use.[50] The definition of absolute iron deficiency in healthy children, from population-based data, includes serum ferritin values less than 10 to 12 ng/mL and TSAT values lower than 10% to 15%.[51] The current KDIGO clinical practice recommends initiation of oral iron (IV iron in patients undergoing hemodialysis) in anemic children with CKD who are not treated with ESA when the TSAT is 20% or lower and the serum ferritin is 100 ng/mL or lower.[4] Additionally, for children receiving ESA therapy, oral (or IV in the case of hemodialysis) iron supplementation should be provided to maintain the TSAT at more than 20% and the ferritin greater than 100 ng/mL.[4] There is no evidence that targeting a higher ferritin of 200 ng/mL, as has been recommended in adults, is appropriate in pediatric patients.[4] Routine use of iron supplementation to target TSAT greater than 30% or ferritin greater than 500 ng/mL is not recommended, given that the risks and benefits of doing so have not been adequately studied in either adults or children.

## KEY POINTS

- Ferritin and TSAT are the most widely used markers of iron stores in children with CKD.
- Goal thresholds in ESA-treated children are TSAT greater than 20% and ferritin greater than 100 ng/mL.

Ferritin and TSAT have limitations and may not accurately reflect iron that can be used in the bone marrow for erythropoiesis. Children with CKD, and in particular children undergoing long-term dialysis, may demonstrate normal or elevated ferritin levels, low TSAT levels, and persistent anemia despite ESA therapy, findings indicative of inflammation-mediated iron-restricted erythropoiesis.[34,52] Ferritin is the main intracellular storage molecule for iron, and it allows for storage of iron while minimizing the risk of oxidation by free iron.[50] Measurement of ferritin concentration in the serum depends on its leakage from the intracellular compartment into the serum, and the process by which ferritin enters the circulation is not completely understood.[50] Ferritin is also an acute phase reactant, and its production is upregulated by inflammatory stimuli, thus confounding its usefulness as an accurate indicator of accessible stored iron.[49,50] Studies in children with CKD have demonstrated that higher serum ferritin values are associated with lower Hb values,[14,48] a finding suggesting that an elevated ferritin level may be a marker of inflammation rather than an accurate indicator of iron stores. Given that TSAT is calculated from serum iron divided by total iron binding capacity, which is a negative acute phase reactant, its value may also be artificially increased by inflammation.[49,50] There is evidence that serum iron, as an indicator of accessible iron stores, may be more closely associated with clinical outcomes in adults undergoing hemodialysis.[53] In a study of children with CKD who were not undergoing dialysis, serum iron lower than 50 µg/dL was more closely associated with lower Hb than either low ferritin or low TSAT, a finding suggesting that low serum iron values in the setting of normal or increased ferritin and low Hb may be useful indicators of iron-restricted erythropoiesis secondary to inflammation and hepcidin-mediated impaired iron trafficking.[48]

## Route of administration

The choice of route of iron therapy (oral vs. IV) should take into account a variety of factors, including the relative severity of iron deficiency and anemia and the response, tolerance, and adherence to earlier treatment with oral iron.[4] Although oral iron supplementation is generally inexpensive and readily available, it may have limited efficacy for maintaining adequate iron stores as a result of poor enteral absorption coupled with issues of adherence. Children undergoing long-term hemodialysis in particular may be poorly responsive to enteral iron supplements secondary to chronic blood loss and inflammation. The efficacy of IV iron preparations in improving measured iron stores, increasing Hb concentration, and decreasing ESA doses required to maintain Hb has been confirmed in studies in children undergoing hemodialysis.[9,54,55] IV iron increases Hb levels in children with CKD who are not undergoing dialysis and who are not treated with ESAs.[56] Various IV iron preparations are available, including iron dextran, iron gluconate, and iron sucrose, but any formulation may be associated with potentially severe acute reactions that require close monitoring.[4,9] The spectrum of toxicity can range from hypotension and dyspnea to anaphylaxis, potentially mediated by immune mechanisms or acute induction of oxidative stress, and toxicity has been observed more commonly with iron dextran preparations.[4] Administration of IV iron preparations should be avoided in patients with active systemic infections out of concern that many pathogens require iron for proliferation.

---

### KEY POINTS

- Oral iron supplementation is safe and efficacious in children with CKD, but children with more advanced CKD or undergoing dialysis may have poor enteral iron absorption.
- IV iron preparations are available when there is a poor response to enteral supplements.

---

## ERYTHROPOIESIS-STIMULATING AGENTS

The development of rHuEPO in the 1980s and its clinical utility for replacing endogenous EPO were critical developments in the management of the anemia of CKD in children. One of the most significant effects of its widespread use was a reduction in the need for regular blood transfusions in patients with advanced CKD, thereby decreasing the occurrence of transfusion-associated viral infections, iron overload, and allosensitization.[4,26,27,57] However, clinical trials performed in adults have raised concerns about the safety and efficacy of using escalating ESA doses to normalize Hb levels. The Normal Hematocrit Trial (in hemodialysis recipients) and the Correction of Hemoglobin and Outcomes in Renal Insufficiency (CHOIR) Trial (in CKD not treated with dialysis) both found that the use of epoetin alfa to target higher hematocrit or Hb levels was associated with increased risk for death and adverse cardiovascular events, including myocardial infarction and stroke.[58,59] Subsequently, the Trial to Reduce Cardiovascular Events With Aranesp Therapy (TREAT) trial, performed in more than 4000 adults with diabetes and CKD, randomized subjects to either darbepoetin alfa to achieve Hb levels greater than 13 g/dL or placebo, with only rescue darbepoetin alfa for Hb lower than 9 g/dL. The intervention group had an increased risk for stroke, thus providing additional evidence that ESA treatment to normalize Hb in CKD may lead to adverse events.[60] None of these trials clarified whether higher Hb level or high ESA dose was the more significant contributor to adverse outcomes, although a prospective study performed in adults undergoing hemodialysis found that patients with naturally occurring higher Hb levels were not at increased risk for death.[61,62] Proposed mechanisms for the adverse outcomes associated with ESA use include trophic effects on vascular endothelial or smooth muscle cells.[63]

In 2011 the US Food and Drug Administration changed ESA product labeling to recommend that the previously identified Hb target range of 10 to 12 g/dL should be replaced by the practice of using the lowest possible ESA dose to prevent red blood cell transfusions, and that ESA dosing should be reduced or interrupted for Hb levels exceeding 11 g/dL.[64] Observational studies in pediatric patients undergoing dialysis have demonstrated associations between increased ESA dose and death.[14,65] However, no randomized controlled trials examining the effects of ESA administration on clinical outcomes in children with CKD have been performed, and the current recommendations regarding safe target Hb levels in children treated with ESAs are still extrapolated from adult studies.

---

### KEY POINT

Trials in adults have found ESA use to be associated with increased incidence of stroke and other adverse outcomes, but no such randomized controlled trials have been performed in children with CKD.

---

## Types of agents

Several types of both short-acting and long-acting ESAs are available worldwide, and new formulations continue to emerge, requiring ongoing attention to relative safety and efficacy in children compared with adults. There is currently no definitive evidence of superiority in patient outcomes for any particular ESA brand.[4] Among rHuEPO types, epoetin alfa is a commonly used form of rHuEPO in the United States, and epoetin beta is more commonly used in Europe.[66] Short-acting epoetin formulations reach maximum efficacy when dosed one to three times weekly and are more effective when given by the subcutaneous route (half-life, 19 to 24 h) rather than the IV (half-life, 6 to 8 h) route.[67] In contrast, darbepoetin alfa, an EPO analogue with a longer half-life than rHuEPO, has maximum efficacy when given every 2 weeks.[4,33,67] Darbepoetin alfa may be administered intravenously or subcutaneously, and although drug clearance, half-life, and bioavailability are similar between adults and children regardless of route of administration, absorption when given subcutaneously may be more rapid in children.[68] Longer dosing interval compared with rHuEPO has made subcutaneous darbepoetin alfa an attractive alternative for anemia management in younger children and is likely to improve adherence. A randomized clinical trial in children with CKD stages 4 and 5 demonstrated that darbepoetin alfa is as safe and effective as rHuEPO for the correction of anemia.[69] A potential limitation of darbepoetin alfa in children is the reported discomfort associated with injection. A randomized controlled trial in children with end-stage renal disease demonstrated that subcutaneous injection of darbepoetin alfa was associated with significantly higher pain perception in children than was subcutaneous epoetin beta.[70] A potential explanation is the more physiologic pH of the buffer in the epoetin beta preparation than in the darbepoetin alfa preparation.[70]

> **KEY POINT**
>
> Darbepoetin alfa is a safe and effective treatment for the anemia of CKD in children, with an advantage of a longer dosing interval compared with rHuEPO.

Additional long-acting ESAs include the continuous EPO receptor activator (CERA) methoxy polyethylene glycol-epoetin beta, which has a half-life of 134 h after subcutaneous administration, thus permitting an extended administration interval of 4 weeks.[67] However, there are limited studies of CERA safety and efficacy in children.

## Initiation, dosing, and monitoring

The KDIGO clinical practice guideline for anemia recommends that the selection of the Hb concentration at which to begin ESA therapy be the result of consideration of the benefits and risks of treatment in individual patients. ESA initiation should be considered for Hb levels persistently lower than 10 g/dL, and Hb levels less than 9 g/dL in patients undergoing dialysis should be avoided. In children

receiving ESA therapy, the goal Hb level should be 11 to 12 g/dL.[4] The goal after ESA initiation is for a rate of increase in Hb concentration of no more than 1 to 2 g/dL per month.[4] The starting dose range for epoetin alfa or epoetin beta is 20 to 50 international units/kg three times weekly (subcutaneously or intravenously) with dose adjustments as necessary to maintain Hb in range to avoid transfusion and not to exceed upper limit of 11-12 g/dL.[4] In children older than 1 year, darbepoetin alfa should be initiated at 0.45 µg/kg intravenously or subcutaneously dosed once weekly, or 0.75 µg/kg dosed every 2 weeks subcutaneously.[4]

> **KEY POINT**
>
> The goal Hb level in children receiving ESA therapy is in the range of 11 to 12 g/dL.

The dosing requirements of rHuEPO may differ substantially between children and adults. Based on registry data, young children require higher rHuEPO doses than adults, ranging from 275 to 350 units/kg/week for infants to 200 to 250 units/kg/week for older children.[28] Children and adolescents undergoing long-term hemodialysis have been found to require higher absolute doses of rHuEPO than adults to maintain target Hb levels, despite lower body weight.[71] In contrast to typical drug dosing in children, which is based on body size to account for decreased volume of distribution, rHuEPO dose requirement appears to be independent of weight.[71,72] It has been shown that an absolute rHuEPO dose of 1000 units given intravenously to both adults and children can increase Hb by 0.4 g/dL, a finding suggesting that dosing schemes based on Hb deficit rather than weight may be useful.[73] The potential mechanisms for increased rHuEPO dose requirement in children are not clear, but they may include increased presence of nonhematopoietic EPO binding sites (e.g., endothelial, kidney, brain, and skeletal muscle cells) resulting in increased drug clearance or increased EPO demand during periods of accelerated body growth.[28,29,73]

> **KEY POINT**
>
> Children may require higher absolute rHuEPO doses than adults.

ESA dose adjustments should be made based on Hb response to treatment, including rate of change, ESA dose, and other pertinent clinical circumstances.[4] ESA dose adjustments after initiation should generally not be made until after the first 4 weeks of therapy, and no more often than every 2 weeks in the outpatient setting, because the effects of therapy are not likely to be seen after shorter intervals.[4] When a decrease in Hb is necessary, ESA dose should be decreased but not necessarily held, given that a pattern of holding and reinitiating ESA therapy can lead to Hb cycling around the desired target range.[74] Long-acting ESAs such as darbepoetin alfa, with its increased half-life and lower binding affinity for the EPO receptor, stimulate erythropoiesis for longer periods of time and thus may cause higher than intended Hb levels in clinical practice. This effect can be avoided by using lower starting doses and making less frequent dose adjustments than in children treated with short-acting ESAs.[67]

---

## KEY POINT

Adjustment of ESA dosing should be controlled to minimize large fluctuations in Hb level.

---

## ONGOING THERAPEUTIC CHALLENGES

In some patients, despite iron supplementation combined with escalating ESA therapy, Hb levels are not corrected to even a minimal goal, or these patients may need very large doses of ESA to increase or maintain Hb.[75] Given the need for efficacious anemia therapy along with concern for the potential adverse effects of escalating ESA doses to achieve higher Hb concentration, addressing ESA hyporesponsiveness has become a key component of anemia management. There is no single accepted definition of ESA hyporesponsiveness, but it is generally characterized as persistent Hb deficit despite 1 month of appropriate weight-based dosing or after 3 months of high-dose ESA treatment (rHuEPO in excess of 400 units/kg weekly or darbepoetin alfa in excess of 1 μg/kg weekly).[75,76] The current KDIGO anemia management guidelines discourage repeated ESA dose escalations beyond double the weight-based dose patients have been either initiated on or maintained on before developing ESA hyporesponsiveness, with maximal doses no greater than four times the initial weight-based dose.[4]

Data from NAPRTCS has demonstrated that more than 40% of children with stage 5 CKD have low Hb levels despite ESA treatment.[10] Clinical risk factors for ESA hyporesponsiveness identified in children undergoing hemodialysis include chronic inflammation, nutritional deficits, and chronic blood loss.[71] Although there are various potential mechanisms underlying ESA hyporesponsiveness, inflammation plays a

central role.[77] Identification of the inflammation-mediated upregulation of hepcidin in patients with CKD, with resulting iron-restricted erythropoiesis, has clarified our understanding of this state.[78-81] Although ESA hyporesponsiveness may be chronic, shorter-term clinical events such as infections or surgical procedures may significantly affect response to ESA therapy. The potential risks and benefits of significant escalation in ESA dose versus red blood cell transfusion must be assessed for individual patients.[4]

---

## SUMMARY

Anemia is prevalent and is associated with adverse outcomes in children with CKD. Although various factors contribute to anemia risk, EPO insufficiency and iron deficiency are the major underlying etiologic factors, and they are the mechanisms most commonly targeted by current therapies. Ongoing therapeutic challenges include hepcidin-mediated iron-restricted erythropoiesis and concerns about the safety and efficacy of escalating ESA doses for refractory anemia. Most recommendations regarding ESA use and dosing are based on data from adult trials; there have been no interventional studies examining the effects of ESA administration on clinical outcomes in children. Nevertheless, ESAs continue to be important components of CKD care in children; use of ESAs should balance the risks and benefits.

---

## ACKNOWLEDGMENT

This work was supported by a grant from the National Institutes of Health National Institute of Diabetes and Digestive Diseases (K23-DK-084116).

## REFERENCES

1. Amaral S, Hwang W, Fivush B, et al. Association of mortality and hospitalization with achievement of adult hemoglobin targets in adolescents maintained on hemodialysis. J Am Soc Nephrol. 2006;17:2878–85.
2. Schaefer F. Cardiac disease in children with mild-to-moderate chronic kidney disease. Curr Opin Nephrol Hypertens. 2008;17:292–7.
3. Mitsnefes MM, Kimball TR, Kartal J, et al. Progression of left ventricular hypertrophy in children with early chronic kidney disease: 2-year follow-up study. J Pediatr. 2006;149:671–5.
4. Kidney Disease: Improving Global Outcomes (KDIGO) Anemia Work Group. KDIGO clinical practice guideline for anemia in chronic kidney disease. Kidney Int. Suppl. 2012;2:279–335.

---

## KEY POINTS

- Hyporesponsiveness to ESA therapy is common.
- The risks and benefits of escalation of ESA dose versus red blood cell transfusion must be balanced for individual patients.

5. Hollowell JG, van Assendelft OW, Gunter EW, et al. Hematological and iron-related analytes—Reference data for persons aged 1 year and over: United States, 1988–94. Data from the Third National Health Examination Survey. Vital Health Stat 11. 2005;(247):1–156.

6. Jackson RT. Separate hemoglobin standards for blacks and whites: A critical review of the case for separate and unequal hemoglobin standards. Med Hypotheses. 1990;32:181–9.

7. Atkinson MA, Pierce CB, Zack RM, et al. Hemoglobin differences by race in children with CKD. Am J Kidney Dis. 2010;55:1009–17.

8. Filler G, Mylrea K, Feber J, et al. How to define anemia in children with chronic kidney disease? Pediatr Nephrol. 2007;22:702–7.

9. Greenbaum LA. Anemia in children with chronic kidney disease. Adv Chronic Kidney Dis. 2005;12:385–96.

10. Atkinson MA, Martz K, Warady BA, et al. Risk for anemia in pediatric chronic kidney disease patients: A report of NAPRTCS. Pediatr Nephrol. 2010;25:1699–706.

11. Staples AO, Wong CS, Smith JM, et al. Anemia and risk of hospitalization in pediatric chronic kidney disease. Clin J Am Soc Nephrol. 2009;4:48–56.

12. Fadrowski JJ, Pierce CB, Cole SR, et al. Hemoglobin decline in children with chronic kidney disease: Baseline results from the chronic kidney disease in children prospective cohort study. Clin J Am Soc Nephrol. 2008;3:457–62.

13. Naito M, Kawashima A, Akiba T, et al. Effects of an angiotensin II receptor antagonist and angiotensin-converting enzyme inhibitors on burst forming units-erythroid in chronic hemodialysis patients. Am J Nephrol. 2003;23:287–93.

14. Borzych-Duzalka D, Bilginer Y, Ha IS, et al. Management of anemia in children receiving chronic peritoneal dialysis. J Am Soc Nephrol. 2013;24:665–76.

15. Robins EB, Blum S. Hematologic reference values for African American children and adolescents. Am J Hematol. 2007;82:611–4.

16. Amaral S, Hwang W, Fivush B, et al. Serum albumin level and risk for mortality and hospitalization in adolescents on hemodialysis. Clin J Am Soc Nephrol. 2008;3:759–67.

17. Warady BA, Ho M. Morbidity and mortality in children with anemia at initiation of dialysis. Pediatr Nephrol. 2003;18:1055–62.

18. Mitsnefes M, Flynn J, Cohn S, et al. Masked hypertension associates with left ventricular hypertrophy in children with CKD. J Am Soc Nephrol. 2010;21:137–44.

19. Matteucci MC, Wuhl E, Picca S, et al. Left ventricular geometry in children with mild to moderate chronic renal insufficiency. J Am Soc Nephrol. 2006;17:218–26.

20. KDOQI clinical practice guideline and clinical practice recommendations for anemia in chronic kidney disease: 2007 update of hemoglobin target. Am J Kidney Dis. 2007;50:471–530.

21. Gerson A, Hwang W, Fiorenza J, et al. Anemia and health-related quality of life in adolescents with chronic kidney disease. Am J Kidney Dis. 2004;44:1017–23.

22. Boehm M, Riesenhuber A, Winkelmayer WC, et al. Early erythropoietin therapy is associated with improved growth in children with chronic kidney disease. Pediatr Nephrol. 2007;22:1189–93.

23. Gouva C, Nikolopoulos P, Ioannidis JP, et al. Treating anemia early in renal failure patients slows the decline of renal function: A randomized controlled trial. Kidney Int. 2004;66:753–60.

24. Furth SL, Cole SR, Fadrowski JJ, et al. The association of anemia and hypoalbuminemia with accelerated decline in GFR among adolescents with chronic kidney disease. Pediatr Nephrol. 2007;22:265–71.

25. Staples AO, Greenbaum LA, Smith JM, et al. Association between clinical risk factors and progression of chronic kidney disease in children. Clin J Am Soc Nephrol. 2010;5:2172–9.

26. Yabu JM, Anderson MW, Kim D, et al. Sensitization from transfusion in patients awaiting primary kidney transplant. Nephrol Dial Transplant. 2013;28:2908–18.

27. Obrador GT, Macdougall IC. Effect of red cell transfusions on future kidney transplantation. Clin J Am Soc Nephrol. 2013;8: 852–60.

28. Koshy SM, Geary DF. Anemia in children with chronic kidney disease. Pediatr Nephrol. 2008;23:209–19.

29. Foley RN. Erythropoietin: Physiology and molecular mechanisms. Heart Fail Rev. 2008;13:405–14.

30. Nangaku M, Eckardt KU. Pathogenesis of renal anemia. Semin Nephrol. 2006;26:261–8.

31. Jelkmann W. Regulation of erythropoietin production. J Physiol. 2011;589:1251–8.

32. Bernhardt WM, Wiesener MS, Scigalla P, et al. Inhibition of prolyl hydroxylases increases erythropoietin production in ESRD. J Am Soc Nephrol. 2010;21:2151–6.

33. Atkinson MA, Furth SL. Anemia in children with chronic kidney disease. Nat Rev Nephrol. 2011;7:635–41.

34. Goodnough LT, Nemeth E, Ganz T. Detection, evaluation, and management of iron-restricted erythropoiesis. Blood. 2010;116:4754–61.

35. Babitt JL, Lin HY. Mechanisms of anemia in CKD. J Am Soc Nephrol. 2012;23:1631–4.

36. Atkinson MA, White CT. Hepcidin in anemia of chronic kidney disease: Review for the pediatric nephrologist. Pediatr Nephrol. 2012;27:33–40.

37. Zaritsky J, Young B, Wang HJ, et al. Hepcidin: A potential novel biomarker for iron status in chronic kidney disease. Clin J Am Soc Nephrol. 2009;4:1051–6.

38. Bamgbola OF, Kaskel F. Role of folate deficiency on erythropoietin resistance in pediatric and adolescent patients on chronic dialysis. Pediatr Nephrol. 2005;20:1622–9.

39. Calo LA, Vertolli U, Davis PA, et al. Carnitine in hemodialysis patients. Hemodial Int. 2012;16:428–34.

40. Raimann JG, Levin NW, Craig RG, et al. Is vitamin C intake too low in dialysis patients? Semin Dial. 2013;26:1–5.

41. Kruse A, Uehlinger DE, Gotch F, et al. Red blood cell lifespan, erythropoiesis and hemoglobin control. Contrib Nephrol. 2008;161:247–54.

42. Rao DS, Shih MS, Mohini R. Effect of serum parathyroid hormone and bone marrow fibrosis on the response to erythropoietin in uremia. N Engl J Med. 1993;328:171–5.

43. Chutia H, Ruram AA, Bhattacharyya H, et al. Association of secondary hyperparathyroidism with hemoglobin level in patients with chronic kidney disease. J Lab Physicians. 2013;5:51–4.

44. Pollock C, Johnson DW, Horl WH, et al. Pure red cell aplasia induced by erythropoiesis-stimulating agents. Clin J Am Soc Nephrol. 2008;3:193–9.

45. Bennett CL, Starko KM, Thomsen HS, et al. Linking drugs to obscure illnesses: Lessons from pure red cell aplasia, nephrogenic systemic fibrosis, and Reye's syndrome. A report from the Southern Network on Adverse Reactions (SONAR). J Gen Intern Med. 2012;27:1697–703.

46. Agarwal R. Iron, oxidative stress, and clinical outcomes. Pediatr Nephrol. 2008;23:1195–9.

47. Fishbane S. Upper limit of serum ferritin: Misinterpretation of the 2006 KDOQI anemia guidelines. Semin Dial. 2008;21:217–20.

48. Atkinson MA, Pierce CB, Fadrowski JJ, et al. Association between common iron store markers and hemoglobin in children with chronic kidney disease. Pediatr Nephrol. 2012;27:2275–83.

49. Wish JB. Assessing iron status: Beyond serum ferritin and transferrin saturation. Clin J Am Soc Nephrol. 2006;1(Suppl 1):S4–8.

50. Kalantar-Zadeh K, Lee GH. The fascinating but deceptive ferritin: To measure it or not to measure it in chronic kidney disease? Clin J Am Soc Nephrol. 2006;1(Suppl 1):S9–18.

51. Looker AC, Dallman PR, Carroll MD, et al. Prevalence of iron deficiency in the United States. JAMA. 1997;277:973–6.

52. Ganz T, Nemeth E. Iron sequestration and anemia of inflammation. Semin Hematol. 2009;46:387–93.

53. Kalantar-Zadeh K, McAllister CJ, Lehn RS, et al. A low serum iron level is a predictor of poor outcome in hemodialysis patients. Am J Kidney Dis. 2004;43:671–84.

54. Morgan HE, Gautam M, Geary DF. Maintenance intravenous iron therapy in pediatric hemodialysis patients. Pediatr Nephrol. 2001;16:779–83.

55. Warady BA, Kausz A, Lerner G, et al. Iron therapy in the pediatric hemodialysis population. Pediatr Nephrol. 2004;19:655–61.

56. Morgan HE, Holt RC, Jones CA, et al. Intravenous iron treatment in paediatric chronic kidney disease patients not on erythropoietin. Pediatr Nephrol. 2007;22:1963–5.

57. Shander A, Sazama K. Clinical consequences of iron overload from chronic red blood cell transfusions, its diagnosis, and its management by chelation therapy. Transfusion. 2010;50:1144–55.

58. Besarab A, Bolton WK, Browne JK, et al. The effects of normal as compared with low hematocrit values in patients with cardiac disease who are receiving hemodialysis and epoetin. N Engl J Med. 1998;339:584–90.

59. Singh AK, Szczech L, Tang KL, et al. Correction of anemia with epoetin alfa in chronic kidney disease. N Engl J Med. 2006;355:2085–98.

60. Pfeffer MA, Burdmann EA, Chen CY, et al. A trial of darbepoetin alfa in type 2 diabetes and chronic kidney disease. N Engl J Med. 2009;361:2019–32.

61. Badve SV, Hawley CM, Johnson DW. Is the problem with the vehicle or the destination? Does high-dose ESA or high haemoglobin contribute to poor outcomes in CKD? Nephrology (Carlton). 2011;16:144–53.

62. Goodkin DA, Fuller DS, Robinson BM, et al. Naturally occurring higher hemoglobin concentration does not increase mortality among hemodialysis patients. J Am Soc Nephrol. 2011;22:358–65.

63. Unger EF, Thompson AM, Blank MJ, et al. Erythropoiesis-stimulating agents: Time for a reevaluation. N Engl J Med. 2010;362:189–92.

64. Kliger AS, Foley RN, Goldfarb DS, et al. KDOQI US commentary on the 2012 KDIGO clinical practice guideline for anemia in CKD. Am J Kidney Dis. 2013;62:849–59.

65. Lestz RM, Fivush BA, Atkinson MA. Association of higher erythropoiesis stimulating agent dose and mortality in children on dialysis. Pediatr Nephrol. 2014;29: 2021–8.

66. Covic A, Cannata-Andia J, Cancarini G, et al. Biosimilars and biopharmaceuticals: What the nephrologists need to know—A position paper by the ERA-EDTA council. Nephrol Dial Transplant. 2008;23:3731–7.

67. Horl WH. Differentiating factors between erythropoiesis-stimulating agents: An update to selection for anaemia of chronic kidney disease. Drugs. 2013;73:117–30.

68. KDOQI clinical practice guidelines and clinical practice recommendations for anemia in chronic kidney disease. Am J Kidney Dis. 2006;47 (Suppl 3):S1–146.

69. Warady BA, Arar MY, Lerner G, et al. Darbepoetin alfa for the treatment of anemia in pediatric patients with chronic kidney disease. Pediatr Nephrol. 2006;21:1144–52.

70. Schmitt CP, Nau B, Brummer C, et al. Increased injection pain with darbepoetin-alpha compared to epoetin-beta in paediatric dialysis patients. Nephrol Dial Transplant. 2006;21:3520–4.

71. Bamgbola OF, Kaskel FJ, Coco M. Analyses of age, gender and other risk factors of erythropoietin resistance in pediatric and adult dialysis cohorts. Pediatr Nephrol. 2009;24:571–9.

72. Port RE, Kiepe D, Van Guilder M, et al. Recombinant human erythropoietin for the treatment of renal anaemia in children: No justification for body-weight-adjusted dosage. Clin Pharmacokinet. 2004;43:57–70.

73. Port RE, Mehls O. Erythropoietin dosing in children with chronic kidney disease: Based on body size or on hemoglobin deficit? Pediatr Nephrol. 2009;24:435–7.

74. Fishbane S, Berns JS. Hemoglobin cycling in hemodialysis patients treated with recombinant human erythropoietin. Kidney Int. 2005;68:1337–43.

75. Gilbertson DT, Peng Y, Arneson TJ, et al. Comparison of methodologies to define hemodialysis patients hyporesponsive to epoetin and impact on counts and characteristics. BMC Nephrol. 2013;14:44.–––.

76. Bamgbola O. Resistance to erythropoietin-stimulating agents: Etiology, evaluation, and therapeutic considerations. Pediatr Nephrol. 2012;27:195–205.

77. Kwack C, Balakrishnan VS. Managing erythropoietin hyporesponsiveness. Semin Dial. 2006;19:146–51.

78. Adamson JW. Hyporesponsiveness to erythropoiesis stimulating agents in chronic kidney disease: The many faces of inflammation. Adv Chronic Kidney Dis. 2009;16:76–82.

79. Yee J. Anemia of chronic kidney disease: Forward to the past. Adv Chronic Kidney Dis. 2009;16:71–3.

80. Young B, Zaritsky J. Hepcidin for clinicians. Clin J Am Soc Nephrol. 2009;4:1384–7.

81. Atkinson MA, White CT. Hepcidin in anemia of chronic kidney disease: Review for the pediatric nephrologist. Pediatr Nephrol. 2012;27:33–40.

## REVIEW QUESTIONS

1. The initial laboratory evaluation for anemia in a child with CKD should include which of the following?
   a. Complete blood count
   b. Reticulocyte count
   c. Ferritin
   d. Transferrin saturation
   e. All of the above

2. Which of the following is *not* associated with the anemia of CKD in children?
   a. Increased risk for hospitalization
   b. Increased fracture risk
   c. Decreased quality of life
   d. Increased risk for mortality
   e. Increased risk for left ventricular hypertrophy

3. The primary site of endogenous erythropoietin production in children is:
   a. Hepatocytes
   b. Renal tubular epithelial cells
   c. Erythroid progenitor cells in bone marrow
   d. Peritubular fibroblasts in the renal cortex
   e. Juxtaglomerular apparatus

4. Which is the primary physiologic stimulus for increased EPO gene expression?
   a. Hypoxia
   b. Anemia
   c. Increased distal tubular sodium reabsorption
   d. Uremia
   e. Decrease in blood pressure

5. Iron-restricted erythropoiesis can include:
   a. Absolute iron deficiency
   b. Depletion of accessible iron stores by ESA-stimulated bone marrow
   c. Inflammation-associated impairment in iron trafficking
   d. a and b only
   e. a, b, and c

6. Children receiving ESA therapy should receive iron supplementation as indicated to maintain:
   a. Ferritin greater than 50 ng/mL and transferrin saturation greater than 20%
   b. Ferritin greater than 100 ng/mL and transferrin saturation greater than 10%
   c. Ferritin greater than 100 ng/mL and transferrin saturation greater than 20%
   d. Ferritin greater than 500 ng/mL and transferrin saturation greater than 30%
   e. Ferritin greater than 100 ng/mL and transferrin saturation greater than 30%

7. All of the following are possible indications for IV iron administration *except*:
   a. Poor enteral iron absorption
   b. Poor adherence to oral iron supplementation regimen
   c. Long-term hemodialysis status
   d. Active systemic infection
   e. ESA hyporesponsiveness

8. Short-acting recombinant human erythropoietin formulations have longer half-lives and are more effective when administered:
   a. Subcutaneously
   b. Intravenously
   c. Enterally
   d. Peritoneally
   e. With hemodialysis

9. Potential advantages of darbepoetin alfa compared with short-acting recombinant human erythropoietin include:
   a. Longer interval between doses
   b. Improved adherence
   c. Decreased pain with administration
   d. a and b only
   e. a, b, and c

10. The goal rate of hemoglobin increase after initiation of an ESA is:
    a. 1 to 2 g/dL per week
    b. 1 to 2 g/dL per month
    c. 1 to 2 g/dL over 3 months
    d. Increase to goal hemoglobin of 11 g/dL over 1 month
    e. Increase to goal hemoglobin of 12 g/dL over 3 months

## ANSWER KEY

1. e
2. b
3. d
4. a
5. e
6. c
7. d
8. a
9. d
10. b

# 33

# Chronic kidney disease bone and mineral disorder

KATHERINE WESSELING-PERRY AND ISIDRO B. SALUSKY

Childhood and adolescence are a crucial time for developing a healthy skeletal and vascular system; alterations in bone modeling and remodeling, or vascular biology in youth carry consequences that severely affect quality of life as well as life span. In childhood, chronic kidney disease (CKD) causes disordered regulation of mineral metabolism with subsequent alterations in bone modeling, remodeling, and growth. These alterations occur early in the course of CKD and, in addition, are associated with the development of cardiovascular calcifications. Because growth failure and short stature are clinically apparent and concerning to patients, families, and physicians alike, optimization of growth and final adult height has been a focus of CKD management in children for decades. However, cardiovascular disease is the leading cause of mortality in both adults and children with kidney disease and abnormal mineral metabolism, bone disease, and its therapies are closely linked to cardiovascular pathologic processes. Together, these alterations are termed CKD mineral and bone disorder (CKD-MBD).[1]

CKD-MBD is defined as a systemic disorder of mineral and bone metabolism resulting from CKD that manifests as either one or a combination of the following: (1) abnormalities of calcium, phosphorus, parathyroid hormone (PTH), or vitamin D metabolism; (2) abnormalities in bone histology, linear growth, or strength; and (3) vascular or other soft tissue calcification. Fibroblast growth factor 23 (FGF23), a recently characterized hormone produced in the bone, has been defined as a key regulator of mineral metabolism and cardiovascular disease in the context of CKD-MBD. *Renal osteodystrophy* is the specific term used to describe the bone pathologic process that occurs as a complication of CKD and is therefore one aspect of the CKD-MBD. Although the definitive evaluation of renal osteodystrophy requires a bone biopsy, this procedure is not routinely performed in the clinical setting. However, bone histomorphometry continues to be the gold standard for the assessment of three essential aspects of bone histology: turnover, mineralization, and volume.[1]

## KEY POINTS

- CKD-MBD is a systemic disorder resulting from CKD that has findings in bone as well as in vascular and other soft tissues.
- Renal osteodystrophy is the bone pathologic process of CKD and therefore is one aspect of CKD-MBD.

## PATHOGENESIS OF SECONDARY HYPERPARATHYROIDISM

Hyperparathyroidism and bone disease associated with CKD are the results of numerous underlying pathophysiologic derangements in mineral metabolism. Although the presence of secondary hyperparathyroidism in CKD has been well known, recent discoveries have shed a new light on its pathogenesis.

## ROLE OF FIBROBLAST GROWTH FACTOR 23

As early as stage 2 CKD (glomerular filtration rate [GFR] between 60 and 90 mL/1.73 m²/min), circulating levels of FGF23 begin to rise in adults and children (Figure 33.1).[2,3] Increased levels of FGF23 are due to a combination of its decreased renal excretion, changes in degradation, and increased osteocytic production.[4-6] The cause of increased osteocytic FGF23 expression has not been completely defined. Whereas oral phosphate loading stimulates FGF23 production, serum phosphorus levels remain within the normal range or are slightly diminished in the early CKD stages and phosphate balance is neutral in patients with CKD stages 3 to 4.[7,8] Therefore, mechanisms other than hyperphosphatemia have been suggested to cause elevated circulating FGF23 levels in CKD. These phosphate-independent mechanisms for stimulation of FGF23 production include a decrease in the expression of membrane-bound Klotho (a co-receptor for FGF23 signaling), iron deficiency–mediated stimulation of FGF23 transcription, increased levels of cleaved αKlotho, a potent stimulator or FGF23 production, and a state of chronic inflammation seen in CKD.[9-12]

---

### KEY POINTS

- FGF23 is a key phosphaturic agent (like PTH).
- FGF23 acts by reducing the renal expression of phosphate cotransporters: NaPi2a and NaPi2c.
- Increases in circulating FGF23 levels are the earliest serologic indication of osteocyte dysfunction in CKD.
- FGF23 is a key regulator of mineral metabolism and cardiovascular disease in patients with CKD.

---

Early increases in FGF23 may be the first sign of altered osteocyte function in CKD.[6,13,14] Later in the course of CKD, increasing serum phosphorus and PTH, decreasing renal FGF23 excretion, and active vitamin D sterol therapy are likely to further increase circulating FGF23 levels.[4,7,15,16] The effects of increasing FGF23 on mineral metabolism are profound. Of these, its most prominent impact is on increasing renal phosphate excretion (phosphaturic action) by (1) reducing the expression of renal phosphate cotransporters NaPi2a and NaPi2c, (2) suppressing renal 1α-hydroxylase activity, and (3) stimulating 24-hydroxylase leading to enhanced metabolism of the biologically active 1,25-dihydroxyvitamin D (1,25[OH]₂D).[17]

With progression of CKD, rising serum FGF23 values result in a decline in circulating 1,25(OH)₂D levels, leading to an inverse relationship of circulating 1,25(OH)₂D levels and FGF23.[13] Available evidence suggests that FGF23 also may regulate PTH secretion. In vitro and in vivo experiments indicate that FGF23, by activating the mitogen-activated protein kinase (MAPK) pathways in the parathyroid gland, also directly suppresses through PTH release (Figure 33.2).[15,18]

## ROLE OF 1,25-DIHYDROXYVITAMIN D

In CKD, reduced circulating 1,25(OH)₂ D contributes to secondary hyperparathyroidism and parathyroid gland hyperplasia through the following ways:

- Decreased intestinal calcium absorption
- Decreased 1,25(OH)₂D binding to the vitamin D receptor (VDR)
- Decreased VDR expression
- Reduced calcium-sensing receptor (CaSR) expression

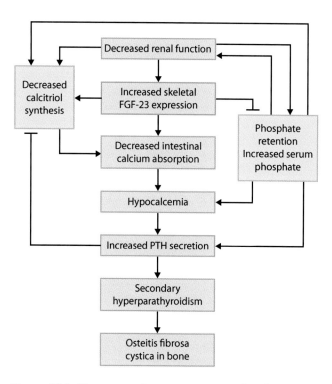

Figure 33.1 Diagrammatic representation of pathogenesis of renal osteodystrophy.

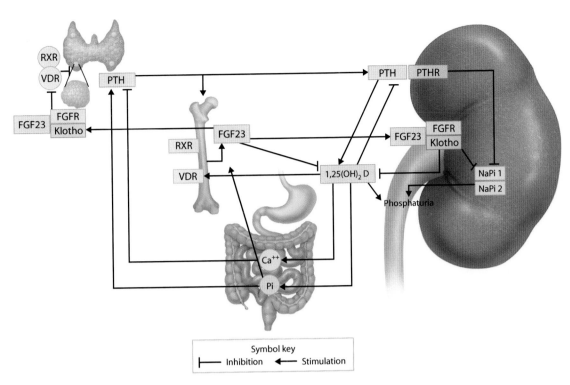

Figure 33.2 Regulatory mechanisms among bone, kidney, parathyroid gland, and gut. Fibroblast growth factor 23 (FGF23), 1,25-dihydroxyvitamin D$_3$, and parathyroid hormone (PTH) regulate each other's expression and secretion and thereby balance mineral ion homeostasis. FGFR, fibroblast growth factor receptor; PTHR, parathyroid hormone receptor; RXR, retinoid-X receptor; VDR, vitamin D receptor. (Redrawn and adapted from concepts in: Lanske B, Densmore MJ, Erben RG. Vitamin D endocrine system and osteocytes. Bonekey Rep. 2014;3:494. doi: 10.1038/bonekey.2013.228. eCollection 2014.)

Administration of 1,25(OH)$_2$D has been shown to suppress *PTH* gene transcription, both in vitro (bovine parathyroid cell culture) and in vivo (intact rats), and to also increase FGF23 production. In conjunction with the VDR, 1,25(OH)$_2$D binds vitamin D response elements in the parathyroid glands that inhibit pre-proPTH gene transcription.[19,20] 1,25(OH)$_2$D administration also appears to increase the number of VDRs in the parathyroid glands in a dose-dependent manner. The number of receptors for calcitriol in parathyroid glands appears to be reduced in animals and humans with CKD, when compared to either patients undergoing renal transplantation or patients with primary hyperparathyroidism.[21–23] In a positive feedback loop, 1,25(OH)$_2$D itself increases *VDR* gene expression in the parathyroid glands, further suppressing *PTH* gene transcription.[24]

1,25(OH)$_2$D$_3$ also increases the expression of the CaSR, the expression of which has been documented to be reduced in hyperplastic parathyroid tissues obtained from patients with secondary hyperparathyroidism.[25] Also, 1,25(OH)$_2$D deficiency in animals is associated with decreased expression of CaSR mRNA (CAR) in parathyroid tissue, whereas 1,25(OH)$_2$D$_3$ therapy increases CAR expression in a dose-dependent manner.[26] Calcitriol also may directly modulate parathyroid cell proliferation by altering the expression of specific replication-associated oncogenes, such as *c-myc* and *c-phos* proto-oncogenes.[27] Thus, low levels of calcitriol may allow parathyroid cells to proliferate while the administration of calcitriol suppresses proliferation of parathyroid cells. It is important to keep in mind, however, that studies in VDR knockout mice have shown that if serum concentrations of calcium and phosphorus are normalized by the use of a rescue diet, parathyroid hyperplasia does not occur.[28,29] Interestingly, it also has been shown that 1,25(OH)$_2$ vitamin D may be important in renal tissue fibrosis. Reductions in 1,25(OH)$_2$ vitamin D levels may prevent or reduce the development of renal tissue fibrosis through a non–VDR dependent mechanism.[30]

## ROLE OF 25-HYDROXYVITAMIN D

Deficiency of 25(OH) vitamin D (25[OH]D) results from multiple factors in patients with CKD. Many are chronically ill, with little outdoor (sunlight) exposure. CKD dietary restrictions, particularly of dairy products, curtail the intake of vitamin D–rich food and lead to decreased dietary calcium intake.[31] Patients with CKD (particularly those with darker skin pigment) display decreased skin synthesis of vitamin D$_3$ in response to sunlight compared with individuals with normal kidney function.[32,33] Proteinuric diseases further exacerbate D deficiency in the CKD population as a result of urinary loss of 25(OH)D bound to vitamin D binding protein.[34,35]

Data also suggest that catabolism of 25(OH)D through 24-hydroxylase is increased in CKD and may play an important role in the development and maintenance of

(25[OH]D) deficiency state.[36] Low levels of 25(OH)D also contribute to the development of secondary hyperparathyroidism—both directly and through limiting the substrate for the formation of 1,25(OH)₂D. Apart from its conversion to 1,25(OH)₂D₃, 25(OH)D also may directly affect tissues. For example, supplementation with ergocalciferol has been shown to decrease serum PTH levels and to delay the development of secondary hyperparathyroidism in patients with CKD.[37–40] Furthermore, 1α-hydroxylase activity is present in the parathyroid glands and 25(OH)D is converted within the gland to 1,25(OH)₂D₃, resulting in PTH supression.[40] By itself, 25(OH)D administration also suppresses PTH synthesis, even when parathyroid gland 1α-hydroxylase is inhibited, indicating that 25(OH)D may directly contribute to PTH suppression.[40] Low levels of 25(OH)D may exacerbate secondary hyperparathyroidism in the context of CKD. Therefore, prevention of vitamin D deficiency has been advocated in early CKD.

## ROLE OF PHOSPHORUS

Even though hyperphosphatemia usually manifests only in late stages of CKD, phosphorus retention and hyperphosphatemia are important triggers in the pathogenesis of secondary hyperparathyroidism. Development of secondary hyperparathyroidism is prevented in experimental animals with CKD when dietary phosphorus intake is lowered in proportion to the GFR.[41] Dietary phosphate restriction also can reduce previously elevated serum PTH levels in patients with moderate renal failure, and aggressive phosphate control in uremic rats not only decreases PTH and FGF23 but also decreases renal fibrosis, left ventricular hypertrophy, and overall mortality.[42–44]

Phosphorus retention and hyperphosphatemia indirectly promote the secretion of PTH in several ways. In the context of hyperphosphatemic, inorganic phosphorus complexes with calcium and lowers serum levels; the ensuing hypocalcemia stimulates PTH release. Phosphorus also enhances the secretion of FGF23, thereby impairing renal 1α-hydroxylase activity, which diminishes the conversion of 25(OH)D to 1,25(OH)₂D₃.[7] Finally, phosphorus can directly enhance PTH synthesis by decreasing cytosolic phospholipase A2 (normally increased by CaSR activation), leading to a decrease in arachidonic acid production and enhancing PTH secretion.[45] Hypophosphatemia also decreases PTH mRNA transcript stability in vitro, suggesting that phosphorus itself affects serum PTH levels, probably by increasing the stability of the PTH mRNA transcript.[46]

## CALCIUM-SENSING RECEPTOR EXPRESSION

Alterations in parathyroid gland *CAR* expression occur in secondary hyperparathyroidism and contribute to parathyroid gland hyperplasia. The CaSR is a seven-transmembrane G protein-coupled receptor with a large extracellular N-terminus, which binds acidic amino acids and divalent cations.[47] Low extracellular calcium levels result in decreased

calcium binding to the receptor, a conformational relaxation of the receptor and a resultant increase in PTH secretion, while activation of the receptor by high levels of serum calcium decrease PTH secretion.[48,49] The expression of the CaSR in hyperplastic parathyroid tissue obtained from patients with renal failure is reduced by 30% to 70%, using immunohistochemical techniques.[25,50]

*CAR* transcription is regulated by vitamin D through two distinct vitamin D response elements in the gene's promoter region. Alterations in vitamin D metabolism in renal failure can account for changes in calcium sensing by the parathyroid glands, and vitamin D may act upstream of *CAR* in preventing parathyroid cell hyperplasia.[51,52] Decreased expression and activity of the CaSR have been linked to decreased responsiveness in PTH secretion to altered calcium levels.[53] Consequently, decreased expression of the CaSR results in an insensitivity to serum calcium levels with subsequent uncontrolled secretion of PTH. Increased stimulation of the CaSR by calcimimetics has been shown to decrease PTH cell proliferation, implicating the CaSR as a regulator of cell proliferation, as well as PTH secretion.[54]

## ROLE OF SKELETAL RESISTANCE TO PARATHYROID HORMONE

Resistance of the skeleton to the hypercalcemic action of PTH is another potential cause of hyperparathyroidism in patients with renal insufficiency (Figure 33.3). It has been demonstrated that the increase in serum calcium in response to infusion of PTH is significantly less in patients with renal failure than in healthy subjects.[55,56] Although the actions of different fragments of the PTH molecule are still uncharacterized, in vitro and in vivo experimental data indicate that one or more amino-terminally truncated PTH(1-84)

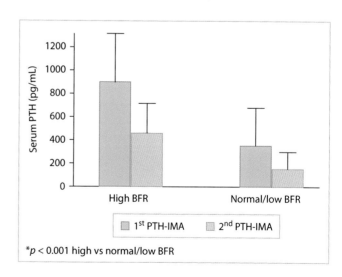

Figure 33.3 Parathyroid hormone (PTH) levels corresponding to high and normal to low turnover bone histology in different stages of chronic kidney disease (CKD). BFR, bone formation rate; 1st PTH-IMA, first-generation immunometric assay; 2nd PTH-IMA, second-generation immunometric assay. See text for details.

fragments antagonize the calcemic actions of PTH(1-84) and diminish bone cell activity, and may, therefore, modulate bone metabolism. Synthetic PTH(7-84), which appears to be similar to naturally occurring circulating amino-terminally truncated PTH fragments, inhibits the formation of tartrate-resistant acid phosphatase (TRAP)-positive bone resorbing cells in vitro and inhibits bone formation in vivo.[57-59]

Nguyen-Yamamoto et al.[60] and Slatopolsky et al.[61] demonstrated that PTH(7-84), with or without a mixture of other carboxyl-terminal PTH-fragments, inhibits the calcemic effect of PTH(1-34) in vivo, indicating that these actions are not mediated through the PTH/PTHrP receptor, but instead via a receptor that interacts only with carboxyl-terminal portions of PTH. In humans, Wesseling-Perry et al.[56] demonstrated that dialysis patients with hyperparathyroid bone disease secondary to increased levels of PTH(1-84), also have increased circulating levels of PTH(7-84) and are resistant to the calcemic actions of PTH(1-34). Thus, a growing body of evidence suggests that at least some of the different carboxyl-terminal PTH fragments have biological activity and circulating amino-terminally truncated PTH fragments may play a role in the skeletal resistance to the full-length PTH molecule.

---

## KEY POINTS

- Some carboxyl-terminal PTH fragments have biological activity.
- Circulating amino-terminally truncated PTH fragments may play a role in skeletal resistance to the full-length PTH molecule.
- First-generation immunoassays for PTH measures not only intact PTH but also some of the fragmented PTH molecules, as well (amino-terminus truncated). These assays overestimate PTH by 40% to 50%.
- Second-generation immunoassays for PTH do not detect large PTH fragments. Clinical application of this finding is still unclear.

---

Over the last few years, a series of observations have highlighted important shortcomings of the first-generation immunometric assays (IMA) for measuring PTH (1st PTH-IMA). Studies by D'Amour et al.[62-64] demonstrated that 1st PTH-IMAs detect not only the intact PTH molecule but also additional PTH fragments truncated at the amino terminus. Indeed, most of the detection antibodies, which are usually directed against epitopes within the amino terminus of the hormone, detect not only PTH(1-84) but also one or several amino-truncated fragments of the PTH molecule, some of which coelute from reverse-phase high-performance liquid chromatography column with synthetic PTH(7-84).[63] By contrast, second-generation immunometric PTH assays (2nd PTH-IMAs) use detection antibodies that interact with epitopes comprising the first four amino

terminal amino acids of human PTH and thus recognize only PTH(1-84) and possibly PTH fragments that are truncated at the carboxyl terminus or modified within the 15 to 20 region, but not PTH(7-84).[48,61,65] PTH levels determined by 1st PTH-IMA overestimate the concentration of PTH(1-84) by 40% to 50% in both healthy individuals with normal renal function and those with varying degrees of CKD.[62,63] Unlike 1st PTH-IMAs, the 2nd PTH-IMAs do not detect these large PTH fragments.[48,61,65-67]

Monier-Faugere et al.[66] suggested that 2nd PTH-IMA and, mainly, the ratio between PTH(1-84) and amino-truncated PTH fragment (calculated from the differences in PTH levels determined between 1st and 2nd PTH-IMAs) could be a better predictor of bone turnover than 1st PTH-IMA. However, these findings were not confirmed by subsequent investigations and available data do not support the claim that 2nd PTH-IMAs provide an advantage over 1st PTH-IMAs for the diagnosis of the different subtypes of renal bone diseases.[67,68] Furthermore, the variation in PTH assays across manufacturers makes interpretation of their values and their relationships to bone turnover difficult to assess. More recently, discrimination of nonoxidized from oxidized forms of PTH has been shown to not only discriminate between active and inactive forms of the molecule but also predict adverse outcomes in dialysis patients.[69] These assays are not currently available for clinical practice, and their value as predictors of the different subtypes of renal osteodystrophy as well as the response to therapeutic interventions remains to be defined. Current guidelines suggest that PTH values, as determined by current commercially available assays, be maintained within a broad range—between two and nine times the range for individuals with normal renal function—in patients treated with maintenance dialysis.[70]

---

## KEY POINT

Current guidelines suggest that in patients on dialysis therapy, PTH values, as determined by current commercially available assays, be maintained within a broad range—between two and nine times the range for individuals with normal renal function.

---

# CONSEQUENCES OF ABNORMAL MINERAL METABOLISM IN CHRONIC KIDNEY DISEASE

## BONE DISEASE

Renal bone disease is a common complication of CKD and is nearly universal at the start of dialysis therapy. Whereas the term *CKD-MBD* refers to the alterations in mineral

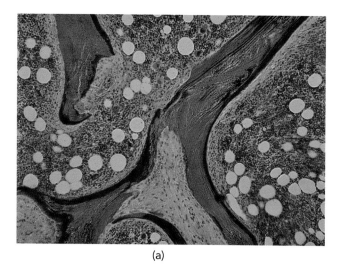

(a)

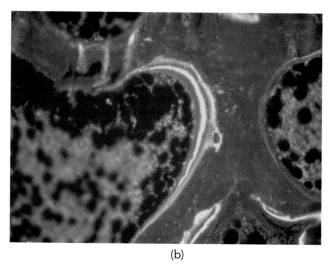

(b)

Figure 33.4 Bone histology, osteitis fibrosa. (a) Under light microscopy, increases in cellular activity, osteoid accumulation, erosion, and fibrosis are visible. (b) An increase in double tetracycline labeling signifies an increase in bone turnover rate.

metabolism and the effects on both the cardiovascular and skeletal systems in the CKD population, the term *renal osteodystrophy* is used specifically to describe the bone pathologic processes defined by bone histomorphometry that occur as a complication of CKD.[70]

## BONE TURNOVER

Traditionally, the lesions of renal bone disease have been characterized according to alterations in bone turnover, ranging from high bone turnover (secondary hyperparathyroidism, osteitis fibrosa) to lesions of low bone turnover (adynamic bone disease and osteomalacia). However, alterations in skeletal mineralization and volume are also common in pediatric patients in CKD[71] and may contribute to outcomes such as fractures, skeletal deformities, and poor growth that persist despite normalization of bone turnover.[72] Bone histomorphometry is the gold standard for the diagnosis of different types of bone diseases associated with CKD, providing measures of bone turnover, mineralization, and volume, and all may be altered in patients with CKD, occurring concomitantly with alterations in circulating levels of PTH, calcium, phosphorus, 1,25D, 25(OH)D, and FGF23.[70]

Abnormalities in bone turnover, driven by circulating PTH concentrations, are prevalent in both adult and pediatric patients with advanced stages of CKD.[73,74] PTH activates the PTH/PTHrP receptor on osteocytes and osteoblasts, thereby directly increasing the cellular activity of osteoblasts and, indirectly, the activity of osteoclasts.[75-77] Elevated bone turnover is evident in patients with moderate-to-advanced stages of CKD, although a substantial proportion of adults with CKD stages 2 to 4 have low bone turnover.[71,79] With progression of CKD, skeletal resistance to PTH develops secondary to multiple factors that include accumulation of circulating PTH fragments and down-regulation of the PTH receptor. At the same time, elevated circulating levels of PTH result in increased resorption of

bone matrix and release of mineral into the circulation.[55,80] Prolonged exposure to elevated PTH levels and increases in bone turnover may lead to peritrabecular fibrous changes in bones. This form of renal osteodystrophy associated with prolonged secondary hyperparathyroidism is often termed *osteitis fibrosa cystica* (Figure 33.4).[73]

A state of low-turnover bone disease (adynamic renal osteodystrophy) defined as decreased bone formation rate in conjunction with decreased cellular activity and an absence of excessive osteoid accumulation, is most common in adult dialysis patients (Figure 33.5). This condition may occur, especially in children treated with maintenance dialysis, as a result of overly aggressive therapy with active vitamin D sterols and calcium salts. In addition to the increased risk for fractures and vascular calcifications observed in adults with adynamic bone, this form of bone disease in children treated with dialysis is associated with a further decline in growth.[80,81]

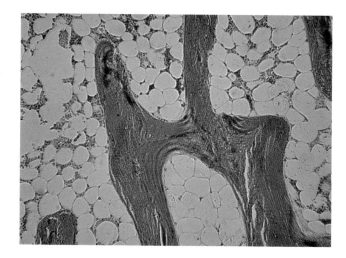

Figure 33.5 Bone histology, adynamic bone. Under light microscopy, decreased cellular activity with minimal osteoid accumulation. Very little or no double tetracycline labeling (not shown) signifies a decrease in bone turnover rate.

Although bone turnover is undoubtedly affected by changes in circulating PTH in advanced CKD, data from animals and humans suggest that changes in bone turnover occur before alterations in circulating mineral, PTH, or vitamin D concentrations are apparent and that these changes are mediated in large part by alterations in osteocyte biology.[6,77,82] Lund et al.[82] demonstrated that renal ablation in mice resulted in low bone turnover if circulating levels of calcium, phosphate, 1,25(OH)$_2$D, and PTH were kept constant, suggesting that some changes in bone turnover, particularly in early CKD, are independent of measurable changes in divalent ion homeostasis.[82] Subsequently, Sabbagh et al.[77] demonstrated similar findings in *Jck* mice, in whom increased osteocytic sclerostin expression was related to changes in bone turnover with progressive CKD.[77] Indeed, sclerostin is an inhibitor of Wnt signaling–mediated bone turnover and its increased expression results in suppression of bone formation and the development of adynamic bone in early stages of CKD.[77] PTH, on the other hand, suppresses sclerostin expression, and, in moderate-to-severe CKD, a rising PTH level inhibits skeletal sclerostin expression, allowing bone formation rates to rise.[77,78]

## BONE MINERALIZATION

As discussed earlier, renal osteodystrophy traditionally has been defined by lesions in bone turnover; however, alterations in skeletal mineralization are also prevalent in children with CKD.[69,78] Increases in unmineralized bone (osteoid) in conjunction with delayed rates of mineral deposition are common. Defective mineralization that is associated with low to normal bone turnover is termed *osteomalacia*. The histomorphometric characteristics of osteomalacia include (1) the presence of wide osteoid seams, (2) an increased number of osteoid lamellae, (3) an increase in the trabecular surface covered with osteoid, and (4) a diminished rate of mineralization or bone formation, as assessed by double tetracycline labeling. Fibrosis is often absent. Defective mineralization in combination with increased bone formation rates is termed *mixed uremic osteodystrophy* and is characterized by wide osteoid seams, prolonged mineralization times, bone marrow fibrosis, and increased bone formation rates.[70] Patients with mixed lesions often display high serum PTH and alkaline phosphatase levels along with lower serum calcium levels.[74]

Although the mechanisms of skeletal mineralization are incompletely understood, factors such as 25(OH)D deficiency and altered FGF23 metabolism have been implicated in their pathogenesis. In the general population, nutritional 25(OH)D deficiency results in osteomalacia and a similar phenotype may occur in patients with CKD. Phosphate depletion, as may occur with frequent dialysis, also may result in osteomalacia. FGF23 may play a role; both overexpression[84–86] and ablation[87,88] of FGF23 in mice with normal renal function are associated with abnormal mineralization of osteoid, although by different mechanisms. The phosphaturic effect of increased FGF23 may cause rickets and osteomalacia through an insufficiency of mineral substrate.

The mechanisms leading to impaired mineralization in FGF23-null animals, which have severe hyperphosphatemia and normal or elevated serum calcium levels, remain uncertain; however, osteomalacia in these animals suggests that FGF23 may play a direct role in skeletal mineral deposition. Although the ramifications of defective mineralization remain to be established, increased fracture rates and bone deformities are prevalent in patients with CKD despite adequate control of bone turnover.[72,89] These complications may be due, in part, to alterations in bone mineralization.

## BONE VOLUME

Because PTH is anabolic at the level of trabecular bone, high levels of serum PTH are typically associated with increases in bone volume, trabecular volume, and trabecular width. However, bone volume also may be low (termed *osteoporosis*), particularly in individuals with underlying age-related bone loss or in those treated with corticosteroids. Low bone volume is rare in the pediatric CKD population.[74]

## EXTRASKELETAL CALCIFICATION

The association between extraskeletal calcifications and CKD has been known for many years,[90] but the link between the two has been clearly defined over the last decade. Currently, vascular calcification is included as part of the definition of CKD-MBD. These lesions have their origins in CKD before dialysis and are also common in childhood CKD (Figure 33.6).[91–93] The mortality rate in adults and children with CKD is markedly higher than that in the general population, and cardiovascular disease is the leading cause of death in this patient population.[94]

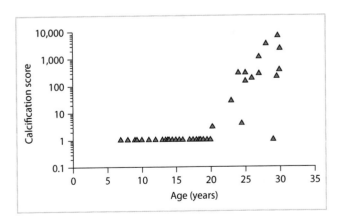

Figure 33.6 Coronary artery calcification scores in 39 children and young adults with end-stage renal disease who were treated by dialysis, according to age. Coronary artery calcification was assessed by electron-beam computed tomography. (Reprinted with permission from: Goodman WG, Goldin J, Kuizon BD, et al. Coronary-artery calcification in young adults with end-stage renal disease who are undergoing dialysis. N Engl J Med. 2000;342:1478–3).

In contrast to the calcified atherosclerotic plaques that develop in the vascular intima with the aging process, uremia facilitates calcification of the tunica media. This form of calcification is associated with decreased distensibility of blood vessels, causing a rigid "lead pipe" pathologic finding that is associated with increased risk for congestive heart failure.[95] Electron beam computed tomography (EBCT), used in the assessment of vascular calcifications in the adult population, and measurements in adults with CKD as well as in young adults who were treated with maintenance dialysis as children have demonstrated that a significant proportion of this population has evidence of vascular calcification.[91] Carotid ultrasound measurement of intimal medial thickness has also been validated for the assessment of cardiovascular pathologic processes in adults and children, with increased thickness being associated with worsening disease.[96,97]

Osteoblasts and vascular smooth muscle cells have a common mesenchymal origin, and vascular tissues in the uremic milieu express osteoblast differentiation factors.[98,99] Core binding factor-1 (Cbfa1; also known as Runx1) is thought to trigger transformation of mesenchymal cell to osteoblasts, and arteries obtained from patients with end-stage renal disease show increased levels of this protein.[98] Upregulation of the sodium-dependent phosphate transporter PIT-1 likely also contributes to increased calcification, and upregulation of promineralization factors such as osteopontin, bone sialoprotein, osteonectin, alkaline phosphatase, type I collagen, and bone morphogenic protein-2 (BMP-2) is potentiated by the uremic milieu.[100-104] By contrast, expression of calcification inhibitors, such as fetuin A, matrix Gla protein, and Klotho, is suppressed.[105-108]

Hypercalcemia, hyperphosphatemia, elevated levels of the calcium-phosphorus ion product, and high doses of vitamin D sterols have been implicated in the pathogenesis of cardiovascular calcification.[91,92] However, as many as 40% of adult patients with CKD stage 3—patients with normal circulating calcium and phosphorus concentrations—have evidence of vascular calcification, suggesting that other factors in the context of CKD contribute to this process.[109,110] Increased circulating levels of FGF23 levels have been implicated in increased cardiovascular mortality in adult dialysis patients.[111] Whether FGF23 contributes to cardiovascular calcification itself remains controversial, but current data suggest a role for the hormone in the development of left ventricular hypertrophy.[111-114] Klotho, the cofactor necessary for mediating the actions of FGF23 on phosphate homeostasis, also has been implicated in vascular calcification. Animals lacking the Klotho gene display elevated levels of phosphorus, $1,25(OH)_2D$ and consequently serum calcium, along with vascular calcification and features of premature aging. CKD is associated with low circulating levels of Klotho, which have been implicated in vascular dysfunction.[109] Because of the complex interplay among calcium, phosphorus, vitamin D, FGF23, and PTH, the contribution of PTH levels to cardiovascular disease and mortality remains controversial.[115]

The pathophysiology of cardiovascular disease in CKD is multifactorial, and thus treatment strategies are also multifaceted and vary according to stage of CKD. Therapies that are effective in early CKD may not be effective in later stages. Lipid-lowering agents decrease mortality in adults with pre-dialysis CKD and in those with stable renal allografts but have not been shown to benefit patients treated with dialysis.[116-118] By contrast, normalization of mineral metabolism (by avoiding hypercalcemia and hyperphosphatemia, limiting calcium intake, and avoiding adynamic bone) is effective at slowing the progression of cardiovascular calcification in patients with CKD and those treated with maintenance dialysis.[119-121] Furthermore, the use of calcium-free binders is associated with a slowing of progression in vascular calcification scores. A recent meta-analysis of clinical trials comparing the long-term consequences of calcium-based binders versus non–calcium-based demonstrated an advantage with the use of calcium-free binders on cardiovascular disease, vascular calcifications, and mortality in patients with CKD.[119,121]

Although high levels of FGF23 have been associated with vascular calcification and mortality, it is unknown whether early control of FGF23 levels, as with the use of phosphate binders in early CKD, might lead to improvements in cardiovascular health.[122-125] Treatment with vitamin D sterols has been associated with improved survival in dialysis patients,[126-129] despite elevated FGF23 levels.[16] Calcimimetic therapy, on the other hand, may provide an additional option for the reduction of PTH, FGF23, and cardiovascular disease. Decreases in parathyroid gland hyperplasia, bone disease, and vascular calcification were found in rodents with renal failure who were treated with calcimimetics.[129-131] Early case reports suggested that calcimimetic therapy also could reduce vascular calcification burden in dialysis patients.[132] A recent prospective trial in 3883 adults with advanced secondary hyperparathyroidism (the EVOLVE trial), however, failed to demonstrate a beneficial effect of calcimimetics on either cardiovascular events or on mortality.[133]

It is critical to monitor the consequences of the vascular calcification process in view of the observations that cardiovascular disease remains the leading cause of death across the spectrum of CKD, including in the dialysis and renal transplant populations. At different stages of CKD, the relative importance of individual risk factors, the value of different biomarkers, and the consequences of the different therapeutic interventions may vary.

## GROWTH RETARDATION

Growth retardation is the hallmark of CKD in children. Growth failure worsens as renal function declines; the average height of children with even mild CKD (GFR 50 to 70 mL/min/1.73 m²) is 1 standard deviation (SD) below the average for healthy children. Moderate CKD (GFR 25 to 49 mL/min/1.73 m²) is associated with a height SD of –1.5, and, at the time of initiation of dialysis, the mean height SD is −1.8. Boys, younger patients, and those with prior renal transplants are at greatest risk for growth failure.[134]

Acidosis has been linked to delayed linear growth in patients with renal tubular acidosis and normal renal function, and its correction often leads to acceleration in growth velocity.[135] Acidotic rats have been found to have decreased growth hormone secretion, serum insulin-like growth factor 1 (IGF-1), and hepatic IGF-1 mRNA expression. Moreover, metabolic acidosis has been shown to inhibit the effects of growth hormone in rats with normal and decreased renal function.[136,137] Growth plate mRNA levels of growth hormone receptor, the IGF-1 receptor, and IGF-1 are downregulated, and IGF-binding proteins are upregulated.[138]

Calcitriol deficiency, secondary hyperparathyroidism, and bone deformities also contribute to growth retardation; however, the optimal target values for PTH in children at all stages of CKD that will maximize growth remain controversial. In children with moderate CKD, some data indicate that normal growth velocity is achieved when PTH levels are maintained within or close to the normal range[139]; others have demonstrated a linear correlation between growth and PTH levels in the same patient population, with those with the highest PTH values displaying the highest growth velocity.[138] Treatment for secondary hyperparathyroidism with large, intermittent doses of calcitriol and calcium-based phosphate binders has been shown to reduce bone formation and suppress osteoblastic activity in both adults and children.[16,141] However, adynamic bone disease may develop and linear bone growth decrease, despite serum PTH levels in the range recommended by the Kidney Disease Outcomes Quality Initiative[142,143] during intermittent vitamin D sterol therapy. Maintaining serum PTH levels between 300 and 500 pg/mL reduces the frequency of these complications, but whether it will have an effect on final height is not known.[16]

The predominant factor leading to growth retardation has not been defined yet, but one commonly used medication, calcitriol, exerts dose-dependent inhibitory effects on cell proliferation of chondrocytes and osteoblasts in vitro. In addition, vitamin D sterols increase expression of a number of IGF binding proteins (IGFBPs). IGFBP-2, -3, -4, and -5 sequester IGF-1 and may exert IGF-1–independent antiproliferative effects through their own receptors.[144]

Growth hormone resistance contributes to impaired linear growth in renal failure. In CKD, poor growth develops despite normal or increased serum growth hormone levels.[145] Uremia has been associated with diminished hepatic growth hormone receptor and IGF-1 mRNA expression, defects in postreceptor growth hormone–mediated signal transduction,[146] reductions in serum growth hormone binding protein levels,[150] and increased synthesis and reduced clearance of IGF binding proteins.[147] Improved growth velocity during recombinant human growth hormone (rhGH) therapy has been ascribed to increased bioavailability of IGF-1 to target tissues. Children who are treated with maintenance dialysis respond less well to rhGH therapy than do children with less severe CKD; the mechanisms for differences in response to growth hormone therapy remain to be determined. Notably, also, bone formation rate increases out of proportion to changes in PTH values during treatment with rhGH, complicating the noninvasive assessment of renal osteodystrophy during therapy.[148] Thus, although growth hormone is effective in improving final height in early CKD stages, the effects are markedly diminished in dialyzed patients and after renal transplantation.

## CARDIOVASCULAR DISEASE

Cardiovascular disease is the most common cause of mortality in patients with all stages of CKD, with young (i.e., 20 and 30 year old) dialysis patients displaying the same rates of mortality from cardiovascular disease as 80-year-old individuals in the general population.[149] Cardiovascular disease is not limited to adults, but is also common in children with CKD. In addition to traditional risk factors for cardiovascular disease (i.e., hypertension and smoking) found in the general population, risk factors for vascular disease in predialysis CKD and dialysis patients include hypercalcemia, hyperphosphatemia, elevated levels of the calcium-phosphorus ion product, and treatment with high doses of calcium salts and vitamin D sterols. However, 40% of adult patients with stage 3 CKD, without these known risk factors, show evidence of vascular calcification and changes in carotid artery wall thickness are apparent in children as early as CKD stage 2.[97,110]

---

### KEY POINTS

- The causes of growth retardation in childhood CKD are multifactorial.
- Growth hormone levels are normal in CKD.
- Growth hormone resistance is seen in patients with CKD.
- Diminished hepatic growth hormone receptors and decreased IGF-1 mRNA expression are common in CKD.
- Pharmacotherapy with rhGH increases bioavailability of IGF-1.
- Response to rhGH is better in children with predialysis CKD than in children who are on dialysis.

---

### KEY POINTS

- Cardiovascular disease is the leading cause of death in CKD.
- Uremia facilitates calcification of the tunica media of the arteries, decreasing distensibility of the vessels, also known as a "lead pipe" pathologic finding.

In contrast to the calcified atherosclerotic plaques that develop in the vascular intima of aging individuals with normal kidney function, uremia facilitates calcification of the tunica media. This form of calcification is associated with decreased distensibility of blood vessels, causing a rigid "lead pipe" pathologic finding that is associated with increased risk for congestive heart failure.[150] EBCT is used in assessment of vascular calcifications in the adult population, and measurements in young adults who were treated with maintenance dialysis as children demonstrated that a significant proportion of this population has evidence of vascular calcification.[93] Carotid ultrasound measurement of intima medial thickness has been validated for the assessment of cardiovascular pathologic processes in children, with increased thickness associated with worsening disease.[97] The prevalence of vascular changes in children with early CKD—patients who not only lack the mineral metabolism-associated risk factors common in the dialysis population but who also lack traditional adult risk factors such as obesity, diabetes, hypertension, and smoking[97]—suggest that factors unique to CKD and independent of circulating mineral content contribute to vascular disease.

The pathophysiology of vascular calcification in patients with CKD differs from that observed in the general population, although the mechanisms by which vascular calcifications develop remain to be fully elucidated. In atherosclerotic plaques, calcium deposition is observed primarily in the intima and vascular deposition of mineral in CKD occurs primarily in the tunica media.[150] In patients with compromised renal function, the entire smooth muscle layer surrounding arteries may be replaced not only by calcium deposits but also by tissue that resembles bone. Osteoblasts and vascular smooth muscle cells have a common mesenchymal origin. In patients with CKD, Cbfa1 is thought to trigger mesenchymal cell to osteoblast transformation. Mice deficient in Cbfa1 fail to mineralize bone, and arteries obtained from patients undergoing renal transplantation show increased levels of the protein.[98,151] Uremia potentiates expression of pro-mineralization factors including the sodium-dependent phosphate transporters PIT-1 and PIT-2, osteopontin, bone sialoprotein, osteonectin, alkaline phosphatase, type I collagen, and bone morphogenic protein-2 (BMP-2) while expression of calcification inhibitors, such as fetuin A and matrix Gla protein, is suppressed in CKD.[150]

Throughout the past several years, elevated circulating values of FGF23 have been linked to cardiovascular disease in patients with all stages of CKD and experimental data have defined a direct role for FGF23, independent of changes in mineral metabolism, on pathologic changes in cardiac myocytes. Although the effects of circulating FGF23 on mineral metabolism require the presence of Klotho as the coreceptor of FGF receptors,[152] some of the effects on the cardiovascular system appear to be Klotho independent. FGF23 levels are often hundreds-fold to thousands-fold higher in patients with renal failure compared to those detected in individuals with normal kidney function, and these values have been associated with an increased prevalence of left ventricular hypertrophy and with premature mortality in adults with all stages of CKD.[111,153] Experimental data have demonstrated that these associations may reflect a direct effect of FGF23 on the myocardium that induces myocyte hypertrophy in a Klotho-independent manner.[114] However, it is important to note that Klotho is expressed in arteries, although not in myocardium, and decreases in vascular Klotho, as occur with progressive CKD, have been linked to loss of vascular elasticity.[9]

## CALCIPHYLAXIS

Calciphylaxis is a unique syndrome characterized by ischemic necrosis of the skin, subcutaneous fat, and muscles. Although calciphylaxis is uncommon in children, it may develop in patients with advanced renal failure not yet treated by dialysis, in those treated with regular dialysis, and even in patients with well-functioning kidney transplants.[154] Two distinct types of the syndrome are recognized: proximal calciphylaxis, which affects the thighs, abdomen, and chest wall and acral calciphylaxis, which involves sites distal to the knees and elbows, such as the toes, fingers, and ankles.[155] The former has a poor prognosis, with death occurring in more than 80% to 90% of affected patients. This syndrome is often accompanied by morbid obesity and hypoalbuminemia. Many patients have severe secondary hyperparathyroidism, and most have a history of severe and uncontrolled hyperphosphatemia, but it has been described in patients with adynamic osteodystrophy.[155,156] Some patients may have defective regulation of coagulation.[157] The appearance of this syndrome in renal transplant recipients receiving glucocorticoids suggests that steroids also may play a role. Patients with calciphylaxis frequently die of secondary infection.

A significant number of patients with calciphylaxis improve after parathyroidectomy, and a few have healed after substantial reductions in levels of serum phosphorus. Parathyroidectomy and aggressive control of serum

---

## KEY POINTS

Factors promoting vascular calcification include:

- Cbfa1
- Sodium-dependent phosphate transporters PIT-1 and PIT-2
- Osteopontin
- Bone sialoprotein
- Osteonectin
- Alkaline phosphatase
- Type I collagen
- Bone morphogenic protein-2 (BMP-2)

phosphate levels therefore are indicated in those with evidence of severe secondary hyperparathyroidism. However, secondary hyperparathyroidism should be well documented before parathyroidectomy, because adynamic bone has been associated with this syndrome. Although ischemic lesions and medial vascular calcifications are common in uremic patients with diabetes, such lesions rarely improve after parathyroidectomy. Calcimimetics, as well as sodium-thiosulfate (a calcium chelating agent) and pamidronate, have been used effectively in some individuals.[158,159] Hyperbaric oxygen therapy also has been advocated, and some patients will require amputation of the extremities as a result of advanced disease process.[159]

## BONE BIOPSY

Although not routinely performed in the clinical setting, a bone biopsy should be considered in all patients with CKD who have fractures with minimal trauma (pathologic fractures), suspected aluminum bone disease, or persistent hypercalcemia despite serum PTH levels between 400 and 600 pg/mL.[142] For bone labeling, a 2-day course of tetracycline is administered at 15 mg/kg/day (divided into twice-daily or thrice-daily doses). Phosphate binders should be withheld during labeling because they may interfere with gut absorption of tetracycline. Fourteen days later, the 2-day course is repeated. For children younger than 8 years old, tetracycline dosage usually is kept below 10 mg/kg/day to avoid toxicity. Histochemical staining procedures may demonstrate deposition of abnormal components such as iron, aluminum, and oxalate within bone.[160]

## MANAGEMENT OF CHRONIC KIDNEY DISEASE AND MINERAL AND BONE DISORDER

To minimize complications in the skeleton and prevent extraskeletal calcification, particular attention must be paid to alterations of bone and mineral metabolism in CKD. The specific aims of management of CKD-MBD are to (1) maintain blood levels of serum calcium and phosphorus near normal limits, (2) prevent hyperplasia of the parathyroid glands and maintain serum PTH at levels appropriate for the stage of CKD, (3) avoid the development of extraskeletal calcifications, and (4) prevent or reverse the accumulation of toxic substances such as FGF23, aluminum and $\beta_2$-microglobulin.

## DIETARY MANIPULATION OF CALCIUM AND PHOSPHORUS

As active vitamin D levels fall during the progression of renal disease, calcium absorption in the gut and kidney diminishes and hypocalcemia evolves in advanced CKD. Patients with untreated CKD commonly ingest as little as 400 to 700 mg of elemental calcium per day in their diet. Calcium-rich foods such as dairy products, unfortunately, also are high in phosphorus. Thus, increasing dietary consumption of calcium to meet daily needs is accompanied by excessive intake of phosphorus, which cannot be excreted in the face of renal failure. As a result, calcium supplementation in the form of calcium-containing salts is often required. The total amount of calcium supplementation provided, however, must be monitored carefully, because values above 1.5 g/day are associated with positive calcium balance in patients with CKD stages 3 and 4 disease[8] and may lead to hypercalcemia and vascular calcification.

The development of hyperphosphatemia occurs in the vast majority of patients with advanced renal insufficiency. Hyperphosphatemia and an elevated calcium-phosphorus ion product have been reported as independent risk factors for vascular calcification and mortality in adult dialysis patients.[119,120] Thus, treatment goals include maintaining serum phosphorus levels within normal limits for age (Table 33.1) and avoiding a calcium-phosphorus ion product above 55. The average phosphorus intake of both adults and children in the U.S. population is approximately 1500 to 2000 mg/day, and 60% to 70% of the dietary intake is absorbed. In early stages of renal failure, mild dietary phosphate restriction is sufficient to prevent hyperphosphatemia and also may modulate the progressive rise in circulating FGF23. However, strict adherence to dietary phosphate restriction is often difficult because low-phosphate diets are unpalatable, especially to older children and adults, and because phosphorus intake is directly linked to protein

Table 33.1 Age appropriate normal values of serum calcium, phosphorus, and alkaline phosphatase

| Age (yr) | S-Phosophorus (mg/dL) | S-Calcium (Total) (mg/dL) | S-Calcium (ionized) (mM) | Alkaline phosphatase (International units) |
|---|---|---|---|---|
| First yr | 4.8–7.4 | 8.8–11.3 | 1.22–1.4 | |
| 1–5 | 4.5–6.5 | 9.4–10.8 | 1.22–1.32 | 100–350 |
| 6–12 | 3.6–5.8 | 9.4–10.3 | 1.15–1.32 | 60–450 |
| 13–20 | 2.3–4.5 | 8.8–10.2 | 1.12–1.30 | 40–180 |

Source: K/DOQI Workgroup. K/DOQI clinical practice guidelines for cardiovascular disease in dialysis patients. Am J Kidney Dis. 45(Suppl 3): S1, 2005. Reproduced with permission

Table 33.2 Dosing of ergocalciferol in vitamin D deficiency

| Serum 25(OH) D (ng/mL) | Definition | Ergocalciferol dose | Duration | Comment |
|---|---|---|---|---|
| <5 | Severe vitamin D deficiency | 8000 international units/day (or 50,000 IU per week) PO × 4 wk, then 4000 international units/day × 8 wk | 3 mo | Measure 25(OH)D levels after 3 mo |
| 5–15 | Mild vitamin D deficiency | 4000 international units/day (or 50,000 IU every two weeks) PO | 3 mo | Measure 25(OH)D levels after 3 mo |
| 16–30 | Vitamin D insufficiency | 2000 international units/day PO | 3 mo | Measure 25(OH)D levels after 3 mo |

Source: K/DOQI Workgroup. K/DOQI clinical practice guidelines for cardiovascular disease in dialysis patients. Am J Kidney Dis. 2005;45(Suppl 3):S1, 2005. Reproduced with permission

intake, with 10 to 12 mg of phosphorus accompanying each gram of protein. Adequate protein intake is necessary for growth in children and for maintenance of lean body mass in adults. Current dietary recommendations suggest that adults with CKD ingest 0.8 to 1 g/kg/day of protein and that children, depending on age, ingest 1 to 2.5 g/kg/day.[142,143] This translates to a minimum phosphate ingestion of 800 mg/day in an 80-kg person.

Patients treated with dialysis require dietary phosphorus restriction, in addition to phosphate-binder therapy, because standard prescription peritoneal dialysis and hemodialysis remove insufficient amounts of phosphate (300 to 400 mg/day for peritoneal dialysis and 800 mg/treatment for hemodialysis) to maintain normal serum phosphorus levels. On the other hand, the use of daily, slow, continuous hemodialysis has been associated with excellent control of serum phosphorus levels, often allowing phosphate-binding agents to be discontinued.[161,162] Indeed, some patients have developed hypophosphatemia and required the addition of phosphorus to the dialysate solution to prevent the long-term consequences of hypophosphatemia.[161,162]

## PHOSPHATE-BINDING AGENTS

Phosphate-binding agents reduce intestinal phosphate absorption by forming poorly soluble complexes with phosphorus in the intestinal tract. Aluminum-containing phosphate binders were used frequently in the past, but long-term treatment led to bone disease, encephalopathy, and anemia.[163] The use of aluminum-containing phosphate binders, therefore, should be restricted to the treatment of patients with severe hyperphosphatemia (greater than 7 mg/dL) associated with hypercalcemia or an elevated calcium-phosphorus ion product, because both conditions will be aggravated by calcium-containing compounds. In such cases, the dose of aluminum hydroxide should not exceed 30 mg/kg/day and the lowest possible dose should be given for only a limited period of approximately 4 to 6 weeks.[164] Plasma aluminum levels should be monitored regularly. Concomitant intake of citrate-containing compounds should be avoided, because citrate enhances intestinal aluminum absorption and increases the risk for acute aluminum intoxication.[165]

To avoid aluminum-related bone disease and encephalopathy, the use of aluminum-free phosphate binders has been advocated. Among these, calcium-containing salts are widely used for control of hyperphosphatemia and also serve as an additional source of supplemental calcium. Several calcium salts, including calcium carbonate, calcium acetate, and calcium citrate, are commercially available. Calcium carbonate is the most commonly used compound, and studies in adults and children have documented its efficacy in controlling serum phosphorus levels.[166] The recommended dose is proportional to the phosphorus content of the meal and is adjusted to achieve acceptable serum levels of calcium and phosphorus.

Large doses of calcium carbonate may lead to hypercalcemia, particularly in patients treated concomitantly with active vitamin D sterols or those with adynamic bone.[167] Hypercalcemia usually is reversible with reductions in the dose of oral calcium salts, dose of vitamin D sterol, and dialysate calcium concentration. To avoid the development and progression of cardiovascular calcifications, it is currently recommended that elemental calcium intake should not exceed 2 g/day, with less than 1500 mg of calcium given as calcium-containing phosphorus binders.[70,142,143] It is important to consider that adult patients with CKD stage 3 or 4 who ingest 1.5 g/day of calcium carbonate are in positive calcium balance. Although requirements in children are not well defined, calcium intake should be considered in light of age-based recommendations.[168]

Comparison studies between calcium carbonate and calcium acetate have demonstrated that an equivalent dose of calcium acetate binds twice as much phosphorus, but the relative incidence of hypercalcemia varies among studies.[169] Calcium citrate is an effective phosphate-binding agent but should be used with caution in patients with renal failure because of enhanced intestinal aluminum absorption when given in combination with aluminum-containing phosphate binders.[170] Calcium ketoglutarate is less calcemic than calcium carbonate and has anabolic benefits, but gastrointestinal side effects and high cost of therapy often limit its use.[171]

To limit the vascular calcification risks associated with the use of calcium salts and the bone and neurologic toxicity associated with aluminum hydroxide, alternative phosphate binders have been developed. Sevelamer hydrochloride (RenaGel), a calcium-free and aluminum-free hydrogel of cross-linked polyallylamine, has been shown to lower serum phosphorus levels, the calcium-phosphorus ion product, and PTH without inducing hypercalcemia in adult patients treated with hemodialysis.[119] Sevelamer also halts the progression of vascular calcifications, although such lesions increase during calcium-containing binder therapy in adult hemodialysis patients.[119] In addition to its effects on serum phosphorus levels, sevelamer has been shown to decrease concentrations of total serum cholesterol and low-density lipoprotein cholesterol, but to increase high-density lipoprotein levels.[172] These effects may offer additional benefits in reducing cardiovascular complications in patients with ESRD. Acidosis may occur in patients treated with sevelamer. A newer formulation of sevelamer, sevelamer carbonate (Renvela), also has been introduced. This new compound is as effective a phosphate binder as sevelamer hydrochloride, with less potential to induce acidosis.[173]

Other alternative phosphate-binding agents include magnesium, iron, and lanthanum compounds. Magnesium carbonate lowers serum phosphorus levels, but magnesium-free dialysate solutions should be used in those treated with dialysis.[174] Large doses, however, result in diarrhea, limiting the use of this compound as a single agent. Iron compounds, such as stabilized polynuclear iron hydroxide and ferric polymaltose complex, have proved effective phosphate binders in short-term studies in adults with CKD.[175]

Clinical trials have demonstrated that lanthanum carbonate (Fosrenol) also effectively controls serum phosphorus and PTH levels without increasing serum calcium values. Lanthanum carbonate lowers serum phosphorus and PTH levels without causing hypercalcemia, adynamic bone disease, or osteomalacia.[176] However, lanthanum is a heavy metal that accumulates in different organs in animals with normal renal function.[177] Lanthanum also accumulates in the bone of dialysis patients, where its presence persists despite discontinuation for as long as 2 years. Additional long-term studies are therefore needed to confirm the absence of toxicity before this agent is recommended for widespread use in pediatric patients with CKD. It is important to also consider the different effects of phosphate binders on FGF23. Indeed, FGF23 levels remained unchanged or increase with calcium-based binders; by contrast, FGF23 levels appear to decrease with calcium-free phosphate binders and a recent meta-analysis demonstrated improved overall mortality and cardiovascular disease with the use of calcium-free versus calcium-based binders across the spectrum of CKD.[121]

# VITAMIN D THERAPY

Despite dietary phosphate restriction, the intake of phosphate-binding agents, the use of an appropriate level of calcium in dialysate solution, and an adequate intake of calcium, progressive osteitis fibrosa cystica secondary to hyperparathyroidism develops in a significant number of uremic patients. Treatment with active vitamin D sterols is aimed at controlling serum PTH levels and the resultant high turnover bone disease. Current evidence indicates that two main issues should be considered with respect to vitamin D therapy: first, treatment of 25(OH)D deficiency, a common finding in patients with renal disease, in itself may reverse hyperparathyroidism. Second, treatment with active vitamin D sterols is useful in pharmacologically reducing PTH levels.

## Assessment and treatment of 25(OH) vitamin D deficiency

Measurement of 25(OH)D levels and treatment of vitamin D deficiency are an important part of the management of hyperparathyroidism in patients with CKD. Although current guidelines are controversial, the National Academy of Medicine, formerly the Institute of Medicine, suggests that 25(OH)D values be maintained above 20 ng/mL.[178] Current recommendations from the National Kidney Foundation stratify vitamin D deficiency into three categories: (1) severe deficiency, defined as serum levels less than 5 ng/mL; (2) mild deficiency, equivalent to serum concentrations of 5 to 15 ng/mL; and (3) vitamin D insufficiency, with levels between 16 and 30 ng/mL.[142] Thus, ergocalciferol treatment should be initiated in patients with CKD when 25(OH)D levels fall below 30 ng/mL (Table 33.2).

## Treatment with active vitamin D sterols

Active vitamin D sterols act through a variety of pathways to decrease PTH production—by increasing calcium absorption in the gut and kidney, by binding to the CaSR, by increasing skeletal sensitivity to PTH, and by altering prepro-PTH transcription. Calcitriol (Rocaltrol®) has been widely used for many years to control secondary hyperparathyroidism in both adults and children. The efficacy of daily oral doses of calcitriol for the treatment of patients with symptomatic renal osteodystrophy has been well documented in several clinical trials.[68,179,180] With appropriate treatment, bone pain diminishes, muscle strength, gait, and posture improve, and osteitis fibrosa frequently resolves partially or completely. Doses of oral calcitriol in most clinical trials have ranged from 0.25 to 1.5 mcg/day. In patients with CKD, initial doses are determined by target PTH levels and specific stage of kidney disease.[181] In dialysis patients, $1,25(OH)_2D_3$ given thrice weekly by intravenous injection or by oral pulse therapy is effective in reducing serum PTH levels.[182] Dosage regimens range from 0.5 to 1 mcg to 3.5 to 4 mcg three times weekly or 2 to 5 mcg twice weekly. Low doses should be used initially, and dosage adjustments should be based on frequent measurements of serum calcium, phosphorus, and PTH levels (Table 33.3).

Oral $1\alpha$-$(OH)D_3$ (alfacalcidol) undergoes 25-hydroxylation in the liver to form calcitriol,[183] and this agent is used widely in Europe, Japan, and Canada. Calcitriol and

Table 33.3 Target ranges of plasma parathyroid hormone by stage of chronic kidney disease in children

| CKD stage | GFR range | Target intact PTH level (pg/mL) |
|---|---|---|
| 3 | 30–59 | 35–70 |
| 4 | 15–29 | 70–110 |
| 5 | <15 or dialysis | 200–300 |

Source: K/DOQI Workgroup. K/DOQI clinical practice guidelines for cardiovascular disease in dialysis patients. Am J Kidney Dis. 2005;45(Suppl 3):S1, 2005. Reproduced with permission
CKD, chronic kidney disease; GFR, glomerular filtration rate; PTH, parathyroid hormone.

$1\alpha$-(OH)D$_3$ are similarly effective for the treatment of secondary hyperparathyroidism in patients with CKD.

Although calcitriol and alfacalcidol are effective in decreasing PTH levels and preventing osteitis fibrosis cystica, treatment with these sterols in combination with calcium-based binders often results in hypercalcemia and hyperphosphatemia and contributes to the development of soft tissue calcification, which limits their use. Thus, new vitamin D analogues have been developed to prevent or minimize intestinal calcium and phosphorus absorption, while suppressing PTH levels as effectively as calcitriol. Three of these new vitamin D analogues are already on the market for use in patients with CKD: 22-oxacalcitriol (maxacalcitol) in Japan; 19-nor-1,25-(OH)$_2$D$_2$ (paricalcitol [Zemplar]); and $1\alpha$-(OH)D$_2$ (doxercalciferol [Hectorol]) in the United States.

19-Nor-1 $\alpha$,25(OH)$_2$D$_2$ (paricalcitol) is effective in controlling serum PTH levels in adult patients with CKD stages 3 and 4, as well as in dialysis patients. The long-term consequences of therapy with paricalcitol in conjunction with the use of calcium-containing binders for vascular calcification and cardiovascular complications remain to be determined. Interestingly, in a large cohort of patients undergoing hemodialysis, higher survival rates were observed in dialyzed patients treated with paricalcitol when compared with those receiving calcitriol.[184]

$1\alpha$-(OH)D$_2$ ($1\alpha$-D$_2$, doxercalciferol), is equipotent to $1\alpha$-(OH)D$_3$ in intestinal calcium absorption and bone calcium mobilization in rats.[185] A comparative trial of calcitriol and doxercalciferol in the control of secondary hyperparathyroidism in pediatric patients revealed no differences between the two vitamin D sterols in the control of secondary hyperparathyroidism or the development of hypercalcemia.[6] Doxercalciferol also effectively controls secondary hyperparathyroidism in adult patients with stable CKD.[186] Similar to paricalcitol, a survival advantage has been observed in adult hemodialysis patients receiving paricalcitol over those treated with calcitriol.[128]

Active vitamin D therapy has been associated with protective effects on both the heart and the kidney. Active vitamin D sterols ameliorate cardiac hypertrophy in animals, and calcitriol therapy improves cardiac systolic function in hemodialysis patients. However, paracalcitrol did not affect cardiac structure when it was prospectively compared

in patients with CKD stages 3 and 4.[187] Administration of active vitamin D sterols reduces proteinuria, fibrosis, and podocyte hypertrophy in subtotally nephrectomized rats, and paricalcitol treatment decreases proteinuria in CKD patients.[188,189] These effects may be mediated by suppression of the renin-angiotensin system (RAS). In vitro studies have demonstrated that calcitriol, paricalcitol, and doxercalciferol all suppress the RAS to a similar degree.[190] 1,25(OH)$_2$D$_3$ has recently been shown to reduce renal fibrosis by a non–VDR-related mechanism.[31] However, all activated vitamin D analogues also may increase FGF23 secretion. Although the consequences of these increased levels in dialyzed patients remain to be completely determined, current evidence suggests that excessive circulating FGF23 is associated with increased mortality rates.[111]

## CALCIMIMETICS

Cinacalcet (Sensipar), an allosteric activator of the calcium-sensing receptor, is now available for the treatment of secondary hyperparathyroidism. This small organic molecule reduces serum PTH levels and has been shown to decrease the calcium-phosphorus ion product in adult patients treated with maintenance dialysis, regardless of the specific phosphate-binding agent.[191] Experiments also have demonstrated that calcimimetics are able to halt the progression of parathyroid cell hyperplasia, and the antiproliferative effect of this agent shows promise for use of the molecule as a medical parathyroidectomy.[191] Calcimimetic therapy may provide an additional option for the reduction of both PTH levels and cardiovascular disease. Indeed, a decrease in parathyroid gland hyperplasia, bone disease, and vascular calcification were found in rodents with renal failure who were treated with calcimimetics.[129–132] Early case reports suggested that calcimimetic therapy could also reduce vascular calcification burden in dialysis patients.[132] However, a 2012 prospective trial in 3883 adults with advanced secondary hyperparathyroidism (the EVOLVE trial) failed to demonstrate a beneficial effect of calcimimetics on either cerebrovascular events or mortality.[133] Owing to the presence of the calcium-sensing receptor on the growth plate, these agents are not approved and should be used with caution in growing children.

## PARATHYROIDECTOMY

In many cases when parathyroid surgery is needed and undertaken, the parathyroid tissue has become monoclonal and demonstrated an autonomous growth.[192] Patients with severe hyperparathyroidism are often unresponsive to vitamin D therapy and develop hypercalcemia without reduction in PTH values or parathyroid gland size (tertiary hyperparathyroidism).[193] Indications for parathyroidectomy are (1) the presence of hyperplasia, hypertrophy, or both of the parathyroid glands (as documented by the presence of biochemical and radiographic features and, if necessary, the findings of osteitis fibrosa cystica on bone biopsy); (2) elevated serum PTH levels unresponsive to vitamin D sterol therapy; (3) persistent hypercalcemia; (4) pruritus unresponsive to dialysis or other medical treatment; (5) progressive extraskeletal calcification; (6) severe skeletal pain or fractures; and (7) calciphylaxis. Aluminum-related bone disease must be ruled out first in patients receiving low-dose calcitriol with persistent hypercalcemia.[194] Other causes of hypercalcemia, such as sarcoidosis, malignancy-related hypercalcemia, intake of calcium supplements, and the presence of adynamic or aplastic bone lesions not related to aluminum, also should be considered.[195]

When the decision has been made to perform parathyroid surgery, it is essential to avoid a marked postoperative fall in serum calcium levels caused by the "hungry bone" syndrome. Because of the severity of the bone disease, this fall can be much more marked and prolonged than after parathyroidectomy for primary hyperparathyroidism. Patients with CKD should receive daily oral calcitriol (0.5 to 1 mcg) or some sort of intravenous active vitamin D sterol for 2 to 6 days before parathyroid surgery and during the postoperative period to stimulate intestinal calcium absorption and to maximize the effectiveness of oral calcium salts. Within 24 to 36 hours after surgery, marked hypocalcemia with serum calcium levels below 7 to 8 mg/dL may develop. This condition may be associated with serious symptoms, including seizures resulting in fractures and tendon avulsion. For reasons that are still unclear, these seizures most often occur during the last 1 to 2 hours of a hemodialysis procedure or immediately thereafter.

To reduce the risk for seizures, an infusion containing calcium gluconate should be started in the operating room, on removal of the parathyroid glands. Calcium gluconate should be initiated at a rate of 100 mg of calcium ion per hour. Serum calcium should be measured every 4 to 6 hours, and the calcium gluconate infusion rate increased if the serum calcium level continues to fall. The infusion rate may exceed 200 mg/h. Enteral calcium carbonate is initiated once the patient is able to tolerate oral intake, and doses as high as 1 g (elemental calcium) given four to six times daily, along with vitamin D sterol in excess of 1 to 2 mcg/day (for calcitriol, doses of other agents vary according to their potency), are often needed for patients with marked hypocalcemia. The intravenous calcium drip is weaned as soon as the oral intake of calcium salts is able to maintain normal serum calcium levels. The duration of intravenous calcium requirements varies greatly across patients—most patients require intravenous therapy for 2 to 3 days, but severe hypocalcemia may persist for several weeks or months, necessitating permanent central catheter access for daily home infusions of 800 to 1000 mg of elemental calcium. Serum phosphorus levels may fall to subnormal levels postoperatively. Supplemental phosphate treatment will markedly aggravate the hypocalcemia, and patients should not be treated with phosphate unless serum phosphorus falls to below 2.0 mg/dL.[196]

Hyperplastic parathyroid glands may be infiltrated with ethanol or calcitriol to cause sclerosis of the parathyroid tissue. This technique has been used at some centers with variable efficacy in reducing hyperplastic tissue.[197,198] This technique is used currently by only a few centers worldwide.

## GROWTH HORMONE THERAPY

rhGH should be considered in children with growth failure that does not respond to optimization of nutrition, correction of acidosis, and control of renal osteodystrophy. Serum phosphorus and PTH levels should be well controlled before the initiation of rhGH in children with CKD. Serum phosphorus levels should be less than 1.5 times the upper limit for age and PTH-IMA-1 levels less than 1.5 times the upper target values for the CKD stage before rhGH therapy is begun.[168] Growth hormone therapy will increase serum PTH levels during the first months of therapy; therefore, serum PTH levels should be monitored monthly. Current recommendations suggest that growth hormone therapy should be discontinued temporarily if PTH levels exceed three times the upper target value for the CKD stage[168]; however, it is important to note that growth hormone also directly increases bone formation rate, independent of PTH values, thus distorting the relationship between PTH and bone formation rate.[148]

## BONE DISEASE AFTER SUCCESSFUL RENAL TRANSPLANTATION

Successful kidney transplantation corrects many of the abnormalities associated with renal osteodystrophy, but disorders of bone and mineral metabolism remain a major problem in such patients. Several factors, including persistent secondary hyperparathyroidism, prolonged immobilization, graft function, and, most important, use of different immunosuppressive agents, have been implicated in the development of bone disease after organ transplantation.

Hypercalcemia is not uncommon after renal transplantation. During the first several months following transplantation, it can be quite severe and patients with severe secondary hyperparathyroidism before renal transplantation are at the greatest risk. More often, hypercalcemia is less severe, with serum calcium levels between 10.5 and 12.0 mg/dL, and usually resolves within the first 12 months.[198] Parathyroidectomy should be considered when serum calcium levels are persistently above 12.5 mg/dL for longer than 1 year after transplantation.[199] Calcimimetic agents may be useful in preventing the need for parathyroidectomy in these patients, but it is important to note that adynamic bone disease may be present in hypercalcemic renal transplant recipients, despite apparently increased PTH values.[200,201]

Hypophosphatemia may occur early in the post-transplant period, mainly in patients with severe secondary hyperparathyroidism, although persistent post-transplant elevation of serum FGF23 levels also may contribute.[202,203] The clinical manifestations are variable; some patients complain of malaise, fatigue, and muscle weakness.[204,205] Phosphorus supplementation should be considered when values are persistently below 2.0 mg/dL, primarily in pediatric patients.

Significant bone loss has been shown to occur as early as 3 to 6 months after kidney transplantation.[206,207] Several factors, including persistent alterations in mineral metabolism, prolonged immobilization, and the use of immunosuppressive agents required to maintain graft function, have been implicated in the development of bone disease after transplantation. Osteonecrosis, or avascular necrosis, is by far the most debilitating skeletal complication associated with organ transplantation. In approximately 15% of patients, osteonecrosis develops within 3 years of renal transplantation.[208,209] The occurrence of osteonecrosis in inpatients after cardiac, hepatic, and bone marrow transplantation suggests that glucocorticoids play a critical role in the pathogenesis of this disorder.[210,211]

In both adult and pediatric kidney recipients, bone histologic changes associated with secondary hyperparathyroidism have been shown to resolve within 6 months after kidney transplantation.[207] However, some patients have persistently elevated rates of bone turnover and others develop adynamic lesions, despite moderately elevated serum PTH levels.[212] Bone biopsy data from pediatric kidney recipients indicate that 67% of patients with stable graft function have features of normal bone formation, 10% have adynamic bone lesions, and 23% have bone lesions characteristic of secondary hyperparathyroidism.[213] Bone resorption typically is increased,[214] leading to a net loss of bone mass over time. Serum PTH levels are unable to discriminate among adynamic, normal, and increased bone turnover in the pediatric transplant population.[213] The use of maintenance corticosteroids has been implicated in these alterations; steroids decrease intestinal calcium absorption, enhance urinary calcium excretion, inhibit osteoblastic activity, decrease bone formation, and increase osteoclastic activity and bone resorption.[215-217] Likewise, cyclosporine has been reported to increase both bone formation and resorption and to reduce cancellous bone volume in the rat.[218,219] By contrast, azathioprine has been shown to have minimal impact on skeletal remodeling.[220] The role of other immunosuppressive agents, such as mycophenolate mofetil, as potential modifiers of bone formation and bone resorption has not been evaluated.

Although bone turnover may return to normal, defective skeletal mineralization is present in many pediatric transplant recipients.[213] Osteoid volume is increased, and mineral apposition rate is markedly reduced.[213] Although the factors responsible for the persistent increase in osteoid formation remain to be fully explained, corticosteroid use may contribute, as may persistent imbalances in PTH, vitamin D, and FGF23 metabolism.[203]

After successful kidney transplantation with standard immunosuppressive regimens (daily corticosteroids, calcineurin inhibitor, and antimetabolite), growth may be accelerated by an improvement in kidney function, but catch-up growth may not be observed even in children who undergo transplantation very early in life.[94] Moreover, height deceleration occurs in approximately 75% of patients who undergo transplantation before the age of 15 years.[221] The cause of persistent growth retardation is not completely understood, but immunosuppressive agents, persistent secondary hyperparathyroidism, altered vitamin D and FGF23 metabolism, and the persistence of defective skeletal mineralization may contribute. Used in children with significant height deficit after kidney transplantation, rhGH has produced a substantial increase in linear growth within the first year of therapy, but the magnitude of growth response may decline thereafter.[222]

Cardiovascular disease continues to be the leading cause of death after renal transplantation. In the post-transplant period, the presence of hypertension is strongly linked to increased intimal medial thickness and poor vessel distensibility in children.[223] Alterations in bone and mineral metabolism also may contribute, because impaired kidney function persists in most patients during the post-transplant period. Indeed, EBCT data indicate that vascular calcifications do not regress post-transplantation and do contribute to the burden of cardiovascular disease in this population.[224] Although FGF23 levels substantially diminished in the immediate period after renal transplantation, values are increased in long-term renal transplant recipients and have been associated with CKD progression and episodes of rejection, and cardiovascular morbidity in adult and pediatric renal transplant recipients.[225,226] Prospective studies are needed to further assess the effects of controlling effects of FGF23 on survival and cardiac disease.

---

### Clinical Vignette 33.1

A 15-year-old boy with a history of prenatally diagnosed posterior urethral valves was followed in the CKD clinic. He had received adequate protein and calorie nutrition since infancy via a gastrointestinal tube. Acidosis was treated with bicarbonate supplementation, and his anemia was corrected with epoetin alfa (Epogen) and iron. His hypertension was well controlled with enalapril. His serum calcium, phosphorus, and PTH levels were maintained within the appropriate range for CKD stage. However, he had growth failure since 18 months of age. Growth hormone therapy was initiated because of his height being persistently below the 3rd percentile. Initially, he experienced some catch-up growth, which subsequently tapered off.

At 5 years of age he received a preemptive transplant from his mother. Growth hormone was reinitiated 6 months after his renal transplant, but he continued to be short for age. At age 15, he lost his allograft to medication noncompliance. Over the next 6 years, he was followed in the chronic dialysis unit and was repeatedly counseled on dietary phosphorus restriction and on compliance with his calcium-based and calcium-free phosphate binders. However, his serum phosphorus concentrations persistently remained between 7 and 9 mg/dL, and his PTH remained above 1000 pg/mL. He had significant genu valgum deformity. At age 21, an EBCT demonstrated extensive coronary artery calcifications.

## TEACHING POINTS

- This case illustrates the complex interplay among mineral metabolism, bone disease, and cardiovascular disease in pediatric CKD.
- Despite optimization of nutrition, mineral metabolism, and acidosis, children with CKD grow poorly. Although growth hormone therapy improves final height in many patients with predialysis CKD, many children have decreased final adult height despite growth hormone therapy.
- Hyperphosphatemia and secondary hyperphosphatemia are particularly problematic in children and adolescents treated with maintenance dialysis; compliance with dietary phosphate restriction and phosphate binder therapy are essential in this population so that active vitamin D sterol therapy can be used to control serum PTH concentrations.
- Long-standing secondary hyperparathyroidism is associated with bone deformities, while long-standing hyperphosphatemia contributes to progressive vascular calcification in both the pediatric and adult populations.

## REFERENCES

1. Moe S, Drueke T, Cunningham J, et al. Definition, evaluation, and classification of renal osteodystrophy: A position statement from Kidney Disease: Improving Global Outcomes (KDIGO). Kidney Int. 2006;69:1945–53.
2. Isakova T, Wahl P, Vargas GS, et al. Fibroblast growth factor 23 is elevated before parathyroid hormone and phosphate in chronic kidney disease. Kidney Int. 2011;79:1370–8.
3. Bacchetta J, Dubourg L, Harambat J, et al. The influence of glomerular filtration rate and age on fibroblast growth factor 23 serum levels in pediatric chronic kidney disease. J Clin Endocrinol Metab. 2010;95:1741–8.
4. Wesseling-Perry K, Pereira RC, Wang H, et al. Relationship between plasma FGF-23 concentration and bone mineralization in children with renal failure on peritoneal dialysis. J Clin Endocrinol Metab. 2009;94:511–7.
5. Bhattacharyya N, Wiench M, Dumitrescu C, et al. Mechanism of FGF23 processing in fibrous dysplasia. J Bone Miner Res. 2012;27:1132–41.
6. Pereira RC, Juppner H, Azucena-Serrano CE, et al. Patterns of FGF-23, DMP1, and MEPE expression in patients with chronic kidney disease. Bone. 2009;45:1161–8.
7. Antoniucci DM, Yamashita T, Portale AA. Dietary phosphorus regulates serum fibroblast growth factor-23 concentrations in healthy men. J Clin Endocrinol Metab. 2006;91:3144–9.
8. Hill KM, Martin BR, Wastney ME, et al. Oral calcium carbonate affects calcium but not phosphorus balance in stage 3-4 chronic kidney disease. Kidney Int. 2013;83:959–66.
9. Lim K, Lu TS, Molostvov G, et al. Vascular Klotho deficiency potentiates the development of human artery calcification and mediates resistance to fibroblast growth factor 23. Circulation. 2012;125:2243–55.
10. Farrow EG, Yu X, Summers LJ, et al. Iron deficiency drives an autosomal dominant hypophosphatemic rickets (ADHR) phenotype in fibroblast growth factor-23 (Fgf23) knock-in mice. Proc Natl Acad Sci U S A. 2011;108:E1146–55.
11. Smith RC, O'Bryan LM, Farrow EG, et al. Circulating alphaKlotho influences phosphate handling by controlling FGF23 production. J Clin Invest. 2012;122:4710–5.
12. Portale AA, Wolf M, Juppner H, et al. Disordered FGF23 and mineral metabolism in children with CKD. Clin J Am Soc Nephrol. 2014;9:344–53.
13. Gutierrez O, Isakova T, Rhee E, et al. Fibroblast growth factor-23 mitigates hyperphosphatemia but accentuates calcitriol deficiency in chronic kidney disease. J Am Soc Nephrol. 2005;16:2205–15.
14. van Husen M, Fischer AK, Lehnhardt A, et al. Fibroblast growth factor 23 and bone metabolism in children with chronic kidney disease. Kidney Int. 2010;78:200–6.
15. Ben-Dov IZ, Galitzer H, Lavi-Moshayoff V, et al. The parathyroid is a target organ for FGF23 in rats. J Clin Invest. 2007;117:4003–8.
16. Wesseling-Perry K, Pereira RC, Sahney S, et al. Calcitriol and doxercalciferol are equivalent in controlling bone turnover, suppressing parathyroid hormone, and increasing fibroblast growth factor-23 in secondary hyperparathyroidism. Kidney Int. 2011;79:112–9.
17. Shimada T, Hasegawa H, Yamazaki Y, et al. FGF-23 is a potent regulator of vitamin D metabolism and phosphate homeostasis. J. Bone Miner Res. 2004;19:429–35.
18. Krajisnik T, Bjorklund P, Marsell R, et al. Fibroblast growth factor-23 regulates parathyroid hormone and 1alpha-hydroxylase expression in cultured bovine parathyroid cells. J Endocrinol. 2007;195:125–31.
19. Silver J, Naveh-Many T, Mayer H, et al. Regulation by vitamin D metabolites of parathyroid hormone gene transcription in vivo in the rat. J Clin Invest. 1986;78:1296–301.

20. Silver J, Russell J, Sherwood LM. Regulation by vitamin D metabolites of messenger ribonucleic acid for preproparathyroid hormone in isolated bovine parathyroid cells. Proc Natl Acad Sci U S A. 1985;82:4270–3.

21. Merke J, Hugel U, Zlotkowski A, et al. Diminished parathyroid 1,25(OH)$_2$D$_3$ receptors in experimental uremia. Kidney Int. 1987;32:350–3.

22. Brown AJ, Dusso A, Lopez-Hilker S, et al. 1,25-(OH)2D receptors are decreased in parathyroid glands from chronically uremic dogs. Kidney Int. 1989;35:19–23.

23. Korkor AB. Reduced binding of [3H]1,25-dihydroxyvitamin D$_3$ in the parathyroid glands of patients with renal failure. N Engl J Med. 1987;316:1573–7.

24. Naveh-Many T, Silver J. Regulation of parathyroid hormone gene expression by hypocalcemia, hypercalcemia, and vitamin D in the rat. J Clin Invest. 1990;86:1313–9.

25. Kifor O, Moore FD, Jr, Wang P, et al. Reduced immunostaining for the extracellular Ca2+-sensing receptor in primary and uremic secondary hyperparathyroidism. J Clin Endocrinol Metab. 1996;81:1598–606.

26. Brown AJ, Zhong M, Finch J, et al. Rat calcium-sensing receptor is regulated by vitamin D but not by calcium. Am J Physiol. 1996;270:F454–60.

27. Kremer R, Bolivar I, Goltzman D, Hendy GN. Influence of calcium and 1,25-dihydroxycholecalciferol on proliferation and proto-oncogene expression in primary cultures of bovine parathyroid cells. Endocrinology. 1989;125:935–41.

28. Li YC, Amling M, Pirro AE, et al. Normalization of mineral ion homeostasis by dietary means prevents hyperparathyroidism, rickets, and osteomalacia, but not alopecia in vitamin D receptor-ablated mice. Endocrinology. 1998;139:4391–6.

29. Panda DK, Miao D, Bolivar I, et al. Inactivation of the 25-hydroxyvitamin D 1alpha-hydroxylase and vitamin D receptor demonstrates independent and interdependent effects of calcium and vitamin D on skeletal and mineral homeostasis. J Biol Chem. 2004;279:16754–66.

30. Ito I, Waku T, Aoki M, et al. A nonclassical vitamin D receptor pathway suppresses renal fibrosis. J Clin Invest. 2013;123:4579–94.

31. Coburn JW, Koppel MH, Brickman AS, Massry SG. Study of intestinal absorption of calcium in patients with renal failure. Kidney Int. 1973;3:264–72.

32. Holick MF. Vitamin D and the kidney. Kidney Int. 1987;32:912–29.

33. Clemens TL, Adams JS, Henderson SL, Holick MF. Increased skin pigment reduces the capacity of skin to synthesise vitamin D$_3$. Lancet. 1982;1:74–6.

34. Koenig KG, Lindberg JS, Zerwekh JE, et al. Free and total 1,25-dihydroxyvitamin D levels in subjects with renal disease. Kidney Int. 1992;41:161–5.

35. Saha H. Calcium and vitamin D homeostasis in patients with heavy proteinuria. Clin Nephrol. 1994;41:290–6.

36. Helvig CF, Cuerrier D, Hosfield CM, et al. Dysregulation of renal vitamin D metabolism in the uremic rat. Kidney Int. 2010;78:463–72.

37. Zisman AL, Hristova M, Ho LT, Sprague SM. Impact of ergocalciferol treatment of vitamin D deficiency on serum parathyroid hormone concentrations in chronic kidney disease. Am J Nephrol. 2007;27:36–43.

38. Chandra P, Binongo JN, Ziegler TR, et al. Cholecalciferol (vitamin D$_3$) therapy and vitamin D insufficiency in patients with chronic kidney disease: A randomized controlled pilot study. Endocr Pract. 2008;14:10–7.

39. Shroff R, Wan M, Gullett A, et al. Ergocalciferol supplementation in children with CKD delays the onset of secondary hyperparathyroidism: A randomized trial. Clin J Am Soc Nephrol. 2012;7:216–23.

40. Ritter CS, Armbrecht HJ, Slatopolsky E, Brown AJ. 25-Hydroxyvitamin D(3) suppresses PTH synthesis and secretion by bovine parathyroid cells. Kidney Int. 2006;70:654–9.

41. Slatopolsky E, Caglar S, Pennell JP, et al. On the pathogenesis of hyperparathyroidism in chronic experimental renal insufficiency in the dog. J Clin Invest. 1971;50:492–9.

42. Portale AA, Booth BE, Halloran BP, Morris RC, Jr. Effect of dietary phosphorus on circulating concentrations of 1,25-dihydroxyvitamin D and immunoreactive parathyroid hormone in children with moderate renal insufficiency. J Clin Invest. 1984;73:1580–9.

43. Llach F, Massry SG. On the mechanism of secondary hyperparathyroidism in moderate renal insufficiency. J Clin Endocrinol Metab. 1985;61:601–6.

44. Finch JL, Lee DH, Liapis H, et al. Phosphate restriction significantly reduces mortality in uremic rats with established vascular calcification. Kidney Int. 2013;84:1145–53.

45. Almaden Y, Canalejo A, Ballesteros E, et al. Regulation of arachidonic acid production by intracellular calcium in parathyroid cells: Effect of extracellular phosphate. J Am Soc Nephrol. 2002;13:693–8.

46. Silver J, Kilav R, Sela-Brown A, et al. Molecular mechanisms of secondary hyperparathyroidism. Pediatr Nephrol. 2000;14:626–8.

47. Brown EM, Gamba G, Riccardi D, et al. Cloning and characterization of an extracellular Ca(2+)-sensing receptor from bovine parathyroid. Nature. 1993;366:575–80.

48. John MR, Goodman WG, Gao P, et al. A novel immunoradiometric assay detects full-length human PTH but not amino-terminally truncated fragments: Implications for PTH measurements in renal failure. J Clin Endocrinol Metab. 1999;84:4287–90.

49. Freichel M, Zink-Lorenz A, Holloschi A, et al. Expression of a calcium-sensing receptor in a human medullary thyroid carcinoma cell line and its contribution to calcitonin secretion. Endocrinology. 1996;137:3842–8.

50. Martin-Salvago M, Villar-Rodriguez JL, Palma-Alvarez A, et al. Decreased expression of calcium receptor in parathyroid tissue in patients with hyperparathyroidism secondary to chronic renal failure. Endocr Pathol. 2003;14:61–70.

51. Canaff L, Hendy GN. Human calcium-sensing receptor gene: Vitamin D response elements in promoters P1 and P2 confer transcriptional responsiveness to 1,25-dihydroxyvitamin D. J Biol Chem. 2002;277:30337–50.

52. Li YC, Pirro AE, Amling M, et al. Targeted ablation of the vitamin D receptor: An animal model of vitamin D-dependent rickets type II with alopecia. Proc Natl Acad Sci U S A. 1997;94:9831–5.

53. Brown AJ, Zhong M, Ritter C, et al. Loss of calcium responsiveness in cultured bovine parathyroid cells is associated with decreased calcium receptor expression. Biochem Biophys Res Commun. 1995;212:861–7.

54. Wada M, Furuya Y, Sakiyama J, et al. The calcimimetic compound NPS R-568 suppresses parathyroid cell proliferation in rats with renal insufficiency: Control of parathyroid cell growth via a calcium receptor. J Clin Invest. 1997;100:2977–83.

55. Massry SG, Stein R, Garty J, et al. Skeletal resistance to the calcemic action of parathyroid hormone in uremia: Role of 1,25 (OH)2 D3. Kidney Int. 1976;9:467–74.

56. Wesseling-Perry K, Harkins GC, Wang HJ, et al. The calcemic response to continuous parathyroid hormone (PTH)(1-34) infusion in end-stage kidney disease varies according to bone turnover: A potential role for PTH(7-84). J Clin Endocrinol Metab. 2010;95:2772–80.

57. D'Amour P, Brossard JH, Rousseau L, et al. Structure of non-(1-84) PTH fragments secreted by parathyroid glands in primary and secondary hyperparathyroidism. Kidney Int. 2005;68:998–1007.

58. Divieti P, John MR, Juppner H, et al. Human PTH-(7-84) inhibits bone resorption in vitro via actions independent of 59

59. Langub MC, Monier-Faugere MC, Wang G, et al. Administration of PTH-(7-84) antagonizes the effects of PTH-(1-84) on bone in rats with moderate renal failure. Endocrinology. 2003;144:1135–8.

60. Nguyen-Yamamoto L, Rousseau L, Brossard JH, et al. Synthetic carboxyl-terminal fragments of parathyroid hormone (PTH) decrease ionized calcium concentration in rats by acting on a receptor different from the PTH/PTH-related peptide receptor. Endocrinology. 2001;142:1386–92.

61. Slatopolsky E, Finch J, Clay P, et al. A novel mechanism for skeletal resistance in uremia. Kidney Int. 2000;58:753–61.

62. Brossard JH, Cloutier M, Roy L, et al. Accumulation of a non-(1-84) molecular form of parathyroid hormone (PTH) detected by intact PTH assay in renal failure: Importance in the interpretation of PTH values. J Clin Endocrinol Metab. 1996;81:3923–9.

63. Lepage R, Roy L, Brossard JH, et al. A non-(1-84) circulating parathyroid hormone (PTH) fragment interferes significantly with intact PTH commercial assay measurements in uremic samples. Clin Chem. 1998;44:805–9.

64. Brossard JH, Yamamoto LN, D'Amour P. Parathyroid hormone metabolites in renal failure: Bioactivity and clinical implications. Semin Dial. 2002;15:196–201.

65. Gao P, Scheibel S, D'Amour P, et al. Development of a novel immunoradiometric assay exclusively for biologically active whole parathyroid hormone 1-84: Implications for improvement of accurate assessment of parathyroid function. J Bone Miner Res. 2001;16:605–14.

66. Monier-Faugere MC, Geng Z, Mawad H, et al. Improved assessment of bone turnover by the PTH-(1-84)/large C-PTH fragments ratio in ESRD patients. Kidney Int. 2001;60:1460–8.

67. Coen G, Bonucci E, Ballanti P, et al. PTH 1-84 and PTH "7-84" in the noninvasive diagnosis of renal bone disease. Am J Kidney Dis. 2002;40:348–54.

68. Salusky IB, Goodman WG, Kuizon BD, et al. Similar predictive value of bone turnover using first- and second-generation immunometric PTH assays in pediatric patients treated with peritoneal dialysis. Kidney Int. 2003;63:1801–8.

69. Tepel M, Armbruster FP, Gron HJ, et al. Nonoxidized, biologically active parathyroid hormone determines mortality in hemodialysis patients. J Clin Endocrinol Metab. 2013;98:4744–51.

70. Kidney Disease: Improving Global Outcomes. Clinical practice guideline for the diagnosis, evaluation, prevention, and treatment of chronic kidney disease-mineral and bone disorder (CKD-MBD). Kidney Int Suppl. 2009;113:S1–130.

71. Wesseling-Perry K, Pereira RC, Tseng CH, et al. Early skeletal and biochemical alterations in pediatric chronic kidney disease. Clin J Am Soc Nephrol. 2012;7:146–52.

72. Groothoff JW, Offringa M, Van Eck-Smit BL, et al. Severe bone disease and low bone mineral density after juvenile renal failure. Kidney Int. 2003;63:266–75.

73. Malluche H, Faugere MC. Renal bone disease 1990: An unmet challenge for the nephrologist. Kidney Int. 1990;38:193–211.

74. Bakkaloglu SA, Wesseling-Perry K, Pereira RC, et al. Value of the new bone classification system in pediatric renal osteodystrophy. Clin J Am Soc Nephrol. 2010;5:1860–6.

75. Atkins D, Peacock M. A comparison of the effects of the calcitonins, steroid hormones and thyroid hormones on the response of bone to parathyroid hormone in tissue culture. J Endocrinol. 1975;64:573–83.

76. Lee K, Deeds JD, Bond AT, et al. in situ localization of PTH/PTHrP receptor mRNA in the bone of fetal and young rats. Bone. 1993;14:341–5.

77. Sabbagh Y, Graciolli FG, O'Brien S, et al. Repression of osteocyte Wnt/beta-catenin signaling is an early event in the progression of renal osteodystrophy. J Bone Miner Res. 2012;27:1757–72.

78. Lobao R, Carvalho AB, Cuppari L, et al. High prevalence of low bone mineral density in pre-dialysis chronic kidney disease patients: Bone histomorphometric analysis. Clin Nephrol. 2004;62:432–9.

79. Sebastian EM, Suva LJ, Friedman PA. Differential effects of intermittent PTH(1-34) and PTH(7-34) on bone microarchitecture and aortic calcification in experimental renal failure. Bone. 2008;43:1022–30.

80. Kuizon BD, Goodman WG, Juppner H, et al. Diminished linear growth during intermittent calcitriol therapy in children undergoing CCPD. Kidney Int. 1998;53:205–11.

81. Kuizon BD, Salusky IB. Intermittent calcitriol therapy and growth in children with chronic renal failure. Miner Electrolyte Metab. 1998;24:290–5.

82. Lund RJ, Davies MR, Brown AJ, Hruska KA. Successful treatment of an adynamic bone disorder with bone morphogenetic protein-7 in a renal ablation model. J Am Soc Nephrol 2004;15:359–69.

83. Rhee Y, Bivi N, Farrow E, et al. Parathyroid hormone receptor signaling in osteocytes increases the expression of fibroblast growth factor-23 in vitro and in vivo. Bone. 2011;49:636–43.

84. De Beur SM, Finnegan RB, Vassiliadis J, et al. Tumors associated with oncogenic osteomalacia express genes important in bone and mineral metabolism. J Bone Miner Res. 2002;17:1102–10.

85. Jonsson KB, Zahradnik R, Larsson T, et al. Fibroblast growth factor 23 in oncogenic osteomalacia and X-linked hypophosphatemia. N Engl J Med. 2003;348:1656–63.

86. Nelson AE, Bligh RC, Mirams M, et al. Clinical case seminar: Fibroblast growth factor 23: A new clinical marker for oncogenic osteomalacia. J Clin Endocrinol Metab. 2003;88:4088–94.

87. Shimada T, Kakitani M, Yamazaki Y, et al. Targeted ablation of FGF23 demonstrates an essential physiological role of FGF23 in phosphate and vitamin D metabolism. J Clin Invest. 2004;113:561–8.

88. Sitara D, Razzaque MS, Hesse M, et al. Homozygous ablation of fibroblast growth factor-23 results in hyperphosphatemia and impaired skeletogenesis, and reverses hypophosphatemia in Phex-deficient mice. Matrix Biol. 2004;23:421–32.

89. Bartosh SM, Leverson G, Robillard D, et al. Long-term outcomes in pediatric renal transplant recipients who survive into adulthood. Transplantation. 2003;76:1195–200.

90. Conger JD, Hammond WS, Alfrey AC, et al. Pulmonary calcification in chronic dialysis patients: Clinical and pathologic studies. Ann Intern Med. 1975;83:330–6.

91. Goodman WG, Goldin J, Kuizon BD, et al. Coronary-artery calcification in young adults with end-stage renal disease who are undergoing dialysis. N Engl J Med. 2000;342:1478–83.

92. Milliner DS, Zinsmeister AR, Lieberman E, et al. Soft tissue calcification in pediatric patients with end-stage renal disease. Kidney Int. 1990;38:931–6.

93. Oh J, Wunsch R, Turzer M, et al. Advanced coronary and carotid arteriopathy in young adults with childhood-onset chronic renal failure. Circulation. 2002;106:100–5.

94. North American Pediatric Renal Transplant Cooperative Study (NAPRTCS) 2008 annual report. https://web.emmes.com/study/ped/annlrept/Annual%20Report%20-2008.pdf. Accessed January 27, 2015.

95. Shanahan CM, Crouthamel MH, Kapustin A, et al. Arterial calcification in chronic kidney disease: Key roles for calcium and phosphate. Circ Res. 2011;109:697–711.

96. Mitsnefes MM, Kimball TR, Kartal J, et al. Cardiac and vascular adaptation in pediatric patients with chronic kidney disease: Role of calcium-phosphorus metabolism. J Am Soc Nephrol. 2005;16:2796–803.

97. Mitsnefes MM. Cardiovascular disease in children with chronic kidney disease. Adv Chronic Kidney Dis. 2005;12:397–405.

98. Moe SM, Duan D, Doehle BP, et al. Uremia induces the osteoblast differentiation factor Cbfa1 in human blood vessels. Kidney Int. 2003;63:1003–11.

99. Shroff RC, McNair R, Skepper JN, et al. Chronic mineral dysregulation promotes vascular smooth muscle cell adaptation and extracellular matrix calcification. J Am Soc Nephrol. 2010;21:103–12.

100. Jono S, McKee MD, Murry CE, et al. Phosphate regulation of vascular smooth muscle cell calcification. Circ Res. 2000;87:E10–17.

101. Ahmed S, O'Neill KD, Hood AF, et al. Calciphylaxis is associated with hyperphosphatemia and increased osteopontin expression by vascular smooth muscle cells. Am J Kidney Dis. 2001;37:1267–76.

102. Bostrom K. Insights into the mechanism of vascular calcification. Am J Cardiol. 2001;88:20E–2E.

103. Moe SM, O'Neill KD, Duan D, et al. Medial artery calcification in ESRD patients is associated with deposition of bone matrix proteins. Kidney Int. 2002;61:638–47.

104. Chen NX, O'Neill KD, Duan D, et al. Phosphorus and uremic serum up-regulate osteopontin expression in vascular smooth muscle cells. Kidney Int. 2002;62:1724–31.

105. Schafer C, Heiss A, Schwarz A, et al. The serum protein alpha 2-Heremans-Schmid glycoprotein/fetuin-A is a systemically acting inhibitor of ectopic calcification. J Clin Invest. 2003;112:357–66.

106. Schinke T, Amendt C, Trindl A, et al. The serum protein alpha2-HS glycoprotein/fetuin inhibits apatite formation in vitro and in mineralizing calvaria cells: A possible role in mineralization and calcium homeostasis. J Biol Chem. 1996;271:20789–96.

107. Sweatt A, Sane DC, Hutson SM, et al. Matrix Gla protein (MGP) and bone morphogenetic protein-2 in aortic calcified lesions of aging rats. J Thromb Haemost. 2003;1:178–85.

108. Koh N, Fujimori T, Nishiguchi S, et al. Severely reduced production of Klotho in human chronic renal failure kidney. Biochem Biophys Res Commun. 2001;280:1015–20.

109. Russo D, Battaglia Y, Buonanno E. Phosphorus and coronary calcification in predialysis patients. Kidney Int. 2010;78:818.

110. Russo D, Palmiero G, De Blasio AP, et al. Coronary artery calcification in patients with CRF not undergoing dialysis. Am J Kidney Dis. 2004;44:1024–30.

111. Gutierrez OM, Mannstadt M, Isakova T, et al. Fibroblast growth factor 23 and mortality among patients undergoing hemodialysis. N Engl J Med. 2008;359:584–92.

112. Jean G, Bresson E, Terrat JC, et al. Peripheral vascular calcification in long-haemodialysis patients: Associated factors and survival consequences. Nephrol Dial Transplant. 2009;24:948–55.

113. Scialla JJ, Lau WL, Reilly MP, et al. Fibroblast growth factor 23 is not associated with and does not induce arterial calcification. Kidney Int. 2013;83:1159–68.

114. Faul C, Amaral AP, Oskouei B, et al. FGF23 induces left ventricular hypertrophy. J Clin Invest. 2011;121:4393–408.

115. Buizert PJ, van Schoor NM, Simsek S, et al. PTH: A new target in arteriosclerosis? J Clin Endocrinol Metab. 2013;98:1583–90.

116. Tonelli M, Keech A, Shepherd J, et al. Effect of pravastatin in people with diabetes and chronic kidney disease. J Am Soc Nephrol. 2005;16:3748–54.

117. Holdaas H, Fellstrom B, Cole E, et al. Long-term cardiac outcomes in renal transplant recipients receiving fluvastatin: The ALERT extension study. Am J Transplant. 2005;5:2929–36.

118. Wanner C, Krane V, Marz W, et al. Atorvastatin in patients with type 2 diabetes mellitus undergoing hemodialysis. N Engl J Med. 2005;353:238-–48.

119. Block GA, Spiegel DM, Ehrlich J, et al. Effects of sevelamer and calcium on coronary artery calcification in patients new to hemodialysis. Kidney Int. 2005;68:1815–24.

120. Block GA, Raggi P, Bellasi A, et al. Mortality effect of coronary calcification and phosphate binder choice in incident hemodialysis patients. Kidney Int. 2007;71:438–41.

121. Jamal SA, Vandermeer B, Raggi P, et al. Effect of calcium-based versus non-calcium-based phosphate binders on mortality in patients with chronic kidney disease: An updated systematic review and meta-analysis. Lancet. 2013;382:1268–77.

122. Oliveira RB, Cancela AL, Graciolli FG, et al. Early control of PTH and FGF23 in normophosphatemic CKD patients: A new target in CKD-MBD therapy? Clin J Am Soc Nephrol. 2010;5:286–91.

123. Gonzalez-Parra E, Gonzalez-Casaus ML, Galan A, et al. Lanthanum carbonate reduces FGF23 in chronic kidney disease stage 3 patients. Nephrol Dial Transplant. 2011;26:2567–71.

124. Isakova T, Barchi-Chung A, Enfield G, et al. Effects of dietary phosphate restriction and phosphate binders on FGF23 levels in CKD. Clin J Am Soc Nephrol. 2013;8:1009–18.

125. Block GA, Wheeler DC, Persky MS, et al. Effects of phosphate binders in moderate CKD. J Am Soc Nephrol. 2012;23:1407–15.

126. Teng M, Wolf M, Ofsthun MN, et al. Activated injectable vitamin D and hemodialysis survival: A historical cohort study. J Am Soc Nephrol. 2005;16:1115–25.

127. Teng M, Wolf M, Lowrie E, et al. Survival of patients undergoing hemodialysis with paricalcitol or calcitriol therapy. N Engl J Med. 2003;349:446–56.

128. Tentori F, Hunt WC, Stidley CA, et al. Mortality risk among hemodialysis patients receiving different vitamin D analogs. Kidney Int. 2006;70:1858–65.

129. Joki N, Nikolov IG, Caudrillier A, et al. Effects of calcimimetic on vascular calcification and atherosclerosis in uremic mice. Bone. 2009;45 (Suppl 1):S30–4.

130. Henley C, Davis J, Miller G, et al. The calcimimetic AMG 641 abrogates parathyroid hyperplasia, bone and vascular calcification abnormalities in uremic rats. Eur J Pharmacol. 2009;616:306–13.

131. Kawata T, Nagano N, Obi M, et al. Cinacalcet suppresses calcification of the aorta and heart in uremic rats. Kidney Int. 2008;74:1270–7.

132. Aladren Regidor MJ. Cinacalcet reduces vascular and soft tissue calcification in secondary hyperparathyroidism (SHPT) in hemodialysis patients. Clin Nephrol. 2009;71:207–13.

133. Chertow GM, Block GA, Correa-Rotter R, et al. Effect of cinacalcet on cardiovascular disease in patients undergoing dialysis. N Engl J Med. 2012;367:2482–94.

134. North American Pediatric Renal Transplant Cooperative Study (NAPRTCS) 2005 Annual Report. http://spitfire.emmes.com/study/ped/resources/annl-rept2005.pdf. Accessed January 27, 2015.

135. Nash MA, Torrado AD, Greifer I, et al. Renal tubular acidosis in infants and children: Clinical course, response to treatment, and prognosis. J Pediatr. 1972;80:738–48.

136. Challa A, Chan W, Krieg RJ, Jr, et al. Effect of metabolic acidosis on the expression of insulin-like growth factor and growth hormone receptor. Kidney Int. 1993;44:1224–7.

137. Challa A, Krieg RJ, Jr, Thabet MA, et al. Metabolic acidosis inhibits growth hormone secretion in rats: Mechanism of growth retardation. Am J Physiol 1993;265:E547–53.

138. Green J, Maor G. Effect of metabolic acidosis on the growth hormone/IGF-I endocrine axis in skeletal growth centers. Kidney Int. 2000;57:2258–67.

139. Borzych D, Rees L, Ha IS, et al. The bone and mineral disorder of children undergoing chronic peritoneal dialysis. Kidney Int. 2010;78:1295–304.

140. Schmitt CP, Ardissino G, Testa S, et al. Growth in children with chronic renal failure on intermittent versus daily calcitriol. Pediatr Nephrol. 2003;18:440–4.

141. Martin KJ, Ballal HS, Domoto DT, et al. Pulse oral calcitriol for the treatment of hyperparathyroidism in patients on continuous ambulatory peritoneal dialysis: Preliminary observations. Am J Kidney Dis. 1992;19:540–5.

142. Kidney Disease: Outcomes Qualtiy Initiative. Clinical practice guidelines for chronic kidney disease: Evaluation, classification, and stratification. Am J Kidney Dis. 2002;39(2 Suppl 1):S1–266.

143. Kidney Disease: Outcomes Qualtiy Initiative. Clinical practice guidelines for bone metabolism and disease in children with chronic kidney disease. Am J Kidney Dis. 2005;46(Suppl 1):1-–122.

144. Miyakoshi N, Richman C, Kasukawa Y, et al. Evidence that IGF-binding protein-5 functions as a growth factor. J Clin Invest. 2001;107:73–81.

145. Kidney Disease: Outcomes Qualtiy Initiative. B, Veldhuis JD, Heinrich U, et al. Deconvolution analysis of spontaneous nocturnal growth hormone secretion in prepubertal children with preterminal chronic renal failure and with end-stage renal disease. Pediatr Res 1995;37:86–93.

146. Schaefer F, Chen Y, Tsao T, et al. Impaired JAK-STAT signal transduction contributes to growth hormone resistance in chronic uremia. J Clin Invest. 2001;108:467–75.

147. Tonshoff B, Cronin MJ, Reichert M, et al. Reduced concentration of serum growth hormone (GH)-binding protein in children with chronic renal failure:

Correlation with GH insensitivity. The European Study Group for Nutritional Treatment of Chronic Renal Failure in Childhood. The German Study Group for Growth Hormone Treatment in Chronic Renal Failure. J Clin Endocrinol Metab. 1997;82:1007–13.

148. Bacchetta J, Wesseling-Perry K, Kuizon B, et al. The skeletal consequences of growth hormone therapy in dialyzed children: A randomized trial. Clin J Am Soc Nephrol. 2013;8:824–32.

149. Foley RN, Parfrey PS, Sarnak MJ. Clinical epidemiology of cardiovascular disease in chronic renal disease. Am J Kidney Dis. 1998;32:S112–S9.

150. Shanahan CM. Mechanisms of vascular calcification in renal disease. Clin Nephrol. 2005;63:146–57.

151. Ducy P, Zhang R, Geoffroy V, et al. Osf2/Cbfa1: A transcriptional activator of osteoblast differentiation. Cell. 1997;89:747–54.

152. Razzaque MS, Sitara D, Taguchi T, et al. Premature aging-like phenotype in fibroblast growth factor 23 null mice is a vitamin D-mediated process. FASEB J. 2006;20:720–2.

153. Gutierrez OM, Januzzi JL, Isakova T, et al. Fibroblast growth factor 23 and left ventricular hypertrophy in chronic kidney disease. Circulation. 2009;119:2545–52.

154. Gipstein RM, Coburn JW, Adams DA, et al. Calciphylaxis in man: A syndrome of tissue necrosis and vascular calcification in 11 patients with chronic renal failure. Arch Intern Med. 1976;136:1273–80.

155. Bleyer AJ, Choi M, Igwemezie B, et al. A case control study of proximal calciphylaxis. Am J Kidney D. 1998;32:376–83.

156. Mawad HW, Sawaya BP, Sarin R, et al. Calcific uremic arteriolopathy in association with low turnover uremic bone disease. Clin Nephrol. 1999;52:160–6.

157. Goldsmith DJ. Calciphylaxis, thrombotic diathesis and defects in coagulation regulation. Nephrol Dial Transplant. 1997;12:1082–3.

158. Mohammed IA, Sekar V, Bubtana AJ, et al. Proximal calciphylaxis treated with calcimimetic 'cinacalcet'. Nephrol Dial Transplant. 2008;23:387–9.

159. Rogers NM, Teubner DJ, Coates PT. Calcific uremic arteriolopathy: Advances in pathogenesis and treatment. Semin Dial. 2007;20:150–7.

160. Hernandez JD, Wesseling K, Pereira R, et al. Technical approach to iliac crest biopsy. Clin J Am Soc Nephrol. 2008;3(Suppl 3):S164–9.

161. Mucsi I, Hercz G, Uldall R, et al. Control of serum phosphate without any phosphate binders in patients treated with nocturnal hemodialysis. Kidney Int. 1998;53:1399–404.

162. Fischbach M, Terzic J, Menouer S, et al. Intensified and daily hemodialysis in children might improve statural growth. Pediatr Nephrol. 2006;21:1746–52.

163. Goodman WG. Aluminum and renal osteodystrophy. In: Bushinsky DA, editor. Renal Osteodystrophy. Philadelphia: Lippincott-Raven; 1998. p. 317.

164. Salusky IB, Foley J, Nelson P, et al. Aluminum accumulation during treatment with aluminum hydroxide and dialysis in children and young adults with chronic renal disease. N Engl J Med. 1991;324:527–31.

165. Coburn JW, Mischel MG, Goodman WG, et al. Calcium citrate markedly enhances aluminum absorption from aluminum hydroxide. Am J Kidney Dis. 1991;17:708–11.

166. Andreoli SP, Dunson JW, Bergstein JM. Calcium carbonate is an effective phosphorus binder in children with chronic renal failure. Am J Kidney Dis. 1987;9:206-–10.

167. Salusky IB, Goodman WG. Adynamic renal osteodystrophy: Is there a problem? J Am Soc Nephrol. 2001;12:1978–85.

168. National Kidney Foundation. KDOQI clinical practice guideline for nutrition in children with CKD: 2008 update. Executive summary. Am J Kidney Dis. 2009;53:S11–104.

169. Wallot M, Bonzel KE, Winter A, et al. Calcium acetate versus calcium carbonate as oral phosphate binder in pediatric and adolescent hemodialysis patients. Pediatr Nephrol. 1996;10:625–30.

170. Cushner HM, Copley JB, Lindberg JS, et al. Calcium citrate, a nonaluminum-containing phosphate-binding agent for treatment of CRF. Kidney Int. 1988;33:95–9.

171. Birck R, Zimmermann E, Wassmer S, et al. Calcium ketoglutarate versus calcium acetate for treatment of hyperphosphataemia in patients on maintenance haemodialysis: A cross-over study. Nephrol Dial Transplant. 1999;14:1475–9.

172. Chertow GM, Burke SK, Dillon MA, et al. Long-term effects of sevelamer hydrochloride on the calcium x phosphate product and lipid profile of haemodialysis patients. Nephrol Dial Transplant. 1999;14:2907–14.

173. Delmez J, Block G, Robertson J, et al. A randomized, double-blind, crossover design study of sevelamer hydrochloride and sevelamer carbonate in patients on hemodialysis. Clin Nephrol. 2007;68:386–91.

174. O'Donovan R, Baldwin D, Hammer M, et al. Substitution of aluminium salts by magnesium salts in control of dialysis hyperphosphataemia. Lancet. 1986;1:880–2.

175. Hergesell O, Ritz E. Stabilized polynuclear iron hydroxide is an efficient oral phosphate binder in uraemic patients. Nephrol Dial Transplant. 1999;14:863–7.

176. D'Haese PC, Spasovski GB, Sikole A, et al. A multicenter study on the effects of lanthanum carbonate (Fosrenol) and calcium carbonate on renal bone disease in dialysis patients. Kidney Int Suppl. 2003;85:S73–8.

177. Slatopolsky E, Liapis H, Finch J. Progressive accumulation of lanthanum in the liver of normal and uremic rats. Kidney Int. 2005;68:2809–13.

178. Ross C A, Taylor CL, Yaktine AL, Del Valle HB. Dietary Reference Intakes for Calcium and Vitamin D. Washington, DC: National Academies Press; 2011.

179. Salusky IB, Goodman WG, Sahney S, et al. Sevelamer controls parathyroid hormone-induced bone disease as efficiently as calcium carbonate without increasing serum calcium levels during therapy with active vitamin D sterols. J Am Soc Nephrol. 2005;16:2501–8.

180. Salusky IB, Kuizon BD, Belin TR, et al. Intermittent calcitriol therapy in secondary hyperparathyroidism: A comparison between oral and intraperitoneal administration. Kidney Int. 1998;54:907–14.

181. National Kidney Foundation. K/DOQI clinical practice guidelines for bone metabolism and disease in chronic kidney disease. Am J Kidney Dis. 2003;42:S1–201.

182. Fukagawa M, Okazaki R, Takano K, et al. Regression of parathyroid hyperplasia by calcitriol-pulse therapy in patients on long-term dialysis. N Engl J Med. 1990;323:421–2.

183. Pierides AM, Ellis HA, Simpson W, et al Variable response to long-term 1alpha-hydroxycholecalciferol in haemodialysis osteodystrophy. Lancet. 1976;1:1092–5.

184. Dobrez DG, Mathes A, Amdahl M, et al. Paricalcitol-treated patients experience improved hospitalization outcomes compared with calcitriol-treated patients in real-world clinical settings. Nephrol Dial Transplant. 2004;19:117–81.

185. Sjoden G, Smith C, Lindgren U, DeLuca HF. 1 alpha-Hydroxyvitamin $D_2$ is less toxic than 1 alpha-hydroxyvitamin $D_3$ in the rat. Proc Soc Exp Biol Med. 1985;178:432–6.

186. Andress DL, Norris KC, Coburn JW, et al. Intravenous calcitriol in the treatment of refractory osteitis fibrosa of chronic renal failure. N Engl J Med. 1989;321:274–9.

187. Thadhani R, Appelbaum E, Pritchett Y, et al. Vitamin D therapy and cardiac structure and function in patients with chronic kidney disease: The PRIMO randomized controlled trial. JAMA. 2012;307:674–84.

188. Schwarz U, Amann K, Orth SR, et al. Effect of 1,25 (OH)2 vitamin $D_3$ on glomerulosclerosis in subtotally nephrectomized rats. Kidney Int. 1998;53:1696–705.

189. Agarwal R, Acharya M, Tian J, et al. Antiproteinuric effect of oral paricalcitol in chronic kidney disease. Kidney Int. 2005;68:2823–8.

190. Nakane M, Ma J, Ruan X, et al. Mechanistic analysis of VDR-mediated renin suppression. Nephron Physiol. 2007;107:35–44.

191. Wada M, Nagano N. Control of parathyroid cell growth by calcimimetics. Nephrol Dial Transplant. 2003;18(Suppl 3):iii13-7.

192. Arnold A, Brown MF, Urena P, et al. Monoclonality of parathyroid tumors in chronic renal failure and in primary parathyroid hyperplasia. J Clin Invest. 1995;95:2047–53.

193. Quarles LD, Yohay DA, Carroll BA, et al. Prospective trial of pulse oral versus intravenous calcitriol treatment of hyperparathyroidism in ESRD. Kidney Int. 1994;45:1710–21.

194. Froment DP, Molitoris BA, Buddington B, et al. Site and mechanism of enhanced gastrointestinal absorption of aluminum by citrate. Kidney Int. 1989;36:978-84.

195. Jorna FH, Tobe TJ, Huisman RM, et al. Early identification of risk factors for refractory secondary hyperparathyroidism in patients with long-term renal replacement therapy. Nephrol Dial Transplant. 2004;19:1168–73.

196. Andress DL, Ott SM, Maloney NA, Sherrard DJ. Effect of parathyroidectomy on bone aluminum accumulation in chronic renal failure. N Engl J Med. 1985;312:468–73.

197. de Barros Gueiros JE, Chammas MC, Gerhard R, et al. Percutaneous ethanol (PEIT) and calcitriol (PCIT) injection therapy are ineffective in treating severe secondary hyperparathyroidism. Nephrol Dial Transplant. 2004;19:657–63.

198. Diethelm AG, Edwards RP, Whelchel JD. The natural history and surgical treatment of hypercalcemia before and after renal transplantation. Surg Gynecol Obstet. 1982;154:481–90.

199. D'Alessandro AM, Melzer JS, Pirsch JD, et al. Tertiary hyperparathyroidism after renal transplantation: Operative indications. Surgery. 1989;106:1049–55.

200. Bergua C, Torregrosa JV, Fuster D, et al. Effect of cinacalcet on hypercalcemia and bone mineral density in renal transplanted patients with secondary hyperparathyroidism. Transplantation. 2008;86:413–7.

201. Borchhardt K, Sulzbacher I, Benesch T, et al. Low-turnover bone disease in hypercalcemic hyperparathyroidism after kidney transplantation. Am J Transplant. 2007;7:2515–21.

202. Bhan I, Shah A, Holmes J, et al. Post-transplant hypophosphatemia: Tertiary 'hyper-phosphatoninism'? Kidney Int. 2006;70:1486–94.

203. Evenepoel P, Naesens M, Claes K, et al. Tertiary 'hyperphosphatoninism' accentuates hypophosphatemia and suppresses calcitriol levels in renal transplant recipients. Am J Transplant. 2007;7:1193–200.

204. Bonomini V, Feletti C, Di FA, Buscaroli A. Bone remodelling after renal transplantation (RT). Adv Exp Med Biol. 1984;178:207–16.

205. Nielsen HE, Melsen F, Christensen MS. Aseptic necrosis of bone following renal transplantation: Clinical and biochemical aspects and bone morphometry. Acta Med Scand. 1977;202:2–32.

206. Grotz WH, Mundinger FA, Gugel B, et al. Bone mineral density after kidney transplantation: A cross-sectional study in 190 graft recipients up to 20 years after transplantation. Transplantation. 1995;59:982–6.

207. Julian BA, Laskow DA, Dubovsky J, et al. Rapid loss of vertebral mineral density after renal transplantation. N Engl J Med. 1991;325:544–50.

208. Slatopolsky E, Martin K. Glucocorticoids and renal transplant osteonecrosis. Adv Exp Med Biol. 1984;171:353–9.

209. Parfrey PS, Farge D, Parfrey NA, et al. The decreased incidence of aseptic necrosis in renal transplant recipients: A case control study. Transplantation. 1986;41:182–7.

210. Isono SS, Woolson ST, Schurman DJ. Total joint arthroplasty for steroid-induced osteonecrosis in cardiac transplant patients. Clin Orthop Relat Res. 1987:201–8.

211. Enright H, Haake R, Weisdorf D. Avascular necrosis of bone: A common serious complication of allogeneic bone marrow transplantation. Am J Med. 1990;89:733–8.

212. Velasquez-Forero F, Mondragon A, Herrero B, Pena JC. Adynamic bone lesion in renal transplant recipients with normal renal function. Nephrol Dial Transplant. 1996;11(Suppl 3):58–64.

213. Sanchez CP, Salusky IB, Kuizon BD, et al. Bone disease in children and adolescents undergoing successful renal transplantation. Kidney Int. 1998;53:1358–64.

214. Lindberg JS, Culleton B, Wong G, et al. Cinacalcet HCl, an oral calcimimetic agent for the treatment of secondary hyperparathyroidism in hemodialysis and peritoneal dialysis: A randomized, double-blind, multicenter study. J Am Soc Nephrol. 2005;16:800–7.

215. Allen DB, Goldberg BD. Stimulation of collagen synthesis and linear growth by growth hormone in glucocorticoid-treated children. Pediatrics. 1992;89:416–21.

216. Root AW, Bongiovanni AM, Eberlein WR. Studies of the secretion and metabolic effects of human growth hormone in children with glucocorticoid-induced growth retardation. J Pediatr. 1969;75:826–32.

217. Wehrenberg WB, Bergman PJ, Stagg L, et al. Glucocorticoid inhibition of growth in rats: Partial reversal with somatostatin antibodies. Endocrinology. 1990;127:2705–8.

218. Aubia J, Serrano S, Marinoso L, et al. Osteodystrophy of diabetics in chronic dialysis: A histomorphometric study. Calcif Tissue Int. 1988;42:297–301.

219. Movsowitz C, Epstein S, Fallon M, et al. Cyclosporin-A in vivo produces severe osteopenia in the rat: Effect of dose and duration of administration. Endocrinology. 1988;123:2571–7.

220. Bryer HP, Isserow JA, Armstrong EC, et al. Azathioprine alone is bone sparing and does not alter cyclosporin A-induced osteopenia in the rat. J Bone Miner Res. 1995;10:132–8.

221. Hokken-Koelega AC, van Zaal MA, van BW, et al. Final height and its predictive factors after renal transplantation in childhood. Pediatr Res. 1994;36:323–8.

222. Fine RN, Yadin O, Nelson PA, et al. Recombinant human growth hormone treatment of children following renal transplantation. Pediatr Nephrol. 1991;5:147–51.

223. Mitsnefes MM, Kimball TR, Border WL, et al. Abnormal cardiac function in children after renal transplantation. Am J Kidney Dis. 2004;43:721–6.

224. Ishitani MB, Milliner DS, Kim DY, et al. Early subclinical coronary artery calcification in young adults who were pediatric kidney transplant recipients. Am J Transplant. 2005;5:1689–93.

225. Wolf M, Molnar MZ, Amaral AP, et al. Elevated fibroblast growth factor 23 is a risk factor for kidney transplant loss and mortality. J Am Soc Nephrol. 2011;22:956–66.

226. Wesseling-Perry K, Tsai EW, Ettenger RB, et al. Mineral abnormalities and long-term graft function in pediatric renal transplant recipients: A role for FGF-23? Nephrol Dial Transplant. 2011;26:3779–84.

## REVIEW QUESTIONS

A 12-year-old boy has come to a pediatrician's office for a school physical. He wakes up several times at night to urinate. On examination, he is found to be a pale boy with a height and a weight that are both below the 3rd percentile. He has Tanner 1 pubertal development and normal blood pressure. Serum electrolytes are sodium, 136 mmol/L; potassium, 3.8 mmol/L; chloride, 108 mmol/; total carbon dioxide, 18 mmol/L; blood urea nitrogen, 40 mg/dL; creatinine, 1.8 mg/dL (stage 3 CKD); phosphorus, 4 mg/dL; calcium, 9.9 mg/dL; parathyroid hormone, 170 pg/mL, and hematocrit, 28%.

1. An appropriate serum PTH level for this child with this degree of renal insufficiency is:
   a. 10 to 65 pg/mL
   b. 65 to 110 pg/mL
   c. 200 to 300 pg/mL
   d. >400 pg/mL

2. Growth hormone therapy should be initiated:
   a. Immediately, to maximize final height potential
   b. After correction of acidosis, anemia, and secondary hyperparathyroidism
   c. After the initiation of dialysis
   d. After successful renal transplantation
   e. Growth hormone therapy is contraindicated in this child

3. An 8-year-old girl presents with reflux nephropathy and growth failure and has the following serum biochemical determinations: Serum creatinine, 2.5 mg/dL (CKD stage 4); calcium, 8.9 mg/dL; phosphorus, 6 mg/dL; and PTH, 140 pg/mL. The first step in serum phosphorus management is:
   a. Initiation of a non–calcium-containing phosphate binder
   b. Nutritional assessment and phosphate restriction
   c. Vitamin D sterol therapy
   d. Growth hormone therapy

4. A 14-year-old boy with obstructive uropathy and stage 3 CKD has been treated with growth hormone therapy for the past 2 years. His growth velocity has been decreasing over the past 6 months. An indication to stop therapy would be:
   a. Serum PTH of 150 pg/mL
   b. Height at percentile corresponding to the mean parental height
   c. Tanner 2 pubertal development
   d. Increasing alkaline phosphatase activity

5. A 10-year-old boy receiving maintenance hemodialysis is treated with calcium carbonate and thrice weekly calcitriol to control his renal osteodystrophy. His serum PTH level is 700 pg/mL; phosphorus, 5 mg/dL; and calcium, 11.5 mg/dL. To ameliorate his hypercalcemia, the next step in his therapy should include:
   a. Dietary calcium restriction
   b. Bone biopsy
   c. Switching to a non–calcium-containing phosphate binder
   d. Increasing the calcitriol therapy

## ANSWER KEY

1. a
2. b
3. b
4. b
5. c

# 34

# Nutrition in chronic kidney disease

SUN-YOUNG AHN AND ROBERT MAK

Maintenance of optimum nutrition continues to be a vital aspect in the care of children with chronic kidney disease (CKD). The nutritional status and requirements for these patients need to be evaluated regularly with the goals of maintaining a normal pattern of growth and body composition and avoiding electrolyte abnormalities, uremic toxicity, and malnutrition.[1] The association between poor linear growth and low body mass index (BMI) with increased risk for mortality in children with CKD underscores the importance of adequate nutrition in this patient population.[2,3] Because rates of linear growth and neurodevelopment are highest during the first 3 years of life, nutrition during this period is especially essential for reducing morbidity and mortality.[4] Indeed, growth failure during infancy in children with CKD has been primarily attributed to malnutrition.[5]

## NUTRITIONAL ASSESSMENT

The Kidney Disease Outcomes Quality Initiative (KDOQI) established clinical practice guidelines for the evaluation of nutritional status in patients with CKD.[6] Children with CKD stages 2 to 5 and 5D (5D: patients on dialysis) should be evaluated at least twice as frequently as same-aged healthy children, with more frequent monitoring to be done in infants (Table 34.1). Parameters to be followed include dietary intake, length and height for age percentiles

or standard deviation score (SDS), length and height velocity-for-age percentiles or SDS, estimated dry weight and weight-for-age percentile or SDS, BMI-for-height age percentile or SDS, head circumference-for-age percentile, or SDS for children younger than 3 years of age, and normalized protein catabolic rate (nPCR) in adolescents with CKD stage 5D. The challenges of using age-matched children for comparison include the short stature and delayed puberty found in most children with CKD. Therefore, comparison by height age (age at which the child's height would be at the 50th percentile) or pubertal stage may be more appropriate.

### KEY POINT

Children with CKD stages 2 to 5 and 5D should be evaluated at least twice as frequently as same-aged healthy children, with more frequent monitoring to be done in infants as well as patients with comorbidities such as cachexia, protein-energy wasting, and growth failure.

## HEIGHT AND LENGTH

The length (children younger than 2 years) or height (children older than 2 years) should be measured regularly and plotted on the length-for-age or height-for-age

Table 34.1 Recommended parameters and frequency of nutritional assessment for children with chronic kidney disease stages 2 to and 5D

| Measure | Minimum interval (Mo) | | | | | | | | | |
| --- | --- | --- | --- | --- | --- | --- | --- | --- | --- | --- |
| | Age 0 to < 1 yr | | | Age 1–3 yr | | | Age > 3yr | | | |
| | CKD 2–3 | CKD 4–5 | CKD 5D | CKD 2–3 | CKD 4–5 | CKD 5D | CKD 2 | CKD 3 | CKD 4–5 | CKD 5D |
| Dietary intake | 0.5–3 | 0.5–3 | 0.5–2 | 1–3 | 1–3 | 1–3 | 6–12 | 6 | 3–4 | 3–4 |
| Height or length-for-age percentile or SDS | 0.5–2 | 0.5–2 | 0.5–1 | 1–6 | 1–3 | 1–2 | 6 | 6 | 6 | 1–3 |
| Height or length velocity-for-age percentile or SDS | 0.5-2 | 0.5–2 | 0.5–1 | 1–6 | 1–3 | 1–2 | 6 | 6 | 6 | 6 |
| Estimated dry weight and weight-for-age percentile or SDS | 0.5–1.5 | 0.5–1.5 | 0.25–1 | 1–3 | 1–2 | 0.5–1 | 3–6 | 3–6 | 1–3 | 0.5–1 |
| BMI-for-height-age percentile or SDS | 0.5–1.5 | 0.5–1.5 | 0.5–1 | 1–3 | 1–2 | 1 | 3–6 | 3–6 | 1–3 | 1–3 |
| Head circumference-for- age percentile or SDS | 0.5–1.5 | 0.5–1.5 | 0.5–1 | 1–3 | 1–2 | 1–2 | N/A | N/A | N/A | N/A |
| nPCR | N/A | N/A | N/A | N/A | N/A | N/A | N/A | N/A | N/A | 1* |

*Source:* KDOQI Clinical Practice Guideline for Nutrition in Children with CKD: 2008 update. Executive summary. Am J Kidney Dis 2009; 53:S11–104. Reprinted with permission.
*Abbreviations:* BMI, body mass index; CKD, chronic kidney disease; N/A, not applicable; nPCR, normalized protein catabolic rate; SDS, standard deviation score.
* Only applies to adolescents receiving hemodialysis.

curves, with percentiles and SDS calculated. Length can be measured using a length board, and height using a wall-mounted stadiometer. The KDOQI guidelines recommend using the 2006 World Health Organization (WHO) Growth Standards as a reference for children from birth to 2 years.[6] After 2 years of age, the Centers for Disease Control and Prevention (CDC) reference curves may be used because of minimal differences with the WHO Growth Standards after this time point. The WHO Growth Standards are based on children from diverse ethnic backgrounds growing under ideal conditions (nonsmoking mothers, high socioeconomic status, breast fed for at least 4 months, receiving regular health care) and therefore represent ideal growth.

## WEIGHT

Assessment of euvolemic (or dry) weight in children with CKD can present a challenge because oliguric and anuric children may be fluid overloaded or polyuric children may be dehydrated. Therefore, a careful clinical examination is warranted, and indicators of volume status including edema, hypertension, pulse rate, skin turgor, or laboratory indices such as sodium or albumin levels, must be evaluated. The euvolemic weight can then be used to calculate the weight-for-age percentile and, SDS, or both. The height-for-age percentiles must be taken into account when looking at the weight-for-age percentiles. BMI takes into consideration both the weight and height and therefore is another parameter that is useful in assessing growth.

## BODY MASS INDEX

As with weight and height, the percentile for SDS or BMI (weight in kg/length in $m^2$) relative to age can be determined based on the WHO Growth Standard for children younger than 2 years, and the CDC reference data for children older than 2 years of age. Children with CKD, however, may have delays in growth or differences in body proportions that render comparisons with healthy children of the same age inaccurate.[7] Therefore, relating BMI to height for age in pubertal or peripubertal children with CKD may provide better comparisons with children of similar height and maturation.[8] When interpreting BMI values, consideration must be given to the fact that the BMI does not reflect body composition and therefore fat mass. A patient who has an appropriate BMI for height or chronologic age may therefore not have an ideal body composition.[9]

## HEAD CIRCUMFERENCE

Infants with CKD may be at greater risk for poor head growth.[10,11] Hence, head circumference should be measured

Table 34.2 Macronutrient distribution ranges

| Macronutrient | Children 1–3 yr (%) | Children 4–18 yr (%) |
|---|---|---|
| Carbohydrate | 45–65 | 45–65 |
| Fat | 30–40 | 25–35 |
| Protein | 5–20 | 10–30 |

Source: Health Canada. http://www.hc-sc.gc.ca/fn-an/alt_formats/hpfb-dgpsa/pdf/nutrition/dri_tables-eng.pdf.

routinely in children with CKD until 3 years of age,[6] along with percentiles, SDS, or both calculated from WHO Growth Standards. No studies have yet shown a correlation between head circumference and nutritional status in children with CKD; however, delayed head growth should prompt a neurodevelopmental evaluation and a thorough evaluation of nutritional status.

## DIETARY ASSESSMENT

It is recommended that dietary intake be assessed with a minimum frequency of every 2 weeks to yearly in children with CKD, depending on the age of the child and stage of disease (Table 34.2). More frequent assessments are recommended for younger children and for children with advanced stages of CKD. Children who depend solely on enteral feeding may benefit from more frequent monitoring. The dietary intake should be assessed with either a prospective 3-day diet diary or three 24-hour diet recalls.[6] Either technique should include one weekend day to represent variations in the diet because of changes in schedules on weekends. Information obtained from either method can then be used by a registered dietitian to estimate the daily intake of energy, macronutrients, vitamins, and minerals and overall dietary adequacy.

## NORMALIZED PROTEIN CATABOLIC RATE

Normalized protein catabolic rate (nPCR), which represents the protein catabolic rate normalized to weight, is used to objectively measure the dietary protein intake in patients on chronic hemodialysis who are in a nutritionally steady state. The nPCR formula is based on the urea generation rate (G; mg/min), which is calculated from the difference in blood urea nitrogen (BUN) level at the end of one hemodialysis session and the beginning of the next session. The urea generation rate can be derived using formal urea kinetic modeling or from the following algebraic equation[6]:

$$G \text{ (mg/min)} = [(C2 \times V2) - (C1 \times V1)]/t$$

where:  C1 = postdialysis BUN (mg/dL)
C2 = predialysis BUN (mg/dL)
V1 = postdialysis total body water (dL; V1 = 5.8 dL/kg × postdialysis weight; kg)

V2 = predialysis total body water (dL; V2 = 5.8 dL/kg × predialysis weight; kg)

t = time (minutes) from the end of the dialysis treatment to the beginning of the following treatment

The nPCR is then calculated by using the modified Borah equation[12]:

$$nPCR = 5.43 \times est\ G/V1 + 0.17$$

where V1 = total body water (L) post dialysis (0.58 × weight; kg)

Whereas a correlation between mean nPCR values and persistent weight loss of at least 2% was shown in adolescents, no link between nPCR values and weight loss was seen in younger patients.[13] Differences in protein metabolism and growth rate may be some reasons that nPCR offers no predictive value for weight loss in younger children. Because values used for Kt/V calculations are the same for nPCR calculations, the nPCR can be calculated monthly together with the Kt/V.

In patients on chronic peritoneal dialysis, the protein equivalent of nitrogen appearance (PNA) can be used to measure the protein intake. The PNA can be obtained by multiplying the total nitrogen appearance (TNA) by 6.25, which is based on the principle that 1 g of nitrogen is generated from 6.25 g of metabolized protein.[14] The TNA in children can, in turn, be calculated using the following formula[15]:

$$TNA\ (g/day) = 0.03 + 1.138\ urea\text{-}N_{urine} + 0.99\ urea\text{-}N_{dialysate}$$
$$+ 1.18\ BSA\ (body\ surface\ area) + 0.965\ protein\text{-}N_{dialysate}$$

where: $N_{urine}$ = urea nitrogen content in urine
$N_{dialysate}$ = urea nitrogen content in dialysate

Limited data exist on PNA in the pediatric population, and optimal normalization methods are not yet established. In adults, the PNA is normalized to ideal body weight.

## SERUM ALBUMIN

Hypoalbuminemia has been linked to increased morbidity and mortality in both adults and children with CKD.[16–8] Therefore, the serum albumin level has customarily been considered a marker of nutritional status. Patients on chronic peritoneal dialysis lose significant amounts of protein through the dialysate, with infants on peritoneal dialysis having almost twofold more peritoneal protein loss per body surface area (m²) compared to older children weighing more than 50 kg. This may lead to impaired growth and loss of growth potential.[19] Serum albumin levels are also decreased in states of inflammation, heavy urinary protein losses (nephrotic syndrome), and volume overload and are therefore not necessarily indicative of poor nutrition. Nevertheless, hypoalbuminemia is a biomarker of

morbidity and mortality in CKD patients and thus albumin levels should be regularly monitored.

## MIDARM MEASUREMENTS

Triceps skinfold thickness (TSF) measures subcutaneous fat and was previously considered to reflect total fat mass. In addition, the midarm muscle area (MAMA) and midarm muscle circumference (MAMC), calculated from the TSF and midarm circumference (MAC), were thought to reflect total muscle mass. However, these measures since have been found to be unreliable because of various factors, including interoperator variability and the unclear relationship between MAMA and total muscle mass resulting from confounding variables such as fluid overload and abnormal fat distribution.[6] They are therefore no longer used in the routine nutritional assessment of patients with CKD.

## BODY COMPOSITION MEASURE

Methods for determining body composition include the dual-energy x-ray (DXA) absorptiometry scan, which estimates fat mass, lean mass, and bone mineral density. DXA, however, cannot distinguish water content and lean body mass in patients with CKD and therefore may not provide accurate measures of lean mass in volume-overloaded subjects.[20] Other methods for measuring body composition include bioelectrical impedance, which estimates body fluid compartment volumes, and in vivo neutron activation, which measures certain total body elements. These methods have yet to be validated in children.[6,9] Most recently, Tsampalieros et al.[21] measured muscle and fat cross-sectional areas, expressed as gender-specific and age-specific Z scores, by quantitative computed tomography in children with CKD, and found significant muscle deficits as these children developed end-stage renal disease (ESRD). Further studies are needed to validate this new methodology and to justify its clinical utility.[21]

## FACTORS CONTRIBUTING TO CACHEXIA AND PROTEIN ENERGY WASTING IN CHRONIC KIDNEY DISEASE

Cachexia or protein energy wasting is prevalent in adult patients with CKD.[22] Mortality in patients on dialysis is eight times higher compared with healthy individuals and higher than in patients with cancer and heart failure. Cachexia, chronic inflammation, and cardiovascular complications are comorbidities in patients with CKD associated with mortality. Ghrelin is an orexigenic hormone with additional effects on the regulation of inflammation and the cardiovascular system. It may play an important role in the pathogenesis of cachexia, inflammation, and cardiovascular complications in CKD. There are three circulating products of the ghrelin gene: acyl ghrelin, des-acyl ghrelin, and obestatin, each with individual distinct functions on appetite regulation. Perturbations of these circulating ghrelin proteins have an impact on the overall orexigenic milieu of CKD.

---

## KEY POINT

Cachexia or protein energy wasting is prevalent in adult patients with CKD. Ghrelin and leptin may play yin-and-yang roles in the pathophysiology of cachexia and cardiovascular complications in CKD.

---

Leptin is an anorexigenic hormone that is secreted from the adipocytes and interacts with ghrelin and other appetite-regulating hormones. Leptin also plays a role in regulating inflammation and the cardiovascular system. Indeed, ghrelin and leptin may play yin-and-yang roles in the pathophysiology of cachexia and cardiovascular complications in CKD.[23] Vitamin D deficiency is common in patients with CKD. Low vitamin D levels upregulate the renin-angiotensin-aldosterone system, increase inflammation, and cause endothelial dysfunction. Epidemiologic studies suggest an association between low vitamin D levels and risk factors for cardiovascular disease, but a causal relationship has not been established.[24] Vitamin D supplementation improves cachexia, inflammation, cardiovascular complications, and mortality in experimental CKD. Further understanding of these interactions in CKD pathophysiology is needed for potential large-scale clinical trials that may have an impact on the quality of life and survival of patients with CKD.

## NUTRITIONAL MANAGEMENT IN CHRONIC KIDNEY DISEASE

Inadequate nutritional intake is prevalent in children with CKD, resulting in poor weight gain and delayed growth.[25] These children often require a program for enteral or parenteral nutritional supplementation to promote growth. The development of such a program requires a team approach in which the role of the dietitian is vital. Several components have to be considered in developing the dietary prescription, including energy, macronutrients, micronutrients, fluid, and electrolytes.

## ENERGY

The caloric or energy requirements for children with CKD are similar to those of healthy children.[26,27] Therefore, the caloric intake for children with CKD should be determined from national recommendations of the estimated energy requirements based on chronologic age and gender.

The caloric intake can then be adjusted based on the individual patient's needs and response. For example, infants with low birth weight and patients with recurrent vomiting may require supplemental calories to maintain growth. On the other hand, patients on peritoneal dialysis who demonstrate excessive weight gain may need reduction of their energy intake to take into account the energy intake from dialysate glucose, which is estimated at 8 to 12 kcal/kg/day.[28,29] Several studies have established that optimizing energy intake results in improved weight gain and linear growth.[25,30-32] Children on chronic dialysis who received nutritional support through gastrostomy tube feedings showed improvement in weight and height SDS,[30] while initiation of enteral feeding before 2 years of age resulted in significant catch-up growth.

---

## KEY POINT

The energy requirements for children with CKD are similar to those of healthy children. Therefore, the starting point for estimating caloric intake for children with CKD can be determined from national recommendations of the estimated energy requirements based on chronologic age and gender.

---

In a study of European children on chronic dialysis, overweight and obesity, rather than underweight, were highly prevalent. Short stature among kidney allograft recipients strongly correlated with overweight, whereas underweight appeared to be a problem only in infants. These findings suggest that nutritional management in children receiving chronic dialysis should focus as much on the prevention and treatment of overweight as on preventing cachexia and protein energy wasting.[33]

Nutritional intake can be optimized by concentrating feeds, selecting foods high in calories, and adding concentrated sources of carbohydrate and fat to the diet. Poor oral intake, recurrent emesis, and poor weight gain and growth should prompt initiation of tube feedings. Tube feedings can relieve the stress that comes with trying to meet nutritional requirements[34] and have a low complication rate.[30] Infants who are totally dependent on tube feedings should be provided oral stimulation exercises to encourage oral intake and also help their transition to complete oral feeding after successful renal transplantation.[35] Several centers have reported the successful transition of all tube-fed patients to complete oral feeding after transplantation.[36,37]

In children who are unable to receive their target nutritional requirements through enteral supplementation, intradialytic parenteral nutrition (IDPN) may be an option. A few pediatric studies have shown that IDPN was successful in inducing weight gain and increasing body mass index in a small group of poorly nourished HD patients.[38-40] Due to

Table 34.3 Recommended dietary protein intake for children with chronic kidney disease stages 3 to 5D

| Age | DRI (g/kg/day) | Recommended for CKD stage 3 (g/kg/day) (100%–140% DRI) | Recommended for CKD stages 4–5 (g/kg/day) (100%–120% DRI) | Recommended for hemodialysis (g/kg/day)* | Recommended for peritoneal dialysis (g/kg/day)† |
|---|---|---|---|---|---|
| 0-6 mo | 1.5 | 1.5-2.1 | 1.5-1.8 | 1.6 | 1.8 |
| 7–12 mo | 1.2 | 1.2–1.7 | 1.2–1.5 | 1.3 | 1.5 |
| 1–3 yr | 1.05 | 1.05–1.5 | 1.05–1.25 | 1.15 | 1.3 |
| 4–13 yr | 0.95 | 0.95–1.35 | 0.95–1.15 | 1.05 | 1.1 |
| 14–18 yr | 0.85 | 0.85-1.2 | 0.85–1.05 | 0.95 | 1.0 |

Source: Kidney Disease Outcomes Quality Initiative, Clinical Practice Guideline for Nutrition in Children with CKD: 2008 update. Executive summary. Am J Kidney Dis. 2009;53:S11–104. Reprinted with permission
* DRI + 0.1 g/kg/day to compensate for dialytic losses.
† DRI + 0.15–0.3 g/kg/day depending on patient age to compensate for peritoneal losses.
CKD, chronic kidney disease; DRI, dietary reference intake.

limited data available, the ideal IDPN composition remains unknown. However, standard amino acids that fulfill the daily protein requirements for the child's age are typically used, together with dextrose and 20% or 30% lipid components. Electrolytes and minerals can be adjusted according to the patient's needs, and trace elements (zinc, copper, selenium, manganese, and chromium) can be added to the IDPN. The IDPN should be infused through the venous limb of the hemodialysis circuit to avoid clearance of the amino acids.

## DISTRIBUTION RATIO OF MACRONUTRIENTS

The distribution of carbohydrate, protein, and fat intake for children with CKD is similar to that recommended for healthy children. For children older than 3 years of age, calories from carbohydrates should make up 45% to 65%, fat 25% to 35%, and protein 10% to 30% of total intake. For children 1 to 3 years of age, the distribution of calories from carbohydrate, fat, and protein should be 45% to 65%, 30% to 40%, and 5% to 20% of total caloric intake, respectively (see Table 34.2).[6] There is no consensus on macronutrient distribution for infants younger than 1 year of age. Therefore, the distribution of carbohydrate, fat, and protein should be consistent with infant formula, which is 36% to 56% carbohydrate, 40% to 54% fat, and 7% to 12% protein.[6] Because of the high risk for cardiovascular disease in children with CKD, unsaturated fat is preferable to saturated or trans-fat and complex carbohydrates to simple sugars.

## PROTEIN

Restricting protein in the diet had been thought to slow the rate of progression of CKD. However, studies in both adults[41,42] and children[43,44] showed no benefit with low-protein diets, with some studies actually indicating potential adverse effects of a diet very low in protein, including

possible increased risks for poor nutritional status and mortality.[41,42]

The KDOQI Nutrition Guidelines recommend maintaining the dietary protein intake at 100% to 140% of the dietary reference intake (DRI) for ideal body weight in children with CKD stage 3. Because nitrogen-containing waste products and phosphorus from protein intake can accumulate with decreasing kidney function, it is suggested that protein intake be reduced to 100% to 120% of the DRI in children with CKD stages 4 to 5. The protein requirements for these children may vary depending on various clinical conditions such as proteinuria and catabolism.

In children with ESRD, the KDOQI Nutrition Guidelines recommend that the starting point for estimating dietary protein intake be at 100% of the DRI for ideal body weight plus supplementation of protein losses that occur with dialysis.[6] For children on hemodialysis, an additional 0.1 g/kg/day is recommended to supplement the intradialytic losses. Because patients on peritoneal dialysis experience loss of protein through the dialysate ultrafiltrate that is inversely related to body weight and peritoneal surface area and protein supplementation differs according to the patient age and ranges from 0.15 to 0.3 g/kg/day (Table 34.3). Infants, who have a larger peritoneal surface area than older children, will therefore require more protein supplementation on a Gram-per-kilogram basis.

---

**KEY POINT**

In children with ESRD, the KDOQI Nutrition Guidelines recommend that the starting point for estimating dietary protein intake be at 100% of the DRI for ideal body weight plus supplementation of protein losses that occur with dialysis.

---

Because of the almost linear relationship between protein and phosphorus intake,[45] sources of protein that are relatively low in phosphorus should be selected when possible. Protein derived from animal flesh contains the lowest amount of phosphorus (11 mg of phosphorus per 1 g of protein), whereas protein derived from plants (legumes and lentils), eggs, or dairy products contains higher amounts of phosphorus (20 mg of phosphorus per 1 g of protein).[6] However, because humans do not have the enzyme phytase to release phosphorus contained in the form of phytic acid in plants, the bioavailability of phosphorus from plants (50%) is lower than that from animal products (greater than 70%).[6,46] In addition, phosphate salts are frequently added to meat products, increasing their phosphorus content. Therefore, dietary protein that is not entirely derived from animal products and that also contains vegetable sources of protein is recommended.

## CARBOHYDRATES

For healthy children of any age, calories from carbohydrate should constitute 45% to 65% of total caloric intake. Simple sugars should be restricted to avoid hypertriglyceridemia, especially in the early post-transplant period when there is a higher risk for developing glucose intolerance and hyperglycemia from corticosteroid and calcineurin inhibitor therapy.

Dietary fiber, which is found in most vegetables, fruits, and whole grains, can help reduce cholesterol levels and therefore decrease the risk for cardiovascular disease.[47] Fiber also can reduce constipation. However, the choice of fiber-containing foods is somewhat limited for children with CKD because of the potassium and phosphorus content in these foods. The KDOQI Nutrition Guidelines list foods containing fiber and their potassium and phosphorus content.[6] Other sources of fiber that can be added to meals or drinks include tasteless powdered forms that do not contain electrolytes (e.g., Benefiber, Unifiber). Children on strict fluid restrictions may be limited in the amount of fiber they can consume because of the water intake required with such a diet.

## FAT

Dyslipidemia is frequently seen in patients with CKD.[48] In a cross-sectional study of children with CKD, 45% had dyslipidemia, among whom 32% had hypertriglyceridemia. There was a positive association between dyslipidemia and a lower GFR, higher BMI, and nephrotic-range proteinuria.[49] Other studies have shown the prevalence of hypertriglyceridemia and hypercholesterolemia to be as high as 63% to 88% and 61% to 93%, respectively, in children on peritoneal dialysis.[50] Dyslipidemia not only potentially accelerates the progression of CKD but is also an important contributor of cardiovascular disease in children with CKD.[51,52] Cardiovascular disease is the leading cause of morbidity and mortality in children with CKD, constituting nearly 25% of total deaths.[53] Therefore, regulating dietary fat intake is an important component of nutritional management in children with CKD.

> **KEY POINT**
>
> Dyslipidemia is frequently seen in patients with CKD. Dyslipidemia not only potentially accelerates the progression of CKD but is also an important contributor of cardiovascular disease in children with CKD.

The KDOQI Dyslipidemia Guidelines recommend that adolescents and postpubertal children with CKD follow the KDOQI dietary and lifestyle recommendations for adults and that prepubertal children follow the recommendations by the National Cholesterol Education Program.[53,54] The American Heart Association consensus statement on dietary recommendations for children and adolescents can be used as a guideline for managing dyslipidemia in patients with CKD.[55]

Children with CKD and dyslipidemia should be strongly encouraged to reduce their intake of total fat, cholesterol, and saturated and *trans*-fatty acids. Heart-healthy fats such as oils produced from plant sources such as canola, corn, soybean, and olives are recommended. These dietary changes should be implemented in conjunction with controlling caloric intake and increasing physical activity.[34] Restricting dietary fat to 30% of the total caloric intake has been shown to have no adverse effects on growth and development.[56] The primary goal for nutritional management in children with CKD is to meet energy, protein, and micronutrient requirements. Dyslipidemia management should be initiated after the patient is well-nourished.[6] For this reason, dietary or lifestyle recommendations should be implemented cautiously or avoided in malnourished children.

The beneficial effects of omega-3 fatty acids on cardiovascular disease and prevention have been widely studied in adults. Omega-3 fatty acids have been reported to reduce serum triglyceride levels, blood pressure, thrombotic risk factors, and inflammation in adult patients.[53,57–59] Recent studies, however, have questioned some of the previous cardioprotective effects reported for adult patients.[60] Studies looking at the effects of omega-3 fatty acids on children with CKD are limited. In a small study of 16 children (7 to 8 years of age) on dialysis, 8 weeks of daily oral fish oil supplementation (3 to 8 g/day) resulted in a 27.5% reduction in triglyceride levels.[61] Because of limited data, there are currently no established recommendations for the use of omega-3 fatty acids to treat hypertriglyceridemia in children with CKD.

> **KEY POINT**
>
> The distribution of carbohydrate, protein, and fat intake recommended for children with CKD is the same as that recommended for healthy children.

## VITAMINS AND TRACE ELEMENTS

Patients with CKD are at increased risk for vitamin and trace element deficiencies as a result of inadequate intake, drug-nutrient interactions, urinary loss of protein-bound vitamins (such as vitamin D binding protein) in proteinuric patients, and loss of water-soluble nutrients through dialysis. A study of 30 children (9.3 ± 7.4 years old) on dialysis reported that the majority of patients had less dietary intake of water-soluble vitamins than the recommended daily allowance (RDA).[62]

25-Hydroxyvitamin D deficiency is commonly seen in pediatric dialysis patients.[63] In contrast, serum concentrations of vitamin A have been found to be normal or elevated without supplementation in patients on dialysis.[64,65] Supplementation with multivitamins may result in normal or higher than normal intake or serum concentrations for some of these vitamins,[62,64,65] which may be explained in part by the fact that the patients receive adult doses of renal multivitamins.

---

### KEY POINT

Patients with CKD are at increased risk for vitamin and trace element deficiencies secondary to inadequate intake, drug-nutrient interactions, urinary loss of protein-bound vitamins in proteinuric patients, and loss of water-soluble nutrients through dialysis.

---

The KDOQI Nutrition Guidelines recommend dietary intake of at least 100% of the DRI for vitamins $B_1$, $B_2$, $B_3$, $B_5$, $B_6$, $B_8$, $B_{12}$, C (ascorbic acid), A (retinol), E ($\alpha$-tocopherol), K, folic acid, copper, and zinc for children with CKD stages 2 to 5. If dietary intake does not meet 100% of the DRI, or if a vitamin or trace element deficiency is present in children with CKD stages 2 to 5, supplementation is recommended. In addition, children with ESRD should receive a water-soluble vitamin supplement. If available, a liquid containing the B vitamins and vitamin C can be used for infants and children unable to swallow tablets. If the liquid form is not available, an adult renal supplement containing the B vitamins and vitamin C can be crushed and dissolved in water. Infants and toddlers are usually given half a tablet and older children are given 1 tablet daily. Serum concentrations of vitamin A and E have been found to be normal or elevated without supplementation in dialysis patients; thus, supplementation of these fat-soluble vitamins, including vitamin K, is usually not recommended in patients with CKD, except in cases in which there is a documented deficiency (e.g., fat malabsorption).[34] For children on erythropoietin-stimulating agents, either oral or intravenous iron supplementation is typically required to replenish iron stores and prevent iron-deficient red blood cell formation.

## CALCIUM, PHOSPHORUS, AND VITAMIN D

Calcium, phosphorus, and vitamin D homeostasis are altered in CKD, leading to metabolic bone disease. The kidneys are responsible for excreting excess phosphorus and converting 25-hydroxyvitamin D to 1,25-dihydroxyvitamin D, the active form of vitamin D. Active vitamin D increases serum calcium levels by promoting calcium absorption from the intestines and inhibits parathyroid hormone (PTH) secretion by the parathyroid glands. As renal function declines, hyperphosphatemia and hypocalcemia develop, eventually leading to renal osteodystrophy. High-turnover osteodystrophy is associated with high PTH levels and can be prevented by close monitoring and management of serum calcium, phosphorus, and PTH levels through dietary measures, vitamin D treatment, and phosphate binders.[66]

---

### KEY POINT

Calcium, phosphorus, and vitamin D homeostasis are altered in CKD, leading to metabolic bone disease. Vitamin D deficiency is also commonly seen in patients with CKD.

---

The KDOQI Bone Guidelines for children with CKD recommend restriction of phosphorus in the diet when serum PTH levels are above the recommended levels for the stage of CKD.[67] Phosphate binders should be initiated when dietary measures fail to control serum phosphorus levels within the goal range. Calcium-based phosphorus binders (e.g., calcium carbonate, calcium acetate) and non–calcium-containing phosphorus binders (e.g., sevelamer carbonate) are available for the treatment of hyperphosphatemia. Target level of calcium and phosphorus are age-based because normal levels of calcium and phosphorus are higher in younger age groups.

Active vitamin D directly inhibits PTH secretion by acting on vitamin D receptors in the parathyroid gland. Dosing for active vitamin D should take into account the reduced activity of chondrocytes and development of adynamic bone disease associated with large doses of vitamin D and oversuppression of PTH secretion.[68] Other limitations of active vitamin D therapy include hypercalcemia and hyperphosphatemia resulting from increased absorption from the gut. Alternative medications that have less of a hypercalcemic effect are now available, including less calcemic active vitamin D analogues (e.g., paricalcitol [Zemplar], doxercalciferol [Hectorol]), and calcimimetics (e.g., cinacalcet hydrochloride [Sensipar]). The latter increases the sensitivity of calcium-sensing receptors to extracellular calcium, thereby reducing PTH levels. However, there are few data supporting the use of calcimimetics in children with CKD.

The KDOQI Bone Guidelines for children with CKD include opinion-based and evidence-based recommendations

Table 34.4 Recommended target ranges for serum parathyroid hormone

| Chronic kidney disease stage | Serum PTH level (pg/mL) |
| --- | --- |
| 2 | 35–70 |
| 3 | 35–70 |
| 4 | 70–110 |
| 5 | 200–300 |

*Source:* National Kidney Foundation: K/DOQI clinical practice guidelines for bone metabolism and disease in children with chronic kidney disease. Am J Kidney Dis 2005; 46: S1-121. Reprinted with permission
*Abbreviation:* PTH, parathyroid hormone.

for target serum PTH levels for each stage of CKD (Table 34.4).[67]

In addition, the recommended calcium-phosphorus product for children 12 years and younger is less than 65 mg$^2$/dL$^2$, and for children older than 12 years of age is less than 55 mg$^2$/dL$^2$.[67] These guidelines were established to minimize the risk for extraskeletal and vascular calcifications in children with CKD. Recent evidence suggests that markers for cardiovascular disease are optimum and growth is maintained when PTH levels are less than twice the upper limit of normal in children on dialysis.[69]

## SUMMARY

The association between mortality and extremes of BMI in children with CKD heightens the importance of careful nutritional management in this patient population. Close assessment, monitoring, and management of nutritional status in CKD may have a critical impact on growth and neurodevelopment, especially in younger children.[4] Therefore, the active involvement of a registered dietitian, health care professionals, and caregivers is essential for providing proper nutritional care to children with CKD. Moreover, further clinical trials are needed to establish evidence-based guidelines for nutritional assessment and management in pediatric CKD.

## REFERENCES

1. Kidney Disease Outcomes Quality Initiative, National Kidney Foundation. Clinical practice guidelines for nutrition in chronic renal failure. Am J Kidney Dis. 2000;35:S1–140.
2. Furth SL, Stablein D, Fine RN, et al. Adverse clinical outcomes associated with short stature at dialysis initiation: A report of the North American Pediatric Renal Transplant Cooperative Study. Pediatrics. 2002;109:909–13.
3. Wong CS, Gipson DS, Gillen DL, et al. Anthropometric measures and risk of death in children with end-stage renal disease. Am J Kidney Dis. 2000;36:811–9.
4. Foster BJ, McCauley L, Mak RH. Nutrition in infants and very young children with chronic kidney disease. Pediatr Nephrol. 2012;27:1427–39.
5. Karlberg J, Schaefer F, Hennicke M, et al. Early age-dependent growth impairment in chronic renal failure. European Study Group for Nutritional Treatment of Chronic Renal Failure in Childhood. Pediatr Nephrol. 1996;10:283–7.
6. Kidney Disease Outcomes Quality Initiative, Clinical Practice Guideline for Nutrition in Children with CKD: 2008 update. Executive summary. Am J Kidney Dis. 2009;53:S11–104.
7. Zivicnjak M, Franke D, Filler G, et al. Growth impairment shows an age-dependent pattern in boys with chronic kidney disease. Pediatr Nephrol. 2007;22:420–9.
8. Schaefer F, Wuhl E, Feneberg R, et al. Assessment of body composition in children with chronic renal failure. Pediatr Nephrol. 2000;14:673–8.
9. Rees L, Shaw V. Nutrition in children with CRF and on dialysis. Pediatr Nephrol. 2007;22:1689–702.
10. Van Dyck M, Proesmans W. Head circumference in chronic renal failure from birth. Clin Nephrol. 2001;56:S13–6.
11. Warady BA, Belden B, Kohaut E. Neurodevelopmental outcome of children initiating peritoneal dialysis in early infancy. Pediatr Nephrol. 1999;13:759–65.
12. Borah MF, Schoenfeld PY, Gotch FA, et al. Nitrogen balance during intermittent dialysis therapy of uremia. Kidney Int. 1978;14:491–500.
13. Juarez-Congelosi M, Orellana P, Goldstein SL. Normalized protein catabolic rate versus serum albumin as a nutrition status marker in pediatric patients receiving hemodialysis. J Ren Nutr. 2007;17:269–74.
14. Kopple JD, Jones MR, Keshaviah PR, et al. A proposed glossary for dialysis kinetics. Am J Kidney Dis. 1995;26:963–81.
15. Edefonti A, Picca M, Damiani B, et al. Models to assess nitrogen losses in pediatric patients on chronic peritoneal dialysis. Pediatr Nephrol. 2000;15:25–30.
16. Leavey SF, Strawderman RL, Jones CA, et al. Simple nutritional indicators as independent predictors of mortality in hemodialysis patients. Am J Kidney Dis. 1998;31:997–1006.
17. Stenvinkel P, Barany P, Chung SH, et al. A comparative analysis of nutritional parameters as predictors of outcome in male and female ESRD patients. Nephrol Dial Transplant. 2002;17:1266–74.
18. Wong CS, Hingorani S, Gillen DL, et al. Hypoalbuminemia and risk of death in pediatric patients with end-stage renal disease. Kidney Int. 2002;61:630–7.

19. Quan A, Baum M. Protein losses in children on continuous cycle peritoneal dialysis. Pediatr Nephrol. 1996;10:728–31.

20. Rashid R, Neill E, Smith W, et al. Body composition and nutritional intake in children with chronic kidney disease. Pediatr Nephrol. 2006;21:1730–8.

21. Tsampalieros A, Kalkwarf HJ, Wetzsteon RJ, et al. Changes in bone structure and the muscle-bone unit in children with chronic kidney disease. Kidney Int. 2013;83:495–502.

22. Mak RH, Cheung WW, Zhan JY, et al. Cachexia and protein-energy wasting in children with chronic kidney disease. Pediatr Nephrol. 2012;27:173–81.

23. Gunta SS, Mak RH. Ghrelin and leptin pathophysiology in chronic kidney disease. Pediatr Nephrol. 2013;28:611–6.

24. Gunta SS, Thadhani RI, Mak RH. The effect of vitamin D status on risk factors for cardiovascular disease. Nat Rev Nephrol. 2013;9:337–47.

25. Ledermann SE, Shaw V, Trompeter RS. Long-term enteral nutrition in infants and young children with chronic renal failure. Pediatr Nephrol. 1999;13:870–5.

26. Marques de Aquino T, Avesani CM, Brasileiro RS, de Abreu Carvalhaes JT. Resting energy expenditure of children and adolescents undergoing hemodialysis. J Ren Nutr. 2008;18:312–9.

27. Pollock C, Voss D, Hodson E, Crompton C. The CARI guidelines: Nutrition and growth in kidney disease. Nephrology (Carlton) 2005;10(Suppl 5):S177–230.

28. Edefonti A, Picca M, Damiani B, et al. Dietary prescription based on estimated nitrogen balance during peritoneal dialysis. Pediatr Nephrol. 1999;13:253–8.

29. Salusky IB, Fine RN, Nelson P, et al. Nutritional status of children undergoing continuous ambulatory peritoneal dialysis. Am J Clin Nutr. 1983;38:599–611.

30. Coleman JE, Watson AR, Rance CH, Moore E. Gastrostomy buttons for nutritional support on chronic dialysis. Nephrol Dial Transplant. 1998;13:2041–6.

31. Reed EE, Roy LP, Gaskin KJ, Knight JF. Nutritional intervention and growth in children with chronic renal failure. J Ren Nutr. 1998;8:122–6.

32. Van Dyck M, Bilem N, Proesmans W. Conservative treatment for chronic renal failure from birth: A 3-year follow-up study. Pediatr Nephrol. 1999;13:865–9.

33. Bonthuis M, van Stralen KJ, Verrina E, et al. Underweight, overweight and obesity in paediatric dialysis and renal transplant patients. Nephrol Dial Transplant. 2013;28(Suppl 4):iv195–iv204.

34. Secker D, Mak R. Nutritional challenges in pediatric chronic kidney disease. In: Geary DF, Schaefer F, editors. Comprehensive Pediatric Nephrology, 1st ed. Philadelphia: Mosby; 2008. pp. 743–59.

35. Dello Strologo L, Principato F, Sinibaldi D, et al. Feeding dysfunction in infants with severe chronic renal failure after long-term nasogastric tube feeding. Pediatr Nephrol. 1997;11:84–6.

36. Coleman JE, Watson AR. Growth posttransplantation in children previously treated with chronic dialysis and gastrostomy feeding. Adv Perit Dial. 1998;14:269–73.

37. Pugh P, Watson AR. Transition from gastrostomy to oral feeding following renal transplantation. Adv Perit Dial. 2006;22:153–7.

38. Goldstein SL, Baronette S, Gambrell TV, et al. nPCR assessment and IDPN treatment of malnutrition in pediatric hemodialysis patients. Pediatr Nephrol. 2002;17:531–4.

39. Krause I, Shamir R, Davidovits M, et al. Intradialytic parenteral nutrition in malnourished children treated with hemodialysis. J Ren Nutr. 2002;12:55–9.

40. Orellana P, Juarez-Congelosi M, Goldstein SL. Intradialytic parenteral nutrition treatment and biochemical marker assessment for malnutrition in adolescent maintenance hemodialysis patients. J Ren Nutr. 2005;15:312–7.

41. Kopple JD, Levey AS, Greene T, et al. Effect of dietary protein restriction on nutritional status in the Modification of Diet in Renal Disease Study. Kidney Int. 1997;52:778 91.

42. Menon V, Kopple JD, Wang X, et al. Effect of a very low-protein diet on outcomes: Long-term follow-up of the Modification of Diet in Renal Disease (MDRD) Study. Am J Kidney Dis. 2009;53:208–17.

43. Chaturvedi S, Jones C. Protein restriction for children with chronic renal failure. Cochrane Database Syst Rev. 2007:(17)006863.

44. Wingen AM, Fabian-Bach C, Schaefer F, Mehls O. Randomised multicentre study of a low-protein diet on the progression of chronic renal failure in children. European Study Group of Nutritional Treatment of Chronic Renal Failure in Childhood. Lancet. 1997;349:1117–23.

45. Boaz M, Smetana S. Regression equation predicts dietary phosphorus intake from estimate of dietary protein intake. J Am Diet Assoc. 1996;96:1268–70.

46. Uribarri J. Phosphorus homeostasis in normal health and in chronic kidney disease patients with special emphasis on dietary phosphorus intake. Semin Dial. 2007;20:295–301.

47. Van Horn L. Fiber, lipids, and coronary heart disease: A statement for healthcare professionals from the Nutrition Committee, American Heart Association. Circulation. 1997;95:2701–4.

48. Keane WF, Tomassini JE, Neff DR. Lipid abnormalities in patients with chronic kidney disease. Contrib Nephrol. 2011;171:135–42.

49. Saland JM, Pierce CB, Mitsnefes MM, et al. Dyslipidemia in children with chronic kidney disease. Kidney Int. 2010;78:1154–63.

50. Querfeld U, Salusky IB, Nelson P, et al. Hyperlipidemia in pediatric patients undergoing peritoneal dialysis. Pediatr Nephrol 1988;2:447–52.
51. Kavey RE, Allada V, Daniels SR, et al. Cardiovascular risk reduction in high-risk pediatric patients: A scientific statement from the American Heart Association Expert Panel on Population and Prevention Science; the Councils on Cardiovascular Disease in the Young, Epidemiology and Prevention, Nutrition, Physical Activity and Metabolism, High Blood Pressure Research, Cardiovascular Nursing, and the Kidney in Heart Disease; and the Interdisciplinary Working Group on Quality of Care and Outcomes Research: Endorsed by the American Academy of Pediatrics. Circulation. 2006;114:2710–38.
52. Schaefer B, Wuhl E. Progression in chronic kidney disease and prevention strategies [educational paper]. Eur J Pediatr. 2012;171:1579–88.
53. Kidney Disease Outcomes Quality Initiative. Clinical practice guidelines for cardiovascular disease in dialysis patients. Am J Kidney Dis. 2005;45:S1–153.
54. American Academy of Pediatrics. National Cholesterol Education Program: Report of the Expert Panel on Blood Cholesterol Levels in Children and Adolescents. Pediatrics. 1992;89:525–84.
55. Gidding SS, Dennison BA, Birch LL, et al. Dietary recommendations for children and adolescents: A guide for practitioners. Consensus statement from the American Heart Association. Circulation. 2005;112:2061–75.
56. Niinikoski H, Lapinleimu H, Viikari J, et al. Growth until 3 years of age in a prospective, randomized trial of a diet with reduced saturated fat and cholesterol. Pediatrics. 1997;99:687–94.
57. Cabo J, Alonso R, Mata P. Omega-3 fatty acids and blood pressure. Br J Nutr. 2012;107(Suppl 2):S195–200.
58. Rangel-Huerta OD, Aguilera CM, Mesa MD, Gil A. Omega-3 long-chain polyunsaturated fatty acids supplementation on inflammatory biomarkers: A systematic review of randomised clinical trials. Br J Nutr. 2012;107(Suppl 2):S159–70.
59. Vedtofte MS, Jakobsen MU, Lauritzen L, Heitmann BL. The role of essential fatty acids in the control of coronary heart disease. Curr Opin Clin Nutr Metab Care. 2012;15:592–6.
60. Calder PC, Yaqoob P. Marine omega-3 fatty acids and coronary heart disease. Curr Opin Cardiol. 2012;27:412–9.
61. Goren A, Stankiewicz H, Goldstein R, Drukker A. Fish oil treatment of hyperlipidemia in children and adolescents receiving renal replacement therapy. Pediatrics. 1991;88:265–8.
62. Pereira AM, Hamani N, Nogueira PC, Carvalhaes JT. Oral vitamin intake in children receiving long-term dialysis. J Ren Nutr. 2000;10:24–9.
63. Dibas BI, Warady BA. Vitamin D status of children receiving chronic dialysis. Pediatr Nephrol. 2012;27:1967–73.
64. Kriley M, Warady BA. Vitamin status of pediatric patients receiving long-term peritoneal dialysis. Am J Clin Nutr. 1991;53:1476–9.
65. Warady BA, Kriley M, Alon U, Hellerstein S. Vitamin status of infants receiving long-term peritoneal dialysis. Pediatr Nephrol. 1994;8:354–6.
66. Goodman WG, Coburn JW. The use of 1,25-dihydroxyvitamin D3 in early renal failure. Annu Rev Med. 1992;43:227–37.
67. Kidney Disease Outcomes Quality Initiative, National Kidney Foundation. Clinical practice guidelines for bone metabolism and disease in children with chronic kidney disease. Am J Kidney Dis. 2005;46:S1–121.
68. Wang M, Hercz G, Sherrard DJ, et al. Relationship between intact 1-84 parathyroid hormone and bone histomorphometric parameters in dialysis patients without aluminum toxicity. Am J Kidney Dis. 1995;26:836–44.
69. Rees L. What parathyroid hormone levels should we aim for in children with stage 5 chronic kidney disease: What is the evidence? Pediatr Nephrol. 2008;23:179–84.

## REVIEW QUESTIONS

1. Which one of the following statements is true?
   a. No association has been found between low body mass index and increased risk for mortality in children.
   b. Growth failure in infants with CKD is mainly due to malnutrition.
   c. Rates of linear growth and neurodevelopment are highest during the second decade of life.
   d. The nutritional status of children with CKD should be evaluated with the same frequency as in same-aged healthy children.
2. Which one of the following parameters is *not* included in the typical nutritional assessment for a child with CKD?
   a. Head circumference-for-age percentile for children younger than 3 years of age
   b. Height-for-age percentile
   c. Weight-for-age percentile
   d. Triceps skinfold thickness
3. Which one of the following statements *most* accurately describes the factors contributing to cachexia in CKD?
   a. Ghrelin is an orexigenic hormone that may play a role in the pathogenesis of cachexia in CKD.
   b. The four circulating gene products of ghrelin include acyl ghrelin, des-acyl-ghrelin, obestatin, and melatonin.

c. Leptin is an anorexigenic hormone secreted from leukocytes.

d. Vitamin supplementation has been shown to have little effect on cachexia in experimental CKD.

4. Which one of the following statements is false?

a. The energy requirements of children with CKD are higher than those of healthy children.

b. The caloric intake for children with CKD should be determined from national recommendations of the estimated energy requirements based on chronologic age and gender.

c. Children on chronic dialysis who receive nutritional support through gastrostomy tube feedings show improvement in weight and height SDS.

d. The energy intake from dialysate glucose is approximately 8 to 12 kcal/kg/day.

5. For children older than 3 years of age, which of the following distributions of calories from carbohydrates, fat, and protein is recommended?

a. Carbohydrates 25% to 35%, fat 45% to 65%, protein 10% to 30%

b. Carbohydrates 10% to 30%, fat 45% to 65%, protein 25% to 35%

c. Carbohydrates 25% to 35%, fat 10% to 30%, protein 45% to 65%

d. Carbohydrates 45% to 65%, fat 25% to 35%, protein 10% to 30%

6. Which of the following macronutrients is lost through the peritoneal dialysate ultrafiltrate?

a. Protein

b. Carbohydrates

c. Lipids

d. None of the above

7. Which of the following statements is true?

a. Dyslipidemia is rare in patients with CKD.

b. Children on PD have low prevalence rates (30% to 40%) of hypertriglyceridemia.

c. Dyslipidemia potentially accelerates the progression of CKD.

d. Restricting dietary fat to 30% of the total caloric intake has adverse effects on growth.

8. Which one of the following vitamin supplements is recommended in children on dialysis?

a. Vitamin A

b. Vitamin E

c. Vitamin B

d. Vitamin K

9. Which one of the following vitamins inhibits PTH secretion and at large doses causes adynamic bone disease?

a. Vitamin A

b. Vitamin E

c. Vitamin C

d. Vitamin D

10. Which of the following medications inhibits PTH secretion by increasing the sensitivity of calcium-sensing receptors to extracellular calcium?

a. Calcitriol

b. Paricalcitol

c. Cinacalcet hydrochloride

d. Doxercalciferol

## ANSWER KEY

1. b
2. d
3. a
4. a
5. d
6. a
7. c
8. c
9. d
10. c

# Renal replacement therapies

# 35

# Continuous renal replacement therapy

AKASH DEEP AND TIMOTHY E. BUNCHMAN

Acute kidney injury (AKI) commonly occurs in critically ill patients, and it affects nearly 30% to 40% of patients admitted to pediatric intensive care units (PICUs). Approximately 5% of patients in PICUs have AKI that requires supportive renal replacement therapy (RRT). Continuous RRT (CRRT) is an important adjunctive therapy in such patients. CRRT, as a technology, has evolved dramatically since the 1980s from an experimental modality to the accepted standard of care for hemodynamically unstable, critically ill pediatric and adult patients.[1–4] CRRT is now considered to be the treatment of choice for critically ill patients, with diagnoses ranging from volume overload to acute renal failure and complex multiorgan dysfunction syndrome (MODS).[5]

to hemodialysis. Since then, the technique introduced by Peter Kramer has evolved and has been modified further to provide both convective and diffusive exchange of solutes for enhanced solute clearance. To achieve predictable and controlled ultrafiltration, pump-assisted systems were developed in early 1990s and replaced arterial blood pressure–driven systems. These pump-assisted techniques have collectively come to be known as continuous venovenous hemofiltration (CVVH). In the past decade, elaborate CVVH devices with added safety, ultrafiltration, and thermal control mechanisms have been introduced in clinical practice. These devices are a far cry from the simple and unconventional design envisioned by Peter Kramer.

## EARLY DEVELOPMENT

In 1977, Kramer et al.[6] demonstrated the efficacy of a unique system for ultrafiltration in patients with fluid overload. The device consisted of a capillary hemofilter that used the patient's systemic arterial blood pressure to drive ultrafiltration. This novel technique, termed continuous arteriovenous hemofiltration (CAVH), was initially adopted as a technology-independent alternative

## INDICATIONS AND APPLICATIONS

In general, clinical indications for initiating CRRT in children are similar to those in the adults (Table 35.1). The most common use of CRRT is in children with AKI associated with fluid overload, severe or persistent hyperkalemia, or severe metabolic acidosis. Hypernatremia or hyponatremia (sodium level of less than or equal to 120 mEq/L or in a symptomatic patient) and uremic encephalopathy are other less common clinical indications of CRRT. Nonrenal indications for CRRT include initial treatment of inborn errors of metabolism and hyperammonemia, prevention or treatment of tumor lysis syndrome, and treatment of intoxications.

CRRT is often considered the therapy of choice for hemodynamically unstable or critically ill patients who would not be considered optimal candidates for either intermittent hemodialysis or peritoneal dialysis. Indeed, the chief advantage of CRRT is its ability to allow correction of metabolic disorders and fluid and electrolyte disturbances with a minimal impact on hemodynamic stability in critically sick patients (Table 35.2). Because CRRT is a continuous therapy conducted over several days, the overall solute clearance achievable with this modality can be superior to that feasible with intermittent hemodialysis.[7–10] Slow and continuous clearance of solutes and intravascular fluid by CRRT in patients with AKI may also be more physiologic and lessen the likelihood of rapid metabolic shifts and the disequilibrium syndrome.

Successful application of CRRT requires patients to be connected to an extracorporeal circuit for prolonged periods and remain immobilized. This is especially important in small children, who may require sedation for the procedure to be conducted safely. CRRT procedures necessitate the placement of an appropriately sized intravascular catheter that can be associated with its own risks, such as blood stream infection, bleeding, and injury to other organs. The CRRT circuits also require the use of anticoagulation, thereby enhancing the risks of systemic bleeding. In the absence of an adequate blood warming mechanism in the CRRT circuits, hypothermia can ensue, and this can be especially consequential in infants.

Current generation of CRRT machines use a roller pump to draw blood from the patient through a venous access into the extracorporeal circuit and then back into the patient. The blood roller pump also generates the positive pressure needed to achieve ultrafiltration of blood within the hemofilter. The vascular access often used in CRRT consists of a double-lumen access

Table 35.1 Indications (AEIOUM) for initiation of continuous renal replacement therapy

**Acute Severe Metabolic Acidosis (A)**
**Electrolyte Abnormalities (E)**
- Hyperkalemia
- Hypernatremia
- Hypocalcemia and hypercalcemia
- Hypophosphatemia and hyperphosphatemia

**Intoxications (I)**
- Low molecular weight, not protein bound
  - Gentamicin
  - Lithium
  - Ethylene glycol
  - Methanol
  - Ethanol
  - Salicylates
  - Acetaminophen
- High molecular weight, protein bound
  - Vancomycin
  - Phenobarbital
  - Carbamazepine
- Theophylline

**Fluid Overload (O)**
- Pulmonary edema not responsive to diuretics
- Oliguria
- Anuria

**Uremia (U)**
**Metabolic and Miscellaneous (M)**
- Inborn errors of metabolism
  - Urea cycle defects
  - Branched-chain amino acidurias
- Tumor lysis syndrome
- Hyperosmolality
- Coagulopathy and need for large volumes of blood products, combined with acute kidney injury
- Uncontrolled hyperthermia: core temperature higher than 39.5° Celsius
- Lactic acidosis

inserted into the venous circulation, such as the internal jugular or femoral vein.

## DIFFUSION AND CONVECTION

Ion transport and solute exchange in CRRT can be achieved by diffusion, convection, or a combination of both. Diffusion, simply put, is the transfer of solute across a semipermeable membrane from an area of high concentration to an area of low concentration.[7–9]

## KEY POINTS

- Fluid overload and AKI in hemodynamically unstable patients are the dominant clinical indications for CRRT.
- Nonrenal indications of CRRT include inborn errors of metabolism, tumor lysis syndrome, and intoxications.
- Some form of anticoagulation, either systemic (heparin) or regional (citrate), is necessary for effective CRRT.

Table 35.2 Advantages and disadvantages of continuous renal replacement therapy

| Advantages | Disadvantages |
| --- | --- |
| • Hemodynamic stability | • Need for intravascular access |
| • Slow fluid and solute removal | • Need for anticoagulation |
| • Greater solute clearance (Kt/V) | • Need for patient immobilization |
| • Runs continuously | • Nutritional clearance |
| • ICU nurses troubleshoot the machines | • Higher cost |

Abbreviations: ICU, intensive care unit; Kt/V, a measure of clearance in which K is dialyzer clearance of urea, t is dialysis time, and V is the volume of distribution of urea.

Diffusion of solutes is directly proportional to the concentration gradient across the semipermeable membrane, the diffusive coefficient of the solute, the temperature, the surface area of the interface, and the distance to traverse across the membrane.[7] Diffusion is effective at clearing low-molecular-weight solutes in CRRT, but solute clearance declines with increasing molecular weight.[9,10] In contrast, convection relates to transfer of solute across a semipermeable membrane in association with a significant amount of water across the membrane.[7-9] In other words, convection involves bulk removal of solutes dissolved in the ultrafiltrate that is removed in the CRRT procedure.[7,8]

## TERMINOLOGY

Since its original description, the technology of conducting CRRT has changed considerably. It is important to understand the principles associated with these techniques to provide optimal clinical care for critically sick patients.

## SLOW CONTINUOUS ULTRAFILTRATION

During the slow continuous ultrafiltration (SCUF) procedure, the CRRT circuit is used merely to ultrafilter plasma water (Figure 35.1A). This is the simplest form of CRRT and may be achieved with either a continuous arteriovenous (AV) system or a continuous venovenous system that uses a CRRT machine. In a poorly monitored circumstance, SCUF may result in a dangerously high fluid removal rate and may lead to shock and severe electrolyte abnormalities. Because solute clearance with SCUF is not substantial, its use as a CRRT modality has declined over the years.

## CONTINUOUS VENOVENOUS HEMOFILTRATION

In CVVH, a sterile replacement electrolyte solution is infused into the CRRT circuit, either in a prefilter or a postfilter location, and the fluid is removed from the patient by ultrafiltration at a rate equal to the replacement fluid infusion if the patient is to stay euvolemic (Figure 35.1B). A positive or negative fluid balance can be achieved by decreasing or increasing the net ultrafiltration rate, respectively. A high ultrafiltration rate that is possible in this procedure provides a convective solute transport.

## CONTINUOUS VENOVENOUS HEMODIALYSIS

Continuous venovenous hemodialysis (CVVHD) is characterized by adding diffusive solute removal by additional dialysis capability in the CRRT circuit. Sterile dialysate solution is infused through the dialyzer, which circulates outside the capillary membrane in a countercurrent manner, similar to hemodialysis (Figure 35.1C). The rate of dialysate flow, however, is substantially lower than that used in hemodialysis. Replacement fluid is not used in the CRRT circuit, but some CRRT machines may require a minimal amount of replacement fluid to be present in the circuit for optimal functioning of the device. Although a custom dialysate solution can be used, several brands of premixed sterile dialysate solutions are commercially available for this purpose. Because some ultrafiltration is done in most patients, the convective solute (and toxin) removal continues in CVVHD, *albeit* at a much slower pace.

## CONTINUOUS VENOVENOUS HEMODIAFILTRATION

Continuous venovenous hemodiafiltration (CVVHDF) uses both convective and diffusive solute removal capabilities in CRRT. In addition to a dialysate set-up similar to that of CVVHD, replacement fluid is infused into the circuit in the predialyzer or the postdialyzer position (Figure 35.1D). Ultrafiltration removes fluid from the patient at a rate that is dictated by the patient's needs, and it provides convective solute removal, whereas the dialysis feature provides diffusive solute removal.

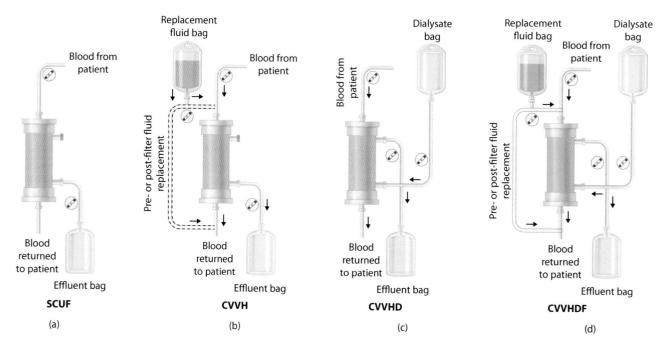

Figure 35.1 Diagrammatic representation of **(a)** slow continuous ultrafiltration (SCUF), **(b)** continuous venovenous hemofiltration (CVVH), **(c)** continuous venovenous hemodialysis (CVVHD), and **(d)** continuous venovenous hemodiafiltration (CVVHDF).

## DEVICES

Several devices are now available commercially for use in CRRT modalities. These devices are based on the principle that a high hydraulic permeability hemofilter connected to the patient's central venous access by tubing is used to ultrafilter plasma in a slow but continuous manner. In most of the available CRRT machines, a peristaltic "arterial pump" helps pump blood into the extracorporeal circuit and also generates the hydrostatic pressure necessary for ultrafiltration in the hemofilter (Figure 35.2). Following ultrafiltration and convective solute exchange in the hemofilter, the blood is returned to the patient through the "venous" port of the vascular access. Some CRRT devices have a pump in the "venous" side of the extracorporeal circuit to control the flow of blood in the circuit. The dialysate used for diffusive solute clearance is pumped into and out of the hemofilter through its side ports. The dialysate is separated from the blood by the hemofilter capillary membrane and flows in a path that is countercurrent to the flow of the blood inside the capillary column. The flow of the dialysate into the hemofilter is controlled with one pump, whereas another pump administers the replacement filter into the extracorporeal circuit at the prehemofilter or posthemofilter location.

Pulsatile or piston action intravenous pumps were used in early versions of CRRT devices to control ultrafiltration rate during the procedure. These pumps can have an error rate of up to 30%, are inaccurate for control of ultrafiltration, and have been largely abandoned.[11] The ultrafiltration control error in the newer CRRT devices is only 1% to 2% of total ultrafiltration, and resultant improved control of therapy goals. The current generation of CRRT devices also provides for plug-in warming modules for the blood pathway, thus reducing the possibility of hypothermia. Some of the commonly used CRRT devices in the United States are shown in Figure 35.3.

## HEMOFILTERS

Hemofilters used in CRRT are similar in design to hemodialyzers, except that the filter capillaries have significantly higher hydraulic permeability. Some CRRT devices permit interchangeability of hemofilters with varying size and permeability characteristics, whereas other devices require the use of specific hemofilter sets.

## CLINICAL APPLICATION OF CLEARANCE TECHNIQUES

CRRT can be performed by using convection (CVVH), diffusion (CVVHD), or a combination of convection and diffusion (CVVHDF). Choosing the appropriate modality is determined by the patient's needs and

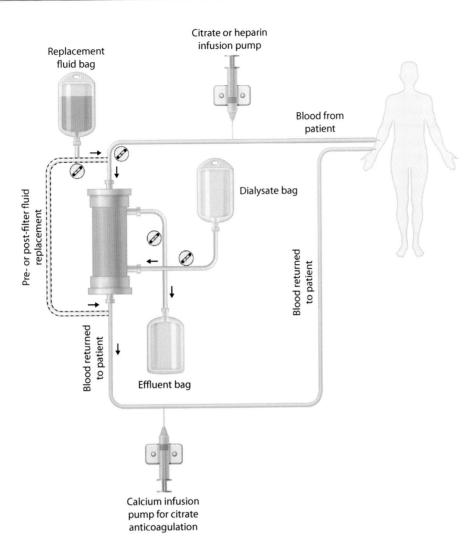

Figure 35.2  Diagrammatic representation of a continuous renal replacement therapy circuit.

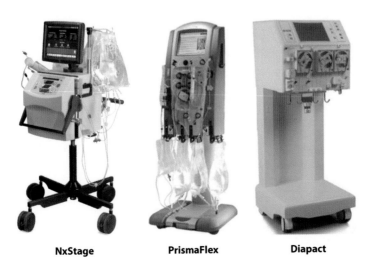

Figure 35.3  Continuous renal replacement therapy machines available for clinical use in the United States. (Reproduced by permission of NexStage, Lawrence, MA; Baxter-Gambro, Deerfiled IL; B. Braun USA, Bethlehem, PA.)

the technical expertise and preferences of the staff. Another technical decision in conducting CRRT relates to the choice of replacement fluid infused in the prefilter or postfilter position. Herein also, superiority of one method over the other has not been clearly established. Historical data in adults suggest that postfilter convection allows for greater solute clearance, but it has a higher risk of clotting because of hemoconcentration within hemofilter capillaries.

A sterile physiologic solution is used as dialysate (diffusive clearance), and a replacement fluid is infused directly into the CRRT circuit (for convective clearance). In septic patients with AKI, there may be a significant improvement in cytokine clearance in a convective mode over the diffusive mode. It is clear that low-molecular-weight substances, such as urea and citrate, are cleared equally by the diffusive and convective modes. As the molecular weight increases and molecular protein binding enhances, the convective mode of CRRT provides some advantage in clearance. Flores et al.[12] demonstrated that in the highly catabolic bone marrow transplant population, there appear to be improved survival rates in patients using the convective mode. Long-term multicenter studies are needed to look at the outcome and efficacy of convection versus diffusion in CRRT.

## KEY POINTS

- SCUF as a CRRT modality is less commonly used at present. This technique can be useful in addressing urgent fluid overload concerns when machine set-up may take time or for managing cardiovascular surgical patients in the operating room.
- CVVH is best suited to remove larger molecules and may be beneficial in patients with sepsis. CVVH uses the convective or bulk removal technique.
- The CVVHD modality is ideally suited for patients with AKI because electrolyte balance and uremic toxin removal can be effectively managed by the process of diffusion.

## VASCULAR ACCESS

The success of CRRT depends greatly on the adequacy of vascular access. Therefore, considerable thought must be given to the selection of site for insertion, as well as size and type of AV access in each patient.

Potential sites for placement of the AV access include the internal jugular vein, the subclavian vein, and the femoral vein. Because of lower risk of vascular stenosis and pneumothorax and its large size, the internal jugular site is a preferred site for placement of AV access. Moreover, placement of catheter is in the right side of the heart, which acts as a reservoir and allows access to the volume of blood needed for successful CRRT.[13] The internal jugular vein site access also allows easier rehabilitation of the patient while receiving CRRT. The femoral vein is a relatively large vessel and is also often used for access for CRRT. However, longer catheters with more "dead space" may be necessary for the tip of the vascular access to reach the common iliac vessel or the inferior vena cava. The subclavian vessel can also be used for vascular access, but because of the risk of pneumothorax, it is a less preferred access site. The size of the vascular access should be proportional to the size of the patient (Table 35.3). Umbilical arterial and venous catheters have been used in neonates in past, but these sites are not preferred because of the less than optimal blood flow achieved.

## KEY POINT

Adequate blood flow and appropriate size and placement of the vascular catheter are the keys to a successful CRRT procedure.

While choosing the site of insertion of vascular access, it is important to avoid placement of the vascular access for CRRT close to other central venous accesses. This is to avoid siphoning of medications, especially inotropes and sedatives, from the patients into the hemofilter during the CRRT procedure.

## BLOOD FLOW RATE

A minimum blood flow rate (BFR) of 30 to 50 mL/min, and ideally a BFR of 400 mL/min/1.73 m$^2$, should be targeted for successful CRRT. This BFR approximates to 10 to 12 mL/kg/min in infants, 4 to 6 mL/kg/min in children, and 2 to 4 mL/kg/min in adolescents. The maximum achievable BFR varies with the CRRT device used. The BFR is often dictated by the adequacy of the vascular access. The risk of a higher BFR is greater hemodynamic instability, but in clinical settings a greater BFR may also result in less circuit clotting.

## DIALYSATE SOLUTION

At the inception of CRRT, the replacement or dialysate solutions used were lactate based, such as peritoneal dialysis solutions or Ringer lactate. Increased plasma lactate concentrations have been reported with the use of such

Table 35.3 Recommended catheter sizes and insertion sites in infants and children

| Patient group/weight | Catheter size and manufacture | Preferred insertion site |
|---|---|---|
| **Neonates**<br>3–5 kg | Two 5-French single lumen inserted separately | Femoral and internal jugular vein(s) |
| | 7-French double lumen, 10 cm (Medcomp) | Internal jugular, femoral veins |
| | 7-French double lumen, 13 cm (Cook) | Femoral vein |
| **Infants/school-age Children**<br>5–15 kg | 7-French triple lumen, 16 cm (Arrow) | Internal jugular, subclavian, or femoral veins |
| 10–30 kg | 8-French double lumen, 11–16 cm (Arrow)<br>9-French double lumen, 12–15 cm (Medcomp)<br>9-French double lumen, 12–15 cm (Medcomp)<br>10-French double lumen, 12–19.5 cm (Mahurkar)<br>11.5- or 12-French double lumen, 12–20 cm (Medcomp, Arrow, Mahurkar) | |
| **Pediatric**<br>>30 kg, but <70 kg | 11.5- or 12-French double lumen, 12–20 cm (Medcomp, Mahurkar) | Internal jugular, subclavian, or femoral veins |

lactate-based solutions, especially in patients with acute hepatic failure.[14–17] Hemodynamic instability and poor cardiac performance have also been raised as concerns with lactate-based dialysate used in CRRT.[16,17]

In contrast, bicarbonate-based dialysate has been shown to result in a significant increase in the arterial pH and a decrease in the base deficit, as well as a trend toward a greater cardiac index, a lower infusion rate of dobutamine, and high oxygen delivery.[18,19] Distinct advantages of bicarbonate-based dialysate in improving cardiovascular functions in CRRT have also been documented in several clinical studies.[20–22] For these reasons, bicarbonate-based dialysate and replacement solutions are now recommended as the standard of care for CRRT. Since the early 2000s, several bicarbonate-based solutions for CVVH or CVVHD have become available commercially.[23] If citrate anticoagulation is used, a calcium free-bicarbonate-based solution may be the optimal choice.[24]

## TIMING OF INITIATION

The optimal timing of CRRT initiation in patients with severe AKI remains uncertain, and this represents an important knowledge gap and a priority for high-quality research. Although a systematic review suggested that "earlier" initiation of CRRT improves survival, reliable data are limited by small study size, single-center experiences, and use of variable definitions to define "early" CRRT initiation. Karvellas et al.[25] performed a systematic review of the effect of CRRT timing on mortality rates in adult critically ill patients and included 15 studies published between 1999 and 2010. In a pooled analysis, early initiation of CRRT was associated with significantly reduced odds of death (odds ratio, 0.45; 95% confidence interval [CI], 0.28, 0.72).[25] This

analysis was, however, limited by the low methodologic quality of the included studies and by statistical heterogeneity. Another randomized controlled trial of CRRT timing (n = 106) found no difference in mortality. However, the study was underpowered to detect a clinically implausible absolute difference in mortality of less than 40%.[26]

## ANTICOAGULATION

One of the key elements that determines the success of CRRT and the longevity of the circuit is prevention of clot formation in the extracorporeal circuit and the hemofilter. Some form of anticoagulation, which maintains the fluidity of blood and the circuit and yet has minimal systemic effects in the patient, is used to achieve this goal. Commonly used anticoagulants during CRRT are listed in Table 35.4.

---

### KEY POINTS

- Early initiation of CRRT improves mortality rates.
- Initiating CRRT after fluid overload of greater than 20% body weight is associated with higher mortality rates.

---

### Saline flushes

Flushing the extracorporeal lines, blood pump, hemofilter, and air detectors with sterile normal saline can allow effective functioning of the CRRT procedure in a patient with bleeding diathesis or when anticoagulation is contraindicated. To

Table 35.4 Commonly used anticoagulants in continuous renal replacement therapy

- Saline flushes
- Heparin (unfractionated heparin)
- Low-molecular-weight heparin
- Citrate regional anticoagulation
- Prostacyclin
- Nafamostat mesylate
- Danaparoid
- Hirudin or lepirudin
- Argatroban (thrombin inhibitor)

adopt this technique, a three-way stopcock is placed at the connection of the "arterial" end of extracorporeal tubing and the vascular access. When performing a normal saline flush, the blood flow in the CRRT circuit is decreased to 100 mL/min to prevent the formation of bubbles in the blood tubing. The three-way stopcock is then closed to the patient and opened to a bag of normal sterile saline. The saline (10 to 20 mL) is then flushed through the CRRT circuit at a flow rate of 100 mL/min. The inner lumen of the tubing and the filter fibers are visually inspected during the procedure for evidence of any clot formation. The volume of normal sterile saline infused during the flush must be recorded as intravenous fluid administered to the patient.

## Heparin

Heparin has long been the mainstay of anticoagulation in CRRT. Typically, the CRRT circuit is primed with 1 to 2 L of normal sterile saline containing 2500 to 5000 units/L of heparin. Then, a prefilter heparin infusion is initiated, usually at 10 to 20 units/kg/h, with a goal activated clotting time (ACT) of 180 to 220 sec. The ACT or activated partial thromboplastin time is used to monitor the adequacy of the heparinization. The ACT test is commonly performed at the bedside, thus decreasing the turn-around time from the laboratory. The heparin dose is highly variable and must be individualized. The main advantage of unfractionated heparin (UFH) is the experience people have when using heparin in various conditions, the short biologic half-life, the availability of an efficient inhibitor, and the possibility to monitor its effect with routine laboratory tests such as the ACT.

In spite of the vast experience in the use of UFH, it has some clinically significant side effects. Heparin is not removed by the CRRT process, thus leading to systemic heparinization of the patient and increasing the risk of bleeding in the patient. Severe bleeding events have been reported in 10% to 50% of patients undergoing CRRT.[27] Heparinization is monitored by measuring ACT every 30 min and adjusting the dose of heparin to keep it in 180 to 200 sec range. If the ACT is very high, then the heparin infusion is stopped altogether until it normalizes to the recommended range. The development of heparin resistance is not uncommon in

critically ill patients, in whom antithrombin (AT) concentrations are often reduced as a result of consumption secondary to sepsis or systemic inflammation. AT degradation by elastase is also enhanced by heparin, and this adds to heparin resistance during critical illnesses.

An uncommon but feared side effect of heparin therapy is the development of heparin-induced thrombocytopenia (HIT). It has been reported to occur in 1% to 5% of patients as a result of development of anti–platelet factor 4-heparin (PF4/H) antibodies.[28] The PF4/H antibody is an immunoglobulin G (IgG) antibody that reacts with the heparin-PF4 complex on the platelet surface and triggers the clotting cascade. HIT usually occurs in the second week (7 to 10 days) after the start of heparin treatment. The presence of thrombocytopenia and frequent circuit clotting in a patient undergoing CRRT should alert the clinician to the possibility of HIT. The diagnosis of HIT can be established by presence of thrombocytopenia and circulating PF4/H antibodies. Discontinuation of heparin and use of an alternate form of anticoagulation, such as citrate, is necessary if the diagnosis of HIT is considered.

Another issue with the use of heparin is its unpredictable pharmacokinetics. The pharmacokinetics of heparin is not only time and dose dependent but also unpredictable, with considerable interpatient and intrapatient variability. Heparin binds not only to AT, but also to numerous other proteins and cells, thereby limiting its availability and reducing its anticoagulant effect. Some of these proteins are acute phase reactants, many of which are elevated in critically ill patients.

Clinicians have tried using various low-molecular-weight heparins (LMWHs) such as dalteparin, enoxaparin, and nadroparin in CRRT. These LMWHs differ in size, half-life, and activity. Because of their reduced chain length, LMWHs have higher anti-Xa and anti-IIa activity than does UFH. The pharmacokinetics of LMWHs is more predictable than that of UFH because of less plasma protein binding. The theoretical advantages include a more reliable anticoagulant response and a lower incidence of HIT. However, because of the stronger anti-Xa effect, reversal with protamine is less effective. Because LMWHs are renally excreted, their effects are prolonged in renal failure. Special coagulation assays are required to monitor anti-Xa activity. Furthermore, LMWHs are more expensive than standard heparin, and no difference in prolonging the hemofilter life has been convincingly demonstrated.

## Citrate anticoagulation

In 1990, Mehta et al.[29] demonstrated the efficacy of citrate anticoagulation for CRRT circuits. Citrate anticoagulation is based on the concept of chelation of calcium to avoid clotting of blood in the CRRT circuit. Calcium is necessary for the activation of factors XI, IX, X, and prothrombin. Thus, chelation of free calcium by citrate inhibits the activation of the intrinsic pathway of coagulation, thereby resulting in anticoagulation.

Table 35.5 Adjustment of citrate infusion by circuit ionized calcium*

| CRRT circuit iCa²⁺ (mmol/L) | Weight >20 kg Action | Weight <20 kg Action |
|---|---|---|
| <0.35 | ↓ rate by 10 mL/h | ↓ rate by 5 mL/h |
| 0.35–0.40 | No change | No change |
| 0.41–0.50 | ↑ rate by 10 mL/h | ↑ rate by 5 mL/h |
| >0.50 | ↑ rate by 20 mL/h | ↑ rate by 10 mL/h |

*Abbreviations:* CRRT, continuous renal replacement therapy; iCa²⁺, ionized circuit calcium.
* Titrate citrate (ACD-A) drip to maintain CRRT circuit iCa²⁺ between 0.35 and 0.40 mmol/L. Physician review of therapy is indicated if ACD-A infusion rate is >200 mL/h.

By infusing citrate in the prefilter position and neutralizing calcium in the postfilter location, regional anticoagulation of the hemofilter, without systemic anticoagulation of the patient, can be achieved. Systemic intravenous calcium infusion needs to be carefully adjusted to prevent hypocalcemia induced by citrate infusion in the extracorporeal circuit. Citrate is removed by CRRT; its clearance has been reported to be equal to that of urea in CRRT, and no significant difference in clearance is noted between CVVH and CVVHD modes.[30]

Bunchman et al.[23,24] adopted citrate infusion protocols designed for use in pediatric patients. They administered ACD-A solution (Baxter Healthcare, Deerfield, IL) in the prefilter location through a three-way stopcock placed at the connection between the arterial bloodline and the vascular access. The ACD-A infusion (mL/h) is initiated at 1.5 times the BFR (mL/min) in the CRRT circuit. Calcium chloride (8000 mg calcium chloride/L of normal sterile saline or 8 mg/mL), or calcium gluconate (24 g of calcium gluconate/L of normal saline or 240 mg/mL) infusion is begun through either a third lumen of a triple-lumen dialysis catheter or through a different central venous line at 0.4 times the ACD-A infusion rate in mL/h. The circuit ionized calcium (iCa) is checked post-filter (after ACD-A infusion) with a target iCa of 0.35 to 0.50 mmol/L. The systemic ionized calcium is checked either through a central line or pre–ACD-A site in the arterial limb of the CRRT circuit, with a target iCa of 1.1 to 1.3 mmol/L.[23,24] The ACD-A and calcium chloride infusions are titrated according to guidelines given in Tables 35.5 and 35.6, respectively.

Complications of citrate anticoagulation include hypocalcemia, metabolic alkalosis, and citrate toxicity. Hypocalcemia is avoidable by following titration guidelines for infusion of the calcium chloride (Table 35.6). Metabolic alkalosis result from hepatic conversion of 1 mole of citrate to 3 moles of bicarbonate. In our experience, all children treated with ACD-A citrate anticoagulation developed metabolic alkalosis.[23,24] Indeed, failure to develop metabolic alkalosis while receiving citrate anticoagulation should lead to a search for underlying metabolic acidosis and a mixed acid-base disorder in the patient. The metabolic alkalosis is treated by decreasing the dialysate flow (in CVVHD mode) by approximately 30% and by substituting the replacement fluid with an equivalent volume (30%) of normal sterile.[24]

Citrate toxicity (or citrate lock) develops if the citrate infusion rate is higher than the combined capacity to remove it by CRRT and the hepatic metabolism in the patient. Citrate toxicity can be suspected by a rising total calcium and a decreasing ionized calcium concentration in the patient. The diagnosis is established by measuring the ratio of the total calcium to ionized calcium (systemic-to-CRRT ionized calcium).[31] A total-to-ionized calcium ratio of more than 2.5 represents citrate toxicity. Patients with hepatic dysfunction are especially prone to this complication. Although the overall prevalence of citrate toxicity was 12% in this single-center experience, it affected 33% of patients with AKI complicating hepatic failure.[31]

Apart from fewer bleeding complications compared with heparin use, citrate anticoagulation may also offer increased

Table 35.6 Adjustment of calcium chloride infusion by patient's peripheral ionized calcium*

| Patient iCa²⁺ (mmol/L) | Weight >20 kg Action | Weight <20 kg Action |
|---|---|---|
| >1.30 | ↓ rate by 10 mL/h | ↓ rate by 5 mL/h |
| 1.10–1.30 | No change | No change |
| 0.90–1.10 | ↑ rate by 10 mL/h | ↑ rate by 5 mL/h |
| <0.90 | ↑ rate by 20 mL/h | ↑ rate by 10 mL/h |

*Abbreviations:* iCa²⁺, ionized circuit calcium.
* Titrate calcium chloride drip rate to maintain the patient's iCa²⁺ between 1.10 and 1.30 mmol/L.

survival of the CRRT circuit. One study found that citrate-anticoagulated circuits lasted a median of 70 h, compared with a median of 40 h for heparin-anticoagulated circuits.[32] The rate of spontaneous circuit failure was 87% in the heparin arm and 57% in the citrate arm of the study.[32] A recent meta-analysis has also confirmed superiority of citrate over heparin anticoagulation in prolonging circuit life.[27] In contrast, in a multicenter prospective, noninterventional study, mean circuit life was similar between heparin- and citrate-anticoagulated systems (42.1 ± 27.1 vs. 44.7 ± 35.9 h, respectively).[33]

## Prostacyclin

Because platelets play an important role in the coagulation cascade, inhibitors of platelet activation have been used for anticoagulation in CRRT, either alone or in combination with heparin. Prostaglandin I-2 ($PGI_2$), also known as prostacyclin, is synthesized endogenously from the arachidonic acid pathway by cyclooxygenase enzymes, and it acts on endothelium and platelets. $PGI_2$ and its synthetic derivative epoprostenol sodium (Flolan) inhibit platelet aggregation and adhesion, and they have been used as anticoagulants.[34] Antiplatelet action occurs at a dose between 2 and 8 ng/kg/min. Prostacyclin can cause hypotension from vasodilation at doses of 20 ng/kg/min. Although the vasodilator half-life is 2 min, the antiplatelet effect lasts for 2 h. Besides antiplatelet and vasodilatory actions, prostacyclin has anti-inflammatory and antimitogenic actions as well.

An important feature of prostacyclin is its heparin-sparing effect, which can be put to use especially in patients with decreased levels of antithrombin-3 (e.g., septic patients) who may have frequent circuit clotting despite treatment with heparin. The addition of prostacyclin to heparin not only potentiates the effect of heparin and results in a decreased need for heparin dose, but also, because of its antiplatelet action, can dramatically improve the hemofilter life. Prostacyclin has been compared with both heparin and citrate as an anticoagulant, with promising results.[35,36]

The most important drawbacks with the use of prostacyclin are its limited clinical experience and the paucity of published reports on its safety and efficacy. Systemic side effects include hypotension and an increase of intracranial pressure, both of which can be prevented or limited by infusion into the extracorporeal circuit, thus reducing the systemic levels related to extracorporeal elimination. Prostacyclin may be considered an anticoagulant in patients with increased risk of bleeding. An important limiting factor of prostacyclin is its high cost.

## COMPLICATIONS

Complications of CRRT can result from technical issues, such as vascular access and device malfunction and failure, as well as those resulting from the clinical impacts of the procedure itself (Table 35.7).

## Technical and equipment malfunction

Complications associated with the vascular catheter, such as kinking, partial or complete obstruction, or displacement, can lead to malfunction or cessation of the CRRT and clotting of the circuit. Circuit down-time due to above listed factors can result in delivery of less than optimal CRRT therapy dose in critically sick patients. In one study, prescribed dose was delivered to only 68% patients due to circuit downtime problems.[37] The CRRT device can experience technical failure or loss of integrity of the extracorporeal tubing set, and air may enter the blood circuit and result in air embolism. Newer CRRT devices, are, however, equipped with air detectors that clamp the blood return line to the patient if air is detected within the tubing set. Errors of ultrafiltration are less common with modern CRRT equipment, but may occur in small infants and newborns if the device controls are manually overridden by the operators. Finally, the efficiency of the hemofilter may deteriorate due to the accumulation of plasma proteins and blood cells along the intravascular side of the capillary filters.

## Bleeding

Anticoagulation-associated bleeding is a well-known complication seen in CRRT.[27] The source of bleeding is often at the catheter exit site, but it can also be internal, usually at the vascular puncture site. Because of systemic heparinization, internal bleeding in the gastrointestinal tract and other vital organs can be severe.

Table 35.7 Complications of continuous renal replacement therapy

| Technical complications | Clinical complications |
| --- | --- |
| • Vascular access failure | • Bleeding |
| • Circuit clotting | • Infection (catheter related and bacteremia) |
| • Occlusion of catheter | • Hypothermia |
| • Inadequate blood flow for clearance | • Nutritional losses |
| • Tubing malfunction or separation | • Hypotension |
| • Air embolism | • Electrolyte disturbance |
| • Loss of clearance over time | |

## Infection

The risk of infection from placement of the AV access can add significantly to morbidity in a critically ill patient. In suspected sepsis, blood should be cultured from the peripheral source, as well as from the dialysis catheter, to distinguish catheter colonization from a bacteremic state.

## Hypotension

Despite the slow nature of CRRT, excessive ultrafiltration and hypotension can occur, especially if set alarms on the CRRT machines are manually overridden without addressing the underlying reason for the alarm. Hypotension is an even more important concern in small infants and neonates because excess ultrafiltration alarms in some CRRT devices are not activated unless 150 mL of fluid removal has occurred over 3 h. Therefore, such critically ill patients need heightened vigil for hypovolemia by the clinical staff.[38]

> ### KEY POINTS
>
> - Potassium phosphate 1 mmol/L provides 1.5 mol/L of potassium.
> - Potassium chloride 1 mmol/L provides 1 mol/L of potassium.

## Electrolyte disturbances

Hypokalemia and hypophosphatemia are common occurrences in CRRT, especially if the dialysate or replacement fluid has not been appropriately reconstituted. This is particularly important when CRRT is used in patients with intoxications or inborn errors of metabolism. Often, these children do not have AKI, and they can have ongoing renal excretion of potassium and phosphorus, in addition to losses encountered during CRRT, with resulting profound hypokalemia or hypophosphatemia, or both. Potassium can be added as potassium chloride or potassium phosphate in the dialysate or in the replacement fluid. Each mmol of potassium phosphate/L provides 1.5 mmol of potassium/L, whereas 1 mmol/L of potassium chloride provides 1 mmol/L of potassium.

The use of citrate anticoagulation and dextrose in the citrate infusion (ACD solution) may deliver significant amounts of glucose, thus enhancing the risk for hyperglycemia in the patient. Similar hyperglycemia can develop with the use of peritoneal dialysis solutions (Dianeal) as dialysate in CRRT.[39]

> ### KEY POINTS
>
> - Hypothermia may occur if the CRRT circuit is not supported by a blood warmer.
> - Neonates and infants are especially susceptible to hypothermia during CRRT.
> - Overriding fluid removal alarms on multiple occasions without addressing them appropriately can result in excessive ultrafiltration and hypotension.

## Hypothermia

Extracorporeal circuits can have a cooling effect on the patient, and the patient's temperature may reach the ambient temperature in the room. This is especially likely if the CRRT device lacks blood-warming capability. The warming units are often add-on appliances to the CRRT devices and need to be purchased separately. As pointed out earlier, extracorporeal cooling of blood may mask the development of a clinical fever in the critically ill patient.

## Nutritional losses

Hypermetabolism and malnutrition are common in AKI. Increased mortality and morbidity, as well as an increased length of hospital stay as a result of malnutrition, have been well established in adults.[40] Given these risks with AKI, the goals of therapy should be to maximize nutrition and to reverse the catabolic state in these patients. Optimal nutritional management of AKI in adults includes increasing the protein content while possibly providing adequate total caloric intake.[41,42] In adult patients with AKI who require CRRT, provision of 1 g/kg/day or more of protein has been associated with a trend toward a higher normalized protein catabolic rate (nPCR), and a smaller nitrogen deficit, as compared with a protein intake of less than 1 g/kg/day.[41] However, even with CRRT, it is often difficult to reverse the catabolic state in patients with AKI.[43]

Significant dialytic clearance of amino acids has been noted during CRRT, especially with the addition of dialysis. Loss of amino acids can range from 1.5% to more than 100% for some amino acids, and an even higher dialytic clearance is associated with the high ultrafiltration rate.[44] Maxvold et al.[45] compared amino acid loss and nitrogen balance in critically ill pediatric patients requiring CVVH and CVVHD who were receiving similar dialysate or replacement fluid rates and total parenteral nutrition. These investigators noted that amino acid loss was slightly greater with CVVH than with CVVHD, and these losses accounted for approximately 12% and 11% of the total daily protein intake, respectively.[45] It has been suggested that amino acid intake should be enhanced by approximately 12 g/1.73 m²/day in addition to the standard recommendation of 1.5 g/kg/day of amino acids (protein) in pediatric patients undergoing CRRT.[45]

Micronutrients also are removed by both diffusive and convective CRRT. A net negative balance of selenium, copper, and thiamine, while having a slightly positive net balance of zinc, has been shown to occur with hemodialfiltration.[46] Trace element supplementation with selenium, and possibly other micronutrients, may be necessary in situations of prolonged CRRT.

## NEONATES

The use of CRRT in the neonatal patient requires close attention to the potential for adverse events. Because of the small intravascular blood volume of these patients, careful attention must be paid to the volume status and the percentage of intravascular blood volume to be contained in the extracorporeal circuit. In order to avoid adverse events, such as hypotension, priming the CRRT circuit with blood is usually necessary in neonates and infants (also see below).

---

**KEY POINTS**

- Anaphylactic reaction to bradykinin release is a concern with hemofilters using the AN69 membrane.
- The risk is highest in neonates, in the presence of metabolic acidosis, or when using stored blood for priming the CRRT circuit.

---

## BLOOD FLOW RATE

The BFR in neonates and young infants is targeted at 5 to 10 mL/kg/min. However, this may lead to blood flow through the extracorporeal CRRT circuit that is too slow and may result in clotting of the CRRT circuit and the need for its frequent replacement. To overcome these problems, the CRRT blood flow should run at a minimum speed of 50 mL/min in neonates, regardless of body weight.

## BLOOD PRIMING AND RISK OF (AN69) MEMBRANE REACTIONS

In neonates and infants, the calculated extracorporeal blood volume of more than 10% of the patient's estimated

intravascular blood requires priming the CRRT circuit with whole blood, in order to prevent volume depletion and hypotension. Priming the circuit with normal saline or 5% albumin should be avoided because of the risk of hemodilution of the patient's hematocrit.

Serious life-threatening hyperkalemia, metabolic acidosis, and hypotension have been reported with priming of the CRRT circuits with stored unbuffered blood.[47,48] These manifestations are believed to represent a specific bioincompatibility associated with hemofilters that use the AN69 membrane. This reaction results from activation of leukocytes and release of bradykinin when stored acidemic blood comes in contact with this membrane.[47] Options to mitigate this potentially lethal side effect are as follows:

- To minimize the impact of the previously described complication, a "bypass maneuver" has been suggested. In this procedure, the patient's blood, after its first pass through the hemofilter, is discarded, while simultaneously providing a blood transfusion of packed red blood cells diluted with normal saline in a ratio of 1:1. The procedure requires placement of two three-way stopcocks on the venous return line of the extracorporeal circuit.[47] The patient's blood containing any activated leukocytes after contact with the hemofilter membrane is drained into a waste bag connected to the proximal three-way stopcock. Blood is transfused to the patient through the distal three-way stopcock. During the procedure, the CRRT device blood pump is set to a flow rate of 10 mL/min, and the packed red blood cell solution is infused at 600 to 900 mL/h (10 to 15 mL/min).[47] Buffering of the packed red blood cells to normalize the pH and neutralize the citrate content to minimize or prevent the bradykinin release has been recommended.[47]
- Buffering of the blood to improve the pH, potassium, and calcium can occur to offset some of the metabolic perturbations of blood bank blood, as listed in Table 35.8.

Table 35.8 Composition of the modified blood prime for AN69 filter

| Component | Volume |
|---|---|
| Packed red blood cells | 300 mL |
| Tris-hydroxy-methyl aminomethane (THAM) | 50 mL |
| Calcium chloride (27%) | 250 mg |
| Heparin (100 Units/mL) | 5–7 mL (500–700 units) |
| Mix equal parts with: | |
| Sterile water | 850 mL |
| Sodium bicarbonate (1 mEq/ mL) | 150 mL |

*Source:* Brophy PD, Mottes TA, Kudelka TL, et al. AN-69 membrane reactions are pH-dependent and preventable. Am J Kidney Dis. 2001;38:173–8.

- It has been reported that dialyzing the blood prime of a CRRT circuit for use in neonates has resulted in nearly physiologic correction of the metabolic acidosis and hyperkalemia commonly seen when using banked blood. The procedure is instituted by recirculation and zero-balance ultrafiltration hemodialysis of the blood prime before connecting the patient to the CRRT circuit.[49] "Z-BUF," another technique of predialysis of the priming blood, uses recirculation of blood after buffering it with 5% albumin in a ratio of 60:40.[50] Dialysate flow rate in the Z-BUF technique prime predialysis is recommended at 2 L/h, and the procedure is conducted for 30 min. Using this technique, these authors found that it nearly normalized the blood pH and serum electrolytes while having virtually no effect on tumor necrosis factor-$\alpha$, interleukin-1$\beta$, and interleukin-6 levels before and after Z-BUF.[50] A significant reduction in bradykinin in the blood prime was also noted.[50]

## OUTCOME

In one large pediatric series, survival rates of 25% and 41% were been reported in children weighing less than 3 kg and in those weighing between 3 and 10 kg, respectively.[51] Overall survival was 38%. The mean BFR in this series was 9.5 ± 4.2 mL/kg/min, and the mean duration of CRRT was 7.6 ± 8.6 days. Survivors weighing more than 3 kg required fewer vasopressor medications than did nonsurvivors, and there was no difference in outcome based on the use of convective or diffusive clearance. The clinical conditions associated with CRRT use in these patients were congenital heart diseases (16.5%), metabolic disorders (16.5%), multiple organ dysfunction syndrome (MODS) (15.3%), sepsis (14.1%), and liver failure (10.6%).

## EXTRACORPOREAL MEMBRANE OXYGENATION

Managing CRRT and extracorporeal membrane oxygenation (ECMO) requires an appreciation of the effect of shunting blood flow from the membrane oxygenator to the hemofilter. CRRT may be accomplished either with a dedicated CRRT machine (CVVHD) or by the insertion of a postpump hemofilter.

## CONTINUOUS ARTERIOVENOUS HEMOFILTRATION CIRCUIT SET-UP

A simpler form of CRRT on an ECMO circuit consists of a CAVH arrangement, using the ECMO pump itself to drive the extracorporeal circulation of blood through the CRRT

hemofilter. In this arrangement, the arterial line is placed in the postpump position, either in the preoxygenator or postoxygenator position, with the venous return line returning to the bladder.

The main concern in this procedure is uncontrolled diversion of blood to the hemofilter, resulting in a "steal" phenomenon from the ECMO circuit. The steal phenomenon can be measured by the difference in ECMO blood flow necessary to maintain the mixed central venous oxygen saturation at the same level before and immediately after diverting blood flow to the hemofilter.[52] Calculating the hemofilter blood flow in this arrangement of CRRT on an ECMO circuit can be done using the following formula:

$$\text{Patient blood flow\%} = \frac{[\text{CaO}_2(\text{postoxygenator}) - \text{CvO}_2(\text{postoxygenator})] \times 100}{[\text{CaO}_2(\text{postoxygenator}) - \text{CvO}_2(\text{Prebladder})]}$$

Hemofilter (CRRT) blood flow% = 100 − Patient blood flow%

where $\text{CaO}_2$ is the arterial oxygen content and $\text{CvO}_2$ is the mixed venous oxygen content.

### KEY POINT

The preferred sites for connecting the CRRT circuit in a patient on ECMO are the prebladder position for the arterial site and the postbladder position for the venous site.

## LOW-PRESSURE CIRCUIT SET-UP

In infants and small children, the blood flow of an ECMO circuit may not result in a steal phenomenon from the CRRT bloodlines. However, with high blood flow of the ECMO circuit in children and adolescents, the steal phenomenon from the CRRT circuit can become evident and lead to poor solute and fluid clearance in the CRRT procedure. The steal phenomenon may also lead to increased "arterial" (access) pressure and alarms in the CRRT device. Similarly, if the venous line of the CRRT device is placed in the postpump

### KEY POINTS

- Inborn errors of metabolism form an important indication for CRRT.
- For rapid correction of hyperammonemia, standard hemodialysis is preferred as the initial therapy. This can be followed by CRRT to prevent a rebound rise of plasma ammonia levels.

position of an ECMO circuit, the high blood flow may overcome the venous pressure in the CRRT circuit, result in the backflow of blood into the CRRT circuit, and cause venous pressure alarms in the CRRT device. Therefore, it is important to place both the "arterial" and "venous" lines of the CRRT in the low-flow sections of the ECMO circuit. Because of the foregoing considerations, the preferred location for placement of CRRT access is in the prebladder to the bladder position or from the bladder to the prebladder position.

## OUTCOME

The outcome of CRRT on ECMO depends more on the underlying disorder requiring treatment with ECMO than on AKI requiring CRRT. One study found that 6 of 27 patients receiving ECMO therapy developed AKI and needed CRRT. Of these patients, only 2 survived.[53] Another retrospective study, of 35 pediatric patients less than 18 years of age who were receiving CRRT with ECMO therapy, found an overall survival of 43%, with 93% of survivors recovering renal function.[54] The latter study also found that the use of vasopressors on ECMO and CRRT portended a poor outcome of patients.

## INBORN ERRORS OF METABOLISM

CRRT has been used effectively to correct metabolic derangements associated with a variety of inborn errors of metabolism. Children with a suspected or confirmed inborn error of metabolism often require extracorporeal therapy to achieve rapid correction of their metabolic disturbance. Accumulation of ammonia is the primary abnormality encountered in urea cycle disorders. In these patients, CRRT modalities can achieve excellent clearance of ammonia and rapid correction of the hyperammonemic coma.[55-63] The extracorporeal clearance of ammonia with CRRT always must be accompanied by the concomitant use of alternative pathway medications to decrease ammonia generation.

Branched-chain amino acidemias, such as maple syrup urine disease, methylmalonic acidemia, propionic acidemia, and isovaleric acidemia, have also been successfully treated using CRRT.[60] As in urea cycle disorders, CRRT provides rapid and ongoing removal of accumulated branched-chain amino acids and their ketoacid metabolites that are responsible for the neurologic sequelae of these disorders. However, hemodialysis may provide better clearance of ammonia in a shorter time and may be considered the initial therapy of choice, especially if the plasma ammonia level is very high. Following hemodialysis, CRRT may provide relief from the rebound of plasma ammonia level that is commonly noted in these patients.

## MULTIPLE ORGAN DYSFUNCTION SYNDROME

MODS is defined as a clinical condition that is characterized by simultaneous failure of two or more organ systems.[64,65] The Prospective Pediatric CRRT (ppCRRT) Registry Group described MODS as the indication in 181 of 294 pediatric patients who underwent CRRT. In this cohort, sepsis (28.7%) and cardiovascular shock (16.0%) were the most common causes of MODS. The overall survival rate from MODS requiring CRRT support was 50.8%.[66] Mean fluid overload at the time of ICU admission and the Pediatric Risk of Mortality 2 (PRISM2) score at the time of initiation of CRRT had a significant impact on survival in these patients.[66] Survival rates were better for patients who had less than 20% fluid overload (survival, 61%) at the time of initiation of CRRT when compared with a greater than 20% fluid overload (survival, 32%).[66] These data support the concepts of goal-directed fluid therapy and early initiation of CRRT in treatment of MODS.

## LIVER DISEASE

It has been well reported that coexisting liver and renal dysfunctions have a significant impact on hospital and intensive care mortality rates. The prevalence of AKI in adult patients with end-stage liver disease and cirrhosis has been estimated to be 10%–50%.[67,68] The cohort of patients with liver disease in ICUs who require RRT includes those with acute liver failure (ALF), acute decompensation of chronic liver disease, post-liver transplant renal failure, metabolic liver disease, and liver disease in patients who develop AKI as a part of multiorgan failure resulting from sepsis.

Significance of renal dysfunction in a patient with liver failure was demonstrated by the observations of du Cheyron et al.,[68] who compared a cohort of cirrhotic patients with mild and severe renal failure and those without renal failure. Patients with AKI had a hazard ratio of 4.1 for mortality, and all were associated with higher Acute Physiology and Chronic Health Evaluation (APACHE) and Sequential Organ Failure Assessment (SOFA) scores, as well as a higher crude mortality rate. The incidence of AKI in patients with ALF and acute decompensation of chronic liver disease varies from 40% to 75%. Defining the etiopathogenesis of ALF and AKI, assessing the need for detoxification therapy, and timing and dosing of CRRT are the key clinical tasks for the clinical team taking care of these patients.

The indications of CRRT in patients with ALF include AKI, metabolic abnormalities, hepatic encephalopathy (HE), the need to remove toxic metabolites resulting from hepatic dysfunction, and maintaining adequate fluid balance to ensure end-organ perfusion. Patients with ALF may have sepsis-like hyperdynamic circulation with vasoplegia and intense arterial vasodilatation resulting from release of endogenous vasodilators. Systemic vascular resistance declines, and despite an increased cardiac output, a reduction in blood pressure is common. The renal autoregulation curve is shifted to the right in these patients, thus rendering renal hemodynamics even more perfusion pressure dependent and creating the environment for development of acute tubular necrosis and AKI.

The potential for recovery of hepatic function, the small organ donor pool, and the risk of death while awaiting liver transplantation have focused clinical efforts on detoxification liver support devices as bridges to transplantation or recovery. CRRT serves several purposes in ALF: (1) treatment of the associated AKI; (2) correction of high levels of ammonia, lactate, and other metabolic disturbances associated with ALF; and (3) manipulation of fluid balance.

In the absence of any relevant data, timing of initiation of renal support in ALF is entirely determined on clinical grounds. It is recommended that CRRT be initiated early in the course of ALF, as soon as the metabolic abnormalities such as hyperammonemia, increased lactate level, metabolic acidosis, and hyponatremia develop. Hyperammonemia is a particularly important factor in deciding the timing of initiation of CRRT in patients with ALF, because it can be associated with HE and intracranial hypertension (ICH). Bernal et al.[69] evaluated the relationships of the admission arterial ammonia concentration and other clinical variables in the development of HE and ICH. Arterial ammonia level was measured on admission to the ICU in 257 patients; 165 of these had ALF and severe HE. An ammonia level greater than 100 μmol/L predicted the onset of severe HE with 70% accuracy. ICH developed in 55% of patients with ALF and an arterial ammonia level greater than 200 μmol/L. After admission, ammonia levels remained high in those patients who developed ICH and fell in those who did not. Being an independent risk factor for the development of both HE and ICH, ammonia measurements could form part of the risk stratification for HE and ICH, and in identifying patients for ammonia-lowering therapies and invasive monitoring.[68]

The presence of renal dysfunction preoperatively, hypotension during and after transplantation, the need for infusion of blood products, and the use of nephrotoxic drugs are potential risk factors for development of AKI after liver transplantation. These patients may also require CRRT support in the immediate post-liver transplant course.

Anticoagulation for CRRT in liver disease needs to be considered carefully. Because patients with ALF usually have high INR, intuitively suggesting that anticoagulation may not be necessary in CRRT. However, it is important to recall that these patients have a deficiency of both procoagulant and anticoagulant factors, and there may also be a concurrent need for blood and blood product infusions in them. Depending on the balance among these competing aspects of coagulation, patients with ALF may be in a hypercoagulable state and result in frequent CRRT circuit or hemofilter clotting. Agrawal et al.[70] retrospectively reviewed CRRT circuit life in three groups of patients with liver disease who were treated with CRRT: ALF, acute on chronic liver disease, and after elective liver transplantation, with two control groups consisting of systemic sepsis and hematologic malignant disease. The mean filter life was low in all patients with liver disease and sepsis, being 11 ± 10.5 h in ALF, 11.6 ± 6.6 h in acute on chronic liver disease, 7.4 ± 5.1 h in liver transplantation, and 9.2 ± 6.5 h in systemic sepsis. After starting anticoagulation in a select group of patients with liver disease, filter life increased from 5.6 ± 3.4 h to 13 ± 5.1 h. There was no increased bleeding or requirement for blood transfusions in the anticoagulation-treated groups. These data suggest that careful anticoagulation may help in preserving CRRT circuit life in patients with advanced liver disease.[70]

## MALIGNANT DISEASE

Tumor lysis syndrome (TLS), characterized by rapid destruction of a large solid tumor or white blood cell burden by chemotherapeutic agents, results in hyperuricemia, hyperkalemia, and hyperphosphatemia with associated hypocalcemia. CRRT has been demonstrated to normalize serum uric acid, potassium, and phosphorus levels in children at risk for development of tumor lysis syndrome.[71]

Another significant oncologic population at risk for development of AKI is the hematopoietic cell transplant recipient. It is estimated that 25% of children with hemopoetic cell malignancies develop TLS after initiation of therapy.[72] The incidence of AKI in these patients, defined as a doubling of the serum creatinine, is reported to be 25% to 50%.[73] The ppCRRT Registry Group reported on the outcomes of 44 pediatric bone marrow transplantation recipients who required CRRT.[12] Overall patient survival to ICU discharge was 40%, with a trend toward improved survival from 2003 to 2004 in the ppCRRT registry (36% and 44%, respectively). In this retrospective cohort study, mean airway pressure at the termination of CRRT was significantly greater (26.06 ± 2.02 vs. 8.44 ± 2.69 mm Hg) in the nonsurvivors compared with survivors. In this analysis, the percentage of fluid overload did not discriminate between survivors and nonsurvivors. The role of CRRT in the management of bone marrow transplant recipients with acute respiratory distress syndrome (ARDS) has been investigated by DiCarlo et al.,[74] who initiated CRRT concomitantly with intubation for ARDS in 6 pediatric bone marrow transplant recipients. These authors achieved a high rate of clearance (50 mL/min/1.73 m²) by performing hemofiltration with a replacement solution at 1800 mL/h and dialysis with a countercurrent dialysate solution at 1800 mL/h (termed as high efficiency CRRT). Eighty percent of these patients survived to hospital discharge with recovery of their native renal function. These findings suggest that early and aggressive use of CRRT in a bid to normalize fluid balance and use of high efficiency CRRT may be important in improving survival of hematopoietic cell transplant recipients who develop either AKI or ARDS.

## HYPEROSMOLAR STATES

Hyperosmolar disorders secondary to hypernatremia have been associated with a mortality rate of up to 70% in pediatric patients.[75] Slow correction of hyperosmolality using CRRT and hypertonic dialysate or replacement fluid has been advocated.[5]

## INTOXICATIONS AND POISONINGS

The ability of extracorporeal therapies to remove an intoxicant is affected by the volume of distribution of the drug. Generally, drugs with volumes of distribution of less than 1 L/kg (total body water) are amenable to dialytic removal.[76] Drugs with large volumes of distribution are less likely to be effectively removed by dialysis, and they are more likely to result in rebound elevations of blood levels following dialytic therapy. High-molecular-weight drugs are also more difficult to dialyze than are low-molecular-weight drugs. High-efficiency hemofilters can overcome this size barrier, to some extent. The degree of protein binding has a negative effect on a drug's dialyzability. However, if protein-binding sites are fully saturated, free drug may be amenable to dialytic clearance.

Numerous medications have been described as being cleared by CRRT. Although an extensive listing of all drugs removed by CRRT is beyond the scope of this chapter, some of the common drugs that can be removed include vancomycin, lithium, ethylene glycol, procainamide, theophylline, methotrexate, phenytoin, carbamazepine, and valproic acid.[77-86]

Use of albumin dialysis has been reported to aid in the removal of highly protein-bound drugs. Askenazi et al.[86] described the use of albumin dialysis using CVVHD to treat an acute, severe carbamazepine overdose. These investigators found a dramatic decrease in the serum half-life of carbamazepine (from 25 to 60 h to 7 to 8 h) by using albumin-dialysis CVVHD.[76] Phenytoin and valproic acid removal has been reported to be enhanced with albumin dialysis, compared with standard high-efficiency CVVHD.[85,87]

## COMBINED CONTINUOUS RENAL REPLACEMENT THERAPY AND PLASMAPHERESIS

The combination of plasmapheresis and CRRT may be occasionally performed in the management of immune-mediated diseases complicated by AKI. In most instances, however, CRRT is discontinued during plasmapheresis and is resumed after the completion of the plasmapheresis. Stopping CRRT may cause citrate accumulation during plasmapheresis, thus leading to hypocalcemia, and it also poses a risk for hemodynamic instability.[88]

Yorgin et al.[89] described the use of concurrent plasmapheresis and CRRT in the treatment of a 14-year-old girl with leukemia. In this instance, the investigators placed a three-way stopcock at both the arterial and venous sides of the double-lumen dialysis catheter.[89] The three-way stopcocks allowed for parallel flow of the arterial blood through both the centrifugation plasmapheresis circuit and the CRRT circuit and parallel return of venous blood flow back to the patient. Alternately, in an in-series configuration, the plasmapheresis circuit draws the patient's blood from the arterial side of the double-lumen catheter, and the plasmapheresis in-port is connected to the venous line of the CRRT circuit. The patient's blood is returned through the venous return line of the plasmapheresis circuit. With this technique, citrate anticoagulation used in the plasmapheresis circuit can then undergo high dialytic clearance.

## OUTCOME

Experience in using concurrent centrifugation plasmapheresis and CRRT is limited. Ponkivar et al.[90] reported the use of this approach in 21 neonates and infants. These authors found that recovery of renal function occurred in 47.6% of patients, with an overall patient survival rate of 42.9%. Complications of concurrent therapy include hemofilter thrombosis, catheter malfunction, hypotension and bradycardia, and pulmonary edema.[90]

## SINGLE-PASS ALBUMIN DIALYSIS

The molecular adsorbent recirculation system (MARS) is an evolving technology for treatment of fulminant liver failure.[91] A meta-analysis of the published literature by Vaid et al.[92] suggested that MARS therapy leads to a significant decrease in the serum bilirubin concentration and West Haven grade of HE. Overall mortality, however, remained unchanged in this analysis. MARS is recommended as a bridge to orthotopic liver transplantation in patients with fulminant liver failure.

Because of the complexity and cost of the MARS circuit, efforts to adopt current CRRT machines to support patients with ALF have been considered. The use of CRRT for this purpose is known as single-pass albumin dialysis (SPAD). The purpose of this therapy is to provide dialytic clearance of protein-bound inflammatory mediators or toxins

Table 35.9 Survival in continuous renal replacement therapy by primary diagnosis

| Clinical parameter | n | Survivors | % Survival |
|---|---|---|---|
| Sepsis | 81 | 48 | 59 |
| Bone marrow transplant | 55 | 25 | 45 |
| Cardiac disease or transplant | 41 | 21 | 51 |
| Renal disease | 32 | 27 | 84 |
| Liver disease or transplant | 29 | 9 | 31 |
| Malignant disease (no tumor lysis syndrome) | 29 | 14 | 48 |
| Ischemia/shock | 19 | 13 | 68 |
| Inborn error of metabolism | 15 | 11 | 73 |
| Drug intoxication | 13 | 13 | 100 |
| Tumor lysis syndrome | 12 | 10 | 83 |
| Pulmonary disease/transplant | 11 | 5 | 45 |
| Other | 7 | 5 | 71 |

Source: Symons JM, Chua AN, Somers MJ, et al. Demographic characteristics of pediatric continuous renal replacement therapy: a report of the Prospective Pediatric Continuous Renal Replacement Therapy Registry. Clin J Am Soc Nephrol.2007;2:732–8.

associated with ALF. In contrast to MARS, SPAD does not involve regeneration of the albumin dialysate, thus resulting in a single-pass of the albumin dialysate, which is then discarded.

In a retrospective analysis, Kortgen et al.[93] demonstrated that MARS and SPAD were comparable in biochemical improvement scores, the need for blood transfusions, overall health score, and mortality rates. Saur et al.[94] evaluated the in vitro clearance of bilirubin, ammonia, and bile acids by using MARS, SPAD, and CVVHDF. Clearance of bile acids was equal with MARS and SPAD, but the clearance of bilirubin was better with SPAD than with MARS. There was no difference in ammonia clearance among MARS, SPAD, and CVVHDF.[94] Ringe et al.[95] retrospectively analyzed data in nine patients with ALF who were treated with SPAD as a bridge to transplantation or as a detoxification method. These investigators found SPAD to be well tolerated and an effective detoxification mechanism in ALF, and it bridged 75% of patients successfully to transplantation. Most of these patients had a very low probability of survival by both Pediatric Index of Mortality 2 (PIM2) and Pediatric End-Stage Liver Disease (PELD) scoring.[95]

In vivo use of SPAD has been reported in case reports and case series to treat ALF secondary to Wilson disease and acute hepatitis.[96,97] Kreymann et al.[96] used a 44 g/L (4.4%) albumin dialysate solution by replacing 1 L of a 4.5-L bicarbonate-based dialysate with 20% albumin. CRRT was performed as CVVHDF, without apparent modification from the standard protocol. These authors found significant clearance of copper and total bilirubin, with a resultant improvement in the patient's HE and electroencephalogram. Collins et al.[97] reported on the use of SPAD in an adolescent girl with ALF secondary to Wilson disease who was bridged successfully to orthotopic liver transplantation. These authors used 5% albumin added to a bicarbonate-based dialysate and ran the dialysate at 1 to 2 L/h of flow.

This patient experienced a reduction in her transfusion requirements, serum copper concentrations, and conjugated bilirubin and improvements in her renal function and HE. Chawla et al.[98] compared bilirubin clearance by using both 1.85% and 5.0% albumin dialysate and found improved total bilirubin clearance using the 5.0% albumin concentration. It appears that a 5% (50 g/L) albumin concentration provides the best clearance in SPAD. Specific cautions in the use of SPAD include the potential for hypernatremia secondary to high sodium content in the commercially available albumin solution. Prevention of hypernatremia may require a custom-made dialysis solution with a reduced sodium chloride concentration.

## PROGNOSTIC FACTORS

Early single-center reports of outcome following CRRT in pediatric patients found an overall survival rate of only 42%.[99] In a retrospective study, Goldstein et al.[100] reported results in 21 pediatric patients receiving CRRT; these investigators took into account the patient's severity of illness score by using the PRISM2 score. They identified the percentage of fluid overload as a predictor of mortality, after controlling for severity of illness. The ppCRRT registry, reporting on 273 pediatric patients, found an overall survival rate of 58%. Patients with hepatic failure or a hepatic transplant had the lowest survival rate (37%), and those with drug intoxication had the highest survival rate (100%).[101] In the ppCRRT analysis, mortality rates in patients weighing less than 10 kg were significantly higher (64%) than in patients with more than 10 kg body weight (43%, P <0.001).[102] Some European studies have demonstrated lower mortality rates with CRRT (36% to 39%) than the ppCRRT data.[103,104] Table 35.9 lists survival by primary disease indication for CRRT.

## SUMMARY

CRRT has evolved since the 1980s as an efficient and safe treatment for AKI in both adult and pediatric patients. Newer dialysate and replacement fluid solutions are available, and now one can safely use bicarbonate as the buffer to minimize cardiovascular instability, as well as to minimize the possibility of confounding the serum lactic acid levels. Anticoagulation for maintenance of the CRRT circuit is critical to providing adequate fluid and electrolyte therapy in the pediatric patient with AKI, and citrate anticoagulation appears to have multiple benefits over heparin anticoagulation. Prostacyclin is an emerging anticoagulant with great promise. Vascular access is critical for proper functioning of a CRRT circuit, and ideally it should use the largest catheter possible. Finally, CRRT may be a useful therapy in other clinical conditions, such as hyperosmolality, intoxications, hematopoietic cell transplantation, tumor lysis syndrome prevention, extracorporeal hepatic support, and plasmapheresis.

## REFERENCES

1. Haq NU, Nolph KD. Past, present, and future of quantified peritoneal dialysis. Semin Dial. 2001;14:263-7.
2. Van Stone JC. Dialysis equipment and dialysate, past, present and the future. Semin Nephrol. 1997;17:214-7.
3. Merrill JP. The use of the artificial kidney in the treatment of uremia. J Urban Health. 1998;75:911-18.
4. Kramer P, Schrader J, Bohnsack W, et al. Continuous arteriovenous haemofiltration: A new kidney replacement therapy. Proc Eur Dial Transplant Assoc. 1981;18:743–9.
5. Maxvold NJ, Bunchman TE. Renal failure and replacement therapy. Crit Care Clin. 2003;19:563-75.
6. Kramer P, Wigger W, Rieger J, et al. Arteriovenous haemofiltration: A new and simple method for treatment of over-hydrated patients resistant to diuretics. Klin Wochenschr .1977;55:1121-2.
7. Bellomo R, Ronco C. An introduction to continuous renal replacement therapy. In: Bellomo R, Baldwin I, Ronco C, Golper T, editors. Atlas of Hemofiltration. Philadelphia: Saunders; 2001. p. 1–9.
8. Forni LG, Hilton PJ. Continuous hemofiltration in the treatment of acute renal failure. N Engl J Med. 1997;336:1303-9.
9. Lebedo I. Principles and practice of hemofiltration and hemodiafiltration. Artif Organs. 1998;22:20-5.
10. Parakininkas D, Greenberg LA. Comparison of solute clearance in three modes of continuous renal replacement therapy. Pediatr Crit Care Med. 2004;5:269-74.
11. Jenkins R, Harrison H, Chen B, et al. Accuracy of intravenous infusion pumps in continuous renal replacement therapies. ASAIO J. 1992;38:808-10.
12. Flores FX, Brophy PD, Symons JM, et al. CRRT after stem cell transplantation: A report from the Prospective Pediatric CRRT Registry Group. Pediatr Nephrol. 2008;23:625–63.
13. Hackbarth R, Bunchman TW, Chua AN, et al. The effect of vascular access location and size on circuit survival in pediatric continuous renal replacement therapy: A report from the PPCRRT registry. Int J Artif Organs. 2007;12:1116–21.
14. Davenport A, Aulton K, Payne PB, et al. Hyperlactatemia and increasing metabolic acidosis due to the use of lactate based fluid during haemofiltration. Intensive Care Med. 1989;15:546-7.
15. Davenport A, Will EJ, Davison AM. The effect of lactate-buffered solutions on the acid-base status of patients with renal failure. Nephrol Dial Transplant. 1989;4:800-4.
16. Davenport A, Aulton K, Payne RB, et al. Hyperlactatemia and increasing metabolic acidosis in hepatorenal failure treated by hemofiltration. Ren Fail. 1990;12:99-101.
17. Davenport A, Will EJ, Davison AM. Hyperlactataemia and metabolic acidosis during haemofiltration using lactate-buffered fluids. Nephron. 1991;59:461-5.
18. Thomas AN, Guy JM, Kishen R, et al. Comparison of lactate and bicarbonate buffered haemofiltration fluids: Use in critically ill patients. Nephrol Dial Transplant. 1997;12:1212-7.
19. Zimmerman D, Cotman P, Ting R, et al. Continuous veno-venous haemodialysis with a novel bicarbonate dialysis solution: Prospective cross-over comparison with a lactate buffered solution. Nephrol Dial Transplant. 1999;14:2387-91.
20. Maxvold NJ, Flynn JT, Smoyer WE, et al. Prospective, crossover comparison of bicarbonate vs lactate-based dialysate for pediatric CVVHD. Blood Purif. 1999;17:27 (abstract).
21. Barenbrock M, Hausberg M, Matzkies F, et al. Effects of bicarbonate- and lactate-buffered replacement fluids on cardiovascular outcome in CVVH patients. Kidney Int. 2000;58:1751-7.
22. McLean AG, Davenport A, Cox D, et al. Effects of lactate-buffered and lactate-free dialysate in CAVHD patients with and without liver dysfunction. Kidney Int. 2000;58:1765-72.
23. Bunchman TE, Maxvold NJ, Barnett J, et al. Pediatric hemofiltration: Normocarb® dialysate solution with citrate anticoagulation. Pediatr Nephrol. 2002;17:150-4.
24. Bunchman TE, Maxvold NJ, Brophy PD. Pediatric convective hemofiltration (CVVH): Normocarb replacement fluid and citrate anticoagulation. Am J Kidney Dis. 2003;42:1248-52.

25. Karvellas CJ, Farhat MR, Sajjad I, et al. A comparison of early versus late initiation of renal replacement therapy in critically ill patients with acute kidney injury: A systematic review and meta-analysis. Crit Care. 2011;15:R72. doi:10.1186/cc10061

26. Bouman CS, Oudemans-Van Straaten HM, Tijssen JG, et al. Effects of early high-volume continuous venovenous hemofiltration on survival and recovery of renal function in intensive care patients with acute renal failure: A prospective, randomized trial. Crit Care Med. 2002;30:2205–11.

27. Bai M, Zhou M, He L, et al. Citrate versus heparin anticoagulation for continuous renal replacement therapy: An updated meta-analysis of RCTs. Intensive Care Med. 2015;41:2098-110.

28. O'Shea SI, Oftel TL, Kovalik EC. Alternative methods of anticoagulation for dialysis-dependent patients with heparin-induced thrombocytopenia. Semin Dial. 2003;16:61-7.

29. Mehta RL, McDonald BR, Aguilar MM, et al. Regional citrate anticoagulation for continuous arteriovenous hemodialysis in critically ill patients. Kidney Int. 1990;38:976-81.

30. Chadha V, Garg U, Warady BA, et al. Citrate clearance in children receiving continuous venovenous renal replacement therapy. Pediatr Nephrol. 2002;17:819-24.

31. Meier-Kriesche HU, Gitomer J, Finkel K, et al. Increased total to ionized calcium ratio during continuous venovenous hemodialysis with regional citrate anticoagulation. Crit Care Med. 2001;29:748-52.

32. Monchi M, Berghams D, Ledoux D, et al. Citrate vs. heparin for anticoagulation in continuous venovenous hemofiltration: A prospective randomized study. Intensive Care Med. 2004;30:260-5.

33. Brophy PD, Somers MJG, Baum MA, et al. Multicentre evaluation of anticoagulation in patients receiving continuous renal replacement therapy (CRRT). Nephrol Dial Transplant. 2005;20:1416–21.

34. Gainza FJ, Quintanilla N, Pijoan JI, et al. Role of prostacyclin (epoprostenol) as anticoagulant in continuous renal replacement therapies: Efficacy, safety and cost analysis. J Nephrol. 2006;19:648–55.

35. Arcangeli A, Rocca B, Salvatori G, et al. Heparin versus prostacyclin in continuous hemodiafiltration for acute renal failure: Effects on platelet function in the systemic circulation and across the filter. Thromb Res. 2010;126:24–31.

36. Balik M, Waldauf P, Plasil P, et al. Prostacyclin versus citrate in continuous hemodiafiltration: An observational study in patients with high risk of bleeding. Blood Purif. 2005;23:325–29.

37. Venkataraman R, Kellum JA, Palevsky P. Dosing patterns for continuous renal replacement therapy at a large academic medical center in the United States. J Crit Care 2002;17:246-250.

38. Ronco C. Fluid balance in CRRT: A call to attention! Int J Artif Organs. 2005;28:763-4.

39. Soysal DD, Karaböcüoğlu M, Citak A, et al. Metabolic disturbances following the use of inadequate solutions for hemofiltration in acute renal failure. Pediatr Nephrol. 2007;22: 715-9.

40. Fiaccadori E, Lombardi M, Leonardi, et al. Prevalence and clinical outcomes associated with preexisting malnutrition in acute renal failure: A prospective cohort study. J Am Soc Nephrol. 1999;10:581-93.

41. Macias WL, Alaka KJ, Murphy MH, et al. Impact of the nutritional regimen on protein catabolism and nitrogen balance in patients with acute renal failure. JPEN J Parenter Enteral Nutr. 1996;20:56-62.

42. Kopple JD. The nutrition management of the patient with acute renal failure. J Parenter Enteral Nutr. 1996;20:3-12.

43. Chima CS, Meyer L, Hummell AC, et al. Protein catabolic rate in patients with acute renal failure on continuous arteriovenous hemofiltration and total parenteral nutrition. J Am Soc Nephrol. 1993;3:1516-21.

44. Davies SP, Reaveley DA, Brown EA, et al. Amino acid clearance and daily losses in patients with acute renal failure treated by continuous arteriovenous hemodialysis. Crit Care Med. 1991;19:1510-5.

45. Maxvold NJ, Smoyer WE, Custer JR, et al. Amino acid loss and nitrogen balance in critically ill children with acute renal failure: A prospective comparison between classic hemofiltration and hemofiltration with dialysis. Crit Care Med. 2000;28:1161-5.

46. Berger MM, Shenkin A, Revelly JP, et al. Copper, selenium, zinc, and thiamine balances during continuous venovenous hemodiafiltration in critically ill patients. Am J Clin Nutr. 2004;80:410-6.

47. Brophy PD, Mottes TA, Kudelka TL, et al. AN-69 membrane reactions are pH-dependent and preventable. Am J Kidney Dis. 2001;38:173-8.

48. Parshuram CS, Cox PN. Neonatal hyperkalemic-hypocalcemic cardiac arrest associated with initiation of blood-primed continuous venovenous hemofiltration. Pediatr Crit Care Med. 2002;3:67-9.

49. Pasko DA, Mottes TA, Mueller BA. Pre dialysis of blood prime in continuous hemodialysis normalizes pH and electrolytes. Pediatr Nephrol. 2003;18:1177-83.

50. Hackbarth RM, Eding D, Smith CG, et al. Zero-balance ultrafiltration (Z-BUF) in blood-primed CRRT circuits achieves electrolyte and acid-base homeostasis prior to patient connection. Pediatr Nephrol. 2005;20:1328-33.

51. Symons JM, Brophy PD, Gregory MJ, et al. Continuous renal replacement therapy in children up to 10 kg. Am J Kidney Dis. 2003;41:984-9.

52. Smoyer WE, Maxvold NJ, Remenapp RT, et al. Pediatric renal replacement therapy. In: Fuhrman BP, Zimmerman JJ, editors. Pediatric Critical Care, 2nd ed. St. Louis: Mosby–Year Book; 1998. p. 767.

53. Sell LL, Cullen ML, Whittlesey GC, et al. Experience with renal failure during extracorporeal membrane oxygenation: Treatment with continuous hemofiltration. J Pediatr Surg. 1987;22:600-2.
54. Meyer RJ, Brophy PD, Bunchman TE, et al. Survival and renal function in pediatric patients following extracorporeal life support with hemofiltration. Pediatr Crit Care Med. 2001;2:238-42.
55. Braun MC, Welch TR. Continuous venovenous hemodiafiltration in the treatment of acute hyperammonemia. Am J Nephrol. 1998;18:531-3.
56. Sperl W, Geiger R, Maurer H, et al. Continuous arteriovenous haemofiltration in hyperammonemia of newborn babies. Lancet. 1990;336:1192-3.
57. Sperl W, Geiger R, Maurer H, et al. Continuous arteriovenous haemofiltration in a neonate with hyperammonaemic coma due to citrullinaemia. J Inherit Metab Dis. 1992;15:158-9.
58. Thompson GN, Butt WW, Shann FA, et al. Continuous venovenous hemofiltration in the management of acute decompensation in inborn errors of metabolism. J Pediatr. 1991;118:879-84.
59. Jouvet P, Poggi F, Rabier D, et al. Continuous venovenous haemodiafiltration in the acute phase of neonatal maple syrup urine disease. J Inherit Metab Dis. 1997;20:463-72.
60. Falk MC, Knight JF, Roy LP, et al. Continuous venovenous haemofiltration in the acute treatment of inborn errors of metabolism. Pediatr Nephrol. 1994;8:330-3.
61. Wong KY, Wong SN, Lam SY, et al. Ammonia clearance by peritoneal dialysis and continuous arteriovenous hemodiafiltration. Pediatr Nephrol. 1998;12:589-91.
62. Picca S, Dionisi-Vici C, Abeni D, et al. Extracorporeal dialysis in neonatal hyperammonemia: Modalities and prognostic indicators. Pediatr Nephrol. 2001;16:862-7.
63. Deodato F, Boenzi S, Rizzo C, et al. Inborn errors of metabolism: An update on epidemiology and on neonatal-onset hyperammonemia. Acta Paediatr Suppl. 2004;93:18-21.
64. Beal AL, Cerra FB. Multiple organ failure syndrome in the 1990s. JAMA. 1994;271:226-33.
65. Proulx F, Fayon M, Farrell CA, et al. Epidemiology of sepsis and multiple organ dysfunction syndrome in children. Chest. 1996;109:1033-7.
66. Goldstein SL, Somers MJ, Baum MA, et al. Pediatric patients with multi-organ dysfunction syndrome receiving continuous renal replacement therapy. Kidney Int. 2005;67:653-8.
67. Russ KB, Stevens TM, Singal AK. Acute Kidney Injury in Patients with Cirrhosis. J Clin Transl Hepatol. 2015;3:195-204.
68. du Cheyron D, Bouchet B, Parienti JJ, et al. The attributable mortality of acute renal failure in critically ill patients with liver cirrhosis. Intensive Care Med. 2005;31:1693-9.
69. Bernal W, Hall C, Karvellas CJ, et al. Arterial ammonia and clinical risk factors for encephalopathy and intracranial hypertension in acute liver failure. Hepatology. 2007;46:1844-52.
70. Agarwal B, Shaw S, Shankar Hari M, et al. Continuous renal replacement therapy (CRRT) in patients with liver disease: Is circuit life different? J Hepatol. 2009;51:504-9.
71. Saccente SL, Kohaut EC, Berkow RL. Prevention of tumor lysis syndrome using continuous veno-venous hemofiltration. Pediatr Nephrol. 1995;9:569-73.
72 Wilson FP, Berns JS. Tumor lysis syndrome: New challenges and recent advances. Adv Chronic Kidney Dis. 2014;21 :18-26.
73. Hingorani SR, Guthrie K, Batchelder A, et al. Acute renal failure after myeloablative hematopoietic cell transplant: Incidence and risk factors. Kidney Int. 2005;67:272-7.
74. DiCarlo JV, Alexander SR, Agarwal R, et al. Continuous veno-venous hemofiltration may improve survival from acute respiratory distress syndrome after bone marrow transplantation or chemotherapy. J Pediatr Hematol Oncol. 2003;25:801-5.
75. McBryde KD, Bunchman TE, Kudelka TL, et al. Hyperosmolar solutions in continuous renal replacement therapy for hyperosmolar acute renal failure: A preliminary report. Pediatr Crit Care Med. 2005;6:220-5.
76. Borkan SC. Extracorporeal therapies for acute intoxications. Crit Care Clin. 2002;18:393-40.
77. Mokhlesi B. Leikin JB, Murray P, et al. Adult toxicology in critical care. Part I. General approach to the intoxicated patient. Chest. 2003;123:577-92.
78. Mokhlesi B. Leikin JB, Murray P, et al. Adult toxicology in critical care. Part II. Specific poisonings. Chest. 2003;123:897-922.
79. Goebel J, Ananth M, Lewy JE. Hemodiafiltration for vancomycin overdose in a neonate with end-stage renal failure. Pediatr Nephrol. 1999;13:423-5.
80. Meyer RJ, Flynn JT, Brophy PD, et al. Hemodialysis followed by continuous hemofiltration for treatment of lithium intoxication in children. Am J Kidney Dis. 2001;37:1044-7.
81. Christiansson LK, Kaspersson KE, Kulling PE, et al. Treatment of severe ethylene glycol intoxication with continuous arteriovenous hemofiltration dialysis. J Toxicol Clin Toxicol. 1995;33:267-70.
82. Domoto DT, Brown WW, Bruggensmith P. Removal of toxic levels of N-acetylprocainamide with continuous arteriovenous hemofiltration or continuous arteriovenous hemodiafiltration. Ann Intern Med. 1987;106:550-2.
83. Okada S, Teramoto S, Matsuoka R. Recovery from theophylline toxicity by continuous hemodialysis with filtration. Ann Intern Med. 2000;133:922.

84. Vilay AM, Mueller BA, Haines H, et al. Treatment of methotrexate intoxication with various modalities of continuous extracorporeal therapy and glucarpidase. Pharmacotherapy. 2010;30:111.

85. Jalan R, Sen S. Extracorporeal albumin dialysis for intoxication from protein-bound agents. Crit Care Med. 2004. 32:1436-7.

86. Askenazi DJ, Goldstein SL, Chang IF, et al. Management of a severe carbamazepine overdose using albumin-enhanced continuous venovenous hemodialysis. Pediatrics. 2004;113:406-9.

87. Churchwell MD, Pasko DA, Smoyer W, et al. Enhanced clearance of highly protein-bound drugs by albumin-supplemented dialysate during modeled continuous hemodialysis. Nephrol Dial Transplant. 2009;24:231–38.

88. Bunchman TE. Plasmapheresis and renal replacement therapy in children. Curr Opin Pediatr. 2002;14:310-4.

89. Yorgin PD, Eklund DK, Al-Uzri A, et al. Concurrent centrifugation plasmapheresis and continuous venovenous hemodiafiltration. Pediatr Nephrol. 2000;14:18-21.

90. Ponikvar R, Kandus A, Urbančič A, et al. Continuous renal replacement therapy and plasma exchange in newborns and infants. Artif Organs. 2002;26:163-8.

91. Lexmond WS, Van Dael CM, Scheenstra R, et al. Experience with molecular adsorbent recirculating system treatment in 20 children listed for high-urgency liver transplantation. Liver Transpl. 2015; 21:369-80.

92. Vaid A, Chweich H, Balk EM, et al. Molecular adsorbent recirculating system as artificial support therapy for liver failure: A meta-analysis. ASAIO J. 2012;58:51–9.

93. Kortgen A, Rauchfuss F, Götz M, et al. Albumin dialysis in liver failure: Comparison of molecular adsorbent recirculating system and single pass albumin dialysis-a retrospective analysis. Ther Apher Dial. 2009;13:419–25.

94. Sauer IM, Goetz M, Steffen I, et al. In vitro comparison of the molecular adsorbent recirculation system (MARS) and single-pass albumin dialysis (SPAD). Hepatology. 2004;39:1408–14.

95. Ringe H, Varnholt V, Zimmering M, et al. Continuous veno-venous single-pass albumin hemodiafiltration in children with acute liver failure. Pediatr Crit Care Med. 2011;12:257–64.

96. Kreymann B, Seige M, Schweigart U, et al. Albumin dialysis: Effective removal of copper in a patient with fulminant Wilson disease and successful bridging to liver transplantation. A new possibility for the elimination of protein-bound toxins. J Hepatol. 1999;31:1080-5.

97. Collins KL, Roberts EA, Adeli K, et al. Single pass albumin dialysis (SPAD) in fulminant wilsonian liver failure: A case report. Pediatr Nephrol. 2008;23:1013–16.

98. Chawla LS, Georgescu F, Abell B, S et al. Modification of continuous venovenous hemodiafiltration with single-pass albumin dialysate allows for removal of serum bilirubin. Am J Kidney Dis. 2005;45:e51–6.

99. Smoyer WE, McAdams C, Kaplan BS, et al. Determinants of survival in pediatric continuous hemofiltration. J Am Soc Nephrol. 1995;6:1401-9.

100. Goldstein SL, Currier H, Graf JM, et al. Outcomes in children receiving continuous venovenous hemofiltration. Pediatrics. 2001;107:1309-12.

101. Symons JM, Chua AN, Somers MJG, et al. Demographic characteristics of pediatric continuous renal replacement therapy: A report of the Prospective Pediatric Continuous Renal Replacement Therapy Registry. Clin J Am Soc Nephrol. 2007;2:732–8.

102. Askenazi DJ, Goldstein SL, Koralkar R, et al. Continuous renal replacement therapy for children ≤10 kg: A report from the Prospective Pediatric Continuous Renal Replacement Therapy Registry. J Pediatr. 2013;162:587–92.

103. López-Herce J, Santiago MJ, Solana MJ, et al. Clinical course of children requiring prolonged continuous renal replacement therapy. Pediatr Nephrol. 2010;25:523–28.

104. Pedersen O, Jepsen SB, and Toft P. Continuous renal replacement therapy for critically ill infants and children. Dan Med J. 2012;59:A4385.

## REVIEW QUESTIONS

## CASE 1

A 6-year-old, 20-kg child with leukemia during induction develops Gram-negative septic shock with multiorgan system failure. The child is intubated on 70% $FIO_2$ and a PEEP of 10 cm. The child is oliguric and is 18% fluid overloaded. The child's laboratory tests include the following: sodium, 140 mmol/L; potassium, 6.9 mmol/L; chloride, 105 mmol/L; bicarbonate, 14 mmol/L; BUN, 100 mg/dL; and lactate, 4.5 mmol/L. A recent ABG showed: pH, 7.23; $pAO_2$ of 90; and $pCO_2$ of 43. The child is receiving norepinephrine for maintaining hemodynamic stability. Current blood pressure is 90/60 mm Hg. The child is to be placed on CRRT.

1. Optimal size and site of placement of the vascular access is:
   a. 11-Fr dual-lumen catheter in subclavian vein.
   b. 8- or 9-Fr dual-lumen catheter in right internal jugular vein

c. 8- or 9-Fr dual-lumen catheter in femoral vein

d. 11-Fr dual-lumen catheter in femoral vein

2. Use of AN 69 membrane based hemofilter in this patient may be associated with the risk of:
   a. Hemofilter clotting more frequently
   b. Poor clearance, if used in convective mode
   c. Anaphylaxis
   d. AN69 membrane has less clinical risk than polysulfone membrane

3. If AN69 membrane hemofilter is used in CRRT, blood prime should be avoided in this patient due to presence of metabolic acidosis and enhanced risk of anaphylaxis.
   a. True
   b. False

4. To allow *optimal* functioning of CRRT, the ideal arterial and venous pressures (as noted on the CRRT monitors) should be:
   a. Greater than 50 mm and less than 400 mm
   b. Greater than −50 mm and less than −400 mm
   c. Greater than −150 mm and less than 200 mm
   d. Greater than −150 mm and less than −200 mm

5. In this septic patient, the *best* modality of CRRT is:
   a. Diffusive method (CVVHD)
   b. Convective method (CVVH)
   c. Slow continuous ultrafiltration (SCUF)
   d. Both convestive and diffusive methods (CVVHDF)

6. Small molecular solutes are removed equally well by convection and diffusion.
   a. True
   b. False

7. To optimize solute clearance, the *optimal* total volume of dialysate and replacement fluid (if using CVVHDF) is:
   a. 2000 mL/h/1.73 m²
   b. 35 mL/kg/h
   c. Either a or b
   d. Neither a nor b

8. Target net fluid ultrafiltration rate to be ordered should be:
   a. 10 mL/h
   b. 1 to 2 mL/kg/h
   c. 10 mL/kg/h
   d. 25 mL/kg/h

## CASE 2

A 14-year-old female patient is admitted with new-onset AKI, oliguria, hyperkalemia, IDDM, dehydration. Her laboratory tests show: serum sodium, 175 mmol/L (uncorrected); glucose, 1300 mg/dL; and BUN, 90 mg/dL.

1. What is this patient's calculated serum osmolality (mOsm/L)?
   a. 280
   b. 380
   c. 480
   d. 542

2. Osmolality (mOsm/L) of the peritoneal dialysate (PD), 1.5% dextrose, low-calcium solution is:
   a. 280
   b. 300
   c. 320
   d. 344

3. Osmolality (mOsm/L) of hemodialysis dialysate is:
   a. 280
   b. 300
   c. 320
   d. 340

4. Osmolality (mOsm/L) of dialysate used in CRRT is:
   a. 280
   b. 300
   c. 320
   d. 340

## CASE 3

A 16-year-old male patient is admitted to the intensive care unit with multimedication overdose. He has AKI and oliguria. He is unresponsive and but is hemodynamically stable. No seizures have been noted. If started on CRRT,

1. The *most important* factor(s) in determining drug clearance is(are):
   a. Protein binding
   b. Molecular weight
   c. Volume of distribution
   d. All of the above

2. The *preferred* form of renal replacement therapy (RRT) in this case is:
   a. PD
   b. CRRT convective
   c. CRRT diffusive
   d. CRRT convective and diffusive
   e. HD standard
   f. HD sigh flux

## CASE 4

A 3-day-old male newborn infant is admitted to the intensive care unit with somnolence, refusal to feed for 2 days, and twitching of the face today. The child weighs 2.9 kg (240 mL intravascular blood volume). Serum electrolytes show: sodium, 140 mmol/L; potassium, 5 mmol/L;, $CO_2$ 14 mmol/L; and arterial blood pH, 7.02. Ammonia level was 1500 µmol/L.

1. The *best* type of renal replacement therapy (RRT) that will lower ammonia most rapidly is:
   a. PD
   b. CRRT
   c. Hemodialysis, standard
   d. Hemodialysis, high flux

## ANSWER KEY

## CASE 1

1. b
2. c
3. a
4. c
5. b
6. a
7. c
8. b

## CASE 2

1. c
2. d
3. a
4. a

## CASE 3

1. d
2. f

## CASE 4

1. c

# Hemodialysis

RAJ MUNSHI AND JORDAN M. SYMONS

Hemodialysis is the most efficient method of artificial renal support. It accomplishes molecular transfer at much higher rates than either peritoneal dialysis (PD) or continuous renal replacement therapy (CRRT). Hemodialysis is highly effective in short-term settings for management of critical volume overload or intoxication, and it serves as an important method for long-term maintenance dialysis. Children require special evaluation and monitoring for successful hemodialysis. This chapter discusses general principles of hemodialysis operation, vascular access, prescription, and management, with emphasis on the unique considerations for pediatric patients.

## HISTORY

The earliest report of a child receiving hemodialysis was a little boy with uremia who was dialyzed by Georg Haas in 1924.[1,2] The child was Haas's second patient to tolerate the procedure, but the child did not survive. Later, Willem Kolff developed the first practical human hemodialysis machine: a rotating drum with 20 m of cellophane tubing in a stationary 100-L tank.[3] The first pediatric application of the Kolff machine came in 1950 in Boston by John Merrill et al.,[4] when they treated a 3½ year old boy with nephrotic syndrome as part of a study that included 42 adults. In 1955, Mateer et al.,[5] at the Children's Hospital of Pittsburgh, described performing hemodialysis in 5 children 15 to 17 years of age by using 50-foot cellophane tubing and a 32-L dialysate bath for 13 h. As with all patients up to this time, ongoing therapy was limited by the necessity for new access for each session. Six years after the advent of the Scribner shunt in 1960, the Seattle group reported long-term hemodialysis in a 15½ year old girl for 18 months.[6] This was followed by the description of 5 adolescents dialyzed by Fine et al. in 1968.[7] Kjellstrand et al.[8] were able to achieve dialysis in patients weighing less than 15 kg. Access was a challenge with smaller patients because there was increased clotting of the Scribner shunt, and these patients were too small for the arteriovenous fistula (AVF) described by Brescia et al. in 1963.[9] The need for better access drove Hickman[10] to develop the central venous catheter that now bears his name. The Hickman catheter allowed a more permanent access for small children requiring hemodialysis.[10] Other technological advances such as volumetric controls allowed for greater efficiency and accuracy in ultrafiltration (UF) and solute removal. Ongoing progress allows us to offer hemodialysis to our pediatric patients as a method for metabolic and volume control in acute kidney injury (AKI), a means to address intoxications, and a bridge toward transplantation in those children with end-stage renal disease (ESRD).

## PHYSIOLOGY OF MOLECULAR MOVEMENT AND REMOVAL

Dialysis involves the movement of molecules between the plasma and the dialysate, which are separated from each other by a semipermeable membrane. In hemodialysis, three processes remove uremic toxins: diffusion, convection, and adsorption. Water removal occurs through UF. A clear understanding of the underlying physical principles that occur in hemodialysis is essential.

*Diffusion* involves the movement of molecules down a concentration gradient (Figure 36.1A). Molecules in plasma are in constant random motion. The smaller the molecule, the faster that motion will be. When a semipermeable membrane separates blood and dialysate, molecules within these solutions randomly make contact with the membrane and move across to the opposite side. Smaller molecules have more contact with the membrane within a given period of time because of their increased rate of motion. If side A has more molecules as compared with side B, there will be increased contact with the membrane on side A and thus increased passage of the molecule from side A to side B. The final result will be movement of molecules from a solution of high concentration to a solution of lower concentration. When the concentration of a molecule within both solutions is equal, there will be zero net movement of that molecule because passage between solutions will be equal.

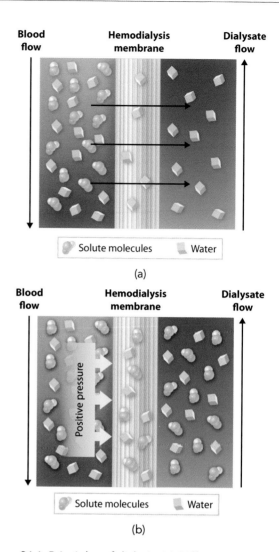

Figure 36.1 Principles of dialysis. **(a)** Diffusion: movement of molecules from an area of high concentration to an area of low concentration. **(b)** Convection: movement of molecules as a result of the pressure-related movement of the solution.

---

## KEY POINTS

- *Diffusion* is the movement of molecules down a concentration gradient.
- *Convection* is the movement of molecules within a solution as a result of the movement of the solution.

---

*Convection* is the movement of molecules within a solution as a result of the movement of the solution (Figure 36.1B). Pressure is applied to solution A, thereby causing movement of the solution across the semipermeable membrane and dragging dissolved molecules with it. Here it is not the random motion of the molecules contacting the membrane causing transfer of the molecule, but rather the force of motion of the solvent taking dissolved solute with it. This process is described as *solvent drag*. In convection, the rate-limiting factor is not the size of the molecule, but the size of the membrane pores. Molecules that are smaller than the membrane pore size move across the membrane, whereas molecules too large to pass are left behind.

Molecular transport across a semipermeable membrane, resulting from diffusion or convection, is limited by the size and distribution of its pores. Small molecules are able to pass through small and large pores, whereas larger molecules are limited to large pores. Molecules larger than the size of the pores on the membrane are not able to pass at all.

As blood flows through the dialyzer, proteins may be *adsorbed* to the dialyzer membrane. Once the dialyzer

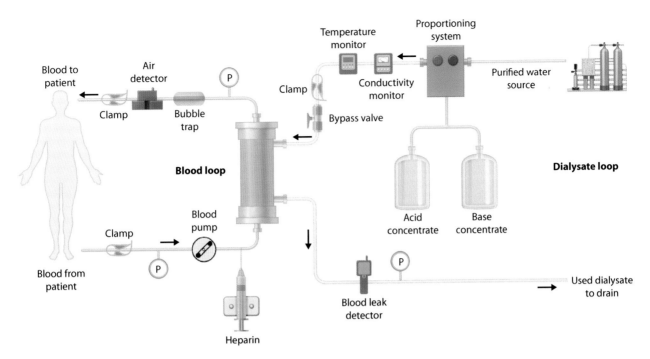

Figure 36.2 Schematic representation of hemodialysis circuit blood loop and dialysate loop. P, pressure monitors.

is discarded, the molecules bound to the membrane are removed from the body.

*Ultrafiltration* (UF) is the passage of water, or any solvent, through a semipermeable membrane down a pressure gradient. This pressure gradient can be generated by mechanical hydrostatic pressure, termed hydrostatic UF, or by osmotic pressure, termed osmotic UF.

## DIALYSIS WATER

The blood of a hemodialysis-treated patient is exposed to a large volume of dialysate during a hemodialysis session. Using a standard dialysate flow rate (Qd) of 500 mL/min, a patient receiving hemodialysis for 3 h each session, three times a week, encounters 270 L of fluid on a weekly basis. Consequently, the water used to generate dialysate must meet rigorous standards for chemical, bacteriologic, and endotoxin content to avoid illness or injury. Municipal water is purified by employing carbon filtration and reverse osmosis. Depending on the chemical composition and hardness of the municipal water, it may be necessary to employ a water softener before it is subjected to reverse osmosis.

### KEY POINTS

- Water used in hemodialysis must meet stringent quality standards.
- Water quality affects morbidity and mortality in patients undergoing hemodialysis.

Guidelines for water purity for dialysis use are updated periodically and published in the United States.[11]

## HEMODIALYSIS MACHINES

The hemodialysis apparatus can be divided into two main components: the blood circuit and the dialysate circuit (Figure 36.2). The blood circuit contains the tubing set, the blood pump, and the hemodialyzer (Figure 36.3A and B). The dialysate circuit contains the proportioning and dialysate delivery system, a complex, integrated network that prepares the dialysate during the procedure. Some devices do not employ a proportioning system to generate dialysate online during the hemodialysis session. In machines that do not have proportioning systems, the dialysate delivery system uses centrally preconstituted final solutions.

## BLOOD CIRCUIT

### Tubing set

The tubing set can be divided into two parts: the arterial and venous segments. The *arterial segment* carries the blood from the patient to the hemodialyzer, and the *venous segment* returns the blood from the hemodialyzer back to the patient. The blood pump generates the blood flow; the revolutions per minute of the blood pump determine the blood flow rate (Qb). Usually, both the arterial and venous segments of the tubing set contain a drip chamber that allows separation of air, which rises to the top as blood flows through it. Some tubing sets have a venous drip chamber

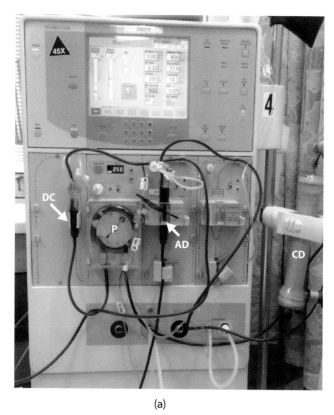
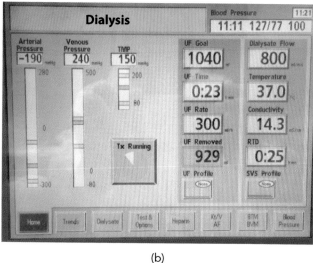

(a)            (b)

Figure 36.3 **(a)** Hemodialysis machine demonstrating the blood pump (P), capillary dialyzer (CD), air detector (AD), and drip chamber in the arterial path (DC). **(b)** Hemodialysis machine monitor showing arterial pressure (–190 mm Hg), venous pressure (240 mm Hg), transmembrane pressure (TMP; 150 mm Hg), ultrafiltration and dialysate. (Courtesy of Fresenius Medical Care North America, Kaysville, UT.)

and not an arterial chamber. Pressure is monitored at multiple sites along the blood path. The pressure in the arterial (prepump) segment is negative, reflecting the pressure generated by the blood pump to draw blood into the tubing. The pressure in the venous (postpump) segment is positive, reflecting the resistance generated by the vascular access. The venous drip chamber also has a level and air detector, followed by a clamp distal to the drip chamber. If an alarm is activated by the pressure, air, or level detector, thus suggesting a safety risk to the patient, the blood return line will be clamped and the blood pump will stop. This clamp functions as the last line of control, and the machine malfunction needs to be addressed before blood can be returned to the patient.

## Blood pump

The blood pump is a "demand-driven" pump, in that blood flow is set at a fixed rate. If the arterial access cannot provide the blood at a specified rate, the arterial line pressures will become more negative. If blood cannot be returned to the patient at a specified rate set by the blood pump, the venous pressures will become progressively more positive. Extremes of pressure may be incompatible with the function of the dialysis procedure, and they may put the dialysis membrane at risk for rupture or clotting.

This situation causes machine alarms and triggers the blood pump to stop.

## Hemodialyzer

The hemodialyzer is a key component of the dialysis apparatus. It is where fluid removal and solute exchange occur across a semipermeable membrane. Historically, dialyzer designs have evolved from a drum, to parallel plates, and now to a hollow fiber capillary system (Figure 36.4). The hollow fiber dialyzers consist of thousands of capillary filters encased in transparent tubular casing and anchored by "potting material" at each end of the dialyzer. These dialyzers have a blood port at each end, one port for the blood inlet and the second port for the outlet. In close proximity to the blood port is the "header," where the blood collects before traveling into the hollow fibers. Within the body of the dialyzer are two dialysate ports, one for the inlet and the second for the outlet. The outlet port also serves as the exit for ultrafiltrate.

Membrane technology used within the dialyzer has evolved from plant-based cellulosic membranes to synthetic membranes. Cellulosic membranes contain free hydroxyl groups that activate complement and other inflammatory markers, thus leading to bioincompatibility.[12] Biocompatibility of the dialyzer membranes improved

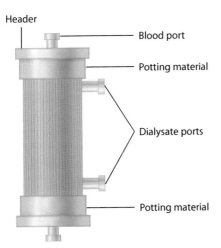

Figure 36.4 Anatomy of a hollow fiber membrane hemodialyzer.

after manufacturers modified the hydroxyl groups through chemical substitution, initially with acetate and later with tertiary amine, to create semisynthetic membranes. Most dialyzer membranes at present are synthetic, which are more biocompatible and also have greater hydraulic permeability. Some dialyzer membranes can also adsorb plasma proteins, immunoglobulins, and complement. Common synthetic membrane materials include polysulfone (PS), polyacrylonitrile (PAN), polycarbonate, polymethylmethacrylate (PMMA), and polyamide.

The main function of the dialyzer is solute and fluid removal. In vitro testing by manufacturers allows reporting of solute clearance for molecules of various sizes, such as urea (molecular weight [MW], 60 Da), vitamin B$_{12}$ (MW, 1355 Da), and β$_2$-microglobulin (MW, 11,000 Da). Knowledge of the clearance parameters of a given dialyzer permits a better understanding of its capabilities and allows a more specific dialysis prescription in patients. Clearance of various solutes (e.g., "uremic toxins," electrolytes) depends on the blood flow, dialysate flow, and dialyzer membrane characteristics that include thickness, surface area, pore size, and pore density.

### DIALYZER CLEARANCE

When limitations of blood flow (Qb) and dialysate flow (Qd) are eliminated, one can isolate the membrane's ability to remove solutes, or its efficiency in clearing certain solutes. This measurement is termed the *mass transfer area coefficient* (KoA). KoA is the theoretical clearance of a solute at

infinite Qb and Qd. Efficiency of a membrane is defined by how rapidly it completely removes urea from a solution (KoA$_{urea}$). Membranes are separated into low- and high-efficiency membranes: those with a KoA$_{urea}$ less than 500 mL/min are characterized as low-efficiency membranes, and those with a KoA$_{urea}$ greater than 500 mL/min are characterized as high-efficiency membranes.

In clinical settings, the restrictions of Qb and Qd cannot be eliminated. The actual clearance (K$_D$) achieved by a given dialyzer depends on operational characteristics beyond KoA and depends on Qb and Qd. K$_D$ is lower with lower Qb or Qd and increases, within limits, with higher flows.

### ULTRAFILTRATION CHARACTERISTICS

The ability of the membrane to remove plasma water is reported as the UF coefficient (K$_{uf}$). The K$_{uf}$ signifies the volume of plasma water removed per hour per mm Hg of transmembrane pressure (TMP). A membrane with a K$_{uf}$ less than 10 mL/h/mm Hg is considered low flux, whereas membranes with K$_{uf}$ greater than 10 mL/h/mm Hg are considered high flux. UF volume achieved within a defined period of time depends on the K$_{uf}$ and the TMP used to generate the ultrafiltrate:

$$UF = K_{uf} \times TMP$$

The term *flux* is also defined by the membrane's ability to clear middle molecules such as β$_2$-microglobulin. A dialyzer is considered low flux if KoA$_{β2\text{-microglobulin}}$ is less than 10 mL/min and high flux if it is greater than 10 mL/min.

### DIALYZER STERILIZATION

Multiple techniques exist for commercial sterilization of the dialyzer and the tubing sets. Options include ethylene oxide (ETO), steam autoclaving, gamma irradiation, and electron beam irradiation. ETO can pose a risk of anaphylaxis for sensitive patients.[13] To avoid this reaction, proper rinsing of the dialyzer must be performed to ensure that all the ETO is removed before use. Electron beam irradiation has been associated with mild thrombocytopenia, especially with polysulfone and other synthetic membranes.[14]

## DIALYZER REUSE

Some centers reuse a dialyzer for an individual patient over several sessions. The reuse procedure requires chemical cleaning, disinfection, and resterilization of the dialyzer after each hemodialysis session. This practice is decreasing and is generally not recommended for the pediatric population.

# DIALYSATE CIRCUIT

## Dialysate

The dialysate is a key component in the dialysis procedure. A patient dialyzing for 4 h at a dialysate flow of 500 mL/min requires 120 L of dialysate. Dialysate flows outside the dialyzer membrane capillaries in a countercurrent direction to the blood path and exchanges electrolytes and toxins. Thus, the purity of the water used to make the dialysate is of paramount importance. Because of the high volume of dialysate, most modern hemodialysis machines use concentrated solution or powders that are mixed by the hemodialysis machine with purified water to generate the dialysate during the session.

Dialysate concentrates are separated into two components, labeled "A" and "B" concentrates. The A concentrate contains the majority of the electrolytes and an acid, whereas the B concentrate contains the base, most often as bicarbonate. The concentrates are kept separate before initiation of the dialysis procedure to prevent precipitation because mixing of sodium bicarbonate ($NaHCO_3$) and calcium chloride ($CaCl_2$) would lead to precipitation of calcium carbonate ($CaCO_3$):

$$CaCl_2 + NaHCO_3 \rightarrow Ca(HCO_3)_2 + NaCl \rightarrow CaCO_3 + H_2O + CO_2$$

Acid is included in the A concentrate to keep the pH of the final dialysate solution lower than 7.4. Lower pH drives the chemical reaction noted earlier to the left, thereby preventing formation of highly insoluble calcium carbonate. Two types of acid are currently in use: acetate and citrate. Acetate comes in two concentrate forms, liquid and powder, that in the final dialysate solution make 4 mEq/L (liquid concentrate) or 8 mEq/L (powder concentrate) of acetic acid. Acetate is metabolized by the body to generate bicarbonate. Acid concentrates containing citrate have citric acid at 2.4 mEq/L, with 0.3 mEq/L of acetic acid in the final concentration.

The composition of typical dialysate delivered in treatment is presented in Table 36.1. Modern dialysis machines have the capability to adjust the concentration of components in the final dialysis by either using a different concentrate for the A component or by adjusting the blend of A and B components with the purified water. Dialysate concentrates for the A component come in various formulations to deliver the desired concentration of potassium (1, 2, 3, or

Table 36.1 Composition of dialysate

| Component | Amount |
|---|---|
| Sodium | 135–145 mEq/L |
| Potassium | 0–4 mEq/L |
| Calcium | 2.5–3.5 mEq/L |
| Magnesium | 0.5–1.5 mEq/L |
| Chloride | 98–112 mEq/L |
| Acetate/citrate | 4–10/2.4 mEq/L |
| Glucose | 0–200 mg/dL |
| Bicarbonate | 35–40 mEq/L |

4 mEq/L) and calcium (1.5, 2.5, or 3.0 mEq/L) in the dialysate. Selection of the initial concentrate permits adjustment of the potassium and calcium in the final dialysate without affecting the concentrations of the other electrolytes. In contrast, adjusting the final concentration of other components of the dialysate, specifically sodium and bicarbonate, is achieved by reprogramming the proportioning system to change the admixture of the concentrates with water. Consequently, this affects the concentration of the other electrolytes in that solution. For example, reduction of the sodium concentration by 4% reduces the final concentration of the other electrolytes by 4%.

## KEY POINT

Adjusting the concentration of sodium and bicarbonate in the dialysate solution alters the concentrations of other electrolytes.

## Dialysate delivery

The dialysate delivery system prepares the final dialysate in the dialysis machine, by using purified water and concentrated solutes. The components that make up the delivery system include the proportioning system, the volumetric control system, and the monitoring system.

Treated or purified water is sent to the machine *proportioning system*, which takes the necessary volume of water to dilute the A and B concentrates to generate the final dialysate. The final dialysate is checked for appropriate mixing by measuring its conductivity, which depends on its electrolyte concentration. Pure water has zero conductivity, whereas water containing solutes (salts) has higher conductivity. The conductivity of the dialysate, measured in millisiemens, is generally one-tenth of its sodium concentration. Thus, at a sodium concentration of 137 mEq/L the conductivity is 13.7 millisiemens. If the conductivity of the dialysate is within range, it will proceed to the dialyzer; failing this test, the dialysate will be diverted away from the dialyzer.

## SAFETY DEVICES

Numerous safety mechanisms are present in modern dialysis machines that test for appropriate pressure, temperature, and dialysate content. Test failure causes an audible and visual alarm on the machine and may divert dialysate away from the patient or halt the dialysis machine completely. These systems are designed to ensure the patient's safety.

The *volumetric control system* protects the patient from excess UF. This is of paramount importance with high-flux dialyzers, which generate higher volumes of ultrafiltrate for a given TMP. UF control in the dialysis machines is achieved by numerous techniques, such as flow sensors, closed loop, or volumetric balancing. All these techniques are designed to provide safe and accurate UF.

The *blood leak detector,* which is located on the dialysate outflow tract, uses photo-optical sensors to detect red blood cells that have migrated from the blood to the dialysate through a fracture in the dialyzer. Some machines may have *pH sensors* on the proportioning system to ensure that both the A and B components are functioning and the final dialysate is well proportioned in its composition.

As described earlier, blood side monitors include arterial and venous pressure monitors, usually located in the drip chambers, and an air detector located in the venous drip chamber. To prevent catastrophic consequences such as blood loss, pressure limits are set to turn the blood pump off and clamp the venous line if the pressure limits are exceeded. The limits are usually −200 mm Hg for the arterial pressure and +200 mm Hg for the venous pressure. If there is venous needle dislodgment or catheter disconnection, the venous pressures will become very low, thus denoting the lack of resistance provided by the intravascular space; the blood pump will stop, and the venous line will be clamped to prevent exsanguination.

## DIALYSIS PRESCRIPTION

Before hemodialysis is initiated, either in the short-term or long-term setting, careful assessment of the patient and clinical circumstances is required. Points include the indication for hemodialysis, appropriate vascular access, suitability of the patient for anticoagulation, assessment of vital signs with particular attention to blood pressure, selection of appropriate blood and dialysate flow rates, determination of the length of the dialysis session, and determinations of the dialysis dose and the UF goal. The guidelines for both short-term and long-term hemodialysis prescription are provided here and are outlined in Table 36.2.

## INDICATIONS FOR SHORT-TERM HEMODIALYSIS

Initiation of short-term dialysis is required when medical management has failed to overcome complications of AKI. Clinical examples include fluid overload, electrolyte imbalance, acidosis, uremia leading to end-organ damage such as pericarditis, and encephalopathy, all refractory to medical intervention. Intoxication is another indication for short-term dialysis that may not be associated with AKI. Regardless of indication, an individualized approach is required when selecting a modality for renal replacement therapy, including consideration of the patient's size, access challenges, severity of illness, comorbidities, electrolyte imbalances, and level of blood urea nitrogen (BUN).

## INDICATIONS FOR LONG-TERM HEMODIALYSIS

Controversy remains regarding the ideal time to initiate long-term dialysis support. The general trend among our colleagues who treat adults is earlier initiation of dialysis. The premise for this shift has been the assumption that an earlier start of dialysis (glomerular filtration rate, 10 to 15 mL/min/1.73 m$^2$) will provide a survival benefit. Observational studies have demonstrated that an earlier start of dialysis may improve survival,[15-17] but this finding was not supported by the Initiating Dialysis Early and Late (IDEAL) study, the only randomized controlled trial.[18]

In the pediatric population, as in adults, there is no single factor on which the clinician can rely to determine when to initiate long-term dialysis. Generally, indications to start dialysis can be separated into absolute and relative indications (Table 36.3). A specific factor that pediatric nephrologists should account for is growth, and some investigators hypothesize that adequate dialysis may reduce growth hormone resistance. The National Kidney Foundation Kidney Disease Outcomes Quality Initiative (KDOQI) guidelines recommend that in a patient without significant manifestation of renal failure, one should consider dialysis initiation if the native creatinine clearance calculated by 24-h urine collection is less than 6 to 7 mL/min/1.73 m$^2$. This lower limit is derived from a weekly Kt/V of 2, the minimum target for standard Kt/V (see later for a discussion of dialysis adequacy and a definition and discussion of Kt/V).

## VASCULAR ACCESS

The hemodialysis procedure requires vascular access to permit the patient's blood to flow through the hemodialysis machine. Without acceptable blood flow, the hemodialysis procedure cannot be successful. An ideal vascular access for hemodialysis is one that provides appropriate blood flow to permit adequate clearance and UF with a low complication rate and reliability to provide the necessary blood flow for repeated hemodialysis sessions. Vascular access methods for hemodialysis include temporary devices (central venous catheters) and permanent subcutaneous access systems,

Table 36.2 Components of the hemodialysis order set

Frequency of dialysis
Individual session length
Type of vascular access to be used:

- Catheter
- Fistula or graft
- Needles for fistula or graft

Dialyzer
Tubing set
Tubing system prime:

- Blood
- Albumin
- Saline
- Self

Blood flow rate
Dialysate flow rate
Dialysate components:

- Sodium program (concentration, modelling)
- Bicarbonate concentration
- Potassium concentration
- Calcium concentration
- Special dialysate formula or components

Anticoagulation:

- Initial heparin dose
- Continuous heparin infusion
- Intermittent heparin dose

Ultrafiltration plan:

- Ultrafiltration goal or target weight
- Ultrafiltration modelling or profile

Monitoring:

- Activated clotting times (frequency and goals)
- Blood pressure monitoring (frequency and goals)
- Special monitoring (as indicated):
  - Cardiac monitor
  - Pulse oximetry
- One-to-one nursing

Dialysis-associated medications (as indicated):

- Erythropoietin
- Iron
- Vitamin D analogue
- Antibiotics
- Special medications

Laboratory tests (as indicated):

- Blood chemistry studies (e.g., predialysis and postdialysis BUN)
- Complete blood count
- Blood cultures
- Special blood tests

Access care and monitoring:

- Catheters:
  - Dressing change plan
  - Indwelling heparin following dialysis
- Fistulas and grafts:
- Pressure and flow monitoring plan|

*Abbreviation:* BUN, blood urea nitrogen.

which include the native AVF and the synthetic arteriovenous graft (AVG).

Currently, the AVF best meets the goals for hemodialysis vascular access and is therefore considered the preferred form of long-term access. The AVF is formed by subcutaneous anastomosis of an artery to an adjacent vein. One study demonstrated that the minimal venous and arterial lumen diameters should be 2.5 and 1.5 mm, respectively.[19] After anastomosis, it takes 2 to 4 months for the vein to dilate and for the venous wall to thicken enough to allow successful repeated needle access. The site of an AVF ideally should be the distal arm by creation of a radiocephalic fistula. This allows for more proximal sites to be used in the future if a complication occurs. In children, distal access in the wrist may not be possible because of size limitations; thus, more proximal access may need to be used for even initial AVF attempts.

An AVG provides the second-best option for permanent hemodialysis vascular access. An AVG differs from a native AVF in that a prosthetic tube, most often of

**KEY POINT**

In patients with ESRD, or at risk for ESRD, central lines should be avoided in the upper extremities to preserve future AVF access sites.

polytetrafluoroethylene (PTFE), bridges between a feeding artery and the recipient vein. The AVG requires less maturation time after its creation before it can be used because dilatation and thickening of the vein are not necessary. Generally, an AVG can be used within 1 to 3 weeks or even sooner if necessary. Because maturation of the native vein is not necessary, AVGs have a lower primary failure rate as compared with AVFs. However, the life span of the AVG is limited when compared with the AVF. The complication rate is also higher in AVGs, with more frequent infections and a greater need for surgical

Table 36.3 Indications for dialysis initiation

**Absolute Indications**

Uremia: life-threatening.

Neurologic: encephalopathy, confusion, asterixis, seizures, myoclonus, wrist and foot drop

Cardiac: pericarditis, pericardial effusion

Hematologic: bleeding diathesis

Hyperkalemia (life-threatening): refractory to medical management

Fluid overload (life-threatening): refractory to medical management

Absence of kidneys (congenital or after bilateral nephrectomy)

Anuria

**Relative Indications**

Uremia: subtle

Fatigue, reduced school or job performance, cognitive dysfunction, intermittent nausea or emesis, sleep dysfunction, and other conditions

Electrolyte imbalance (e.g., hyponatremia, hyperkalemia, hyperphosphatemia, hypercalcemia) difficult to medically manage

Malnutrition secondary to advanced chronic kidney disease

Growth failure secondary to advanced chronic kidney disease

Table 36.4 Acute dialysis catheter choices

| Patient size | Catheter choice |
| --- | --- |
| Neonate | 7-French double-lumen |
| | 5-French single-lumen (requires two separate catheters) |
| 3–6 kg | 7-French double-lumen |
| 6–30 kg | 8-French double-lumen |
| 15–30 Kg | 9-French double-lumen |
| >30 kg | 10-French double-lumen |
| | 12.5-French double-lumen |

and causes less patient discomfort as compared with the femoral site. In contrast, subclavian access is associated with increased risk of vascular stenosis that would result in loss of potential sites for AVF formation in the ipsilateral arm. Femoral access is a poor choice for long-term hemodialysis because of limitations on ambulation and a higher potential for complications, but it is a frequently used site for short-term hemodialysis given the relative ease of insertion. In neonates, umbilical catheters may also be used if other access sites have failed, but these catheters are often not successful as a result of poor flow dynamics, and they are not recommended.

## ANTICOAGULATION

intervention to address problems with thrombosis, stenosis, and occlusion.

Central venous access for short-term or long-term hemodialysis can be achieved through a double-lumen catheter (most common) or through two single-lumen catheters. The hemodialysis catheter must be large and stiff enough to permit the required Qb for hemodialysis; standard central venous catheters designed for infusion of intravenous fluids are not acceptable. General recommendations based on weight or body surface area are available as an estimate of the catheter size that can be inserted (Table 36.4), but the largest catheter that can be safely inserted should be selected. Multiple central locations that permit needed high Qb can be considered for placement of the dialysis catheter. Potential sites for central venous cannulation include the jugular, femoral, and subclavian veins. The most desirable site for insertion of a double-lumen hemodialysis catheter is the right internal jugular vein. This vein provides access to a high–blood flow area in the superior vena cava and right atrium, permits a straight venous path for the operator from insertion site to the target location, can be readily used for insertion of either tunneled or nontunneled catheters, allows ambulation, is less susceptible to complicating venous stenosis that could limit future permanent vascular,

Exposure of blood to foreign surfaces results in clotting. To prevent clotting, anticoagulants are required when performing hemodialysis. Unfractionated heparin (UFH) is the most commonly used anticoagulant for dialysis. UFH works by activating antithrombin and inhibiting clotting factors, particularly factor Xa and thrombin. UFH is associated with platelet activation and aggregation, but by inactivating clotting factors on the platelet membrane, which limit binding and activation, it counterbalances this effect. The onset of action for UFH is within 3 to 5 min, and its half-life is 0.5 to 2 h.

Dosing of UFH for hemodialysis includes an initial bolus of 10 to 30 units/kg, which is administered through the venous access before connecting the patient, or into the arterial port before the hemodialyzer. Continuous infusion rates per session range from 10 to 20 units/kg/h. The dose of heparin is adjusted to obtain an activated clotting time of 150 to 200 sec (1.5 to 2 times normal). Alternatively, whole blood activated partial thromboplastin time (aPTT) can be followed with a goal of 80% greater than baseline during dialysis and 40% above baseline at the end of dialysis to prevent bleeding. Other techniques for dosing UFH include giving a large initial bolus without a maintenance infusion. Smaller additional boluses are administered as needed if clotting is seen. UFH can be used to coat the dialyzer by rinsing the dialyzer with 3000 to 5000 units of UFH/L of saline. The dialyzer is subsequently rinsed with equal amounts of saline without heparin before connecting the patient. Side effects of UFH include pruritus, allergy, osteoporosis, hyperlipidemia, thrombocytopenia, and excessive bleeding.

## ALTERNATIVES TO HEPARIN

Low molecular weight heparin (LMWH), which is a smaller fraction of UFH, retains its ability to activate antithrombin and bind and inactivate factor Xa, but it does not bind thrombin. Because of its longer half-life, LMWH can be administered as a single dose at the start of dialysis. The usual dose is 125 to 250 anti-Xa units/kg. Anti–factor Xa is monitored with a goal of 0.4 to 0.8 international units/mL to ensure that an appropriate therapeutic level is attained. It is believed that some of the side effects of UFH such as pruritus and hyperlipidemia are reduced with LMWH. LMWH is also associated with reduced activation of platelets and leukocytes. The risk of heparin-induced thrombocytopenia (HIT) is lower, although for patients found to have HIT from UFH, LMWH use is contraindicated.

---

### KEY POINT

LMWH is contraindicated in patients with a history of HIT.

---

Another common alternative to heparin in the United States is the use of citrate. Citrate functions as an anticoagulant because of its ability to chelate calcium, which is an essential cofactor in the clotting cascade and for platelet activation. Citrate can be administered as an infusion, or citrate-containing dialysate may be used. Infusions are mostly used in CRRT, and numerous protocols exist to administer regional citrate appropriately and safely as an anticoagulant in CRRT.[20,21]

Dialysate solutions that have substituted some of the acetate in the acid bath with citrate have been found to function well as anticoagulants. The citrate in the dialysate binds calcium locally at the dialyzer membrane environment, thereby preventing clotting within the dialyzer. The dialysate citrate concentration is usually 2.4 mEq/L of citric acid. Monitoring of ionized calcium is not required in hemodialysis because the concentration of citrate is low, and thus the patient is not at risk for developing hypocalcemia. Citrate-containing dialysate appears to be effective as an anticoagulant, but some centers have found that additional reduced doses of systemic heparin are required.[22]

Other anticoagulation methods much less frequently used include heparinoids, direct thrombin inhibitors, prostacyclins, and other prostanoids. Each class of anticoagulant has specific risks and benefits.[20]

## ANTICOAGULATION IN BLEEDING DIATHESIS

Many critically ill patients who require short-term dialysis may have a bleeding diathesis that precludes the use of systemic anticoagulation. Anticoagulation-free dialysis can be performed successfully by maximizing blood flow and performing prefilter intermittent saline flushes (10- to 20-mL flushes every 15 to 20 min). In younger patients with small vascular access, a high Qb may be difficult to achieve, wherein a dialyzer with a smaller surface area can be used to increase the relative Qb per fiber bundle.

### BLOOD FLOW RATE

The maximum Qb is determined by the vascular access. Large double-lumen hemodialysis catheters (larger than 12 French) provide a Qb of at least 200 mL/min. By contrast, smaller-caliber catheters (e.g., 8 French) may produce a Qb of only 75 to 100 mL/min. Permanent vascular access (AVFs and AVGs) provides vastly superior Qbs of 300 mL/min or higher. Higher blood flow improves the efficiency of the hemodialysis session and permits greater mass transfer in a given period of time.

### DIALYSATE FLOW RATE

The standard Qd is 500 mL/min. Some dialysis machines permit variation of the Qd, allowing flows as high as 800 mL/min. This also increases dialysis efficiency, but it has less impact than changes in Qb. If Qd is 150 to 250 mL/min faster than Qb, increasing Qd further will have a negligible effect on clearance.

### EXTRACORPOREAL BLOOD VOLUME CONSIDERATIONS

Traditional physiologic principles suggest that the total extracorporeal volume of the blood circuit (tubing and dialyzer) should not exceed 10% of the patient's blood volume. Pediatric tubing sets and dialyzers with small priming

---

### KEY POINTS

- Total extracorporeal volume of the blood circuit should not exceed 10% of the patient's blood volume.
- In infants, priming of the circuit with blood or 5% albumin may be needed to avoid hypovolemia.

---

volumes have been developed for smaller patients. Despite best efforts, extracorporeal volume may exceed these limits in infants. In this setting, priming of the circuit with blood or colloid may be necessary to prevent hypotension during dialysis initiation.

## DIALYZER SELECTION

The clinician selects the dialyzer with consideration of the biocompatibility of the membrane, priming volume, clearance, and UF characteristics. A dialyzer with a larger surface area and greater permeability permits greater mass transfer and UF, but the volume of blood required to fill such a dialyzer may be too large for a small child. Slow blood flow reduces the efficiency of mass transfer and may increase the likelihood of clotting. Choosing a dialyzer based on biocompatibility remains controversial. Some studies have documented reduced complement activation with biocompatible membranes, but improved clinical outcomes have not been convincingly achieved.[23] Consequently, the choice of dialyzer depends on a balance of multiple factors noted earlier and should be individualized.

## DURATION OF DIALYSIS

Greater time on dialysis permits greater mass transfer of both small and middle molecules. In addition, longer time may allow more successful UF because the rate of fluid removal can be lowered, thus reducing the likelihood of hypotension and symptoms related to rapid depletion of the vascular compartment volume. Extended time on dialysis for the patient undergoing long-term dialysis may result in lost time in school and fewer opportunities for play and thus may have a negative impact on quality of life.

## MASS TRANSFER EQUATION

Use of the mass transfer equation can guide the clinician's choice of dialyzer, blood pump speed, and session length. The mass transfer equation describes the changing blood concentration of a given molecule based on the dialysis session parameters (Figure 36.5):

$$C_t/C_0 = e^{-Kt/V}$$

where $C_t$ and $C_0$ are the concentrations of the molecule in question at time t (end of the session) and at session start (time zero), respectively; K is the clearance coefficient for the molecule in question; t is session length in minutes; and V is volume of distribution for the given molecule, in milliliters.

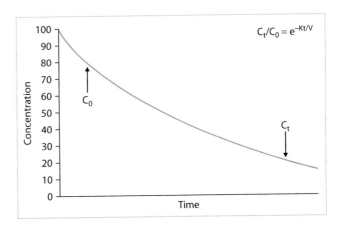

Figure 36.5 The mass transfer equation describes the concentration of a molecule within the patient during the dialysis session. $C_0$, concentration of molecule at time zero; $C_t$, concentration at time t; K, dialyzer clearance coefficient for molecule in question; t, time in minutes; and V, volume of distribution of molecule in question, in milliliters.

BUN is the most commonly used molecular marker for determining the dialysis prescription; therefore, K would be the $K_D$ for urea. The foregoing formula is particularly useful in gauging the dialysis prescription in the circumstances of short-term hemodialysis or with initiation of long-term hemodialysis.

## EXAMPLE

Consider a new patient weighing 40 kg with a starting BUN concentration of 100 mg/dL. The clinician anticipates a blood pump speed of 200 mL/min and selects a dialyzer that has a $K_D$ for urea of 180 mL/min at the given blood pump speed, based on the manufacturer's published data. Urea distributes within the total body water, which can be estimated as 60% of the body weight, or 24,000 mL in this case. Initial hemodialysis sessions often target lower levels of mass transfer to prevent the complications of dialysis dysequilibrium (see later). A 30% reduction of urea to a final target value of 70 mg/dL is reasonable in this case. To determine the length of the hemodialysis session with these parameters, the mass transfer equation can be rearranged to solve for t:

$$t \text{ (minutes)} = -\ln (C_t / C_0) \times (V / K)$$

$$t \text{ (minutes)} = -\ln (70 / 100) \times (24{,}000 / 180)$$

$$t \text{ (minutes)} = -\ln (0.7) \times 133.3$$

*[natural log determination from scientific calculator]*

$$t \text{ (minutes)} = -(-0.357) \times 133.3$$

$$t \text{ (minutes)} = 0.357 \times 133.3$$

$$t \text{ (minutes)} = 48$$

The mass transfer equation provides the clinician with a useful tool to manipulate the hemodialysis prescription. One can adjust the value of K by choosing an appropriate dialyzer or changing blood pump speed. This, along with adjusting the dialysis session time, can provide the desired level of mass transfer necessary for the given clinical situation. Measurement of BUN levels immediately before and after the dialysis session permits evaluation of the predicted mass transfer and subsequent fine tuning of the prescription.

The initial hemodialysis prescription for a new, highly uremic patient should provide urea reduction of no greater than 30%. The patient undergoes hemodialysis for 3 or 4 consecutive days, each day with progressively higher levels of mass transfer, until a full dose of greater than 70% urea reduction is achieved.

---

## KEY POINT

To reduce the possibility of dialysis dysequilibrium, urea reduction in the first acute dialysis session should be restricted to approximately 30%.

---

The ongoing dialysis prescription and schedule depend on the clinical situation. In the short-term setting, only one or two hemodialysis sessions may be required for the treatment of intoxication, whereas other patients with AKI may be served best by daily hemodialysis to limit metabolic fluctuation, maintain relative volume stability, and permit delivery of fluids, medications, and nutrition. Other patients with more persistent AKI, or those with chronic renal failure who require maintenance dialysis, may receive hemodialysis on an alternate-day or three times a week schedule. Individual clinical needs may necessitate hemodialysis more frequently.

## ULTRAFILTRATION

Each hemodialysis session requires a UF plan. UF control devices on modern hemodialysis machines permit precise levels of fluid removal throughout the hemodialysis session. The clinician must make a judgment about the level of UF that the patient can tolerate in the given session time. The hemodialysis machine can then be programmed to remove fluid from the patient at the desired rate. Careful monitoring of blood pressure, heart rate, and general patient status is required as the intravascular compartment volume contracts. This is especially true with smaller pediatric patients, in whom minor fluctuations in intravascular volume can have significant hemodynamic consequences. Blood volume monitoring devices (e.g., Crit-Line, Fresenius Medical Care North America, Kaysville, UT), which noninvasively measure the change in the patient's hematocrit during dialysis,

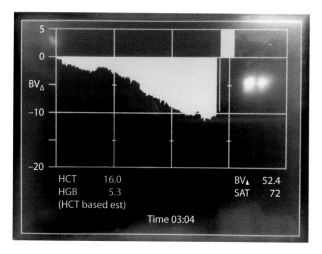

Figure 36.6 Screen shot from non-invasive blood volume monitor showing ultrafiltration data in a patient with newly diagnosed end-stage renal disease with anemia and pulmonary edema secondary to fluid overload. The patient has undergone ultrafiltration during the hemodialysis procedure to achieve approximately 10% reduction of intravascular volume. BV-delta, change in blood volume; HCT, hematocrit; HGB, hemoglobin; SAT, oxygen saturation. (Courtesy of Crit-Line, Fresenius Medical Care North America, Kaysville, UT.)

can be useful in monitoring fluid removal during dialysis (Figure 36.6).[24,25]

## EFFECTIVENESS OF THE DIALYSIS PROCEDURE

## DIALYSIS DOSE

The goals of dialysis are to rebalance serum solute concentrations, remove toxins, and attain a euvolemic state. Currently, we substitute BUN for the uremic toxins because of the ease of BUN testing and its ability to provide information about nutritional status. Determining the optimal dose of maintenance hemodialysis remains difficult. Using data from the National Cooperative Dialysis Study (NCDS), Gotch and Sargent[26] developed a method using the removal of urea as a proxy for the dose of hemodialysis. Despite controversy, using urea as an acceptable marker for small molecule clearance remains a standard method for measuring the quantity of dialysis delivered to the patient. The formal urea kinetic model, as well as various simplified estimating equations, allows the calculation of a mathematical derivative, known as Kt/V. Kt/V is a dimensionless ratio that represents the volume of plasma cleared (Kt) divided by the urea distribution volume (V) and is familiar as a component of the mass transfer equation. One may evaluate Kt/V and the movement of urea using a single-pool model or a more complex double-pool (equilibrated) model, which takes into account urea kinetics between cells and the vascular compartment. Based on the early evaluation of the NCDS data and subsequent studies,[27] minimum levels of Kt/V have been established for adult populations.[28]

Current KDOQI guidelines for thrice-weekly maintenance hemodialysis recommend single-pool Kt/V (spKt/V) greater than 1.2, with a goal of greater than 1.4. These recommendations are based on studies in adults that demonstrate spKt/V lower than 1.2 to be associated with underdialysis and poor outcome.[27,29] The term "single pool" implies that the urea is sequestered mainly in the plasma and that equilibration of urea between various compartments of the body occurs almost instantaneously. In reality, equilibration takes 30 to 60 min to occur; consequently, spKt/V overestimates the amount of urea clearance. To correct for this, one can measure BUN 30 to 60 minutes after dialysis to calculate the *equilibrated Kt/V* (eKt/V). This value is likely more accurate, but it has not been correlated with outcome, as has been done for spKt/V.

The goal spKt/V of 1.2 to 1.4 assumes thrice-weekly hemodialysis. More frequent dialysis results in lower peak urea concentration before dialysis and requires a lower Kt/V value to yield similar results. Conversely, less frequent dialysis requires a higher Kt/V value. *Standard Kt/V* (stdKt/V) permits calculation of comparable Kt/V when dialysis is performed two to seven times a week. Three formulas can be used to calculate stdKt/V: those of Gotch and Sargent,[30] Leypoltd et al.,[31] and the Frequent Hemodialysis Network trial[32] formula. The formulas are complicated, but online calculators are available for use at: http://www.davita.com/ktvcalculator. The stdKt/V of 2.0 is considered the minimum dose of dialysis for all treatment modalities.

The *urea reduction ratio (URR)* is a much less complex technique that can be used to measure delivered dialysis dose. The calculation of URR is based on the simple ratio of the predialysis and postdialysis BUN levels, as follows:

$$\{(BUNpre - BUNpost) / (BUNpre)\} \times 100$$

This measurement of urea clearance is simple, but it has many limitations. The URR does not account for urea generation during dialysis or for the urea removed by UF because UF does not change the concentration of urea. It also does not provide any information regarding the patient's nutritional status. Urea kinetic modeling by Kt/V addresses many of these issues.

Although Kt/V allows a measurement to target minimally acceptable dialysis, the level of dialysis that is optimal remains unclear. Growing clinical data in small numbers of patients suggest that more frequent hemodialysis with schedules employing short daily sessions or long nocturnal sessions leads to improved biochemical parameters and a greater sense of patients' well-being.[33,34] There is also evidence that dialysis three times a week that achieves an spKt/V of 2.0 results in improved growth without growth hormone therapy.[35] It seems likely that a multipronged approach, considering urea kinetics, phosphate clearance, blood pressure control, nutritional status, overall patient health, and other parameters, will be necessary to define the optimal level of hemodialysis.

## TECHNIQUE OF SAMPLING

The accuracy of Kt/V and URR measurements depends on appropriate sample collection. Dialysis staff must obtain blood samples for BUN before and after the dialysis session by using a standardized technique. The predialysis BUN sample must be obtained using a method that will avoid dilution of the blood that could lead to a spuriously low BUN value. The recommended method for obtaining the postdialysis sample is the "slow flow/stop pump" technique. Dialysate flow is minimized, UF is discontinued, and blood flow is reduced to 50 to 100 mL/min in the vascular access for 15 sec. The blood sample is obtained from the arterial limb, either with continued slow flow through the system or after fully stopping the blood pump.[36] This approach minimizes the effects of recirculation and urea rebound, which can lead to spurious results.

## INADEQUATE DIALYSIS

Numerous factors can reduce dialysis adequacy and lead to insufficient mass transfer, volume overload, and symptoms. The clinician must evaluate the patient, laboratory values, and dialysis adequacy studies (Kt/V or URR) to determine whether dialysis is adequate. The finding of inadequate dialysis warrants an investigation into its possible causes.

## RECIRCULATION

Recirculation describes the phenomenon whereby blood that has passed through the dialysis circuit is promptly drawn back into the "arterial end" of the blood loop on return into the vascular access. Thus, instead of returning to systemic circulation, the dialyzed blood constantly recirculates within the dialysis circuit. This reduces dialysis efficiency and can lead to inadequate delivery of prescribed dialysis dose. Recirculation can occur when attempting hemodialysis through a catheter using a Qb that is too high, when needle placement in an AVF or AVG is inappropriate, or when flow through the permanent vascular access is suboptimal. Low flow through an AVF or AVG is of particular concern because it can presage thrombosis of the vascular access. The dialysis team can evaluate the vascular access for recirculation by using an ultrasound dilution device or through blood sampling using a slow flow/stop pump technique[36] that obtains blood for BUN from the arterial line, venous line, and systemic circulation. The percentage of recirculation is characterized by a simple equation:

$$Recirculation = (Systemic\ BUN - Arterial\ BUN) / (Systemic\ BUN - Venous\ BUN) \times 100$$

A vascular access with significant recirculation (greater than 5% to 10%) should be evaluated for low internal blood flow.

# UNDERPRESCRIPTION

Underdialysis may occur if the prescribed dose of dialysis is insufficient. The clinician should review all aspects of the dialysis prescription and ensure that they are optimized. This includes using the largest possible dialyzer, the highest Qb permitted by the vascular access, and sufficient time undergoing dialysis. As previously noted, many of these parameters are limited in the pediatric population because of the size of the patient and technical constraints of the vascular access. Careful attention to the prescription, optimized for the individual patient, helps to avoid underdialysis.

Once a prescription is optimized, the delivered dose must be evaluated on a regular basis. When the delivered dose falls to less than target levels (e.g., Kt/V less than 1.2), a systematic evaluation of the technical aspects of the dialysis procedure should be undertaken to determine whether there is an identifiable cause for inadequate dialysis delivery. Published guidelines[36] describe a sophisticated algorithm for hemodialysis dose troubleshooting. Conceptually, the investigation should center on the components of the prescription under the clinician's control, namely, the clearance (K) and the effective time on dialysis (t). Other factors that may have an effect on the calculated delivered dose include blood recirculation in the vascular access and errors in obtaining the blood sample for adequacy study.

# DIMINISHED CLEARANCE

Because clearance on hemodialysis is a function of the dialyzer permeability surface area product (KoA), Qb, and Qd, the clinician should consider various factors that will cause the KoA, Qb, or Qd to differ from the values originally prescribed. Incorrect dialyzer, dialyzer volume loss from the reuse procedure, inappropriate dialysis machine settings, excessive dialyzer clotting, and machine miscalibration or malfunction are potential causes for clearance that is less than expected.

Perhaps the most common fundamental issue leading to diminished clearance in pediatric hemodialysis is lower than expected Qb, which is often a result of problems with the vascular access. Many pediatric patients are dialyzed with a central venous catheter as the vascular access, which can be particularly prone to problems with blood flow related to smaller caliber, thrombosis, kinking, and malposition. AVFs created in pediatric patients take longer to mature and may not achieve the high Qb values seen in adults. Poorly positioned needles or stenosis in the AVF or in an AVG can cause suboptimal blood flow and inadequate dialysis. Elevated pressures in the dialysis blood circuit causing machine alarms or clinical events such as hypotension may force the dialysis staff to reduce the Qb. Careful assessment of the vascular access and other factors with an effect on Qb is required when the delivered hemodialysis dose is inadequate.

# DIMINISHED EFFECTIVE DIALYSIS TIME

The patient's time on dialysis may be shortened by patient-related issues such as late arrival for the session or request for early termination. Misinterpretation of orders or incorrect programming of the dialysis machine can also lead to a shortened session that delivers less dialysis than intended. Clinical events such as hypotension, nausea, or cramps may cause staff to terminate a dialysis session early. Technical problems with the machine or vascular access may cause temporary cessation of the dialysis session, which, if not compensated for by extending the session, will lead to reduced effective dialysis time. The clinician must perform a review of session parameters and engage in discussion with dialysis unit staff to determine causes of diminished effective dialysis time.

# COMPLICATIONS

Complications in patients undergoing hemodialysis can be related to the hemodialysis procedure, the vascular access, or renal failure. Complications related to renal failure are addressed elsewhere in this text.

# COMPLICATIONS RELATED TO THE HEMODIALYSIS PROCEDURE

Hemodialysis represents a fundamentally nonphysiologic procedure involving extracorporeal perfusion, rapid removal of volume and small molecules from the vascular compartment, fluid shifts, changes in osmolality, and exposure of the patient's blood to foreign materials and solutions. Nevertheless, hemodialysis can be performed safely and effectively with close attention to the patient and knowledge of technology. Safety has been increased by the development of biocompatible materials, use of multiple patient safety devices, implementation of carefully designed protocols, and appropriate observation by trained staff. However, complications do arise during the hemodialysis procedure, and the clinician must be aware of potential complications and of the methods to evaluate, treat, and prevent their occurrence.

## Intradialytic hypotension

Low blood pressure during the hemodialysis session is a common complication. Potential causes of intradialytic hypotension are listed in Table 36.5. A common cause is overly aggressive UF that exceeds the vascular refilling rate. Hypotension can be treated by slowing the UF rate, providing intravenous saline to the patient, and placing the patient in the head-down (Trendelenburg) position. Careful clinical evaluation and planning of UF goals can avoid this complication.

**Table 36.5** Etiology of dialysis-induced hypotension

**Patient-Related Factors**
- Impaired plasma refilling (? decreased UF coefficient of vascular wall)
- Decreased cardiac reserve (diastolic or systolic dysfunction)
- Impaired venous compliance
- Autonomic dysfunction (diabetic, uremic)
- Arrhythmias
- Anemia
- Drug therapy (vasodilators, β blockers, calcium channel blockers)
- Alteration of vasoactive substances in the blood
- Eating during treatment (increased splanchnic blood flow)
- Low dry-weight estimation

**Procedure-Related Factors**
- Decreased plasma osmolality (relatively large surface area membrane, high starting BUN)
- Excess absolute volume and rate of fluid removal (large interdialytic weight gain)
- Change in serum electrolyte (hypocalcemia, hypokalemia)
- Dialysate: acetate, too warm dialysate
- Membrane blood interaction
- Hypoxia

**Uncommon Causes**
- Pericardial tamponade
- Myocardial infarction
- Aortic dissection
- Internal hemorrhage
- Septicemia
- Air embolism
- Pneumothorax
- Hemolysis

*Abbreviations:* BUN, blood urea nitrogen; UF, ultrafiltration

## Muscle cramps

Painful muscle contractions, most often seen near the end of the dialysis session, are frequent complications of hemodialysis therapy. These contractions are often seen in patients who require high rates of UF and are presumed to be related to relative intravascular volume depletion and subsequent hypoperfusion of the muscles. Electrolyte shifts during dialysis therapy are also implicated.[37] Similar to the approach with hypotension, maneuvers to permit refilling of the vascular compartment may alleviate painful cramps. Medications such as quinine have been used successfully to treat muscle cramping,[38] but they have not been validated in pediatric patients.

## Dialysis disequilibrium

The dialysis disequilibrium syndrome is a neurologic disorder thought to be related to acute cerebral edema in the setting of hemodialysis. Symptoms can range from minor issues (headache, nausea, restlessness) to more severe findings (myoclonus, disorientation, blurred vision, seizure, coma) and even death.[37] Despite the knowledge of this potentially fatal complication since the 1960s, the precise mechanism remains elusive. One theory of dialysis dysequilibrium suggests that the increased efficiency of urea clearance from the blood to dialysate, as compared with movement of urea from brain cells and interstitium to blood, creates a transient gradient of higher osmolality in brain cells, a condition in which water would move into the brain and cerebral edema occurs. This effect is exacerbated for patients with significantly elevated BUN. Consequently, dialysis dysequilibrium has most often been seen in a first hemodialysis session or in the setting of a very high predialysis BUN. Limiting urea reduction to 30% in this setting seems to reduce the risk of dysequilibrium.

## Allergic reactions

Exposure of blood to foreign materials during dialysis can lead to adverse reactions. Severe anaphylactoid reactions are uncommon, but sterilants and components of the dialysis membrane have been implicated as potential causes.[37] These reactions often occur early in the dialysis session and may be associated with dyspnea, feeling of warmth, angioedema, urticaria, and recurrence with similar dialysis equipment.[39] The hemodialysis session should be discontinued immediately when such a reaction is suspected. Oxygen and therapy for acute allergy (e.g., antihistamines, epinephrine, corticosteroids) may also be indicated. Future dialysis sessions should avoid the use of the offending materials. Milder reactions, such as back pain and chest discomfort, can also occur. The cause is unclear, and therapy is usually symptomatic.[37] Differentiation from more severe complications such as cardiac ischemia requires careful clinical evaluation.

The combination of angiotensin-converting enzyme (ACE) inhibitors and polyacrylonitrile (PAN) membranes has been associated with anaphylactic reactions.[40] PAN membranes activate Hageman factor and lead to the formation of kallikrein, with subsequent liberation of kinins such as bradykinin. ACE degrades bradykinin; thus, ACE inhibitors lead to accumulation of bradykinin, leading to anaphylactic reactions.

## Air embolism

Air entry into the blood loop of the hemodialysis circuit can cause significant injury or death. This serious complication is relatively uncommon as a result of numerous patient safety devices built into the hemodialysis machines. The blood pump stops when air enters the blood loop accidentally and prevents the entry of air into the patient through the vascular access. Air potentially can enter the hemodialysis blood circuit through loose connections or cracks in the tubing system. Clinical findings depend on the amount of air that has entered the patient and the status of the patient before air entry. Arterial air embolism results in occlusion and distal ischemia; venous air embolism can lead to obstruction of right ventricular outflow through the pulmonary venous system. Symptoms are often nonspecific, and a high index of suspicion is needed to recognize this complication. When air embolism is suspected, the dialysis session is terminated with care to prevent any further air entry. The patient is placed flat and supine and is provided with oxygen and volume expansion as necessary.[41] Evacuation of the air from the vascular system requires special expertise. Careful adherence to safety procedures in the dialysis unit can prevent this potentially devastating complication.

---

### KEY POINT

If there is concern for air embolism, terminate the dialysis session, place the patient flat and supine, and provide oxygen and volume expansion.

---

## Bleeding

Hemodialysis-treated patients are at increased risk for bleeding because of extracorporeal perfusion of blood through the hemodialysis circuit, uremia-associated platelet dysfunction, and systemic heparinization during the hemodialysis session. A minor manifestation may be prolonged oozing from AVF or AVG puncture sites; adjustment to the heparin prescription may be indicated in such circumstances. Careful titration of heparin dose and skilled nursing care can minimize the risks of more severe bleeding. Treatment of hemorrhage is supportive and includes volume expansion and correction of the acute cause. Neutralization of heparin with protamine sulfate can be considered,[37] but it carries risks of allergic reactions.

## Dialysate concentrate

The acetate in the acid A bath is available in two concentrations and generates dialysate concentrations of 4 mEq/L (liquid concentrate) or 8 mEq/L (powder concentrate) of acetic acid. Acetate is metabolized into bicarbonate. The use of a higher concentration of acetate without reducing the B (sodium bicarbonate) concentrate can lead to metabolic alkalosis because acetate is metabolized to bicarbonate. The alkalosis results in transcellular shifting of potassium into cells, thereby placing the patient at risk for cardiac arrhythmias secondary to hypokalemia. On March 29, 2012, the Food and Drug Administration issued a class 1 recall on acetate-containing solutions. In patients with predialysis serum bicarbonate greater than 27 mEq/L, a higher concentration of acetic acid was linked to increased cardiovascular morbidity and mortality.

## COMPLICATIONS RELATED TO VASCULAR ACCESS

Dialysis catheters and permanent vascular access for hemodialysis (AVFs and AVGs) share several potential complications, with some complications unique to the type of access.

## Hemodialysis catheters

Bleeding complications can occur at the time of hemodialysis catheter insertion or, more rarely, at a later time in response to catheter erosion through a vessel. Placement of a catheter in a central vein promotes stenosis, which can complicate venous drainage from the affected limb and can limit the success of permanent vascular access placed at a later time within the drainage field of the stenotic vessel. Poor catheter function with diminished blood flow can result from catheter migration, kinking, side-hole occlusion at the catheter tip, fibrin sheath formation, or thrombosis. Repositioning of the patient, instillation of thrombolytic agents into the catheter, and surgical replacement of the catheter may be required to reestablish effective blood flow. Infection can complicate vascular catheter use; the presence of the foreign body within the patient's vascular space predisposes to bacterial infection. Aggressive use of parenteral antibiotics can salvage an infected catheter; patients with recalcitrant infections may require catheter removal and replacement.

## Permanent vascular access

Primary AVFs may fail to mature after creation. This is of particular concern in children, whose vascular caliber is smaller than in adults. Careful preoperative evaluation of the patient's vascular potential, coupled with an experienced surgeon, maximizes successful fistula creation. AVGs avoid the issue of maturation, but they can be complicated by a higher failure rate. Complications of both AVGs and AVFs include infection, edema of the limb, and vascular steal syndrome. These complications are seen somewhat more frequently in AVGs. Permanent vascular access can also be complicated by stenosis, which may be amenable to angioplasty or surgical revision.

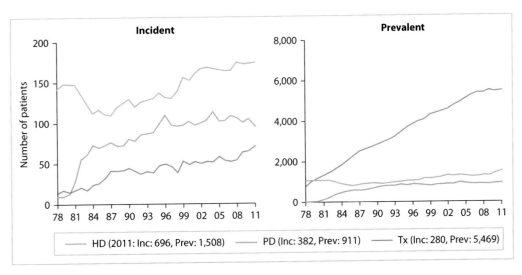

Figure 36.7  Incident and point prevalent patients with end-stage renal disease, 0 to 19 years old, by treatment modality in the United States. HD, hemodialysis; Inc, incidence; PD, peritoneal dialysis; Prev, prevalence; Tx, transplantation. (From US Renal Data System. USRDS 2013 Annual Data Report: Atlas of Chronic Kidney Disease and End-Stage Renal Disease in the United States. Bethesda, MD: National Institutes of Health, National Institute of Diabetes and Digestive and Kidney Diseases; 2013.)

## OUTCOME OF HEMODIALYSIS IN CHILDREN

Use of hemodialysis in the short-term setting has waned somewhat with the growing use of CRRT,[42] but hemodialysis remains an important modality in the acute setting, sometimes in conjunction with CRRT.[43] For children with ESRD, hemodialysis remains the most common modality for patients initiating renal replacement therapy[44] (Figure 36.7). The outcome for children undergoing long-term maintenance hemodialysis is somewhat more difficult to determine than for adults because most pediatric patients who undergo dialysis move on to renal transplantation. Cardiovascular disease is the primary cause of death, and patients younger than 10 years old are at the highest risk of morbidity and mortality. Fluid overload, uncontrolled hypertension, heart failure, and death continue to be major concerns. Pediatric patients undergoing hemodialysis have increased cardiovascular and overall mortality at 1 year when compared with pediatric patients undergoing PD and pediatric transplant recipients. Five-year survival is lower in pediatric patients undergoing hemodialysis (75%) than pediatric transplant recipients (95%) or those undergoing PD (81%).[44]

In contrast to adult patients, hospitalization rates related to cardiovascular disease and infection are on the rise, despite similar use of cardiovascular drugs. Hemodialysis-treated patients 0 to 9 years of age have higher rates of hospital admission because of catheter infection as compared with patients those receiving PD. Readmission rates for bacteremia and septicemia in pediatric patients are highest among hemodialysis-treated patients. Vascular access infections are more frequent in patients with catheters than in patients with AVFs or AVGs.[44]

## SUMMARY

Hemodialysis remains an important technique for renal replacement therapy in children. Its efficiency makes it the clear preference for selected short-term indications. Well-established guidelines permit successful use in the long-term setting. Ongoing issues related to vascular access and determination of optimal dose require continued investigation. Promising new data on maintenance hemodialysis schedules that employ more frequent sessions may lead to improved outcomes for children with ESRD.

## REFERENCES

1. Haas G. Versuche der Blutauswaschung am Lebenden mit Hilfe der Dialyse. Klin Wochenschr. 1925;4:13.
2. Scharer K, Fine RN. The history of dialysis therapy in children. In: Warady BA, Schaefer FS, Fine RN, Alexander SR, editors. Pediatric Dialysis. Dordrecht, Kluwer Academic Publisher; 2004. p. 3.
3. Kolff WJ, Berk HTJ, et al. Artificial kidney, dialyzer with great area. Geneeskd Gids. 1943;21:409.
4. Merrill JP, Smith, S, 3rd, Callahan EJ, 3rd, Thorn GW. The use of an artificial kidney. II. Clinical experience. J Clin Invest. 1950;29:425–38.
5. Mateer FM, Greenman L, Danowski TS. Hemodialysis of the uremic child. AMA Am J Dis Child. 1955;89:645–55.
6. Hutchings RH, Hickman R, Scribner BH. Chronic hemodialysis in a pre-adolescent. Pediatrics. 1966;37:68–73.

7. Fine RN, DePalma JR, Lieberman E, Donnel GN, Gordon A, Maxwell MH. Extended hemodialysis in children with chronic renal failure. J Pediatr. 1968;73:706–13.

8. Kjellstrand CM, Shideman, JR, Santiago, EA, et al. Technical advances in hemodialysis of very small pediatric patients. Proc Clin Dial Transplant Forum. 1971;1:124–32.

9. Brescia M, Cimino JE, Appel K, Hurwich BJ. Chronic hemodialysis using venipuncture and a surgically created arteriovenous fistula. N Engl J Med. 1966;275:1089–92.

10. Mahan JD, Mayer M, Nevins TE. The Hickman catheter: A new hemodialysis access device for infants and children. Kidney Int. 1983;24:694–97.

11. Ward RA. New AAMI standards for dialysis fluids. Nephrol News Issues. 2011;25:33–6.

12. Aljama P, Bird PA, Ward MK, et al. Hemodialysis-induced leucopenia and activation of complement: Effects of different membranes. Proc Eur Dial Transplant Assoc. 1978;15:144–53.

13. Caruana RJ, Hamilton RW, Pearson FC. Dialyzer hypersensitivity syndrome: Possible role of allergy to ethylene oxide. Report of 4 cases and review of the literature. Am J Nephrol. 1985;5:271–4.

14. Kiali M, Djurdev O, Farah M, et al. Use of electron-beam sterilized hemodialysis membranes and the risk of thrombocytopenia. JAMA. 2011;306:1679–87.

15. Bonomini V, Feletti C, Stefoni S, Vangelista A. Early dialysis and renal transplantation. Nephron. 1986;44:267–71.

16. Bonomini V, Vangelista A, Stefoni S. Early dialysis in renal substitutive programs. Kidney Int Suppl. 1978;8:S112–6.

17. Tattersall J, Greenwood R, Farrington K. Urea kinetics and when to commence dialysis. Am J Nephrol. 1995;15:283–9.

18. Cooper BA, Branley P, Bulfone L, et al. A randomized, controlled trial of early versus late initiation of dialysis. N Engl J Med. 2010;363:609–19.

19. Silva MB, Jr, Hobson RW, 2nd, Pappas PJ, et al. A strategy for increasing use of autogenous hemodialysis access procedures: Impact of preoperative noninvasive evaluation. J Vasc Surg. 1998;27:302–7.

20. Davenport A. Alternatives to standard unfractionated heparin for pediatric hemodialysis treatments. Pediatr Nephrol. 2012;27:1869–97.

21. Thijssen S, Kruse A, Raimann J, et al. A mathematical model of regional citrate anticoagulation in hemodialysis. Blood Purif. 2005;29:197–203.

22. Hanevold C, Lu S, Yonekawa K. Utility of citrate dialysate in management of acute kidney injury in children. Hemodial Int. 2011;14(Suppl 1):S2–6.

23. Hoenich NA, Woffindin C, Matthews JN, et al. Clinical comparison of high-flux cellulose acetate and synthetic membranes. Nephrol Dial Transplant. 1994;9:60–6.

24. Jain SR, Smith L, Brewer ED, Goldstein SL. Non-invasive intravascular monitoring in the pediatric hemodialysis population. Pediatr Nephrol. 2001;16:15–8.

25. Michael M, Brewer ED, Goldstein SL. Blood volume monitoring to achieve target weight in pediatric hemodialysis patients. Pediatr Nephrol. 2004;19:432–37.

26. Gotch FA Sargent JA. A mechanistic analysis of the National Cooperative Dialysis Study (NCDS). Kidney Int. 1985;28:526–34.

27. Owen WF, Jr, Lew NL, Liu Y, et al. The urea reduction ratio and serum albumin concentrations as predictors of mortality in patients undergoing hemodialysis. N Engl J Med. 1993;329:1001–6.

28. Rocco MV. Revisions to KDOQI guidelines released at the NKF 2006 spring clinical meetings. Nephrol News Issues. 2006;20:40, 42.

29. Daugirdas JT. Simplified equations for monitoring kt/V, PCRn, eKt/V and ePCRn. Adv Ren Replace Ther. 1995;2:295–304.

30. Gotch FA. The current place of urea kinetic modeling with respect to different dialysis modalities. Nephrol Dial Transplant. 1998;13:10–14.

31. Leypoltd JK, Jaber BL, Zimmerman DL. Predicting treatment dose for novel therapies using urea standard kt/V. Semin Dial. 2004;17:142–5.

32. Suri RS, Garg AX, Chertow GM, et al. Frequent Hemodialysis Network (FHN) randomized trials: Study design. Kidney Int. 2007;71:349–59.

33. Lindsay RM, Nesrallah G, Suri R, et al. Is more frequent hemodialysis beneficial and what is the evidence? Curr Opin Nephrol Hypertens. 2004;13:631–5.

34. Raimann JG, Thijssen S, Ramos R, Levin NW. More frequent hemodialysis: What do we know? Where do we stand? Contrib Nephrol. 2011;171:10–6.

35. Tom A, McCauley L, Bell L, et al. Growth during maintenance hemodialysis: Impact of enhanced nutrition and clearance. J Pediatr. 1999;134:464–71.

36. I. NKF-K/DOQI clinical practice guidelines for hemodialysis adequacy: Update 2000. Am J Kidney Dis. 2001;37(Suppl 1):S7–64.

37. Sarkar SR, Kaitwatcharachai C, Levin NW. Complications during hemodialysis. In: Nissenson AR, Fine RN, editors. Clinical Dialysis. 4th ed. New York: McGraw-Hill; 2005. p. 237.

38. Mandal AK, Abernathy T, Nelluri SN, Stitzel V. Is quinine effective and safe in leg cramps? J Clin Pharmacol. 1995;35:588–93.

39. Daugirdas JT, Ing TS. First-use reactions during hemodialysis: A definition of subtypes. Kidney Int Suppl. 1988;24:S37–43.

40. Schulman G, Hakim R, Arias R, et al. Bradykinin generation by dialysis membranes: Possible role in anaphylactic reaction. J Am Soc Nephrol. 1993;3:1563–9.

41. Muth CM, Shank ES. Gas embolism. N Engl J Med. 2000;342:476–82.

42. Warady BA, Bunchman T. Dialysis therapy for children with acute renal failure: Survey results. Pediatr Nephrol. 2000;15:11–13.

43. Meyer RJ, Flynn JT, Brophy PD, et al. Hemodialysis followed by continuous hemofiltration for treatment of lithium intoxication in children. Am J Kidney Dis. 2001;37:1044–7.

44. US Renal Data System. USRDS 2013 Annual Data Report: Atlas of Chronic Kidney Disease and End-Stage Renal Disease in the United States. Bethesda, MD: National Institutes of Health, National Institute of Diabetes and Digestive and Kidney Diseases; 2013.

## REVIEW QUESTIONS

1. A 16-year-old boy with a history of end-stage renal disease from focal segmental glomerulosclerosis has a failing renal allograft and will need to return to dialysis within the next 6 months. He and his family choose hemodialysis as their preferred modality. He is highly sensitized, and although he will be listed for renal transplant again, you anticipate that his waiting time will be at least 1 to 2 years. Of the following, the *most appropriate* recommendation for hemodialysis vascular access is:
   a. Arteriovenous fistula
   b. Arteriovenous graft
   c. Femoral venous catheter
   d. Internal jugular venous catheter
   e. Subclavian venous catheter

2. You are determining the appropriate hemodialysis prescription for a new patient in your hemodialysis unit. When choosing a dialyzer, you obtain the manufacturer's specifications regarding the $K_{uf}$. Of the following, the *most accurate* statement about $K_{uf}$ is that it defines:
   a. The maximum theoretical limit for ultrafiltration at infinite transmembrane pressure
   b. The maximum theoretical limit for urea clearance at infinite blood and dialysate flow rate
   c. The minimum required transmembrane pressure necessary to prevent back-filtration
   d. The volume of blood cleared of urea in 1 min at a given blood flow rate
   e. The volume of fluid that will cross the membrane in 1 h at a given transmembrane pressure

3. A 12-year-old patient presenting to the emergency department with several weeks of fatigue, malaise, and weight loss is found to have renal failure with BUN 110 mg/dL and Cr 11.7 mg/dL. Renal ultrasound demonstrates small, echogenic kidneys bilaterally. You believe that the patient likely has had undiagnosed renal dysplasia and now has end-stage renal disease. The patient is tired and thin but alert without signs of volume overload. You make arrangements to initiate hemodialysis. Of the following, the *most appropriate* consideration in the initial hemodialysis prescriptions would be:
   a. Ensure vascular access that can provide blood flow of at least 300 mL/min.
   b. Avoid heparin anticoagulation for the first week.
   c. Preferentially choose a polysulfone dialyzer membrane.
   d. Target urea clearance of no more than 30%.
   e. Use a dialyzer with a high KoA.

4. During the dialysis process, several factors are responsible for molecular transport. Of the following, the *most accurate* statement regarding the physical principles of molecular transport that are active in hemodialysis is:
   a. Adsorption favors movement of smaller molecules over larger molecules.
   b. Convection favors movement of smaller molecules over larger molecules.
   c. Diffusion favors movement of smaller molecules over larger molecules.
   d. Ultrafiltration favors movement of smaller molecules over larger molecules.
   e. Under most circumstances in hemodialysis, small and large molecules transport equally.

5. The hemodialysis apparatus is complex and has multiple components designed to provide safe and effective therapy to the patient. Of the following, the option that *best* describes the two main components of the dialysis apparatus is:
   a. The blood circuit and the dialysate circuit
   b. The hemodialyzer and the vascular access
   c. The arterial segment and the venous segment
   d. The proportioning system and the ultrafiltration controller
   e. The "A" concentrate and the "B" concentrate

6. An 11-year-old girl is admitted to the intensive care unit with meningococcemia and renal failure as a secondary effect of her multiorgan dysfunction syndrome. Her potassium level has risen to 7.2 mEq/L, with changes on her electrocardiogram suggesting evidence for cardiac effects. You are preparing to perform emergency hemodialysis to correct the hyperkalemia. Of the following, the *most appropriate* option for vascular access would be:
   a. Arteriovenous fistula
   b. Arteriovenous graft
   c. Bilateral single-lumen cephalic vein catheters
   d. Femoral double-lumen venous catheter
   e. Subclavian double-lumen venous catheter

7. A 19-year-old male patient has been receiving hemodialysis for acute kidney injury for 8 weeks because of complications following liver transplantation. He has tolerated his sessions well, but he remains intubated in the intensive care unit. Over the last week, his platelet count has dropped, and the intensive care unit

team is concerned that he may have heparin-induced thrombocytopenia. They ask whether there are options to perform his hemodialysis sessions but limit his heparin exposure. Of the following, the method *most likely* to ensure effective hemodialysis sessions and also address the concern for heparin-induced thrombocytopenia would be to:

a. Change unfractionated heparin to low-molecular-weight heparin.
b. Eliminate heparin and use citrate-containing dialysate.
c. Give a heparin bolus at the start of hemodialysis but avoid use of continuous infusion.
d. Perform hemodialysis without anticoagulation.
e. Use half the previous dose of unfractionated heparin.

8. A 10-month-old boy with end-stage renal disease from posterior urethral valves who is maintained on peritoneal dialysis develops fungal peritonitis and must make a temporary transition to hemodialysis. He weighs 7.7 kg and is polyuric. Of the following, the *most accurate* statement about plans for hemodialysis is that:

a. Extended session length is likely required to achieve ultrafiltration goals.
b. Heparin cannot be used as the anticoagulant.
c. High metabolic needs will obligate use of a dialyzer with a high KoA.
d. Outcome data indicate that the single-pool Kt/V target for this age group is 1.6.
e. The patient will likely need blood prime of the hemodialysis circuit.

9. You are preparing the prescription for a 10-year-old girl with end-stage renal disease from renal dysplasia who will initiate hemodialysis. The patient has a new right-sided 10-French internal jugular catheter that you anticipate will deliver a blood flow rate of 150 mL/min. You have chosen a hemodialyzer with $K_D$ for urea of 120 mL/min at that blood flow rate. The patient weighs 35 kg; she does not appear volume overloaded. You would like to target a urea clearance of approximately 30% for this first session. Of the following, the dialysis time that will *most likely* give a urea clearance closest to the target of 30% is:

a. 30 min
b. 60 min
c. 90 min
d. 120 min
e. 180 min

10. You are reviewing the dialysis adequacy studies for your unit and notice that a patient has Kt/V this month of 1.1. The patient has been doing well on hemodialysis, growing, thriving and participating in school. Results of blood testing have been stable. Previous values for Kt/V over the last 6 months have been 1.4 to 1.6. His current prescription is as follows:

    Dialyzer: KoA 1100 mL/min
    Vascular access: 12-French right-sided internal jugular catheter
    Blood flow rate: 250 mL/min
    Session length: 3 h
    Schedule: Tuesday, Thursday, Saturday

Of the following, the *most appropriate* next step to address the low Kt/V for this patient would be to:

a. Adjust the dialysis schedule to Monday, Tuesday, Thursday, and Saturday.
b. Change to a larger dialyzer with KoA 1400 mL/min.
c. Increase dialysis time to 4 h/session.
d. Refer the patient for urgent placement of an arteriovenous fistula.
e. Review session characteristics and repeat Kt/V measurement.

## ANSWER KEY

1. a
2. e
3. d
4. c
5. a
6. d
7. b
8. e
9. b
10. e

37

# Peritoneal dialysis

BRADLEY A. WARADY

Peritoneal dialysis (PD) has been recognized as an important modality for renal replacement therapy (RRT) since it was first used to treat children with acute kidney injury (AKI) in the 1960s. Its relative ease of administration has also been crucial to the successful treatment of infants and young children with end-stage renal disease (ESRD). This chapter provides an overview of PD that is pertinent to the clinical application of this RRT modality.

## HISTORY

The peritoneal cavity has been used for the treatment of serious illness in children since the second decade of the 20th century. In 1918, Blackfan and Maxcy[1] described the successful use of intraperitoneal injections of saline solution in dehydrated infants, a method that is still used today in rural areas of some developing countries. The first reports of the use of PD to treat children with renal failure were published by Bloxsom and Powell in 1948[2] and by Swan and Gordon in 1949.[3] These articles appeared when the worldwide reported clinical experience with PD was fewer than 100 patients.[4] As detailed by Swan and Gordon,[3] the technique allowed large volumes of dialysate to flow continuously by gravity from 20-L carboys through a rigid metal catheter that had been surgically implanted into the upper abdomen. Dialysate was constantly drained from the peritoneal cavity by water suction through an identical catheter implanted in the pelvis. Today, this technique is termed continuous peritoneal lavage, and in some ways it foretold the current emphasis on continuous as opposed to intermittent PD therapies.

Swan and Gordon maintained fluid balance in their young patients by adjusting the dialysate dextrose concentration between 2 and 4 g/100 mL, as is generally done today. Excellent solute removal was achieved with an average daily dialysate delivery of 33 L. Dialysate temperature was regulated by adjusting the number of illuminated 60-watt incandescent light bulbs in a box placed over the dialysate inflow path. Although two of the three children treated for AKI by Swan and Gordon survived after 9 and 12 days of continuous peritoneal lavage, this technique did not attract much interest among physicians treating children with renal failure during this period, and it was more than a decade before the use of PD in children was again reported. During the 1950s, the development of disposable nylon catheters and commercially prepared dialysis solutions made PD a practical short-term treatment for AKI.[5] Successful adaptation of this technique, now known as acute intermittent PD (acute IPD), for use in infants and children with AKI was first reported by Segar et al. in 1961[6] and later by Etteldorf et al. in 1962.[7]

Although PD was successful in treating AKI, early attempts at PD appeared to offer little in the treatment of children with ESRD. These early acute IPD techniques required reinsertion of the dialysis catheter for each treatment, thus making prolonged use in small patients essentially impossible.[8] The development of a "permanent" peritoneal catheter was first proposed by Palmer et al.[9,10] and was later perfected by Tenckhoff and Schecter.[11] This made long-term IPD an accessible form of RRT for adult and pediatric patients with ESRD. Boen et al.[12] and Tenckhoff et al.[13] independently devised automated dialysate delivery systems that could be used in the patient's home. With this development, long-term IPD became a practical and potentially desirable alternative to long-term hemodialysis (HD) for children with ESRD.

A new era in the history of PD as a treatment for children with ESRD was heralded in 1972 by the description of a "novel portable/wearable equilibrium dialysis technique" by Popovich et al.,[14] which is currently known as continuous ambulatory PD (CAPD). Pediatric nephrologists were quick to recognize the potential advantages of CAPD in young patients. Advantages of CAPD over HD in children included the maintenance of nearly steady-state biochemical control, avoidance of disequilibrium syndrome, greatly reduced dietary and fluid restrictions, and freedom from repeated dialysis needle punctures. CAPD also allowed children of all ages to receive dialysis at home and have nearly normal school attendance and other childhood activities. CAPD and, later, automated PD (APD) made possible the routine treatment of very young infants with ESRD, thereby extending the option of RRT to a patient population previously considered too young to be suitable for long-term treatment (Figures 37.1 to 37.5).

CAPD was first used in a child in 1978 in Toronto.[15,16] Since that time, CAPD and its many modifications (which together can be called continuous PD or CPD) have become the dialysis treatment modalities most commonly prescribed for children with ESRD throughout much of the world.[17]

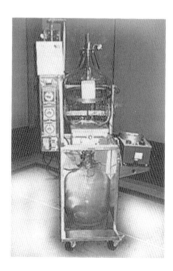

Figure 37.1 Early automatic peritoneal dialysis cycler designed by Boen et al. (1960s).

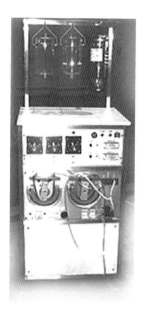

Figure 37.2 Drake-Willock peritoneal dialysis cycler machine (1970s).

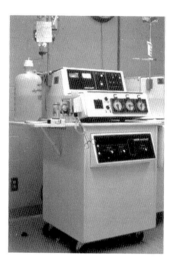

Figure 37.3 Physio-Control peritoneal dialysis cycling machine.

## EPIDEMIOLOGY

Dramatic growth in the use of CPD as maintenance dialysis treatment for children occurred worldwide during the 15 years following its introduction to pediatric dialysis. By 1993, ESRD patient registry reports showed that CPD was the most commonly prescribed long-term dialysis modality for children less than 15 years of age in the United States, Canada, Australia, New Zealand, the United Kingdom, the former West Germany, Israel, and the Netherlands.[18-20]

Data on CPD use in North American children have been compiled within the registry of the North American

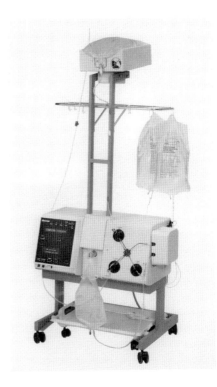

Figure 37.4 Baxter PacX automated peritoneal dialysis cycler (1984). (Courtesy of Baxter Healthcare, Deerfield, Illinois.)

Pediatric Renal Trials and Collaborative Studies (NAPRTCS). The NAPRTCS has collected data on pediatric dialysis from more than 100 pediatric dialysis centers located in the United States, Canada, Mexico, and Costa Rica. Between 1992 and 2010, the NAPRTCS enrolled 7039 pediatric dialysis-treated patients 1 day to 20 years old.[21] Of these, the initial modality selected for 4430 (62.9 %) patients was CPD, most commonly performed with an automated cycling machine. Although most patients in all age groups were prescribed CPD, the preference for CPD over HD was most pronounced among younger patients. Eighty-five percent of infants and young children 0 to 5 years of age were treated with CPD, compared with 65% of children 6 to 12 years and 51% of patients more than 12 years of age.

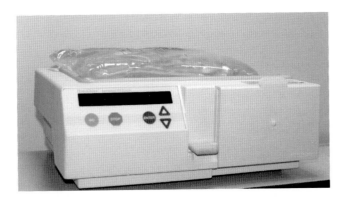

Figure 37.5 Baxter HomeChoice Pediatric peritoneal dialysis cycler (2002). (Courtesy of Baxter Healthcare, Deerfield, Illinois.)

Noteworthy is the finding that the overall percentage of incident patients prescribed CPD decreased to 55.7% in 2008 to 2010.

Participation in the NAPRTCS is restricted to specialized pediatric dialysis centers staffed by pediatric nephrologists, a fact that may influence observations such as dialysis modality choice. Furth et al.,[22] in fact, showed that older children treated in nonpediatric units are more likely to receive maintenance HD than CPD. To that end, information from the 2013 edition of the United States Renal Data System (USRDS) Annual Data Report (ADR), which addresses RRT for all children (0 to 19 years old) in the United States with ESRD, regardless of the site of care (pediatric vs. adult dialysis units), revealed that at the time of ESRD diagnosis, 695 (49.2%) of the 1410 patients were initiated on HD, 396 (28%) were started on PD, and 280 (19.9%) received a preemptive renal transplant.[23] Earlier data from 12 pediatric registries in Europe also revealed similar statistics, with 48% of incident patients receiving HD, 34% PD, and 18% preemptive transplantation.[24] More recent data from 14 pediatric centers in Europe demonstrated slightly different results, with 50% of patients commencing therapy with PD and 34% with HD.[25] Patient and family choice and the age and size of the patient were the predominant factors influencing modality selection.

As would be expected with a pediatric cohort, data on modality status of prevalent patients with ESRD from the USRDS revealed that of 7983 patients, the majority (69%) had a kidney transplant, whereas 11% were maintained on PD.[23]

## PRINCIPLES

The peritoneal solute exchange process is the sum of two simultaneous and interrelated transport mechanisms: diffusion and convection. Diffusion refers to the movement of solute down a concentration gradient, whereas convection refers to movement of solutes that are "transported" in a fluid flux, the magnitude of which is determined by the ultrafiltration rate.[26]

Several theories, each progressively more complex and more accurate, have been developed to model the movement of water and solute across the peritoneal membrane. A comprehensive model, known as the three-pore model provides the basis for widely held beliefs regarding solute transport mechanics. As the name suggests, the model postulates three types of peritoneal membrane pores:

1. Ultrasmall transcellular water pores or channels (aquaporins), which comprise 1% to 2% of the total pore area, but account for 40% of water flow, and are driven by osmotic forces.
2. Small pores, which are 4 to 6 nm in diameter and comprise 90% of total pore area. These pores are subject to both concentration gradients (diffusive forces) and osmotic gradients (convective forces).

3. Large pores, which are 200 to 300 nm in diameter and comprise the remaining 5% to 7% of total pore area. These pores allow larger molecules, such as albumin, to be transported from the peritoneal capillaries, possibly driven by hydrostatic forces within the capillary bed.

---

### KEY POINTS

- The three-pore model describes the movement of water and solute across the peritoneum.
- Diffusion refers to the movement of solute down a concentration gradient, whereas convection refers to movement of solutes that are "transported" in a fluid flux.

---

Although water moves through all three pores, only the small and large pores allow convective solute transfer.[27-30]

## MASS TRANSFER AREA COEFFICIENT

The term *mass transfer area coefficient* (MTAC) characterizes the diffusive permeability of the peritoneal membrane and the functional peritoneal surface area, and it is for the most part independent of dialysis mechanics.[26,31] Some studies in adult patients have provided evidence that the functional and not the anatomic peritoneal surface area participates in solute and water exchange, and the functional component accounts for only 25% to 30% of total peritoneal surface area.[32] The MTAC has also been variably defined as the area available for solute transport divided by the sum of resistances to peritoneal diffusion and represents the clearance rate (expressed in milliliters/min), which would be obtained in the absence of ultrafiltration or solute accumulation in the dialysate.[33] The MTAC, as applied to the current three-pore model of transperitoneal solute and water flux, equals the product of the free-diffusion coefficient for the solute, the fractional area available for diffusion (which is a percentage of the area of the unrestricted pores), and the term $A_0/\delta_X$, which characterizes the diffusion distance across the peritoneum.[34] To date, very few studies have measured MTACs in pediatric patients.[35-38] In the largest such study, Warady et al.[38] found evidence of enhanced transport in the youngest patients, likely to result from differences in permeability, effective surface area, or possibly maturational changes of the peritoneum. In contrast, MTAC data in children using a three-pore model demonstrate values for children to be similar to those of adults, when the data are scaled to body surface area (BSA).[39]

## ULTRAFILTRATION AND CONVECTION

Ultrafiltration represents the bulk movement of water along with permeable solutes across the peritoneum. The removal of fluid during an exchange reflects the interaction of the hydraulic permeability of the peritoneal membrane with the permeability of the membrane to the osmotically active solutes on either side of the membrane. In PD, the osmotically active agents in the dialysate fluid are either crystalloids, such as glucose, or colloids, such as icodextrin. In designing the dialysis prescription in terms of ultrafiltration, children receiving CAPD with 1.5% or 4.25% dextrose as the osmotic agent should expect the drainage volume to exceed the infused volume of dialysate by 15% to 25%, and 30% to 40%, respectively.[40] Conversely, children receiving APD with shorter dwell time of 30 to 40 min, using 1.5% and 4.25% dextrose dialysis solutions, should be expected to have drain volumes to exceed infused volumes by 4% to 8% and 12% to 18%, respectively.[40]

Convective mass transfer, which depends on fluid removal and peritoneal membrane permeability, contributes little to the movement of small solutes but is responsible for most of the large solute removal. Permeability to a specific solute can be characterized by the sieving coefficient, calculated by dividing the concentration of the solute in the ultrafiltrate by its concentration in plasma water. Studies by Pyle[41] demonstrated that the contribution of convection in a 4-h CAPD exchange with 4.25% dextrose is 12% for urea, 45% for inulin, and 86% for total protein.

Early studies and most clinical experience suggest that adequate ultrafiltration is often difficult to achieve in infants and young children. Schaefer et al.[27] suggested that the reduced ultrafiltration rate observed in infancy may actually be related to a greater total fluid "reuptake" or reabsorption from the peritoneal cavity. The reuptake phenomenon in these patients may be the result of increased lymphatic reabsorption rate (see later) or greater intraperitoneal pressure (IPP) in infants that generates a reversed transcapillary flux of fluid along hydrostatic and oncotic pressure gradients.[27]

Finally, the availability of icodextrin, a glucose polymer with an average molecular weight of 16,200 Da, allows the use of an osmotic agent that is characterized by an iso-osmotic and sustained colloid osmotic effect through the small pores. This agent improves ultrafiltration in patients undergoing CAPD and APD during long dwells, which may be essential for continuing CPD in patients experiencing loss of ultrafiltration. In a manner similar to the adult experience, de Boer et al.[42] found that 7.5% icodextrin is capable of maintaining ultrafiltration during a 12-h dwell in children, with the ultrafiltration capacity comparable to what could be obtained with 3.86% dextrose.[43] Because of its delayed ultrafiltration pattern compared with dextrose-based solutions, and out of concern for the potential side effects of its low-molecular-weight metabolites, icodextrin-containing solutions should be used only once daily during the long dwell.[44] Icodextrin has been reported to be less successful in some studies in infants, and this requires further evaluation.[45]

## PERITONEAL FLUID AND LYMPHATIC ABSORPTION

During PD, dialysate fluid is continuously removed from the peritoneal cavity, both directly into the tissues surrounding the peritoneal cavity as a result of the intraperitoneal hydraulic pressure and by the lymphatic vessels.[46] Whereas lymphatic absorption is believed by some investigators to account for only 20% to 30% of fluid reabsorption, the data on lymphatic absorption in children are especially conflicting.[47,48]

## PRINCIPLES OF THE PERITONEAL EQUILIBRATION TEST

The peritoneal equilibration test (PET) was developed by Twardowski et al.[49] as a means of characterizing solute transport rates across the peritoneum in patients on PD. The reference curves, based on the kinetics of solute equilibration between dialysate and plasma (D/P ratio) after a 2-L exchange volume, irrespective of the patient's size, made it possible to categorize adult patients into those with high, high-average, low-average, and low peritoneal membrane solute transport rates. Such PET data provide important information on which to base the PD prescription in both adults and children.[50]

Adoption of a standardized PET procedure in children resulted from an appreciation of (1) the age-independent relationship between BSA and peritoneal membrane surface area and (2) the recommended use of an exchange volume scaled to BSA in studying peritoneal transport kinetics.[38,51--53] In the largest pediatric study to date, the Pediatric Peritoneal Dialysis Study Consortium (PPDSC) evaluated 95 children by using a test exchange volume of 1100 mL/m² BSA to develop reference kinetic data (D/P and D/D0 ratios), which can be used to categorize an individual pediatric patient's peritoneal membrane solute transport capacity (Figures 37.6 and 37.7).[38] Similar reference data have been generated from pediatric studies in Europe with a test exchange volume of 1000 mL/m² BSA.[53] Details of the 4-h PET procedure in children are provided in Table 37.1. More recently, several publications have proposed the use of a 2-h PET procedure in children, the so-called short PET, as previously described by Twardowski et al. The shortened study is less labor and cost intensive, and it may promote more frequent use of this test in clinical practice.[54,55]

---

### KEY POINT

The PET characterizes solute transport rates across the peritoneum and aids the prescription process.

---

Because the transport capacity of a patient's peritoneal membrane is such an important factor to consider in determining the dialysis prescription, a PET evaluation should be conducted soon after the initiation of dialysis.[50,56] However, a PET performed within the first week after the initiation of CPD may yield higher transport results than a PET performed several weeks later.[57] Accordingly, whereas it may be most convenient to perform the initial PET at the conclusion

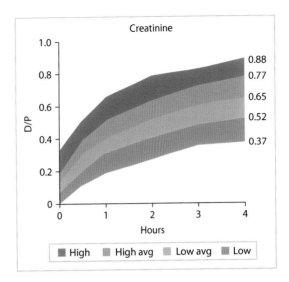

Figure 37.6 Peritoneal equilibration test results for creatinine. Shaded areas represent high, high-average, low-average, and low transport rates. The four categories are bordered by the maximal, mean +1 standard deviation (SD), mean, mean −1 SD, and minimal values for the population. Avg, average; D/P, dialysate-to-plasma ratio. (From Warady BA, Alexander SR, Hossli S, et al. Peritoneal membrane transport function in children receiving long-term dialysis. J Am Soc Nephrol. 1996;7:2385.)

of CPD training, the results after 1 to 2 months of CPD may more accurately reflect peritoneal transport properties.[50,57]

The PET evaluation should be repeated when knowledge of the patient's current membrane transport capacity

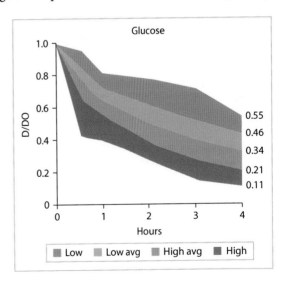

Figure 37.7 Peritoneal equilibration test results for glucose. Shaded areas represent high, high-average, low-average, and low transport rates. The four categories are bordered by the maximal, mean +1 standard deviation (SD), mean, mean −1 SD, and minimal values for the population. Avg, average; D/DO, dialysate glucose–to–initial dialysate glucose concentration ratio. (From Warady BA, Alexander SR, Hossli S, et al. Peritoneal membrane transport function in children receiving long-term dialysis. J Am Soc Nephrol. 1996;7:2385.)

Table 37.1 Peritoneal equilibration test procedure in children

- Dwell period: 4 h
- Fill volume: 1100 mL/m² body surface area*
- 2.3% to 2.4% anhydrous glucose dialysis solution (Europe)
- 2.5% dextrose dialysis solution (North America, Japan)
- Test exchange after prolonged (8 h) dwell, if possible as follows:
  - Drain the overnight dwell.
  - Record the length of the dwell and the volume drained. Also note the dextrose concentration and volume infused.
  - Infuse the calculated fill volume, note infusion time.
  - Keep patient in supine position.
  - Drain less than 10% of dialysate solution into the drain bag at 0, 120, and 240 min.
  - Invert bag for mixing and obtain sample. Reinfuse any remaining effluent.
  - Obtain blood sample after 120 min.
- Measure creatinine and glucose in each sample.
- Calculate dialysate-to-plasma (D/P) creatinine and dialysate glucose–to–baseline dialysate glucose (D/DO) concentration ratios.
- Determine transporter state by comparing creatinine and glucose equilibration curves with pediatric reference percentiles (Figures 37.6 and 37.7).

* In early infancy, volume may not be tolerable; in these cases, conduct the peritoneal equilibration test with regular daily exchange volume for evaluation.

is necessary for determination of the patient's optimal CPD prescription. Examples of this would be when there is evidence of decreased ultrafiltration capacity, such as unexplained volume overload, worsening of hypertension, or erythropoiesis stimulating agent (ESA)–resistant anemia. The other such indication for a repeat PET is impaired solute removal, such as that characterized by unexplained signs or symptoms of uremia, especially when the patient may have had repeated peritonitis episodes that can alter transport characteristics.[58]

## PATIENT SELECTION

CPD can be attempted in any child whose peritoneal cavity is intact and will admit an adequate volume of dialysate. Experience has shown that CPD can be used successfully in children with the following conditions: polycystic kidney disease (usually after bilateral nephrectomy), prune belly syndrome, bilateral Wilms tumor, recent abdominal surgical procedures (if no draining wounds are present), or with

Table 37.2 Absolute contraindications to peritoneal dialysis in children

- Omphalocele
- Gastroschisis
- Bladder exstrophy
- Diaphragmatic hernia
- Obliterated peritoneal cavity

vesicostomy, cutaneous ureterostomy, colostomy, or ventriculoperitoneal shunt.[59-61] Absolute contraindications to PD are given in Table 37.2.

CPD is the therapy of choice for the treatment of ESRD in infants.[61-64] It is widely recognized that CPD can be an effective maintenance therapy in babies who develop ESRD as early as the first few days or weeks of life.[65] Of course, the provision of home CPD, especially to infants, does mandate an evaluation of the patient's family by the treating facility to determine the likelihood of success. In addition, participation of the patient's caregivers in a formal training program and assessment of their readiness to accept the substantial responsibilities associated with home dialysis, which is often referred to as the "burden of care", are other prerequisites for starting patients on CPD.[66]

## KEY POINTS

- Peritoneal dialysis can be attempted in virtually any child whose peritoneal cavity is intact and will admit an adequate volume of dialysate.
- A pediatric PD program must include a multidisciplinary team to provide the necessary support to the patient and family.

Finally, a successful pediatric PD program must also be able to provide the necessary multidisciplinary services required by the child and family on an ongoing basis. These services are provided by a team consisting of nephrologists, nurse specialists, urologists, general surgeons, renal dietitians, renal social workers, psychologists, psychiatrists, child development specialists, child life therapists, speech pathologists, and chaplains. Compared with adult patients, children require a significantly greater investment of time and resources from the CPD team.[62,67,68]

## PERITONEAL DIALYSIS ACCESS

A reliable peritoneal catheter is the cornerstone of successful CPD. Goals for PD access should include the attainment of rapid dialysate flow rates, the absence of fluid leaks, and a low incidence of catheter-related infections.

## PERITONEAL DIALYSIS CATHETER

In general, most long-term PD catheters are constructed of soft material, such as silicone rubber or polyurethane. The catheters can be thought of as having two separate regions: the intraperitoneal portion and the extraperitoneal portion. The intraperitoneal portion contains holes or slots to allow the passage of dialysate. The shape of the intraperitoneal portion typically is straight or curled; the curled configuration is often associated with less pain with dialysate inflow and a decreased predisposition to omental wrapping of the catheter. The most common catheters with these characteristics used by pediatric patients have been the straight and curled Tenckhoff catheters (Figures 37.8 and 37.9).[21,69,70]

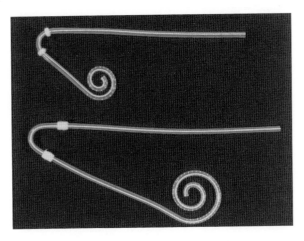

Figure 37.8 Swan-neck, double-cuff Tenckhoff peritoneal catheters with curled intraperitoneal portion.

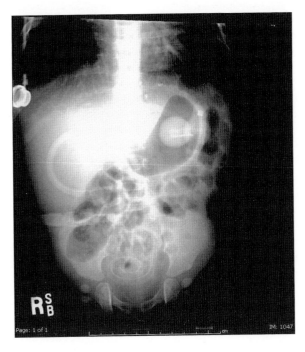

Figure 37.9 Radiologic appearance of the peritoneal dialysis catheter location. Note the curled intraperitoneal portion within the pelvis.

The extraperitoneal portion of each of these catheters has one or two Dacron cuffs to prevent fluid leaks and bacterial migration and to fix the catheter's position. The shape of this portion of the catheter is also variable and may be straight or have a preformed angle (e.g., swan-neck or pail handle) to help create a downward-directed catheter exit site. The catheter characteristics themselves may influence the risk of peritonitis (see later), although this remains controversial.[21,71-73]

## IMPLANTATION SITE

The catheter implantation technique and the immediate postoperative care ultimately influence the longevity of the PD access. Adoption of a lateral placement technique through the body of the rectus muscle has resulted in a decrease in catheter leakage (Figures 37.10 and 37.11).[69,74,75] Although an open surgical technique is used most often, there is a growing experience with laparoscopic placement of PD catheters in children, a technique that may result in rapid postoperative recovery and greater catheter longevity.[76] Irrespective of the implantation procedure, the catheter exit site should be directed lateral or downward, and the provision of preoperative antibiotics within 60 min the skin incision is recommended to decrease the incidence of postoperative peritonitis.[72,77,78] Most current recommendations suggest the preferential use of a first-generation cephalosporin in adults and children at the time of catheter placement.

It is believed that infants and young children with a vesicostomy, ureterostomy, or colostomy may benefit from placement of the catheter exit site as far from the stoma as possible to prevent contamination and infection. Placement of the exit site on the chest wall and with a downward orientation has successfully limited the number of infections in such high-risk situations in children and adults.[62,79,80]

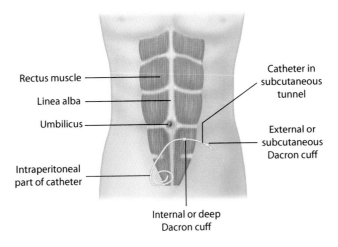

Rectus muscle

Linea alba

Umbilicus

Intraperitoneal part of catheter

Catheter in subcutaneous tunnel

External or subcutaneous Dacron cuff

Internal or deep Dacron cuff

Figure 37.10 A diagrammatic representation of the surface anatomy of the abdomen used for placement of a peritoneal dialysis catheter.

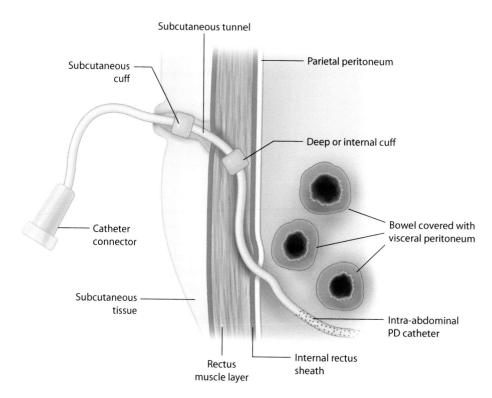

Figure 37.11 A diagrammatic representation of the S-shaped track of the peritoneal dialysis (PD) catheter through the subcutaneous tissue and the rectus muscle. Such an insertion configuration minimizes the possibility of a peritoneal fluid leak.

## IMMEDIATE POSTOPERATIVE CARE

Following catheter insertion, catheter immobilization is imperative to prevent trauma to the healing exit site, but exit site sutures should not be placed because of the risk of subsequent infection.[78] Whenever possible, a delay of 10 to 14 days before using the long-term catheter is desirable to allow for completion of healing and a decreased risk of leakage.[81] Ideally, exit site care conducted during the immediate postoperative period should be performed weekly with mask and gloves and should be performed by trained dialysis staff. The initial low frequency of dressing changes is designed to prevent contamination of the exit site with bacteria and to decrease the likelihood of manipulation of the catheter, which increases the risk of exit site trauma.[82] The exit site should be cleansed with a nonirritating agent such as poloxamer 188, chlorhexidine, or normal saline and the exit site should be evaluated weekly for the quality of healing. Application of a topical antibiotic ointment or cream at the time of the weekly dressing change has been recommended by some clinicians.[77,83]

## LONG-TERM CARE

There is little consensus regarding the optimal approach to long-term exit site care after healing is complete.[84] However, it does appear that cleansing the catheter exit site is best performed with sterile gauze and a sterile antiseptic solution, preferably chlorhexidine, sodium hypochlorite, or octenidine. It has also been recommended that a topical antibiotic be placed at the catheter exit site as a component of long-term exit site care.[77,78,85] After cleansing, the catheter should be well immobilized. Most pediatric patients are prescribed a dressing over the exit site that is changed as part of daily or alternate-day exit site care.

## COMPLICATIONS

### PERITONITIS

The single most significant complication in children maintained on CPD is peritonitis.[78,86-88] Present data make it clear that children have a significantly greater rate of peritonitis than adults, and many children experience an episode of peritonitis during their first year of CPD treatment.[21] Reductions in observed peritonitis rates have been reported in both adults and children by treatment of *Staphylococcus aureus* nasal carriage and the application of topical antibiotics (e.g., mupirocin or gentamicin) at the catheter exit site, as well as by important technical developments, such as disconnect systems and the flush-before-fill technique.[89-91] Systemic antibiotic use should be considered following touch contamination and before gastrointestinal or dental procedures.[78] The important contribution of prolonged dialysis training, with an emphasis on proper hand hygiene, to the prevention of peritonitis has been well demonstrated.[92]

## Incidence

In the 2011 NAPRTCS annual report, data on 4248 episodes of peritonitis revealed an annualized peritonitis rate of 0.64, or 1 infection every 18.8 patient-months.[21] The rate of peritonitis was highest in the youngest patients (0 to 1 years of age), who had an annualized peritonitis rate of 0.79, or 1 infection every 15.3 patient-months, in contrast to an annualized rate of 0.57 or 1 episode every 21.2 patient-months in children more than 12 years of age. A significant improvement in the overall annualized infection rate from 0.79 in 1992 to 1996 to 0.44 in recent years is noteworthy. In this same report, the annualized peritonitis rate was noted to be best with the following strategies: use of Tenckhoff catheters with straight intraperitoneal segments, double cuffs on the catheter, swan-neck tunnels, and downward-pointed exit sites.

## Infecting organisms

Data from the International Pediatric Peritoneal Dialysis Network (IPPN) demonstrated that peritonitis in children is the result of Gram-positive organisms in 44% of episodes, Gram-negative organisms in 25%, and fungi (e.g., *Candida* species) in approximately 2% of episodes. The remaining 31% of episodes were culture negative in the IPPN registry. Of the Gram-positive organisms, coagulase-negative *Staphylococcus* was most common; *Pseudomonas* species was the most common Gram-negative organism in the United States, whereas other Gram-negative organisms were most common in other countries.[88]

## Treatment

The current approach to the treatment of bacterial peritonitis relies primarily on the intraperitoneal administration of antibiotics (Table 37.3). Key prophylactic and treatment recommendations have been incorporated into the "Consensus Guidelines for the Treatment of Catheter-Related Infections and Peritonitis in Pediatric Patients Receiving Peritoneal Dialysis: 2012 Update," under the auspices of the International Society for Peritoneal Dialysis.[78] This set of 22 guidelines includes recommendations for empiric antibiotic therapy as well as for treatment of Gram-positive and Gram-negative peritonitis (Figures 37.12 to 37.14). The guidelines also emphasize that the center-specific antibiotic susceptibility pattern should help guide the selection of empiric therapy because of the geographic variation in the distribution of causative organisms.[84]

The most crucial element in the treatment of fungal peritonitis is removal of the PD catheter.[93] The duration of antifungal treatment following catheter removal should be 2 to

3 weeks or longer after complete resolution of the clinical symptoms of infection. Whereas the peritoneal penetration of amphotericin B with systemic administration is poor, fluconazole is characterized by excellent bioavailability and peritoneal penetration, and fluconazole is currently the drug of choice for treatment of infection with most *Candida* species.[94-96] Ideally, susceptibility testing should also be performed when yeast is detected.

## SCLEROSING ENCAPSULATING PERITONITIS

Sclerosing encapsulating peritonitis (SEP) is a rare but a serious clinical complication of CPD that is characterized by the presence of continuous, intermittent, or recurrent bowel obstruction associated with gross thickening of the peritoneum.[97,98] Although primarily diagnosed in adults, SEP may also occur in children, typically those who have received CPD for more than 5 years. SEP is associated with a high mortality rate. The presence of peritoneal membrane thickening, peritoneal calcifications, or bowel adhesions on abdominal computed tomography (CT) scan in association with ultrafiltration failure is highly suggestive of the diagnosis, and it may be considered an indication to discontinue CPD. SEP has also been diagnosed in kidney transplant recipients, and this finding suggests a need for prolonged surveillance of all patients who have received long-term PD.[99,100] It is hoped that greater use of biocompatible dialysis solutions will be associated with less peritoneal membrane injury and a decreased incidence of SEP.[101,102]

## EXIT SITE AND TUNNEL INFECTION

Catheter exit site and tunnel infections, most often caused by *Staphylococcus* or *Pseudomonas,* are associated with a significantly increased risk for the development of peritonitis.[103] As noted previously, the initial approach to prevention occurs at the time of catheter placement, usually in the form of a single dose of a first-generation cephalosporin, unless the patient is known to be colonized with a methicillin-resistant organism.[77,78,91] Preventive measures should continue in the immediate postoperative period and should include the delayed (2 to 6 weeks) initiation of dialysis to facilitate wound healing and minimize the risk of dialysate leakage. The catheter should also be securely immobilized

Table 37.1 Antibiotic dosing recommendations for the treatment of peritonitis

| Antibiotic Type | Continuous* Loading dose | Continuous* Maintenance dose | Intermittent therapy* |
|---|---|---|---|
| **Aminoglycosides (IP)[†]** | | | |
| Gentamicin | 8 mg/L | 4 mg/L | — |
| Netilmicin | 8 mg/L | 4 mg/L | Anuric: 0.6 mg/kg |
| Tobramycin | 8 mg/L | 4 mg/L | Nonanuric: 0.75 mg/kg |
| Amikacin | 25 mg/L | 12 mg/L | — |
| **Cephalosporins (IP)** | | | |
| Cefazolin | 500 mg/L | 125 mg/L | 20 mg/kg |
| Cefepime | 500 mg/L | 125 mg/L | 15 mg/kg |
| Cefotaxime | 500 mg/L | 250 mg/L | 30 mg/kg |
| Ceftazidime | 500 mg/L | 125 mg/L | 20 mg/kg |
| **Glycopeptides (IP)[‡]** | | | |
| Vancomycin | 1,000 mg/L | 25 mg/L | 30 mg/kg: repeat dosing: 15 mg/kg every 3–5 days |
| Teicoplanin[§] | 400 mg/L | 20 mg/L | 15 mg/kg every 5–7 days |
| **Penicillins (IP)[†]** | | | |
| Ampicillin | — | 125 mg/L | — |
| **Quinolones (IP)** | | | |
| Ciprofloxacin | 50 mg/L | 25 mg/L | — |
| **Others** | | | |
| Aztreonam (IP) | 1,000 mg/l | 250 mg/L | — |
| Clindamycin (IP) | 300 mg/L | 150 mg/L | — |
| Imipenem-cilastin (IP) | 250 mg/L | 50 mg/L | — |
| Linezolid (PO) | <5 yr: 30 mg/kg daily, divided into 3 doses 5–11 yr: 20 mg/kg daily, divided into 2 doses ≥12 yr: 600 mg/dose, twice daily | — | |
| Metronidazole (PO) | 30 mg/kg daily, divided into 3 doses (maximum, 1.2 g daily) | — | |
| Rifampin (PO) | 10–20 mg/kg daily, divided into 2 doses (maximum, 600 mg daily) | — | |
| **Antifungals** | | | |
| Fluconazole (IP, IV, or PO) | 6–12 mg/kg every 24–48 h (maximum, 400 mg/daily) | — | |
| Caspofungin (IV only) | 70 mg/m$^2$ on day 1 (maximum: 70 mg daily) | 50 mg/m$^2$ daily (maximum, 50 mg daily) | — |

*Source:* Warady BA, Bakkaloglu S, Newland J, et al. Consensus guidelines for the prevention and treatment of catheter-related infections and peritonitis in pediatric patients receiving peritoneal dialysis: 2012 update. Perit Dial Int. 2012;32(Suppl 2):S32–86.

*Abbreviations:* IP, intraperitoneally; IV, intravenously; PO, orally.

* For continuous therapy, the exchange with the loading dose should dwell for 3 to 6 h; all subsequent exchanges during the treatment course should contain the maintenance dose. For intermittent therapy, the dose should be applied once daily in the long-dwell, unless otherwise specified.

[†] Aminoglycosides and penicillins should not be mixed in dialysis fluid because of the potential for inactivation.

[‡] In patients with residual renal function, glycopeptide elimination may be accelerated. If intermittent therapy is used in such a setting, the second dose should be time based on a blood level obtained 2 to 4 days after the initial dose. Redosing should occur when the blood level is <15 mg/L for vancomycin, or <8 mg/L for teicoplanin. Intermittent therapy is not recommended for patients with residual renal function unless serum levels of the drug can be monitored in a timely manner.

[§] Teicoplanin is not currently available in the United States.

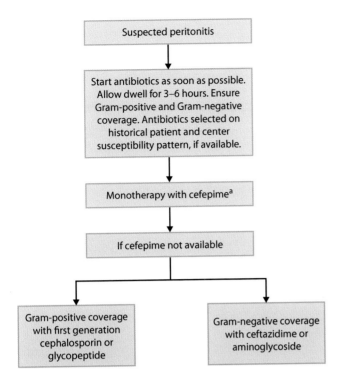

Figure 37.12 Empiric therapy of peritonitis. [a]If the center's rate of methicillin-resistant *Staphylococcus aureus* (MRSA) exceeds 10%, or if the patient has a history of MRSA infection or colonization, glycopeptide (vancomycin or teicoplanin) should be added to cefepime or should replace the first-generation cephalosporin for Gram-positive coverage. Glycopeptide use can also be considered if the patient has a history of allergy to penicillins and cephalosporins. (From Warady BA, Bakkaloglu S, Newland J, et al. Consensus guidelines for the prevention and treatment of catheter-related infections and peritonitis in pediatric patients receiving peritoneal dialysis: 2012 update. Perit Dial Int. 2012;32[Suppl 2]:S52.)

without the use of surgical sutures.[78] Regular assessment of the exit site and catheter tunnel and proper hand hygiene are additional important practice elements.

As noted earlier, attention to *S. aureus* nasal carriage in patients undergoing CPD is recommended because a substantial body of literature supports an association between nasal carriage and the development of catheter-related infections and peritonitis.[77,104] In families of children undergoing CPD, concern related to *S. aureus* nasal carriage extends to caretakers, given that as many as 45% of families with children undergoing CPD have been found to have one or more members with evidence of nasal carriage.[2] The use of mupirocin, intranasally or at the catheter exit site, has been associated with a decreased rate of exit site infections.[77,85,105] The occasional development of a *Pseudomonas* exit site infection in association with mupirocin use has prompted many investigators to recommend the prophylactic application of gentamicin ointment instead.[77,106]

Prompt diagnosis and effective therapy of exit site and tunnel infections (Table 37.4) are crucial to prevent peritonitis. Objective criteria for diagnosis have been developed based on experiences in children and adults. The isolation of a pathogen is not necessary if the clinical findings of an infection are readily apparent.[78,107]

Once the condition is diagnosed, antibiotic therapy should be chosen according to the susceptibilities of the cultured organism. The duration of treatment should be 2 to 4 weeks, and at least 7 days following complete resolution of the infection.[78] Treatment for at least 3 weeks is recommended for exit site infections secondary to *S. aureus* or *Pseudomonas aeruginosa.*

## HERNIA

The incidence of hernias in children undergoing PD (8% to 57%) is inversely proportional to the patient's age, with the highest frequency of inguinal hernias occurring in patients less than 1 year of age.[108–110] Apart from age, other risk factors include increased IPP and the presence of anatomically weak sites in the abdominal wall. The most common presentation of a hernia is a painless swelling, with less frequent occurrence of discomfort or disfigurement.[109] More than 75% of hernias in patients on CPD require surgical repair, a procedure that typically is followed immediately by abstaining from CPD, followed by low-volume dialysis for several days.

## FLUID LEAKS

Early fluid leaks that occur after catheter implantation (less than 30 days) usually manifest at the catheter exit site.[111–113] In contrast, later leaks may manifest as abdominal wall or genital edema, scrotal swelling, and apparent ultrafiltration failure. Potential risk factors for leaks include initiation of CPD immediately after catheter insertion, a median PD catheter insertion site, and weakness of the abdominal wall.

The diagnosis of a fluid leak is typically made by detecting the high glucose content of dialysate from fluid found at the exit site, by radiologic imaging with a T2-weighted magnetic resonance imaging scan (MRI) with an empty and filled abdominal cavity, or by CT with a contrast agent added in the dialysate.[111] Whereas leaks may be managed in some patients by the use of smaller exchange volumes, other patients may require a change from CAPD to APD and overnight cycling, or possibly catheter revision. Prevention of fluid leaks is preferable and may be best achieved by delayed initiation of CPD following catheter placement and application of fibrin glue at the deeper cuff at the time of catheter implantation.

## HYDROTHORAX

Hydrothorax, or the accumulation of dialysis fluid within the pleural space, is an uncommon complication of CPD with an incidence of 1.6% to 10%. Although the pathophysiology is not clear, contributing factors may include a disorder

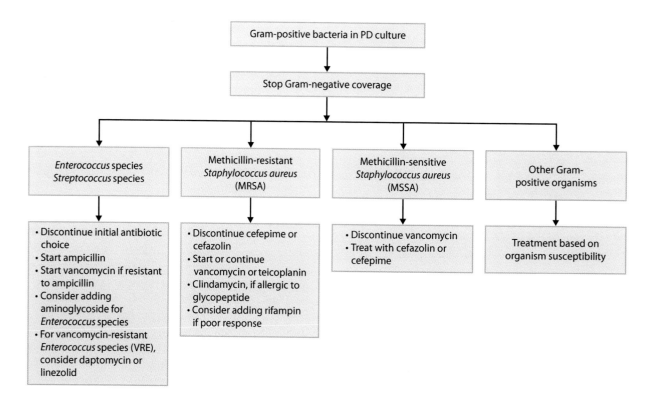

Figure 37.13 Treatment of peritonitis with Gram-positive organism on culture. MRSA, methicillin-resistant *Staphylococcus aureus*; MSSA, methicillin-sensitive *S. aureus*; PD, peritoneal dialysis; VRE, vancomycin-resistant enterococci. (From Warady BA, Bakkaloglu S, Newland J, et al. Consensus guidelines for the prevention and treatment of catheter-related infections and peritonitis in pediatric patients receiving peritoneal dialysis: 2012 update. Perit Dial Int. 2012;32[Suppl 2]:S54.)

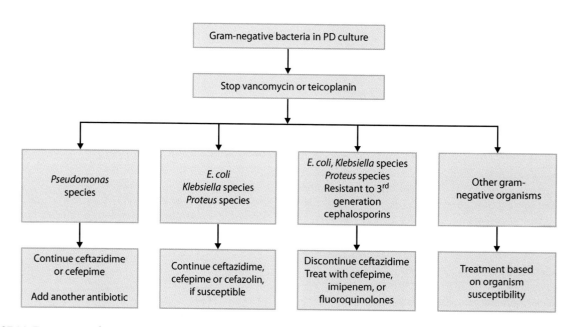

Figure 37.14 Treatment of peritonitis with Gram-negative organism on culture. PD, peritoneal dialysis. (From Warady BA, Bakkaloglu S, Newland J, et al. Consensus guidelines for the prevention and treatment of catheter-related infections and peritonitis in pediatric patients receiving peritoneal dialysis: 2012 update. Perit Dial Int. 2012;32[Suppl 2]:S56.)

Table 37.4 Oral antibiotics used in exit site and tunnel infection

| Antibiotic | Recommended dose | Dose frequency | Per-dose maximum |
|---|---|---|---|
| Amoxicillin | 10–20 mg/kg/day | Daily | 1000 mg |
| Cephalexin | 10–20 mg/kg/day | Daily or 2 times daily | 1000 mg |
| Ciprofloxacin | 10–15 mg/kg/day | Daily | 500 mg |
| Clarithromycin | 7.5 mg/kg/day | Daily or 2 times daily | 500 mg |
| Clindamycin | 30 mg/kg/day | 3 times daily | 600 mg |
| Dicloxacillin | | | |
| <40 kg | 25–50 mg/kg/day | 4 times daily | 500 mg |
| >40 kg | 125–500 mg/dose | | |
| Erythromycin (as base) | 30–50 mg/kg/day | 3 or 4 times daily | 500 mg |
| Fluconazole | 6 mg/kg/day | Every 24–48 h | 400 mg |
| Levofloxacin | 10 mg/kg | Every 48 h | Day 1: 500 mg; then 250 mg |
| Linezolid | | | |
| <5 yr | 10 mg/kg/dose | 3 times daily | 600 mg |
| 5–11 yr | 10 mg/kg/dose | 2 times daily | |
| ≥12 yr | 600 mg/dose | 2 times daily | |
| Metronidazole | 30 mg/kg/day | 3 times daily | 500 mg |
| Rifampin* | 10–20 mg/kg/day | 2 times daily | 600 mg |
| Trimethoprim | 5–10 mg/kg/day | Daily | 80 mg |

*Source:* Warady BA, Bakkaloglu S, Newland J, et al. Consensus guidelines for the prevention and treatment of catheter-related infections and peritonitis in pediatric patients receiving peritoneal dialysis: 2012 update. Perit Dial Int. 2012;32(Suppl 2):S32–86.
* Should not be used as monotherapy, or used routinely in areas in which tuberculosis is endemic.

of lymphatic drainage, a pleura-peritoneal pressure gradient, congenital diaphragmatic defects, and increased IPP.[114] Hydrothorax may be detected incidentally on routine chest radiograph or may manifest soon after the initiation of CPD as shortness of breath. The hydrothorax is more common on the right side, quite possibly because the heart and pericardium prevent fluid movement across the left hemidiaphragm.[115] In addition to the physical examination and chest radiograph, diagnosis of a hydrothorax may be made by thoracentesis and detection of fluid with the characteristic high glucose content of dialysate (greater than 300 to 400 mg/dL or pleural fluid to serum glucose concentration gradient greater than 50 mg/dL) or by scintigraphy, MRI, or CT. The subsequent continuation of PD has occurred following temporary cessation of PD (and the institution of HD), the use of APD and small nocturnal exchange volumes associated with a lower IPP, or obliteration of the pleural space with a variety of materials.[116,117] When a clear anatomic defect is noted, operative repair is characteristically successful.[117,118]

## PERITONEAL DIALYSIS ADEQUACY

Providing adequate solute clearance with CPD requires the physician to be cognizant of the patient's BSA, peritoneal membrane solute transport capacity (as determined by the PET), and residual renal function (RRF) when designing the dialysis prescription.[102,119] Several computer-based dialysis modeling programs have been validated in children and can assist the prescription process.[120,121]

Although data that correlate solute removal and clinical outcome in children are lacking, current recommendations are that the minimal "delivered" dose of total (peritoneal and kidney) small solute clearance should be a volume of plasma cleared (Kt) of urea divided by the urea distribution volume, of at least 1.8/week.[50]

The total weekly $Kt/V_{urea}$ is calculated as follows:

$$Weekly\ Kt/V_{urea} = \frac{(D_{ur} \cdot V_D)(U_{ur} \cdot V_u)}{P_{ur} \cdot V} \cdot 7$$

$D_{ur}$, $U_{ur}$, and $P_{ur}$ are the dialysate, urinary and plasma concentrations of urea, $V_D$ and $V_U$ are the 24-h dialysate and urine volumes, and V is the urea distribution volume.

In the calculation of $Kt/V_{urea}$, it is most important to use an accurate estimate of V, which is considered to be equivalent to the total body water (TBW) volume. A set of anthropometric TBW prediction equations has been developed and validated in the pediatric PD-treated population.[122] The gender-specific formulas are as follows:

Boys: $TBW = 0.10 \times (HtWt)^{0.68} - 0.37 \times weight$

Girls: $TBW = 0.14 \times (HtWt)^{0.65} - 0.35 \times weight$

Apart from weekly $Kt/V_{urea}$, the clinical status of the pediatric patient should also be monitored closely as an important qualitative means of determining whether the patient is receiving adequate dialysis. A variety of clinical, metabolic, and psychosocial aspects of care should also be taken into consideration to determine a patient's well-being (Table 37.5).[123] Attention to volume status is imperative in view of the frequent presence of hypertension and left ventricular hypertrophy noted in children receiving CPD.[124] Figure 37.15 provides an evaluation algorithm for management of adequacy targets in patients undergoing CPD.

---

### KEY POINT

Assessment of PD adequacy in children should take the total Kt/V and the patient's clinical status into consideration.

---

### OUTCOME

An assessment of patient outcome must take into account short-term and long-term measures. Data on the health-related quality of life (HRQOL) of children with ESRD

**Table 37.5** Clinical, metabolic, and psychosocial considerations in assessing the adequacy of long-term peritoneal dialysis treatment in pediatric patients

- Hydration status
- Nutritional status
- Dietary intake of energy, protein, salts and trace elements
- Electrolyte and acid-base balance
- Calcium phosphate homeostasis
- Control of anemia
- Blood pressure control
- Growth and mental development
- Level of psychosocial rehabilitation

*Source:* Verrina E, Perri K. Technical aspects and prescription of peritoneal dialysis in children. In: Warady BA, Schaefer F, Alexander S, editors. Pediatric Dialysis, 2nd ed. New York: Springer; 2012. p. 169–203.

reveals that the HRQOL parameters of children undergoing dialysis are inferior to those of children with a successful kidney transplant. Risk factors for an impaired HRQOL should regularly be sought by repeated assessments and addressed if present.[125,126]

In a review of the pediatric USRDS mortality data derived from 1990 to 2010, mortality rates for both children and adolescents had decreased significantly over those decades,

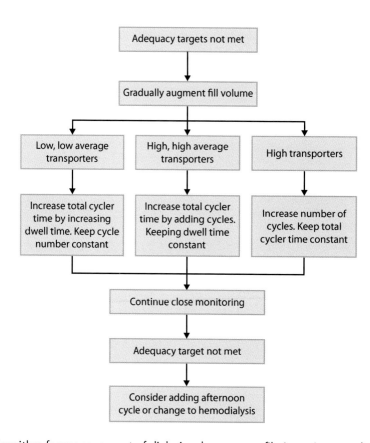

Figure 37.15 Evaluation algorithm for management of dialysis adequacy profile in patients undergoing peritoneal dialysis.

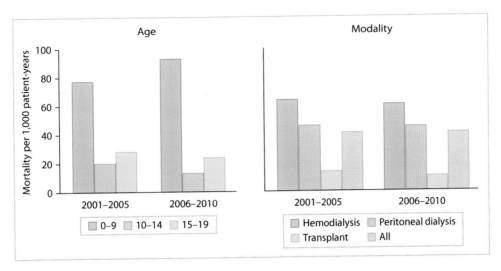

Figure 37.16 One-year adjusted all-cause mortality rates in pediatric patients (from day 1), by age and modality. (From United States Renal Data System [USRDS] 2013 Annual Data Report: Atlas of Chronic Kidney Disease and End-Stage Renal Disease in the United States. Bethesda, MD: National Institutes of Health, National Institute of Diabetes and Digestive and Kidney Diseases; 2013.)

with the highest mortality rates still evident in patients who initiated dialysis at less than 5 years of age.[127] Additionally, the 2013 annual report of the USRDS continued to demonstrate that most PD-treated patients receive a kidney transplant over the course of 5 years, the outcome of PD-treated patients is inferior compared with transplant recipients, and cardiovascular disease and infection are the primary causes of death.[23] The 1-year adjusted all-cause mortality rate was 60.4 per 1000 patient-years for children undergoing HD, 45 for those undergoing PD, and 10.4 for transplant recipients (Figure 37.16). For those patients who initiated ESRD therapy in 2002 to 2006, the overall probability of surviving 5 years was 0.75 for patients undergoing HD, 0.80 for those undergoing PD, and 0.96 for transplant patients. In fact, the expected remaining lifetime (years) for patients with incident ESRD who were 0 to 14 years old and were undergoing dialysis was only 16.0 years, compared with 57.6 years for the transplant population of the same age and 72.8 years for the general population. These data emphasize that irrespective of the positive aspects of dialysis, one should aim to minimize the time a child spends on dialysis before transplantation whenever possible. Clinical Vignette 37.1 describes a child undergoing dialysis in whom transplantation is being considered.

---

### KEY POINT

Mortality rates of patients undergoing HD and PD are higher than in kidney transplant recipients.

---

### Clinical Vignette 37.1

D.W. is a 6-year-old boy who has developed end-stage kidney disease secondary to the presence of posterior urethral valves. Subsequent to a discussion between the dialysis team and his family regarding renal replacement therapy options, a swan-neck peritoneal dialysis catheter was placed. Automated peritoneal dialysis was initiated following the training of his parents to provide home therapy. His dialysis prescription included seven exchanges nightly after his peritoneal equilibration test evaluation revealed him to be a low-average transporter. An assessment of his clearance revealed his total Kt/V to be 1.9, and his overall well-being was felt to be good. Patient's course on dialysis was unremarkable until he developed an episode of *Staphylococcus aureus* peritonitis in association with an exit site infection with the same organism. Treatment consisted of intraperitoneal vancomycin with complete resolution of the infections. His parents are currently being evaluated as possible transplant donors.

### TEACHING POINTS

This clinical course of the patient in Clinical Vignette 37.1 illustrates the usual clinical course of a patient with end-stage renal disease. The decision for placement of the peritoneal dialysis catheter is made after discussions are held between the patient's family and the dialysis team. The pros and cons of all forms of renal replacement therapy (peritoneal dialysis, hemodialysis, and renal transplantation) are reviewed during this discussion. Dialysis prescription is empirically started and is modified after the peritoneal equilibration test data are available. Eventual transplantation is the goal for all pediatric patients who are receiving dialysis therapies.

# REFERENCES

1. Blackfan K, Maxcy K. The intraperitoneal injection of saline solution. Am J Dis Child. 1918;15:19.
2. Bloxsom A, Powell N. The treatment of acute temporary dysfunction of the kidneys by peritoneal irrigation. Pediatrics. 1948;1:52–7.
3. Swan H, Gordon HH. Peritoneal lavage in the treatment of anuria in children. Pediatrics. 1949;4:586–95.
4. Odel H, Ferris D, Power M. Peritoneal lavage as an effective means of extra-renal excretion. Am J Med. 1950;9:63–77.
5. Maxwell MH, Rockney RE, Kleeman CR, et al. Peritoneal dialysis. 1. Technique and applications. JAMA. 1959;170:917–24.
6. Segar WE, Gibson RK, Rhamy R. Peritoneal dialysis in infants and small children. Pediatrics 1961;27:603–13.
7. Etteldorf JN, Dobbins WT, Sweeney MJ, et al Intermittent peritoneal dialysis in the management of acute renal failure in children. J Pediatr. 1962;60:327–39.
8. Feldman W, Baliah T, Drummond KN. Intermittent peritoneal dialysis in the management of chronic renal failure in children. Am J Dis Child. 1968;116:30–6.
9. Palmer RA, Quinton WE, Gray JE. Prolonged peritoneal dialysis for chronic renal failure. Lancet. 1964;1:700–2.
10. Palmer RA, Newell JE, Gray EJ, et al. Treatment of chronic renal failure by prolonged peritoneal dialysis. N Engl J Med. 1966;274:248–54.
11. Tenckhoff H, Schechter H. A bacteriologically safe peritoneal access device. Trans Am Soc Artif Intern Organs. 1968;14:181–7.
12. Boen ST, Mion CM, Curtis FK, et al. Periodic peritoneal dialysis using the repeated puncture technique and an automatic cycling machine. Trans Am Soc Artif Intern Organs. 1964;10:409–14.
13. Tenckhoff H, Meston B, Shilipetar G. A simplified automatic peritoneal dialysis system. Trans Am Soc Artif Intern Organs. 1972;18:436–40.
14. Popovich R, Moncrief J, Decherd J, et al. The definition of a novel portable/wearable equilibrium dialysis technique (Abstract). Trans Am Soc Artif Intern Organs. 1976;5:64.
15. Oreopoulos DG, Katirtzoglou A, Arbus G, et al. Dialysis and transplantation in young children. Br Med J. 1979;1:1628–9.
16. Balfe JW, Irwin M. Continuous ambulatory peritoneal dialysis in children. In: Legrain M, editor. Continuous Ambulatory Peritoneal Dialysis. Amsterdam: Excerpta Medica; 1980. p. 131--6.
17. Schaefer F, Warady BA. Peritoneal dialysis in children with end-stage renal disease. Nat Rev Nephrol. 2011;7:659–68.
18. Warady BA, Hebert D, Sullivan EK, et al. Renal transplantation, chronic dialysis, and chronic renal insufficiency in children and adolescents: The 1995 Annual Report of the North American Pediatric Renal Transplant Cooperative Study. Pediatr Nephrol. 1997;11:49–64.
19. Honda M, Iitaka K, Kawaguchi H, et al. The Japanese National Registry data on pediatric CAPD patients: A ten-year experience. A report of the Study Group of Pediatric PD Conference. Perit Dial Int. 1996;16:269–75.
20. Alexander S, Warady B. The demographics of dialysis in children. In: Warady B, Schaefer F, Fine R, Alexander S, editors. Pediatric Dialysis. Dordrecht: Kluwer; 2004. p. 35.
21. North American Pediatric Renal Trials and Collaborative Studies (NAPRTCS) Annual Dialysis Report. Rockville, MD: Emmes Corporation; 2011.
22. Furth SL, Powe NR, Hwang W, et al. Does greater pediatric experience influence treatment choices in chronic disease management? Dialysis modality choice for children with end-stage renal disease. Arch Pediatr Adolesc Med. 1997;151:545–50.
23. US Renal Data System (USRDS) 2013 Annual Data Report: Atlas of Chronic Kidney Disease and End-Stage Renal Disease in the United States. Bethesda, MD: National Institutes of Health, National Institute of Diabetes and Digestive and Kidney Diseases; 2013.
24. van der Heijden BJ, van Dijk PC, Verrier-Jones K, et al. Renal replacement therapy in children: Data from 12 registries in Europe. Pediatr Nephrol. 2004;19:213–21.
25. Watson AR, Hayes WN, Vondrak K, et al. Factors influencing choice of renal replacement therapy in European paediatric nephrology units. Pediatr Nephrol. 2013;28:2361–8.
26. Rippe B, Stelin G. Simulations of peritoneal solute transport during CAPD: Application of two-pore formalism. Kidney Int. 1989;35:1234–44.
27. Schaefer F, Haraldsson B, Haas S, et al. Estimation of peritoneal mass transport by three-pore model in children. Kidney Int. 1998;54:1372–9.
28. Fischbach M, Haraldsson B. Dynamic changes of the total pore area available for peritoneal exchange in children. J Am Soc Nephrol. 2001;12:1524–9.
29. Flessner MF. The peritoneal dialysis system: Importance of each component. Perit Dial Int. 1997;17(Suppl 2):S91–7.
30. Flessner MF. Peritoneal ultrafiltration: Physiology and failure. Contrib Nephrol. 2009;163:7-14.

31. Popovich R, Moncrief J, Okutan M, et al. A model of the peritoneal dialysis system. Proceedings of the 25th Annual Conference on Engineering in Medicine and Biolology. 1972. p. 172.

32. Morgenstern B. Structure and function of the pediatric peritoneal membrane. In: Richard F, Alexander S, Warady B, editors. CAPD/CCPD in Children. Norwell, MA: Kluwer; 1998:73–85.

33. Krediet R. The physiology of peritoneal solute, water, and lymphatic transport. In: Khanna R, Krediet R, editors. Nolph and Gokal's Textbook of Peritoneal Dialysis, 3rd ed. New York: Springer; 2009. p. 137–72.

34. Haraldsson B. Assessing the peritoneal dialysis capacities of individual patients. Kidney Int. 1995;47:1187–98.

35. Morgenstern BZ, Baluarte HJ. Peritoneal dialysis kinetics in children. In: Fine RN, editor. Chronic Ambulatory Peritoneal Dialysis (CAPD) and Chronic Cycling Peritoneal Dialysis in Children. Boston: Martinus Nijhoff; 1987. p. 47–61.

36. Popovich R, Pyle W, Rosenthal D, et al. Kinetics of peritoneal dialysis in children. In: Moncrief J, Popovich R, editors. CAPD Update. New York: Masson; 1981. p. 227.

37. Geary D, Harvey E, Balfe J. Mass transfer area coefficients in children. Perit Dial Int. 1994;14:30–3.

38. Warady BA, Alexander SR, Hossli S, et al. Peritoneal membrane transport function in children receiving long-term dialysis. J Am Soc Nephrol. 1996;7:2385–91.

39. Bouts AH, Davin JC, Groothoff JW, et al. Standard peritoneal permeability analysis in children. J Am Soc Nephrol. 2000;11:943–50.

40. Gruskin AB, Rosenblum H, Baluarte HJ, et al. Transperitoneal solute movement in children. Kidney Int Suppl. 1983;15:S95–100.

41. Pyle W. Mass transfer in peritoneal dialysis. PhD thesis, University of Texas at Austin. Ann Arbor, MI: University Microfilms International; 1987.

42. de Boer AW, Schroder CH, van Vliet R, et al. Clinical experience with icodextrin in children: Ultrafiltration profiles and metabolism. Pediatr Nephrol. 2000;15:21–4.

43. Schroder CH. New peritoneal dialysis fluids: Practical use for children. Pediatr Nephrol. 2003;18:1085–8.

44. Finkelstein F, Healy H, Abu-Alfa A, et al. Superiority of icodextrin compared with 4.25% dextrose for peritoneal ultrafiltration. J Am Soc Nephrol. 2005;16:546–54.

45. Dart A, Feber J, Wong H, Filler G. Icodextrin re-absorption varies with age in children on automated peritoneal dialysis. Pediatr Nephrol. 2005;20:683–5.

46. Mactier RA, Khanna R, Moore H, et al. Kinetics of peritoneal dialysis in children: Role of lymphatics. Kidney Int. 1988;34:82–8.

47. Rippe B. Is lymphatic absorption important for ultrafiltration? Perit Dial Int. 1995;15:203–4.

48. Schroder CH, Reddingius RE, van Dreumel JA, et al. Transcapillary ultrafiltration and lymphatic absorption during childhood continuous ambulatory peritoneal dialysis. Nephrol Dial Transplant. 1991;6:571–3.

49. Twardowski Z, Nolph K, Khanna R, et al. Peritoneal equilibration test. Perit Dial Bull. 1987;7:378.

50. KDOQI clinical practice guidelines and clinical practice recommendations for 2006 updates: Hemodialysis adequacy, peritoneal dialysis adequacy and vascular access. Am J Kidney Dis. 2006;28:S1.

51. Kohaut EC, Waldo FB, Benfield MR. The effect of changes in dialysate volume on glucose and urea equilibration. Perit Dial Int. 1994;14:236–9.

52. Sliman GA, Klee KM, Gall-Holden B, et al. Peritoneal equilibration test curves and adequacy of dialysis in children on automated peritoneal dialysis. Am J Kidney Dis. 1994;24:813–8.

53. Schaefer F, Langenbeck D, Heckert KH, et al. Evaluation of peritoneal solute transfer by the peritoneal equilibration test in children. Adv Perit Dial. 1992;8:410–5.

54. Warady BA, Jennings J. The short PET in pediatrics. Perit Dial Int. 2007;27:441–5.

55. Cano F, Sanchez L, Rebori A, et al. The short peritoneal equilibration test in pediatric peritoneal dialysis. Pediatr Nephrol. 2010;25:2159–64.

56. Geary D, Warady B. The peritoneal equilibration test in children. In: Fine R, Alexander S, Warady B, editors. Chronic Ambulatory Peritoneal Dialysis (CAPD) and Chronic Cycling Peritoneal Dialysis (CCPD) in Children, 2nd ed. Boston: Kluwer Group; 1998.

57. Rocco MV, Jordan JR, Burkart JM. Changes in peritoneal transport during the first month of peritoneal dialysis. Perit Dial Int. 1995;15:12–7.

58. Borzych-Duzalka D, Bilginer Y, Ha IS, et al. Management of anemia in children receiving chronic peritoneal dialysis. J Am Soc Nephrol. 2013;24:665–76.

59. Dolan NM, Borzych-Duzalka D, Suarez A, et al. Ventriculoperitoneal shunts in children on peritoneal dialysis: A survey of the International Pediatric Peritoneal Dialysis Network. Pediatr Nephrol. 2013;28:315–9.

60. Warady B, Alexander S, Schaefer F. Peritoneal dialysis in children. In: Khanna R, Krediet R, editors. Nolph and Gokal's Textbook of Peritoneal Dialysis. New York: Springer; 2009. p. 803–59.

61. Zaritsky J, Warady BA. Peritoneal dialysis in infants and young children. Semin Nephrol. 2011;31:213–24.

62. Zurowska AM, Fischbach M, Watson AR, et al. Clinical practice recommendations for the care of infants with stage 5 chronic kidney disease (CKD5). Pediatr Nephrol. 2013;28:1739–48.

63. Hölttä T, Holmberg C, Rönnholm K. Peritoneal dialysis during infancy. In: Warady B, Schaefer F, Alexander S, editors. Pediatric Dialysis, 2nd ed. New York: Springer; 2012. p. 219–29.

64. Vidal E, Edefonti A, Murer L, et al. Peritoneal dialysis in infants: The experience of the Italian Registry of Paediatric Chronic Dialysis. Nephrol Dial Transplant. 2012;27:388–95.

65. Lantos JD, Warady BA. The evolving ethics of infant dialysis. Pediatr Nephrol. 2013;28:1943–7.

66. Watson AR. Stress and burden of care in families with children commencing renal replacement therapy. Adv Perit Dial. 1997;13:300–4.

67. Jones L, Aldridge M. Organization and management of a pediatric dialysis program. In: Warady B, Schaefer F, Alexander S, editors. Pediatric Dialysis, 2nd ed. New York: Springer; 2012. p. 53–72.

68. Watson AR. Psychosocial support for children and families requiring renal replacement therapy. Pediatr Nephrol. 2014; 29:1169–74.

69. Warady B, Andrews W. Peritoneal dialysis access. In: Geary D, Schaefer F, editors. Comprehensive Pediatric Nephrology. Philadelphia: Mosby Elsevier; 2008. p. 823–34.

70. Rinaldi S, Sera F, Verrina E, et al. Chronic peritoneal dialysis catheters in children: A fifteen-year experience of the Italian Registry of Pediatric Chronic Peritoneal Dialysis. Perit Dial Int. 2004;24:481–6.

71. Furth SL, Donaldson LA, Sullivan EK, et al. Peritoneal dialysis catheter infections and peritonitis in children: A report of the North American Pediatric Renal Transplant Cooperative Study. Pediatr Nephrol. 2000;15:179–82.

72. White CT, Gowrishankar M, Feber J, et al. Clinical practice guidelines for pediatric peritoneal dialysis. Pediatr Nephrol. 2006;21:1059–66.

73. Lo WK, Lui SL, Li FK, et al. A prospective randomized study on three different peritoneal dialysis catheters. Perit Dial Int. 2003;23(Suppl 2):S127–31.

74. Lindley RM, Williams AR, Fraser N, et al. Synchronous laparoscopic-assisted percutaneous endoscopic gastrostomy and peritoneal dialysis catheter placement is a valid alternative to open surgery. J Pediatr Urol. 2012;8:527–30.

75. Cribbs RK, Greenbaum LA, Heiss KF. Risk factors for early peritoneal dialysis catheter failure in children. J Pediatr Surg. 2010;45:585–9.

76. Daschner M, Gfrorer S, Zachariou Z, et al. Laparoscopic Tenckhoff catheter implantation in children. Perit Dial Int. 2002;22:22–6.

77. Piraino B, Bernardini J, Brown E, et al. ISPD position statement on reducing the risks of peritoneal dialysis-related infections. Perit Dial Int. 2011;31:614–30.

78. Warady BA, Bakkaloglu S, Newland J, et al. Consensus guidelines for the prevention and treatment of catheter-related infections and peritonitis in pediatric patients receiving peritoneal dialysis: 2012 update. Perit Dial Int. 2012;32(Suppl 2):S32–86.

79. Chadha V, Jones LL, Ramirez ZD, et al. Chest wall peritoneal dialysis catheter placement in infants with a colostomy. Adv Perit Dial. 2000;16:318–20.

80. Warchol S, Ziolkowska H, Roszkowska-Blaim M. Exit-site infection in children on peritoneal dialysis: Comparison of two types of peritoneal catheters. Perit Dial Int. 2003;23:169–73.

81. Rahim KA, Seidel K, McDonald RA. Risk factors for catheter-related complications in pediatric peritoneal dialysis. Pediatr Nephrol. 2004;19:1021–8.

82. Twardowski ZJ, Prowant BF. Current approach to exit-site infections in patients on peritoneal dialysis. Nephrol Dial Transplant. 1997;12:1284–95.

83. Bender FH, Bernardini J, Piraino B. Prevention of infectious complications in peritoneal dialysis: Best demonstrated practices. Kidney Int Suppl. 2006:S44–54.

84. Schaefer F, Feneberg R, Aksu N, et al. Worldwide variation of dialysis-associated peritonitis in children. Kidney Int. 2007;72:1374–9.

85. Chua AN, Goldstein SL, Bell D, et al. Topical mupirocin/sodium hypochlorite reduces peritonitis and exit-site infection rates in children. Clin J Am Soc Nephrol. 2009;4:1939–43.

86. Warady BA, Sullivan EK, Alexander SR. Lessons from the peritoneal dialysis patient database: A report of the North American Pediatric Renal Transplant Cooperative Study. Kidney Int Suppl. 1996;53:S68–71.

87. Tranaeus A. Peritonitis in pediatric continuous peritoneal dialysis. In: Fine RN AS, Warady BA, editors. CAPD/CCPD in Children. Norwell, MA: Kluwer; 1998. p. 301–47.

88. Warady BA, Feneberg R, Verrina E, et al. Peritonitis in children who receive long-term peritoneal dialysis: A prospective evaluation of therapeutic guidelines. J Am Soc Nephrol. 2007;18:2172–9.

89. Warady BA, Ellis EN, Fivush BA, et al. "Flush before fill" in children receiving automated peritoneal dialysis. Perit Dial Int. 2003;23:493–8.

90. Strippoli GF, Tong A, Johnson D, et al. Catheter-related interventions to prevent peritonitis in peritoneal dialysis: A systematic review of randomized, controlled trials. J Am Soc Nephrol. 2004;15:2735–46.

91. Bakkaloglu SA. Prevention of peritonitis in children: Emerging concepts. Perit Dial Int. 2009;29(Suppl 2):S186–9.

92. Holloway M, Mujais S, Kandert M, et al. Pediatric peritoneal dialysis training: Characteristics and impact on peritonitis rates. Perit Dial Int. 2001;21:401–4.

93. Warady BA, Bashir M, Donaldson LA. Fungal peritonitis in children receiving peritoneal dialysis: A report of the NAPRTCS. Kidney Int. 2000;58:384–9.

94. Wong SF, Leung MP, Chan MY. Pharmacokinetics of fluconazole in children requiring peritoneal dialysis. Clin Ther. 1997;19:1039–47.

95. Reuman PD, Neiberger R, Kondor DA. Intraperitoneal and intravenous fluconazole pharmokinetics in a pediatric patient with end stage renal disease. Pediatr Infect Dis J. 1992;11:132–3.

96. Blowey DL, Garg UC, Kearns GL, et al. Peritoneal penetration of amphotericin B lipid complex and fluconazole in a pediatric patient with fungal peritonitis. Adv Perit Dial. 1998;14:247–50.

97. Honda M, Warady BA. Long-term peritoneal dialysis and encapsulating peritoneal sclerosis in children. Pediatr Nephrol. 2010;25:75–81.

98. Vidal E, Edefonti A, Puteo F, et al. Encapsulating peritoneal sclerosis in paediatric peritoneal dialysis patients: The experience of the Italian Registry of Pediatric Chronic Dialysis. Nephrol Dial Transplant. 2013;28:1603–9.

99. da Silva N, Rocha S, Rocha L, et al. Posttransplantation encapsulating peritoneal sclerosis in a pediatric patient. Pediatr Nephrol. 2012;27:1583–8.

100. Korte MR, Habib SM, Lingsma H, et al. Posttransplantation encapsulating peritoneal sclerosis contributes significantly to mortality after kidney transplantation. Am J Transplant. 2011;11:599–605.

101. Schmitt CP. Peritoneal dialysis solutions. In: Warady B, Schaefer F, Alexander SR, editors. Pediatric Dialysis, 2nd ed. New York: Springer; 2012. p. 205-18.

102. Verrina E, Cappelli V, Perfumo F. Selection of modalities, prescription, and technical issues in children on peritoneal dialysis. Pediatr Nephrol. 2009;24:1453–64.

103. Chadha V, Schaefer F, Warady B. Peritonitis and exit-site infections. In: Warady B, Schaefer F, Alexander S, editors. Pediatric Dialysis, 2nd ed. New York: Springer; 2012. p. 231–56.

104. Piraino B. Staphylococcus aureus infections in dialysis patients: Focus on prevention. ASAIO J. 2000;46:S13–7.

105. Uttley L, Vardhan A, Mahajan S, et al. Decrease in infections with the introduction of mupirocin cream at the peritoneal dialysis catheter exit site. J Nephrol. 2004;17:242–5.

106. Bernardini J, Bender F, Florio T, et al. Randomized, double-blind trial of antibiotic exit site cream for prevention of exit site infection in peritoneal dialysis patients. J Am Soc Nephrol. 2005;16:539–45.

107. Schaefer F, Klaus G, Muller-Wiefel DE, et al. Intermittent versus continuous intraperitoneal glycopeptide/ceftazidime treatment in children with peritoneal dialysis-associated peritonitis: The Mid-European Pediatric Peritoneal Dialysis Study Group (MEPPS). J Am Soc Nephrol. 1999;10:136–45.

108. von Lilien T, Salusky IB, Yap HK, et al. A frequent complication in children treated with continuous peritoneal dialysis. Am J Kidney Dis. 1987;10:356–60.

109. Aranda RA, Romao Junior JE, Kakehashi E, et al. Intraperitoneal pressure and hernias in children on peritoneal dialysis. Pediatr Nephrol. 2000;14:22–4.

110. Bakkaloglu A. Non-infectious compolications of peritoneal dialysis in children. In: Warady BA, Schaefer F, Alexander S, editors. Pediatric Dialysis, 2nd ed. New York: Springer; 2012. p. 257–71.

111. Levin NW, Zasuwa G. Relationship between dialyser type and signs and symptoms. Nephrol Dial Transplant. 1993;8(Suppl 2):30–9.

112. Rockel A, Klinke B, Hertel J, et al. Allergy to dialysis materials. Nephrol Dial Transplant. 1989;4:646–52.

113. Purello D'Ambrosio F, Savica V, Gangemi S, et al. Ethylene oxide allergy in dialysis patients. Nephrol Dial Transplant. 1997;12:1461–3.

114. Hothi D, Harvey E. Common complications of haemodialysis. In: Warady B, Schaefer F, Alexander S, editors. Pediatric Dialysis, 2nd ed. New York: Springer; 2012:345–74.

115. Boeschoten EW, Krediet RT, Roos CM, et al. Leakage of dialysate across the diaphragm: An important complication of continuous ambulatory peritoneal dialysis. Neth J Med. 1986;29:242–6.

116. Coppo R, Amore A, Cirina P, et al. Bradykinin and nitric oxide generation by dialysis membranes can be blunted by alkaline rinsing solutions. Kidney Int. 2000;58:881–8.

117. Hakim RM, Schafer AI. Hemodialysis-associated platelet activation and thrombocytopenia. Am J Med. 1985;78:575–80.

118. Silver SM, DeSimone JA, Jr, Smith DA, et al. Dialysis disequilibrium syndrome (DDS) in the rat: Role of the "reverse urea effect." Kidney Int. 1992;42:161–6.

119. Fischbach M, Warady BA. Peritoneal dialysis prescription in children: Bedside principles for optimal practice. Pediatr Nephrol. 2009;24:1633–42; quiz 40, 42.

120. Warady BA, Watkins SL, Fivush BA, et al. Validation of PD Adequest 2.0 for pediatric dialysis patients. Pediatr Nephrol. 2001;16:205–11.

121. Verrina E, Amici G, Perfumo F, et al. The use of the PD Adequest mathematical model in pediatric patients on chronic peritoneal dialysis. Perit Dial Int. 1998;18:322–8.

122. Morgenstern BZ, Wuhl E, Nair KS, et al. Anthropometric prediction of total body water in children who are on pediatric peritoneal dialysis. J Am Soc Nephrol. 2006;17:285–93.

123. Verrina E, Perri K. Technical aspects and prescription of peritoneal dialysis in children. In: Warady BA Schaefer F, Alexander S, editors. Pediatric Dialysis, 2nd ed. New York: Springer; 2012. p. 169–203.

124. Bakkaloglu SA, Borzych D, Soo Ha I, et al. Cardiac geometry in children receiving chronic peritoneal dialysis: Findings from the International Pediatric Peritoneal Dialysis Network (IPPN) registry. Clin J Am Soc Nephrol. 2011;6:1926–33.

125. Gerson A, Hwang W, Fiorenza J, et al. Anemia and health-related quality of life in adolescents with chronic kidney disease. Am J Kidney Dis. 2004;44:1017–23.

126. Goldstein SL, Graham N, Burwinkle T, et al. Health-related quality of life in pediatric patients with ESRD. Pediatr Nephrol. 2006;21:846–50.

127. Mitsnefes MM, Laskin BL, Dahhou M, et al. Mortality risk among children initially treated with dialysis for end-stage kidney disease, 1990-2010. JAMA. 2013;309:1921–9.

## REVIEW QUESTIONS

1. The greatest percentage of prevalent pediatric patients receives which of the following renal replacement modalities?
   a. Peritoneal dialysis
   b. Hemodialysis
   c. Kidney transplant

2. Which of the following peritoneal membrane pores comprise 90% to total pore area?
   a. Aquaporins
   b. Small pores
   c. Large pores

3. Convective mass transfer is responsible for only a small portion of large solute removal.
   a. True
   b. False

4. The PET test should be performed with which one of the following solutions for all older children and adolescents undergoing PD?
   a. Icodextrin
   b. The regular clinical fill volume for that patient
   c. 1100 mL/m$^2$ of a mixture of 2.5% and 4.25% PD solution
   d. 1100 mL/m$^2$ of 2.5% PD solution

5. Which one of the following is not an absolute contraindication to long-term PD?
   a. Gastroschisis
   b. Ventriculoperitoneal shunt
   c. Omphalocele
   d. Obliterated peritoneal cavity

6. Which of the following measures has not led to a decreased rate of peritonitis in children and adults? (Choose one)
   a. Topical application of antibiotic at catheter exit site
   b. Flush before fill technique
   c. Disconnect systems
   d. Use of Tenckhoff catheter with curled intraperitoneal portion

7. Which of the following is not true about hernias that develop in pediatric patients undergoing PD? (Choose one)
   a. The incidence is directly proportional to the patient's age.
   b. More than 75% require surgical repair.
   c. Raised IPP is a risk factor for hernia development.
   d. Surgical repair should be followed by no/low-volume dialysis.

8. The achievement of PD adequacy should take all but which one of the following factors into consideration?
   a. Peritoneal membrane solute transport capacity
   b. Frequency of peritonitis
   c. Patient's body surface area
   d. Residual renal function

9. The term "V" in Kt/V is equivalent to which one of the following?
   a. Volume of the peritoneal dialysis solution
   b. Total blood volume
   c. Total body water
   d. Volume of ultrafiltrate

10. An important cause of mortality in pediatric patients undergoing PD includes which one of the following?
    a. Cardiovascular disease
    b. Inadequate Kt/V
    c. Poor catheter function
    d. Loss of residual kidney function

## ANSWER KEY

1. c
2. b
3. b
4. d
5. b
6. d
7. a
8. b
9. c
10. a

# 38

# Renal transplantation

## ASHA MOUDGIL AND STANLEY C. JORDAN

Renal transplantation is generally regarded as the treatment of choice for end-stage renal disease (ESRD) in children and adolescents. Although long-term dialysis therapy is possible, it is generally considered a bridge to renal transplantation for pediatric patients with ESRD. Compared to chronic dialysis, renal transplantation offers survival advantage, improved nutrition and linear growth, decreased hospitalization rate, and improved quality of life.[1] Preemptive renal transplantation provides an opportunity for the child and the family to bypass dialysis altogether and remains a viable option for patients with a suitable living donor. Renal transplantation requires lifelong immunosuppressive therapy, and adherence to treatment is paramount. Additionally, transplant recipients are at risk for complications of chronic immunosuppression and ongoing chronic kidney disease (CKD) both of which require close monitoring. This chapter outlines the key concepts of kidney transplantation process in children including long-term post-transplant management.

## INDICATIONS AND CONTRAINDICATIONS TO TRANSPLANTATION

Most children with ESRD are considered good candidates for renal transplantation, because the spectrum of comorbidities seen in adults is often absent. Although there is no clear agreement on the contraindications to renal transplantation in children, the generally practiced absolute and relative contraindications to renal transplantation are listed in Table 38.1.[2,3]

Patients with ESRD secondary to immune-mediated diseases should wait until the underlying disease is in remission. Those with childhood malignancies should be free of recurrence for a period of 2 to 5 years, based on the site and type of malignancy.[3] Children with oxalosis and other genetic disorders, such as methylmalonic acidemia, should be considered for a combined liver and kidney transplant.[4–6] Patients with human immunodeficiency virus (HIV) infection can

Table 38.1 Contraindications to renal transplantation in children

**Absolute Contraindications**

- Acute infection
- Untreated malignancy
- Oxalosis and other genetic syndromes that might benefit from a combined liver and kidney transplant
- Life-limiting coexisting medical conditions: Advanced cardiac, pulmonary, neurologic, or other systemic disease
- Multiorgan failure
- Progressive neurologic illness
- Pregnancy

**Relative Contraindications**

- Uncontrolled HIV infection
- Untreated hepatitis C infection
- Untreated hepatitis B infection
- MAI, BKV, and other infections
- Ventilator dependent children*
- Recurrent FSGS in previous transplant
- Active immune-mediated glomerulonephritis (SLE, Good-Pasteur's syndrome, ANCA-associated GN)
- Persistent vegetative state*
- Extreme obesity and malnutrition
- Psychosocial concerns, including poor adherence with medical regimen

* Some centers would consider these as absolute contraindications.
*Abbreviations:* ANCA, Antineutrophil cytoplasmic antibody; BKV, BK virus; FSGS, focal segmental glomerulosclerosis; GN, glomerulonephritis; HIV, human immunodeficiency virus, MAI, *Mycobacterium avium-intracellulare*; SLE, systemic lupus erythematosus.

undergo transplantation, provided infection is under control and they meet other selection criteria.[7] Those with evidence of chronic hepatitis C and B infection should be evaluated by a hepatologist before listing. Evaluation should include a liver biopsy for staging of the disease and consideration for treatment with antiviral therapy on dialysis before transplantation. Post-transplant immunosuppressive regimens in these patients should be chosen carefully because induction with T-cell depleting agents can result in fulminant progression of hepatitis C and B infections.[8]

As a result of advancements in medical technology there is an increase in the number of children with ESRD who have survived extreme prematurity, complex malformations, and associated comorbidities. Some of these children have physical, neurodevelopmental, or both disabilities and are medically fragile. Increasingly, children dependent on external life-sustaining support for feeding, ventilation, or both are receiving dialysis care and need consideration for

transplantation. Although the Centers for Medicare and Medicaid Condition of Participation (482.90) mandates that transplant centers must have a fair and nondiscriminatory patient selection process for determining transplant candidacy, no clear guidelines exist for transplant candidacy for medically fragile children.[9] A careful evaluation should be done of the child's overall comorbidities and their impact on survival by seeking the advice of medical teams with expertise in these difficult conditions. Involvement of the family and an ethicist, along with a patient advocate from the community, is essential in considering the risks and benefits of renal transplantation in such children.[10]

Nonadherence to medical treatment is an important challenge to successful outcome of renal transplantation.[11] Nonadherence of the patient on dialysis is considered a relative contraindication to renal transplantation in many centers. However, there is limited consensus on defining nonadherence to medical therapy, which can be poor phosphorus control or fluid balance, poor compliance with prescribed home dialysis, or frequent unanticipated absences from in-center hemodialysis.

## DONOR SOURCE

As in the adults, children can receive renal transplantation from living or deceased donors. Living renal transplant donation can be from either an individual who is related to the child (parents or siblings older than 18 years of age) or an unrelated person.[12] Living donor (related and unrelated) allografts have a longer half-life compared to those obtained from the deceased donors.[1,13] This is thought to be the result of a relatively healthy organ and elimination of cold ischemia time. Increased cold ischemia time increases the risk for acute rejection as a result of enhanced expression of human leukocyte antigens (HLAs) and adhesion molecules on the surface of endothelial and renal tubular cells.[14]

## ORGAN PROCUREMENT AND ALLOCATION FOR CHILDREN

### ORGAN PROCUREMENT PROCESS

The U.S. Congress passed the *National Organ Transplant Act* in 1984 and established the Organ Procurement and Transplantation Network (OPTN) to facilitate and regulate organ transplantation in the

United States. The United Network for Organ Sharing (UNOS), an independent nonprofit organization, was established in 1984 and is under federal contract to operate OPTN since 1986.[15] UNOS is divided into 11 operational regions, with each region having a number of organ procurement organizations that are responsible for the procurement of organs from deceased donors and their shipment to the recipient hospitals. UNOS is responsible for allocation of deceased organs to all potential recipients in the United States and has standard policies and procedures that are periodically updated as new research becomes available.[16] All living donors and potential recipients are also listed on the UNOS website (known as UNET) to track all transplants occurring in the United States and for outcome research.

## DECEASED ORGAN ALLOCATION

After the evaluation and decision that the patient should receive a deceased organ renal transplant, the first step is to list potential recipients on the UNOS waiting list. There are no set qualifying criteria for pediatric patients to be listed on the UNOS waiting list. Generally, patients are eligible for listing when they enter chronic dialysis or have measured or estimated glomerular filtration rate (GFR) of less than 20 mL/min/1.73 m$^2$. However, children can be listed at higher GFR if clinically warranted and at the discretion of the transplant center. Information on the HLA typing and unacceptable HLA antigens (presence of specific antibodies to HLA molecules in the recipient sera) is entered in the UNOS database. These unacceptable antigens are used to estimate calculated panel reactive antibodies (CPRA), and the result is considered for point allocation of deceased donor organs. Once listed, the potential recipient starts accumulating time on the waiting list.

UNOS employs point-based allocation policies developed through collaborative efforts between the transplant community, the Scientific Renal Transplant Registry (SRTR), and OPTN.[16] These allocation policies are based on scientific evidence to optimize outcomes in transplant recipients and are revised periodically as new data become available. UNOS allocates points based on a number of recipient and donor factors (the detailed discussion is beyond the scope of this chapter). Zero antigen–mismatched kidneys are mandated to be shared across the geographic and time zones in the United States.

Once an organ becomes available, donor information is entered in UNET. The list of prospective blood group–compatible recipients having no anti-HLA antibodies directed at HLA molecules of this particular donor (virtual cross-match negative) is generated.

An offer is made to the first recipient with the most points. Allocation preferences are given to multivisceral transplants, highly sensitized patients, recipients who have been organ donors in the past, and pediatric recipients. Over the years, the organ allocation process has been refined. No points are assigned for medical urgency.

## ALLOCATION OF ORGANS TO PEDIATRIC RECIPIENTS

Children are given priority for high-quality kidneys. Kidneys from deceased donors are classified using the Kidney Donor Profile Index (KDPI). The KDPI score (1 to 100) is based on the age, weight, height, ethnicity, serum creatinine, history and duration of hypertension and diabetes, cause of death, presence of hepatitis C, and whether the donation is after cardiac death (DCD).[17] Kidneys with lower KDPI score have better long-term survival. Because there are allocation advantages for deceased donors in children, it is important to list eligible pediatric patients before their 18th birthday to give them access to high-quality organs.

## DATA ANALYSIS

A number of scientific registries maintain ESRD databases and transplant outcomes.[1,15] These include the United States Renal Data System (USRDS), SRTR, and the North American Pediatric Renal Trials and Collaborative Study (NAPRTCS). All transplant centers are mandated to send information pertaining to all transplant recipients to the UNOS periodically. The SRTR in collaboration with UNOS plays a critical role in policy development through ongoing data analysis and development of statistical, analytic, and simulation models.[18] NAPRTCS, a consortium of pediatric ESRD and transplant centers was established in 1987 with the scientific objectives of capturing information about current practice and trends in immunosuppressive therapy in children.[1] Participation in NAPRTCS is voluntary.

## IMMUNOLOGIC BARRIERS TO TRANSPLANTATION

A number of immunologic barriers to successful transplantation exist, of which the most important are blood group antigens, HLA mismatches and preexisting anti-HLA antibodies before transplant, and development of de novo donor-specific antibodies (DSA) following transplant.[19]

## BLOOD GROUP

ABO compatibility between donor and recipient is generally considered an absolute prerequisite for successful transplantation.[20] ABO antigens are expressed on the surface of endothelial cells, in addition to red blood cells (RBCs). Blood group antibodies (anti-A, anti-B, and anti-AB) are naturally occurring isoagglutinins that bind to the endothelium, causing cell swelling, destruction, and irreversible graft loss known as hyperacute rejection (HAR). The rules that govern blood transfusion also apply to solid organ transplantation. Individuals with type O blood group are considered universal donors, and those with type AB blood group are regarded as universal recipients. Experience in solid organ transplantation, including kidneys, across blood group barriers has begun to evolve in many centers in the United States and Japan. In these studies, blood group isoagglutinins are removed by plasmapheresis, or immunoadsorption, followed by intense immunosuppression.[21] Rh blood group antigen matching is traditionally not considered a requirement for successful renal transplantation.

## HUMAN LEUKOCYTE ANTIGEN TYPING

Genetic differences among individuals are recognized by differences in the composition of major histocompatibility complex antigens, also known as *HLA antigens*.[22] HLA antigens help differentiate self from nonself and fight invading organisms. The genes encoding these antigens are present on the short arm of chromosome 6. Based on their structural differences, HLA antigens are divided into class I (A, B, and C) and class II (DR, DQ, DP). HLA class I antigens are present on all nucleated cells. RBCs lack HLA antigens. HLA class II antigens are present on macrophages, dendritic cells, endothelial cells, and B cells. T cells, renal tubular epithelial cells, and endothelial cells increase expression of class II molecules on stimulation with cytokines such as interferon-gamma (IFN-$\gamma$).

Histocompatibility genes are extremely polymorphic and are expressed as codominant alleles. The concentration of HLA genes in one defined area of the chromosome allows these genes to be inherited as a packet, or haplotype. Individuals inherit 1-haplotype from each parent. Children are 1-haplotype matched with their biologic parents. Siblings can be complete HLA matched, 1-haplotype matched, or completely mismatched, depending on the recombination of their haplotypes.

The HLA type of an individual can be determined by conventional serologic methods or DNA-based typing. Once the HLA typing is determined, the number of matched and mismatched antigens between the recipient and the prospective donor can be calculated. The number of mismatches, or nonshared HLA antigens, between the donor and the recipient may differ from the number of shared antigens or matches because of some yet unidentified HLA antigens or inheritance of two copies of the same HLA allele. From the renal transplant perspective, currently only six antigen pairs (A, B, and DR), inherited from each parent, are considered in the allocation process. However, by DNA typing other alleles (*A, B, C, DRA1, DRB1, DRB3/4/5, DQB1, DQA1, DPB1, and DPA1*) can be identified. HLA mismatching determines the extent of anticipated allogeneic response.[14] Recently, DQ and DP antigen mismatches between donor and recipients have been identified to play an important role in the development of de novo DSAs after transplant.[23]

Identical twins are fully matched or are zero mismatched. Generally these perfectly matched recipients do not require post-transplant immunosuppression. The first successful human transplant was done between identical twins. Availability of potent immunosuppressive therapy has, to some extent, attenuated the effect of HLA matching on short-term allograft survival and the incidence of acute rejection. However, HLA matching, in particular DR matching, continues to have an effect on long-term renal allograft survival. HLA identical grafts have a longer half-life compared to those that are less well matched. The high degree of polymorphism makes complete HLA matching between two random individuals an exceedingly rare event.

Current clinical practice in the United States is to share all six antigen matched or zero mismatched kidneys from deceased donors in the entire national recipient waiting list pool and across the geographic regions of the country.[16] Fewer than 20% of kidneys transplanted in the United States from deceased organ donors are zero mismatched and transported across the country. The potential benefits of sharing these kidneys come at a price of increased cold ischemia time associated with organ transport, sometimes over several time zones.

## ANTI–HUMAN LEUKOCYTE ANTIGEN ANTIBODIES

Anti-HLA antibodies can exist before transplant or develop after transplant. Transplant recipients can develop anti-HLA antibodies as a result of sensitization events that include blood transfusions, previous transplants, pregnancies, and, rarely, infections. With widespread use of recombinant erythropoietin in ESRD patients, allosensitization as a result of blood transfusion has decreased considerably. When present, preexisting anti-HLA antibodies bind to HLA antigens expressed on the surface of allograft endothelial cells and can cause HAR and immediate graft loss. These antibodies are particularly deleterious if they are directed at HLA class I antigens and are able to activate the complement cascade by binding to complement proteins. Anti-HLA antibodies developing after transplant (de novo) are specific to the donor, are known as DSA, and can result in an accelerated graft loss. DSA can develop as a result of nonadherence, inadequate immunosuppression, or viral infections.[24]

Testing for anti-HLA antibodies has undergone remarkable technologic enhancements.[19] The oldest and least sensitive method for testing anti-HLA antibodies is the complement-dependent cytotoxicity assay. The complement-dependent cytotoxicity assay involves testing donor's T and B cells for lympholysis by anti-HLA antibodies in the recipient's serum, in the presence of complement. Enzyme-linked immunosorbent assay (ELISA) and flow cytometry have provided an increasing order of sensitivity for detection of anti-HLA antibodies. Cells from the donor as well as HLA antigen–coated beads can be used for ELISA or flow cytometry. Antibodies to specific HLA antigens can be characterized by flow cytometry or Luminex technology, using single HLA antigens coated on spherical particles known as single antigen beads. In recipients with anti-HLA antibodies to specific HLA antigens, transplant from donors with these HLA antigens should be avoided and these antigens are listed as unacceptable antigens on the UNOS-UNET. Donors carrying unacceptable HLA antigens are automatically excluded from the organ offer. These unacceptable antigens are used to define CPRA as described in the following section.

## CALCULATED PANEL REACTIVE ANTIBODIES

Adopted by UNOS in 2006, the CPRA procedure is based on a calculation of the reaction frequency of a listed set of unacceptable mismatches for a patient, against a panel of 10,000 recently added deceased donors.[25] The CPRA is derived from HLA antigen/allele group and haplotype frequencies for different racial and ethnic groups in proportion to their representation in the national deceased donor population. The CPRA values are rounded to the nearest one hundredth percentage and give a measure of the chances of a patient finding a compatible donor from the donor pool. The use of CPRA is made much easier by use of solid-phase assays such as Luminex assays, especially those involving the use of single antigen beads. These assays allow precise characterization of anti-HLA antibodies. The strength of the mean fluorescence intensity (MFI) is used to assess immunologic risk and to help decide whether or not a particular antigen should be listed as unacceptable on the UNET.

## CROSS-MATCH

Cross-match determines the compatibility between a specific recipient and a donor and is the final pretransplantation immunologic screening step. The test involves testing recipient's serum against donor T and B cells to detect any preformed antibodies against donor's lymphocytes. Until recently, cross-matching was routinely done by complement-dependent cytotoxicity assay. Immunoglobulin (IgM) autoantibodies in a recipient's serum can give a false-positive result in this assay. These antibodies can be inactivated by pretreatment of serum with dithiothreitol (DTT), which disrupts the S-S bonds in IgM. A negative cross-match after DTT treatment excludes alloantibodies, whereas a positive T-cell cross-match is indicative of preformed alloantibodies and is a contraindication to transplantation from that specific donor. The sensitivity of the cross-match is enhanced many-fold by antihuman globulin ELISA assay and flow-cytometry cross-match. These tests are especially useful for highly sensitized patients and those undergoing retransplant. Most transplant centers use flow-cytometry cross match routinely.

## IMMUNOBIOLOGY OF ALLOGRAFT REJECTION

Allograft rejection is an orchestrated process.[14] The physical process of reimplanting and reperfusing organs for transplantation initiates ischemia-reperfusion injury. The recipient's innate immune system can recognize these markers of tissue injury and result in upregulation of the inflammatory response genes. The consequence of such a response is an increased production of the proinflammatory cytokines, such as interleukin (IL)-1, IL-6, tumor necrosis factor-alpha (TNF)-α, and type I interferon, all of which trigger release of antigens from the graft. Additionally, there is increased expression of adhesion molecules by the endothelial cells that promote their adhesion with the inflammatory cells. Donor antigens released from the graft are taken up by the antigen-presenting cells (APCs) of either donor or recipient origin. Recipient APCs (macrophages, dendritic cells, B lymphocytes) process donor antigens into small peptides that are subsequently presented on their cell surface in association with HLA class I or II molecules. These APCs then leave the graft and migrate to secondary lymphoid tissues, where they activate naive recipient T-cells that have specific receptors for HLA-allopeptide complexes (indirect allorecognition). Additionally, recipient T cells can directly recognize donor APCs bearing HLA molecules loaded with self-peptide (direct allorecognition). CD4+ T lymphocytes recognize HLA class II and CD8+ T lymphocytes recognize HLA class I associated allopeptides. Direct pathway of antigen presentation plays an important role early on after transplant, whereas indirect pathway plays a more prominent role later on. The ability of T cells to recognize and respond to alloantigens is identical to their ability to respond to foreign antigens and infectious agents.

---

## KEY POINTS

- Precise characterizations of anti-HLA antibodies have become feasible with solid-phase assays such as Luminex and availability of single HLA antigen–coated beads.
- Specific unacceptable antigens are listed on the UNET for each recipient and help determine CPRA.
- Flow cross-match is the most sensitive assay currently available and is most widely used.

---

Within secondary lymph nodes, T-cells respond to alloantigens presented by APCs in a sequence of three signals

(Figure 38.1). Signal I, or antigenic signal, is the interaction between HLA-allopeptide complex and CD4+ T-cell receptor. Signal II is a costimulatory signal mediated by a number of pathways. These include CD40/CD40 ligand interaction that increases γ-IFN, which upregulates B7 expression and subsequently the B7-CD28 interaction, a powerful costimulator of T-cell activation. When T cells receive both signals I and II, there is an activation of a number of enzymes, followed by an increase in cytosolic calcium. Cytosolic calcium binds to calcineurin that turns on the nuclear factor activating transcription (NFAT) and mitogen activated protein kinases (MAPKs), which promote synthesis of interleukin-2 (IL-2) and γ-IFN. IL-2 enhances synthesis of other cytokines, including IL-3, IL-4, IL-5, IL-6, and TNF-α.

Signal III consists of secreted IL-2 interacting with the IL-2 receptor present on the surface of these T-cells. This interaction stimulates a series of enzymatic reactions and drives the cell into division, resulting in clonal expansion and differentiation of graft reactive CD4+ lymphocytes. However, before cell division, de novo synthesis of purine and pyrimidine nucleotides occurs in T cells. If T cells receive only signal I without signal II, they undergo apoptotic cell death.

Activated CD4+ T cells provide help to CD8+ T cells, B cells, macrophages, natural killer (NK) cells, and platelets through secreted cytokines. CD8+ T cells, also known as cytotoxic T cells, secrete granzyme and perforins that cause cell death in the allografts. IL-3, IL-4, and IL-5 stimulate B cells that produce antibodies against donor antigens. IL-1

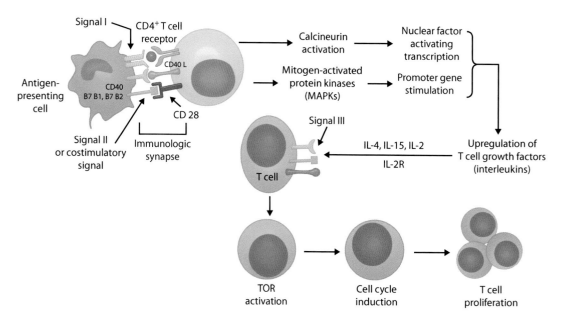

Figure 38.1 Signal pathways to T-cell activation. Signal I: Interaction between antigen-presenting cells presenting allopeptides and CD4+ T-cell receptor of the recipient. Signal II: includes a number of costimulatory pathways, of which the most important are interaction between B7-1/B7-2 and CD28, and CD40 and CD40 ligand. On receiving both signal I and II, there is an increase in cytosolic calcium that activates calcineurin and promotes synthesis of interleukin-2 (IL-2) and other cytokines. Mitogen-activated protein kinases are also activated in the T cells on receiving signals I and II, leading to promoter gene stimulation. IL-2 and other cytokines generated from T-cell activation act on the T-cells' surface (as signal III), sending downstream signals to activate the target of rapamycin (TOR), which induces immune cells into cell cycle division and causes T-cell proliferation. CD40L = CD40 ligand.

and TNF–α facilitate activation of macrophages and other inflammatory cells, and IL-6 stimulates platelets. These activated T cells and other inflammatory cells (B cells, macrophages, and platelets) leave the lymph nodes and enter the circulation to infiltrate the allograft causing allograft destruction and inflammation (Figure 38.2). IL-6 also appears to be critical in reversing the action of regulatory T (Treg) cells that might prevent allograft rejection. Allografts containing disparate HLA antigens generate a stronger signal I and are more likely to experience rejection compared to those more closely related to the recipient's HLA.

> ## KEY POINTS
>
> - Donor exchange programs and desensitization protocols offer opportunities for transplantation in highly sensitized individuals.
> - Graft loss can result in a highly sensitized state in pediatric patients.

## IMMUNOSUPRESSIVE THERAPIES

Immunosuppressive drugs help overcome immunologic barriers to transplantation and are essential for transplant survival.[26] The drugs or procedures used before or at the time of transplantation to suppress unwanted allograft-directed immune responses are referred to as *induction* *therapies.* The medications are used for long-term maintenance of the immunosuppressed state in the recipient for graft survival. Induction therapies are more potent than the maintenance immunosuppressive medications.

## INDUCTION THERAPIES

Induction therapies include antibodies, high-dose intravenous (IV) methylprednisolone, plasmapheresis, and splenectomy. Induction antibodies can be directed at T cells, B cells, or the complement cascade and can be monoclonal or polyclonal. Antibodies target the cell surface molecules of the immune-competent cells and do not enter into the cells.[27] Antibodies can be depleting or nondepleting antibodies. Depleting antibodies cause cell death, whereas nondepleting antibodies interfere with cell function.

### Polyclonal antibodies

Polyclonal antibodies include antithymocyte globulin raised in horses (ATG) and rabbits (Thymoglobulin) and IV immunoglobulin (IVIg). Both ATG and Thymoglobulin contain antibodies against multiple T-cell surface antigens (CD2, CD3, CD4, CD5, CD8, CD11, CD18, CD28, CD45, and T-cell receptor) and cause extensive T-cell depletion. IVIg downregulates production of antibodies in addition to neutralizing preexisting antibodies. IVIg also causes upregulation of Fc-gamma (Fcγ) receptor IIB on B cells and is a modifier of complement activation and injury.[28] Thymoglobulin is commonly used for induction in renal

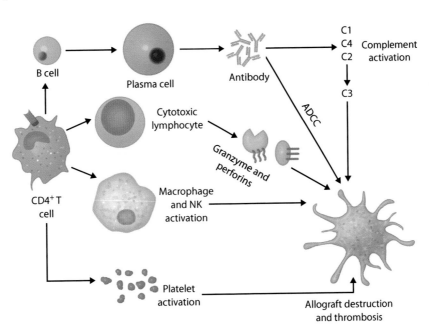

Figure 38.2 Orchestration of different cells in causing allograft destruction. Activated CD4+ T cells secrete cytokines that stimulate a number of cells participating in graft destruction. Activated B cells mature into plasma cells that secrete alloantibodies, causing complement-mediated allograft damage. Activated cytotoxic lymphocytes secrete granzyme and perforins that cause direct damage to the allograft cells. Activated macrophages and natural killer (NK) cells also participate in graft destruction. Activated platelets add thrombotic component to the graft destruction. ADCC, antibody-dependent cellular toxicity.

transplant recipients because of superior performance compared with that of ATG.

## Monoclonal antibodies

Monoclonal antibodies include anti–IL-2R antibody (basiliximab), anti-CD52 monoclonal antibody (alemtuzumab), anti-CD20 antibody (rituximab), and anti–membrane attack complex antibody (eculizumab). Basiliximab binds to the α-chain of IL-2 receptor, making it unavailable for IL-2 binding and subsequent cell division (blocking signal III) and is a nondepleting antibody. Alemtuzumab is a humanized monoclonal antibody that targets the CD52 antigen on lymphocytes, monocytes, macrophages, and NK cells, causing extensive lymphocyte depletion. Rituximab binds to C20 on pre-B and B cells causing their depletion but does not affect plasma cells. Basiliximab, Thymoglobulin, or alemtuzumab are used for standard induction, whereas IVIg and rituximab are used in highly sensitized recipients. Eculizumab is used for induction in patients with ESRD secondary to atypical hemolytic uremic syndrome (HUS).[29] Plasmapheresis is used for recurrent focal segmental glomerulosclerosis FSGS, in highly sensitized recipients, and for prevention of atypical HUS. Splenectomy is rarely used for ABO-incompatible and highly sensitized transplant recipients. Characteristics, doses, and side effects of commonly used induction therapies are shown in Tables 38.2 and 38.3.

These pharmacologic agents are capable of acting on targets inside the cells (Figure 38.3) and maintain a state of immunosuppression for long-term viability of the allograft. These agents include calcineurin inhibitors (CNIs), such as cyclosporine A (CsA) and tacrolimus; antiproliferative agents such as mycophenolate mofetil (MMF); azathioprine and sirolimus; and corticosteroids (prednisone, prednisolone, and methylprednisolone). A summary of these drugs is given in Table 38.4.

## Calcineurin inhibitors

CsA and tacrolimus bind to cyclophilin and FK binding proteins, respectively, and inhibit the activity of the enzyme intracellular calcineurin in T cells. Nuclear factor activating transcription (NFAT) translocation to the nucleus is consequently blocked, preventing transcription of IL-2 and other cytokine genes.

## Antiproliferative agents

Azathioprine and MMF act as antiproliferative agents by inhibiting de novo purine synthesis that is necessary for cell division. Mycophenolic acid (MPA), the active metabolite of MMF, is a potent, selective, noncompetitive, and reversible inhibitor of inosine monophosphate dehydrogenase, an enzyme required for de novo purine synthesis. MPA inhibits T- and B-lymphocyte proliferation that is critically

Table 38.2 Pharmacologic agents available for induction therapy of renal transplants

| Name | Antibody type | Origin | Target and mechanism of action |
|---|---|---|---|
| Antithymocyte globulin (Thymoglobulin)* | Polyclonal | Rabbit | T-cell receptor, CD3, CD4, CD8, CD2, CD18, CD25, CD44, CD45, CD28, CD11A, B7 integrin, CD54, HLA class I and DR, and β2 microglobulin-depleting antibody |
| Intravenous immunoglobulin G, or IVIg (Gammagard, Carimune, Gamunex) | Polyclonal | Human | Multiple putative mechanisms: Immunomodulation, upregulation of Fcγ III receptor on B cells, modifier of complement activation and injury, nondepleting antibody |
| Basiliximab (Simulect) | Monoclonal | Mouse, chimeric | CD25 on T cells, nondepleting antibody |
| Alemtuzumab (Campath) | Monoclonal | Rat, humanized | CD52 on mononuclear cells, depleting antibody |
| Rituximab (Rituxan) | Monoclonal | Mouse, chimeric | CD20 on pre-B and B cells, depleting antibody |
| Eculizumab (Soliris) | Monoclonal | Mouse, humanized | Complement C5, blocks formation of membrane attack complex |

* Brand names of the drugs are given in parentheses.
*Abbreviations:* CD, Cluster determinant (cluster of antigens that characterize a cell surface marker with which antibodies react); Fcγ, Fc-gamma receptors that bind to Fc region of the antibody.

Table 38.3 Dose, duration, and side effects of induction therapies available for clinical use in renal transplantation

| Induction Therapy | Dose | Route and duration | Side effects |
|---|---|---|---|
| Antithymocyte globulin (Thymoglobulin) | 1.5 mg/kg/d | IV over 6–8 house via central line for 4–7 days | Fever, chills, anaphylaxis, leukopenia, thrombocytopenia, Increased risk for CMV and PTLD |
| Basiliximab (Simulect) | 10 mg or 12 mg/m² for < 35 kg, 20 mg for > 35 kg | IV, day 0 and 4 | Same as placebo |
| Alemtuzumab (Campath) | 0.3–0.4 mg/kg/dose | IV or s/c, 1-2 doses | First-dose reaction, allergic reaction, and increased incidence of infections |
| Methylprednisolone (Solumedrol) | 10–15 mg/kg | IV push in the OR | Salt and water retention, gastric ulceration, insomnia, impaired wound healing, growth retardation, cataract, osteopenia |
| Intravenous Immunoglobulin G, or IVIG | 2 gm/kg/dose | IV infusion over 4 hours, variable duration | Headache, aseptic meningitis, chills, rarely acute renal failure in preparations containing sucrose |
| Rituximab (Rituxan) | 375–750 mg/m²/dose | IV infusion, 1–4 doses | Fever, chills, anaphylaxis, hypogammaglobulinemia, increased risk for bacterial infections |
| Eculizumab (Soliris) | Loading dose 1200 mg, then 900 mg weekly. See package insert for weight based guidelines. | IV, variable duration | Increased risk for infection with encapsulated bacteria |

*Abbreviations:* CMV, Cytomegalovirus; OR, operating room; PTLD, post-transplant lymphoproliferative disorder.

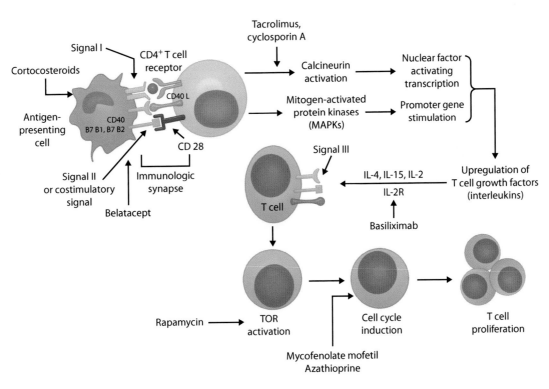

Figure 38.3 Mechanism of action of common immunosuppressive medications used in clinical practice. Corticosteroids have inhibitory action on the antigen APCs. Belatacept inhibits the interaction between CD28 on T cells and the costimulatory ligands (B7-1/B7-2) (blocking signal II). Immunoglobulin G and Thymoglobulin (not shown) have antibodies to the multiple cell surface receptors on T cells. Cyclosporine A and tacrolimus inhibit calcium-activated calcineurin, blocking interleukin-2 (IL-2) gene promotor action and synthesis of IL-2. Basiliximab blocks interaction of IL-2 with IL-2R (blocking signal III). Rapamycin binds to TOR and blocks the entry of cells into the cell cycle after IL-2 binds to IL-2R. Mycofenolate mofetil and azathioprine inhibit purine synthesis required for cell division. CD40L, CD40 ligand.

Table 38.4 Maintenance immunosuppressive drugs

| Name of the drug | Dose | Side effects |
| --- | --- | --- |
| Prednisone | 2 mg/kg/day to be tapered to 0.5 mg/kg/day in 2 wk, 0.1–0.15 mg/kg/day over 6 mo | Excessive weight gain, hypertension, hyperglycemia, cushingoid features, acne, growth suppression, osteoporosis, gastric ulceration, impaired wound healing, mood change, cataracts |
| Cyclosporine A | 6–8 mg/kg/day at the onset, adjust dose according to levels | Nephrotoxicity, hypertension, hirsutism, gingival hyperplasia, tremors |
| Tacrolimus | 0.1–0.15 mg/kg/day, adjust dose according to levels | Nephrotoxicity, tremors, diabetes mellitus, hair loss, increased absorption in diarrhea |
| Azathioprine | 2 mg/kg/day | Myelosuppression, hepatotoxicity |
| Mycophenolate mofetil | 1200 mg/m$^2$/day to a maximum of 1500 mg BID | Myelosuppression, diarrhea |
| Sirolimus | Loading dose 6 mg/day followed by 2–5 mg/day, adjust according to levels | Hypertriglyceridemia, mucosal ulcers, thrombocytopenia, pneumonia |

dependent on de novo purine synthesis. Additionally, MPA also alters the expression of cell surface adhesion molecules by inhibiting glycosylation of lymphocyte and monocyte glycoproteins. Sirolimus, also known as rapamycin, acts on the molecular target of rapamycin (mTOR) and blocks the ability of cells to enter the cell cycle.

## Corticosteroids

Corticosteroids primarily act on the APCs and inhibit their ability to produce IL-1 and other cytokines.[30] Many cytokine genes, including IL-2 have a glucocorticoid response element (GRE) in the 5′ regulatory region that serves as a target for corticosteroid and intracellular glucocorticoid receptor complex. Binding of this complex with GRE blocks transcription of cytokines. High-dose methylprednisolone causes lympholysis and therefore is useful for the treatment of acute allograft rejection.

## NOVEL IMMUNOSUPPRESSIVE DRUGS

Currently, a few immunosuppressive agents are in different phases of clinical trials.[31] Belatacept (costimulation inhibitor, CTLA4Ig) was recently approved for use in Epstein-Barr virus (EBV)-positive adults by the U.S. Food and Drug Administration; it has potential benefits because of lack of nephrotoxicity and neurotoxicity and might replace chronic CNI therapy. Belatacept therapy provides GFR advantage and decreases the risk for post-transplant hypertension and metabolic complications. Initial data from the controlled clinical trials are encouraging, but the current recommendation is not to use this drug in EBV-naive individuals at the time of transplant because of high risk for developing post-transplant lymphoproliferative disorder (PTLD).[32] Other studies with

Belatacept induction combined with Thymoglobulin show promise for development of CNI-free and steroid-free protocols with low rejection rates. At this point, no data are available in children. A multicenter randomized conversion study is currently underway in the United States and Europe and will evaluate the efficacy and safety of Belatacept immunosuppression in EBV-seropositive children with a stable renal transplant (NCT 01791491).[33]

If efficacious, Belatacept would eliminate the use of chronic nephrotoxic CNI therapy as maintenance immunosuppression in children. Major concerns with Belatacept include higher risk for early rejection in the CNI-free environment and the increased risk for infectious complications, including CMV, EBV, and polyoma BKV nephropathy.

ASKP1240 is a fully human monoclonal antibody directed against CD40. It inhibits CD40/CD40L complex among B cells, T cells, APCs, and endothelial cells. Prolonged allograft survival has been noted in primate transplants, and human phase II studies are underway.[31] TOL101 is a murine monoclonal IgM antibody against αβ subunit of T-cell receptor. As TOL101 is not active against γδ T-cell receptor, it inhibits T-cell proliferation while preserving tolerogenic effects of γδ T-cell receptors. TOL101 is currently in phase I/II trial.[31]

## PRETRANSPLANT EVALUATION OF RECIPIENT

The pretransplant evaluation is aimed to ensure and enhance patient's suitability as a transplant recipient and identify any potential contraindications to transplant. Table 38.5 lists the principles of pretransplant evaluation applicable to children.

Table 38.5 Principles of pretransplant evaluation process in pediatric recipients

1. History and physical examination
   Determine the cause of end-stage renal disease
   Identify comorbidities
   Genitourinary, lower spine, perineum, and neurologic examination
   Nutrition evaluation and optimization
   All age-appropriate immunizations, including Pneumovax-23 and meningitis
2. Psychosocial evaluation and counseling of the child and family
3. Immunologic evaluation: ABO and human leukocyte antigen (HLA) typing, screening for anti-HLA antibodies
4. Evaluation for exposure to infections: Antibodies to viral infections (cytomegalovirus, Epstein-Barr virus, herpes simplex virus, human immunodeficiency virus, varicella zoster virus, hepatitis B and C), hepatitis B surface antigen, serologic tests for syphilis, chest x-ray, and tuberculin testing
5. Urologic evaluation: Urinalysis and urine culture, ultrasonography including postvoid images of the bladder, vesicocystourethrogram. Voiding diary, uroflow, urodynamics, and, rarely, cystoscopy in patients with complicated urologic problems
6. Optional: Neurocognitive evaluation, hematologic evaluation if suspected to be at risk for thrombosis, cardiac, pulmonary, dental, and ophthalmologic as indicated
7. Financial screening and counseling

## UROLOGIC EVALUATION AND PREPARATION

Approximately a third of children undergoing renal transplantation have some form of structural abnormalities or dysfunction of the urinary tract, such as posterior urethral valve (PUV), vesicoureteric reflux, prune belly syndrome, neurogenic bladder, Hinman syndrome, and exstrophy of the bladder. The abnormal high-pressure bladder can contribute to allograft failure. Consequently, urologic evaluation and management is an important preparatory step for children being evaluated for renal transplantation. Such an evaluation may include examination of the lower urinary tract anatomy by contrast vesicocystourethrogram (VCUG), assessment of bladder compliance and emptying function by postvoid ultrasound, uroflow studies, and urodynamic studies. Any necessary urinary tract reconstructive surgery should be done in advance of transplantation.

## DETERMINING CAUSE OF END-STAGE RENAL DISEASE

Establishing the cause of ESRD is important, because many diseases have the potential for recurrence in the transplant. These include FSGS, atypical HUS, and membranoproliferative glomerulonephritis (MPGN). In these cases strategies should be developed to optimize the timing of transplant and monitor for recurrence and treatment. The potential for recurrence of primary glomerular diseases is not considered a contraindication to transplantation. Children with Alport syndrome can develop anti–glomerular basement membrane (GBM) antibodies after transplant secondary to the absence of $\alpha$-3, -4 and -5 subtypes of collagen IV in their native kidney basement membrane. Similarly, children with congenital nephrotic syndrome secondary to nephrin mutations can develop antinephrin antibodies, causing damage to the allograft.

## IDENTIFYING COMORBID CONDITIONS

Pretransplant evaluation should be aimed at identifying clinical, physiologic, psychological, and socioeconomic conditions that may have an impact on the successful outcome of a renal transplant. Patients should be screened for chronic infections, which may require treatment and planning before renal transplantation. Native nephrectomies for chronic infection of the kidneys, severe nephrotic syndrome (congenital nephrotic syndrome or idiopathic FSGS), polyuria with severe fluid and electrolyte wasting, polycystic kidneys, intractable hypertension, large renal masses, or nephrolithiasis may be necessary in some children. Careful review of other comorbid conditions should be done to assess whether these require special provisions after transplant or may serve as relative or absolute contraindications to transplantation.

## IMMUNOLOGIC EVALUATION

Immunologic evaluation includes determining the blood group and HLA typing and identifying specific anti-HLA antibodies. The final step is to perform a cross-match with the prospective donor as described earlier.

## GENERAL HEALTH MAINTENANCE

Age-appropriate immunizations, including hepatitis B, varicella, Pneumovax, meningitis, and human papillomavirus (HPV) immunizations should be provided to children before transplantation procedure because response to immunizations may be blunted after transplantation.[34] Immunity to live viral vaccines (measles, mumps, rubella, and varicella) should be documented, and children should be revaccinated if not immune because live virus vaccines are contraindicated after renal transplant. Growth and nutritional status should be optimized, because both malnutrition and obesity result in increased risks for complications after transplantation.

## PSYCHOSOCIAL EVALUATION

Psychosocial evaluation and planning are paramount to success of transplant. Nonadherence to medical therapy is an important barrier to allograft survival, particularly in adolescents. Therefore, a careful assessment of the child and family's ability to adhere to long-term immunosuppression and medical therapy should be conducted and documented. There is an increased prevalence of mood and adjustment disorders in the children and family members of those with chronic illness. Referral to psychiatrist and or counseling may be desired. The family support system may need to be strengthened to ensure an optimal long-term outcome.

## DONOR EVALUATION

## LIVING DONOR EVALUATION

It is generally recommended that a physician not familiar with the child's needs should evaluate living donors to ensure that they are medically suitable for a donation kidney. An outline of donor workup is shown in Table 38.6. The UNOS Ad Hoc Living Donor Committee has published living kidney donor evaluation guidelines.[35]

## DECEASED DONOR EVALUATION

All deceased donors undergo comprehensive evaluation and management after the decision for donation is made. The goal is to identify any conditions that may preclude

Table 38.6 Evaluation of living donors

1. Detailed history and physical examination
2. Psychosocial screening and counseling
3. Renal function tests, including 24-hour urine collection for protein and creatinine measurement, liver function tests, screening for diabetes
4. Age-appropriate screening for cardiovascular health and malignancies
5. ABO, Rh, and human leukocyte antigen typing
6. Screening for infections: Antibodies to viral infections (human immunodeficiency virus, cytomegalovirus, Epstein-Barr virus, hepatitis B and C), hepatitis B surface antigen, serologic tests for syphilis, chest x-ray, and tuberculin testing and screening for infection pertaining to the geographic area of origin
7. Renal and renovascular anatomy: Renal ultrasound, renal angiography or spiral computed tomography scan or magnetic resonance imaging of kidneys with magnetic resonance angiography and magnetic resonance venography

donation or require special provisions after transplant. There are standardized protocols for donor management for optimization of organ function after transplant. The details of management are beyond the scope of this chapter. The deceased donors are divided into brain-dead donors or those from whom donation is obtained after cardiac death (DCD). DCD donors pose an increased risk for delayed graft function (DGF); pulsatile preservation may decrease this risk.

## SURGICAL PROCEDURE

## LIVING DONOR NEPHRECTOMY

Kidney from a live donor can be procured by open donor nephrectomy (ODN) or laparoscopic donor nephrectomy (LDN). LDN was first used to procure kidneys for transplant in 1995.[36] LDN is offered at most of the transplant centers in the United States. LDN has shortened the hospital stay and recovery time for donors and has decreased the need for analgesia. Short-term graft outcomes for kidneys obtained by LDN are comparable to those obtained by ODN. Analysis of UNOS data shows a higher incidence of DGF and acute rejection in young recipients (0 to 5 years) of kidneys obtained by LDN, raising a concern for the use of this practice in this age group. However, there is a need to update these data with increased experience gained with LDN countrywide.

## DECEASED DONOR NEPHRECTOMY

Kidneys are obtained from deceased donors by standard ODN procedure. Renal artery or arteries are on a patch of aorta known as the Carroll patch. The left renal vein is longer than the right renal vein. Extreme care is taken to preserve blood supply to the lower part of the ureter to prevent ischemia as ureteric supply comes from multiple vessels. After nephrectomy, the kidney is placed in cold preservative solution or placed on a pump with which the cold preservative solution is pumped into the renal artery. Cold ischemia time is the time gap between placement of kidney into the cold preservative solution and the time it is taken out for implantation into the recipient. Warm ischemia time is the timegap between removal of the kidney from the preservative solution and the time when blood starts to perfuse into the recipient renal artery. The shorter the cold and warm ischemia times, the better is the organ function. The warm ischemia time is much more detrimental to organ function than cold ischemia time.

## ORGAN IMPLANTATION PROCEDURE

The renal allograft is placed extraperitoneally in the iliac fossa in children weighing greater than 20 kg.[37] The donor renal artery and vein are connected to the child's common iliac or external iliac artery and vein, using an end-to-side anastomosis technique. In infants and young children less than 20 kg, the donor kidney is placed intraperitoneally in the abdomen and the renal artery and vein of the allograft are connected to the side of the aorta and inferior vena cava, close to the bifurcation (Figure 38.4).

These general surgical principles are applied to both living and deceased donor renal transplants. Meticulous detail to the vascular anastomosis technique is required in children. This is especially important in young infants, in whom the vessel size is considerably smaller than in adults and older children. In the case of multiple arteries in the living donor, they can be anastomosed separately or joined together in side-to-side anastomosis and then connected to the recipient vessels. Multiple renal arteries in deceased donors are usually on the common aortic (Carroll) patch.

The ureter is generally connected to the bladder using ureteroneocystostomy. Attention should be paid to preserve the arterial supply of the lower segment of the ureter, because interruption of the blood supply to this segment may result in ureteral ischemia and consequent urinary leaks or ureteral stricture.

## PERIOPERATIVE TRANSPLANT MANAGEMENT

### FLUID AND ELECTROLYTES

Children may need to be dialyzed before renal transplantation if they are hyperkalemic or severely fluid overloaded,

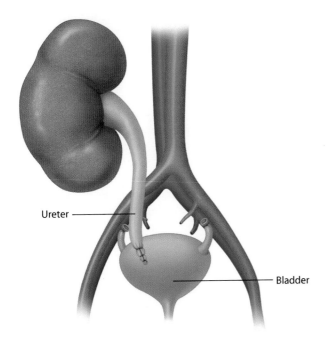

Figure 38.4 Surgical anastomoses and placement of an extraperitoneal renal allograft. Donor renal artery and vein are connected to the lower end of recipient's aorta and inferior vena cava, respectively.

particularly if they receive an organ from a deceased donor that may not be expected to function right away. Hypovolemia should be avoided at all costs. Except in polyuric children, preoperative IV fluids are not necessary in most cases. Close attention needs to be paid to intravascular volume in the operating room by infusion of crystalloid and colloid solutions in particular at the time of vascular anastomosis because an adult kidney can sequester up to 250 mL of the recipient's blood volume. This may represent a significant change in total blood volume in an infant or a small child (blood volume of a 10-kg child is 80 mL/kg, 800 mL) and cause hypotension if not appropriately replaced. As a result, appropriate intraoperative fluid management is critical in infants and young children.[37]

Central venous pressure (CVP) should be maintained between 10 to 15 cm $H_2O$ before removal of the aortic cross clamps to ensure good blood flow to the allograft, because hypoperfusion can promote allograft thrombosis. Vasopressors such as dopamine may be required to help maintain adequate blood pressure. Mannitol (0.5 to 1 g/kg) and furosemide (1 to 2 mg/kg) at the time of removal of the cross clamp are often used to induce diuresis in the transplanted organ. Occasionally, an intra-arterial vasodilator such as verapamil may be given to overcome renal arterial vasospasm.

Postoperative fluid and electrolyte management includes replacement of insensible losses and urine output with an appropriately constituted fluid. Five percent dextrose is used for insensible losses, and replacement of urine output can be achieved with a fluid with an electrolyte composition approximating that of urine electrolytes. Usually, 1/2 normal saline with 20 mEq of sodium bicarbonate per liter can be used as initial urine replacement. Further adjustments in the composition of the replacement fluids should be based on the serum and urine electrolyte analysis. To facilitate function of the transplanted organ, CVP is generally maintained at 8 to 10 cm $H_2O$ in the first 24 hours.

Fluid and electrolyte status needs to be monitored and managed carefully in patients with DGF. Dialysis should be used judiciously as aggressive fluid removal during dialysis can result in hypovolemia and superimposed acute tubular necrosis (ATN), further impeding the recovery of graft function.

### IMMUNOSUPPRESSIVE MANAGEMENT

The goal of immunosuppressive therapy is to prevent allograft rejection, while avoiding complications of excessive immunosuppression such as infections and malignancy. Immunosuppressive therapy is most intense in the first few weeks to months.

Most centers use some form of induction therapy that may include basiliximab in standard-risk and Thymoglobulin or alemtuzumab in high-risk transplant recipients (highly sensitized, retransplants, and patients with DGF) or in steroid avoidance protocols. Infants and young children may benefit from induction therapies because they have more intense allograft-directed immune responses and usually metabolize immunosuppressive medications at a faster rate than adults.

CsA, tacrolimus, prednisone, azathioprine, MMF, and sirolimus are used in various combinations for maintenance immunosuppression and are initiated around transplant surgery. Steroids have been traditionally used in most immunosuppression protocols. IV steroids are often used intraoperatively and for the first few postsurgery days, followed by oral therapy after adequate gastrointestinal function is achieved. A combination of CNI (CsA or tacrolimus) and antiproliferative agents (azathioprine, MMF, or sirolimus) is initiated soon after transplantation. To avoid nephrotoxicity in patients with DGF, CNI use is avoided until satisfactory allograft function is apparent. The use of CsA as a primary immunosuppressive agent has been largely replaced by tacrolimus in recent years.[13] Similarly, MMF has replaced azathioprine. Sirolimus is being used selectively in pediatric renal transplantation.

Because of a high toxicity profile associated with long-term steroid use, attempts have been made to eliminate steroid use in maintenance immunosuppressive protocols. In the earlier studies, steroid withdrawal was associated with a high incidence of acute rejection. Steroid withdrawal or avoidance has been successful in protocols using tacrolimus in combination with MMF. Steroid avoidance studies have shown no increased risk for acute rejection and benefits in reducing post-transplant dyslipidemia and hypertension, although growth advantage is not always realized, especially in postpubertal children.[38] Leukopenia and anemia are more prevalent in children on steroid avoidance protocols. Although short-term data are useful, long-term effects on graft survival are lacking. A combination of tacrolimus and MMF with or without steroids is the most commonly used maintenance immunosuppressive regimen in both adults and children.[13]

---

### KEY POINTS

- Most children receive some form of induction therapy.
- Steroid withdrawal protocols may improve growth and metabolic parameters.
- A combination of tacrolimus and MMF with and without steroids is the most commonly prescribed maintenance immunosuppressive regimen.

---

In steroid-based protocols, steroids are gradually tapered, and by the end of 3 months most children receive low-dose prednisone at 0.1 to 0.2 mg/kg/day either daily or on alternate days. Generic formulations have become available for tacrolimus, CsA, and MMF. Although shown to be bioequivalent in healthy volunteers, data in children after transplant is lacking. Transplant physicians should be familiar with the mechanism of action of various drugs, drug interactions, dosages, and side effect profiles of the immunosuppressive agents. Inadvertent use of drugs that interact with immunosuppressive medications can result in significant complications and morbidity. Prevention and treatment of infections should be an integral part of immunosuppressive management and should be incorporated in the protocols.

## ANTI-INFECTIVE PROPHYLAXIS

Anti-infective prophylaxis is important in preventing opportunistic infections. The American Society of Transplantation has published guidelines for the prevention and management of infections after solid-organ transplantation.[39] Trimethoprim-sulfamethoxazole (TMP-SMX) is used for prophylaxis against *Pneumocystis jiroveci* (formerly *Pneumocystis carinii*) pneumonia (PCP) and urinary tract infection (UTI). The usual dose is 5 mg/kg/day (based on the trimethoprim component with a maximum daily dose of 320 mg) given on thrice-weekly schedule, such as Monday-Wednesday-Friday or on three consecutive days per week. Duration of PCP prophylaxis is usually for 4 to 6 months but may need to be prolonged, depending on the intensity of immunosuppression and therapy of acute rejection episodes.

In children allergic to TMP-SMX or those with G6PD deficiency, inhaled (>6 years of age) or IV pentamidine (<6 years of age) can be used once a month. The dose of inhaled pentamidine is 300 mg via Respirgard II inhaler and for IV pentamidine is 4 mg/kg/dose. Alternatively, dapsone or atovaquone could be used in children allergic to TMP-SMX. TMP-SMX also serves as prophylaxis for nocardia and toxoplasmosis. Suppressive therapy can be continued in children at high risk for UTI. Nystatin (2 to 5 mL) as swish and swallow three or four times per day is prescribed for 4 to 6 weeks following transplantation for fungal prophylaxis.

---

### KEY POINTS

- Post-transplant infections are an important cause of morbidity and hospitalizations in transplant recipients.
- Prospective monitoring and prompt treatment of infections is an important therapeutic strategy, especially when immunosuppression is augmented.

---

Cytomegalovirus (CMV) prophylaxis is necessary for patients at high risk (donor CMV IgG positive/recipient CMV IgG negative) or moderate risk (recipient CMV IgG positive) for developing CMV infection. Oral valganciclovir dose in milligrams (7 × BSA × CrCl, calculated using a modified Schwartz formula). is often used for 3 to 6 months. If the calculated Schwartz creatinine clearance exceeds 150 mL/min/1.73 m², then a maximum value of 150 mL/min/1.73m² should be used in the equation. Herpes simplex virus (HSV) infections can be prevented by low-dose acyclovir in children who are not receiving valganciclovir.

## TRANSPLANTATION IN HIGHLY SENSITIZED RECIPIENTS

It is extremely difficult to find compatible organs for highly sensitized patients. In recent years, these individuals have been successfully transplanted using varying desensitization protocols including high-dose IVIg, rituximab, plasmapheresis, bortezomib, or eculizumab.[20] There are few data in children on the use of such protocols. However, there are increasing numbers of highly sensitized pediatric patients awaiting renal transplantation who may benefit from these interventions.

Transplant centers need to develop an infrastructure of an advanced HLA laboratory, plasmapheresis unit, and renal pathology services before considering ABO or HLA incompatible transplantation and using desensitization protocols. Donor exchange programs between incompatible donor-recipient pairs are becoming popular to transplant individuals with positive cross-match against their respective donors. However, it is likely exchange programs alone will not be successful in transplanting the very highly HLA-sensitized patients. These patients will likely need a combination of desensitization and paired exchange. There are several national donor exchange programs available. UNOS is currently piloting a kidney paired exchange program with the ultimate intent of making it available nationwide.[40]

## POST-TRANSPLANT MONITORING

Transplant recipients need close monitoring, particularly in the first few months of transplant, to assess renal function, adequacy of tacrolimus drug levels, monitoring for infections, adherence with medications and their side effects, and other complications, including PTLD.[41] The risk for acute rejection has decreased significantly from 50% to 60% to less than 10% in the first 6 months of transplantation. Surveillance for malignancy should be included in long-term management. Frequency of monitoring decreases with time as the risks for rejection and infection wane. However, the risks for late acute rejection episodes, development of de novo DSA, and nonadherence increase with time.

There are no immunologic markers for adequacy of immunosuppression. Therefore, judgment regarding adequacy of immunosuppression is usually based on careful clinical evaluation for acute rejection and infections. Measurement of cytokines (granzyme and perforins), or chemokines in the urine by polymerase chain reaction (PCR) has been shown to correlate with acute rejection.[42] The gene profiling of blood and biopsy tissue by microarray technology also holds some promise in differentiating cases of acute rejection from those with stable graft function.[43] These tests, however, are not used widely for routine clinical purposes and their value relative to careful assessment of renal function over time coupled with renal allograft biopsies is unclear.

## COMPLICATIONS OF TRANSPLANTATION

### DELAYED GRAFT FUNCTION

DGF refers to transplants that fail to function after blood flow through the allograft is established. There are varied definitions of DGF, of which the most commonly employed is the need for dialysis in the immediate postoperative period.[44] DGF is more common in organs transplanted from deceased donors because of factors during terminal stages of death, especially in those with increased cold ischemia time. DGF is more prevalent in organs obtained from DCD donors because of an increase in warm ischemia time. A higher incidence of DGF also has been observed in young recipients (0 to 5 years of age) transplanted with laparoscopically procured kidneys.[45] Other well-known causes include acute renal arterial or venous thrombosis, ATN, and HUS. Urinary obstruction secondary to blood clots, urine leakage, and obstructed Foley catheter may mimic DGF (Table 38.7). DGF increases the risk for acute rejection and has deleterious effects on long-term graft survival. During DGF, there is an increased expression of HLA class II molecules on the graft endothelium; thus increasing propensity for acute rejection.[14]

Prompt management of primary DGF is crucial to prevent graft loss. Urinary obstruction and graft blood flow can be assessed by Doppler renal ultrasound, and function can be assessed by MAG-3 nuclear renal scan. Presence of an adequate renal blood flow with a lagging excretory function is suggestive of ATN. Surgical exploration may be necessary if vascular thrombosis is suspected. ATN is managed conservatively. Dialysis should be performed carefully, and hypotension should be avoided as it may impede recovery from DGF. CNI and other nephrotoxic drugs should not be used, and sirolimus should be avoided because it delays recovery from DGF.[46] Induction therapy may need to be intensified to prevent acute rejection. If the allograft is found to be nonviable by MAG-3 scan or biopsy, an allograft nephrectomy is recommended.

### SURGICAL COMPLICATIONS

Surgical complications include renal arterial or venous thrombosis, lymphocele, perirenal serous fluid collection, hematoma, urinary leaks, and obstruction at the uretero-vesical junction (UVJ). Patients at risk for thrombosis include those on peritoneal dialysis, those younger than 2 years of age, recipients of deceased donors under 5 years of age, and those with cold ischemia time greater than 24 hours. Patients with severe nephrotic syndrome may be at increased risk for thrombosis. Placement of an adult kidney

Table 38.7 Differential diagnosis of post-transplant graft dysfunction

| Clinical state | Diagnostic possibilities |
|---|---|
| Acute increase in serum creatinine (20% above baseline or an increase of ≥ 0.3 mg/dL) | Acute rejection |
| | Acute calcineurin inhibitor nephrotoxicity |
| | Dehydration |
| | Urinary obstruction |
| | Pyelonephritis |
| | BK virus infection |
| Slow increase in serum creatinine (creatinine creep) | Interstitial fibrosis and tubular atrophy |
| | Chronic calcineurin inhibitor nephrotoxicity |
| | Urinary tract obstruction or functional bladder dysfunction |
| | Recurrent or de novo glomerulonephritis |
| | BK virus nephropathy |
| | Renal artery stenosis |
| Hypertension | Fluid overload in the peritransplant period |
| | Side effects of steroids, calcineurin inhibitor |
| | Acute rejection |
| | Transplant renal artery stenosis |
| | Interstitial fibrosis and tubular atrophy |
| | Recurrent and de novo glomerulonephritis |
| | Diseased native kidneys |
| | Excessive weight gain and obstructive sleep apnea |
| Proteinuria | Recurrent and de novo glomerulonephritis |
| | Interstitial fibrosis and tubular atrophy |
| | Chronic calcineurin inhibitor nephrotoxicity |
| | Acute rejection |
| | Transplant glomerulopathy |

in children less than 2 years of age results in unique hemodynamic challenges. High aortic blood flow is necessary to prevent arterial thrombosis in infants and children transplanted with adult-sized kidneys.[47]

Several disorders of coagulation causing deficiency of protein C, protein S, antithrombin III, and plasminogen and genetic mutations for factor V Leiden, prothrombin, and methyl-tetrahydrofolate reductase have been described in the general population.[48] Patients with antiphospholipid antibodies are also at high risk for thrombosis. The role of these predisposing factors in post-transplant thrombosis is emerging.[48]

Lymphocele, perirenal serous fluid, or blood collections are common surgical complications in the immediate post-transplant period. Increased incidence of lymphocele also has been noted with the use of sirolimus.[46] Lymphoceles may resolve spontaneously. However, large fluid collections can cause urinary obstruction. Percutaneous aspiration or surgical drainage may be needed in such cases. Urinary leaks are uncommon because of the current practice of using lower doses of steroids and closer attention to urologic surgical techniques. Urinary obstruction at the UVJ may be a manifestation of ureteral ischemia, CMV infection, polyoma BKV infection, or acute rejection. Ureteral stents may

be used for prevention and treatment of UVJ obstruction.[50] UTIs are more common in patients who have stents but can be prevented by the use of TMP-SMX prophylaxis.

## ALLOGRAFT REJECTION

Allograft rejection can be hyperacute, acute, or chronic. HAR occurs because of preformed antibodies to the ABO and HLA antigens. The onset of HAR occurs within minutes to an hour of perfusing the allograft. The allograft shows signs of mottling, followed by vascular thrombosis, and allograft failure. Less commonly, it can manifest as primary nonfunction of the graft. The incidence of HAR has become an extremely rare event in recent years, in particular in primary transplant recipients, as a result of wide availability of sensitive techniques for detecting preformed anti-HLA antibodies and cross-match. Once established, HAR is not amenable to therapy and graft loss is the usual outcome.

### Acute rejection

Acute allograft rejection can occur any time after transplantation. In the early immunosuppression era, acute rejection occurring within the first 3 to 6 months of transplantation known as early acute rejection was a common occurrence. With the advent of potent induction and maintenance immunosuppressive medications, the incidence of early acute rejection has dropped significantly to less than 10% for those transplanted in recent years compared to 68.9% before 1990.[1] However, significant numbers of pediatric patients are experiencing acute rejection after 6 months of transplant, known as late acute rejection. Acute rejection occurring within 1 week of transplantation is known as accelerated acute rejection and has a relatively poor outcome. This also should suggest the possibility of antibody-mediated rejection (AMBR) mediated by DSA reactive with donor HLA or antibodies directed at non-HLA autoantigens on the transplant endothelium. Early diagnosis and treatment of acute rejection are most important for both short-term and long-term graft survival. The relationship between acute rejection and poor long-term graft survival has been clearly demonstrated. In children, tacrolimus-based therapy is known to be associated with fewer episodes of acute rejection when compared to CsA-based therapy.[51]

The classical clinical features of acute rejection, including fever, oliguria, hypertension, proteinuria, and graft tenderness, are rarely observed with current immunosuppression unless a patient is nonadherent with medical therapy. More commonly, children present with an increase in serum creatinine on routine blood monitoring. An increase in serum creatinine of 20% above baseline or greater than 0.3 mg/dL should raise a concern for acute rejection. The differential diagnosis of acute rejection includes dehydration, CNI toxicity, urinary obstruction, and BKV nephropathy (see Table 38.7). A definitive diagnosis of acute rejection is made by biopsy of the transplant kidney. Acute rejection can be T-cell mediated (TCMR) or ABMR or a combination. The Banff classification (Table 38.8) is most widely used for the diagnosis of acute rejection.[52] The characteristic pathologic features of TCMR are interstitial inflammation and tubulitis (Figure 38.5).

Table 38.8 Banff diagnostic criteria

| | Classification | Characteristics |
|---|---|---|
| 1 | Normal histology | |
| 2 | Antibody-mediated rejection (ABMR) | Positive C4d staining and circulating donor-specific antibodies with renal dysfunction<br>*Acute ABMR:* Three histologic variants<br>• ATN like picture<br>• Capillaritis (glomerulitis, neutrophils, and/or mononuclear cells (MNC) in the peritubular capillaries (PTC)<br>• Arterial involvement (transmural inflammation and fibrinoid change)<br>*Chronic ABMR:* Evidence of chronic tissue injury such as glomerular double contours, PTC basement membrane multilayering, IFTA, or fibrous intimal thickening in arteries |
| 3 | Borderline T-cell–mediated rejection (borderline TCMR) | • *Mild tubulitis* (1–4 MNC/tubular cross section (t1), with moderate interstitial inflammation (25%–50% parenchyma affected (i2), or severe interstitial inflammation (i3)<br>• *Foci of moderate tubulitis* (4–10 MNC/tubular cross section (t2), or severe tubulitis (>10 MNC/tubular cross section (t3), with no/trivial interstitial inflammation (<10% parenchyma affected (i0), or minimal interstitial inflammation (<25% parenchyma affected (i1) |
| 4 | T-cell mediated rejection (TCMR) | *Acute TCMR*<br>• *IA:* At least 25% of parenchyma showing interstitial infiltration (i2 and i3) and foci of moderate tubulitis (t2)<br>• *IB:* Just like class IA except there is more severe tubulitis (t3)<br>• *IIA:* Mild-to-moderate intimal arteritis (<25% of luminal area, v1)<br>• *IIB:* Severe intimal arteritis (>25% of the luminal area, v2)<br>• *III:* Transmural (e.g., the full vessel wall thickness) arteritis, v3<br>*Chronic TCMR:* Same as acute TCMR with chronic changes of IFTA |
| 5 | Interstitial fibrosis and tubular atrophy (IFTA) | *Grade I:* <25% of cortical area<br>*Grade II:* 25%–50% of cortical area<br>*Grade III:* 50%–75% of cortical area<br>*Grade IV:* >75% |
| 6 | Renal damage not related to rejection | Changes related to recurrent FSGS, CNI toxicity, or recurrent glomerulonephritis |

*Source:* Solez K, Colvin RB, Racusen LC, et al. Banff 07 classification of renal allograft pathology: updates and future directions. Am J Transplant. 2008;8:753–60; Mengel M, Sis B, Haas M, et al. Banff 2011 Meeting report. New concepts in antibody-mediated rejection. Am J Transplant. 2012;12:563–70; Solez K, Racusen LC. The Banff classification revisited. Kidney Int. 2013;83:201–6.

*Abbreviations:* ATN, acute tubular necrosis; CNI, calcineurin inhibitor; FSGS, focal segmental glomerulosclerosis; IFTA, interstitial fibrosis and tubular atrophy; MCN, mononuclear cells.

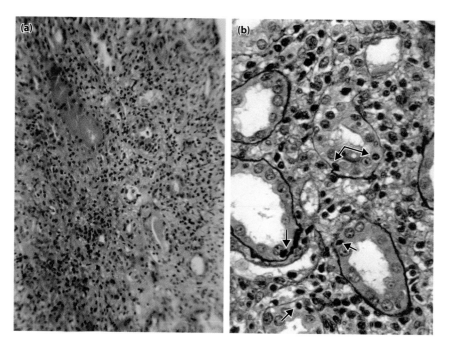

Figure 38.5 Acute renal transplant rejection. (a) Light microscopy photomicrograph of renal transplant biopsy showing acute cellular rejection. Extensive lymphocyte infiltration of the interstitium and tubules is seen. (b) Higher magnification photomicrograph showing lymphocytes infiltrating into the tubular epithelial lining (arrows).

ABMR is characterized by the presence of a combination of features that include detection of de novo DSA, presence of glomerulitis and peritubular caplilliritis, and C4d in the peritubular capillaries (Figure 38.6) and graft dysfunction. It is important to recognize that the most recent Banff recommendations do not require C4d positivity for diagnosis of ABMR. However, the diagnosis of ABMR does require the presence of DSA and evidence of inflammation in glomeruli and peritubular capillaries.[53] Borderline or grade 1A acute rejection is usually treated with IV methylprednisolone (10 to 15 mg/kg/day for 3 to 5 days). Thymoglobulin (1.5 mg/kg/day for 5 to 7 days) or alemtuzumab (0.3–0.4 mg/kg/dose, 1-2 doses) can be used for steroid-resistant acute rejection or higher grade acute rejection episodes.[54,55] A switch to tacrolimus from CsA or increasing the dose of tacrolimus also can be used to treat borderline acute rejection. Therapies including plasmapheresis, rituximab, IVIg, bortezomib, and eculizumab are currently being used for the treatment of ABMR.[56] Late acute rejection may be associated with the development of de novo DSA, nonadherence to medical therapy, and high coefficient of variation of tacrolimus levels and is less amenable to therapy.[57]

## CHRONIC ALLOGRAFT FAILURE RESULTING FROM IMMUNOLOGIC CAUSES

Chronic allograft failure can occur secondary to immunologic or nonimmunologic causes and is histologically characterized by thickening and narrowing of the lumen of

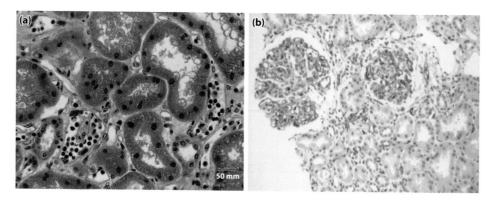

Figure 38.6 Acute antibody-mediated allograft rejection. (a) Peritubular capillaritis showing infiltration by mononuclear cells and polymorphonuclear cells into peritubular capillaries suggestive of acute antibody-mediated rejection. (b) Immunoperoxidase staining showing c4d positive staining in the peritubular capillary walls. C4d is normally present in glomerular capillaries, which serve as an internal control.

the blood vessels and interstitial fibrosis and tubular atrophy (IFTA). Acute rejection including ABMR and chronic ABMR are immunologic causes of IFTA. IFTA can be mild, moderate, or severe. Transplant glomerulopathy, a form of chronic ABMR, is characterized by thickening of glomerular capillary walls and increased mesangial matrix and cellularity (Figure 38.7).[58] Both IFTA and transplant glomerulopathy have a significant negative impact on long-term allograft survival and are commonly associated with the presence of DSA. Because there are no well-established therapies for IFTA and transplant glomerulopathy, the most important strategy is to prevent it by monitoring patient adherence with medication.

## INFECTIONS

Infections constitute the most common reason for hospitalization after renal transplantation.[39] Infectious complications after transplantation usually follow a predictable pattern. In the first month after transplant, infectious complications are related to technical and mechanical problems, such as wound infections, UTI, pneumonia, and fungal infections. Between 1 and 6 months post-transplant, common infectious events involve viral pathogens, such as CMV, EBV, HSV, human herpes virus (HHV), varicella zoster virus, parvovirus (PV) B19, polyoma BKV, PCP, and fungal infections. Beyond 6 months, the patterns of infections in patients on stable maintenance immunosuppression and with good allograft function are similar to those seen in the general population. Patients who develop opportunistic infections more than 6 months post-transplant are generally those who have higher serum creatinine, are receiving higher doses of maintenance steroids, or have had recurrent acute rejection episodes requiring intensification of immunosuppression.

Hepatitis B and C infections may become a clinical concern in long-term survivors of kidney transplants. This may be due to reactivation of these viruses in the recipient or occur

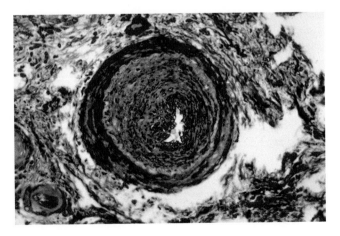

Figure 38.7 Chronic transplant glomerulopathy characterized by arterial luminal narrowing caused by intimal and medial fibrosis and disruption and duplication of internal elastic lamina. The surrounding interstitium shows changes of fibrosis.

as a result of infection acquired in the peritransplant period. Tuberculosis is a serious problem in developing countries because of the high risk for exposure and the immunosuppressed state of these patients. A number of donor-derived infections, including deaths resulting from the West Nile and rabies viruses have been reported in transplant recipients of organs from deceased donors. Proper screening of donors by sensitive assays, including nucleic acid testing, and a high index of suspicion for infections prevalent in the community and prompt treatment are necessary.

UTI in the allograft may be related to abnormal bladder function or vesicouretric reflux in the transplanted ureter. Most patients present with symptoms of fever, malaise, dysuria, and graft tenderness, and some may present with elevated creatinine. However, no difference in the long-term outcome of patients with and without pyelonephritis has been noted.

Risk factors for different HHV infections, clinical features, diagnosis, treatment, and prevention are shown in Table 38.9. Of these, CMV and BKV infections have long-term deleterious effects on the allograft. Figure 38.8 shows renal biopsy sample of a child showing viral inclusions in tubular cells suggestive of BKV nephropathy.

## HYPERTENSION

Of pediatric kidney transplant recipients, 50% to 80% develop hypertension.[1] In the immediate post-transplant period, hypertension may be related to fluid overload, high-dose steroids, and acute rejection. Presence of diseased native kidneys, side effect of medications (CNI and prednisone), acute rejection, recurrent glomerulonephritis, and renal artery stenosis may be the cause of hypertension beyond the first few weeks post-transplantation. NAPRTCS data and other studies suggest that hypertension and use of antihypertensive drugs are significant risk factors for subsequent graft failure. Pediatric patients treated with antihypertensive drugs during the first month after transplantation are noted to have worse linear growth over the first two post-transplant years compared to those who do not require antihypertensive medications.[1]

Post-transplant hypertension is a major amplifier of the CKD-cardiovascular disease continuum and should be managed aggressively.[59] Hypertension is managed with a low-sodium diet and antihypertensive medications. Reduction of corticosteroid dose also may improve blood pressure control. Calcium channel blockers are particularly useful in the treatment of hypertension in the early post-transplant period because of their ability to counteract vasoconstrictive effects of CNI. However, the use of calcium channel blockers may be associated with development of significant edema.

Angiotensin-converting enzyme inhibitors (ACEIs) may be useful in the long-term management of hypertension and in prolonging the life of the allograft because of their inhibitory effect on expression of transforming growth factor-β and other growth factors, IFTA, and their ability to ameliorate proteinuria.[60] However, ACEI

Table 38.9 Post-transplant infections

| Disease | Risk factors | Clinical features | Diagnosis | Treatment | Prevention |
|---|---|---|---|---|---|
| Cytomegalovirus (CMV) | D+/R– Polyclonal antibodies Induction Recurrent acute rejections | Viral syndrome Pneumonia Hepatitis Myelosuppression Colitis | q-PCR, Pp 65 Ag assay | IV GCV+/– Cytogam Valganciclovir | Valganciclovir Monitoring by PCR |
| HHV-6 and HHV-7 | Net state of immunosuppression | Myelosuppression Hepatitis Pneumonia Encephalitis Exacerbates | q-PCR | No data | No data |
| HHV-8 | Net state of immunosuppression | Kaposi sarcoma | q-PCR | Chemotherapy | No data |
| Varicella zoster virus (VZV) | Net state of immunosuppression | Disseminated zoster, pneumonia | DFA for VZV | IV acyclovir until lesions crusted | |
| Parvovirus B19 (PVB19) | Net state of immunosuppression | Aplastic anemia | q-PCR, PVB19 IgM, bone marrow | IVIg | No data |
| BK virus | Net state of immunosuppression | Graft dysfunction Hemorrhagic cystitis | q-PCR, renal biopsy, decoy cells in urine | Decrease IS Cidofovir, Lefllunomide Quinolones | Avoidance of excessive immunosuppression Monitoring by PCR |
| *Pneumocystis jiroveci*, also known as *Pneumocystis carinii* pneumonia (PCP) | Net state of immunosuppression | Interstitial pneumonitis | DFA on sputum/BAL | IV TMP-SMX | TMP-SMX Aerosolized or IV Pentamidine Dapsone Atovaquone |

*Abbreviations:* BAL, Bronchoalveolar lavage; DFA, direct fluorescent antibody; GCV ganciclovir; IV, intravenous; IVIg, intravenous immunoglobulin G; PCR, polymerase chain reaction; q-PCR, quantitative PCR; TMP-SMX, trimethoprim-sulfamethoxazole.

drugs are difficult to use in renal transplant recipients because they may cause increases in serum creatinine and serum potassium and anemia, especially if used in the early post-transplant period. Renal artery stenosis is best treated by percutaneous transluminal angioplasty or surgical correction.[61]

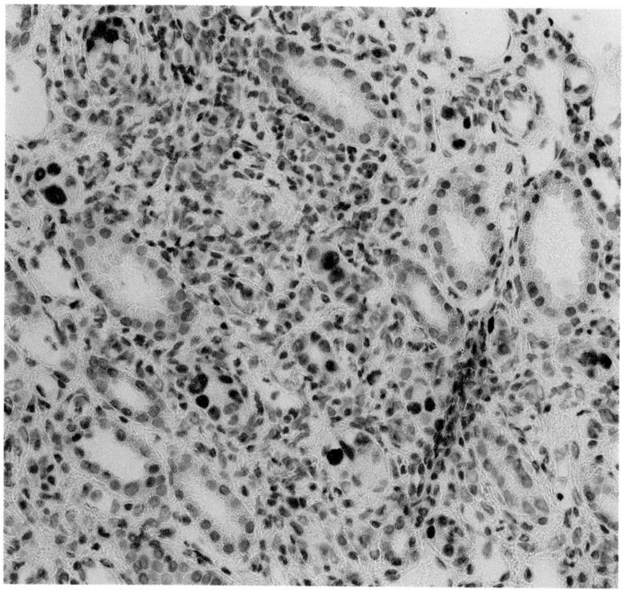

Figure 38.8 Renal biopsy of a child showing BK virus nephropathy. The renal tubular cells show viral inclusions. Immunoperoxidase staining with antibodies to SV40.

## HEMATOLOGIC COMPLICATIONS

Hematologic complications of transplantation include anemia, erythrocytosis, and, rarely, leukopenia and thrombocytopenia. Anemia after transplant may be related to bone marrow suppression secondary to MMF, azathioprine, sirolimus, CsA, or tacrolimus.[62] The incidence of hematologic complications is higher in patients on steroid-free protocols. Aplastic anemia can occur secondary to PVB19 and CMV infections. Hemolytic anemia may result from recurrent or acquired HUS. Hemolytic anemia can result from the administration of high-dose IVIg in patients with A, B, and AB blood groups.[63]

Erythrocytosis is sometimes seen after transplant in children. The risk factors include male gender, retention of native kidneys, smoking, renal artery stenosis, and rejection-free course.[62] Erythrocytosis can be treated with ACEIs and rarely by phlebotomy. Neutropenia and thrombocytopenia may occur after transplant as a side effect of medications, viral infections, or residual hyperparathyroidism.[62]

# GROWTH RETARDATION

Although an acceleration of growth velocity is commonly seen in the majority of children following successful renal transplantation, growth retardation may continue to be a concern in some. Post-transplant growth velocity is better in children who receive transplant at young age (younger than 5 years), have good allograft function, are on minimal (prednisone dose < 0.15 mg/kg/day) or no steroids, or are on alternate-day steroids.

Children with continued post-transplant growth retardation may benefit from recombinant growth hormone therapy. Growth hormone therapy is usually not considered in the first year following transplantation, because children may demonstrate a spontaneous growth spurt. When growth hormone therapy is used, linear growth is best in the first year of therapy with a somewhat slower growth seen in the second and third years.[64,65]

Treatment with growth hormone should continue until full potential for growth is realized or puberty is reached. Treatment with growth hormone can lead to glucose intolerance, slipped capital femoral epiphysis, and intracranial hypertension. However, the incidence of these complications is not higher than in the control ESRD population.[64] An increased risk for acute rejection with growth hormone therapy in early clinical studies has not been substantiated.[64] Patients with one or more episodes of acute rejection before initiation of growth hormone therapy may be at a higher risk for acute rejection afterward. Close monitoring of renal function and acute rejection is therefore desirable. The dose of CsA or tacrolimus may need to be increased after initiation of growth hormone.[64,65]

# RECURRENCES OF PRIMARY DISEASES IN ALLOGRAFTS

Several diseases that cause ESRD have potential to recur in allografts. These include FSGS, atypical HUS, MPGN, IgA nephropathy, Wegener granulomatosis, lupus nephritis, and Henoch-Schönlein purpura.[41,66]

## Focal segmental glomerulosclerosis

Recurrence of FSGS is seen in 30% to 40% of those undergoing primary transplant and approximately 80% of those undergoing repeat transplants.[67] Graft failure occurs in 50% of these cases. Clinical manifestations include massive proteinuria, hypoalbuminemia, and often the full-blown picture of nephrotic syndrome. Recurrence of FSGS may happen immediately or weeks to months after transplantation. Predictors of recurrence include patients who have had a rapid progression to ESRD from the time of initial diagnosis (less than 3 years), poor response to therapy, white race, and presence of mesangial proliferation in the biopsy sample. Patients with FSGS secondary to genetic mutations have a low risk for recurrence. Live donor transplant recipients may have a higher rate of recurrence, but this is not considered a contraindication to live donor transplantation. However, if a primary transplant has been lost to FSGS recurrence, a second living donor for a repeat transplantation should be considered with great caution, careful patient and family preparation, and informed consent of the donor and the family.

A protein permeability factor has been isolated in the sera of patients with FSGS and is reported to predict recurrence and the severity of FSGS in the transplant. The precise nature of this factor has not been identified. Several therapeutic interventions have been suggested in small single-center trials and anecdotal reports. These include plasmapheresis, high-dose CsA, pulse methylprednisolone, immunoadsorption with protein-A columns, cyclophosphamide, and rituximab. Although intensive plasmapheresis treatment for the first 6 to 8 weeks is generally considered, an occasional patient has been treated with long-term plasmapheresis.[67] Galactose was able to reduce the plasma permeability factor but did not induce complete or partial remission in two children with post-transplant recurrent FSGS.[68] Recently, treatment with abatacept (a costimulatory inhibitor targeted at B7-1) was noted to be useful in four patients with recurrent FSGS and B7-1 expression on the podocytes.[69]

## Hemolytic-uremic syndrome

Atypical HUS usually recurs in the allograft, resulting in graft failure. Shiga-toxin–associated HUS without underlying complement abnormalities does not recur. Plasmapheresis and eculizumab have been used successfully to treat atypical HUS recurring after transplant, the latter being more successful. Ideally, eculizumab should be used prophylactically to prevent recurrence.[29]

Recurrent, as well as de novo, HUS in renal transplants has been linked to the use of CsA and tacrolimus.[70] Recurrence of HUS may be present without evidence of hemolysis or thrombocytopenia in more than half of the cases. Typically, recurrent HUS manifests shortly after starting treatment with CsA or tacrolimus, with features of declining urine output, increasing serum creatinine level, and hematuria or proteinuria. A renal biopsy establishes the diagnosis. Discontinuation of CNI and plasmapheresis may help salvage some grafts. However, overall prognosis remains poor. Substitution of CSA for tacrolimus (or vice versa) has been recommended by some. Successful use of sirolimus in this situation also has been reported. De novo transplant micoangiopathy may manifest in a similar manner, but is usually a manifestation of ABMR.

## Membranoproliferative glomerulonephritis

MPGN, especially type II, has the potential to recur in transplants.[66] MPGN type I has recurrence rate of 30% to 40%, whereas MPGN type II may recur in 90% of allografts and may be caused by uncontrolled stimulation of complement cascade. These patients are usually asymptomatic and may show some proteinuria and hematuria. Usually, recurrence leads to slow deterioration of allograft function. Plasmapheresis, high-dose steroids, rituximab, and eculizumab may be useful in salvaging graft function in patients with rapid deterioration.

Recurrent IgA nephropathy, lupus nephritis, and Wegener granulomatosis usually do not cause allograft failure.

## De novo glomerulonephritis

De novo glomerulonephritis, including membranous glomerulonephritis, IgA nephropathy, FSGS, collapsing glomerulopathy, steroid-resistant nephrotic syndrome in patients with Finnish type congenital nephrotic syndrome, and anti-GBM disease in patients with Alport syndrome can be seen after renal transplantation.[71-73]

Post-transplant recurrence of nephrotic syndrome occurs in approximately 25% children with Finnish type congenital nephrotic syndrome secondary to *NPHS1* gene mutations.[74] Manifestation with proteinuria, hypoalbuminemia, and edema may start immediately or as late as 3 years post-transplant. Precedent infection with CMV or EBV may be seen in some.

The histologic lesion is often minimal-change disease, and glomerular endothelial cell swelling has been noted in some. Response to steroids and cyclophosphamide is poor, and graft loss occurs in more than 50% of cases. Antinephrin antibodies have been shown to play a role in the recurrence of nephrotic syndrome.[73] Plasma exchange in combination with cyclophosphamide or rituximab may be useful.

Anti-GBM disease can occur in approximately 5% of patients with Alport syndrome who demonstrate complete absence of the α-3, -4 or -5 portion of type IV collagen in the basement membrane. Crescentic glomerulonephritis with linear IgG deposits in the GBM may occur and lead to rapid graft loss.[73]

## SIDE EFFECTS OF PHARMACOTHERAPY

Immunosuppressive medications have significant side effects, which are listed in Table 38.4. Tacrolimus and cyclosporine (CNIs) are nephrotoxic medications and can cause acute increase in creatinine. Renal biopsy showing isometric vacuoles in the tubules (Figure 38.9) is diagnostic of CNI toxicity. Side effects and toxicities of therapies can become an important concern in transplant patients. This may lead to nonadherence and delayed episodes of acute rejection, particularly in the teenagers.

## METABOLIC COMPLICATIONS

A number of metabolic complications can be seen in children following renal transplantation. These include hypomagnesemia, hypophosphatemia, hypercalcemia, hyperkalemia, renal tubular acidosis, bone and mineral disorders, and dyslipidemia. Hypomagnesemia commonly

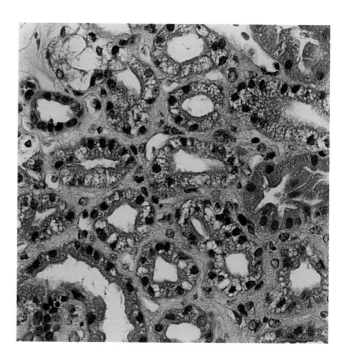

Figure 38.9 Calcineurin inhibitor (CNI)-induced acute tubulopathy. Proximal renal tubules showing isometric vacuoles that are characteristic of CNI toxicity. The vacuoles are small and evenly distributed throughout the cytoplasm of the affected tubular cells.

occurs from renal tubular magnesium wasting as a result of the use of CsA, tacrolimus, or diuretics.[41] Oral replacement with magnesium oxide is needed to control hypomagnesemia. Hypomagnesemia has been noted to be a risk factor for new onset of diabetes after renal transplantation (NODAT). Hyperkalemia and renal tubular acidosis may be a manifestation of CNI toxicity, acute rejection urinary obstruction, or use of ACEIs. Isolated hyperkalemia may be associated with TMP-SMX therapy.[41]

## Bone and mineral disorders

The pathogenesis of post-transplantation bone disease is multifactorial and includes the persistent manifestations of pretransplantation CKD mineral and bone disorder, peritransplantation changes in the fibroblast growth factor 23 (FGF23)–parathyroid hormone–vitamin D axis, metabolic perturbations such as persistent hypophosphatemia, hypomagnesemia, hypercalcemia, and the effects of immunosuppressive therapies.[75] Vitamin D deficiency is prevalent in children after renal transplantation. Hypophosphatemia resulting from residual hyperparathyroidism and increased FGF23 is commonly seen following renal transplantation. Hyperparathyroidism resolves slowly post-transplant and may require therapy with cinacalcet (Sensipar). In rare cases, parathyroidectomy may be needed.

Hypophosphatemia may persist long term in approximately 25% of patients even after a successful transplant, the pathogenesis of which is not well understood.[75] Post-transplant fractures occur more commonly at peripheral sites than at central sites. Although there is significant loss of bone density after transplantation, the evidence linking post-transplantation bone loss and subsequent fracture risk is circumstantial. Presently, there is no optimal therapy for post-transplant bone disease. Combined pharmacologic therapy that targets multiple components of the disordered pathways has been used. Although bisphosphonate or 1,25 dihydroxyvitamin D therapy can preserve bone mineral density after transplantation, there is no evidence that these agents decrease fracture risk. Bisphosphonates pose potential risks for adynamic bone disease.[76]

## Dyslipidemia

A number of lipid abnormalities are being recognized in children after transplant that include elevated blood levels of total cholesterol, low-density lipoprotein cholesterol, very-low-density lipoprotein cholesterol, and triglycerides and decrease in levels of high-density lipoprotein cholesterol. Theses lipid abnormalities may be seen in as many as 50% of children.[77] The contributing factors include use of steroids, CsA, tacrolimus, sirolimus, excessive weight gain, and insulin-dependent diabetes mellitus (IDDM). Dyslipidemia is an important contributor to cardiovascular morbidity and mortality and may contribute to functional deterioration of the graft in the adult population. There is a paucity of data on adverse effects of dyslipidemia and their management in children.[77]

## Obesity

Excessive weight gain and its consequences are important considerations in transplant recipients. The factors responsible for obesity in the general population combined with the use of steroids may play a part. Excessive weight gain may be responsible for sleep apnea, nocturnal enuresis, hypertension, dyslipidemia, and glucose intolerance.[41] NAPRTCS data have shown an increasing prevalence of obesity in pediatric transplant recipients. Obese children between the ages of 6 and 12 years in this study were at higher risk for death compared to nonobese patients, and death was more likely due to cardiopulmonary disease.[78] Early and intense nutritional counseling should be undertaken to prevent this serious complication.

## Diabetes mellitus

Approximately 5% of children develop NODAT after transplantation. The risk is somewhat higher with the use of tacrolimus compared to CsA; both of these medications are toxic to islet cells. Other contributing factors may be the repeated use of pulse steroid therapy, family history of diabetes, excessive weight gain, and hypomagnesemia. Steroids cause insulin resistance. Rigorous management of NODAT is essential for long-term patient and graft survival.[41]

## CHRONIC ALLOGRAFT DYSFUNCTION

Chronic allograft dysfunction histologically characterized by IFTA, ultimately leads to allograft failure and the return of patients to dialysis.[79] Both immune and nonimmune factors contribute to IFTA. The immune-mediated factors were mentioned earlier, and nonimmune factors include DGF, chronic nephrotoxicity related to CsA or tacrolimus, hypertension, hyperglycemia, hyperlipidemia, donor and recipient size mismatch, recipient weight, donor age, CMV and BKV infections, and recurrent and de novo glomerular lesions.

## MALIGNANCY

The risk for malignancy is increased with the intensity and duration of immunosuppression. Malignancies are uncommon in the pediatric age group, but may become a problem as survival of these children increases with successful transplantation. The most important malignancy observed in children is PTLD.

PTLD includes a spectrum of conditions that range between infectious mononucleosis and malignant neoplasia. A large body of literature exists demonstrating the pivotal role of EBV in most cases of PTLD in pediatric solid organ transplant recipients; approximately 85% to 90% of cases of PTLD are EBV driven.

Most cases of PTLD occur in children who are seronegative for EBV at the time of transplantation.[80,81] Primary EBV infection after transplantation can potentially come from several sources, including donor organ, perioperative use of blood products, and subsequent community acquisition of the virus. Its incidence varies from 1% to 10% (usually close to 1%) in most series. The risk for PTLD is bimodal, being highest in the first year post-transplantation and increases again after 7 years of transplantation. However, patients remain at risk indefinitely. The spectrum of clinical features include nonspecific viral syndrome, weight loss, sore throat, abdominal pain, lymphadenopathy, tonsillar enlargement, hepatosplenomegaly, focal neurologic signs, and allograft dysfunction (Figures 38.10 and 38.11).

Diagnostic evaluation of patients with suspected PTLD and management is outlined in Tables 38.10 and 38.11. Strategies to prevent PTLD include close monitoring for EBV replication by PCR and appropriate adjustment of immunosuppressive therapies. The role of antiviral agents and IVIg infusions in preventing PTLD in children with high viral load needs formal clinical trials. Treatment of PTLD includes reducing immunosuppression and use of rituximab in the early stages, and rituximab in combination of chemotherapy may be used in late stages of PTLD.[81] Surgical resection and radiation therapy may be needed in localized cases.

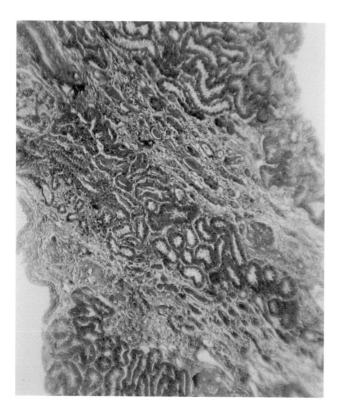

Figure 38.10 Chronic calcineurin inhibitor (CNI) nephrotoxicity. Renal biopsy shows strip fibrosis of the renal interstitium, with normal-appearing tubules between areas of interstitial fibrosis.

**Table 38.11** Therapeutic approach to a patient with post-transplant lymphoproliferative disorder

1. Reduction of immunosuppression: Useful in early and polymorphic post-transplant lymphoproliferative disorder (PTLD)
2. Antiviral therapy with valganciclovir: Unproved benefit but widely used
3. Cytomegalovirus immunoglobulin G
4. Anti–B-cell antibodies such as rituximab, useful in polymorphic PTLD persisting after reduction of immunosuppression
5. Interferon-alpha: May cause severe rejection and usually not recommended
6. Chemotherapy in combination with rituximab: Burkitt lymphoma, refractory PTLD, monomorphic PTLD, and late-onset disease
7. Surgery ± radiation: Reserved for bowel obstruction, localized lesions, or those compressing critical structures
8. Experimental therapies: Autologous or human leukocyte antigen matched Epstein-Barr virus–specific cytotoxic T-cell infusions

**Table 38.10** Diagnostic evaluation of patient with suspected post-transplant lymphoproliferative disorder

1. Complete blood count with differential
2. Serum electrolytes, blood urea nitrogen, creatinine, liver function tests, lactate dehydrogenase, uric acid, serum immunoglobulins
3. Chest radiograph, computed tomography (CT) scan of chest, abdomen, and pelvis
4. Stool for occult blood
5. Biopsy of the lymph nodes and or allograft with immunophenotyping of the cells by immunohistochemistry and flow cytometry, molecular studies for clonality, Epstein-Barr virus (EBV) demonstration in the biopsy tissue by in situ hybridization
6. EBV viral load in blood by quantitative polymerase chain reaction
7. Other investigations: Bone scan; bone marrow aspirate; brain CT, magnetic resonance imaging, positron-emission tomography scan; lumbar puncture; gastrointestinal endoscopies, as indicated

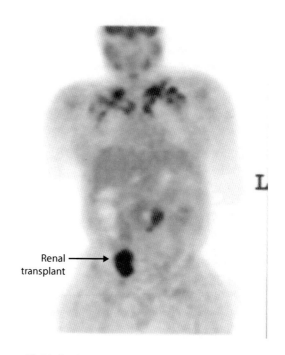

Renal transplant

Figure 38.11 Positron-emission tomography scan of a child with post-transplant lymphoproliferative disorder. The patient presented with abdominal pain, and a mass was detected in the para-aortic area of the abdomen. This scan shows positive pickup by the tumor mass as well as lymph nodes of the mediastinum and cervical region. Kidney transplant is also visualized.

## NONADHERANCE IN TRANSPLANTATION

Nonadherence to the medical regimen is widely prevalent in children. Nonadherence is seen in approximately half of the recipients of deceased organs, and its prevalence increases in adolescents. It may be responsible for 25% of graft loss in children. It may vary from occasional nonadherence to complete nonadherence. Occasional nonadherence could be secondary to forgetfulness, misunderstanding of instructions, or change in routine. Measuring nonadherence is difficult and cumbersome. Often, patients and families would not admit to nonadherence, and, if they do, the extent is usually understated. Manual or electronic pill counting or assessment of refills may be helpful in determining nonadherence but is labor intensive.

Increased coefficient of variation of tacrolimus levels and de novo development of DSA have been suggested as objective markers of nonadherence.[57] Risk factors include disorganized family structure, adolescence, and history of previous graft loss as a result of nonadherence. Parents and children should be reminded to pay special attention while traveling, around vacation times, and when children first leave home to be independent. Counseling, continuing education, planning medication timings, using a pillbox, automated reminders using cellphone alarms and text messaging, involving children and their caretakers in decision-making processes and frequent clinic visits are some of the strategies to improve adherence to medications.[11,83,84] In addition, there are several online tools available to children and adolescents to help increase adherence to medications.

## TRANSITION OF CARE

A systematic transition of children to adult care is paramount to success of the allograft, because a chaotic transition may lead to allograft failure.[84] A systematic analysis of the adolescent readiness skills including psychosocial evaluation, financial planning, health knowledge, and self-management skills should be undertaken and a close communication with the adult providers should be maintained until smooth transition occurs.

## SUMMARY

Renal transplantation is a most rewarding endeavor because it transforms the lives of chronically ill children to near normal in a matter of weeks to months, with an improvement in their growth, neurodevelopment, and quality of life. Short-term graft survival has improved significantly in young children.[85] However, it remains poor in adolescents.[13,85] This is likely due to a large degree of nonadherence. Meticulous attention to the proper management of immunosuppressive medications, infections, and CKD-related complications is needed to improve long-term patient and graft survival (Table 38.12). The benefits of transplantation come at a price of life-long treatment with immunosuppressive medications with concomitant side effects. The ongoing challenges include prevention and treatment of late acute rejection, de novo DSA, finding reliable noninvasive immune-monitoring tools, successful transplantation of highly sensitized patients and those with recurrent FSGS, decreasing the cardiovascular morbidity and mortality and improving bone-mineral disorders in the long-term survivors, dealing with the organ shortage, improving adherence particularly in adolescents, psychosocial rehabilitation of the children and their families, and, finally, the elusive goal of tolerance.

Table 38.12 Principles of long-term management of kidney transplant patients

- Minimize immunosuppression without causing acute rejection
- Diagnose and treat late acute rejection promptly
- Screen for de novo donor-specific antibodies development
- Diagnose and improve nonadherence
- Optimize blood pressure control
- Screen and treat dyslipidemia
- Screen and treat albuminuria
- Screen and treat anemia
- Screen and treat new onset of diabetes after renal transplantation
- Maintain optimal weight, growth, and nutrition
- Optimize cardiovascular outcome
- Optimize bone and mineral health
- Maintain age-appropriate immunizations for child and family, including special immunizations recommended for immunosuppressed children
- Screen for infections and malignancy
- Screen for psychological disorders and provide appropriate timely help
- Optimize child's and family's quality of life
- Planned transition of care

### Clinical Vignette 38.1

A 13-year-old African-American boy with ESRD secondary to posterior urethral valves who had been on chronic hemodialysis for 6 months was referred for renal transplantation. He underwent valve fulguration in the neonatal period. There was no history of any other surgeries or blood transfusions. There was no history of other comorbidities. He was one of eight siblings, four of them above 18 years of age. His parents were in mid-40s and were otherwise healthy. His weight and height were at 10th percentile and blood pressure was normal. Immunizations were up to date, he was immune to varicella and hepatitis B. His blood group was A+ and CPRA was 0%. He tested negative for antibodies to human HIV and hepatitis C and was seropositive for CMV and EBV.

He had a daily urine output of approximately 1.5 L while on hemodialysis. Urodynamic study before transplantation indicated adequate bladder capacity and no significant postvoid residual. The family was educated about merits of living-related transplant and the role of adherence in the transplant survival. After completing workup and receiving additional vaccines with Pneumovax-23, meningitis, and HPV and undergoing dental and cardiac evaluation, he was placed on the deceased donor list.

None of the family members volunteered to donate a kidney for him, and he received a kidney from a 20-year-old donor who had died in a motor vehicle accident. The donor's terminal creatinine was 0.9 mg/dL. The recipient was 1B and 1DR matched (four-antigen mismatched) with the donor. Flow cross-match was negative. Both recipient and donor were positive for antibodies to CMV and EBV. The cold ischemia time was 12 hours and warm ischemia time was 30 minutes. The donor kidney had three arteries (two were on the Carroll patch and one was found to be separate), two veins, and a single ureter.

Intraoperatively, the child received a single dose of anti-IL2R antibody (daclizumab, 1 mg/kg) and 10 mg/kg IV methylprednisolone. Post-operatively, he continued to make urine but had a relatively slow drop in creatinine. However, he did not require dialysis postoperatively. An ultrasound of the transplant kidney showed ischemia of the lower third of the allograft, corresponding to the blood supply of the lower pole artery.

Because of slow recovery of graft function, and ischemia of the transplant, his induction therapy was changed to Thymoglobulin for 5 days. His creatinine came down from 11.0 mg/dL before transplant to 1.8 mg/dL over a period of 5 days. Tacrolimus and MMF were started on postoperative day 4 and continued as maintenance immunosuppression along with tapering doses of prednisone. He was discharged home on the 7th day with a serum creatinine of 1.6 mg/dL that came down to 1.3 mg/dL over the next month. He received antifungal prophylaxis with nystatin for 8 weeks and CMV prophylaxis with valganciclovir and TMP-SMX prophylaxis for PCP and UTI for 6 months post-transplant. On routine follow-up visits, he was noted to have stable graft function (serum creatinine ranging from 1.3 to 1.5 mg/dL, normal blood pressure, low-grade proteinuria (2+ protein on dipstick and random urine protein-to-creatinine ratio of 0.5), and therapeutic tacrolimus levels.

At 11 months post-transplantation, he came to the emergency department with abdominal pain, mostly on the right side (over his transplant kidney). He denied any history of fever, dysuria, nausea, or vomiting and missing any medications. He was noted to have stable vital signs; he was afebrile. There were no clinical signs of dehydration, and his blood pressure was elevated at 135/85 mm Hg. Laboratory testing showed the serum creatinine to be markedly elevated at 9.8 mg/dL; the electrolytes were normal, although the serum bicarbonate level was low at 14 (normal anion gap metabolic acidosis). The tacrolimus level was undetectable. Ultrasound of the transplant kidney showed a slight increase in the kidney size from baseline ultrasound obtained in the immediate post-transplant period, the resistive index was increased to 0.85, and there was no evidence of hydronephrosis. He was suspected to have acute rejection, which was confirmed by renal biopsy to be Banff grade 1B. There was no evidence of glomerulitis or peritubular capillaritis. The biopsy was negative for C4d by immunofluorescence assay. In addition, there was mild IFTA. A biopsy sample was negative for BKV by immunoperoxidase stain. Plasma viral load for BKV, EBV, and CMV by quantitative PCR was negative. DSAs were detected against DR53 and DQ8 antigens with peak MFI of 5000 and 8000, respectively; C1Q binding was negative for these antibodies.

He was treated with IV methylprednisolone (10 mg/kg/day) for 3 days, followed by 7 days of Thymoglobulin for steroid-resistant acute rejection. In addition, he was treated with two doses of IVIg (2 g/kg/dose), given 4 weeks apart, and one dose of rituximab (750 mg/m$^2$) given after 2 weeks of first dose of IVIG. He also was given fungal prophylaxis with nystatin for 8 weeks and TMP-SMX and valganciclovir for 6 months for PCP and CMV prophylaxis, respectively. His creatinine came down to 2.5 mg/dL at the end of therapy. There was improvement in DSA titers when checked 4 weeks after completion of therapy.

The patient admitted to missing his medications, because his mom was not supervising him anymore. He and his family were counseled extensively, and he was closely monitored in the transplant clinic, seen every 2 to 4 weeks. He had two more episodes of acute allograft rejection at 4 and 8 months later. He responded partially to pulse methylprednisolone. His subsequent biopsy results showed progressively increasing IFTA in addition to acute rejection, and he returned to hemodialysis 25 months after transplant. He underwent transplant nephrectomy for intractable pain over the graft and hematuria. He became highly sensitized with CPRA of 100% and broad sensitizations against multiple class I and II antigens and has been on hemodialysis for 5 years.

## TEACHING POINTS

- The patient described in this case highlights several key issues related to pediatric transplantation.
- The patient had no comorbidities and had a panel reactive antibody level of 0%, which is typical of most children with ESRD.
- His late acute rejection episodes after transplant highlight the impact of poor transplant medication adherence on long-term transplant outcome.
- Late acute rejections resulting from nonadherence are highly prevalent in the adolescent population and lead to development of de novo DSA and graft loss as seen in this child. Moreover, there are no clear predictors of poor post-transplant adherence in the pretransplant state, as demonstrated by this case. A highly sensitized state, as seen in this child can, unfortunately be the outcome of a failed transplant state.
- Ischemia of the lower third of the allograft in this patient resulted from thrombosis of the inferior pole artery and he suffered graft injury from it.
- Arterial thrombosis can be a significant surgical concern in children, especially with multiple renal arteries.

## REFERENCES

1. North American Pediatric Renal Trials and Collaborative Study. 2010 Annual transplant report. 2010 Available at https://web.emmes.com/study/ped/annlrept/2010_Report.pdf.
2. Moudgil A. Primer on renal transplantation. Indian J Pediatr. 2012;79:1076–83.
3. Kasiske BL, Cangro CB, Hariharan S, et al. The evaluation of renal transplantation candidates: Clinical practice guidelines. Am J Transplant 2001;1(Suppl 2):3–95.
4. Lubrano R, Perez B, Elli M. Methylmalonic acidemia and kidney transplantation. Pediatr Nephrol. 2013;28:2067–8.
5. McGuire PJ, Lim-Melia E, Diaz GA, et al. Combined liver-kidney transplant for the management of methylmalonic aciduria: A case report and review of the literature. Mol Genet Metab. 2008;93:22–9.
6. Rumsby G, Cochat P. Primary hyperoxaluria. N Engl J Med. 2013;369:2163.
7. El Sayegh S, Keller MJ, Huprikar S, Murphy B. Solid organ transplantation in HIV-infected recipients. Pediatr Transplant. 2004;8:214–21.
8. Morales JM, Aguado JM. Hepatitis C and renal transplantation. Curr Opin Organ Transplant. 2012;17:609–15.
9. 42 CFR 482.90. Condition of participation: Patient and living donor selection. Available at http://www.ecfr.gov/cgi-bin/text-idx?SID=63359829bd75a679b008b46384d49373&node=42:5.0.1.1.1&rgn=div5#42:5.0.1.1.1.5.6.11. Accessed August 31, 2015.
10. Goldberg A, Amaral S, Moudgil A. Developing a framework for evaluating kidney transplantation candidacy in children with multiple co-morbidities. Pediatr Nephrol. 2015;30:5–13.
11. Rianthavorn P, Ettenger RB. Medication non-adherence in the adolescent renal transplant recipient: A clinician's viewpoint. Pediatr Transplant. 2005;9:398–407.
12. Kasiske BL, Ramos EL, Gaston RS, et al. The evaluation of renal transplant candidates: Clinical practice guidelines. JASN. 1995;6:1–34.
13. Matas AJ, Smith JM, Skeans MA, et al. OPTN/SRTR 2011 annual data report: Kidney. Am J Transplant 2013;13(Suppl 1):11–46.
14. Wood KJ, Goto R. Mechanisms of rejection: Current perspectives. Transplantation. 2012;93:1–10.
15. United Network for Organ Sharing. Available at http://www.unos.org/.
16. Organ Allocation. 2013. Available at http://www.unos.org/donation/index.php?topic=organ_allocation.
17. KDPI Calculator. 2013. Available at http://optn.transplant.hrsa.gov/resources/allocationcalculators. Accessed August 31, 2015.
18. Organ Procurement and Transplantation Network. Available at http://optn.transplant.hrsa.gov/. Accessed August 31, 2015.
19. Gebel HM, Liwski RS, Bray RA. Technical aspects of HLA antibody testing. Curr Opin Organ Transplant. 2013;18:455–62.
20. Becker LE, Susal C, Morath C. Kidney transplantation across HLA and ABO antibody barriers. Curr Opin Organ Transplant. 2013;18:445–54.
21. Takahashi K, Saito K. ABO-incompatible kidney transplantation. Transplant Rev (Orlando). 2013;27:1–8.
22. Duquesnoy RJ, Claas FH. 14th International HLA and Immunogenetics Workshop: Report on the structural basis of HLA compatibility. Tissue Antigens. 2007;69(Suppl 1):180–4.
23. Ling M, Marfo K, Masiakos P, et al. Pretransplant anti-HLA-Cw and anti-HLA-DP antibodies in sensitized patients. Human Immunol. 2012;73:879–83.
24. Ginevri F, Nocera A, Comoli P, et al. Posttransplant de novo donor-specific HLA antibodies identify pediatric kidney recipients at risk for late antibody-mediated rejection. Am J Transplant. 2012;12:3355–62.
25. Cecka JM. Calculated PRA (CPRA): The new measure of sensitization for transplant candidates. Am J Transplant 2010;10:26–9.

26. Halloran PF. Immunosuppressive drugs for kidney transplantation. N Engl J Med. 2004;351:2715–29.

27. Moudgil A, Puliyanda D. Induction therapy in pediatric renal transplant recipients: An overview. Paediatr Drugs. 2007;9:323–41.

28. Jordan SC, Toyoda M, Kahwaji J, Vo AA. Clinical aspects of intravenous immunoglobulin use in solid organ transplant recipients. Am J Transplant. 2011;11:196–202.

29. Zuber J, Le Quintrec M, Krid S, et al. Eculizumab for atypical hemolytic uremic syndrome recurrence in renal transplantation. Am J Transplant. 2012;12:3337–54.

30. Matasic R, Dietz AB, Vuk-Pavlovic S. Dexamethasone inhibits dendritic cell maturation by redirecting differentiation of a subset of cells. J Leukocy Biol. 1999;66:909–14.

31. Vincenti F. Are calcineurin inhibitors-free regimens ready for prime time? Kidney Int. 2012;82:1054–60.

32. Kinnear G, Jones ND, Wood KJ. Costimulation blockade: Current perspectives and implications for therapy. Transplantation. 2013;95:527–35.

33. Phase II Pharmacokinetics, efficacy, and safety of belatacept in pediatric renal transplant recipients: 2013. Available at http://clinicaltrials.gov/ct2/show/NCT01791491. Accessed September 4, 2015.

34. Abuali MM, Arnon R, Posada R. An update on immunizations before and after transplantation in the pediatric solid organ transplant recipient. Pediatr Transplant. 2011;15:770–7.

35. Kasiske BL, Bia MJ. The evaluation and selection of living kidney donors. Am J Kidney Dis. 1995;26:387–98.

36. Piros L, Langer RM. Laparoscopic donor nephrectomy techniques. Curr Opin Organ Transplant. 2012;17:401–5.

37. Shapiro M, Sarwal MM. Pediatric kidney transplantation. Pediatr Clin North Am. 2010;57:393–400.

38. Sarwal MM, Ettenger RB, Dharnidharka V, et al. Complete steroid avoidance is effective and safe in children with renal transplants: A multicenter randomized trial with three-year follow-up. Am J Transplant. 2012;12:2719–29.

39. The American Society of Transplantation infectious diseases guidelines, ed 3. Am J Transplant. 2013;13:1–371.

40. Kidney paired donation pilot program. Available at http://optn.transplant.hrsa.gov/. Accessed September 4, 2015.

41. Kidney Disease Improving Global Outcomes. Clinical practice guideline for the care of kidney transplant recipients. Am J Transplant. 2009;9(Suppl 3):S1–155

42. Hartono C, Muthukumar T, Suthanthiran M. Noninvasive diagnosis of acute rejection of renal allografts. Curr Opin Organ Transplant. 2010;15:35–41.

43. Halloran PF, Pereira AB, Chang J, et al. Potential impact of microarray diagnosis of T cell-mediated rejection in kidney transplants: The INTERCOM study. Am J Transplant. 2013;13:2352–63.

44. Siedlecki A, Irish W, Brennan DC. Delayed graft function in the kidney transplant. Am J Transplant. 2011;11:2279–96.

45. Troppmann C, McBride MA, Baker TJ, Perez RV. Laparoscopic live donor nephrectomy: A risk factor for delayed function and rejection in pediatric kidney recipients? A UNOS analysis. Am J Transplant. 2005;5:175–82.

46. Cravedi P, Ruggenenti P, Remuzzi G. Sirolimus for calcineurin inhibitors in organ transplantation: Contra. Kidney Int. 2010;78:1068–74.

47. Salvatierra O Jr, Millan M, Concepcion W. Pediatric renal transplantation with considerations for successful outcomes. Semin Pediatr Surg. 2006;15:208–17.

48. Coppola A, Tufano A, Cerbone AM, Di Minno G. Inherited thrombophilia: Implications for prevention and treatment of venous thromboembolism. Semin Thromb Hemost. 2009;35:683–94.

49. Kfoury E, Taher A, Saghieh S, et al. The impact of inherited thrombophilia on surgery: A factor to consider before transplantation? Mol Biol Rep. 2009;36:1041–51.

50. Wilson CH, Rix DA, Manas DM. Routine intraoperative ureteric stenting for kidney transplant recipients. Cochrane Database Syst Rev. 2013;(6)004925.

51. Coelho T, Tredger M, Dhawan A. Current status of immunosuppressive agents for solid organ transplantation in children. Pediatr Transplant. 2012;16:106–22.

52. Solez K, Colvin RB, Racusen LC, et al. Banff 07 classification of renal allograft pathology: Updates and future directions. Am J Transplant. 2008;8:753–60.

53. Sis B, Jhangri GS, Riopel J, et al. A new diagnostic algorithm for antibody-mediated microcirculation inflammation in kidney transplants. Am J Transplant. 2012;12:1168–79.

54. Upadhyay K, Midgley L, Moudgil A. Safety and efficacy of alemtuzumab in the treatment of late acute renal allograft rejection. Pediatr Transplant. 2012;16:286–93.

55. van den Hoogen MW, Hesselink DA, van Son WJ, et al. Treatment of steroid-resistant acute renal allograft rejection with alemtuzumab. Am J Transplant. 2013;13:192–6.

56. Roberts DM, Jiang SH, Chadban SJ. The treatment of acute antibody-mediated rejection in kidney transplant recipients-a systematic review. Transplantation. 2012;94:775–83.

57. Eid L, Tuchman S, Moudgil A. Late acute rejection: Incidence, risk factors, and effect on graft survival and function. Pediatr Transplant. 2014;18:155–62.

58. Husain S, Sis B. Advances in the understanding of transplant glomerulopathy. Am J Kid Dis 2013;62:352–63.

59. Wheeler DC, Becker GJ. Summary of KDIGO guideline. What do we really know about management of blood pressure in patients with chronic kidney disease? Kidney Int. 2013;83:377–83.

60. Hocker B, Tonshoff B. Treatment strategies to minimize or prevent chronic allograft dysfunction in pediatric renal transplant recipients: An overview. Paediatr Drugs. 2009;11:381–96.

61. Touma J, Costanzo A, Boura B, et al. Endovascular management of transplant renal artery stenosis. J Vasc Surg. 2014;59:1058–65

62. Marinella MA. Hematologic abnormalities following renal transplantation. Int Urol Neph. 2010;42:151–64.

63. Kahwaji J, Barker E, Pepkowitz S, et al. Acute hemolysis after high-dose intravenous immunoglobulin therapy in highly HLA sensitized patients. CJASN. 2009;4:1993–7.

64. Wu Y, Cheng W, Yang XD, et al. Growth hormone improves growth in pediatric renal transplant recipients: A systemic review and meta-analysis of randomized controlled trials. Pediatr Nephrol. 2013;28:129–33.

65. Fine RN, Stablein D, Cohen AH, et al. Recombinant human growth hormone post-renal transplantation in children: A randomized controlled study of the NAPRTCS. Kidney Int. 2002;62:688–96.

66. Ponticelli C, Glassock RJ. Posttransplant recurrence of primary glomerulonephritis. CJASN. 2010;5:2363–72.

67. Vinai M, Waber P, Seikaly MG. Recurrence of focal segmental glomerulosclerosis in renal allograft: An in-depth review. Pediatr Transplant. 2010;14:314–25.

68. Sgambat K, Banks M, Moudgil A. Effect of galactose on glomerular permeability and proteinuria in steroid-resistant nephrotic syndrome. Pediatr Nephrol. 2013;28:2131–5.

69. Yu CC, Fornoni A, Weins A, et al. Abatacept in B7-1-positive proteinuric kidney disease. N Engl J Med. 2013;369:2416-–23.

70. Caires RA, Marques ID, Repizo LP, et al. De novo thrombotic microangiopathy after kidney transplantation: Clinical features, treatment, and long-term patient and graft survival. Transplantation Proc. 2012;44:2388–90.

71. Ponticelli C, Glassock RJ. De novo membranous nephropathy (MN) in kidney allografts: A peculiar form of alloimmune disease? Transpl Int. 2012;25:1205–10.

72. Swaminathan S, Lager DJ, Qian X, et al. Collapsing and non-collapsing focal segmental glomerulosclerosis in kidney transplants. Nephrol Dial Transplant. 2006;21:2607–14.

73. Kashtan CE. Renal transplantation in patients with Alport syndrome. Pediatr Transplant. 2006;10:651–7.

74. Benoit G, Machuca E, Antignac C. Hereditary nephrotic syndrome: A systematic approach for genetic testing and a review of associated podocyte gene mutations. Pediatr Nephrol. 2010;25:1621–32.

75. Kidney Disease Improving Global Outcomes. Clinical practice guideline for the diagnosis, evaluation, prevention, and treatment of chronic kidney disease-mineral and bone disorder (CKD-MBD). Kidney Int. 2009;76(Suppl 113):S3–S121.

76. Kalantar-Zadeh K, Molnar MZ, Kovesdy CP, et al. Management of mineral and bone disorder after kidney transplantation. Curr Opin Nephrol Hypertens. 2012;21:389–403.

77. Wanner C, Tonelli M, for Improving Global Outcomes Lipid Guideline Development Work Group. KDIGO clinical practice guideline for lipid management in CKD: Summary of recommendation statements and clinical approach to the patient. Kidney Int. 2014;85:1303–9.

78. Foster BJ, Martz K, Gowrishankar M, et al. Weight and height changes and factors associated with greater weight and height gains after pediatric renal transplantation: A NAPRTCS study. Transplantation. 2010;89:1103–12.

79. Pascual J, Perez-Saez MJ, Mir M, et al. Chronic renal allograft injury: Early detection, accurate diagnosis and management. Transplant Rev (Orlando). 2012;26:280–90.

80. Dharnidharka VR, Lamb KE, Gregg JA, et al. Associations between EBV serostatus and organ transplant type in PTLD risk: An analysis of the SRTR National Registry Data in the United States. Am J Transplant. 2012;12:976–83.

81. Green M, Michaels MG. Epstein-Barr virus infection and posttransplant lymphoproliferative disorder. Am J Transplant. 2013;13:41–54

82. Prendergast MB, Gaston RS. Optimizing medication adherence: An ongoing opportunity to improve outcomes after kidney transplantation. CJASN. 2010;5:1305–11.

83. Shellmer DA, Dabbs AD, Dew MA. Medical adherence in pediatric organ transplantation: What are the next steps? Curr Opin Organ Transplant. 2011;16:509–14.

84. Watson AR, Harden PN, Ferris ME, et al. Transition from pediatric to adult renal services: A consensus statement by the International Society of Nephrology (ISN) and the International Pediatric Nephrology Association (IPNA). Kidney Int. 2011;80:704–7.

85. Moudgil A, Dharnidharka VR, Lamb KE, et al. Best allograft survival from share-35 kidney donors occurs in middle-aged adults and young children: An analysis of OPTN data. Transplantation. 2013;95:319–25.

86. Mengel M, Sis B, Haas M, et al. Banff 2011 Meeting report: New concepts in antibody-mediated rejection. Am J Transplant. 2012;12:563–70.

87. Solez K, Racusen LC. The Banff classification revisited. Kidney Int. 2013;83:201–6.

## REVIEW QUESTIONS

1. A 5-year-old previously healthy child developed acute kidney injury as a result of septic shock. He received continuous renal replacement therapy for 1 month and then transitioned to peritoneal dialysis as his kidneys failed to recover. He received a number of blood transfusions during his stay in the ICU. His parents ask about the option of kidney transplant. He has otherwise completely recovered and weighs 15 kg. He is CMV IgG positive and EBV IgG negative. The *most* important challenge posed for kidney transplant in this child is:
   a. Size of 15 kg
   b. Potential for sensitization because of number of blood transfusions
   c. EBV negative status
   d. CMV positive status

2. A 10-year-old with ESRD secondary to FSGS underwent living kidney transplant from a family friend. The kidney worked immediately with good urine output and decrease in creatinine. At 36 hours later, he developed severe oliguria and creatinine started to increase. The next step in workup of graft dysfunction includes which of the following?
   a. Urinalysis and urine for ratio of protein to creatinine
   b. Renal ultrasound with Doppler
   c. MAG-3 renal scan
   d. VCUG

3. A 15-year-old girl underwent kidney transplant 4 years ago for ESRD secondary to renal dysplasia with stable serum creatinine level of 0.6 mg/dL. For the past year, she often missed clinic appointments, and her tacrolimus trough levels are quite variable, including some undetectable levels. She has come to the clinic after 8 months and after repeated reminders. On questioning, she denies missing any medications. During clinic visit, she is asymptomatic but her serum creatinine level is 1.1 mg/dL and her tacrolimus level is therapeutic. You plan for renal biopsy. The *most* likely finding on biopsy would be:
   a. Acute rejection
   b. Tacrolimus toxicity
   c. BKV nephropathy
   d. Urinary tract infection

4. A 9-year-old with ESRD secondary to PUV presents for kidney transplant. He has daytime increased frequency and nighttime incontinence. VCUG shows a small-capacity trabeculated bladder. The next step in preparation of this child for transplant includes:
   a. Ultrasound and urinalysis and urine culture
   b. Urodynamic studies, bladder augmentation, and use of a Mitrofanoff procedure for catheterization before transplant

   c. Bladder augmentation and use of a Mitrofanoff procedure for catheterization after transplant
   d. No special preparation needed, because bladder would enlarge after transplant

5. A 6-year-old girl with blood group A+ with ESRD secondary to renal dysplasia, CPRA of 40% is being worked up for living-related transplant. She has four potential donors. Which one is the *best* donor for this child?
   a. A 30-year-old mom with blood group O+, flow cross-match is negative, and there are no donor specific antibodies.
   b. A 32-year-old dad with blood group A+, child has moderately strong donor-specific antibody to DR53, flow B-cell cross-match is positive, and CDC cross-match is negative.
   c. A 22-year-old unrelated six-antigen mismatched donor with blood group O+, flow cross-match negative, and there are no donor-specific antibodies.
   d. A 3-year-old brother with five-antigen mismatch, blood group O+, flow cross-match is negative, and there are no donor-specific antibodies.

6. A 16-year-old girl who received a kidney renal transplant approximately 4 months ago was doing well, with a baseline creatinine level of 0.7 mg/dL. She was on tacrolimus 1 mg capsule (4 mg PO BID) and mycophenolate mofetil (CellCept) 500 mg PO BID. You receive a call from her mother stating that she has been accidentally taking 4 (5 mg) capsules of tacrolimus for the past 2 days. When seen in the emergency room, you expect to see:
   a. Hypertension, tremors, and headache
   b. Increase in creatinine, high serum potassium, low $CO_2$ and magnesium, and high tacrolimus level in blood
   c. A and B
   d. Stable creatinine, normal serum K and $CO_2$, and high magnesium and tacrolimus level

7. A 12-year-old kidney transplant recipient presents to the clinic with unexplained weight loss and intermittent vague abdominal pain for the past 2 to 3 months. He had ESRD secondary to nephronophthisis and received a kidney transplant 8 years ago from a deceased donor. He has been stable until recently and has not had any acute rejections. He has no fever and denies any other symptoms. His physical examination is normal, except for weight loss of 6 kg. His BP is normal and his creatinine is at its baseline of 0.6 mg/dL and urinalysis is normal. You would like to start the workup of his weight loss, and the tests that would be *most* useful are:
   a. CMV and BKV viral loads
   b. Interferon-γ release assay for tuberculosis
   c. LDH, uric acid, EBV viral load

d. CT scan of abdomen, chest, and pelvis

e. Hemoglobin A$_{1c}$

8. A 9-year-old child transplanted with his father's kidney 9 days ago is seen for post-transplant follow-up in the clinic. You notice that he has a swelling near the allograft and in the suprapubic area, which is mildly tender to touch. He had ESRD secondary to renal dysplasia, his Foley catheter was removed on postoperative day 5, and he was discharged home on postoperative day 6 with a serum creatinine of 0.7 mg/dL. His serum creatinine today is 1.3 mg/dL. Renal ultrasound with Doppler shows good perfusion and normal renal transplant morphology and resistive index. An anechoic fluid collection is present next to his transplant and in the pelvis, which was not present 4 days ago. Which tests would help in determining the cause of acute renal dysfunction in this child?

a. Renal biopsy

b. Pharmacokinetics of tacrolimus

c. MAG-3 renal scan and VCUG

d. Needle aspiration of fluid and measurement of creatinine in this fluid

e. c and d

9. A 4-year-old child who received a CMV mismatched kidney transplant comes to clinic 3 months after transplant with a history of low-grade fever for 2 days. He had received induction with Thymoglobulin for 4 days and is on steroid withdrawal protocol. His CBC shows a white cell count of 1.5 K and a platelet count of 120 K, decreased from 4.2 K and 240 K, respectively, 1 week ago. His creatinine has increased by 0.2 mg/dL from the baseline. You make a diagnosis of CMV infection based on elevated CMV viral load. The next *best* step in management of this child is:

a. Decrease MMF and continue the remainder of management because he is already receiving valganciclovir.

b. Admit for intravenous ganciclovir and monitor renal function and CMV viral load.

c. Perform renal biopsy to rule out acute rejection before starting any therapy.

d. Suspect resistant CMV infection and discontinue all immunosuppression.

10. The impact of delayed graft function on the outcome of kidney transplants is:

a. It would increase the risk for acute rejection.

b. It has a negative impact on long-term graft survival.

c. You need to increase the intensity of immunosuppression.

d. a, b, and c

e. It does not increase acute rejection or have an impact on graft survival.

## ANSWER KEY

1. b
2. a
3. a
4. b
5. a
6. c
7. d
8. e
9. b
10. d

# Hypertension

# 39

# Hypertension in children and adolescents

KAREN MCNIECE REDWINE

Hypertension has become an epidemic among adult populations. Worldwide, uncontrolled hypertension is the number one attributable cause of death,[1] and it is the leading disease burden.[2] In fact, hypertension contributes to almost three times the attributable risk for cardiovascular mortality as all other risk factors combined, including smoking, abnormal glucose, and poor diet quality (approximately 41% versus less than 14%).[3] Only in the last few decades, however, has the impact of hypertension in children been recognized. The precursors for adult cardiovascular disease clearly begin in childhood. Blood pressure (BP) tracks from childhood into adulthood.[4,5] In addition, traditional adult cardiovascular risk factors such as elevated BP, increased body mass index (BMI), and dyslipidemia have been associated with atherosclerotic changes in children as young as 2 years old.[6,7] Thus, hypertension should no longer be considered an adult disease. This chapter provides an overview of the epidemiology, pathophysiology, etiology, detection, and diagnostic evaluation of hypertension in children. Therapy of pediatric hypertension is discussed in Chapter 40.

## EPIDEMIOLOGY

The prevalence of hypertension increases with age. Although hypertension was originally reported to be rare during the first 2 decades of life (less than 1%),[8] more recent data suggest that between 3.2% and 5.1%

of children and adolescents have hypertension.[9–15] Therefore, it is one of the most prevalent chronic diseases of childhood.[16] In addition, 15% of adolescents have prehypertension.[9,13] This increase in pediatric hypertension has been attributed in part to a rising rate of obesity observed since the 1990s. Both hypertension and prehypertension increase as BMI increases, and up to 30% of overweight adolescents have a diagnosable BP disorder (Figure 39.1).[13] Along with this increasing rate of obesity has come a shift in prevailing hypertensive diagnoses from those associated with secondary causes to essential hypertension, especially among adolescents.

> ## KEY POINT
>
> Although secondary hypertension is more common in children than adults, obesity-related "essential" hypertension has become the most common form of pediatric hypertension.

## DEFINITION OF HYPERTENSION

BP values used to define hypertension in adults are derived from numerous studies associating BP level with cardiovascular sequelae.[17] Similar studies have not been performed in children because it takes decades for these events to occur. Consequently, abnormal BP values in children are based on

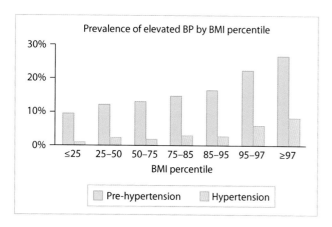

Figure 39.1 Prevalence of hypertension and prehypertension by body mass index (BMI) percentile after three measurements in 6790 adolescents in Houston, Texas. (Adapted from McNiece KL, Poffenbarger TS, Turner JL, et al. Prevalence of hypertension and pre-hypertension among adolescents. J Pediatr. 2007;150:640–4, 4e1.)

normative percentiles generated from pooled data of multiple large cross-sectional studies of "healthy" populations.[18] Normative values of BP in children are based on gender, height, and age because all three have been shown to affect developmental changes in BP independently (Tables 39.1 and 39.2).

BP values lower than the 90th percentile are considered normal. Children with either systolic or diastolic BP between the 90th and 95th percentiles have prehypertension. However, adolescents with BP higher than 120/80 mm Hg and lower than the 95th percentile should also be considered prehypertensive, regardless of the 90th percentile. Recognizing prehypertension is important, to intervene early with nonpharmacologic measures to prevent the development of persistent hypertension.

Children with systolic or diastolic BP persistently higher than the 95th percentile have hypertension. It is currently recommended that hypertension in children be staged to assess the need for more immediate evaluation and treatment. Patients with BP values between the 95th and 99th percentiles plus 5 mm Hg have stage 1 hypertension. BP greater than the 99th percentile plus 5 mm Hg represents stage 2 hypertension and warrants more rapid intervention (Table 39.3). Unless

### KEY POINTS

- BP readings between the 90th and 95th percentiles are designated as prehypertension.
- Hypertension in children is defined as having a blood pressure greater than the 95th percentile for gender, height, and age on three separate occasions.

a patient has severe or symptomatic hypertension, elevated values must be confirmed on at least three occasions to reduce the statistical bias associated with the current classification system.

Occasionally, patients have consistently elevated BP readings (greater than the 95th percentile) in the physician's office, but BP is normal (less than the 90th percentile) at home. Termed "white coat hypertension," this phenomenon is best diagnosed with 24-h ambulatory BP monitoring. Although the significance of white coat hypertension in children has yet to be determined, this may not be an entirely benign condition and represents an intermediate pathophysiologic state between normal BP and hypertension.[19] Ambulatory BP monitoring may also be useful for identifying several other BP abnormalities, including masked hypertension, nocturnal hypertension, and decreased diurnal variation. However, because of the specialized equipment required and complexities of this procedure in children, ambulatory monitoring should be performed only by physicians who have experience with its use and interpretation.[18]

## PATHOPHYSIOLOGY

It is helpful to consider the two main determinants of BP, cardiac output and peripheral vascular resistance, when discussing the pathophysiology of hypertension (Table 39.4). Clinical disorders that increase either determinant raise BP. Although both cardiac output and peripheral vascular resistance can increase independently through various mechanisms, they also have a dependent relationship. For example, if the initiating hypertensive event is caused by a rise in cardiac output, a compensatory rise in peripheral vascular resistance develops over time. Even if the inciting event resolves and cardiac output returns to normal, BP may remain elevated in response to the ongoing elevated peripheral vascular resistance

### KEY POINT

Blood pressure is determined by the product of cardiac output and peripheral vascular resistance. An increase in either leads to hypertension.

Cardiac output is a product of stroke volume and heart rate. Most mechanisms of persistent hypertension are predominantly associated with an increased stroke volume and only slight increases in heart rate. Despite this observation, elevated heart rate has important prognostic significance for cardiovascular disease.[20] Increased stroke volume is usually caused by increased intravascular volume. This may occur with either excessive fluid retention or shifting of fluid from the extravascular space to the intravascular space.[21,22]

Table 39.1 Blood pressure levels for boys by age and height percentile

| Age (yr) | BP Percentile | Systolic BP (mm Hg) | | | | | | | Diastolic BP (mm Hg) | | | | | | |
|---|---|---|---|---|---|---|---|---|---|---|---|---|---|---|---|
| | | Percentile of height | | | | | | | Percentile of height | | | | | | |
| | | 5th | 10th | 25th | 50th | 75th | 90th | 95th | 5th | 10th | 25th | 50th | 75th | 90th | 95th |
| 1 | 50th | 80 | 81 | 83 | 85 | 87 | 88 | 89 | 34 | 35 | 36 | 37 | 38 | 39 | 39 |
| | 90th | 94 | 95 | 97 | 99 | 100 | 102 | 103 | 49 | 50 | 51 | 52 | 53 | 53 | 54 |
| | 95th | 98 | 99 | 101 | 103 | 104 | 106 | 106 | 54 | 54 | 55 | 56 | 57 | 58 | 58 |
| | 99th | 105 | 106 | 108 | 110 | 112 | 113 | 114 | 61 | 62 | 63 | 64 | 65 | 66 | 66 |
| 2 | 50th | 84 | 85 | 87 | 88 | 90 | 92 | 92 | 39 | 40 | 41 | 42 | 43 | 44 | 44 |
| | 90th | 97 | 99 | 100 | 102 | 104 | 105 | 106 | 54 | 55 | 56 | 57 | 58 | 58 | 59 |
| | 95th | 101 | 102 | 104 | 106 | 108 | 109 | 110 | 59 | 59 | 60 | 61 | 62 | 63 | 63 |
| | 99th | 109 | 110 | 111 | 113 | 115 | 117 | 117 | 66 | 67 | 68 | 69 | 70 | 71 | 71 |
| 3 | 50th | 86 | 87 | 89 | 91 | 93 | 94 | 95 | 44 | 44 | 45 | 46 | 47 | 48 | 48 |
| | 90th | 100 | 101 | 103 | 105 | 107 | 108 | 109 | 59 | 59 | 60 | 61 | 62 | 63 | 63 |
| | 95th | 104 | 105 | 107 | 109 | 110 | 112 | 113 | 63 | 63 | 64 | 65 | 66 | 67 | 67 |
| | 99th | 111 | 112 | 114 | 116 | 118 | 119 | 120 | 71 | 71 | 72 | 73 | 74 | 75 | 75 |
| 4 | 50th | 88 | 89 | 91 | 93 | 95 | 96 | 97 | 47 | 48 | 49 | 50 | 51 | 51 | 52 |
| | 90th | 102 | 103 | 105 | 107 | 109 | 110 | 111 | 62 | 63 | 64 | 65 | 66 | 66 | 67 |
| | 95th | 106 | 107 | 109 | 111 | 112 | 114 | 115 | 66 | 67 | 68 | 69 | 70 | 71 | 71 |
| | 99th | 113 | 114 | 116 | 118 | 120 | 121 | 122 | 74 | 75 | 76 | 77 | 78 | 78 | 79 |
| 5 | 50th | 90 | 91 | 93 | 95 | 96 | 98 | 98 | 50 | 51 | 52 | 53 | 54 | 55 | 55 |
| | 90th | 104 | 105 | 106 | 108 | 110 | 111 | 112 | 65 | 66 | 67 | 68 | 69 | 69 | 70 |
| | 95th | 108 | 109 | 110 | 112 | 114 | 115 | 116 | 69 | 70 | 71 | 72 | 73 | 74 | 74 |
| | 99th | 115 | 116 | 118 | 120 | 121 | 123 | 123 | 77 | 78 | 79 | 80 | 81 | 81 | 82 |
| 6 | 50th | 91 | 92 | 94 | 96 | 98 | 99 | 100 | 53 | 53 | 54 | 55 | 56 | 57 | 57 |
| | 90th | 105 | 106 | 108 | 110 | 111 | 113 | 113 | 68 | 68 | 69 | 70 | 71 | 72 | 72 |
| | 95th | 109 | 110 | 112 | 114 | 115 | 117 | 117 | 72 | 72 | 73 | 74 | 75 | 76 | 76 |
| | 99th | 116 | 117 | 119 | 121 | 123 | 124 | 125 | 80 | 80 | 81 | 82 | 83 | 84 | 84 |
| 7 | 50th | 92 | 94 | 95 | 97 | 99 | 100 | 101 | 55 | 55 | 56 | 57 | 58 | 59 | 59 |
| | 90th | 106 | 107 | 109 | 111 | 113 | 114 | 115 | 70 | 70 | 71 | 72 | 73 | 74 | 74 |
| | 95th | 110 | 111 | 113 | 115 | 117 | 118 | 119 | 74 | 74 | 75 | 76 | 77 | 78 | 78 |
| | 99th | 117 | 118 | 120 | 122 | 124 | 125 | 126 | 82 | 82 | 83 | 84 | 85 | 86 | 86 |
| 8 | 50th | 94 | 95 | 97 | 99 | 100 | 102 | 102 | 56 | 57 | 58 | 59 | 60 | 60 | 61 |
| | 90th | 107 | 109 | 110 | 112 | 114 | 115 | 116 | 71 | 72 | 72 | 73 | 74 | 75 | 76 |
| | 95th | 111 | 112 | 114 | 116 | 118 | 119 | 120 | 75 | 76 | 77 | 78 | 79 | 79 | 80 |
| | 99th | 119 | 120 | 122 | 123 | 125 | 127 | 127 | 83 | 84 | 85 | 86 | 87 | 87 | 88 |
| 9 | 50th | 95 | 96 | 98 | 100 | 102 | 103 | 104 | 57 | 58 | 59 | 60 | 61 | 61 | 62 |
| | 90th | 109 | 110 | 112 | 114 | 115 | 117 | 118 | 72 | 73 | 74 | 75 | 76 | 76 | 77 |
| | 95th | 113 | 114 | 116 | 118 | 119 | 121 | 121 | 76 | 77 | 78 | 79 | 80 | 81 | 81 |
| | 99th | 120 | 121 | 123 | 125 | 127 | 128 | 129 | 84 | 85 | 86 | 87 | 88 | 88 | 89 |
| 10 | 50th | 97 | 98 | 100 | 102 | 103 | 105 | 106 | 58 | 59 | 60 | 61 | 61 | 62 | 63 |
| | 90th | 111 | 112 | 114 | 115 | 117 | 119 | 119 | 73 | 73 | 74 | 75 | 76 | 77 | 78 |
| | 95th | 115 | 116 | 117 | 119 | 121 | 122 | 123 | 77 | 78 | 79 | 80 | 81 | 81 | 82 |
| | 99th | 122 | 123 | 125 | 127 | 128 | 130 | 130 | 85 | 86 | 86 | 88 | 88 | 89 | 90 |
| 11 | 50th | 99 | 100 | 102 | 104 | 105 | 107 | 107 | 59 | 59 | 60 | 61 | 62 | 63 | 63 |
| | 90th | 113 | 114 | 115 | 117 | 119 | 120 | 121 | 74 | 74 | 75 | 76 | 77 | 78 | 78 |
| | 95th | 117 | 118 | 119 | 121 | 123 | 124 | 125 | 78 | 78 | 79 | 80 | 81 | 82 | 82 |
| | 99th | 124 | 125 | 127 | 129 | 130 | 132 | 132 | 86 | 86 | 87 | 88 | 89 | 90 | 90 |
| 12 | 50th | 101 | 102 | 104 | 106 | 108 | 109 | 110 | 59 | 60 | 61 | 62 | 63 | 63 | 64 |
| | 90th | 115 | 116 | 118 | 120 | 121 | 123 | 123 | 74 | 75 | 75 | 76 | 77 | 78 | 79 |
| | 95th | 119 | 120 | 122 | 123 | 125 | 127 | 127 | 78 | 79 | 80 | 81 | 82 | 82 | 83 |

(continued)

Table 39.1 Blood pressure levels for boys by age and height percentile (Continued)

| Age (yr) | BP Percentile | Systolic BP (mm Hg) Percentile of height | | | | | | | Diastolic BP (mm Hg) Percentile of height | | | | | | |
|---|---|---|---|---|---|---|---|---|---|---|---|---|---|---|---|
| | | 5th | 10th | 25th | 50th | 75th | 90th | 95th | 5th | 10th | 25th | 50th | 75th | 90th | 95th |
| | 99th | 126 | 127 | 129 | 131 | 133 | 134 | 135 | 86 | 87 | 88 | 89 | 90 | 90 | 91 |
| 13 | 50th | 104 | 105 | 106 | 108 | 110 | 111 | 112 | 60 | 60 | 61 | 62 | 63 | 64 | 64 |
| | 90th | 117 | 118 | 120 | 122 | 124 | 125 | 126 | 75 | 75 | 76 | 77 | 78 | 79 | 79 |
| | 95th | 121 | 122 | 124 | 126 | 128 | 129 | 130 | 79 | 79 | 80 | 81 | 82 | 83 | 83 |
| | 99th | 128 | 130 | 131 | 133 | 135 | 136 | 137 | 87 | 87 | 88 | 89 | 90 | 91 | 91 |
| 14 | 50th | 106 | 107 | 109 | 111 | 113 | 114 | 115 | 60 | 61 | 62 | 63 | 64 | 65 | 65 |
| | 90th | 120 | 121 | 123 | 125 | 126 | 128 | 128 | 75 | 76 | 77 | 78 | 79 | 79 | 80 |
| | 95th | 124 | 125 | 127 | 128 | 130 | 132 | 132 | 80 | 80 | 81 | 82 | 83 | 84 | 84 |
| | 99th | 131 | 132 | 134 | 136 | 138 | 139 | 140 | 87 | 88 | 89 | 90 | 91 | 92 | 92 |
| 15 | 50th | 109 | 110 | 112 | 113 | 115 | 117 | 117 | 61 | 62 | 63 | 64 | 65 | 66 | 66 |
| | 90th | 122 | 124 | 125 | 127 | 129 | 130 | 131 | 76 | 77 | 78 | 79 | 80 | 80 | 81 |
| | 95th | 126 | 127 | 129 | 131 | 133 | 134 | 135 | 81 | 81 | 82 | 83 | 84 | 85 | 85 |
| | 99th | 134 | 135 | 136 | 138 | 140 | 142 | 142 | 88 | 89 | 90 | 91 | 92 | 93 | 93 |
| 16 | 50th | 111 | 112 | 114 | 116 | 118 | 119 | 120 | 63 | 63 | 64 | 65 | 66 | 67 | 67 |
| | 90th | 125 | 126 | 128 | 130 | 131 | 133 | 134 | 78 | 78 | 79 | 80 | 81 | 82 | 82 |
| | 95th | 129 | 130 | 132 | 134 | 135 | 137 | 137 | 82 | 83 | 83 | 84 | 85 | 86 | 87 |
| | 99th | 136 | 137 | 139 | 141 | 143 | 144 | 145 | 90 | 90 | 91 | 92 | 93 | 94 | 94 |
| 17 | 50th | 114 | 115 | 116 | 118 | 120 | 121 | 122 | 65 | 66 | 66 | 67 | 68 | 69 | 70 |
| | 90th | 127 | 128 | 130 | 132 | 134 | 135 | 136 | 80 | 80 | 81 | 82 | 83 | 84 | 84 |
| | 95th | 131 | 132 | 134 | 136 | 138 | 139 | 140 | 84 | 85 | 86 | 87 | 87 | 88 | 89 |
| | 99th | 139 | 140 | 141 | 143 | 145 | 146 | 147 | 92 | 93 | 93 | 94 | 95 | 96 | 97 |

Source: National High Blood Pressure Education Program Working Group on High Blood Pressure in Children and Adolescents. The Fourth Report on the Diagnosis, Evaluation, and Treatment of High Blood Pressure in Children and Adolescents. Bethesda, MD: National Heart Lung and Blood Institute; 2005.
Abbreviation: BP, blood pressure.

Table 39.2 Blood pressure levels for girls by age and height percentile

| Age (yr) | BP Percentile | Systolic BP (mm Hg) Percentile of height | | | | | | | Diastolic BP (mm Hg) Percentile of height | | | | | | |
|---|---|---|---|---|---|---|---|---|---|---|---|---|---|---|---|
| | | 5th | 10th | 25th | 50th | 75th | 90th | 95th | 5th | 10th | 25th | 50th | 75th | 90th | 95th |
| 1 | 50th | 83 | 84 | 85 | 86 | 88 | 89 | 90 | 38 | 39 | 39 | 40 | 41 | 41 | 42 |
| | 90th | 97 | 97 | 98 | 100 | 101 | 102 | 103 | 52 | 53 | 53 | 54 | 55 | 55 | 56 |
| | 95th | 100 | 101 | 102 | 104 | 105 | 106 | 107 | 56 | 57 | 57 | 58 | 59 | 59 | 60 |
| | 99th | 108 | 108 | 109 | 111 | 112 | 113 | 114 | 64 | 64 | 65 | 65 | 66 | 67 | 67 |
| 2 | 50th | 85 | 85 | 87 | 88 | 89 | 91 | 91 | 43 | 44 | 44 | 45 | 46 | 46 | 47 |
| | 90th | 98 | 99 | 100 | 101 | 103 | 104 | 105 | 57 | 58 | 58 | 59 | 60 | 61 | 61 |
| | 95th | 102 | 103 | 104 | 105 | 107 | 108 | 109 | 61 | 62 | 62 | 63 | 64 | 65 | 65 |
| | 99th | 109 | 110 | 111 | 112 | 114 | 115 | 116 | 69 | 69 | 70 | 70 | 71 | 72 | 72 |
| 3 | 50th | 86 | 87 | 88 | 89 | 91 | 92 | 93 | 47 | 48 | 48 | 49 | 50 | 50 | 51 |
| | 90th | 100 | 100 | 102 | 103 | 104 | 106 | 106 | 61 | 62 | 62 | 63 | 64 | 64 | 65 |
| | 95th | 104 | 104 | 105 | 107 | 108 | 109 | 110 | 65 | 66 | 66 | 67 | 68 | 68 | 69 |
| | 99th | 111 | 111 | 114 | 115 | 115 | 116 | 117 | 73 | 73 | 74 | 74 | 75 | 76 | 76 |
| 4 | 50th | 88 | 88 | 90 | 91 | 92 | 94 | 94 | 50 | 50 | 51 | 52 | 52 | 53 | 54 |
| | 90th | 101 | 102 | 103 | 104 | 106 | 107 | 108 | 64 | 64 | 65 | 66 | 67 | 67 | 68 |
| | 95th | 105 | 106 | 107 | 108 | 110 | 111 | 112 | 68 | 68 | 69 | 70 | 71 | 71 | 72 |
| | 99th | 112 | 113 | 114 | 115 | 117 | 118 | 119 | 76 | 76 | 76 | 77 | 78 | 79 | 79 |

Table 39.2 Blood pressure levels for girls by age and height percentile (Continued)

| Age (yr) | BP Percentile | Systolic BP (mm Hg) Percentile of height | | | | | | | Diastolic BP (mm Hg) Percentile of height | | | | | | |
|---|---|---|---|---|---|---|---|---|---|---|---|---|---|---|---|
| | | 5th | 10th | 25th | 50th | 75th | 90th | 95th | 5th | 10th | 25th | 50th | 75th | 90th | 95th |
| 5 | 50th | 89 | 90 | 91 | 93 | 94 | 95 | 96 | 52 | 53 | 53 | 54 | 55 | 55 | 56 |
| | 90th | 103 | 103 | 105 | 106 | 107 | 109 | 109 | 66 | 67 | 67 | 68 | 69 | 69 | 70 |
| | 95th | 107 | 107 | 108 | 110 | 111 | 112 | 113 | 70 | 71 | 71 | 72 | 73 | 73 | 74 |
| | 99th | 114 | 114 | 116 | 117 | 118 | 120 | 120 | 78 | 78 | 79 | 79 | 80 | 81 | 81 |
| 6 | 50th | 91 | 92 | 93 | 94 | 96 | 97 | 98 | 54 | 54 | 55 | 56 | 56 | 57 | 58 |
| | 90th | 104 | 105 | 106 | 108 | 109 | 110 | 111 | 68 | 68 | 69 | 70 | 70 | 71 | 72 |
| | 95th | 108 | 109 | 110 | 111 | 113 | 114 | 115 | 72 | 72 | 73 | 74 | 74 | 75 | 76 |
| | 99th | 115 | 116 | 117 | 119 | 120 | 121 | 122 | 80 | 80 | 80 | 81 | 82 | 83 | 83 |
| 7 | 50th | 93 | 93 | 95 | 96 | 97 | 99 | 99 | 55 | 56 | 56 | 57 | 58 | 58 | 59 |
| | 90th | 106 | 107 | 108 | 109 | 111 | 112 | 113 | 69 | 70 | 70 | 71 | 72 | 72 | 73 |
| | 95th | 110 | 111 | 112 | 113 | 115 | 116 | 116 | 73 | 74 | 74 | 75 | 76 | 76 | 77 |
| | 99th | 117 | 118 | 119 | 120 | 122 | 123 | 124 | 81 | 81 | 82 | 82 | 83 | 84 | 84 |
| 8 | 50th | 95 | 95 | 96 | 98 | 99 | 100 | 101 | 57 | 57 | 57 | 58 | 59 | 60 | 60 |
| | 90th | 108 | 109 | 110 | 111 | 113 | 114 | 114 | 71 | 71 | 71 | 72 | 73 | 74 | 74 |
| | 95th | 112 | 112 | 114 | 115 | 116 | 118 | 118 | 75 | 75 | 75 | 76 | 77 | 78 | 78 |
| | 99th | 119 | 120 | 121 | 122 | 123 | 125 | 125 | 82 | 82 | 83 | 83 | 84 | 85 | 86 |
| 9 | 50th | 96 | 97 | 98 | 100 | 101 | 102 | 103 | 58 | 58 | 58 | 59 | 60 | 61 | 61 |
| | 90th | 110 | 110 | 112 | 113 | 114 | 116 | 116 | 72 | 72 | 72 | 73 | 74 | 75 | 75 |
| | 95th | 114 | 114 | 115 | 117 | 118 | 119 | 120 | 76 | 76 | 76 | 77 | 78 | 79 | 79 |
| | 99th | 121 | 121 | 123 | 124 | 125 | 127 | 127 | 83 | 83 | 84 | 84 | 85 | 86 | 87 |
| 10 | 50th | 98 | 99 | 100 | 102 | 103 | 104 | 105 | 59 | 59 | 59 | 60 | 61 | 62 | 62 |
| | 90th | 112 | 112 | 114 | 115 | 116 | 118 | 118 | 73 | 73 | 73 | 74 | 75 | 76 | 76 |
| | 95th | 116 | 116 | 117 | 119 | 120 | 121 | 122 | 77 | 77 | 77 | 78 | 79 | 80 | 80 |
| | 99th | 123 | 123 | 125 | 126 | 127 | 129 | 129 | 84 | 84 | 85 | 86 | 86 | 87 | 88 |
| 11 | 50th | 100 | 101 | 102 | 103 | 105 | 106 | 107 | 60 | 60 | 60 | 61 | 62 | 63 | 63 |
| | 90th | 114 | 114 | 116 | 117 | 118 | 119 | 120 | 74 | 74 | 74 | 75 | 76 | 77 | 77 |
| | 95th | 118 | 118 | 119 | 121 | 122 | 123 | 124 | 78 | 78 | 78 | 79 | 80 | 81 | 81 |
| | 99th | 125 | 125 | 126 | 128 | 129 | 130 | 131 | 85 | 85 | 86 | 87 | 87 | 88 | 89 |
| 12 | 50th | 102 | 103 | 104 | 105 | 107 | 108 | 109 | 61 | 61 | 61 | 62 | 63 | 64 | 64 |
| | 90th | 116 | 116 | 117 | 119 | 120 | 121 | 122 | 75 | 75 | 75 | 76 | 77 | 78 | 78 |
| | 95th | 119 | 120 | 121 | 123 | 124 | 125 | 126 | 79 | 79 | 79 | 80 | 81 | 82 | 82 |
| | 99th | 127 | 127 | 128 | 130 | 131 | 132 | 133 | 86 | 86 | 87 | 88 | 88 | 89 | 90 |
| 13 | 50th | 104 | 105 | 106 | 107 | 109 | 110 | 110 | 62 | 62 | 62 | 63 | 64 | 65 | 65 |
| | 90th | 117 | 118 | 119 | 121 | 122 | 123 | 124 | 76 | 76 | 76 | 77 | 78 | 79 | 79 |
| | 95th | 121 | 122 | 123 | 124 | 126 | 127 | 128 | 80 | 80 | 80 | 81 | 82 | 83 | 83 |
| | 99th | 128 | 129 | 130 | 132 | 133 | 134 | 135 | 87 | 87 | 88 | 89 | 89 | 90 | 91 |
| 14 | 50th | 106 | 106 | 107 | 109 | 110 | 111 | 112 | 63 | 63 | 63 | 64 | 65 | 66 | 66 |
| | 90th | 119 | 120 | 121 | 122 | 124 | 125 | 125 | 77 | 77 | 77 | 78 | 79 | 80 | 80 |
| | 95th | 123 | 123 | 125 | 126 | 127 | 129 | 129 | 81 | 81 | 81 | 82 | 83 | 84 | 84 |
| | 99th | 130 | 131 | 132 | 133 | 135 | 136 | 136 | 88 | 88 | 89 | 90 | 90 | 91 | 92 |
| 15 | 50th | 107 | 108 | 109 | 110 | 111 | 113 | 113 | 64 | 64 | 64 | 65 | 66 | 67 | 67 |
| | 90th | 120 | 121 | 122 | 123 | 125 | 126 | 127 | 78 | 78 | 78 | 79 | 80 | 81 | 81 |
| | 95th | 124 | 125 | 126 | 127 | 129 | 130 | 131 | 82 | 82 | 82 | 83 | 84 | 85 | 85 |
| | 99th | 131 | 132 | 133 | 134 | 136 | 137 | 138 | 89 | 89 | 90 | 91 | 91 | 92 | 93 |
| 16 | 50th | 108 | 108 | 110 | 111 | 112 | 114 | 114 | 64 | 64 | 65 | 66 | 66 | 67 | 68 |
| | 90th | 121 | 122 | 123 | 124 | 126 | 127 | 128 | 78 | 78 | 79 | 80 | 81 | 81 | 82 |
| | 95th | 125 | 126 | 127 | 128 | 130 | 131 | 132 | 82 | 82 | 83 | 84 | 85 | 85 | 86 |

(continued)

Table 39.2 Blood pressure levels for girls by age and height percentile (Continued)

| Age (yr) | BP Percentile | Systolic BP (mm Hg) Percentile of height | | | | | | | Diastolic BP (mm Hg) Percentile of height | | | | | | |
|---|---|---|---|---|---|---|---|---|---|---|---|---|---|---|---|
| | | 5th | 10th | 25th | 50th | 75th | 90th | 95th | 5th | 10th | 25th | 50th | 75th | 90th | 95th |
| 17 | 99th | 132 | 133 | 134 | 135 | 137 | 138 | 139 | 90 | 90 | 90 | 91 | 92 | 93 | 93 |
| | 50th | 108 | 109 | 110 | 111 | 113 | 114 | 115 | 64 | 65 | 65 | 66 | 67 | 67 | 68 |
| | 90th | 122 | 122 | 123 | 125 | 126 | 127 | 128 | 78 | 79 | 79 | 80 | 81 | 81 | 82 |
| | 95th | 125 | 126 | 127 | 129 | 130 | 131 | 132 | 82 | 83 | 83 | 84 | 85 | 85 | 86 |
| | 99th | 133 | 133 | 134 | 136 | 137 | 138 | 139 | 90 | 90 | 91 | 91 | 92 | 93 | 93 |

*Source:* National High Blood Pressure Education Program Working Group on High Blood Pressure in Children and Adolescents. The Fourth Report on the Diagnosis, Evaluation, and Treatment of High Blood Pressure in Children and Adolescents. Bethesda, MD: National Heart Lung and Blood Institute; 2005.
*Abbreviation:* BP, blood pressure.

Sodium retention from excess intake or increased renal tubular reabsorption is a major contributor to increased intravascular fluid. Activation of the renin-angiotensin-aldosterone system (Figure 39.2) and hyperinsulinemia both contribute to the development of hypertension through this pathway.[23,24] Cardiac output also increases with increased sympathetic tone, which directly increases cardiac contractility and heart rate and stimulates renin release to expand intravascular volume further.

Changes in peripheral vascular resistance can occur with either functional or structural abnormalities. Increased angiotensin II, elevated sympathetic activity, increased endothelins (e.g., prostaglandin $H_2$ [$PGH_2$]), decreased endothelial relaxation factors (e.g., nitric oxide), and genetic abnormalities in vascular cell receptors are all associated with increased vascular smooth muscle contractility and thus raise peripheral vascular resistance.[25] Investigators have also suggested that uric acid, which is known to be elevated in some hypertensive children, may play a role in the pathogenesis of the renal arteriolar changes seen in essential hypertension.[26-28] These changes in vascular compliance are frequently associated with inflammation, and collectively they lead to endothelial dysfunction and vascular remodeling. Although this process may be reversible in some patients,[29] over time it typically progresses to intimal fibrosis and atherosclerosis, which is more likely to be permanent. The complexities by which these multiple factors interact to lead to long-standing hypertension remain elusive, particularly with respect to the development of essential hypertension.

Table 39.3 Classification of blood pressure in children with therapy recommendations

| BP classification | BP compared with 2004 Working Group normative values (percentile for age, gender, and height) | Treatment recommendations |
|---|---|---|
| Normal BP | <90th | Encouragement of healthy diet, sleep, and physical activity |
| Prehypertension | 90th to <95th or if BP ≥120/80 mmHg even if <90th | Weight management counseling if overweight; introduction of physical activity and diet management; initiation of pharmaceutical therapy if compelling indications* exist |
| Stage 1 hypertension | 95th to 99th + 5 mm Hg (on ≥3 separate occasions) | Weight management counseling if overweight; introduction of physical activity and diet management; initiation of pharmaceutical therapy if lifestyle modifications fail or compelling indications* exist |
| Stage 2 hypertension | >99th + 5 mm Hg (on ≥3 separate occasions) | Weight management counseling if overweight; introduction of physical activity and diet management; initiation of pharmaceutical therapy |

*Source:* National High Blood Pressure Education Program Working Group on High Blood Pressure in Children and Adolescents. The Fourth Report on the Diagnosis, Evaluation, and Treatment of High Blood Pressure in Children and Adolescents. Bethesda, MD: National Heart Lung and Blood Institute; 2005.
*Abbreviation:* BP, blood pressure.
* Compelling indications include chronic kidney disease, diabetes mellitus, heart failure, and presence of left ventricular hypertrophy.

Table 39.4  Pathophysiology of hypertension

**Increased Cardiac Output**

Increased intravascular volume

↑ Salt intake

↑ Renal sodium reabsorption

↑ Renin or aldosterone

↑ Insulin

↑ Sympathetic tone

Increased contractility

**Increased Peripheral Vascular Resistance**

Increased vascular contractility

↑ Angiotensin II

↑ Sympathetic activity

↑ Endothelin (PGH₂)

↓ Endothelial relaxation factors (NO)

Structural changes

Endothelial dysfunction

Intimal fibrosis

Atherosclerosis

*Abbreviations:* PGH$_2$, prostaglandin H$_2$; NO, nitric oxide.

## TECHNIQUE OF MEASURING BLOOD PRESSURE

Using proper BP measurement technique is essential when diagnosing hypertension. Incorrect technique can lead to either an erroneous diagnosis of hypertension or failure to identify a child with hypertension. Casual BP measurements should be obtained with the patient in a comfortable seated position, back supported, and feet firmly on the floor after at least 5 min of rest.[30,31] Alternatively, for infants and young children, BP may be measured with the patient supported in a caregiver's lap or lying down.[32] Readings should always be taken in the upper arm with the arm resting at heart level, the method used for generating current normative data. Readings obtained in a leg may be 10 to 20 mm Hg higher than arm pressures. Thus, hypertension should never be diagnosed based on elevated leg pressures, unless there are extenuating circumstances.

Selecting an appropriately sized cuff is critical when measuring BP. Commercial standards are not uniform, and cuff labeling is not always appropriate (e.g., not all 10-year-old children should have their BP measured with the "child

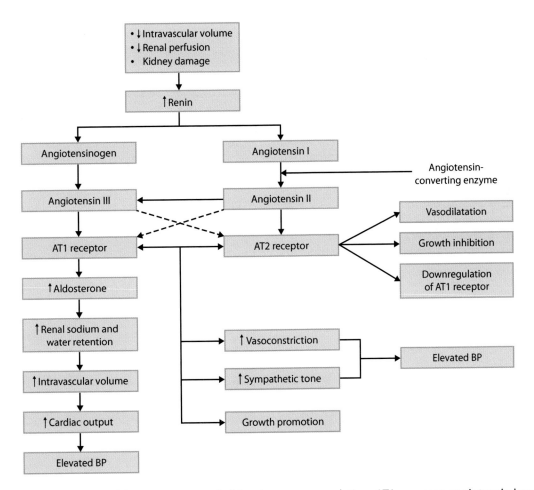

Figure 39.2  Renin-angiotensin-aldosterone system in blood pressure regulation. AT1 receptor, angiotensin I receptor; AT2 receptor, angiotensin II receptor; BP, blood pressure.

Table 39.5 Recommended dimensions for blood pressure cuff bladders

| Age range | Width (cm) | Length (cm) | Maximum arm circumference (cm)* |
|---|---|---|---|
| Newborn | 4 | 8 | 10 |
| Infant | 6 | 12 | 15 |
| Child | 9 | 18 | 22 |
| Small adult | 10 | 24 | 26 |
| Adult | 13 | 30 | 34 |
| Large adult | 16 | 38 | 44 |
| Thigh | 20 | 42 | 52 |

*Source:* National High Blood Pressure Education Program Working Group on High Blood Pressure in Children and Adolescents. The Fourth Report on the Diagnosis, Evaluation, and Treatment of High Blood Pressure in Children and Adolescents. Bethesda, MD: National Heart Lung and Blood Institute; 2005.

* Calculated so that the largest arm would still allow the bladder to encircle the arm by at least 80%.

Table 39.6 Korotkoff sounds for auscultatory blood pressure measurement

| Korotkoff sounds | | Sound characteristics |
|---|---|---|
| First sound | $K_1$ | Snapping sound first heard; indicates systolic BP |
| Second sound | $K_2$ | Muffled sound or murmur; no clinical significance |
| Third sound | $K_3$ | Louder and crisp tapping sound; no clinical significance |
| Fourth sound | $K_4$ | Softer or muted sound, ~5–10 mm Hg above diastolic BP; has been used as indicator of diastolic BP; not recommended in children |
| Fifth sound | $K_5$ | Disappearance of sound; indicates diastolic BP |

*Abbreviation:* BP, blood pressure.

cuff"). Thus, the BP cuff should be chosen based on the actual size of the child's arm and the size of the bladder in the cuff. The BP cuff bladder width should be at least 40% of the midarm circumference (point midway between the olecranon and the acromion), and the length should be at least 80% of the circumference of the arm without overlapping.[18] Using a cuff that is too small can produce erroneously high BP values, whereas too large a cuff may generate results slightly lower than the patient's actual BP. The larger cuff size should be chosen for patients whose midarm circumference measures in the transition zone between cuff sizes, even if the cuff seems too large. The BP cuff size recommendations of *The Fourth Report on the Diagnosis, Evaluation, and Treatment of High Blood Pressure in Children and Adolescents* are given in Table 39.5.[18]

Several noninvasive techniques exist for measuring BP. The gold standard is auscultatory measurement using a mercury manometer.[33] However, mercury manometers have been phased out in many settings out of environmental concerns over mercury exposure. Aneroid manometers may also be used to obtain similar auscultatory measurements. Routine maintenance and recalibration, however, are critical for aneroid manometers to maintain their accuracy.[34,35]

## AUSCULTATORY METHOD

Irrespective of the measuring device, the auscultatory technique requires listening for Korotkoff sounds (Table 39.6) over the brachial artery while slowly deflating the BP cuff. The bell of the stethoscope should be used because it allows the listener to hear softer sounds more clearly. Systolic BP is recorded at $K_1$ (Korotkoff phase 1), which is the onset of sound. This may be followed by a long pause (termed the auscultatory gap) before sounds begin a rhythmic tapping. Diastolic BP is defined at $K_5$, the point at which sound disappears completely. Although $K_4$ (muffling of sounds) is no longer recommended to define diastolic BP, it may be useful in young children in whom $K_5$ is close to zero.[18]

## AUTOMATED DEVICES

Most automated BP devices use oscillometric techniques to measure BP. These monitors have some advantages over standard auscultatory methods, such as increased ease of use and decreased observer error and bias. However, they do not measure systolic and diastolic BP in the same way that the current normative values were obtained. Rather than determining Korotkoff sounds, oscillometric monitors measure mean arterial pressure by capturing the amplitude of oscillation generated by the compressed arterial wall as the BP cuff deflates. Proprietary calculations, which vary among manufacturers, are then used to calculate systolic and diastolic BP from this measured mean arterial pressure.[36] The relationship between mean arterial pressure and systolic and diastolic BP is highly influenced by vascular compliance. Because vascular compliance is typically higher in children than in adults, it is important to choose an oscillometric device that has been validated in children. Overall, oscillometric measurements are similar to those obtained with auscultatory techniques; however, systolic BP tends to be slightly higher, particularly with the first reading.[37,38] For this reason, it is recommended that any BP reading greater than the 90th percentile that is obtained by oscillometric techniques be confirmed using auscultatory methods. Routine maintenance of this equipment according to the manufacturer's recommendations is also important to preserve its accuracy.

## CLINICAL MANIFESTATIONS

Most patients with essential hypertension are identified at a routine physical examination or during a physician's visit for another complaint. Although typically asymptomatic, some of these patients may complain of headaches, dizziness, fatigue, or other mild cardiovascular symptoms. Patients with secondary hypertension present more frequently with symptoms related to their underlying disease (e.g., hematuria with glomerulonephritis or hot flashes and weight loss with hyperthyroidism), rather than symptoms of high BP.

> ### KEY POINT
>
> Mild hypertension may be asymptomatic or may lead to nonspecific symptoms, whereas more severe hypertension may produce life-threatening clinical manifestations.

## HYPERTENSIVE EMERGENCIES

Although less common, severe hypertension can manifest with life-threatening signs and symptoms. Neurologic symptoms are the most common manifestations of hypertensive emergencies in children, although heart failure and renal insufficiency have also been reported.[39] Most children with hypertensive emergencies have a secondary form of hypertension, but reports describing the prevalence of hypertensive crises vary widely (e.g., 20% to 50% in patients with renovascular hypertension).[40,41]

Hypertensive encephalopathy typically manifests with headache that progresses to mental status changes and seizures. Other reported symptoms include facial palsy (particularly Bell palsy),[42] visual changes that may progress to blindness,[39,43] and coma. These symptoms are caused by a disruption in the normal autoregulatory mechanisms of cerebral blood flow that occurs in acute hypertension.[44] With severe, abrupt increases in BP, the cerebral vasculature is unable to constrict adequately to maintain consistent cerebral blood flow. This leads to cerebral hyperperfusion and subsequent edema.[45] When BP increases slowly, these cerebral autoregulatory mechanisms are able to adapt.[46] Thus, hypertensive encephalopathy is most commonly seen in patients with a sudden rise in BP, such as children with acute glomerulonephritis, and rarely in patients with chronic hypertension.

The most common lesion seen with brain imaging of children with hypertensive encephalopathy is the posterior reversible encephalopathy syndrome (PRES) that affects the parieto-occipital white matter (Figure 39.3). These changes can be seen on computed tomography (CT)

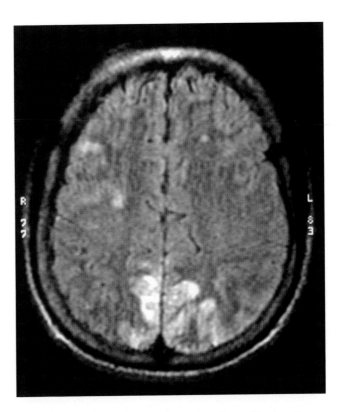

Figure 39.3. Magnetic resonance imaging of brain of an adolescent patient with posterior reversible encephalopathy syndrome (PRES) caused by sudden and severe hypertension.

scan or magnetic resonance imaging (MRI) of the brain. PRES manifests with clinical findings of headache, change in sensorium, confusion, and focal seizures. Apart from severe and sudden elevations in BP, PRES can also be seen in systemic lupus erythematosus and eclampsia. Imaging abnormalities in PRES may persist for weeks after clinical symptoms resolve.[45]

> ### KEY POINT
>
> PRES is a unique clinical and radiologic manifestation seen in patients who develop sudden and severe elevation of BP.

The long-term outcomes of patients following a hypertensive emergency are related in part to appropriate management strategies. Early case series reported significant sequelae of hypertensive encephalopathy, with more than 50% of survivors having long-term neurologic deficits. However, since the introduction of intravenous infusions of antihypertensive medications, which have allowed for a slower reduction in BP, outcomes have been more favorable.[47,48] To compare different treatment strategies, Deal et al.[39] retrospectively investigated the outcomes of 110 severely hypertensive pediatric patients surrounding this change in practice. The initial 57 patients were treated using bolus medications with the intent of normalizing BP in 12 to 24 hours. Of these patients, 13 (23%) developed significant complications, including acute renal failure, both transient and permanent visual loss, and transverse ischemic myelopathy. Subsequently, continuous infusions were used to treat 53 patients, with a goal of gradual BP reduction over 96 hours. Only 2 patients (4%) developed transient acute renal failure, and no neurologic complications were observed.

Thus, although patients presenting with hypertensive emergency require immediate evaluation and intervention, care should be taken not to lower BP too rapidly. Rapid lowering of BP increases the potential for complications associated with hypoperfusion, including ischemic neuropathy of the optic nerve, transverse ischemic myelopathy, and renal impairment.[49-53]

## ETIOLOGY OF HYPERTENSION IN CHILDREN

Hypertension may be either primary (essential) or secondary to an underlying medical condition (Table 39.7, Table 39.8, and Table 39.9). Traditionally, most cases of childhood hypertension were considered secondary. However, the number of children with essential hypertension has risen dramatically in parallel with the obesity epidemic that has occurred since the 1990s. Despite this trend, it is important that practitioners continue to assess patients for secondary causes, particularly in patients who are very young, severely hypertensive, and of normal weight.

### KEY POINTS

- Secondary hypertension is more common in young children and in those with severe hypertension.
- Renal and renovascular diseases are common secondary causes of hypertension in children.

## SECONDARY HYPERTENSION

### Renal Parenchymal Disease

The most common causes of secondary hypertension are related to underlying kidney disease. Up to 50% of children with chronic kidney disease have elevated BP.[54] Congenital abnormalities of the kidneys and urinary tract (CAKUT), chronic glomerulonephritides, polycystic kidney diseases, pyelonephritic renal scars, and external compression of the kidney by a tumor mass are common renal parenchymal diseases associated with hypertension (Figure 39.4).[55] The rise in BP seen in these diseases may be related to intravascular volume expansion from decreased sodium excretion, aberrant activity of the renin-angiotensin-aldosterone system, reduced production of vasodilators, activation of the adrenergic system, or a combination of these factors.[56]

### Renovascular Disease

Renovascular disease is unusual in that it may be surgically correctable. Renal artery stenosis accounts for approximately 8% to 10% of children with secondary hypertension referred to tertiary centers.[57,58] Most of these cases are caused by unilateral fibromuscular dysplasia of the main renal artery (Figure 39.5). Bilateral disease or intrarenal branch artery stenosis can also occur. More extensive involvement is more likely to be seen in children with clinical disorders associated with renal artery stenosis, including neurofibromatosis,[59-63] Marfan syndrome,[64] Takayasu disease,[65] and Klippel-Trénaunay-Weber syndrome.[66]

### Coarctation of Aorta

Coarctation of the aorta is another potentially curable vascular-mediated cause of hypertension (Figure 39.6). Its reported incidence has ranged from as low as 2% to as high as 33% in case series of hypertensive infants. More than 90% of children with coarctation have narrowing of the thoracic aorta just below the origin of the left subclavian artery.[67] However, coarctation may occur at any point along the aorta. When it involves the abdominal aorta, it may extend into branching arteries such as the renal arteries, celiac artery, and mesenteric arteries.[57,68,69] This constellation, known as midaortic syndrome, may be caused by fibromuscular dysplasia or may be part of the vascular pathologic features seen in neurofibromatosis,[62] Takayasu disease,[65] or Williams syndrome.[70] Children whose coarctation goes undiagnosed beyond the first several years of life may have residual hypertension even after surgical correction of the aortic defect.

### Endocrine Disorders

#### HYPERTHYROIDISM

Hyperthyroidism is the most common endocrine disorder that causes hypertension. Although hypertension may be an incidental finding in these patients, some may have significant symptoms of hyperthyroidism, such as tachycardia, weight loss, and anxiety. Because triiodothyronine ($T_3$) is a

Table 39.7 Causes of elevated blood pressure in children and adolescents

**Fictitious Hypertension**
- Too small blood pressure cuff
- Lower extremity measurement

**Renal Diseases**
- Renal dysplasia
- Hemolytic uremic syndrome
- Glomerulonephritis
  - Postinfectious glomerulonephritis
  - Rapidly progressive glomerulonephritis
  - Henoch-Schönlein purpura nephritis
  - Glomerulonephritis with systemic disease (e.g., SLE)
  - Membranoproliferative glomerulonephritis
- Tubulointerstitial nephritis
- Acute tubular necrosis
- Reflux nephropathy
- Renal trauma
- Inherited parenchymal disease (ADPKD, ARPKD)
- Obstructive uropathy (UPJ, UVJ obstruction)
- Chronic renal failure
- Nephrotic syndrome (if hypervolemic)

**Vascular Disorders**
- Coarctation of the aorta
- Renal artery stenosis
- Renal artery thrombosis and embolization
- Renal artery compression

**Neurologic Causes**
- Seizures
- Increased intracranial pressure (tumor, hydrocephalus)
- Guillain-Barré syndrome
- Poliomyelitis
- Dysautonomia
- Spinal cord injury

**Low-Renin Hypertension**
- Gordon syndrome
- Apparent mineralocorticoid excess
- Glucocorticoid-remediable aldosteronism
- Liddle syndrome

**Endocrine Disorders**
- Congenital adrenal hyperplasia
  - 11β-hydroxylase deficiency
  - 17α-hydroxylase deficiency
- Conn syndrome
- Cushing disease
- Hyperthyroidism
- Adrenal hemorrhage

**Renal Tumors**
- Wilms tumor
- Hamartoma
- Hemangiopericytoma

**Catecholamine-Secreting Tumors**
- Pheochromocytoma
- Neuroblastoma
- Paraganglioma

**Neonatal Disorders**
- Congenital rubella
- Bronchopulmonary dysplasia
- Birth asphyxia
- Closure of abdominal wall defects
- Maternal drug use (cocaine and heroin)
- Idiopathic arterial calcification
- Closure of abdominal wall defects
- Maternal drug use (cocaine and heroin)
- Idiopathic arterial calcification

**Miscellaneous Conditions**
- Prolonged TPN
- Pain
- Pneumothorax
- Sickle cell anemia
- Hypercalcemia
- Lead poisoning
- Orthopedic procedures (traction)

**Diet**
- Caffeine
- Alcohol
- Licorice

*Abbreviations:* ADPKD, autosomal dominant polycystic kidney disease; ARPKD, autosomal recessive polycystic kidney disease; SLE, systemic lupus erythematosus; TPN total parenteral nutrition; UPJ, ureteropelvic junction; UVJ, ureterovesicular junction.

peripheral vasodilator, diastolic hypertension is uncommon in these patients, and isolated systolic hypertension is the usual finding.

## ADRENAL DISEASES

Disorders associated with aldosterone excess are uncommon but recognizable causes of hypertension in children. Isolated overproduction of aldosterone may be seen with primary adrenal hyperplasia and aldosterone-producing adenomas. Both conditions are rare in children, however. Aldosterone indirectly activates amiloride-sensitive epithelial sodium channels (ENaC) located on the apical surface of principal cells in the renal cortical collecting duct. Activation of these channels causes sodium retention, with subsequent volume expansion, hypokalemia, and metabolic alkalosis.[71] Plasma renin activity is low to normal in these patients

Table 39.8 Common causes of hypertension by characteristic age of presentation

**Neonate**
- Renal dysplasia
- Obstructive nephropathy
- UAC-associated thrombosis
- Bronchopulmonary dysplasia
- Coarctation of the aorta
- Birth asphyxia
- Autosomal recessive PKD

**Child**
- Congenital renal malformations
- Reflux nephropathy
- Coarctation of the aorta
- Glomerulonephritides
- Renal artery stenosis
- Wilms tumor
- Neuroblastoma

**Adolescent**
- Obesity or essential hypertension
- Glomerulonephritis
- Renal artery stenosis
- Endocrine disorders
- Autosomal dominant PKD
- Illicit drug use

*Abbreviations:* PKD, polycystic kidney disease; UAC, umbilical artery catheter.

Table 39.9 Medications associated with hypertension

| Drug class | Examples |
|---|---|
| Corticosteroid | Prednisone, methylprednisolone |
| Nonsteroidal anti-inflammatory | Ibuprofen, naproxen |
| Estrogen | Oral contraceptives |
| Sympathomimetic | Nasal decongestants, diet pills (pseudoephedrine, phenylephrine) |
| Erythropoiesis-stimulating agent | Erythropoietin, darbepoetin |
| Illicit drug | Cocaine, amphetamines |
| Psychotropic | Buspirone, clozapine, fluoxetine, lithium, tricyclic antidepressants |
| Anticonvulsant | Carbamazepine |
| Herbal | Ephedra, ginseng, ma huang, ginger, St. John's wort |

because of the associated volume expansion. The distinction between adrenal hyperplasia and adrenal adenoma may be difficult because most adenomas are small (less than 1 cm),[72] and hyperplasia of the remainder of the adrenal gland is also common in the presence of an adenoma.[73]

Aldosterone excess also occurs in patients with glucocorticoid-remediable aldosteronism (GRA). GRA is an autosomal dominant disorder wherein DNA encoding aldosterone synthase is coupled to the regulatory sequences conferring adrenocorticotropic hormone (ACTH) responsiveness.[74] Thus, ACTH becomes the main controlling agent of aldosterone production, rather than angiotensin II or potassium. Consequently, patients with GRA have aldosterone-mediated hypertension that can be suppressed with glucocorticoids.

Overproduction of other mineralocorticoids causes hypertension in several rare forms of congenital adrenal hyperplasia (CAH), including 11β-hydroxylase, 3β-hydroxysteroid dehydrogenase, 17β-hydroxylase, and cholesterol desmolase deficiencies.[75–77] 21-Hydroxylase deficiency, which accounts for approximately 90% of all cases of CAH, is not associated with hypertension, except as a side effect of therapy with corticosteroids and mineralocorticoids.

Cushing syndrome leads to hypertension through activation of the mineralocorticoid receptors by cortisol. Aldosterone is approximately 300 times more potent than cortisol at activating mineralocorticoid receptors. However, in high enough concentrations, cortisol can produce an aldosterone-like effect.[78,79] The specific affinity of mineralocorticoid receptors for aldosterone is provided by the enzyme 11β-hydroxysteroid dehydrogenase 2 (11β-HSD2), which is found locally at the receptor site. 11β-HSD2 breaks down cortisol to cortisone, thereby removing its ability to activate the receptor. When levels exceed the threshold concentration of this enzyme (as is seen in Cushing syndrome), cortisol is able to bind to these receptors and stimulate sodium reabsorption. Genetic deficiencies in 11β-HSD2 also lead to hypertension in the autosomal recessive disorder known as apparent mineralocorticoid excess (AME).[80,81]

## Genetic Disorders

Liddle syndrome and Gordon syndrome are monogenic causes of hypertension. Liddle syndrome is an autosomal dominant condition in which a mutation in the ENaC channel leads to persistent activation and sodium reabsorption.[82,83] This creates a clinical picture similar to that of hyperaldosteronism, but plasma renin and aldosterone levels are very low.[84]

Gordon syndrome (pseudohypoaldosteronism type II) is an autosomal dominant syndrome caused by mutations in the WNK1 and WNK4 kinase family, both of which are involved in regulating the activity of the thiazide-sensitive sodium-chloride (Na-Cl) cotransporter in the distal nephron.[85,86] Hyperactivity of this receptor, as seen in Gordon syndrome, leads to a clinical picture of salt reabsorption

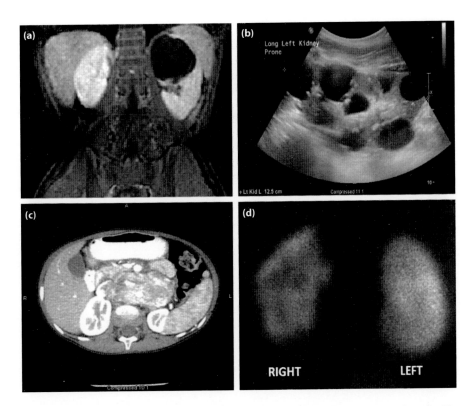

Figure 39.4  Renal parenchymal causes of hypertension. **(a)** Large renal pelvic diverticulum identified by magnetic resonance urography in a thin 14-year-old patient with hypertension. **(b)** Polycystic kidney disease seen on renal ultrasound in a 6-year-old child with hypertension and tuberous sclerosis. **(c)** Large retroperitoneal mass found on computed tomography in an 8-year-old child presenting with hypertension from mass effect. **(d)** Dimercaptosuccinic acid renal scan of a patient with severe hypertension. The upper pole of the right kidney shows multiple photopenic areas, representing renal scars.

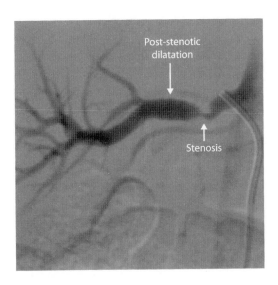

Figure 39.5  Renovascular hypertension. Renal angiogram in a patient with hypertension secondary to fibromuscular dysplasia affecting the midsegment of the right renal artery. Poststenotic dilatation of the renal artery is also seen.

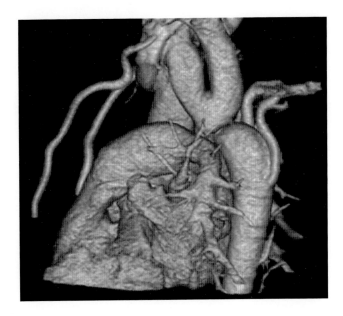

Figure 39.6  Severe coarctation of the descending aorta visualized on three-dimensional reconstruction images obtained with computed tomography angiography in an 11-year-old child with hypertension and diminished lower extremity pulses.

with subsequent low-renin hypertension. Unlike in other forms of monogenic hypertension, patients with Gordon syndrome develop hyperkalemia and metabolic acidosis.[84]

---

### KEY POINTS

- Liddle syndrome is characterized by a mutation in the ENaC channel that leads to its persistent activation and sodium reabsorption.
- Gordon syndrome (pseudohypoaldosteronism type II) is caused by mutations in the WNK1 or WNK4 kinase that regulates the thiazide-sensitive Na-Cl cotransporter in the distal tubule.
- Plasma renin and aldosterone levels in Little syndrome and Gordon syndrome are low in response to excess sodium reabsorption and intravascular volume expansion.

---

## Neoplasms

Intra-abdominal tumors may cause hypertension through compression of the renal vasculature or parenchyma, thus causing inappropriate renin release (Page kidney). Tumors may also raise BP by the direct release of vasoactive substances such as renin (Wilms tumor) or catecholamines (pheochromocytomas). Of these tumors, pheochromocytoma is the most likely to be identified when hypertension is the presenting complaint. Pheochromocytomas are uncommon in childhood; only 10% pheochromocytomas occur in this age group. These tumors are usually benign and originate in the chromaffin cell tissue in the adrenal medulla or other locations along the sympathetic chain (Figure 39.7). Rarely, they may also arise from atypical sites such as the bladder and heart.[87] The unregulated release of metanephrine or normetanephrine from these tumors leads to the classical symptoms of headaches, sweating, and palpitations with tachycardia.[88,89] Other common symptoms include anxiety, nausea and vomiting, unintentional weight loss,

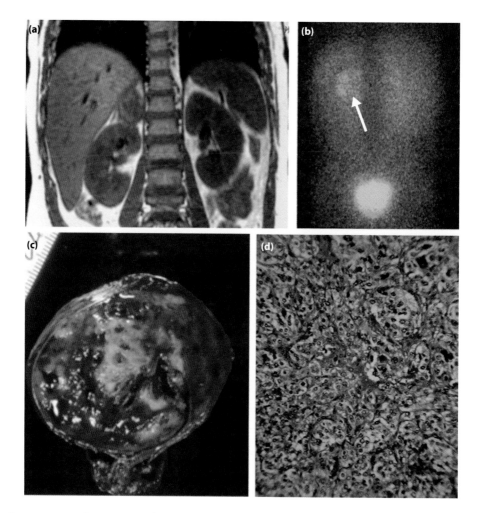

Figure 39.7 Pheochromocytoma in a patient who presented with low-grade fever, weight loss, tachycardia, and hypertension. (a) Magnetic resonance imaging of the abdomen showing tumor in the right adrenal gland. (b) Meta-iodobenzylguanidine scan demonstrating radiotracer uptake in the tumor area (arrow). (c) Cut surface of the tumor removed surgically showing numerous necrotic areas within a yellow background of the mass. (d) Microscopic section (hematoxylin and eosin stain) showing tumor cells with large eccentric nuclei, arranged in rests that are surrounded by a fine fibrovascular membrane-like structure.

being excessively sensitive to warm environment, increased body temperature (low-grade fever), pallor, and acrocyanosis. Whereas symptoms in children with these tumors are often intermittent, elevated BP is more frequently sustained, with periodic spikes of severe hypertension.[88] A 24-h urine collection for determining daily catecholamines and metanephrines excretion is typically recommended for diagnostic evaluation. Serum catecholamine determination may be less accurate, especially if the secretion of these neurohormones is periodic. Plasma metanephrines, however, are more sensitive when samples are obtained correctly through an indwelling catheter.[90]

---

### KEY POINT

Pheochromocytoma can occur as an isolated tumor or in association with neurofibramatosis, von Hippel-Lindau disase, or multiple endocrine neoplasia type II.

---

Localization of a pheochromocytoma may be challenging. A 131-iodine or 123-iodine meta-iodobenzylguanidine (MIBG) scan is the initial scan typically recommended to identify tumors of neural crest origin, but the radionuclide scan may miss even large tumors.[91,92] Labeled somatostatin is an alternate way of identifying catecholamine-secreting tumors missed by MIBG scans.[93] MRI or CT is then needed to delineate tumor borders preoperatively. Localization of a tumor with these modes of imaging should not be considered definitive because finding multiple tumor foci is not uncommon, especially with syndromes associated with pheochromocytomas such as neurofibromatosis,[94,95] von Hippel–Lindau disease,[96] and multiple endocrine neoplasia (MEN).[97,98]

Surgical removal of the tumor is the definitive treatment for pheochromocytoma. BP control initially with α blockade with phenoxybenzamine followed by β blockade if necessary, should be achieved for at least 1 week preoperatively.[99] β-Blocking agents should not be used alone in these patients because this approach results in unopposed stimulation of vascular α receptors, which can precipitate a hypertensive crisis. Calcium channel blockers may also be used safely if BP remains elevated despite α blockade.[100]

## ESSENTIAL HYPERTENSION

The prevalence of essential hypertension among children and adolescents has risen dramatically since the 1990s in parallel with rising rates of obesity. Although the exact cause and mechanisms behind its development have yet to be elucidated, essential hypertension is likely the result of complex interactions between both genetic and environmental factors. Excess weight is the most strongly associated risk factor because approximately 30% of obese adolescents have elevated BP.[101] A lack of exercise and

dietary choices, independent of weight, have also been identified as risk factors for hypertension. In adults, a diet high in salt[102,103] and low in fresh fruits, vegetables, and calcium,[102] along with a sedentary lifestyle,[104] is associated with high BP. Evidence supporting the role of sodium in the development of hypertension in children is strong, although the role of other nutrients such as potassium and calcium is unclear.[105,106]

Race and ethnicity also have some influence on the incidence of hypertension. A larger percentage of African Americans in the United States have hypertension as compared with whites, Hispanics, and Native Americans.[107–109] This finding is likely related to a higher incidence of several genetic polymorphisms that have been associated with the development of essential hypertension. However, environmental factors, such as poverty or demanding environments, which have also been correlated with higher BP, may also contribute to these differences.[110]

## NEONATAL HYPERTENSION

Hypertension is uncommon in infants, but it does affect 1% to 2% of newborns admitted to the neonatal intensive care unit.[111–113] Umbilical artery catheter–associated thromboembolism, which may originate from either the aorta or the renal arteries, is a unique cause of hypertension in this population (Figure 39.8). Congenital lesions of both the vasculature and renal parenchyma (e.g., coarctation of the aorta, renal artery stenosis, polycystic kidney disease, and obstructive uropathy) must also be considered in this age group. In fact, in one series approximately 50% of infants diagnosed with hypertension were found to have an underlying renal anomaly.[113] Bronchopulmonary dysplasia, extracorporeal membrane oxygenation (ECMO), patent ductus arteriosus, intraventricular hemorrhage, and acute renal failure are other well-recognized risk factors for neonatal hypertension.[111–116] Finally, iatrogenic causes of neonatal hypertension include medications, maternal drug use, and complications associated with prolonged parenteral

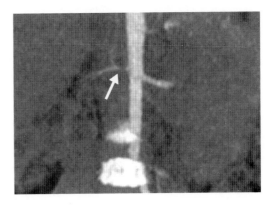

Figure 39.8 Computed tomography angiogram defining residual renal artery stenosis (arrow) in a 1-year-old child with a history of an umbilical artery catheter–associated thrombus.

nutrition. Close monitoring of BP at follow-up is important for all children with a complicated neonatal course because many of these children do not develop hypertension until several months after discharge from the intensive care unit.[117]

## EVALUATION OF A CHILD WITH HYPERTENSION

Evaluation of a child identified as hypertensive should be aimed at identifying potential secondary causes, detecting underlying hypertensive target organ damage, and ascertaining other risk factors for cardiovascular disease. The urgency with which this evaluation is undertaken depends on the severity of the child's illness. Young patients, those with severe BP elevation, and those with symptoms related to hypertension deserve more immediate evaluation with concomitant therapeutic interventions. Less urgent evaluation is appropriate in older children and those with milder BP elevations.

## KEY POINT

Evaluation of the hypertensive child should focus on identifying secondary causes, hypertensive target organ damage, and other comorbidities related to cardiovascular disease.

## HISTORICAL DATA

A detailed history focused on identifying symptoms of severe hypertension, as well as clues to an underlying cause, should be obtained from all patients with hypertension (Table 39.10). A thorough past medical, family, diet, and sleep history may provide clues to the underlying cause of an individual patient's hypertension. Most patients are either asymptomatic or describe nonspecific symptoms such as mild headaches, fatigue, and sleep disturbances. Patients with severe hypertension, however, may complain of significant headaches, visual changes, and chest pain. Urinary symptoms and swelling may suggest acute glomerulonephritis, whereas weight loss and sweating may indicate an endocrine abnormality or neoplasm. Past medical history of an umbilical artery catheter or multiple urinary tract infections suggests an underlying renal abnormality. Loud snoring and sleep disturbances may be present in children with sleep apnea, a potential cause of hypertension. In addition, certain prescribed and illicit drugs may cause hypertension.

## PHYSICAL EXAMINATION

A complete physical examination should be performed, with special attention to findings suggestive of an underlying hypertensive disorder or hypertensive target organ damage (Table 39.11). On initial presentation, four extremity BPs should be obtained to screen for coarctation of the aorta, which should be suspected if upper extremity BPs exceed lower extremity measurements. Lower extremity pulses are typically diminished in these children. The

Table 39.10 Historical clues in the diagnosis of hypertension

| Historical finding | Possible significance |
| --- | --- |
| **Complaint and Review of Systems** | |
| Headaches, dizziness, epistaxis, visual changes | Nonspecific |
| Abdominal pain, dysuria, frequency, urgency, nocturia, enuresis | Underlying renal disease |
| Joint pains or swelling, edema, rashes | Autoimmune-mediated disease or glomerulonephritis |
| Weight loss, sweating, flushing, palpitations | Pheochromocytoma or hyperthyroidism |
| Muscle cramps, weakness, constipation | Hypokalemia associated with hyperaldosteronism |
| Delayed puberty | Congenital adrenal hyperplasia |
| Snoring | Sleep apnea |
| Prescription, over-the-counter, or illicit drug use | Drug-induced hypertension |
| **Past Medical History** | |
| Umbilical artery catheterization | Renal artery thrombosis/renal embolus |
| Thyroid cancer, neurofibromatosis, Von Hippel–Lindau disease | Pheochromocytoma |
| **Family History** | |
| Hypertension | Inherited forms of hypertension (AME, Gordon syndrome, Liddle syndrome, GRA), essential hypertension |
| Renal disease | Polycystic kidney disease, Alport syndrome |
| Tumors | Familial pheochromocytoma, MEN II |
| Early complications of hypertension or atherosclerosis | Predictive of hypertensive course |

*Abbreviations:* AME, apparent mineralocorticoid excess; GRA, glucocorticoid-remediable aldosteronism, MEN II, multiple endocrine neoplasia type II.

Table 39.11 Physical examination abnormalities in children with hypertension

| Clinical abnormality | Diagnostic implication |
| --- | --- |
| **Vital Signs** | |
| Bradycardia | Increased intracranial pressure |
| Drop in BP from upper to lower extremities | Coarctation of the aorta |
| Tachycardia | Hyperthyroidism, pheochromocytoma, neuroblastoma, primary hypertension |
| **Constitutional** | |
| Growth retardation | Chronic kidney disease |
| Obesity | Essential hypertension |
| Truncal obesity | Cushing disease, insulin resistance |
| **Head and Neck** | |
| Adenotonsillar hypertrophy | Sleep disorders |
| Elfin facies | Williams syndrome |
| Fundal changes (papilledema, AV nicking) | Chronic or severe hypertension |
| Moon facies | Cushing disease |
| Proptosis or goiter | Hyperthyroidism |
| Webbed neck | Turner syndrome |
| **Cardiovascular** | |
| Apical heave | Left ventricular hypertrophy |
| Disparity in pulses | Coarctation of the aorta |
| Friction rub | SLE, collagen vascular disease, uremia |
| **Lungs** | |
| Crackles or rales | Heart failure with chronic hypertension |
| **Abdomen** | |
| Bruit | Renal artery stenosis, abdominal coarctation |
| Hepatomegaly | Heart failure |
| Masses | Obstructive nephropathy, Wilms tumor, neuroblastoma, pheochromocytoma, polycystic kidney disease |
| **Genitalia** | |
| Ambiguous, virilized | Congenital adrenal hyperplasia |
| **Extremities** | |
| Edema | Acute or chronic kidney disease |
| Joint swelling | Autoimmune disease |
| Rachitic changes | Chronic kidney disease |
| **Dermatologic** | |
| Acanthosis nigricans | Insulin resistance or metabolic syndrome |
| Needle tracks | Drug-induced hypertension |
| Neurofibromas | Neurofibromatosis |
| Rashes | Vasculitis or nephritis |
| Striae, acne | Cushing disease |
| Tubers, ash-leaf spots, adenoma sebaceum | Tuberous sclerosis |
| **Neurologic** | |
| Encephalopathy | Severe hypertension |
| Cranial nerve palsy | Severe hypertension |

*Abbreviations:* AV, arteriovenous; BP, blood pressure; SLE, systemic lupus erythematosus.

remainder of the cardiac examination, including the presence of abnormal heart sounds or an abdominal bruit, may also provide diagnostic clues. The head and neck examination may reveal proptosis, tonsillar hypertrophy, or papilledema, whereas the dermatologic examination my reveal striae, neurofibromas, or acanthosis nigricans. A neurologic examination may show signs of severe hypertension such as Bell palsy or hemiparesis.

## LABORATORY AND IMAGING STUDIES

Laboratory evaluation should include electrolytes to screen for monogenic forms of hypertension, blood urea nitrogen and creatinine to assess kidney function, and a complete blood count to evaluate for anemia, which is associated with chronic kidney disease and other chronic illnesses (Table 39.12). A urinalysis to detect hematuria or proteinuria should also be performed in all patients. The urine microalbumin-to-creatinine ratio may be obtained to identify more

subtle renal abnormalities. Although microalbuminuria is common in adult patients with isolated chronic hypertension, it is less common in children who do not have underlying diabetes. Plasma renin activity (PRA) levels are useful to screen patients for underlying causes of secondary hypertension. PRA levels are typically normal or mildly elevated in children with renal parenchymal or renovascular disease. They tend to be more significantly elevated in children with pheochromocytoma (increased sympathetic output directly stimulates renin release).[118] Conversely, renin levels are low in children with volume expansion and hyperaldosteronism. Specific laboratory studies, such as thyroid studies or urine catecholamines, are indicated in patients with specific symptoms or when particular diagnostic conditions are suspected. Finally, patients with essential hypertension should also be evaluated for hypercholesterolemia and metabolic syndrome.

An echocardiogram is indicated in all patients with hypertension to evaluate for congenital anomalies and left ventricular hypertrophy (LVH), a sensitive measure of target organ

Table 39.12 Clinical evaluation of confirmed hypertension

| Study or procedure | Purpose | Target population |
|---|---|---|
| **Evaluation for Identifiable Causes** | | |
| History, including sleep history, family history, risk factors, diet, and habits such as smoking and drinking alcohol; physical examination | History and physical examination help focus subsequent evaluation | All children with persistent BP ≥95th percentile |
| BUN, creatinine, electrolytes, urinalysis | Renal parenchymal disease; hypokalemia and alkalosis may point to mineralocorticoid excess disorders | All children with persistent BP ≥95th percentile |
| CBC | Anemia, consistent with chronic renal disease | All children with persistent BP ≥95th percentile |
| Renal ultrasound | Renal scar, congenital anomaly, or disparate renal size, polycystic kidney disease | All children with persistent BP ≥95th percentile |
| **Evaluation for Comorbidity** | | |
| Fasting lipid panel, fasting glucose | Identify hyperlipidemia, identify metabolic abnormalities | Overweight patients with BP at 90th–94th percentile; all patients with BP ≥95th percentile; family history of hypertension or cardiovascular disease; child with chronic renal disease |
| Drug screen | Identify substances that could cause hypertension | History suggestive of possible contribution by substances or drugs |
| Polysomnography | Identify sleep disorder in association with hypertension | History of loud, frequent snoring |
| **Evaluation for Target-Organ Damage** | | |
| Echocardiogram | Identify LVH and other indications of cardiac involvement | Patients with comorbid risk factors* and BP 90th–94th percentile; all patients with BP ≥95th percentile |
| Retinal examination | Identify retinal vascular changes | Patients with comorbid risk factors* and BP 90th–94th percentile; all patients with BP ≥95th percentile |

Table 39.12 Clinical evaluation of confirmed hypertension (Continued)

| Study or procedure | Purpose | Target population |
|---|---|---|
| **Further Evaluation as Indicated** | | |
| Ambulatory BP monitoring | Identify white coat hypertension, abnormal diurnal BP pattern, BP load | Patients in whom white coat hypertension is suspected, and when other information on BP pattern is needed |
| Plasma renin determination | Identify low renin, suggesting mineralocorticoid-related disease | Young children with stage 1 hypertension and any child or adolescent with stage 2 hypertension; positive family history of severe hypertension |
| Renovascular imaging: Isotopic scintigraphy (renal scan) Magnetic resonance angiography Duplex Doppler flow studies Three-dimensional CT Arteriography: DSA or classic | Identify renovascular disease | Young children with stage 1 hypertension and any child or adolescent with stage 2 hypertension |
| Plasma and urine steroid levels | Identify steroid-mediated hypertension | Young children with stage 1 hypertension and any child or adolescent with stage 2 hypertension |
| Plasma and urine catecholamines | Identify catecholamine-mediated hypertension | Young children with stage 1 hypertension and any child or adolescent with stage 2 hypertension |

*Source:* National High Blood Pressure Education Program Working Group on High Blood Pressure in Children and Adolescents. The Fourth Report on the Diagnosis, Evaluation, and Treatment of High Blood Pressure in Children and Adolescents. Bethesda, MD: National Heart Lung and Blood Institute; 2005.

*Abbreviations:* BP, blood pressure; BUN, blood urea nitrogen; CBC, complete blood count; CT, computed tomography; DSA, digital subtraction angiography; LVH, left ventricular hypertrophy.

* Comorbid risk factors also include diabetes mellitus and kidney disease.

damage. The presence of LVH should prompt more aggressive medical management. LVH can improve with therapy.[119-121] Thus, serial testing (annually or semiannually) may be useful for monitoring therapeutic control of hypertension.

A renal ultrasound scan should be performed in all patients with hypertension to identify parenchymal lesions, such as small scarred kidneys, polycystic kidney disease, or other structural anomalies. Compared with its use in adults, Doppler ultrasound is less sensitive in identifying subtle renal artery stenosis in children. Although both CT and MRI are reasonable secondary screening tools for renal artery stenosis, angiography remains the gold standard for diagnosis and treatment.[122-125] Other renal imaging techniques, such as dimercaptosuccinic acid (DMSA) renal scintigraphy to identify renal scarring, may also prove useful in detecting underlying renal disorders.

## TARGET ORGAN DAMAGE

With the rising prevalence of hypertension among children and adolescents, concerns regarding the morbidity and ultimate mortality of this condition are becoming increasingly relevant. For adults, hypertension is an independent risk factor for myocardial infarction, heart failure, stroke, and chronic kidney disease.[126] In fact, the World Health Organization[127] reported that poor BP control was the number one attributable risk for death in the world, and it accounted for 62% of cerebrovascular disease and 49% of ischemic heart disease observed. Hypertension is also the second leading cause of end-stage renal disease among adults requiring dialysis in the United States.[128]

The long-term effects of high BP on children are difficult to define, given the long time period between diagnosis and a definable adverse event such as heart attack or stroke. However, measurable damage to the heart, blood vessels,

---

### KEY POINT

Target organ abnormalities are common in children with hypertension and may include damage to the heart, vasculature, or kidneys.

retina, and kidneys has been documented in young people with elevated BP. Monitoring these subclinical changes may ultimately prove to be a better indicator of hypertension severity and BP control than periodic BP measurements, which are inherently variable.

LVH is the most commonly identified target organ abnormality among hypertensive children. Its reported prevalence has been as high as 40% among children with newly diagnosed hypertension; however, this prevalence varies significantly depending on the definition of LVH.[129-133] Although the adult cut-point of more than 51 g/m[2.7] has been recommended as a conservative definition for LVH in children and adolescents,[18] pediatric-based normal values may ultimately be more appropriate.[134] LVH is an independent risk factor for cardiovascular disease in adults, in whom it predicts both morbidity and mortality.[135,136] The process by which the increased afterload associated with hypertension increases the risk for cardiovascular disease is unknown. Several proposed mechanisms include abnormalities in diastolic function,[137] increased vulnerability of the cardiovascular system to ischemia because of increased oxygen consumption,[138] and induction of electrophysiologic abnormalities which increase the risk for arrhythmias and sudden death.[139] Subtle abnormalities in left ventricular diastolic function identified through tissue Doppler imaging have been reported in hypertensive children, thereby providing support for at least one of these mechanisms.[140] Left atrial enlargement has also been associated with hypertension in children, but its significance remains undetermined.[141]

Vascular changes have also been identified in children with hypertension. Increased carotid artery intima-medial thickness is a marker of generalized atherosclerosis in adults and correlates with incident coronary artery disease, myocardial infarction, and stroke.[142] Carotid artery intima-medial thickness is increased in hypertensive children and is independently associated with BMI and left ventricular mass index.[133,143] In addition, measures of arterial stiffness, such as pulse wave velocity, worsen in children as BP levels increase from normal to sustained hypertension.[144] Finally, hypertensive retinopathy may occur in children and occasionally produces the presenting symptom. Although estimates in children are limited, retinal abnormalities may occur in up to 50% of infants[145] and 20% of older children[146] with hypertension.

Microalbuminuria (30 to 300 mg albumin/g creatinine in a first morning urine specimen) is indicative of early renal damage in adults with hypertension, and it is independently associated with adverse cardiovascular events.[147-149] However, this association with hypertension has not been shown in children without underlying diabetes or chronic kidney disease.[150] The reason may be an increased prevalence of proteinuria in children or a decreased sensitivity of the test to detect lower levels of injury. Children found to have microalbuminuria should be considered at risk for progression of hypertensive renal disease. Further research

is needed, however, to identify more sensitive markers of hypertensive nephropathy and effective intervention strategies to prevent the development of end-stage renal disease.

## SUMMARY

The prevalence of hypertension in children and adolescents has risen significantly since the 1990s. The diagnosis requires attention to proper measurement techniques, consideration of underlying causes, and evaluation of target-organ damage and other cardiovascular risk factors. Early detection is essential to minimize the long-term health consequences of hypertension. Clinical Vignette 39.1 describes an adolescent patient with hypertension.

### Clinical Vignette 39.1

A 14-year-old African-American male patient presented to his pediatrician's office for his annual physical examination before joining the junior varsity football team. He denied any current concerns, although his mother reported that she thought he was overly tired and remembered that he complained of some dizziness during football practice toward the end of the season last year. He was born at term and had otherwise been relatively healthy for most of his life except for being slightly overweight. He was not taking any medications and denied any illicit drug use. He ate a "typical teenage" diet, and his favorite foods were pizza, nachos, and fried chicken. He ate few fresh fruits and vegetables and consumed approximately three caffeinated beverages a day. Both his father and paternal grandfather had hypertension diagnosed in their 40s and 60s, respectively. His mother was recently diagnosed with diabetes mellitus.

Physical examination revealed a moderately overweight male patient in no distress. His height was at the 75th percentile for age, and his body mass index was 29. Vital signs were temperature 98.6° F, pulse 85/min, respiration 20/min, and blood pressure (BP) 142/86 mm Hg. He had mild acanthosis nigricans on the back of his neck, but the remainder of his physical examination was normal. BP in four extremities was as follows:

Right upper extremity: 140/76 mm Hg
Left upper extremity: 132/86 mm Hg
Right lower extremity: 143/82 mm Hg
Left lower extremity: 146/88 mm Hg

Ninety-fifth percentile and 99th percentile of BP for height, age, and gender for this patient were 130/83 mm Hg and 138/91 mm Hg, respectively.

## TEACHING POINTS

Because the patient in Clinical Vignette 39.1 was asymptomatic, he was instructed to return to the office for blood pressure checks two more times over the next month. His average blood pressure over all these readings was 136/78 mm Hg. He was diagnosed with stage 1 hypertension. Serum electrolytes, renal function, complete blood count, urinalysis, urine microalbumin, insulin, and renal ultrasound findings were normal. His fasting triglycerides were elevated, and an echocardiogram showed left ventricular hypertrophy (LVH). A dilated retinal examination by an ophthalmologist was normal. No underlying cause for his hypertension was discerned, and the diagnosis of essential hypertension was made. The presence of LVH suggests an increased risk for cardiovascular disease in the future and is an indication for pharmacologic therapy in addition to lifestyle modifications.

# REFERENCES

1. Chockalingam A, Campbell NR, Fodor JG. Worldwide epidemic of hypertension. Can J Cardiol. 2006;22:553–5.
2. Lim SS, Mokdad AH. Socioeconomic inequalities and infectious disease burden. Lancet. 2012;379:1080–1.
3. Go AS, Mozaffarian D, Roger VL, et al. Heart disease and stroke statistics—2013 update: A report from the American Heart Association. Circulation. 2013;127:e6–e245.
4. Bao W, Threefoot SA, Srinivasan SR, Berenson GS. Essential hypertension predicted by tracking of elevated blood pressure from childhood to adulthood: The Bogalusa Heart Study. Am J Hypertens. 1995;8:657–65.
5. Lauer RM, Clarke WR. Childhood risk factors for high adult blood pressure: The Muscatine Study. Pediatrics. 1989;84:633–41.
6. Berenson GS, Srinivasan SR, Bao W, et al. Association between multiple cardiovascular risk factors and atherosclerosis in children and young adults: The Bogalusa Heart Study. N Engl J Med. 1998;338:1650–6.
7. Zieske AW, Malcom GT, Strong JP. Natural history and risk factors of atherosclerosis in children and youth: The PDAY study. Pediatr Pathol Mol Med. 2002;21:213–37.
8. Kher KK. Hypertension. In: Kher KK, Makker SP, editors. Clinical Pediatric Nephrology. New York: McGraw-Hill; 1992. p. 323–76.
9. Acosta AA, Samuels JA, Portman RJ, Redwine KM. Prevalence of persistent prehypertension in adolescents. J Pediatr. 2012;160:757–61.
10. Antal M, Regoly-Merei A, Nagy K, et al. Representative study for the evaluation of age- and gender-specific anthropometric parameters and blood pressure in an adolescent Hungarian population. Ann Nutr Metab. 2004;48:307–13.
11. Genovesi S, Giussani M, Pieruzzi F, et al. Results of blood pressure screening in a population of school-aged children in the province of Milan: Role of overweight. J Hypertens. 2005;23:493–7.
12. Kardas P, Kufelnicka M, Herczynski D. Prevalence of arterial hypertension in children aged 9–14 years, residents of the city of Lodz. Kardiol Pol. 2005;62:211–6; discussion 6–7.
13. McNiece KL, Poffenbarger TS, Turner JL, et al. Prevalence of hypertension and pre-hypertension among adolescents. J Pediatr. 2007;150:640–4, 4e1.
14. Saleh EA, Mahfouz AA, Tayel KY, et al. Hypertension and its determinants among primary-school children in Kuwait: An epidemiological study. East Mediterr Health J. 2000;6:333–7.
15. Sorof JM, Lai D, Turner J, et al. Overweight, ethnicity, and the prevalence of hypertension in school-aged children. Pediatrics. 2004;113:475–82.
16. Portman RJ, McNiece KL, Swinford RD, et al. Pediatric hypertension: Diagnosis, evaluation, management, and treatment for the primary care physician. Curr Probl Pediatr Adolesc Health Care. 2005;35:262–94.
17. James PA, Oparil S, Carter BL, et al. 2014 Evidence-based guideline for the management of high blood pressure in adults: Report from the panel members appointed to the Eighth Joint National Committee (JNC 8). JAMA. 2014;311:507–20.
18. National High Blood Pressure Education Program Working Group on High Blood Pressure in Children and Adolescents. The Fourth Report on the Diagnosis, Evaluation, and Treatment of High Blood Pressure in Children and Adolescents. Bethesda, MD: National Heart Lung and Blood Institute; 2005.
19. Urbina E, Alpert B, Flynn J, et al. Ambulatory blood pressure monitoring in children and adolescents: Recommendations for standard assessment: A scientific statement from the American Heart Association Atherosclerosis, Hypertension, and Obesity in Youth Committee of the Council on Cardiovascular Disease in the Young and the Council for High Blood Pressure Research. Hypertension. 2008;52:433–51.
20. Julius S, Palatini P, Nesbitt SD. Tachycardia: An important determinant of coronary risk in hypertension. J Hypertens Suppl. 1998;16:S9–15.
21. Bauer JH, Brooks CS. Volume studies in men with mild to moderate hypertension. Am J Cardiol. 1979;44:1163–70.
22. London GM, Safar ME, Weiss YA, et al. Volume-dependent parameters in essential hypertension. Kidney Int. 1977;11:204–8.

23. He FJ, MacGregor GA. Salt, blood pressure and the renin-angiotensin system. J Renin Angiotensin Aldosterone Syst. 2003;4:11–6.

24. Weinberger MH. Sodium and blood pressure 2003. Curr Opin Cardiol. 2004;19:353–6.

25. Jones JE, Natarajan AR, Jose PA. Cardiovascular and autonomic influences on blood pressure. In: Portman RJ, Sorof JM, Ingelfinger JR, editors. Pediatric Hypertension. Totowa, NJ: Humana Press; 2004. p. 23.

26. Feig DI, Madero M, Jalal DI, et al. Uric acid and the origins of hypertension. J Pediatr. 2013;162:896–902.

27. Gruskin AB. The adolescent with essential hypertension. Am J Kidney Dis. 1985;6:86–90.

28. Johnson RJ, Segal MS, Srinivas T, et al. Essential hypertension, progressive renal disease, and uric acid: A pathogenetic link? J Am Soc Nephrol. 2005;16:1909–19.

29. Brunner H, Cockcroft JR, Deanfield J, et al. Endothelial function and dysfunction. Part II. Association with cardiovascular risk factors and diseases: A statement by the Working Group on Endothelins and Endothelial Factors of the European Society of Hypertension. J Hypertens. 2005;23:233–46.

30. Mourad A, Carney S, Gillies A, et al. Arm position and blood pressure: A risk factor for hypertension? J Hum Hypertens. 2003;17:389–95.

31. Netea RT, Lenders JW, Smits P, Thien T. Both body and arm position significantly influence blood pressure measurement. J Hum Hypertens. 2003;17:459–62.

32. Gillman MW, Cook NR. Blood pressure measurement in childhood epidemiological studies. Circulation. 1995;92:1049–57.

33. Jones DW, Appel LJ, Sheps SG, et al. Measuring blood pressure accurately: New and persistent challenges. JAMA. 2003;289:1027–30.

34. Bailey RH, Knaus VL, Bauer JH. Aneroid sphygmomanometers: An assessment of accuracy at a university hospital and clinics. Arch Intern Med. 1991;151:1409–12.

35. Canzanello VJ, Jensen PL, Schwartz GL. Are aneroid sphygmomanometers accurate in hospital and clinic settings? Arch Intern Med. 2001;161:729–31.

36. Ramsey M, 3rd. Blood pressure monitoring: Automated oscillometric devices. J Clin Monit. 1991;7:56–67.

37. Barker ME, Shiell AW, Law CM. Evaluation of the Dinamap 8100 and Omron M1 blood pressure monitors for use in children. Paediatr Perinat Epidemiol. 2000;14:179–86.

38. Park MK, Menard SW, Yuan C. Comparison of blood pressure in children from three ethnic groups. Am J Cardiol. 2001;87:1305–8.

39. Deal JE, Barratt TM, Dillon MJ. Management of hypertensive emergencies. Arch Dis Child. 1992;67:1089–92.

40. Daniels SR, Loggie JM, McEnery PT, Towbin RB. Clinical spectrum of intrinsic renovascular hypertension in children. Pediatrics. 1987;80:698–704.

41. Watson AR, Balfe JW, Hardy BE. Renovascular hypertension in childhood: A changing perspective in management. J Pediatr. 1985;106:366–72.

42. Harms MM, Rotteveel JJ, Kar NC, Gabreels FJ. Recurrent alternating facial paralysis and malignant hypertension. Neuropediatrics. 2000;31:318–20.

43. Browning AC, Mengher LS, Gregson RM, Amoaku WM. Visual outcome of malignant hypertension in young people. Arch Dis Child. 2001;85:401–3.

44. Strandgaard S, Olesen J, Skinhoj E, Lassen NA. Autoregulation of brain circulation in severe arterial hypertension. Br Med J. 1973;1:507–10.

45. Schwartz RB, Mulkern RV, Gudbjartsson H, Jolesz F. Diffusion-weighted MR imaging in hypertensive encephalopathy: Clues to pathogenesis. AJNR Am J Neuroradiol. 1998;19:859–62.

46. Tuor UI. Acute hypertension and sympathetic stimulation: Local heterogeneous changes in cerebral blood flow. Am J Physiol. 1992;263:H511–8.

47. Uhari M, Saukkonen AL, Koskimies O. Central nervous system involvement in severe arterial hypertension of childhood. Eur J Pediatr. 1979;132:141–6.

48. Trompeter RS, Smith RL, Hoare RD, et al. Neurological complications of arterial hypertension. Arch Dis Child. 1982;57:913–7.

49. Adelman RD, Coppo R, Dillon MJ. The emergency management of severe hypertension. Pediatr Nephrol. 2000;14:422–7.

50. Hulse JA, Taylor DS, Dillon MJ. Blindness and paraplegia in severe childhood hypertension. Lancet. 1979;2:553–6.

51. Isles CG. Hypertensive emergencies: Malignant hypertension and hypertensive encephalopathy. In: Swales JD, editor. Textbook of Hypertension. Oxford: Blackwell Scientific; 1994. p. 1233.

52. Ledingham JG, Rajagopalan B. Cerebral complications in the treatment of accelerated hypertension. Q J Med. 1979;48:25–41.

53. Taylor D, Ramsay J, Day S, Dillon M. Infarction of the optic nerve head in children with accelerated hypertension. Br J Ophthalmol. 1981;65:153–60.

54. Flynn JT, Mitsnefes M, Pierce C, et al. Blood pressure in children with chronic kidney disease: A report from the Chronic Kidney Disease in Children study. Hypertension. 2008;52:631–7.

55. Tullus K. Secondary forms of hypertension. In: Flynn JT, Ingelfinger JR, Portman RJ, editors. Pediatric Hypertension, 2nd ed. New York: Humana Press; 2011.

56. Martinez-Maldonado M. Hypertension in end-stage renal disease. Kidney Int Suppl. 1998;68:S67–72.

57. Deal JE, Snell MF, Barratt TM, Dillon MJ. Renovascular disease in childhood. J Pediatr. 1992;121:378–84.

58. Loirat C, Pillion G, Blum C. Hypertension in children: Present data and problems. Adv Nephrol. 1982;11:65.

59. Fossali E, Signorini E, Intermite RC, et al. Renovascular disease and hypertension in children with neurofibromatosis. Pediatr Nephrol. 2000;14:806–10.

60. Greene JF, Jr, Fitzwater JE, Burgess J. Arterial lesions associated with neurofibromatosis. Am J Clin Pathol. 1974;62:481–7.

61. Halpern M, Currarino G. Vascular lesions causing hypertension in neurofibromatosis. N Engl J Med. 1965;273:248.

62. Leumann EP. Blood pressure and hypertension in childhood and adolescence. Ergeb Inn Med Kinderheilkd. 1979;43:109–83.

63. Mena E, Bookstein JJ, Holt JF, Fry WJ. Neurofibromatosis and renovascular hypertension in children. Am J Roentgenol Radium Ther Nucl Med. 1973;118:39–45.

64. Loughridge LW. Renal abnormalities in the Marfan syndrome. Q J Med. 1959;28:531–44.

65. Wiggelinkhuizen J, Cremin BJ. Takayasu arteritis and renovascular hypertension in childhood. Pediatrics. 1978;62:209–17.

66. Proesmans W, Van Damme B, Marchal G, et al. Klippel-Trenaunay syndrome with systemic hypertension and chronic renal failure. Ann Pediatr (Paris). 1982;29:671 [in French].

67. Londe S. Causes of hypertension in the young. Pediatr Clin North Am. 1978;25:55–65.

68. O'Neill JA, Jr, Berkowitz H, Fellows KJ, Harmon CM. Midaortic syndrome and hypertension in childhood. J Pediatr Surg. 1995;30:164–71; discussion 71–2.

69. Sumboonnananda A, Robinson BL, Gedroyc WM, et al. Middle aortic syndrome: Clinical and radiological findings. Arch Dis Child. 1992;67:501–5.

70. Wiltse HE, Goldbloom RB, Antia AU, et al. Infantile hypercalcemia syndrome in twins. N Engl J Med. 1966;275:1157–60.

71. Stewart PM. Mineralocorticoid hypertension. Lancet. 1999;353:1341–7.

72. Rossi GP, Sacchetto A, Chiesura-Corona M, et al. Identification of the etiology of primary aldosteronism with adrenal vein sampling in patients with equivocal computed tomography and magnetic resonance findings: Results in 104 consecutive cases. J Clin Endocrinol Metab. 2001;86:1083–90.

73. Lack E, Travis W, Oertel J. Adrenal cortical nodules, hyperplasia, and hyperfunction. In: Lack EE, editor. Pathology of the Adrenal Glands. New York: Churchill Livingstone; 1990. p. 75.

74. Lifton RP, Dluhy RG, Powers M, et al. Hereditary hypertension caused by chimaeric gene duplications and ectopic expression of aldosterone synthase. Nat Genet. 1992;2:66–74.

75. Dluhy RG. Screening for genetic causes of hypertension. Curr Hypertens Rep. 2002;4:439–44.

76. New MI, Seaman MP. Secretion rates of cortisol and aldosterone precursors in various forms of congenital adrenal hyperplasia. J Clin Endocrinol Metab. 1970;30:361–71.

77. New MI, Wilson RC. Steroid disorders in children: Congenital adrenal hyperplasia and apparent mineralocorticoid excess. Proc Natl Acad Sci U S A. 1999;96:12790–7.

78. Ulick S. Cortisol as mineralocorticoid. J Clin Endocrinol Metab. 1996;81:1307–8.

79. Whitworth JA, Mangos GJ, Kelly JJ. Cushing, cortisol, and cardiovascular disease. Hypertension. 2000;36:912–6.

80. Dave-Sharma S, Wilson RC, Harbison MD, et al. Examination of genotype and phenotype relationships in 14 patients with apparent mineralocorticoid excess. J Clin Endocrinol Metab. 1998;83:2244–54.

81. Cooper M, Stewart PM. The syndrome of apparent mineralocorticoid excess. QJM. 1998;91:453–5.

82. Hansson JH, Nelson-Williams C, Suzuki H, et al. Hypertension caused by a truncated epithelial sodium channel gamma subunit: Genetic heterogeneity of Liddle syndrome. Nat Genet. 1995;11:76–82.

83. Shimkets RA, Warnock DG, Bositis CM, et al. Liddle's syndrome: Heritable human hypertension caused by mutations in the beta subunit of the epithelial sodium channel. Cell. 1994;79:407–14.

84. Yiu VW, Dluhy RP, Lifton RP, Guay-Woodford LM. Low peripheral plasma renin activity as a critical marker in pediatric hypertension. Pediatr Nephrol. 1997;11:343–6.

85. Mansfield TA, Simon DB, Farfel Z, et al. Multilocus linkage of familial hyperkalaemia and hypertension, pseudohypoaldosteronism type II, to chromosomes 1q31-42 and 17p11-q21. Nat Genet. 1997;16:202–5.

86. Wilson FH, Disse-Nicodeme S, Choate KA, et al. Human hypertension caused by mutations in WNK kinases. Science. 2001;293:1107–12.

87. Whalen RK, Althausen AF, Daniels GH. Extra-adrenal pheochromocytoma. J Urol. 1992;147:1–10.

88. Deal JE, Sever PS, Barratt TM, Dillon MJ. Phaeochromocytoma: Investigation and management of 10 cases. Arch Dis Child. 1990;65:269–74.

89. Stackpole RH, Melicow MM, Uson AC. Pheochromocytoma in children: Report of 9 case and review of the first 100 published cases with follow-up studies. J Pediatr. 1963;63:314–30.

90. Lenders JW, Pacak K, Eisenhofer G. New advances in the biochemical diagnosis of pheochromocytoma: Moving beyond catecholamines. Ann N Y Acad Sci. 2002;970:29–40.

91. Shapiro B, Copp JE, Sisson JC, et al. Iodine-131 metaiodobenzylguanidine for the locating of suspected pheochromocytoma: Experience in 400 cases. J Nucl Med. 1985;26:576–85.

92. Shulkin BL, Shapiro B, Francis IR, et al. Primary extra-adrenal pheochromocytoma: Positive I-123 MIBG imaging with negative I-131 MIBG imaging. Clin Nucl Med. 1986;11:851–4.

93. van der Harst E, de Herder WW, Bruining HA, et al. [(123)I]metaiodobenzylguanidine and [(111)In]octreotide uptake in begnign and malignant pheochromocytomas. J Clin Endocrinol Metab. 2001;86:685–93.

94. Chapman RC, Kemp VE, Taliaferro I. Pheochromocytoma associated with multiple neurofibromatosis and intracranial hemangioma. Am J Med. 1959;26:883–90.

95. Glushien AS, Mansuy MM, Littman DS. Pheochromocytoma: Its relationship to the neurocutaneous syndromes. Am J Med. 1953;14:318–27.

96. Sever PS, Roberts JC, Snell ME. Phaeochromocytoma. Clin Endocrinol Metab. 1980;9:543–68.

97. Keiser HR, Beaven MA, Doppman J, et al. Sipple's syndrome: Medullary thyroid carcinoma, pheochromocytoma, and parathyroid disease. Studies in a large family. NIH conference. Ann Intern Med. 1973;78:561–79.

98. Lips KJ, Van der Sluys Veer J, Struyvenberg A, et al. Bilateral occurrence of pheochromocytoma in patients with the multiple endocrine neoplasia syndrome type 2A (Sipple's syndrome). Am J Med. 1981;70:1051–60.

99. Prys-Roberts C. Phaeochromocytoma: Recent progress in its management. Br J Anaesth. 2000;85:44-57.

100. Ulchaker JC, Goldfarb DA, Bravo EL, Novick AC. Successful outcomes in pheochromocytoma surgery in the modern era. J Urol. 1999;161:764–7.

101. Sorof J, Daniels S. Obesity hypertension in children: A problem of epidemic proportions. Hypertension. 2002;40:441–7.

102. Sacks FM, Svetkey LP, Vollmer WM, et al. Effects on blood pressure of reduced dietary sodium and the Dietary Approaches to Stop Hypertension (DASH) diet: DASH-Sodium Collaborative Research Group. N Engl J Med. 2001;344:3–10.

103. Vollmer WM, Sacks FM, Ard J, et al. Effects of diet and sodium intake on blood pressure: Subgroup analysis of the DASH-sodium trial. Ann Intern Med. 2001;135:1019–28.

104. Whelton SP, Chin A, Xin X, He J. Effect of aerobic exercise on blood pressure: A meta-analysis of randomized, controlled trials. Ann Intern Med. 2002;136:493–503.

105. Simons-Morton DG, Hunsberger SA, Van Horn L, et al. Nutrient intake and blood pressure in the Dietary Intervention Study in Children. Hypertension. 1997;29:930–6.

106. Simons-Morton DG, Obarzanek E. Diet and blood pressure in children and adolescents. Pediatr Nephrol. 1997;11:244–9.

107. Cornoni-Huntley J, LaCroix AZ, Havlik RJ. Race and sex differentials in the impact of hypertension in the United States: The National Health and Nutrition Examination Survey I Epidemiologic Follow-up Study. Arch Intern Med. 1989;149:780–8.

108. Eisner GM. Hypertension: Racial differences. Am J Kidney Dis. 1990;16:35–40.

109. Treiber FA, Musante L, Strong WB, Levy M. Racial differences in young children's blood pressure: Responses to dynamic exercise. Am J Dis Child. 1989;143:720–3.

110. Southard DR, Coates TJ, Kolodner K, et al. Relationship between mood and blood pressure in the natural environment: An adolescent population. Health Psychol. 1986;5:469–80.

111. Blowey DL, Duda PJ, Stokes P, Hall M. Incidence and treatment of hypertension in the neonatal intensive care unit. J Am Soc Hypertens. 2011;5:478–83.

112. Seliem WA, Falk MC, Shadbolt B, Kent AL. Antenatal and postnatal risk factors for neonatal hypertension and infant follow-up. Pediatr Nephrol. 2007;22:2081–7.

113. Singh HP, Hurley RM, Myers TF. Neonatal hypertension: Incidence and risk factors. Am J Hypertens. 1992;5:51–5.

114. Abman SH, Warady BA, Lum GM, Koops BL. Systemic hypertension in infants with bronchopulmonary dysplasia. J Pediatr. 1984;104:928–31.

115. Becker JA, Short BL, Martin GR. Cardiovascular complications adversely affect survival during extracorporeal membrane oxygenation. Crit Care Med. 1998;26:1582–6.

116. Boedy RF, Goldberg AK, Howell CG, Jr, et al. Incidence of hypertension in infants on extracorporeal membrane oxygenation. J Pediatr Surg. 1990;25:258–61.

117. Friedman AL, Hustead VA. Hypertension in babies following discharge from a neonatal intensive care unit: A 3-year follow-up. Pediatr Nephrol. 1987;1:30–4.

118. Plouin PF, Chatellier G, Rougeot MA, et al P. Plasma renin activity in phaeochromocytoma: Effects of beta-blockade and converting enzyme inhibition. J Hypertens. 1988;6:579–85.

119. Kupferman JC, Aronson Friedman L, Cox C, et al. BP control and left ventricular hypertrophy regression in children with CKD. J Am Soc Nephrol. 2014;25:167–74.

120. Litwin M, Niemirska A, Sladowska-Kozlowska J, et al. Regression of target organ damage in children and adolescents with primary hypertension. Pediatr Nephrol. 2010;25:2489–99.

121. Matteucci MC, Chinali M, Rinelli G, et al. Change in cardiac geometry and function in CKD children during strict BP control: A randomized study. Clin J Am Soc Nephrol. 2013;8:203–10.

122. Binkert CA, Debatin JF, Schneider E, et al. Can MR measurement of renal artery flow and renal volume predict the outcome of percutaneous transluminal renal angioplasty? Cardiovasc Intervent Radiol. 2001;24:233–9.

123. Debatin JF, Spritzer CE, Grist TM, et al. Imaging of the renal arteries: Value of MR angiography. AJR Am J Roentgenol. 1991;157:981–90.

124. Marcos HB, Choyke PL. Magnetic resonance angiography of the kidney. Semin Nephrol. 2000;20:450–5.

125. Shahdadpuri J, Frank R, Gauthier BG, et al. Yield of renal arteriography in the evaluation of pediatric hypertension. Pediatr Nephrol. 2000;14:816–9.

126. Chobanian AV, Bakris GL, Black HR, et al. Seventh report of the Joint National Committee on Prevention, Detection, Evaluation, and Treatment of High Blood Pressure. Hypertension. 2003;42:1206–52.

127. World Health Organization, editor. The World Health Report 2002: Reducing Risks, Promoting Healthy Life. Geneva: World Health Organization; 2002.

128. US Renal Data System (USRDS) 2013 Annual Data Report: Atlas of Chronic Kidney Disease and End-Stage Renal Disease in the United States. Bethesda, MD: National Institutes of Health, National Institute of Diabetes and Digestive and Kidney Diseases; 2013.

129. Belsha CW, Wells TG, McNiece KL, et al. Influence of diurnal blood pressure variations on target organ abnormalities in adolescents with mild essential hypertension. Am J Hypertens. 1998;11:410–7.

130. Brady TM, Fivush B, Flynn JT, Parekh R. Ability of blood pressure to predict left ventricular hypertrophy in children with primary hypertension. J Pediatr. 2008;152:73–8, 8 e1.

131. Hanevold C, Waller J, Daniels S, et al. The effects of obesity, gender, and ethnic group on left ventricular hypertrophy and geometry in hypertensive children: A collaborative study of the International Pediatric Hypertension Association. Pediatrics. 2004;113:328–33.

132. McNiece KL, Gupta-Malhotra M, Samuels J, et al. Left ventricular hypertrophy in hypertensive adolescents: Analysis of risk by 2004 National High Blood Pressure Education Program Working Group staging criteria. Hypertension. 2007;50:392–5.

133. Sorof JM, Alexandrov AV, Cardwell G, Portman RJ. Carotid artery intimal-medial thickness and left ventricular hypertrophy in children with elevated blood pressure. Pediatrics. 2003;111:61–6.

134. Khoury PR, Mitsnefes M, Daniels SR, Kimball TR. Age-specific reference intervals for indexed left ventricular mass in children. J Am Soc Echocardiogr. 2009;22:709–14.

135. Levy D, Garrison RJ, Savage DD, et al. Prognostic implications of echocardiographically determined left ventricular mass in the Framingham Heart Study. N Engl J Med. 1990;322:1561–6.

136. Messerli FH, Sundgaard-Riise K, Reisin ED, et al. Dimorphic cardiac adaptation to obesity and arterial hypertension. Ann Intern Med. 1983;99:757–61.

137. Snider AR, Gidding SS, Rocchini AP, et al. Doppler evaluation of left ventricular diastolic filling in children with systemic hypertension. Am J Cardiol. 1985;56:921–6.

138. Inou T, Lamberth WC, Jr, Koyanagi S, et al. Relative importance of hypertension after coronary occlusion in chronic hypertensive dogs with LVH. Am J Physiol. 1987;253:H1148–58.

139. Zehender M, Meinertz T, Hohnloser S, et al. Prevalence of circadian variations and spontaneous variability of cardiac disorders and ECG changes suggestive of myocardial ischemia in systemic arterial hypertension. Circulation. 1992;85:1808–15.

140. Agu NC, McNiece Redwine K, Bell C, et al. Detection of early diastolic alterations by tissue Doppler imaging in untreated childhood-onset essential hypertension. J Am Soc Hypertens. 2014;8:303–11.

141. Daniels SR, Witt SA, Glascock B, et al. Left atrial size in children with hypertension: The influence of obesity, blood pressure, and left ventricular mass. J Pediatr. 2002;141:186–90.

142. Heiss G, Sharrett AR, Barnes R, et al. Carotid atherosclerosis measured by B-mode ultrasound in populations: Associations with cardiovascular risk factors in the ARIC study. Am J Epidemiol. 1991;134:250–6.

143. Lande MB, Carson NL, Roy J, Meagher CC. Effects of childhood primary hypertension on carotid intima media thickness: A matched controlled study. Hypertension. 2006;48:40–4.

144. Urbina EM, Khoury PR, McCoy C, et al. Cardiac and vascular consequences of pre-hypertension in youth. J Clin Hypertens (Greenwich). 2011;13:332–42.

145. Skalina ME, Annable WL, Kliegman RM, Fanaroff AA. Hypertensive retinopathy in the newborn infant. J Pediatr. 1983;103:781–6.

146. Williams KM, Shah AN, Morrison D, Sinha MD. Hypertensive retinopathy in severely hypertensive children: Demographic, clinical, and ophthalmoscopic findings from a 30-year British cohort. J Pediatr Ophthalmol Strabismus. 2013;50:222–8.

147. Garg JP, Bakris GL. Microalbuminuria: Marker of vascular dysfunction, risk factor for cardiovascular disease. Vasc Med. 2002;7:35–43.

148. Gerstein HC, Mann JF, Yi Q, et al. Albuminuria and risk of cardiovascular events, death, and heart failure in diabetic and nondiabetic individuals. JAMA. 2001;286:421–6.

149. Jensen JS, Feldt-Rasmussen B, Strandgaard S, et al. Arterial hypertension, microalbuminuria, and risk of ischemic heart disease. Hypertension. 2000;35:898–903.

150. Radhakishun NN, van Vliet M, von Rosenstiel IA, et al. Limited value of routine microalbuminuria assessment in multi-ethnic obese children. Pediatr Nephrol. 2013;28:1145–9.

## REVIEW QUESTIONS

1. According to current guidelines, the initial evaluation of all children with confirmed hypertension should include all of the following *except:*
   a. Renal ultrasound
   b. Electrocardiogram
   c. Urinalysis
   d. Complete history and physical
   e. Echocardiogram

2. All of the following low-renin hypertensive disorders are associated with hypokalemia *except:*
   a. Liddle syndrome
   b. Adrenal hyperplasia
   c. Apparent mineralocorticoid excess
   d. Glucocorticoid-remediable aldosteronism
   e. Gordon syndrome

3. Renin secretion is increased by all of the following *except:*
   a. Decreased intravascular volume
   b. Activation of the sympathetic nervous system
   c. Increased aldosterone secretion
   d. Hypotension
   e. Renal artery stenosis

4. Oscillometric blood pressure monitors directly measure:
   a. Pulse pressure
   b. Systolic blood pressure
   c. Diastolic blood pressure
   d. Mean arterial pressure
   e. Diurnal blood pressure variation

5. A previously healthy 14-year-old male patient is seen for a routine school physical examination. His blood pressure at this visit is 132/70 (95th percentile: 130/83). He is asymptomatic, and the rest of his physical examination is normal. The *next* step in his evaluation and management should be:
   a. Urinalysis
   b. Renal ultrasound.
   c. Repeat blood pressure in 1 to 2 weeks.
   d. Reassurance that his blood pressure is normal
   e. Initiation of antihypertensive medication

6. All of the following are associated with a higher risk for hypertension in the neonatal period *except:*
   a. Umbilical artery catheterization
   b. Large for gestational age
   c. Bronchopulmonary dysplasia
   d. Patent ductus arteriosus
   e. Maternal drug use

7. CT imaging of a child with hypertensive encephalopathy will *most commonly* show changes in the:
   a. Parieto-occipital white matter
   b. Hypothalamus
   c. Pituitary gland
   d. Prefrontal cortex
   e. Optic nerve

8. All of the following may raise the blood pressure of a child with chronic hypertension who is being treated for an acute asthma exacerbation and allergy symptoms *except:*
   a. Prednisone
   b. Albuterol
   c. Phenylephrine
   d. Ibuprofen
   e. Cetirizine

9. Normal blood pressure levels in children are based on the child's:
   a. Age
   b. Gender
   c. Body mass index
   d. Height
   e. a, b, and d

10. Children whose BP is greater than the 90th percentile (or greater than 120/80 mm Hg) but less than the 95th percentile should be classified as prehypertensive. However, these children should be treated as if they were hypertensive if they have any of the following conditions *except:*
    a. Left ventricular hypertrophy
    b. Diabetes mellitus
    c. Renal dysplasia
    d. Short stature
    e. Retinopathy

## ANSWER KEY

1. b
2. e
3. c
4. d
5. c
6. b
7. a
8. e
9. e
10. d

# 40

# Management of hypertension

JOSEPH T. FLYNN

Management of hypertension in adults is guided by evidence derived from the results of large-scale clinical trials that have examined the Beffects of specific antihypertensive agents on cardiovascular morbidity and mortality.[1] In contrast, the management of hypertensive children and adolescents is still largely empiric. This is mainly because of the lack of long-term outcome data regarding the efficacy and safety of nonpharmacologic and pharmacologic approaches to treatment of hypertension in children and adolescents.[2]

Even though a rigorous evidence base is missing, the question of how to manage a child or teen with hypertension is one faced by pediatric nephrologists and other practitioners every day. The purpose of this chapter is to update the reader on current approaches to the treatment of hypertensive children and adolescents, including the special cases of hypertensive neonates, hypertensive urgencies and emergencies, pheochromocytomas, and renal artery stenosis.

## MANAGEMENT APPROACH BY STAGE OF HYPERTENSION

Staging of hypertension is a concept well known to those who care for hypertensive adults,[3] but has only been applied to the management of hypertensive children and adolescents since publication of the 2004 "Fourth Report" from the National High Blood Pressure Education Program.[4] It is now recommended that, as in adults, elevated blood pressure in children and adolescents be staged to help guide the evaluation and management of pediatric patients with hypertension. Table 40.1 gives the pediatric staging criteria and the recommended management approaches for each stage.

As can be seen in Table 40.1, intervention is recommended even for children or adolescents with blood pressures that fall into the prehypertensive range. Such children should be counseled regarding lifestyle changes (weight loss, exercise, and dietary modification as appropriate) and should be seen within 6 months for a repeat blood pressure check and assessment of how well they are adhering to the recommended measures. At the other end of the scale, children or adolescents with stage 2 hypertension should have their blood pressure checked and a workup initiated within a week and are candidates for immediate institution of pharmacologic therapy. This staging system should be viewed as a framework within which to apply the specific approaches discussed in subsequent sections of this chapter.

### KEY POINT

A patient's blood pressure elevation should be staged according to Fourth Report criteria to help guide evaluation and management.

## NONPHARMACOLOGIC MANAGEMENT

Nonpharmacologic interventions have long been emphasized in consensus recommendations as the starting point for treatment of hypertension in children and adolescents. This is reflected in the recently issued "Integrated Guidelines for Cardiovascular Health and Risk Reduction in Children and Adolescents" from the National Heart, Lung and Blood Institute,[5] which emphasizes the potential benefits of nonpharmacologic measures in not only reducing blood

TABLE 40.1 Classification of hypertension in children and adolescents, with measurement frequency and therapy recommendations

| Stage | SBP or DBP percentile* | Frequency of BP measurement | Therapeutic lifestyle changes | Pharmacologic therapy |
|---|---|---|---|---|
| Normal | <90th | Recheck at next scheduled physical examination | Encourage healthy diet, sleep, and physical activity | — |
| Prehypertension | 90th to < 95th or if BP exceeds 120/80 mm Hg even if below 90th percentile up to < 95th percentile† | Recheck in 6 mo | Weight management counseling if overweight, introduce physical activity and diet management§ | None unless compelling indications such as CKD, diabetes mellitus, heart failure, LVH |
| Stage 1 hypertension | 95th percentile to the 99th percentile plus 5 mm Hg | Recheck in 1–2 wk or sooner if the patient is symptomatic; if persistently elevated on two additional occasions, evaluate or refer to source of care within 1 mo | Weight management counseling if overweight, introduce physical activity and diet management§ | Initiate therapy based on indications in Table 40.2 or if compelling indications, as above |
| Stage 2 hypertension | >99th percentile plus 5 mm Hg | Evaluate or refer to source of care within 1 wk or immediately if the patient is symptomatic | Weight management counseling if overweight, introduce physical activity and diet management§ | Initiate therapy‡ |

Source: The fourth report on the diagnosis, evaluation, and treatment of high blood pressure in children and adolescents. National Institutes of Health National Heart, Lung, and Blood Institute, Bethesda, MD: NIH; 2004, revised 2005. p. 14. Reproduced

Abbreviations: BP, blood pressure; CKD, chronic kidney disease; DBP, diastolic blood pressure; LVH, left ventricular hypertrophy; SBP, systolic blood pressure.

* For sex, age, and height measured on at least three separate occasions; if systolic and diastolic categories are different, categorize by the higher value.
† This occurs typically at 12 years old for SBP and at 16 years old for DBP.
‡ More than one drug may be required.
§ Parents and children trying to modify the eating plan to the DASH eating plan could benefit from consultation with a pediatric dietitian to get them started.

pressure in children with prehypertension or hypertension but also in improving the overall cardiovascular health in children with one or more risk factors for cardiovascular disease.

## Weight loss and exercise

Although the magnitude of change in blood pressure may be modest, weight loss, aerobic exercise, and dietary modifications have been shown to successfully reduce blood pressure in children and adolescents. Tracking studies provide the first line of evidence supporting the concept that weight reduction has the potential to control blood pressure in children. Blood pressure clearly tracks from childhood through adolescence and into adulthood,[6] and the rise in blood pressure in these studies is typically associated with an increase in body mass index (BMI).[7] Because of the strong correlation between weight and blood pressure, excessive weight gain is likely to be associated with elevated blood pressure over time. This can be seen in data linking increased blood pressure in American children over the past decade with the

increase in childhood obesity.[8] It then follows that maintenance of normal weight in childhood should prevent the development of hypertension in adulthood.

Several studies have demonstrated that weight loss in obese adolescents lowers blood pressure.[9,10] Weight loss not only decreases blood pressure but also improves other cardiovascular risk factors such as dyslipidemia and insulin resistance.[11,12] In studies in which a reduction in BMI of approximately 10% was achieved, short-term reductions in blood pressure were in the range of 8 to 12 mm Hg. Unfortunately, weight loss is notoriously difficult and usually unsuccessful, especially in the primary care setting.[13] However, identifying a medical complication of obesity such as hypertension can perhaps provide the necessary motivation for patients and families to make appropriate lifestyle changes. This need for family-based intervention was recognized by the authors of the Fourth Report[4] and has been repeated by others.

With respect to exercise, sustained training over 3 to 6 months has been shown to result in a reduction of 6 to 12 mm Hg for systolic blood pressure and 3 to 5 mm Hg for diastolic blood pressure.[14] However, cessation of regular exercise is generally promptly followed by a rise in blood pressure to pre-exercise levels. Aerobic exercise activities such as running, walking, or cycling are usually preferred to static forms of exercise in the management of hypertension.[15] Many children already may be participating in one or more appropriate activities and may need only to increase the frequency, intensity, or both of these activities (usually to at least 40 to 60 minutes per session, 4 or 5 times per week) to produce a reduction in their blood pressure.

It is important to emphasize that hypertension is not considered a contraindication to participation in competitive sports, so long as the child's blood pressure is "controlled."[16] Anecdotal experience suggests that treatment of hypertension in the competitive teen athlete may actually improve performance. However, it may be appropriate to restrict participation while the child's or adolescent's hypertension is being evaluated. Once a diagnosis has been made and treatment initiated, sports participation can be allowed. Indeed, the potential long-term benefits in terms of blood pressure reduction and weight control probably outweigh any possible risks of participation.

## Diet

The role of dietary changes in the management of hypertension has received a great deal of attention, most of which has focused on sodium. Although it is controversial whether excessive sodium intake may cause hypertension,[17] once hypertension has been established, "salt sensitivity" becomes more common and reduction in sodium intake is likely to be of benefit.[17–19] Other nutrients that have been examined in patients with hypertension include potassium and calcium, both of which have been shown to have antihypertensive effects.[19,20] Therefore, a diet low in sodium and enriched in potassium and calcium may be more effective in reducing blood pressure than a diet that restricts sodium only. An example of such a diet is the DASH diet (Dietary Approaches to Stop Hypertension), which has been shown to have an antihypertensive effect in adults with hypertension, even in those receiving antihypertensive medication.[21] The DASH diet was studied in a group of hypertensive adolescents, and was found to successfully lower systolic blood pressure when combined with counseling from a pediatric dietitian.[22] The DASH diet also incorporates measures designed to reduce dietary fat intake, an important strategy given the frequent presence of both hypertension and

elevated lipids in children and adolescents and the imperative to begin prevention of adult cardiovascular disease at as an early an age as possible.[5,11,23]

## PHARMACOLOGIC MANAGEMENT

### Historical perspective

The number of antihypertensive medications that have been systematically studied in children has increased markedly over the past two decades as a result of financial incentives provided to the pharmaceutical industry under the auspices of the 1997 *Food and Drug Modernization Act* (FDAMA) and successive legislation.[24] Thus, although the 2000 *Physicians' Desk Reference* contained pediatric dosing information approved by the U.S. Food and Drug Administration (FDA) for a minority of antihypertensive medications commonly used in children,[25] numerous antihypertensive medications are available now that have FDA-approved pediatric labeling. Although some antihypertensive medications continue to be used off label in children,[24] today's clinician should be able to prescribe agents with evidence-based dosing recommendations for most hypertensive youth.

### Indications for pharmacotherapy

Experience in adults indicates that although blood pressure in some hypertensive patients may decline without treatment, in most it will likely persist and even progress over time.[26] This implies that once a hypertensive patient has started medication, lifetime treatment is likely necessary. This is readily accepted for adults given the known long-term adverse consequences of untreated or undertreated hypertension. However, because the long-term consequences of untreated hypertension in an asymptomatic, otherwise healthy child or adolescent remain unknown,[2] the decision to prescribe antihypertensive medications in a child or adolescent should not be made lightly. Some have even questioned whether antihypertensive medications should be prescribed for children and adolescents at all.[27] Therefore, a clear-cut indication for initiating pharmacotherapy should be established before commencing such treatment in children and adolescents.

Indications for use of antihypertensive medications in children and adolescents are listed in Table 40.2. Other indications for use of antihypertensive medications based on the premise of reducing future risk for developing cardiovascular disease or end-stage renal disease also have been proposed. For example, the presence of multiple cardiovascular risk factors (elevated blood pressure, hyperlipidemia, tobacco use, etc.) increases cardiovascular risk in an exponential rather than additive fashion.[23,28] Thus, antihypertensive therapy might be initiated if the hypertensive child or adolescent is known to have dyslipidemia or impaired glucose tolerance. Similarly, elevated nocturnal blood pressure, blunted nocturnal dipping on ambulatory blood pressure monitoring, or both increase the likelihood of developing hypertensive target-organ damage and other adverse cardiovascular outcomes,[29,30] so nocturnal hypertension also might be considered by some as a reasonable indication for pharmacologic therapy.

## Choice of antihypertensive agent

Recommendations for choice of antihypertensive medications in adults are based on evidence from large-scale studies of hypertension treatment.[1] Many of these studies have compared the effects of different classes of antihypertensive agents on cardiovascular morbidity and mortality. Fortunately, traditional "hard" cardiovascular end points such as myocardial infarction are exceedingly rare in the pediatric age group, making it unlikely that similar studies will ever be conducted in children. Given this, the choice of initial antihypertensive agent for use in children remains empiric. Consideration for selection of antihypertensive medications has been summarized and includes the underlying cause of hypertension and the presence or absence of concurrent medical conditions.[31]

Diuretics and β-adrenergic blockers, which were recommended as initial therapy in the First and Second Task Force reports,[32,33] have a long track record of safety and efficacy in hypertensive children and are still appropriate for pediatric use, although they are now mostly used as second-line

Table 40.2 Indications for antihypertensive drug therapy in children

- Stage 2 hypertension
- Symptomatic hypertension
- Secondary hypertension
- Hypertensive target-organ damage
- Diabetes (types 1 and 2)
- Persistent hypertension despite nonpharmacologic measures

agents. Similarly, newer classes of agents, including angiotensin-converting enzyme inhibitors (ACEIs), calcium channel blockers, and angiotensin receptor blockers (ARBs), have now been shown to be safe and well tolerated in hypertensive children in industry-sponsored trials and may be prescribed if indicated.[31] As noted in a survey of North American pediatric nephrologists, these newer agents, particularly calcium channel blockers and ACE inhibitors, have become the most widely used initial agents in the pediatric age group.[34]

## KEY POINT

All classes of antihypertensive agents may be considered for use in hypertensive children and adolescents when medications are indicated.

A notable point to make here is the importance of using ACEIs or ARBs in children with hypertensive chronic kidney disease (CKD). These classes of agents have been shown to result in better BP control than use of other drugs[35] and have the potential to reduce the rate of progression of CKD, especially if used in a regimen that includes lower blood pressure targets.[36] For these reasons, the most recent Kidney Disease Improving Global Outcomes (KDIGO) recommendations for treatment of hypertension in nondialysis CKD state that "We suggest that an ARB or ACE-I be used in children with ND [nondialysis] CKD in whom treatment with BP-lowering drugs is indicated."[37]

## Approach to prescribing

As illustrated in Figure 40.1, antihypertensive drugs in children and adolescents are generally prescribed in a stepped-care manner. The patient is started on the lowest recommended dose of the initial agent, and the dose is increased until the highest recommended dose is reached or the child experiences adverse effects from the medication. At this point a second drug from a different class should be added, until the desired goal blood pressure is reached. Many antihypertensive drugs now have specific FDA-approved pediatric labeling, so generalists should restrict their choices to those agents. Recommended doses for selected antihypertensive agents for use in hypertensive children and adolescents are given in Table 40.3.

Our usual approach is to begin with a long-acting calcium channel blocker or ACEI and then add either a diuretic or β-blocker as the second agent. Many children and adolescents with "uncomplicated" primary hypertension may require two or more drugs to achieve target blood pressure. Children with secondary hypertension, particularly those with renal disease, almost always require multidrug regimens to achieve adequate blood pressure control. Combination antihypertensive preparations are widely available and offer advantages that may improve adherence

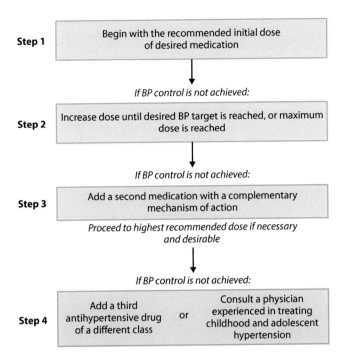

**Step 1** — Begin with the recommended initial dose of desired medication

*If BP control is not achieved:*

**Step 2** — Increase dose until desired BP target is reached, or maximum dose is reached

*If BP control is not achieved:*

**Step 3** — Add a second medication with a complementary mechanism of action

*Proceed to highest recommended dose if necessary and desirable*

*If BP control is not achieved:*

**Step 4** — Add a third antihypertensive drug of a different class    or    Consult a physician experienced in treating childhood and adolescent hypertension

Figure 40.1 Stepped-care approach to prescribing antihypertensive drugs in children.

to treatment.[38] Thus far, only one such preparation has been studied in children,[39] so it is difficult to recommend their widespread use at this time. However, they may be very useful in certain children, particularly those who require an ACEI or angiotensin receptor antagonist plus a diuretic; many preparations offering this combination are available.[38]

## Goals of therapy

There are no clinical trial data available to guide the therapy of childhood hypertension; therefore, treatment goals issued by consensus organizations have been based on expert opinion. The 2004 Fourth Report recommended that for children with uncomplicated primary hypertension and no hypertensive target-organ damage, the target blood pressure should be below the 95th percentile for age, gender, and height, whereas for children with secondary hypertension, diabetes, or hypertensive target-organ damage, target blood pressure should be below the 90th percentile for age, gender, and height.[4] The 2009 European Society of Hypertension (ESH) pediatric guidelines recommended a goal of less than the 90th percentile for primary hypertension and less than the 75th percentile for nonproteinuric CKD and less than the 50th percentile for proteinuric CKD.[40] It should be noted that the Fourth Report goals are based on casual BP readings, whereas the ESH goals are based on mean ambulatory blood pressure. To further complicate matters, the KDIGO blood pressure guideline[37] endorsed a goal of below the 50th percentile for proteinuric CKD based on casual blood pressure measurements. How to reconcile these different recommendations is currently unclear. It does seem reasonable to try to achieve a blood pressure between the 90th and 95th

percentiles for patients with primary hypertension, and the ESCAPE trial results[36] certainly suggest that a lower blood pressure goal is appropriate for children with CKD.

## LONG-TERM ISSUES IN HYPERTENSION TREATMENT

Treatment of childhood hypertension obviously does not end with the decision to prescribe antihypertensive medication. Ongoing monitoring of blood pressure, surveillance for medication side effects, periodic monitoring of electrolytes (in children treated with ACEIs, ARBs, or diuretics), counseling regarding other cardiovascular risk factors, and continued emphasis on therapeutic lifestyle changes also should be incorporated into the management plan. Home blood pressure measurement can be helpful in ensuring that blood pressure control has been achieved. In some patients, repeat ambulatory blood pressure monitoring (ABPM) may be necessary if office blood pressure measurements appear to indicate "resistant hypertension." ABPM also should be performed periodically in children with hypertensive CKD to assess for nocturnal or masked hypertension or both. Hypertensive target organ damage such as left ventricular hypertrophy, if present, should be reassessed periodically.[4]

It may be appropriate to consider withdrawal of drug therapy in selected children and adolescents. This involves an attempt at gradual reduction in medication after an extended course of good blood pressure control, with the eventual goal of completely discontinuing drug therapy. Although no comparable studies have been performed yet in children, experience in adults suggests that a substantial percentage of patients may remain normotensive for a time after withdrawal of active treatment.[26] Children with uncomplicated primary hypertension, especially obese adolescents who successfully lose weight and maintain their weight loss, are the best candidates for this "step-down" approach. These children should receive continued blood pressure monitoring after drug therapy is withdrawn and should continue nonpharmacologic treatment.

> ### KEY POINT
>
> In patients with chronic kidney disease, a lower achieved blood pressure may slow progression, so lower treatment goals have been recommended.

## SPECIAL CLINICAL ISSUES

### Hypertension in infancy

Even fewer data are available on the efficacy and safety of antihypertensive agents in infants than for older children. Although some recent industry-sponsored clinical trials have been extended to children younger than 6 years of age,[41] no industry-sponsored trial has included infants

Table 40.3 Recommended doses for selected antihypertensive agents for use in hypertensive children and adolescents

| Class | Drug | Starting dose | Interval | Maximum dose* |
|---|---|---|---|---|
| Aldosterone receptor antagonists | Eplerenone | 25 mg/day | QD–BID | 100 mg/day |
| | Spironolactone[†] | 1 mg/kg/day | QD–BID | 3.3 mg/kg/day up to 100 mg/day |
| Angiotensin receptor blockers | Candesartan[†] | 1–6 yr: 0.2 mg/kg/day; | QD | 1–6 yr: 0.4 mg/kg/day |
| | | 6–17 yr: <50 kg 4–8 mg QD | | >50 kg: 8–16 mg QD |
| | | >50 kg: 8–16 mg QD | | >50 kg: 32 mg/daily |
| | Losartan[†] | 0.75 mg/kg/day (up to 50 mg QD) | QD | 1.4 mg/kg/day (maximum, 100 mg QD) |
| | Olmesartan[†] | 20–35 kg: 10 mg QD | QD | 20–35 kg: 20 mg QD |
| | | ≥35 kg: 20 mg QD | | ≥35 kg: 40 mg QD |
| | Valsartan[†] | <6 yr: 5–10 mg/day | QD | <6 yr: 80 mg QD |
| | | 6–17 yr: 1.3 mg/kg/day (up to 40 mg QD) | | 6–17 yr: 2.7 mg/kg/day (up to 160 mg QD) |
| ACEIs | Benazepril[†] | 0.2 mg/kg/day (up to 10 mg/day) | QD | 0.6 mg/kg/day (up to 40 mg/day) |
| | Captopril[†] | 0.3–0.5 mg/kg/dose | BID–TID | 0.6 mg/kg/day (up to 450 mg/day) |
| | Enalapril[‡] | 0.08 mg/kg/day | QD–BID | 0.6 mg/kg/day (up to 40 mg/day) |
| | Fosinopril | 0.1 mg/kg/day (up to 10 mg/day) | QD | 0.6 mg/kg/day (up to 40 mg/day) |
| | Lisinopril[†] | 0.07 mg/kg/day (up to 5 mg/day) | QD | 0.6 mg/kg/day (up to 40 mg/day) |
| | Quinapril | 5–10 mg/day | QD | 80 mg/day |
| α- and β-Adrenergic antagonists | Carvedilol[†] | 0.1 mg/kg/dose (up to 6.25 mg BID) | BID | 0.5 mg/kg/dose up to 25 mg BID |
| | Labetalol[†] | 2–3 mg/kg/day | BID | 10–12 mg/kg/day (up to 1.2 g/day) |
| β-Adrenergic antagonists | Atenolol[†] | 0.5–1 mg/kg/day | QD | 2 mg/kg/day up to 100 mg day |
| | Bisoprolol/HCTZ | 2.5/6.25 mg daily | QD | 10/6.25 mg daily |
| | Metoprolol | 1–2 mg/kg/day | BID | 6 mg/kg/day (up to 200 mg/day) |
| | Propranolol[‡] | 1 mg/kg/day | BID–QID | 8 mg/kg/day (up to 640 mg/day) |
| Calcium channel blockers | Amlodipine[†] | 0.06 mg/kg/day | QD | 0.3 mg/kg/day (up to 10 mg/day) |
| | Felodipine | 2.5 mg/day | QD | 10 mg/day |
| | Isradipine[†] | 0.05–0.15 mg/kg/dose | TID–QID | 0.8 mg/kg/day up to 20 mg/day |
| | Extended-release nifedipine | 0.25–0.5 mg/kg/day | QD–BID | 3 mg/kg/day (up to 120 mg/day) |
| Central α-agonist diuretics | Clonidine[†] | 5–20 mcg/kg/day | QD–BID | 25 mcg/kg/day (up to 0.9 mg/day) |
| | Amiloride | 5–10 mg/day | QD | 20 mg/day |
| | Chlorthalidone | 0.3 mg/kg/day | QD | 2 mg/kg/day (up to 50 mg/day) |
| | Furosemide[‡] | 0.5–2 mg/kg/dose | QD – BID | 6 mg/kg/day |
| | HCTZ | 0.5–1 mg/kg/day | QD | 3 mg/kg/day (up to 50 mg/day) |
| Vasodilators | Hydralazine | 0.25 mg/kg/dose | TID – QID | 7.5 mg/kg/day (up to 200 mg/day) |
| | Minoxidil | 0.1–0.2 mg/kg/day | BID – TID | 1 mg/kg/day (up to 50 mg/day) |

*Abbreviations:* ACEI, angiotensin converting enzyme inhibitor; BID, twice daily; HCTZ, hydrochlorothiazide; QD, once daily; QID, four times daily; TID, three times daily.

* The maximum recommended adult dose should not be exceeded.
† Information on preparation of a stable extemporaneous suspension is available for these agents.
‡ Available as a FDA approved commercially supplied oral solution approved by the U.S. Food and Drug Administration.

younger than 1 year of age. Therefore, use of antihypertensive medications in infants is by necessity based on expert opinion and data derived from experience in older patients.

Indications for starting antihypertensive drugs in infants are driven by clinical circumstances. In general, critically ill premature infants with persistent blood pressure elevation substantially above published normative values should be promptly treated. More stable neonates should probably be treated if the majority of blood pressure readings over a 24- to 36-hour period are elevated. Recently compiled normative data for preterm infants may be useful in determining which infants should be treated.[42,43] For older infants, particularly those who have been discharged from the nursery and are being followed as outpatients, blood pressure should be confirmed to be elevated over several weeks before drug treatment is initiated.

> ## KEY POINT
>
> Given the uncertainties regarding diagnosis thresholds for hypertension in infants, it is recommended to defer treatment in asymptomatic patients until sustained blood pressure elevation has been demonstrated.

As in older patients, therapy of hypertensive infants should be tailored to the severity of the hypertension and the infant's overall clinical status.[42] For example, critically ill infants with severe hypertension should be treated with an intravenous agent administered by continuous infusion, because this will allow the greatest control over the magnitude and rapidity of the blood pressure reduction. On the other hand, relatively well infants with mild hypertension may be treated with oral antihypertensive agents. Recommended doses for both intravenous and oral antihypertensive drugs in infants can be found in Table 40.4.

Most classes of antihypertensive drugs that are used in older children have been applied to the treatment of hypertensive infants,[44] and probably most can be safely used when treatment is indicated. The exceptions to this, at least on theoretical grounds, are probably ACEIs. The renin-angiotensin system is crucial to normal renal development both prenatally and postnatally. Experimental data indicate that exposure of the immature kidney to ACE inhibition may impair the completion of normal development and even cause histopathologic lesions.[45,46] Thus, it may be appropriate to avoid ACEIs in infants until they have reached a corrected post-menstrual (post-conceptual) age of 44 weeks.

## Severe acute hypertension

The pathophysiology, management, and outcome of severe acute hypertension in children and adolescents have been reviewed in detail elsewhere.[47] Perhaps the most important aspect to highlight here is that hypertensive encephalopathy occurs frequently in children and adolescents with severe hypertension, particularly in younger children. Given this, it is clear that blood pressure reduction in such patients should be performed in a slow, controlled fashion to prevent ischemic strokes and other complications arising through loss of normal autoregulatory processes.[47–49]

Although evidence-based recommendations are lacking, the usual goal in treatment of a hypertensive emergency is to reduce the blood pressure by no more than 25% over the first 8 hours, with a gradual return to normal or goal blood pressure over 24 to 48 hours.[47] Given the need for controlled blood pressure reduction, treatment of hypertensive emergencies in children and adolescents should be initiated with a continuous infusion of an intravenous antihypertensive, with nicardipine and labetalol finding the greatest popularity in many centers.[50–52] Other commonly used intravenous agents given by infusion include esmolol and sodium nitroprusside; use of the latter agent is limited by the accumulation of thiocyanide.[48]

> ## KEY POINT
>
> Intravenous antihypertensive medications are preferred in most patients with severe acute hypertension.

For less severe degrees of blood pressure elevation, or if the child's symptoms permit, oral antihypertensive agents can be used. Options include isradipine, hydralazine, and clonidine, among others. Short-acting nifedipine has fallen out of favor because of safety concerns,[53] and its use was not endorsed in the Fourth Report. Recommended doses for drugs used to treat severe hypertension in children and adolescents can be found in Table 40.5.

## Pheochromocytoma

Although rare as a cause of hypertension in childhood,[54] pheochromocytomas present a unique set of management challenges. Many children with pheochromocytomas initially present with severe, symptomatic hypertension of unknown cause.[55] Such children require careful immediate stabilization and gradual blood pressure reduction, as described in the preceding section, until such time as the necessary studies can be obtained to establish the diagnosis. Although theoretically the α- and β-blocking agent labetalol may seem uniquely well suited for treatment of hypertension caused by a pheochromocytoma, in practice a continuous infusion of any of the intravenous antihypertensives listed in Table 40.4 could be used for initial blood pressure management. Phentolamine has also been advocated in such patients,[56] although pediatric experience with this agent is extremely limited.

Table 40.4 Recommended doses for selected antihypertensive agents for treatment of hypertensive infants

| Class | Drug | Route | Dose | Interval | Comments |
|---|---|---|---|---|---|
| ACE inhibitors* | Captopril | Oral | <3 m: 0.01–0.5 mg/kg/dose | TID | 1.First dose may cause rapid drop in BP, especially if receiving diuretics |
| | | | Max 2 mg/kg/day > 3m: 0.15–0.3 mg/kg/dose Max 6 mg/kg/day | | 2. Monitor serum creatinine and K+ |
| | Enalapril | Oral | 0.08–0.6 mg/kg/day | QD–BID | |
| | Lisinopril | Oral | 0.07–0.6 mg/kg/day | QD | |
| α-and β-Antagonists | Labetalol | Oral | 0.5–1 mg/kg/dose up to 10 mg/kg/day | BID–TID | Heart failure, BPD relative contraindications |
| | | IV | 0.20–1 mg/kg/dose (bolus) | Q4-6 hr | |
| | | IV | 0.25–3 mg/kg/hr | Infusion | |
| | Carvedilol | Oral | 0.1 mg/kg/dose up to 0.5 mg/kg/dose | BID | May be useful in heart failure |
| β-Antagonists | Esmolol | IV | 100–500 mcg/kg/min | Infusion | Very short-acting, constant infusion necessary. |
| | Propranolol | Oral | 0.5–1 mg/kg/dose Max 8–10 mg/kg/day | TID | Monitor heart rate; avoid in BPD |
| Calcium channel blockers | Amlodipine | Oral | 0.05–0.3 mg/kg/dose up to 0.6 mg/kg/day | QD | All may cause mild reflex tachycardia |
| | Isradipine | Oral | 0.05–0.15 mg/kg/dose up to 0.8 mg/kg/day | QID | |
| | Nicardipine | IV | 0.5-4 mcg/kg/min | Infusion | |
| Central α-agonist | Clonidine | Oral | 5–10 mcg/kg/day up to 25 mcg kg/day | TID | May cause mild sedation |
| Diuretics | Chlorothiazide | Oral | 5–15 mg/kg/dose | BID | Monitor electrolytes |
| | Hydrochlorothiazide | Oral | 1–3 mg/kg/dose | QD | |
| | Spironolactone | Oral | 0.5–1.5 mg/kg/dose | BID | |
| Vasodilators | Hydralazine | Oral | 0.25–1 mg/kg/dose up to 7.5 mg/kg/day | TID–QID | Tachycardia and fluid retention are common side effects |
| | | IV | 0.15–0.6 mg/kg/dose | q4 hr | |
| | Minoxidil | Oral | 0.1–0.2 mg/kg/dose | BID–TID | Tachycardia and fluid retention common side effects; prolonged use causes hypertrichosis |
| | Sodium nitroprusside | IV | 0.5–10 mcg/kg/min | Infusion | Thiocyanate toxicity can occur with prolonged (>72 h) use or in renal failure |

Abbreviations:  BID, twice daily; BPD, bronchopulmonary dysplasia; IV, intravenous; Q, every; QD, once daily; QID, four times daily; TID, three times daily

Table 40.5 Antihypertensive drugs for management of acute severe hypertension in children

**Useful for severely hypertensive patients with life-threatening symptoms**

| Drug | Class | Dose | Route | Comments |
|---|---|---|---|---|
| Esmolol | β-Adrenergic blocker | 100–500 mcg/kg/min | IV infusion | Very short-acting—constant infusion preferred. May cause profound bradycardia. |
| Hydralazine | Direct vasodilator | 0.2–0.6 mg/kg/dose | IV, IM | Should be given q4hr when given IV bolus. |
| Labetalol | α- and β-Adrenergic blocker | *Bolus:* 0.20–1.0 mg/kg/dose, up to 40 mg/dose *Infusion:* 0.25–3.0 mg/kg/hr | IV bolus or infusion | Asthma and overt heart failure are relative contraindications. |
| Nicardipine | Calcium channel blocker | *Bolus:* 30 mcg/kg up to 2 mg/dose *Infusion:* 0.5–4 mcg/kg/min | IV bolus or infusion | May cause reflex tachycardia. |
| Sodium nitroprusside | Direct vasodilator | 0.5–10 mcg/kg/min | IV infusion | Monitor cyanide levels with prolonged (>72 hr) use or in renal failure; or coadminister with sodium thiosulfate. |

**Useful for severely hypertensive patients with less significant symptoms**

| Drug | Class | Dose | Route | Comments |
|---|---|---|---|---|
| Clonidine | Central α-agonist | 0.05–0.1 mg/dose, may be repeated up to 0.8 mg total dose | po | Side effects include dry mouth and drowsiness. |
| Enalaprilat | ACE inhibitor | 5–10 mcg/kg/dose up to 1.25 mg/dose | IV bolus | May cause prolonged hypotension and acute renal failure, especially in neonates. |
| Fenoldopam | Dopamine receptor agonist | 0.2–0.8 mcg/kg/min | IV infusion | Produced modest reductions in BP in a pediatric clinical trial in patients up to 12 years. |
| Hydralazine | Direct vasodilator | 0.25 mg/kg/dose up to 25 mg/dose | PO | Extemporaneous suspension stable for only 1 week |
| Isradipine | Calcium channel blocker | 0.05–0.1 mg/kg/dose up to 5 mg/dose | PO | Stable suspension can be compounded. |
| Minoxidil | Direct vasodilator | 0.1–0.2 mg/kg/dose up to 10 mg/dose | PO | Most potent oral vasodilator; long-acting. |

*Abbreviations:* ACE, angiotensin-converting enzyme; BP, blood pressure; M, intramuscular; IV, intravenous; kg, kilogram; mcg, microgram; mg, milligram; PO, oral.

Once the diagnosis of pheochromocytoma has been made, the child's blood pressure should be stabilized until the tumor can be surgically removed. Phenoxybenzamine, a potent α-adrenergic blocker, is usually recommended as the primary agent for this phase of management.[56,57] The phenoxybenzamine dose is increased gradually (every 48 hours) until the desired blood pressure is achieved. β-Adrenergic blockade is frequently advocated as adjunctive therapy to counter tachycardia in patients treated with phenoxybenzamine. Recently, some authors have recommended use of the peripheral α-blocker doxazosin because of a more favorable side-effect profile compared to phenoxybenzamine.[58]

**KEY POINT**

Medical management of pheochromocytoma-related hypertension should begin with α-blockade, with β-blockade added later.

Definitive treatment of pheochromocytoma requires either open or laparoscopic removal of the tumor. In addition to strict blood pressure control, as discussed earlier, preoperative management also includes volume replacement and monitoring for arrhythmias produced by surges of catecholamine release from the tumor.[55–58] Intraoperatively, blood pressure surges and arrhythmias may occur as a result of manipulation of the tumor. These complications can be treated with use of rapidly acting intravenous antihypertensive agents and β-adrenergic blockade. Volume resuscitation may be required immediately following removal of the tumor.[57] Although successful tumor removal should result in cure of the child's hypertension, periodic monitoring of plasma catecholamines and metanephrines should be performed to detect potential tumor recurrence.

## Renovascular hypertension

Although the term renovascular hypertension can be used to describe hypertension caused by a variety of conditions, it most often implies hypertension secondary to renal artery stenosis (RAS). Children with RAS may have acute presentations with severe, symptomatic hypertension, or they may be asymptomatic.[59] As in other forms of secondary hypertension, initial BP control can be achieved with any of a variety of nonspecific agents, particularly vasodilators. Addition of a diuretic can greatly improve blood pressure control, because a component of volume overload is usually present in patients with RAS, especially with unilateral disease.

The use of ACEIs in patients with RAS is controversial. They are clearly contraindicated in bilateral RAS and or in RAS with a single kidney (including RAS in transplanted kidneys) because of the likelihood of provoking acute kidney injury.[60] However, they may be very effective in cases in which RAS is unilateral and surgery or angioplasty is unable to be performed, or when intrarenal stenoses are present that are not amenable to surgery or angioplasty. In such cases, serial ultrasonography to follow renal growth, serial nuclear scans, or both to follow renal perfusion may be helpful in determining whether to continue ACE inhibition.

---

### KEY POINT

In patients with renovascular hypertension, antihypertensive medications are used frequently—in the initial management until anatomic correction is achieved and long term when there is residual hypertension or vascular lesions that cannot be corrected.

---

As hypertension caused by RAS is potentially curable, the chief issue in managing children with renovascular hypertension is whether and when they should undergo angioplasty or surgical revascularization.[59] Although percutaneous transluminal angioplasty (PCTA) offers the advantage of being less invasive than surgical revascularization, results in children with renovascular hypertension may not be as good as in adults, primarily because RAS in children is typically caused by fibromuscular dysplasia and may be associated with either multiple stenoses or intrarenal branch vessel stenoses. This contrasts with RAS in adults, which is typically related to buildup of atherosclerotic plaque at the origin of the renal arteries. In a series of 48 PCTA procedures performed in 33 children, some of whom required multiple procedures because of restenosis or bilateral disease, most children had improvement of blood pressure following PCTA, although only 9 were normotensive off all medications.[61]

Surgical revascularization, while admittedly more invasive than PCTA, seems to offer a greater likelihood of complete cure of the child's hypertension. At the University of Michigan, for example, 79% of children who underwent various revascularization procedures were considered cured.[62] Surgery is preferred to PCTA in children with multiple stenoses and also can be successful when PCTA has failed.

Finally, although PCTA and surgery for RAS have been performed in very young children[63,64] when renovascular hypertension is diagnosed in infants or toddlers, it may be prudent to manage these children medically until they have grown sufficiently so that a definitive procedure can be safely performed. In such children, careful follow-up with serial renal ultrasonography to assess renal growth and serial echocardiograms to monitor for the development of left ventricular hypertrophy can be crucial in determining when surgery or PCTA should be undertaken.

---

### SUMMARY

The management of pediatric hypertension begins by staging the hypertension based on standard tables, evaluating the patient for the presence of symptoms or target organ damage, and determining if there is an underlying medical condition that warrants more aggressive treatment. Most patients are initially treated with nonpharmacologic intervention initially, although severe, symptomatic hypertension may warrant intravenous medications in an intensive care unit. There are increasing data on the safety and efficacy of antihypertensive medications in children, but few comparative or long-term data are available to guide use of a specific agent. However, in some instances a specific agent is indicated.

---

## REFERENCES

1. James PA, Oparil S, Carter BL, et al. 2014 Evidence-based guideline for the management of high blood pressure in adults: Report from the Panel Members Appointed to the Eighth Joint National Committee (JNC 8). JAMA. 2014;311:507–20.
2. Kay JD, Sinaiko AR, Daniels SR. Pediatric hypertension. Am Heart J. 2001;142:422–32.

3. Chobanian AV, Bakris GL, Black HR, et al. The Seventh Report of the Joint National Committee on Prevention, Detection, Evaluation, and Treatment of High Blood Pressure. The JNC 7 report. JAMA 2003;289:2560–72.

4. National High Blood Pressure Education Program Working Group on High Blood Pressure in Children and Adolescents. The fourth report on the diagnosis, evaluation, and treatment of high blood pressure in children and adolescents. Pediatrics. 2004;114:555–576.

5. Expert Panel on Integrated Guidelines for Cardiovascular Health and Risk Reduction in Children and Adolescents; National Heart, Lung, and Blood Institute. Expert panel on integrated guidelines for cardiovascular health and risk reduction in children and adolescents: Summary report. Pediatrics. 2011;128(Suppl 5):S213–56.

6. Lauer RM, Clarke WR. Childhood risk factors for high adult blood pressure: The Muscatine study. Pediatrics 1989;84:633–641.

7. Luepker RV, Jacobs DR, Prineas RJ, Sinaiko AR. Secular trends of blood pressure and body size in a multi-ethnic adolescent population: 1986 to 1996. J Pediatr. 1999;134:668–74.

8. Muntner P, He J, Cutler JA, et al. Trends in blood pressure among children and adolescents. JAMA. 2004;291:2107–13.

9. Rocchini AP, Katch V, Anderson J, et al. Blood pressure in obese adolescents: Effect of weight loss. Pediatrics. 1988;82:16–23.

10. Figueroa-Colon R, Franklin FA, Lee JY, et al. Feasibility of a clinic-based hypocaloric dietary intervention implemented in a school setting for obese children. Obes Res. 1996;4:419–29.

11. Williams CL, Hayman LL, Daniels SR, et al. Cardiovascular health in childhood: A statement for health professionals from the Committee on Atherosclerosis, Hypertension, and Obesity in the Young (AHOY) of the Council on Cardiovascular Disease in the Young, American Heart Association. Circulation. 2002;106:143–60.

12. Reinehr T, Andler W. Changes in the atherogenic risk factor profile according to degree of weight loss. Arch Dis Child. 2004;89:419–22.

13. Epstein LH, Myers MD, Raynor HA, et al. Treatment of pediatric obesity. Pediatrics. 1998;101:554–70.

14. Alpert BS. Exercise as a therapy to control hypertension in children. Int J Sports Med. 2000;21(Suppl 2):S94–6.

15. Alpert BS, Fox ME. Hypertension. In: Goldberg B, editor. Sports and Exercise for Children with Chronic Health Conditions. Champaign, IL: Human Kinetics; 1995. p. 197–205.

16. American Academy of Pediatrics Council on Sports Medicine and Fitness. Policy statement: Athletic participation by children and adolescents who have systemic hypertension. Pediatrics. 2010;125:1287–94.

17. Chrysant GS, Bakir S, Oparil S. Dietary salt reduction in hypertension: What is the evidence and why is it still controversial? Prog Cardiovasc Dis. 1999;42:23–38.

18. Weinberger MH. Salt sensitivity of blood pressure in humans. Hypertension. 1996;27:481–90.

19. Cutler JA. The effects of reducing sodium and increasing potassium intake for control of hypertension and improving health. Clin Exp Hypertens. 1999;21:769–83.

20. Gillman MW, Oliveria SA, Moore LL, et al. Inverse association of dietary calcium with systolic blood pressure in young children. JAMA. 1992;267:2340–3.

21. Appel LJ, Moore TJ, Obarzanek E, et al. A clinical trial of the effects of dietary patterns on blood pressure. N Engl J Med. 1997;336:1117–24.

22. Couch SC, Saelens BE, Levin L, et al. The efficacy of a clinic-based behavioral nutrition intervention emphasizing a DASH-type diet for adolescents with elevated blood pressure. J Pediatr. 2008;152:494–501.

23. Kavey REW, Daniels SR, Lauer RM, et al. American Heart Association guidelines for primary prevention of atherosclerotic cardiovascular disease beginning in childhood. Circulation. 2003;107:1562–6.

24. Welch WP, Yang W, Taylor-Zapata P, Flynn JT. Antihypertensive drug use by children: Are the drugs labeled and indicated? J Clin Hypertens (Greenwich). 2012;14:388–95.

25. Flynn JT. Pediatric use of antihypertensive medications: Much more to learn. Curr Ther Res Clin Exp. 2001;62:314–28.

26. Kaplan NM. Primary hypertension: Natural history and evaluation. In: Kaplan NM, Victor RG, editors. Kaplan's Clinical Hypertension, 10th ed. Philadelphia: Lippincott Williams & Wilkins; 2010. p. 108–40.

27. Moyer VA; U.S. Preventive Services Task Force. Screening for primary hypertension in children and adolescents: U.S. Preventive Services Task Force recommendation statement. Pediatrics. 2013;132:907–14.

28. Yusuf HR, Giles WH, Croft JB, et al. Impact of multiple risk factor profiles on determining cardiovascular disease risk. Prev Med. 1998;27:1–9.

29. Clement DL, De Buyzere ML, De Bacquer DA, et al. Prognostic value of ambulatory blood-pressure recordings in patients with treated hypertension. N Engl J Med. 2003;348:2407–15.

30. Flynn JT, Urbina EM. Pediatric ambulatory blood pressure monitoring: Indications and interpretations. J Clin Hypertens (Greenwich). 2012;14:372–82.

31. Ferguson M, Flynn JT. Rational use of antihypertensive medications in children. Pediatr Nephrol. 2014;29:979–88.

32. Blumenthal S, Epps RP, Heavenrich R, et al. Report of the task force on blood pressure control in children. Pediatrics. 1977;59(5 2 suppl):I–II, 797–820.

33. Task Force on Blood Pressure Control in Children. Report of the Second Task Force on Blood Pressure Control in Children: 1987. National Heart, Lung, and Blood Institute, Bethesda, Maryland. Pediatrics. 1987;79:1–25.

34. Woroniecki RP, Flynn JT. How are hypertensive children evaluated and managed? A survey of North American pediatric nephrologists. Pediatr Nephrol. 2005;20:791–7.

35. Flynn JT, Mitsnefes M, Pierce C, et al. Blood pressure in children with chronic kidney disease: A report from the Chronic Kidney Disease in Children study. Hypertension. 2008;52:631–7.

36. Wuhl E, Trivelli A, Picca S, et al. Strict blood-pressure control and progression of renal failure in children. N Engl J Med. 2009;361:1639–50.

37. Kidney Disease Improving Global Outcomes (KDIGO) Blood Pressure Work Group. KDIGO clinical practice guideline for the management of blood pressure in chronic kidney disease. Kidney Int Suppl. 2012;2:337–414.

38. Wells T, Stowe C. An approach to the use of antihypertensive drugs in children and adolescents. Curr Ther Res Clin Exp 2001; 62:329-350.

39. Sorof JM, Cargo P, Graepel J, et al. Beta-blocker/thiazide combination for treatment of hypertensive children: A randomized double-blind, placebo-controlled trial. Pediatr Nephrol. 2002;17:345–50.

40. Lurbe E, Cifkova R, Cruickshank JK, et al. Management of high blood pressure in children and adolescents: Recommendations of the European Society of Hypertension. J Hypertens. 2009;27:1719–42.

41. Schaefer F, van de Walle J, Zurowska A, et al. Efficacy, safety and pharmacokinetics of candesartan cilexetil in hypertensive children from 1 to less than 6 years of age. J Hypertens. 2010;28:1083–90.

42. Dionne JM, Abitbol CL, Flynn JT. Hypertension in infancy: Diagnosis, management and outcome. Pediatr Nephrol. 2012;27:17–32.

43. Dionne JM, Abitbol CL, Flynn JT. Erratum to: Hypertension in infancy: Diagnosis, management and outcome. Pediatr Nephrol. 2012;27:159–60.

44. Blowey DL, Duda PJ, Stokes P, Hall M. Incidence and treatment of hypertension in the neonatal intensive care unit. J Am Soc Hypertens. 2011;5:478–83.

45. Guron G, Sundelin B, Wickman A, Friberg P. Angiotensin-converting enzyme inhibition in piglets induces persistent renal abnormalities. Clin Exp Pharmacol Physiol. 1998;25:88–91.

46. Yoo KH. The effect of ACE inhibition on the neonatal kidney: Developmental and signaling considerations [abstract]. Pediatr Nephrol. 2004;19:C58.

47. Flynn JT, Tullus K. Severe hypertension in children and adolescents: Pathophysiology and treatment. Pediatr Nephrol 2009;24:1101–12.

48. Vaughan CJ, Delanty N. Hypertensive emergencies. Lancet. 2000;356:411–7.

49. Schwartz RB. Hyperperfusion encephalopathies: Hypertensive encephalopathy and related conditions. Neurologist. 2002;8:22–34.

50. Deal JE, Barratt TM, Dillon MJ. Management of hypertensive emergencies. Arch Dis Child. 1992;67:1089–92.

51. Flynn, JT, Mottes TA, Brophy PB, et al. Intravenous nicardipine for treatment of severe hypertension in children. J Pediatr. 2001;139:38–43.

52. Thomas CA, Moffett BS, Wagner JL, et al. Safety and efficacy of intravenous labetalol for hypertensive crisis in infants and small children. Pediatr Crit Care Med. 2011;12:28–32.

53. Flynn JT. Safety of short-acting nifedipine in children with severe hypertension. Expert Opin Drug Saf. 2003;2:133–9.

54. Newman KD, Ponsky T. The diagnosis and management of endocrine tumors causing hypertension in childhood. Ann NY Acad Sci. 2002;970:150–8.

55. Kohane DS, Ingelfinger JR, Nimkin K, Wu C-L. Case 16-2005: A nine-year-old girl with headaches and hypertension. N Engl J Med. 2005;352:2223–31.

56. Brouwers FM, Lenders JWM, Eisenhofer G, Pacak K. Pheochromocytoma as an endocrine emergency. Rev Endocrine Metab Dis. 2003;4:121–8.

57. Williams DT, Dann S, Wheeler MH. Phaeochromocytoma: Views on current management. Eur J Surg Oncol. 2003;29:483–90.

58. Pacak K. Preoperative management of the pheochromocytoma patient. J Clin Endocrinol Metab. 2007;92:4069–79.

59. Tullus K, Brennan E, Hamilton G, et al. Renovascular hypertension in children. Lancet. 2008;371:1453–63.

60. Burnier M, Waeber B, Nussberger J, Brunner HR. Effect of angiotensin converting enzyme inhibition in renovascular hypertension. J Hypertens Suppl. 1989;7:S27–31.

61. Shroff R, Roebuck DJ, Gordon I, et al. Angioplasty for renovascular hypertension in children: 20-year Experience. Pediatrics. 2006;118:268–75.

62. Stanley JC, Zelenock GB, Messina LM, Wakefield TW. Pediatric renovascular hypertension: A thirty-year experience of operative treatment. J Vasc Surg. 1995;21:212–26.

63. Coutrel JV, Soto B, Niaudet P et al. Percutaneous transluminal angioplasty of renal artery stenosis in children. Pediatr Radiol 1998;28:59–63.

64. Hofbeck M, Singer H, Rupprecht T, et al. Successful percutaneous transluminal angioplasty for treatment of renovascular hypertension in a 15-month-old child. Eur J Pediatr. 1998;157:512–4.

# REVIEW QUESTIONS

1. A 16-year-old obese boy with hypertension and type 2 diabetes has been referred to you for evaluation. His office blood pressure is 145/82 mm Hg. He has LVH on an echocardiogram and a mildly elevated urinary microalbumin-to-creatinine ratio. The referring physician prescribed hydrochlorothiazide 50 mg daily. Your recommendation should be:
   a. Order ambulatory blood pressure monitoring to assess his blood pressure control.
   b. Add metoprolol 100 mg daily to further reduce his blood pressure.
   c. Start regular aerobic exercise and a low-sodium diet.
   d. Stop the hydrochlorothiazide and start lisinopril 10 mg daily.

2. An 8-year-old girl has been found to have confirmed office hypertension. Her weight and BMI are both at the 97th percentile for age, and her height is at the 40th percentile. Which of the following changes should be made to her daily routine?
   a. Restriction of caloric intake to 1500 calories/day
   b. Supplementation with potassium chloride
   c. 30 minutes of brisk walking around the block with her mother after school
   d. Scheduling for an assessment of obesity in a pediatric endocrinology clinic

3. A 12 year-old girl treated with quinapril for primary hypertension needs the following issues addressed at her quarterly follow-up appointments:
   a. Use of contraception
   b. CBC monitoring
   c. Edema assessment
   d. a and b
   e. a, b, and c

4. When deciding whether to start an antihypertensive medication, the following is the most important consideration:
   a. The age of the child
   b. The presence of obesity
   c. The presence of left ventricular hypertrophy
   d. The success of lifestyle modification

5. A 12-year-old girl with pheochromocytoma has been referred to you by the oncology service for assistance with blood pressure management until surgery, which is scheduled to take place in 2.5 weeks. Which of the following strategies should be employed to control her BP?
   a. Sodium restriction and bedrest
   b. Start treatment with oral labetalol
   c. Start treatment with oral propranolol
   d. Sodium restriction and start phenoxybenzamine
   e. Start treatment with doxazosin

6. An 8-year-old boy presents to the emergency department after having two tonic-clonic seizures. Blood pressures obtained by ambulance personnel were 150 to 168/95 to 118 mm Hg. Ativan has been given and seizures have stopped. Which of the following measures would not be appropriate?
   a. Reduction of blood pressure with sublingual nifedipine to 110/70 mm Hg
   b. Insertion of an arterial monitoring line
   c. Obtain a comprehensive medical history
   d. Order nicardipine from the pharmacy

7. A 12-year-old boy is referred from the urology department with new-onset blood pressure elevation in the setting of known reflux nephropathy. In the clinic, his blood pressure measurements fulfill criteria for stage 2 hypertension. Initial evaluations are notable for an estimated GFR of 65 mL/min/1.73 m² and 3+ proteinuria by dipstick. Which of the following drug classes would be considered most appropriate in this setting?
   a. Nondihydropyridine calcium channel blockers
   b. Loop diuretics
   c. Angiotensin receptor antagonists
   d. Direct-acting vasodilators
   e. β-Adrenergic blockers

8. Which of the following medication classes should be avoided as primary therapy in the hypertensive female athlete?
   a. Angiotensin-converting enzyme inhibitors
   b. Diuretics
   c. β-blockers
   d. Calcium channel blockers
   e. a and b

9. Recommendations for staging hypertension in children and adolescents provide guidance for clinicians in evaluating and managing patients with elevated blood pressure. The new staging system recommends immediate institution of antihypertensive medications for patients with blood pressure in which of the following stages?
   a. Stage 2 hypertension
   b. Normal blood pressure
   c. Stage 1 hypertension
   d. Pre-hypertension
   e. a and c

10. You receive a phone call from a neonatologist in a neighboring community. She has been caring for a now 6-week-old, former 28 weeks of gestation premature infant. She is concerned about some high blood pressure readings and wants your recommendations regarding treatment. What additional information do you need to make the *best* recommendation?
    a. The infant's current weight and length
    b. The infant's medication list
    c. Details about how the infant's blood pressure is being measured

d.  a and b

d.  b and c

11.  An otherwise healthy 16-year-old boy presents with office blood pressure readings of 160/100 mm Hg in both upper extremities. He is not obese, but there is a strong family history of cardiovascular disease. He initially denies any symptoms, but at the end of the visit, his mother tells you that he occasionally complains of his legs aching during soccer, and that he sometimes has abdominal pain after eating. What medication should you prescribe while you are waiting for test results to come back?

a.  Lisinopril

b.  Felodipine

c.  Valsartan

d.  Metoprolol

## ANSWERS

1.  d
2.  c
3.  d
4.  c
5.  e
6.  a
7.  c
8.  e
9.  a
10.  e
11.  b

# Inherited renal disorders

# 41

# Tubulopathies

DETLEF BOCKENHAUER

Assuming a glomerular filtration rate of 100 mL/min, the kidneys of an average adult each day filter approximately 150 L of plasma each day, containing approximately 20 mol of sodium ($Na^+$), the equivalent of more than a kilogram of table salt. Thus, without tubules, we all would have to drink 150 L a day and eat a kilogram of salt to keep up with urinary losses. The enormity of these numbers demonstrates the importance of proper tubular function. Typically, more than 99% of filtered salt and water are reabsorbed. Yet, the tubules not only need to accomplish the massive bulk transport of water and solutes, they also need to finely regulate the precise amount of reabsorption to balance variable intake and extrarenal losses, to maintain volume and electrolyte homoeostasis.

## ORGANIZATION OF TUBULES

The enormous feat of complex tubular functions is accomplished by a whole orchestra of tubular transporters arranged along the entire nephron. Each transporter plays a specific role in coordinating a portion of tubular function. Much has been learned about the individual transport processes through observations of patients in whom one or more of these transport processes is defective, or patients with tubulopathies.

Both from a functional and a histoanatomic perspective, the nephron can be divided into four different segments (Figure 41.1):

1. Proximal tubule (PT)
2. Loop of Henle
3. Distal convoluted and connecting tubule (DCT)
4. Collecting duct (CD)

Disorders of the loop of Henle are mainly restricted to the thick ascending limb (TAL). In general, high-capacity bulk transport occurs in the PT, whereas the fine tuning of reabsorption occurs mostly in the distal end, the CD. Disorders of each segment tend to have a distinctive "fingerprint" of clinical and biochemical abnormalities that informs the diagnosis (Table 41.1).

### KEY POINT

The renal tubule can be separated morphologically and functionally into four main segments: PT, loop of Henle, DCT, and CD.

## DISORDERS OF THE PROXIMAL TUBULE

### PHYSIOLOGY

The PT is not only the site of high-capacity transport, but it is also the exclusive site of reabsorption for several solutes, such as low-molecular-weight (LMW) proteins, amino and organic acids, glucose, and phosphate.[1] Because a sizeable proportion of albumin is also filtered, PT dysfunction is associated with moderately elevated urinary albumin levels, which can lead to confusion with glomerular disorders.[2] Albumin, like LMW proteins and a host of other solutes, is taken up by the proximal tubular epithelial cells

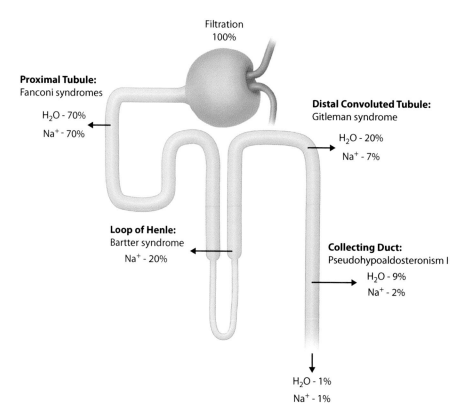

**Figure 41.1** Schematic of a nephron with respect to salt and water ($H_2O$) reabsorption. Shown is a schematic of a nephron depicting the four main segments for sodium ($Na^+$) reabsorption. The indicated percentages for sodium and water reabsorption are rough estimates and may vary with clinical conditions.

through the promiscuous receptors megalin and cubilin, which are then internalized with the cargo into endosomes (Figure 41.2).[3]

Defects in PT can range from very specific dysfunction, such as isolated renal glucosuria, caused by impaired function of the $Na^+$-glucose cotransporter SGLT2 (SLC5A2),[4] to a generalized dysfunction of the PT. Clinically, cases of generalized PT dysfunction with glucosuria, acidosis, and hypophosphatemic rickets were first described in the 1930s by De Toni,[5] Debre et al.,[6] and Fanconi,[7] and consequently this constellation of symptoms is referred to as De Toni–Debre-Fanconi syndrome, or just renal Fanconi syndrome. It can be acquired or inherited, either isolated or in the context of systemic disorders, such as mitochondrial cytopathies or nephropathic cystinosis (Table 41.2).[8]

## CYSTINOSIS

Cystinosis, albeit a rare disorder with an estimated incidence of approximately less than 1 in 100,000, is the most common inherited cause of renal Fanconi syndrome in children.[9] The underlying gene, *CTNS*, encodes a transporter involved in exporting cysteine from lysosomes.[10]

Consequently, impaired CTNS function leads to intracellular cystine accumulation.[11] However, how exactly this accumulation leads to cellular damage has yet to be clarified, although several hypothesis have been proposed, such as increased apoptosis, impaired energy production, and altered glutathione metabolism.[12]

## Clinical features and diagnosis

Although cystinosis is a multiorgan disorder, the renal manifestations initially dominate, potentially because of the high cystine turnover in the PT from amino acid and LMW protein reabsorption. Measurement of urinary excretion of several LMW proteins, such as $\alpha_1$- and $\beta_2$-microglobulins, can be used as markers for LMW proteinuria, but retinol-binding protein has been shown to have the highest sensitivity and specificity[13] for proximal tubular proteinuria.

Presentation is usually in the first 2 years of life with polyuria or polydipsia, failure to thrive, and rickets. Biochemical testing reveals the typical features of renal Fanconi syndrome (Table 41.3). However, because cystinosis affects most cells, other renal segments can be affected: glomerular

Table 41.1 Selected tubulopathies, associated genes, and pertinent clinical and biochemical characteristics*

| Tubular Segment | Diseases | Genes | Mode | Proteins | Pertinent clinical characteristics | K⁺ | Cl⁻ | HCO₃⁻ | Mg²⁺ | Urine Ca²⁺ |
|---|---|---|---|---|---|---|---|---|---|---|
| PT | Isolated Renal Fanconi | EHHADH / SCL12A1 | AD / AR | L-PBE / NaPI-IIa | See Table 41.2 | ↓ | ↑↓ | → | ↑ | ↓ |
| TAL | Bartter type 1 | SLC12A1 | AR | NKCC2 cotransporter (furosemide sensitive) | Typically antenatal onset, nephrocalcinosis | ↓ | ↓ | ↑ | ↑ | ↑ |
| TAL | Bartter type 2 | KCNJ1 | AR | K channel ROMK | Typically antenatal onset, nephrocalcinosis, neonatal hyperkalemia | ↓↑ | ↓ | ↑ | ↑ | ↑ |
| TAL | Bartter type3 | CLCNKB | AR | Cl channel ClCNKB | — | ↓↓ | ↓↓ | ↑↑ | ↑↑ | ↑↑ |
| TAL | Bartter type 4 | BSND | AR | Barttin | Sensorineural deafness | ↓↓ | ↓ | ↑↑ | ↑→ | ↑↑ |
| DCT | Gitelman | SLC12A3 | AR | NCC (thiazide-sensitive) | — | ↓→ | ↓ | ↑← | →↓ | ↓ |
| DCT | EAST | KCNJ10 | AR | K channel Kir4.1 | Epilepsy, ataxia and sensorineural deafness | ↓→ | ↓ | ↑← | ↓ | → |
| CD | PHA1 | SCNN1A / SCNN1B / SCNN1G / NR3C2 | AR / AR / AR / AD | EnaC sodium channel subunits A,B,G / Mineralocorticoid receptor | Recessive forms may have cystic fibrosis—like lung disease and eczema; dominant form improves with age | ↑↑ | ↑↓ | ↓ | ↑ | ↓ |
| DCT | PHA2 (Gordon) | WNK1 / WNK4 / CUL3 / KLHL3 | AD / AD / AD / AD/AR | WNK-kinases / Cullin3 / Kelch-like 3 | — | ↑ | ↑ | ↓ | ↑ | ↓ |
| CD | Liddle | SCNN1B / SCNN1G | AD / AD | EnaC sodium channel subunits B,G | — | ↓↑ | ↑↓ | ↑↑ | ↑ | ↑↓ |
| CD | GRA | CYP11B1/2 | AD | Aldosterone synthase | — | ↓↑ | ↑↓ | ↑↑ | ↑↑ | ↑← |
| CD | AME | HSD11B2 | AR | 11β-hydroxysteroid dehydrogenase | — | →↓ | ↑↓ | ↑↓ | ↑↑ | ↑← |
| CD | HEP | NR3C2 | AD | Mineralocorticoid receptor | — | ↓↑ | ↓ | ↑← | ↑ | ↑↓ |

*Abbreviations:* AD, autosomal dominant; AME, apparent mineralocorticoid excess; AR, autosomal recessive; CD, collecting duct; DCT, distal convoluted tubule; GRA, glucocorticoid-remediable hypertension; HEP, hypertension with exacerbation in pregnancy; PHA, pseudohypoaldosteronism; PT, proximal tubule; TAL, thick ascending limb of the loop of Henle.

Note: [↑], level elevated; [↓], level decreased; [→], normal; combination of [↑] and [→], normal or elevated; combination of [↓] and [→], level normal or low.

* The upper eight rows (un-bold) list disorders of salt wasting (hypovolemia, low/normal blood pressure), whereas the lower five rows (**bold**) list disorders of salt retention (hypervolemia, hypertension). Bartter type 1 and 2 (TAL) and AME (CD) have identical biochemical profiles, but Bartter syndrome is associated with hypovolemia and hypertension, whereas AME is associated with hypervolemia and hypertension.

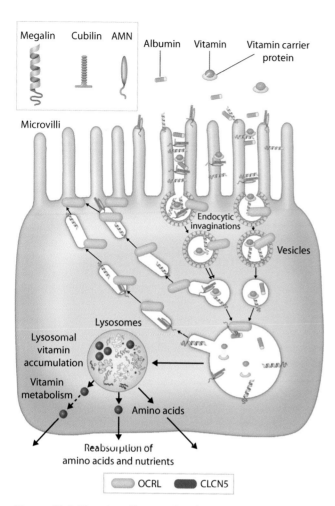

Figure 41.2 Uptake of low-molecular-weight protein in the proximal tubule. Low-molecular-weight proteins and many other solutes bind to the receptors megalin or cubilin and are subsequently incorporated into endosomes. The proteins are degraded in lysosomes, a process that involves CLCN5. The receptors (megalin and cubilin) are recycled back to the apical membrane. OCRL is involved in regulation of the endosomal trafficking. AMN, amnionless.

function deteriorates with time, and other tubular features, such as secondary nephrogenic diabetes insipidus, have also been reported.[14]

Once suspected, the diagnosis is easily established by slit-lamp examination of the eyes, which demonstrates characteristic cystine crystals in virtually all children older than 16 months of age.[15] The absence of crystals before this age does not exclude the diagnosis. The diagnosis can be confirmed by measurement of an increased leukocyte cystine content or genetic testing, or both. Most children with typical clinical features of cystinosis have identifiable biallelic mutations in *CTNS*.[16]

Later in life, other types of organ dysfunction can become apparent, such as hypothyroidism, myopathy with swallowing dysfunction, retinal blindness, diabetes mellitus, male hypogonadism, and pulmonary and central nervous system dysfunction.[9]

## Table 41.2 Causes of renal Fanconi syndrome

### Isolated Inherited Renal Fanconi syndrome
- Autosomal dominant
- Autosomal recessive
- X-linked

### Multiorgan Disorders
- Cystinosis
- Tyrosinemia
- Lowe syndrome
- Galactosemia
- Fructosemia
- Wilson disease
- Mitochondrial cytopathies
- Fabry disease (in addition to glomerular involvement)

### Acquired Fanconi Syndrome
- Antiretroviral agents (tenofovir)
- Chemotherapy (ifosfamide, cisplatin)
- Cyclosporine
- Valproic acid
- Aminoglycosides
- Heavy metal poisoning
- Glue sniffing
- Aristolochic acid (Chinese herb nephropathy)

## Treatment and prognosis

Treatment used to be just supportive, by replacing renal fluid and solute losses, enhancing nutrition, and treating the rickets. Patients developed end-stage renal disease (ESRD) in the

## Table 41.3 Clinical and biochemical features of renal Fanconi syndrome

### Clinical Features
- Polyuria or polydipsia
- Rickets
- Failure to thrive

### Biochemical Features
- Hypokalemia
- Hypophosphatemia with renal phosphate wasting (low TMP/GFR)
- Metabolic non-anion gap acidosis
- Elevated parathyroid hormone
- Hypercalciuria
- Glucosuria
- Low-molecular-weight proteinuria
- Amino aciduria
- Organic aciduria

*Abbreviations:* TMP/GFR, tubular maximum reabsorption for phosphate

first or second decade of life, along with other organ manifestations. Death typically occurred before the third decade of life. The prognosis, however, was transformed with the introduction of cysteamine treatment in the 1980s. Cysteamine acts by entering the lysosomes and reducing cystine to cysteine, which can then exit the lysosome through a different transporter.[17]

---

## KEY POINTS

- Cystinosis manifests clinically with failure to thrive, features of Fanconi syndrome, and photophobia.
- Leukocyte cysteine level and gene testing establish the diagnosis.
- Cysteamine treatment delays ESRD and other complications and prolongs life expectancy.

---

Cysteamine is prescribed in a dose of 60 to 90 mg/kg/day, or 1.3 to 1.95 g/m$^2$/day, given in divided in 6-hourly doses. With appropriate cysteamine treatment early in life, growth is improved, ESRD can often be deferred into the third decade of life or beyond, and other organ manifestations can be similarly delayed.[18] Side effects include a thiol-like taste and odor, which can induce vomiting. Dosage should be gradually increased so that the patient can become used to it. In rare instances, vascular elbow lesions, consistent with angioendotheliomatosis, have been reported; these lesions appear to be associated with excess cysteamine administration and improve with dose reduction.[19] The eye crystals, which can cause photophobia and pain, are not affected by systemic cysteamine treatment, but they dissolve with long-term topical application of cysteamine eye drops (6 to 12 times per day).[15] Clinical Vignette 41.1 describes a case of cystinosis in a young child.

---

### Clinical Vignette 41.1

A 2-year-old boy presented with a several-month history of failure to thrive and bowing of his legs. The parents reported that he had little interest in food, but he constantly drank water.

Physical examination revealed a malnourished child with height below the third percentile and weight well below the third percentile. Vital signs were normal. He had clinical signs of rickets with widened wrists, a rickety rosary, and tibial bowing. Laboratory studies revealed metabolic acidosis, hypokalemia, hypophosphatemia, and elevated creatinine. Urine tests showed glucosuria, phosphate wasting, highly elevated levels of retinol-binding protein, albuminuria, and generalized aminoaciduria. Slit-lamp examination of his eyes showed corneal crystals, suggesting the diagnosis of cystinosis. The diagnosis of cystinosis was confirmed by an elevated leukocyte cystine content and genetic testing.

---

## LOWE SYNDROME

Lowe syndrome is a rare multiorgan disorder with an estimated prevalence of less than 1 in 500,000.[20] It was first described in 1952 by Charles Lowe et al.[21] as the combination of "organic-aciduria, decreased renal ammonia production, hydrophthalmos, and [intellectual impairment]." It is an X-linked recessive disorder, and in 1992 the underlying gene was cloned and named *OCRL*.[22] *OCRL* encodes a phosphatidylinositol 4,5-bisphosphate 5-phosphatase located in the Golgi apparatus.[23] Phosphatidylinositol phosphates (PIPs) serve as important recognition molecules for intracellular membranes and thus are important for intracellular trafficking.[24] In addition to the phosphatase domain, the OCRL protein contains several other domains involved in endosomal trafficking by protein-protein interactions.[25] This protein has been shown to interact directly with clathrin[26,27] and IPIP[27] (inositol phosphatase interacting protein of 27 kDa) A and B (also referred to as Ses1 and 2), two important regulators of endosomal trafficking.[28,29]

---

## KEY POINTS

- Lowe syndrome is characterized by congenital cataracts, intellectual impairment, and selective proximal tubular dysfunction.
- LMW proteinuria (retinol-binding protein and β$_2$-microglobulin) is common.
- Hypercalciuria is common.

---

## Clinical features and diagnosis

Lowe syndrome is characterized by the triad of congenital cataracts, mental impairment, and proximal tubular dysfunction, yet incomplete phenotypes are increasingly recognized in patients without obvious eye findings or mental impairment.[30,31] Clearly, there is overlap with Dent disease (see later).

Patients are typically recognized at birth because of the cataracts, the muscular hypotonia, and, if tested, the LMW proteinuria. The developmental delay becomes apparent later. The diagnosis can be confirmed by genetic testing.

Lowe syndrome is often cited as a cause of renal Fanconi syndrome; however, although proximal tubulopathy is clearly part of the syndrome, it is usually selective.[32] Given the importance of endosomal trafficking for proximal tubular uptake of LMW proteins and a host of other solutes, it is not surprising that LMW proteinuria (retinol-binding protein and β$_2$-microglobulin) is the predominant renal feature in Lowe syndrome. Hypercalciuria with or without nephrocalcinosis is also typically present. In contrast, phosphate wasting and metabolic acidosis are inconsistent features, and glucosuria is rarely seen.[33]

Other clinical features may include glaucoma, seizures, growth retardation, areflexia, nontender joint swelling and arthropathy, subcutaneous nodules, and platelet dysfunction with increased risk for hemorrhage.[20,34,35] Because circulating vitamin D is bound to an LMW binding protein and is taken up into the proximal tubular epithelial cell through megalin-dependent endocytosis before 1-α-hydroxylation, this process is impaired in Lowe syndrome, as in all other diseases with LMW proteinuria, and rickets can develop.[36]

Behavioral abnormalities within the autistic spectrum are also frequently seen and can be very stressful to the families.[37] Cryptorchidism is seen in approximately one-third of patients, but usually testes descend without medical intervention.[34]

How exactly mutations in *OCRL* cause these variable symptoms is not fully clear. Beyond the role in endocytosis and intracellular trafficking, *OCRL* has also been implicated in a wide range of cellular processes, including regulation of the actin skeleton, cell migration, cell polarity, cell-cell interaction, cytokinesis, mitochondrial function, and cilia formation.[38,39]

## Treatment and prognosis

No specific treatment is available for Lowe syndrome, and management is entirely supportive. In those patients with evidence of acidosis or phosphate wasting, bicarbonate and phosphate supplementation is indicated. Parathyroid hormone (PTH) levels should be checked and, if elevated, treated carefully with 1-α-hydroxylated forms of vitamin D. Oversupplementation could, of course, worsen the hypercalciuria. In those patients with nephrocalcinosis or stones, citrate supplementation should be considered.

The bleeding diathesis can be ameliorated by tranexamic acid (Lysteda), and this should be considered prophylactically before surgical interventions. Carnitine is also lost in the urine, and supplementation in deficient patients can restore normal levels.[40] Lowe syndrome is associated with progressive impairment of kidney function, and ESRD typically occurs in the fourth to fifth decade of life.

## DENT DISEASE

Dent disease is an X-linked recessive disorder characterized by LMW proteinuria (e.g., retinol-binding protein and $\beta_2$-microglobulin) and hypercalciuria, with or without nephrocalcinosis and development of renal stones. Like Lowe syndrome, Dent disease is definable as a selective proximal tubulopathy. Metabolic acidosis is not present, and, indeed, patients have been shown to have normal urinary acidification.[41] Phosphate wasting, aminoaciduria, and glucosuria are rarely present.

## Genetics

The first causative gene was identified as *CLCN5* in 1996.[42] *CLCN5* encodes a chloride ($Cl^-$)–proton antiporter expressed in the PT and involved in endosomal acidification.[43] This likely explains the LMW proteinuria (see Figure 41.2). The hypercalciuria is more difficult to explain. Some evidence suggests that hypercalciuria is partly enteral, rather than being caused by direct impairment of proximal calcium ($Ca^{2+}$) reabsorption:

- Adults are normocalciuric when fasting.[44,45]
- Thiazides, which stimulate proximal tubular $Ca^{2+}$ reabsorption, can lower urinary $Ca^{2+}$ excretion in patients with Dent disease.[46,47]
- Circulating levels of PTH are typically below the mean of the normal range.

Consistent with this evidence, sophisticated observations in a mouse model of Dent disease identified low total levels of vitamin D, yet with an increased ratio of fully hydroxylated vitamin D compared with 25-OH vitamin D.[43] This mouse model did not actually exhibit hypercalciuria, so these results must be interpreted with caution. However, although hypercalciuria is a defining criterion of Dent disease, it can be absent in some patients.[48]

Mutations in *CLCN5* are found in approximately 60% of patients with the clinical features of Dent disease, and in 2004, a second gene was identified in a pedigree in whom linkage to the *CLCN5* locus had been excluded.[49] Surprisingly, affected members of this family were found to have mutations in *OCRL*, the gene responsible for Lowe syndrome (see earlier).[49] Mutations in *OCRL* have since been found in several other affected families, including one of the two boys originally described by Dent and Friedman,[50] and *OCRL* mutations account for approximately 15% of all cases with the clinical diagnosis of Dent disease.[31] These patients are often referred to as having Dent2 disease.

---

### KEY POINTS

- Dent disease is characterized by LMW proteinuria (e.g., retinol-binding protein and $\beta_2$-microglobulin) and hypercalciuria.
- PTH level is typically suppressed.
- Thiazide diuretics may improve hypercalciuria.

---

### KEY POINTS

- *CLCN5* gene mutations account for majority of patients with Dent disease.
- *OCRL* gene mutation, which causes Lowe disease, is seen some (15%) patients with Dent disease (known as Dent2).

The identification of *OCRL* mutations in Dent disease created a genetic dilemma: how can mutations in one gene cause two different diseases? Mutation analysis does not provide an immediate answer. Although there is some clustering of mutations, in that frameshift and nonsense mutations underlying Dent disease are found in the first 7 exons, whereas those associated with the clinical phenotype of Lowe syndrome are usually in exons 8 to 23. This does not provide an obvious explanation because these mutations should lead to complete loss of function.[31] Use of an alternative start methionine in exon 8 has been hypothesized, but such variants have not actually been demonstrated, neither on the mRNA nor the protein level.[51]

Clinical observations suggest a spectrum of severity associated with *OCRL* mutations that can range from isolated renal involvement consistent with Dent disease to the multiorgan disorder of Lowe.[52] Thus, patients classified as having Dent2 disease can have some mental impairment, as well as growth failure and elevated muscle enzymes.[52] This finding has been further supported by the report of two brothers with the same mutation, one diagnosed with Dent2 disease and the other with Lowe syndrome.[31]

## Treatment and prognosis

No specific treatment of Dent disease exists. A low-Na+ diet is recommended to minimize hypercalciuria. Thiazides should be considered in patients with nephrocalcinosis and stones. Even though intestinal $Ca^{2+}$ absorption clearly contributes to the hypercalciuria, calcium intake should not be restricted because this is associated with higher oxalate absorption and increased stone risk.[53,54] Citrate supplementation can decrease the tendency for $Ca^{2+}$ precipitation.[55]

Severe stone disease is extremely rare in childhood and should be managed in conjunction with a urologist.

Progression to ESRD occurs in a large subset of patients with Dent disease, typically in the fourth to fifth decade of life. The mechanism is unclear and not necessarily related to the stone burden because progressive decline in kidney function has also been observed in patients without nephrocalcinosis.[56]

## DISORDERS OF THICK ASCENDING LIMB OF LOOP OF HENLE

## PHYSIOLOGY

The TAL is involved in three key functions:

1. Salt reabsorption
2. Urinary dilution or generation of the interstitial concentration gradient
3. $Ca^{2+}$ and magnesium ($Mg^{2+}$) reabsorption

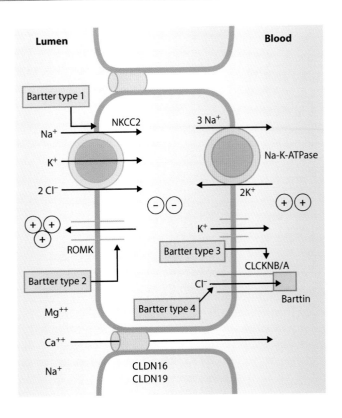

Figure 41.3 Molecular pathogenesis of Bartter syndrome types. Schematic of an epithelial cell in the thick ascending limb of Henle. Apical sodium (Na+) uptake is mediated by the furosemide-sensitive Na+, potassium (K+), 2 chloride (Cl−) cotransporter NKCC2 (SLC12A1), which is mutated in Bartter syndrome type 1. This transporter can function only when it is fully loaded (i.e., it has bound 1 Na+, 1 K+, and 2 Cl− ions). Because the concentration of these electrolytes is similar to those in plasma (given that absorption in the preceding proximal tubule is isotonic), the availability of K+ becomes rate limiting. To ensure an adequate supply, K+ is recycled by the apical K+ channel ROMK (KCNJ1), mutated in Bartter syndrome type 2. Together, these two transporters contribute to a transepithelial voltage gradient (indicated by the unequal number of plus signs), which drives paracellular reabsorption of calcium (Ca2+) and magnesium (Mg2+). Basolateral exit of Cl− is mediated by the Cl− channel CLCKNB, mutated in Bartter syndrome type 3 and probably CLCKNA, both of which require the subunit Barttin, which is mutated in Bartter syndrome type 4. ATPase, adenosine triphosphatase. (Adapted from Kleta R, Bockenhauer D. Bartter syndromes and other salt-losing tubulopathies. Nephron Physiol. 2006;104:73–80.)

Molecularly, these three functions are all linked (Figure 41.3). Because the TAL is water impermeable, salt reabsorption through the furosemide-sensitive cotransporter NKCC2 (SLC12A1) leads to urinary dilution and generates the interstitial concentration gradient needed for urinary concentration in the CD. Although NKCC2 transport is electroneutral (1 Na+, 1 potassium [K+], 2 Cl−), recycling of K+ through the K+ channel ROMK (KCNJ1) generates the electrical gradient that drives paracellular reabsorption of $Ca^{2+}$, $Mg^{2+}$, and $Na^+$. $Na^+$ and $Cl^-$ can exit the cell on the basolateral side through the $Na^+/K^+$–adenosine triphosphatase (ATPase) and the $Cl^-$ channel CLCNKB, respectively, thereby completing the transcellular salt reabsorption. Defects in this transcellular transport lead to Bartter syndrome, whereas defects in the paracellular transport lead to familial hypomagnesemia with hypercalciuria and nephrocalcinosis (see Chapter 13).

---

### KEY POINTS

Disorders of TAL transport are:

- Bartter syndrome
- Familial hypomagnesemia with hypercalciuria

---

Importantly, the macula densa is part of the TAL, and thus tubuloglomerular feedback is impaired in Bartter syndrome, with resultant elevated levels of prostaglandin, especially prostaglandin $E_2$, renin, and aldosterone.[57] This situation is further compounded by the hypovolemia secondary to the renal salt losses.

## BARTTER SYNDROME

The incidence of Bartter syndrome is not fully known, but it has been estimated to be approximately 1 in 1,000,000.[58] However, based on the frequency of mutations in two of the known underlying genes (*SLC12A1* and *KCNJ1*; see later) in members of the Framingham Heart Study, the incidence would be estimated to be approximately 1 in 100,000.[59] Some of the difference may reflect the early lethality of the disease.

So far, four different genes have been shown to cause Bartter syndrome independently (see Table 41.1). All these gene defects are directly involved in the transcellular salt reabsorption in TAL (see Figure 41.3) and lead to four different clinical variants of Bartter syndrome, designated types 1 to 4.

1. **Type 1 Bartter syndrome:** *NKCC2 (SLC12A1)*, the apical furosemide-sensitive $Na^+$-$K^+$-2 $Cl^-$ cotransporter.[60]
2. **Type 2 Bartter syndrome:** *ROMK (KCNJ1)*, the apical $K^+$ channel that recycles $K^+$ back into the tubular lumen. This channel is also expressed in the CD (see later), where it mediates $K^+$ secretion.[61]
3. **Type 3 Bartter syndrome:** *CLCNKB*, the basolateral $Cl^-$ channel that mediates $Cl^-$ exit from the epithelial TAL cell into the interstitium.[62]
4. **Type 4 Bartter syndrome:** *BSND*, a necessary subunit for *CLCNKB*, as well as for the related $Cl^-$ channel CLCNKA. *BSND*, together with the 2 $Cl^-$ channels, is also expressed in the inner ear.[63]

### Clinical features and diagnosis

Because salt transport in this segment involves the furosemide-sensitive transporter NKCC2, Bartter syndrome clinically resembles the effects of loop diuretic administration.

Hyperreninemia and hyperaldosteronism are universally seen in all patients because of associated volume depletion, and hypertrophy of the juxtaglomerular apparatus is evident on renal biopsy. Even so, blood pressure is normal or even low. Salt craving is commonly seen in these patients. Often these patients prefer to eat potato chips and salted pickles. Each of the four types of Bartter syndrome has typical clinical characteristics, which can direct diagnosis and genetic testing. Nevertheless, the severity and spectrum of symptoms can be quite variable.[64–68]

### BARTTER SYNDROME TYPES 1 AND 2

Bartter type 1 and type 2 are typically associated with the antenatal form of the disease, manifesting with polyhydramnios and prematurity. However, gene mutations associated with these two types have also been identified in patients presenting later in life. Because ROMK is also mediating $K^+$ secretion in the CD, these patients typically present with hyperkalemia initially, until other $K^+$ channels can compensate, and then hypokalemia ensues. The patient discussed later in Clinical Vignette 41.2 has a typical case of Bartter syndrome type 2. The excretion of $K^+$ in these patients can be markedly impaired, sometimes resulting in the misdiagnosis of these patients as having pseudohypoaldosteronism type 1.[69]

Because the combination of electroneutral $Na^+$-$K^+$-2$Cl^-$ cotransport through NKCC2 and recycling of $K^+$ through ROMK establishes the electrical gradient that drives paracellular transport of $Ca^{2+}$ and $Mg^{2+}$, patients with type 1 and 2 Bartter syndrome typically have hypercalciuria, hypermagnesuria, and nephrocalcinosis. Polyuria is most pronounced in these two forms of Bartter syndrome. Often, patients have markedly impaired urinary concentrating ability consistent with a secondary form of nephrogenic diabetes insipidus.[14,70] Indeed, some of these patients are initially misdiagnosed as having nephrogenic diabetes insipidus.[71,72]

### BARTTER SYNDROME TYPE 3

Bartter syndrome type 3 is the cause of what is sometimes called "classical Bartter syndrome," with onset during childhood and matching the initial description of the syndrome by Frederick Bartter.[73] Nevertheless, patients are born with a history of polyhydramnios and prematurity, rarely needing amniocentesis. Patients with Bartter syndrome type 3

---

### KEY POINTS

- Bartter types 1, 2, and 4 usually have antenatal or neonatal presentation of the disease.
- Bartter type 2 may be characterized by hyperkalemia, rather than hypokalemia, in the neonatal period.
- Bartter type 3 is the "classic Bartter syndrome."
- Bartter 4 has associated deafness.
- Gene defects in a significant minority of patients with Bartter syndrome have yet to be identified.

typically have the most marked serum electrolyte abnormalities.[64] The reason may be the expression of the channel also in the DCT, thus affecting salt reabsorption in this segment. Indeed, some patients with Bartter syndrome type 3 can have a clinical picture closely resembling Gitelman syndrome, with marked hypomagnesemia.[65]

### BARTTER SYNDROME TYPE 4

Bartter syndrome type 4 has usually severe antenatal onset, and because of the expression of *BSND* in the inner ear, these patients also have profound congenital deafness. Nevertheless, milder variants associated with mutations that likely provide residual function have been described.[74] Although *CLCKNB* is also expressed in the inner ear, it is not associated with deafness, presumably because of compensation from *CLCNKA*. Similar compensation in the kidney may also explain the usually milder phenotype of type 3 Bartter syndrome compared with type 4. This notion is supported by the finding of a severe type 4–like form of Bartter syndrome in a child with homozygous mutations in both *CLCNKA* and *CLCNKB*.[75]

Despite the identification of the four genes, a substantial minority of patients with a clinical diagnosis of Bartter syndrome will not have causative mutations identified, thus suggesting further genetic heterogeneity. However, not all patients with hypokalemic, hypochloremic alkalosis and low blood pressure have Bartter syndrome. A similar clinical picture can sometimes be seen in autosomal dominant hypocalcemia caused by heterozygous gain-of-function mutations in the $Ca^{2+}$-sensing receptor CaSR,[76] a finding demonstrating the importance of the CaSR in the regulation of TAL activity.[76,77]

Mitochondrial cytopathies have also been reported rarely to phenocopy Bartter syndrome.[78–80] Persistent furosemide intake obviously mimics Bartter syndrome. More commonly, however, the plasma biochemical profile of Bartter syndrome is seen in nonrenal salt-wasting states, so-called pseudo-Bartter syndromes (Table 41.4).[81–84] The distinction can easily be made by assessing urinary $Cl^-$ excretion, which is elevated in renal salt wasting, but very low with extrarenal salt wasting. This can be difficult sometimes in babies with congenital $Cl^-$ diarrhea, when the clear diarrheal fluid in the diaper is confused with urine.[85]

## Treatment and prognosis

The mainstays of treatment are prostaglandin synthesis inhibition and electrolyte supplementation. Indomethacin is commonly used for the former, as well as other nonsteroidal agents, such as ibuprofen.[86,87] The main complications are gastric ulcer and bleeding, and coadministration of inhibitors of gastric acid production should always be considered. Selective cyclooxygenase-2 (COX-2) inhibitors have been used successfully to avoid these gastrointestinal complications, but their adoption into routine practice has been hindered by the withdrawal of most of these agents from the market because of increased cardiovascular complications.[88–90] Antenatal

**Table 41.4 Causes of pseudo-Bartter syndrome in children**

- Cystic fibrosis
- Persistent vomiting (infantile hypertrophic pyloric stenosis)
- Eating disorders (induced vomiting)
- Neonates of mothers with eating disorders
- Congenital chloride diarrhea
- Mitochondrial cytopathies
- Diuretic overuse and surreptitious intake
- Long-standing laxative use
- Prostaglandin use in neonates with patent ductus arteriosus
- Aminoglycoside use and toxicity
- Magnesium depletion

administration of indomethacin has been described in cases of severe polyhydramnios, but it should be considered carefully with respect to potential complications (e.g., closure of the ductus arteriosus).[91] Similarly, early administration in premature infants can be associated with severe complications, such as necrotizing enterocolitis.[92,93]

Hypokalemia is part of the syndrome and can be marked ($K^+$ less than 2.0 mmol/L), especially in Bartter syndrome types 3 and 4. The relevance and treatment of this hypokalemia are controversial: long-term electrocardiographic monitoring in patients with Bartter syndrome revealed few potentially dangerous abnormalities in one study, yet there are several anecdotal reports of sudden cardiac death and rhabdomyolysis in children with hypokalemic tubulopathies.[94–96] In an attempt to normalize plasma $K^+$ levels, often enormous doses of $K^+$ supplements are prescribed; these can be difficult to manage for the patient and lead to gastrointestinal problems, such as vomiting and ulcers.

The primary defect in Bartter syndrome is impaired $Na^+$ reabsorption, and $K^+$ wasting reflects the renal response to maintain volume homeostasis. Consequently, generous salt supplementation (up to 10 mmol/kg) can help ameliorate the hypokalemia.[86,88] Indeed, most patients with this syndrome have a craving for salty foods, but even with a high-salt Western diet, it is difficult to achieve the necessary supplementation with food alone. Recognizing the importance of volume homeostasis, the use of $K^+$-sparing diuretics and inhibitors of the renin-angiotensin system to increase $K^+$ levels may lead to serious hypovolemia, especially when there are extra volume losses, such as during a gastrointestinal illness.

---

### KEY POINTS

- $Na^+$ supplementation is key in the treatment of Bartter syndrome.
- Treatment with adequate salt intake may help in the management of hypokalemia.

## Prognosis

The overall prognosis for Bartter syndrome itself is good, although those patients with the antenatal form may have complications of the prematurity.[64,97] Some patients, especially those with Bartter syndrome type 3, develop proteinuria and focal glomerulosclerosis later in life, with progressive chronic kidney disease.[98,99] Associated growth hormone deficiency has also been reported in Bartter syndrome type 3, and it may be related to the severe electrolyte imbalance.[99,100] Clinical Vignette 41.2 describes a case of Bartter syndrome type 2 in a neonate.

### Clinical Vignette 41.2

A 3-day-old newborn boy in the neonatal intensive care unit was noted to have large urine output of 250 to 300 mL/kg/day, with concomitant weight loss of more than 15% of the birth weight. The baby was born at 25 weeks of gestation as a result of premature contractions, which occurred during an amniocentesis procedure. The pregnancy had been complicated by severe polyhydramnios, and there had been two previous amniocentesis procedures performed, each draining between 3 and 5 L. Serum chemistry studies revealed hypernatremia ($Na^+$, 151 mmol/L), hyperkalemia ($K^+$, 6.4 mmol/L), metabolic alkalosis ($HCO_3^-$, 28 mmol/L), and elevated creatinine (58 mmol/L, or 0.65 mg/dL).

Intravenous fluids were administered to maintain fluid balance, and serum plasma sodium levels were normalized. The baby failed to gain weight adequately, and over the following weeks a gradual correction of hyperkalemia was noted; eventually, he developed hypokalemia ($K^+$, 3.1 mmol/L). A diagnosis of Bartter syndrome type 2 was made, and treatment with indomethacin and salt supplementation was commenced. This led to a substantial reduction in urine output and an improvement in weight gain. An ultrasound scan of the kidney revealed marked nephrocalcinosis.

## DISORDERS OF DISTAL CONVOLUTED TUBULE

### PHYSIOLOGY

The DCT is involved in two key functions:

1. Salt reabsorption
2. $Ca^{2+}$ and $Mg^{2+}$ reabsorption

As in all the other nephron segments, the molecular basis for transport of these three ions is linked (Figure 41.4). All these ions are transported transcellularly (i.e. across the epithelial cell). $Na^+$ and $Cl^-$ are transported across the apical membrane by the thiazide-sensitive $Na^+Cl^-$ cotransporter

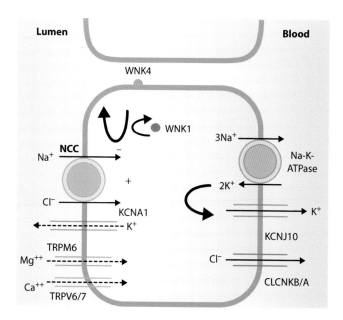

Figure 41.4 Schematic of the distal convoluted tubule epithelial cell ion transport. $Na^+$ is reabsorbed by the apical thiazide-sensitive $Na^+$-$Cl^-$ cotransporter NCC, mutations in which cause Gitelman syndrome. The driving force for $Na^+$ uptake is generated by the basolateral $Na^+$-$K^+$–adenosine triphosphatase ($Na^+$-$K^+$-ATPase), as in all other segments, and this transporter also provides a basolateral exit pathway. The function of this pump is critically dependent on an adequate supply of $K^+$. This is provided by the basolateral $K^+$ channel KCNJ10, mutated in EAST syndrome. Recycling of $K^+$ through this channel also provides the voltage gradient for basolateral $Cl^-$ exit through CLCNKB, mutated in Bartter syndrome type 3. Because of this expression in the distal convoluted tubule, Bartter syndrome type 3 can mimic Gitelman syndrome. Apical entry for $Mg^{2+}$ and $Ca^{2+}$ is provided by the ion channels TRPM6 and TRPV6 and 7, respectively. The necessary voltage gradient is provided by apical $K^+$ exit through $K^+$ channels, such as KCNA1. (Adapted from Kleta R, Bockenhauer D. Bartter syndromes and other salt-losing tubulopathies. Nephron Physiol. 2006;104:73–80.)

NCC (SLC12A3) and exit the cell by the basolateral $Na^+$/$K^+$-ATPase and $Cl^-$ channel CLCNKB. Apical $K^+$ channels including KCNA1 provide the electrical gradient, which enables $Mg^{2+}$ and $Ca^{2+}$ uptake through TRPM6/7 and TRPV5, respectively. Basolateral exit for $Ca^{2+}$ is provided by an $Na^+$/$Ca^{2+}$ exchanger NCX1 and a $Ca^{2+}$ pump PMCA1b.[101] Exit for $Mg^{2+}$ occurs through CNNM2.[102] Most of these molecular players have been identified through genetic investigations of inherited disorders, and more genes may be discovered in the future, thereby identifying additional transport molecules.

### GITELMAN SYNDROME

Gitelman syndrome is a recessive disease caused by inactivating mutations in NCC.[103] Not surprisingly, because *CLCKNB* is also expressed in DCT, it is a rare disorder, with an estimated incidence based on the frequency of heterozygous mutations in NCC in the general population of approximately 1 in 10,000 to 1 in 50,000, although the incidence may be higher in some populations.[59,104,105] Bartter syndrome type 3 can often resemble the clinical picture of Gitelman syndrome.

## Clinical features and diagnosis

Gitelman syndrome is characterized by the combination of hypokalemic, hypochloremic alkalosis with hypomagnesemia and hypocalciuria (see Table 41.1), and the diagnosis can be confirmed by genetic testing. Gitelman syndrome is often described as the benign variant of Bartter syndrome, and many patients are discovered incidentally because of cramps, dizziness, aches, and fatigue.[107] Moreover, severe complications such as rhabdomyolysis and cardiac arrhythmias have been reported.[95,96,108] In later adult years, systemic calcifications, such as chondral and scleroidal calcinosis, may occur.[109,110]

---

### KEY POINTS

- Gitelman syndrome resembles Bartter syndrome and is characterized by hypochloremic metabolic alkalosis and hypokalemia.
- Gitelman syndrome is characterized by hypomagnesemia and hypocalciuria.
- Bartter syndrome, on the other hand, has normal magnesium level and hypercalciuria or normocalciuria.

---

## Treatment and prognosis

The mainstay of treatment of Gitelman syndrome is electrolyte supplementation. As in the case of Bartter syndrome (see earlier), it is important to recognize that the hypokalemia is a secondary consequence of impaired salt reabsorption, and consequently NcCl supplementation is important. In addition, $K^+$ and $Mg^{2+}$ supplementation are used, but normal plasma levels are difficult to achieve, and blood results obviously vary with respect to timing after the last dose.

The use of prostaglandin synthesis inhibitors in Gitelman syndrome has not been well established, and indeed urinary prostaglandin values are usually normal or only moderately elevated.[111,112] As in Bartter syndrome, the use of $K^+$-sparing diuretics and inhibitors of the renin-angiotensin system should be carefully considered with respect to the risk of hypovolemia. Clinical Vignette 41.3 describes a case of Gitelman syndrome in a young child.

---

### Clinical Vignette 41.3

A 5-year-old boy was referred for persistent and unexplained hypokalemia. This was first noted during a diarrheal illness 1 month earlier and was confirmed twice in absence of diarrhea. A subsequent aldosterone level was elevated at 1280 pmol/L. Past medical history and family history were unremarkable. Physical examination revealed a well-appearing boy with a weight and height in the 75th percentile for age and blood pressure of 90/60 mm Hg. Plasma biochemistry studies revealed hypokalemia ($K^+$, 2.8 mmol/l), hypochloremia ($Cl^-$, 97 mmol/L), metabolic alkalosis ($HCO_3^-$, 30 mmol/L), and hypomagnesemia ($Mg^{2+}$, 0.56 mmol/L, or 1.36 mg/dL). A 24-h urine collection demonstrated $Ca^{2+}$ excretion of less than 0.025 mmol/kg/day (less than 1 mg/kg/day) of $Ca^{2+}$.

The diagnosis of Gitelman syndrome was based on the findings of hypokalemic metabolic alkalosis, hypomagnesemia, and hypocalciuria and confirmed by genetic testing.

---

## EPILEPSY, ATAXIA, SENSORINEURAL DEAFNESS, AND A RENAL SALT-LOSING TUBULOPATHY (EAST) SYNDROME

EAST syndrome is a recessive disorder caused by mutations in the $K^+$ channel KCNJ10 (Kir4.1); EAST is an acronym for epilepsy, ataxia, sensorineural deafness, and tubulopathy.[113] The disorder has also been described as SeSAME syndrome.[114] It is an extremely rare disorder, with fewer than 50 patients worldwide described in the literature.

## Clinical features and diagnosis

Patients exhibit the typical biochemical profile of impaired salt reabsorption in DCT (i.e., a Gitelman-like tubulopathy). However, the neurologic symptoms dominate, and most patients present in the first year of life with generalized seizures.[115] Later, ataxia and developmental delay are noted. The severity of all cardinal symptoms can vary markedly, even within families, with some patients confined to wheelchairs because of the movement disorder.

## Treatment and prognosis

Treatment is entirely supportive and involves antiepileptic medications, as well as electrolyte supplementation. The neurologic symptoms are independent of the electrolyte imbalance, and thus attempts to normalize plasma electrolytes have no apparent influence on seizure frequency.[115]

## PSEUDOHYPOALDOSTERONISM TYPE 2: GORDON SYNDROME

Pseudohypoaldosteronism type 2 (PHA2) is a rare inherited disorder of $Na^+$ retention in the DCT. So far, four causative genes have been identified. The first two to be reported were the WNK kinases 1 and 4, which regulate the activity of the thiazide-sensitive $Na^+Cl^-$ cotransporter NCC.[116]

Subsequently, two further genes, *CUL3* and *KLHL3*, have been described, which are likely involved in ubiquitination of either the WNK kinases or NCC.[117] Mutations in all four genes are dominantly inherited, although *KLHL3* is also associated with recessive inheritance.

## Clinical features and diagnosis

PHA2 is often referred to as the "mirror image of Gitelman syndrome" because patients exhibit the opposite symptoms.[118] Physiologically, this makes sense, given that Gitelman syndrome is caused by impaired function of NCC, whereas PHA2 is caused by overactivity of the transporter. Thus, patients have hypertension and hyperkalemic, hyperchloremic metabolic acidosis with hypercalciuria. Renin is typically suppressed, and aldosterone levels can vary, but they are usually low with respect to the degree of hyperkalemia. Symptoms may not be obvious in younger children, and the diagnosis should not be excluded in at-risk children before they have reached adolescence, unless it is confirmed by genetic testing.

## Treatment and prognosis

Once the diagnosis is established, treatment with thiazide diuretics is indicated. This treatment normalizes all symptoms and thus reduces the risk of the hypertension-related complications.

## DISORDERS OF COLLECTING DUCT

## PHYSIOLOGY

Although only approximately 5% of filtered Na+ is reabsorbed in this segment, the CD is critically important because this is the segment were salt reabsorption is highly regulated to adjust urine composition to physiologic needs. Na+ is reabsorbed transcellularly, first entering the principal cell on the apical side through the epithelial Na+ channel ENaC and exiting on the basolateral side through Na+/K+-ATPase (Figure 41.5). The charge movement from Na+ uptake can be balanced by K+ secretion via the K+ channel ROMK (also expressed in TAL; see earlier), paracellular Cl− reabsorption, and proton secretion from the intercalated cells. In this way, volume, K+ and acid-base balance are all molecularly linked in this segment.

## PSEUDOHYPOALDOSTERONISM TYPE 1

Pseudohypoaldosteronism type 1 (PHA1) is a very rare disorder. Clinically and molecularly, it is separated into two distinct entities: the severe autosomal recessive form caused by loss-of-function mutations in one of the subunits of ENaC[119]; and the milder dominant form, caused by heterozygous loss-of-function mutations in the mineralocorticoid receptor (see Table 41.1).[119,120]

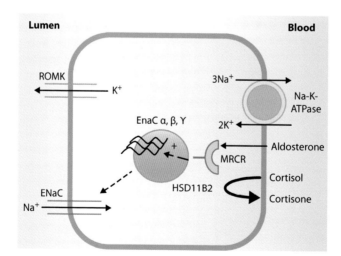

Figure 41.5 Schematic of the collecting duct epithelial cell ion transport. Na+ is reabsorbed in the collecting duct by the epithelial Na+ channel, ENaC. ENaC can be blocked by the diuretic amiloride and is mutated in the recessive form of pseudohypoaldosteronism type 1 (PHA1). Uptake of Na+ creates a favorable gradient for K+ secretion (by ROMK) and proton secretion (from the adjacent intercalated cells; not shown). Expression of ENaC in the membrane is controlled by the mineralocorticoid receptor (MRCR), which is mutated in the dominant form of PHA1. Gain-of-function mutations in this pathway lead to low-renin forms of hypertension, such as Liddle syndrome (ENaC) or hypertension with exacerbation in pregnancy (MRCR). Specificity of the MRCR for mineralocorticoids is provided by HSD11B2, which metabolizes cortisol, which can activate MRCR to cortisol. Loss of function of HSD11B2 leads to apparent mineralocorticoid excess with pathologic activation of MRCR by cortisol. ATPase, adenosine triphosphatase. (Adapted from Kleta R, Bockenhauer D. Bartter syndromes and other salt-losing tubulopathies. Nephron Physiol. 2006;104:73–80.)

## Clinical features and diagnosis

Patients with the recessive form usually present in the neonatal period or early in infancy with severe dehydration and failure to thrive. Laboratory investigations reveal hyponatremia and marked hyperkalemic acidosis, with dramatically elevated renin and aldosterone levels.[121] In some instances, even antenatal presentation with polyhydramnios has been reported.[122,123] Because ENaC mediates salt reabsorption not only in the kidney, but also in the skin, colon, and tracheal and oropharyngeal epithelium, patients have increased salt losses from sweat, skin, saliva, and the gut. Moreover, cystic fibrosis–like pulmonary involvement from impaired $Na^+$-dependent liquid reabsorption in the trachea can be seen.[124] The high salt content of the sweat can cause skin inflammation resembling miliaria rubra.[125]

In contrast to the systemic manifestations seen in recessive PHA1, the dominant form manifests only with renal involvement, reflecting the restricted expression of the underlying mineralocorticoid receptor. Patients typically present in infancy with failure to thrive, and biochemical investigations reveal the typical electrolyte profile of PHA1 (see earlier and Box 41.2). Symptoms typically improve with time, and in adulthood, even aldosterone levels may have normalized.[121]

## Treatment and prognosis

The treatment of PHA1 hinges on salt replacement. In the dominant form, supplementation with NaCl is usually sufficient to normalize electrolytes and allow the child to thrive, and treatment can usually be stopped after a few years. Consequently, the prognosis for the dominant form is excellent. In contrast, the recessive form is often characterized by life-threatening episodes of severe hypovolemia and hyperkalemia. Mortality rates are high, if these episodes are not recognized early and treated aggressively by volume supplementation with normal saline. Hyperkalemia can be dramatic ($K^+$ greater than 10 mmol/L), but the condition responds well to volume expansion. Baseline supplementation with large doses (10 to 20 mmol/kg/day each) of NaCl and $NaHCO_3$ is often needed. NaCl supplementation with doses as high as 50 mmol/kg/day has been reported, but it may be difficult to administer orally.[126] $Na^+/K^+$ exchange

resins, such as sodium polystyrene sulfate, can provide a steady source of $Na^+$ and help stabilize $K^+$ levels.

The diagnosis of PHA1 is easily made by the typical biochemical profile, with inappropriately high $Na^+$ and low $K^+$ excretion in the urine. The systemic (recessive) form can be confirmed by the high $Na^+$ and $Cl^-$ content of the sweat. Genetic testing demonstrating either recessive mutations in one of the ENaC subunits or a heterozygous mutation in *NR3C2* will help establish a definitive diagnosis. Clinical Vignette 41.4 illustrates a case of recessive PHA1 in a neonate.

---

### Clinical Vignette 41.4

A 6-day-old girl presented acutely with irritability, vomiting, and lethargy. Pregnancy was uncomplicated, and the child was born at term with a birth weight of 2.66 kg. Parents were first cousins, and there is a history of early child loss in the extended family. Physical examination: weight, 2.35 kg; blood pressure, 56/palpation; poor skin turgor.

Serum chemistry studies revealed moderate hyponatremia ($Na^+$, 128 mmol/L), severe hyperkalemia ($K^+$, 8.8 mmol/L), and metabolic acidosis ($HCO_3^-$, 12 mmol/L), with severely elevated levels of renin and aldosterone. After repeated normal saline boluses and bicarbonate administration, her clinical status and her serum chemistry results improved. She received oral supplementation with sodium chloride, sodium bicarbonate, and sodium polystyrene sulfonate. However, she had repeated hospitalizations for respiratory infections. Bronchoalveolar lavage revealed colonization with *Pseudomonas aeruginosa*. A sweat test showed elevated sweat $Na^+$ concentration (135 mmol/L).

---

## MISCELLANEOUS TUBULOPATHIES

Glucocorticoid-remediable aldosteronism (GRA), Liddle syndrome (LS), hypertension with exacerbation in pregnancy (HEP), and apparent mineralocorticoid excess (AME) are all very rare disorders. All these disorders represent mirror images of PHA1 and are characterized by overactive $Na^+$ reabsorption by ENaC in the CD, thus leading to hypervolemia with hypertension. As discussed earlier, PHA1 is caused by loss-of-function mutations in the mineralocorticoid receptor or ENaC, whereas HEP and LS are caused by gain of function in these proteins.[127,128] In GRA, unequal meiotic crossover results in a chimeric gene that fuses regulatory sequences of steroid 11β-hydroxylase to coding sequences of aldosterone synthase.[129] Consequently, adrenocorticotropic hormone (ACTH) then drives aldosterone production. As expected for these gain-of-function disorders, LS, HEP, and GRA are inherited dominantly, whereas AME, representing loss of function of the

---

### KEY POINT

Early diagnosis and treatment of disorders of excess sodium reabsorption are critical to avoid potentially devastating consequences of uncontrolled and severe hypertension.

$11\beta$-hydroxysteroid dehydrogenase type 2 *(HSD11B2)*, is autosomal recessive.[130]

The study of AME has provided interesting insights: the mineralocorticoid receptor itself is not specific for mineralocorticoids, but it is also sensitive to glucocorticoids, such as cortisol. To establish specificity, cortisol is metabolized in the principal cells of the CD by HSD11B2 and consequently, impaired function of this enzyme leads to pathologic activation of the receptor by cortisol, which is present in plasma at roughly 1000-fold the concentration of aldosterone.[131] A similar problem with specificity of the receptor is seen in HEP, in which the mutation makes the mineralocorticoid receptor more susceptible to activation by progesterone, thus explaining the exacerbation in pregnancy.

## Clinical features and diagnosis

The clinical picture of these disorders is dominated by hypertension with the biochemical picture of hypokalemic, hypochloremic metabolic alkalosis (hypermineralocorticoid state). Hypertension may be mild or even absent during early childhood in the dominant disorders, but it is usually severe in AME, in which it is associated with early and severe complications, such as stroke and death. *HSD11B2* is also important in the placenta, and AME thus typically manifests antenatally, with the fetus being small for gestational age. Renin levels are suppressed in all four disorders, as is aldosterone, except for GRA, which manifests with excess aldosterone. The hypervolemia leads to decreased $Na^+$ reabsorption in the PT with consequent hypercalciuria and is associated with a urinary concentrating defect and polyuria.[14,71]

The presence of hypertension with the biochemical profile of hypokalemic, hypochloremic metabolic alkalosis and suppressed renin should always prompt consideration of any of these disorders. Even in the dominantly inherited forms, the diagnosis may not have been established despite a strong family history of hypertension, early cardiovascular complications, or unexplained early death. Genetic testing can confirm the diagnosis.

## Treatment and prognosis

Because all four disorders ultimately lead to excess $Na^+$ reabsorption by ENaC, treatment concentrates on blockade of this pathway by ENaC blockers, such as amiloride. Antagonists of the mineralocorticoid receptor may also be helpful, except in LS, because the defect in LS is downstream of the receptor. GRA, as the name implies, can also be treated by glucocorticoid administration, which suppresses ACTH, the driver of the excess aldosterone production in this disorder.

The prognosis depends mostly on timely establishment of the diagnosis and initiation of the correct treatment. Without this treatment, patients are liable to experience the potentially severe cardiovascular consequences of uncontrolled hypertension.[132]

## SUMMARY

Disorders of renal tubules, or tubulopathies, comprise a diverse group of conditions that are characterized by defects in the transport of water and electrolytes. Bartter syndrome and Fanconi syndrome are examples of tubulopathies seen in infants and children. Clinical suspicion of a tubulopathy in a child can involve a variety of symptoms, including failure to thrive, polyuria, and severe abnormalities of electrolytes and acid-base metabolism. Characterization of the gene defects involved in the pathogenesis of various tubulopathies since the 1990s has led to a better understanding of the clinical and biochemical abnormalities seen in these patients. Although treatment of these patients is characteristically simple, relief of the electrolyte abnormalities may be difficult to achieve because of massive urinary losses of specific electrolytes. Development of targeted therapies that influence various channel transports in the nephron may provide therapeutic alternatives in these patients.

## REFERENCES

1. Bokenkamp A, Ludwig M. Disorders of the renal proximal tubule. Nephron Physiol. 2011;118:1–6.
2. Birn H, Christensen EI. Renal albumin absorption in physiology and pathology. Kidney Int. 2006;69:440–9.
3. Christensen EI, Gburek J. Protein reabsorption in renal proximal tubule-function and dysfunction in kidney pathophysiology. Pediatr Nephrol. 2004;19:714–21.
4. Santer R, Kinner M, Lassen CL, et al. Molecular analysis of the SGLT2 gene in patients with renal glucosuria. J Am Soc Nephrol. 2003;14:2873–82.
5. De Toni G. Remarks on the relationship between renal rickets (renal dwarfism) and renal diabetes. Acta Pediatr. 1933;16:479–84.
6. Debre R, Marie J, Cleret F, Messimy R. Rachitisme tardif coexistant avec une nephrite chronique et une glycosurie. Arch Med Enfants. 1934;37:597–606.
7. Fanconi G. Der fruehinfantile nephrotisch-glykosurische Zwergwuchs mit hypophosphataemischer Rachitis. Jahrbuch fuer Kinderheilkd. 1936;147:299–338.
8. Bockenhauer D, van't Hoff W. Fanconi syndrome. In: Geary DF, Schaefer F, editors. Comprehensive Pediatric Nephrology. Philadelphia: Mosby Elsevier; 2008. p. 433–50.
9. Gahl WA, Thoene JG, Schneider JA. Cystinosis. N Engl J Med. 2002;347:111–21.
10. Town M, Jean G, Cherqui S, et al. A novel gene encoding an integral membrane protein is mutated in nephropathic cystinosis. Nat Genet. 1998;18:319–24.

11. Schneider JA, Bradley K, Seegmiller JE. Increased cystine in leukocytes from individuals homozygous and heterozygous for cystinosis. Science. 1967;157:1321–2.

12. Wilmer MJ, Emma F, Levtchenko EN. The pathogenesis of cystinosis: Mechanisms beyond cystine accumulation. Am J Physiol Renal Physiol. 2010;299:F905–16.

13. Norden AG, Scheinman SJ, Deschodt-Lanckman MM, et al. Tubular proteinuria defined by a study of Dent's (CLCN5 mutation) and other tubular diseases. Kidney Int. 2000;57:240–9.

14. Bockenhauer D, van't Hoff W, Dattani M, et al. Secondary nephrogenic diabetes insipidus as a complication of inherited renal diseases. Nephron Physiol. 2010;116:p23–9.

15. Gahl WA, Kuehl EM, Iwata F, et al. Corneal crystals in nephropathic cystinosis: Natural history and treatment with cysteamine eyedrops. Mol Genet Metab. 2000;71:100–20.

16. Anikster Y, Shotelersuk V, Gahl WA. CTNS mutations in patients with cystinosis. Hum Mutat. 1999;14:454–8.

17. Thoene JG, Oshima RG, Crawhall JC, et al. Cystinosis: Intracellular cystine depletion by aminothiols in vitro and in vivo. J Clin Invest. 1976;58:180–9.

18. Nesterova G, Gahl WA. Cystinosis: The evolution of a treatable disease. Pediatr Nephrol. 2013;28:51–9.

19. Besouw MT, Bowker R, Dutertre JP, et al. Cysteamine toxicity in patients with cystinosis. J Pediatr. 2011;159:1004–11.

20. Loi M. Lowe syndrome. Orphanet J Rare Dis. 2006;1:16.

21. Lowe CU, Terrey M, Mac LE. Organic-aciduria, decreased renal ammonia production, hydrophthalmos, and mental retardation: A clinical entity. AMA Am J Dis Child. 1952;83:164–84.

22. Attree O, Olivos IM, Okabe I, et al. The Lowe's oculocerebrorenal syndrome gene encodes a protein highly homologous to inositol polyphosphate-5-phosphatase. Nature. 1992;358:239–42.

23. Zhang X, Jefferson AB, Auethavekiat V, Majerus PW. The protein deficient in Lowe syndrome is a phosphatidylinositol-4,5-bisphosphate 5-phosphatase. Proc Natl Acad Sci U S A. 1995;92:4853–6.

24. Toker A. The synthesis and cellular roles of phosphatidylinositol 4,5-bisphosphate. Curr Opin Cell Biol. 1998;10:254–61.

25. Pirruccello M, De Camilli P. Inositol 5-phosphatases: Insights from the Lowe syndrome protein OCRL. Trends Biochem Sci. 2012;37:134–43.

26. Erdmann KS, Mao Y, McCrea HJ, et al. A role of the Lowe syndrome protein OCRL in early steps of the endocytic pathway. Dev. Cell. 2007;13:377–90.

27. Mao Y, Balkin DM, Zoncu R, et al. A PH domain within OCRL bridges clathrin-mediated membrane trafficking to phosphoinositide metabolism. EMBO J. 2009;28:1831–42.

28. Swan LE, Tomasini L, Pirruccello M, et al. Two closely related endocytic proteins that share a common OCRL-binding motif with APPL1. Proc Natl Acad Sci U S A. 2010;107:3511–6.

29. Noakes CJ, Lee G, Lowe M. The PH domain proteins IPIP27A and B link OCRL1 to receptor recycling in the endocytic pathway. Mol Biol Cell. 2011;22:606–23.

30. Pasternack SM, Bockenhauer D, Refke M, et al. A premature termination mutation in a patient with Lowe syndrome without congenital cataracts: Dropping the "O" in OCRL. Klin Padiatr. 2013;225:29–33.

31. Hichri H, Rendu J, Monnier N, et al. From Lowe syndrome to Dent disease: Correlations between mutations of the OCRL1 gene and clinical and biochemical phenotypes. Hum Mutat. 2011;32:379–88.

32. Kleta R. Fanconi or not Fanconi? Lowe syndrome revisited. Clin J Am Soc Nephrol. 2008;3:1244–5.

33. Bockenhauer D, Bokenkamp A, van't Hoff W, et al. Renal phenotype in Lowe syndrome: A selective proximal tubular dysfunction. Clin J Am Soc Nephrol. 2008;3:1430–6.

34. Recker F, Reutter H, Ludwig M. Lowe syndrome/Dent-2 disease: A comprehensive review of known and novel aspects. J Pediatr Genet. 2013; 2 (2):53-68. DOI: 10.3233/PGE-13049.

35. Lasne D, Baujat G, Mirault T, et al. Bleeding disorders in Lowe syndrome patients: Evidence for a link between OCRL mutations and primary haemostasis disorders. Br J Haematol. 2010;150:685–8.

36. Nykjaer A, Dragun D, Walther D, et al. An endocytic pathway essential for renal uptake and activation of the steroid 25-(OH) vitamin $D_3$. Cell. 1999;96:507–15.

37. Arron K, Oliver C, Moss J, et al. The prevalence and phenomenology of self-injurious and aggressive behaviour in genetic syndromes. J Intellect Disabil Res. 2011;55:109–20.

38. Gobernado JM, Lousa M, Gimeno A, Gonsalvez M. Mitochondrial defects in Lowe's oculocerebrorenal syndrome. Arch Neurol. 1984;41:208–9.

39. Madhivanan K, Mukherjee D, Aguilar RC. Lowe syndrome: Between primary cilia assembly and Rac1-mediated membrane remodeling. Commun Integr Biol. 2012;5:641–4.

40. Gahl WA, Bernardini I, Dalakas M, et al. Oral carnitine therapy in children with cystinosis and renal Fanconi syndrome. J Clin Invest. 1988;81:549–60.

41. Wrong OM, Norden AG, Feest TG. Dent's disease; a familial proximal renal tubular syndrome with low-molecular-weight proteinuria, hypercalciuria, nephrocalcinosis, metabolic bone disease, progressive renal failure and a marked male predominance. QJM. 1994;87:473–93.

42. Lloyd SE, Pearce SH, Fisher SE, et al. A common molecular basis for three inherited kidney stone diseases. Nature. 1996;379:445–9.

43. Piwon N, Gunther W, Schwake M, thet al. ClC-5 Cl⁻-channel disruption impairs endocytosis in a mouse model for Dent's disease. Nature. 2000;408:369–73.

44. Igarashi T, Hayakawa H, Shiraga H, et al. Hypercalciuria and nephrocalcinosis in patients with idiopathic low-molecular-weight proteinuria in Japan: Is the disease identical to Dent's disease in United Kingdom? Nephron. 1995;69:242–7.

45. Reinhart SC, Norden AG, Lapsley M, et al. Characterization of carrier females and affected males with X-linked recessive nephrolithiasis. J Am Soc Nephrol. 1995;5:1451–61.

46. Nijenhuis T, Vallon V, van der Kemp AW, et al. Enhanced passive Ca²⁺ reabsorption and reduced Mg²⁺ channel abundance explains thiazide-induced hypocalciuria and hypomagnesemia. J Clin Invest. 2005;115:1651–8.

47. Raja KA, Schurman S, D'Mello RG, et al. Responsiveness of hypercalciuria to thiazide in Dent's disease. J Am Soc Nephrol. 2002;13:2938–44.

48. Ludwig M, Utsch B, Balluch B, et al. Hypercalciuria in patients with CLCN5 mutations. Pediatr Nephrol. 2006;21:1241–50.

49. Hoopes RR, Jr, Shrimpton AE, Knohl SJ, et al. Dent disease with mutations in OCRL1. Am J Hum Genet. 2005;76:260–7.

50. Dent CE, Friedman M. Hypercalcuric rickets associated with renal tubular damage. Arch Dis Child. 1964;39:240–9.

51. Shrimpton AE, Hoopes RR, Jr, Knohl SJ, et al. OCRL1 mutations in Dent 2 patients suggest a mechanism for phenotypic variability. Nephron Physiol. 2009;112:27–36.

52. Bokenkamp A, Bockenhauer D, Cheong HI, et al. Dent-2 disease: A mild variant of Lowe syndrome. J Pediatr. 2009;155:94–9.

53. Curhan GC, Willett WC, Rimm EB, Stampfer MJ. A prospective study of dietary calcium and other nutrients and the risk of symptomatic kidney stones. N Engl J Med. 1993;328:833–8.

54. Lemann J, Jr, Pleuss JA, Worcester EM, et al. Urinary oxalate excretion increases with body size and decreases with increasing dietary calcium intake among healthy adults. Kidney Int. 1996;49:200–8.

55. Colussi G, De Ferrari ME, Brunati C, Civati G. Medical prevention and treatment of urinary stones. J Nephrol. 2000;13 Suppl 3:S65–70.

56. Scheinman SJ. X-linked hypercalciuric nephrolithiasis: Clinical syndromes and chloride channel mutations. Kidney Int. 1998;53:3–17.

57. Gill JR, Jr. The role of chloride transport in the thick ascending limb in the pathogenesis of Bartter's syndrome. Klin Wochenschr. 1982;60:1212–4.

58. Rudin A. Bartter's syndrome: A review of 28 patients followed for 10 years. Acta Med Scand. 1988;224:165–71.

59. Ji W, Foo JN, O'Roak BJ, et al. Rare independent mutations in renal salt handling genes contribute to blood pressure variation. Nat Genet. 2008;40:592–9.

60. Simon DB, Karet FE, Hamdan JM, et al. Bartter's syndrome, hypokalaemic alkalosis with hypercalciuria, is caused by mutations in the Na-K-2Cl cotransporter NKCC2. Nat Genet. 1996;13:183–8.

61. Simon DB, Karet FE, Rodriguez-Soriano J, et al. Genetic heterogeneity of Bartter's syndrome revealed by mutations in the K⁺ channel, ROMK. Nat Genet. 1996;14:152–6.

62. Simon DB, Bindra RS, Mansfield TA, et al. Mutations in the chloride channel gene, CLCNKB, cause Bartter's syndrome type III. Nat Genet. 1997;17:171–8.

63. Estevez R, Boettger T, Stein V, et al. Barttin is a Cl⁻ channel beta-subunit crucial for renal Cl⁻ reabsorption and inner ear K⁺ secretion. Nature. 2001;414:558–61.

64. Brochard K, Boyer O, Blanchard A, et al. Phenotype-genotype correlation in antenatal and neonatal variants of Bartter syndrome. Nephrol Dial Transplant. 2009;24:1455–64.

65. Jeck N, Konrad M, Peters M, et al. Mutations in the chloride channel gene, CLCNKB, leading to a mixed Bartter-Gitelman phenotype. Pediatr Res. 2000;48:754–8.

66. Konrad M, Vollmer M, Lemmink HH, et al. Mutations in the chloride channel gene CLCNKB as a cause of classic Bartter syndrome. J Am Soc Nephrol. 2000;11:1449–59.

67. Peters M, Jeck N, Reinalter S, et al. Clinical presentation of genetically defined patients with hypokalemic salt-losing tubulopathies. Am J Med. 2002;112:183–90.

68. Pressler CA, Heinzinger J, Jeck N, et al. Late-onset manifestation of antenatal Bartter syndrome as a result of residual function of the mutated renal Na⁺-K⁺-2Cl⁻ co-transporter. J Am Soc Nephrol. 2006;17:2136–42.

69. Nozu K, Fu XJ, Kaito H, et al. A novel mutation in KCNJ1 in a Bartter syndrome case diagnosed as pseudohypoaldosteronism. Pediatr Nephrol. 2007;22:1219–23.

70. Bockenhauer D, Cruwys M, Kleta R, et al. Antenatal Bartter's syndrome: Why is this not a lethal condition? QJM. 2008;101:927–42.

71. Bockenhauer D, Bichet DG. Inherited secondary nephrogenic diabetes insipidus: Concentrating on humans. Am J Physiol Renal Physiol. 2013;304:F1037–42.

72. Bettinelli A, Ciarmatori S, Cesareo L, et al. Phenotypic variability in Bartter syndrome type I. Pediatr Nephrol. 2000;14:940–5.

73. Bartter FC, Pronove P, Gill JR, Jr, Maccardle RC. Hyperplasia of the juxtaglomerular complex with hyperaldosteronism and hypokalemic alkalosis: A new syndrome. Am J Med. 1962;33:811–28.

74. Brum S, Rueff J, Santos JR, Calado J. Unusual adult-onset manifestation of an attenuated Bartter's syndrome type IV renal phenotype caused by a mutation in BSND. Nephrol Dial Transplant. 2007;22:288–9.

75. Schlingmann KP, Konrad M, Jeck N, et al. Salt wasting and deafness resulting from mutations in two chloride channels. N Engl J Med. 2004;350:1314–9.

76. Watanabe S, Fukumoto S, Chang H, et al. Association between activating mutations of calcium-sensing receptor and Bartter's syndrome. Lancet. 2002;360:692–4.

77. Hebert SC. Bartter syndrome. Curr Opin Nephrol Hypertens. 2003;12:527–32.

78. Goto Y, Itami N, Kajii N, et al. Renal tubular involvement mimicking Bartter syndrome in a patient with Kearns-Sayre syndrome. J Pediatr. 1990;116:904–10.

79. Niaudet P, Rotig A. Renal involvement in mitochondrial cytopathies. Pediatr Nephrol. 1996;10:368–73.

80. Emma F, Pizzini C, Tessa A, et al. "Bartter-like" phenotype in Kearns-Sayre syndrome. Pediatr Nephrol. 2006;21:355–60.

81. Koshida R, Sakazume S, Maruyama H, et al. A case of pseudo-Bartter's syndrome due to intestinal malrotation. Acta Paediatrica Jpn. 1994;36:107–11.

82. Mathot M, Maton P, Henrion E, et al. Pseudo-Bartter syndrome in a pregnant mother and her fetus. Pediatr Nephrol. 2006;21:1037–40.

83. Vanhaesebrouck S, Van Laere D, Fryns JP, Theyskens C. Pseudo-Bartter syndrome due to Hirschsprung disease in a neonate with an extra ring chromosome 8. Am J Med Genet A. 2007;143A:2469–72.

84. Horvatovich K, Orkenyi M, Biro E, et al. Pseudo-Bartter syndrome in a case of cystic fibrosis caused by C1529G and G3978A compound heterozygosity. Orv Hetil. 2008;149:325–8 [in Hungarian].

85. Choi M, Scholl UI, Ji W, et al. Genetic diagnosis by whole exome capture and massively parallel DNA sequencing. Proc Natl Acad Sci U S A. 2009;106:19096–101.

86. Kleta R, Bockenhauer D. Bartter syndromes and other salt-losing tubulopathies. Nephron Physiol. 2006;104:73–80.

87. Seyberth HW. An improved terminology and classification of Bartter-like syndromes. Nat Clin Pract Nephrol. 2008;4:560–7.

88. Kleta R, Basoglu C, Kuwertz-Broking E. New treatment options for Bartter's syndrome. N Engl J Med. 2000;343:661–2.

89. Reinalter SC, Jeck N, Brochhausen C, et al. Role of cyclooxygenase-2 in hyperprostaglandin E syndrome/antenatal Bartter syndrome. Kidney Int. 2002;62:253–60.

90. Dogne JM, Hanson J, Supuran C, Pratico D. Coxibs and cardiovascular side-effects: From light to shadow. Curr Pharm Des. 2006;12:971–5.

91. Konrad M, Leonhardt A, Hensen P, et al. Prenatal and postnatal management of hyperprostaglandin E syndrome after genetic diagnosis from amniocytes. Pediatrics. 1999;103:678–83.

92. Proesmans W, Devlieger H, Van Assche A, et al. Bartter syndrome in two siblings: Antenatal and neonatal observations. Int J Pediatr Nephrol. 1985;6:63–70.

93. Ataoglu E, Civilibal M, Ozkul AA, et al. Indomethacin-induced colon perforation in Bartter's syndrome. Indian J Pediatr. 2009;76:322–3.

94. Blomstrom-Lundqvist C, Caidahl K, Olsson SB, Rudin A. Electrocardiographic findings and frequency of arrhythmias in Bartter's syndrome. Br Heart J. 1989;61:274–9.

95. Cortesi C, Lava SA, Bettinelli A, et al. Cardiac arrhythmias and rhabdomyolysis in Bartter-Gitelman patients. Pediatr Nephrol. 2010;25:2005–8.

96. Cortesi C, Bettinelli A, Emma F, et al. Severe syncope and sudden death in children with inborn salt-losing hypokalaemic tubulopathies. Nephrol Dial Transplant. 2005;20:1981–3.

97. Puricelli E, Bettinelli A, Borsa N, et al. Long-term follow-up of patients with Bartter syndrome type I and II. Nephrol Dial Transplant. 2010;25:2976–81.

98. Su IH, Frank R, Gauthier BG, et al. Bartter syndrome and focal segmental glomerulosclerosis: A possible link between two diseases. Pediatr Nephrol. 2000;14:970–2.

99. Bettinelli A, Borsa N, Bellantuono R, et al. Patients with biallelic mutations in the chloride channel gene CLCNKB: Long-term management and outcome. Am J Kidney Dis. 2007;49:91–8.

100. Akil I, Ozen S, Kandiloglu AR, Ersoy B. A patient with Bartter syndrome accompanying severe growth hormone deficiency and focal segmental glomerulosclerosis. Clin Exp Nephrol. 2010;14:278–82.

101. Dimke H, Hoenderop JG, Bindels RJ. Hereditary tubular transport disorders: Implications for renal handling of $Ca^{2+}$ and $Mg^{2+}$. Clin Sci (Lond). 2010;118:1–18.

102. Stuiver M, Lainez S, Will C, et al. CNNM2, encoding a basolateral protein required for renal $Mg^{2+}$ handling, is mutated in dominant hypomagnesemia. Am J Hum Genet. 2011;88:333–43.

103. Simon DB, Nelson-Williams C, Bia MJ, et al. Gitelman's variant of Bartter's syndrome, inherited hypokalaemic alkalosis, is caused by mutations in the thiazide-sensitive Na-Cl cotransporter. Nat Genet. 1996;12:24–30.

104. Fava C, Montagnana M, Rosberg L, et al. Subjects heterozygous for genetic loss of function of the thiazide-sensitive cotransporter have reduced blood pressure. Hum Mol Genet. 2008;17:413–8.

105. Tago N, Kokubo Y, Inamoto N, et al. A high prevalence of Gitelman's syndrome mutations in Japanese. Hypertens Res. 2004;27:327–31.

106. Schepkens H, Lameire N. Gitelman's syndrome: An overlooked cause of chronic hypokalemia and hypomagnesemia in adults. Acta Clin Belg. 2001;56:248–54.

107. Cruz DN, Shaer AJ, Bia MJ, et al. Gitelman's syndrome revisited: An evaluation of symptoms and health-related quality of life. Kidney Int. 2001;59:710–7.

108. Pachulski RT, Lopez F, Sharaf R. Gitelman's not-so-benign syndrome. N Engl J Med. 2005;353:850–1.

109. Garcia Nieto V, Cantabrana A, Muller D, Claverie-Martin F. Chondrocalcinosis and hypomagnesaemia in a patient with a new mutation in the gene of the thiazide-sensitive Na-Cl cotransporter. Nefrologia. 2003;23:504–9 [in Spanish].

110. Gupta R, Hu V, Reynolds T, Harrison R. Sclerochoroidal calcification associated with Gitelman syndrome and calcium pyrophosphate dihydrate deposition. J Clin Pathol. 2005;58:1334–5.

111. Schmidt H, Kabesch M, Schwarz HP, Kiess W. Clinical, biochemical and molecular genetic data in five children with Gitelman's syndrome. Horm Metab Res. 2001;33:354–7.

112. Seyberth HW, Schlingmann KP. Bartter- and Gitelman-like syndromes: Salt-losing tubulopathies with loop or DCT defects. Pediatr Nephrol. 2011;26:1789–802.

113. Bockenhauer D, Feather S, Stanescu HC, et al. Epilepsy, ataxia, sensorineural deafness, tubulopathy, and KCNJ10 mutations. N Engl J Med. 2009;360:1960–70.

114. Scholl UI, Choi M, Liu T, et al. Seizures, sensorineural deafness, ataxia, mental retardation, and electrolyte imbalance (SeSAME syndrome) caused by mutations in KCNJ10. Proc Natl Acad Sci U S A. 2009;106:5842–7.

115. Cross JH, Arora R, Heckemann RA, et al. Neurological features of epilepsy, ataxia, sensorineural deafness, tubulopathy syndrome. Dev Med Child Neurol. 2013;55:846–56.

116. Wilson FH, Disse-Nicodeme S, Choate KA, et al. Human hypertension caused by mutations in WNK kinases. Science. 2001;293:1107–12.

117. Boyden LM, Choi M, Choate KA, et al. Mutations in kelch-like 3 and cullin 3 cause hypertension and electrolyte abnormalities. Nature. 2012;482:98–102.

118. Roser M, Eibl N, Eisenhaber B, et al. Gitelman syndrome. Hypertension. 2009;53:893–7.

119. Chang SS, Grunder S, Hanukoglu A, et al. Mutations in subunits of the epithelial sodium channel cause salt wasting with hyperkalaemic acidosis, pseudohypoaldosteronism type 1. Nat Genet. 1996;12:248–53.

120. Geller DS, Rodriguez-Soriano J, Vallo Boado A, et al. Mutations in the mineralocorticoid receptor gene cause autosomal dominant pseudohypoaldosteronism type I. Nat Genet. 1998;19:279–81.

121. Riepe FG. Clinical and molecular features of type 1 pseudohypoaldosteronism. Horm Res. 2009;72:1–9.

122. Narchi H, Santos M, Kulaylat N. Polyhydramnios as a sign of fetal pseudohypoaldosteronism. Int J Gynaecol Obstet. 2000;69:53–4.

123. Wong GP, Levine D. Congenital pseudohypoaldosteronism presenting in utero with acute polyhydramnios. J Matern Fetal Med. 1998;7:76–8.

124. Kerem E, Bistritzer T, Hanukoglu A, et al. Pulmonary epithelial sodium-channel dysfunction and excess airway liquid in pseudohypoaldosteronism. N Engl J Med. 1999;341:156–62.

125. Martin JM, Calduch L, Monteagudo C, et al. Clinico-pathological analysis of the cutaneous lesions of a patient with type I pseudohypoaldosteronism. J Eur Acad Dermatol Venereol. 2005;19:377–9.

126. Guran T, Degirmenci S, Bulut IK, et al. Critical points in the management of pseudohypoaldosteronism type 1. J Clin Res Pediatr Endocrinol. 2011;3:98–100.

127. Geller DS, Farhi A, Pinkerton N, et al. Activating mineralocorticoid receptor mutation in hypertension exacerbated by pregnancy. Science. 2000;289:119–23.

128. Hansson JH, Schild L, Lu Y, et al. A de novo missense mutation of the beta subunit of the epithelial sodium channel causes hypertension and Liddle syndrome, identifying a proline-rich segment critical for regulation of channel activity. Proc Natl Acad Sci U S A. 1995;92:11495–9.

129. Lifton RP, Dluhy RG, Powers M, et al. Hereditary hypertension caused by chimaeric gene duplications and ectopic expression of aldosterone synthase. Nat Genet. 1992;2:66–74.

130. Stewart PM, Krozowski ZS, Gupta A, et al. Hypertension in the syndrome of apparent mineralocorticoid excess due to mutation of the 11 beta-hydroxysteroid dehydrogenase type 2 gene. Lancet. 1996;347:88–91.

131. Palermo M, Quinkler M, Stewart PM. Apparent mineralocorticoid excess syndrome: An overview. Arq Bras Endocrinol Metabol. 2004;48:687–96.

132. Lifton RP. Genetic dissection of human blood pressure variation: Common pathways from rare phenotypes. Harvey Lect. 2004;100:71–101.

## REVIEW QUESTIONS

1. Hyperkalemia can be associated in the newborn period in which of the following types of Bartter syndrome?
   a. Type 1
   b. Type 2

c. Type 3

d. Type 4

2. Which type of Bartter syndrome is associated with hearing loss?

a. Type 1

b. Type 2

c. Type 3

d. Type 4

3. Barter syndrome is associated with:

a. Normocalciuria

b. Hypercalciuria

c. Hypocalciuria

d. a or b

e. a or c

4. Gitelman syndrome is characterized by:

a. Hypocalciuria

b. Hypercalciuria

c. Normocalciuria

d. None of the above

5. Hypomagnesemia is a feature of:

a. Bartter syndrome

b. Gitelman syndrome

c. Both Bartter syndrome and Gitelman syndrome

d. Neither Bartter syndrome nor Gitelman syndrome

6. Gordon syndrome or pseudohypoaldosteronism-2 is a mirror image of Gitelman syndrome. Both these defects result from a malfunction or disregulation in which of the following transport channels?

a. CLCNKB

b. ENaC

c. ROMK

d. NCC

7. Pseudohypoaldosteronism 1 (PHA1) results from loss-of-function mutations in:

a. The mineralocorticoid receptor or ENaC

b. CLCNKB

c. NKCC2

d. CLCN5

8. Liddle syndrome results from:

a. Loss-of-function mutation of ENaC

b. Gain-of-function mutation of HSD11B2

c. Gain-of-function mutation of ENaC

d. Loss-of-function mutation of TRPM6

9. Transport of low-molecular-weight protein from the tubular lumen in the proximal tubules is facilitated by binding to apical receptors megalin and cubilin.

a. True

b. False

10. Which of the following are features of renal Fanconi syndrome?

a. Hypercalciuria

b. Glucosuria

c. Low-molecular-weight proteinuria

d. Albuminuria

e. All of the above

## ANSWER KEY

1. b

2. d

3. d

4. a

5. b

6. d

7. a

8. c

9. a

10. e

# Renal tubular acidosis

JOHN W. FOREMAN

In renal tubular acidosis (RTA), defective renal tubular function leads to metabolic acidosis, despite normal daily acid production from metabolism and dietary intake. RTA is typically characterized by hyperchloremic metabolic acidosis (HCMA). It can occur sporadically or as a heritable disorder, either as an autosomal dominant or recessive trait, or as part of a more generalized tubular disorder, such as Fanconi syndrome. In its early descriptions, RTA was defined by numerous terms, such as *Lightwood disease* and *infantile tubular acidosis*. Consensus around the classification of RTA into distal and proximal types emerged only after demonstration of defects in urinary acidification and bicarbonate reabsorption in such patients.[1]

## KIDNEY IN ACID-BASE BALANCE

The typical Western diet generates approximately 1 mmol/kg/day of H$^+$ in an adult, and 1 to 3 mEq/kg/day in children and infants.[2,3] Infants and young children generate more daily acid than adults, in part because laying of new bone consumes the buffers (hydroxyl ion) OH$^-$ and phosphate to make hydroxyapatite.[3] Three sequentially acting mechanisms eliminate the new acid generated by daily metabolic activity. The first line of buffering is accomplished by the circulating bicarbonate (HCO$_3^-$) to form carbonic acid (H$_2$CO$_3$), which is converted to water (H$_2$O) and carbon dioxide (CO$_2$) by erythrocyte carbonic anhydrase (CA). The CO$_2$ is eliminated by the second line of buffering process via

the lungs. However, to continue the above two processes, the kidney must regenerate an equivalent amount of HCO$_3^-$, without which the internal milieu will be depleted of bicarbonate reserves (Figure 42.1). In addition, some acids (inorganic acids) must be excreted by the kidney, because these cannot be completely metabolized to CO$_2$ and undergo pulmonary elimination. The renal tubular acid excretion, or net acid excretion (NAE), is composed of (1) titratable acid (TA) production, mainly in the form of monobasic phosphate (H$_2$PO$_4^-$) and (2) ammonium ions (NH$_4^+$). This relationship in is shown as:

$$NAE = TA + NH_4^+ \tag{42.1}$$

### KEY POINTS

- Dietary intake generates approximately 1 mEq/kg of hydrogen ions daily in adults.
- Infants and children produce more acid (1 to 3 mEq/kg/day)

However, any HCO$_3^-$ lost in urine reduces the NAE as represented in Equation 42.2.

$$NAE = TA + NH_4^+ - HCO_3^- \tag{42.2}$$

Organic anions are potential sources of HCO$_3^-$ when completely metabolized. However, if these organic acids are

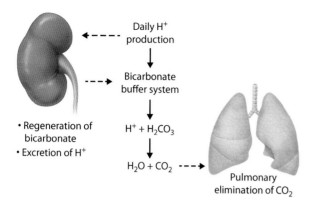

Figure 42.1 Buffering mechanisms involved in elimination of daily metabolic acid load ($H^+$). Kidneys play an important role in the homeostasis by generating new bicarbonate and also elimination of hydrogen ions.

lost in the urine, such as in metabolic disorders, the NAE by the kidney is diminished. This relationship can be expressed by the following equation:

$$NAE = TA + NH_4 - HCO_3^- - \text{Metabolizable anions} \quad (42.3)$$

At a urine pH of less than 6.5, little to no $HCO_3^-$ is present in the urine. Organic acids are not routinely assayed in urine, but their presence can be suspected if there is a significant difference (greater than 100 mOsm/L) between the measured urine osmolality and the calculated osmolality, using the following equation:

$$\text{Calculated } U_{osm} = 2 \times U_{Na} + 2 \times U_K + U_{Urea}/2.8 + U_{Glucose}/18 \quad (42.4)$$

Kidneys generate new bicarbonate ions by recombining $CO_2$ with $H_2O$ in the renal tubular cell (proximal and distal) cytoplasm to form $H^+$ and $HCO_3^-$, a process that is catalyzed by carbonic acid II (CA II). The newly generated $HCO_3^-$ is transported into the blood, replacing the lost $HCO_3^-$ in the initial buffering process. The $H^+$ thus formed is eliminated as buffered monobasic phosphate ($H_2PO_4^-$), or TA, and

### KEY POINTS

- Generated $H^+$ is initially buffered by circulating bicarbonate and bone.
- Eventual elimination of daily acid load occurs via lungs as $CO_2$ and the kidneys via ammonium and as titratable acidity.
- Kidneys also perform the important task of reabsorbing filtered bicarbonate, mainly in the proximal tubules.
- Kidneys also help generate new bicarbonate molecules that replenish the serum bicarbonate lost in initial buffering of $H^+$

as ammonium ($NH_4^+$). The urinary concentration of monobasic phosphate can be modulated over a small range, but $NH_4^+$ generation and excretion can increase by several-fold, especially under the conditions of acidosis. Therefore, the dominant response of the kidneys to acidosis is characterized by an increased $NH_4^+$ production and elimination.

## RENAL HANDLING OF BICARBONATE

In a normal adult, approximately 4500 mEq of bicarbonate is reclaimed daily from the glomerular filtrate (180 L/day glomerular filtrate × 25 mEq/L plasma bicarbonate concentration = 4500 mEq). Approximately 80% to 90% of the filtered load of bicarbonate is reabsorbed in the proximal tubule (Figure 42.2). This is accomplished by the secretion of $H^+$ into the tubular lumen, in exchange for $Na^+$, via the luminal membrane sodium/hydrogen exchanger (NHE$_3$), and to a minor extent by the $H^+$-ATPase pump (Figure 42.3).[4,5] The $H^+$ ion transported into the proximal tubule lumen combines with the filtered bicarbonate to form carbonic acid ($H_2CO_3$). Carbonic acid is further catalyzed to $CO_2$ and $H_2O$, a reaction that is rapidly catalyzed by the luminal carbonic anhydrase IV (CA IV) present on

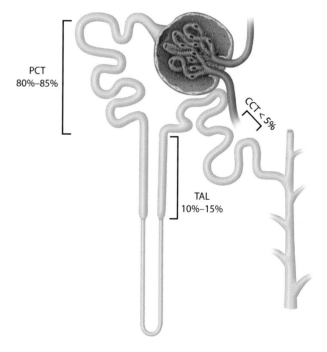

Figure 42.2 Nephron sites of bicarbonate reabsorption. Most filtered bicarbonate is reabsorbed in the proximal nephron, leaving little to none in the excreted urine. CCT, cortical collecting tubule; PCT, proximal convoluted tubule; TAL, thick ascending limb of loop of Henle.

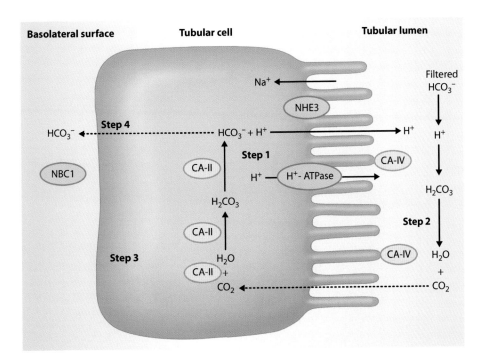

Figure 42.3 A diagrammatic representation of the metabolic process of recapturing filtered bicarbonate in the proximal tubular cells. In the first step, $H^+$ generated in the proximal tubular cell is transported into the tubular lumen via the $Na^+/H^+$ exchanger 3 (NHE3) and the $H^+$-ATPase. In the second step, $H^+$ combines with the filtered $HCO_3^-$ to form $CO_2$ and water (facilitated by apical carbonic anhydrase (CA IV). $CO_2$ diffuses back into the proximal tubular cell, where it recombines with $H_2O$ in step three to reform $HCO_3^-$. Carbonic anhydrase II (CA II) in the cytosol facilitates these steps. In the fourth step, $HCO_3^-$ exits the cell and into the blood via basolateral surface through the $Na^+$-$HCO_3^-$ cotransporter (NBC1).

the apical membrane of the proximal tubule and thick ascending limb of the loop of Henle (TAL). $CO_2$ diffuses into the tubular cell and recombines with $H_2O$, to form bicarbonate, a reaction that is catalyzed by CA II in the cytosol. The $HCO_3^-$ generated in this process exits the tubular cell via the $Na^+$, $HCO_3^-$ exchanger (NBC1), which is coded for by the gene *SLC 4A4*. Three molecules of bicarbonate and one molecule of sodium (Na) are driven out of the tubular cell at this location by NBC1. Additionally, the Na,K-ATPase on the basolateral membrane transports three $Na^+$ ions out of the cell in exchange for two $K^+$ ions, leading to an electrochemical gradient with a negative potential charge relative to the lumen. This electrical gradient favors $Na^+$ entry into the cell from the tubular luminal fluid.[6] Factors that enhance proximal tubular $HCO_3^-$ reabsorption include increased filtered bicarbonate load, low peritubular pH, high $pCO_2$, angiotensin II (ATII), extracellular volume contraction, and potassium depletion.

The TAL reabsorbs the majority of $HCO_3^-$ escaping the proximal tubule. Apical $Na^+/H^+$ exchange (NHE3) mediates most of $H^+$ secretion into the lumen in this nephron segment. The $HCO_3^-$ regenerated in the TAL cell can exit via several transporters including $Na^+/HCO_3^-$ and $K^+/HCO_3^-$ cotransporters and the $Cl^-/HCO_3^-$ exchanger on the basolateral surface. (Figure 42.4). The distal nephron is responsible for reabsorption of the remainder of the filtered $HCO_3^-$ still present (less than 5%) in the tubular fluid (urine).

## KEY POINTS

- Filtered bicarbonate is predominantly reabsorbed in the proximal tubule (approximately 90%).
- Remainder of bicarbonate (approximately 10% to 15%) is reabsorbed in the thick ascending limb of the loop of Henle.
- NCB1 transports bicarbonate across the basolateral surface from the proximal tubular cell.
- CA IV present in the luminal brush border facilitates bicarbonate reabsorption into the tubular cells from the lumen.

## DISTAL TUBULAR ACIDIFICATION

The distal nephron dominantly participates in the acidification of urine, in addition to mopping up any filtered bicarbonate still present in the tubular fluid. Elimination of hydrogen and potassium ions occurs in an integrated manner in this nephron segment. The distal nephron consists of three distinct functional segments: the cortical collecting tubule (CCT), the outer medullary collecting tubule (OMCT), and the inner medullary collecting tubule (IMCT).[7] Two distinct types of cells that have been identified in the distal collecting

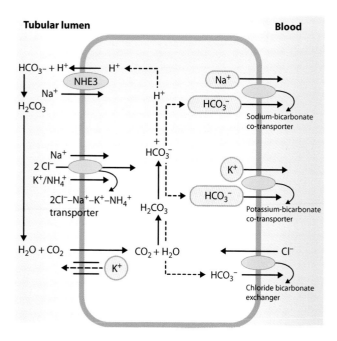

Figure 42.4 Electrolyte transport processes in the thick ascending limb (TAL) of the loop of Henle involved in recapture of the filtered bicarbonate that escapes the proximal tubule. The filtered HCO₃⁻ is reabsorbed by combining with the H⁺ secreted into the tubular lumen via the Na⁺/H⁺ exchanger 3 (NHE3). Re-synthesis of bicarbonate occurs in the tubular cells from CO₂. HCO₃⁻ exits the cell along the basolateral surface via multiple transporters: Na⁺/HCO₃⁻ cotransporter, K⁺/HCO₃⁻ cotransporter, and the Cl⁻/HCO₃⁻ exchanger. NH₄⁺ can enter the tubular cell in place of K⁺ on the 2Cl⁻/Na⁺,K⁺ transporter for recycling in the medullary interstitium.

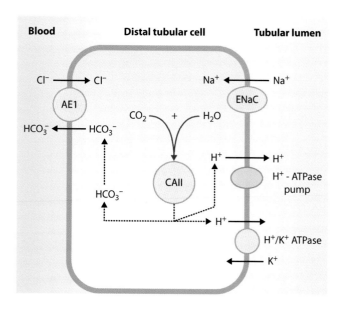

Figure 42.5 H⁺ ion excretion process in the cortical collecting tubular (CCT) segment of distal nephron. H⁺ is generated from CO₂ by carbonic anhydrase II (CA II) in the α-intercalated cell and exits towards the tubular lumen via the H⁺-ATPase pump, or the H⁺/K⁺ exchanger. HCO₃⁻ exits the cell via the anion exchanger 1 (AE1). Na⁺ enters the cell via the epithelial sodium channel (ENaC) generating a lumen to cell negative gradient.

(AE1) that transports the Cl⁻ ion for the HCO₃⁻ ion leaving tubular cells.

tubule have been assigned specific functional roles. Principal cells deal with Na⁺ reabsorption and K⁺ secretion into the tubular ultrafiltrate, and α-intercalated cells found exclusively in the CCT are involved in urinary acidification by H⁺ secretion. However, this traditional concept has been challenged. It has been suggested that the separation of function between these two cell types in the distal tubule may not be as clearly defined as previously thought.[8,9] Both cell types are believed to be crosstalking and are involved in transport of electrolytes, as well as hydrogen ions.[10]

The CCT is a low-capacity segment in which acidification is regulated by Na⁺ reabsorption that generates a lumen negative membrane potential. The OMCT, on the other hand, has a high-capacity for H⁺ secretion but does not transport Na⁺. The IMCT has a low capacity for H⁺ secretion and is regulated by systemic acid-base status and K⁺ balances both in terms of net H⁺ secretion and NH₄⁺ transport. Most H⁺ secretion in this nephron segment occurs via the H⁺-ATPase pump and to a smaller extent by the H⁺/K⁺-ATPase pump (Figure 42.5). Residual bicarbonate reabsorption from the tubular lumen occurs by a mechanism that is similar to one seen in the proximal tubule. Bicarbonate reformulated in the tubular cells exits via the basolateral anion exchanger

**KEY POINTS**

- H⁺ ion secretion occurs in the α-intercalated cells in the cortical collecting tubule.
- H⁺ primarily exits from the tubular cells into the lumen via H⁺-ATPase pump. Some is transported via the H⁺/K⁺-ATPase pump.
- Aldosterone plays a vital role, via its receptors in the distal tubule to enhance H⁺ and K⁺ secretion in the outer and inner medullary collecting tubules.

Mineralocorticoids (aldosterone) play a central role in H⁺ secretion in the distal nephron by Na⁺-dependent and Na⁺-independent mechanisms. Mineralocorticoids exert their tubular effects through the mineralocorticoid receptor present in the distal collecting tubules. The downstream targets of mineralocorticoid receptor activation by aldosterone are the epithelial Na⁺ channel (ENaC), the renal outer medullary K⁺ channel (ROMK), and the serum and glucocorticoid–regulated kinase (SGK).[11] In the CCT, aldosterone increases Na⁺ absorption and H⁺ secretion. Mineralocorticoids also directly stimulate H⁺ secretion in the OMCT and IMCT. Low systemic pH and high pCO₂ augment H⁺ secretion in the distal nephron.

# AMMONIA PRODUCTION AND EXCRETION

H+ ion secreted by the distal nephron is buffered by NH$_3$ (ammonia) in the tubular lumen to form NH$_4$+ (ammonium). NH$_3$ serves as an important buffer system in this location. Most ammonia is synthesized in the proximal tubular cells from the amino acid glutamine (Figure 42.6). The end products of glutamine metabolism are two NH$_3$+ ions and α-ketoglutarate (α-KG). Further metabolism of α-KG yields two "new" HCO$_3$− ions that are transported out of the cell across the basolateral membrane into the systemic circulation.[12]

Ammonia formed in the proximal tubular cells is highly permeable across cell membranes and can diffuse into the tubular lumen. Conventional thinking has been that NH$_3$, being noncharged, moves from the cytosol to the tubular lumen passively across the apical border. In this line of thinking, luminal NH$_3$ is thought to combine with secreted H+ to form NH$_4$+. Being charged, NH$_4$+ is relatively impermeate across the lipid bilayer of the tubular cells and is trapped within the tubular luminal fluid (urine). More recent observations suggest that both NH$_3$ and NH$_4$+ are preferentially moved from the proximal tubular cell into the tubular lumen via Na+/H+ exchanger, NHE3.[13] Any NH$_4$+ that enters systemic circulation is metabolized in the liver to urea.

As tubular fluid leaves the proximal tubule, a number of processes lead to high medullary ammonia-ammonium concentrations. First, with the abstraction of H$_2$O from the thin descending limb of the loop of Henle, the tubular fluid becomes alkalinized by concentrating luminal HCO$_3$−, which favors NH$_3$ efflux into the interstitium. Second, in the TAL, most of the tubular NH$_4$+ is actively reabsorbed into the tubular cells from the luminal fluid by the Na+/2Cl−/K+ cotransporter by substituting for K+. Third, negative charge in the tubular lumen facilitates NH$_4$+ movement into the interstitium. Fourth, similar to the proximal tubular mechanism, NH$_4$+ transport across the basolateral surface is facilitated by Na+/H+ exchanger, NHE4.[13] The consequences of these complicated biologic maneuvers are twofold: (1) tubular fluid reaching the distal nephron has very little NH$_3$ or NH$_4$+, and (b) the renal interstitium has a high concentration of NH$_4$+, mirroring the concentration gradient observed in the medulla with urea.

The high interstitial NH$_4$+ and NH$_3$ concentration facilitates its diffusion into the collecting duct, especially the IMCT, where it is "trapped" by the secretion of H+ to form NH$_4$+. NH$_4$+ also can enter the collecting tubule lumen by substituting for K+ on the Na+/K+-ATPase. This interaction of K+ and NH$_4$+ on the Na+/2Cl−/K+ cotransporter and Na+/K+-ATPase is another mechanism by which plasma K+ regulates

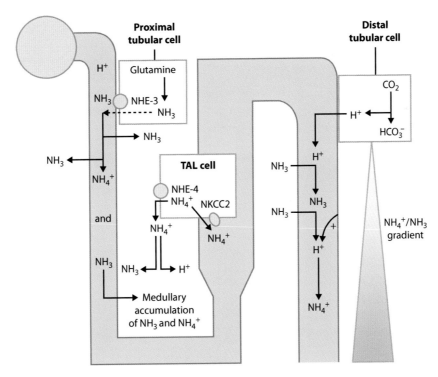

Figure 42.6 Renal ammonia metabolism. NH$_4$+ is generated from glutamine in the proximal tubule cell. As the tubular fluid travels down the thin limb of the loop, water abstraction concentrates the luminal HCO$_3$−, increasing the luminal pH favoring NH$_3$. NH$_3$ diffuses out of the lumen and into the medullary interstitium. The 2Cl−, Na+, K+ transporter can also actively transport NH$_4$+ out of the lumen. Both of these processes lead to NH$_4$+/NH$_3$ accumulation in the medulla and an increasing concentration favors ammonia entry into the medullary collecting duct. TAL, thick ascending limb.

## KEY POINTS

- Ammonia ($NH_3$) formed in the proximal tubule reaches the distal tubule via the lumen, as well as from diffusion from the renal medullary interstitium.
- $NH_3$ traps $H^+$ in the distal tubule to form $NH_4$, which is excreted in urine.

$NH_4^+$ excretion. In summary, the net excretion of $NH_4^+$, and thus acid excretion, depends on $NH_3$ formation in the proximal tubule lumen, the development of the high interstitial medullary $NH_3$ gradient, and its trapping as $NH_4^+$ in the collecting duct by $H^+$ secretion.

Acidosis stimulates glutamine release from muscles, uptake by the proximal tubule cells, and metabolism to $NH_4^+$. Acidosis also increases glucocorticoid levels, which in turn stimulates ammoniagenesis. Hypokalemia also stimulates ammoniagenesis and hyperkalemia inhibits it. ATII increases proximal tubule secretion of $NH_4^+$.

## CLASSIFICATION AND CLINICAL SPECTRUM OF RENAL TUBULAR ACIDOSIS

For clinical purposes, RTA is classified into four subtypes listed in Table 42.1. Distal RTA (DRTA) was the first one to be distinctly identified and is termed RTA type 1, and proximal RTA (PRTA), which is less commonly encountered, is known as RTA type 2. RTA type 3 has pathophysiologic and clinical features of both PRTA and DRTA, and RTA type 4 is associated with hyporeninemic-hypoaldosteronemic states, or associated with distal tubular resistance to aldosterone. Genetically inherited forms of RTA, with specific and recognizable phenotypes are increasingly being identified (Table 42.2), and these will continue to constitute an increasing clinical subgroup of RTA.

Clinical presentation of RTA in children is often protean and nonspecific. These manifestations include anorexia, vomiting, constipation, polyuria, and polydipsia. Failure to thrive is commonly present in infants and younger children.w HCMA, or normal anion gap metabolic acidosis, is the hallmark of all forms of untreated RTA. Normal anion metabolic acidosis also can be seen in clinical conditions other than RTA, and these need to be considered in the evaluation process (Table 42.3).

Table 42.1 Classification of renal tubular acidosis based on site and type of acidification defect

| | RTA type 1 (Distal) | RTA type 2 (Proximal) | RTA type 3 (Mixed) | RTA type 4 (Hyperkalemic) |
|---|---|---|---|---|
| Defect site | Distal tubule | Proximal tubule | Proximal and distal tubule | Distal tubule and proximal tubule |
| Type of defect | Distal tubular $H^+$ excretion | Filtered $HCO_3^-$ reabsorption defect | Distal tubular $H^+$ excretion. Proximal tubular filtered $HCO_3^-$ reabsorption | Distal tubular $H^+$ and $K^+$ excretion. Proximal tubular $NH_3$ synthesis secondary to hyperkalemia |
| Age of onset | Early infancy | Early infancy | Variable | Variable |
| Growth retardation | Yes | Yes | Yes | Uncommon, may be part of underlying disease |
| Bone disease | Osteopenia | Rickets common | Osteopetrosis in inherited form | Absent |
| Nephrocalcinosis | Common | No | No | No |
| Serum bicarbonate (mmol/L) | Low (15–19) | Low (10–15) | Low (15–19) | Low (15–19) |
| Serum potassium | Very low to low | Low to normal | Low to normal | High |
| Urine pH | >5.5 | <5.5, untreated or severe acidosis. > 5.5 if treated or modest acidosis. | >5.5 | <5.5 |
| FE $HCO_3$ | ≤5% | >10%–15% | 5%–15% | 5%–10% |
| Ammonium excretion | Decreased | Normal | Decreased | Decreased |
| Urine anion gap | Positive | Negative | Positive | Positive |

Abbreviations: FE, fractional excretion; RTA, renal tubular acidosis.

Table 42.2 Inherited forms of renal tubular acidosis

| | OMIM | Gene product and gene | Distinctive clinical features |
|---|---|---|---|
| **RTA type 1 (DRTA)** | | | |
| Autosomal dominant | 179800 | AE1 (SCL4A1) | • Nephrocalcinosis<br>• Nephrolithiasis<br>• Older age of onset<br>• RTA can be incomplete |
| Autosomal recessive | 267300 | β₁ subunit of H⁺-ATPase (ATP6V1B1) | • Deafness in early infancy<br>• Nephrocalcinisis is prominent<br>• Profound hypokalemia |
| Autosomal recessive | 602722 | α4 subunit of H⁺-ATPase (ATP6V0A4) | • Growth retardation<br>• Deafness with later onset<br>• Other features as noted in above (ATP6V1B1) |
| **RTA type 2 (PRTA)** | | | |
| Autosomal recessive | 604278 | NBC1 (SLC4A4) | • Ocular abnormalities (glaucoma, band keratopathy)<br>• Mental retardation<br>• Basal ganglia calcification<br>• Enamel defects |
| Autosomal dominant or pseudodominant | 179830 | Not established yet | • Only one family described<br>• Most have only short stature |
| **RTA Type 3** | | | |
| Autosomal recessive | 259730 | CA II (CA2) | • Osteopetrosis<br>• Blindness<br>• Deafness (conductive) |
| **RTA Type 4** | | | |
| Disorders of adrenal steroid biosynthesis | | | • Discussed in the text |

Table 42.3 Causes of non–anion gap metabolic acidosis

**Associated with hypokalemia**

- Distal RTA
- Proximal RTA
- Diarrheal losses of bicarbonate
- Ureteroileostomy
- Ureterosigmoidostomy
- Toluene abuse (glue sniffing)
- Sjögren syndrome
- Drugs
  - Amphotericin B
  - Acetazolamide
  - Aminoglycosides
  - Sodium valproate,
  - Topiramate
  - Zonisamide
  - 6-Mercaptopurine
  - Ifosfamide
- Heavy metals (lead, cadmium, mercury)

**Associated with normokalemia**
- TPN use with amino acids
- Diagnostic or therapeutic intake of ammonium chloride or hydrochloric acid

**Associated with hyperkalemia**

- RTA type 4
- Sickle cell disease
- Obstructive uropathy
- Systemic lupus erythematosis
- Gordon syndrome
- Chronic interstitial nephritis
- Drugs
  - Cyclosporine
  - Tacrolimus
  - Spironolactone
  - Triamterene
  - Trimethoprim
  - Angiotensin-converting enzyme inhibitors
  - Angiotensin receptor blocker
  - Nonsteroidal anti-inflammatory drugs
  - Amiloride
  - Pentamidine

Nephrocalcinosis, nephrolithiasis, and musculoskeletal pain are more commonly seen in older children and adults with RTA type 1. Patients with RTA, especially type 1, can present with life-threatening metabolic acidosis and hypokalemia. Rickets may be seen in DRTA but are more common in patients with Fanconi syndrome associated with PRTA. Genetically inherited variants of RTA may be seen in the context of other organ dysfunction, such as nerve deafness or osteopetrosis. RTA can be a feature of aldosterone deficiency and hyporeninemia from diabetes mellitus with renal insufficiency and a variety of interstitial diseases (RTA type 4).

## RENAL TUBULAR ACIDOSIS TYPE 1

DRTA was the first to be recognized, and has been historically named RTA type 1.[14–16] Childhood presentation of RTA type 1 includes vomiting, failure to thrive, life-threatening metabolic acidosis, and hypokalemia. Less commonly, children with RTA type 1 present with nephrocalcinosis, renal calculi (at times as staghorn calculi), or bone disease. Children can develop rickets and in adults may have osteomalacia. Adults with RTA type 1 commonly present with renal calculi or with musculoskeletal complaints. Causes of RTA type 1 are listed in Table 42.4.

### Inherited forms

RTA type 1 can be inherited as an autosomal dominant or recessive trait. Autosomal recessive form is the most common form of inherited RTA type 1. Mutations affecting the $\beta_1$ and $\alpha_4$ subunits of the $H^+$-ATPase pump on the $\alpha$-intercalated cell (Figure 42.7) result in autosomal recessive RTA type 1.[17–19] The *ATP6V1B1* gene on chromosome 2 encodes the $\beta_1$ subunit. The $\beta_1$ subunit of the $H^+$-ATPase pump is also important in maintaining the cochlear endolymph pH at 7.4, and patients with this genetic defect usually have early onset of severe bilateral sensineural hearing loss. Other features include profound hypokalemia, growth

Table 42.4 Causes of renal tubular acidosis type 1 or distal renal tubular acidosis

**Genetic**

- Autosomal dominant (AE1 deficiency)
- Autosomal recessive
- With deafness ($\beta_1$ subunit of $H^+$-ATPase)
- Without deafness ($\alpha_4$ subunit $H^+$-ATPase)
- Ovalocytosis with AE1 mutation (Thailand)

**Hereditary diseases**

- Ehlers-Danlos syndrome
- Sickle cell disease
- Familial hypercalciuria
- Type 1 glycogen storage disease
- Carnitine palmitoyl transferase deficiency
- Medullary cystic disease
- Nephronophthisis

**Hypercalciuria with nephrocalcinosis**

- Primary hyperparathyroidism
- Hyperthyroidism
- Medullary sponge kidney
- X-linked hyperphosphatemia
- Fabry disease
- Vitamin D intoxication
- Wilson disease
- Hereditary fructose intoxication
- Idiopathic hypercalciuria

**Autoimmune disease**

- Sjögren syndrome
- Hyperglobulinemic purpura
- Systemic lupus erythematosus

**Drug- and toxin-induced DRTA**

- Amphotericin
- Cyclamate
- NSAIDs nephropathy
- Lithium
- Foscarnet

**Tubulointerstitial disease**

- Chronic pyelonephritis
- Obstructive nephropathy
- Acute and chronic renal transplant rejection
- Leprosy
- Hyperoxaluria
- Vesicoureteral reflux nephropathy

**Functional (Decreased sodium delivery)**

- Volume contraction (UNa <10 mEq/L)
- Edema forming states
- Nephrotic syndrome
- Cirrhosis
- Congestive heart failure

failure, and nephrocalcinosis, which can be seen even in neonates. Mutation affecting *ATP6V0A4* gene on chromosome 7 that encodes the $\alpha_4$ subunit of the $H^+$-ATPase pump also causes autosomal recessive form of RTA type 1. Children with this gene mutation have preserved hearing during early childhood, but mild-to-moderate hearing impairment becomes evident as children get older.

Autosomal dominant RTA type 1 is the result of a defect in the $HCO_3^-/Cl^-$ exchanger AE1 because of the mutations in the *SLC4A1* gene, located on chromosome 17.[20–22] These patients often present with renal stones, nephrocalcinosis, and incomplete RTA type 1.[19] Apart from the distal nephron, the AE1 exchanger is also expressed in the red blood cells. Some patients with the autosomal dominant form of RTA type 1 secondary to the *AE1* gene mutation may also have hemolytic anemia due to of spherocytosis.

A few studies from Thailand have reported the recessive form RTA type 1 and ovalocytosis with mutations in AE1 that facilitates bicarbonate-chloride transport in the α-intercalated cells of the distal collecting duct cells.[22,23] This disorder has been exclusively reported only from Southeast Asia. Other genetically transmitted diseases associated with RTA type 1 include Ehlers-Danlos syndrome,[24] hereditary elliptocytosis,[25] sickle cell disease,[26] familial hypercalciuria,[27,28] type 1 glycogen storage disease,[29] carnitine palmitoyltransferase type I deficiency,[30] and medullary cystic disease.[31]

## Pathophysiology

Impaired $H^+$ ion secretion in the CCT and MCT leads to decreased ammonium and titratable acid excretion and an increased bicarbonate excretion (not reabsorbed in distal nephron), all of which cause metabolic acidosis. The hallmark of RTA type 1 is the inability to excrete appropriate amounts of $H^+$ and an inability to lower urine pH below 5.5 in face of systemic acidosis. In young children with RTA type 1, the fractional excretion (FE) $HCO_3^-$ may be higher than usually seen in adults and can range from 5% to 15%, leading to potentially life-threatening acidosis.[14,16] Because of higher FE $HCO_3^-$ in children compared to adults, treatment of RTA type 1 requires a larger dose in children, especially to maintain normal growth. After age 4 to 5 years, there is usually a decrease in the alkali requirement to levels seen in adults. Acidosis in RTA type 1 is associated with significant renal sodium wasting, leading to increased renin and aldosterone secretion, and hypokalemia that can be profound. Correction of the acidosis usually leads to a reduction in these electrolyte losses. Volume contraction and salt wasting are especially common in patients with nephrocalcinosis and tubulointerstitial disease.

The chronic metabolic acidosis leads to buffering of $H^+$ by the bone and impaired bone mineralization. This causes rickets in children and osteomalacia in adults.[14–16,32] Correction of the metabolic acidosis reverses this type of bone disease.[33] Chronic acidosis in RTA type 1 is also associated with decreased renal citrate production and hypocitraturia.[34] Combined with increased urinary calcium, hypocitraturia in these patients predisposes to nephrocalcinosis and nephrolithiasis (Figure 42.8).[14,16] Nephrocalcinosis further worsens NAE by impairing transfer of $NH_4^+$ from the loop of Henle into the collecting duct. Ongoing nephrocalcinosis and recurrent calcium phosphate and calcium oxalate stone disease can cause progressive loss of renal function. Alkali therapy decreases urinary calcium excretion and increases citrate excretion, reducing the risk for further nephrocalcinosis and stone formation. However, nephrocalcinosis, if present before alkali therapy is instituted, does not resolve with correction of acidosis. Chronic metabolic acidosis also interferes with growth, and failure to thrive and short stature are common findings in children with untreated RTA-type 1.[14–16]

Autoimmune disorders, especially Sjögren syndrome, have been associated with RTA type 1.[36–38] Nephrocalcinosis from any cause also can also lead to RTA type 1, by itself.

---

**KEY POINTS**

- Most cases of RTA type 1 have no clearly identifiable cause and are considered idiopathic.
- Genetic defects causing RTA type 1 are being increasingly recognized.
- Some inherited forms of RTA type 1 have associated sensorineural deafness.
- Hypercalciuria and nephrocalcinosis are common in RTA type 1.

---

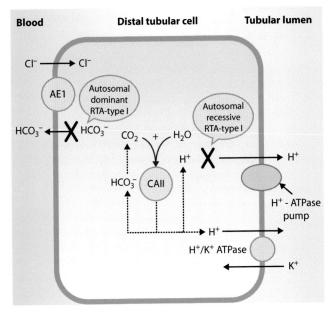

Figure 42.7 Inherited defects in distal tubular hydrogen ion transport that result in renal tubular acidosis (RTA) type 1.

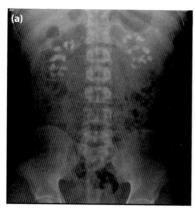
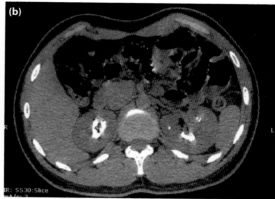

Figure 42.8 (a) Abdominal radiograph of a 17-year-old male patient with renal tubular acidosis type 1 demonstrating nephrocalcinosis affecting the renal pyramids. (b) CAT scan of the abdomen demonstrating medullary site of nephrocalcinosis in the same patient.

Buckalew et al.[27] described a large family in which the hypercalciuria and nephrocalcinosis preceded the development of RTA type 1. Medullary sponge kidney is associated with RTA type 1, suggesting that cystic dilatation of the collecting tubules can impair acid excretion.[31] Chronic medullary injury from sickle cell disease is also associated with RTA type 1.[26]

A functional defect and transient RTA type 1 may be observed in clinical states with markedly reduced distal Na+ delivery. In conditions such as nephrotic syndrome, congestive heart failure, or cirrhosis, urine Na+ concentration is below 10 mmol/L, resulting in impairment of voltage-dependent H+ secretion in the CCT and an inability to lower the urine pH below 5.5.[39-41] Expanding volume in such patients, or increasing distal sodium delivery with furosemide or a nonreabsorbable anion-like sulfate restores the distal nephron's ability to acidify and excrete ammonium.

Strife et al.[41] described a group of young children who had a transient mild HCMA but were able to lower their urine pH below 5.5. Most had poor linear growth, and two of the seven patients described also had nephrocalcinosis. Although they could generate a low urine pH, they were unable to raise their urine $pCO_2$ above blood $pCO_2$, indicating rate-dependent RTA as proposed by Batlle at al.[42] On follow-up, none of these patients with rate-dependent RTA progressed to more severe RTA, and a number have been able to discontinue alkali supplementation altogether.

A number of medications have been implicated in impaired distal H+ excretion. Amphotericin B alters the permeability of the distal nephron, allowing back-leak of H+ from lumen to blood.[43] This dissipates the H+ gradient (gradient defect RTA) and limits H+ excretion. Lithium carbonate impairs H+ secretion, but this usually does not result in disease.[44] Large doses of cyclamate and nonsteroidal anti-inflammatory drugs (NSAIDs) impair distal tubular H+ secretion.[45,46] Foscarnet also has been shown to decrease distal acidification.[47] Tubulointerstitial diseases also can cause RTA type 1. These include transplant rejection,[48-50] obstructive uropathy,[51,52] vesicoureteral reflux,[53] hyperoxaluria,[54] leprosy,[55] and pyelonephritis, especially if associated with urolithiasis.[56]

## Treatment

Patients with RTA type 1 usually require 1 to 3 mEq/kg/day of alkali supplementation to correct the metabolic acidosis, often also resolving kaliuresis and naturesis, as well.[15,16] Infants and young children require larger doses of alkali supplementation for optimal growth, usually 2 to 4 mEq/kg/day, but at times more than 5 mEq/kg/day.[14-16,57] Larger doses are needed because of increased endogenous acid production and bicarbonate loss in young children with RTA type 1. Some patients require potassium supplementation, in addition to alkali therapy. When patients with RTA type 1 present with severe metabolic acidosis and hypokalemia, initial therapy should be directed at correcting hypokalemia before treating acidosis. Correcting the acidosis first may worsen hypokalemia and cause respiratory depression.

## Prognosis

With adequate treatment, normal growth can be achieved and bone disease prevented or reversed. Early treatment is necessary to prevent nephrocalcinosis that can lead to renal insufficiency. After age 4 to 5 years, there is less bicarbonate loss and lower doses of alkali become necessary to correct metabolic acidosis (1 to 2 mmol/kg/day).

## RENAL TUBULAR ACIDOSIS TYPE 2

Patients with RTA type 2, or PRTA, may present with an isolated defect of bicarbonate reabsorption, or as a generalized proximal tubular dysfunction (Fanconi syndrome) characterized by aminoaciduria, phosphaturia, and glycosuria, in addition to bicarbonaturia. Common causes of RTA type 2 are listed in Table 42.5. Fanconi syndrome can result from inherited error of metabolism, such as cystinosis, tyrosinemia, galatosemia, Wilson disease, Lowe syndrome, and mitochondrial myopathies, as well as many drugs and toxins. Transient isolated RTA type 2 also has been described in newborns, especially in premature and extremely premature infants.[58,59]

## Inherited forms

An autosomal recessive RTA type 2 has been well described. In addition to the features of RTA type 2, these patients also have mental retardation and ocular abnormalities, such as glaucoma and corneal opacities. It is caused by a genetic defect in defect in the NBC1 cotransporter (sodium-bicarbonate cotransporter 1) (Figure 42.9).[61-63] The *SLC4A4* gene, which encodes for NBC1, is located on chromosome 4. A much less common autosomal dominant form of RTA type 2 has been described by Brenes et al.[60] All patients in this group were asymptomatic, other than having short stature. A genetic defect in these patients has not been clearly identified.

CA II is essential for both bicarbonate reabsorption and hydrogen ion secretion in the renal tubules. Deficiency of CA II results in a unique disorder consisting of osteopetrosis and RTA with features of both RTA type 2 and RTA type 1.[64] These patients also may have brain ventricular fluid or cerebrospinal fluid abnormalities or both, since CA II also plays a role in cerebrospinal fluid turnover in the lateral ventricles.

### Table 42.5 Causes of renal tubular acidosis type 2

**Sporadic**
- Idiopathic
- Transient (infants)
- Cyanotic heart disease
- Renal vascular accident

**Genetic**
- Autosomal dominant
- Autosomal recessive with mental retardation and ocular disease (NBC1 deficiency)
- Leigh syndrome
- Metachromatic leukodystrophy

**Carbonic anhydrase inhibition**
- Topiramide (Topamax)
- Acetazolamide
- Sulfanilamide
- Mafenide

## Pathophysiology

The pathophysiology of RTA type 2, except in the inherited variants of CA II and NBC1 deficiency, remains unclear. In the autosomal recessive form of RTA type 2, the basolateral NBC1 cotransporter is deficient.[63] This exchanger is necessary for transporting $HCO_3^-$ out of the proximal tubule cell in exchange for $Cl^-$ and its impaired activity inhibits luminal reabsorption of filtered $HCO_3^-$. NBC1 is also highly expressed in corneal endothelium, and its defective function

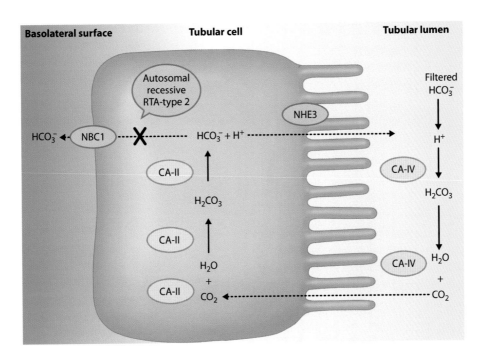

Figure 42.9 Site of defect in recessive form of renal tubular acidosis (RTA) type 2. CA II, carbonic anhydrase II. CA IV, carbonic anhydrase IV; NHE3, sodium-hydrogen ion exchanger 3 ( also known as sodium-hydrogen antiporter 3); NBC1, sodium-bicarbonate cotransporter 1.

is associated with corneal opacities, cataracts, and glaucoma.[26] In CA II deficiency, cytosolic carbonic anhydrase is defective and unable to generate adequate $H^+$ and $HCO_3^-$ for transepithelial transport of the filtered $HCO_3^-$.[21,25] CA II is also present in the $\alpha$-intercalated cell in the CCT leading to impaired generation of $H^+$ for transport into the distal nephron leading to RTA type 1 as well.

Other possible mechanisms for RTA type 2 include an abnormality in the $Na^+/H^+$ exchanger on the lumen membrane or CA IV on the luminal membrane. An abnormality at either of these sites would impair reclamation of the filtered bicarbonate, causing excessive amounts of $HCO_3^-$ to escape the proximal tubule. This excess $HCO_3^-$ would overwhelm the limited capacity of distal nephron, which is able to reclaim only up to 15% of the filtered load, leading to bicarbonaturia along with the loss of $Na^+$ and $K^+$. The bicarbonaturia leads to a fall in plasma $HCO_3^-$ and thus a fall in the filtered load. At some point the filtered load decreases to the extent that the nephron is able to reclaim virtually the entire filtered load of bicarbonate. The serum $HCO_3^-$ concentration at which this occurs is termed the *renal threshold* for bicarbonate. In such a steady-state, the distal nephron is now able to acidify urine and the urine pH can be <5.5.

### KEY POINTS

- Most cases of RTA type 2 have no clearly identifiable cause and are considered idiopathic.
- Genetic defects in the NCB1 exchanger have been shown to cause RTA type 2.
- Bicarbonaturia is the hallmark of RTA type 2.
- Fanconi syndrome is characterized by glucosuria, phosphaturia, aminoaciduria, and bicarbonaturia.

## Clinical manifestations

RTA type 2 usually manifests with clinical features of growth failure in infants and children.[58] Recurrent vomiting is another common symptom. Untreated patients have severe metabolic acidosis with serum $HCO_3^-$ in the range of 10 to 15 mMol/L, mild hypokalemia, and the urine pH is often below 5.5. This paradoxical finding results from the fact that as serum bicarbonate declines during severe metabolic acidosis, filtered bicarbonate load diminishes to within the range of proximal tubular threshold for bicarbonate. This results in reabsorption of most of the filtered bicarbonate, leaving little of it in the tubular fluid. Since the distal tubular hydrogen ion secretion is intact in such patients, urine can be adequately acidified and urine pH can be lowered to < 5.5. However, once patients receive alkali supplementation and serum bicarbonate level improves, filtered bicarbonate load again increases and exceeds the proximal tubular bicarbonate reabsorptive threshold, resulting in an alkaline urine pH (often >7). Polyuria resulting from solute diuresis is

common. Aldosterone and renin levels are elevated because of the associated renal sodium and water loss, and intravascular volume depletion. Hypokalemia in RTA type 2 results from potassium secretion by the principal cells in the CCT secondary to elevated aldosterone levels. Metabolic acidosis often causes vomiting, decreased appetite, and caloric intake, eventually leading to failure to thrive. With the correction of metabolic acidosis, failure to thrive can be reversed. Isolated RTA type 2 is not associated with abnormalities of serum calcium, phosphorus, or vitamin D. Nephrolithiasis and nephrocalcinosis are absent in RTA type 2, because citrate excretion is unaffected or may even be increased.

RTA type 2 may be associated with a more global disorder of proximal tubule functions, known as Fanconi syndrome. Fanconi syndrome is characterized by glucosuria, aminoaciduria, and phosphaturia, in addition to bicarbonaturia.[59] Rickets and osteomalacia secondary to renal phosphate losses and abnormal vitamin D metabolism are common in patients with Fanconi syndrome. A number of inborn errors of metabolism are associated with Fanconi syndrome, including cystinosis, tyrosinemia, hereditary fructose intolerance, Wilson disease, galactosemia, and Lowe syndrome (Table 42.6). Several drugs can result in Fanconi syndrome (Table 42.7).

## Treatment

The goal of RTA type 2 treatment is the normalization of serum $HCO_3^-$. However, as serum $HCO_3^-$ is corrected, urinary $HCO_3^-$ losses also increase. Thus, 2 to 20 mEq/kg/day of alkali supplementation, either as bicarbonate or as an anion that can be metabolized to form bicarbonate, is necessary for

Table 42.6 Causes of Fanconi syndrome

**Inherited causes**
Cystinosis
Hereditary fructose intolerance
Tyrosinemia
Wilson disease
Lowe syndrome
Glycogenesis
Dent disease
Mitochondrial cytopathies
Drugs (see Box 42.3)

**Toxins and poisons**
Glue sniffing (toluene), diachrome, Chinese herbal medicine (*Aristolochia*), heavy metal poisoning (lead, cadmium)

**Dysproteinemias**
Sjögren's syndrome, light-chain proteinuria, amyloidosis, multiple myeloma

**Miscellaneous**
Nephrotic syndrome, renal transplantation, mesenchymal tumors Idiopathic

Table 42.7 Causes of drug-induced renal Fanconi syndrome

| Drug Class | Drugs | Indications for use |
|---|---|---|
| Alkylating agents | Ifosfamide | Cancer |
| Aminoglycoside antibiotics | Gentamicin, amikacin | Gram-negative bacterial infection |
| Anti-epileptics | Sodium valproate | Seizures, bipolar disorder |
| Anti-protozoals | Suramin | Trypanosomiasis |
| Dicarboxylic acids | Fumaric acid | Psoriasis |
| Iron chelators | Desferrioxamine | Iron overload (e.g., in sickle cell or thalassemia) |
| NRTIs | Didanosine, stavudine | HIV |
| NtRTIs | Tenofovir, adefovir, cidofovir | HIV, hepatitis B, and CMV |
| Platinum compounds | Cisplatin/carboplatin | Cancer |
| Salicylates | Aspirin | Analgesia, anti-inflammatory |
| Tetracycline antibiotics | Degraded tetracycline | Bacterial infection |
| Tyrosine kinase inhibitors | Imatinib mesylate | Chronic myeloid leukemia |

*Source:* Hall AM, Bass P, Unwin RJ. Drug-induced renal Fanconi syndrome. QJM. 2014;107:261–9. Reproduced with permission.

*Abbreviations:* CMV, cytomegalovirus; HIV, human immunodeficiency virus; NRTI, nucleoside reverse-transcription inhibitor; NtRTI, nucleotide analogue reverse-transcription inhibitor.

correction of metabolic acidosis in RTA type 2 (Table 42.8). Given that the ability of the nephron to reabsorb bicarbonate is impaired, it may not be possible to fully overcome the effect of bicarbonate losses. Alkali administration should be divided into multiple, frequent doses. Sodium restriction or hydrochlorothiazide (1.5 to 2 mg/kg/day) may decrease alkali requirements by increasing proximal $HCO_3^-$ reabsorption. Potassium losses often increase with alkali replacement. Therefore, some or all of the replacement alkali should be given as the potassium salt, such as potassium citrate.

The primary treatment of Fanconi syndrome is to treat the underlying cause with available specific therapies. This would include cysteamine for cystinosis, 2-(2-nitro-4-trifluoromethylbenzoyl)-1,3-cyclohexanedione (NTBC) for tyrosinemia, penicillamine for Wilson disease, avoidance of galactose in galatosemia, and avoidance of fructose in hereditary fructose intolerance. In patients in whom the primary disease cannot be corrected, supplemental phosphate (Neutra-Phos or Phospha 250 Neutral), vitamin D (calcitriol), sodium, and potassium supplements must be given in addition to bicarbonate.

## Prognosis

Isolated RTA type 2 can be transient, and supplemental alkali for a period to preserve growth is all that is necessary. In others, the RTA type 2 is life-long disorder, and supplemental alkali is necessary to preserve bone mineralization. The prognosis of children with Fanconi syndrome depends on the underlying cause. Wilson disease, tyrosinemia, galatosemia, and hereditary fructose intolerance can have a relatively good prognosis with early intervention. Early therapy with cysteamine in children with cystinosis is beneficial, although the long-term prognosis for preservation of renal function is unclear.[64] To date, there is no, or only incomplete, therapy, directly aimed at patients with Lowe syndrome or mitochondrial myopathies. Patients with acquired Fanconi syndrome have an outcome dependent on the extent of injury at the time the disorder is discovered, with some patients having only transient disease and others permanent.

## RENAL TUBULAR ACIDOSIS TYPE 3

After the description of RTA types 1 and 2, it was recognized that some infants and young children had inability to acidify their urine in the face of severe acidosis and also had significant urinary bicarbonate losses, in the range of 5% to 10% of the filtered load.[14,16,65] A few of these infants had a fractional bicarbonate loss as high as 15%. This combined pattern suggesting a proximal and distal nephron dysfunction, and was termed RTA type 3. It was recognized later that the bicarbonate loss improved after the child was 4 to 5 years old and the abnormality was then consistent with RTA

Table 42.8 Commonly available alkali replacements

| Name | Composition | Amount of alkali |
|---|---|---|
| Sodium bicarbonate tablets | Sodium bicarbonate | |
| 325 mg | | 4 mEq |
| 650 mg | | 8 mEq |
| Bicitra, Oracit, Cytra-2, Shohl solution | Sodium citrate | 1 mEq/mL |
| Citra-K solution | Potassium citrate | 2 mEq/mL |
| Citra-3 solution | Sodium and potassium citrate | 2 mEq/mL |
| Cytra-K packet | Potassium citrate | 30 mEq/packet |
| Urocit-K tablet | Potassium citrate | 5- and 10-mEq tablets |

type 1 or DRTA. Whether this disorder primarily reflects proximal or distal tubular dysfunction is still unclear, and its existence has been questioned by some.

An autosomal recessive disorder characterized by osteopetrosis, mental retardation, cerebral calcifications (marble brain disease), and metabolic acidosis has been described in association with deficiency of cytosol CA II and is caused by loss of function mutation in *CA2* gene.[66] CA II is in the cytoplasm of a number of cells, including proximal and distal tubule cells, as well as osteoclasts. Defective CA II function impairs the ability of these cells to form $HCO_3^-$ and $H^+$ from $H_2O$ and $CO_2$, a process that facilitates reclamation of filtered bicarbonate in the proximal tubule. In the distal tubular cells, absence of CA II impairs acidification and bicarbonate regeneration (Figure 42.9). $H^+$ secretion by the osteoclast is also important for bone remodeling and may be an important pathogenic factor in the development of the bone disease in osteopetrosis (Figure 42.10). These patients can have conductive nerve deafness. Metabolic acidosis in these patients is a combination of defective $HCO_3^-$ reclamation and $H^+$ excretion—RTA type 3.

---

## KEY POINTS

- RTA type 3 has features of both RTA types 1 and 2.
- Some have questioned the existence of clinically distinct RTA type 3.
- Osteopetrosis and RTA type 3 resulting from a genetic defect in intracellular CA II are well recognized.

---

## RENAL TUBULAR ACIDOSIS TYPE 4

RTA type 4 or hyperkalemic RTA is an uncommon form of RTA that can be seen in diverse clinical disorders. The distinguishing feature of RTA type 4 is the presence of hyperkalemia, in addition to a mild normal anion gap metabolic acidosis. These patients are able to acidify the urine pH below 5.5. Patients with RTA type 4 have underlying aldosterone deficiency or tubular resistance to it. Infants with RTA type 4 often present with failure to thrive. Causes of RTA type 4 are listed in Table 42.9.

---

## KEY POINTS

- RTA type 4 results from hyporeninemia and hypoaldosteronemic states.
- Hyperkalemia is the hallmark of RTA type 4.
- Hyperkalemia reduces proximal tubular $NH_3$ generation, leading to decreased acid excretion.

---

## Pathophysiology

RTA type 4 is caused by hyperkalemia associated with aldosterone deficiency or tubular resistance (Figure 42.11). Hyperkalemia decreases proximal tubule ammonia production and competes with $NH_4^+$ for the $Na^-/2Cl^-/K^+$ transporter in the ascending limb of the loop of Henle, reducing the medullary ammonium gradient. Hyperkalemia also impairs the entry of $NH_4^+$ into the MCT cell from the

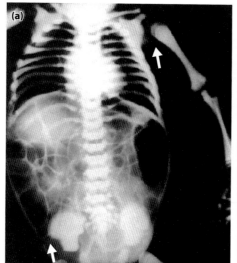
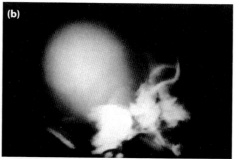

Figure 42.10 Skeletal radiographs of a 10-day-old newborn with loss of function carbonic anhydrase (CA) mutation leading to renal tubular acidosis (RTA) type 3 and osteopetrosis. **(a)** There is a generalized increase in bone density. Typical features of osteopetrosis are the "bone in bone" appearance seen in the left humerus and iliac crests (a, arrows), and the severely sclerotic appearance of the skull base relative to the calvarium **(b)**. Soft tissue calcification is evident in **(c)**. (Reproduced with permission from: Borthwick KJ, Kandemir N, Topaloglu R, et al. J Med Genet. 2003;40:115–21.)

Table 42.9  Causes of renal tubular acidosis type 4

**Aldosterone deficiency**

- Addison disease
- Bilateral adrenalectomy
- Congenital adrenal hyperplasia
- 21-Hydroxylase deficiency
- 3β-Hydroxysteriod dehydrogenase
- Cortisterone methyloxidase I and II deficiency
- Congenital lipoid adrenal hyperplasia (StAR deficiency)
- Angiotensin-converting enzyme inhibitors

**Hyporeninemia and hypoaldosteronism**

- Diabetic nephropathy
- Acquired immunodeficiency syndrome nephropathy
- Gouty nephropathy
- Tubulointerstial nephritis
- Nonsteroidal anti-inflammatory drugs
- β-Blockers
- Hypoaldosteronism of critical illness
- Heparin

**Pseudohypoaldosteronism II**

- Gordon syndrome (WNK 1 and 4 mutations, Kelch-like 3, Cullin 3)

**Aldosterone resistance**

- Autosomal dominant pseudohypoaldosteronism I (aldosterone receptor defect)
- Autosomal recessive pseudohypoaldosteronism I (ENaC defect)
- Tubulointerstitial disease
- Fetal alcohol syndrome
- Sickle cell nephropathy
- Renal transplant rejection
- Obstructive uropathy
- Renal dysplasia
- Analgesic nephropathy
- Nephrocalcinosis and nephrolithiasis
- Systemic lupus erythematosus

**Drugs that interfere with aldosterone receptor**

- Spironolactone

**Drugs that inhibit ENaC**

- Amiloride
- Trimethoprim
- Triamterene
- Pentamidine

**Drugs that interfere with $Na^+,K^+$ ATPase**

- Cyclosporine
- Tacrolimus

---

medullary interstitium via the $K^+$ secretory site on the basolateral membrane $Na^+,K^+$-ATPase. The net effect is decreased $NH_4^+$ and NAE.[67] Aldosterone deficiency or resistance decreases $H^+$ secretion in the collecting duct by decreasing the number and function of $H^+$-ATPase pumps. Aldosterone is also important for increasing the negativity of the lumen of the CCT by enhancing the absorption of $Na^+$ via the apical membrane epithelial sodium channel (ENaC) and the basolateral membrane $Na^+,K^+$-ATPase. The increased lumen negativity facilitates $H^+$ secretion into the lumen of CCT.

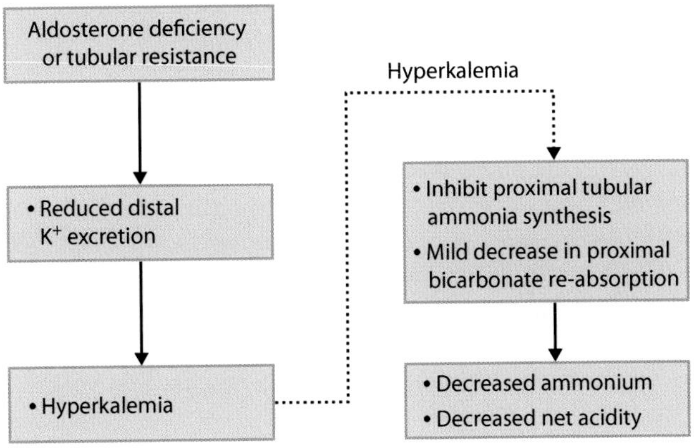

## Inherited forms

### STEROID BIOSYNTHESIS DEFECTS

Several autosomal recessive genetic disorders of adrenal steroid synthesis leading to decreased or absent aldosterone synthesis can result in RTA type 4 in infants and children. The most common defect of adrenal steroid synthesis is 21-hydroxylase deficiency (CYP21), coded for by the genes on chromosome 6 (Online Mendelian Inheritance in Man [OMIM] #613815).[68,69] Rarely, the cortisol and sex steroid pathways are entirely normal and there is an isolated aldosterone deficiency. This results from the defect in the enzyme aldosterone synthase (CYP11B2) also known as corticosterone methyloxidase, which is involved in the final step of aldosterone synthesis and converts deoxycorticosterone to aldosterone. Two distinct subtypes of aldosterone synthase deficiency have been characterized and are known as type I (OMIM #124080) and type II (OMIM #124080) defects. These enzymatic defects have similar phenotypic expression but have varied biochemical identifiers. Other rare defects in steroid biosynthesis involve 3β-hydroxysteroid dehydrogenase, coded on chromosome 1 and congenital lipoid adrenal hyperplasia or StAR deficiency, coded on chromosome 8.[70,71]

Figure 42.11  Pathophysiology of renal tubular acidosis (RTA) type IV (hyporeninemia-hypoaldosteronemia).

## PSEUDOHYPOALDOSTERONISM

Autosomal dominant pseudohypoaldosteronism I (PHA I) is associated with hyperkalemia, salt wasting, elevated renin and aldosterone levels, and hypotension. Autosomal dominant PHAI is caused by a mutation in the mineralocorticoid receptor in the collecting tubule.[72] The mutant mineralocorticoid receptor is unable to respond to aldosterone properly, and this leads to a decrease in the activity of the ENaC. This in turn decreases luminal $Na^+$ absorption and the transepithelial potential difference. The decreased potential difference reduces $K^+$ and $H^+$ secretion.[72] Supplemental mineralocorticoid therapy will not correct the defect. However, carbenoxolone, an 11 β-hydroxysteroid dehydrogenase inhibitor, can raise intracellular cortisol levels and overcome the functional defect in the mineralocorticoid receptor. The clinical features become less severe as the child ages.

Autosomal recessive PHAI is caused by a defective ENaC.[72,73] Infants with recessive PHAI have severe hyperkalemia, salt wasting, RTA type 4, and hypotension. Renin and aldosterone levels are elevated. Newborns with recessive PHAI may have respiratory distress due to impaired $Na^+$ and water reabsorption from the alveoli resulting from defective ENaC in the alveolar membranes.[74]

Gordon syndrome, or pseudoaldosteronism II (PHAII), is a rare autosomal dominant disorder characterized by hypertension, hyperkalemia, low renin, low aldosterone levels, RTA type 4, and mild volume expansion.[75] Previously, PHAII was thought to result from an early distal tubule "chloride shunt." It is now known to be caused by mutations in WNK4, Kelch-like 3, and Cullin 3 proteins.[76] WNK4, coded on chromosome 17, inhibits the NaCl cotransporter in the DCT and the ROMK channel, and the paracellular permeability of $Cl^-$. Mutations in WNK4 increase the activity of the NaCl cotransporter and paracellular $Cl^-$ permeability, but inhibit ROMK activity, leading to volume expansion, hyperkalemia, and voltage dependent type IV RTA. Abnormalities in Kelch-like 3 and Cullin 3 proteins may interfere with the ubiquitination and degradation of distal nephron proteins involved with NaCl absorption and K secretion.[77] How WNK1 mutations cause Gordon syndrome is unclear. Thiazide diuretics correct the hyperkalemia, acidosis, and hypertension.

## Acquired hypoaldosteronism and aldosterone resistance

Acquired diseases of the adrenal gland can lead to RTA type 4, including autoimmune adrenal failure, tuberculosis, fungal infection, or acquired immunodeficiency syndrome (AIDS). Isolated hypoaldosteronism can occur in critically ill patients and is thought to be related to inhibition of aldosterone synthetase by hypoxia, cytokines, atrial natriuretic peptide, and heparin.[78] Hypoaldosteronism leads to hyperkalemia and RTA type 4. Hyporeninemic, hypoaldosteronism typically occurs in older patients with renal insufficiency from diabetic nephropathy, AIDS, systemic lupus erythematosus (SLE) and tubulointerstitial nephritis.[79] The hyporeninemia does not respond to the usual measures to stimulate renin secretion, but low aldosterone levels increase with the infusion of angiotensin II.

Tubulointerstitial diseases may also cause unresponsiveness to aldosterone, leading to hyperkalemia and metabolic acidosis from decreased ammonium excretion. Such tubulointerstitial diseases include analgesic abuse, sickle cell disease, nephrolithiasis, nephrocalcinosis, acute and chronic transplant rejection, and SLE. Infants with fetal alcohol syndrome may have mild RTA type 4.[80] Obstructive uropathy and renal dysplasia are also common causes of RTA type 4 and relative tubular unresponsiveness to aldosterone in children.[52,53,81,82]

A number of drugs can cause RTA type 4. NSAIDs can cause hyperkalemia and metabolic acidosis by inhibiting renin release.[83] β-Blockers similarly inhibit renin release and alter potassium distribution. Heparin can be directly toxic to the zona glomerulosa and inhibit aldosterone synthase.[84] Angiotensin-converting enzyme inhibitors and angiotensin receptor blockers lead to hypoaldosteronism and can cause hyperkalemia and acidosis, especially in patients with renal insufficiency. Spironolactone is a competitive inhibitor of aldosterone and also can cause hyperkalemia and metabolic acidosis.[85] Amiloride, triamterene, trimethoprim, and pentamidine inhibit the ENaC channel in the collecting duct principal cell.[86-88] This lowers the transepithelial potential difference reducing the secretion of $H^+$ and $K^+$. The resulting hyperkalemia reduces ammonium production and excretion. Cyclosporine and tacrolimus cause hyperkalemia and metabolic acidosis through inhibition of basolateral $Na^+,K^+$-ATPase.[89,90] This decreases intracellular $K^+$ concentration and the transepithelial potential, lowering the driving force for $K^+$ secretion in the CCT.

## Diagnosis of renal tubular acidosis type 4

The responsiveness of the CCT to aldosterone in the setting of hyperkalemia can be evaluated by the transtubular gradient for potassium (TTKG), that is the potassium gradient between the peritubular capillary and the CCT lumen.[91] The TTKG is defined as:

$$TTKG = \frac{UrineK \times Serum\ Osmolality}{Serum\ K \times Urine\ Osmolality} \quad (42.5)$$

A TTKG of 8 or greater indicates that adequate aldosterone is present and that the CCT is responding appropriately in the hyperkalemic patient. A value less than 8 suggests aldosterone deficiency or tubular unresponsiveness. Patients with aldosterone deficiency will increase their TTKG after several days of therapy with fludrocortisone, whereas those with tubular insensitivity fail to do so. Although the TTKG is a useful clinical test, it tends to underestimate the $K^+$ secretory capacity in the hyperkalemic patient with dilute urine.

## Treatment of renal tubular acidosis type 4

Treatment in RTA type 4 is based on the underlying cause. A careful history of drug use is important to identify potential offending pharmaceutical or toxic agents. Evaluation of plasma renin activity, aldosterone secretion, and TTKG is useful to distinguish aldosterone deficiency from tubular unresponsiveness. Patients with glucocorticoid and mineralocorticoid deficiency need replacement steroids. Patients with hyporeninemic, hypoaldosteronism may benefit from a loop diuretic and cation exchange resin to increase potassium excretion. Supraphysiologic doses of fludrocortisone may be helpful, but can cause volume overexpansion and hypertension.

Infants with PHAI should get salt supplements to correct the volume depletion. In contrast, patients with PHAII should be treated with thiazide diuretics and salt restriction. Patients with tubular resistance to aldosterone and hyperkalemia should be treated with dietary $K^+$ restriction and loop diuretics to increase $K^+$ secretion and augment transepithelial potential difference. Cation exchange resins to decrease the hyperkalemia also may be helpful. Supplemental alkali should be used to treat the acidosis as discussed previously.

# CLINICAL TOOLS FOR EVALUATION

## Anion gap

The first step in evaluating a patient for RTA is to look for HCMA by determining the anion gap (AG) in the serum of patients with acidosis.

$$AG = Na^+ - (HCO_3^- + Cl^-) \qquad (42.6)$$

AG between 6 and 16 is normal; AG exceeding 16 is elevated.

Normal serum AG varies over a wide range because of the large span of normal values of electrolytes used in this calculation. Whether or not serum potassium is used in this calculation also determines the normal value of serum AG. Most laboratories, however, do not include potassium in this calculation. Readers should familiarize themselves with normal values in their clinical laboratory. The serum $HCO_3^-$ should be measured soon after obtaining the serum. Factors that can lead to a falsely low $HCO_3^-$ concentration include allowing the sample to remain in contact with red cells for a prolonged period, obtaining the blood by "heel prick," and a prolonged tourniquet time. Serum albumin accounts for the bulk of the anion gap, therefore changes in the serum albumin should be taken into consideration when calculating anion gap. For every 1 g/dL decrease in the serum albumin below normal, the anion gap will decrease by approximately 2.5 mEq/L.[92]

## Urine pH

Measuring urine pH is the traditional method for initial evaluation of patients suspected to have RTA. Urine pH >6.5 in face of metabolic acidosis is considered as a presumptive evidence of RTA. Some authors have, however, downplayed the importance of urine pH in the diagnosis of RTA.[93] These investigators have argued that ammonium generation is a better index for understanding the pathophysiology as well as diagnosis of RTA. It is important to note that the normal urine pH varies quite widely, depending on diet consumed. Furthermore, patients with chronic acidosis and normal renal tubular function can have a low urine pH between 5.4 and 6.4.[94,95] Therefore, an elevated urine pH (>6.5) should be considered abnormal only if associated with metabolic acidosis. Urine pH is measured ideally by glass electrode, since urine dipsticks are relatively inaccurate.

## Urine anion gap

As mentioned previously, urinary ammonium excretion is the prime renal defense against an acid load. Therefore, determining the rate of urine $NH_4^+$ excretion is the next critical step in deciding whether there is a renal tubular acidification defect. Direct measurements of urine ammonium generally are not available to the clinician. Carlisle et al.[93] have shown that an estimate of urine ammonium can be made by determining the urine net charge or urine anion gap (UAG). The urine cations, $Na^+$, $K^+$, $NH_4^+$, calcium ($Ca^{2+}$), and magnesium ($Mg^{2+}$), must balance the urine anions, which are $Cl^-$, $HCO_3^-$, $PO_4^-$, $SO_4^-$, and organic anions. Urine $Ca^{2+}$, $Mg^{2+}$, $PO_4^-$, and $SO_4^-$ usually are in relatively low and fixed concentrations such that they can be ignored. If the urine pH is below 6.5, the urine $HCO_3^-$ concentration will be very low. In absence of an inborn error of metabolism, urine organic acid concentration will also be very low. Therefore, under most circumstances, the major ions in urine are $Na^+$, $K^+$, $NH_4^+$, and $Cl^-$, all of which can be easily measured and UAG calculated as follows:

$$\text{UAG or Urine net charge} = Na^+ + K^+ - Cl^- \qquad (42.7)$$

Carlisle et al.[93] demonstrated that when the concentration of $Cl^-$ exceeds that of $Na^+ + K^+$, then $NH_4^+$ concentration must be high and the renal tubule is responding appropriately to the acidosis. Therefore, under normal circumstances, UAG is either zero or slightly positive (less than 10 mmol/L). The expectation is that with metabolic acidosis, ammonium excretion will increase and will be excreted as ammonium chloride, increasing urine chloride concentration. This would make the UAG negative (−10 to −20). In case of RTA type 1, in which $H^+$ secretion by the distal nephron is defective, UAG remains positive, despite presence of metabolic acidosis. This contrasts with extrarenal losses of bicarbonate, such as in diarrheal disorders, in which renal ammonium generation is normal and therefore UAG is negative.

Another indirect method of assessing renal ammonium excretion is by assessing the urinary osmolal gap.[96] Urinary osmolal gap is calculated by subtracting calculated urine osmolality from measured urine osmolality (See Equation 42.4). Urine osmolal gap divided by 2 (to account for accompanying anion) approximates urinary ammonium excretion (in milliequivalents/L). Normal urinary ammonium excretion varies from 5 to 50 mEq/L. If this result is greater than 75 mEq/L, the kidney is responding appropriately to metabolic acidosis by generating significant amounts of ammonium. Urinary ammonium of less than 25 mEq/L in face of metabolic acidosis should be considered evidence of an inappropriately poor renal response and suggestive of the diagnosis of RTA type 1. Estimating ammonium excretion using the urine urinary osmolal gap is especially helpful in situations where a large amount of unmeasured organic anion present, such as hippurate to (glue-sniffing) or β-hydroxybutyrate (diabetic ketoacidosis) are present in urine. In these situations the UAG may be positive, even though the kidney is excreting appropriate amounts of ammonium that can be detected by the calculating the urine osmolal gap.

## Fractional excretion of bicarbonate

To test the tubular ability to reclaim the filtered load of $HCO_3^-$, the fractional excretion of $HCO_3^-$ can be determined after the serum $HCO_3^-$ has been restored to normal (22 to 25 mEq/L) by simultaneously measuring the serum creatinine and $HCO_3^-$ and the urine creatinine and $HCO_3^-$.

$$FE\ HCO_3^- = \frac{U_{HCO_3^-}}{U_{creatinine}} \times \frac{P_{creatinine}}{P_{HCO_3^-}} \times 100 \qquad (42.8)$$

Normally this value should be less than 5%. With RTA type 2, the FE $HCO_3^-$ exceeds 15%, and in the RTA type 1 FE $HCO_3^-$ is less than 15%, usually 5% to 10%.[1] Urine $HCO_3^-$ is calculated by measuring the urine pH and $pCO_2$ on a standard blood gas analyzer. Bicarbonate is calculated from the Henderson-Hasselbalch equation as follows:

$$HCO_3^- = 10^{(pH-pK)} \times 0.03 \times pCO_2 \qquad (42.9)$$

In the above formula one can assume the pK to be close to 6.1. Most blood gas analysis machines can provide calculated urine $HCO_3^-$ values directly, without the need to calculate it from Equation 42.9.

## Urine-blood pCO$_2$

The urine $pCO_2$ concentration in alkaline urine has been used to test the distal nephron's ability to secrete $H^+$.[97] In the distal tubular lumen, the $H^+$ combines with $HCO_3^-$ and the resulting $H_2CO_3$ only slowly decomposes into $H_2O$ and $CO_2$ because carbonic anhydrase IV absent from the luminal membrane, unlike in the proximal tubule. This slow decomposition means that $CO_2$ remains in urine where it can be measured. The countercurrent system in the medulla also helps maintain a high urine $pCO_2$.

To perform this test, the urine pH and $HCO_3^-$ concentration are raised to greater than 7.5 and 85 mEq/L, respectively by infusing $HCO_3^-$ (2.5 mEq/Kg) or administering acetazolamide 17 mg/kg. Urine and blood $pCO_2$ is then measured.[98] A normal response is that urine $pCO_2$ that exceeds the blood $pCO_2$ by 30 mm Hg. If this difference is less than 30 mm Hg, distal hydrogen ion pumping is defective and is suggestive of RTA type I or DRTA. In contrast, urine $pCO_2$ exceeds the blood $pCO_2$ by 30 mm Hg in patients with RTA type II ( PRTA), since distal hydrogen ion secretion is intact in these patients.

## Acid loading

The classic test for RTA is to determine the NAE (see Equation 42.1) during spontaneous acidosis or after acid loading. Most children with untreated RTA have metabolic acidosis, making acid loading unnecessary. Acid loading can be useful in equivocal cases. Traditionally, ammonium chloride ($NH_4Cl$) is given orally in a dose of 150 to 300 mg/kg.[99,100] The urine is then collected for 4 to 8 hours and the urine pH, titratable acid (defined as the amount of NaOH need to raise the urine pH to 7.4), and urine ammonium are measured. Oral $CaCl_2$ (2 mg/kg) and intravenous arginine hydrochloride (150 mEq $H^+/m^2$ or 300 mL/$m^2$ of a 10% arginine solution) have also been used for acid loading.[101,102] A normal response is a lowering of urine pH to less than 5.2 and an increase of TA to above 33 µEq/min/1.73 $m^2$, and ammonium to above 46 µEq/min/1.73 $m^2$.

## Furosemide and sodium sulfate challenge test

A simple way of testing the distal tubule's ability to acidify the urine is to give 1 to 2 mg/kg of furosemide orally or intravenously, especially in combination with fludrocortisone. Furosemide causes an increase in distal $Na^+$ and $Cl^-$ delivery.[103] The $Na^+$ is reabsorbed but the poorly reabsorbed $Cl^-$ causes a lumen negative transepithelial potential difference and increased $H^+$ secretion.[11] Expected normal response is a fall in urine pH to below 5.5 and a doubling of the urinary excretion of net acid and potassium 2 to 5 hours after administration

Sodium sulfate infusion (¼ to ½ g/kg) also can be used to assess distal $H^+$ secretion. Sulfate is poorly reabsorbed in the distal nephron, increasing the lumen negative, transepithelial potential difference. This facilitates $H^+$ secretion and a fall in urine pH below 5.[104] An abnormal response to either sodium sulfate or furosemide suggests either a secretory (hydrogen pump) or voltage-dependent defect.

## Approach to evaluation of a child for possible renal tubular acidosis

The initial step in the evaluation of a child suspected to have RTA is to document the presence of hyperchloremic normal anion gap metabolic acidosis (Figure 42.12). The history and physical examination should also be supportive of the diagnosis, and extrarenal bicarbonate loss, such as with ongoing diarrhea, should be ruled out. Arterial blood gas analysis is generally not necessary in most patients with suspected RTA. But if obtained, the test would document a low blood pH and $CO_2$. Next, the serum electrolytes should be obtained to document evidence for low bicarbonate, hyperchloremia, hypokalemia, and anion gap should

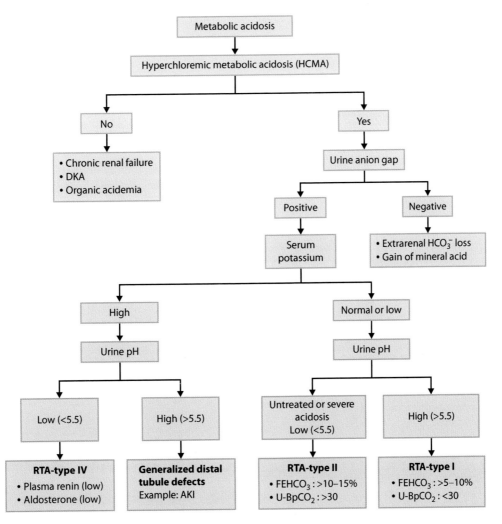

Figure 42.12 Algorithm for evaluation of a child suspected to have RTA. HCMA, hyperchloremic metabolic acidosis. DKA, diabetic ketoacidosis.

be determined and corrected for serum albumin. Urine pH should be obtained order to document an inappropriately elevated urine pH in face of metabolic acidosis. If the anion gap is between 6 and 16 mEq/L (normal anion gap metabolic acidosis), RTA is a diagnostic possibility. If the anion gap is elevated, some other cause of metabolic acidosis must be sought, such as renal failure, diabetic ketoacidosis, or another organic acidosis.

The next step in the evaluation of normal anion gap acidosis, or hyperchloremic metabolic acidosis (HCMA), is to measure the urine net charge (urine anion gap) to determine if there is an appropriate increase in urine ammonium excretion. If the net charge is negative, then the cause of the acidosis is extrarenal, such as gastrointestinal loss of $HCO_3^-$. If the anion gap is positive, the patient has RTA.

To determine the type of RTA, the following steps are helpful. Measure serum $K^+$. If the serum $K^+$ is high, the low urine $NH_4^+$ concentration is a consequence of hyperkalemia and the patient can be diagnosed to have RTA type 4. Measurement of serum renin and aldosterone and the TTKG are useful to determine whether the hyperkalemia is from hypoaldosteronism or distal tubular resistance to the hormone. Metabolic

acidosis in RTA type 4 is usually modest, with serum bicarbonate is the range of 16–18 mEq/L. Urine pH is <5.5, since urinary acidification is normal in these patients.

If the serum $K^+$ is low, the next step is to determine the urine pH and fractional excretion of $HCO_3^-$ with alkali loading. Urine pH in RTA II or PRTA can be variable, being low (<5.5) during severe and spontaneous metabolic acidosis. This results from the fact that filtered bicarbonate load decreases as acidosis becomes more severe, and the proximal tubules are able to reabsorb most of the tubular load of bicarbonate. As patients are treated with alkali and serum bicarbonate level rises, filtered bicarbonate load increases and urine pH rise to >5.5, and is often >6.5. A low urine pH during spontaneous acidosis along. A high urinary fractional excretion of $HCO_3^-$ (greater than 10% to 15%) is another important feature of RTA II. The presence of glucosuria, hypophosphatemia, and aminoaciduria, along with the HCMA and hypokalemia, suggests a global proximal tubule disorder, Fanconi syndrome. A urine pH greater than 5.5 in the face of metabolic acidosis, hyperchloremia, hypokalemia, and FEHCO$_3^-$ of 5% to 10% is suggestive of RTA type I, or DRTA. suggests DRTA. An FE HCO$_3^-$ above

10% is common in infants and young children with DRTA. Further confirmation of RTA type I or DRTA can be made by demonstrating a low urine-blood (U-B) $pCO_2$ during $HCO_3^-$ loading or after acetazolamide.

## CLINICAL VIGNETTES

### Clinical Vignette 42.1

An 8-month-old infant was noted to be failing to thrive. Serum electrolytes showed a Na+, 140; K+, 3.5; Cl–, 114; and $HCO_3^-$, 14 mEq/L. The urinalysis had no glucosuria or proteinuria. Urine amino acids were normal. He was started on supplemental alkali and his serum $HCO_3^-$ rose to 24 mEq/L after giving him 8 mEq/kg/day. His urine pH rose to 8, and his urinary fractional $HCO_3^-$ excretion was 18%.

### TEACHING POINTS

- This patient had HCMA with a normal anion gap. During spontaneous acidosis, the urine pH was low.
- With correction of the acidosis the fractional $HCO_3^-$ excretion was very high, suggesting PRTA. The lack of aminoaciduria, glucosuria, and proteinuria indicates that this is isolated PRTA.

### Clinical Vignette 42.2

A 6-year-old presents to the emergency room with a blood pH of 7.10. His serum electrolytes are Na+, 136; K+, 2.5; Cl–, 116; and $HCO_3^-$, 8 mEq/L. His urine electrolytes are Na+, 72; K+, 31; Cl–, 70 mEq/L; and urine pH, 6.2. A renal ultrasound showed nephrocalcinosis. He required 3 mEq/kg/day of alkali to maintain a normal serum $HCO_3^-$ and at this point his urinary fractional $HCO_3^-$ excretion was 3%. A U-B $pCO_2$ test showed a difference of only 2 mm Hg.

### TEACHING POINTS

- This patient again had HCMA with a normal anion gap. The positive net urine charge indicates RTA.
- The alkaline urine pH in the face of marked acidosis suggests DRTA and the low U-B $pCO_2$ confirms it.
- Nephrocalcinosis is common in untreated DRTA.

### Clinical Vignette 42.3

A 3-month-old infant presents to the emergency room with dehydration from diarrhea and a blood pH of 7.2. The serum electrolytes show Na+, 135 mEq/L; K+, 3.5 mEq/L; Cl–, 110 mEq/L; and $HCO_3^-$, 11 mEq/L. His urine electrolytes were Na+, 3 mEq/L; K+, 6 mEq/L; Cl–, 16 mEq/L; and urine pH, 6.0.

### TEACHING POINTS

- Again this patient had normal anion gap acidosis. The urine pH was relatively alkaline in the face of significant acidosis.
- However, the urine net charge was negative indicating increased ammonium excretion and an appropriate response to the acidosis. The alkaline urine is secondary to decreased Na+ delivery to the CCT for H+ excretion.
- With restoration of the extracellular volume, a U-B $pCO_2$ test was normal with a difference of 30 mm Hg.

## SUMMARY

- The human kidney maintains aid-base balance by excreting acid generated from the diet and absorbing the bicarbonate filtered by the glomerulus. In the average adult the acid production is 1 mEq/kg/day, but it is higher in children, averaging 1 to 3 mEq/kg/day. It also can respond to increases in acid production by increasing acid excretion, mainly as ammonium.
- RTA occurs when the kidney fails to excrete the normal acid load or reabsorb the filtered bicarbonate. Type I RTA arises from an abnormality in the distal nephron that impairs acid excretion and is characterized by the inability to lower the urine pH. In type II RTA, the proximal tubule incompletely reabsorbs the filtered bicarbonate and is characterized by a high FE $HCO_3^-$ when the serum $HCO_3^-$ is normal. Type III is a combination of types I and II. Type IV is caused by hyperkalemia that decreases ammonia production and excretion. The first line of treatment for all types of RTA is treatment of the underlying disease or stopping the offending medication. If that is not possible, administration of bicarbonate to restore the serum bicarbonate to normal and preventing secondary impacts of metabolic acidosis should be the clinical goal. Patients with proximal renal tubular acidosis Type II RTA may require phosphate supplementation to prevent bone disease associated with hypophosphatemia.

## REFERENCES

1. Rodriguez-Soriano J, Edelmann CM, Jr. Renal tubular acidosis. Annu Rev Med. 1969;20:363–82.
2. Remer T, Manz F. Estimation of the renal net acid excretion by adults consuming diets containing variable amounts of protein. Am J Clin Nutr. 1994;59:1356–61.
3. Manz F, Kalhoff H, Remer T. Renal acid excretion in early infancy. Pediatr Nephrol. 1997;11:231–43.

4. Dubose TD, Jr. Reclamation of filtered bicarbonate. Kidney Int. 1990;38:584–9.

5. Wang T, Hropot M, Aronson PS, Giebisch G. Role of NHE isoforms in mediating bicarbonate reabsorption along the nephron. Am J Physiol Renal Physiol. 2001;281:F1117–22.

6. Boron WF. Acid-base transport by the renal proximal tubule. J Am Soc Nephrol. 2006;17:2368–82.

7. Rilly RF, Ellison DH. Mammalian distal tubule: Physiology, pathophysiology, and molecular anatomy. Physiol Rev. 2000;80:277–313.

8. Eladari D, Chambrey R, Peti-Peterdi J. A new look at electrolyte transport in the distal tubule. Annu Rev Physiol. 2012;74:325–49.

9. Kleyman TR, Satlin LM, Hallows KR. Opening lines of communication in the distal nephron. J Clin Invest. 2013;123:4139–41.

10. Gueutin V, Vallet M, Jayat M, et al. Renal β-intercalated cells maintain body fluid and electrolyte balance. J Clin Invest. 2013;123:4219–31.

11. Thomas W, Harvey BJ. Mechanisms underlying rapid aldosterone effects in the kidney. Annu Rev Physiol. 2011;73:335–57.

12. Weiner ID, Verlander JW. Renal ammonia metabolism and transport. Compr Physiol. 2013;3:201–20.

13. Weiner ID, Verlander JW. Role of $NH_3$ and NH4+ transporters in renal acid-base transport. Am J Physiol Renal Physiol. 2011;300:F11–23.

14. Rodriguez Soriano J, Vallo A, Castillo G, Olveros R. Natural history of primary distal renal tubular acidosis treated since infancy. J Pediatr. 1982;101:669–76.

15. Cauana RJ, Buckalew VM, Jr. The syndrome of distal (type 1) renal tubular acidosis: Clinical and laboratory findings in 58 cases. Medicine. 1988;67:84–99.

16. Caldas A, Broyer M, Dechaux M, Kleinknecht C. Primary distal tubule acidosis in childhood: Clinical study and long-term follow up of 28 patients. J Pediatr. 1992;121:233–41.

17. Karet FE, Finberg KE, Nelson RD, et al. Mutations in the gene encoding B1 subunit of the H⁺-ATPase cause renal tubular acidosis with sensorineural deafness. Nat Genet. 1999;21:8–90.

18. Karet FE, Finberg KE, Nayir A, et al. Localization of a gene for autosomal recessive distal renal tubular acidosis with normal hearing (rdRTA2) to 7q33-34. Am Hum Genet. 1999;65:1656–65.

19. Bruce LJ, Cope, Jones GK, et al. Familial distal renal tubular acidosis is associated with mutations in the red cell anion exchanger (Band 3), AE1 gene. J Clin Invest. 1997;100:1693–707.

20. Jarolim P, Shayakul C, Prabakaran D, et al. Autosomal distal renal tubular acidosis is associated in three families with heterozygosity for the R589H mutation in the AE1 (Band 3) Cl⁻/HCO3⁻ exchanger. J Biol Chem. 1998;273:6380–8.

21. Karet FE, Gainza FJ, Gyory AZ, et al. Mutations in the chloride-bicarbonate exchanger gene AE1 cause autosomal dominant but not recessive distal renal tubular acidosis. Proc Natl Acad Sci U S A. 1997;95:6337–42.

22. Tanphaichitr VS, Sumboonnanonda A, Ideguchi H, et al. Novel AE1 mutations in recessive distal renal tubular acidosis: Loss of function is rescued by glycophorin A. J Clin Invest. 1998;2173–9.

23. Vasuvattakul S, Yenchitsomanus PT, Vachuanichsanong P, et al. Autosomal recessive distal renal tubular acidosis associated with Southeast Asian ovalocytosis. Kidney Int. 1999;56:1674–82.

24. Levine AS, Michael AF, Jr. Ehlers-Danlos syndrome with renal tubular acidosis and medullary sponge kidneys. J Pediatr. 1967;71:107–13.

25. Baehner RI, Gilchrist GS, Anderson FJ. Hereditary elliptocytosis and primary renal tubular acidosis in a single family. Am J Dis Child. 1968;115:414–9.

26. Pham PT, Pham PC, Wilkinson AH, et al. Renal abnormalities in sickle cell disease. Kidney Int. 2000;57:1–8.

27. Buckalew VM, Jr, Pyrvis ML, Schulman MG, et al. Hereditary renal tubular acidosis: Report of a 64 member kindred with variable clinical expression including idiopathic hypercalciuria. Medicine. 1974;53:229–54.

28. Hamed JA, Czerwinski AW, Coates B, et al. Familial absorptive hypercalciuria and renal tubular acidosis. Am J Med. 1979;67:385–91.

29. Restano I, Kaplan BS, Stanley C, Baker L. Nephrolithiasis, hypocitraturia, and a distal renal tubular acidification defect in type 1 glycogen storage disease. J Pediatr. 1993;122:392–6.

30. Falik-Borenstein ZC, Jordan SC, Saudubray J-M, et al. Renal tubular acidosis in carnitine palmitoyltransferase type I deficiency. N Engl J Med 1992;327:24–7.

31. Fabris A1, Anglani F, Lupo A, et al. Medullary sponge kidney: State of the art. Nephrol Dial Transplant. 2013;28:1111–9.

32. Brenner RJ, Spring DB, Sebastian A, et al. Incidence of radiographically evident bone disease, nephrocalcinosis, and nephrolithiasis in various types of renal tubular acidosis. N Engl J Med. 1982;307:217–21.

33. Mutalen C, Montoreano R, Labarrere C. Early skeletal effects of alkali therapy upon the osteomalacia of renal tubular acidosis. J Clin Endocrinol Metab. 1976;42:875–81.

34. Norman ME, Feldman NI, Cohn RM, et al. Urinary citrate in the diagnosis of renal tubular acidosis. J Pediatr. 1978;92:394–400.

35. Morris RC Jr, Frudenberg HH. Impaired renal acidification in patients with hypergammaglobulinemia. Medicine. 1967;46:57–69.

36. Caruana RJ, Barish CF, Buckalew VM, Jr. Complete distal renal tubular acidosis in systemic lupus: Clinical and laboratory findings. Am J of Kid Dis. 1985;6:59–63.

37. Talal N. Sjögren syndrome, lymphoproliferation and renal tubular acidosis. Ann Intern Med. 1971;74:633–4.

38. Cohen EP, Bastani B, Cohen MR, et al. Absence of H$^+$-ATPase in cortical collecting tubules of a patient with Sjögren's syndrome and distal renal tubular acidosis. J Am Soc Nephrol. 1992;3:264–72.

39. Batlle DC, von Riotte A, Schlueter W. Urinary sodium in the evaluation of hyperchloremic metabolic acidosis. N Engl J Med. 1987;316:140–4.

40. Izraeli s, Rachmel A, Frishberg Y, et al. Transient renal acidification defect during acute infantile diarrhea: The role of urinary sodium. J Pediatr. 1990;117:711–6.

41. Strife CF, Clardy CW, Varade WS, et al. Urine to blood carbon dioxide tension gradient and maximal depression of urine pH to distinguish rate-dependent from classic distal renal tubule acidosis in children. J Pediatr. 1993;122:60–5.

42. Batlle DC, Grupp M, Gaviria M, Kurtzman NA. Distal renal tubular acidosis with intact capacity to lower urine pH. Am J Med. 1982;72:751–6.

43. McCurdy DK, Frederick M, Elkington JR. Renal tubule acidosis due to amphotericin B. N Engl J Med. 1968;278:124–31.

44. Batlle D, Gaviria M, Grupp M, et al. Distal nephron function in patients receiving chronic lithium therapy. Kidney Int. 1982;21:477–85.

45. Yong JM, Sanderson KV. Photosensitive dermatitis and renal tubular acidosis after ingestion of calcium cyclamate. Lancet. 1969;2:1273–5.

46. Steele TW, Gyory AZ, Edwards KD. Renal function in analgesic nephropathy. Br Med J. 1969;2:213–6.

47. Navarro JF, Quereda C, Quereda C, et al. Nephrogenic diabetes insipidus and renal tubular acidosis secondary to foscarnet therapy. Am J of Kidney Dis. 1996;27:431–4.

48. Gyory AZ, Stewart JH, George CRP, et al. Renal tubular acidosis, acidosis due to hyperkalemia, hypercalcemia, disordered citrate metabolism, and other tubular dysfunction following human renal transplantation. Q J Med. 1969;38:231.

49. Better OS, Chasnowitz C, Naveh Y, et al. Syndrome of incomplete renal tubular acidosis after cadaveric renal transplantation. Ann Intern Med. 1969;71:39–46.

50. Jordan J, Cohen EP, Roza A, et al. An immunochemical study of H$^+$-ATPase in kidney transplant rejection. J Lab Clin Med. 1996;127:310–4.

51. Berlyne GM. Distal tubular function in chronic hydronephrosis. Q J Med. 1961;30:339–55.

52. Hutcheon RA, Kaplan BS, Drummond KN. Distal renal tubular acidosis in children with chronic hydronephrosis. J Pediatr. 1976;89:372–6.

53. Guizar JM, Kornhauser C, Malacaro M, et al. Renal tubular acidosis in children with vesicoureteral reflux. J Urol. 1996;156:193–5.

54. Vainder M, Kelly J. Rebal tubular dysfunction secondary to jejunoileal bypass. JAMA. 1976;235:1257–8.

55. Drutz DJ, Gutman RA. Renal tubular acidosis in leprosy. Ann Intern Med. 1971;75:475–6.

56. Cochran M, Peacock M, Smith DA, Nordin BEC. Renal tubular acidosis of pyelonephritis with renal stone disease. Br Med J. 1968;2:721–9.

57. McSherry E, Morris RC, Jr. Attainment and maintenance of normal stature with alkali therapy in infants and children with classic renal tubular acidosis. J Clin Invest. 1978;61:509–27.

58. Rodriguez Soriano J, Boichis H, Stark H, Edelmann CM, Jr. Proximal renal tubular acidosis: A defect in bicarbonate reabsorption with normal urinary acidification. Pediatr Res. 1967;1:81–98.

59. Foreman JW. Roth KS. Human renal Fanconi syndrome: Then and now. Nephron.1989;51:301–6.

60. Brenes LG, Brenes JN, Hernandez MM. Familial proximal renal tubular acidosis. Am J Med. 1977;63:244–52.

61. Winsnes A, Monn E, Stokke O, Feyling T. Congenital, persistent proximal type of renal tubule acidosis in two brothers. Acta Paediatr Scand 1979;60;861–8.

62. Igarashi T, Ishii T, Watanabe K, et al. Persistent isolated proximal renal tubular acidosis: A systemic disease with a distinct clinical entity. Pediatr Nephrol. 1994;8:70–1.

63. Igarashi T, Inatomi J, Sekine T, et al. Mutations in SLC4A4 cause permanent isolated proximal tubular acidosis with ocular abnormalities. Nat Genet. 1999;23:264–266.

64. Kleta R, Bernardini I, Ueda M, et al. Long-term follow-up of well-treated nephropathic cystinosis patients. J Pediatr. 2004;145:555-60.

65. McSherry E, Sebastian A, Morris RC Jr. Renal tubular acidosis in infants: The several kinds, including bicarbonate-wasting, classic renal tubular acidosis. J Clin Invest. 1972 51:499-514.

66. Sly WS, Whyte MP, Sundaram V, et al. Carbonic anhydrase II deficiency in 12 families with the autosomal recessive syndrome of osteopetrosis with renal tubular acidosis and cerebral calcification. N Engl J Med. 1985;313:139–5.

67. Karet FE. Mechanisms in hyperkalemic renal tubular acidosis. J Am Soc Nephrol 2009;20:251–4.

68. Oetliker O, Zurbrugg RP. Renal regulation of fluid, electrolytes and acid-base homeostasis in the salt losing form of congenital adrenal hyperplasia (SL-CAH).

ECF volume a compensating factor in aldosterone deficiency. Clin Endocrinol Metab. 1978;46:543–51

69. New MI. Inborn errors of steroidogenesis. Mol Cell Endocrinol. 2003;211:75–83.

70. Stratakis CA, Bossis I. Genetics of the adrenal gland. Rev Endocr Metab Dis. 2004;5:53–68

71. Geller DS, Rodriguez Soriano J, Vallo Boado A, et al. Mutations in the mineralocorticoid receptor gene cause autosomal pseudohypoaldosteronism type 1. Nat Genet. 1998;19:279–81.

72. Chang SS, Grunder S Hanukoglu A, et al. Mutations in the subunits of the epithelial sodium channel cause salt wasting with hyperkalemia acidosis, pseudohypoaldosteronism type 1. Nat Genet. 1996;l12:248–53.

73. Grunder S, Firsou D, Chang SS, et al. A mutation causing pseudohypoaldosteronism type 1 identifies a conserved glycine that is involved in the gating of the epithelial sodium channel. EMBO J. 1997;16:899–907.

74. Barker PM, Nguyen MS, Gatzy JT, at al. Role of gamma ENaC subunit in lung liquid clearance and electrolyte balance in newborn mice: Insights into perinatal adaptation and pseudohypoaldosteronism. J Clin Invest. 1998;102:1634–40.

75. Achard JM, Disse-Nicoderm S, Fiquet-Kempf B, et al. Phenotypic and genetic heterogeneity of familial hyperkalemic hypertension (Gordon syndrome). Clin Exp Pharmacol Physiol. 2001;28:1048–52.

76. Wilson FH, Disse-Nicoderm S, Choate KA, et al. Human hypertension caused by mutations in WNK kinases. Science 2001;293:1107–11.

77. Boyden LM, Choi M, Choate KM, et al. Mutations in Kelch-like 3 and Cullin 3 cause hypertension and electrolytes abnormalities. Nature 2012;482:98–102.

78. Davenport MW, Zipser RD. Association of hypotension with hyperreninemic hypoaldosteronism in the critically patient. Ach Intern Med. 1983;143:735–75.

79. DeFronzo RA. Hyperkalemia and hyporeninemic hypoaldosteronism. Kidney Int. 1980;17:118–34.

80. Assadi FK, Ziai M. Impaired renal acidification in infants with fetal alcohol syndrome. Pediatr Res. 1985;19:850–3.

81. Alon U, Kodroff MB, Broecker B, et al. Renal tubular acidosis in neonatal unilateral kidney diseases. J Pediatr. 1984;104:855–60.

82. Batlle DC, Arruda JAL, Kurtzman NA. Hyperkalemic distal renal tubular acidosis associated with obstructive uropathy. N Engl J Med. 1981;304:373–80.

83. Henrich WL. Nephrotoxicity of nonsteroidal anti-inflammatory agents. Am J Kidney Dis. 1983;2:478–84.

84. O'Kelly R, Magee F, McKenna TJ. Routine heparin therapy inhibits adrenal aldosterone production. J Clin Endocrinol Metab. 1983;56:108–12.

85. Hulter HN, Bonner EL, Jr, Glynn RD, Sebastian A. Renal and acid-base effects of chronic spironolactone administration. Am J Physiol. 1891;240:F381–7.

86. Ponce SP, Jennings AE, Madias NE, et al. Drug-induced hyperkalemia. Medicine (Baltimore). 1985;64:357–70.

87. Valazquez H, Perazella MN, Wright FS, et al. Renal mechanisms of trimethoprim induced hyperkalemia. Ann Intern Med. 1993;119:296–302.

88. Kleyman TR, Roberts C, Ling BN. A mechanism for pentamidine-induced hyperkalemia: Inhibition of distal sodium nephron sodium transport. Ann Intern Med. 1995;122:103–6.

89. Kamel DS, Ethier JH, Quaggin S, et al. Studies to determine the basis of the hyperkalemia in recipients of a renal transplant who are treated with cyclosporine. J Am Soc Nephrol. 1991;2:1279–84.

90. Sands JM, McMahan SJ, Tumlin JA. Evidence that the inhibition of $Na^+/K^+$-ATPase activity by FK506 involves a calcineurin. Kidney Int. 1994;46:647–52.

91. West ML, Marsden PA, Richardson MA, et al. New clinical approach to evaluate disorders of potassium excretion. Miner Electrolyte Metab. 1986;12:234–38.

92. Kraut JA, Madias N. Serum anion gap: Its uses and limitations in clinical medicine. Clin J Am Soc Nephrol. 2007;2:162–74.

93. Carlisle EJF, Donnelly SM, Halperin ML. Renal tubular acidosis (RTA): Recognize the ammonium defect and pHorget the urine pH. Pediatr Nephrol. 1991;5:242–48.

94. Schloeder FX, Stinebaugh BJ. Defect of urinary acidification during fasting. Metabolism. 1966;15:17–25.

95. Madison LL, Seldin DW. Ammonium excretion and renal enzymatic adaptation in human subjects, as disclosed by administration of precursor amino acids. J Clin Invest. 1958;37:1615–27.

96. Kraut JA, Madias NE. Differential diagnosis of nongap metabolic acidosis: Value of a systematic approach. Clin J Am Soc Nephrol. 2012;7:671-9.

97. Halperin ML, Goldstein MB, Haig A, et al. Studies on the pathogenesis of type I (distal) renal tubular acidosis as revealed by the urinary $pCO_2$. J Clin Invest. 1974;53:669–677.

98. Alon U, Hellerstein S, Warady BA. Oral acetazolamide in the assessment of (urine-blood) $pCO_2$. Pediatr Nephrol. 1991;5:307–11.

99. Edelmann CM, Jr, Biochis H, Rodriguez Soriano J, Stark H. The renal response of children to acute ammonium chlorise acidosis. Pediatr Res. 1967;1:452–60.

100. Edelmann CM, Jr, Rodriguez Soriano J, Biochis H, et al. Renal bicarbonate and hydrogen ion excretion in normal infants. J Clin Invest. 1967;46:1309–17.

101. Oster JR, Hotchkiss, Carbon M, et al. A short duration renal acidification test using calcium chloride. Nephron. 1975;14:281–92.

102. Loney LC, Norling LL, Robson A. The use of arginine hydrochloride infusion to assess urinary acidification. J Pediatr. 1982;100:95–8.

103. Lash JP, Arruda JAL. Laboratory evaluation of renal tubular acidosis. Clin Lab Med. 1993;13:117–29.
104. Rastogi SP, Crawford C, Wheeler R, et al. Effect of furosemide in urinary acidification in distal renal tubular acidosis. J Lab Clin Med. 1984;271–82.

## REVIEW QUESTIONS

1. The normal acid production of children is:
   a. <1 mEq/kg/day
   b. 1 to 3 mEq/kg/day
   c. 4 to 6 mEq/kg/day
   d. >6 mEq/kg/day

2. The *most* important way of excreting acid during increased acid production is:
   a. Increased ammonium excretion
   b. Increased phosphate excretion
   c. Increased urea excretion
   d. Decreased bicarbonate excretion

3. Proximal tubule bicarbonate reabsorption occurs because of which of the following?
   a. Ammonia generation from glutamine
   b. Hydrogen ion excretion by the $K^+/H^+$ ATPase
   c. AE1 in the basolateral membrane
   d. Carbonic anhydrase on the brush border membrane

4. For adequate distal tubule acid excretion, there must be adequate:
   a. Sodium reabsorption
   b. Potassium absorption
   c. Ammonium absorption
   d. Sodium excretion

5. Ammoniagenesis occurs in the:
   a. Thick ascending limb
   b. Cortical collecting tubule
   c. Medullary collecting tubule
   d. Proximal tubule

6. Fanconi syndrome involves RTA type:
   a. Type I
   b. Type II
   c. Type III
   d. Type IV

7. In RTA, the urine anion gap is:
   a. Positive
   b. Negative
   c. Neutral

8. Type 1 is associated with a mutation in the gene coding for:
   a. NBC1
   b. 2Cl/Na/K
   c. AE1
   d. CA

9. An abnormal $\beta_1$ subunit of $H^+$-ATPase is associated with:
   a. Skeletal dysplasia
   b. Early onset deafness
   c. Cardiac defect
   d. Mental retardation

10. The *main* abnormality of RTA type 4 is:
    a. Hyperkalemia causing decreased ammoniagenesis
    b. Hypokalemia causing decreased ammoniagenesis
    c. Hyperkalemia causing increased ammoniagenesis
    d. Hypokalemia causing increased ammoniagenesis

11. Nephrocalcinosis is associated with:
    a. Type I RTA
    b. Type II RTA
    c. Type IV RTA
    d. None of above

12. The anticonvulsant medication, topiramate, is associated with:
    a. Type I RTA
    b. Type II RTA
    c. Type III RTA
    d. Type IV RTA

13. The type of RTA requiring the largest dose of supplemental alkali to correct the acidosis is:
    a. Type I
    b. Type II
    c. Type IV

14. The *major* urinary buffer of titratable acid is:
    a. Citrate
    b. Phosphate
    c. Urate
    d. Creatinine

15. A simple way of testing the distal nephron's ability to acidify the urine is to administer orally:
    a. Phosphate
    b. Citrate
    c. Furosemide
    d. Hydrochlorothiazide

## ANSWER KEY

1. b
2. a
3. d
4. a
5. d
6. b
7. a
8. c
9. b
10. a
11. a
12. b
13. b
14. b
15. c

# 43

# Cystic kidney disease

LISA M. GUAY-WOODFORD

Renal cysts are observed in a variety of kidney diseases. Many of these disorders are inherited as single gene defects, and some are associated with extrarenal manifestations or represent manifestations of syndromes. Different ages of onset, variability in kidney disease progression, and a diverse array of extrarenal manifestations help distinguish these disorders. On the whole, renal cystic disorders are relatively rare diseases, although a few, such as autosomal recessive polycystic kidney disease (ARPKD), juvenile nephronophthisis (NPHP), and hepatocyte nuclear factor-1β (HNF1B)–related renal disease, are common enough to cause considerable pediatric morbidity and mortality. In contrast, autosomal dominant polycystic kidney disease (ADPKD), one of the most common human genetic diseases, typically has relatively mild clinical manifestations during childhood. Table 43.1 provides a clinicopathologic classification of the cystic renal diseases.

## CELLULAR MECHANISM OF CYST FORMATION

With the identification of disease-causing genes, proteins involved in renal cystic diseases have been localized, often in multimeric complexes, at discrete subcellular locations in renal epithelial cells, including the primary apical cilium, intercellular junctions, and focal adhesions.[1] In addition, defects in several common signaling pathways have been defined in renal cystic epithelia. Taken together, these data suggest that cyst formation may involve the abnormal integration of signal transduction pathways that lead to altered cell proliferation and apoptosis.[2]

## KEY POINT

Renal cysts result from abnormal integration of signal transduction in the epithelial cells that alters cell proliferation and apoptosis.

## AUTOSOMAL RECESSIVE POLYCYSTIC KIDNEY DISEASE

ARPKD is one of the most common form of renal cystic disease encountered in children. It was previously known as infantile polycystic kidney disease, a term no longer in use. With the advent of high-resolution ultrasound, many cases of ARPKD are diagnosed prenatally. While the true incidence of the disease is not certain because many patients die in the neonatal period, ARPKD is estimated to occur in 1 in 20,000 live births.

Table 43.1 Classification of cystic kidney diseases

| Disorder | Affected genes |
|---|---|
| **Nongenetic renal cystic disease** | |
| Simple renal cysts | NA |
| Multilocular cysts | NA |
| **Polycystic kidney disease** | |
| Autosomal recessive polycystic kidney disease | PKHD1 |
| Autosomal dominant polycystic kidney disease | PKD1, PKD2 |
| **Cystic diseases of the renal medulla** | |
| Juvenile nephronophthisis | NPHP1-NPHP18 |
| Medullary cystic kidney disease | MUC1, UMOD |
| Medullary sponge kidney | NA |
| **Other renal cystic diseases** | |
| HNF1B-related renal cystic disease | TCF2 |
| Glomerulocystic kidney disease | PKD1, TCF2, UMOD |

*Abbreviation:* NA, not applicable.

Table 43.2 Clinical manifestations of autosomal recessive polycystic kidney disease in children

**Prenatal**
- Abnormal prenatal ultrasound scan, large kidneys with increased echogenicity

**Postnatal**
- Respiratory distress
- Enlarged kidneys
- Hyponatremia
- Systemic hypertension
- Renal failure
- Pyuria
- Urinary tract infection
- Proteinuria
- Failure to thrive
- Hepatomegaly
- Portal hypertension
- Esophageal varices

**Family History**
- Renal cystic disease in a sibling
- Normal renal ultrasound scan in parents

## CLINICAL MANIFESTATIONS

ARPKD (Mendelian Inheritance in Man [MIM] 173900) is a severe, typically early-onset form of cystic disease. Patients with ARPKD have a spectrum of clinical phenotypes that depend in part on the age at presentation.[3] Most patients are identified either in utero or at birth with enlarged echogenic kidneys and oligohydramnios. At birth, the most severely affected neonates have a critical degree of pulmonary hypoplasia that may be incompatible with survival. The estimated perinatal mortality rate is 30%. In patients who survive the first month of life, 1-year survival rates of 92% to 95% have been reported.[3,4] Renal function, although frequently compromised, is rarely a cause of neonatal death.

---

### KEY POINTS

- ARPKD is the most common inherited renal cystic disease encountered in children.
- Oligohydramnios and large kidneys are common manifestations of ARPKD in neonates.
- Pulmonary hypoplasia is a cause of neonatal morbidity and mortality in ARPKD.
- Some ARPKD patients may manifest Potter syndrome.

---

For those patients who survive the first few weeks of life, the major morbidities include severe systemic hypertension, renal impairment, and portal hypertension (Table 43.2).[3,5,6] Hyponatremia occurs in a subset of neonates, presumably secondary to defects in free water excretion.[3] Systemic hypertension usually develops during the first 6 months of life, often associated with a transient improvement in glomerular filtration rate (GFR) resulting from renal maturation. Subsequently, there is a progressive, but variable decline in renal function.[7]

A subset of patients with late-onset ARPKD has a liver-predominant phenotype with few or no manifestations of kidney disease.[6] These patients present with portal hypertension, hepatosplenomegaly, esophageal or gastric varices, and hypersplenism with associated thrombocytopenia, anemia, and leukopenia. Hepatocellular function is usually preserved. Ascending suppurative cholangitis, a serious complication, can cause fulminant hepatic failure in such patients.[8,9]

Other associated features of ARPKD include an increased incidence of culture-confirmed urinary tract infections,

---

### KEY POINTS

- Hyponatremia is common in ARPKD neonates.
- Hypertension and chronic kidney disease (CKD) evolve over time in ARPKD.
- Liver disease (hepatic fibrosis) can be a prominent clinical finding in some patients.

---

very rare occurrence of intracranial aneurysms (ICAs), and growth retardation, although the pathophysiology of the growth retardation is poorly defined.[3,10]

## GENETICS

All typical forms of ARPKD are caused by mutations in a single gene, *PKHD1*, which encodes multiple alternatively spliced isoforms predicted to form both membrane-bound and secreted proteins.[11] To date, more than 700 pathogenic mutations have been catalogued in the ARPKD Mutation Database,[12] of which approximately half are missense changes. Although a missense mutation in exon 3, c.107C>T (p.Thr36Met), accounts for approximately 20% of all mutant alleles,[5] no other mutational hotspots have been described. Indeed, ARPKD mutations have been identified along the entire length of the *PKHD1* gene, and many of these mutations are unique to single families.[13]

## MOLECULAR PATHOGENESIS

The largest protein product of *PKHD1*, termed the fibrocystin-polyductin complex (FPC), localizes, at least in part, to the primary cilium and the centrosome in renal epithelial cells.[14] The basic defects observed in ARPKD suggest that the FPC mediates the terminal differentiation of the collecting duct and the biliary tract. However, the exact function of the numerous isoforms has not been defined, and the widely variable clinical spectrum may partially depend on the nature and number of splice variants that are disrupted by specific *PKHD1* mutations.

---

### KEY POINTS

- ARPKD involves dysfunction of the cilia-centrosome complex, and is classified under the group of conditions designated as ciliopathies.
- Because of associated congenital hepatic fibrosis, ARPKD is often grouped under the disorders known as hepatorenal fibrocystic diseases.

---

ARPKD is one of several renal cystic diseases that are associated with congenital hepatic fibrosis, thus prompting these disorders to be described as hepatorenal fibrocystic diseases[15] (Table 43.3). The primary cilium appears to play a central role in the pathogenesis of ARPKD and other hepatorenal fibrocystic diseases.[16] Hence this subset of clinical disorders is now grouped under the broader term of "ciliopathies," in which dysfunction of the cilia-centrosome complex appears to underpin the development of a wide array of phenotypes, including renal cystic disease.[17]

## ANATOMIC PATHOLOGY

Kidneys in ARPKD are grossly enlarged, but they usually retain their reniform appearance. These enlarged kidneys may appear to occupy the entire abdominal cavity in the affected neonates. The outer surface of the kidneys demonstrate cysts that are usually small. The cysts in ARPKD represent fusiform dilatation of the collecting tubules (Figure 43.1). These dilated collecting tubules (cysts) run perpendicular to the cortical surface (Figure 43.2) in cut section of the kidney.

## DIAGNOSTIC EVALUATION

### Imaging

In utero ARPKD kidneys are hyperechogenic by ultrasound evaluation and display decreased corticomedullary differentiation as a result of the hyperechogenic medulla (Figure 43.3A). These ultrasound findings are generally observable by the mid-second trimester. With high-resolution ultrasound, the radial array of dilated collecting ducts may be observed. A hypoechoic cortical rim may be seen many infants (Figure 43.3B). In comparison, autosomal dominant polycystic kidney disease (ADPKD) kidneys tend to be moderately enlarged in utero, with a hyperechogenic cortex and relatively hypoechogenic medulla resulting in increased cortico-medullary differentiation.

Kidney size in ARPKD typically peaks at 1 to 2 years of age, then gradually declines relative to the child's body size, and stabilizes by 4 to 5 years.[18] As patients age, medullary echogenicity increases, with scattered cysts that are smaller than 2 cm, and progressive interstitial fibrosis. A hypoechoic cortical rim may be seen many infants (Figure 43.3B). The resulting sonographic pattern may be confused with ADPKD, and contrast-enhanced computed tomography (CT) can better delineate the renal architecture. Bilateral pelvicaliectasis (Figure 43.3C) and renal calcifications have been reported.[6,19] In adults with medullary ectasia alone, the cystic lesion may be confused with medullary sponge kidney (MSK).

By ultrasound evaluation, liver may be either normal in size or enlarged. It is usually less echogenic than the kidneys. Presence of prominent intrahepatic bile duct dilatation suggests associated Caroli syndrome (Figure 43.4). With age, the portal fibrosis tends to progress, and in older children, ultrasound typically shows hepatosplenomegaly and a patchy increase in hepatic echogenicity.[20,21]

### Genetic testing

Gene-based testing is clinically available. At present, the mutation detection rate is only 80% to 87%.[5,22] Therefore, sequence analysis is largely reserved for prenatal testing and preimplantation genetic diagnosis.[23]

Table 43.3 Hepatorenal fibrocystic diseases

| Disease | Gene(s) | Renal disease | Hepatic disease | Associated features |
|---|---|---|---|---|
| ARPKD | *PKHD1* | Collecting duct dilatation | CHF, Caroli disease | Growth retardation |
| ADPKD | *PKD1, PKD2* | Cysts along entire nephron | Biliary cysts, CHF | Minimal in children |
| Nephronophthisis (NPHP) | *NPHP1-NPHP18* | Cysts at the corticomedullary junction | CHF | Tapetoretinal degeneration, situs inversus |
| Joubert syndrome (JBTS) | *JBTS1-JBTS22* | Cystic dysplasia, NPHP | CHF, Caroli disease | Cerebellar vermis hypoplasia or aplasia with episodic hyperpnea, abnormal eye movements, intellectual disability |
| Bardet-Biedl syndrome (BBS) | *BBS1-BBS19* | Cystic dysplasia, NPHP | CHF | Retinal degeneration, obesity, postaxial polydactyly, hypogonadism in male patients, intellectual disability |
| Meckel-Gruber syndrome (MKS) | *MKS1-MKS11* | Cystic dysplasia | CHF | Occipital encephalocele, polydactyly |
| Oral-facial-digital syndrome, Type I | *OFD1* | Glomerular cysts | CHF (rare) | Malformations of the face, oral cavity, and digits |
| Glomerulocystic disease | *PKD1, HNF1B(TCF2), UMOD* | Enlarged; normal or hypoplastic kidneys | CHF (with *PKD1* mutations) | Diabetes, hyperuricemia |
| Jeune syndrome (asphyxiating thoracic dystrophy [ATD]) | *IFT80 (ATD2) DYNC2H1 (ATD3) ATD1, ATD4, ATD5* | Cystic dysplasia | CHF, Caroli disease | Short stature, skeletal dysplasia, small thorax, short limbs; polydactyly, hypoplastic pelvis |
| Renal-hepatic-pancreatic dysplasia | *NPHP3, NEK8* | Cystic dysplasia | Intrahepatic biliary dysgenesis | Pancreatic cysts, dysplasia, or fibrosis; splenic abnormalities, situs inversus |
| Zellweger syndrome | *PEX1-3, 5-6, 10-11, 13, 14, 16, 19, 26* | Renal cortical microcysts | Intrahepatic biliary dysgenesis | Hypotonia, seizures, agenesis or hypoplasia of corpus callosum, characteristic facies, skeletal abnormalities, neonatal death |

*Source:* Adapted from Somlo S, Guay-Woodford L. Polycystic kidney disease. In: Lifton RP, Somlo S, Giebisch GH, Seldin DW, editors. Genetic Diseases of the Kidney. New York: Academic Press; 2009. p. 393–424.

*Abbreviations:* ARPKD, autosomal recessive polycystic kidney disease; ADPKD, autosomal dominant polycystic kidney disease; CHF : congenital hepatic fibrosis.

## GENETIC COUNSELING

Most patients with ARPKD are compound heterozygotes, and the functional effect of any particular mutant allele can be difficult to define. In general, patients with two truncating mutations have a severe phenotype, leading to perinatal demise.[13] However, there are notable exceptions, such as a child homozygous for a large *PKHD1* deletion who survives well past the neonatal period.[24] Although

## KEY POINTS

- Genetic testing in ARPKD is generally reserved for prenatal testing and preimplantation genetic diagnosis.
- Phenotypic variability in ARPKD may be expected as a result of genetic modifiers.

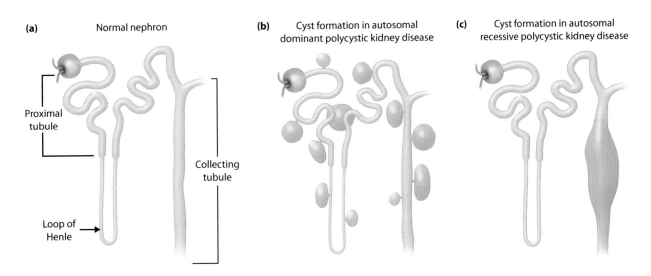

Figure 43.1 Mechanisms of cyst formation in polycystic kidney disease. (a) Normal nephron. (b) In autosomal dominant polycystic kidney disease, cystic outgrowths arise in every segment of the tubule and rapidly close off from the nephron of origin. (c) In autosomal recessive polycystic kidney disease, cysts are derived from collecting tubules, which remain connected to the nephron of origin. (Redrawn with permission from Wilson PD. Polycystic kidney disease. N Engl J Med. 2004;350:151–64.)

most missense mutations are associated with milder disease, some missense mutations result in severe phenotypes when combined with a truncating mutation, or occurring in the homozygous state.[13] In addition, significant phenotypic variability in a subset of families suggests that genetic modifiers modulate disease expression. These data can complicate genetic counseling, and caution must be exercised in predicting the clinical outcome of future affected children.[25]

## MANAGEMENT AND PROGNOSIS

Neonatal pulmonary hypoplasia, often complicated by pneumothoraces, is a major cause of neonatal mortality in ARPKD.[26] Aggressive interventions such as unilateral or bilateral nephrectomies and continuous hemofiltration have been advocated for neonatal management. However, these recommendations are based on limited set of small case reports and case series. Evidence-based clinical practice will require prospective, controlled studies.

For those children who survive the perinatal period, hypertension is a dominant clinical issue, with a prevalence of 55% to 75% and an onset that typically precedes the decline in GFR. Angiotensin-converting enzyme (ACE) inhibitors, angiotensin receptor blockers (ARB), adrenergic antagonists, and loop diuretics are effective antihypertensive agents. The management of children with ARPKD who have a declining GFR should follow the standard guidelines established for chronic kidney disease in the pediatric patients.[27] Given the relative urinary concentrating defect, children with ARPKD should be monitored for dehydration during intercurrent illnesses associated with fever, tachypnea, nausea, vomiting, or diarrhea.

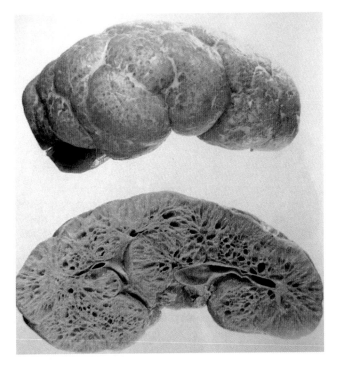

Figure 43.2 Autosomal recessive polycystic kidney disease. (From Kissane JM. Renal cysts in pediatric patients. Pediatr Nephrol. 1990;4:69–77.)

Most patients with ARPKD progress to end-stage renal disease (ESRD), but the age at onset is highly variable, and partly depends on the age at initial presentation. For example, 25% of patients diagnosed in the perinatal period required renal replacement therapy by 11 years, whereas only 25% of those who presented after 1 month of age required renal replacement therapy by age 32 years.[7]

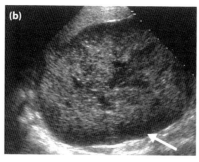
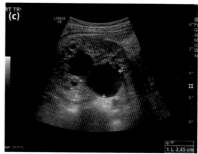

Figure 43.3 Autosomal recessive polycystic kidney disease (ARPKD). **(a)** Renal sonogram of a fetus at 34 weeks demonstrating large kidneys bilaterally, almost filling the entire abdomen. Echogenicity of the kidneys is increased. **(b)** Renal ultrasound scan of a 6-month-old infant showing increased echogenicity of the medullary cortex. The arrow points to the hypoechoic cortical rim. **(c)** Hydronephrosis seen in the transverse section of the right kidney in a 3-year-old girl with ARPKD.

A subset of ARPKD patients develop portal hypertension and the associated complications of hypersplenism and esophageal varices.[20] Platelet counts, serial abdominal ultrasound scans (assessing liver and splenic size), and Doppler flow studies provide surrogate markers for portal hypertension severity.[21] Medical management includes sclerotherapy or variceal banding; whereas surgical approaches such as portocaval or splenorenal shunting may be indicated in some patients.[20] Ascending cholangitis is a leading cause of morbidity and mortality in patients with ARPKD.[28] Meticulous evaluation is required for suspected bacterial cholangitis, and if indicated, aggressive antibiotic therapy should be initiated.

## KIDNEY TRANSPLANTATION

Because ARPKD is a recessive disorder, either parent may be a suitable kidney donor. However, subtle renal and liver sonographic abnormalities have been described in ARPKD parents,[29] thus warranting particular caution in donor evaluation. Native nephrectomies may be indicated in patients

> ### KEY POINTS
>
> - Because ARPKD is a recessive disorder, either parent can be considered as a renal transplant donor for the affected child.
> - Liver disease in the recipient and in the organ donors should be carefully investigated.
> - Liver-kidney transplant may be appropriate in patients with significant liver disease, in addition to ESRD.

with massively enlarged kidneys in order to allow space for allograft placement within the abdominal cavity.

In some patients, combined kidney-liver transplantation may be appropriate.[30] Indications include the combination of renal failure and either recurrent cholangitis or significant complications of portal hypertension (e.g., recurrent variceal bleeding, refractory ascites, and the hepatopulmonary syndrome).[20]

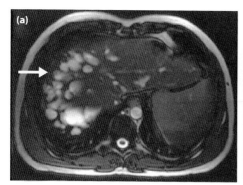
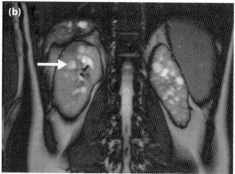

Figure 43.4 Caroli syndrome. **(a)** Axial T2-weighted MRI scans showing intrahepatic biliary dilatation (arrow). **(b)** Coronal T2-weighted MRI scans showing bilaterally enlarged kidneys with extensive cystic disease (white arrow) that simulate findings in ARPKD. (Reproduced with permission from from Kurschat CE, Müller RU, Franke M, et al. An approach to cystic kidney diseases: the clinician's view. Nat Rev Nephrol. 2014;10:687–99.)

Effective management of systemic and portal hypertension, coupled with successful renal replacement therapy and transplantation options, has allowed for long-term patient survival. Therefore, the prognosis in ARPKD, particularly for those children who survive the first month of life, is far less bleak than previously thought, and aggressive medical therapy is warranted.

## AUTOSOMAL DOMINANT POLYCYSTIC KIDNEY DISEASE

## CLINICAL MANIFESTATIONS

ADPKD (MIM 173900) is a multisystem disorder characterized by bilateral and multiple renal cysts, as well as a variety of extrarenal manifestations. These extrarenal features include cysts in the bile ducts, pancreatic ducts, seminal vesicles, and arachnoid membrane, as well as noncystic abnormalities, such as ICAs and elongation and dilatation of intracranial arteries (dolichoectasia) aortic root dilatation and aneurysms, mitral valve prolapse, and abdominal wall hernias.[31]

> ### KEY POINTS
>
> - ADPKD is a multisystem disorder. Cystic lesions can be seen in multiple organs.
> - 1% to 2% patients may present early in infancy with features that are indistinguishable from those of ARPKD.
> - Incidental finding of renal cysts is a common presentation during childhood.

The typical symptomatic presentation of ADPKD and major morbidities occur in adults. However, ADPKD is also diagnosed in fetuses, infants, children, and adolescents. Most of the time, the diagnosis is made in the at-risk children as an incidental imaging finding, or by presymptomatic sonographic screening. However, renal manifestations and limited extrarenal manifestations do occur in children with ADPKD (Table 43.4).[32] In addition, a form of very early-onset ADPKD occurs in 1% to 2% of affected children and may be clinically indistinguishable from ARPKD.[33]

## GENETICS

Mutations in *PKD1* account for approximately 85% of ADPKD cases, and mutations in *PKD2* account for the remainder.[34] De novo mutations account for up to 10% of cases. The high mutability of *PKD1* likely explains why de novo mutations arise much more frequently in this gene and why private mutations (i.e., unique to a single family) are more common in *PKD1*.[22,35]

Although the disease is transmitted as an autosomal dominant trait, it is recessive on a cellular level[36]; that is, ADPKD is genetically a "two-hit" disease, analogous to what has been described for tumor suppressor genes. Cysts form only when both copies of the gene are mutated and *PKD* gene activity is reduced below a cellular threshold. Although not precisely defined, this threshold likely differs in cells of different nephron segments and may even change over time depending on developmental stage.

> ### KEY POINTS
>
> - Mutations in the *PKD1* gene comprise approximately 85% cases of ADPKD, and *PKD2* gene mutation accounts for 15% cases.
> - De novo mutations are relatively common in ADPKD, and are seen in up to 10% cases..
> - Pathogenesis of ADPKD is considered to be a "two-hit" disease.

## MOLECULAR PATHOGENESIS

After decades of investigation, it is well established that increased cell proliferation, fluid secretion, and loss of normal renal parenchyma are the key elements that cause loss of renal function in ADPKD. The identification of the disease-causing genes and of the proteins they encode has provided key pathogenic insights. The *PKD1* gene encodes a membrane receptor polycystin-1 (PC1), and *PKD2* encodes a nonselective cation channel permeable to calcium designated polycystin-2 (PC2). Together, these proteins function as a receptor-channel complex on the cell surface.[37] The complex, as well as virtually every other cystoprotein (i.e., a protein encoded by a gene whose mutation results in renal cystic disease), localizes to the primary apical cilium. The PC1/PC2 complex has been postulated to function as a flow sensor that triggers the release of intracellular calcium stores[38] and regulates a cascade of integrated signaling pathways that regulate cellular growth, fluid secretion, and tubular morphology.

## ANATOMIC PATHOLOGY

The kidneys in ARPKD can be normal to very large in size. In advanced cases, the cysts are large and conspicuous in the cut section of the kidney, giving it a "Swiss cheese" appearance (Figure 43.5). The cysts in ADPKD arise from every segment of the nephron (see Figure 43.1b) and have a narrow attachment to the nephron, from which the cysts eventually lose communication.[1]

Table 43.4 The incidence of renal and extrarenal manifestations of autosomal dominant polycystic kidney disease in adults and children

| Manifestation | ADPKD in adults | ADPKD in children |
|---|---|---|
| Hematuria (micro and macro) | 35%–50% | 10% |
| Concentrating defects | 100% | 60% |
| Proteinuria | 18% | 14% |
| Microalbuminuria | 25% | 30% |
| Nephrolithiasis | 20% | Unknown |
| Flank or abdominal pain | 60% | 10% |
| Hepatic cysts revealed by MRI | 83% | 55% by age 25 yr |
| Colonic diverticula | 82% | Unknown |
| Cerebral aneurysms | 5%–7% | Rare |
| Prolapse of the mitral valve | 26% | 12% |
| Hypertension before eGFR decline | 60% | 22% |
| Hyperlipidemia | Unknown | 54% |

Source: Rizk D, Chapman A. Treatment of autosomal dominant polycystic kidney disease (ADPKD): the new horizon for children with ADPKD. Pediatr Nephrol. 2008;23:1029–36. Reproduced with permission.

ADPKD, autosomal dominant polycystic kidney disease; eGFR, estimated glomerular filtration rate; MRI, magnetic resonance imaging.

## DIAGNOSTIC EVALUATION

A screening algorithm for children at risk for ADPKD and for patients with confirmed ADPKD is provided in Figure 43.6.

> ## KEY POINTS
>
> - The membrane receptor PC1/PC2 complex on the primary apical cilium of the epithelial cell is a flow sensor and facilitates intracellular calcium release.
> - Intracellular calcium release triggers signal pathways that regulate cell growth, fluid secretion, and morphology of renal tubules.
> - Defective function of the PC1/PC2 complex contributes to tubular cell abnormalities in ADPKD.

## Imaging

Renal sonography is the main diagnostic tool in ADPKD. It is widely available, has a relatively low cost, is well tolerated by patients, and lacks known adverse effects. Sonographic imaging shows increased echogenicity of the renal parenchyma with many cysts distributed throughout (Figure 43.7). Magnetic resonance imaging (MRI) may provide better delineation of renal cysts, especially if hemorrhage within the cysts needs to be confirmed (Figure 43.8). Sonographic screening in asymptomatic children is controversial because of the limited sensitivity of ultrasonography, particularly in children younger than 5 years of age.[39] A study involving sonographic analysis of 420 at-risk children 15 years or younger demonstrated this point. Investigators detected bilateral renal cysts in 193 (46%) and cysts were

(a)

(b)

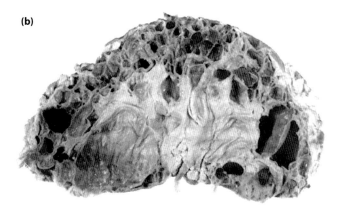

Figure 43.5 Autosomal dominant polycystic kidney disease. (a) Kidney surface showing extensive and large cysts throughout. (b) Cut section of the kidney showing cysts distributed throughout the cortex and medulla of the kidney. (Reproduced with permission from Kissane JM. Renal cysts in pediatric patients. Pediatr Nephrol. 1990;4:69–77.)

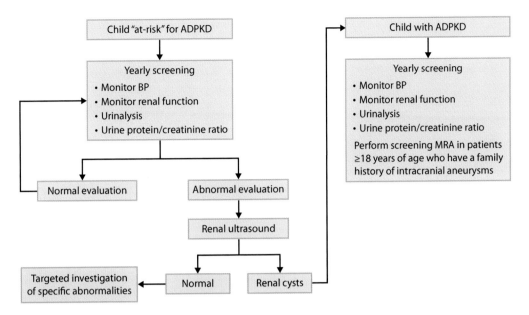

Figure 43.6  Algorithm for screening and monitoring of children with autosomal dominant polycystic kidney disease (ADPKD). BP, blood pressure; MRA, magnetic resonance angiography.

absent in 227 (54%) of participants.[39] Of these, bilateral cysts were evident in 150 out of 193 (77%) and unilateral cysts observed in 43 out of 193 (22%) subjects (Figure 43.9).[39]

In another single-center study, the manifestations of ADPKD in cohorts of children whose disease was diagnosed by screening ultrasound were compared with disease manifestations in children presenting with symptoms. The proportions of children with nephromegaly, hypertension, microalbuminuria, and decreased estimated GFR (eGFR), were similar in both groups.[40] These data reinforce the prevailing wisdom that at-risk children should have regular surveillance for hypertension and urinary abnormalities.

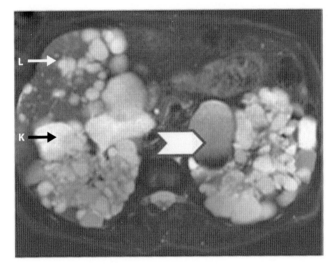

Figure 43.8  Autosomal dominant polycystic kidney disease. Coronal T2-weighted magnetic resonance imaging (MRI) scans showing renal (K) and liver (L) cysts (arrows). One renal cyst in the left kidney is hemorrhagic (arrowhead). (Reproduced with permission from  Kurschat CE, Müller RU, Franke M, et al. An approach to cystic kidney diseases: the clinician's view. Nat Rev Nephrol. 2014;10:687–99.)

New onset of flank or abdominal pain, hypertension, or urinary abnormalities in these at-risk children should prompt sonographic evaluation. Screening for extrarenal features of the disease is not recommended during childhood.

## Genetic testing

Several key caveats merit consideration before undertaking gene-based testing, including the current expense of sequencing *PKD1*, a large, complex gene with multiple *PKD1*

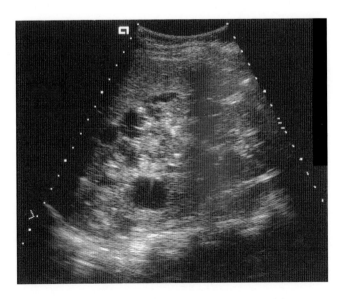

Figure 43.7  Renal ultrasound scan in a 17-year-old patient with autosomal dominant polycystic kidney disease. Numerous cysts are evident in the parenchyma, and the echogenicity of the kidney tissue is increased.

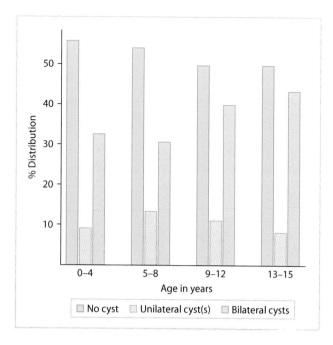

Figure 43.9 Distribution of renal cysts by age in 420 children at risk for autosomal dominant polycystic kidney disease. The data compiled from the initial ultrasonographic examination. Distribution within each age group are as follows: age 0 to 4 years, 59% with no cysts, 9% with unilateral cysts, 33% with bilateral cysts; age 5 to 8 years, 57% with no cysts, 15% with unilateral cysts, 30% with bilateral cysts; age 9 to 13 years, 50% with no cysts, 10% with unilateral cysts, 40% with bilateral cysts; and age 13 to 15 years, 50% with no cysts, 8% with unilateral cysts, 42% with bilateral cysts. (Reproduced with permission from Reed B, Nobakht E, Dadgar S, et al. Renal ultrasonographic evaluation in children at risk of autosomal dominant polycystic kidney disease. Am J Kidney Dis. 2010;56:50–6.)

homologues (i.e., pseudogenes that must be distinguished from the actual gene)[41], the limited detection rate for *PKD1* mutations (approximately 85%), imprecision in predicting the pathogenicity of missense variants,[22,35] and the minimal predictive value of a specific sequence variation.

Despite these limitations, under certain circumstances a DNA-based diagnosis may be informative. For example, very early-onset ADPKD can result from a combination of mutations in *PKD1* and hypomorphic (limited loss-of-function) alleles of other genes that cause cystic kidney disease.[42] Therefore, genetic testing should be considered to evaluate the contribution of other "cystogenes" to the clinical disease expression. In addition, limited numbers of pedigrees have been described in which an affected child presented with an ARPKD-like phenotype resulting from the inheritance of incompletely penetrant *PKD1* alleles from each parent.[43] Finally, in children with massively enlarged kidneys and associated neurologic deficits, genetic testing may identify deletions involving both the *PKD1* gene and the adjacent tuberous sclerosis 2 *(TSC2)* gene, the *TSC2/PKD1* contiguous gene syndrome, which is associated with a much poorer renal outcome.[44]

## GENETIC COUNSELING

Genetic counseling in childhood is limited. Prenatal screening, albeit feasible, is not often requested, and in the one study that examined family attitudes, less than 5% would terminate a pregnancy for ADPKD.[45] Therefore, genetic counseling must be tailored to the specific patient and family, be directed toward explaining genetic risk and genetic tests, and discuss when to test (e.g., for interested adolescents before transitioning to adult care).

## MANAGEMENT AND PROGNOSIS

Most children with ADPKD are asymptomatic throughout childhood, and even in adulthood, clinical issues may arise only intermittently. Management in pediatric patients focuses on five principal issues.

First, hypertension and cardiovascular health are foremost longterm clinical concerns in these patients. Most patients with ADPKD develop hypertension, and cardiovascular disease is the leading cause of death in adults. One study demonstrated that children with ADPKD and hypertension have larger kidney volumes and higher left ventricular mass indices as compared with their normotensive counterparts.[46] Therefore, blood pressure control in children with ADPKD is of paramount importance. ACE inhibitors and ARBs are the therapeutic mainstays, with treatment goals the same as for other hypertensive patients.[47]

The second issue involves renal function. Although decline in renal function is uncommon during childhood,

---

**KEY POINTS**

- Gene testing may be helpful in the diagnosis of early-onset ADPKD in neonates and infants.
- *PKD1* and the tuberous sclerosis 2 *(TSC2)* genes are adjacent to each other. Deletions in both genes may be detected in some patients with tuberous scle-rosis who may have large cystic kidneys.

---

**KEY POINTS**

- Most children with ADPKD are asymptomatic.
- Hypertension is common in patients with ADPKD and can lead to cardiovascular morbidity and mortality in adulthood.
- Back pain in ADPKD results from large kidneys and may be the earliest presenting symptom in some patients.
- Urinary tract infection with localization in a cyst can be difficult to treat. Drugs that penetrate ADPKD cysts need to be selectively used.
- ICAs occur but tend to cluster in 5-10% of ADPKD families.

glomerular hyperfiltration (GH) is prevalent and is associated with more rapid disease progression.[48] A few small studies suggest that ACE inhibitor therapy reduces GH, but the long-term impact has yet to be determined.[49]

The third issue focuses on evaluation and management of abdominal or back pain, which can be challenging, particularly in adolescents with ADPKD.[50,51] For acute episodes, diagnostic considerations should include cyst infection, rupture, or hemorrhage; and renal stones. Treatment is directed at the underlying diagnosis. Chronic pain is much more vexing; it correlates poorly with renal size and, like most other types of chronic pain, can be difficult to manage. After excluding acute events, non–narcotic-based treatments are the preferred approach; acupuncture and other nonpharmacologic approaches can provide reasonable relief. Early referral to pain management specialists also may be helpful.

The fourth issue involves urinary tract infections. Most are easily treated, but cyst infections can be particularly difficult to diagnose and treat. Often, persistent fever or high clinical suspicion may provide the only clues.[52] Positron emission tomography (PET) scan may be helpful in establishing cyst infection in ADPKD. Antibiotics that penetrate cysts well include trimethoprim-sulfamethoxazole, fluoroquinolones, clindamycin, vancomycin, and metronidazole.

The fifth issue relates to ICAs, one of the most feared extrarenal manifestations of ADPKD.[53] ICAs often manifest at an earlier age in patients with ADPKD than in the general population. These aneurysms are reported to rupture at a smaller size, and ICA rupture can sometimes be the presenting symptom in otherwise asymptomatic individuals.[54] Fortunately, only a small fraction (approximately 8%) of patients with ADPKD develop this problem, so standard practice is to reserve screening for a small subset of patients. Among pediatric patients with ADPKD, screening candidates include those with symptoms suggestive of ICA (unusual, but reported in patients with ADPKD who are less than 18 years of age) and 18-year-old patients from families with a known history of ICA and ADPKD.

## CYSTIC DISEASES OF RENAL MEDULLA

Renal cysts that primarily affect renal medulla can be seen in association with several disorders (see Table 43.1), many of which are syndromic or multisystem conditions.

## JUVENILE NEPHRONOPHTHISIS

Juvenile nephronophthisis (NPHP; MIM 256100) comprises a group of autosomal recessive tubulointerstitial diseases associated with renal cysts.[55] At least in some reports, it is one of the most frequent inherited causes of ESRD in children and adolescents.[56]

## Clinical manifestations

Initial reports described three distinct forms of NPHP (infantile, juvenile, and adolescent), based on the age of onset of ESRD. In the infantile form, the age of onset of ESRD consistently occurs before 5 years of age, whereas in juvenile NPH (the most common form), ESRD occurs at a mean age of 13 years. However, more recent studies have demonstrated no clear genotype-phenotype correlation for this spectrum of presentations, and these disorders should be referred to with the single designation, NPHP.[57,58]

---

### KEY POINTS

- NPHP is a common cause of ESRD in children.
- Clinical presentation can occur early in infancy, but onset of the disease during early adolescence is most common.
- Persistent nocturnal enuresis and polyuria are well-known presenting manifestations.
- Renal dysfunction, hypertension, growth retardation, and anemia out of proportion to renal dysfunction are usual at onset.
- Hypertension is not a common presenting feature of NPHP, save in the small subset of infantile variety.

---

Decreased urinary concentrating capacity is quite common in NPHP and usually precedes the decline in renal function, with typical onset between 4 and 6 years of age. Polyuria and polydipsia are common, often resulting in night-time and even day-time wetting. Salt wasting develops in most patients with renal impairment, and sodium supplementation is often commonly required until the onset of ESRD. One-third of patients become anemic before the onset of renal impairment, and this has been attributed to a defect in the functional regulation of erythropoietin production by peritubular fibroblasts.[59] Growth retardation, out of proportion to the degree of renal impairment, is a common finding.

Slowly progressive decline in renal function is typical of NPHP. Although symptoms can be detected after the age of 2 years, they may progress insidiously, such that 15% of affected patients are recognized as having NPHP only after ESRD has developed. The disease is not known to recur in renal allografts.

Children with the infantile variant, which results primarily from mutations in *NPHP2* or *NPHP3*,[57] develop symptoms in the first few months of life and rapidly progress to ESRD, usually before the age of 2 years, but invariably by 5 years of age. Severe hypertension is common in this subset of patients with NPHP. In general, patients with NPHP rarely develop flank pain, hematuria, hypertension, urinary tract infections, or renal calculi.

## Associated extrarenal abnormalities

Extrarenal abnormalities have been described in approximately 10% to 15% of patients with NPHP.[60] The most frequently associated anomaly is retinal dystrophy secondary to tapetoretinal degeneration (Senior-Loken syndrome). Severely affected patients present with coarse nystagmus, early blindness, and a flat electroretinogram (Leber amaurosis). Patients with moderate retinal dystrophy typically have mild visual impairment and retinitis pigmentosa. Other extrarenal anomalies include oculomotor apraxia (Cogan syndrome), cerebellar vermis aplasia (Joubert syndrome), and cone-shaped epiphyses of the bones. Congenital hepatic fibrosis occurs in some NPHP patients, but the associated bile duct proliferation is mild and qualitatively different from that found in ARPKD.

## Genetics

Mutations in 18 distinct genes have been identified in patients with NPHP. Defects in *NPHP1* account for 21% of NPHP cases with large, homozygous deletions detected in 80% of affected family members and in 65% of sporadic cases. Mutations in each of the remaining *NPHP* genes cause no more than 3% of NPHP-related disease.[56] Clinical disease expression seems to be exacerbated by oligogenic inheritance (i.e., patients carrying two mutations in a single *NPHP* gene, as well as a single-copy mutation in an additional *NPHP* gene).[61] In addition, multiple allelism, or distinct mutations in a single gene, appears to explain the continuum of multiorgan phenotypic abnormalities observed in NPHP, Meckel syndrome, and Joubert syndrome.[62] Most of the protein products of the NPHP-associated genes are expressed in the cilia-centrosome complex.[56,63] NPHP is included among the hepatorenal fibrocystic disease subset of the ciliopathies.

---

**KEY POINTS**

- NPHP is an autosomal recessive disorder.
- Most of the proteins associated with NPHP-related genes are expressed in the cilia-centrosome complex.
- *NPHP1* gene defects account for about 20% of the cases of NPHP. Homozygous deletions are common in *NPHP1* families (80%). This information can be useful in genetic counseling.
- Known defects in NPHP-related genes account for only about 35% to 40% cases.

---

## Diagnostic evaluation

### IMAGING

In a child with NPHP and renal impairment, ultrasound examination typically reveals normal-sized or small kidneys with increased echogenicity and loss of corticomedullary differentiation.[58] On occasion, cysts can be detected at the corticomedullary junction or in the medulla. Thin-section CT scanning may be more sensitive than ultrasound in detecting these cysts.

### GENETIC TESTING

Molecular testing can be useful in establishing the diagnosis of *NPHP1*-related disease.[64] However, to date defects in 18 different genes have been described in patients with NPHP, but these defects together account for the disease in only 30% to 40% of patients with NPHP.[65] Newer strategies using next-generation sequencing technologies should allow high-throughput mutation detection for known *NPHP* genes, as well as facilitate the identification of new NPHP-associated genes.

## Genetic counseling

For those patients with *NPHP1*-related disease, identification of a homozygous deletion in the index child can be quite useful in genetic counseling regarding future pregnancies. Otherwise, the large number of disease-associated genes and their contribution in the aggregate to less than 50% of the observed NPHP cases limit the utility of genetic testing in clinical diagnosis. In these families, genetic counseling relies on the probability that for a recessive trait, each fetus has a 25% of being affected.

## Management and prognosis

Current treatment of NPHP is entirely supportive. With progressive decline in renal function, treatment should follow standard guidelines for chronic kidney disease. Renal replacement therapy, including transplantation, is indicated for patients who progress to ESRD. A 2006 report from the North American Pediatric Renal Trials and Collaborative Studies (NAPRTCS) group revealed that NPHP renal transplant recipients have excellent outcomes when compared with all other patients registered in the NAPRTCS database.[66]

## MEDULLARY CYSTIC KIDNEY DISEASE

Medullary cystic kidney disease (MCKD) is a rare an autosomal dominant disorder that is histopathologically indistinguishable from NPHP.

## Clinical features

Key features of MCKD include formation of renal cysts at the corticomedullary junction, a urinary concentrating defect, salt wasting, and a progressive decline in renal function. Two distinct forms of MCKD have been described: MCKD type 1 (MCKD1; MIM 174000), which is a renal-specific disorder, and MCKD type 2 (MCKD2; MIM 603860), which is also associated with hyperuricemia and gout. In both disorders, hypertension appears to be a sequela of the disease, and it occurs after the onset of kidney failure. Progression to ESRD typically occurs in adulthood in both disorders, although the onset can range from 20 to 70 years of age, and patients with MCKD1 typically have a later onset of ESRD.

## Genetics

MCKD1 results from variants in the mucin (MUC1) gene, whereas defects in the uromodulin (UMOD) gene account for most cases of MCKD2. UMOD mutations have also been identified in families with the following: (1) familial juvenile hyperuricemic nephropathy (FJHN; MIM 162000), a dominantly transmitted disorder characterized by MCKD, hyperuricemia, and gout; and (2) familial glomerulocystic disease with hyperuricemia (MIM 609886).

---

### KEY POINTS

- MCKD is an autosomal dominant disorder.
- MCKD1 is caused by a mucin gene (MUC1) defect.
- MCKD2 is caused by defect in the uromodulin (UMOD) gene.
- UMOD gene defects have also been noted in patients with familial juvenile hyperuricemic nephropathy and familial glomerulocystic disease with hyperuricemia.

---

## Diagnostic evaluation

The diagnosis is suspected in patients with a positive family history of kidney disease and the clinical features described earlier. Renal ultrasound examination may reveal normal or small kidneys, but medullary cysts are typically not observed. Genetic testing can confirm the diagnosis.

## Genetic counseling

MCKD is inherited as an autosomal dominant trait. Therefore, each child of an affected patient has a 50% chance of inheriting the mutation. Asymptomatic siblings of an affected child should be considered at 50% risk during childhood and should undergo annual surveillance for hypertension and renal dysfunction. If the disease-causing mutation has been identified in an affected family member, diagnostic testing can be offered to other at-risk family members, including at-risk siblings and in the prenatal context. However, prenatal testing of at-risk pregnancies is not commonly practiced.

## Management and prognosis

Treatment follows standard guidelines for managing chronic kidney disease and its sequelae, which can include hypertension, anemia, and gout. Annual surveillance of blood pressure and renal function is advised for affected patients. With progression to ESRD, renal replacement therapy becomes the mainstay of management. All related potential kidney donors should be evaluated to identify the family-specific MUC1 or UMOD mutation. Only those persons without the mutation are suitable candidate donors. Based on small cohort studies, it appears that these patients do well after transplantation, and the disease does not recur.[67]

# MEDULLARY SPONGE KIDNEY

Medullary sponge kidney (MSK) is a relatively common disorder in adults that occasionally manifests in adolescents. It is typically asymptomatic unless it is complicated by nephrolithiasis, hematuria, or infection. Renal stones and granular debris are composed of either pure apatite (calcium phosphate) or a mixture of apatite and calcium oxalate. Several factors contribute to stone formation, including urinary stasis within the ectatic ducts, hypercalciuria, and hypocitraturia.

---

### KEY POINTS

- MSK is commonly seen in adults but can be detected in adolescents.
- Although MSK is often asymptomatic, renal stones, (calcium phosphate) may be manifest.
- MSK is believed to be a developmental disorder affecting the renal pyramids.

---

Hematuria, unrelated to either coexisting stones or infection, may be recurrent. It is usually asymptomatic, unless extensive bleeding causes clot-induced colic. Urinary tract infection may occur in association with nephrolithiasis or as an independent event. In those patients with stones, infections are more likely to occur in female patients than in male patients.

Decreased renal concentrating ability and impaired distal urinary acidification are common clinical features. Although the acidification defect is not associated with overt systemic acidosis, bone mineralization defects are well described.[68]

## Molecular pathogenesis

The occasional presence of embryonal tissue in the affected papillae and the coexistence of other urinary tract anomalies suggest that MSK results from a developmental defect in the medullary pyramids, with more recent data suggesting that MSK is caused by a disruption at the "ureteric bud-metanephric mesenchyme" interface.[69] In addition, MSK occurs more frequently in patients with other developmental anomalies or tumors (e.g., congenital hemihypertrophy, Beckwith-Wiedemann syndrome, CAKUT [congenital abnormalities of the kidneys and urinary tract] syndrome, and Wilms tumor).[68]

## Diagnostic evaluation

In patients with MSK, abdominal plain radiographs often reveal radiopaque concretions in the medulla. Historically, the diagnosis has been established by excretory urography, with the "bouquet of flowers" or "paintbrush" sign reflecting retention of contrast media in the ectatic collecting ducts. However, CT has been almost completely supplanted urography for routine clinical imaging.[70] Nonenhanced CT may help distinguish MSK from papillary necrosis or even ADPKD.

## Genetic counseling

MSK is generally considered to be a sporadic disorder, but more recent studies have provided evidence for familial clustering involving autosomal dominant inheritance with reduced disease penetrance and variable disease expression.[71] In addition, genetic analyses of 55 patients with MSK identified 2 novel variants in the glial cell–derived neurotrophic factor (GDNF) gene, a finding suggesting a role for this gene in MSK pathogenesis.[72] The implications of these data for genetic counseling are currently unclear.

## Management and prognosis

No therapy is indicated for asymptomatic patients with MSK or for those patients with hematuria in the absence of stones or infection. If the tubular ectasia is unilateral and segmental, partial nephrectomy may alleviate recurrent nephrolithiasis and urinary tract infection.

Given that hypercalciuria and hypocitraturia are key factors contributing to nephrolithiasis, potassium citrate and high fluid intake are the mainstays of treatment for patients with stones. Recurrent stone formers may benefit from thiazide diuretics or inorganic phosphate therapy. However, oral phosphates should not be used in patients with previous urinary tract infections caused by urease-producing organisms. Patients who form and pass stones recurrently may require lithotripsy or surgical intervention.

Urinary tract infection should be treated with standard antibiotic regimens, and for some patients, prolonged therapy may be warranted. Urease-producing organisms, such as coagulase-negative staphylococci, are particularly problematic as urinary pathogens in MSK. Positive urine culture results, even with relatively insignificant colony counts, should be vigorously pursued. With proper management of the clinical complications, the long-term prognosis is excellent. Progression to renal impairment is unusual.

## HEPATOCYTE NUCLEAR FACTOR-1B–RELATED RENAL DISEASE

Hepatocyte nuclear factor-1β (HNF1B), a transcription factor encoded by the HNF1B (or TCF2) gene, is involved in the early development of the kidney, pancreas, liver, and genital tract. HNF1B-related disease is pleiotropic, with expression sometimes restricted to the kidney and sometimes involving both renal and nonrenal manifestations.[73] There is a striking phenotypic heterogeneity within families.

## CLINICAL MANIFESTATIONS

Renal involvement in HNF1B-related disease is quite heterogeneous. During fetal life and childhood, the predominant phenotype is characterized by either hyperechogenic kidneys or bilateral renal cystic hypodysplasia. In adults, renal involvement is widely variable, including renal cysts (mostly few cortical cysts), a solitary kidney, pelvicaliceal abnormalities, hypokalemia and hypomagnesemia from tubular dysfunction, and, more rarely, Fanconi syndrome and chromophobe renal carcinoma. Adult-onset disease is associated with slowly progressive renal decline.

The extrarenal phenotype consists of maturity-onset diabetes of the young, type 5 (MODY5), exocrine pancreas failure and pancreatic atrophy, diverse genital tract abnormalities in female patients or infertility in male patients, and, rarely, mild mental retardation. HNF1B-related disease is now recognized as the second most prevalent dominantly inherited kidney disease,[73] and HNF1B mutations are among the most common causes of bilateral hyperechogenic kidneys in the fetus.[74]

## GENETICS

The HNF1B transcription factor regulates several renal cystogenes, including PKHD1, PKD1, PKD2, and UMOD. In addition, HNF1B modulates expression of three genes involved in magnesium homeostasis: ATP1A1, FXYD2, and CLDN16.[75] In mice, antenatal HNF1B inactivation causes downregulation of all these genes, suggesting mechanisms that contribute to the observed renal cystic disease and hypomagnesemia. In contrast, when compared with controls, human patients had no significant difference in the urinary mRNA levels of HNF1B or other renal cystic genes. Thus, the pathogenesis of the human renal cystic disease phenotype remains unclear. However, a significant alteration in ATP1A1 expression was observed in patients with HNF1B-related disease, consistent with its role in magnesium homeostasis.

---

### KEY POINTS

- HNF1B-related disease is the second most common form of dominantly inherited renal disease
- HNF1B-related disease can be detected in fetuses and neonates and can mimic ARPKD
- HNF1B defects can result in diverse manifestations, which can include renal multicystic dysplastic kidneys, and solitary kidneys.

---

## DIAGNOSTIC EVALUATION

Mutations in HNF1B are dominantly inherited and typically involve complete heterozygous deletion of the TCF2 gene.[74] De novo mutations occur in more than one-half of tested kindreds.[73,76] The diagnosis of HNF1B-related renal disease requires a high index of suspicion.

## GENETIC COUNSELING

Effective genetic counseling must take into consideration the striking phenotypic heterogeneity within families and the high rate of spontaneous mutations in the *HNF1B* gene.

## MANAGEMENT AND PROGNOSIS

Management is directed toward the specific clinical manifestations. For patients who progress to ESRD, renal replacement therapy becomes the primary therapeutic option. In individuals with ESRD and diabetes (MODY5) combined kidney-pancreas transplantation should be considered.

## GLOMERULOCYSTIC KIDNEY DISEASE

Glomerulocystic kidney disease (GCKD) consists of diverse clinical disorders with unifying pathologic findings of Bowman space dilatation (Figure 43.10). These dilated Bowman capsules are widely distributed throughout the renal cortex, and glomeruli within them may appear rudimentary or even collapsed by light microscopy.

## CLINICAL FEATURES

Cystic glomeruli are evident in five different clinical contexts (Table 43.5): (1) isolated, nonsyndromic GCKD; (2) associated with single-gene disorders, such as ADPKD; (3) associated with heritable malformation syndromes, such as tuberous sclerosis, Meckel-Gruber syndrome, oral-facial-digital syndrome type I (OFD1), the short-rib polydactyly syndromes, and Zellweger cerebrohepatorenal syndrome;

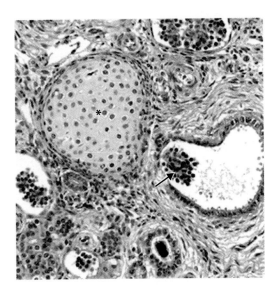

Figure 43.10 Glomerulocystic kidney disease in a patient with multicystic dysplastic kidney. Histologic sample demonstrating glomerular cysts (arrow) and a focus of cartilage (asterisk). (Reproduced with permission from Bissler JJ, Siroky BJ, Yin H. Glomerulocystic kidney disease. Pediatr Nephrol. 2010;25:2049–56.)

(4) associated with trisomies 9, 13, and 18; and (5) dysplastic kidneys or urinary tract obstruction.[77]

## GENETICS

Isolated GCKD can occur as a sporadic condition, as a familial disorder, or as the infantile manifestation of ADPKD. Glomerular cysts can be distributed from the subcapsular zone to the inner cortex.[78] Familial hypoplastic GCKD (also called the renal cysts and diabetes syndrome; MIM 137920) appears to be a distinct form of GCKD caused by mutations in *HNF1B*.[79] As noted earlier, intrafamilial disease expression is widely variable with variable associations of hypoplastic GCKD, gynecologic abnormalities, and MODY5.

## DIAGNOSTIC EVALUATION

The typical ultrasound pattern in GCKD involves increased echogenicity of the renal cortex with minute cysts, smaller than those evident in ADPKD. The appearance and distribution of the renal cysts by MRI may further validate the diagnosis of GCKD.[80] Young infants with either familial or sporadic forms of GCKD may also have renal medullary dysplasia and biliary dysgenesis.[77]

### KEY POINTS

- GCKD is characterized by microcysts in the subcortical region.
- Enlarged Bowman capsules with rudimentary or collapsed glomeruli are the pathologic hallmarks.
- GCKD is a diverse disorder that can be sporadic, familial, or associated with syndromic malformations or urinary tract obstruction.

## GENETIC COUNSELING

GCKD is typically transmitted as an autosomal dominant trait, save for when associated with rare, recessive syndromic disorders. In addition, several sporadic cases of nonsyndromal GCKD have been described, suggesting either new spontaneous mutations or a recessively transmitted disorder.[77]

## MANAGEMENT AND PROGNOSIS

Management is directed toward the specific underlying disorder and its associated clinical manifestations.

## NONGENETIC RENAL CYSTIC DISEASE

## SIMPLE RENAL CYSTS

Simple renal cysts (SRCs) are the most commonly acquired renal cystic lesion. They occur rarely in children (less than 1.0%), but become increasingly frequent with age. Men are

Table 43.5 Disorders associated with glomerular cysts

| | Disorder | Gene |
|---|---|---|
| **Single gene disorders** | | |
| | Autosomal dominant polycystic kidney disease | *PKD1* |
| | Autosomal dominant glomerulocystic kidney disease | *UMOD* |
| | Familial hypoplastic glomerulocystic kidney disease | *HNF1B* |
| **Syndromic disorders** | | |
| | Tuberous sclerosis complex | *TSC1, TSC2* |
| | Meckel-Gruber syndrome (MKS) | *MKS1-MKS11* |
| | Oral-facial-digital syndrome, type I | *OFD1* |
| | Short rib-polydactyly syndrome, type IIA and type IIB | *NEK1, DYNC2H1* |
| | Zellweger syndrome | *PEX1-3, 5-6, 10-11, 13, 14, 16, 19, 26* |
| | Renal-hepatic-pancreatic dysplasia (Ivemark II) | *NPHP3, NEK8* |
| | Glutaric acidemia type II | *ETFA, ETFB, ETFDH* |
| **Chromosomal disorders** | | |
| | Trisomy 9, 13, 18 | — |
| **Renal dysplasia** | | — |
| **Urinary tract obstruction** | | |

affected more commonly than women.[81,82] In children, SRCs are usually asymptomatic; although in some children they cause flank or abdominal pain. In some adolescents, there appears to be a relationship between SRCs and hypertension.[83]

## Molecular pathogenesis

SRCs likely originate from the distal convoluted tubule or collecting ducts and may arise from renal tubular diverticula, but the pathogenic mechanisms are unknown. They are usually spherical and unilocular. They can occur in the cortex, where they can protrude from the cortical surface (exophytic cysts), in the corticomedullary junction, or in the medulla. By definition, they do not communicate with the renal pelvis. The cyst walls are lined with a single layer of flattened epithelium, and cyst fluid is essentially an ultra-filtrate of plasma.

## Diagnostic evaluation

SRCs are usually discovered as an incidental finding during radiologic evaluation of the abdomen. The critical clinical issue in children is to distinguish single or multiple SRCs from cysts associated with ADPKD and other cystic diseases. This distinction can usually be made on the basis of the patient's age, family history, and renal imaging patterns.[81,84] The ultrasound features of SRCs include smooth walls, no septa, and no intracystic debris (Figure 43.11A). If the ultrasound pattern is indeterminate, CT scanning should be performed.

A classification system for renal cysts based on their appearance and enhancement on CT was described by Bosniak and is widely used (Table 43.6).[85] SRCs or benign cysts (class I) have homogeneous attenuation, no contrast enhancement,

thin and smooth cyst walls, and no associated calcifications, unless earlier infection has occurred (Figure 43.11C).

## Management and prognosis

In children, SRCs are rarely symptomatic. Rarely, SRCs occasionally can be associated with flank pain or renin-dependent hypertension. Such symptomatic cysts can be effectively treated by ultrasound-guided percutaneous puncture, drainage, and instillation of a sclerosing agent into the cyst cavity.[86,87] The prognosis is excellent.

## MULTILOCULAR CYSTS

Solitary multilocular cysts are generally benign neoplasms that arise from the metanephric blastema. These solitary cysts have also been termed multilocular cystic nephroma (CN), benign cystic nephroma, and papillary cystadenoma. By definition, the cystic structures are unilateral, solitary, and multilocular. The cystic locules do not communicate with each other or with the renal pelvis. These locules are lined with a simple epithelium, and the interlocular septa do not contain differentiated renal epithelia structures.[18]

## Molecular pathogenesis

Multilocular cysts represent a spectrum,[88] from CN to cystic partially differentiated nephroblastoma (CPDN), in which the septa contain foci of blastemal cells. It is not clear whether a multilocular cyst represents a congenital abnormality in nephrogenesis, a hamartoma, a partially or completely differentiated Wilms tumor, or a benign variant of Wilms tumor.

A bimodal age distribution has been described, with approximately half the cases occurring in children less than

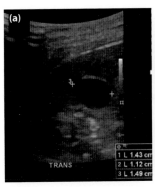
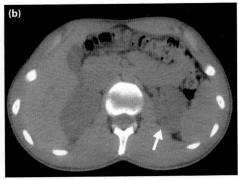
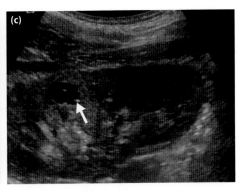

Figure 43.11 **(a)** Ultrasound scan of a simple renal cyst showing a smooth-walled outline and no echogenic focus in the cyst itself (Bosniak category I). **(b)** Computed tomography (CT) scan of the same patient as in (a) showing the smooth-walled cyst posteriorly projecting slightly from the cortical surface (arrow). **(c)** Ultrasound scan of the kidney showing a renal cyst with an irregular but sharply marginated outline (arrow). An echogenic focus exists within the cyst itself (Bosniak category II). The CT scan did not demonstrate any lesion or growth within the cyst. During 5 years of follow up, the patient's ultrasound findings have remained unchanged.

4 years of age and the remaining cases detected in adults.[89] The childhood-onset disease (mostly CPDN) is usually found in boys, whereas multilocular cysts presenting in adulthood (mostly CN) occur more commonly in women.

---

### KEY POINTS

- SRCs are less common in children and increase in occurrence with age.
- The contour of the cysts is thin walled on ultrasound or CT scan.
- Multilocular cysts are large and can occupy the entire pole of the kidney. The cystic lobules do not communicate with each other or with the renal pelvis.
- Multilocular cysts need to be differentiated from a renal neoplasm.

---

## Diagnostic evaluation

An abdominal or flank mass is the most common clinical presentation because these cysts are typically quite large and often replace an entire pole. Associated hematuria, calculi, urinary tract obstruction, and infection occur in rare instances. The diagnosis can be made either by ultrasonography or with CT.

## Management and prognosis

Almost all multilocular cysts are complex renal cysts, which in adults are suspicious for malignancy (Bosniak class III).[84] CPDNs in children may contain blastema and incompletely differentiated metanephric tissue, but usually they have a benign course. In adults, associated foci of renal cell carcinoma or sarcoma must be excluded.[90] For diagnostic accuracy, as well as treatment, enucleation or partial surgical resection is recommended.[91] The typical prognosis of solitary multilocular cysts is excellent.

Table 43.6 Bosniak classification of renal cysts for neoplastic risk

| Bosniak category | Ultrasound and CT cyst features |
|---|---|
| I | Simple benign cyst with a hairline thin wall that does not contain septa, calcification, or solid components; measures as water density and does not enhance with contrast material. |
| II | Benign cyst that may contain a few hairline thin septa. Fine calcification may be present in the wall or septa; high-attenuation lesions of <3 cm that are sharply marginated and do not enhance |
| IIF | Cysts containing more hairline thin septa; minimal enhancement of a hairline thin septum or wall visible, minimal thickening of the septa or wall. Cyst containing calcification that could be nodular and thick but there is no contrast enhancement. Entirely intrarenal nonenhancing high-attenuation renal lesions of ≥3 cm that are well marginated are also included in this category. Malignant potential higher than Bosniak category II. |
| III | Indeterminate cystic masses that have thickened irregular walls or septa in which enhancement can be seen. Should be considered potentially malignant. |
| IV | Clearly malignant cystic lesions that contain enhancing soft tissue components. |

*Source:* Adapted from Warren KS, McFarlane J. The Bosniak classification of renal cystic masses. BJU Int. 2005;95:939–42. ; Bosniak MA. The current radiologic approach to renal cysts. Radiology: 1986;158:1-10.

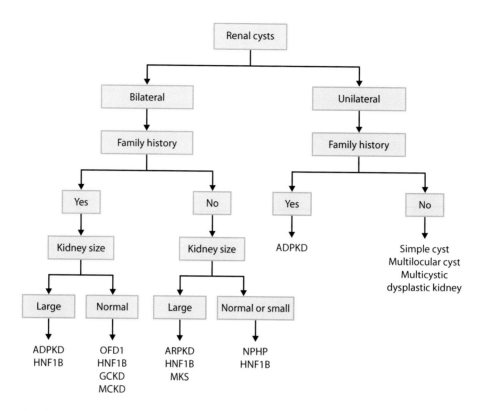

Figure 43.12 Algorithm for screening infants and children with renal cysts. ADPKD, autosomal dominant polycystic kidney disease; GCK, glomerulocystic kidney; HNF1B, hepatocyte nuclear factor-1β–related renal disease; MCKD, medullary cystic kidney disease; MCDK, multicystic dysplastic kidney; MSK, medullary sponge kidney; NPHP, nephronophthisis; OFD1, oral-facial-digital syndrome, type I.

## DIAGNOSTIC EVALUATION OF RENAL CYSTIC DISORDERS

As described earlier, disorders associated with renal cysts may be inherited or acquired. Their manifestations may be confined to the kidney or expressed systemically. Renal cysts may be single or multiple, and the associated renal impact may range from clinical insignificance to progressive parenchymal destruction with resultant renal insufficiency. For those disorders associated with systemic manifestations, such as oral-facial-digital syndrome, type 1 (OFD1) and ADPKD, the associated extrarenal features may provide other important differential diagnostic clues. However, in some patients with atypical presentations, more extensive imaging studies or genetic testing may be required to establish the diagnosis.

The algorithm provided in Figure 43.12 outlines an initial guide to diagnosis, based on family history, the laterality of the cystic findings, and kidney size on renal imaging (Figure 43.13). Distinguishing features of key pediatric renal cystic diseases are provided in Table 43.7. Genetic testing resources for inherited renal cystic diseases are available at GeneTests (http://www.genetests.org) and at the National Institutes of Health (NIH) Genetic Testing Registry (http://www.ncbi.nlm.nih.gov/gtr).

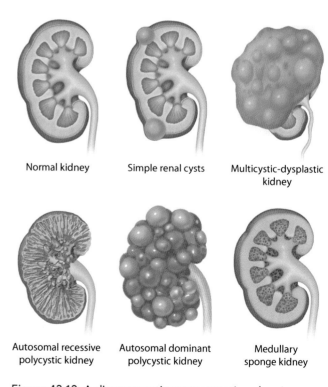

Figure 43.13 A diagrammatic representation showing common types cystic renal diseases during childhood.

Table 43.7 Clinical features of pediatric renal cystic disease

| Feature | Autosomal recessive polycystic kidney disease | Autosomal dominant polycystic kidney disease | Nephronophthisis | Hepatocyte nuclear factor-1β | Glomerulocystic kidney disease |
|---|---|---|---|---|---|
| Clinical onset (yr) | Perinatal | Infancy Older childhood | NPHP2/3: 0–5 NPHP: 10–18 | Infancy Older childhood | Infancy Older childhood |
| Enlarged kidneys | Yes | Occurs | NPHP2: yes NPHP3: some cases NPHP: no | Unusual | Unusual |
| Renal disease | Multiple cysts | Multiple cysts | NPHP2: multiple cysts NPHP: few cysts at corticomedullary junction | Multiple cortical cysts | Multiple cortical cysts |
| Cyst infection | Uncommon | Occurs | No | No | No |
| BP | Normal or increased | Normal or increased | NPHP2: increased NPHP: normal | Normal or increased | Normal or increased |
| Renal function | Normal or impaired | Normal | Normal or impaired | Normal | Normal |
| Nephrocalcinosis or nephrolithiasis | Nephrocalcinosis up to 25% | Nephrolithiasis | No | No | No |
| Congenital hepatic fibrosis | Yes | 10% to 15% infantile ADPKD | Rare | No | No |
| Pancreas lesions | No | No | No | MODY5 | No |
| CNS involvement | No | No | (Joubert)* | No | No |
| **Genetics of Pediatric Renal Cystic Disease** | | | | | |
| Disease gene | *PKHD1* | *PKD1, PKD2* | *NPHP1-NPHP18* | *HNF1B* | *PKD1, HNF1B, UMOD* |
| Genetic testing† | Yes | Yes | Yes | Yes | Yes |

*Source:* Adapted from Guay-Woodford L. Other cystic diseases. In: Feehally J, Johnson R, editors. Comprehensive Clinical Nephrology. 4th ed. London: Mosby; 2010. p. 543–59.

*Abbreviations:* ADPKD, autosomal dominant polycystic kidney disease; BP, blood pressure; CNS, central nervous system; MODY5, maturity-onset diabetes of the young, type 5; NPHP, nephronophthisis.

* Joubert syndrome (JBTS; MIM 213300) is a genetically heterogeneous (JBTS 1–22), autosomal recessive disorder characterized by developmental defects in the cerebellum (cerebellar vermis aplasia) and the eye (coloboma), as well as retinitis pigmentosa, congenital hypotonia, and either ocular motor apraxia or irregularities in breathing patterns during the neonatal period. The disease can be associated with NPHP, and mutations in several *NPHP* genes have been described in patients with JBTS.

† Genetic testing: listed at GeneTests (http://www.genetests.org) and the NIH Genetic Testing Registry (http://www.ncbi.nlm.nih.gov/gtr).

## FUTURE THERAPEUTIC DIRECTIONS

The discovery of the single-gene defects that cause renal cystic diseases and the generation of corresponding animal models have provided important insights into disease pathobiology. Preclinical studies in animal models have implicated a central role for primary apical cilium signaling in suppressing cell proliferation, cyst formation, and progression (Figure 43.14). Ciliary dysfunction contributes to increased intracellular accumulation of cyclic adenosine monophosphate (cAMP) and activation of mammalian target of rapamycin (mTOR), key signatures of renal cystic epithelia. These insights have spurred the identification of potential molecular targets for therapeutic intervention within these pathways, as well as other signaling pathways.

The ultimate goal of preclinical studies is to translate knowledge of disease mechanisms into effective therapy. However, the ability to assess clinically significant changes in outcome is predicated on having defined predictive and prognostic endpoints for disease progression. In experimental animals, renal cystic disease progression can be quantitated by serial histologic examination, and more recently, by serial live animal imaging.[92] However, for most human renal cystic diseases, clinical trial design has been hampered by the lack of defined biomarkers to track disease progression meaningfully. Therefore, imperatives for designing clinical translational studies in ARPKD, NPHP,

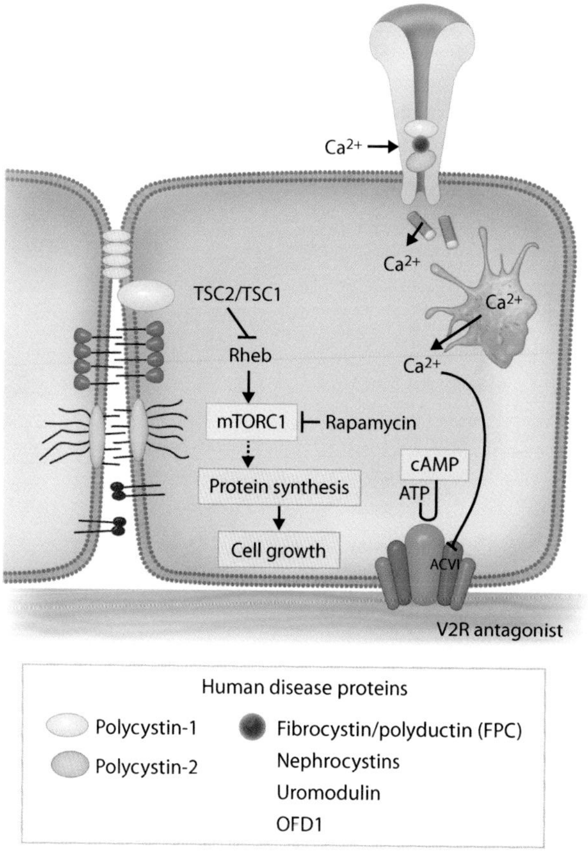

Figure 43.14 Ciliary dysfunction in the pathogenesis of renal cysts. The cilium concentrates and organizes numerous channels, receptors, and effectors, such as transcription factors and proteolytic fragments of cystoproteins. Cilia play a critical role in transmitting information on the external milieu back into the cell and ultimately regulating cellular and tubular differentiation and homeostasis. Cilia appear to play a role in maintaining this balance through sensing the extracellular milieu, by responding to mechanical cues and modulating different signaling cascades. Ciliary dysfunction contributes to increased intracellular accumulation of cyclic adenosine monophosphate (cAMP) and activation of mammalian target of rapamycin (mTOR), features common to cystic epithelia in human and rodent models of renal cystic disease. Almost all cystoproteins, including (but not limited to) the polycystins, fibrocystin/polyductin (FPC), the nephrocystins, uromodulin, and the OFD1 protein, localize to the cilia-centrosome complex, a finding suggesting that this complex is critical in the pathogenesis of renal cystic disease. ACVI, Adenylate cyclase VI; ATP, adenosine triphosphate; Ca2+, calcium; V2R, V2 receptor.

and other renal cystic disorders are the identification and validation of reliable, noninvasive biomarkers to monitor the effectiveness of potential therapies.

ADPKD is the one renal cystic disease for which an early predictive marker has been defined. Specifically, total kidney volume (TKV) is now widely accepted as an early predictor of ADPKD progression, based on the findings of the NIH-sponsored Consortium for Radiologic Imaging Studies of Polycystic Kidney Disease (CRISP) study.[93,94] This longitudinal study developed a highly reproducible, MRI-based imaging protocol that demonstrated that rates of increase in kidney volume correlated with changes in renal function. Several trials directed at slowing disease progression have used TKV measurements as a surrogate for ADPKD progression.

Three randomized, controlled, blinded trials have been reported. The first two tested rapamycin analogues (inhibitors of the mTOR signaling pathway) in ADPKD.[95,95] In

the first study,[95] no benefit was observed with respect to renal volume or function in subjects with well-preserved function. In the second study, renal volumes were better preserved in subjects taking the study drug, but renal function was not, a finding suggesting that changes in volume and function may be disassociated.[96] The third study tested tolvaptan, an inhibitor of the vasopressin-2 receptor.[97] Tolvaptan slowed the rate of cyst growth; it had a modestly positive effect on renal function, and treated subjects experienced fewer and less severe pain episodes. Although these data are encouraging, several issues prompted the US Food and Drug Administration (FDA) to defer approval of tolvaptan for ADPKD treatment.[98] These issues included (1) rodent studies demonstrating that the drug benefits attenuate over time,[99] (2) the development of liver enzyme abnormalities in a small but significant fraction of patients taking tolvaptan, and (3) dropout of approximately 25% of the treatment group (twice the placebo rate) because of side effects. Although the outcomes of these initial clinical trials are disappointing, the data suggest that additional, well-designed studies of targeted therapies, perhaps using composite clinical outcome markers that include TKV, may be able to demonstrate a positive impact on attenuating the disease course in ADPKD.

## SUMMARY

Cystic renal diseases are diverse disorders, many of which are genetically transmitted. These disorders are also diverse in their age of presentation, clinical manifestations, and progression to ESRD. With the growing use of fetal ultrasound evaluation, these disorders are increasingly diagnosed prenatally. Although ARPKD is the most common genetically inherited cystic disorder in children, ADPKD can also be clinically significant during childhood. Several syndromes are associated with renal cysts and must be considered in the evaluation of children found to have cysts on ultrasound evaluation. Cystic diseases are now classified as ciliopathies because ciliary dysfunction in renal eipthelia is a major contributor to disease pathogenesis in most of these conditions. Treatment modalities for most renal cystic diseases are limited at the present time, and these disorders often progress to ESRD. Future development of drugs that reduce cyst size, attenuate interstitial fibrosis, and prevent progressive decline in renal function could reduce the evolution of ESRD in these patients.

## REFERENCES

1. Wilson PD. Polycystic kidney disease. N Engl J Med. 2004;350:151–64.
2. Arts HH, Knoers NV. Current insights into renal ciliopathies: What can genetics teach us? Pediatr Nephrol. 2013;28:863–74.
3. Guay-Woodford LM, Desmond RA. Autosomal recessive polycystic kidney disease: The clinical experience in North America. Pediatrics. 2003;111:1072–80.
4. Bergmann C, Senderek J, Windelen E, et al. Clinical consequences of PKHD1 mutations in 164 patients with autosomal-recessive polycystic kidney disease (ARPKD). Kidney Int. 2005;67:829–48.
5. Bergmann C, Kupper F, Dornia C, et al. Algorithm for efficient PKHD1 mutation screening in autosomal recessive polycystic kidney disease (ARPKD). Hum Mutat. 2005;25:225–31.
6. Adeva M, El-Youssef M, Rossetti S, et al. Clinical and molecular characterization defines a broadened spectrum of autosomal recessive polycystic kidney disease (ARPKD). Medicine (Baltimore). 2006;85:1–21.
7. Gunay-Aygun M, Font-Montgomery E, Lukose L, et al. Correlation of kidney function, volume and imaging findings, and PKHD1 mutations in 73 patients with autosomal recessive polycystic kidney disease. Clin J Am Soc Nephrol. 2010;5:972–84.
8. Kashtan CE, Primack WA, Kainer G, et al. Recurrent bacteremia with enteric pathogens in recessive polycystic kidney disease. Pediatr Nephrol. 1999;13:678–82.
9. Davis ID, Ho M, Hupertz V, et al. Survival of childhood polycystic kidney disease following renal transplantation: The impact of advanced hepatobiliary disease. Pediatr Transplant. 2003;7:364–9.
10. Chalhoub V, Abi-Rafeh L, Hachem K, et al. Intracranial aneurysm and recessive polycystic kidney disease: The third reported case. JAMA Neurol. 2013;70:114–6.
11. Onuchic LF, Furu L, Nagasawa Y, et al. PKHD1, the polycystic kidney and hepatic disease 1 gene, encodes a novel large protein containing multiple immunoglobulin-like plexin-transcription-factor domains and parallel beta-helix 1 repeats. Am J Hum Genet. 2002;70:1305–17.
12. Mutation Database Autosomal Recessive Polycystic Kidney Disease (ARPKD/PKHD1). 2013. Available at http://www.humgen.rwth-aachen.de. Accessed October 1, 2015.
13. Rossetti S, Harris PC. Genotype-phenotype correlations in autosomal dominant and autosomal recessive polycystic kidney disease. J Am Soc Nephrol. 2007;18:1374–80.
14. Menezes LF, Cai Y, Nagasawa Y, et al. Polyductin, the PKHD1 gene product, comprises isoforms expressed in plasma membrane, primary cilium, and cytoplasm. Kidney Int. 2004;66:1345–55.
15. Kerkar N, Norton K, Suchy FJ. The hepatic fibrocystic diseases. Clin Liver Dis. 2006;10:55–71, v–vi.
16. Yoder BK. Role of primary cilia in the pathogenesis of polycystic kidney disease. J Am Soc Nephrol. 2007;18:1381–8.
17. Hildebrandt F, Benzing T, Katsanis N. Ciliopathies. N Engl J Med. 2011;364:1533–43.
18. Guay-Woodford L. Other cystic diseases. In: Feehally J, Johnson R, editors. Comprehensive Clinical Nephrology, 4th ed. London: Mosby; 2010. p. 543–59.
19. Capisonda R, Phan V, Traubuci J, et al. Autosomal recessive polycystic kidney disease: Outcomes from a single-center experience. Pediatr Nephrol. 2003;18:119–26.
20. Srinath A, Shneider BL. Congenital hepatic fibrosis and autosomal recessive polycystic kidney disease. J Pediatr Gastroenterol Nutr. 2012;54:580–7.
21. Gunay-Aygun M, Font-Montgomery E, Lukose L, et al. Characteristics of congenital hepatic fibrosis in a large cohort of patients with autosomal recessive polycystic kidney disease. Gastroenterology. 2013;144:112–21 e2.

22. Rossetti S, Consugar MB, Chapman AB, et al. Comprehensive molecular diagnostics in autosomal dominant polycystic kidney disease. J Am Soc Nephrol. 2007;18:2143–60.

23. Gigarel N, Frydman N, Burlet P, et al. Preimplantation genetic diagnosis for autosomal recessive polycystic kidney disease. Reprod Biomed Online. 2008;16:152–8.

24. Zvereff V, Yao S, Ramsey J, et al. Identification of PKHD1 multiexon deletions using multiplex ligation-dependent probe amplification and quantitative polymerase chain reaction. Genet Test Mol Biomarkers. 2010;14:505–10.

25. Guay-Woodford LM, Knoers NV. Genetic testing: Considerations for pediatric nephrologists. Semin Nephrol. 2009;29:338–48.

26. Beaunoyer M, Snehal M, Li L, et al. Optimizing outcomes for neonatal ARPKD. Pediatr Transplant. 2007;11:267–71.

27. Van De Voorde RG, Mitsnefes MM. Hypertension and CKD. Adv Chronic Kidney Dis. 2011;18:355–61.

28. Telega G, Cronin D, Avner ED. New approaches to the autosomal recessive polycystic kidney disease patient with dual kidney-liver complications. Pediatr Transplant. 2013;17:328–35.

29. Gunay-Aygun M, Turkbey BI, Bryant J, et al. Hepatorenal findings in obligate heterozygotes for autosomal recessive polycystic kidney disease. Mol Genet Metab. 2011;104:677–81.

30. Chapal M, Debout A, Dufay A, et al. Kidney and liver transplantation in patients with autosomal recessive polycystic kidney disease: A multicentric study. Nephrol Dial Transplant. 2012;27:2083–8.

31. Torres VE, Harris PC, Pirson Y. Autosomal dominant polycystic kidney disease. Lancet. 2007;369:1287–301.

32. Rizk D, Chapman A. Treatment of autosomal dominant polycystic kidney disease (ADPKD): The new horizon for children with ADPKD. Pediatr Nephrol. 2008;23:1029–36.

33. Boyer O, Gagnadoux MF, Guest G, et al. Prognosis of autosomal dominant polycystic kidney disease diagnosed in utero or at birth. Pediatr Nephrol. 2007;22:380–8.

34. Harris PC. 2008 Homer W. Smith Award: Insights into the pathogenesis of polycystic kidney disease from gene discovery. J Am Soc Nephrol. 2009;20:1188–98.

35. Garcia-Gonzalez MA, Jones JG, Allen SK, et al. Evaluating the clinical utility of a molecular genetic test for polycystic kidney disease. Mol Genet Metab. 2007;92:160–7.

36. Qian F, Watnick TJ, Onuchic LF, et al. The molecular basis of focal cyst formation in human autosomal dominant polycystic kidney disease type I. Cell. 1996;87:979–87.

37. Torres VE, Harris PC. Polycystic kidney disease in 2011: Connecting the dots toward a polycystic kidney disease therapy. Nat Rev Nephrol. 2012;8:66–8.

38. Nauli SM, Alenghat FJ, Luo Y, et al. Polycystins 1 and 2 mediate mechanosensation in the primary cilium of kidney cells. Nat Genet. 2003;33:129–37.

39. Reed B, Nobakht E, Dadgar S, et al. Renal ultrasonographic evaluation in children at risk of autosomal dominant polycystic kidney disease. Am J Kidney Dis.2010;56:50–6.

40. Mekahli D, Woolf AS, Bockenhauer D. Similar renal outcomes in children with ADPKD diagnosed by screening or presenting with symptoms. Pediatr Nephrol. 2010;25:2275–82.

41. Harris PC, Rossetti S. Molecular diagnostics of ADPKD coming of age. Clin J Am Soc Nephrol. 2008;3:1–2.

42. Bergmann C, Bruchle NO, Frank V, et al. K. Perinatal deaths in a family with autosomal dominant polycystic kidney disease and a PKD2 mutation. N Engl J Med. 2008;359:318–9.

43. Vujic M, Heyer CM, Ars E, et al. Incompletely penetrant PKD1 alleles mimic the renal manifestations of ARPKD. J Am Soc Nephrol. 2010;21:1097–102.

44. Harris PC. The TSC2/PKD1 contiguous gene syndrome. Contrib Nephrol. 1997;122:76–82.

45. Sujansky E, Kreutzer SB, Johnson AM, et al. Attitudes of at-risk and affected individuals regarding presymptomatic testing for autosomal dominant polycystic kidney disease. Am J Med Genet. 1990;35:510–5.

46. Cadnapaphornchai MA, McFann K, Strain JD, et al. Prospective change in renal volume and function in children with ADPKD. Clin J Am Soc Nephrol. 2009;4:820–9.

47. National High Blood Pressure Education Working Group on High Blood Pressure in Children and Adolescents. The fourth report on the diagnosis, evaluation, and treatment of high blood pressure in children and adolescents. Pediatrics. 2004;114(Suppl):555–76.

48. Helal I, Reed B, McFann K, et al. Glomerular hyperfiltration and renal progression in children with autosomal dominant polycystic kidney disease. Clin J Am Soc Nephrol. 2011;6:2439–43.

49. Wong H, Vivian L, Weiler G, Filler G. Patients with autosomal dominant polycystic kidney disease hyperfiltrate early in their disease. Am J Kidney Dis. 2004;43:624–8.

50. Bajwa ZH, Sial KA, Malik AB, et al. Pain patterns in patients with polycystic kidney disease. Kidney Int. 2004;66:1561–9.

51. Hogan MC, Norby SM. Evaluation and management of pain in autosomal dominant polycystic kidney disease. Adv Chronic Kidney Dis. 2010;17:e1–e16.

52. Suwabe T, Ubara Y, Sumida K, et al. Clinical features of cyst infection and hemorrhage in ADPKD: New diagnostic criteria. Clin Exp Nephrol. 2012;16:892–902.

53. Somlo S, Guay-Woodford L. Polycystic kidney disease. In: Lifton RP, Somlo S, Giebisch GH, Seldin DW, editors. Genetic Diseases of the Kidney. New York: Academic Press; 2009. p. 393–424.

54. Kanne JP, Talner LB. Autosomal dominant polycystic kidney disease presenting as subarachnoid hemorrhage. Emerg Radiol. 2004;11:110–2.

55. Benzing T, Schermer B. Clinical spectrum and pathogenesis of nephronophthisis. Curr Opin Nephrol Hypertens. 2012;21:272–8.

56. Wolf MT, Hildebrandt F. Nephronophthisis. Pediatr Nephrol. 2011;26:181–94.

57. Tory K, Rousset-Rouviere C, Gubler MC, et al. Mutations of NPHP2 and NPHP3 in infantile nephronophthisis. Kidney Int. 2009;75:839–47.

58. Salomon R, Saunier S, Niaudet P. Nephronophthisis. Pediatr Nephrol. 2009;24:2333–44.

59. Ala-Mello S, Kivivuori SM, Ronnholm KA, et al. Mechanism underlying early anaemia in children with familial juvenile nephronophthisis. Pediatr Nephrol. 1996;10:578–81.

60. Saunier S, Salomon R, Antignac C. Nephronophthisis. Curr Opin Genet Dev. 2005;15:324–31.

61. Hoefele J, Wolf MT, O'Toole JF, et al. Evidence of oligogenic inheritance in nephronophthisis. J Am Soc Nephrol. 2007;18:2789–95.

62. Chaki M, Hoefele J, Allen SJ, et al. Genotype-phenotype correlation in 440 patients with NPHP-related ciliopathies. Kidney Int. 2011;80:1239–45.

63. Sang L, Miller JJ, Corbit KC, et al. Mapping the NPHP-JBTS-MKS protein network reveals ciliopathy disease genes and pathways. Cell. 2011;145:513–28.

64. Heninger E, Otto E, Imm A, et al. Improved strategy for molecular genetic diagnostics in juvenile nephronophthisis. Am J Kidney Dis. 2001;37:1131–9.

65. Halbritter J, Diaz K, Chaki M, et al. High-throughput mutation analysis in patients with a nephronophthisis-associated ciliopathy applying multiplexed barcoded array-based PCR amplification and next-generation sequencing. J Med Genet. 2012;49:756–67.

66. Hamiwka LA, Midgley JP, Wade AW, et al. Outcomes of kidney transplantation in children with nephronophthisis: An analysis of the North American Pediatric Renal Trials and Collaborative Studies (NAPRTCS) Registry. Pediatr Transplant. 2008;12:878–82.

67. Soloukides AP, Moutzouris DA, Papagregoriou GN, et al. Renal graft outcome in autosomal dominant medullary cystic kidney disease type 1. J Nephrol. 2013;26:793–8.

68. Fabris A, Anglani F, Lupo A, Gambaro G. Medullary sponge kidney: State of the art. Nephrol Dial Transplant. 2013;28:1111–9.

69. Gambaro G, Danza FM, Fabris A. Medullary sponge kidney. Curr Opin Nephrol Hypertens. 2013;22:421–6.

70. Maw AM, Megibow AJ, Grasso M, et al. Diagnosis of medullary sponge kidney by computed tomographic urography. Am J Kidney Dis. 2007;50:146–50.

71. Fabris A, Lupo A, Ferraro PM, et al. Familial clustering of medullary sponge kidney is autosomal dominant with reduced penetrance and variable expressivity. Kidney Int. 2013;83:272–7.

72. Torregrossa R, Anglani F, Fabris A, et al. Identification of GDNF gene sequence variations in patients with medullary sponge kidney disease. Clin J Am Soc Nephrol. 2010;5:1205–10.

73. Chauveau D, Faguer S, Bandin F, et al. HNF1B-related disease: Paradigm of a developmental disorder and unexpected recognition of a new renal disease. Nephrol Ther. 2013;9:393–7.

74. Decramer S, Parant O, Beaufils S, et al. Anomalies of the TCF2 gene are the main cause of fetal bilateral hyperechogenic kidneys. J Am Soc Nephrol. 2007;18:923–33.

75. Faguer S, Decramer S, Devuyst O, et al. Expression of renal cystic genes in patients with HNF1B mutations. Nephron Clin Pract. 2012;120:c71–8.

76. Ulinski T, Lescure S, Beaufils S, et al. Renal phenotypes related to hepatocyte nuclear factor-1beta (TCF2) mutations in a pediatric cohort. J Am Soc Nephrol. 2006;17:497–503.

77. Bissler JJ, Siroky BJ, Yin H. Glomerulocystic kidney disease. Pediatr Nephrol. 2010;25:2049–56.

78. Lennerz JK, Spence DC, Iskandar SS, et al. Glomerulocystic kidney: One hundred-year perspective. Arch Pathol Lab Med. 2010;134:583–605.

79. Bingham C, Hattersley AT. Renal cysts and diabetes syndrome resulting from mutations in hepatocyte nuclear factor-1beta. Nephrol Dial Transplant. 2004;19:2703–8.

80. Oliva MR, Hsing J, Rybicki FJ, et al. Glomerulocystic kidney disease: MRI findings. Abdom Imaging. 2003;28:889–92.

81. Eknoyan G. A clinical view of simple and complex renal cysts. J Am Soc Nephrol. 2009;20:1874–6.

82. Nascimento AB, Mitchell DG, Zhang XM, et al. Rapid MR imaging detection of renal cysts: Age-based standards. Radiology. 2001;221:628–32.

83. Hong S, Lim JH, Jeong IG, et al. What association exists between hypertension and simple renal cyst in a screened population? J Hum Hypertens. 2013;27:539–44.

84. Israel GM, Bosniak MA. An update of the Bosniak renal cyst classification system. Urology. 2005;66:484–8.

85. Warren KS, McFarlane J. The Bosniak classification of renal cystic masses. BJU Int. 2005;95:939–42.

86. Akinci D, Gumus B, Ozkan OS, et al. Single-session percutaneous ethanol sclerotherapy in simple renal cysts in children: Long-term follow-up. Pediatr Radiol. 2005;35:155–8.

87. Skolarikos A, Laguna MP, de la Rosette JJ. Conservative and radiological management of simple renal cysts: A comprehensive review. BJU Int. 2012;110:170–8.

88. Silver IM, Boag AH, Soboleski DA. Best cases from the AFIP: Multilocular cystic renal tumor: Cystic nephroma. Radiographics. 2008;28:1221–5.

89. Freire M, Remer EM. Clinical and radiologic features of cystic renal masses. AJR Am J Roentgenol. 2009;192:1367–72.

90. Moch H. Cystic renal tumors: New entities and novel concepts. Adv Anat Pathol. 2010;17:209–14.

91. Boybeyi O, Karnak I, Orhan D, et al. Cystic nephroma and localized renal cystic disease in children: Diagnostic clues and management. J Pediatr Surg. 2008;43:1985–9.

92. Sun Y, Zhou J, Stayner C, et al. Magnetic resonance imaging assessment of a murine model of recessive polycystic kidney disease. Comp Med. 2002;52:433–8.

93. Chapman AB, Guay-Woodford LM, Grantham JJ, et al. Renal structure in early autosomal-dominant polycystic kidney disease (ADPKD): The Consortium for Radiologic Imaging Studies of Polycystic Kidney Disease (CRISP) cohort. Kidney Int. 2003;64:1035–45.

94. Grantham JJ, Chapman AB, Torres VE. Volume progression in autosomal dominant polycystic kidney disease: The major factor determining clinical outcomes. Clin J Am Soc Nephrol. 2006;1:148–57.

95. Serra AL, Poster D, Kistler AD, et al. Sirolimus and kidney growth in autosomal dominant polycystic kidney disease. N Engl J Med. 2010;363:820–9.

96. Walz G, Budde K, Mannaa M, et al. Everolimus in patients with autosomal dominant polycystic kidney disease. N Engl J Med. 2010;363:830–40.

97. Torres VE, Chapman AB, Devuyst O, et al. Tolvaptan in patients with autosomal dominant polycystic kidney disease. N Engl J Med. 2012;367:2407–18.

98. Anonymous. Summary Minutes of the Drug Safety and Risk Management Advisory Committee. Available at http://www.fda.gov/downloads/AdvisoryCommittees/CommitteesMeetingMaterials/Drugs/CardiovascularandRenalDrugsAdvisoryCommittee/UCM373520.pdf. Accessed October 1, 2015.

99. Meijer E, Gansevoort RT, de Jong PE, et al. Therapeutic potential of vasopressin V2 receptor antagonist in a mouse model for autosomal dominant polycystic kidney disease: Optimal timing and dosing of the drug. Nephrol Dial Transplant. 2011;26:2445–53.

## REVIEW QUESTIONS

1. Extrarenal complications of ARPKD can include:
   a. Congenital hepatic fibrosis
   b. Caroli syndrome
   c. Growth retardation
   d. Intracranial aneurysms
   e. All of the above

2. All of the conditions below are included in hepatocellular fibrocystic disorders, *except:*
   a. ARPKD
   b. ADPKD
   c. Multicystic dysplastic kidney (MCDK)
   d. Nephronophthisis (NPHP)
   e. Joubert syndrome (JBTS)

3. In which of the pediatric age groups can ADPKD manifest?
   a. Fetus
   b. Infant
   c. Child
   d. Adolescent
   e. All of the above

4. Small, contracted kidneys are characteristically seen in seen in which of the following cystic disease(s)?
   a. HNF1B-related disease
   b. ARPKD
   c. Nephronophthisis
   d. Medullary sponge kidney
   e. None of the above

5. A causal relationship between hypertension and renal cystic disease has been proposed in each of the following disorders *except:*
   a. ARPKD
   b. ADPKD
   c. NPHP
   d. MCKD
   e. Simple cysts

6. Gene-based testing is a clinically informative tool for which disorder?
   a. ARPKD
   b. ADPKD
   c. NPHP
   d. MCKD
   e. All of the above

7. Medullary sponge kidney is a single-gene disorder in a subset of patients.
   a. True
   b. False

8. Which disorder is the *most common* cause of hyperechoic kidneys in a fetus?
   a. ARPKD
   b. ADPKD
   c. NPHP

   d.  HNF1B-related disease
   e.  Glomerulocystic kidney disease
9.  Glomerular cysts can be observed in which disorders?
   a.  ADPKD
   b.  MCKD2
   c.  HNF1B-related disease
   d.  Trisomy 18
   e.  All of the above
10.  Simple cysts can lead to clinical symptoms in childhood.
   a.  True
   b.  False

**ANSWER KEY**

1  e
2.  c
3.  e
4.  c
5.  d
6.  e
7.  a
8.  a
9.  e
10.  a

# 44

# Ciliopathies and nephronophthisis

JOHN SAYER, SHREYA RAMAN, AND SHALABH SRIVASTAVA

Nephronophthisis (NPHP), which literally means "disappearance of nephrons," is an autosomal recessively inherited renal disease leading to end-stage renal disease (ESRD). NPHP belongs to a group of disorders that are now classed as *ciliopathies* with the underlying morphologic and functional defect in the primary cilium, basal body, or centrosome.

Ciliopathies are a relatively new class of disorders, in which the pathologic process lies in the cilium and basal body complex. They encompass a wide spectrum of diseases involving almost any organ system. Interest in the cilium as an organelle, described in 1675 by Anthony van Leeuwenhoek, has gathered such momentum that a new journal dedicated to the cilia and its associated diseases was launched in 2012.[1,2] The primary cilium is a hairlike organelle that is present on virtually all somatic cells. It functions as a cellular antenna through which it allows the cell to remain constantly in contact with its environment.

Ciliopathies result from mutation in genes encoding component proteins of the basal body, transition zone, or ciliary axoneme. Table 44.1 lists examples of the diseases caused by such mutations and the proposed consequent functional defect in the cilium and basal body. In its most severe form, the loss of ciliary structure may cause the loss of planar cell polarity (PCP) in renal tubular cells and in less severe case result in cellular disruption and disordered signal transduction. The various signaling cascades intimately related to the primary cilium are discussed later. The result of these abnormalities is not only renal tubular cell dysfunction and renal cyst formation, but also abnormal development and organ function throughout the body.

Table 44.1 Examples of ciliopathy diseases, their genes, and their proposed functional role

| Disease | Gene(s) | Affected function |
|---|---|---|
| Bardet-Biedl syndrome | BBS1/BBS2/ BBS5/BBS7/ BBS8 | Ciliary function |
| | BBS3 | Vesicle trafficking |
| | BBS4 | Microtubule transport |
| | BBS6 | Cilia/chaperone |
| Alström syndrome | ALMS1 | Ciliogenesis |
| Joubert syndrome | AHI1 | Ciliogenesis |
| Meckel-Gruber syndrome | MKS1 | Ciliogenesis |
| | MKS2/MKS3 | Transmembrane/ ciliary protein |
| | MKS4 | Basal body function |
| Nephronophthisis | NPHP1 | Ciliary function |
| Short-rib thoracic dysplasia (Jeune asphyxiating thoracic dystrophy) | IFT80 | IFT subcomplex B |
| Ellis–van Creveld | EVC1/EVC2 | Ciliary |

## CILIARY STRUCTURE

The primary cilium has a 9 + 0 microtubular structure and arises from the mother centriole, the older of the two centrioles (Figure 44.1). Centrioles are microtubule-based cylindrical structures surrounded by pericentriolar material (PCM). The PCM forms a scaffold around the centriole and has been shown to be involved in intracellular transport to the ciliary base. The cilium is assembled by the transfer of actin subunits from the cytoplasm by transport proteins. After assembly, the cilium is in contact with the cellular cytoplasm via a specialized transition zone, which along with transition fibers acts as a gatekeeper to the cilium (see Figure 44.1). There are approximately 600 proteins within the cilium and their transport in and out of the cilium is closely regulated by specific ciliary localization sequence.[3,4] Intraflagellar transport (IFT) of proteins is mediated by kinesin 2 and IFT B motor complexes involved in the anterograde movement of molecules and dynein and IFT A complexes and is involved in the retrograde movement of proteins.[5]

It is important to understand that the cilium consists of clearly defined subciliary compartments that are anatomically and functionally distinct. The ciliary axoneme is separated from the cell by a transition zone. The component

proteins of the transition zone are organized into modules.[6] The interaction of transition zone proteins between and within these modules defines its function and allows prediction of disease phenotypes. Even within the NPHP ciliopathy, there is a significant degree of genetic heterogeneity.[7] The role of modifier genes, oligogenicity, and mutation load is an area of intense research and may be responsible for the huge phenotypic variability seen in certain ciliopathies.[8,9]

## CILIARY SIGNALING CASCADES

### Hedgehog signaling

The Hedgehog (Hh) signaling pathway (Figure 44.2) is an ancient signaling cascade that is involved in development, organogenesis, growth, and intracellular and intercellular

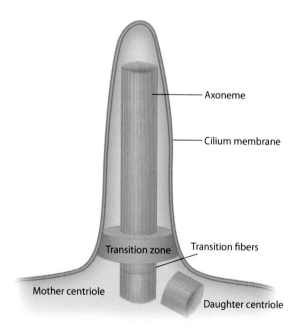

Figure 44.1 Structure of the cilium. The ciliary axoneme comprises nine microtubule doublets. The mother centriole comprises nine microtubule triplets, arranged in a cylinder. Cells contain two centrioles, the mother and the daughter. The mother centriole is the older of the two and provides a template for the nine microtubule doublets to form the ciliary axoneme. The transition fibers and transition zone form a ciliary gate that mediates entry and exit of molecules into the cilium.

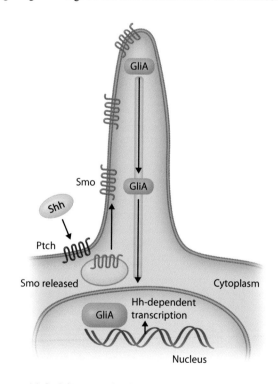

Figure 44.2 Ciliary Hedgehog signaling. The cilia mediate Hedgehog (Hh) signaling. In the absence of the ligand Sonic hedgehog (Shh), Patched (Ptch) represses the function of Smoothened (Smo) and there is no activation of Gli transcription factor. In the presence of Hh, Smo is released and moves into the cilium. At the ciliary tip, Smo promotes activation of Gli (GliA), which enters the nucleus and promotes Hh-dependent gene transcription.

signaling. Excess Sonic hedgehog (Shh) pathway activation can lead to severe developmental defects, extra digits, and tumor formation.[10] The Glioma (Gli) family of proteins are the terminal mediators of the Shh, and they localize to the primary cilia.[11] In the absence of Shh, Patched (Ptch) inhibits Smoothened (Smo) and there is no Gli3 activation. When Shh binds to its receptor Ptch, Smo enters the cilium and induces activation of Gli3, which then translocates to the nucleus, where it regulates gene expression.[5] The transport of the Shh pathway proteins within the cilium depends on the IFT machinery.[12,13]

## Wnt signaling

The noncanonical PCP pathway is a Wnt signaling pathway that is responsible for targeted cell migration, mitotic spindle orientation, and PCP.[14] Mutations in the components of the Wnt pathway lead to neural tube defects and have been implicated in the development of a cystic kidney phenotype.[15] May-Simera and Kelly[16] published an excellent review exploring the role of this pathway in ciliopathies.

## Platelet-derived growth factor receptor-alpha (PDGFR-α)

The cilium responds to chemosensory and mechanosensory stimulus by multiple signaling pathways involving PDGFR-α and its downstream effectors of the MEK/ERK cascade. A review of the ciliary signaling pathways mentioned previously and novel pathways such as the Hippo pathway can be found in a recent paper by Basten and Giles.[17]

## CLASSIFICATION OF NEPHRONOPHTHISIS

Historically, NPHP was classified by its clinical presentations and was also based on the age of onset of ESRD (Table 44.2). Modern-day molecular genetics allows a more precise diagnosis to be made.[18] It is now clear that single-gene disorders leading to NPHP may have a spectrum of presentations and

Table 44.2 Clinical classification of nephronophthisis

| Type | Median age of onset of ESRD | Most frequent genetic correlate |
|---|---|---|
| Infantile | <1 yr | NPHP2 and NPHP3 |
| Juvenile | 13 yr | NPHP1 |
| Adolescent | 19 yr | NPHP3 originally described |
| Late onset | 3rd to 6th decade | NPHP1 and others |

*Abbreviation:* ESRD, end-stage renal disease.

disease severity. Indeed, mutations in NPHP genes may give rise to isolated NPHP or to overlapping syndromes, including Senior-Loken syndrome (SLS), Joubert syndrome (JBTS), and Meckel-Gruber syndrome (MKS) (Table 44.3). Mutations in *NPHP6* may even cause Bardet-Biedl syndrome (BBS) phenotype.[19]

Table 44.3 Genetic causes of nephronophthisis and related syndromes

| Gene Name | Alias | Related syndromes |
|---|---|---|
| NPHP1 | SLSN1/JBTS4 | NPHP/SLS/JBTS |
| NPHP2 | INVS | NPHP |
| NPHP3 | MKS7 | NPHP/MKS |
| NPHP4 | SLSN4 | NPHP/SLS |
| NPHP5 | IQCB1/SLSN5 | NPHP/SLS |
| NPHP6 | CEP290/JBTS5/BBS14/MKS4 | NPHP/JBTS/MKS/BBS/LCA |
| NPHP7 | GLIS2 | NPHP |
| NPHP8 | RPGRIP1L/JBTS7/MKS5 | NPHP/JBTS/MKS |
| NPHP9 | NEK8 | NPHP |
| NPHP10 | SDCCAG8/BBS16 | NPHP/BBS |
| NPHP11 | TMEM67/MKS3/JBTS6 | NPHP/JBTS/MKS |
| NPHP12 | TTC21B/JBTS11 | NPHP/JBTS/JATD |
| NPHP13 | WDR19 | NPHP/JATD |
| NPHP14 | ZNF423/JBTS19 | NPHP/JBTS |
| NPHP15 | CEP164 | NPHP |
| NPHP16 | ANKS6 | NPHP |
| JBTS1 | INPP5E | JBTS |
| JBTS2 | TMEM216/MKS2 | JBTS/MKS |
| JBTS3 | AHI1 | JBTS/NPHP |
| JBTS8 | ARL13B | JBTS |
| JBTS9 | CC2D2A/MKS6 | JBTS/MKS |
| JBTS10 | OFD1 | JBTS/OFD |
| JBTS12 | KIF7 | JBTS |
| JBTS13 | TCTN1 | JBTS |
| JBTS14 | TMEM237 | JBTS |
| JBTS15 | CEP41 | JBTS |
| JBTS16 | TMEM138 | JBTS |
| JBTS17 | C5ORF42 | JBTS |
| JBTS18 | TCTN3 | JBTS |
| JBTS20 | TMEM231/MKS11 | JBTS/MKS |
| JBTS21 | CSPP1 | JBTS/JATD |
| JBTS22 | PDE6D | JBTS |
| MKS1 | MKS1 | MKS/BBS |
| MKS8 | TCTN2 | MKS |
| MKS9 | B9D | MKS |
| MKS10 | B9D2 | MKS |

*Abbreviations:* BBS, Bardet-Biedl syndrome; JATD, Jeune asphyxiating thoracic dystrophy; JBTS, Joubert syndrome; LCA, Leber congenital amaurosis; MKS, Meckel-Gruber syndrome; OFD, oral-facial-digital syndrome; SLS, Senior-Loken syndrome.

Table 44.4 Nephronophthisis may be associated with extrarenal manifestations and various eponymous syndromes

| NPHP-associated syndrome | Extrarenal features |
| --- | --- |
| Arima syndrome | Agenesis of the cerebellar vermis, ocular abnormalities, variable liver disease |
| COACH syndrome | Cerebellar vermis hypo/aplasia, oligophrenia (mental retardation), ataxia, ocular coloboma, and hepatic fibrosis |
| Cogan oculomotor apraxia | Defective or absent horizontal voluntary eye movements |
| Jeune asphyxiating thoracic dystrophy (JATD) (short-rib thoracic dysplasia) | Chondrodysplasia characterized by a severely constricted thoracic cage, short-limbed short stature, and polydactyly. Variable hepatic disease, retinal degeneration, pancreatic cysts |
| Joubert syndrome (JBTS) | Hypoplasia of the cerebellar vermis; neurologic symptoms, including dysregulation of breathing pattern and developmental delay. Variable retinal dystrophy, renal anomalies |
| Meckel-Gruber syndrome (MKS) | CNS malformation (including occipital encephalocele) and hepatic abnormalities, including portal fibrosis or ductal proliferation. Variable polydactyly, most often postaxial |
| RHYNS syndrome | Retinitis pigmentosa, hypopituitarism and mild skeletal dysplasia |
| Senior-Loken syndrome (SLS) | Leber congenital amaurosis |
| Sensenbrenner syndrome (cranioectodermal dysplasia) | Skeletal abnormalities, including craniosynostosis, narrow rib cage, short limbs, brachydactyly, and ectodermal defects. Variable hepatic fibrosis, heart defects, and retinitis pigmentosa |

## CLINICAL PRESENTATION

NPHP is a clinically and genetically heterogeneous disease (see Tables 44.2 and 44.3). The clinical presentation can vary from a very mild urinary concentrating defect to intrauterine death. The average age of presentation is approximately 6 years. The child usually presents with polydipsia, polyuria, secondary enuresis or nocturia, and generalized lethargy.[20] An inability to concentrate the urine usually precedes renal dysfunction, and ESRD ensues usually under the age of 25 years. The diagnosis of NPHP should be questioned if ESRD has not developed by the age of 25 years.[21] However, late adulthood presentation is possible

(see later). Extrarenal manifestations occur in 15% of cases and may help determine a clinical diagnosis of the disease (Table 44.4). Although NPHP is the most common genetic cause for ESRD in children and young adults, its reported incidence is widely variable (Table 44.5).[22–25]

### Infantile nephronophthisis

The rare infantile form of NPHP is characterized by early and widespread development of tubulointerstitial nephritis with cortical cysts, enlarged kidneys, and ESRD before 2 years of age. It is histologically distinct from juvenile NPHP.[26] Genetically, *NPHP2* and *NPHP3* are the most common causes of infantile NPHP. *NPHP2* encodes for inversin, and *NPHP3* encodes for nephrocystin-3.[27–29] Situs inversus and other cardiac defects may be associated with infantile NPHP.

### Juvenile nephronophthisis

Juvenile NPHP is the most common form of inherited kidney disease leading to chronic kidney disease in children.[30] Mutations in *NPHP1* account for approximately 20% of cases of NPHP.[7] *NPHP1* encodes for the primary ciliary protein nephrocystin-1 and is expressed in the human collecting duct.[31]

### Adult-onset nephronophthisis

There are a few case reports of onset of renal failure in the 3rd to 6th decade of life along with extra renal manifestations of NPHP.[32–34] It is important to perform accurate assessment of a patient's vision and neurologic status to

Table 44.5 Demographics and pathology of nephronophthisis

| Inheritance | Autosomal recessive |
| --- | --- |
| Incidence | 1:50,000 to 1:900,000 |
| Geographic distribution | Worldwide |
| Macroscopic renal pathology | Normal or reduced kidney size with corticomedullary cysts arising from collecting ducts and distal tubule |
| Renal microscopy | Corticomedullary cysts, tubulointerstitial nephritis, and tubular basement membrane disruption |

- NPHP may present as an isolated lesion or as a part of a complex of symptoms involving multiple organs.
- Common findings of NPHP include a urine concentrating defect, normal to small kidneys on ultrasound, and anemia more severe than would be expected by the degree of renal impairment.

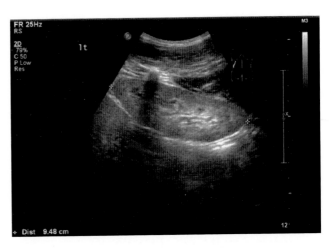

Figure 44.3 Renal ultrasound appearance of nephronophthisis (NPHP). Renal ultrasound scan of a patient with NPHP showing loss of corticomedullary differentiation, normal renal size, and few corticomedullary cysts.

assess for the extrarenal manifestations of NPHP. These patients have been reported to have pendular nystagmus, retinal degeneration, and a reduction in vision. They have also been reported to have ataxia. These features along with chronic interstitial nephritis should lead the physician toward a genetic analysis for NPHP mutations.

## DIAGNOSIS

### CLINICAL EVALUATION

To establish a clinical diagnosis of NPHP, a detailed history and clinical examination including looking for extrarenal associations (abnormal eye movements, retinopathy, ataxia, polydactyly, cardiac malformations) is necessary. A detailed family history must be obtained.[18] Fundoscopic evaluation should be performed by an ophthalmologist. The majority of patients with NPHP present with renal disease and its manifestations. However, as described earlier, ciliary dysfunction may lead to multiorgan involvement. Patients with extrarenal manifestations require referral to appropriate specialists for management.

### RENAL FUNCTION AND ANCILLARY DATA

Investigations should include renal and liver function tests, hemoglobin determination, and urine concentration ability. Key diagnostic features are elevated serum creatinine level with reduced urine osmolarity (typically < 400 mOsm/kg). Anemia that is out of proportion to the degree of chronic kidney disease (CKD) is a frequent finding in patients with NPHP. Regular review is required to appropriately manage CKD and ESRD.

### RADIOLOGIC INVESTIGATIONS

The most informative and practical modality for radiologic assessment is ultrasound of the kidney. The important features are loss of corticomedullary differentiation, presence of corticomedullary cysts, and reduced or normal renal size (Figure 44.3). Indeed, a patient with previously undetected CKD, small kidneys on ultrasound, and anemia that is disproportionate to the degree of renal dysfunction may be

presumed to have NPHP until proved otherwise. Hepatic ultrasound may provide information about extrarenal involvement.

Brain magnetic resonance imaging (MRI) may be performed, if indicated, to assess for intracranial abnormalities. The pathognomonic "molar tooth sign" (Figure 44.4) is seen in JBTS and represents a deep interpeduncular fossa; narrow isthmus; thickened, elongated, and maloriented superior cerebellar peduncles; and cerebellar vermis hypoplasia.[35]

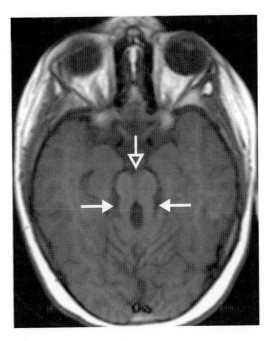

Figure 44.4 Molar tooth sign (within arrowheads). This finding is strongly associated with Joubert syndrome. (Reproduced with permission from: Brancati F, Dallapiccola B, Valente EM. Joubert syndrome and related disorders. Orphanet J Rare Dis. 2010;5:20. doi:10.1186/1750-1172-5-20.)

## GENETIC TESTING

After genetic counseling, genetic testing to seek a molecular diagnosis should be undertaken, and this may avoid the need for renal biopsy. Targeted *NPHP1* mutational analysis (including searching for whole gene deletion) will detect approximately 20% of cases.[36] However, given the huge genetic heterogeneity, high-throughput polymerase chain reaction (PCR), and next-generation sequencing and whole exome approaches are providing a more efficient means of genetic diagnosis than individual gene sequencing.[27,37–39] At this point, however, more than half of NPHP cases remain unsolved in terms of a molecular genetic defect.[27]

## RENAL PATHOLOGIC FINDINGS

Traditionally, a diagnosis of NPHP has relied on a pathologic evaluation (Table 44.5 and Figure 44.5). Typically, the kidneys are normal or reduced in size. This is in contrast to autosomal dominant polycystic kidney disease, in which there are grossly enlarged kidneys and predominantly cortical cysts. In NPHP, the presence of corticomedullary cysts is not universal and depends on the underlying genetic defect. In NPHP, the histopathologic changes are characterized by diffuse interstitial fibrosis, tubular basement membrane thickening, tubular atrophy, corticomedullary cyst formation, and periglomerular fibrosis.[24,28] Karyomegalic interstitial nephritis described by Mihatsch et al.[40] has histopathologic features similar to those of NPHP, apart from the presence of karyomegaly. The autosomal dominant condition medullary cystic kidney disease also may mimic NPHP histologically.[36]

## TREATMENT

Presently there is no cure for NPHP and related ciliopathies. Clinicians must focus on optimizing the delivery of renal replacement therapy, ideally with renal transplantation where possible. However, with a growing understanding of the pathophysiology of NPHP, therapeutic interventions are possible in the future. Management of extrarenal manifestations requires input from specialists and multidisciplinary care teams, to ensure the best possible quality of life for these patients.

## PROGNOSIS

Infantile forms of NPHP have a guarded prognosis, given the challenges and difficulties of managing ESRD, especially if it occurs before 5 years of age. The prognosis for children and young adults with other forms of NPHP is variable, depending on the age of onset of CKD or ESRD and presence of extrarenal manifestations. Following transplantation, there is no recurrent disease in the allograft and patients with nonsyndromic forms of NPHP do well. Where severe extrarenal manifestations are present, such as in JBTS, the prognosis largely depends on the degree of associated brain anomalies.

## SUMMARY

The nephronophthises are a group of diseases that result from abnormal function of the primary cilium. This structure is essential for transducing environmental signals into the cell, and its disruption results in organ maldevelopment and malfunction. Although the primary manifestations in the kidney are renal concentrating defects and cyst formation, systemic loss of cilia can affect the form and function of many organs. Further, the mutation of different proteins in the cilium may have different effects, so that multiple mutations have been identified, each of which causes a unique pattern of systemic pathologic processes. Given that NPHP is a genetically determined disease, treatment is directed entirely toward ameliorating symptoms.

## ACKNOWLEDGMENTS

Dr. Shalabh Srivastava is a Kidney Research UK Clinical Training Fellow. Dr. John Sayer is funded by Kidney Research UK, Kids Kidney Research, the Medical Research Council (MR/M012212/1), and The Northern Counties Kidney Research Fund.

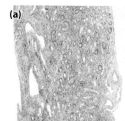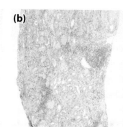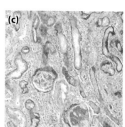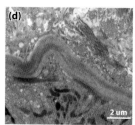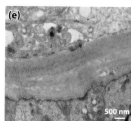

Figure 44.5 Renal histopathology and electron microscopy features of nephronophthisis (NPHP). **(a)** and **(b)** Hematoxylin- and eosin-stained sections of renal tissue demonstrating cyst formation, tubular atrophy, and interstitial infiltrates. **(c)** Periodic acid–Schiff stain showing tubular basement membrane disruption. **(d)** and **(e)** Electron microscopy images demonstrating tubular basement membrane thickening and lamellation.

## Clinical Vignette 44.1

A 5-year-old girl presented to the nephrology department with symptoms of being tired and lethargic. Her medical history revealed developmental delay and possible seizures as a neonate. She had no breathing abnormalities during the perinatal period and no history of gaze palsy. She was still wearing diapers at night because of nocturnal enuresis, and the mother reported polydipsia from an early age. Her parents were consanguineous (first-degree cousins). She had one healthy sibling 7 years of age, and there was no other family history of renal disease. Fundoscopic examination was normal and showed no coloboma or retinal dystrophy. Her serum creatinine level was 4 mg/dL and hemoglobin was 7 g/dL. MRI of the brain revealed hypertrophy of the superior cerebellar peduncles and dysplasia of the cerebellar vermis. Renal ultrasound showed small kidneys bilaterally with loss of corticomedullary differentiation. No renal cysts were seen. Urine biochemistry revealed a urine osmolarity of 320 mOsm/kg and serum biochemistry confirmed CKD stage 5 (eGFR 12 mL/min).

## TEACHING POINTS

- This child presented with a cerebral-renal syndrome. She had evidence of CKD and severe anemia, in addition to neurologic symptoms.
- A search for additional clinical features suggestive of a ciliopathy should be performed. These include documenting polydactyly (may be already corrected surgically) and other skeletal abnormalities, ataxia, cardiac malformations, and liver dysfunction.
- A formal ophthalmologic examination should be performed, because retinal changes may be subtle.
- A detailed family history may reveal other family members at risk.
- An obstetric history from the mother (oligohydramnios, miscarriages, etc.) may be informative.
- Baseline investigations should include renal and liver function tests, hemoglobin determination, urine concentrating ability, renal and hepatic ultrasound scans, and cerebral imaging.
- Brain imaging should be reviewed to look for the pathognomonic "molar tooth" sign of JBTS syndrome.
- A renal biopsy should be withheld in cases in which there is evidence of CKD or ESRD. Instead, genetic testing should be performed. Mutations in *NPHP1* are the most common molecular genetic findings in NPHP and may be associated with both brain and eye phenotypes.
- Whole exome sequencing approaches may be the most efficient way of obtaining a definitive molecular genetic diagnosis if the *NPHP1* gene testing is negative.
- Clinical management should focus on the treatment of CKD and impending ESRD, with optimization of blood pressure, anemia, and bone health.
- Assessment and preparation for dialysis and transplantation are important needs to be addressed. Extrarenal clinical manifestations should be managed by referral to appropriate specialists.

# REFERENCES

1. Dobell C. Antony van Leeuwenhoek and his 'Little Animals'. New York: Harcourt, Brace; 1932.
2. Beales P, Jackson PK. Cilia: The prodigal organelle. Cilia. 2012;1:1.
3. Pazour GJ, Agrin N, Leszyk J, Witman GB. Proteomic analysis of a eukaryotic cilium. J Cell Biol. 2005;170:103–13.
4. Garcia-Gonzalo FR, Reiter JF. Scoring a backstage pass: Mechanisms of ciliogenesis and ciliary access. J Cell Biol. 2012;197:697–709.
5. Scholey JM, Anderson KV. Intraflagellar transport and cilium-based signaling. Cell. 2006;125:439–42.
6. Szymanska K, Johnson CA. The transition zone: An essential functional compartment of cilia. Cilia. 2012;1:10.
7. Wolf MT, Hildebrandt F. Nephronophthisis. Pediatr Nephrol. 2011;26:181–94.
8. Eley L, Gabrielides C, Adams M, et al. Jouberin localizes to collecting ducts and interacts with nephrocystin-1. Kidney Int. 2008;74:1139–49.
9. Novarino G, Akizu N, Gleeson JG. Modeling human disease in humans: The ciliopathies. Cell. 2011;147:70–9.
10. McMahon AP, Ingham PW, Tabin CJ. Developmental roles and clinical significance of hedgehog signaling. Curr Top Dev Biol. 2003;53:1–114.
11. Haycraft CJ, Banizs B, Aydin-Son Y, et al. Gli2 and Gli3 localize to cilia and require the intraflagellar transport protein polaris for processing and function. PLoS Genet. 2005;1:e53.
12. Huangfu D, Liu A, Rakeman AS, et al. Hedgehog signalling in the mouse requires intraflagellar transport proteins. Nature. 2003;426:83–7.
13. Liu A, Wang B, Niswander LA. Mouse intraflagellar transport proteins regulate both the activator and repressor functions of Gli transcription factors. Development. 2005;132:3103–11.
14. McNeill H. Planar cell polarity and the kidney. J Am Soc Nephrol. 2009;20:2104–11.
15. Saburi S, Hester I, Fischer E, et al. Loss of Fat4 disrupts PCP signaling and oriented cell division and leads to cystic kidney disease. Nat Genet. 2008;40:1010–5.
16. May-Simera HL, Kelley MW. Cilia, Wnt signaling, and the cytoskeleton. Cilia. 2012;1:7.

17. Basten SG, Giles RH. Functional aspects of primary cilia in signaling, cell cycle and tumorigenesis. Cilia. 2013;2:6.

18. Simms RJ, Hynes AM, Eley L, Sayer JA. Nephronophthisis: A genetically diverse ciliopathy. Int J Nephrol. 2011;2011:527137.

19. Leitch CC, Zaghloul NA, Davis EE, et al. Hypomorphic mutations in syndromic encephalocele genes are associated with Bardet-Biedl syndrome. Nat Genet. 2008;40:443–8.

20. Krishnan R, Eley L, Sayer JA. Urinary concentration defects and mechanisms underlying nephronophthisis. Kidney Blood Press Res. 2008;31:152–62.

21. Hildebrandt F, Zhou W. Nephronophthisis-associated ciliopathies. J Am Soc Nephrol. 2007;18:1855–71.

22. Hildebrandt F, Otto E, Rensing C, et al. A novel gene encoding an SH3 domain protein is mutated in nephronophthisis type 1. Nat Genet. 1997;17:149–53.

23. Potter DE, Holliday MA, Piel CF, et al. Treatment of end-stage renal disease in children: A 15-year experience. Kidney Int. 1980;18:103–9.

24. Waldherr R, Lennert T, Weber HP, et al. The nephronophthisis complex: A clinicopathologic study in children. Virchows Arch A Pathol Anat Histol. 1982;394:235–54.

25. Ala-Mello S, Koskimies O, Rapola J, Kaariainen H. Nephronophthisis in Finland: Epidemiology and comparison of genetically classified subgroups. Eur J Hum Genet. 1999;7:205–11.

26. Salomon R, Saunier S, Niaudet P. Nephronophthisis. Pediatr Nephrol. 2009;24:2333–44.

27. Halbritter J, Porath JD, Diaz KA, et al. Identification of 99 novel mutations in a worldwide cohort of 1,056 patients with a nephronophthisis-related ciliopathy. Hum Genet. 2013;132:865–84.

28. Otto EA, Schermer B, Obara T, et al. Mutations in INVS encoding inversin cause nephronophthisis type 2, linking renal cystic disease to the function of primary cilia and left-right axis determination. Nat Genet. 2003;34:413–20.

29. Olbrich H, Fliegauf M, Hoefele J, et al. Mutations in a novel gene, NPHP3, cause adolescent nephronophthisis, tapeto-retinal degeneration and hepatic fibrosis. Nat Genet. 2003;34:455–9.

30. Antignac C, Arduy CH, Beckmann JS, et al. A gene for familial juvenile nephronophthisis (recessive medullary cystic kidney disease) maps to chromosome 2p. Nat Genet. 1993;3:342–5.

31. Eley L, Moochhala SH, Simms R, et al. Nephrocystin-1 interacts directly with Ack1 and is expressed in human collecting duct. Biochem Biophys Res Commun. 2008;371:877–82.

32. Georges B, Cosyns JP, Dahan K, et al. Late-onset renal failure in Senior-Loken syndrome. Am J Kidney Dis. 2000;36:1271–5.

33. Apostolou T, Nikolopoulou N, Theodoridis M, et al. Late onset of renal disease in nephronophthisis with features of Joubert syndrome type B. Nephrol Dial Transplant. 2001;16:2412–5.

34. Hoefele J, Nayir A, Chaki M, et al. Pseudodominant inheritance of nephronophthisis caused by a homozygous NPHP1 deletion. Pediatr Nephrol. 2011;26:967–71.

35. Nag C, Ghosh M, Das K, Ghosh T. Joubert syndrome: The molar tooth sign of the mid-brain. Ann Med Health Sci Res. 2013;3:291–4.

36. Simms RJ, Eley L, Sayer JA. Nephronophthisis. Eur J Hum Genet. 2008;17:406–16.

37. Chaki M, Airik R, Ghosh AK, et al. Exome capture reveals ZNF423 and CEP164 mutations, linking renal ciliopathies to DNA damage response signaling. Cell. 2012;150:533–48.

38. Gee HY, Otto EA, Hurd TW, et al. Whole-exome resequencing distinguishes cystic kidney diseases from phenocopies in renal ciliopathies. Kidney Int. 2014;85:880–7.

39. Sayer JA, Simms RJ. The challenges and surprises of a definitive molecular genetic diagnosis. Kidney Int. 2014;85:748–9.

40. Mihatsch MJ, Gudat F, Zollinger HU, et al. Systemic karyomegaly associated with chronic interstitial nephritis: A new disease entity? Clin Nephrol. 1979;12:54–62.

## REVIEW QUESTIONS

1. Clinical features of a ciliopathy may include:
   a. Renal cysts
   b. Retinal disease
   c. Cerebral malformations
   d. All of above
   e. None of above

2. Nephronopthisis may be associated with which of the following syndromes?
   a. Joubert syndrome
   b. Long QT syndrome
   c. Medullary cystic kidney disease
   d. Senior-Loken syndrome
   e. a and d
   f. b and c

3. The most common genetic cause of nephronophthisis is:
   a. NPHP1
   b. NPHP4
   c. SDCCAG8
   d. NPHP5

4. A molecular genetic diagnosis can be made in what percentage of cases of NPHP?
   a. 25%
   b. 40%
   c. 60%
   d. 10%
5. The histologic features of nephronophthisis may include:
   a. Glomerular basement membrane thinning
   b. Interstitial fibrosis
   c. Karyomegaly
   d. Cortical microcysts
   e. b and d
   f. a and c

## ANSWER KEY

1. d
2. e
3. a
4. c
5. e

# 45

# Alport syndrome and thin basement membrane nephropathy

MICHELLE N. RHEAULT AND CLIFFORD E. KASHTAN

Alport syndrome (AS) and thin basement membrane nephropathy (TBMN) are related inherited disorders of glomerular basement membranes (GBMs) that manifest with hematuria in childhood. AS is characterized clinically by progressive deterioration of kidney function with cochlear and ocular involvement, leading to end-stage renal disease (ESRD) and deafness in many affected individuals.

Familial hematuria associated with renal disease was described by several English investigators in the early 20th century. Cecil Alport recognized that these patients also exhibited deafness and that symptoms were more severe in the affected males.[1] The underlying genetic cause was identified in 1990 when Barker et al.[2] discovered mutations in *COL4A5*, the gene encoding the α5 chain of type IV collagen, in several kindreds affected by X-linked Alport syndrome (XLAS). In 1994, mutations in both alleles of the related type IV collagen genes *COL4A3* and *COL4A4* were identified as causative for autosomal recessive Alport syndrome (ARAS).[3]

TBMN, formerly known as benign familial hematuria, has been recognized since the early 1970s as a cause of familial hematuria.[4] TBMN is usually not associated with extrarenal clinical manifestations and is generally a nonprogressive disorder. However, a subset of patients have been found to develop overt proteinuria and hypertension.[5] Heterozygous mutations in *COL4A3* and *COL4A4* were identified in some patients with TBMN in 1996, but the genetic basis in others remains unclear.[6]

## ALPORT SYNDROME

### EPIDEMIOLOGY

The prevalence of AS has been estimated at 1:50,000 live births.[7] The prevalence of TBMN is estimated at 1% to 2% of the population.[8] There does not appear to be an ethnic predisposition to development of AS or TBMN. In children undergoing kidney biopsy for persistent microscopic hematuria, approximately 12% to 27% are diagnosed with AS and 15% to 50% are diagnosed with TBMN.[9–11] According to the US Renal Data System (USRDS), 1.3% of pediatric ESRD patients and 0.4% of adult ESRD patients have a primary diagnosis of AS.[12]

### KEY POINTS

- AS and TBMN are common causes of persistent microscopic hematuria in childhood.
- TBMN is estimated to affect 1% to 2% of the population.

### GLOMERULAR BASEMENT MEMBRANE COLLAGEN NETWORK

Transmission electron microscopy of the normal GBM exhibits an electron-dense lamina densa surrounded on each side by more electron-lucent layers known as the lamina rara interna and externa. Both podocytes and endothelial cells secrete components of the GBM during glomerulogenesis and are responsible for maintenance of its structure and function.[13,14] Similar to other basement membranes, the GBM is composed of type IV collagen, laminin, entactin/nidogen, and heparan sulfate proteoglycan. However, the isoforms of each protein class that are present in the GBM are often unique compared to those in other basement membranes in the body.[15]

There are six isoforms of type IV collagen, $\alpha$1(IV)-$\alpha$6(IV), encoded by six genes, COL4A1 to COL4A6. The type IV collagen genes are arranged in pairs on three chromosomes: COL4A1 to COL4A2 on chromosome 13, COL4A3 to COL4A4 on chromosome 2, and COL4A5 to COL4A6 on the X chromosome. Each gene pair is oriented in a head-to-head manner with intervening promoter and transcriptional regulatory sites allowing for coordinated transcription.[16,17] All $\alpha$(IV) chains share similar structural features, including a noncollagenous aminoterminal sequence of approximately 20 amino acids (7S), a collagenous domain of approximately 1400 amino acids with multiple Gly-X-Y repeats, and a noncollagenous carboxyterminal (NC1) domain of approximately 230 amino acids. The type IV collagen $\alpha$ chains wind around one another to form triple helixes or trimers. Despite multiple combinatorial possibilities, only three type IV collagen trimers are found in mammalian basement membranes: $\alpha$1$\alpha$1$\alpha$2(IV), $\alpha$3$\alpha$4$\alpha$5(IV), and $\alpha$5$\alpha$5$\alpha$6(IV). Trimer formation is directed by sequence and structure within each NC1 domain.[18] The 7S and NC1 domains are then responsible for linking trimers together to form three-dimensional collagen IV networks.[19] The $\alpha$1$\alpha$1$\alpha$2(IV) network is found in all basement membranes, whereas the $\alpha$3$\alpha$4$\alpha$5(IV) network has a more limited distribution in GBM, Bowman capsule, distal and collecting tubules, alveoli, inner ear, and eye, and some other basement membranes.[20,21] The $\alpha$5$\alpha$5$\alpha$6(IV) trimer is present in the Bowman capsule and distal and collecting tubule basement membranes, as well as some skin, alimentary canal, and vascular basement membranes, but is not present in GBM.

During glomerulogenesis, the primary type IV collagen network switches from a predominantly $\alpha$1$\alpha$1$\alpha$2(IV) network in GBM of primitive glomeruli to a predominantly $\alpha$3$\alpha$4$\alpha$5(IV) network in the mature GBM.[22] The $\alpha$3$\alpha$4$\alpha$5(IV) network is more highly cross-linked and may be more resistant to proteases than the $\alpha$1$\alpha$1$\alpha$2(IV) network, which may account for some of the unique properties of the GBM.[23,24] Absence or disruption of the $\alpha$3$\alpha$4$\alpha$5(IV) network with persistence of the embryonal $\alpha$1$\alpha$1$\alpha$2(IV) network is the primary abnormality in AS.

## COLLAGEN DEFECT IN ALPORT SYNDROME

The $\alpha$3(IV), $\alpha$4(IV), and $\alpha$5(IV) chains must associate into trimers to be deposited into basement membranes. If any one of the chains is absent, the other collagen chains are degraded, and $\alpha$3$\alpha$4$\alpha$5(IV) network is not deposited in basement membranes.[23] If the $\alpha$3$\alpha$4$\alpha$5(IV) network is absent, $\alpha$1$\alpha$1$\alpha$2(IV) network remains as the dominant collagen network. This has significant consequences for the composition, structure, and function of the GBM and other affected basement membranes in individuals with mutations in any of the associated genes. For example, severe COL4A5 mutations that result in failure to synthesize $\alpha$5(IV) chains (deletions, frame shift mutations, premature stop codons, etc.) prevent the formation of $\alpha$3$\alpha$4$\alpha$5(IV) trimers (Figure 45.1). The $\alpha$3(IV) and $\alpha$4(IV) chains are then degraded before deposition in the basement membrane and $\alpha$3$\alpha$4$\alpha$5(IV) network is absent. Similarly, severe mutations in COL4A3 or COL4A4 lead to absence of the entire $\alpha$3$\alpha$4$\alpha$5(IV) network in the basement membranes. Mutations in the collagenous domain of COL4A3 to COL4A5, particularly the glycine residues that allow for triple helix formation, lead to the formation of abnormally folded trimers that are susceptible to degradation before being incorporated into basement membranes. Finally, minor missense mutations may allow for abnormal $\alpha$3$\alpha$4$\alpha$5(IV) network formation that is deposited into basement membranes.

## GENETICS OF ALPORT SYNDROME AND THIN BASEMENT MEMBRANE NEPHROPATHY

There are three distinct genetic forms of AS that are clinically similar: X-linked, autosomal recessive, and autosomal dominant. XLAS is caused by mutations in COL4A5 on the X-chromosome and has been known to account for approximately 80% of the affected patients. ARAS is caused by mutations in COL4A3 or COL4A4. Autosomal dominant Alport syndrome (ADAS) rarely has been reported in the literature and is caused by heterozygous mutations in COL4A3 or COL4A4.[25] With the advent of next-generation sequencing, recent studies are finding a much higher percentage of patients with AS who demonstrate autosomal dominant inheritance than was previously recognized, with

---

### KEY POINTS

- AS is most often inherited as an X-linked disorder, but autosomal recessive and autosomal dominant forms also can be observed.
- Affected individuals with AS demonstrate absence or dysfunction of the normal $\alpha$3$\alpha$4$\alpha$5(IV) network within the GBM.
- Mutations that block synthesis of a full-length $\alpha$5(IV) chain prevent $\alpha$3(IV) and $\alpha$4(IV) from forming trimers, resulting in their degradation. The $\alpha$3$\alpha$4$\alpha$5(IV) GBM network cannot be formed, causing a severe Alport phenotype.

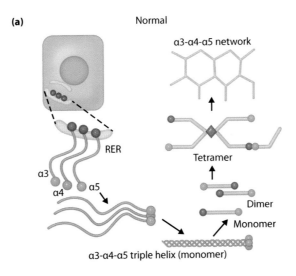

**(a)** Normal

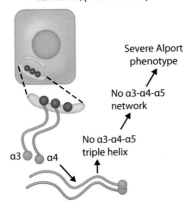

**(b)** Effect of a "severe" COL4A5 mutation: deletion, frameshift, premature stop

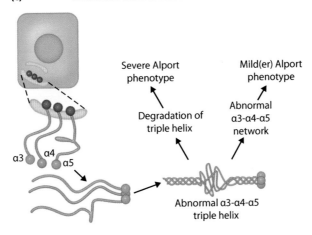

**(c)** Effects of a COL4A5 missense mutation

Figure 45.1 Models of assembly of collagen IV α3α4α5 networks. **(a)** In normal individuals, α3(IV), α4(IV), and α5(IV) chains form trimers, which then self-associate through carboxyterminal and aminoterminal interactions to form networks. **(b)** Mutations that block synthesis of a full-length α5(IV) prevent α3(IV) and α4(IV) from forming trimers, resulting in their degradation. The α3α4α5(IV) network cannot be constructed, and the result is a severe Alport phenotype. **(c)** The effect of missense *COL4A5* mutations is variable. Formation of abnormal α3α4α5(IV) trimers can result in their degradation, causing a severe Alport phenotype. Some missense mutations are compatible with formation of α3α4α5(IV) trimers that can self-associate into networks. Partial degradation may result in basement membranes that are relatively deficient in their content of this network or the network may function abnormally, resulting in a milder Alport phenotype. (Reprinted with permission from: Kashtan, CE. Alport syndrome and thin basement membrane disease. Curr Diagn Pathol. 2000;8:349–60.)

up to 31% in one report.[26] Future large studies using this technique will likely help to clarify the population genetics of this disorder. Over 600 pathogenic mutations in *COL4A5* have been identified in families with XLAS, and these span the entire 51 exons of the gene with no identified hot spots.[27] Approximately 10% to 15% of *COL4A5* mutations occur as spontaneous events in the proband and these patients have a negative family history of the disease. All males with pathogenic *COL4A5* mutations are affected with the disease, and clinical expression in heterozygous females is variable. Unlike XLAS, ARAS affects males and females equally. Affected patients may be homozygous or compound heterozygous for their mutations.

TBMN and ADAS are both caused by heterozygous mutations in *COL4A3* or *COL4A4*.[28,29] It is not clear why some individuals with these mutations have asymptomatic hematuria whereas others have progressive and multisystem disease. TBMN is not always linked to *COL4A3* and *COL4A4* mutations, and other causative genetic loci may be identified in the future.[30]

# CLINICAL FEATURES OF ALPORT SYNDROME

## Renal manifestations

Microscopic hematuria is the hallmark finding in AS and is present in 100% of males and more than 90% of heterozygous females with XLAS and all males and females with ARAS.[31,32] Intermittent gross hematuria is not unusual, particularly in affected children with XLAS and ARAS. Untreated affected males with XLAS, some females with XLAS, and both males and females with ARAS, exhibit progression of kidney disease from isolated microscopic hematuria to microalbuminuria, overt proteinuria, progressive renal dysfunction, and eventual ESRD.[33]

Large deletions, nonsense mutations, and frame shift mutations in *COL4A5* are associated with more rapid progression to ESRD. Affected males with such mutations have a 90% probability of ESRD by age 30 years.[31] Missense mutations are associated with less severe disease with only a 50% probability of ESRD by age 30.[31] There is no genotype-phenotype correlation for females with heterozygous *COL4A5* mutations, and disease severity appears to be influenced by X-inactivation and other yet unknown factors.[32,34] The risk for ESRD for heterozygous females is 12% by age 40 and approximately 30% by age 60.[32]

---

**KEY POINT**

Heterozygous females with *COL4A5* mutations (carriers) are at risk for developing proteinuria, sensorineural hearing loss, and ESRD.

---

## Cochlear manifestations

The α3α4α5(IV) network is normally found in the cochlea in the basement membrane between the organ of Corti and the basilar membrane and within the spiral ligament.[35] The mechanism of hearing loss in AS is unknown but may be related to dysfunction of the spiral ligament or alterations in cochlear micromechanics.[37,36]

Audiologic abnormalities in AS are typically apparent by late childhood as high tone (2000- to 8000-Hz range) hearing loss detectable by audiometry. Newborn hearing screening is normal. Hearing loss is progressive over time with 80% to 90% of XLAS males demonstrating sensorineural deafness by 40 years of age.[31] Heterozygous females with *COL4A5* mutations have a 10% risk for sensorineural deafness by age 40 and 20% by age 60.[32] Sensorineural hearing loss is common in ARAS as well, with 66% of individuals affected in a recent study.[37] Similar to the case in kidney disease, affected individuals with severe mutations such as large rearrangements, nonsense mutations, splice site mutations, or frameshift mutations have more severe hearing loss at earlier ages.[31]

## Ocular manifestations

The α3α4α5(IV) network is present in the lens capsule, retina, and cornea of the eye.[38] Ocular findings resulting from absence or dysfunction of the α3α4α5(IV) network in these locations are present in 40% to 60% of patients with AS, and the spectrum of disease appears to be similar in XLAS and ARAS.[31,37] Findings in affected patients include anterior lenticonus, dot and fleck maculopathy, or posterior polymorphous dystrophy. Anterior lenticonus, the protrusion of the central portion of the lens into the anterior chamber, is pathognomonic of AS.[38,39] Lenticonus is absent at birth and manifests during the second and third decades of life in approximately 13% to 25% of affected individuals.[31,38] Anterior lenticonus has been described only rarely in heterozygous females with *COL4A5* mutations.[32] A maculopathy consisting of whitish or yellowish flecks in a perimacular distribution, likely because of abnormality of the internal limiting membrane, is found in 14% to 85% of affected individuals and does not appear to be associated with any abnormality in vision.[38,40] Posterior polymorphous dystrophy has been more rarely observed in individuals with AS and may be due to abnormalities in the Descemet membrane.[41] Recurrent corneal erosions also have been described, likely secondary to abnormalities in the corneal basement membrane.[42]

## Renal pathology

There are no pathognomonic abnormalities present on kidney biopsy by light microscopy or routine immunofluorescence microscopy. Electron microscopy (EM) in young children typically shows diffuse thinning of the glomerular capillary wall. The glomerular capillary walls of older children and adolescents exhibit areas of diffuse thickening and splitting of the basement membrane with a "basket-weave" appearance

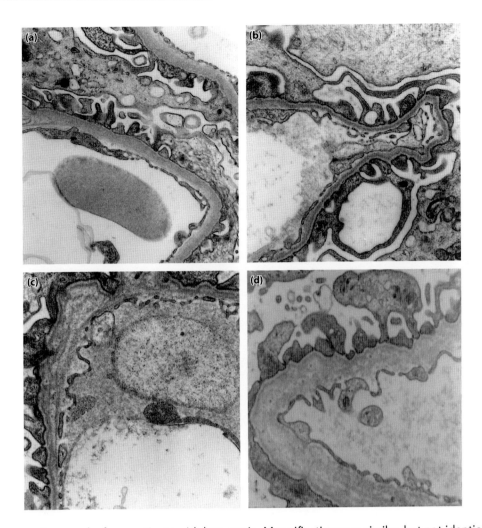

Figure 45.2 Electron micrographs from patients with hematuria. Magnifications are similar, but not identical. **(a)** Normal glomerular basement membrane (GBM). **(b)** Attenuated GBM in a patient with thin basement membrane nephropathy. **(c)** This female with a heterozygous *COL4A5* mutation exhibits both thin and split lamellated GBM. **(d)** This male with XLAS shows diffuse thickening and lamellation of GBM. (Reprinted with permission from: Kashtan, CE. Alport syndrome and thin basement membrane disease. Curr Diagn Pathol. 2000;8:349–60.)

of the lamina densa (Figure 45.2). The subepithelial aspect of the GBM frequently appears irregular or scalloped. Areas of thickening and basket weaving are usually associated with overlying effacement of foot processes. By immunohistology, approximately 80% of affected males with XLAS demonstrate absence of the α3(IV), α4(IV), and α5(IV) chains from the GBM, Bowman capsules, and distal/collecting tubule basement membranes (Figure 45.3).[43] Females with heterozygous mutations in *COL4A5* may demonstrate a patchy or mosaic expression pattern for α3α4α5(IV) in the GBM consistent with X-inactivation. The GBM of males and females with ARAS typically lacks the α3(IV), α4(IV), and α5(IV) chains. Bowman capsules and distal/collecting tubule basement membranes lack the α3(IV) and α4(IV) chains, but the α5(IV) chain is present in Bowman capsules and distal/collecting tubule basement membranes as part of the α5α5α6(IV) network. Thus, immunostaining of kidney biopsy specimens for type IV collagen can be used to distinguish XLAS and ARAS. Patients with ADAS typically show normal renal basement membrane expression of the α3α4α5(IV) network.

Skin biopsy shows absence of the α5α5α6(IV) network in approximately 80% of males with XLAS, and mosaic expression of this network in 60% to 70% of XLAS females. For individuals with ARAS or ADAS, α5(IV) will be present in skin as part of the α5α5α6(IV) network.[44]

## THIN BASEMENT MEMBRANE NEPHROPATHY

TBMN is the most common cause of persistent microscopic hematuria in children and adults.[45] Affected individuals typically demonstrate persistent microscopic hematuria with rare episodes of gross hematuria, although for some the hematuria may be intermittent. The penetrance of hematuria is only approximately 70%.[46] Proteinuria is rare in childhood but is observed in a significant proportion of adult patients, up to 63% in one series.[47] Chronic kidney disease (CKD) or ESRD is observed in fewer than 5% of affected adults.[47] The presence of proteinuria and CKD in

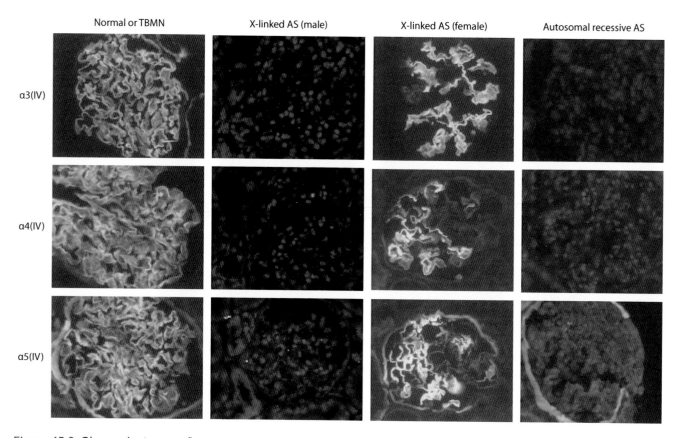

| Normal or TBMN | X-linked AS (male) | X-linked AS (female) | Autosomal recessive AS |

Figure 45.3 Glomerular immunofluorescence microscopy in X-lined Alport syndrome (XLAS) and autosomal recessive (ARAS). α3(IV), α4(IV), and α5(IV) chains are expressed in the glomerular basement membrane in patients with normal glomeruli and thin basement membrane nephropathy. All three chains are missing in affected males with XLAS. A mosaic pattern is present for heterozygous females with XLAS secondary to X-inactivation. In ARAS, α3(IV), α4(IV), and α5(IV) chains are absent from the glomerulus; however, α5(IV) is visible in the Bowman capsule as part of the α5α5α6(IV) network. (Reprinted with permission from: Kashtan, CE. The nongenetic diagnosis of thin basement membrane nephropathy. Semin Nephrol. 2005;25:159–62.)

individuals diagnosed with TBMN may represent misclassification of patients who more accurately should be designated as having ADAS or XLAS. Future large genetic and natural history studies will hopefully clarify the prognosis for affected patients. Extrarenal manifestations are only sporadically reported.

Kidney biopsy in patients with TBMN demonstrates normal light and immunofluorescence microscopy, including immunostaining for type IV collagen chains. EM shows diffuse thinning of the GBM that may be identical in appearance to that seen in early stages of AS. The thickness of the GBM varies with age, gender, and EM technique and should be interpreted based on individual criteria for each histologic laboratory.[48,49]

## DIAGNOSTIC CONSIDERATIONS

The diagnosis of AS or TBMN is often suspected in patients with persistent microscopic hematuria and a family history of hematuria. Although difficult to distinguish at times,

features that may help in differentiating these two disorders are listed in Table 45.1. The likelihood of AS increases with a family history of AS or renal failure; the presence of sensorineural hearing loss; the presence of anterior lenticonus, maculopathy, or both; and lamellation of the GBM or abnormalities of type IV collagen immunostaining on kidney or skin biopsy.[50] The diagnosis of AS can be confirmed by genetic testing that demonstrates a pathogenic mutation(s) in COL4A3, COL4A4, or COL4A5. The results of genetic studies can improve the accuracy of genetic counseling and provide prognostic information. Genetic testing is at least 90% sensitive for XLAS.[51] All at-risk family members of a patient with a new diagnosis of XLAS, including females, should be screened for hematuria on at least two occasions and offered genetic testing to confirm their disease status.[50] Genetic counseling is recommended for the affected families.

Genetic confirmation in patients with TBMN is generally not necessary, unless the clinical course is atypical. Genetic testing for mutations in COL4A3 to COL4A5 should be considered in individuals with proteinuria or renal impairment or when AS cannot be excluded based on family history.

Table 45.1 Alport syndrome versus thin basement membrane nephropathy

| | XLAS | | ARAS | ADAS | TBMN |
|---|---|---|---|---|---|
| | Males | Females | | | |
| Gene | COL4A5 | | COL4A3 or COL4A4 | COL4A3 or COL4A4 | COL4A3 or COL4A4, other |
| Clinical findings | | | | | |
| Hematuria (%) | 100 | >90 | 100 | 100 | 100 |
| ESRD | 100% | ~30% by age 60 | 100% | ? | Rare |
| Sensorineural deafness | 80%–90% | 20% by age 60 | ? | ? | None |
| Ocular findings | ~40% | ~15% | ~40% | ? | None |
| Biopsy findings | | | | | |
| GBM width | Thick and thin* | Thick and thin* | Thick and thin* | Diffusely thin | |
| Lamellated GBM | Diffuse* | Focal† | Diffuse* | Diffuse* | Focal or absent |
| α5(IV) chains in GBM | Absent‡ | Mosaic‡ | Absent | Present | Present |
| α5(IV) chains in Bowman capsule and dTBM | Absent‡ | Mosaic‡ | Present | Present | Present |
| α5(IV) chains in skin BM | Absent§ | Mosaic§ | Present | Present | Present |

ADAS, autosomal dominant Alport syndrome; ARAS, autosomal recessive Alport syndrome; dTBM, distal tubular basement membranes; ESRD, end-stage renal disease; GBM, glomerular basement membrane; TBMN, thin basement membrane nephropathy; XLAS, X-linked Alport syndrome.

* In young children with AS, GBM width may initially be diffusely thinned with only rare or focal areas of lamellation, whereas older children and adults will demonstrate diffuse lamellation and thickening of the GBM.

† Females with XLAS often demonstrate thin or lamellated GBM interspersed with areas of normal-appearing GBM. They may, however, have GBM that appears identical to individuals with TBMN.

‡ Approximately 20% of males with XLAS, 30% to 40% of females with XLAS, and some patients with ARAS have normal type IV collagen immunostaining on renal biopsy. Normal renal immunostaining for type IV collagen cannot by itself exclude a diagnosis of AS.

§ Approximately 20% of males with XLAS and 30% to 40% of females with XLAS have normal α5(IV) expression in skin basement membranes.

## MONITORING AND TREATMENT

Individuals with AS should have formal ophthalmologic and hearing examinations performed at the time of diagnosis and at regular intervals thereafter to ensure early detection of extrarenal abnormalities. They should be monitored regularly for the presence of microalbuminuria, overt proteinuria, hypertension, and renal dysfunction. The goal of treatment in AS is to slow the progression of kidney disease and delay the need for renal replacement therapy. Treatment with an angiotensin-converting enzyme inhibitor (ACEI) is recommended for affected individuals with proteinuria, including heterozygous females (Table 45.2).[33,52] ACEI therapy should be considered for those with microalbuminuria and a family history of ESRD younger than 30 years of age or a severe COL4A5 mutation (deletion, splice site, or nonsense mutation).[33] Data are insufficient to recommend treatment for individuals with microscopic hematuria only. Retrospective data from a large European database suggests that treatment of AS with ACEIs is associated with a significant delay in the need for renal replacement therapy.[53] Early treatment with ACEIs also has been shown to improve lifespan in a mouse model of ARAS by more than 100%.[54] A prospective clinical trial of ACEIs in patients with AS is underway.[55]

### KEY POINT

Treatment of proteinuric AS patients with ACEIs may slow the progression of the disease and delay renal replacement therapy.

Individuals with TBMN should be monitored yearly for disease progression, including evaluation for proteinuria, hypertension, and renal impairment. The presence of proteinuria should prompt treatment with an ACEI, similar to treatment in patients with AS.[33,50]

## TRANSPLANTATION IN ALPORT SYNDROME

Patients with AS have graft survival rates as good as or better than those with other inherited renal diseases.[56] Females

Table 45.2 Recommendations for intervention based on urinary findings and anticipated disease course

| | Family history of early ESRD (<30 yr) or severe* COL4A5 mutation | | Family history of late ESRD (>30 years) or less severe† COL4A5 mutation | |
| | Males | Females | Males | Females |
| --- | --- | --- | --- | --- |
| Hematuria | Intervention before onset of microalbuminuria is not recommended at this time | No | No | No |
| Hematuria + microalbuminuria | Consider intervention | Consider intervention | No | No |
| Hematuria + proteinuria | Yes | Yes | Yes | Yes |

Source: Kashtan CE, Ding J, Gregory M, et al. Clinical practice recommendations for the treatment of Alport syndrome: a statement of the Alport Syndrome Research Collaborative. Pediatr Nephrol. 2013;28:5–11. Reprinted with permission
ESRD, end-stage renal disease.
* Deletion, nonsense, or splice site mutation.
† Missense mutation.

with heterozygous mutations in COL4A5 should be discouraged as living donors because of the risk for progressive kidney disease.[50,57] Of males with XLAS, 3% to 5% develop anti-GBM disease after transplantation secondary to the presence of antibodies predominantly against the α5(IV) NC1 domain.[58,59] Anti-GBM disease following transplantation is associated with rapid allograft loss and is likely to recur in subsequent grafts.[58]

## SUMMARY

Both AS and TBMN can manifest clinically with persistent microscopic hematuria and, in the case of AS, progress to proteinuria and ESRD. The past two decades have seen enormous developments in understanding the genetic defects that lead to AS and TBMN. Research efforts in the future will continue to focus on delaying or preventing ESRD in AS by two general approaches: (1) Correction of the underlying defect by gene or cell therapy and (2) interference with downstream events that promote cell injury and fibrosis. The demonstration that renal manifestations of AS can be ameliorated by nonspecific therapies such as angiotensin blockade is likely to stimulate investigation of novel antifibrotic agents in this disorder. Clinical evaluation of new therapies will require collaborative networks built on national registries and patient advocacy groups, combined with support from government, industry, and philanthropic sources.

## Clinical Vignette 45.1

An otherwise healthy girl presented with gross hematuria and dysuria at the age of 2 years. Urinalysis demonstrated 3+ blood, trace protein, and packed red blood cells on microscopic examination. Urine culture was negative. Blood pressure, physical examination, and renal ultrasound were all normal. Family history was negative for hematuria, chronic kidney disease, dialysis, kidney transplant, consanguinity, or deafness. She had normal values for blood urea nitrogen and creatinine (0.4 mg/dL), albumin, electrolytes, complete blood count, complement C3, complement C4, antistreptolysin O antibody titer, anti-DNAse B antibody titer, antinuclear antibody screen, and antineutrophil cytoplasmic antibody titer. Urine calcium-to-creatinine ratio also was normal (0.06 mg/mg). She continued to have intermittent grossly bloody urine with persistent microscopic hematuria over the next 3 months, and a kidney biopsy was performed. Light microscopy demonstrated three fetal-appearing glomeruli with otherwise normal-appearing tissue. EM demonstrated thin GBMs diffusely with no evidence for splitting, thickening, or basket weaving. No immune deposits were identified. Unfortunately, no tissue was available for immunofluorescence examination. Because of the inconclusive biopsy findings, genetic testing was sent to evaluate for mutations in COL4A3, COL4A4, and COL4A5. She was found to have a homozygous mutation in COL4A3 with transition C*T at nucleotide 4981 with an amino acid change of arginine to cysteine at codon 1661 in a conserved residue in the NC1 domain, confirming a diagnosis of autosomal recessive AS. Formal hearing and vision screening were normal. She was started on an ACEI after she developed mild proteinuria at the age of 5 years (ratio of urine protein to creatinine, 0.57 mg/mg).

## TEACHING POINTS

- This case highlights the importance of keeping AS in the differential diagnosis for girls who present with hematuria. Both X-linked and autosomal recessive AS were possible diagnoses in this case. Autosomal dominant AS is an unlikely cause of gross hematuria in a child.
- Confirmation of a genetic diagnosis allows for informed counseling of the family about the possibility of disease in other family members and in subsequent pregnancies.
- Another important highlight of this case is that children affected with autosomal recessive AS may not have a family history of hematuria or kidney disease that would be more typically seen in children with X-linked AS.

## REFERENCES

1. Alport AC. Hereditary familial congenital haemorrhagic nephritis. Br Med J. 1927;1:504–6.
2. Barker DF, Hostikka SL, Zhou J, et al. Identification of mutations in the COL4A5 collagen gene in Alport syndrome. Science. 1990;248:1224–7.
3. Mochizuki T, Lemmink HH, Mariyama M, et al. Identification of mutations in the alpha 3(IV) and alpha 4(IV) collagen genes in autosomal recessive Alport syndrome. Nat Genet. 1994;8:77–81.
4. Rogers PW, Kurtzman NA, Bunn SM, Jr., White MG. Familial benign essential hematuria. Arch Intern Med. 1973;131:257–62.
5. van Paassen P, van Breda Vriesman PJ, et al. Signs and symptoms of thin basement membrane nephropathy: A prospective regional study on primary glomerular disease—The Limburg Renal Registry. Kidney Int. 2004;66:909–13.
6. Lemmink HH, Nillesen WN, Mochizuki T, et al. Benign familial hematuria due to mutation of the type IV collagen alpha4 gene. J Clin Invest. 1996;98:1114–8.
7. Levy M, Feingold J. Estimating prevalence in single-gene kidney diseases progressing to renal failure. Kidney Int. 2000;58:925–43.
8. Haas M. Thin glomerular basement membrane nephropathy: Incidence in 3471 consecutive renal biopsies examined by electron microscopy. Arch Pathol Lab Med. 2006;130:699–706.
9. Trachtman H, Weiss RA, Bennett B, Greifer I. Isolated hematuria in children: Indications for a renal biopsy. Kidney Int. 1984;25:94–9.
10. Schroder CH, Bontemps CM, Assmann KJ, et al. Renal biopsy and family studies in 65 children with isolated hematuria. Acta Paediatr Scand. 1990;79:630–6.
11. Piqueras AI, White RH, Raafat F, Moghal N, Milford DV. Renal biopsy diagnosis in children presenting with haematuria. Pediatr Nephrol. 1998;12:386–91.
12. U.S. Renal Data System. USRDS 2013 Annual Data Report: Atlas of Chronic Kidney Disease and End-Stage Renal Disease in the United States. Bethesda, MD: USRDS; 2013.
13. Abrahamson DR. Origin of the glomerular basement membrane visualized after in vivo labeling of laminin in newborn rat kidneys. J Cell Biol. 1985;100:1988–2000.
14. Abrahamson DR, Hudson BG, Stroganova L, et al. Cellular origins of type IV collagen networks in developing glomeruli. J Am Soc Nephrol. 2009;20:1471–9.
15. Miner JH. The glomerular basement membrane. Exp Cell Res. 2012;318:973–8.
16. Poschl E, Pollner R, Kuhn K. The genes for the alpha 1(IV) and alpha 2(IV) chains of human basement membrane collagen type IV are arranged head-to-head and separated by a bidirectional promoter of unique structure. EMBO J. 1988;7:2687–95.
17. Segal Y, Zhuang L, Rondeau E, et al. Regulation of the paired type IV collagen genes COL4A5 and COL4A6: Role of the proximal promoter region. J Biol Chem. 2001;276:11791–7.
18. Khoshnoodi J, Cartailler JP, Alvares K, et al. Molecular recognition in the assembly of collagens: Terminal noncollagenous domains are key recognition modules in the formation of triple helical protomers. J Biol Chem. 2006;281:38117–21.
19. Hudson BG. The molecular basis of Goodpasture and Alport syndromes: Beacons for the discovery of the collagen IV family. J Am Soc Nephrol. 2004;15:2514–27.
20. Kalluri R, Gattone VH, 2nd, Hudson BG. Identification and localization of type IV collagen chains in the inner ear cochlea. Connect Tissue Res. 1998;37:143–50.
21. Hudson BG, Reeders ST, Tryggvason K. Type IV collagen: Structure, gene organization, and role in human diseases: Molecular basis of Goodpasture and Alport syndromes and diffuse leiomyomatosis. J Biol Chem. 1993;268:26033–6.
22. Miner JH, Sanes JR. Collagen IV alpha 3, alpha 4, and alpha 5 chains in rodent basal laminae: Sequence, distribution, association with laminins, and developmental switches. J Cell Biol. 1994;127:879–91.

23. Gunwar S, Ballester F, Noelken ME, et al. Glomerular basement membrane: Identification of a novel disulfide-cross-linked network of alpha3, alpha4, and alpha5 chains of type IV collagen and its implications for the pathogenesis of Alport syndrome. J Biol Chem. 1998;273:8767–75.

24. Zeisberg M, Khurana M, Rao VH, et al. Stage-specific action of matrix metalloproteinases influences progressive hereditary kidney disease. PLoS Med. 2006;3:e100.

25. Pescucci C, Mari F, Longo I, et al. Autosomal-dominant Alport syndrome: Natural history of a disease due to COL4A3 or COL4A4 gene. Kidney Int. 2004;65:1598–603.

26. Fallerini C, Dosa L, Tita R, et al. Unbiased next generation sequencing analysis confirms the existence of autosomal dominant Alport syndrome in a relevant fraction of cases. Clin Genet. 2014;86:252–7.

27. Crockett DK, Pont-Kingdon G, Gedge F, et al. The Alport syndrome COL4A5 variant database. Hum Mutat. 2010;31:e1652–7.

28. Rana K, Wang YY, Buzza M, et al. The genetics of thin basement membrane nephropathy. Semin Nephrol. 2005;25:163–70.

29. Jefferson JA, Lemmink HH, Hughes AE, et al. Autosomal dominant Alport syndrome linked to the type IV collage alpha 3 and alpha 4 genes (COL4A3 and COL4A4). Nephrol Dial Transplant. 1997;12:1595–9.

30. Rana K, Wang YY, Powell H, et al. Persistent familial hematuria in children and the locus for thin basement membrane nephropathy. Pediatr Nephrol. 2005;20:1729–37.

31. Jais JP, Knebelmann B, Giatras I, et al. X-linked Alport syndrome: Natural history in 195 families and genotype-phenotype correlations in males. J Am Soc Nephrol. 2000;11:649–57.

32. Jais JP, Knebelmann B, Giatras I, et al. X-linked Alport syndrome: Natural history and genotype-phenotype correlations in girls and women belonging to 195 families: A European Community Alport Syndrome Concerted Action study. J Am Soc Nephrol. 2003;14:2603–10.

33. Kashtan CE, Ding J, Gregory M, et al. Clinical practice recommendations for the treatment of Alport syndrome: A statement of the Alport Syndrome Research Collaborative. Pediatr Nephrol. 2013;28:5–11.

34. Rheault MN, Kren SM, Hartich LA, et al. X-inactivation modifies disease severity in female carriers of murine X-linked Alport syndrome. Nephrol Dial Transplant. 2010;25:764–9.

35. Zehnder AF, Adams JC, Santi PA, et al. Distribution of type IV collagen in the cochlea in Alport syndrome. Arch Otolaryngol Head Neck Surg. 2005;131:1007–13.

36. Harvey SJ, Mount R, Sado Y, et al. The inner ear of dogs with X-linked nephritis provides clues to the pathogenesis of hearing loss in X-linked Alport syndrome. Am J Pathol 2001;159:1097–104.

37. Storey H, Savige J, Sivakumar V, et al. COL4A3/COL4A4 mutations and features in individuals with autosomal recessive Alport syndrome. J Am Soc Nephrol. 2013;24:1945–54.

38. Colville DJ, Savige J. Alport syndrome: A review of the ocular manifestations. Ophthalmic Genet. 1997;18:161–73.

39. Nielsen CE. Lenticonus anterior and Alport's syndrome. Acta Ophthalmol (Copenh). 1978;56:518–30.

40. Perrin D, Jungers P, Grunfeld JP, et al. Perimacular changes in Alport's syndrome. Clin Nephrol. 1980;13:163–7.

41. Teekhasaenee C, Nimmanit S, Wutthiphan S, et al. Posterior polymorphous dystrophy and Alport syndrome. Ophthalmology. 1991;98:1207–15.

42. Burke JP, Clearkin LG, Talbot JF. Recurrent corneal epithelial erosions in Alport's syndrome. Acta Ophthalmol (Copenh). 1991;69:555–7.

43. Kashtan CE, Kleppel MM, Gubler MC. Immunohistologic findings in Alport syndrome. Contrib Nephrol. 1996;117:142–53.

44. Gubler MC, Knebelmann B, Beziau A, et al. Autosomal recessive Alport syndrome: Immunohistochemical study of type IV collagen chain distribution. Kidney Int. 1995;47:1142–7.

45. Tryggvason K, Patrakka J. Thin basement membrane nephropathy. J Am Soc Nephrol. 2006;17:813–22.

46. Savige J, Rana K, Tonna S, et al. Thin basement membrane nephropathy. Kidney Int. 2003;64:1169–78.

47. Gregory MC. The clinical features of thin basement membrane nephropathy. Semin Nephrol. 2005;25:140–5.

48. Vogler C, McAdams AJ, Homan SM. Glomerular basement membrane and lamina densa in infants and children: An ultrastructural evaluation. Pediatr Pathol. 1987;7:527–34.

49. Cosio FG, Falkenhain ME, Sedmak DD. Association of thin glomerular basement membrane with other glomerulopathies. Kidney Int. 1994;46:471–4.

50. Savige J, Gregory M, Gross O, et al. Expert guidelines for the management of Alport syndrome and thin basement membrane nephropathy. J Am Soc Nephrol. 2013;24:364–75.

51. Hertz JM, Thomassen M, Storey H, Flinter F. Clinical utility gene card for: Alport syndrome. Eur J Hum Genet. 2012;20.

52. Webb NJ, Shahinfar S, Wells TG, et al. Losartan and enalapril are comparable in reducing proteinuria in children with Alport syndrome. Pediatr Nephrol. 2013;28:737–43.

53. Gross O, Licht C, Anders HJ, et al. Early angiotensin-converting enzyme inhibition in Alport syndrome delays renal failure and improves life expectancy. Kidney Int. 2012;81:494–501.

54. Gross O, Beirowski B, Koepke ML, et al. Preemptive ramipril therapy delays renal failure and reduces renal fibrosis in *COL4A3*-knockout mice with Alport syndrome. Kidney Int. 2003;63:438–46.

55. Gross O, Friede T, Hilgers R, et al. Safety and efficacy of the ACE-inhibitor ramipril in Alport syndrome: The double-blind, randomized, placebo-controlled, multicenter phase III EARLY PRO-TECT Alport Trial in Pediatric Patients. ISRN Pediatr 2012;436046.

56. Temme J, Kramer A, Jager KJ, et al. Outcomes of male patients with Alport syndrome undergoing renal replacement therapy. Clin J Am Soc Nephrol. 2012;7:1969–76.

57. Gross O, Weber M, Fries JW, Muller GA. Living donor kidney transplantation from relatives with mild urinary abnormalities in Alport syndrome: Long-term risk, benefit and outcome. Nephrol Dial Transplant. 2009;24:1626–30.

58. Browne G, Brown PA, Tomson CR, et al. Retransplantation in Alport post-transplant anti-GBM disease. Kidney Int. 2004;65:675–81.

59. Kashtan CE. Renal transplantation in patients with Alport syndrome. Pediatr Transplant. 2006;10:651–7.

## REVIEW QUESTIONS

1. In a patient with persistent microscopic hematuria, which of the following findings is suggestive of a diagnosis of Alport syndrome rather than thin basement membrane nephropathy?
   a. Male gender
   b. Family history of hematuria
   c. Failed newborn hearing screen
   d. Anterior lenticonus
   e. Elevated cholesterol

2. X-linked Alport syndrome is caused by mutations in which gene?
   a. COL4A3
   b. COL4A4
   c. COL4A5
   d. MYH9
   e. PAX2

3. Heterozygous females with *COL4A5* mutations are at risk for:
   a. Microscopic hematuria
   b. Proteinuria
   c. End-stage renal disease
   d. Deafness
   e. All of the above

4. ACEIs are NOT indicated for treatment of which patient?
   a. Male with XLAS and proteinuria
   b. Male with XLAS and microalbuminuria with family history of ESRD at age 20
   c. Male with XLAS and microalbuminuria with family history of ESRD at age 50
   d. Female with XLAS and proteinuria
   e. Female with ARAS and proteinuria

5. This type of mutation in *COL4A5* is associated with a milder Alport phenotype:
   a. Missense mutation
   b. Large deletion
   c. Splice site mutation
   d. Nonsense mutation
   e. Large rearrangement

6. The following ophthalmologic findings are frequently observed in patients with Alport syndrome, *except*:
   a. Anterior lenticonus
   b. Myopia
   c. Corneal erosion
   d. Maculopathy
   e. Posterior polymorphous dystrophy

7. α5(IV) may be absent from the GBM and present in the Bowman capsule in which disorder?
   a. Males with XLAS
   b. Females with XLAS
   c. TBMN
   d. ARAS
   e. ARAS and ADAS

8. TBMN can be caused by mutations in:
   a. COL4A3
   b. COL4A4
   c. COL4A5
   d. Both a and b
   e. Both a and c

## ANSWERS

1. d
2. c
3. e
4. c
5. a
6. b
7. e
8. d

# 46

# Renal disease in syndromic disorders

PATRICK NIAUDET

Renal disease occurs in a very large number of syndromic disorders in which anomalies involving other organs are also present. More than 500 such syndromes have been described. Congenital renal anomalies, such as renal hypoplasia, renal dysplasia, renal cysts, or congenital abnormalities of the urinary tract, accompany many syndromic disorders. Other kidney-related symptoms, such as nephrotic syndrome or hematuria, may also be observed in the syndromic disorders.

Syndromic disorders with renal disease may have a genetic basis. Mutated genes expressed in different organs and tissues, correspondingly, give rise to diverse clinical manifestations in these organs. The proteins encoded by these genes have many functions, including structural, signaling, and regulation. As an example, mutations of some type-IV collagen genes that are involved in the structure of basement membranes in the kidney and cochlea lead to the Alport syndrome, a progressive hematuric nephropathy associated with sensorineural hearing loss. Another example concerns the ciliopathies, wherein the genes coding for proteins expressed in the primary cilia may lead to different clinical entities such as Jeune, Joubert, Bardet-Biedl, or Meckel-Gruber syndromes, as well as nephronophthisis and polycystic kidney diseases.

Some of the selected syndromes that are observed more frequently by pediatric nephrologists are discussed in this chapter (Tables 46.1 and 46.2). For more details on the subject, the reader may refer to other references.[1-3]

## ALAGILLE SYNDROME

Alagille syndrome (Online Mendelian Inheritance in Man [OMIM] 118450, 610205), also called arteriohepatic dysplasia, is characterized by a paucity of interlobular bile ducts with chronic cholestasis present in the neonatal period or during the first months of life and various other congenital malformations.[4] The prevalence is approximately 1 in 70,000. Alagille syndrome is an autosomal dominant disorder with incomplete penetrance and variable expressivity. Liver disease is present in 95% of cases of Alagille syndrome. Other manifestations include the following: heart anomalies, most commonly pulmonary artery stenosis and tetralogy of Fallot; skeletal anomalies such as butterfly vertebrae; eye anomalies, including posterior embryotoxon (prominent Schwalbe line) and dysmorphic facies, consisting of prominent forehead, broad nasal bridge, straight nose, triangular facies, and

Table 46.1 Syndromes associated with renal disease

| Syndrome | Mutated gene | Renal and urologic anomalies | Extrarenal anomalies |
|---|---|---|---|
| Alagille syndrome | JAG1 | Renal dysplasia, mesangiolipidosis | Paucity of intrahepatic bile duct, cardiac defect, vertebral anomalies |
| Bardet-Biedl syndrome | BBS1 to BBS14 | Renal dysplasia, calyceal malformations | Retinopathy, polydactyly, obesity, diabetes, male hypogonadism |
| Beckwith-Wiedemann syndrome | p57KIP2 | Large kidneys, cysts, dysplasia | Somatic overgrowth, embryonal tumors |
| Branchio-oto-renal syndrome | EYA1 | Renal agenesis, dysplasia | Deafness, branchial arch defects |
| CHARGE syndrome | CHD7 and SEMA3E | Solitary kidney, duplex kidneys, renal hypoplasia, nephrolithiasis, ureteropelvic junction obstruction, vesicoureteral reflux | Coloboma, heart malformation, choanal atresia, mental retardation, genital anomalies |
| Di George syndrome | Microdeletion at 22q11 | Renal agenesis, dysplasia, and vesicoureteric reflux | Heart anomalies, branchial arch defects |
| Fraser syndrome | FRASI | Renal agenesis, dysplasia | Digital and ocular malformations |
| Kallmann syndrome | KAL1 | Renal agenesis, dysplasia | Hypogonadotropic hypogonadism, anosmia |
| Meckel syndrome | MKSI-6 | Cystic renal dysplasia | Central nervous system malformations, polydactyly |
| Oral-facial-digital syndrome | OFD1 | Glomerular cysts | Facial and digital anomalies |
| Renal-coloboma syndrome | PAX2 | Renal hypoplasia, vesicoureteral reflux | Coloboma of the optic nerve |
| Renal cyst and diabetes | TCF2 | Renal cysts, dysplasia, hypoplasia | Diabetes, genital anomalies |
| Simpson-Golabi-Behmel syndrome | GPC3 | Renal cysts, dysplasia | Somatic overgrowth, craniofacial and vertebral anomalies, cardiac defect, cryptorchidism |
| Smith-Lemli-Opitz syndrome | DHCR7 | Renal cysts, dysplasia, urinary tract obstruction, vesicoureteral reflux | Failure to thrive, craniofacial malformations |
| Townes-Brocks syndrome | SALL1 | Renal hypoplasia, dysplasia, agenesis, vesicoureteric reflux, posterior urethral valve | Limb malformation, hearing loss, imperforate anus |
| VACTERL association | ? | Renal dysplasia | Vertebral defects, anal atresia, tracheoesophageal fistula, esophageal atresia, limb anomalies |

deep-set eyes (Figure 46.1). Systemic vascular abnormalities have been reported, including carotid and cerebral arteries and moyamoya syndrome predisposing to stroke. The mid-aortic syndrome and renal artery stenosis may be responsible for severe hypertension and renal failure.[5,6] Renal and urologic anomalies, such as cysts and ureteropelvic obstruction, have been reported. Mesangiolipidosis, with accumulation of lipid vacuoles in the mesangial matrix, in mesangial cells and in the glomerular basement membranes have been reported (Figure 46.2).[7]

Alagille syndrome results from defects in the Notch signaling pathway, which is important in angiogenesis. Mutations in the JAG1 gene are responsible for the disease in more than 90% of patients. JAG1 encodes the JAGGED1 cell surface protein, a ligand for the Notch receptors. Knockout mice for JAG1 die early from vascular defects. More than 400 mutations have been reported in the JAG1 gene, which consists of 26 exons on chromosome 20p12. Approximately 60% are de novo mutations, and germline mosaicism has been observed in 8% of cases. Mutations in the NOTCH2

Table 46.2 Syndromic disorders associated with nephrotic syndrome

| Syndrome | Mutated gene | Renal anomalies | Extrarenal anomalies |
| --- | --- | --- | --- |
| Pierson syndrome | LAMB2 | Renal failure, diffuse mesangial sclerosis | Microcoria, neurologic anomalies |
| Denys–Drash syndrome | WT1 | Renal failure, diffuse mesangial sclerosis | Wilms tumor, pseudohermaphroditism |
| Frasier syndrome | WT1 | Renal failure in adult life, focal segmental glomerulosclerosis | Male pseudohermaphroditism with normal female external genitalia |
| Nail-patella syndrome | LMX1B | Progression to renal failure in 30% of cases with nephropathy | Nail dysplasia, hypoplastic or absent patellas |
| Schimke immuno-ossous dysplasia | SMARCAL1 | Progression to renal failure, focal segmental glomerulosclerosis | Spondyloepiphyseal dysplasia, T-cell deficiency, cerebral ischemic lesions |
| Mitochondrial cytopathies | Mitochondrial DNA or nuclear DNA | Proximal tubulopathy, nephrotic syndrome | Myopathy, hearing loss, neurologic deterioration, diabetes mellitus |
| Galloway syndrome | WDR73 | Renal failure, focal and segmental glomerulosclerosis or diffuse mesangial sclerosis | Microcephaly with psychomotor retardation, ocular abnormalities, hiatal hernia |

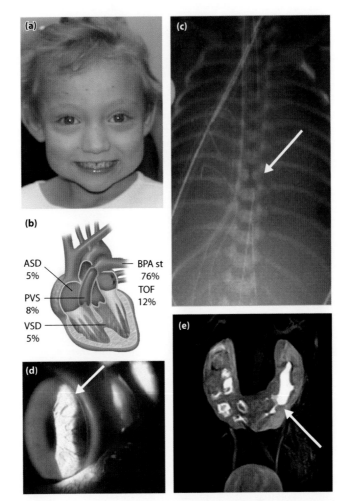

Figure 46.1 Alagille syndrome. (a) Characteristic facies in a patient with Alagille syndrome: broad forehead, pointed chin, and deep-set eyes. Note also the scleral icterus and excoriations on the forehead. Written consent for publication of this image was obtained from the patient's responsible relative by the original authors. (b) Diagram of classic cardiac abnormalities and their frequency in Alagille syndrome. ASD, atrial septal defect; BPA st, branch pulmonary artery stenosis; PVS, pulmonary valve stenosis; TOF, tetralogy of Fallot; VSD, ventricular septal defect. (c) Radiograph showing butterfly vertebra (arrow). (d) Slit-lamp examination of the eye revealing posterior embryotoxon (arrow). (e) Magnetic resonance imaging scan showing the fused poles of a horseshoe kidney (arrow) in a patient with Alagille syndrome. (From Kamath BM, Spinner NB, Rosenblum ND. Renal involvement and the role of Notch signaling in Alagille syndrome. Nat Rev Nephrol. 2013;9:409–18.)

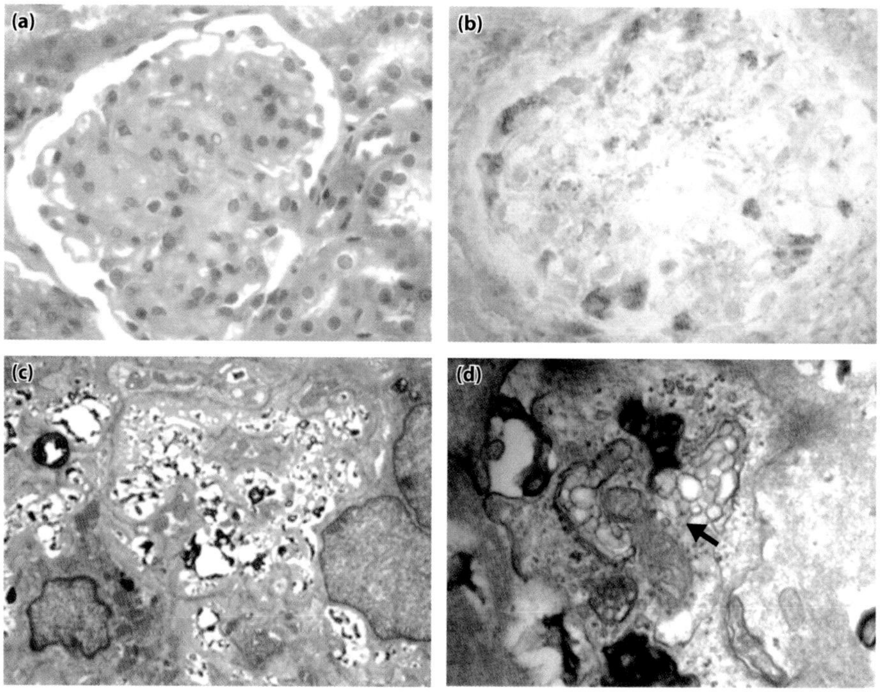

Figure 46.2 Renal pathology in Alagille syndrome. **(a)** Mesangiolipidosis, characterized by an increase in the mesangial matrix and the presence of mesangial foam cells (hematoxylin-eosin-safran stain, 400×). **(b)** Lipid deposits were confirmed by Sudan black stain (400×). **(c)** Electronic microscopy showed numerous clear vacuoles containing osmiophilic lamellated inclusions in the mesangial cells and matrix (5000×). **(d)** Higher magnification electron microscopy image of mesangial cell cytoplasm showed lipid vacuoles (arrow) with a mean diameter of 46 nm (44,000×). (From Benoit G, Sartelet H, Levy E, et al. Mesangiolipidosis in Alagille syndrome: relationship with apolipoprotein A-I. Nephrol. Dial Transplant. 2007;22:2072–5.)

gene that encodes the NOTCH2 transmembrane protein have been reported in two families.

## BARDET-BIEDL SYNDROME

The Bardet-Biedl syndrome (OMIM 209900) is an autosomal recessive disorder characterized by retinal dystrophy, truncal obesity, hypogenitalism in men or genital abnormalities in women, learning disabilities, postaxial polydactyly, and renal anomalies (Figure 46.3).[8] Retinal dystrophy leads to a progressive decline of visual acuity and blindness at a mean age of 15 years.[9] Learning disabilities may be in part explained by visual impairment, and less than half of the patients are mentally retarded. Some patients show speech disorders or behavior problems. Other signs and symptoms may be present such as anosmia, dental anomalies, congenital heart defects, and diabetes mellitus.

Renal symptoms are nonspecific.[10] Polyuria and polydipsia, related to a concentrating defect, are present in one-third of cases. Urinary tract infections are frequent. Tubular defects may be observed, such as tubular acidosis, glucosuria, or hyperaminoaciduria. Chronic renal failure is a major complication, and 10% of patients progress to end-stage renal disease (ESRD) during childhood. Blood hypertension is frequently observed, sometimes early in life.

Ultrasonography shows enlarged hyperechogenic kidneys after birth.[11,12] Cysts may be present. Later in life, an inversion of corticomedullary differentiation may be observed. These anomalies tend to disppear after age 2 years. Renal histologic examination shows nonspecific tubulointerstitial changes, cysts, and dysplasia. Glomerular lesions may appear later as a consequence of nephron reduction.

Mutations in at least 14 genes have been described in patients with this syndrome.[13] The genes most frequently involved are *BBS1* on chromosome 11q13, *BBS10* on chromosome 12q, *BBS2* on chromosome 16q21, and *BBS9* on chromosome 7p14.[14] Disordered function of the cilia is a fundamental defect in this syndrome. Indeed, BBS genes code for proteins of the primary cilia, basal body, or centrosome. The age of first symptoms and the severity of symptoms are not related to the genotype. Furtheremore, there is a high variability of symptoms within and among affected families.[15]

## BECKWITH-WIEDEMANN SYNDROME

The Beckwith-Wiedemann syndrome (BWS) (OMIM 130650) is a congenital overgrowth syndrome with a predisposition to tumor development. The estimated prevalence is 1 in 13,700, and it affects female and male patients equally.[16]

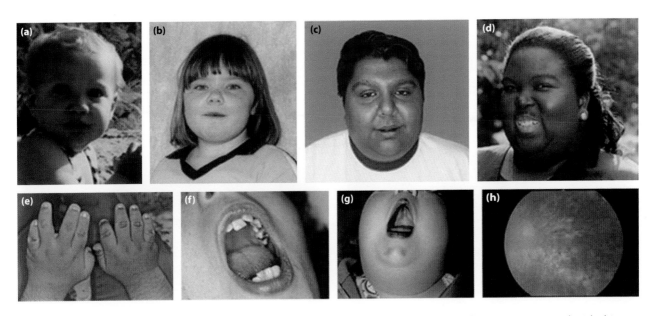

Figure 46.3 Bardet-Biedl syndrome. Images of patients demonstrating the dysmorphic features associated with this syndrome. (a) to (d) Typical facial features. These are often subtle and are not always present. Features include deep-set eyes, hypertelorism, downward-slanting palpebral fissures, a flat nasal bridge, small mouth, malar hypoplasia, and retrognathia. (e) Brachydactyly and scars from excision of accessory digits. (f) Dental crowding. (g) High-arched palate. (h) Funduscopy demonstrating rod-cone dystrophy. (From Forsythe E, Beales PL. Bardet-Biedl syndrome. Eur J Hum Genet. 2013;21:8–13.)

Most cases are sporadic, but autosomal dominant transmission with variable expressivity and incomplete penetrance is observed in 15% of cases. Clinical features include omphalocele, macroglossia, and macrosomia, with height and weight greater than the 97th percentile, asymmetric overgrowth of certain regions of the body, visceromegaly, and tumors (Figure 46.4).[17] Neonatal hypoglycemia may be observed. Patients develop embryonic tumors such as Wilms tumor, hepatoblastoma, neuroblastoma, or rhabdomyosarcoma. Renal symptoms consist of nephromegaly, duplicated collecting system, nephrocalcinosis, renal cysts, and medullary sponge kidney.

### KEY POINTS

- Patients with BWS present with omphalocele, macroglossia, macrosomia, and visceromegaly.
- They are at high risk of embryonic tumors.

Dysregulation of the expression of multiple imprinted growth regulatory genes in the chromosome 11p15.5 region has been reported.[18] Epigenomic or genomic alterations in this 11p15.5 region are detected in most patients. The distal domain I contains the imprinted genes *IGF2* (paternal monoallelic expression) and *H19* (maternal monoallelic expression), which play important roles in growth and development. The proximal domain 2 contains two genes, *KCNQ1OT1* and *CDKN1C* that are both implicated in the BWS.

## BRANCHIO-OTO-RENAL SYNDROME

Branchio-oto-renal (BOR) syndrome (OMIM 113650, 610896) is an autosomal dominant disorder that combines branchial defects with lateral cervical fistulas or cysts, ear pits, hearing loss, and renal anomalies (Figure 46.5).[19] The incidence of BOR syndrome is 1 in 40,000 infants. In this syndrome, penetrance is incomplete, and patients may have only one or two features of the syndrome.[20] Renal anomalies are not observed in all patients and may differ among members of the same family. Renal findings include renal agenesis or hypoplasia (which may be unilateral or bilateral), vesicoureteral reflux, ureteropelvic junction obstruction, or ureteral duplication.[21,22] If renal hypoplasia is present, it may vary in severity and may progress to end-stage renal failure. Ear abnormalities include periauricular pits, anomalies of the middle and external ear, and hypoplasia of the cochlea, resulting in hearing loss.

More than 80 mutations in the *EYA1* gene on chromosome 8q13.3 have been identified in patients with BOR syndrome.[22–24] The *EYA1* gene encodes for a transcription cofactor that is expressed in the metanephric mesenchyme during kidney development.[25] The *EYA1* gene interacts with members of the SIX family, which encodes transcription factors that control expression of *PAX2* and *GDNF* in the metanephric mesenchyme. *Eya1*[+/-] mice may show renal hypoplasia or unilateral renal agenesis, whereas *Eya1*[-/-] mice lack both ureters and kidneys.[25] Mutations in *SIX1* (chromosome 14q23.1) and *SIX5* genes have also been reported in families with the BOR syndrome.[26–28]

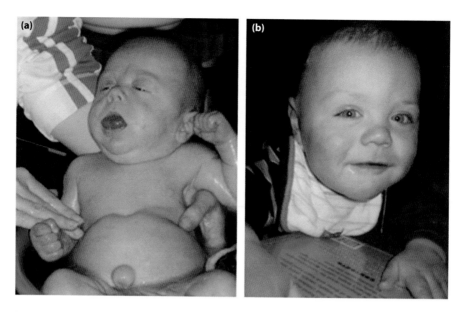

Figure 46.4 Beckwith-Wiedemann syndrome. **(a)** A 1-month-old boy showing macroglossia and umbilical hernia. **(b)** Photograph taken 1 year after a tongue reduction surgical procedure. (From Weksberg R, Shuman C, Beckwith JB. Beckwith-Wiedemann syndrome. Eur J Hum Genet. 2010;18:8–14.)

## CHARGE SYNDROME

Infants with the CHARGE (coloboma of the retina or the iris, heart anomalies, choanal atresia, mental retardation, and genital and ear anomalies) syndrome[29] (OMIM 214800) often have renal or urologic anomalies, such as unilateral renal agenesis, renal hypoplasia, duplex kidneys, ureteropelvic junction obstruction, or vesicoureteral reflux.[30]

Most cases of CHARGE syndrome are related to mutations of the gene coding for the chromodomain helicase DNA-binding protein-7 (CHD7).[31,32] These are heterozygous mutations, suggesting that haploinsufficiency of the gene is responsible for CHARGE syndrome. Most cases are caused

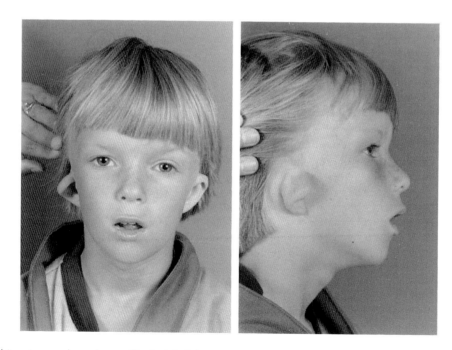

Figure 46.5 Branchio-oto-renal syndrome. Typical facial appearance. Note the cup-shaped ear deformity. Bilaterally symmetric ear deformities also can be seen. (From Smith RJ, Schwartz C. Branchio-oto-renal syndrome. J Commun Disord. 1998;31:411–21.)

by de novo mutations, although rare familial cases have been reported.[33]

## COCKAYNE SYNDROME

Cockayne syndrome (OMIM 216400, 133540, 216411) is an autosomal recessive disorder characterized by neurologic anomalies with progressive dementia, microcephaly, growth retardation, premature aging, sensorineural deafness, retinopathy, cataract, and sun sensitivity.[34] There is wide variability in the severity of clinical manifestations. Renal manifestations consist of hypertension, proteinuria, and renal failure, which occurs in 10% of patients. Ultrastructural lesions include thickened glomerular basement membranes.[35]

Cockayne syndrome results from a defect in the ability to perform transcription-coupled repair of active genes after ultraviolet irradiation. Two complementation groups (CS-A and CS-B) have been identified, and 80% of patients belong to the second group.[36] The *CSA* gene encodes a WD repeat protein that interacts with the *CSB* protein and RNA polymerase II transcription factor IIH.[37] The *CSB* protein is a helicase involved in the repair of active genes.[38]

## DI GEORGE SYNDROME

Di George syndrome (OMIM 188400) is characterized by conotruncal cardiac anomalies, a hypoplastic thymus, hypocalcemia secondary to parathyroid hypoplasia, and developmental disabilities, learning disabilities, or both.[39,40] The most frequent cardiac anomalies include interrupted aortic arch, truncus arteriosus, tetralogy of Fallot, atrial or ventricular septal defects, and vascular rings. The first three of them are responsible for cyanotic heart disease. The thymus may be absent or hypoplastic. The severity of the immunodeficiency is related to the size of the thymus and varies between severe combined immunodeficiency and mild recurrent infections. Hypocalcemia may be life-threatening in the newborn, who can present with tetany, seizures, and laryngospasm. This condition is accompanied by hyperphosphatemia and a low parathyroid hormone (PTH) level.

Renal and urologic anomalies are observed in 36% of patients and consist of unilateral renal agenesis, multicystic kidney, megaureter, vesicoureteric reflux, and renal ectopy.[39,41] Systematic renal ultrasound is recommended in these patients to detect such anomalies which can be asymptomatic. In the majority of cases, Di George syndrome is caused by hemizygous 22q11.2 deletion at chromosome 22q11.2 which can be detected by fluorescence in situ hybridization. The inheritance is autosomal dominant, but most cases are caused by de novo mutations.[42]

## FRASER SYNDROME

Fraser syndrome (OMIMI 219000) is an autosomal recessive disease characterized by cryptophthalmos, cutaneous syndactyly, genital malformations with ambiguous genitalia, craniofacial anomalies, and malformations of the larynx (stenosis or atresia) and the kidneys. Cryptophthalmos is bilateral or less frequently unilateral. Other ocular malformations include coloboma, microphthalmia, or anophthalmia. Bilateral renal agenesis was reported in 23% of 117 cases.[43] Patients who survive may have unilateral renal agenesis or renal cystic dysplasia.

Fraser syndrome occurs in 1 in 10,000 live births. Mutations in the *FRAS1* and *FREM2* genes have been described in patients with this syndrome.[44,45] Both genes are involved in kidney development in the embryo.

## GOLDENHAR SYNDROME (OCULO-AURICULO-VERTEBRAL SYNDROME)

Goldenhar syndrome (OMIM 164210), also referred to as first and second branchial arch syndrome, is characterized by unilateral craniofacial and vertebral malformations. They consist of preauricular skin tags, dermal epitubular tumors, cleft palate, mandibular hypoplasia, ear microtia, and facial asymmetry.[46] Vertebral anomalies consist of hemivertebrae or absence of vertebrae and scoliosis. The incidence of this syndrome is 1 in 5,000 to 1 in 25,000 live births. Most cases are sporadic, but an autosomal dominant mode of inheritance is possible with variable penetrance.

In addition to cardiac and pulmonary malformations, renal and urologic anomalies are observed in up to 50% of the patients: renal ectopy, unilateral renal agenesis, vesicoureteric reflux, ureteropelvic junction obstruction, and multicystic dysplasic kidney.[47]

## HEPATIC NUCLEAR FACTOR-1β-- RELATED DISEASE (RENAL CYSTS AND DIABETES SYNDROME)

Heterozygous mutations of the TCF2 gene encoding the hepatic nuclear factor-1β are responsible for an autosomal dominant disease named renal cysts and diabetes (RCAD) syndrome (OMIM 137920).

The renal disease may be discovered on antenatal ultrasound examination with enlarged hyperechogenic kidneys, renal cysts, unilateral or bilateral multicystic kidney disease, or unilateral renal agenesis.[48] During childhood, kidney size decreases while renal cysts increase in size. Progression to renal failure is observed during childhood in one-half of the patients.[49] Renal histologic examination shows glomerular cysts or cysts in any part of the nephron and often renal dysplasia. Renal cell carcinoma may develop later in life.[50]

Several extrarenal manifestations may be present. Maturity-onset diabetes of the young type 5, with slow aggravation of insulin production, no autoantibodies, and persistent C-peptide, may be the first sign before the renal disease is recognized.[51] The diabetes usually begins in adolescence but may have a neonatal onset.[52] Exocrine pancreas deficiency may also develop in adult patients. Asymptomatic cholestasis with increased gamma-glutamyl transferase but without liver histologic anomalies is observed in 40% to 80% of adult cases. Other anomalies include hypomagnesemia, hyperuricemia, and genital tract anomalies. An increased incidence of autism and schizophrenia has been reported in these patients.[53,54]

> ## KEY POINT
>
> Mutations of *TCF2* gene are responsible for a renal cystic disease which progresses to ESRD in 50% of cases.

*TCF2* gene is located on chromosome 17q12 and codes for a transcription factor, HNF1β, that controls the expression of several genes involved in development in the liver, kidney, intestine, and pancreas. Deletion of the whole gene is observed in 50% to 60% of patients, whereas other patients show small mutations. De novo mutations occur in more than 50% of cases. The severity of the renal disease associated with *TCF2* mutations is extremely variable and is not correlated with the genotype.[55]

## KALLMANN–DE MORSIER SYNDROME

Kallmann syndrome (OMIM 308700) is defined by the association of hypogonadotropic hypogonadism and anosmia or hyposmia. Some patients also present with cleft lip, heart defects, obesity, and mental retardation.[56] Renal malformations include unilateral renal agenesis and, less frequently, hydronephrosis or vesicoureteric reflux.

The association of hypogonadotropic hypogonadism and anosmia is explained by the embryologic origin of olfactory sensory neurons and gonadotropin-releasing hormone (GnRH)–producing neurons whose precursors migrate together during development from the nasal placode to the telencephalon. This migration is regulated by neurotransmitters, extracellular matrix proteins, and growth factors. Kallmann syndrome is genetically heterogeneous. Anomalies have been found in six different genes (*KAL1, FGFR1, FGF8, CHD7, PROK2, PROKR2*), explaining one-third of cases.[57,58] The *KAL1* gene is located on the X chromosome and encodes anosmin-1, an extracellular matrix protein that is involved in neuronal development, migration,

and organogenesis. Anosmin-1 was detected in the basement membranes of mesonephric tubules and duct, as well as in branches of the ureteric bud.[59] Of patients with *KAL1* gene mutations, 40% show renal anomalies, most often unilateral renal agenesis.[60]

## MAYER-ROKITANSKY-KUSTER-HAUSER SYNDROME

Mayer-Rokitansky-Kuster-Hauser (MRKH) syndrome (OMIM 277000) is characterized by müllerian duct aplasia in XX individuals with female phenotype. Patients have uterovaginal atresia or hypoplasia and present with primary amenorrhea at adolescence while they have normal breast development and pubarche.[61] Some patients have renal, skeletal, and cardiac malformations, also described as MURCS association (aplasia or hypoplasia of müllerian ducts [MU], congenital renal dysplasia [R], and cervicothoracic dysplasia [CS]).

Renal malformations include unilateral renal agenesis, renal ectopy, renal hypoplasia, horseshoe kidney, and hydronephrosis. Bilateral renal agenesis associated with absence of the uterus and oviducts has been reported in a medically aborted fetus.[62] In familial cases, the syndrome appears to be transmitted as an autosomal dominant trait with incomplete penetrance and variable expressivity. At present, no specific gene has been identified in MRKH syndrome.

## MECKEL-GRUBER SYNDROME

Meckel-Gruber syndrome (MKS, MIM 249000) is a rare and lethal autosomal recessive syndrome characterized by cystic dysplastic kidneys, occipital encephalocele, hepatic ductal dysplasia, and postaxial polydactyly.[63,64] Other anomalies may be observed, such as anophthalmia or microphthalmia and cardiac and genitalia malformations. Other renal anomalies include renal hypoplasia or aplasia and horseshoe kidneys.

The incidence of MKS varies from 1 in 13,250 to 1 in 140,000 live births and is higher in Belgian (1 in 3000) and Finnish (1 in 9000) populations.[63] MKS is caused by mutations in several different genes, including *B9D1, B9D2, MKS1, MKS3 (TMEM67), NPHP3, CEP290, RPGRIP1L, CC2D2A,* and *TMEM216.*[65] These genes, like other genes associated with renal ciliopathies, encode proteins that regulate ciliogenesis and control renal development and homeostasis

## MITOCHONDRIAL DISORDERS

Mitochondrial disorders are genetic defects of oxidative phosphorylation that can affect different organs or tissues.[66,67] Oxidative phosphorylation takes place in the mitochondrial

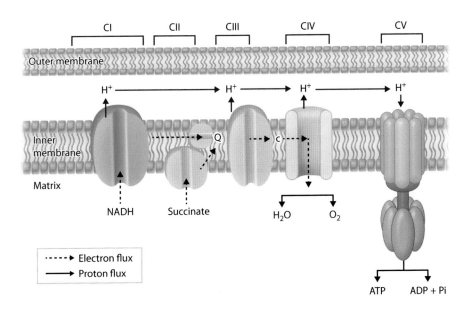

Figure 46.6 Oxidative phosphorylation occurs within the respiratory chain that is composed of four protein complexes (I to IV). These proteins transfer electrons and protons through the inner mitochondrial membrane generating the electrochemical gradient for adenosine triphosphate (ATP) synthesis, which is performed by the ATP synthase (complex V). ADP, adenosine diphosphate; $H^+$, hydrogen Ion; $H_2O$, water; NADH, nicotinamide adenine dinucleotide (reduced form); $O_2$, oxygen; Pi, inorganic orthophosphate.

inner membrane and consists of the oxidation of fuel molecules by oxygen and the concomitant energy transduction into adenosine triphosphate (Figure 46.6). The mitochondrial respiratory chain is a complex metabolic pathway. It is made of approximately 100 polypeptides, most of which are encoded in the nucleus, whereas 13 are encoded in the mitochondria. Mitochondrial DNA is maternally inherited, and its mutations are transmitted by the mother.[68] During cell division, mitochondria are randomly partitioned in daughter cells. Therefore, in cases when normal DNA and mutant DNA are present in the mother's cells, some lineages may have only mutant mitochondrial DNA or normal mitochondrial DNA, whereas others may have both mutant and normal DNA, a condition called heteroplasmy (Figure 46.7). Mitochondrial disorders have long been regarded as neuromuscular diseases. However, other organs, including heart, liver, pancreas, hematopoietic system, and kidney, depend on a mitochondrial energy supply and can therefore be affected during the course of these disorders (Table 46.3). Several clinical entities encompassing mitochondrial disorders have been described according to the clinical presentation (Table 46.4). Renal involvement and symptoms are more common in children than in adults.[69]

The most frequent renal manifestation of mitochondrial disorders is proximal tubulopathy resulting in a more or less complete and severe form of De Toni-Debre-Fanconi syndrome with urinary losses of amino acids, glucose, proteins, phosphate, uric acid, calcium, bicarbonate, potassium, sodium, and water.[70–73] The proximal tubulopathy is often moderate, with isolated hyperaminoaciduria in the absence of clinical manifestations. Some patients, however, have metabolic acidosis, hypophosphatemia, hypercalciuria, glycosuria, and tubular proteinuria and may develop growth

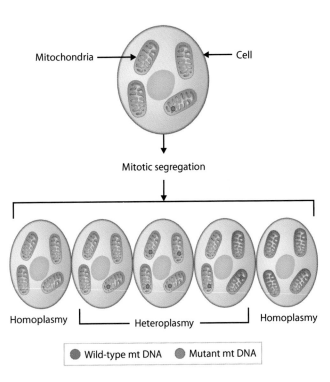

Figure 46.7 All human cells contain several mitochondria. In most cases, mitochondrial DNA (mtDNA) copies are identical, a condition called homoplasmy. When a mutation arises, it creates a mixture of normal and mutant mtDNA called heteroplasmy. During mitotic cell division, mitochondria are randomly partitioned to daughter cells. If normal DNA and mutant DNA are present in mother cells, daughter cells may drift to purely normal mtDNA or purely mutant mtDNA, or they may remain heteroplasmic.

Table 46.3 Clinical symptoms observed in patients with mitochondrial cytopathies

| Affected organ or system | Symptoms |
|---|---|
| Central nervous system | Apnea, lethargy, hypotonia, coma in the neonatal period |
| | Hypotonia, psychomotor regression, cerebellar ataxia, strokelike episodes, myoclonus, seizures, dementia, spasticity, headache, hemiparesis in infants and children |
| Muscle | Myopathy, poor head control, limb weakness, myalgia, exercise intolerance |
| Liver | Liver enlargement, hepatocellular dysfunction |
| Heart | Cardiomyopathy, heart block |
| Kidney | Proximal tubulopathy, nephrotic syndrome, renal failure, tubulointerstitial nephritis |
| Gut | Vomiting, diarrhea, villous atrophy, colonic pseudo-obstruction, exocrine pancreas dysfunction |
| Endocrine | Diabetes mellitus, growth hormone deficiency, hypoparathyroidism, hypothyroidism |
| Bone marrow | Sideroblastic anemia, neutropenia, thrombocytopenia |
| Ear | Hearing loss |
| Eye | Progressive external ophthalmoplegia, pigmentary retinal degeneration, ptosis, diplopia, cataract |

retardation, rickets, or dehydration. Most patients develop tubular symptoms before the age of 2 years. Renal biopsy demonstrates nonspecific abnormalities of the tubular epithelium, with dilatations and obstructions by tubular casts, de-differentiation, or atrophy of the tubular cells also seen. Giant mitochondria are often observed within the tubular cells by light and electron microscopy. Extrarenal symptoms are always present and include myopathy, neurologic symptoms, Pearson syndrome, diabetes mellitus, or cardiac problems.

Children with mitochondrial disorders may present with steroid-resistant nephrotic syndrome and focal segmental glomerular sclerosis. A triad of steroid-resistant nephrotic syndrome, hypoparathyroidism, and sensorineural deafness has been reported.[74] Some patients may even present with congenital nephrotic syndrome.[75] Coenzyme $Q_{10}$ deficiency was reported in siblings with severe encephalopathy, nephrotic syndrome, and renal failure. Mutations of the COQ2 gene have been found in these patients. Coenzyme $Q_{10}$ supplementation may improve neurologic and renal symptoms.[76,77] Mutations of the PDSS2 and COQ6 genes involved in coenzyme $Q_{10}$ synthesis have been reported in

children with early-onset nephrotic syndrome progressing to end-stage renal failure.[78]

A tubulointerstitial nephropathy has been described in a few patients with mitochondrial disorders.[79,80] The clinical presentation is characterized by polyuria secondary to impaired urinary concentrating ability without proximal tubular defects and by progression to end-stage renal failure. These patients present with extrarenal symptoms consisting of hearing loss, cardiomyopathy, myopathy, growth retardation, mental retardation, or pigmentary retinopathy.

The defect in the respiratory chain alters the redox status in the plasma and leads to increases in the ketone bodies ($\alpha$-OH butyrate–to-acetoacetate molar ratio) within the mitochondria, along with an increase in the lactate-to-pyruvate molar ratio in the cytoplasm and a secondary elevation of plasma lactate level. Therefore, screening for mitochondrial disorders includes the determination of lactate, pyruvate, ketone bodies, and their molar ratios. Gas chromatography-mass spectrometry can detect high amounts of lactate and Krebs cycle intermediates in the urine in patients with proximal tubulopathy.

Table 46.4 Clinicopathologic entities in mitchondrial cytopathies

| Mitochondrial cytopathy | Clinical manifestations |
|---|---|
| Kearns-Sayre syndrome | Progressive external ophthalmoplegia, retinal pigmentary degeneration, cerebellar ataxia, heart block |
| Myoclonus epilepsy and ragged-red fibers (MERRF) | Encephalomyopathy with myoclonus, epilepsy, ataxia, myopathy, hearing loss, dementia |
| Leber hereditary optic neuropathy (LHON) | Blindness, cardiac dysrhythmia |
| Mitochondrial encephalomyopathy, lactic acidosis, and stroke-like episodes (MELAS) | Headache, vomiting, lactic acidosis, myopathy with ragged-red fibers, seizures, dementia, deafness |
| Leigh disease | Subacute necrotizing encephalomyopathy, ataxia, respiratory troubles with weak cry, deafness, blindness |
| Chronic progressive external ophthalmoplegia (CPEO) and mitochondrial myopathy | Ocular myopathy, retinal pigmentary degeneration, central nervous system dysfunction |
| Alpers disease | Progressive infantile poliodystrophy, hepatic failure |

Polarographic and spectrophotometric studies allow identification of the biochemical nature of the mitochondrial defect.[81] Polarography measures oxygen consumption by mitochondria in the presence of various oxidative substrates. The only limitation of this technique is that it requires fresh tissue. Spectrophotometric studies assess isolated or combined respiratory chain complexes. When the disease is expressed in organs difficult to access, such as the kidney, accessible peripheral tissues, including skeletal muscle, cultured skin fibroblasts, and circulating lymphocytes, should be tested.

Any mode of inheritance (autosomal recessive, dominant, X-linked, maternal, or sporadic) can be observed in mitochondrial disorders.[82] Mutations in both mitochondrial and nuclear genes have been identified in patients with mitochondrial disorders associated with renal disease. However, the molecular definition is complicated by the dual genetic control of respiratory chain proteins and by the high number of genes involved in the biogenesis and assembly of the respiratory chain. Therefore, mutations are identified in only very few cases. The A-3243-G change in the tRNALeu gene is one of the most commonly encountered mitochondrial DNA (mtDNA) mutation (MELAS mutation).[83] This mutation is maternally inherited and is heteroplasmic. It can be associated with a large variety of clinical phenotypes, including nephrotic syndrome. Large mtDNA deletions have been described in several patients with renal disease. There are only few examples of mitochondrial kidney diseases associated with nuclear gene mutations.[73]

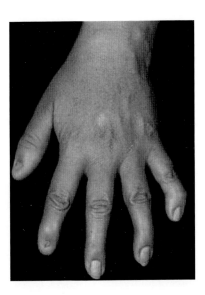

Figure 46.8 Nail-patella syndrome. Left hand in nail-patella syndrome showing dysplasia of the nails. The severity of dysplasia decreases from the thumb to the fifth finger. Clinodactyly of the fifth finger and triangular lunulae are also present.

### KEY POINTS

- A mitochondrial disorder should be considered in any patient with unexplained disease, especially when two or more seemingly unrelated symptoms are present.
- Proteinuria is observed in 30% of patients with NPS. ESRD occurs in approximately 10% of cases.

## NAIL-PATELLA SYNDROME

The nail-patella syndrome (NPS) or osteo-onychodysplasia (OMIM 161200) is an autosomal dominant disease characterized by hypoplastic or absent patella, dystrophic fingernails and toenails, and dysplasia of the elbows and iliac horns.[84,85] Renal symptoms are present in approximately 50% of patients. The estimated incidence of NPS is 22 per million population.[86]

Nail abnormalities are present in 80% to 90% of patients with NPS and are observed at birth.[87] The nails may be absent but more often are hypoplastic or dysplastic. Abnormalities predominate on the fingernails and consist of discoloration, longitudinal pterygium, splitting, and triangular lunulae (Figure 46.8). Abnormalities of the knees and elbows are found in almost all patients. The patella may be absent or hypoplastic, often with fragmentation, causing lateral slippage during knee flexion. The radial heads and the distal ends of the humerus are typically hypoplastic, leading to subluxation and limitations of extension, pronation, and supination of the forearm. Iliac horns, observed in 30% to 70% of the patients, are pathognomonic radiologic features of the disease (Figure 46.9). They consist of asymptomatic symmetric bone formations arising from the anterosuperior iliac crest.

The degree of renal involvement varies among families and also within members of the same family. The most frequent symptoms are proteinuria, sometimes with the nephrotic syndrome, hematuria, and hypertension.

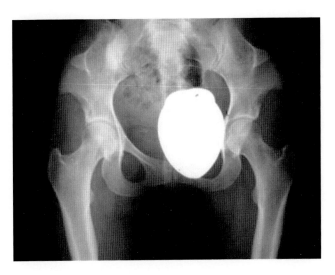

Figure 46.9 Nail-patella syndrome. x-ray film of the hip and iliac bones showing the characteristic iliac horns.

Urine-concentrating ability may be impaired. ESRD develops in approximately 10% of cases.[88] Patients with heavy proteinuria or impaired renal function may show basement membrane thickening and nonspecific lesions of focal segmental glomerular sclerosis. Electron microscopy shows pathognomonic and consistent lesions of the glomerular basement membrane.[89] These lesions consist of irregular and lucent rarefactions within the lamina densa, containing clusters of cross-banded collagen fibrils.

NPS is caused by mutations of the *LMX1B* gene located on chromosome 9.[90,91] LMX1B is a transcription factor of the LIM-homeodomain type, which plays an important role for limb development in vertebrates. More than 140 mutations in this gene have been identified in patients with NPS. *LMX1B* is expressed in the podocyte. The study of homozygous knockout mice has shown that this gene regulates the transcription of four genes: *COL4A3, COL4A4, CD2AP,* and *NPHS2*.[92-94] Investigators have suggested that there may be two allelic mutations of the gene: one responsible for the NPS without nephropathy and one responsible for the NPS with nephropathy. It has been calculated that, for a parent with the NPS whose family has nephropathy, the risk of having a child with nephropathy is 24%, and the risk of having a child who will progress to ESRD is 7%.[95]

## OCHOA SYNDROME (UROFACIAL SYNDROME)

Ochoa syndrome (OMIM 236730, 615112) is characterized by voiding dysfunction and an abnormal facial expression on smiling or crying.[96] The facial dysmorphism is related to an inversion of facial expression on smiling or crying (Figure 46.10). Children present with urinary incontinence and incomplete voiding of the bladder leading to urinary tract infections. Vesicoureteric reflux is frequently associated, and patients may progress to chronic renal failure. Patients may also have severe constipation.

Ochoa syndrome is inherited as an autosomal recessive trait. Most patients who have been studied carry biallelic mutations of *HPSE2* or, less commonly, of *LRIG2* genes, encoding for heparanase 2 and leucin-rich repeats and immunoglobulin-likedomains 2.[97] These two proteins are detected in the fetal bladder nerves and may facilitate neural growth in the bladder and bladder function.

## ORAL-FACIAL-DIGITAL SYNDROMES

Oral-facial-digital (OFD) syndromes are characterized by malformations of the oral cavity, the face, and the digits.[98] Several different forms of the syndrome have been described.

OFD1 (OMIM 311200) is the most frequent. It is lethal before birth in males. There is a high phenotypic variability

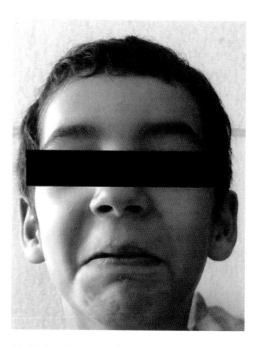

Figure 46.10 Urofacial syndrome (Ochoa syndrome). Characteristic inversion of the facial expression with smiling. (From Stamatiou K, Tyritzis S, Karakos C, et al. Urofacial syndrome: a subset of neurogenic bladder dysfunction syndromes? Urology. 2011;78:911–3.)

in females. Female patients present with oral malformations (clefts of the palate and tongue-gingival frenulae, abnormal dentition), craniofacial anomalies (facial asymmetry, hypertelorism, micrognathia, pseudocleft upper lip), abnormal hair, and digital malformations (brachydactyly, syndactyly, clinodactyly, and polydactyly). Neurologic anomalies are observed in 40% (intracerebral cysts, agenesis of the corpus callosum, cerebellar anomalies), and variable degrees of mental retardation occur in one-half of the patients. Renal disease consists of bilateral renal cysts, mostly glomerular cysts. Patients with renal cystic disease may progress to renal failure.[99]

The *OFD1* gene is located on the Xp22 region and encodes a centrosomal protein localized in the basal body of the primary cilia.[100] Many cases result from de novo mutations.

## RENAL-COLOBOMA SYNDROME

Renal-coloboma syndrome, also named papillorenal syndrome (OMIM 120330), is an autosomal dominant disorder characterized by renal hypoplasia and optic nerve coloboma.[101] Renal malformations include oligomeganephronic hypoplasia, vesicoureteral reflux, and, less often, multicystic dysplasia and ureteropelvic junction obstruction. Ophthalmologic examination shows an optic disc split and vascular anomalies associated with variable visual impairment.[102] Some patients have a large coloboma of the optic nerve, whereas other patients present with optic nerve dysplasia without visual impairement (Figure 46.11). Other

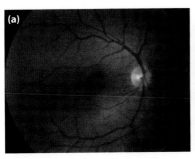
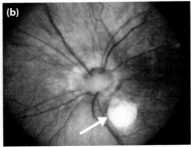
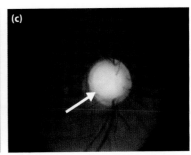

Figure 46.11 Renal-coloboma syndrome (RCS). Fundus photographs. (a) Normal fundus. Note that the typical optic nerve is smaller and compact, and the retinal vessels emerge from the center of the disc. (b) Right retinal coloboma in a patient with RCS (arrow). (c) Right retina from a patient with showing an optic disc coloboma in RCS (arrow). The optic disc is enlarged and excavated. The retinal vessels emerge from the edge of the disc, rather than the center. (From Schimmenti LA. Renal coloboma syndrome. Eur J Hum Genet. 2011;19:1207–12.)

features include sensorineural hearing loss, Arnold Chiari malformation, seizures, and joint laxity.[103]

More than 50 heterozygous mutations in the *PAX2* gene have been described in patients with the renal-coloboma syndrome.[104,105] Identified mutations have mostly been located in the second and third exons of the *PAX2* gene, which is located on chromosome 10q24-25.[104] The *PAX2* gene encodes a transcription factor involved in the development of the kidneys and eyes. Studies in mice found that heterozygous *PAX2* mutations (1Neu) are associated with increased apoptosis and reduced branching of the ureteric bud.[106] *PAX2* mutations have been identified in a few patients with oligomeganephronia and limited or no optic nerve anomalies.[107,108]

## SIMPSON-GOLABI-BEHMEL SYNDROME

Simpson-Golabi-Behmel syndrome (SGBS, OMIM 312870) is a rare X-linked congenital syndrome characterized by prenatal and postnatal overgrowth, craniofacial anomalies, organomegaly, increased risk of tumors, moderate intellectual deficiency, and variable congenital malformations.[109] Two types of the disorder have been described: a less severe form (SGBS type I) and a severe form (SGBS type II).

The glypican 3 (*GPC3*) gene located on Xq26 encodes a heparan sulfate proteoglycan, an extracellular matrix protein, that plays an important role in cell growth during development.[110] Mutations in this gene have been identified mostly in patients with SGBS type I, the most frequent form of SGB syndrome. Renal anomalies are observed in 50% of patients with *GPC3* mutations and consist of duplicated collecting duct, megaureter, vesicoureteral reflux, and ureteropelvic junction obstruction. Patients may have renal dysplasia, renal cysts, and nephromegaly and may develop Wilms tumor.[111] A second locus on chromosome Xp22 is associated with SGBS type II.

## TOWNES-BROCKS SYNDROME

Townes-Brocks syndrome (OMIM 107480), also named anus-hand-ear syndrome, is an autosomal dominant disorder characterized by the association of imperforate anus, preaxial polydactyly and triphalangeal thumbs, external ear anomalies, sensorineural hearing loss, renal and heart anomalies, and variable expressivity (Figure 46.12).[112] Most patients have normal intelligence. Renal malformations consist of unilateral or bilateral hypoplasic or dysplasic kidneys, renal agenesis, multicystic kidney, horseshoe kidney, vesicoureteral reflux, and posterior urethral valves. These

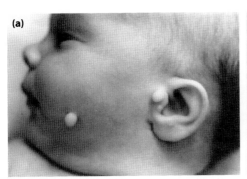
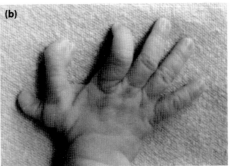

Figure 46.12 Townes-Brocks syndrome. (a) Dysplastic ear with a preauricular tag and a cheek tag. (b) Preaxial polydactyly and bifid distal phalanx of the thumb with ulnar deviation. (From Powella CM, Michaelisb RC. Townes-Brocks syndrome. J Med Genet. 1999;36:89–93.)

malformations may be responsible for renal failure, including end-stage renal failure.

Townes-Brocks syndrome occurs in 1 in 200,000 live births. More than 60 mutations have been identified in the *SALL1* gene on chromosome 16q12.1, which codes for a zinc finger transcription factor that is involved in kidney development.[113,114] *SALL1* is essential for ureteric bud invasion, the first step of metanephros development.[115] De novo mutations are observed in 50% of cases. Approximately 65% of patients have point mutations and 5% deletions.[116] A significant proportion of patients with the typical malformations does not have a *SALL1* mutation.

## VATER AND VACTERL ASSOCIATIONS

VATER association, initially described in 1973, is characterized by congenital malformations including Vertebral defects, Anal atresia, Tracheo-Esophageal fistula, and Renal anomalies.[117] VACTERL association also includes Cardiac malformations and Limb abnormalities.[118] VACTERL association occurs in 1 in 10,000 to 1 in 40,000 liveborn infants. The diagnosis is made if three of the foregoing symptoms are present in early life.

Renal anomalies have been reported in 50% to 80% of cases and include unilateral or bilateral renal agenesis, horseshoe kidney, and cystic or dysplastic kidneys. Some patients may progress to renal failure.[119]

## SUMMARY

Genetic and syndromic disorders can be associated renal malformations, the presence of renal cysts, hypercalciuria, nephrocalcinosis, and proteinuria. Progressive loss of renal function, chronic kidney disease, and ESRD can also result from some of these disorders. Recognition of syndromes that are associated with renal disease requires the input of a genetics team in addition to the nephrologist. Complex surgical management in disorders such as VATER or VACTERL association requires the involvement of urologic and other surgical expertise. Genetic diagnosis of many syndromic disorders is possible now, and the array of available diagnostic tests for clinical use is ever increasing. This chapter provides an overview of the common syndromes and genetic diseases associated with renal manifestations. The reader is referred to the broader literature on the subject for a deeper understanding, if needed.

## REFERENCES

1. Lin F, Patel V, Igarashi P. Renal dysgenesis. In: Lifton RP, Somlo S, Giebish GH, Seldin DW, editors. Genetic Diseases of the Kidney. New York: Academic Press; 2009. p. 463–93.

2. Limwongse C. Syndromes and malformations of the urinary tract. In: Avner E, Harman, WE, Niaudet, P, Yoshikawa, N, editors. Pediatric Nephrology, 6th ed. New York: Springer; 2010. p. 121–56.

3. Spitzer AA, editor. Inheritance of Kidney and Urinary Tract Diseases. Boston: Kluwer Academic Publishers; 1989.

4. Turnpenny PD, Ellard S. Alagille syndrome: Pathogenesis, diagnosis and management. Eur J Hum Genet. 2012;20:251–7.

5. Berard E, Sarles J, Triolo V, et al. Renovascular hypertension and vascular anomalies in Alagille syndrome. Pediatr Nephrol. 1998;12:121–4.

6. Salem JE, Bruguiere E, Iserin L, et al. Hypertension and aortorenal disease in Alagille syndrome. J Hypertens. 2012;30:1300–6.

7. Habib R, Dommergues JP, Gubler MC, et al. Glomerular mesangiolipidosis in Alagille syndrome (arteriohepatic dysplasia). Pediatr Nephrol. 1987;1:455–64.

8. Green JS, Parfrey PS, Harnett JD, et al. The cardinal manifestations of Bardet-Biedl syndrome, a form of Laurence-Moon-Biedl syndrome. N Engl J Med. 1989;321:1002–9.

9. Beales PL, Elcioglu N, Woolf AS, et al. New criteria for improved diagnosis of Bardet-Biedl syndrome: Results of a population survey. J Med Genet. 1999;36:437–46.

10. Putoux A, Attie-Bitach T, Martinovic J, Gubler MC. Phenotypic variability of Bardet-Biedl syndrome: Focusing on the kidney. Pediatr Nephrol. 2012;27:7–15.

11. Imhoff O, Marion V, Stoetzel C, et al. Bardet-Biedl syndrome: A study of the renal and cardiovascular phenotypes in a French cohort. Clin J Am Soc Nephrol. 2011;6:22–9.

12. Dippell J, Varlam DE. Early sonographic aspects of kidney morphology in Bardet-Biedl syndrome. Pediatr Nephrol. 1998;12:559–63.

13. Janssen S, Ramaswami G, Davis EE, et al. Mutation analysis in Bardet-Biedl syndrome by DNA pooling and massively parallel resequencing in 105 individuals. Hum Genet. 2011;129:79–90.

14. Zaghloul NA, Katsanis N. Mechanistic insights into Bardet-Biedl syndrome, a model ciliopathy. J Clin Invest. 2009;119:428–37.

15. Schurman SJ, Scheinman SJ. Inherited cerebrorenal syndromes. Nat Rev Nephrol. 2009;5:529–38.

16. Pettenati MJ, Haines JL, Higgins RR, et al. Wiedemann-Beckwith syndrome: Presentation of clinical and cytogenetic data on 22 new cases and review of the literature. Hum Genet. 1986;74:143–54.

17. Weksberg R, Shuman C, Beckwith JB. Beckwith-Wiedemann syndrome. Eur J Hum Genet. 2010;18:8–14.

18. Choufani S, Shuman C, Weksberg R. Molecular findings in Beckwith-Wiedemann syndrome. Am J Med. Genet. C Semin Med Genet. 2013;163C:131–40.

19. Melnick M, Bixler D, Silk K, et al. Autosomal dominant branchiootorenal dysplasia. Birth Defects Orig Artic Ser. 1975;11:121–8.

20. Chen A, Francis M, Ni L, et al. Phenotypic manifestations of branchio-oto-renal syndrome. Am J Med Genet. 1995;58:365–70.

21. Fraser FC, Ling D, Clogg D, Nogrady B. Genetic aspects of the BOR syndrome: Branchial fistulas, ear pits, hearing loss, and renal anomalies. Am J Med Genet. 1978;2:241–52.

22. Rodriguez Soriano J. Branchio-oto-renal syndrome. J Nephrol. 2003;16:603–5.

23. Orten DJ, Fischer SM, Sorensen JL, et al. Branchio-oto-renal syndrome (BOR): Novel mutations in the EYA1 gene, and a review of the mutational genetics of BOR. Hum Mutat. 2008;29:537–44.

24. Abdelhak S, Kalatzis V, Heilig R, et al. A human homologue of the Drosophila eyes absent gene underlies branchio-oto-renal (BOR) syndrome and identifies a novel gene family. Nat Genet. 1997;15:157–64.

25. Xu PX, Adams J, Peters H, et al. Eya1-deficient mice lack ears and kidneys and show abnormal apoptosis of organ primordia. Nat Genet. 1999;23:113–7.

26. Hoskins BE, Cramer CH, Silvius D, et al. Transcription factor SIX5 is mutated in patients with branchio-oto-renal syndrome. Am J Hum Genet. 2007;80:800–4.

27. Kochhar A, Orten DJ, Sorensen JL, et al. SIX1 mutation screening in 247 branchio-oto-renal syndrome families: A recurrent missense mutation associated with BOR. Hum Mutat. 2008;29:565.

28. Ruf RG, Xu PX, Silvius D, et al. SIX1 mutations cause branchio-oto-renal syndrome by disruption of EYA1-SIX1-DNA complexes. Proc Natl Acad Sci U S A. 2004;101:8090–5.

29. Verloes A. Updated diagnostic criteria for CHARGE syndrome: A proposal. Am J Med Genet A. 2005;133A:306–8.

30. Ragan DC, Casale AJ, Rink RC, et al. Genitourinary anomalies in the CHARGE association. J Urol. 1999;161:622–5.

31. Jongmans MC, Admiraal RJ, van der Donk KP, et al. CHARGE syndrome: The phenotypic spectrum of mutations in the CHD7 gene. J Med Genet. 2006;43:306–14.

32. Vissers LE, van Ravenswaaij CM, Admiraal R, et al. Mutations in a new member of the chromodomain gene family cause CHARGE syndrome. Nat Genet. 2004;36:955–7.

33. Lalani SR, Safiullah AM, Fernbach SD, et al. Spectrum of CHD7 mutations in 110 individuals with CHARGE syndrome and genotype-phenotype correlation. Am J Hum Genet. 2006;78:303–14.

34. Nance MA, Berry SA. Cockayne syndrome: Review of 140 cases. Am J Med Genet. 1992;42:68–84.

35. Hirooka M, Hirota M, Kamada M. Renal lesions in Cockayne syndrome. Pediatr Nephrol. 1988;2:239–43.

36. Mallery DL, Tanganelli B, Colella S, et al. Molecular analysis of mutations in the CSB (ERCC6) gene in patients with Cockayne syndrome. Am J Hum Genet. 1998;62:77–85.

37. Henning KA, Li L, Iyer N, et al. The Cockayne syndrome group A gene encodes a WD repeat protein that interacts with CSB protein and a subunit of RNA polymerase II TFIIH. Cell. 1995;82:555–64.

38. Selby CP, Sancar A. Cockayne syndrome group B protein enhances elongation by RNA polymerase II. Proc Natl Acad Sci U S A. 1997;94:11205–9.

39. Ryan AK, Goodship JA, Wilson DI, et al. Spectrum of clinical features associated with interstitial chromosome 22q11 deletions: A European collaborative study. J Med Genet. 1997;34:798–804.

40. Bassett AS, McDonald-McGinn DM, Devriendt K, et al. Practical guidelines for managing patients with 22q11.2 deletion syndrome. J Pediatr. 2011;159:332–9 e1.

41. Devriendt K, Swillen A, Fryns JP, et al. Renal and urological tract malformations caused by a 22q11 deletion. J Med Genet. 1996;33:349.

42. Saitta SC, Harris SE, Gaeth AP, et al. Aberrant interchromosomal exchanges are the predominant cause of the 22q11.2 deletion. Hum Mol Genet. 2004;13:417–28.

43. Slavotinek AM, Tifft CJ. Fraser syndrome and cryptophthalmos: Review of the diagnostic criteria and evidence for phenotypic modules in complex malformation syndromes. J Med Genet. 2002;39:623–33.

44. Jadeja S, Smyth I, Pitera JE, et al. Identification of a new gene mutated in Fraser syndrome and mouse myelencephalic blebs. Nat Genet. 2005;37:520–5.

45. McGregor L, Makela V, Darling SM, et al. Fraser syndrome and mouse blebbed phenotype caused by mutations in FRAS1/Fras1 encoding a putative extracellular matrix protein. Nat Genet. 2003;34:203–8.

46. Rollnick BR, Kaye CI, Nagatoshi K, et al. Oculoauriculovertebral dysplasia and variants: Phenotypic characteristics of 294 patients. Am J Med Genet. 1987;26:361–75.

47. Ritchey ML, Norbeck J, Huang C, et al. Urologic manifestations of Goldenhar syndrome. Urology. 1994;43:88–91.

48. Decramer S, Parant O, Beaufils S, et al. Anomalies of the TCF2 gene are the main cause of fetal bilateral hyperechogenic kidneys. J Am Soc Nephrol. 2007;18:923–33.

49. Ulinski T, Lescure S, Beaufils S, et al. Renal phenotypes related to hepatocyte nuclear factor-1beta (TCF2) mutations in a pediatric cohort. J Am Soc Nephrol. 2006;17:497–503.

50. Lebrun G, Vasiliu V, Bellanne-Chantelot C, et al. Cystic kidney disease, chromophobe renal cell carcinoma and TCF2 (HNF1 beta) mutations. Nat Clin Pract Nephrol. 2005;1:115–9.

51. Bellanne-Chantelot C, Chauveau D, Gautier JF, et al. Clinical spectrum associated with hepatocyte nuclear factor-1beta mutations. Ann Intern Med. 2004;140:510–7.

52. Yorifuji T, Kurokawa K, Mamada M, et al. Neonatal diabetes mellitus and neonatal polycystic, dysplastic kidneys: Phenotypically discordant recurrence of a mutation in the hepatocyte nuclear factor-1beta gene due to germline mosaicism. J Clin Endocrinol Metab. 2004;89:2905–8.

53. Moreno-De-Luca D, Mulle JG, Kaminsky EB, et al. Deletion 17q12 is a recurrent copy number variant that confers high risk of autism and schizophrenia. Am J Hum Genet. 2010;87:618–30.

54. Loirat C, Bellanne-Chantelot C, Husson I, et al. Autism in three patients with cystic or hyperechogenic kidneys and chromosome 17q12 deletion. Nephrol. Dial Transplant. 2010;25:3430–3.

55. Heidet L, Decramer S, Pawtowski A, et al. Spectrum of HNF1B mutations in a large cohort of patients who harbor renal diseases. Clin J Am Soc Nephrol. 2010;5:1079–90.

56. Karstensen HG, Tommerup N. Isolated and syndromic forms of congenital anosmia. Clin Genet. 2012;81:210–5.

57. Hardelin JP, Dode C. The complex genetics of Kallmann syndrome: KAL1, FGFR1, FGF8, PROKR2, PROK2, et al. Sex Dev. 2008;2:181–93.

58. Dode C, Teixeira L, Levilliers J, et al. Kallmann syndrome: Mutations in the genes encoding prokineticin-2 and prokineticin receptor-2. PLoS Genet. 2006;2:e175.

59. Hardelin JP, Julliard AK, Moniot B, et al. Anosmin-1 is a regionally restricted component of basement membranes and interstitial matrices during organogenesis: Implications for the developmental anomalies of X chromosome-linked Kallmann syndrome. Dev Dyn. 1999;215:26–44.

60. Kirk JM, Grant DB, Besser GM, et al. Unilateral renal aplasia in X-linked Kallmann's syndrome. Clin Genet. 1994;46:260–2.

61. Morcel K, Camborieux L, Guerrier D. Mayer-Rokitansky-Kuster-Hauser (MRKH) syndrome. Orphanet J Rare Dis. 2007;2:13.

62. Devriendt K, Moerman P, Van Schoubroeck D, et al. Chromosome 22q11 deletion presenting as the Potter sequence. J Med Genet. 1997;34:423–5.

63. Alexiev BA, Lin X, Sun CC, Brenner DS. Meckel-Gruber syndrome: Pathologic manifestations, minimal diagnostic criteria, and differential diagnosis. Arch Pathol Lab Med. 2006;130:1236–8.

64. Blankenberg TA, Ruebner BH, Ellis WG, et al. Pathology of renal and hepatic anomalies in Meckel syndrome. Am J Med Genet Suppl. 1987;3:395–410.

65. Arts HH, Knoers NV. Current insights into renal ciliopathies: What can genetics teach us? Pediatr Nephrol. 2013;28:863–74.

66. Di Donato S. Multisystem manifestations of mitochondrial disorders. J Neurol. 2009;256:693–710.

67. DiMauro S, Schon EA. Mitochondrial respiratory-chain diseases. N Engl J Med. 2003;348:2656–68.

68. Anderson S, Bankier AT, Barrell BG, et al. Sequence and organization of the human mitochondrial genome. Nature. 1981;290:457–65.

69. Niaudet P, Rotig A. Renal involvement in mitochondrial cytopathies. Pediatr Nephrol. 1996;10:368–73.

70. Au KM, Lau SC, Mak YF, et al. Mitochondrial DNA deletion in a girl with Fanconi's syndrome. Pediatr Nephrol. 2007;22:136–40.

71. Majander A, Suomalainen A, Vettenranta K, et al. Congenital hypoplastic anemia, diabetes, and severe renal tubular dysfunction associated with a mitochondrial DNA deletion. Pediatr Res. 1991;30:327–30.

72. Niaudet P, Heidet L, Munnich A, et al. Deletion of the mitochondrial DNA in a case of de Toni-Debre-Fanconi syndrome and Pearson syndrome. Pediatr Nephrol. 1994;8:164–8.

73. de Lonlay P, Valnot I, Barrientos A, et al. A mutant mitochondrial respiratory chain assembly protein causes complex III deficiency in patients with tubulopathy, encephalopathy and liver failure. Nat Genet. 2001;29:57–60.

74. Barakat AY, D'Albora JB, Martin MM, Jose PA. Familial nephrosis, nerve deafness, and hypoparathyroidism. J Pediatr. 1977;91:61–4.

75. Goldenberg A, Ngoc LH, Thouret MC, et al. Respiratory chain deficiency presenting as congenital nephrotic syndrome. Pediatr Nephrol. 2005;20:465–9.

76. Montini G, Malaventura C, Salviati L. Early coenzyme Q10 supplementation in primary coenzyme Q10 deficiency. N Engl J Med. 2008;358:2849–50.

77. Rotig A, Appelkvist EL, Geromel V, et al. Quinone-responsive multiple respiratory-chain dysfunction due to widespread coenzyme Q10 deficiency. Lancet. 2000;356:391–5.

78. Emma F, Bertini E, Salviati L, Montini G. Renal involvement in mitochondrial cytopathies. Pediatr Nephrol. 2012;27:539–50.

79. Rotig A, Goutieres F, Niaudet P, et al. Deletion of mitochondrial DNA in patient with chronic tubulointerstitial nephritis. J Pediatr. 1995;126:597–601.

80. Tzen CY, Tsai JD, Wu TY, et al. Tubulointerstitial nephritis associated with a novel mitochondrial point mutation. Kidney Int. 2001;59:846–54.

81. Rustin P, Chretien D, Bourgeron T, et al. Biochemical and molecular investigations in respiratory chain deficiencies. Clin Chim Acta. 1994;228:35–51.

82. Rotig A, Munnich A. Genetic features of mitochondrial respiratory chain disorders. J Am Soc Nephrol. 2003;14:2995–3007.

83. Goto Y, Nonaka I, Horai S. A mutation in the tRNA(Leu)(UUR) gene associated with the MELAS subgroup of mitochondrial encephalomyopathies. Nature. 1990;348:651–3.

84. Sweeney E, Fryer A, Mountford R, et al. Nail patella syndrome: A review of the phenotype aided by developmental biology. J Med Genet. 2003;40:153–62.

85. McIntosh I, Dunston JA, Liu L, et al. Nail patella syndrome revisited: 50 years after linkage. Ann Hum Genet. 2005;69:349–63.

86. Levy M, Feingold J. Estimating prevalence in single-gene kidney diseases progressing to renal failure. Kidney Int. 2000;58:925–43.

87. Dunston JA, Lin S, Park JW, et al. Phenotype severity and genetic variation at the disease locus: An investigation of nail dysplasia in the nail patella syndrome. Ann Hum Genet. 2005;69:1–8.

88. Lemley KV. Kidney disease in nail-patella syndrome. Pediatr Nephrol. 2009;24:2345–54.

89. Ben-Bassat M, Cohen L, Rosenfeld J. The glomerular basement membrane in the nail-patella syndrome. Arch Pathol. 1971;92:350–5.

90. Chen H, Lun Y, Ovchinnikov D, et al. Limb and kidney defects in Lmx1b mutant mice suggest an involvement of LMX1B in human nail patella syndrome. Nat Genet. 1998;19:51–5.

91. Vollrath D, Jaramillo-Babb VL, Clough MV, et al. Loss-of-function mutations in the LIM-homeodomain gene, LMX1B, in nail-patella syndrome. Hum Mol Genet. 1998;7:1091–8.

92. Morello R, Zhou G, Dreyer SD, et al. Regulation of glomerular basement membrane collagen expression by LMX1B contributes to renal disease in nail patella syndrome. Nat Genet. 2001;27:205–8.

93. Miner JH, Morello R, Andrews KL, et al. Transcriptional induction of slit diaphragm genes by Lmx1b is required in podocyte differentiation. J Clin Invest. 2002;109:1065–72.

94. Heidet L, Bongers EM, Sich M, et al. *In vivo* expression of putative LMX1B targets in nail-patella syndrome kidneys. Am J Pathol. 2003;163:145–55.

95. Looij BJ, Jr, te Slaa RL, Hogewind BL, van de Kamp JJ. Genetic counselling in hereditary osteo-onychodysplasia (HOOD, nail-patella syndrome) with nephropathy. J Med Genet. 1988;25:682–6.

96. Ochoa B. Can a congenital dysfunctional bladder be diagnosed from a smile? The Ochoa syndrome updated. Pediatr Nephrol. 2004;19:6–12.

97. Woolf AS, Stuart HM, Roberts NA, et al. Urofacial syndrome: A genetic and congenital disease of aberrant urinary bladder innervation. Pediatr Nephrol. 2014;29:513–8.

98. Gurrieri F, Franco B, Toriello H, Neri G. Oral-facial-digital syndromes: Review and diagnostic guidelines. Am J Med Genet A. 2007;143A:3314–23.

99. Odent S, Le Marec B, Toutain A, et al. Central nervous system malformations and early end-stage renal disease in oro-facio-digital syndrome type I: A review. Am J Med Genet. 1998;75:389–94.

100. Macca M, Franco B. The molecular basis of oral-facial-digital syndrome, type 1. Am J Med Genet C Semin Med Genet. 2009;151C:318–25.

101. Sanyanusin P, Schimmenti LA, McNoe LA, et al. Mutation of the PAX2 gene in a family with optic nerve colobomas, renal anomalies and vesicoureteral reflux. Nat Genet. 1995;9:358–64.

102. Dureau P, Attie-Bitach T, Salomon R, et al. Renal coloboma syndrome. Ophthalmology. 2001;108:1912–6.

103. Eccles MR, Schimmenti LA. Renal-coloboma syndrome: A multi-system developmental disorder caused by PAX2 mutations. Clin Genet. 1999;56:1–9.

104. Schimmenti LA, Cunliffe HE, McNoe LA, et al. Further delineation of renal-coloboma syndrome in patients with extreme variability of phenotype and identical PAX2 mutations. Am J Hum Genet. 1997;60:869–78.

105. Bower M, Salomon R, Allanson J, et al. Update of PAX2 mutations in renal coloboma syndrome and establishment of a locus-specific database. Hum Mutat. 2012;33:457–66.

106. Porteous S, Torban E, Cho NP, et al. Primary renal hypoplasia in humans and mice with PAX2 mutations: Evidence of increased apoptosis in fetal kidneys of Pax2(1Neu)$^{+/-}$ mutant mice. Hum Mol Genet. 2000;9:1–11.

107. Salomon R, Tellier AL, Attie-Bitach T, et al. PAX2 mutations in oligomeganephronia. Kidney Int. 2001;59:457–62.

108. Nishimoto K, Iijima K, Shirakawa T, et al. PAX2 gene mutation in a family with isolated renal hypoplasia. J Am Soc Nephrol. 2001;12:1769–72.

109. Neri G, Gurrieri F, Zanni G, Lin A. Clinical and molecular aspects of the Simpson-Golabi-Behmel syndrome. Am J Med Genet. 1998;79:279–83.

110. Grisaru S, Rosenblum ND. Glypicans and the biology of renal malformations. Pediatr Nephrol. 2001;16:302–6.

111. Cottereau E, Mortemousque I, Moizard MP, et al. Phenotypic spectrum of Simpson-Golabi-Behmel syndrome in a series of 42 cases with a mutation in GPC3 and review of the literature. Am J Med Genet C Semin Med Genet. 2013;163C:92–105.

112. Powell CM, Michaelis RC. Townes-Brocks syndrome. J Med Genet. 1999;36:89–93.

113. Kohlhase J, Wischermann A, Reichenbach H, et al. Mutations in the SALL1 putative transcription factor gene cause Townes-Brocks syndrome. Nat Genet. 1998;18:81–3.

114. Miller EM, Hopkin R, Bao L, Ware SM. Implications for genotype-phenotype predictions in Townes-Brocks syndrome: Case report of a novel SALL1 deletion and review of the literature. Am J Med Genet A. 2012;158A:533–40.

115. Nishinakamura R, Takasato M. Essential roles of Sall1 in kidney development. Kidney Int. 2005;68:1948–50.

116. Borozdin W, Steinmann K, Albrecht B, et al. Detection of heterozygous SALL1 deletions by quantitative real time PCR proves the contribution of a SALL1 dosage effect in the pathogenesis of Townes-Brocks syndrome. Hum Mutat. 2006;27:211–2.

117. Quan L, Smith DW. The VATER association. Vertebral defects, anal atresia, T-E fistula with esophageal atresia, radial and renal dysplasia: A spectrum of associated defects. J Pediatr. 1973;82:104–7.

118. Solomon BD. VACTERL/VATER Association. Orphanet J Rare Dis. 2011;6:56.

119. Ahn SY, Mendoza S, Kaplan G, et al. Chronic kidney disease in the VACTERL association: Clinical course and outcome. Pediatr Nephrol. 2009;24:1047–53.

## REVIEW QUESTIONS

1. Children affected with *one* of the following syndromes are at higher risk of developing Wilms tumor.
   a. Branchio-oto-renal syndrome
   b. Renal-coloboma syndrome
   c. Townes-Brocks syndrome
   d. Beckwith-Wiedemann syndrome
   e. Cockayne syndrome

2. Which of the following anomalies is *not* observed in patients with HNF1B-mutation?
   a. Cholestasis
   b. Hypomagnesemia
   c. Multicystic kidney disease
   d. Vertebral malformations
   e. Diabetes mellitus

3. Children affected with *one* of the following syndromes may develop proteinuria and a nephrotic syndrome.
   a. CHARGE syndrome
   b. Nail-patella syndrome
   c. Ochoa syndrome
   d. Fraser syndrome
   e. Simpson-Golabi-Behmel syndrome

4. Concerning mitochondrial disorders, which of the following assertions is *not applicable*?
   a. They are secondary to defects of oxidative phosdphorylation.
   b. Mitochondrial DNA is inherited from the father.
   c. The most frequent renal manifestation is proximal tubulopathy.
   d. Patients may present with hyperlactatemia.
   e. Patients may develop a nephrotic syndrome.

5. All of the following are seen in patients with Alagille syndrome, *except:*
   a. Chronic cholestasis
   b. Pulmonary artery stenosis
   c. Posterior embryotoxon
   d. Hearing loss
   e. Vascular abnormalities

6. Which of the following *does not apply* to nail-patella syndrome?
   a. It is an autosomal dominant disease.
   b. Iliac horns are a pathognomonic radiologic feature of the disease.
   c. Urinary tract malformations are frequently observed in nail-patella syndrome.
   d. Nail-patella syndrome is caused by mutations of the LMX1B gene.
   e. End-stage renal disease develops in 10% to 15% of cases.

## ANSWER KEY

1. d
2. d
3. b
4. b
5. d
6. c

# PART J

# Urologic disorders

# 47

# Hydronephrosis and obstructive uropathies

IHOR V. YOSYPIV

Congenital obstructive uropathy is characterized by compromised urine flow or transport that begins in utero and can impair fetal renal development and function. This group of disorders forms one of the most important and identifiable causes of chronic kidney disease (CKD) in infants and children.[1] Congenital obstructive uropathy constitutes a part of the spectrum of the congenital anomalies of the kidney and urinary tract (CAKUT), which occurs in 1 of 1000 live births and counts for 50% to 56% of CKD and end-stage renal disease (ESRD) in children of all ages.[2-4]

Because urinary tract obstruction during fetal life has serious consequences for the structural and functional development of kidneys and the urinary tract, there is a clear need for early diagnosis, for appropriate and timely interventions, and to monitor progression and response to therapy. This chapter reviews the causes and pathophysiology of urinary tract obstruction, discusses antenatal and postnatal clinical manifestations, and examines clinical management.

## CLASSIFICATION

Obstructive uropathy can be classified based on the site of obstruction and whether it is acute or chronic. Because congenital obstructive uropathies are developmental in origin from fetal life, all of them can be considered to be chronic. This is in contrast to older children and adults, in whom urinary obstruction is often acute in timing and is likely to be reversible.

Based on the site of obstruction (Figure 47.1), congenital obstructive uropathies can be classified as upper urinary tract obstruction and lower urinary tract obstruction (LUTO). The upper urinary tract obstruction encompasses the renal pelvis and the upper part of the ureters. Ureteropelvic junction (UPJ) obstruction typifies this type of urinary obstruction. LUTO, on the other hand, involves lower ureters, urinary bladder, and the urethra. Ureterovesicular junction (UVJ) obstruction can be present unilaterally or bilaterally, with the corresponding side of urinary tract involvement. On the other hand, lesions of the bladder and urethra usually affect both sides of the urinary tract. Posterior urethral valves (PUVs) are common examples of LUTO that often affect both sides of the urinary tracts. Urethral stenosis and atresia also cause bilateral urinary tract effects.

### KEY POINTS

- CAKUT accounts for 50% to 56% of ESRD and CKD in children.
- Congenital obstructive uropathy affects the development and functions of fetal kidneys.
- Based on the site of urinary obstruction, obstructive uropathy can be classified as upper urinary tract obstruction or (LUTO).
- Urinary obstruction may be acute or chronic.

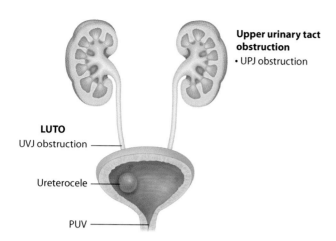

**Upper urinary tact obstruction**
• UPJ obstruction

**LUTO**
UVJ obstruction

Ureterocele

PUV

Figure 47.1 Location of most common sites of congenital urinary tract obstruction. LUTO, lower urinary tract obstruction; PUV, posterior urethral valves. UPJ, ureteropelvic junction; UVJ, ureterovesical junction.

## EPIDEMIOLOGY

The most common cause of prenatally detected hydronephrosis is UPJ obstruction, which occurs in 1 in 1500 live births.[3-5] Obstruction is bilateral in 20% to 25% of cases of UPJ obstruction, with 3:1 male predominance.[6] Ureterovesical junction (UVJ) obstruction accounts for 20% of cases of neonatal hydronephrosis, has a 4:1 male predominance and is bilateral in 25% of cases.[6] The incidence of PUV that occurs exclusively in males is 1 in 5000 to 8000.[3,7] Because both kidneys are affected, the presence of PUV carries the greatest risk for development of ESRD. Therefore, intervention is potentially most urgent in patients with PUV.[8] The prevalence of ureterocele, a cystic dilatation of the terminal ureter within the bladder, the urethra, or both, is 1 in 5000 newborns, with 3:1 female predominance.[6] Bilateral ureteroceles occur in 20% to 50% of cases.[6] Approximately 50% of all cases of congenital hydronephrosis have no evidence of physical obstruction or abnormality in the structural components of the lower urinary tract (LUT). In these cases, the presence of functional urinary tract obstruction is assumed.

## PATHOPHYSIOLOGY

Obstruction of the urinary tract causes rapidly detectable changes in ureteric function and anatomy and leads to numerous closely linked cellular and molecular responses in the kidneys that result in (1) changes in developmental physiology of the kidneys, (2) induction of inflammatory and fibrosis induction pathways, and (3) apoptosis. The underlying mechanisms that account for congenital structural or functional obstructive uropathy are poorly understood. Although numerous genes have been postulated to play a

role in the normal and abnormal development of the urinary tract, none has been shown to be responsible for the common lesions associated with congenital obstructive uropathy in humans. The potential role played by some of the well-characterized mechanisms in the pathogenesis of congenital obstructive uropathy is discussed in the following section.

> ## KEY POINTS
>
> • Approximately 50% cases of congenital hydronephrosis have no recognizable cause.
> • UPJ obstruction is the most common cause of unilateral prenatal hydronephrosis (1:5000 live births).
> • PUV occurs in 1:5000 to 8000 male births.
> • Patients with PUV are at the greatest risk for CKD and ESRD because of potential bilateral renal injury.

## URETERAL PRESSURE AND RENAL BLOOD FLOW

The structural and functional changes occurring at the level of the ureter in the presence of obstruction depend on its extent and duration of obstruction, the rate of urine formation, and the presence or absence of infection. An acute increase in the intraluminal baseline ureteral pressure is followed, within several hours, by a decline in the intraluminal ureteral pressure to values slightly above normal.[9] The fall in ureteral pressure is attributable to decreased renal blood flow (RBF) and glomerular filtration rate (GFR). In addition, an increase in the ureteral cross-sectional muscle area, ureteral length and diameter, and an alteration of ureteral peristalsis are also observed.

RBF in the affected kidney decreases after unilateral ureteral obstruction (UUO) in experimental models.[9] In some experimental models of UUO, despite a substantial rise in the ureteral pressure, there is an initial rise in RBF that lasts up to 1½ hours. Subsequently, the renal blood flow continues to decline as the ureteric pressure rises and this decline persists even after the ureteric pressure reduces.[10] In the unobstructed contralateral kidney, however, RBF increases and is a mirror image of the changes noted in the kidney with ureteral obstruction (Figure 47.2).[10] This may represent an early hemodynamic compensatory mechanism. In experimental models, RBF and GFR have been noted to be persistently decreased by as much as 40% from baseline even after release of the obstruction, suggesting a long-lasting impact of urinary obstruction on renal structure and function.[11]

### Renin-angiotensin system activation in obstructive uropathy

Numerous experimental studies have demonstrated an important role for the renin-angiotensin system (RAS) in

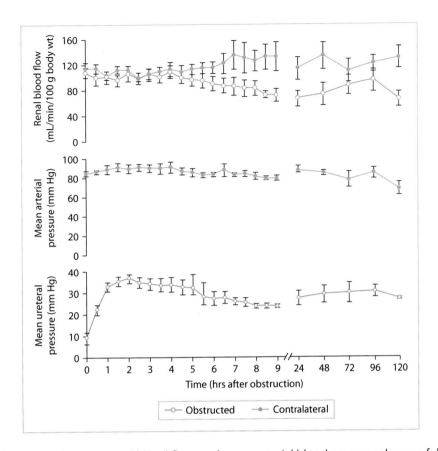

Figure 47.2 Ureteral pressure changes, renal blood flow, and mean arterial blood pressure changes following unilateral ureteral obstruction in lambs. Mean ureteral pressure increased from a baseline of 9 to 37 mm Hg (P < 0.001) 2 hours after obstruction but gradually decreased to 24 mm Hg after 24 hours and remained elevated for 5 days. Renal blood flow in the obstructed kidney remained unchanged for the first 5 hours, then there was a downward trend and it remained significantly lower for 5 days after obstruction. Blood flow in the contralateral kidney tended to increase after 5 hours and it remained above baseline for 5 days. Blood flow is represented as mean percent change ± standard error of the mean after obstruction. (Reproduced with permission from: Kim KM, Bogaert GA, Nguyen HT, et al. Hemodynamic changes after complete unilateral ureteral obstruction in the young lamb. J Urol. 1997;158:1090–3.)

modulating renal and collecting system development. Mice with angiotensinogen *(Agt)*, *renin*, angiotensin-converting enzyme *(ACE)*, or angiotensin II receptor type 1 *(AT1)* receptor gene mutations exhibit severe medullary hypoplasia and hydronephrosis.[12] Emerging evidence suggests that *RAS* gene mutations may be associated with diverse types of CAKUT in humans. Mutations in the genes encoding *Agt*, *renin*, *ACE*, or *AT1* receptor have been associated with renal tubular dysgenesis (RTD, Online Mendelian Inheritance in Man [OMIM] 267430) in one study.[13] These patients with RTD exhibit severe hypotension, thickening of renal arterial walls, reduced number of proximal tubules, collapsed collecting ducts, and interstitial fibrosis, but do not manifest severe medullary hypoplasia and hydronephrosis that are observed in mice with *Agt, renin, ACE,* or *AT1* receptor mutations.[12] The reasons for different renal phenotypes observed in mice but not in humans with *RAS* gene mutations are not clear. It is possible that differences in timing for completion of nephrogenesis, unique renal morphology in mice with a single papilla, or variability in renal tissue *RAS* activity in relation to critical periods of metanephric organogenesis may contribute these species-specific phenotypic expressions. Although clinical studies have suggested an association of other types of CAKUT with mutations in components of the *RAS* in children, this has not been confirmed in others.[12,14]

## Influencing genes in obstructive uropathy

Mice with targeted deletion of a disintegrin and metalloproteinase with thrombospondin motifs 1(ADAMTS1), lysosomal membrane protein LIMP-2/L GP85, calcineurin, sonic hedgehog cell surface effector smoothened (Smo) or transgenic megabladder mice develop urinary tract obstruction in the postnatal period.[15-19] Functional obstruction observed in *Smo*-deficient mice is due to ureter dyskinesia from loss

---

### KEY POINTS

- RAS plays an important role in renal development.
- Genes affecting ureteral muscle development may play a role in congenital obstructive uropathy.

of ureteral pacemaker cells.[19] Targeted deletion of *Smad4*, a signaling molecule critical for transcriptional responses to transforming growth factor-β (TGF-β and bone morphogenic protein 4 (BMP4) signaling in the ureteral and bladder mesenchyme during embryogenesis, results in bilateral UPJ obstruction and hydronephrosis from functional obstruction secondary to abnormal pyeloureteral peristalsis during embryogenesis.[20] Subsequent bending and luminal constriction of the ureter at the UPJ account for the transition from a functional into a more damaging and permanent physical obstruction. These observations suggest that early intervention of milder obstruction may prevent more irreversible damage to the urinary tract.[20] Emerging evidence points to an important role for epigenetic regulators in the pathophysiology of obstructive uropathy. In this regard, conditional ablation of *Brg1*, a member of Swi/Snf transcription complex, in mouse ureter results in hydroureter as a result of reduced smooth muscle cell development.[21] These observations, furthermore, point to the critical role played by ureteral muscular development and peristalsis in the pathogenesis of some cases of congenital hydronephrosis.

## Impact of obstructive uropathy on renal development

Clinical and experimental evidence indicates that urinary obstruction during early development has deleterious consequences on the structure and function of the developing kidney. Compared to the adult kidney, the developing kidney is highly susceptible to injury from obstruction to urine flow.[22] A variety of experimental models have been used to investigate the pathophysiology of congenital obstructive uropathy. UUO or urethral obstruction in fetal sheep results in hydronephrosis, renal dysplasia, and marked changes in renal growth.[23] UUO in the fetal rhesus monkey disrupts branching of the ureteric bud, an embryonic precursor of the renal collecting system (pelvis, ureter, collecting ducts).[24] Over the past two decades, much has been learned from studies of the developing rat and mouse.[25] Whereas nephrogenesis in humans is complete by the 36th week of gestation, nephrogenesis in the rat and mouse proceeds after birth.[3] Thus, surgical obstruction of the ureter in the neonatal rat or mouse is analogous to ureteral obstruction in the mid to late trimester of the human fetus.

Transient complete UUO in the neonatal rat impairs growth of the obstructed kidney, which correlates well with the duration of obstruction (Figure 47.3).[26] This suggests that a delay in the relief of severe obstruction can permanently impair the growth potential of the kidney. Chronic partial UUO in the neonatal rat also impairs renal growth, an effect that depends on the severity of obstruction.[27] There appears to be a critical reduction in ureteral diameter (65%) that, if exceeded, results in impaired renal growth. Because renal growth is a major determinant of long-term renal function, a better understanding of the "critical" ureteral stenosis in humans may permit the development of a better definition of clinically significant obstruction.

Chronic UUO delays maturation of all the major components of the nephron, from the glomerulus to the collecting duct, as well as the microvasculature and renal interstitium.[28] As a consequence of obstruction, there are also major hemodynamic changes with profound renal vasoconstriction mediated by the RAS (already highly activated in the developing kidney compared to the adult kidney).[29-34] Although the renal vasoconstriction is modulated by endogenous vasodilators such as prostaglandins and nitric oxide, the net balance favors vasoconstriction.[35,36] There is increased renin production by afferent arterioles and an upregulation of molecules induced by activation of the RAS.[32,37,38]

### KEY POINTS

- Urinary obstruction affects renal development.
- Tubulointerstitial fibrosis and atrophy in obstructive uropathy result from induction of numerous cytokines in response to stretch stress injury.

Chronic severe obstructive uropathy is characterized by the development of tubular atrophy and interstitial fibrosis, both of which contribute to impaired renal growth (Figure 47.4). Tubular atrophy results from progressive destruction of tubular epithelial cells by apoptosis, or programmed cell death.[39,40] Chronic partial UUO in the neonatal rat leads to apoptosis of epithelial cells in the dilated collecting ducts and the characteristic atrophic tubules with thickened basement membranes.[27] Stimuli leading to tubular apoptosis include mechanical stretch of epithelial cells in dilated tubules and altered gene expression.[28,40-44] Renal tubular expression of epidermal growth factor (EGF), which is a survival factor, is reduced by UUO, and expression of TFG-β1 (a proapoptotic factor) is increased by UUO.[28] The balance of survival and death signals is tipped in favor of cell death, leading to progressive loss of renal mass.[45]

Chronic UUO also has profound effects on the renal interstitium, leading to infiltration by macrophages and fibroblasts, which release cytokines such as TGF-β1 (Figure 47.5).[44] Activated macrophages and their products can induce both tubular apoptosis and progressive interstitial fibrosis.[46] This can involve the transformation of interstitial fibroblasts to myofibroblasts that express α-smooth muscle actin, and release additional fibrogenic molecules.[28] Most remarkable is the recent discovery that mechanical stretching of tubular cells and changes in the local production of growth factors, cytokines, and chemokines can lead to transformation of renal tubular epithelial cells to assume mesenchymal characteristics.[47,48] Tubular cells undergoing epithelial-mesenchymal transformation can differentiate into fibroblasts that augment the progression of interstitial fibrosis.[49] The multiple interacting processes depicted in Figure 47.3 are dynamic and

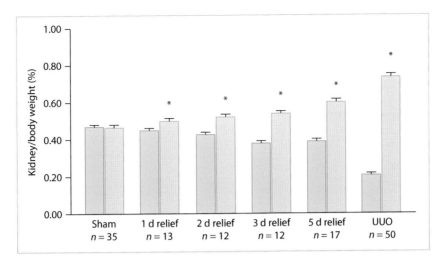

Figure 47.3 The ratio of kidney to body weight of obstructed (pink) and contralateral (blue) kidneys of neonatal rats 28 days following sham operation, following relief of 1 to 5 days of unilateral ureteral obstruction (UUO) and following persistent complete UUO. *$P < 0.05$ versus sham. (Reproduced with permission from: Chevalier RL, Thornhill BA, Wolstenholme JT, et al. Unilateral ureteral obstruction in early development alters renal growth: dependence on the duration of obstruction. J Urol. 1999;161:309–14.)

activated by the persistence of significant urinary tract obstruction. Recent studies demonstrate that pharmacologic antagonism of TGF-β1 receptor aggravates obstructive renal injury from UUO in neonatal mice, indicating caution for pediatric use of TGFβ1 inhibitors.[50] A more thorough understanding of these interactions may lead to improved therapies for obstructive uropathy by interfering with tubular apoptosis, macrophage infiltration, or epithelial-mesenchymal transformation. Once this process has progressed to tubular atrophy and extensive interstitial fibrosis, the impairment of renal growth becomes irreversible.

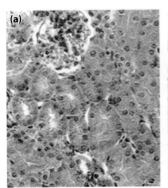
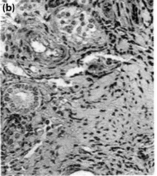

Figure 47.4 Renal interstitial collagen and tubular atrophy after sham operation or in chronic obstructive nephropathy during postnatal development. Light microscopy of kidney from neonatal mice (a) following sham operation and (b) chronic unilateral ureteral obstruction showing marked interstitial fibrosis and tubular atrophy. (Reproduced with permission from: Fern RJ, Yesko CM, Thornhill BA, et al. Reduced angiotensinogen expression attenuates renal interstitial fibrosis in obstructive nephropathy in mice. J Clin Invest. 1999;103:39–46.)

## NEPHRON LOSS IN OBSTRUCTIVE UROPATHY

Even transient complete UUO during nephrogenesis or during nephron maturation can lead to a permanent loss of nephrons mass in the obstructed kidney.[51,52] Chronic partial UUO in the neonatal rat also reduces nephron number, although the loss of nephrons takes place over a longer period.[27] As with any loss of renal mass, chronic UUO leads to compensatory growth of the contralateral kidney (see Figure 47.3). This "counterbalance" is very finely tuned and develops after even short periods of ureteral obstruction.[26,53] Because the severity of urinary tract obstruction in clinical practice is usually asymmetrically distributed between the two kidneys, adaptive growth by the remaining nephrons may occur in both kidneys. Current limitations in detecting such adaptive growth lie in the relative lack of precision in imaging techniques, as well as in the measurement of differential renal function.[54]

## TUBULAR DYSFUNCTION IN OBSTRUCTIVE UROPATHY

Chronic obstructive uropathy leads to impaired tubular function, which can have significant clinical implications. Downregulation of sodium transporters and aquaporins and distortion of the medullary architecture contribute to limited renal concentrating capacity.[55,56] These factors also contribute to the phenomenon of postobstructive diuresis that often follows the relief of severe bilateral urinary tract obstruction (such as PUV).[56] Because positive sodium balance is necessary for normal somatic growth in infancy, impaired growth is another consequence of reduced renal sodium reabsorption in obstructive uropathy.[57] Thus, infants may require sodium supplements to prevent volume

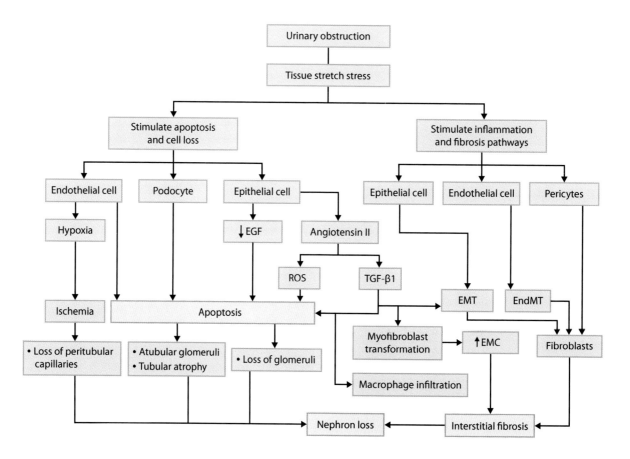

Figure 47.5 Schematic representation of the pathogenesis of obstructive nephropathy. Downstream obstruction to urine flow causes mechanical stretching and dilation of tubules, leading to apoptosis and epithelial-mesenchymal transition (EMT) of the tubular epithelial cells. Affected epithelial cells downregulate epidermal growth factor (EGF) and activate the local renin-angiotensin system (angiotensin II) that stimulates the expression of transforming growth factor- $\beta_1$ (TGF-$\beta_1$) and the generation of reactive oxygen species (ROS). This leads to interstitial macrophage recruitment and the generation of monocyte chemoattractant protein-1 (MCP-1), adhesion molecules, and tumor necrosis factor-$\alpha$ (TNF$\alpha$). This contributes to apoptosis of epithelial and endothelial cells, podocytes, leading to renal hypoxia and ischemia, loss of peritubular capillaries and glomeruli, proximal tubular disruption, tubular atrophy and atubular glomeruli. Phenotypic transition occurs in EMT, endothelial cells (EndMTs), pericytes, as they become fibroblasts, which in turn develop into myofibroblasts that express $\alpha$-smooth muscle actin ($\alpha$-SMA). Myofibroblasts contribute to expansion of the extracellular matrix (ECM) and progressive fibrosis. The end result is progressive loss of all components of the nephron.

contraction and optimize somatic growth. Somatic growth also may be limited in obstructive uropathy by abnormal distal tubular potassium and hydrogen ion secretion as a result of type 4 renal tubular acidosis (RTA).[58] These tubular defects can lead to hyperkalemia and metabolic acidosis, even with unilateral obstruction, and may persist even after surgical relief of the obstruction.[59,60]

### KEY POINTS

- Nephron loss and tubular dysfunction are common accompaniments of congenital obstructive uropathy.
- Renal salt wasting and metabolic acidosis resulting from distal RTA are common in obstructive uropathy.

## CLINICAL FEATURES

## PRENATAL DETECTION

Most cases of congenital obstructive uropathy are detected by prenatal ultrasonography, usually performed between 16 and 20 weeks of gestation. Measurement of the anteroposterior diameter of the renal pelvis obtained in the maximal transverse plane (usually near hilum region) in ultrasound has been used as an index of the severity of hydronephrosis (Figure 47.6). There is lack of consensus on grading the fetal and neonatal hydronephrosis, but the criteria developed by the Society for Fetal Urology (SFU) provide a clinically applicable platform (Figure 47.7).[61]

The risk for clinically significant urinary tract obstruction is increased when the fetal renal pelvic diameter exceeds 6 mm at less than 20 weeks, 8 mm at 20 to 30 weeks,

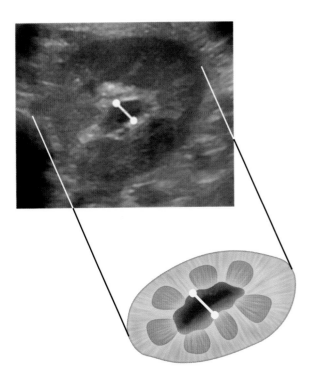

Figure 47.6 Renal ultrasound showing anatomic points used to determine the anteroposterior diameter (APD) of renal pelvis in ultrasound evaluation of hydronephrosis. The kidney is seen in a transverse image at the level of renal hilum. White bar represents the APD of pelvis.

or 10 mm at more than 30 weeks of gestation.[62] However, the diagnosis of fetal hydronephrosis based on renal pelvic dimensions can be misleading. Not only is the reliability of the measurement operator-dependent, the high urine flow of the fetus can cause relative distention of the pelvis and

normal dimensions following fetal voiding, even with a partially obstructed ureter.

Equally important in the prenatal diagnosis of obstructive uropathy is to determine whether the lesion is unilateral or bilateral, the presence of ureteral dilatation, whether the bladder is dilated or has a thickened wall, and if other organ system abnormalities are present. Dilatation of renal calyces also should be looked for in the ultrasound evaluation, because greater severity of calyceal dilatation indicates a clinically significant hydronephrosis.[63] Suspected fetal hydronephrosis should be confirmed by postnatal ultrasonography. It is important to note that not all cases of fetal hydronephrosis are due to urinary obstruction. Other diagnoses that can mimic neonatal hydronephrosis include vesicoureteral reflux (VUR), megacalicosis, and multicystic dysplastic kidney (Table 47.1 and Table 47.2).

Table 47.1 Causes of dilated urinary tract in the fetus and neonates

**True Hydronephrosis**

- Transient
- Ureteropelvic junction obstruction
- Vesicoureteral reflux
- Ureterocele
- Posterior urethral valves
- Nonobstructive hydronephrosis

**Hydronephrosis Mimickers**

- Multicystic dyplastic kidney
- Megaureter
- Megacalycosis
- Large renal cysts

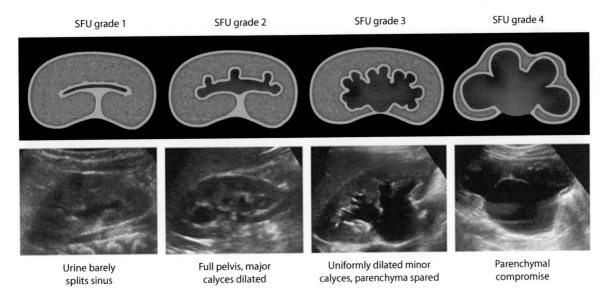

| SFU grade 1 | SFU grade 2 | SFU grade 3 | SFU grade 4 |
| --- | --- | --- | --- |
| Urine barely splits sinus | Full pelvis, major calyces dilated | Uniformly dilated minor calyces, parenchyma spared | Parenchymal compromise |

Figure 47.7 Society for Fetal Urology (SFU) grading system for antenatal hydronephrosis. (Reproduced with permission from: Timberlake MD, Herndon CDA. Mild to moderate postnatal hydronephrosis: grading systems and management. Nat Rev Urol. 2013;10:649–5.)

Table 47.2 Prenatal ultrasound findings of obstructive uropathies and other CAKUT disorders

| Cause | Incidence (%) | Prenatal ultrasound findings |
|---|---|---|
| Transient/physiologic | 50–70 | Isolated hydronephrosis, most often mild |
| Ureteropelvic junction (UJP) obstruction | 10–30 | Moderately (10–15 mm) or severely (>15 mm) dilated renal pelvis in the absence of any dilation of ureter or bladder |
| Vesicoureteral reflux (VUR) | 10–40 | Variation in the degree of antidiuretic during the time of ultrasound evaluation (in general, there are no specific ultrasound findings that are pathognomonic) |
| Ureterovesical junction (UVJ) obstruction | 5–15 | Hydronephrosis and dilated ureter to level of the UVJ |
| Multicystic dysplastic kidney (MCDK) | 2–5 | Varying sizes of randomly located renal cysts, a large noncommunicating central cyst, and nonrenoform shape |
| Posterior urethral valves (PUVs) | 1–5 | A combination of posterior urethral dilatation (keyhole sign), a full bladder with thickened wall, oligohydramnios or anhydramnios, unilateral or bilateral hydronephrosis, increased renal echogenicity |
| Ureterocele | 1–3 | A cystic mass in the bladder, and hydroureteronephrosis to the level of the obstructing ureterocele |
| Less common causes: Ectopic ureter, urethral atresia, prune belly syndrome, polycystic kidney diseases, and renal cysts | <1 | |

Source: Yamaçake KG, Nguyen HT. Current management of antenatal hydronephrosis. Pediatr Nephrol. 2013;28:237–43. Reproduced with permission

Radiologic findings of PUV in fetal ultrasound evaluation are characterized by a thickened bladder wall, bilaterally dilated ureters, and the so-called keyhole sign (Figure 47.8).

In addition to a direct impact on the bilateral renal development and function in the fetus, LUTO, such as PUV, also has a clinically significant impact on pulmonary development. Severe oligohydramnios resulting from reduced fetal urine output in PUV leads to pulmonary hypoplasia that can be even more life-threatening in the immediate postnatal period than renal failure itself. Therefore, estimation of amniotic fluid volume is critical in the evaluation of any fetus suspected of CAKUT. Severe cases of PUV can develop Potter syndrome, characterized by oligohydramnios, pulmonary hypoplasia, and typical facial appearance of a broad nasal bridge, low-set ears and epicanthic folds. Severe cases of LUTO also may develop fetal urinomas or urinary ascites, resulting from rupture of urinary bladder or other parts of the dilated urinary tract. In one study the incidence of urinomas in PUV was reported to be 15%.[64] Postnatally, these patients may have pseudoazotemia secondary to reabsorption of urea nitrogen present in leaked urine in the peritoneal cavity. Concurrent renal maldevelopment, such as dysplasia, is common in patients with LUTO (Figure 47.9), which leads to progressive CKD and ESRD in these children.

Fetal urinary sodium and osmolality can be used to predict fetal outcome in suspected bladder outlet obstruction. Normally, fetal urine sodium concentration is less than 90 mmol/L at 20 to 30 weeks of gestation.[65] Higher fetal urinary sodium values are indicative of deranged tubular functions associated with renal maldevelopment. Similarly, fetal urine osmolality should be less than 200 mOsm/L, and higher values are consistent with significant renal impairment.[66] The sensitivity and specificity of fetal urine chemistries are not ideal, and the results lack predictive value.

## POSTNATAL PRESENTATION

A palpable abdominal mass is a common manifestation of obstructive uropathy in an infant or child. Such a mass may represent a large hydronephrotic kidney or an enlarged bladder resulting from LUTO, such as PUV. In older children, other symptoms may include flank pain, incontinence, urinary dribbling, urinary tract infection (UTI),

---

### KEY POINTS

- Nephron loss and tubular dysfunction are common accompaniments of congenital obstructive uropathy.
- Renal salt wasting and metabolic acidosis secondary to distal RTA can be seen in obstructive uropathy.
- Pulmonary hypoplasia can be the consequence of fetal urinary obstruction and poor urine output into the amniotic fluid.

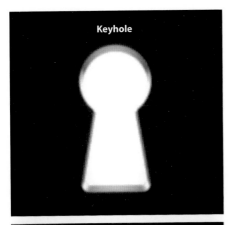

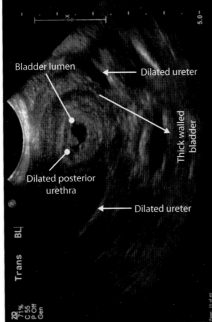

Figure 47.8 Fetal ultrasound showing the characteristic findings of "keyhole" sign.

or hematuria as a result of injury to the dilated urinary tract. Patients with imperforate anus or other organ system anomalies should be suspected of having obstructive uropathy. Patients with abnormalities such as preauricular tags or pits, Townes-Brocks syndrome, or branchio-oto-renal syndrome have a higher incidence of renal anomalies, including obstructive uropathy. LUTO is more common in male newborns and should be suspected in a neonate with antenatal diagnosis of bilateral hydronephrosis, or other clinical findings noted in Table 47.3.

Dietl crisis is a unique clinical presentation consisting of recurrent abdominal pain or flank pain seen in patients with undiagnosed UPJ obstruction. These painful crises are

Table 47.3 Clinical features suggestive of lower urinary tract obstruction in neonates, infants, and older children

**Neonate**
- Male predominance
- Bilateral antenatal hydronephrosis
- Oligohydramnios
- Fetal or neonatal urinary ascites
- Hematuria following birth (trauma to the enlarged urinary system)

**Infants and Children**
- Male predominance
- Urinary tract infection
- Urinary incontinence
- Large and thickened bladder mass
- Flank pain
- Visible hematuria (with or without trauma)

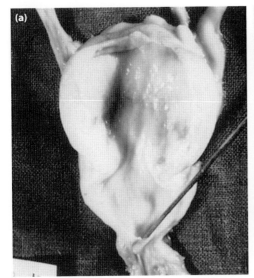

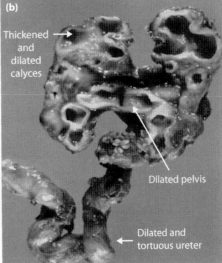

Figure 47.9 (a) Autopsy specimen of urinary bladder demonstrating posterior urethral valves (probe in place). Cut section of kidney (b) demonstrating dilated renal pelvicalyceal system and dilated ureter in lower urinary tract. Sparse and poorly differentiated renal tissue is noted. (Figure [a] courtesy of Barry Belman, MD; Figure [b] courtesy of Kathleen Patterson, MD.)

usually precipitated by increased fluid intake, in vigorous exercise, or when the bladder is full.

## DIAGNOSTIC EVALUATION

### Postnatal ultrasound

Several diagnostic algorithms have been proposed for evaluation of antenatal hydronephrosis.[66] The initial diagnostic study for patients with antenatal diagnosis of hydronephrosis, or for any infant with a suspicious prenatal ultrasound, should be to obtain a postnatal ultrasound of the kidneys, ureters, and bladder. In general, ultrasonography in newborns should be performed in a well-hydrated state several days after birth, because the degree of hydronephrosis may be underestimated if urine flow rate is low. Infants with LUTO, on the other hand, should have immediate imaging studies to determine the state of urinary dilatation and degree of hydronephrosis.

### Diuretic renography

Intravenous pyelography is indicated only in a rare circumstance in an older infant or child, in whom a better definition of urinary tract anatomy may be needed in preparation for surgical intervention. Most pediatric centers use radionuclide diuretic renography in place of conventional intravenous pyelography to determine the site of urinary obstruction (Figure 47.10). An added advantage of renography is that it provides information on the relative

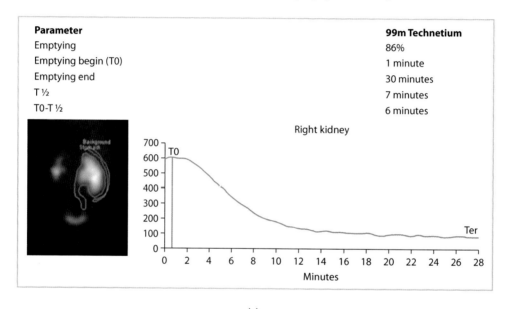

| Parameter | 99m Technetium |
|---|---|
| Emptying | 86% |
| Emptying begin (T0) | 1 minute |
| Emptying end | 30 minutes |
| T ½ | 7 minutes |
| T0–T ½ | 6 minutes |

(a)

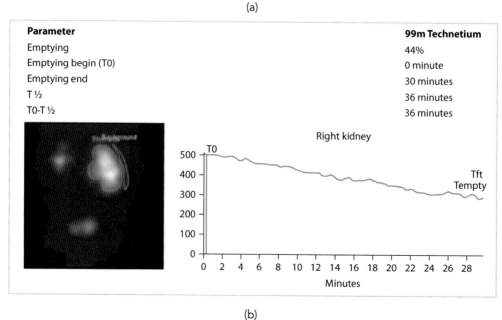

| Parameter | 99m Technetium |
|---|---|
| Emptying | 44% |
| Emptying begin (T0) | 0 minute |
| Emptying end | 30 minutes |
| T ½ | 36 minutes |
| T0–T ½ | 36 minutes |

(b)

Figure 47.10 (a) Diuretic renography showing normal excretion pattern, half-life 7 $T\frac{1}{2}$ minutes. (b) Pattern of prolonged $T\frac{1}{2}$ (>36 minutes) in a patient with ureteropelvic junction obstruction.

contribution of each kidney to total renal function. This study should be performed with a bladder catheter in place in the newborn. Unless there is an urgent need, such as in suspected LUTO, diuretic urography also should be delayed until the infant is several weeks of age, because maturation of renal concentration capacity significantly improves the imaging quality.[67]

## Contrast cystogram

Contrast voiding cystourethrography (VCUG) is indicated if the diagnosis of PUV is being considered in a male newborn or VUR is suspected (Figure 47.11). Radionuclide cystogram may provide a lesser degree of radiation to pelvic organs compared to that with contrast VCUG and may be considered in females suspected to have VUR. Interestingly, in patients with UPJ obstruction, VUR is often seen on the opposite-side urinary tract. Magnetic resonance imaging (MRI) offers some promise of enhanced resolution, better anatomic delineation, and functional information in some patients (Figure 47.12).[68] Although the combination of ultrasonography and renography provides useful diagnostic information in an infant with suspected obstructive uropathy, the decision for surgical correction or timing of such surgery is a clinical one that should involve the pediatric nephrologist, urologist, and radiologist.

## MANAGEMENT

## PRENATAL MANAGEMENT

Fetuses with unilateral hydronephrosis should be monitored with serial ultrasound examinations throughout pregnancy, for not only the degree of hydronephrosis but also the volume of amniotic fluid. Fetuses with bilateral hydronephrosis and oligohydramnios should be suspected to have LUTO and are at risk for the development of pulmonary hypoplasia. In utero fetal surgical interventions, with the aim of improving renal and pulmonary outcome, and overall fetal survival in severely affected fetuses have been attempted since early 1980s. Such interventions consist of either repeated fetal vesicocentesis procedures or placement of a vesicoamniotic shunt. The aim of such treatments is to decompress the urinary tract and increase the amniotic

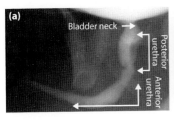
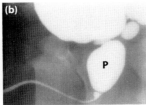

Figure 47.11 Contrast vesicocystourethrogram.
**(a)** Showing normal urethral anatomy. **(b)** Radiologic findings in a patient with posterior urethral valves (P).

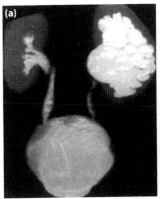
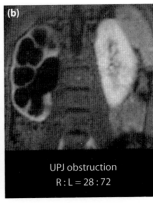

UPJ obstruction
R : L = 28 : 72

Figure 47.12 Magnetic resonance imaging **(a)** showing maximum intensity projection reconstruction after gadopentetic acid (Gd-DTPA) infusion in a patient with left ureteropelvic junction (UPJ) obstruction. Magnetic resonance image demonstrating differential renal function in post–Gd-DTPA **(b)** in UPJ obstruction (R/L ratio, 28:72). (Reproduced with permission from: Perez-Brayfield MR, Kirsch AJ, Jones RA, et al. A prospective study comparing ultrasound, nuclear scintigraphy and dynamic contrast enhanced magnetic resonance imaging in the evaluation of hydronephrosis. J Urol. 2003;170:1330–34.)

fluid volume to prevent associated pulmonary hypoplasia. The results of such interventions, however, have been largely disappointing, with a high incidence of displacement of the catheter, amnionitis, and fetal loss.[69,70]

Despite prenatal vesicoamniotic shunts for LUTO, ESRD developed in 30% of patients after a mean follow-up of only 5.8 years.[71] Even in fetuses with successful retention of the diversion catheter through the pregnancy and normal postnatal pulmonary functions, long-term renal function may still be poor.[64] This is likely due to aberrant renal development in the first trimester, before the kidneys and urinary tract are reliably identified by maternal sonography. Unfortunately, an international prospective randomized trial on the percutaneous vesicoamniotic shunting versus conservative management for fetal lower urinary tract obstruction (PLUTO) had to be terminated early for lack of adequate recruitment of patients.[70]

### KEY POINT

Fetal vesicoamniotic shunt placement, although technically feasible, has not succeeded in improving renal survival in antenatal diagnosis of urinary tract obstruction.

## POSTNATAL MANAGEMENT

The postnatal management of the infant with obstructive uropathy depends on the specific findings from the imaging evaluations described earlier. A management pathway, based on SFU grading, has been suggested recently by Timberlake and Herndon, and is shown in Figure 47.13.[72]

## Ureteropelvic junction obstruction

For the infant with unilateral UPJ obstruction, mild obstruction (without caliectasis) may be followed with sequential renal ultrasound examinations, because many of these patients will undergo progressive and spontaneous improvement of the obstruction.[73] There is considerable controversy about the management of infants with moderate-to-severe UPJ obstruction. Some centers have reported good results with close monitoring over the long term, and others recommend early surgical correction.[73–78]

Based on the principles of pathogenesis outlined earlier and to avoid ongoing renal damage, the truly "conservative" approach in significant UPJ obstruction is to consider an early pyeloplasty.[77,78] Difficulties of subjecting infants to repeated diuretic renography, noncompliance with a rigorous schedule of imaging studies, and the potential for irreversible loss of renal function should be taken into account in the clinical decision-making process.[79] Although most

pediatric urologists are reluctant to postpone surgical correction in infants with bilateral UPJ obstruction, Onen et al.[80] advocated nonoperative management with close follow-up during the first 2 years of life. Significant concerns associated with observational approach in bilateral UPJ obstruction, especially the difficulty in compliance with a rigorous imaging schedule, have been stressed by Peters.[81]

## Lower urinary tract obstruction

In infants with bilateral hydronephrosis, and in any male infant suspected to have LUTO, a voiding cystogram should be obtained promptly to rule out the possibility of PUV. If the diagnosis of PUV is established, the bladder should be continually drained with a sterile 5-Fr feeding tube and serial plasma creatinine concentration should be measured until it stabilizes.

Many cases of LUTO are associated with VUR or with secondary ureteral obstruction resulting from kinking of the dilated ureters. Pending a complete radiologic evaluation, it is prudent to treat infants with prophylactic antibiotics to minimize the possibility of UTI and septicemia. Oral

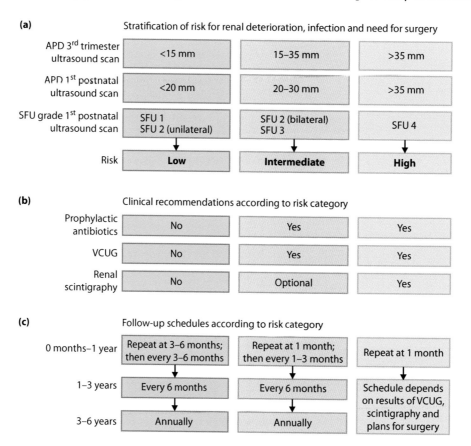

Figure 47.13 Risk-stratification algorithm for postnatal hydronephrosis. Risk category for each patient will also be influenced by factors that include gender, circumcision status, presence of a solitary kidney, bilateral hydronephrosis, the presence of impaired renal function, and whether bladder outlet obstruction is suspected. (a) Stratification of patients by risk for renal deterioration, infection, and need for surgery on the basis of the renal ultrasonography findings. (b) Clinical recommendations according to risk category. (c) Follow-up ultrasonography schedule according to risk category. APD, anteroposterior diameter; SFU, Society for Fetal Urology; VCUG, Contrast voiding cystourethrography. (Reproduced with permission from: Timberlake MD, Herndon CDA. Mild to moderate postnatal hydronephrosis: grading systems and management. Nat Rev Urol. 2013;10:649–5.)

amoxicillin, 25 mg/kg daily, should be used in the neonate or infant (unless there are specific contraindications).

To optimize growth, infants with obstructive uropathy may require increased sodium intake or alkali therapy after surgical relief of obstruction, to manage natriuresis or distal RTA seen in these patients.[82] Hyperkalemia may be a feature of distal RTA in some patients and needs to be treated with low-potassium formula feeds and with potassium exchange resins.[58,59]

---

### KEY POINTS

- Neonates with LUTO need relief of obstruction by either cutaneous vesicostomy or PUV ablation.
- Not all patients with unilateral UPJ obstruction need surgical relief. Many can be followed by renal ultrasound and radionuclide scans.
- Medical management includes attention to maintaining fluid, electrolyte, and acid-base balance.
- Prophylactic antibiotics to prevent UTI are generally recommended.

---

Primary ablation of the PUV is challenging in neonates because of the small urethral caliber, but may be possible in some centers. If valve ablation is not technically feasible in the neonate, a cutaneous vesicostomy may be the bridging drainage procedure of choice, especially in the low-birth-weight neonates. Definitive PUV ablation and closure of the vesicostomy can be attempted at a later age. Bladder dysfunction is common in older children with a history of PUV. Dysfunctional bladder and associated postvoid residual urinary volume in the bladder may lead to recurrent UTIs and persistently dilated urinary tracts. Use of α-adrenergics, has been advocated by some to decrease the postvoid residues, but pediatric use of these drugs in this indication has not yet been approved by the US Food and Drug Administration in the United States. A clean intermittent catheterization trial to keep the bladder in a decompressed state may be considered as the initial intervention in such patients. If successful, Mitrofanoff appendicovesicostomy and augmentation of the bladder may be an option for others with severe bladder dysfunction associated with PUV, especially those being considered for renal transplantation.

## LONG-TERM IMPACT OF OBSTRUCTIVE UROPATHIES

Over time, some patients with UPJ obstruction often develop glomerular sclerosis, likely from ongoing hyperfiltration injury.[83,84] Similar morphologic changes have also been noted 1 year after release of transient complete UUO in the neonatal rat.[54] Immediate surgical intervention for relief of urinary obstruction is not generally necessary in most neonates, and follow-up by ultrasound and radionuclide scans is an acceptable strategy, especially in those with mild-to-moderate hydronephrosis.[72] Nevertheless, approximately 20% to 25% of babies born with UPJ require surgical intervention within the first year of life because of progressive increase in hydronephrosis. Kumar et al.[84] reported that in 762 infants with antenatally diagnosed hydronephrosis, 103 patients (13.5%) had severe hydronephrosis (anteroposterior diameter [APD] of >15 mm). UPJ obstruction was confirmed in 48 cases, of which 10 (20.8%) required surgical intervention within the first year of life.[84]

It is important to note that renal function may not normalize despite pyeloplasty in patients with severe UPJ obstruction.[86,87] In a long-term follow-up study of children after pyeloplasty for unilateral UPJ obstruction, Boubaker et al.[87] noted that despite renal function (measured by radio-nuclide renography) improvement in all but one patient, 14 of 33 patients developed CKD.[7]

---

### KEY POINT

Patients with obstructive uropathy need to be monitored for evolution of CKD over the long-term horizon.

---

For patients with PUV and other types of bladder outlet obstruction, continued monitoring of renal function is essential. Despite surgical correction of the obstruction, many of the prenatally diagnosed PUV patients develop CKD in the second decade of life (Figure 47.14). Roth et al.[88] reported that over a mean follow up of 11.3 ± 2.1 years, 7 of the 10 (70%) patients surgically treated for PUV as infants developed ESRD. In a Finnish study, Heikkilä et al.[89] followed 193 boys treated for PUV as infants into adulthood

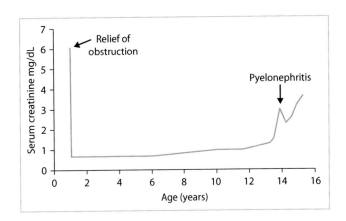

Figure 47.14 Progression of chronic kidney disease in a patient with posterior urethral valve (PUV). Serum creatinine concentration is plotted against time in years. After surgical relief of PUV, patient's serum creatinine remained below 1 mg/dL for a decade before he developed pyelonephritis. Despite effective treatment of infection he continued to have worsening renal function and developed end-stage renal disease. (Figure courtesy of Robert Chevalier, MD.)

(median age 31 years). Of these, 44 (22.8%) patients progressed to ESRD. Lifetime risk for ESRD in these patients was 28.5% (standard error 3.8%).

In another study of 312 children with CAKUT followed for a median of 6 years (2 to 30 years), the risk for ESRD was highest in patients with PUV (Figure 47.15).[8] Correlation of the timing of diagnosis of PUV with outcome has been evaluated in several studies. Diagnosis after age 1 year is associated with better renal function outcome and risk for ESRD.[90] It has been suggested that prenatal presentation may represent more severe form of the obstructive uropathy and this may be associated with a significant degree of renal dysplasia in these patients.[91] Some studies have noted that a nadir serum creatinine greater than 1 mg/dL after PUV surgery, presence of bladder dysfunction, and VUR may be additional factors associated with risk for ESRD.[92]

## CLINICAL FOLLOW-UP

Clinical follow-up of infants and children with obstructive uropathy should include regular monitoring of blood pressure, urinalysis, renal function by plasma creatinine concentration or cystatin C, and renal ultrasound (Table 47.4). Urine culture may be considered, if clinically indicated, and individualized strategies to minimize urinary tract infections need to be considered. Renal ultrasound permits evaluation of renal growth, as well as assessing the progress of hydronephrosis. Monitoring the rate of growth of the normal contralateral kidney, representing compensatory hypertrophy, has been suggested as an index of functional impairment of the obstructed kidney.[93,94] It is important to emphasize that serial measurements are necessary to detect the subtle changes in renal dimensions over time.[95,96] Radionuclide renal scans with diuretics may be indicated

for following renal function and determining the degree of urinary obstruction in some patients.

The patient family should also be counseled to maintain adequate hydration and sodium repletion in the patient, particularly during hot weather. Use of nephrotoxic drugs, such as nonsteroidal anti-inflammatory compounds, should be avoided. Likelihood of progression of renal disease and development of CKD, regardless of the time of diagnosis and surgical intervention, should be discussed with the parents of children with congenital urinary obstruction. Although patients with obstructive uropathy often suffer from urinary sodium wasting secondary to tubulointerstitial dysfunction, children with intermittent complete obstruction resulting from severe UPJ stenosis can develop hypertension.[97] Hypertension in such cases may result from progressive interstitial fibrosis or glomerular sclerosis. Hypertension is, by itself, a determinant of progression of renal disease; therefore, it is critical to monitor blood pressure and to treat hypertension appropriately.

**Table 47.4** Principles of follow-up of congenital obstructive uropathy

- Monitor blood pressure and prevent hypertension
- Monitor urinary protein excretion and urinalysis
- Monitor renal function (serum creatinine or cystatin-C concentration)
- Renal ultrasound
- Prevent urinary infection
- Avoid dehydration
- Avoid use of nonsteroidal anti-inflammatory drugs

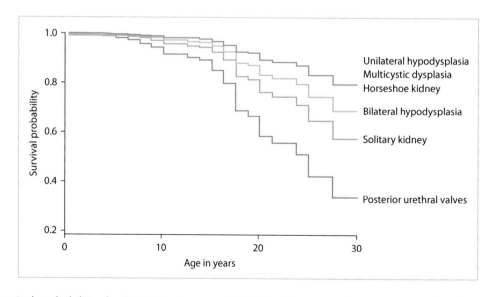

Figure 47.15 Survival probabilities by CAKUT category, adjusted for the concomitant presence of vesicoureteral reflux, time varying values of serum creatinine (mg per 100 mL) and proteinuria (X1 g/day vs. less), and referral period (before 1990 vs. 1990 and thereafter). (Reproduced with permission from: Sanna-Cherchi S, Ravani P, Corbani V, et al. Renal outcome in patients with congenital anomalies of the kidney and urinary tract. Kidney Int. 2009;76:528–33.)

# PREVENTING PROGRESSION

Emerging evidence suggests that the patient's genotype is a significant determinant of renal disease progression and *ACE* gene polymorphisms can have a profound impact on the rate of renal disease progression.[98] Angiotensin II and hypertension are risk factors for proteinuria associated with progressive renal disease, and proteinuria itself may further accelerate glomerular and tubular injury.[99] Since the intrarenal RAS is highly activated in obstructive uropathy, inhibition of angiotensin by ACE inhibitors or angiotensin receptor blockers (ARBs) can have a salutary effect on both the hemodynamic and the fibrotic consequences of chronic urinary tract obstruction (Table 47.5). Inhibition of angiotensin can impair normal renal development and maturation through the period of infancy, especially in premature infants.[100,101] In addition, RAS inhibition can markedly reduce intraglomerular pressure and GFR in neonates and infants, necessitating close monitoring.[102,103]

# PROTEOMIC TOOLS FOR MONITORING PROGRESSION

Renal histology and ultrasonographic findings in infants and children with obstructive uropathy correlate poorly with renal function.[104] It is also well accepted that plasma creatinine concentration and urine protein excretion are relatively insensitive markers for CKD resulting from obstructive uropathy. Abnormalities in serum concentrations in these patients are noted only with significantly advanced renal disease. Prospective urinary proteome analysis in neonates with congenital obstructive uropathy is a promising technology that may allow early detection and a more accurate follow-up of progression of CKD in these patients.[1,105]

As shown in Figure 47.5, TGF-β1 plays a central role in the pathophysiology of obstructive uropathy, and the expression of this cytokine is increased in dysplastic renal tubules.[106] Urinary excretion of TGF-β1 may be able to identify patients with early renal tissue injury secondary to urinary tract obstruction, even when it is unilateral (Figure 47.16).[107] L1 cell adhesion molecule (L1CAM) is another biomolecular marker that might be important in correlating renal injury with renal functional impairment. In boys with PUV, urinary TGF-β1 and L1CAM have been shown to be significantly increased and correlated negatively with GFR.[108] Other candidate biomarkers in the urine include monocyte chemoattractant protein-1 (MCP-1), which is increased in patients with UPJ obstruction and EGF, which is decreased in UPJ obstruction.[109] An inverse correlation of SFU grade of hydronephrosis and urinary EGF has been demonstrated, suggesting a possible use as a predictor of progression in obstruction.[110] Urinary kidney injury molecule-1 (KIM-1) and neutrophil gelatinase–associated lipocalin also may be potential predictors of progression of obstructive uropathy, even when renal function by conventional techniques is normal.[111]

Table 47.5 Therapeutic consequences of renin-angiotensin system inhibition in congenital obstructive uropathy

**Advantages**
- Control hypertension
- Reduce proteinuria
- Attenuate fibrosis

**Disadvantages**
- Impair renal development
- Reduce glomerular filtration rate
- Exacerbate sodium wasting

## SUMMARY

Given the broad spectrum of CAKUT in children and the variable clinical impact of different forms of obstructive uropathy, ranging from mild clinically asymptomatic cases to severe kidney injury manifesting before or after birth, each patient with obstructive uropathy requires individualized clinical management. Because morbidity in mild cases of obstructive uropathy may not manifest until later in life, these patients should be closely followed throughout life. Medical monitoring should include diet, nutritional status, growth, blood pressure, renal function, proteinuria, and urinary tract imaging. Close partnership between the pediatric nephrologist and pediatric urologist is essential to integrating medical and surgical management, as well as transition to appropriate specialists when the patient reaches adulthood. New biomarkers are needed to better assess disease progression and therapeutic strategies to slow progression of renal injury. Genetic counseling is recommended for all patients with familial cases of isolated obstructive uropathy, obstructive uropathy associated with other types of CAKUT, or newly diagnosed forms of obstructive uropathy that suggest the presence of genetic anomalies. Introduction of more sensitive array-based methods that allow screening for multiple gene mutations and unraveling a complex network of molecular interactions will help determine and predict occurrence and consequences of obstructive uropathy. Finally, establishment of shared large biorepositories of patients with obstructive uropathy/CAKUT for molecular, genetic, and translational studies will have a major impact on designing novel strategies to predict, prevent, and manage these malformations.

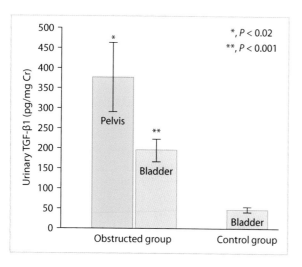

Figure 47.16 Mean urinary transforming growth factor-β (TGF-β₁) concentration in children with upper tract urinary obstruction versus controls, as corrected for creatinine (Cr). Bladder urine TGF-β₁ in obstructed group was fourfold that in control group. In the obstructed group, mean renal pelvic urine TGF-β₁ was twofold that in bladder urine. Bars represent mean ± standard error of the mean SEM. (Reproduced with permission from: Furness PD, III, Maizels M, Han SW, et al. Elevated bladder urine concentration of transforming growth factor-beta1 correlates with upper urinary tract obstruction in children. J Urol. 1999;162:1033–6.)

---

### Clinical Vignette 47.1

A male infant with antenatal diagnosis of bilateral hydronephrosis and oligohydramnios was born at 37 weeks of gestation and birth weight of 2.7 kg. On day 1 of birth he developed right-sided pneumothorax and voided normally. Postnatal ultrasound demonstrated bilateral severe left hydroureter. A VCUG established the diagnosis of PUV. He also had bilateral severe VUR, grade 5/5 on the left side and 4/5 on the right side. At 2 weeks his blood urea nitrogen (BUN) was 30 mg/dL, serum creatinine 1.8 mg/dL, and serum electrolytes normal. Transurethral PUV ablation was done successfully at 2 weeks of life. He was started on Similac PM 60/40 formula, alkali supplements, and calcitriol. Prophylactic antibiotics for prevention of UTI consisted of amoxicillin initially and trimethoprim-sulfamethoxazole subsequently. The patient was followed in the outpatient clinic.

Height and weight remained at approximately the 2nd percentile. He developed one episode of UTI at 4 years of age. The patient was lost to follow-up at 5 years of age. At 8 years of age he presented with urinary incontinence at school and being "smelly" in the classroom. He also had nocturnal enuresis. Examination showed height in the 2nd percentile and weight in 4th percentile. Blood pressure was normal for age (110/67 mm Hg). A large bladder mass filling the suprapubic area up to the umbilicus was noted on abdominal palpation. A VCUG test

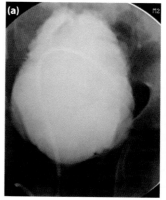 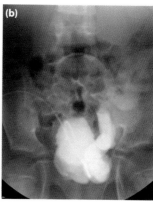

Figure 47.17 Contrast voiding cystourethrogram (VCUG) shows (a) a large urinary bladder with a highly trabeculated wall and (b) dilated posterior urethra.

demonstrated a large urinary bladder with a highly trabecular wall (Figure 47.17). Severe VUR persisted bilaterally, being worse on the left side. Electrolytes demonstrated sodium, 139 mmol/L; potassium, 4.5 mmol/L; chloride, 102 mmol/L; bicarbonate, 19 mmol/L; BUN, 24 mg/dL; creatinine, 1.7 mg/dL; calcium 8.6 mg/dL; phosphorus 5.4 mg/dL; and parathyroid hormone, 294 pg/mL. Estimated GFR (using the Schwartz equation) was 38 mL/min/1.73 m². Urodynamic studies showed bladder capacity of 340 mm³/mL; voiding pressure was elevated at 98 cm $H_2O$ and after voiding. The patient was restarted on erythropoietin for anemia, growth hormone for poor linear growth, calcitriol, alkali supplementation, and nutritional counseling. The patient was trained to do intermittent clean urethral catheterization, which provided relief from incontinence and symptoms of being "smelly" in the classroom. Nocturnal enuresis has also improved. At 11 years of age, he underwent a Mitrofanoff appendicovesicostomy procedure to facilitate urinary catheterization. At 12.5 years of age, his GFR declined and he was started on peritoneal dialysis.

### TEACHING POINTS

- This case traces the clinical course of a patient with PUV from antenatal diagnosis to the point of initiation of dialysis. The diagnosis of PUV was suspected because of bilateral hydronephrosis, and the diagnosis was confirmed postnatally by renal ultrasound and a VCUG.
- Despite a successful PUV ablation at 2 weeks of age, the patient continued to have abnormal renal function and CKD. Unfortunately, he was lost to follow-up and later presented with symptoms of bladder dysfunction (incontinence), in addition to CKD, growth failure, and anemia.
- Treatment of bladder dysfunction with intermittent catheterization resulted in improvement of clinical symptoms, but his CKD continued to progress.

- This case demonstrates the need for long-term follow-up of patients with obstructive uropathy, and interventions for treatment of CKD that may be necessary throughout the childhood and adolescence.

# REFERENCES

1. Chevalier RL, Peters CA. Congenital urinary tract obstruction: Proceedings of the State-Of-The-Art Strategic Planning Workshop—National Institutes of Health, Bethesda, MD, 11–12 March 2002. Pediatr Nephrol. 2003;18:576–606.

2. Collins A J, Foley R N, Herzog C, et al. US renal data system 2012 annual data report. Am J Kidney Dis. 2013;61:A7, e1–476.

3. Song R, Yosypiv IV. Genetics of congenital anomalies of the kidney and urinary tract. Pediatr Nephrol. 2011;26:353–64.

4. Lebowitz RL. Neonatal hydronephrosis: 146 cases. Radiol Clin North Am. 1977;15:49–54.

5. Flashner SC. Ureteroplevic junction. In: Kelalis PP, King LR, Belman AB, editors. Clinical Pediatric Urology. Philadelphia: Saunders; 1992. pp 693–705.

6. Woodward M, Frank D. Postnatal management of antenatal hydronephrosis. BJU Int. 2002;89:149–56.

7. Brown T, Mandell J, Lebowitz RL. Neonatal hydronephrosis in the era of sonography. Am J Radiol 1992; 148:959–964.

8. Sanna-Cherchi S, Ravani P, Corbani V, et al. Renal outcome in patients with congenital anomalies of the kidney and urinary tract. Kidney Int. 2009;76:528–33.

9. Kim KM, Bogaert GA, Nguyen HT, et al. Hemodynamic changes after complete unilateral ureteral obstruction in the young lamb. J Urol. 1997;158:1090–3.

10. Moody TE, Vaughan ED, Gillenwater JY. Relationship between renal blood flow and ureteral pressure during 18 hours of total unilateral ureteral occlusion: limplications for changing sites of increased renal resistance. Invest Urol. 1975;13,246–51.

11. Chaabane W, Praddaude F, Buleon M, et al. Renal functional decline and glomerulotubular injury are arrested but not restored by release of unilateral ureteral obstruction (UUO). Am J Physiol Renal Physiol. 304:F432–F439, 2013.

12. Yosypiv IV. Renin-angiotensin system in ureteric bud branching morphogenesis: Insights into the mechanisms. Pediatr Nephrol. 2011;26:1499–512.

13. Gribouval O, Gonzales M, Neuhaus T, et al. Mutations in genes in the renin-angiotensin system are associated with autosomal recessive renal tubular dysgenesis. Nat Genet 2005;37:964–8.

14. Hiraoka M, Taniguchi T, Nakai H et al. No evidence for AT2R gene derangement in human urinary tract anomalies. Kidney Int 2001; 59:1244.

15. Yokoyama H, Wada T, Kobayashi K, et al. A disintegrin and metalloproteinase with thrombospondin motifs (ADAMTS)-1 null mutant mice develop renal lesions mimicking obstructive nephropathy. Nephrol Dial Transplant. 2002;17:39–41.

16. Gamp AC, Tanaka Y, Lüllmann-RauchR, et al. LIMP-2/LGP85 deficiency causes ureteric pelvic junction obstruction, deafness and peripheral neuropathy in mice. Hum Mol Genet 2003;12:631–46.

17. Chang CP, McDill BW, Neilson JR, et al. Calcineurin is required inurinary tract mesenchyme for the development of the pyeloureteral peristaltic machinery. J Clin Invest 2004;113:1051–8.

18. Singh S, Robinson M, Nahi F, et al. Identification of a unique transgenic mouse line that develops mega bladder, obstructive uropathy, and renal dysfunction. J Am Soc Nephrol 2007; 18:461–71.

19. Cain JE, Islam E, Haxho F, et al. GLI3 repressor controls functional development of the mouse ureter. J Clin Invest. 2011;121:1199–2006.

20. Tripathi P, Wang Y, Casey AM, et al. Absence of canonical SMAD signaling in ureteral and bladder mesenchyme causes ureteropelvic junction obstruction. J Am Soc Nephrol. 2012;23:618–28.

21. Weiss RM, Guo S, Shan A, et al. Brg1 determines urothelial cell fate during ureter development. J Am Soc Nephrol. 2013;24:618–26.

22. Chevalier RL. Perinatal obstructive nephropathy. Semin Nephrol. 2004cx;28:124–129.

23. Peters CA. Animal models of fetal renal disease. Prenat Diagn. 2001;21:917–22.

24. Matsell DG, Mok A, Tarantal AF. Altered primate glomerular development due to in utero urinary tract obstruction. Kidney Int. 2002;61:1263–9.

25. Chevalier RL. Pathophysiology of obstructive nephropathy in the newborn. Semin Nephrol. 1998;18:585–9.

26. Chevalier RL, Thornhill BA, Wolstenholme JT, et al. Unilateral ureteral obstruction in early development alters renal growth: Dependence on the duration of obstruction. J Urol. 1999;161:309–14.

27. Thornhill BA, Burt LA, Chen C et al. Variable chronic partial ureteral obstruction in the neonatal rat: A new model of ureteropelvic junction obstruction. Kidney Int. 2005;67:42–7.

28. Chung KH, Chevalier RL. Arrested development of the neonatal kidney following chronic ureteral obstruction. J Urol. 1996;155:1139–1144.

29. Chevalier RL, Peach MJ. Hemodynamic effects of enalapril on neonatal chronic partial ureteral obstruction. Kidney Int. 1985;28:891–896.

30. Chevalier RL, Gomez RA. Response of the renin-angiotensin system to relief of neonatal ureteral obstruction. Am J Physiol. 1988;255:F1070–7.

31. El-Dahr SS, Gomez RA, Gray MS et al. In situ localization of renin and its mRNA in neonatal ureteral obstruction. Am J Physiol. 1990;258:F854–9.

32. Norwood VF, Carey RM, Geary KM et al. Neonatal ureteral obstruction stimulates recruitment of renin- secreting renal cortical cells. Kidney Int. 1994;45:1333–8.

33. Yoo KH, Norwood VF, El-Dahr SS et al. Regulation of angiotensin II AT1 and AT2 receptors in neonatal ureteral obstruction. Am J Physiol. 1997; 273:R503–8.

34. Chevalier RL, Thornhill BA, Wolstenholme JT. Renal cellular response to ureteral obstruction: Role of maturation and angiotensin II. Am J Physiol. 1999;277:F41–6.

35. Chevalier RL, Jones CE. Contribution of endogenous vasoactive compounds to renal vascular resistance in neonatal chronic partial ureteral obstruction. J Urol. 1986;136:532–8.

36. Chevalier RL, Thornhill BA, Gomez RA. EDRF modulates renal hemodynamics during unilateral ureteral obstruction in the rat. Kidney Int. 1992;42:400–5.

37. Yoo KH, Thornhill BA, Chevalier RL. Angiotensin stimulates TGF-beta 1 and clusterin in the hydronephrotic neonatal rat kidney. Am J Physiol. 2000;278:R640–6.

38. Chevalier RL, Cachat F. Role of angiotensin II in chronic ureteral obstruction. In: Wolf G, editor. The Renin-Angiotensin System and Progression of Renal Diseases. Basel: Karger, 2001; p. 250–255.

39. Gobe GC, Axelsen RA. Genesis of renal tubular atrophy in experimental hydronephrosis in the rat. Lab Invest. 1987;56:273–7.

40. Chevalier RL, Chung KH, Smith CD, et al. Renal apoptosis and clusterin following ureteral obstruction: The role of maturation. J Urol. 1996;156:1474–80.

41. Cachat F, Lange-Sperandio B, Chang AY, et al. Ureteral obstruction in neonatal mice elicits segment-specific tubular cell responses leading to nephron loss. Kidney Int. 2002;63:564–9.

42. Silverstein DM, Thornhill BA, Leung JC, et al. Expression of connexins in the normal and obstructed developing kidney. Pediatr Nephrol. 2003;18:216–122.

43. Silverstein DM, Travis BR, Thornhill BA, et al. Altered expression of immune modulator and structural genes in neonatal unilateral ureteral obstruction. Kidney Int. 2003;64:25–9.

44. Chevalier RL, Thornhill BA, Forbes MS, et al. Mechanisms of renal injury and progression of renal disease in congenital obstructive nephropathy. Pediatr Nephrol. 2010;25:687–97

45. Kiley SC, Thornhill BA, Tang SS, et al. Growth factor-mediated phosphorylation of propapoptotic BAD reduces tubule cell death in vitro and in vivo. Kidney Int. 2002;63:33–8.

46. Lange-Sperandio B, Cachat F, Thornhill BA, et al. Selectins mediate macrophage infiltration in obstructive nephropathy in newborn mice. Kidney Int 2002; 61:516-521

47. El Nahas AM. Plasticity of kidney cells: Role in kidney remodeling and scarring. Kidney Int. 2003;64:1553–9.

48. Liu Y. Epithelial to mesenchymal transition in renal fibrogenesis: Pathologic significance, molecular mechanism, and therapeutic intervention. J Am Soc Nephrol. 2004;15:1–6.

49. Iwano M, Plieth D, Danoff TM, et al. Evidence that fibroblasts derive from epithelium during tissue fibrosis. J Clin Invest. 2002;110:341–7.

50. Galarreta CI, Thornhill BA, Forbes MS, et al. Transforming growth factor-$\beta$1 receptor inhibition preserves glomerulotubular integrity during ureteral obstruction in adults but worsens injury in neonatal mice. Am J Physiol Renal Physiol. 2013;304:F481–90.

51. Chevalier RL, Kim A, Thornhill BA, Wolstenholme JT. Recovery following relief of unilateral ureteral obstruction in the neonatal rat. Kidney Int. 1999;55:793–9.

52. Chevalier RL, Thornhill BA, Chang AY, et al. Recovery from release of ureteral obstruction in the rat: Relationship to nephrogenesis. Kidney Int. 2002;61:2033–8.

53. Chevalier RL. Counterbalance in functional adaptation to ureteral obstruction during development. Pediatr Nephrol. 1990; 4:442–6.

54. Chevalier RL, Thornhill BA, Chang AY. Unilateral ureteral obstruction in neonatal rats leads to renal insufficiency in adulthood. Kidney Int. 2000;58:1987–92.

55. Li C, Wang W, Kwon TH, et al. Downregulation of AQP1, -2, and -3 after ureteral obstruction is associated with a long-term urine-concentrating defect. Am J Physiol. 2001;281:F163–70.

56. Li CL, Wang WD, Kwon TH, et al. Altered expression of major renal Na transporters in rats with bilateral ureteral obstruction and release of obstruction. Am J Physiol Renal Physiol. 2003;285:F889–94.

57. Chevalier RL. The moth and the aspen tree: Sodium in early postnatal development. Kidney Int. 2001;59:1617–21.

58. Batlle DC, Arruda JAL, Kirtzman NA. Hyperkalemic distal renal tubular acidosis associated with obstructive uropathy. New Engl J Med. 1981;304:373–9.

59. Alon UA, Kodroff MB, Broecker BH et al. Renal tubular acidosis type 4 in neonatal unilateral kidney diseases. J Pediatr. 1984;104:855–861.

60. Marra G, Goj V, Appiani AC, et al. Persistent tubular resistance to aldosterone in infants with congenital hydronephrosis corrected neonatally. J Pediatr. 1987;110:868–73.

61. Nguyen HT, Herndon CD, Cooper C, et al. The Society for Fetal Urology consensus statement on the evaluation and management of antenatal hydronephrosis. J Pediatr Urol. 2010;6:212–31.

62. Siemens D, Prouse K, MacNiely A. Antenatal hydronephrosis: Thresholds of renal pelvic diameter to predict insignificant postnatal pelviectasis. Tech Urol. 1998;4:198–203.

63. Lee RS, Borer JG. Perinatal Urology. In: Campbell-Walsh Urology. - 10th ed. Editor-in-chief, Wein AJ; Editors, Kavoussi LR, Novick AC, Partin AW, Peters CA. Elsevier Health Sciences, Philadelphia, USA. 2012, pp. 3048–3066.

64. Heikkilä J, Taskinen S, Rintala R. Urinomas associated with posterior urethral valves. J Urol. 2008;180:1476–8.

65. Johnson MP, Bukowski TP, Reitleman C, et al. In utero surgical treatment of fetal obstructive uropathy: A new comprehensive approach to identify appropriate candidates for vesicoamniotic shunt therapy. Am J Obstet Gynecol. 1994;170:1770–76.

66. de Kort EH, Bambang Oetomo S, Zegers SH. The long-term outcome of antenatal hydronephrosis up to 15 millimetres justifies a noninvasive postnatal follow-up. Acta Paediatr. 2008; 97:708-713

67. Conway JJ, Maizels M. The "well tempered" diuretic renogram: A standard method to examine the asymptomatic neonate with hydronephrosis or hydroureteronephrosis. J Nucl Med. 1992;33:2047–52.

68. Riccabona M. Obstructive diseases of the urinary tract in children: Lessons from the last 15 years. Pediatr Radiol. 2010;40:947–55.

69. Morris R, Malin G, Khan K, et al. Systematic review of the effectiveness of antenatal intervention for the treatment of congenital lower urinary tract obstruction. BJOG 2010;117:382–90.

70. Morris RK, Malin GL, Quinlan-Jones E, et al. Percutaneous vesicoamniotic shunting versus conservative management for fetal lower urinary tract obstruction (PLUTO): A randomized trial. Lancet. 2013;382:1496–506.

71. Biard JM, Johnson MP, Carr MC, et al. Long-term outcomes in children treated by prenatal vesicoamniotic shunting for lower urinary tract obstruction. Obstet Gynecol. 2005;106:503–8.

72. Timberlake MD, Herndon CDA. Mild to moderate postnatal hydronephrosis: Grading systems and management. Nat Rev Urol. 2013;10:649–5.

73. Koff SA, Campbell K. Nonoperative management of unilateral neonatal hydronephrosis. J Urol. 1992;148:525–30.

74. King LR, Coughlin PWF, Bloch EC, et al. The case for immediate pyeloplasty in the neonate with ureteropelvic junction obstruction. J Urol 1984;132:725–9.

75. Chertin B, Fridmans A, Knizhnik M, et al. Does early detection of ureteropelvic junction obstruction improve surgical outcome in terms of renal function? J Urol 1999;162:1037–42.

76. Ulman I, Jayanthi VR, Koff SA. The long-term follow-up of newborns with severe unilateral hydronephrosis initially treated nonoperatively. J Urol. 2000;164:1101–7.

77. Palmer LS, Maizels M, Cartwright PC, et al. Surgery versus observation for managing obstructive grade 3 to 4 unilateral hydronephrosis: A report from the society for fetal urology. J Urol. 1998;159:222–7.

78. DiSandro MJ, Kogan BA. Ureteropelvic junction obstruction. Urol Clin No Am. 1998; 25:187–92.

79. Eskild-Jensen A, Jorgensen TM, Olsen LH, et al. Renal function may not be restored when using decreasing differential function as the criterion for surgery in unilateral hydronephrosis. BJU Int. 2003;92:779–84.

80. Onen A, Jayanthi VR, Koff SA. Long-term follow up of prenatally detected severe bilateral newborn hydronephrosis initially managed nonoperatively. J Urol. 2002;168:1118–22.

81. Peters CA. Editorial: The long-term follow up of prenatally detected severe bilateral newborn hydronephrosis initially managed nonoperatively. J Urol. 2002;168:1121–26.

82. Terzi F, Assael BM, Claris AA, et al. Increased sodium requirement following early postnatal surgical correction of congenital uropathies in infants. Pediatr Nephrol. 1990;4:581–6.

83. Zhang PL, Peters CA, Rosen S. Ureteropelvic junction obstruction: Morphological and clinical studies. Pediatr Nephrol. 2000;14:820–6.

84. Kumar S, Walia S, Ikpeme O, et al. Postnatal outcome of prenatally diagnosed severe fetal renal pelvic dilatation. Prenat Diagn. 2012;32:519–22.

85. Stock JA, Krous HF, Heffernan J, et al. Correlation of renal biopsy and radionuclide renal scan differential function in patients with unilateral ureteropelvic junction obstruction. J Urol. 1995;154:716–21.

86. Capolicchio G, Leonard MP, Wong C, et al. Prenatal diagnosis of hydronephrosis: Impact on renal function and its recovery after pyeloplasty. J Urol. 1999;162:1029–34.

87. Boubaker A, Prior JO, Meyrat B, et al. Unilateral uretero pelvic junction obstruction in children: Long-term follow up after unilateral pyeloplasty. J Urol. 2003;170:575–9.

88. Roth KS, Carter WH, Jr, Chan JCM. Obstructive nephropathy in children: Long-term progression after relief of posterior urethral valve. Pediatrics 2001; 107:1004-1009.

89. Heikkilä J, Holmberg C, Kyllönen L, et al. Long-term risk of end stage renal disease in patients with posterior urethral valves. J Urol. 2011;186:2392–6.

90. Kibar Y, Ashley RA, Roth CC, et al. Timing of posterior urethral valve diagnosis and its impact on clinical outcome. J Pediatr Urol. 2011;7:538–42.

91. Kousidis G, Thomas DF, Morgan H, et al. The long-term outcome of prenatally detected posterior urethral valves: A 10 to 23-year follow-up study. BJU Int. 2008;102:1020–4.

92. DeFoor W, Clark C, Jackson E, et al. Risk factors for end stage renal disease in children with posterior urethral valves. J Urol. 2008;180:1705–8.

93. Koff SA, Peller PA, Young DC, et al. The assessment of obstruction in the newborn with unilateral hydronephrosis by measuring the size of the opposite kidney. J Urol. 1994;152:596–601.

94. Garcia-Pena BM, Keller MS, Schwartz DS et al. The ultrasonographic differentiation of obstructive versus nonobstructive hydronephrosis in children: A multivariate scoring system. J Urol. 1997;158:560–6.

95. Brandell RA, Brock JW, III, Hamilton BD, et al. Unilateral hydronephrosis in infants: Are measurements of contralateral-renal length useful? J Urol. 1996;156:188–94.

96. Koff SA. Letter. Unilateral hydronephrosis in infants: Are measurements of contralateral renal length useful? J Urol. 1997;157:962–3.

97. Wanner C, Luscher TF, Schollmeyer P, Vetter W. Unilateral hydronephrosis and hypertension: Cause or coincidence? Nephron. 1987;45:236–9.

98. Hohenfellner K, Wingen A-M, Nauroth O, et al. Impact of ACE I/D gene polymorphism on congenital renal malformations. Pediatr Nephrol. 2001;16:356–61.

99. Hebert LA, Wilmer WA, Falkenhain ME et al. Renoprotection: One or many therapies? Kidney Int. 2001;59:1211–6.

100. Guron G, Friberg P. An intact renin-angiotensin system is a prerequisite for normal renal development. J Hypertens. 2000;18:123–8.

101. Guron G, Marcussen N, Nilsson A, et al. Postnatal time frame for renal vulnerability to enalapril in rats. J Am Soc Nephrol. 2000;10:155–9.

102. O'Dea RF, Mirkin BL, Alward CT, et al. Treatment of neonatal hypertension with captopril. J Pediatr. 1988;113:403–8.

103. Chevalier RL, Thornhill BA, Belmonte DC, et al. Endogenous angiotensin II inhibits natriuresis following acute volume expansion in the neonatal rat. Am J Physiol. 1996;270:R393–7.

104. Elder JS, Stansbrey R, Dahms BB, et al. Renal histological changes secondary to ureteropelvic junction obstruction. J Urol. 1995;154:719–24.

105. Chevalier RL. Biomarkers of congenital obstructive nephropathy: Past, present and future. J Urol. 2004;172:852–6.

106. Yang SP, Woolf AS, Quinn F, et al. Deregulation of renal transforming growth factor-beta 1 after experimental short-term ureteric obstruction in fetal sheep. Am J Pathol. 2001;159:109–113.

107. Furness PD, III, Maizels M, Han SW, et al. Elevated bladder urine concentration of transforming growth factor-b1 correlates with upper urinary tract obstruction in children. J Urol. 1999;162:1033–38.

108. Trnka P, Ivanova L, Hiatt MJ, et al. Urinary biomarkers in obstructive nephropathy. Clin J Am Soc Nephrol. 2012;7:1567–75.

109. Grandaliano G, Gesualdo L, Bartoli F, et al. MCP-1 and EGF renal expression and urine excretion in human congenital obstructive nephropathy. Kidney Int. 2000;58:182–8.

110. Li Z, Zhao Z, Liu X, et al. Prediction of the outcome of antenatal hydronephrosis: Significance of urinary EGF. Pediatr Nephrol. 2012;27:2251–9.

111. Wasilewska A, Taranta-Janusz K, Dębek W, et al. KIM-1 and NGAL: New markers of obstructive nephropathy. Pediatr Nephrol. 2011;26:579–86.

## REVIEW QUESTIONS

1. The *most* common cause of antenatal obstructive uropathy is:
   a. Posterior urethral valves
   b. Vesicoureteric reflux
   c. Ureterovesicular junction obstruction
   d. Ureteropelvic junction obstruction

2. Routine antenatal ultrasound detects most cases of antenatal hydronephrosis.
   a. False
   b. True

3. In prenatally detected hydronephrosis, no evidence of urinary tract obstruction is seen in:
   a. 10%
   b. 90%
   c. 50%
   d. 30%

4. A prenatal ultrasound in a male fetus demonstrate bilateral hydronephrosis and a thickened bladder wall. A diagnosis of posterior urethral valves is being entertained. The most important clinical concern in the neonatal period in this patient will be:
   a. Reduced nephron mass
   b. Urinary tract infection
   c. Pulmonary hypoplasia
   d. Diaphragmatic hernia

5. Risk for CKD and ESRD risk in patients with posterior urethral valves is determined by:
   a. Severity of hydronephrosis
   b. Severity of renal dysplasia
   c. Frequency of urinary tract infections
   d. Amniotic fluid sodium concentration

6. A male baby at the age of 37 weeks of gestation is born via cesarean section delivery and requires mechanical ventilation after resuscitation. His mother had poor prenatal follow-up, and there is no record of her having had any prenatal ultrasound evaluations. The patient developed right-sided pneumothorax on day 2. He did not urinate for 12 hours, urinary bladder catheterization was done, and an

indwelling catheter was left in place. Renal ultrasound showed bilateral hydronephrosis, bilateral hydroureters and a distended urinary bladder with thickened wall. The *most* important next investigative step in this patient should be:

a. Monitor renal ultrasound for worsening of hydronephrosis
b. Monitor serum creatinine for renal function
c. A DMSA renal scan
d. A nuclear cystogram
e. A contrast vesicocystourethrogram

7. Following are the features of lower urinary tract obstruction in neonates, *except:*
a. Hematuria following birth
b. Bilateral antenatal hydronephrosis
c. Hypospadias
d. Fetal or neonatal urinary ascites

8. Urinary incontinence is a clinical manifestation of lower urinary tract obstruction:
a. True
b. False

9. Of prenatally detected cases of pyelectasis/hydronephrosis, 50% to 70% are due to:
a. Ureteropelvic junction obstruction
b. Vesicoureteric reflux
c. Transient or physiologic neonatal changes
d. Potter syndrome

10. Which of the following disorders can mimic hydronephrosis in an antenatal sonogram?
a. Multicystic dysplastic kidney
b. Megaureter
c. Large renal cysts
d. All of the above

11. A 6-year-boy complains of right-side abdominal pain every time he goes out with his parents for dinner or when parents give him a small carton of juice to drink. He was seen today in the emergency room with severe right flank pain. Because of concern about a renal colic, the staff started him on ½ normal saline an intravenous infusion at 1.5 times maintenance. Within a half-hour after infusion being started, his flank pain worsened, requiring morphine for adequate pain control. His urinalysis showed: pH 6.5, specific gravity 1.015, no protein, no blood, nitrate negative, and leukocytes negative. Renal ultrasound shows a severe right-side hydronephrosis. The child has which of the following?
a. Acute appendicitis
b. Renal colic
c. Dietl crisis
d. Recurrent colonic volvulus

12. Diagnosis of posterior urethral valves in a male after 1 year of age is associated with:
a. Better overall prognosis for renal function and ESRD compared to neonatal diagnosis
b. Worse overall prognosis for renal function and ESRD compared to neonatal diagnosis

## ANSWERS

1. d
2. b
3. c
4. c
5. b
6. e
7. c
8. a
9. c
10. d
11. c
12. a

# 48

# Vesicoureteral reflux

TEJ K. MATTOO

Vesicoureteral reflux (VUR) denotes the retrograde flow of urine from bladder to the kidneys, most commonly the result of anatomic abnormality of vesicoureteral junction with shortening of intravesical submucosal length of the ureter. VUR may be an isolated abnormality (primary VUR) that is diagnosed mostly after urinary tract infection (UTI). Primary VUR is predominantly seen in white children. Indeed, 81% of the 607 patients in the Randomized Intervention in Children with VUR (RIVUR) study were white.[1] Primary VUR is also diagnosed during postnatal follow-up of antenatally diagnosed hydronephrosis or screening a sibling of a patient with VUR. VUR also occurs in association with other congenital anomalies of the kidney and urinary tract, including renal dysplasia, and can occur in association with obstructive uropathy or neurogenic bladder (secondary VUR).

## EPIDEMIOLOGY

The prevalence of primary VUR varies from 1.3% of healthy children to 8% to 50% of children evaluated after UTI.[2-5] In newborns and infants, the incidence of VUR diagnosed after UTI is 36% to 49%.[6-8] Children with VUR detected after UTI are predominantly females, although in some studies no gender difference or even male predominance has been reported.[3,4,9,10-12] VUR is less common in African-American children.[13,14] High prevalence of VUR in whites is well known and was also documented in the RIVUR study.[1] Moreover, only approximately one-third as many

African-American as white girls with UTI have VUR, but there are no significant differences in age or mode of presentation between the two races.[13,16] Interestingly, in comparison to white children, VUR is generally less severe in African-American children.[17]

In patients with prenatally detected hydronephrosis, postnatal evaluation reveals the presence of VUR in 10% to 30% of infants and the incidence is higher in boys.[18,19] The reported incidence of VUR in asymptomatic siblings of index cases is 32% to 45%.[20,21] The incidence of VUR in the offspring of parents with known VUR in one study was 66%, suggesting high likelihood of parent-to-child transmission.[22]

## KEY POINT

Vesicoureteral reflux is less common in African-American children.

## DIAGNOSIS AND GRADING

The diagnosis of VUR is based on the demonstration of reflux of urine from the bladder to the upper urinary tract by either contrast voiding cystourethrogram (VCUG) or radionuclide cystogram (RNC). Contrast VCUG is preferable, particularly in males and as the initial study, because it allows more precise grading of VUR and helps evaluate lower genitourinary tract anatomy.

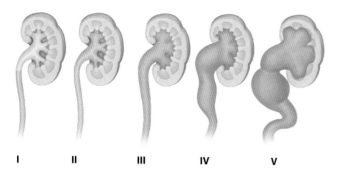

I   II   III   IV   V

Figure 48.1 International Reflux Study grading system for vesicoureteral reflux. Grade I: Reflux into nondilated ureter. Grade II: Reflux into the renal pelvis and calyces without dilatation. Grade III: Mild/moderate dilatation of ureter and pelvicalyceal system. Grade IV: Dilation of the renal pelvis and calyces with moderate ureteral tortuosity, blunting of fornices. Grade V: Gross dilatation of the ureter, pelvis, and calyces; ureteral tortuosity; loss of papillary impressions. (Reproduced with permission from: Gargollo PC, Diamond DA. Therapy Insight: what nephrologists need to know about primary vesicoureteral reflux. Nat Clin Pract Nephrol. 2007;3:551–63.)

The grading system used most widely for classifying the severity of VUR was proposed by the International Reflux Study in Children (IRSC).[23] It classifies VUR into the following five grades based on appearance in contrast VCUG (Figures 48.1 and 48.2):

*Grade I:* Reflux into the ureter
*Grade II:* Reflux into the renal pelvis, without any dilation of the calyces
*Grade III:* Reflux to the renal pelvis with mild dilation of the renal pelvis
*Grade IV:* Reflux to the renal pelvis with greater dilation of the renal pelvis
*Grade V:* Reflux includes reflux to the renal pelvis with ureteral and pelvic dilation

Intrarenal reflux (IRR) is the condition in which the contrast flows backward from the renal pelvis into the collecting tubules (pyelotubular backflow). IRR is usually present in conjunction with high-grade VUR (Figure 48.3).

The degree of reflux seen in the VCUG may be modified by how aggressively the bladder is filled during VCUG, by both volume and as rapidity. Sometimes, ureteral dilatation may be present without calyceal dilation, leading to difficulties with grading. The severity of VUR in RNC (Figure 48.4) is usually classified as mild (grades I and II), moderate (grade III), and severe (grades IV and V).

## NATURAL HISTORY

Primary VUR generally improves with time; this is attributed to the lengthening of the submucosal segment of the ureter.[24] The reported rate of improvement is not consistent because of differences in patient selection, definition of resolution, duration of follow-up, and use of single versus two negative VCUGs to confirm resolution of VUR. The Birmingham Reflux Study, which used single negative VCUG, reported approximately 50% cessation of VUR after 5-year follow-up in medically managed moderate-to-severe VUR.[25] In the International Reflux Study in Children (IRCS), which used two consecutive negative VCUGs, the corresponding number was 25.0%.[26] In a study by Wennerstrom et al.,[4] the end point of reflux grade I or less was reached in approximately 75% of children after 10 years of follow-up. The rate of resolution is higher in younger children. In a 5-year follow-up study in children younger than 5 years old, including 60% younger than 2 years, grade I VUR resolved in 82%, grade II in 80%, and grade III in 46% of the ureters.[6]

The important factors identified with resolution of VUR are nonwhite race, lower grades of reflux, absence of renal damage, and lack of voiding compared to high-grade VUR. The IRSC reported that VUR disappeared in more than 80%

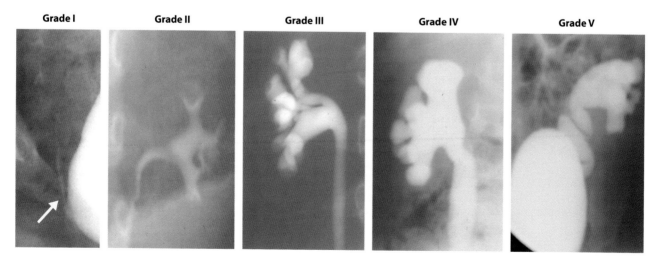

Grade I   Grade II   Grade III   Grade IV   Grade V

Figure 48.2 VUG images showing different grades of VUR, scored by the International Reflux Study grading system. (Figures courtesy of Dr. Eglal Shalaby-Rana, Children's National Medical Center, Washington, DC.)

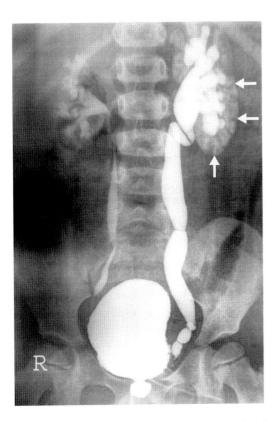

Figure 48.3 Intrarenal reflux. (Figure reproduced with permission from: Yüksel S. Intrarenal reflux. Clinical Kidney Journal 2008; 1: 188-189.)

of undilated and approximately 40% of dilated ureters.[3] Schwab et al.[28] reported that grades I to III VUR resolve at a rate of 13% per year for the first 5 years of follow-up and 3.5% per year during subsequent years, whereas grades IV and V VUR resolve at a rate of 5% per year. In the IRSC, resolution of VUR was significantly better in grade III versus grade IV VUR.[29] A systematic review of published literature

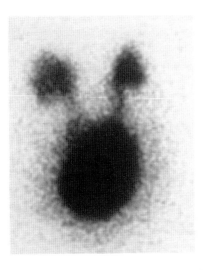

Figure 48.4 Radionuclide cystogram showing bilateral severe vesicoureteral reflux. (Figure courtesy of Dr. Eglal Shalaby-Rana, Children's National Medical Center, Washington, DC.)

on the resolution of VUR concluded that increasing age at presentation and bilateral VUR decrease the probability of resolution, and bilateral grade IV VUR has a particularly low chance of spontaneous resolution.[30] In one study, the mean time until spontaneous resolution in black children was 14.6 months, which was significantly shorter than the mean of 21.4 months in white children.[16]

VUR diagnosed because of antenatal hydronephrosis has a high a high rate of spontaneous resolution (59% by age 4 years), even in those with grades IV and V reflux.[31]

Review of the natural history of VUR in siblings indicated that 52% had resolution of the reflux at follow-up of 18 months, with yearly resolution rates of 28%.[32]

---

### KEY POINT

VUR diagnosed in response to antenatal hydronephrosis has a high rate of spontaneous resolution.

---

## CLINICAL MANIFESTATIONS

## URINARY TRACT INFECTION

By itself, VUR is usually asymptomatic, but an increased risk for febrile UTI (acute pyelonephritis) in these patients is well established.[33,34] Indeed, initial discovery of VUR in many of these patients occurs after a febrile UTI. The majority of children diagnosed with VUR after UTI are girls, but there is no gender difference in infants younger than 6 months of age.[35]

## DYSFUNCTIONAL ELIMINATION SYNDROME

The symptoms of dysfunctional elimination syndrome (DES) include daytime wetness, urgency, frequency, infrequency, constipation, or fecal incontinence in toilet-trained children with no underlying anatomic or neurologic abnormality.[36-38] Toilet-trained children diagnosed with VUR following a UTI have a high association (43%) with DES.[38] Voiding dysfunction in these children is likely to predispose them to recurrent UTI, worsening or delaying resolution of VUR and increasing risk for renal scarring.[39,40] In a study by Koff et al.,[38] DES, besides increasing the rate of breakthrough UTI, delayed resolution of reflux. DES also adversely affected the results of surgical ureteric reimplantation in this study. In another study that involved use of a questionnaire in 310 children enrolled in the European branch of the IRSC, a strong negative correlation was seen between recurrences of UTIs, as well as disappearance of VUR, and non-neuropathic bladder or sphincter dysfunction (equivalent of DES).[41]

Constipation, as an isolated finding or as part of the DES, results in compression of the bladder and bladder neck, increasing bladder storage pressure and postvoid residual urine volume. Also, distended colon, soiling, or both provides an abundant reservoir of pathogens.[42–44] By these mechanisms, constipation increases the likelihood of urinary incontinence, bladder overactivity, dyscoordinated voiding, a large capacity and poorly emptying bladder, recurrent UTI, and deterioration of VUR.[45] In a study that involved 366 children, constipation, encopresis, or both was reported in 30% cases, daytime wetting in 89%, nighttime wetting in 79%, and recurrent UTI in 60% of the patients. VUR was present in 20% of the patients.

## RENAL SCARRING

Renal scarring seen in conjunction with VUR is termed *reflux nephropathy* (RN). Although most commonly seen in patients with acute or chronic pyelonephritis (Figure 48.5), RN also may be of congenital origin. Differences between the two forms of RN are outlined in Table 48.1.

The risk for renal scarring following acute pyelonephritis is 5% to 10%.[46,47] In children with VUR and UTI, however, the incidence of renal scarring is significantly higher, at 30% to 56%.[48–50] A systematic review of 23 studies that included a total of 2106 children with renal scarring after pyelonephritis from across the world revealed the incidence of RN to be 48.5%.[9] The prevalence of renal scarring in healthy populations is not known. In a study in healthy children and adolescents who were evaluated for newly diagnosed hypertension, the dimercaptosuccinic acid (DMSA) renal scans revealed renal scarring in 33 (21%) of 159 patients.[51] In a study in adults with hypertension, radionuclide VCUG

---

**KEY POINT**

Reflux nephropathy may be congenital or acquired secondary to scarring from UTIs.

---

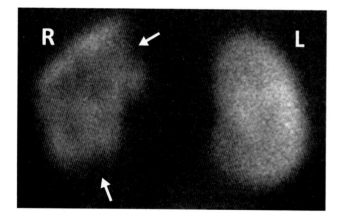

Figure 48.5 Dimercaptosuccinic acid (DMSA) renal scan demonstrating upper and lower pole scarring (arrows) in the right kidney (R). The left kidney (L) is normal. (Figures courtesy of Dr. Eglal Shalaby-Rana, Children's National Medical Center, Washington, DC.)

---

Table 48.1 Congenital versus acquired reflux nephropathy in children

|  | **Acquired RN** | **Congenital RN** |
|---|---|---|
| Time of occurrence | Postnatal | Prenatal |
| UTI before diagnosis | Common | Uncommon |
| Age distribution | All pediatric age groups | Mostly in younger children |
| Gender distribution | Predominantly females | Predominantly males |
| Grade of VUR | Mostly high-grade | Mostly high-grade |
| Dysplastic features on renal histopathology | No | Yes |

*Source:* Adapted from Mattoo TK. Vesicoureteral reflux and reflux nephropathy. Adv Chronic Kidney Dis. 2011;18: 348–54.

*Abbreviations:* RN, reflux nephrology; UTI, urinary tract infection; VUR, vesicoureteral reflux

---

revealed VUR in 30 of 157 (19.1%) of the patients.[52] Of the 30 patients, 7 (23%) had bilateral VUR that was graded as severe. Congenital RN in association with VUR has been reported in 30% to 60% of such children, most of whom are diagnosed during follow-up for antenatal hydronephrosis.[53–55]

The relative risk for renal scarring in children with VUR after acute pyelonephritis is 2.6 (95% confidence interval [CI], 1.7 to 3.9) compared to those with no VUR.[33] Children with VUR grades III or higher are more likely to develop scarring than children with lower VUR grades (relative risk [RR], 2.1; 95% CI, 1.4 to 3.2]).[33] Renal injury is more common in infants because of their unique kidney papillary morphology.[56,57] The International Reflux Study reported that renal injury is more frequent in children younger than 2 years old, particularly in the presence of high-grade VUR.[58] A comprehensive literature review on febrile UTI in children by the Committee on Quality Improvement (Subcommittee on Urinary Tract Infection) of the American Academy of Pediatrics identified children younger than 2 years old as being at highest risk for renal injury with febrile UTI.[59] The risk is aggravated by diagnostic challenges, nonspecific clinical presentation, difficulties in getting urine specimens, and a higher prevalence and severity of VUR in smaller children. Other factors that affect the probability of renal scarring in children with VUR and UTI include delayed treatment of UTI, recurrent UTI, and bacterial virulence.[60–64] Finally, there is evidence that genetic factors predispose patients with VUR to scarring, as demonstrated by studies of angiotensin-converting enzyme (ACE) gene polymorphisms.[65,66]

The complications of renal scarring are well known but poorly defined because of their insidious onset, slow progression, and a lack of well-designed prospective studies in children, as well as in adults. Hypertension and proteinuria are the most common reported complications. Other complications include focal segmental glomerulosclerosis (FSGS), urine concentration defects, hyperkalemia, and acidosis.[44,45]

## HYPERTENSION

Hypertension occurs in 17% to 30% of pediatric patients and 3% to 38% of adult patients with renal scarring.[9,48,67,68] Simoes e Silva et al.[69] found that 3% of patients with VUR developed hypertension during childhood, but survival analysis of data suggested that 50% of patients with unilateral or bilateral renal damage were expected to develop sustained hypertension later in adult life. In a follow-up lasting 15 years in pediatric patients with renal scarring, approximately 13% of patients at ages 20 to 31 years were noted to be hypertensive.[70] In another 5-year prospective study of patients with long-standing RN, there was no correlation between blood pressure and plasma renin activity, plasma creatinine concentration, or degree of scarring.[71] Some studies have, however, reported no increase in BP after many years of follow-up.[72,73]

## PROTEINURIA

Overt proteinuria, which has been reported in 21% of adult patients with RN, is rare in pediatric patients.[74] Significant degrees of microalbuminuria, an indicator of glomerular damage at a very early stage, have been reported in patients with renal scarring and precede the development of overt proteinuria.[75] Patients with RN also have increased urinary excretion of low-molecular-weight proteins (LMWPs) such as $\beta_2$-microglobin, retinol-binding protein, $\alpha_1$-microglobin, and N-acetyl-$\beta$-D-glucosaminase. Microalbuminuria occurs around the same time or soon after the appearance of LMWPs in urine. Urinary albumin excretion increases with the severity of renal scarring.[75,76] FSGS is known to occur in patients with RN.[76] FSGS is progressive and can occur in nonscarred parts of the kidney or in the normal contralateral kidney in patients with unilateral RN.[77]

> ### KEY POINT
>
> Hypertension and proteinuria are the most common complications of renal scarring.

## CHRONIC KIDNEY DISEASE

Renal scarring is responsible for 5% to 10% of pediatric and adult cases of end-stage renal disease. According to 2008 North American Pediatric Renal Trials and Collaborative Studies (NAPRTCS) report, RN is the fourth most common cause of chronic kidney disease (CKD) in 8.4% of the children and is present in 5.2% of transplanted patients and 3.5% of dialysis patients.[78] In the Chronic Kidney Disease in Children (CKiD) study following a cohort of 586 children aged 1 to 16 years with an estimated glomerular filtration rate (GFR) of 30 to 90 mL/min/1.73m$^2$, RN was the underlying cause of CKD in 87 (14.8%) patients, constituting 19% of the patients with a nonglomerular etiology of CKD.[79]

## ADULTS DIAGNOSED IN CHILDHOOD

Adults who develop renal scarring secondary to VUR are at risk for developing renal disease and hypertension as adults. In a study of 21 adults (mean age, 23.9 years) with gross VUR diagnosed in infancy, proteinuria and renal insufficiency were diagnosed in 3 of the 13 patients (23%) with unilateral RN and 2 of the 4 patients (50%) with bilateral RN.[80] In another study of 127 adults (mean age, 41 years) with VUR diagnosed during childhood, 44 (35%) had unilateral renal scarring and 30 (24%) had bilateral renal scarring.[81] Of these, 30 patients (24%) had albuminuria and 14 (11%) had hypertension. Of the 30 patients with bilateral renal scars, 25 (83%) had an abnormal GFR.[81] Renal scarring also may cause pregnancy-related complications such as recurrent pyelonephritis, hypertension, toxemia of pregnancy, babies with low birth weight, and miscarriage.[82-84]

## MANAGEMENT

The two main treatment modalities that have been practiced for more than three decades in the management of VUR are long-term antimicrobial prophylaxis and surgical correction. A third, more recent option is surveillance, with no routine prophylaxis or surgical intervention. Surgical correction of VUR was common until the concept of antimicrobial prophylaxis for childhood UTI was introduced in 1975.[85] Numerous subsequent studies established that medical management of VUR is as good as the surgical treatment, and there is no significant outcome difference between the two treatment approaches.[25,58,86-89]

## ANTIMICROBIAL PROPHYLAXIS

The antimicrobial agents most appropriate for prophylaxis include trimethoprim-sulfamethoxazole (TMP-SMX), trimethoprim alone, nitrofurantoin, and cephalexin. For infants younger than 2 months, ampicillin or amoxicillin is preferable for prophylaxis. The prophylactic dose of antimicrobials is one-fourth to half of the therapeutic dose for acute infection.[59,90] The dosage for commonly used antimicrobials is shown in Table 48.2. In toilet-trained children, the medication is generally administered at bedtime, although this recommendation is not evidence-based.

Follow-up of patients with VUR-associated UTI requires close monitoring, early detection and prompt treatment of UTI, change of antimicrobial prophylaxis if the patient has recurrent breakthrough UTI, and monitoring of the VUR by periodic VCUG or RNC examinations. The timing of follow-up VCUG is not well defined, but studies have suggested time intervals of 12 to 24 months. The duration of antimicrobial prophylaxis and the potential surgical

Table 48.2 Prophylactic antimicrobial agents

| Antibiotic | Dose |
|---|---|
| Trimethoprim (TMP)-sulfamethoxazole | 2 mg TMP/kg/day daily |
| Nitrofurantoin | 1-2 mg/kg/dose daily |
| Cephalexin | 10 mg/kg/dose daily |
| Amoxicillin | 10 mg/kg/dose daily |

Source: Adopted from Saadeh SA, Mattoo TK. Managing urinary tract infections. Pediatr Nephrol. 2011;26:1967–76.

intervention depends on the age of the patient, severity of the VUR, frequency of UTI, and degree of renal scarring, if present. Cessation of antimicrobial prophylaxis after age 5 to 7 years, even if the low-grade VUR persists, has been recommended by some.[91]

---

**KEY POINT**

Management options for VUR include surgical correction, antibiotic prophylaxis, and surveillance.

---

## Limitations of prophylactic antimicrobials

Long-term antimicrobial prophylaxis has its limitations. Antimicrobial prophylaxis is not always effective, and breakthrough UTI rates in children with VUR range from 25% to 38%.[25,92] Antimicrobial resistance is a major concern with long-term antimicrobial prophylaxis. In one study, children who received the medication for more than 4 weeks in the preceding 6 months had more resistant *Escherichia coli* than those not on such treatment (odds ratio [OR], 13.9; 95% CI,

8.2 to 23.5).[93] Approximately 10% of children on long-term prophylaxis have adverse reactions, most of which occur within the first 6 months. These include gastrointestinal symptoms, skin rashes, hepatotoxicity, and hematologic complications with TMP-SMX, and mostly gastrointestinal symptoms with nitrofurantoin. More adverse reactions such as marrow suppression and rarely Stevens-Johnson syndrome also may occur with TMP-SMX.[94,95] Compliance for daily administration of the medication over a prolonged period also remains a concern. In one study, 97% of the parents reported compliance with low-dose daily antimicrobial prophylaxis and yet excretion of the antimicrobial agent in urine was found in only 31% of the patients' urine.[96]

---

**KEY POINT**

Antibiotic prophylaxis increases the risk for resistant organisms.

---

## Controversies in prophylactic antimicrobial use

Systematic reviews of published literature have raised serious questions about the role of antimicrobial prophylaxis in VUR.[97-99] A Cochrane review in 2006 identified eight randomized studies (618 children) that compared antibiotics with placebo or no treatment to prevent recurrent UTI. This analysis demonstrated that prophylactic antibiotics decreased the risk for positive urine culture compared to a placebo. However, the authors concluded that more evidence in the form of properly randomized double-blind trials was necessary to support the routine use of antibiotic prophylaxis in preventing recurrent UTI.[100]

Table 48.3 Recent randomized trials on antimicrobial prophylaxis in vesicoureteral reflux with urinary tract infection

| Author (yr) | Patient age | Total number of patients in study | VUR status | Number of patients with VUR | VUR grade | Follow-up (mo) |
|---|---|---|---|---|---|---|
| Garin et al. (2006) | 1 mo–18 yr | 218 | ±VUR | 113 | I–III | 12 |
| Roussey-Kesler et al. (2008) | 1 mo–3 yr | 225 | +VUR | 225 | I–III | 18 |
| Pennesi et al. (2008) | 0–30 mon | 100 | + VUR | 100 | II–IV | 24–48 |
| Montini et al. (2008) | 2 mo–7 yr | 338 | ±VUR | 128 | I–III | 12 |
| Craig et al. (2009) | 0–18 yr | 576 | ±VUR | 243 | I–V | 12 |
| Swedish Reflux Trial (2010) | 1–2 yr | 203 | +VUR | 203 | III–IV | 24 |
| RIVUR Study | 2–71 mo (6 yr) | 607 | +VUR | 607 | I–IV | 24 |

Source: Adopted from Saadeh SA, Mattoo TK. Managing urinary tract infections. Pediatr Nephrol. 2011;26:1967–76.

Several randomized trials (see Table 48.3) have investigated the utility of antimicrobial prophylaxis for UTI.[88,101–105] Overall, these studies included patients from 0–18 years of age, with grades 0-V VUR. Three studies included children with and without VUR.[101,104,105] Garin et al.[101] and Montini et al.[104] reported no benefit with prophylaxis in children with and without VUR (grades I to III), The study by Craig et al.,[105] which was placebo-controlled, showed a reduction in the absolute risk for UTI (6 percentage points) that did not vary with any stratifying variable (age, sex, reflux status, history of more than one UTI, or susceptibility of the causative organism for TMP-SMX).[105] The other randomized trials of antimicrobial prophylaxis for UTI included only patients with VUR grades I to IV, and patient age ranged from 0 to 3 years.[88,102,103] Roussey-Kesler et al.[102] did not show any benefit to antibiotic prophylaxis in low-grade VUR, except in boys with grade III reflux. Pennesi et al.[103] found no difference in UTI recurrence between prophylaxis and no prophylaxis in all patients younger than 30 months of age.[103] The Swedish Reflux Trial included 203 children (1 to 2 years of age) with grades III or IV reflux openly randomized into three groups.[88] Treatment groups were assigned to low-dose antibiotic prophylaxis, endoscopic therapy, and a surveillance group. The study demonstrated that the rate of UTI recurrence in girls older than 1 year with dilating VUR was higher than in boys and that this rate can be decreased with antibiotic prophylaxis and endoscopic treatment. There was no difference between the prophylaxis and endoscopic treatment groups. Of patients in the surveillance group, 57% had a UTI recurrence during follow-up. The study also showed that girls had a significantly higher rate of new renal damage on DMSA scan than in boys at 2 years. The renal damage was most common in the surveillance group and showed a strong association with recurrent febrile UTI.[89]

## Randomized Intervention for Children with Vesicoureteral Reflux Study and antimicrobial prophylaxis

In 2011, the American Academy of Pediatrics revised its recommendations regarding investigations and use of prophylactic antibiotics after first UTI.[106] These recommendations suggested renal ultrasound be the sole investigation after first UTI. After treatment with antibiotics for 14 days, use of antimicrobial prophylaxis was not recommended for prevention of UTI. VCUG after the first UTI was also discouraged in these recommendations, unless hydronephrosis, potential scarring, high-grade VUR, or obstructive uropathy was suggested on the renal ultrasound evaluation. VCUG was, however, recommended in cases of recurrent febrile UTIs.

The Randomized Intervention for Children with Vesicoureteral Reflux (RIVUR) study recruited 607 children with VUR who were diagnosed after a first or second

febrile or symptomatic UTI.[107] Efficacy of TMP-SMX prophylaxis in preventing recurrence of UTI, renal scarring, and antibiotic resistance was assessed over 2 years. The group of 302 children were assigned to the prophylaxis arm, and 305 children received placebo. Of the 302 children, 39 (12.8%) developed recurrent infections in the prophylaxis (treatment) group compared 72 of 305 (25.4%) children in the placebo group who developed recurrent infections. Renal scarring did not differ between the prophylaxis group and the placebo group, being 11.9% and 10.2%, respectively in the two groups. The investigators concluded that the data support use of antibiotic prophylaxis in children with documented VUR. The data also provide some support to the argument for obtaining VCUG in patients who have febrile UTI (acute pyelonephritis).

## SURGICAL MANAGEMENT

The surgical intervention has the advantage of a "quick fix" in most cases and is recommended in patients with high-grade VUR, breakthrough febrile UTIs while on prophylaxis, allergy to prophylactic antimicrobials, poor adherence, worsening of renal scarring, and sometimes parental preference.[108] Some of the commonly used methods are described in the following section.

### Endoscopic treatment

Currently, of all the surgical options, endoscopic treatment that involves subureteral or intraureteral injection of dextranomer hyaluronidase (Deflux) is offered in most cases (Figures 48.6 and 48.7). The reported success rate for this procedure is 83%, compared to 98.1% for open surgical reimplantation.[34] Meta-analysis of all of the endoscopic modalities used for VUR revealed that the cure rates per ureter for grades I and II was 78.5%, grade III was 72%, grade IV was 63%, and grade V was 51%.[109] A success rate of 68% was noted for patients failing first injection and 34% for those failing a second injection. Reduced success rates have been reported in patients with duplicated systems and those with neurogenic bladders.[109] Postoperative ureteral obstruction and calcification of the implant of dextranomer/hyaluronic acid, which mimics distal ureteral calculus, have been noted as complications of the procedure.[110,111] Improved success rate and the minimally invasive nature have led to a substantial increase in the number of endoscopic procedures.[112]

---

**KEY POINT**

The success rate of endoscopic repair of VUR decreases with increasing grade of VUR.

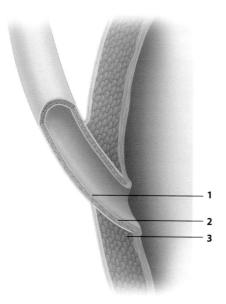

Figure 48.6 The endoscopic method currently achieving the highest success rates for treatment of vesicoureteral reflux (VUR) is the double hydrodistention implantation technique (HIT). The needle is passed into the ureteric orifice (UO) and inserted at the midureteral tunnel at the 6 o'clock position. Sufficient bulking agent is injected to produce a bulge, which initially coapts the detrusor tunnel, while a second implant within the most distal intramural tunnel leads to coaptation of the UO. Sites 1 and 2 comprise the double HIT method, and site 3 (STING) is rarely used. (Reproduced with permission from: Läckgren G, Kirsch AJ. Surgery: illustrated surgical atlas endoscopic treatment of vesicoureteral reflux. BJU Int. 2010;105:1332–47.)

## Laparoscopic ureteral reimplantation

Laparoscopic ureteral reimplantation has the benefit of providing results that are less invasive than with open surgery. Overall success with correction of VUR is similar to that with the open procedures.[113] Complications include ureteral injury, ureteral leak, and ureteral stricture.[113,114]

## Open surgical technique

The gold standard for the surgical management of VUR remains the open approaches. The most commonly performed open technique is the Cohen cross-trigonal reimplantation (Figure 48.8).[115] The success rates of this procedure for the correction of VUR are consistently approximately 98%, to the point that most clinicians have stopped performing follow-up studies to confirm reflux resolution.[116,117] Contralateral VUR is noted in 19% of patients who have had unilateral ureteral reimplantation, with the majority resolving over the ensuing 2 years, and are thought to be the result of trigonal changes following ureteral reimplantation.[118] Ureteral stricture resulting from ischemia of the distal ureter also has been reported in surgically corrected patients. Endoscopic access to the ureter following ureteral reimplantation can be difficult, which should be kept in mind if a patient needs the procedure for stone removal later in life. Sung and Skoog[119] extensively reviewed the open surgical techniques for ureteric reimplantation.

## MANAGING VOIDING AND BOWEL DYSFUNCTION

Treatment of constipation by dietary measures, behavioral therapy, and laxatives helps reduce UTI recurrence and facilitates the resolution of enuresis and uninhibited bladder contractions.[43,120] The treatment of voiding dysfunction or DES includes the use of laxatives and timed frequent voiding, every 2 to 3 hours. Pelvic floor exercises, behavioral modification, anticholinergic medication, or a combination of these may be required. A combined conservative medical and computer game–assisted pelvic floor muscle retraining decreased the incidence of breakthrough UTI and facilitated VUR resolution in children with voiding dysfunction and VUR.[121] Similar results of improved outcome with medical management have been reported by others.[122,123]

(a)

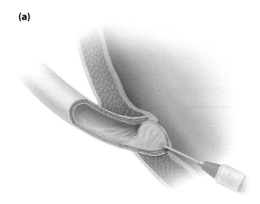

(b)

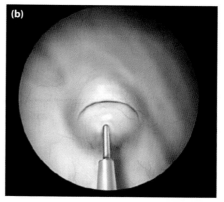

Figure 48.7 Endoscopic injection technique developed by Kirsch et al. In most patients a combination of the intraureteric injection and the STING is used to achieve an optimal bolus. (Reproduced with permission from: Läckgren G, Kirsch AJ. Surgery: illustrated surgical atlas endoscopic treatment of vesicoureteral reflux. BJU Int. 2010;105:1332–47.)

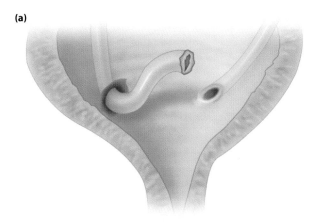

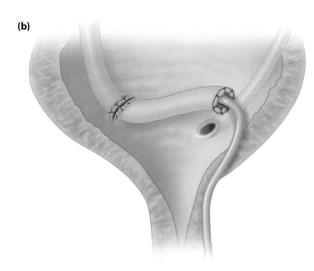

Figure 48.8 The Cohen procedure is the most widely used technique for surgical correction of vesicoureteral reflux. **(a)** The ureters (the procedure is often bilateral) are mobilized intravesically. **(b)** Two separate submucosal tunnels are created so that each ureter opens on the opposite side from its hiatus. (Reproduced with permission from: Capozza N, Caione P. Vesicoureteral reflux: surgical and endoscopic treatment. Pediatr Nephrol. 2007;22:1261–5.)

## HYPERTENSION AND PROTEINURIA

Appropriate management of hypertension and proteinuria is important to slow progression of renal disease. Although a large number of antihypertensive drugs are available for clinical use, ACE inhibitors (ACEIs) or angiotensin II receptor blockers (ARBs) are preferred because of their renoprotective effect. Studies have revealed that ACEIs, besides lowering the blood pressure, reduce proteinuria resulting from RN.[124] Therapy with ACEI may be particularly beneficial for patients with RN, especially those born with D alleles of the ACE gene.[125] In some patients with very poorly functioning scarred kidney and a healthy second kidney, the removal of a poorly functioning kidney may help cure hypertension.

## SUMMARY

VUR increases the risks for UTI and renal scarring, which can lead to CKD and hypertension. Management strategies continue to evolve, with options that include open surgical repair, endoscopic repair, antibiotic prophylaxis, and surveillance. A variety of variables influence the management strategy for the individual patient, including the severity of the VUR, the presence of UTIs and scarring, and the age of the patient. Prophylactic antibiotics have been used in prevention of UTI in patients with VUR for over three decades. For various reasons, including the risk of antibiotic resistance, the use of prophylactic antibiotics in VUR has come under increasing criticism. The RIVUR study, however, has provided support for use of prophylactic antibiotics in prevention of UTIs in patients with VUR.

## REFERENCES

1. Carpenter MA, Hoberman A, Mattoo TK, et al. The RIVUR Trial: Profile and baseline clinical associations of children with vesicoureteral reflux. Pediatrics. 2013;132:e34–45.
2. Ransley PG. Vesicoureteric reflux: Continuing surgical dilemma. Urology. 1978;12:246–55.
3. Smellie J, Edwards D, Hunter N, et al. Vesicoureteric reflux and renal scarring. Kidney Int Suppl. 1975;4:S65–72.
4. Wennerstrom M, Hansson S, Jodal U, Stokland E. Disappearance of vesicoureteral reflux in children. Arch Pediatr Adolesc Med. 1998;152:879–83.
5. Dick PT, Feldman W. Routine diagnostic imaging for childhood urinary tract infections: A systematic overview. J Pediatr. 1996;128:15–22.
6. Arant BS, Jr. Medical management of mild and moderate vesicoureteral reflux: Followup studies of infants and young children—A preliminary report of the Southwest Pediatric Nephrology Study Group. J Urol. 1992;148:1683–7.
7. Rolleston GL, Shannon FT, Utley WL. Follow-up of vesico-ureteric reflux in the newborn. Kidney Int Suppl. 1975;4:S59–64.
8. Rolleston GL, Shannon FT, Utley WL. Relationship of infantile vesicoureteric reflux to renal damage. Br Med J. 1970;1:460–3.
9. Skoog SJ, Belman AB, Majd M. A nonsurgical approach to the management of primary vesicoureteral reflux. J Urol. 1987;138:941–6.
10. Dwoskin JY, Perlmutter AD. Vesicoureteral reflux in children: A computerized review. J Urol. 1973;109:888–90.
11. Scott JE. The management of ureteric reflux in children. Br J Urol. 1977;49:109–18.

12. Snodgrass W. The impact of treated dysfunctional voiding on the nonsurgical management of vesicoureteral reflux. J Urol. 1998;160:1823–5.

13. Drachman R, Valevici M, Vardy PA. Excretory urography and cystourethrography in the evaluation of children with urinary tract infection. Clin Pediatr (Phila). 1984;23:265–7.

14. Askari A, Belman AB. Vesicoureteral reflux in black girls. J Urol. 1982;127:747–8.

15. Kunin CM. A ten-year study of bacteriuria in schoolgirls: Final report of bacteriologic, urologic, and epidemiologic findings. J Infect Dis. 1970;122:382–93.

16. Skoog SJ, Belman AB. Primary vesicoureteral reflux in the black child. Pediatrics. 1991;87:538–43.

17. Chand DH, Rhoades T, Poe SA, et al. Incidence and severity of vesicoureteral reflux in children related to age, gender, race and diagnosis. J Urol. 2003;170:1548–50.

18. Zerin JM, Ritchey ML, Chang AC. Incidental vesicoureteral reflux in neonates with antenatally detected hydronephrosis and other renal abnormalities. Radiology. 1993;187:157–60.

19. Marra G, Barbieri G, Dell'Agnola CA, et al. Congenital renal damage associated with primary vesicoureteral reflux detected prenatally in male infants. J Pediatr. 1994;124:726–30.

20. Jerkins GR, Noe HN. Familial vesicoureteral reflux: A prospective study. J Urol. 1982;128:774–8.

21. Van den Abbeele AD, Treves ST, Lebowitz RL, et al. Vesicoureteral reflux in asymptomatic siblings of patients with known reflux: Radionuclide cystography. Pediatrics. 1987;79:147–53.

22. Noe HN, Wyatt RJ, Peeden JN, Jr, Rivas ML. The transmission of vesicoureteral reflux from parent to child. J Urol. 1992;148:1869–71.

23. Lebowitz RL, Olbing H, Parkkulainen KV, et al. International system of radiographic grading of vesicoureteric reflux. International Reflux Study in Children. Pediatr Radiol. 1985;15:105–9.

24. Hutch JA. Theory of maturation of the intravesical ureter. J Urol. 1961;86:534–8.

25. Birmingham Reflux Study Group. Prospective trial of operative versus non-operative treatment of severe vesicoureteric reflux in children: Five years' observation. Br Med J. 1987;295:237–41.

26. Tamminen-Mobius T, Brunier E, Ebel KD, et al. Cessation of vesicoureteral reflux for 5 years in infants and children allocated to medical treatment. The International Reflux Study in Children. J Urol. 1992;148:1662–6.

27. Silva JM, Diniz JS, Lima EM, et al. Predictive factors of resolution of primary vesico-ureteric reflux: A multivariate analysis. BJU Int. 2006;97:1063–8.

28. Schwab CW, Jr, Wu HY, Selman H, et al. Spontaneous resolution of vesicoureteral reflux: A 15-year perspective. J Urol. 2002;168:2594–9.

29. Smellie JM, Jodal U, Lax H, et al. Outcome at 10 years of severe vesicoureteric reflux managed medically: Report of the International Reflux Study in Children. J Pediatr. 2001;139:656–63.

30. Elder JS, Peters CA, Arant BS, Jr, et al. Pediatric Vesicoureteral Reflux Guidelines Panel summary report on the management of primary vesicoureteral reflux in children. J Urol. 1997;157:1846–51.

31. Upadhyay J, McLorie GA, Bolduc S, et al. Natural history of neonatal reflux associated with prenatal hydronephrosis: Long-term results of a prospective study. J Urol. 2003;169:1837–41; discussion 41; author reply 41.

32. Connolly LP, Treves ST, Zurakowski D, Bauer SB. Natural history of vesicoureteral reflux in siblings. J Urol. 1996;156:1805–7.

33. Shaikh N, Ewing AL, Bhatnagar S, Hoberman A. Risk of renal scarring in children with a first urinary tract infection: A systematic review. Pediatrics. 2010;126:1084–91.

34. Peters CA, Skoog SJ, Arant BS, et al. Summary of the AUA guideline on management of primary vesicoureteral reflux in children. J Urol. 2010;184:1134–44.

35. Chen JJ, Pugach J, West D, et al. Infant vesicoureteral reflux: A comparison between patients presenting with a prenatal diagnosis and those presenting with a urinary tract infection. Urology. 2003;61:442–6, discussion 6–7.

36. Shaikh N, Hoberman A, Wise B, et al. Dysfunctional elimination syndrome: Is it related to urinary tract infection or vesicoureteral reflux diagnosed early in life? Pediatrics. 2003;112:1134–7.

37. Norgaard JP, van Gool JD, Hjalmas K, et al. Standardization and definitions in lower urinary tract dysfunction in children. International Children's Continence Society. Br J Urol. 1998;81(Suppl 3):1–16.

38. Koff SA, Wagner TT, Jayanthi VR. The relationship among dysfunctional elimination syndromes, primary vesicoureteral reflux and urinary tract infections in children. J Urol. 1998;160:1019–22.

39. Seruca H. Vesicoureteral reflux and voiding dysfunction: A prospective study. J Urol. 1989;142:494–8; discussion 501.

40. Koff SA. Relationship between dysfunctional voiding and reflux. J Urol. 1992;148:1703–5.

41. van Gool JD, Hjalmas K, Tamminen-Mobius T, Olbing H. Historical clues to the complex of dysfunctional voiding, urinary tract infection and vesicoureteral reflux. The International Reflux Study in Children. J Urol. 1992;148:1699–702.

42. Rushton HG. Wetting and functional voiding disorders. Urol Clin North Am. 1995;22:75–93.

43. O'Regan S, Yazbeck S, Schick E. Constipation, bladder instability, urinary tract infection syndrome. Clin Nephrol. 1985;23:152–4.

44. Neumann PZ, DeDomenico IJ, Nogrady MB. Constipation and urinary tract infection. Pediatrics. 1973;52:241–5.

45. Chase JW, Homsy Y, Siggaard C, et al. Functional constipation in children. J Urol. 2004;171:2641–3.

46. Winberg J, Andersen HJ, Bergstrom T, et al. Epidemiology of symptomatic urinary tract infection in childhood. Acta Paediatrica Suppl. 1974;252:1–20.

47. Pylkkanen J, Vilska J, Koskimies O. The value of level diagnosis of childhood urinary tract infection in predicting renal injury. Acta Paediatr Scand. 1981;70:879–83.

48. Faust WC, Diaz M, Pohl HG. Incidence of post-pyelonephritic renal scarring: A meta-analysis of the dimercapto-succinic acid literature. J Urol. 2009;181:290–7; discussion 7–8.

49. Rushton HG. The evaluation of acute pyelonephritis and renal scarring with technetium 99m-dimer-captosuccinic acid renal scintigraphy: Evolving concepts and future directions. Pediatr Nephrol. 1997;11:108–20.

50. Doganis D, Siafas K, Mavrikou M, et al. Does early treatment of urinary tract infection prevent renal damage? Pediatrics. 2007;120:e922–8.

51. Ahmed M, Eggleston D, Kapur G, et al. Dimercaptosuccinic acid (DMSA) renal scan in the evaluation of hypertension in children. Pediatr Nephrol. 2008;23:435–8.

52. Barai S, Bandopadhayaya GP, Bhowmik D, et al. Prevalence of vesicoureteral reflux in patients with incidentally diagnosed adult hypertension. Urology. 2004;63:1045–8; discussion 8–9.

53. Yeung CK, Godley ML, Dhillon HK, et al. The characteristics of primary vesico-ureteric reflux in male and female infants with pre-natal hydronephrosis. Br J Urol. 1997;80:319–27.

54. Ismaili K, Hall M, Piepsz A, et al. Primary vesicoureteral reflux detected in neonates with a history of fetal renal pelvis dilatation: A prospective clinical and imaging study. J Pediatr. 2006;148:222–7.

55. Sweeney B, Cascio S, Velayudham M, Puri P. Reflux nephropathy in infancy: A comparison of infants presenting with and without urinary tract infection. J Urol. 2001;166:648–50.

56. Ransley PG, Risdon RA. Renal papillary morphology in infants and young children. Urol Res. 1975;3:111–3.

57. Verber IG, Meller ST. Serial 99mTc dimercaptosuc-cinic acid (DMSA) scans after urinary infections presenting before the age of 5 years. Arch Dis Child 1989;64:1533–7.

58. Piepsz A, Tamminen-Mobius T, Reiners C, et al. Five-year study of medical or surgical treatment in children with severe vesico-ureteral reflux dimercaptosuccinic acid findings. International Reflux Study Group in Europe. Eur J Pediatr. 1998;157:753–8.

59. American Academy of Pediatrics, Committee on Quality Improvement. Subcommittee on Urinary Tract Infection. Practice parameter: The diagnosis, treatment, and evaluation of the initial urinary tract infection in febrile infants and young children. Pediatrics. 1999;103:843–52.

60. Miller T, Phillips S. Pyelonephritis: The relationship between infection, renal scarring, and antimicrobial therapy. Kidney Int. 1981;19:654–62.

61. Jodal U. The natural history of bacteriuria in childhood. Infect Dis Clin North Am. 1987;1:713–29.

62. Jakobsson B, Berg U, Svensson L. Renal scarring after acute pyelonephritis. Arch Dis Child. 1994;70:111–5.

63. Lomberg H, Hellstrom M, Jodal U, et al. Virulence-associated traits in Escherichia coli causing first and recurrent episodes of urinary tract infection in children with or without vesicoureteral reflux. J Infect Dis. 1984;150:561–9.

64. de Man P, Claeson I, Johanson IM, et al. Bacterial attachment as a predictor of renal abnormalities in boys with urinary tract infection. J Pediatr. 1989;115:915–22.

65. Ozen S, Alikasifoglu M, Saatci U, et al. Implications of certain genetic polymorphisms in scarring in vesicoureteric reflux: Importance of ACE polymorphism. Am J Kid Dis. 1999;34:140–5.

66. Hohenfellner K, Hunley TE, Brezinska R, et al. ACE I/D gene polymorphism predicts renal damage in congenital uropathies. Pediatr Nephrol. 1999;13:514–8.

67. Zhang MJ, Hoelzer D, Horowitz MM, et al. Long-term follow-up of adults with acute lymphoblastic leukemia in first remission treated with chemo-therapy or bone marrow transplantation. The Acute Lymphoblastic Leukemia Working Committee. Ann Int Med. 1995;123:428–31.

68. Kohler J, Tencer J, Thysell H, Forsberg L. Vesicoureteral reflux diagnosed in adulthood: Incidence of urinary tract infections, hypertension, proteinuria, back pain and renal calculi. Nephrol Dialysis Transplant. 1997;12:2580–7.

69. Simoes e Silva AC, Silva JMP, Diniz JSS, et al. Risk of hypertension in primary vesicoureteral reflux. Pediatr Nephrol. 2007;22:459–62.

70. Goonasekera CD, Shah V, Wade AM, et al. 15-year follow-up of renin and blood pressure in reflux nephropathy. Lancet 1996;347:640–3.

71. Savage JM, Koh CT, Shah V, et al. Five year prospective study of plasma renin activity and blood pressure in patients with longstanding reflux nephropathy. Arch Dis Child. 1987;62:678–82.

72. Wolfish NM, Delbrouck NF, Shanon A, et al. Prevalence of hypertension in children with primary vesicoureteral reflux. J Pediatr. 1993;123:559–63.

73. Wennerstrom M, Hansson S, Hedner T, et al. Ambulatory blood pressure 16–26 years after the first urinary tract infection in childhood. J Hypertens. 2000;18:485–91.

74. Zhang Y, Bailey RR. A long term follow up of adults with reflux nephropathy. N Z Med J. 1995;108:142–4.

75. Karlen J, Linne T, Wikstad I, Aperia A. Incidence of microalbuminuria in children with pyelonephritic scarring. Pediatr Nephrol (Berlin) 1996;10:705–8.
76. Craig JC, Irwig LM, Knight JF, Roy LP. Does treatment of vesicoureteric reflux in childhood prevent end-stage renal disease attributable to reflux nephropathy? Pediatrics 2000;105:1236–41.
77. Kincaid-Smith P. Glomerular lesions in atrophic pyelonephritis and reflux nephropathy. Kidney Int Suppl. 1975;4:S81–3.
78. North American Pediatric Renal Transplant Cooperative Studies. 2008 Annual Report, Boston, NAPRTCS; 2008.
79. Furth SL, Abraham GA, Jerry-Fluker J, et al. Metabolic abnormalities, CVD risk factors and GFR decline in children with CKD. Clin J Am Soc Nephrol. 2011;6:2132–40.
80. Bailey RR, Lynn KL, Smith AH. Long-term followup of infants with gross vesicoureteral reflux. J Urol. 1992;148:1709–11.
81. Lahdes-Vasama T, Niskanen K, Ronnholm K. Outcome of kidneys in patients treated for vesicoureteral reflux (VUR) during childhood. Nephrol Dial Transplant. 2006;21:2491–7.
82. el-Khatib M, Packham DK, Becker GJ, Kincaid-Smith P. Pregnancy-related complications in women with reflux nephropathy. Clin Nephrol. 1994;41:50–5.
83. Jungers P, Houillier P, Chauveau D, et al. Pregnancy in women with reflux nephropathy. Kidney Int. 1996;50:593–9.
84. Hollowell JG. Outcome of pregnancy in women with a history of vesico-ureteric reflux. BJU Int. 2008;102:780–4.
85. Gruneberg RN, Leakey A, Bendall MJ, Smellie JM. Bowel flora in urinary tract infection: Effect of chemotherapy with special reference to cotrimoxazole. Kidney Int Suppl. 1975;4:S122–9.
86. Smellie JM, Tamminen-Mobius T, Olbing H, et al. Five-year study of medical or surgical treatment in children with severe reflux: Radiological renal findings. The International Reflux Study in Children. Pediatr Nephrol. 1992;6:223–30.
87. Jodal U, Smellie JM, Lax H, Hoyer PF. Ten-year results of randomized treatment of children with severe vesicoureteral reflux: Final report of the International Reflux Study in Children. Pediatr Nephrol. 2006;21:785–92.
88. Brandstrom P, Esbjorner E, Herthelius M, et al. The Swedish reflux trial in children. III. Urinary tract infection pattern. J Urol. 2010;184:286–91.
89. Brandstrom P, Neveus T, Sixt R, et al. The Swedish reflux trial in children. IV. Renal damage. J Urol. 2010;184:292–7.
90. Shakil A, Reed L, Wilder L, Strand WR. Clinical inquiries: Do antibiotics prevent recurrent UTI in children with anatomic abnormalities? J Fam Pract. 2004;53:498–500.
91. Cooper CS, Chung BI, Kirsch AJ, et al. The outcome of stopping prophylactic antibiotics in older children with vesicoureteral reflux. J Urol. 2000;163:269–72; discussion 72–3.
92. Tamminen-Mobius T, Brunier E, Ebel KD, et al. Cessation of vesicoureteral reflux for 5 years in infants and children allocated to medical treatment. The International Reflux Study in Children. J Urol. 1992;148:1662–6.
93. Allen UD, MacDonald N, Fuite L, et al. Risk factors for resistance to "first-line" antimicrobials among urinary tract isolates of Escherichia coli in children. Can Med Assoc J. 1999;160:1436–40.
94. Karpman E, Kurzrock EA. Adverse reactions of nitrofurantoin, trimethoprim and sulfamethoxazole in children. J Urol. 2004;172:448–53.
95. Uhari M, Nuutinen M, Turtinen J. Adverse reactions in children during long-term antimicrobial therapy. Pediatr Infect Dis J. 1996;15:404–8.
96. Bollgren I. Antibacterial prophylaxis in children with urinary tract infection. Acta Paediatr Suppl. 1999;88:48–52.
97. Williams G, Lee A, Craig J. Antibiotics for the prevention of urinary tract infection in children: A systematic review of randomized controlled trials. J Pediatr. 2001;138:868–74.
98. Wheeler D, Vimalachandra D, Hodson EM, et al. Antibiotics and surgery for vesicoureteric reflux: A meta-analysis of randomised controlled trials. Arch Dis Child. 2003;88:688–94.
99. Gordon I, Barkovics M, Pindoria S, et al. Primary vesicoureteric reflux as a predictor of renal damage in children hospitalized with urinary tract infection: A systematic review and meta-analysis. J Am Soc Nephrol. 2003;14:739–44.
100. Williams GJ, Wei L, Lee A, Craig JC. Long-term antibiotics for preventing recurrent urinary tract infection in children. Cochrane Database Syst Rev. 2006;(3):001534.
101. Garin EH, Olavarria F, Garcia Nieto V, et al. Clinical significance of primary vesicoureteral reflux and urinary antibiotic prophylaxis after acute pyelonephritis: A multicenter, randomized, controlled study. Pediatrics. 2006;117:626–32.
102. Roussey-Kesler G, Gadjos V, Idres N, et al. Antibiotic prophylaxis for the prevention of recurrent urinary tract infection in children with low grade vesicoureteral reflux: Results from a prospective randomized study. J Urol. 2008;179:674–9.

103. Pennesi M, Travan L, Peratoner L, et al. Is antibiotic prophylaxis in children with vesicoureteral reflux effective in preventing pyelonephritis and renal scars? A randomized, controlled trial. Pediatrics. 2008;121:e1489–94.

104. Montini G, Rigon L, Zucchetta P, et al. Prophylaxis after first febrile urinary tract infection in children? A multicenter, randomized, controlled, noninferiority trial. Pediatrics. 2008;122:1064–71.

105. Craig JC, Simpson JM, Williams GJ, et al. Antibiotic prophylaxis and recurrent urinary tract infection in children. N Engl J Med. 2009;361:1748–59.

106. Subcommittee on Urinary Tract Infection, Steering Committee on Quality Improvement and Management. Urinary tract infection: Clinical practice guideline for the diagnosis and management of the initial UTI in febrile infants and children 2 to 24 months. Pediatrics. 2011;128:595–610.

107. Randomized Intervention for Children with Vesicoureteral Reflux Trial Investigators. Antimicrobial prophylaxis for children with vesicoureteral reflux. N Engl J Med. 2014;370:2367–76.

108. Diamond DA, Mattoo TK. Endoscopic treatment of primary vesicoureteral reflux. N Engl J Med. 2012;366:1218–26.

109. Elder JS, Diaz M, Caldamone AA, et al. Endoscopic therapy for vesicoureteral reflux: A meta-analysis. I. Reflux resolution and urinary tract infection. J Urol. 2006;175:716–22.

110. Vandersteen DR, Routh JC, Kirsch AJ, et al. Postoperative ureteral obstruction after subureteral injection of dextranomer/hyaluronic acid copolymer. J Urol. 2006;176:1593–5.

111. Nelson CP, Chow JS. Dextranomer/hyaluronic acid copolymer (Deflux) implants mimicking distal ureteral calculi on CT. Pediatr Radiol. 2008;38:104–6.

112. Lendvay TS, Sorensen M, Cowan CA, et al. The evolution of vesicoureteral reflux management in the era of dextranomer/hyaluronic acid copolymer: A Pediatric Health Information System database study. J Urol. 2006;176:1864–7.

113. Kutikov A, Guzzo TJ, Canter DJ, Casale P. Initial experience with laparoscopic transvesical ureteral reimplantation at the Children's Hospital of Philadelphia. J Urol. 2006;176:2222–5; discussion 5–6.

114. Lakshmanan Y, Fung LC. Laparoscopic extravesicular ureteral reimplantation for vesicoureteral reflux: Recent technical advances. J Endourol. 2000;14:589–93; discussion 593–4.

115. Kaplan WE, Firlit CF. Management of reflux in the myelodysplastic child. J Urol. 1983;129:1195–7.

116. Kennelly MJ, Bloom DA, Ritchey ML, Panzl AC. Outcome analysis of bilateral Cohen cross-trigonal ureteroneocystostomy. Urology. 1995;46:393–5.

117. Bisignani G, Decter RM. Voiding cystourethrography after uncomplicated ureteral reimplantation in children: Is it necessary? J Urol. 1997;158:1229–31.

118. Hoenig DM, Diamond DA, Rabinowitz R, Caldamone AA. Contralateral reflux after unilateral ureteral reimplantation. J Urol. 1996;156:196–7.

119. Sung J, Skoog S. Surgical management of vesicoureteral reflux in children Pediatr Nephrol. 2012;27:551–61

120. O'Regan S, Yazbeck S, Hamberger B, Schick E. Constipation a commonly unrecognized cause of enuresis. Am J Dis Child. 1986;140:260–1.

121. Herndon CD, Decambre M, McKenna PH. Interactive computer games for treatment of pelvic floor dysfunction. J Urol. 2001;166:1893–8.

122. Upadhyay J, Bolduc S, Bagli DJ, et al. Use of the dysfunctional voiding symptom score to predict resolution of vesicoureteral reflux in children with voiding dysfunction. J Urol. 2003;169:1842–6; discussion 6; author reply 6.

123. Schulman SL, Quinn CK, Plachter N, Kodman-Jones C. Comprehensive management of dysfunctional voiding. Pediatrics. 1999;103:E31.

124. Praga M, Hernandez E, Montoyo C, et al. Long-term beneficial effects of angiotensin-converting enzyme inhibition in patients with nephrotic proteinuria. Am J Kidney Dis. 1992;20:240–8.

125. Ohtomo Y, Nagaoka R, Kaneko K, et al. Angiotensin converting enzyme gene polymorphism in primary vesicoureteral reflux. Pediatr Nephrol. 2001;16:648–52.

126. Risdon RA. The small scarred kidney in childhood. Pediatr Nephrol. 1993;7:361–4.

## REVIEW QUESTIONS

1. Which of the following is associated with a higher incidence of primary vesicoureteral reflux diagnosed after urinary tract infection?
   a. Older age
   b. Male gender
   c. African American race
   d. Family history of vesicoureteral reflux in parent or sibling

2. Which of the following is a risk factor for renal scarring after a UTI?
   a. African American race
   b. High grade vesicoureteral reflux
   c. Absence of vesicoureteral reflux
   d. Diarrhea
   e. Pyuria

3. Hypertension is most directly associated with which of the following?
   a. History of urinary tract infections
   b. Vesicoureteral reflux
   c. Use of Deflux
   d. Renal scarring

4. Which of the following is a risk factor for unsuccessful endoscopic repair of vesicoureteral reflux?
   a. Neurogenic bladder
   b. Congenital reflux
   c. History of UTI
   d. Caucasian race
   e. Grade I or II reflux

5. The success rate of open surgical repair of vesicoureteral reflux is approximately:
   a. 65%
   b. 75%
   c. 85%
   d. 90%
   e. 98%

6. Which of the following is the preferred agent for treating hypertension in a patient with reflux nephropathy?
   a. Calcium channel blocker
   b. Beta blocker
   c. ACE inhibitor
   d. Thiazide diuretic

## ANSWER KEY

1. d
2. b
3. d
4. a
5. e
6. c

# 49

# Urinary tract infection

BRITTANY GOLDBERG AND BARBARA JANTAUSCH

Urinary tract infection (UTI) is a common childhood infection, being second in frequency only to respiratory infections. In many children, these infections recur, causing significant morbidity, hospitalizations, and long-term health effects, such as renal scars, hypertension, and chronic kidney disease (CKD). Although bacterial UTIs are well recognized in children and adults, fungal, viral, and parasitic infections of the urinary tract are also encountered with an increasing frequency, especially in immunocompromised and susceptible subpopulations. The increasing prevalence of antimicrobial resistance in bacteria introduces an additional level of complexity to the management of patients with UTIs.

## KEY POINTS

- Asymptomatic bacteriuria is more common among girls.
- Lifetime risk for symptomatic UTI is 3 to 5 times higher in girls than in boys.
- Approximately 2% of boys and 3% to 8% of girls will develop a UTI during their lifetime.
- During first 3 months of life, male infants have a higher incidence of UTI than females.

## EPIDEMIOLOGY

Large-scale urinary screening studies of school children suggests the prevalence of bacteriuria in asymptomatic children to be 0.7% to 1.95% in girls and 0.04% to 0.2% in boys.[1,2] It has been estimated that 2% to 5% of girls would develop bacteriuria by the time they graduate from high school.[2,3] The American Association of Pediatrics (AAP) clinical practice guidelines estimates the prevalence of UTI to be approximately 5% in children 2 to 24 months of age.[4] The lifetime risk for symptomatic UTI is 3 to 5 times higher in girls than boys. In numerous epidemiologic studies, the overall risk for UTI has been reported as 1.1% to 1.8% in boys and 3.3% to 7.8% in girls.[5-7]

In the first 3 months of life, UTI is more common in males than in females. The male-to-female ratio of children with UTI in this age group ranges from 2:1 to 5:1.[8-10] The reasons for male predilection for UTI in neonates remains unclear, but follows a similar trend noted for other infections and sepsis in this age group. Circumcision has been noted to reduce the risk for UTI in male infants.[11] Bacteremia associated with UTI is also common in neonates and young infants. Ginsburg and McCracken[12] reported the incidence of bacteremia in hospitalized infants younger than 8 weeks with UTI to be as high as 31%. A recent study found the incidence of bacteremia in febrile infants aged 29 to 60 days with UTI to be only 6.5%.[13] Others also have reported a lower incidence (approximately 10%) of bacteremia in unselected nonhospitalized infants with UTI.[14]

## BACTERIOLOGY

Gram-negative enteric bacteria of the Enterobacteriaceae family cause most UTIs in children of all ages. This includes *Escherichia coli*, which is responsible for 80% to 85% of all UTIs in children. *Klebsiella, Proteus, Citrobacter, Enterobacter* species, and *Morganella morganii,* the other members of the Enterobacteriaceae family, are less frequent causes of UTI.[12,15-17] *Pseudomonas aeruginosa,* Gram-positive organisms such as *Enterococcus, Staphylococcus,* and *group B streptococci* also can cause UTI in children. *Group B streptococcus* is almost exclusively seen as a cause of UTI in neonates, whereas *Staphylococcus saprophyticus* is seen commonly in adolescent girls.[18,19] *Staphylococcus aureus* is an uncommon cause of UTI and may be the result of hematogenous spread to the kidney. Infection with *S. aureus* often results in focal renal lesions, such as intrarenal and perinephric abscesses.[20,21]

Since their discovery in the 1980s, bacteria that produce extended-spectrum β-lactamase (ESBL) have increased in prevalence among nosocomial and community-acquired UTIs. ESBL bacteria primarily include Gram-negative organisms, particularly *Klebsiella* and *E. coli.*[22] Prevalence of ESBL bacteria varies among geographic regions, with regional rates of resistant organisms surpassing 50% in some areas.[23] A study by Moland et al. found that 11.3% of *Klebsiella pneumoniae,* 2.6% of *E. coli,* 1.6% of *Serratia marcescens,* 1.4% of *Proteus,* and 3.5% of *Citrobacter koseri* were categorized as ESBL.[24] Another review of ESBL bacteria at a tertiary children's hospital found that 78% of ESBL bacterial cultures were isolated in urine.[25] The overall incidence of ESBL bacteria among Enterobacteriaceae was found to be 7%, with *E. coli* responsible for 78% of ESBL isolates and *Klebsiella* accounting for 12.7%.

---

### KEY POINTS

- Ascending infection accounts for most cases of UTI.
- Most UTIs are caused by Gram-negative bacteria, such as *E. coli* and *Klebsiella.*
- *Group B streptococci* may cause UTI in neonates.
- *S. aureus* is an uncommon cause of UTI that may result in renal abscess.

---

## PATHOGENESIS

Infection can reach the urinary tract via the ascending route or by the hematogenous route. Hematogenous spread of infection to the urinary tract accounts for fewer than 1%

of UTIs and commonly occurs in association with sepsis, particularly that caused by *S. aureus.*[20,21] Resultant infection leads to focal renal lesions, such as pyelonephritis, intraparenchymal abscess, and perinephric abscess. In most cases, UTI results from an ascending infection, where the Gram-negative enteric flora ascends via the urethra to invade the urinary tract and cause asymptomatic bacteruria, acute cystitis, or acute pyelonephritis.

Virulence of the infecting organism is an important aspect of establishing infection within the host urinary tract. Predisposition to UTIs also can result from structural abnormalities of the urinary tract, such as vesicoureteral reflux (VUR), or from functional derangements of the bladder. Identification and treatment of these underlying disorders is an integral component of the management plan for affected children.

## BACTERIAL VIRULENCE FACTORS

Specific microbiologic properties of *E. coli,* known as virulence factors, are now recognized to be involved in enhancing the invasiveness of these organisms. Strains possessing these virulence factors are able to spread to the urinary tract and result in more serious infections. Interestingly, *E. coli* strains isolated from patients with asymptomatic bacteriuria have been found to carry virulence genes that are similar to pathogenic strains, but appear to down-regulate expression of these genes when they establish colonization.[26]

---

### KEY POINT

The increasing prevalence of ESBL Gram-negative bacteria is changing antibiotic resistance patterns in communities.[26]

---

### Adhesins or fimbriae

Adhesins, or fimbriae, are microscopic appendages present on the surface of *E. coli* that allow bacterial adherence to the uroepithelial cell.[27] Fimbriae allow *E. coli* to bind to specific glycolipid receptors on uroepithelial cells and permit evasion of host defense mechanisms for colonization of the urinary tract. Type I fimbriae, type II fimbriae (also known as *P* fimbriae), and the Dr hemagglutinin are the three types of clinically significant fimbriae expressed by uropathogenic *E. coli.*

Recent studies have demonstrated significant differences in fimbrial expression between commensal *E. coli* strains and pathogenic *E. coli.* Pyelonephritis isolates have more fimbrial types than commensal isolates.[28] Type I fimbriae exhibit mannose-sensitive hemagglutination and attach to bladder epithelial cells.[29] *P* fimbriae demonstrate mannose-resistant hemagglutination and are associated with acute pyelonephritis.[30] *E. coli* that express the Dr hemagglutinin, a fimbria-like adhesin, are associated with the development of cystitis.[31]

## Hemolysin and cytotoxic protein

*E. coli* strains that produce hemolysin, a cytotoxic protein that lyses erythrocytes and other cells, are associated with the development of acute pyelonephritis. The effects of hemolysin on host cells are thought to contribute to the inflammation and tissue injury associated with hemolytic *E. coli*.[32] Similarly, colicin, another cytotoxic protein, is also thought to contribute to *E. coli* virulence.[33]

## Serotypes and bacterial virulence

*E. coli* contain three major antigens that are identified through antibody serotyping and are associated with invasiveness, virulence, and the ability to evade phagocytosis and complement-mediated lyses. These are the O antigen present in the outer membrane of the cell wall, K antigen, the capsular antigen, and H antigen, or the flagellar antigen. More than 150 O antigens and in excess of 80 K and H antigens have been identified.[32,34] *E. coli* strains with certain O antigen serogroups (1, 2, 4, 6, 7, 8, 16, 18, 25, and 75) are associated with the development of pyelonephritis.[35-37] *E. coli* strains are typically named after their O and H serotypes.

## Bacterial genetics

Many of the genes encoding for the virulence factors in *E. coli* are located on distinct pieces of DNA called *pathogenicity islands* (PAIs) that are present in the genome of pathogenic bacteria and are not found in avirulent bacteria strains. Genes encoding for hemolysin or *P* fimbriae production are characteristically found in PAIs. PAIs can be deleted from the chromosome and also can be transferred to other bacteria by helper phages.[38,39] Many pathogenic strains of *E. coli* may carry more than one PAI, although the implication for virulence is unclear.[40]

## HOST FACTORS

Some children are prone to developing UTI and may have frequent recurrences. Several anatomic, functional, and behavioral factors can render children prone to UTI. Although it is possible that a solitary risk factor may render many children susceptible to UTI, multiple risk factors often are operative in others.

## Inflammatory response

The inflammatory response generated by the host in the kidney and the urinary tract to the invading bacteria is an essential determinant of the severity and outcome of UTI. Once uropathogenic *E. coli* attach to the uroepithelial cells, they initiate inflammation by stimulating uroepithelial cells to produce cytokines and chemokines, such as interleukin-6 (IL-6) and IL-8.[41-43] Urinary IL-6 and IL-8 concentrations are elevated in children with UTI.[44-46] IL-8 has also been found to be elevated in noninfectious renal conditions such as VUR and non-VUR congenital abnormalities, suggesting that IL-8 is a nonspecific marker of renal injury.[47] IL-8 also may provide insight into the severity of renal scarring after UTI.[48] Recent genomics studies have also identified IL-10 upregulation in response to UTI.[49]

Infection with *P* fimbriated *E. coli* is associated with the presence of elevated concentrations of these inflammatory mediators in urine and is also involved in neutrophil recruitment within the infected urinary tract.[46] *P* fimbriae activate epithelial cells to release cytokines and chemokines by using the Toll-like receptor 4 (TLR-4) pathway for signal transduction.[50] IL-8, also designated CXC chemokine, recruits neutrophils and other inflammatory cells to migrate to the site of infection within the urinary tract.[51] IL-8 orchestrates neutrophil recruitment by binding to two high-affinity IL-8 receptors, CXCR1 and CXCR2, expressed on the surface of uroepithelial cells. Expression of these receptors increases with infection, leading to higher IL-8 binding and greater neutrophil migration across infected epithelial cells. Neutrophils exit the blood vessels, cross the lamina propria and the epithelial barrier, and enter the urinary lumen, resulting in pyuria (Figure 49.1).[52] IL-8 levels have been found to be significantly elevated in patients with urosepsis, and urine samples demonstrated increased recruitment of neutrophils in chemotaxic assays, suggesting that local production of cytokines contributes to the migration of neutrophils to infected urine.[53] The overall cytokine response to UTI is complex, involves multiple different cytokines, and may reflect disease severity. Bacterial endotoxins also facilitate chemotaxis by activating the complement pathway.[54]

The neutrophils recruited by the cytokines kill bacteria and help clear the infection. Chemokine receptor CXCRI expression and CXCRI-specific mRNA were found to be low on the neutrophils of children with recurrent UTI, compared to those of matched controls.[55] CXCR1 receptor expression was also significantly lower in a cohort of UTI-prone children compared to age-matched controls without a significant history of UTIs.[56] Polymorphisms in *TLR-4* genes also have been implicated in susceptibility to UTIs.[57-59] These findings suggest that molecular factors in the host may contribute to susceptibility to acute pyelonephritis.

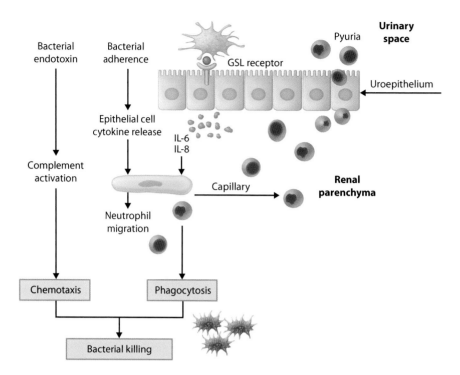

Figure 49.1 Host response to urinary tract infection. GSL, Glycosphingolipid.

## Host response and renal scarring

Renal parenchymal scarring as a result of acute pyelonephritis is intimately related to the host response to infection. Bladder inoculation of *E. coli* in IL-8 receptor knockout (KO) mice triggered a chemokine response and neutrophil recruitment, but the neutrophils accumulated under the epithelium and failed to cross the mucosal barrier and kill bacteria.[55] Although control mice successfully cleared the infection in this study, the KO mice developed edema of kidneys, neutrophil abscesses, and subsequent renal scarring. This animal model underscores the importance of chemokine receptors in the host's ability to successfully clear infection, and suggests a potential molecular basis for the progression of acute pyelonephritis to renal scarring.

Despite encouraging data in the animal models, studies in children have provided conflicting results regarding the correlation between IL-8 levels and renal scarring. Tramma et al.[60] compared children with and without renal scars following UTI. Six months after UTI, no children had detectable levels of IL-8 in their urine. Another study performed within 3 weeks of UTI demonstrated significantly increased levels of IL-8 in patients with renal scarring.[61,62] It seems that although IL-8 may play a role in immediate inflammatory responses, it is unclear what molecular mechanisms lead to the chronic inflammatory responses that may contribute to renal scarring.

Procalcitonin is emerging as a potential marker for the diagnosis of acute pyelonephritis and renal scarring in children. A prospective study of 100 Italian children found that patients who developed renal scars on DMSA scintigraphy had significantly elevated procalcitonin levels compared to children with normal or mild renal involvement. The study concluded that procalcitonin values 0.8 ng/mL or greater had a sensitivity of 83.3% and specificity of 93.6% in predicting acute pyelonephritis.[63] Similarly, meta-analysis of procalcitonin in the pediatric literature found that procalcitonin correlated with both renal scarring and acute pyelonephritis.[64] Procalcitonin has not yet been incorporated into clinical algorithms for management decisions in pediatric patients with UTI.

> ### KEY POINTS
>
> - IL-6 and IL-8 may serve as markers of renal injury during infection.
> - Procalcitonin may be a predictive biomarker for the development of pyelonephritis and renal scarring.
> - The host chemokine response also may contribute to the development of renal scarring.

## Blood group

In addition to underlying structural urogenital anomalies, an individual's blood group also may influence predisposition to UTI.[65–67] Blood group antigens are genetically determined carbohydrate moieties present on erythrocytes and epithelial cells, including uroepithelial cells. Blood group antigens may influence the binding of fimbriated bacteria to carbohydrate receptors present on uroepithelial cell surfaces by producing a specific receptor site for bacteria or blocking an exposed receptor site. Women with recurrent UTIs have an increased frequency of Lewis blood-group nonsecretor and recessive phenotypes.[65] Jantausch et al.[66] reported that the relative risk for UTI was 3.2 in children with the Lewis (Le) (a-b-) phenotype. Sheinfeld et al.[67] in a study of children with genitourinary structural anomalies, correlated uroepithelium nonsecretor phenotype with a history of UTI. These children had low or undetectable levels of ABO and Le-b reactivity in their uroepithelium compared to children without a history of UTI, whose uroepithelium demonstrated strong ABO and/or Le-b immunoreactivity. Other studies have cast doubt on the role of blood group antigens in the pathogenesis of UTI.[68-70]

## URINARY ANATOMY

Because of known predisposition of females to UTI, a short urethra in girls in comparison to boys has long been proposed to be a factor in facilitating spread of ascending infection. Although intuitively plausible, published evidence for this hypothesis is almost nonexistent. A small urethral diameter in girls has also been cited as a reason for susceptibility of some girls to UTI. Works of Graham et al.[71] and Immergut and Wahman,[72] however, convincingly demonstrated that the internal urethral diameter does not differ significantly between the bacteriuric and nonbacteriuric girls. In conclusion, although commonly cited, the role of normal urethral anatomy in facilitating movement of bacteria upstream into the urinary bladder is largely unclear.

---

### KEY POINTS

- Most UTIs are the result of ascending infections.
- Hematogenous spread occurs in a minority of infections.
- Structural abnormalities of the urinary tract may predispose to infection.

---

## Prepuce and circumcision

Circumcision is practiced as a religious and sociocultural ritual in many parts of the world. In the religious context, circumcision is widely practiced in the Jewish and Muslim faiths. Incidence of circumcision in the United States peaked at 85% in 1965.[73] In a cross-sectional study, the Centers for Disease Control and Prevention estimated

that the incidence of routine newborn male circumcision in the United States was between 54.7% and 56.9%.[74] The rate of circumcision in African-American neonates used to be 10% to 15% lower than in white neonates, but recent data suggest that the circumcision rate is similar in the two races.[73,75,76] Geographic variation also exists within circumcision incidence in the United States. States in which Medicaid covers routine circumcision were found to have circumcision rates that were 24% higher than states without Medicaid coverage.[74] The circumcision rate in countries outside the United States is low. In Europe, circumcision is generally practiced for medical reasons only, and rates vary from 2 percent in Denmark to about 3.1 percent in the United Kingdom.[77-79]

The role of circumcision in preventing UTI has been recognized since the 1980s. Ginsburg et al.[12] noted that 75% of boys with febrile UTI in the first 8 weeks of life were noncircumcised. In a retrospective analysis of 5261 infants younger than 1 year of age, Wiswell and Roscelli[80] showed that the incidence of UTI in females and circumcised males was 0.47 and 0.21, respectively, whereas 4.21% of uncircumcised males had a confirmed UTI. These authors subsequently expanded their studies to suggest a 20- to 29-fold increase in febrile UTI in uncircumcised males compared to circumcised infants.[80-82] Schoen et al.[83] reviewed the incidence of UTI in 28,812 neonates in the Kaiser Permanente system in California. The incidence of UTI during the first year of life in the noncircumcised infants group was 2.15% compared to 0.22% in circumcised infants—a 9.1-fold increase of UTI in noncircumcised infants. A Cochrane review of UTIs found that there were no randomized controlled trials examining the effect of circumcision on infection.[84] A meta-analysis of existing literature found the summary odds ratio to be 0.13 for the seven included studies and estimated that the number of subjects needed to treat (circumcise) to prevent one UTI was 111.[85] These authors inferred that the evidence is insufficient to support routine circumcision of all male infants, but that males at increased risk for UTI or with a history of recurrent UTI may benefit from circumcision. Over all, the incidence of UTI in uncircumcised infants is reported to be 3 to 7 times higher than in circumcised infants.[11,14,83,86-88]

The mechanism by which the intact prepuce predisposes to UTI is unclear. One possible explanation is that the prepuce allows enteropathogenic bacteria to harbor and multiply in an uncircumcised male.[89,90] Urethral swabs in male infants before and after circumcision found that 89.5% of males grew bacteria before circumcision and only 33.9% of swabs grew bacteria after circumcision.[91] Culture independent investigations of bacterial flora before and after circumcision have shown a similar decrease in the diversity of penile microbiota, although it is unclear what impact this finding may have on disease risk.[92] Enhanced adherence capability of the uropathogenic organisms to the nonkeratinized mucosa of the prepuce also has been cited as leading to a higher incidence of UTI in uncircumcised male infants.[93] Colonization by highly virulent strains of *E.coli* appears to be facilitated by presence of the prepuce in young infants.[94] The molecular mechanism for this predisposition, especially in absence of urinary tract malformations, is unclear.

## Routine neonatal circumcision: View of the American Academy of Pediatrics

The AAP's Task Force on Circumcision issued a revised policy statement on male circumcision in September 2012. This statement points out that based on available evidence, the health benefits of newborn male circumcision outweigh the risks of the procedure.[95] However, universal circumcision has not been recommended. If parents choose to have male neonates circumcised, access to the procedure has been advocated.

---

### KEY POINTS

- The 2012 AAP statement indicates that the health benefits of newborn male circumcision outweigh the risks of the procedure, but does not recommend universal circumcision in males.
- Parental choice for access to circumcision has been advocated by AAP.
- Males at an increased risk for infection may benefit from circumcision.

---

## ELIMINATION DYSFUNCTION

Voiding and bowel dysfunction often occur together and are usually termed *elimination dysfunction*. These children have an abnormal micturition and stooling pattern associated with normal urinary tract anatomy and intact neurogenic control of the urinary tract and bowel. The association between voiding and bowel dysfunctions and UTI is well known.[7,96–100] Patients with elimination dysfunction also have been independently noted to have a high incidence of VUR, which can also predispose to UTIs.[97–100] Clinical manifestations of elimination dysfunction in children include urinary frequency and urgency, prolonged voiding intervals, daytime wetting, perineal and penile pain, holding maneuvers, or posturing to prevent wetting, constipation, and encopresis.[99] Predisposition to UTI in these patients is thought to be due to incomplete bladder emptying, leading to accumulation and proliferation of uropathogenic bacteria in the bladder. Voiding dysfunction and its management are discussed further in Chapter 52.

## Urinary obstruction

In an unselected childhood population with UTI, the incidence of urinary obstruction has been reported to be as

high as 10%.[5] In the more recent literature, however, urinary obstruction accounts for fewer than 1% of children with UTI caused by *E. coli*.[9,101] On the other hand, urinary obstruction is more commonly (15%) seen in children with UTI caused by *Proteus, Enterococcus, Klebsiella,* or coagulase-negative staphylococcal infections.[102] In the era of prenatal ultrasound evaluation, most patients with obstructed urinary tracts are detected early, even before the onset of first UTI. However, children with posterior urethral valves may first come to medical attention because of febrile UTI or urosepsis. Obstruction at the ureteropelvic junction or along the ureteric length also can lead to a predisposition to UTI.

## Vesicoureteral reflux

Retrograde flow of the urine from the urinary bladder into the ureters is prevented during micturition by a functional valve mechanism at the level of the ureterovesicular junction (UVJ). Incompetence of the UVJ valve leads to flow of urine upstream into the ureter and the kidney, or VUR. The association between VUR and predisposition to UTI is well established. VUR is discussed in Chapter 48.

---

### KEY POINTS

- Voiding dysfunction and urinary obstruction predispose children to UTIs.
- VUR is an important predisposition to UTI in children.

---

## CLINICAL MANIFESTATIONS

Manifestations of UTI vary with age, site of infection within the urinary tract, and severity of infection. From a clinical perspective, infection of the urinary tract may be discussed as a nonfebrile UTI or acute cystitis and febrile UTI or acute pyelonephritis.

## CYSTITIS

Among preschoolers, cystitis is more commonly seen in girls than in boys. Of the 157 children under the age of 6 years identified with first-time symptomatic nonfebrile UTI by Marild and Jodal,[7] 130 were girls, and only 27 were boys. The peak incidence of nonfebrile UTI in preschool girls in this study was 9.4 cases per 1000 at-risk children and occurred in the third year of life. Thereafter, the incidence gradually declined to a stable level of 2.5 cases per 1000 at-risk children. In contrast, the peak incidence of nonfebrile UTI in preschool boys in this study was only was 2.8 per 1000 at-risk children and was noted during the first year of life.[7]

In children who can verbalize (usually more than 3 to 4 years of age), dysuria and suprapubic pain are common manifestations of cystitis.[101] Symptoms of dysuria may be difficult to ascertain in younger children. In boys between 6 and 12 years of age with bacteriologically proved UTI, Hallett et al.[102] found dysuria or urinary frequency (82%), enuresis (66%), and abdominal pain (39%) to be the most common symptoms. Urinary incontinence is another common symptom of cystitis, especially in girls. Parental observations may range from a general reluctance of the child to urinate, to excessive crying and abdominal pain. Parents may report the urine to have a foul odor, but these symptoms may be subjective and not reported.

Gross hematuria has been reported to be a common manifestation of bacterial cystitis in children. Bergstrom et al.[8] noted macroscopic hematuria as a clinical symptom in 26% of children with UTI. Hematuria was more common in males (43%) than in females (9%) in this study. In another study, Ingelfinger et al.[103] reported that of the 158 children with macroscopic hematuria seen in the emergency room, UTI was the underlying cause in 26% of cases. Cystitis has been reported in children who self-inject or manipulate the urethra.[104] Hematuria is also a common manifestation (60%) in such children.

## ACUTE PYELONEPHRITIS (FEBRILE URINARY TRACT INFECTION)

Association of fever in a patient with a positive urinary culture suggests renal parenchymal infection or acute pyelonephritis. Other symptoms of acute pyelonephritis include abdominal pain and costovertebral angle pain and tenderness, which are more commonly present in older children and adolescents. In younger children and infants, in addition to fever, other nonlocalizing symptoms such as excessive crying, irritability, vomiting, feeding problems, and lethargy are often present. Dysuria is an uncommon manifestation of febrile UTI in children younger than 1 year of age, but up to a quarter of older children may complain of this symptom.[105] Febrile UTI, or acute pyelonephritis associated with manifestations of sepsis is referred to as *urosepsis* and is particularly common in children with clinically significant urinary tract anomalies, such as obstructive disease, or VUR.

Bacteremia is present in 4% to 9% of infants and children younger than 1 year of age with UTI.[106,107] Fever may be the only symptom in many patients with UTI associated with bacteremia, especially early in their presentation. Symptoms of chills and rigors may also be seen in these patients, but clinical symptoms alone are poor predictors of bacteremia.[105] Meningitis may be present in patients with urosepsis, especially in those younger than 3 months of age.[107] Although ESBL-producing bacteria have come to represent an increasing percentage of community-acquired UTIs, no difference in clinical presentation has been noted in children with ESBL and non-ESBL bacterial pneumonia.[108]

Acute renal failure is an uncommon manifestation of acute pyelonephritis. Such patients may require dialysis therapy, and complete renal recovery after successful treatment of the infection is possible.[109]

## URINARY TRACT INFECTION IN NEONATES AND INFANTS

The diagnosis of UTI needs to be considered in neonates and infants younger than 3 months of age with sepsis or unexplained fever. Although girls are generally at higher risk for UTI, the majority of UTIs in infants younger than 3 months of age are in males.[110-112] In infants with known urinary tract abnormalities, such as hydronephrosis, obstructive uropathy, or VUR, diagnosis of UTI should be considered and ruled out during febrile episodes. Fever may be absent in some patients, especially in neonates. Winberg et al.[5] found fever as an accompanying symptom in only 42% of neonates with acute pyelonephritis. Hypothermia, hypotension, shock, jaundice, failure to thrive, diarrhea, vomiting, feeding problems, irritability cyanosis, polyuria, and metabolic acidosis also have been reported as presenting manifestations in neonates and infants younger than 3 months of age with acute pyelonephritis.[9,113]

Febrile UTI in neonates may be associated with sterile cerebrospinal fluid (CSF) pleocytosis. A multicenter retrospective review of 1190 infants aged 29 to 60 days with febrile UTIs showed that 214 (18.0%) had CSF white blood cell (WBC) counts of 10/$\mu$L or higher.[114] The dominant risk factor associated with sterile CSF pleocytosis was elevated peripheral WBC count, leading the study authors to propose a possible inflammatory mechanism for the development of sterile pleocytosis.

## RENAL ABSCESS

Renal abscesses are an uncommon complication of UTI. Two retrospective studies of pediatric patients identified only 13 patients over 20 years.[115,116] Renal abscesses can be divided into two anatomic categories: intrarenal and perirenal abscesses. Intrarenal abscesses include cortical and corticomedullary abscesses. Renal cortical abscesses are often a consequence of hematogenous spread from infection elsewhere in the body.[116,117] Corticomedullary abscesses, on the other hand, are more likely to be associated with a urinary tract abnormality and are often the result of an ascending infection. A perinephric abscess is characterized by infection between the renal capsule and Gerota fascia. These abscesses often develop after an intrarenal abscess ruptures and spreads infection into the perinephric space, but also may develop as a complication from a primary infection elsewhere in the body.

Clinical presentation of renal abscesses is often insidious, and most symptoms can be nonspecific. Fever, nausea, vomiting, abdominal pain, and localized flank pain are reported as the most common manifesting symptoms.[116,118,119] Although Wippermann et al.[116] did not find an association between renal abscess and underlying urologic abnormalities, five of the six patients described by Angel et al.[119] were found to have abnormal anatomy that may have contributed to the development of a renal abscess. Among adults, diabetes mellitus, urolithiasis, and immunosuppression have been reported to be risk factors for renal abscesses.[120,121] Diagnosis of renal abscess can be made by renal ultrasound (Figure 49.2), or computed tomography (CT) scan of the abdomen, which may demonstrate a partially filled cystic lesion. Treatment consists of surgical drainage of the abscess under ultrasound guidance and antibiotic therapy for 3 weeks or longer, as dictated by the patient's clinical state.

## DIAGNOSIS

The aims of investigation in a child with UTI are to: (1) confirm the diagnosis, (2) identify the infecting organism, (3) localize the site of infection and identify children with acute pyelonephritis, and (4) recognize patients with urinary tract malformations.

## URINALYSIS

Urinalysis is often the initial laboratory study performed in patients with a presumptive diagnosis of UTI, especially in

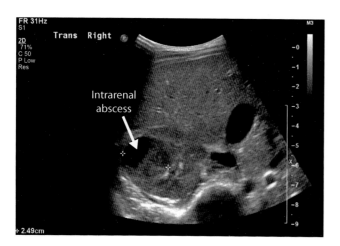

Figure 49.2 Ultrasound of the kidney showing an intrarenal abscess. The abscess demonstrates fluid and debris within it (arrow). Aspirated fluid from the abscess grew *Escherichia coli.*

the office or emergency room setting. Collection methodology of urine for examination has significant implications for sensitivity and specificity of findings. Urinalysis can be collected by any method, including perineum bag, but the sample should be processed promptly. A specimen kept at room temperature should be analyzed within 1 hour, or in 4 hours if refrigerated.[4,122] Urine dipsticks are frequently used in the primary care setting, in which the rapid return of results is desirable for clinical decision making. Most urine dipsticks provide leukocyte esterase and nitrite values. Hematuria and proteinuria may be detected in UTI, but sensitivity and specificity are poor.[123]

## URINE COLOR AND SMELL

Turbid urine may be an indication of pyuria and UTI. Clarity of urine has been shown to have a negative predictive value for absence of UTI in some reports.[124] In contrast, Bulloch et al. found that 3 of 29 children with UTI and positive urine culture were found to have clear urine.[125] In general, clarity of urine has limitations as a discerning indicator for absence of UTI.

Parents often report an abnormal smell to be suggestive of onset of UTI in children. In a study of 110 patients, 52% of parents reported that their child's urine smelled different from usual, but only 6.4% of children had a positive urine culture.[126] These observations indicate that urine smell is also a poor screening test for UTI. Neither color nor odor is taken into consideration for diagnosis in the AAP UTI Practice Guideline.[4]

## URINE MICROSCOPY

### Bacteriuria

Detection of any bacteria in the uncentrifuged urine slide stained by Gram stain has been used as the gold standard for the presumptive diagnosis of UTI. In a meta-analysis of published studies in children, Gorelick and Shaw[127] reported that presence of any bacteria in the Gram-stained urine slide demonstrated a true positive rate of 0.97 (high sensitivity) and false positive rate of only 0.05 (high specificity). The AAP practice guideline for UTI suggests that by combining the findings of pyuria and bacteriuria results, a greater sensitivity and specificity of the tests may be achieved.[4] The limitations of this test for a wider acceptability in clinical practice are that it is time-consuming and requires expertise in performing the Gram stain and identifying the organisms in the urine sample.

### Pyuria

Pyuria or light microscopy visualization of more than 5 white blood cells per high-power field (WBCs/hpf) in centrifuged urinary sediment is considered as presumptive evidence of UTI.[4] Presence of 10 WBCs/hpf has been noted to have a true positive rate of 0.77 and a true negative rate of 0.11.[127]

Pyuria alone cannot be used as the sole diagnostic criteria for UTI, but it is unusual to diagnose UTI in the absence of pyuria. Variables such as centrifuge speed, centrifugation time, volume of urine centrifuged, and volume of urine used for resuspension can influence the quantitation of pyuria. Sterile pyuria, or urinary WBC excretion, without concurrent evidence of bacterial infection or UTI may be seen in some clinical conditions (Table 49.1). Other limitations include neutropenia, in which the patient may not be able to mount a urinary WBC response. Infection with organisms such as *Proteus* species, that produce alkaline urine, leads to disruption of urinary WBCs in urine and an apparent absence of pyuria in the face of UTI.

---

## KEY POINTS

- The finding of single bacteria in an uncentrifuged urine sample stained with Gram stain is presumptive of UTI with high sensitivity and specificity.
- Pyuria detection requires urine centrifugation.
- Presence of pyuria is not sufficient to diagnose UTI.
- The nitrite test has high specificity but modest sensitivity.
- The nitrite test identifies only Gram-negative bacterial UTI.

---

Table 49.1 Clinical conditions that may be associated with sterile pyuria

1. Partially treated urinary tract infection
2. Interstitial nephritis
3. Renal tubular acidosis
4. Glomerulonephritis, especially acute postinfectious glomerulonephritis
5. Renal cystic diseases
6. Renal stone disease
7. Hydronephrosis
8. Appendicitis
9. Dehydration
10. Meatal or urethral irritation, especially in males
11. Vaginitis in females
12. Neonates
13. Renal tuberculosis
14. Exercise
15. Kawasaki's disease

## Leukocyte esterase

Testing for leukocyte esterase may overcome some of the limitations of urinary microscopy in identifying leukocyturia. Leukocyte esterase is present in the neutrophils and can be assayed in the urine by dipstick strips. For patients with a suspected UTI, the sensitivity of this test is 94%, with an average specificity of 72%.[4] False-negative tests can be caused by the presence of ascorbic acid, high urinary protein, glycosuria, presence of urobilinogen, gentamicin, nitrofurantoin, cephalexin, and boric acid. A false-positive test can result from presence of imipenem and clavulanic acid in the urine.

## Nitrite test

This test is based on the fact that bacterial enzyme nitrate reductase can convert urinary nitrate to nitrite, which can be detected by several chemical methods. The nitrite test has now been incorporated in commercially available dipstick test strips. Specificity is estimated to be 90% to 100%, although sensitivity is significantly lower at 16% to 82%.[123]

Although a good screening test, nitrite testing cannot be relied on as a confirmatory test for UTI. Kunin et al.[128] found that the test was positive in 65.4% patients with culture-positive UTI if performed one time. The nitrite test does not identify patients with Gram-positive infections because they lack the nitrate reductase enzyme. Also, conversion of the urinary nitrate to nitrite requires sufficient time (usually 3 to 4 hours in the bladder) even in presence of Gram-negative infection. In patients with UTI and urinary frequency, the reaction time may be less than optimal, leading to poor conversion of nitrate and a falsely negative test. The 2011 AAP guidelines suggest that in infants with frequent urination, nitrite testing may be particularly insensitive.[4] High urine specific gravity reduces the sensitivity of this test, and high urinary ascorbic acid may also produce a negative test in the presence of a small amount of nitrite.

## URINE CULTURE

### Urine collection

Culturing urine remains the gold standard for confirming the diagnosis of UTI. Potential contamination of the urine sample is a well-recognized problem that can make interpretation of the culture results difficult. Collection of urine in infants by a collection device, such as the U-Bag (Hollister, Libertyville, IL), is associated with a high rate of bacterial contamination (56% to 69%) and is not an acceptable collection method for urine culture.[129] A positive culture from a bagged specimen cannot be used as confirmatory evidence of a UTI.[4]

To reduce the risk for bacterial contamination, urine for culture is collected by clean catch, catheterization, or suprapubic aspiration in neonates. The clean catch method involves cleaning the external genitalia with mild antiseptic and collecting urine in midstream into a sterile container. This method is generally acceptable for adolescents and cooperative children. Suprapubic urine aspiration involves percutaneous insertion of a needle into the urinary bladder and aspirating urine into a sterile syringe. This method is reserved for use in neonates and infants younger than 2 months of age, when the urinary bladder is a pelvic organ. The single most important factor in success of the procedure is whether the bladder is palpable at the time of the aspiration. The success rate can be further enhanced by the use of ultrasound guidance. Catheterization of the urethra to obtain urine is the preferred method for collection in a noncooperative patient, in whom clean catch collection of urine is not possible. If a delay in the inoculation of the culture is expected, urine specimens should be refrigerated to prevent the overgrowth of bacteria at ambient temperature.

## Bacterial count

> **KEY POINTS**
>
> - A positive urine culture obtained from bagged specimens is inadequate to confirm the presence of UTI.
> - Suprapubic aspiration (neonates) and catheterization are the preferred methods for urine culture.

A growth of more than $10^5$ colony-forming units (CFU)/mL of a single species of bacteria in a catheterized urine sample is considered positive evidence of UTI (Table 49.2).[12] Any growth of a single organism in a sample obtained by suprapubic aspiration is regarded as a strong indication of UTI. From his study of catheterized urine cultures in patients younger than 24 months of age, Hoberman et al.[130] concluded that UTI can be diagnosed accurately by a colony count of 50,000 CFU/mL in this age group. The AAP guidelines also endorse a colony count of 50,000 CFU/mL of a single organism in association with evidence of pyuria as the cutoff for a positive culture.[4]

Colony counts lower than those listed in Table 49.2 may be considered diagnostic of UTI in some clinical circumstances. These include patients currently receiving

Table 49.2 Microbiologic criteria for positive urine culture

| Method of collection | Threshold for diagnosis of urinary tract infection* |
|---|---|
| Suprapubic aspiration | 1,000 CFU/mL |
| Catheterization of bladder | 50,000 CFU/mL† |
| Midstream clean catch | 50,000 CFU/mL† |
| Bagged urine culture | Unreliable |

* Assumes single organism is identified.
† Presence or absence of pyuria should be used to differentiate between true infection and colonization.

antibiotic therapy, patients with complete ureteral obstruction preventing the flow of infected urine and bacteria into the bladder, patients with urinary frequency who may have a reduced dwell time of urine in the bladder, and patients infected with organisms that are well known to have lower colony counts in urine culture, such as *S. saprophyticus*.[18,19,29] On the other hand, certain organisms are not considered clinically relevant in children under 2 years of age. These include *Lactobacillus* species, coagulase-negative staphylococci, and *Corynebacterium* species.[4]

> **KEY POINTS**
>
> - *S. saprophyticus* can be pathogenic with low CFU counts, especially in a symptomatic patient (usually adolescent girls).
> - *Lactobacillus* species, *Corynebacterium* species, and coagulase-negative staphylococci are not usual urinary pathogens. These can be ignored in urine culture in otherwise healthy children.

## RADIOLOGIC IMAGING

The purpose of radiologic investigations in patients with UTI is twofold: (1) to search for any malformations of the urinary tract that may predispose to UTI and (2) to establish the diagnosis of acute pyelonephritis, when other evidence may be lacking. A consensus regarding the types of imaging studies necessary in patients with first UTI is still lacking.

## Ultrasound

Renal ultrasound has been considered an essential investigation in patients with first-time febrile UTI.[131] But recommendations regarding the use of renal ultrasound in the management of children with UTI continues to evolve. In a review of the radiologic investigations of 309 children younger than 2 years of age, renal ultrasound was normal in 88% and provided no additional diagnostic advantage in most patients.[132] Change in therapy as a result of ultrasound findings would have been indicated in fewer than 1% of cases. In another study of radiologic imaging in 124 children with first febrile UTI, ultrasound detected only one patient with urologic

> **KEY POINTS**
>
> - Renal ultrasound detects very few abnormalities in children with UTI.
> - Renal scarring cannot be effectively detected by renal ultrasound.
> - AAP recommends renal ultrasound in all children with UTI.

abnormality.[133] Others also have pointed out the poor performance of renal ultrasound in children with UTI to detect significant abnormalities that would alter the management course.[134,135] Additionally, renal ultrasound also performs poorly in detecting renal scars.

The guidelines from the National Institute for Health and Clinical Excellence (NICE) in the United Kingdom recommend that all infants under 6 months of age should undergo a renal ultrasound.[136] A critical appraisal of the NICE guidelines seems to indicate that limiting ultrasounds to children under 6 months of age does not significantly change patient management.[137] In contrast, the AAP guidelines make no such age differentiation and recommends that all children with a febrile UTI undergo a renal ultrasound.[4] Ultrasound may be the initial investigation of choice when suspicion of complications, such as renal or perinephric abscess are being considered in a patient with acute pyelonephritis. It is important to point out that the clinical need should guide the investigative decision regarding the use of renal ultrasound in patients with UTI, especially those with atypical manifestations or clinical courses.

## Vesicocystourethrography and radionuclide cystography

Traditionally, vesicocystourethrography (VCUG) or radionuclide cystography (RNC) have been used to assess VUR. Since recent studies has cast doubt on the utility of antibiotic prophylaxis in the management of VUR, the role of the routine VCUG is also being challenged. Contrast VCUG with fluoroscopic guidance allows visualization of the anatomy of the bladder and urethra. RNC is an acceptable alternative to contrast VCUG, particularly in females, when bladder outlet and urethral obstructive lesions are unlikely. The advantage of nuclear cystogram is that it exposes children to only approximately 1% to 2% percent of the radiation dose used in contrast fluoroscopy VCUG.

---

**KEY POINTS**

- In past, VCUG has been used to detect VUR in most patients with a febrile UTI.
- Selective use of VCUG is now emerging.
- AAP recommends VCUG after a second UTI.

---

A growing body of evidence supports a more selective use of VCUG in the evaluation of febrile UTIs.[138-141] In a retrospective review of 2036 children who had imaging following a UTI, VCUG detected abnormalities in only 42 patients (4.9%), leading the authors to conclude that VCUG could safely be reserved for patients with additional risk factors.[138] The NICE guidelines suggest avoiding routine VCUGs for

the identification of VUR.[136] The AAP guidelines recommend that VCUG can be delayed until the second episode of UTI, because the risk for radiation exposure and discomfort from the procedure outweigh the potential benefits for the majority of patients.[4]

Timing of VCUG or RNC in a patient with newly diagnosed febrile UTI also has been recently re-evaluated. So as not to overdiagnose transient VUR associated with UTI, the general recommendation in the past has been to defer VCUG/RNC for 4 to 6 weeks after the diagnosis of UTI. In several recent studies, however, it has been shown that the incidence of VUR in cystograms obtained within 1 week of diagnosis of UTI is not different from cystograms performed later in the clinical course of febrile UTI (1 to 4 weeks).[142-145] It has also been demonstrated that the patients undergoing early VCUG evaluation (less than 1 week) did not have any worsening of their clinical condition.[142] The AAP guidelines do not comment regarding optimal timing of VCUG or RNC studies.[4]

## Dimercaptosuccinic acid renal scan

Intravenous pyelography has, in the past, been used as the gold standard for detection of pyelonephritic scars following acute pyelonephritis. In the last two decades, nuclear scan, using technetium-99m–dimercaptosuccinic acid (DMSA) has evolved as an attractive alternative to intravenous pyelogram for evaluation of pyelonephritic renal scars or reflux nephropathy.[146] Furthermore, DMSA renal scan obtained early in the course of a febrile UTI also can help in the diagnosis of acute pyelonephritis, in cases in which other evidence may be lacking.[146,147] DMSA renal scan is discussed further in Chapter 7.

Preference for diagnostic use of DMSA renal scan in the investigation of febrile UTI is highly institution dependent. The AAP Subcommittee on Urinary Tract Infection has not recommended DMSA scan as a required imaging investigation of children less than 2 years.[148] Recently, a "top-down" approach replacing cystograms with DMSA renal scans as the initial investigation has been advocated for investigation of febrile UTI in children.[149,150] A meta-analysis of the top-down approach, however, concluded that the DMSA scan did not perform well in identifying VUR.[151] VUR and its management are discussed further in Chapter 48.

## RECURRENT URINARY TRACT INFECTION

After the first episode of UTI, recurrent UTI may be seen in 30% to 40% of patients, especially in those with anatomic urinary tract anomalies such as VUR, urinary obstruction, or bladder divirticulum.[152-154] Female sex, age younger than 6 months, dysfunctional elimination, and bladder instability are other risk factors for recurrent UTIs.

## TREATMENT OF URINARY TRACT INFECTION

The aims of antimicrobial treatment for UTI are (1) to clear the acute infection, (2) prevent urosepsis, and (3) reduce the likelihood of renal damage. The principles for selection of antibiotic therapy for UTI are similar to the guidelines used in choosing antibiotics for other serious infections, which are bacterial susceptibility, a narrow antimicrobial spectrum antibiotic selection, tolerance of therapy by patients, a low toxicity profile of therapy, and cost-effectiveness.

### INITIAL THERAPY

Initial antibiotic therapy of UTI is often empiric. The susceptibility pattern of the infecting organism grown in urine culture should be used subsequently to guide transition to an appropriate antimicrobial agent. The choice of empiric antibiotics is dictated by the sensitivity pattern of the organisms in the community, especially in view of the increasing resistance of uropathogens to antimicrobial agents over the last two decades, particularly ESBL organisms.[155] Up to 40% to 58% of uropathogens are known to be resistant to ampicillin or amoxicillin, and 5% to 36% are resistant to trimethoprim-sulfamethoxazole (TMP-SMX).[156-158] Antibiotic resistance, however, varies across geographic regions, and local antibiotic resistance patterns should be considered in choice of empiric antibiotic therapy.

TMP-SMX, second- and third-generation cephalosporins, and amoxicillin/clavulanate are generally used as the initial empiric therapy for the treatment of UTI in the United States.[159] Table 49.3 details dosing regimens for commonly used antibiotics to treat UTI. The US Food and Drug Administration also has approved ciprofloxacin as an option for complicated UTI or pyelonephritis in children.[160] Antibiotics doses in children should not exceed the maximum daily adult dosage.

---

### KEY POINTS

- Antimicrobial resistance patterns vary widely with geographic region.
- TMP-SMX, second- and third-generation cephalosporins, and Augmentin (amoxicillin) are generally the first-line agents for empiric treatment of UTI.
- Ciprofloxacin may be used in complicated urinary infections or to treat multidrug resistant organisms, but should not be routinely used as empiric therapy.

---

## FEBRILE URINARY TRACT INFECTION

### First three months

Neonates (younger than 1 month of age) with febrile UTI should be hospitalized and treated with intravenous therapy at least initially. Bacteremia and meningitis should be excluded by obtaining blood for culture and examining the CSF. Inpatient intravenous antibiotic therapy is recommended because of the inability of young infants to adequately absorb oral antibiotics, the immaturity of the young infant's immune system, and the consequent increased risk for disseminated infection.

Initial parenteral therapy is generally recommended for all infants up to 3 months of age with UTI, especially if they are ill appearing.[161] Empiric parenteral antibiotic therapy for infants younger than 3 months of age can consist of the combination of ampicillin and gentamicin, which provides coverage for *group B streptococci, Enterococcus,* and Gram-negative organisms. Alternatively, cefotaxime as a monotherapy or the combination of cefotaxime and gentamicin can be considered.[161,162] Emerging evidence suggests that infants may be safely transitioned to oral therapy without increased risk for treatment failure. Parenteral therapy should continue until the infants improve clinically (usually 3 to 7 days) before switching to oral therapy. Oral antibiotic therapy is continued to complete a total of 14 days of antibiotic treatment.[163]

Outpatient management may be considered in carefully selected 1- to 3-month-old infants with febrile UTI, provided they do not appear acutely ill, do not have bacteremia or meningitis, and are able to be followed closely.[156,161] Efficacy of oral cefixime (16 mg/kg on first day and then 8 mg/kg/day for remainder of duration) with intravenous cefotaxime (200 mg/kg/day) was compared in one study of infants with UTI.[156] The study found the two treatment regimens to be equally effective, with urine culture becoming negative after 24 hours in both treatment arms. It needs to be cautioned that the number of patients in the 4- to 7-week age group in this study was small (13 total, 4 oral, and 9 intravenous treatment). Apart from cefixime, other third-generation cephalosporins, such as cefdinir and ceftibuten, also can be antibiotic choices. Outpatient treatment with ceftriaxone or gentamicin given every 24 hours also can be an acceptable alternative in such patients.[161] Parenteral therapy should be continued until the infant is afebrile for 24 hours, with the remainder of the 14-day total course of therapy completed with oral antibiotics.

## Infants and children

Although intravenous antibiotic therapy has been the standard in the 3- to 24-month-old children, oral antibiotics, particularly the third-generation cephalosporins may be equally effective in these children. Effectiveness of oral antibiotic therapy in treating febrile UTI in children 1 to 24 months of age has been well established.[156] Total duration of therapy should be between 7 and 14 days.[4]

Table 49.3 Empiric antibiotic treatment for common urinary pathogens

| Organism | Oral antibiotic therapy | Intravenous antibiotic therapy |
|---|---|---|
| **Gram-negative bacteria** | | |
| Enterobacteriaceae | Amoxicillin 30 mg/kg/day divided q 8–12 h | Cefazolin 50 mg/kg/day divided q 8 h |
| | Amoxicillin-clavulanate 45 mg/kg/day divided q 12 h | Cefuroxime 150 mg/kg/day divided q 8 h |
| | Cephalexin 50 mg/kg/day divided q 6–8 h | Cefotaxime 150 mg/kg/day divided q 8 h |
| | Cefprozil 30 mg/kg/day divided q 12 h | Ceftriaxone 50 mg/kg/day q 24 h |
| | Cefuroxime axetil 20–30 mg/kg/day divided q 12 h | Gentamicin 6 mg/kg/day divided q 8 h in children, 7.5 mg/kg/day divided q 8 h in neonates |
| | Cefixime 8 mg/kg/day once daily | |
| | TMP-SMZ 8–12 mg TMP/kg/day divided q 12 h | |
| ESBL organisms | Use susceptibility results to guide therapy | Meropenem 60 mg/kg/day divided q 8 h |
| *Pseudomonas aeruginosa* | Ciprofloxacin 20-40 mg/kg/day PO divided q 12 h, maximum dose 1.5 g/24 hr. | Ceftazidime 150 mg/kg/day divided q 8 h, *or* Ticarcillin-clavulanate 200–300 mg/kg/day divided q 6 h |
| **Gram-positive bacteria** | | |
| Enterococcus | Ampicillin 200 mg/kg/day divided q 6 h, if organism is susceptible. | Ampicillin 200 mg/kg/day divided q 6 h, *or* Vancomycin 40 mg/kg/day divided q 6–8 h |
| *Group B streptococci* | Penicillin G 150,000–200,000 units/kg/day divided q 6 h, or Ampicillin 200 mg/kg/day divided q 6 h | Ampicillin 200 mg/kg/day divided q 6 h Oxacillin 100 mg/kg/day divided q 6 h, *or* Vancomycin 40 mg/kg/day divided q 6–8 h |
| *Staphylococcus aureus* | Use susceptibility to guide therapy. | Use susceptibility results to guide therapy |
| *Staphylococcus saprophyticus* | Use susceptibility results to guide therapy. | |

Oral cefixime also can be used to treat older children and adolescents with febrile UTI. Alternatively, a short course of intravenous antibiotic therapy (2 to 4 days), followed by oral antibiotic therapy may be used. In children treated with intravenous antibiotics, single daily dosing of aminoglycosides is reported to be as safe and effective as every 8 hour dosing.[164,165] The AAP guidelines state that evidence distinguishing among treatment durations of 7, 10, or 14 days is lacking, and a treatment range of 7 to 14 days is appropriate for the management of UTIs.[4] Children with additional risk factors, such as underlying urinary abnormalities, may require a prolonged course of parenteral therapy.

## KEY POINTS

- Neonates with UTI should be hospitalized for intravenous therapy.
- Infants under 1 month of age should have a complete sepsis evaluation to evaluate for concomitant bacteremia or meningitis.
- Oral therapy may be considered in uncomplicated patients.
- The treatment of pyelonephritis is generally 14 days.
- Infection with ESBL organisms may require prolonged parenteral therapy in an otherwise healthy child.

## CYSTITIS

Oral antibiotic treatment is generally adequate for treatment of uncomplicated cystitis. A short course of antibiotics (3 days) has been shown to be effective for treatment of adults with uncomplicated cystitis and normal urinary tract anatomy. Short-course oral antibiotics also have been shown to be safe and effective in treating cystitis in children with normal urinary tracts.[166,167] In these studies, there were no significant differences in the recurrence rate of UTI, or development of resistant organisms at the end of treatment with short antibiotic therapy. Three days of oral TMP-SMX has been found as effective as conventional therapy (longer than 5 days) in treatment of cystitis.[164,167] A meta-analysis of studies of comparing short-course therapy (less than 3 days) to long-course therapy (longer than 10 days), however, found insufficient evidence to safely endorse short-course therapy.[168]

Single-dose amoxicillin has been found to be an ineffective treatment of cystitis and is not recommended.[166,167] Madrigal et al. noted an unacceptably high recurrence rate of UTI (20.5%) in children treated with a single dose of TMP-SMX, compared to a recurrence rate of 5.6% and 8%, for children treated with a 3-day and 7-day course of treatment with TMP-SMX, respectively.[169]

## TREATMENT OF EXTENDED-SPECTRUM β-LACTAMASE URINARY TRACT INFECTION

The increasing prevalence of multidrug-resistant uropathogens has posed clinicians with new therapeutic dilemmas. Selection of appropriate antimicrobial therapy should, eventually, be guided by the susceptibility results of the urine culture. ESBL isolates are resistant to all β-lactam antibiotics, including penicillins, monobactams, and cephalosporins. ESBL organisms remain susceptible to carbapenems and cephamycins.[170] Ciprofloxacin may be a possible therapeutic option; however, plasmid-mediated gene transfer also may result in resistance to fluoroquinolones, aminoglycosides, and TMP-SMX. If the index of suspicion for an ESBL organism is particularly high, such as in patients with prolonged or complex hospital course, previous antibiotic use, indwelling medical devices, invasive procedures, or history of ESBL infections, empiric coverage of ESBLs with a carbapenem antibiotic may be indicated.

## COMPLICATIONS OF URINARY TRACT INFECTION

## RENAL SCARS

Acute pyelonephritis has the potential to cause tubulointerstitial damage and renal scar formation. Host response, tubular injury, and ischemia during acute pyelonephritis result in the formation of renal parenchymal scars. Using DMSA renal scan, renal parenchymal abnormalities suggestive of acute pyelonephritis are detected in the acute phase (less than 15 days) in 50% to 85% of children with the first episode of acute pyelonephritis.[171-173] A meta-analysis of 33 published studies meeting inclusion criteria found that overall prevalence of renal scarring after 5 months was only 15% (confidence interval [CI], 11% to 18%) in patients who had a febrile UTI.[174] Such scars are sometimes denoted as "primary scars," are common in boys.[173] Girls, on the other hand, are more prone to developing recurrent UTI and secondary renal scars. Because renal scarring following febrile

UTI occurs in some patients, whereas others are spared, the roles played by mediators of inflammation and genetic predisposition have been proposed.[175,176] However, a meta-analysis of the literature was unable to definitively link specific genetic polymorphisms with an increased risk for renal scarring.[177] Urinary tract abnormalities, especially severity of VUR, influence renal scarring, being more common in grade III or higher.[174,178,179] The number of acute pyelonephritis events also has a bearing on the incidence of renal scarring. Jodal reported that renal scars were seen in only 9% of children with one episode of acute pyelonephritis, whereas 58% of children with four or more episodes of pyelonephritis developed chronic scars.[180]

Pyelonephritic renal scars are usually present in the upper and lower poles of the kidney, possibly because of the type of papillae present in these regions. Patients with severe bilateral renal scarring can develop decreased creatinine clearance compared to those with unilateral or mild scarring.[181,182] It is possible that compensatory hypertrophy in the contralateral kidney leads to a normal glomerular filtration rate (GFR) in patients with unilateral damage. Reports that early and effective treatment of acute pyelonephritis prevents acute renal parenchymal damage but the impact on development of renal scars is conflicting.[183,184]

## HYPERTENSION

The prevalence of hypertension in patients with history of UTI has been reported to be 1.2% to 35%.[184-189] In some studies, a higher prevalence of hypertension has been reported in patients with renal scars, and the relative risk for hypertension has been estimated to be 2.9 times higher in those with renal scars compared to those without renal scarring.[186] Hypertension in these patients is believed to be mediated by renin released by the ischemic renal scar tissue.

## CHRONIC KIDNEY DISEASE

Chronic pyelonephritis is an uncommon cause of ESRD in children.[185,190] Smellie et al. followed 226 children with VUR and UTI into adulthood over 10 to 41 years and noted that CKD developed in 10% of patients in whom renal functions were assessed, and ESRD evolved in 1.9% percent.[191] The 2013 report of the US Renal Data System (USRDS) lists chronic pyelonephritis and reflux nephropathy as the primary diagnosis of ESRD in 3.5% in the 2000 to 2006 cohort and 2.5% in the 2007 to 2011 cohort.[192] According to the 2011 annual report of the North American Pediatric Transplant Cooperative (NAPRTCS) database, chronic pyelonephritis and interstitial nephritis account for 1.4% all patients on dialysis.[193] A review of the published literature on the relationship of UTI and CKD led Salo et al.[194] to conclude that UTI without associated structural abnormalities does not lead to CKD and ESRD. It is possible that a decreasing trend in CKD resulting from febrile UTI (chronic pyelonephritis) reflects early diagnosis and improved management of these patients.

## FUNGAL URINARY TRACT INFECTION

Fungal UTI in children is primarily caused by *Candida* species and is most frequently seen in neonates or older children in the intensive care unit (ICU), in immunocompromised patients, and in those with prolonged indwelling urinary drainage catheters. Bryant et al.[195] reported a prevalence of 0.5% candiduria among 8790 infants admitted to the neonatal ICU (NICU). *Candida* species was the pathogen recovered in 42% of neonates with hospital-acquired UTI in the NICU.[196] Candida UTI is more commonly seen in preterm and low-birth-weight babies and may present with nonspecific symptoms of fever, feeding intolerance, respiratory distress, lethargy, apnea, and abdominal distention.[197,198] Oliguria or anuria can be seen as a result of obstruction of the urinary tract by a fungus ball (Figure 49.3). Renal involvement also can manifest as rising serum creatinine and nonoliguric renal failure.

## DIAGNOSIS

Growth of greater than $10^4$ CFU/mL *Candida* organism in a single urine culture obtained in a catheterized urine sample is generally considered as diagnostic of candidal UTI.[196-198] Abnormalities in renal ultrasound and CT scan are common in patients with funguria. Renal fungus balls or a fungal abscess are reported in 35% to 40% of patients on renal imaging studies.[195,196] Because of its portability, ultrasonography can be used as the initial investigative tool for detecting renal lesions, but CT scan and or magnetic resonance imaging also may be necessary in some cases.

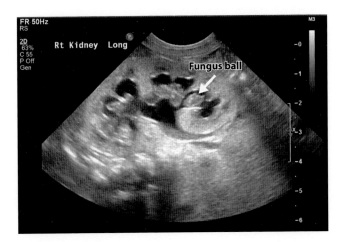

Figure 49.3 Renal ultrasound showing dilated calyces, pelvis, and proximal ureter. An echogenic fungus ball (arrow) is seen. The patient's blood and urine grew *Candida parapsilosis*.

## TREATMENT

Positive blood culture for fungus or candidemia has been reported in 30% to 50% in neonates with candiduria.[195,196] Therefore, systemic antifungal therapy is recommended in the treatment of patients with fungal UTI. Amphotericin B monotherapy is the preferred therapy for candiduria in neonates in the United States.[199] Intravenous amphotericin B is administered at a dose of 1 mg/kg/day. Amphotericin B is preferred to the lipid formulations of amphotericin B in neonates with renal candidiasis, because lipid formulations penetrate renal tubules poorly.[197,199] Renal function and serum electrolytes should be monitored closely in these patients, and the amphotericin B dose should be decreased if serum creatinine rises. Hypokalemia resulting from renal tubular acidosis may require potassium supplementation.

The Infectious Disease Society of America (IDSA) guidelines for the treatment of candidiasis, recommends no treatment for patients with asymptomatic cystitis.[200] Because of the risk for dissemination, treatment may be considered irrespective of symptoms in high risk patients such as neonates, patients undergoing urologic procedures, or neutropenic patients. For symptomatic cystitis and pyelonephritis, IDSA recommends fluconazole therapy for 2 weeks, with amphotericin as an alternative therapeutic option.[200] The site of infection within the urinary tract and the clinical response determine the length of treatment of funguria. Treatment for at least 3 weeks after negative blood and urine cultures is generally recommended. Surgical intervention is reserved for patients with fungus balls causing severe obstruction of the urinary tract, or those with renal abscess requiring drainage.

### KEY POINTS

- Fungal UTIs are primarily caused by *Candida* species.
- Admission to an ICU, prolonged indwelling catheters and an immunocompromised condition predispose to fungal UTIs.
- Growth of greater than 10,000 CFU/mL from a catheterized urine sample is diagnostic of candidal UTI.
- Fluconazole or amphotericin may be used to treat candidal UTIs. Infants generally should be treated with amphotericin.

Irrigation of the urinary bladder by an aqueous solution of amphotericin B has been used for the treatment of uncomplicated fungal infection of the lower urinary tract. Amphotericin is used in a concentration of 50 mcg/mL in sterile water. Such therapy has, however, come into question recently. Lack of controlled studies to evaluate the dose and duration of therapy, as well as availability of oral fluconazole as a treatment option, has decreased the attractiveness of amphotericin B bladder irrigation for the treatment of funguria.[201] Bladder irrigation has a high relapse rate and generally should be reserved for refractory infections with resistant organisms. The IDSA guideline does not recommend bladder irrigation for uncomplicated cystitis; its potential role in the treatment of fluconazole-resistant *Candida* infections has been suggested.[200]

# VIRAL HEMORRHAGIC CYSTITIS

Viral hemorrhagic cystitis is commonly seen in immunocompromised patients and is especially common in patients with bone marrow transplantation (BMT). Viral hemorrhagic cystitis in BMT occurs either 1 to 2 weeks after transplantation (early onset) or 4 to 6 months later (late onset). Viruses associated with late-onset hemorrhagic cystitis are adenovirus, polyoma BK virus, cytomegalovirus, human herpesvirus-6, and simian virus 40 (SV40).[202-206] A prospective study of 102 children who underwent allogenic stem cell transplantation found that 25.5% of patients developed hemorrhagic cystitis, of which 80.8% were due to BK virus, 15.4% to adenovirus, and 3.8% to JC virus.[207]

Gross hematuria, severe suprapubic pain, and dysuria are common symptoms of viral hemorrhagic cystitis. Diagnosis of viral cystitis in an immunocompromised host is made by quantitative polymerase chain reaction (PCR) obtained in the urine. Serologic methods are less reliable in immunocompromised hosts, who may not be able to mount a good antibody response.[208] Ultrasound examination of the urinary bladder in hemorrhagic cystitis shows a thickened bladder wall. This finding may resemble the ultrasound features seen in rhabdomyosarcoma of the bladder.

---

## KEY POINTS

- Hemorrhagic cystitis can be the result of chemotherapy, viral infection or radiation.
- Late-onset hemorrhagic cystitis may occur in BMT patients with adenovirus, BK virus, cytomegalovirus, or JC virus.
- Diagnosis of viral cystitis may be made by quantitative PCR from the urine.
- Viral cystitis is generally self-limited, but may be treated with cidofovir in immunocompromised patients.

---

Viral cystitis is self-limiting and resolves in approximately 2 to 3 weeks. Persistence of ultrasound findings or symptoms is an indication for cystoscopy and biopsy of the bladder wall. Symptomatic therapy is usually sufficient in hemorrhagic cystitis. Cidofovir, a newer antiviral agent, has been used in the treatment of polyoma BK, as well as adenoviral hemorrhagic cystitis, but well-controlled studies are lacking.[209-211] The propensity of cidofovir to cause nephrotoxicity limits its use to the most severe cases at this time.

## Asymptomatic bacteriuria

Bacteriuria present in children without any clinical manifestations of UTI has been well known. Such asymptomatic bacteriuria (ABU) can occur in all age groups and is more common in girls than boys.[212] Wettergren et al.[10] described ABU in 2.5% of unselected boys and 0.9% of girls in infancy. In their landmark epidemiologic study, Kunin et al.[1] screened 9878 school children in Virginia. They reported the prevalence of ABU to be 1.1% in girls and only 0.04% in boys. Similarly, in screening of 13,464 schoolgirls aged 4 to 18 years in Newcastle, the prevalence of asymptomatic bacteriuria was noted to be 1.9%.[212,213] In contrast, the prevalence of asymptomatic bacteriuria in boys was only 0.2%.

The spectrum of organisms isolated in patients with ABU is similar to that associated with symptomatic UTIs. *E. coli* was noted to be the most common organism (91.7%) in the Newcastle study, followed by *Klebsiella* species (5.2%), *Proteus mirabilis* (1.2%), *Streptococcus faecalis, group B streptococci,* and coagulase-positive *Staphylococcus* (0.4% in each group).[213] Although it was initially thought that *E. coli* causing ABU are less virulent, further research has revealed highly variable virulence properties of ABU *E. coli.* Some strains of *E. coli* associated with ABU do seem to be less adherent to epithelial cells compared to disease-causing strains. Among ABU *E. coli* that do adhere to epithelial cells, there may be a reduced host proinflammatory cytokine response compared to uropathogenic *E. coli* strains.[214]

Although patients are asymptomatic at the time of initial detection, close evaluation of these children may reveal a history of nonspecific symptoms, such as urgency, abdominal pain, nocturia, frequency of urination, or generally poor health. Complete absence of recent symptoms has been reported in 24% to 56% of cases and a history of UTI can be demonstrated in 13% to 21% cases.[1,213] Minor structural abnormalities of the urinary tract, such as caliectasis, hydronephrosis, and abnormalities in renal size have been noted in 10% of 20% cases.[1,213]

Management of ABU had been controversial. Kunin recommended treatment to reduce morbidity associated with UTI.[2] Savage et al. demonstrated that antibiotic therapy did not alter long-term recurrence or eradication of bacteriuria.[215] Lindberg et al.[216] also noted that despite clearance of bacteriuria by antibiotics, there was no difference in recurrence rate in the treated and untreated groups over 3 years of observation.[216] The Newcastle Covert Bacteriuria Study Group also showed similar results on treatment with antibiotics.[212] Based on these observations, patients with ABU need not be treated with antibiotics, unless symptomatic infections are demonstrated.

The long-term outlook of patients with ABU is generally optimistic. Of children, 40% to 50% become culture negative in 2 to 5 years without any antibiotic therapy.[217] Although up to 15% of patients with ABU may have renal scars when investigated, new scar formation is unusual.[212,215]

## SUMMARY

Infections of the urinary tract are a common childhood disorder that can lead to significant morbidity and hospitalizations. Our understanding of the structural and molecular predispositions to UTI makes it possible to develop a unified diagnostic and therapeutic approach that can be practiced in tertiary care centers and in the community. Such a unified management approach may result in a lowered long-term risk for renal damage. Recent data suggest that the renal scarring resulting from UTI may be determined by host inflammatory response, presence of urinary tract abnormalities, and the bacterial virulence. UTI and chronic pyelonephritis is, by itself, an uncommon cause of CKD and ESRD.

### Clinical Vignette 49.1

A previously healthy 3-month-old male infant presented to his pediatrician with a 3-day history of fever. Besides a mild cough, he was otherwise asymptomatic. His pediatrician obtained a urinalysis, which showed 20 WBCs, positive nitrites, and positive leukocyte esterase. A urine culture was obtained via catheterization, and the patient started on oral amoxicillin. Three days later the urine culture demonstrated greater than 100,000 CFU/mL of *E. coli* resistant to all β-lactam antimicrobial agents, but sensitive to ciprofloxacin, carbapenems, and nitrofurantoin. The child was admitted to a local hospital and given 2 days of intravenous ciprofloxacin before being transitioned to oral ciprofloxacin.

After approximately 5 days of oral ciprofloxacin at home, the patient developed a red rash along his torso and extremities. He returned to his pediatrician and was diagnosed to have an allergy to fluoroquinolones. The pediatrician transitioned the boy to nitrofurantoin and discharged him home. Shortly after finishing his course of nitrofurantoin, the patient became febrile again and returned to his pediatrician. He was otherwise doing well, although his oral intake is slightly decreased from his baseline. The pediatrician obtained a repeat urine culture, which again demonstrated greater than 100,000 CFU/mL

of ESBL *E. coli.* The patient was admitted for further therapy. He was treated with intravenous meropenem, and his fever quickly defervesced in the next 36 hours.

### TEACHING POINTS

- This case describes an otherwise healthy young boy who presents with a UTI resulting from an ESBL organism. The initial choice of ciprofloxacin is appropriate, despite the patient's young age, because he has an infection with a multidrug resistant organism.
- His subsequent development of a presumed fluoroquinolone allergy is unfortunate, because it limits his therapeutic options to parenteral agents. Although the initial organism was susceptible to nitrofurantoin, this agent is not indicated for the treatment of pyelonephritis in children and it is not surprising that the child relapsed.
- In view of the development of allergy to ciprofloxacin, the only appropriate therapeutic option is an intravenous carbapenem, preferably meropenem.
- Despite his excellent and rapid clinical recovery, this patient must receive 14 days of therapy with intravenous meropenem, but may be eligible for intravenous therapy at home. A patient's eligibility for home therapy should be made on an individual basis.
- This child should undergo a renal ultrasound while hospitalized, and a VCUG also may be indicated. Generally, it seems that VCUG is not indicated until the second episode of UTI, although abnormalities on renal ultrasound could trigger a more through radiologic evaluation.
- Given that the patient did not receive appropriate therapy after developing a fluoroquinolone allergy, it may not be necessary to obtain additional imaging to explain his subsequent relapse. The timing of further imaging studies is controversial, and it may be appropriate to obtain the VCUG once he has recovered from his current infection.

## REFERENCES

1. Kunin CL, Zacha E, Paquin AJ. Urinary tract infection in children. I. Prevalence of bacteriuria and associated urologic findings. N Engl J Med. 1962;266:1287–96.
2. Kunin CM. The natural history of recurrent bacteriuria in schoolgirls. N Engl J Med. 1970;282:1443–8.
3. Raz R. Asymptomatic bacteriuria: Clinical significance and management. Int J Antimicrob Agents. 2003;22:45–7.
4. Roberts KB. Urinary tract infection: Clinical practice guideline for the diagnosis and management of the initial UTI in febrile infants and children 2 to 24 months. Pediatrics. 2011;128:595–610.

5. Winberg J, Anderson HJ, Bergstrom T, et al. Epidemiology of symptomatic urinary tract infection in childhood. Acta Paediatr Scand. 1974;252:1–20.

6. Hellstrom A, Hanson E, Hansson S, et al. Association between urinary symptoms at 7 years old and previous urinary tract infection. Arch Dis Child. 1991;66:232–4.

7. Marild S, Jodal U. Incidence rate of first-time symptomatic urinary tract infection in children under 6 years of age. Acta Paediatr. 1998;87:549–52.

8. Bergstrom T, Larson H, Loncoln K, et al. Studies of urinary tract infections in infancy and childhood. XII. Eighty consecutive patients with neonatal infections. J Pediatr. 1972;80:858–66.

9. Drew JH, Acton CM. Radiological findings in newborn infants with urinary tract infection. Arch Dis Child. 1976;51:628–30.

10. Wettergren B, Jodal U, Jonasson G. Epidemiology of bacteriuria during the first year of life. Acta Paeditr Scand. 1985;74:925–33.

11. To T, Agha M, Dick PT, et al. Cohort study on circumcision of newborn boys and subsequent risk of urinary-tract infection. Lancet. 1998;352:1813-6.

12. Ginsburg CM, McCracken Jr, GH. Urinary tract infections in young infants. Pediatrics. 1982;69:409–12.

13. Schnadower D, Kuppermann N, Macias CG, et al.; American Academy of Pediatrics Pediatric Emergency Medicine Collaborative Research Committee. Febrile infants with urinary tract infections at very low risk for adverse events and bacteremia. Pediatrics. 2010;126:1074–83.

14. Newman TB, Bernzweig JA, Takayama JI, et al. Urine testing and urinary tract infection in febrile infants seen in office settings. Arch Pediatr Adolesc Med. 2002;156:44–54.

15. Hoberman A, Wald ER. Treatment of urinary tract infection. Pediatr Infect Dis J. 1999;18:1020–1.

16. Majd M, Rushton HG, Jantausch B, et al. Relationship among vesicoureteral reflux, P-fimbriated *Escherichia coli* and acute pyelonephritis in children with febrile urinary tract infection. J Pediatr. 1991;19:578–85.

17. Zorc JJ, Levine DA, Platt SL, et al. Clinical and demographic factors associated with urinary tract infection in young febrile infants. Pediatrics. 2005;116:644–8.

18. Didier C, Streicher MP, Chognot D, et al. Late-onset neonatal infections: Incidences and pathogens in the era of antenatal antibiotics. Eur J Pediatr. 2012;171:681–7.

19. Abrahamsson K, Hansson S, Jodal U. *Staphylococcus saprophyticus* urinary tract infections in children. Eur J Pediatr. 1993;152:69–71.

20. Dougherty FE, Gottlieb RP, Gross GW. Neonatal renal abscess caused by *Staphylococcus aureus*. Pediatr Infect Dis J. 1991;10:463–6.

21. Wippermann CF, Schofer O, Beetz R. Renal abscess in childhood: Diagnostic and therapeutic progress. Pediatr Infect Dis J. 1991;10:446–50.

22. Bush K. Extended-spectrum beta-lactamases in North America, 1987-2006. Clin Microbiol Infect. 2008;14:134–43.

23. Bertrand X, Dowzicky MJ. Antimicrobial susceptibility among Gram-negative isolates collected from intensive care units in North America, Europe, the Asia-Pacific Rim, Latin America, the Middle East, and Africa between 2004 and 2009 as part of the Tigecycline Evaluation and Surveillance Trial. Clin Ther. 2012;34:124–37.

24. Moland ES, Hanson ND, Black JA, et al. Prevalence of newer beta-lactamases in Gram-negative clinical isolates collected in the United States from 2001 to 2002.J Clin Microbiol. 2006;44:3318–24.

25. Chandramohan L, Revell PA. Prevalence and molecular characterization of extended-spectrum-β-lactamase-producing Enterobacteriaceae in a pediatric patient population. Antimicrob Agents Chemother. 2012;56:4765–70.

26. Plos K, Carter T, Hull S, et al. Frequency and organization of pap homologous DNA in relation to clinical origin of uropathogenic *Escherichia coli*. J Infect Dis. 1990;161:518–24.

27. Korhonen TK, Vaisanen V, Kallio P, et al. The role of pili in the adhesion of *Escherichia coli* to human urinary tract epithelial cells. Scand J Infect Dis. 1982;33:26–31.

28. Spurbeck RR, Stapleton AE, Johnson JR, et al. Fimbrial profiles predict virulence of uropathogenic *Escherichia coli* strains: Contribution of ygi and yad fimbriae. Infect Immun. 2011;79:4753–63.

29. Schilling JD, Mulvey MA, Huttgren SJ. Structure and function of *Escherichia coli* type I pilli: New insight into the pathogenesis of urinary tract infections. J Infect Dis. 2001;183:S36–40.

30. Kallenius G, Mollby R, Svenson SB. Occurrence of P-fimbriated *Escherichia coli* in urinary tract infections. Lancet. 1981;2:1369–72.

31. Nowicki B, Svanborg-Eden C, Hull R. Molecular analysis and epidemiology of the Dr hemagglutinin of uropathogenic *Escherichia coli*. Infect Immun. 1989;57:446–51

32. Rama G, Chhina DK, Chhina RS, et al. Urinary tract infections-microbial virulence determinants and reactive oxygen species. Comp Immunol Microbiol Infect Dis. 2005;28:339–49.

33. Azpiroz MF, Poey ME, Laviña M. Microcins and urovirulence in *Escherichia coli*. Microb Pathog. 2009;47:274–80.

34. Kunin C. Detection, Prevention and Management of Urinary Tract Infections, ed 4. Philadelphia: Lea & Febiger; 1987. p. 130.

35. Orskov I, Orskov F, Birch-Andersen A, et al. O, K, H and fimbrial antigens in *Escherichia coli* serotypes associated with pyelonephritis and cystitis. Scand J Infect Dis. 1982;33:18–25.

36. Lomberg H, Hellstrom M, Jodal U. Virulence-associated traits in *Escherichia coli* causing first and recurrent episodes of urinary tract infection in children with or without vesicoureteral reflux. J Infect Dis. 1984;150:561–9.

37. Emamghorashi F, Farshad S, Kalani M, et al. The prevalence of O serogroups of *Escherichia coli* strains causing acute urinary tract infection in children in Iran. Saudi J Kidney Dis Transpl. 2011;22:597–601.

38. Hacker J, Bender L, Oh M, et al. Deletions of chromosomal regions coding for fimbriae and hemolysin occur in vivo and in vitro in various extraintestinal *Escherichia coli* isolates. Microb Pathog. 1990;8:213–25.

39. Middendorf B, Blum-Oehler G, Dobrindt U. The pathogenicity islands (PAIs) of the uropathogenic *Escherichia coli* strain 536: Island probing of PAI II5 36. J Infect Dis. 2001;183:S17–20.

40. Sabaté M, Moreno E, Pérez T, et al. Pathogenicity island markers in commensal and *uropathogenic Escherichia coli* isolates. Clin Microbiol Infect. 2006;12:880–6.

41. Svanborg C, Bergsten G, Fischer H, et al. The "innate" host response protects and damages the infected urinary tract. Ann Med 2001;33:563–S70

42. Hedges S, Svensson M, Svanborg C. Interleukin-6 response of epithelial cell lines to bacterial stimulation in vitro. Infect Immun. 1992;60:1295–301.

43. Agace WW, Hedges SR, Ceska M. Interleukin-8 and the neutrophil response to mucosal Gram-negative infection. J Clin Invest. 1993;92:780–5.

44. Jantausch B, O'Donnell R, Wiedermann B. Urinary interleukin-6 and interleukin-8 in children with urinary tract infection. Pediatr Nephrol. 2000;15:236–40.

45. Benson M, Jodal U, Agace W, et al. Interleukin (IL)-6 and IL-8 in children with febrile urinary tract infection and asymptomatic bacteriuria. J Infect Dis. 1996;174:1080–4.

46. Wullt B, Bergsten G, Samuelsson M, et al. The role of P fimbriae for colonization and host response induction in the human urinary tract. J Infect Dis. 2001;183:S43–6.

47. Bitsori M, Karatzi M, Dimitriou H, et al. Urine IL-8 concentrations in infectious and non-infectious urinary tract conditions. Pediatr Nephrol. 2011;26:2003–7.

48. Sheu JN, Chen SM, Meng MH, et al. The role of serum and urine interleukin-8 on acute pyelonephritis and subsequent renal scarring in children. Pediatr Infect Dis J. 2009;28:885–90.

49. Duell BL, Carey AJ, Tan CK, et al. Innate transcriptional networks activated in bladder in response to uropathogenic *Escherichia coli* drive diverse biological pathways and rapid synthesis of IL-10 for defense against bacterial urinary tract infection. J Immunol. 2012;188:781–92.

50. Frendeus B, Wachtler C, Hedlund M, et al. *Escherichia coli* P fimbriae utilize the Toll-like receptor 4 pathway for cell activation. Mol Microbiol. 2001;40:37–51.

51. Luster AD. Chemokines: Chemotactic cytokines that mediate inflammation. N Engl J Med. 1998;338:436–45.

52. Svanborg C, Frendeus B, Godaly G, et al. Toll-like receptor signaling and chemokine receptor expression influence the severity of urinary tract infection. J Infect Dis. 2001;183:S61–5.

53. Olszyna DP, Opal SM, Prins JM, et al. Chemotactic activity of CXC chemokines interleukin-8, growth-related oncogene-alpha, and epithelial cell-derived neutrophil-activating protein-78 in urine of patients with urosepsis. J Infect Dis. 2000;182:1731–7.

54. Otto G, Burdick M, Strieter R, et al. Chemokine response to febrile urinary tract infection. Kidney Int. 2005;68:62–70.

55. Frendeus B, Godaly G, Hang L, et al.: Interleukin-8 receptor deficiency confers susceptibility to acute experimental pyelonephritis and may have a human counterpart. J Exp Med. 2000;192:881–90.

56. Lundstedt AC, Leijonhufvud I, Ragnarsdottir B, et al. Inherited susceptibility to acute pyelonephritis: A family study of urinary tract infection. J Infect Dis. 2007;195:1227–34.

57. Hawn TR, Scholes D, Wang H, et al. Genetic variation of the human urinary tract innate immune response and asymptomatic bacteriuria in women. PLoS One. 2009;4:e8300

58. Karoly E, Fekete A, Banki NF, et al. Heat shock protein 72 (HSPA1B) gene polymorphism and Toll-like receptor (TLR) 4 mutation are associated with increased risk of urinary tract infection in children. Pediatr Res. 2007;61:371–4.

59. Yin X, Hou T, Liu Y, et al. Association of Toll-like receptor 4 gene polymorphism and expression with urinary tract infection types in adults. PLoS One. 2010;5:e14223

60. Tramma D, Hatzistylianou M, Gerasimou G, et al. Interleukin-6 and interleukin-8 levels in the urine of children with renal scarring. Pediatr Nephrol. 2012;27:1525–30

61. Haraoka, M, Senoh K, Ogata N, et al. Elevated interleukin-8 levels in the urine of children with renal scarring and/or vesicoureteral reflux. J Urol 1996;155:678–80

62. Gokce I, Alpay H, Biyikli N, et al. Urinary levels of interleukin-6 and interleukin-8 in patients with vesicoureteral reflux and renal parenchymal scar. Pediatr Nephrol. 2010;25:905–12.

63. Pecile P, Miorin E, Romanello C, et al. Procalcitonin: A marker of severity of acute pyelonephritis among children. Pediatrics. 2004;114:e249–54.

64. Leroy S, Fernandez-Lopez A, Nikfar R, et al. Association of procalcitonin with acute pyelonephritis and renal scars in pediatric UTI. Pediatrics. 2013;131:870–9.

65. Sheinfeld J, Schaeffer AJ, Condin-Cordo C, et al. Association of the Lewis blood-group phenotype with recurrent urinary tract infection in women. N Engl J Med. 1989;320:773–7.

66. Jantausch B, Criss VR, O'Donnell R et al. Association of Lewis blood group phenotypes with urinary tract infection in children. J Pediatr. 1994;124:863–8.

67. Sheinfeld J, Cordon-Cardo C, Fair WR, et al.: Association of type 1 blood group antigens with urinary tract infections in children with genitourinary structural abnormalities. J Urol. 1990;144:469–73.

68. Albarus MH, Salzano FM, Goldraich NP. Genetic markers and acute febrile urinary tract infection in the 1st year of life. Pediatr Nephrol. 1997;11:691–4.

69. Kanematsu A, Yamamoto S, Yoshino K, et al. Renal scarring is associated with nonsecretion of blood type antigen in children with primary vesicoureteral reflux. J Urol. 2005;174:1594–7.

70. Scholes D, Hooton TM, Roberts PL, et al. Risk factors for recurrent urinary tract infection in young women. J Infect Dis. 2000;182:1177–82.

71. Graham JB, King LR, Kropp KA. The significance of distal urethral narrowing in young girls. J Urol 1967;97:1045–9.

72. Immergut MA, Wahman GE. The urethral caliber of female children with urinary tract infection. J Urol. 1968;99:189–90.

73. Laumann, EO, Masi CM, Zuckerman EW. Circumcision in the United States: Prevalence, prophylactic effects, and sexual practice. JAMA. 1997;277:1052–7.

74. Trends in in-hospital newborn male circumcision: United States, 1999–2010. Morb Mortal Wkly Rep (MMWR) 2011;60;1167–8.

75. Kozak LJ, Owings MF, Hall MJ. National Hospital Discharge Survey: 2002 annual summary with detailed diagnosis and procedure data. Vital Health Stat 13. 2005;158:1–199.

76. Xu F, Markowitz LE, Sternberg MR, et al. Prevalence of circumcision and herpes simplex virus type 2 infection in men in the United States: The National Health and Nutrition Examination Survey (NHANES) 1999-2004. Sex Transm Dis. 2007;34:479–84

77. Frisch M, Friis S, Krager-Kjaer S, et al. Falling incidence of penile cancer in an uncircumcised population (Denmark 194390). B Med J. 1995;311:1471.

78. Rickwood AM, Kenny SE, Donnell SC. Towards evidence based circumcision of English boys: Survey of trends in practice. B Med J. 2000;321:792–3.

79. Cathcart P, Nuttall M, van der Meulen J, et al. Trends in paediatric circumcision and its complications in England between 1997 and 2003. Br J Surg. 2006;93:885–90.

80. Wiswell TE, Roscelli JD. Corroborative evidence for the decrease incidence of urinary tract infections in circumcised male infants. Pediatrics. 1986;78:96–99.

81. Wiswell TE, Hachey WE. Urinary tract infections and the uncircumcised state: An update Clin Pediatr. 1993;32:130–4.

82. Wiswell TE, Geschke DW. Risks from circumcision during the first month of life compared with those for non-circumcised. Pediatrics. 1989;83:1011–15.

83. Schoen EJ, Colby CJ. Newborn circumcision decreases incidence and costs of urinary tract infections during the first year of life. Pediatrics. 2000;105:789–93.

84. Jagannath VA, Fedorowicz Z, Sud V, et al. Routine neonatal circumcision for the prevention of urinary tract infections in infancy. Cochrane Database Syst Rev. 2012;(11)009129.

85. Singh-Grewal D, Macdessi J, Craig J. Circumcision for the prevention of urinary tract infection in boys: A systematic review of randomised trials and observational studies. Arch Dis Child. 2005;90:853–8

86. Herzog LW. Urinary tract infections and circumcision. A case control study. Am J Dis Child. 1989;143:348–50

87. Craig JC, Knight JF, Sureshkumar P, et al. Effect of circumcision on incidence of urinary tract infection in preschool boys. J Pediatr. 1996;128:23–7.

88. Nayir A. Circumcision for the prevention of significant bacteriuria in boys. Pediatr Nephrol. 2001;16:1129–34

89. Wiswell TE, Miller GM, Gelston, HM, Jr, et al.: Effect of circumcision status on periurethral bacterial flora during the first year of life. J. Pediatr. 1988;113:442–6

90. Wiswell TE: John K. Lattimer Lecture. Prepuce presence portends prevalence of potentially perilous periurethral pathogens. J Urol. 1992;148:739–42.

91. Laway MA, Wani ML, Patnaik R, et al. Does circumcision alter the periurethral uropathogenic bacterial flora. Afr J Paediatr Surg. 2012;9:109–12

92. Price LB, Liu CM, Johnson KE, et al. The effects of circumcision on the penis microbiome. PLoS ONE 2010;5:e8422

93. Fussell EN, Kaack MB, Cherry R, et al. Adherence of bacteria to human foreskin. J Urol. 1988;140:997–1001

94. Bonacorsi S, Lefevre S, Clermont O. *Escherichia coli* strains causing urinary tract infection in uncircumcised infants resemble urosepsis-like adult strains. J Urol. 2005;173:195–7.

95. American Academy of Pediatrics Task Force on Circumcision. Male circumcision. Pediatrics. 2012;130:e756–85

96. Loening-Baucke V. Urinary incontinence and urinary tract infection and their resolution with treatment of chronic constipation of childhood. Pediatrics. 1997;100:228–32.

97. McKenna PH, Herndon CDA. Voiding dysfunction associated with incontinence, vesicoureteral reflux and recurrent urinary tract infections. Curr Opin Urol. 2000;10:599–606.

98. Koff SA, Wagner TT, Jayanthi VR. The relationship among dysfunctional elimination syndromes, primary vesicoureteral reflux and urinary tract infections in children. J Urol. 1998;160:1019–22.

99. Elder JS, Diaz M. Vesicoureteral reflux: The role of bladder and bowel dysfunction. Nat Rev Urol. 2013;10:640–8.

100. Honkinen O, Lehtonen O-P, Ruuskanen O, et al. Cohort study of bacterial species causing urinary tract infection and urinary tract abnormalities in children. B Med J. 1999;318:770–1.

101. Hobermann A, Wald ER. Urinary tract infections in febrile children. Pediatr Infect Dis. 1997;16:11–7.

102. Hallett RJ, Pead L, Maskell R. Urinary tract infection in boys, a three-year prospective study. Lancet. 1976;2:1107–10.

103. Ingelfinger JR, Davis AE, Grupe WE. Frequency and etiology of gross hematuria in a general pediatric setting. Pediatrics. 1977;59:557–61.

104. Labbé J: Self-induced urinary tract infection in school-aged boys. Pediatrics. 1990;86:703–6.

105. Honkinen O, JahnukainenT, Mertsola, J, et al.: Bacteremic urinary tract infection in children. Pediatr Infect Dis J. 2000;19:630–4

106. Hoberman A, Han-Pu C, Keller DM, et al. Prevalence of urinary tract infection in febrile infants. J Pediatr. 1993;123:17–23.

107. Bachur R, Caputo GL. Bacteremia and meningitis among infants with urinary tract infections. Pediatr Emerg Care. 1995;11:280–4.

108. Özçakar ZB, Yalçınkaya F, Kavaz A, et al. Urinary tract infections owing to ESBL-producing bacteria: Microorganisms change: Clinical pattern does not. Acta Paediatr. 2011;100:e61–4.

109. Turner ME, Weinstein J, Kher K. Acute renal failure secondary to pyelonephritis. Pediatrics. 1996;97:742–3.

110. Kanellopoulos TA, Salakos C, Spiliopoulou I, et al. First urinary tract infection in neonates, infants and young children: A comparative study. Pediatr Nephrol. 2006; 21:1131–7.

111. Hansson S, Martinell J, Stokland E, et al. The natural history of bacteriuria in childhood. Infect Dis Clin North Am. 1997;11:499–512.

112. Ismaili K, Lolin K, Damry N, et al. Febrile urinary tract infections in 0- to 3-month-old infants: A prospective follow-up study. J Pediatr. 2011;158:91–4.

113. Littlewood JM. 66 infants with urinary tract infection in first month of life. Arch Dis Child. 1972;47:218–26.

114. Schnadower D, Kuppermann N, Macias CG, et al. Sterile cerebrospinal fluid pleocytosis in young febrile infants with urinary tract infections. Arch Pediatr Adolesc Med. 2011;165:635–41.

115. Angel C, Shu T, Green J, et al. Renal and perirenal abscesses in children: Proposed physiopathologic mechanisms and treatment algorithm. Pediatr Surg Int. 2003;19:35–9.

116. Wippermann CF, Schofer O, Beetz R, et al. Renal abscess in childhood: Diagnostic and therapeutic progress. Pediatr Infect Dis J. 1991;10:446–50.

117. Dembry LM, Andriole VT. Renal and perirenal abscesses. Infect Dis Clin North Am. 1997;11:663–80.

118. Wang, YT, Lin KY, Chen MJ, et al. Renal abscess in children: A clinical retrospective study, Acta Paediatr. 2003;44:197–201.

119. Angel T, Shu J, Green E, et al. Renal and perirenal abscesses in children: Proposed physiopathologic mechanisms and treatment algorithm. Pediatr Surg Int. 2003;19:35–9.

120. Shu T, Green JM, Orihuela E. Renal and perirenal abscesses in patients with otherwise anatomically normal urinary tracts. J Urol. 2004;172:148–50.

121. Coelho RF, Schneider-Monteiro ED, Mesquita JL, et al. Renal and perinephric abscesses: Analysis of 65 consecutive cases. World J Surg. 2007;31:431–6.

122. Delanghe J, Speeckaert M. Preanalytical requirements of urinalysis. Biochem Med (Zagreb). 2014;24:89–104.

123. Downs SM. Technical report: Urinary tract infections in febrile infants and young children. Pediatrics. 1999;103:e54.

124. Rawal K, Senguttuvan P, Morris M, et al. Significance of crystal clear urine. Lancet. 1990;335:1228.

125. Bulloch B, BausherJC, Pomerantz WJ, et al.: Can urine clarity exclude the diagnosis of urinary tract infection? Pediatrics 2000;106.e60.

126. Struthers S, Scanlon J, Parker K, et al.: Parental reporting of smelly urine and urinary tract infection. Arch Dis Child. 2003;88:250–2.

127. Gorelic MD, Shaw KN. Screening tests for urinary tract infection in children: A meta-analysis. Pediatrics. 1999;104:e54.

128. Kunin CN, DeGroot JE, Uehling D, et al.: Detection of urinary tract infection in 3-5 year old girls by mothers using a nitrite strip indicator. Pediatrics. 1976;57:829–35.

129. Al-Ori F, McGillivray D, Tange S, et al. Urine culture from bag specimens in young children: Are the risks too high? J Pediatr. 2000;137:221–6.

130. Hoberman A, Wald ER, Reynolds EA, et al. Pyuria and bacteriuria in urine specimens obtained by catheter from young children with fever. J Pediatr. 1994;124:513–9.

131. Giorgi LJ, Bratslavsky G, Kogan BA. Febrile urinary tract infections in infants: Renal ultrasound remains necessary. J Urol. 2005;173:568–70

132. Hoberman A, Charron M, Hickey RW, et al. Imaging studies after a first febrile urinary tract infection in young children. N Engl J Med. 2003;348:195–202.

133. Alon US, Ganapathy S. Should renal ultrasonography be done routinely in children with first urinary tract infection? Clin Pediatr. 1999;38:21–5.

134. Zamir W, Sakran Y, Horowitz, A et al. Urinary tract infection: Is there a need for routine renal ultrasonography? Arch Dis Child. 2004;89:466–8.

135. Massanyi EZ, Preece J, Gupta A, et al. Utility of screening ultrasound after first febrile UTI among patients with clinically significant vesicoureteral reflux. Urology. 2013;82:905–9.

136. Mori R, Lakhanpaul M, Verrier-Jones K. Diagnosis and management of urinary tract infection in children: Summary of NICE guidance. BMJ. 2007;335:395–7.

137. Deader R, Tiboni SG, Malone PS, et al. Will the implementation of the 2007 National Institute for Health and Clinical Excellence (NICE) guidelines on childhood urinary tract infection (UTI) in the UK miss significant urinary tract pathology? BJU Int. 2012;110:454–8.

138. Hannula A, Venhola M, Renko M, et al. Vesicoureteric reflux in children with suspected and proven urinary tract infection. Pediatr Nephrol. 2010;25:1463–9.

139. Berry CS, Vander Brink BA, Koff SA, et al. Is VCUG still indicated following the first episode of urinary tract infection in boys? Urology. 2012;80:1351–5.

140. Lee JH, Kim MK, Park SE. Is a routine voiding cystourethrogram necessary in children after the first febrile urinary tract infection? Acta Paediatr. 2012;101:e105–9.

141. Pennesi M, L'Erario I, Travan L, et al., Managing Children under 36 months of age with febrile urinary tract infection: A new approach. Pediatr Nephrol. 2012;4:611–5.

142. Spencer JD, Bates CM, Mahan JD, et al. The accuracy and health risks of a voiding cystourethrogram after a febrile urinary tract infection. J Pediatr Urol. 2012;8:72–6.

143. Craig JC, Knight JF, Sureshkumar P, et al. Vesicoureteral reflux and timing of micturating cystourethrography after urinary tract infection. Arch Dis Child. 1997;76:275–7.

144. Mahant S, To T, Friedman J. Timing of voiding cystourethrogram in the investigation of urinary tract infections in children. J Pediatr. 2001;139:568–71.

145. Doganis D, Mavrikou M, Delis D, et al. Timing of voiding cystourethrography in infants with first time urinary infection. Pediatr Nephrol. 2009;24:319–22.

146. Gil Rushton H. The evaluation of acute pyelonephritis and renal scarring with technetium 99m-dimercaptosuccinic acid renal scintigraphy: Evolving concepts and future directions. Pediatr Nephrol. 1997;11:108–20.

147. Zhang X, Xu H, Zhou L, et al. Accuracy of early DMSA scan for VUR in young children with febrile UTI. Pediatrics. 2014;133:e30–8.

148. American Academy of Pediatrics, Committee on Quality Improvement, Subcommittee on Urinary Tract Infection. Practice parameter: The diagnosis, treatment, and evaluation of the initial urinary tract infection in febrile infants and young children. Pediatrics. 1999;103:843–52.

149. Hansson S, Dhamey M, Sigstro O, et al. Dimercapto-succinicacid scintigraphy instead of voiding cystourethrography for infants with urinary tract infection. J Urol. 2004;172:1071–4.

150. Tsai JD, Huang CT, Lin PY, et al. Screening high-grade vesicoureteral reflux in young infants with a febrile urinary tract infection. Pediatr Nephrol. 2012;27:955–63.

151. Mantadakis E, Vouloumanou EK, Georgantzi GG, et al. Acute Tc-99m DMSA scan for identifying dilating vesicoureteral reflux in children: A meta-analysis. Pediatrics. 2011;128:e169–79.

152. Winberg J, Bergstrom T, Jacobsson B. Morbidity, age and sex distribution, recurrences and renal scarring in symptomatic urinary tract infection in childhood. Kid Int Suppl. 1975; 8:101–6.

153. Rushton HG. Urinary tract infections in children. Pediatr Clin N Am. 1997;44:1133–69.

154. Hellerstein S. Recurrent urinary tract infections in children. Pediatr Infect Dis. 1982;1:271–81.

155. Ladhani S, Gransden W. Increasing antibiotic resistance among urinary tract isolates. Arch Dis Child. 2003;88:444–5.

156. Hoberman A, Wald ER, Hickey RW, et al. Oral versus initial intravenous therapy for urinary tract infections in young febrile children. Pediatr. 1999;104:79–86.

157. Byington CL, Rittichier KK, Bassett KE, et al. Serious bacterial infections in febrile infants younger than 90 days of age: The importance of ampicillin-resistant pathogens. Pediatrics. 2003;111:964–8.

158. Ismaili K, Wissing KM, Lolin K, et al. Characteristics of first urinary tract infection with fever in children: A prospective clinical and imaging study. Pediatr Infect Dis J. 2011;30:371–4.

159. Wald ER. Urinary tract infection in infants and children: A comprehensive overview. Curr Opin Pediatr. 2004;16:85–8.

160. American Academy of Pediatrics. Red Book: 2012 Report of the Committee on Infectious Diseases, ed 29. Pickering LK, editor. Elk Grove Village, IL: American Academy of Pediatrics; 2012.

161. Hellerstein S. Antibiotic treatment for urinary tract infections in pediatric patients. Minerva Pediatr. 2003;55:395–406.

162. Beetz R. Evaluation and management of urinary tract infections in the neonate. Curr Opin Pediatr. 2012;24:205–11.

163. Brady PW, Conway PH, Goudie A. Length of intravenous antibiotic therapy and treatment failure in infants with urinary tract infections. Pediatrics. 2010;126:196–203.

164. Bloomfield P, Hodson EM, Craig JC. Antibiotics for acute pyelonephritis in children. Cochrane Database Syst Rev. 2003;(3):003772.

165. Hodson EM, Willis NS, Craig JC. Antibiotics for acute pyelonephritis in children. Cochrane Database of Systematic Reviews 2007;(4):003772.

166. Tran D, Muchant DG, Aronoff SC. Short-course versus conventional length antimicrobial therapy for uncomplicated lower urinary tract infections in children: A meta-analysis of 1279 patients. J Pediatr. 2001;139:93–9.

167. Michael M, Hodson EM, Craig JC, et al. Short versus standard duration oral antibiotic therapy for acute urinary tract infection in children. Cochrane Database Syst Rev. 2003;(1)003966.

168. Keren R, Chan E. A meta-analysis of randomized, controlled trials comparing short and long-course antibiotic therapy for urinary tract infections in children. Pediatrics. 2002;09:e70-0.

169. Madrigal G, Odio CM, Mohs E, et al. Single dose antibiotic therapy is not as effective as conventional regimens for management of acute urinary tract infections in children. Pediatr Infect Dis J. 1988;7:316–9.

170. Malloy, A, Campos JM. Extended-spectrum beta-lactamases. PIDJ. 2011;30:1092–3.

171. Benador D, Benador N, Slosman D, et al. Are younger children at risk of renal sequelae after pyelonephritis? Lancet. 1997;349:17–9.

172. Fernández-Menández JM, Malaga S, Matesanz JL, et al.: Risk factors in the development of early technetium-99m dimercaptosuccinic acid renal scintigraphy lesions during first urinary tract infection in children. Acta Paediatr. 2003;92:21–6.

173. Wennerström, M, Hansson, S, Jodal, U, et al. Primary and acquired renal scarring in boys and girls with urinary tract Infection. J Pediatr. 2000;136:30–4.

174. Shaikh N, Ewing AL, Bhatnagar S, et al. Risk of renal scarring in children with a first urinary tract infection: A systematic review. Pediatrics. 2010;126:1084–91.

175. Cotton SA, Gbadegesin RA, Williams S, et al. Role of TGF-beta1 in renal parenchymal scarring following childhood urinary tract infection. Kidney Int. 2002;61:61–7.

176. Hussein A, Askar E, Elsaeid M, et al. Functional polymorphisms in transforming growth factor-beta-1 (TGFbeta-1) and vascular endothelial growth factor (VEGF) genes modify risk of renal parenchymal scarring following childhood urinary tract infection. Nephrol Dial Transplant. 2010;25:779–85.

177. Zaffanello M, Tardivo S, Cataldi L, et al. Genetic susceptibility to renal scar formation after urinary tract infection: A systematic review and meta-analysis of candidate gene polymorphisms. Pediatr Nephrol. 2011;26:1017–29.

178. Poulsen EU, Johannesen NL, Nielsen JB, et al.: Vesico-ureteral reflux. II. The long term outcome of kidney function in non-surgical treatment. Scand J Urol Nephrol Suppl. 1989;125:29–34.

179. Soylu A, Demir BK, Türkmen M, et al. Predictors of renal scar in children with urinary infection and vesicoureteral reflux. Pediatr Nephrol. 2008;23:2227–32.

180. Jodal U. The natural history of bacteriuria in childhood. Infect Dis Clin North Am. 1987;1:713–29.

181. Yiee JH, DiSandro M, Wang MH, et al. Does severity of renal scarring on DMSA scan predict abnormalities in creatinine clearance? Urology. 2010;76:204–8.

182. Wennerström M, Hansson S, Jodal U, et al. renal function 16 to 26 years after the first urinary tract infection in childhood. Arch Pediatr Adolesc Med. 2000;154:339–45.

183. Hiraoka M, HashimotoG, Tsuchida S, et al.: Early treatment of urinary infection prevents renal damage on cortical scintigraphy. Pediatr Nephrol. 2003;18:115–8.

184. Doganis D, Siafas K, Mavrikou M, et al. Does early treatment of urinary tract infection prevent renal damage? Pediatrics. 2007;120:e922–8.

185. Toffolo A, Ammenti A, Montini G. Long-term clinical consequences of urinary tract infections during childhood: A review. Acta Paediatr. 2012;101:1018–31.

186. Elder JS, Peters CA, Arant BS, Jr, et al. Pediatric vesicoureteral reflux guidelines panel summary report on the management of primary vesicoureteral reflux in children. J Urol. 1997;157:1846–51.

187. Wennerström M, Hansson S, Hedner T, et al.: Ambulatory blood pressure 16-26 years after the first urinary tract infection in childhood. J Hyperten. 2000;18:485–91.

188. Beetz R, Schulte-Wissermann H, Troger J, et al.: Long-term follow-up of children with surgically treated vesicorenal reflux: Postoperative incidence of urinary tract infections, renal scars and arterial hypertension. Eur Urol. 1989;16:366–71.

189. Jacobson SH, Eklof O, Eriksson CG, et al.: Development of hypertension and uraemia after pyelonephritis in childhood: 27 year follow up. B Med J. 1989;299:703–6.

190. Sreenarasimhaiah S, Hellerstein S. Urinary tract infections per se do not cause end-stage kidney disease. Pediatr Nephrol. 1998;12:210–3.

191. Smellie JM, Prescod NP, Shaw PJ, et al.: Childhood reflux and urinary infection: A follow-up of 10–41 years in 226 adults. Pediatr Nephrol. 1998;12:727–36.

192. U.S. Renal Data System. USRDS 2013 Annual data report: Atlas of chronic kidney disease and end-stage renal disease in the United States. Bethesda, MD: National Institutes of Health, National Institute of Diabetes and Digestive and Kidney Diseases; 2013. pp. 295–306.

193. North American Pediatric Renal Transplant Cooperative Study. 2011 annual report: Dialysis. https://web.emmes.com/study/ped/annlrept/annualrept2011.pdf . Accessed September 9, 2014.

194. Salo J, Ikäheimo R, Tapiainen T, et al. Childhood urinary tract infections as a cause of chronic kidney disease. Pediatrics. 2011;128:840–7.

195. Bryant K, Maxfield C, Rabalais G, et al. Renal candidiasis in neonates with candiduria. Pediatr Infect Dis J. 1999;18:959–63.

196. Phillips JR, Karlowicz MG. Prevalence of Candida species in hospital-acquired urinary tract infections in a neonatal intensive care unit. Pediatr Infect Dis J. 1997;16:190–4.

197. Karlowicz MG. Candidal renal and urinary tract infection in neonates. Semin Perinatol. 2003;27:393–400.

198. Robins JL, Davies HD, Barton M, et al. Characteristics and outcome of infants with candiduria in neonatal intensive care: A Paediatric Investigators Collaborative Network on Infections in Canada study BMC Infect D 2009;9:183.

199. Rowen JL, Tate JM; Neonatal Candidiasis Study Group. Management of neonatal candidiasis. Pediatr Infect Dis J. 1998;17:1007–11.

200. Pappas PG, Kauffman CA, Andes D, et al. Clinical practice guidelines for the management of candidiasis: 2009 Update by the Infectious Diseases Society of America. Clin Infect Dis. 2009;48:503–35.

201. Drew RH, Arthur RR, Perfect JR. Is it time to abandon the use of amphotericin B bladder irrigation? Clin Infect Dis. 2005;40:1465–70.

202. Azzi A, Fanci R, Bosi A, et al. Monitoring of polyomavirus BK viruria in bone marrow transplantation patients by DNA hybridization assay and by polymerase chain reaction: An approach to assess the relationship between BK viruria and hemorrhagic cystitis. Bone Marrow Transplant. 1994;14:235–40.

203. Erard V, Storer B, Corey L, et al. BK virus infection in hematopoietic stem cell transplant recipients: Frequency, risk factors, and association with postengraftment hemorrhagic cystitis. Clin Infect Dis. 2004;39:1861–5.

204. Kim YJ, Kim DW, Lee DG, et al. Human herpesvirus-6 as a possible cause of encephalitis and hemorrhagic cystitis after allogeneic hematopoietic stem cell transplantation. Leukemia. 2002;16:958–9.

205. Comar M, D'Agaro P, Andolina M, et al. Hemorrhagic cystitis in children undergoing bone marrow transplantation: A putative role for simian virus 40. Transplantation. 2004;78:544–8.

206. Lee H-J, Pyo J-W, Choi E-H, et al. Isolation of adenovirus type 7 from the urine of children with acute hemorrhagic cystitis. Pediatr Infect Dis J. 1996;15:633–4.

207. Gorczynska E, Turkiewicz D, Rybka K, et al. Incidence, clinical outcome, and management of virus-induced hemorrhagic cystitis in children and adolescents after allogeneic hematopoietic cell transplantation. Biol Blood Marrow Transplant. 2005;11:797–804.

208. Paduch DA, Viral lower urinary tract infections. Curr Urol Rep. 2007;8:324–35.

209. Nagafuji K, Aoki K, Henzan H, et al.: Cidofovir for treating adenoviral hemorrhagic cystitis in hematopoietic stem cell transplant recipients. Bone Marrow Transplant. 2004;34:909–14.

210. Cesaro S, Hirsch HH, Faraci M, et al.; European Group for Blood and Marrow Transplantation. Cidofovir for BK virus-associated hemorrhagic cystitis: A retrospective study. Clin Infect Dis. 200949:233–40.

211. Yusuf U, Hale GA, Carr J, et al. Cidofovir for the treatment of adenoviral infection in pediatric hematopoietic stem cell transplant patients. Transplantation. 2006;81:1398–404.

212. Newcastle Asymptomatic Bacteriuria Group. Asymptomatic bacteriuria in schoolchildren in Newcastle upon Tyne. Arch Dis Child. 1975;50:90–102.

213. Newcastle Covert Bacteriuria Research Group. Covert bacteriuria in schoolgirls in Newcastle upon Tyne: 5-year follow-up. Arch Dis Child. 1981;56:585–92.

214. Mabbett AN, Ulett GC, Watts RE, et al. Virulence properties of asymptomatic bacteriuria *Escherichia coli*. Int J Med Microbiol. 2009;299:53–63.

215. Savage DCL, Howie G, Adler K, et al.: Controlled trial of therapy in covert bacteriuria of childhood. Lancet. 1978;1:358–61.

216. Lindberg U, Claesson I, Hanson LÅ, et al.: Asymptomatic bacteriuria in schoolgirls. VIII. Clinical course during a 3-year follow-up. J Pediatr. 1978;92:194–9.

217. Cardiff-Oxford Bacteriuria Study Group. Sequelae of covert bacteriuria in schoolgirls. Lancet. 1978;1:889–93.

## REVIEW QUESTIONS

1. Which bacteria are responsible for most UTIs in children?
   a. *E. coli*
   b. *S. aureus*
   c. *Klebsiella* species
   d. Group B streptococci
   e. *Staphylococcus saprophyticus*

2. The 2012 AAP Task Force on Circumcision states that all male infants should undergo circumcision.
   a. True
   b. False

3. Which symptoms or laboratory test results differentiate cystitis from acute pyelonephritis?
   a. Abdominal pain
   b. Excessive crying
   c. Hematuria
   d. Fever
   e. Dysuria

4. According to the 2011 AAP UTI Practice Guideline, what is the minimum colony count diagnostic of urinary tract infection?
   a. 100,000 CFU/mL
   b. 50,000 CFU/mL
   c. 20,000 CFU/mL
   d. 10,000 CFU/mL

5. All children under 2 years of age should have a renal ultrasound after diagnosis of UTI.
   a. True
   b. False

6. A 6-year-old girl with a history of spina bifida requiring routine urinary catheterization has a history of multiple episodes of UTI. She has been on multiple courses of antibiotics and was recently admitted after failing outpatient therapy on cefixime. You are suspicious she may have developed an ESBL infection. What is the *best* choice of empiric therapy for this child?
   a. Ceftriaxone
   b. Ceftazidime
   c. Meropenem
   d. Ampicillin-sulbactam

7. A male infant is born at 25 weeks' gestation and develops candiduria at two weeks of age while in the neonatal intensive care unit. Which antimicrobial agent should be empirically started?
   a. Fluconazole
   b. Micafungin
   c. Itraconazole
   d. Amphotericin

8. Which of the following viruses may cause cystitis in an immunocompromised patient?
   a. Adenovirus
   b. BK virus
   c. HHV-6
   d. CMV
   e. All of the above

9. Which of the following therapies is indicated in a 16-year-old girl with *Proteus mirabilis* bacteriuria found during a routine health screen?
   a. Cefixime
   b. Trimethoprim-sulfamethoxazole
   c. Ciprofloxacin
   d. Amoxicillin
   e. No therapy.

10. *E. coli* associated with asymptomatic bacteriuria have fewer virulence factors than pathogenic *E. coli*.
    a. True
    b. False

## ANSWER KEY

1. a
2. b
3. d
4. b
5. a
6. c
7. d
8. e
9. e
10. b

# 50

# Pediatric renal tumors

EUGENE MINEVICH, ARMANDO J. LORENZO, W. ROBERT DEFOOR, AND MARTIN A. KOYLE

Tumors of the kidney account for fewer than 8% of childhood neoplasms. Although the great majority of these are embryonal (mostly Wilms) tumors, other malignancies also may be seen. Both the primary lesion and the effects of therapy have implications for the treating pediatric nephrologists. A clinicopathologic classification of renal tumors in children shown in Table 50.1 provides a framework for discussion in this chapter. It is likely that emerging genetic and molecular data may be instrumental in therapeutic and prognostic classification of these malignancies in the future.

## WILMS TUMOR (NEPHROBLASTOMA)

Wilms tumor (WT), or nephroblastoma, is the most common primary malignant renal neoplasm of childhood. The multidisciplinary approach to this tumor by the National Wilms Tumor Study Group (NWTSG, now under the Children's Oncology Group [COG]) and the International Society of Pediatric Oncology (SIOP), has become an example for successful cancer treatment. Owing to refinements in surgery, chemotherapy, and radiation therapy, the overall cure rate for WT exceeds 85%. Studies of tumor genetics have laid the foundation for our understanding of tumor suppressor genes and genomic imprinting.

## EPIDEMIOLOGY

The annual incidence of WT is 8 cases per million children younger than 15 years, representing 6.3% of cases of childhood cancer.[1] In the United States, approximately 450 new cases are diagnosed each year, making WT the fourth most common pediatric cancer by specific histologic type.[1] Girls have a slightly increased risk for the tumor with a male-to-female ratio of 0.92 to 1.00. The mean age at diagnosis is 44 months for unilateral disease and 31 months for bilateral disease. WT in the adult population is rare, although numerous cases have been reported.[2]

The majority of WT cases are sporadic and unilateral. Familial WT is uncommon, occurring in only 1.5% of the affected patients.[3] Most cases of familial WT occur in distant relatives rather than parents or siblings. Sixteen percent of cases of familial WT are bilateral, compared with 7% of sporadic cases. Children with bilateral disease present at a younger age, and their mothers tend to be older. Genitourinary anomalies (hypospadias, cryptorchidism, renal fusion anomalies) are present in 4.5% of patients with WT.[4]

## GENETICS AND EMBRYOLOGY

WT is thought to result from an abnormal proliferation of metanephric blastema, without normal differentiation into tubules or glomeruli. Although WT was one of the original paradigms of the Knudson and Strong two-hit model of cancer formation, it has become apparent that several genetic events participate in Wilms tumorigenesis.[5] The first suppressor gene *WT1* (the only WT gene isolated to date) was identified as a direct result of the study of children with WT who also had aniridia, genitourinary anomalies, and mental retardation (WAGR syndrome).[6] Cytogenetic analysis of children with WAGR syndrome revealed deletions at chromosome 11p13, which was later found to encompass a

Table 50.1 Clinicopathologic classification of renal tumors in children

**Nephroblastic Tumors**
- Nephroblastoma (Wilms tumor)
- Nephroblastomatosis and nephrogenic rests

**Mesenchymal Tumors**
- Clear cell sarcoma
- Rhabdoid tumor
- Congenital mesoblastic nephroma

**Metanephric Tumors**
- Metanephric adenoma
- Metanephric adenofibroma
- Metanephric stromal tumor

**Renal Epithelial Tumors**
- Papillary renal cell carcinoma
- Renal medullary carcinoma
- Renal tumor associated with Xp11.2 translocation

**Mixed Tumors**
- Angiolipoma

Table 50.2 Clinical and genetic conditions associated with increased risk for Wilms tumor

**High risk (>20%)**
- WAGR syndrome (Wilms-aniridia-genitourinary-mental retardation) (*WT1* deletions)
- Denys-Drash syndrome (truncating and pathogenic missense *WT1* mutations)
- Familial Wilms tumor
- Perlman syndrome
- Mosaic variegated aneuploidy
- Fanconi anemia (D1/biallelic *BRCA2* mutations)

**Moderate risk (5% to 20%)**
- Fraser syndrome (*WT1* intron 9 splice mutations)
- Beckwith-Wiedemann syndrome (11p15 uniparental disomy, isolated H19 hypermethylation)
- Simpson-Golabi-Behmel syndrome (*GPC3* mutations/deletions)

**Low risk (<5%)**
- Isolated hemihypertrophy
- Bloom syndrome
- Li-Fraumeni syndrome, Li-Fraumeni-like association
- Hereditary hyperparathyroidism–jaw tumor syndrome
- Mulibrey nanism
- Trisomy 18 or Edwards syndrome
- Trisomy 13 or Patau syndrome
- 2q37 deletions

*Source:* Modified from Scott RH, Stiller, CA, Walker L, et al. Syndromes and constitutional chromosomal abnormalities associated with Wilms tumour. J Med Genet. 2006;43:705–15. Reproduced with permission.

contiguous set of genes, including *PAX6* (the gene responsible for aniridia) and *WT1*.[7,8] *WT1* encodes a transcription factor critical to normal kidney and gonadal development; its deletion in experimental models has been shown to result in major genitourinary maldevelopment.[9] Although germinal deletions or mutations in *WT1* have been documented in almost all patients with WAGR syndrome and the related Denys-Drash syndrome (nephropathy, WT, and pseudohermaphroditism), only a small number of patients with sporadic WT carry *WT1* mutations.[10,11]

---

**KEY POINTS**

Overgrowth syndromes are associated with increased risk for WT, which include:
- Beckwith-Wiedemann syndrome
- Isolated hemihypertrophy
- Perlman syndrome (facial gigantism, renal dysplasia, islet hypertrophy, mental retardation, and WT)
- Sotos syndrome (cerebral gigantism)

---

A second WT predisposing gene *(WT2)* has been identified on chromosome 11p15.[12] This locus has been proposed based on studies of patients with both WT and Beckwith-Wiedemann syndrome (BWS). BWS is an overgrowth syndrome characterized by high birth weight, macroglossia, organomegaly, hemihypertrophy, neonatal hypoglycemia, abdominal wall defects, and ear pits and creases. Patients with BWS have a 5% to 10% risk for development of WT but are also predisposed to other malignant tumors, such as hepatoblastoma, neuroblastoma, and rhabdomyosarcoma.[13] Finally, mutations in the *p53* gene are observed in most cases of anaplastic histologic features of WT, implicating a role for this gene in progression from favorable to anaplastic histologic type.[14] Diverse genetic disorders that may be associated with an increased risk for WT are listed in Table 50.2.

## PATHOLOGY

Wilms tumors can be variable in size, and margins are usually well circumscribed that separate it from normal kidney. Cut surface usually appears tan and may be lobulated (Figure 50.1).

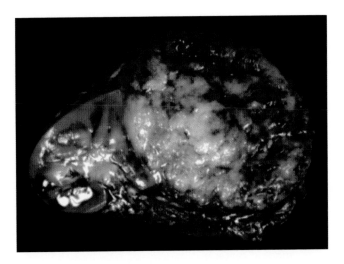

Figure 50.1 Cut section of the kidney showing Wilms tumor affecting the lower pole of the kidney. Tumor is well demarcated and shows tan-brown cut surface with a few hemorrhages.

Hemorrhages may be present in the tumor mass. The classic histologic pattern (Figure 50.2) is composed of epithelial, blastemal, and stromal elements (triphasic). Approximately 90% of all renal tumors have favorable histologic findings. Up to 7% of WTs have unfavorable histologic features, which are characterized by diffuse anaplastic changes, a feature that predicts poor outcome. Anaplasia is defined as cells with nuclei having a diameter greater than normal, with increased nuclear

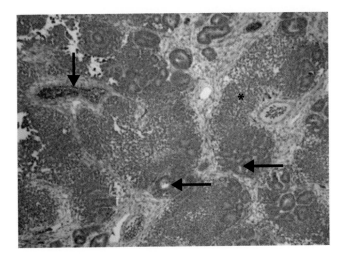

Figure 50.2 Light microscopy of Wilms tumor showing the classic or triphasic microscopic findings. Three elements of the tumor pathologic tissue (triphasic) consist of densely packed tumor cells with scant cytoplasm and large nuclei (asterisk), mesenchymal stroma consisting of fibroblast-like structures, and epithelial elements forming primitive renal tubules within islands of tumor cells (arrows). Primitive glomeruli may be in seen in some cases. Several primitive blood vessels are seen within the tumor in this patient (arrow head).

content or polyploid mitosis. Finally, clear cell sarcoma of the kidney and rhabdoid tumor of the kidney previously included in the WT category of unfavorable histologic findings are in fact clearly separate malignant entities.

Nephrogenic rests (NRs) are foci of embryonal kidney cells that persist abnormally into postnatal life. Histologically, these structures are similar to those of WT. They are present in approximately 1% of newborn kidneys and usually regress or differentiate by early childhood.[15] Because NRs are present in the kidneys of approximately 40% of patients with WT, it is presumed that the rests represent WT precursors.[16] *Nephroblastomatosis* is the diffuse or multifocal presence of nephrogenic rests.[17] NRs are subdivided as *intralobar* (ILNR) and *perilobar* (PLNR) according to their position in the renal lobe.[15] ILNRs are less common and are associated with WT syndromes discovered earlier in life (e.g., WAGR, Drash syndrome). PLNRs are associated with bilateral tumors and syndromes that present later (e.g., BWS and hemihypertrophy).

## CLINICAL PRESENTATION

The vast majority of patients with WT present with an asymptomatic palpable abdominal mass. They also may present with abdominal pain, gross hematuria, hepatomegaly, varicocele, or lower extremity edema. Hypertension may result from either renal tissue compression by the tumor leading to renal ischemia (known as Page kidney) or by renin production by the tumor itself.[18] A small number of patients who have bleeding into their tumor may present with signs of hypotension, anemia, and fever. Rarely, patients with advanced-stage disease may present with respiratory symptoms related to the presence of lung metastases. More recently, WT has been diagnosed in utero with fetal ultrasonography.[19]

Every child should have a complete physical examination. Because of the concerns of rupture of the tumor capsule and local spread, care should be exercised not to palpate the tumor repeatedly or deeply. High-risk patients, such as those with syndromes or isolated physical findings having a high association with WT (aniridia, hemihypertrophy, BWS, WAGR syndrome), require regular, periodic screening by renal ultrasound to ensure that any asymptomatic tumor is identified before it becomes clinically manifested, and to provide the opportunity for nephron-sparing surgery.[20] Laboratory evaluation should include complete blood cell count, chemistry profile including renal function tests, routine electrolytes with calcium, urinalysis, and coagulation studies. Radiologic studies form an essential part of initial diagnostic evaluation, and are discussed below.

## EVALUATION

Radiographic imaging is performed to evaluate the dimensions and location of the abdominal mass, to characterize

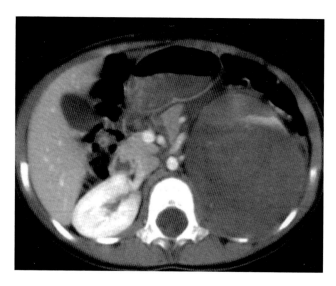

Figure 50.3 Computerized axial tomography showing a large Wilms tumor in the left kidney.

Table 50.3 Surveillance recommendations for patients at high risk for developing Wilms tumor

- Surveillance should be offered to children at greater than 5% risk for Wilms tumor.
- Surveillance should be offered only after review by a clinical geneticist.
- Surveillance should be carried out by renal ultrasonography every 3 to 4 months.
- Surveillance should continue until 5 years in all conditions except Beckwith-Wiedemann syndrome, Simpson-Golabi-Behmel syndrome, and some familial Wilms tumor pedigrees, in which it should continue until age 7 years.
- Surveillance can be undertaken at a local medical center with experience in pediatric ultrasonography.
- Screen-detected lesions should be managed at a tertiary care specialized center.

*Source:* Modified from RH, Walker L, Olsen/E, et al. Surveillance for Wilms tumour in at-risk children: pragmatic recommendations for best practice. Arch Dis Child. 2006;91:995–9. Reproduced with permission.

tumor origin, determine local extension, evaluate the contralateral kidney, and determine venous involvement of the malignancy. Renal ultrasonography (US) with Doppler technique is usually employed initially, because it can confirm the location as well as the nature of the tumor (cystic vs. solid). US also can provide good dynamic imaging of the renal vein and inferior vena cava. Abdominal computerized tomography (CT) and occasionally magnetic resonance imaging (MRI) can provide additional delineation data on the tumor's origin and extension, lymph node involvement, bilateral kidney involvement, invasion into major vessels, or liver metastases (Figure 50.3). Newly improved and efficient three-dimensional volume-rendering software is now available for visual reconstruction of tumor anatomy.[21] Chest radiographs, chest CT scan, or both should be obtained to evaluate the chest and identify any pulmonary metastases, which, if present, upstages the patient and hence the treatment.[22] Patients with conditions that have increased risk for WT should undergo periodic surveillance by renal US. Suggested guidelines for surveillance are given in Table 50.3.

## STAGING

The staging of WT is critical to determining therapy and prognosis. The most widely accepted system in North America is the one developed by the National Wilms' Tumor Study Group (NWTSG) and extended by the Children's Oncology Group (COG). The NWTSG/COG approach allows pathologic and surgical staging to predict tumor behavior and tailor subsequent adjuvant therapy. Consequently, in North America, most patients with suspected WT undergo nephrectomy with lymphadenectomy immediately. Exceptions include patients with bilateral renal tumors, neoplasms in a solitary kidney, and the presence of tumor thrombus extending above the level of

the hepatic veins, situations that are managed with initial chemotherapy. The NWTS-V staging of WT is shown in Table 50.4. The NWTSG has further classified WT patients into low-risk and high-risk patients according to the presence of favorable versus unfavorable histologic findings based on the postnephrectomy histology.

## TREATMENT APPROACHES

The approach to a patient with WT varies in Europe, compared to the North American approach.[23] Although most Societe Internationale D'oncologie Pediatrique (SIOP) centers make a presumptive diagnosis of WT based on imaging studies alone, in the United Kingdom, a needle biopsy may be performed to avoid misdiagnosis and to ascertain histology. The SIOP centers administer prenephrectomy chemotherapy, realizing that there may be as much as a 5% misdiagnosis rate and hence incorrect treatment. Over the past 30 years, these centers have shown that preoperative therapy decreases the incidence of tumor rupture during surgery.[24,25] Chemotherapy also downstages the tumor and in cases of metastases decreases the need for postoperative radiotherapy. Chemotherapy may shrink the tumor and eliminate overt signs of tumor spread. Chemotherapy clearly affects the final staging process and thus can sometimes confuse interpretation of results with the North American data. Despite the differences in approaches on either side of the Atlantic, both produce equally high rates of overall treatment success. Hence, there is no obvious better approach and both philosophies gain knowledge from one another synergistically. Nephrectomy, via a transperitoneal approach, is the initial

Table 50.4 National Wilms Tumor Study clinicopathologic staging of Wilms tumor

| Stage | Clinicopathologic staging |
|---|---|
| 1 | Tumor limited to kidney and completely excised. No penetration of the renal capsule or involvement of renal sinus vessels. |
| 2 | Tumor extends beyond the kidney but is completely excised with negative margins and lymph nodes. At least one of the following has occurred: penetration of the renal capsule, invasion of the renal sinus vessels, biopsy of the tumor before removal (except for fine needle aspirate, which may qualify as stage 1), or spillage of tumor locally during removal. |
| 3 | Gross or microscopic residual tumor remains postoperatively (including inoperable tumor, positive surgical margins, diffuse tumor spillage involving peritoneal surfaces, regional lymph not metastasis, or transected tumor thrombus. |
| 4 | Hematogenous metastasis or lymph node metastasis outside the abdominal or pelvic cavities. |
| 5 | Bilateral renal tumors at diagnosis. |

*Source:* Neville HL, Ritchey ML: Wilms' tumor: overview of National Wilms' Tumor Study Group results. Urol Clin North Am. 2000;27:435–42. Reproduced with permission.

treatment for unilateral disease if the mass can be completely resected. This is usually done via a chevron incision.

Current recommendations are to administer preoperative chemotherapy only to children with bilateral disease and those with inoperable tumor at presentation, intravascular tumor extension above the hepatic veins, and a tumor involving a solitary kidney. Pretreatment dramatically reduces tumor thrombus for patients with caval extension and tumor burden, which will substantially reduce the surgical morbidity.[26–28] Patients with bilateral disease, solitary kidney, or renal insufficiency or abnormalities of the non-involved kidney should be considered for a renal-sparing protocol, if at all possible.[29]

Partial nephrectomy of unilateral WT has been explored by some investigators to avoid late occurrence of renal dysfunction and the risk for metachronous WT.[30,31] They argue that nephrectomy for unilateral WT increases the risk for hypertension, proteinuria, glomerulosclerosis, and renal insufficiency owing to injuries from hyperfiltration and adjunctive chemotherapy or radiotherapy.[32–34] Most WTs are too large for a partial nephrectomy at initial presentation; therefore, preoperative chemotherapy is usually necessary if renal-sparing surgery is to be considered.

Current protocols do allow for flank approaches to the tumor, but the role of laparoscopy is being debated.[35] Whereas in the past, contralateral exploration was mandatory, modern imaging, which is able to uncover the smallest of contralateral tumors, and with the knowledge that the majority of these patients will receive adjuvant therapy that will likely have an impact on nonvisible lesions, this practice is no longer necessary.[36] In North America, however, lymph node sampling is mandatory, and, if it is not done, patients are automatically upstaged to stage 3, with the inherent need for more aggressive chemotherapy. In those with presumed bilateral disease, the current practice is to administer up-front chemotherapy without initial surgical exploration or biopsy. Of note is that in North America, just as when lymph nodes are not submitted for pathologic examination, any biopsy mandates upstaging to a stage 3.[37]

The major complications of surgical therapy have continued to decrease. A recent review of the records of patients in NWTS-IV found an 11% incidence of surgical complications after nephrectomy.[38] The most common complications were hemorrhage and small bowel obstruction. Risk factors associated with increased surgical complications are higher local tumor stage, intravascular extension, *en bloc* resection of other visceral organs, and incorrect preoperative diagnosis.[39]

---

**KEY POINTS**

- European data suggest that presurgical chemotherapy may shrink the tumor and decrease the likelihood of tumor rupture during surgery.
- With modern imaging techniques, exploration or biopsy of the contralateral kidney is not necessary.
- Lymph node sampling during surgery provides important information for staging. Omission of this surgical step can adversely affect treatment decisions.

---

## TREATMENT OF NEPHROGENIC REST TUMOR

Surgical management becomes more controversial in the case of unilateral or bilateral multiple NRs, as seen in patients with nephroblastomatosis. The histologic appearance may be indistinguishable from that of WT. Thus, the growth pattern of the lesion as seen on serial imaging may be the best indication of the need for a nephrectomy. Accordingly, serial imaging is important in planning the appropriate intervention and avoiding unnecessary surgery. However, in children presenting with diffuse hyperplastic PLNR, seen as a ring surrounding the entire kidney, surgery should be considered because of the high risk for WT. Most of these cases will manifest with bilateral disease, and partial nephrectomy after chemotherapy is a consideration.

## POSTSURGICAL MANAGEMENT

Consecutive trials of the NWTSG, beginning in the late 1960s, provided critical insights into the role of adjuvant therapy for WT. The intergroup studies sought to refine adjuvant therapy regimens, with each study intensifying the therapy provided to high-risk patients and decreasing or modifying the therapy to lower risk patients.[40] NWTSG-I and NWTSG-II revealed that postoperative radiation was unnecessary in stage 1 disease and that the combined use of vincristine and dactinomycin was more efficacious than either drug alone. NWTSG-III showed that patients with stage 2 tumors with favorable histologic findings can be treated without abdominal irradiation if vincristine and dactinomycin are administered. This study also revealed that the addition of doxorubicin to the two-drug regimen improves outcome in stage 3 and 4 disease with favorable histologic findings. The remainder of the study focused on postoperative radiation treatment.

The last of the NWTSGs showed that pulse-intensive therapy is equally efficacious, less toxic, and more cost-effective than the conventional regimen, with overall 4-year survival rates of patients with favorable histologic findings approaching 90%.[41] The ongoing NWTSG-V was designed to find possible roles of gene expression in identifying patients at greater risk for relapse.[40] The role of adjuvant chemotherapy in providing benefit to children younger than 24 months who have small stage 1 tumors with favorable histologic features is being explored in this protocol. The current treatment algorithm of WT based on its stage and histology is shown in Table 50.5.

---

### KEY POINTS

- WT is sensitive to chemotherapy and radiotherapy.
- Postoperative radiotherapy is not routinely recommended in stage 1 and 2 disease.
- Combined chemotherapy with vincristine and dactinomycin is more efficacious than either drug alone.

---

## BILATERAL WILMS TUMOR

Bilateral WT occurs in approximately 5% to 10% of patients with WT. These children pose a therapeutic challenge because of difficulty in obtaining local control while sparing renal parenchyma. Compared to patients with unilateral WT, patients with bilateral tumors have an increased rate of renal failure, estimated to be 3.8% among patients treated in the NWTSG-IV.[42] The most common cause of renal failure in this patient group is need for nephrectomy because of tumor progression or recurrence, and not therapy-related effects.

In a child with bilateral WT, as noted previously, performing biopsies on both kidneys is no longer mandated. If tumor is identified in both kidneys, patients should be given preoperative chemotherapy that is appropriate for the tumor stage and histology. After 6 weeks of chemotherapy, the patient should be reassessed with abdominal CT to determine the feasibility of resection. If the tumor size has decreased, partial nephrectomy may be performed. If persistent tumor is discovered, additional chemotherapy, in addition to radiation is appropriate. Definitive surgery should not be delayed beyond 12 weeks after initiation of chemotherapy. Patients undergoing initial biopsy followed by postoperative chemotherapy had survival equivalent (83% at 2 years) to that of patients undergoing initial surgical resection.[43] Rarely, bilateral nephrectomies are necessary, and a mandatory waiting period of 2 years should be considered before kidney transplantation in such cases.

## RECURRENT WILMS TUMOR

With refinement of treatment modalities the cure rate for WT is in excess of 85%.[44] However, 10% to 15% of patients with favorable histologic findings, as well as 50% of patients with anaplastic tumors, experience primary progression or tumor recurrence. Most relapses are diagnosed within the first 2 years after the original diagnosis. The most common sites of recurrence are the lung, tumor bed, liver, bone, and lymph nodes. Approximately 1% of children presenting initially with unilateral WT develop metachronous bilateral disease.[31] Patients with NRs (particularly PLNRs) and especially those children who were younger than 12 months at diagnosis have a statistically significant increased risk for developing a contralateral tumor. As a result, some authors recommended more frequent surveillance for this group of patients.[31]

With aggressive therapy, up to 80% of patients with favorable prognostic features can be cured. Factors associated with favorable prognosis after recurrence include favorable histologic features, initial treatment with only vincristine and dactinomycin, relapse to the lungs only, relapse in the abdomen of a patient who did not receive abdominal irradiation, and relapse more than 12 months after the original diagnosis.[45,46]

---

### KEY POINTS

- Recurrence rate of WT in the contralateral kidney is low (1%).
- Most recurrences occur within 2 years of the initial diagnosis.
- Common sites of recurrences are lungs, tumor bed, and liver.

Table 50.5 Treatment protocol for Wilms Tumor: National Wilms Tumor Study—V

| Stage, histology | Surgery | Chemotherapy | Radiotherapy* |
|---|---|---|---|
| Stage 1 or 2 with FH<br>Stage 1 with anaplasia | Nephrectomy | Dactinomycin<br>Vincristine (18 wk) | No |
| Stage 3 or 4 with FH<br>Stage 2–4 with focal anaplasia | Nephrectomy | Dactinomycin<br>Doxorubicin<br>Vincristine (24 wk) | Yes |
| Stage 2–4 with diffuse anaplasia<br>Stage 1–4 CCSK | Nephrectomy | Vincristine<br>Doxorubicin<br>Cyclophosphamide<br>Etoposide (24 wk) | Yes |
| Stage I–4 RTK | Nephrectomy | Cyclophosphamide<br>Carboplatin Etoposide (24 wk) | Yes |

*Source:* Modified from: Neville HL, Ritchey ML. Wilms' tumor: overview of National Wilms' Tumor Study Group results. Urol Clin North Am. 2000;27:435–42. Reproduced by permission.

*Abbreviations:* FH, favorable history; CCSK, clear cell sarcoma of kidney; RTK, rhabdoid tumor of kidney.

* Current radiotherapy dosage is approximately 1080 cGy for the abdomen and 1200 cGy for the lung. Only patients with stage 4 with lung metastases receive whole lung radiotherapy

To improve the outcomes, many different chemotherapy regimens have been attempted. These include salvage chemotherapy with ifosfamide, platinum, and etoposide, with a response rate up to 72%.[46,47] In addition, some patients have been treated with high-dose chemotherapy followed by autologous hematopoietic stem-cell rescue.[48]

## LATE EFFECTS OF TREATMENT

Numerous organ systems can be affected by the late sequelae of anticancer therapy. The late effects of WT treatment have received considerable attention because WT usually is curable, with an increasing number of long-term survivors. Renal function can be affected by several modalities of treatment, including nephrectomy, chemotherapy (especially the one used to treat recurrent disease), and radiation. Although most WT survivors have only one kidney, only 0.25% of patients were found to have end-stage renal disease (ESRD).[42] The median interval from diagnosis to onset of ESRD was 21 months. Renal failure is most prevalent in patients with bilateral WT.

Another recognized long-term effect of WT therapy is congestive heart failure (CHF), which was found to have a cumulative frequency of 4.4% 20 years after diagnosis of WT in patients initially treated with doxorubicin.[49] Risk factors for CHF included increasing cumulative doxorubicin dose and radiation to the lung and left hemiabdomen. An analysis of pregnancy outcome among WT survivors revealed that women who received flank radiation therapy were at increased risk for fetal malposition, premature labor, low birth weight, and occurrence of congenital malformations.[50] Gonadal irradiation can produce hypogonadism and temporary azoospermia in boys.[51] In females, the main therapeutic modality shown to cause ovarian dysfunction is radiation.[52] Finally, the cumulative incidence of second malignancy in WT survivors was 1.6% 15 years after diagnosis of primary tumor.[53]

## CLEAR CELL SARCOMA

Clear cell sarcoma of the kidney (CCSK) is now considered a separate tumor, distinct from WT. The peak incidence is between 3 and 5 years of age. Unlike WT, CCSK is associated with bone and brain metastases in 40% to 60% cases. Bilateral involvement thus far has not been reported, nor has the presence of congenital anomalies associated with WT been noted. The classic histologic pattern consists of a cellular lesion of polygonal cells with round or oval nuclei having a delicate chromatin pattern and indistinct nucleoli.[54] NWTSG-V recommends treating CCSK at all stages with the same regimen used for WT with diffuse anaplasia (excluding stage 1). Expected 4-year survival is 75%.[55] Important predictors of improved survival are lower stage, younger age at diagnosis, and absence of tumor necrosis.[56]

## RHABDOID TUMOR OF KIDNEY

Rhabdoid tumor of the kidney (RTK) is another tumor that was formerly categorized as an unfavorable histologic pattern of WT. It accounts for 2% of the renal tumors in the NWTSG database.[57] RKT is characterized by large cells with abundant acidophilic cytoplasm, frequently with a discrete zone of pale eosinophilia, which is made of fibrillary inclusion bodies. Nuclei are large with very prominent nucleoli.

The tumor is typically large, often replacing the entire kidney. It manifests early in life (median age 11 months), with more than 50% of patients younger than 1 year of age. Metastases may be found not only in the lungs and liver, but also in the brain (unlike WT).[58] In addition, RTK can be associated with second primary tumors in the brain (10% to 15%), the most common being medulloblastoma.[59] RTK is the most aggressive and lethal childhood renal tumor, with an overall mortality of 80%.[58] The current treatment protocol consists of nephrectomy, followed by chemotherapy

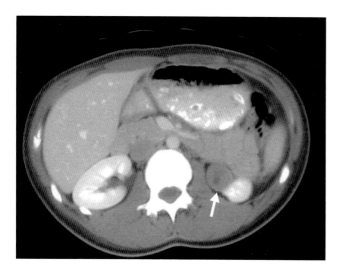

Figure 50.4. Computerized axial tomography showing a renal cell carcinoma in the left kidney.

with carboplatinum, etoposide, and cyclophosphamide for 24 weeks, along with radiotherapy.

## RENAL CELL CARCINOMA

Renal cell carcinoma (RCC) is an uncommon renal epithelial malignant tumor in children. It represents 2% to 5% of primary renal malignant tumors of childhood (Figures 50.4 to 50.6).[60] Childhood RCC may resemble the adult clear cell and papillary subtypes.[61] RCC has been reported in infancy, but most patients are older, with a mean age of 9 to 15 years. Most children present with abdominal mass (24% to 55%), hematuria (42%), and pain (32%). Children also may have hypertension, fever, weight loss, and polycythemia.[62] Approximately 25% of children with RCC have distant metastatic disease at presentation, most commonly to the lung, liver, and bone. Imaging studies cannot differentiate

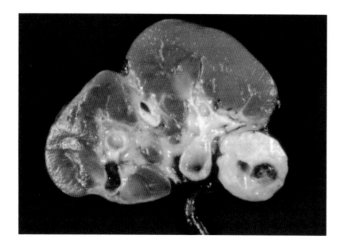

Figure 50.5 Cut section of the kidney showing well-circumscribed renal cell carcinoma with fatty yellow coloration of the tumor.

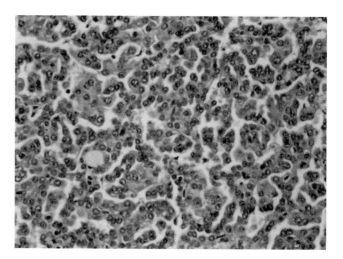

Figure 50.6 Light microscopy of renal cell carcinoma showing tumor cells arranged in nests, with small nuclei and clear cytoplasm.

RCC from other renal tumors. (Figure 50.4). Renal cell carcinomas are usually smaller than Wilms tumor in size, but may be large in some (Figure 50.5). Histologic examination shows tumor cells with small nuclei and clear cytoplasm arranged in nests (Figure 50.6).

The most significant prognostic variable for survival of pediatric patients with RCC is accomplishing a complete resection and histologically low-stage disease.[63] Survival for patients presenting with stage 1 disease is greater than 90%, approximately 50% for patients with stage 2 and 3 disease and almost 0% for patients with stage 4 disease.[64] The tumor is not responsive to radiotherapy, and there is no effective chemotherapy for nonlocalized or relapsed disease.

## CONGENITAL MESOBLASTIC NEPHROMA

Congenital mesoblastic nephroma (CMN) is the most common renal tumor in infants, with a mean age at diagnosis of 3.5 months.[65] CMN occurs in two forms: the typical, or fibromatous, type is seen almost exclusively in infants under 3 months of age and is benign. The second one, or atypical (cellular) variety, is usually seen in older children but also occurs in infants. The latter type is potentially malignant and capable of recurrence and metastasis.[66,67] Hypertension may occur from renin hypersecretion.[68] Hypercalcemia also has been reported, owing to tumor secretion of prostaglandin.[66] Nephrectomy alone is an adequate treatment option for infants younger than 3 months of age and perhaps even in older patients with typical fibrous histologic findings and complete tumor resection. Chemotherapy with a WT regimen should be considered for patients with incomplete resection, cellular features, or a high mitotic index and certainly for any patient with evidence of metastasis or recurrence. Partial nephrectomy should not be performed because the risk for local recurrence is high owing to the tumor's tendency to infiltrate surrounding renal parenchyma.

# ANGIOMYOLIPOMA

Angiomyolipoma is a benign hamartoma-like mass composed of smooth muscle, blood vessels, and fat. This lesion is seen almost exclusively in children with tuberous sclerosis, which is characterized by mental retardation, seizures, glial nodules in the brain, adenoma sebaceum, phakoma of the retina, and hamartomas of the liver, heart, bone, or kidney. It is estimated that 80% of patients with tuberous sclerosis complex have angiomyolipomas and that the frequency increases with age.[69] Tumors are frequently bilateral and multifocal. Females appear to be more susceptible to multiple and larger tumors than males.[70] Hormonal influences (progesterone receptors in the smooth muscle cells of angiomyolipomas) may offer an explanation to the gender differences in tumor growth at puberty.

Most angiomyolipomas less than 4 cm do not pose a clinical concern. Larger tumors are at risk for hemorrhage.[71] Management should be nonoperative, with periodic reimaging for small asymptomatic lesions. Nephron-sparing approaches are recommended for children with large or symptomatic tumors. Angioinfarction of amenable lesions or partial nephrectomy should be considered.

## SUMMARY

Renal tumors in children are rare. Advances in management have been the result of cooperative studies enrolling patients from different centers. This strategy is bound to be the basis for future improvements in diagnosis and therapy. The introduction of nephron-sparing procedures and minimally invasive surgery is expected to change current surgical management. Long-term complications from surgery, chemotherapy, and radiation need to be addressed as survivors grow into adulthood.

## REFERENCES

1. Miller RW, Young JL, Jr., Novakovic B. Childhood cancer. Cancer. 1995;75(Suppl 1):395–405.
2. Hentrich MU, Meister P, Brack NG, et al. Adult Wilms' tumor: Report of two cases and review of the literature. Cancer. 1995;75:545–51.
3. Breslow NE, Olson J, Moksness J, et al. Familial Wilms' tumor: A descriptive study. Med Pediatr Oncol. 1996;27:398–403.
4. Breslow NE, Beckwith JB. Epidemiological features of Wilms' tumor: Results of the National Wilms' Tumor Study. J Natl Cancer Inst. 1982;68:429–36.
5. Knudson AG, Jr., Strong C. Mutation and cancer: A model for Wilms' tumor of the kidney. J Natl Cancer Inst. 1972;48:313–24.
6. Koufos A, Hansen MF, Lampkin BC, et al. Loss of alleles at loci on human chromosome 11 during genesis of Wilms' tumour. Nature. 1984;309:170–2.
7. Ton CC, Hirvonen H, Miwa H, et al. Positional cloning and characterization of a paired box- and homeobox-containing gene from the aniridia region. Cell. 1991;67:1059–74.
8. Call KM, Glaser T, Ito CY, et al. Isolation and characterization of a zinc finger polypeptide gene at the human chromosome 11 Wilms' tumor locus. Cell. 1990;60:509–20.
9. Coppes MJ, Haber DA, Grundy PE. Genetic events in the development of Wilms' tumor. N Engl J Med. 1994;331:586–90.
10. Gessler M, Konig A, Arden K, et al. Infrequent mutation of the WT1 gene in 77 Wilms' tumors. Hum Mutat. 1994;3:212–22.
11. Diller L, Ghahremani M, Morgan J, et al. Constitutional WT1 mutations in Wilms' tumor patients. J Clin Oncol. 1998;16:3634–40.
12. Mannens M, Slater RM, Heyting C, et al. Molecular nature of genetic changes resulting in loss of heterozygosity of chromosome 11 in Wilms' tumours. Hum Genet. 1988;81:41–8.
13. DeBaun MR, Tucker MA. Risk of cancer during the first four years of life in children from the Beckwith-Wiedemann Syndrome Registry. J Pediatr. 1998;132:398–400.
14. Bardeesy N, Falkoff D, Petruzzi MJ, et al. Anaplastic Wilms' tumour, a subtype displaying poor prognosis, harbours p53 gene mutations. Nat Genet. 1994;7:91–7.
15. Beckwith JB, Kiviat NB, Bonadio JF. Nephrogenic rests, nephroblastomatosis, and the pathogenesis of Wilms' tumor. Pediatr Pathol. 1990;10:1–36.
16. Bove KE, McAdams AJ. The nephroblastomatosis complex and its relationship to Wilms' tumor: A clinicopathologic treatise. Perspect Pediatr Pathol. 1976;3:185–223.
17. Beckwith JB. Precursor lesions of Wilms tumor: Clinical and biological implications. Med Pediatr Oncol. 1993;21:158–68.
18. Ganguly A, Gribble J, Tune B, et al. Renin-secreting Wilms' tumor with severe hypertension: Report of a case and brief review of renin-secreting tumors. Ann Intern Med. 1973;79:835–7.
19. Suresh I, Suresh S, Arumugam R, et al. Antenatal diagnosis of Wilms tumor. J Ultrasound Med. 1997;16:69–72.
20. Romão RL, Pippi SJL, Shuman C, et al. Nephron sparing surgery for unilateral Wilms tumor in children with predisposing syndromes: Single center experience over 10 years. J Urol. 2012;188(Suppl 4):1493–8.
21. Gunther P, Schenk JP, Wunsch R, et al. Abdominal tumours in children: 3-D visualisation and surgical planning. Eur J Pediatr Surg. 2004;14:316–21.

22. Wootton-Gorges SL, Albano EA, et al. Chest radiography versus chest CT in the evaluation for pulmonary metastases in patients with Wilms' tumor: A retrospective review. Pediatr Radiol. 2000;30:533–7; discussion 537–9.

23. D'Angio GJ. Pre- or post-operative treatment for Wilms tumor? Who, what, when, where, how, why— And which. Med Pediatr Oncol. 2003;41:545–9.

24. D'Angio GJ. Pre- or postoperative therapy for Wilms' tumor? J Clin Oncol. 2008;26:4055–7.

25. Powis M, Messahel B, Hobson R, et al. Surgical complications after immediate nephrectomy versus preoperative chemotherapy in non-metastatic Wilms' tumour: Findings from the 1991-2001. United Kingdom Children's Cancer Study Group UKW3 Trial. Pediatr Surg. 2013;48:2181–6.

26. Montgomery BT, Kelalis PP, Blute ML, et al. Extended followup of bilateral Wilms tumor: Results of the National Wilms Tumor Study. J Urol. 1991;146:514–8.

27. Ritchey ML, Pringle KC, Breslow NE, et al. Management and outcome of inoperable Wilms tumor: A report of National Wilms Tumor Study 3. Ann Surg. 1994;220:683–90.

28. Ritchey ML, Kelalis PP, Haase GM, et al. Preoperative therapy for intracaval and atrial extension of Wilms tumor. Cancer. 1993;71:4104–10.

29. Horwitz JR, Ritchey ML, Moksness J, et al. Renal salvage procedures in patients with synchronous bilateral Wilms' tumors: A report from the National Wilms' Tumor Study Group. J Pediatr Surg. 1996;31:1020–5.

30. Moorman-Voestermans CG, Aronson DC, Staalman CR, et al. Is partial nephrectomy appropriate treatment for unilateral Wilms' tumor? J Pediatr Surg. 1998;33:165–70.

31. Coppes MJ, Arnold M, Beckwith JB, et al. Factors affecting the risk of contralateral Wilms tumor development: A report from the National Wilms Tumor Study Group. Cancer. 1999;85:1616–25.

32. Welch TR, McAdams AJ. Focal glomerulosclerosis as a late sequela of Wilms tumor. J Pediatr. 1986;108:105–9.

33. Di Tullio MT, Casale F, Indolfi P, et al. Compensatory hypertrophy and progressive renal damage in children nephrectomized for Wilms' tumor. Med Pediatr Oncol. 1996;26:325–8.

34. Smith GR, Thomas PR, Ritchey M, et al. Long-term renal function in patients with irradiated bilateral Wilms tumor. National Wilms' Tumor Study Group. Am J Clin Oncol. 1998;21:58–63.

35. Romao RL, Weber B, Gerstle JT, et al. Comparison between laparoscopic and open radical nephrectomy for the treatment of primary renal tumors in children: Single-center experience over a 5-year period. J Pediatr Urol. 2014;10:488–94.

36. Koo AS, Koyle MA, Hurwitz RS, et al. The necessity of contralateral surgical exploration in Wilms tumor with modern noninvasive imaging technique: A reassessment. J Urol. 1990;144:416–7; discussion 422.

37. Martin LW, Reyes PM, Jr. An evaluation of 10 years' experience with retroperitoneal lymph node dissection for Wilms' tumor. J Pediatr Surg. 1969;4:683–7.

38. Ritchey ML, Shamberger RC, Haase G, et al. Surgical complications after primary nephrectomy for Wilms' tumor: Report from the National Wilms' Tumor Study Group. J Am Coll Surg. 2001;192:63–8.

39. Ritchey ML, Kelalis PP, Breslow N, et al. Surgical complications after nephrectomy for Wilms' tumor. Surg Gynecol Obstet. 1992;175:507–14.

40. Neville HL, Ritchey ML. Wilms' tumor: Overview of National Wilms' Tumor Study Group results. Urol Clin North Am. 2000;27:435–42.

41. Green DM, Breslow NE, Evans I, et al. Relationship between dose schedule and charges for treatment on National Wilms' Tumor Study-4: A report from the National Wilms' Tumor Study Group. J Natl Cancer Inst Monogr. 1995;21–5.

42. Ritchey ML, Green DM, Thomas PR, et al. Renal failure in Wilms' tumor patients: A report from the National Wilms' Tumor Study Group. Med Pediatr Oncol. 1996;26:75–80.

43. Blute ML, Kelalis PP, Offord KP, et al. GJ, Bilateral Wilms tumor. J Urol. 1987;138:968–73.

44. Green DM, Thomas PR, Shochat S. The treatment of Wilms tumor: Results of the National Wilms Tumor Studies. Hematol Oncol Clin North Am. 1995;9:1267–74.

45. Grundy P, Breslow N, Green DM, et al. Prognostic factors for children with recurrent Wilms' tumor: Results from the Second and Third National Wilms' Tumor Study. J Clin Oncol. 1989;7:638–47.

46. Dome JS, Liu T, Krasin M, et al. Improved survival for patients with recurrent Wilms tumor: The experience at St. Jude Children's Research Hospital. J Pediatr Hematol Oncol. 2002;24:192–8.

47. Abu-Ghosh AM, Krailo MD, Goldman SC, et al. Ifosfamide, carboplatin and etoposide in children with poor-risk relapsed Wilms' tumor: A Children's Cancer Group report. Ann Oncol. 2002;13:460–9.

48. Pein F, Michon J, Valteau-Couanet D, et al. High-dose melphalan, etoposide, and carboplatin followed by autologous stem-cell rescue in pediatric high-risk recurrent Wilms' tumor: A French Society of Pediatric Oncology study. J Clin Oncol. 1998;16:3295–301.

49. Green DM, Grigoriev YA, Nan B, et al. Congestive heart failure after treatment for Wilms' tumor: A report from the National Wilms' Tumor Study group. J Clin Oncol. 2001;19:1926–34.

50. Green DM, Peabody EM, Nan B, et al. Pregnancy outcome after treatment for Wilms tumor: A report from the National Wilms Tumor Study Group. J Clin Oncol. 2002;20:2506–13.

51. Kinsella TJ, Trivette G, Rowland J, et al. Long-term follow-up of testicular function following radiation therapy for early-stage Hodgkin's disease. J Clin Oncol 1989;7:718–24.

52. Stillman RJ, Schinfeld JS, Schiff I, et al. Ovarian failure in long-term survivors of childhood malignancy. Am J Obstet Gynecol. 1981;139:62–6.

53. Breslow NE, Takashima JR, Whitton JA, et al. Second malignant neoplasms following treatment for Wilm's tumor: A report from the National Wilms' Tumor Study Group. J Clin Oncol. 1995;13:1851–9.

54. Schmidt D, Beckwith JB. Histopathology of childhood renal tumors. Hematol Oncol Clin North Am. 1995;9:1179–200.

55. D'Angio GJ, Breslow N, Beckwith JB, et al. Treatment of Wilms' tumor: Results of the Third National Wilms' Tumor Study. Cancer. 1989;64:349–60.

56. Argani P, Perlman EJ, Breslow NE, et al. Clear cell sarcoma of the kidney: A review of 351 cases from the National Wilms Tumor Study Group Pathology Center. Am J Surg Pathol. 2000;24:4–18.

57. Tomlinson GE, Breslow NE, Dome J, et al. Rhabdoid tumor of the kidney in the National Wilms' Tumor Study: Age at diagnosis as a prognostic factor. J Clin Oncol. 2005;23:7641–5.

58. Weeks DA, Beckwith JB, Mierau GW, et al. Rhabdoid tumor of kidney: A report of 111 cases from the National Wilms' Tumor Study Pathology Center. Am J Surg Pathol. 1989;13:439–58.

59. Malik R. Rhabdoid tumor of the kidney. Med Pediatr Oncol. 1988;16:203–5.

60. Eckschlager T, Kodet R. Renal cell carcinoma in children: A single institution's experience. Med Pediatr Oncol. 1994;23:36–9.

61. Renshaw AA, Granter SR, Fletcher JA, et al. Renal cell carcinomas in children and young adults: Increased incidence of papillary architecture and unique subtypes. Am J Surg Pathol. 1999;23:795–802.

62. Carcao MD, Taylor GP, Greenberg ML, et al. Renal-cell carcinoma in children: A different disorder from its adult counterpart? Med Pediatr Oncol. 1998;31:153–8.

63. Aronson DC, Medary I, Finlay JL, et al. Renal cell carcinoma in childhood and adolescence: A retrospective survey for prognostic factors in 22 cases. J Pediatr Surg. 1996;31:183–6.

64. Indolfi P, Spreafico F, Collini P, et al. Metastatic renal cell carcinoma in children and adolescents: A 30-year unsuccessful story. J Pediatr Hematol Oncol; 2012;34:e277–81.

65. Howell CG, Othersen HB, Kiviat NE, et al. Therapy and outcome in 51 children with mesoblastic nephroma: A report of the National Wilms' Tumor Study. J Pediatr Surg. 1982;17:826–31.

66. Shen SC, Yunis EJ. A study of the cellularity and ultrastructure of congenital mesoblastic nephroma. Cancer. 1980;45:306–14.

67. Vujanic GM, Delemarre JF, Moeslichan S, et al. Mesoblastic nephroma metastatic to the lungs and heart: Another face of this peculiar lesion—Case report and review of the literature. Pediatr Pathol. 1993;13:143–53.

68. Cook HT, Taylor GM, Malone P, et al. Renin in mesoblastic nephroma: An immunohistochemical study. Hum Pathol. 1988;19:1347–51.

69. O'Hagan AR, Ellsworth R, Secic M, et al. Renal manifestations of tuberous sclerosis complex. Clin Pediatr (Phila). 1996;35:483–9.

70. Fittschen A, Wendlik I, Oeztuerk S, et al. Prevalence of sporadic renal angiomyolipoma: A retrospective analysis of 61,389 in- and out-patients. Abdom Imaging. 2014;39:1009–13.

71. Dickinson M, Ruckle H, Beaghler M, et al. Renal angiomyolipoma: Optimal treatment based on size and symptoms. Clin Nephrol. 1998;49:281–6.

## REVIEW QUESTIONS

## CASE 1

A 2-day-old boy is found to have a hard, palpable abdominal mass on routine newborn examination. The pregnancy and delivery were unremarkable. There is no relevant family history. Both parents and an older 7-year-old sibling are healthy. No other abnormalities are encountered on physical examination. The baby appears well. He underwent an abdominal ultrasound and, subsequently, a CT scan of the abdomen, shown.

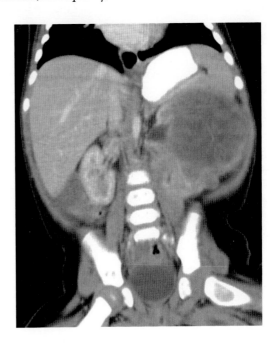

1. Based on the presentation and findings on imaging studies, the findings on the left kidney are *most* likely to represent:
   a. Wilms tumor
   b. Congenital mesoblastic nephroma
   c. Clear cell sarcoma
   d. Renal cell carcinoma
   e. Multilocular cystic nephroma

2. The *best* next step in management is:
   a. Percutaneous biopsy
   b. Open biopsy
   c. Chemotherapy (Wilms tumor protocol) and repeat imaging in 6 weeks
   d. Partial nephrectomy
   e. Radical nephrectomy

## CASE 2

A 3-year-old boy presents with rapid increase in abdominal girth. He has been healthy and has no significant medical or surgical history. His family history is unremarkable. Physical examination demonstrated a normal blood pressure for age, no dismorphic features, and a palpable abdominal mass. CT evaluation is shown below.

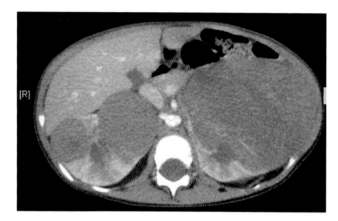

3. Based on these findings, all of the following are indicated *except:*
   a. Chest CT scan
   b. Doppler ultrasound of the renal vein and vena cava
   c. Port placement for chemotherapy
   d. Bilateral nephrectomies
   e. Screen for predisposition syndromes
4. Which of the following are associated with a predisposition to Wilms tumor?
   a. Macroglossia
   b. Aniridia
   c. Hemihypertrophy
   d. Cryptorchidism
   e. All of the above
5. Which of the following surgical principles regarding the management of renal masses consistent with Wilms tumor is *true:*

a. Ipsilateral adrenalectomy is always indicated.
b. Removal almost always includes radical resection of adjacent structures, such as spleen, tail of pancreas, bowel segment, and liver segment.
c. Early intraoperative tumor rupture demands aborting the procedure and proceeding with chemotherapy and radiation.
d. Ipsilateral lymph node sampling always should be done.
e. Nephron-sparing surgical procedures should not be offered.

## CASE 3

A 14-year-old patient with tuberous sclerosis has the following findings on a routine CAT scan imaging study.

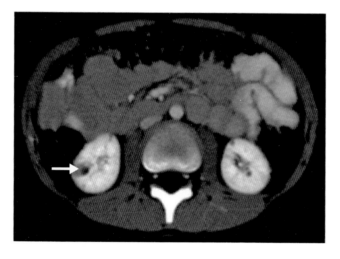

6. Which one of the following is an *accepted* step in management for the lesion highlighted with an arrow?
   a. Serial imaging with ultrasound
   b. Reimage every 3 months with CT scan
   c. Open biopsy
   d. Radical nephrectomy
   e. Partial nephrectomy and lymph node dissection

## ANSWER KEY

1. b
2. e
3. d
4. e
5. d
6. a

# 51

# Urolithiasis in children

URI S. ALON AND TARAK SRIVASTAVA

Urolithiasis has become more common in children over the past few decades, probably as a result of rapid changes in the society's dietary habits and socioeconomic status. Epidemiologic studies indicate an increasing trend of calcium oxalate and/or calcium phosphate stones in the upper urinary tract in children in industrialized countries, rather than the infection-related ammonium urate stones in the bladder of the past century and now seen mostly in less affluent countries.

Urolithiasis is a disorder "shared" by the urologist and the nephrologist. The role of the urologist is to extract the stone from the urinary tract and correct anatomic abnormalities of the genitourinary tract as indicated, whereas the role of the nephrologist is to identify the cause for the stone and plan a management strategy to prevent stone recurrence.

## EPIDEMIOLOGY

Changes in global socioeconomic conditions and the subsequent changes in dietary habits have affected not only the incidence but also the site and chemical composition of calculi.[1,2] At the beginning of the last century, bladder calculus from ammonium urate was relatively frequent in Europe, but over time it has changed to the more common renal-ureteral calculus made up of calcium oxalate, phosphate, or both, probably related to a diet rich in proteins, refined carbohydrates, and sodium and low in potassium and citrate.[1–4] Bladder stones are still common in the developing world, whereas in industrialized countries upper tract stones predominate. The majority of bladder stones seen in developed, affluent countries are a result of bladder dysfunction or bladder reconstruction. In the United States the incidence of urolithiasis is highest among whites, especially in the "stone belt" in the Southeast, peaking in July, August, and September. This has been linked to higher exposure to sunlight and consequently increased production of vitamin D and calcium absorption from the intestine on one hand and higher incidence of dehydration on the other.[2] Kidney stone formation was described among lifeguards in Israel for the same reason.[5] In recent years an increase in pediatric urolithiasis has been observed. Lattimer et al.[6] in 1951 reported no cases of urolithiasis in 21,835 patients at the Babies Hospital in New York. In later studies, the incidence of urolithiasis in children was reported as 1 in 6000 and 1 in 7600 hospitalized children.[7,8] Malek et al.[9] in 1975 described 78 cases of urolithiasis in 145,000 hospitalized children (1 in 1850); 32% of the calculi were from infection, with a greater incidence in boys (2:1 ratio) and an even distribution of patients in all age groups. Stapleton et al.[10] described 112 children with urolithiasis. Of these, 94% were white, 59% were boys, and calcium oxalate stones predominated. Milliner and Murphy[11] observed that only 19 of 221 children in the Mayo Clinic had bladder or urethral calculi whereas the rest of the urolithiasis cases were present in the upper urinary tract and ureters, unlike the distribution in developing countries, in which bladder stones are more frequent.[11] Osorio and Alon[12] found the incidence of hypercalciuria to be significantly lower in African-American children compared with white children. Penido et al.[13] showed a threefold increase in urolithiasis incidence in a pediatric nephrology clinic between 1999 and 2011. Our observation also has been validated by Routh et al.[14] and Sas et al.[15] who showed the incidence of kidney stones in children has increased over the past decade. Thus, epidemiologic studies have shown an increasing trend ("stone wave") associated with a change in social conditions and in eating habits; however, the importance of genetic predisposition as recognized by racial distribution and family history of urolithiasis cannot be disregarded.

## PATHOGENESIS

Stone formation is a complex process. In a simple solution, such as water, a solute will precipitate out of a solution once its saturation point, or the solubility product of ions, is reached. In contrast to water, in a complex solution such as urine a situation of supersaturation of stone promoters such as calcium, oxalate, and uric acid occurs as a result of the presence of many other ions and molecules in the urine that allow these promoter ions to remain in solution even at higher concentrations. Some of the better known substances that inhibit stone formation, include citrate, pyrophosphate, magnesium, and glycosaminoglycans. Other inhibitors in this category described in the literature are Tamm-Horsfall protein, uropontin, nephrocalcin, FK506 binding protein 12 (FKBP-12), bikunin, lithostathine, and others. The point at which urine will no longer hold a substance in solution is called the *formation product,* and it also may be influenced by urine pH. At the formation product, spontaneous nucleation takes place to form new crystals. The nucleation can be homogeneous or heterogeneous. The former refers to the joining of similar ions into crystals. Heterogeneous nucleation results when one crystal grows around another type of crystal, for example, calcium oxalate crystallizing around a uric acid or cystine crystal. Sloughed epithelial cells and other materials also can provide the nidus around which heterogeneous nucleation can occur. Thus, for stone formation or crystallization to materialize, either intermittent or continuous urinary

supersaturation must occur. Supersaturation is affected by water intake and urine flow rate. High urine flow rate induced by increased fluid intake reduces urine supersaturation. This holds true for all stone types and thus is one of the mainstays of therapy for urolithiasis. Insufficient urine flow is one of the more common causes of pediatric urolithiasis, and unfortunately even after diagnosis only a minority of patients adheres to high fluid intake.[13,16,17] To form a stone, multiple crystals need to combine together, a process called *aggregation,* which is thought to take place in the tubules or the collecting system. It seems that to allow this process to take place, crystals have to anchor to the urinary epithelium for a limited time and not be washed away by urine, by a process that is yet not fully understood.[2,18] The presence of anatomic abnormalities that impede urine flow and of urinary tract infections (UTIs), which change the milieu in the urinary tract system, are also known contributors to stone formation.

Nanobacteria, which have the ability to produce carbonate apatite on their cell wall, also have been implicated in stone formation. These bacteria may act as a nidus for kidney stones and in one study were isolated from 97% of the kidney stones.[19] The urinary proteome contains over 1500 proteins, but only a small subset of these proteins have been associated with stone formation.[20] These stone matrix proteins are under intense study for their role in stone formation at the present time.[21-23] Thus, many factors play a role in stone formation: presence of promoters, lack of inhibitors, urine flow rates, anatomic abnormalities, nanobacteria, stone matrix proteins, UTIs, and homogeneous or heterogeneous nucleation, all of which have to be considered when planning a therapeutic strategy to prevent formation of recurrent stones.

## CLINICAL MANIFESTATIONS

The two most characteristic manifesting symptoms of urolithiasis are pain and hematuria. Less common manifestations are UTI and acute renal failure. In other cases, stones can be detected as an incidental finding by imaging studies of the abdomen or urinary tract done for another purpose. These asymptomatic stones may at times cause obstructive uropathy.

Acute renal colic presents abruptly as a severe paroxysmal pain in waves on the affected side, associated, at times, with nausea and vomiting. The child with renal colic will usually writhe in pain or move constantly to try to find a position of comfort. The pain can occur anywhere from the flank down to the ipsilateral groin. This visceral type of pain is caused by distention of the proximal urinary collecting system from distal obstruction or from passage of the stone (or associated blood clot and debris). The location of the pain may give information about the possible location of the stone. Stones within the kidney or in the proximal ureter produce flank pain. As the stone moves down,

---

### KEY POINTS

Pathogenesis of stone formation requires:

- Supersaturation of promoters (affected by water intake).
- Decreased urinary concentration of inhibitors.
- Appropriate pH needs for the ions to precipitate.
- Nidus for crystals to deposit around.
- Stasis, urinary tract abnormalities, and infection may further promote stone formation.

the pain radiates around the front of the abdomen into the lower quadrant. Referred pain often occurs in the ipsilateral groin, testicle, and labia as the stone reaches the ureterovesicle junction. Urolithiasis and UTI are closely related. Calculi may develop as a consequence of UTI and form struvite or carbonate apatite stones *(vide infra)*. Urolithiasis places the child at risk for UTI, and the infection may be the initial presentation for stones. Presentation with UTI is more common in younger children, whereas acute renal colic is more common in older children. Lower ureter and bladder stones may manifest with hematuria, dysuria, or urgency, thus mimicking a UTI. Stones may also move within the ureter without any associated resistance or obstruction, causing painless hematuria, which can be either macroscopic or microscopic. The finding of hematuria with urolithiasis is relatively consistent throughout childhood. Macroscopic or microscopic hematuria has been observed in as many as 90% of children with urolithiasis.

## CLINICAL EVALUATION

At the initial visit, the medical history should focus on risk factors for stone formation and complications such as UTI, voiding dysfunction, and surgical procedures on the urinary tract. A positive family history for stone disease can be obtained in 22% (Turkey) to 75% (United States) of children with urolithiasis.[24,25] Clinical features suggestive of a hereditary cause for stone disease in childhood are shown in Table 51.1.

**Table 51.1** Clinical features indicating possible hereditary cause of pediatric urolithiasis

- Infantile or early childhood presentation
- Parental consanguinity
- Family history of urolithiasis
- Multiple, bilateral, and/or recurrent stones
- Coexistence of tubular dysfunction manifested by polyuria, acidosis, growth retardation, and/or renal failure
- Presence of nephrocalcinosis
- Dysmorphic and extrarenal manifestations suggestive of a syndrome

A wide variety of medical conditions can be associated with urolithiasis in children, including gastrointestinal disorders associated with malabsorption, cystic fibrosis, myelodysplasia, and immobilization. Recurrent skeletal fractures may indicate the presence of hyperparathyroidism or other bone diseases. A history of prematurity (especially with use of furosemide), use of supplemental vitamin D, and enteral or parenteral nutrition formulas high in calcium and/or phosphorus should be obtained. The dietary history must search for any dietary excesses or deficiencies and intake of medications, vitamins, and supplements. Medications such as steroids, chemotherapy drugs, anticonvulsants, loop diuretics, acetazolamide, other carbonic anhydrase inhibitors, uricosuric drugs, and antacids have been associated with urolithiasis (Table 51.2). Ketogenic diets used to treat

**Table 51.2** Medications associated with urolithiasis (listed alphabetically)

**Calcium stone formation**
- Acetazolamide
- Amphotericin B
- Antacids (calcium and noncalcium antacids)
- Glucocorticoids
- Loop diuretics
- Theophylline
- Topiramate
- Vitamin D
- Zonisamide

**Uric acid stone formation**
- Acetohexamide
- Allopurinol (xanthine stones)
- Ascorbic acid
- Benzbromarone
- Calcium ipodate
- Chlorprothixene
- Cinchophen
- Dicumarol
- Estrogen
- Glycerol guaiacholate
- Halofenate
- Iodopyracet
- Iopanoic acid
- Ketogenic diet
- Meglumine iodipamide
- Outdated tetracyclines
- Phenylbutazone
- Phenolsulfonphthalein
- Probenecid
- Salicylates
- Sodium diatrizoate
- Zoxazolamine

**Medications that may precipitate into stones**
- Acyclovir
- Ceftriaxone
- Felbamate
- Indinavir
- Sulfadiazine
- Triamterene

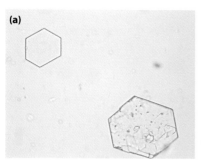 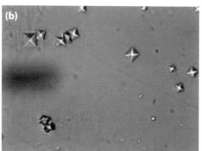 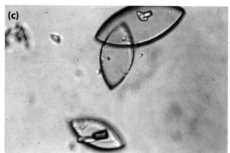

Figure 51.1 Urine microscopy showing (a) clear hexagonal cysteine crystals, (b) calcium oxalate crystals (envelope shaped), and (c) uric acid crystals.

intractable seizures in children are associated with uric acid stones.[26] Excess salt and insufficient potassium intake may contribute to stone formation.[12]

Urogenital tract abnormalities predispose to the formation of infected stones. Therefore, a careful urologic evaluation of patients with infected stones is mandatory. Children on clean intermittent catheterization via a Mitrofanoff conduit, exstrophy-epispadias complex, and bladder augmentation frequently develop urolithiasis.[27–29]

The examination should search for chronic diseases, including failure to thrive (distal renal tubular acidosis [RTA]), hypertension (renal disease), skeletal findings of rickets, soft tissue calcification (hypercalcemia), and abnormal external genitalia.

Urinalysis should always be part of the evaluation process in the physician's office, and any abnormality might present a clue to the source of stone formation. As mentioned in later discussion, urine specific gravity provides a good idea about the patient's hydration. Attention should be paid to urine pH and the presence of crystals, which can provide a clue to diagnosis, but only cystine crystals are pathognomonic (Figure 51.1). On rare occasions, the presence of proteinuria may indicate a need to search for a tubular disorder.[30] At times, when infection-related stones are suspected or indicated by urinalysis, urine culture might be needed as well.

## LABORATORY AND RADIOLOGIC EVALUATION

The laboratory evaluation is based on three components: stone analysis, biochemical profile of the urine (stone risk analysis), and blood tests. All efforts must be made to obtain the stone, either by straining the urine or by the medical team extracting it. However, in many cases the stone is not captured, and in others, even if its composition is known, further analysis is needed to define the metabolic abnormality leading to its formation. For instance, calcium oxalate stones can be caused by excess calcium or oxalate in the urine, or diminished citrate or urine flow, or any combination of these.

A timed 24-hour urine collection should be performed for volume, creatinine, calcium, sodium, potassium, uric acid, oxalate, citrate, phosphorus, and magnesium (Table 51.3). In certain circumstances, measurements may need to be done for cystine, glycerate, glycolate, 2,8-dihydroxy adenine, orotic acid, xanthine, hypoxanthine, ornithine, lysine, and arginine. Urinary calcium excretion is increased during acute pyelonephritis and with immobilization. The 24-hour urine sample should be evaluated ideally after the patient is free of stones, free of infection, and on his or her usual diet with normal fluid intake. The accuracy of the collection is validated by calculating creatinine excretion (creatinine index) expressed as mg/kg/24 h.[13] An important component of the diagnostic urine evaluation is the assessment of urinary volume (vide infra). In geographic regions where calcium oxalate and phosphate stones constitute the vast majority of stones, we recommend a step-wise approach to analyzing urine chemistry. First, only urine calcium excretion is assessed, with the rest of the urine sample kept refrigerated. Only when hypercalciuria is ruled out are other chemistries analyzed.[17]

In situations in which it may be difficult to collect a 24-hour urine sample, random urine samples may be used (Table 51.4). It should be emphasized that normative data for random urine specimens using creatinine as denominator were established in children with normal muscle mass and should not be used in patients with significantly increased or decreased muscle mass because of the effect on urine creatinine. In such cases, another denominator such as urine osmolality can be used. The normal value for the calcium-to-osmolality ratio [urine calcium (mg/dL)/osmolality (mOsmol/kg $H_2O$) × 10] is established at less than 0.25.[31]

## KEY POINTS

- 24-Hour urine collection must include creatinine expressed as mg/kg/24 h to validate accurate collection.
- When analyzing a random urine sample, urine creatinine can serve as denominator only in those with normal muscle mass.

Table 51.3 Normal 24-hour urinary excretion rates in children studied for urolithiasis

| Normal values for 24 hour urine collection samples | |
| --- | --- |
| Volume | 20–25 mL/kg/24 h |
| Creatinine excretion | 15–20 mg/kg/24 h in adolescent male |
| | 12–15 mg/kg/24 h in adolescent female |
| Creatinine clearance | >90 mL/min/1.73 m² |
| Uric acid excretion | <815 mg/1.73 m²/24 h |
| | <35 mg/kg/24 h |
| Calcium excretion | <4 mg/kg/24 h |
| Sodium excretion | <3 mEq/kg/24 h |
| Potassium excretion | >3 mEq/kg/24 h |
| Magnesium excretion | >88 mg/1.73 m²/24 h |
| Oxalate excretion | <52 mg/1.73 m2/24 h |
| | <2 mg/kg/24 h |
| Citrate excretion | >180 mg/g creatinine in children |
| | >128 mg/g creatinine in adult males |
| | >300 mg/g creatinine in adult females |
| Protein excretion | <4 mg/m²/h |
| Cystine excretion | <60 mg/1.73 m²/24 h |
| Urine glycolate | 0.19 ± 0.07 mmol/24 h |
| Xanthine* | 20–60 µmol/24 hr |
| Hypoxanthine* | 20–100 µmol/24 h |

*Mayo Clinic laboratories.

Table 51.4 Normal urine excretion rates in random urine samples corrected for urinary creatinine excretion*

| Normal values for random urine samples | |
| --- | --- |
| Calcium/creatinine (mg/mg) | <0.2 |
| Oxalate/creatinine (mg/mg) | <0.05 |
| Uric acid/creatinine (mg/mg) | <0.65 (10–14 yr) |
| | <0.60 (14–17 yr) |
| Uric acid/GFR | <0.56 |
| Tubular phosphate reabsorption/ GFR (mg/dL) | 4.1 ± 0.6 (12–16 yr) |
| | 3.3 ± 0.3 (>16 yr) |
| Magnesium/creatinine (mg/mg) | >0.05 |
| Sodium/potassium (mEq/mEq) | <2.5 |
| Citrate/creatinine (mg/mg) | >0.18 in children |
| | >0.14 in adult males |
| | >0.30 in adult females |
| Cystine/creatinine (mg/mg) | <0.075 |
| Glycolate/creatinine (mmol/mmol) | <0.013 (>12 yr) |
| L-Glycerate/creatinine (µmol/mmol) | <28 |

* Note that these values can be utilized only in children with normal muscle mass.

Table 51.5 Urinary stone composition and structure

**Calcium oxalate**
- Calcium oxalate monohydrate (whewellite)
- Calcium oxalate dihydrate (weddellite)

**Calcium phosphates**
- Calcium phosphate, carbonate form (carbonate apatite)
- Calcium phosphate, hydroxyl form (hydroxyl apatite)
- Calcium hydrogen phosphate dihydrate (brushite)
- Tricalcium phosphate (whitlockite)

**Purines**
- Uric acid
- Xanthine
- Sodium acid urate
- Ammonium acid urate
- 2,8-Dihydroxyadenine
- Orotic acid

**Cystine**
- Cystinuria

**Drugs**
- Acyclovir
- Indinavir
- Triamterene
- Ceftriaxone
- Felbamate
- Sulfadiazine
- Silicate

**Miscellaneous**
- Magnesium ammonium phosphate hexahydrate (struvite)
- Magnesium phosphate (newberyite)

The four most common types of stones are calcium oxalate, calcium phosphate, uric acid, and struvite (Box 51.5). The initial blood work for all patients undergoing examination for stones includes tests for renal function, electrolytes, calcium, phosphorus, magnesium, uric acid, and parathyroid hormone. Subsequent blood work may be needed for vitamin D levels, enzyme assays, and genetic studies.

Plain abdominal radiographs detect only radiopaque stones and have a low sensitivity (62%) and specificity (67%) for making the diagnosis of urolithiasis.[32] Radiolucent stones that are not detectable by plain x-ray of the abdomen include uric acid stones, cysteine stones, and those caused by antiretroviral drug indinavir. Ultrasound can be used to detect such stones. Plain x-ray of the abdomen as well as the traditional intravenous pyelography have been replaced in recent years by ultrasonography and computed tomography

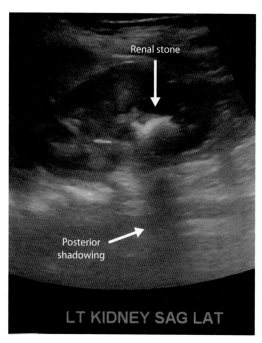

Figure 51.2 Renal ultrasound evaluation of left kidney demonstrating a stone (upper arrow) and the associated posterior shadowing (lower arrow).

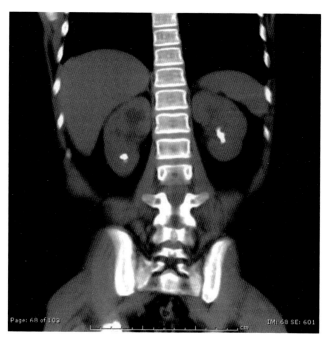

Figure 51.3 A computed axial tomography scan of abdomen showing bilateral nonobstructing renal stones.

(CT).[2,33,34] Ultrasound evaluation presents the advantage of not exposing the child to ionizing radiation. Apart from the stone itself, a renal sonogram also usually reveals a posterior shadowing, a conical (dark) area that represents the segment where ultrasound waves are unable to penetrate through the density of the renal stone (Figure 51.2). The disadvantages of the renal ultrasound are that it is operator dependent and that stones in ureters may be difficult to locate, especially in patients with significant intestinal gaseous dilatation. A noncontrast spiral CT, readily available in most emergency rooms 24 hours per day, is now replacing other imaging techniques during acute episodes of urolithiasis (Figure 51.3). In patients requiring repeat studies we recommend maximal use of ultrasonography to minimize exposure to CT-related radiation.

Nephrocalcinosis (Figure 51.4) may be seen in many patients with high risk for stone disease or recurrent stones. Medullary nephrocalcinosis is often associated with renal tubular acidosis (RTA-1 or distal RTA), hypercalciuria,

primary hyperparathyroidism, sickle cell disease, medullary sponge kidney, hypervitaminosis D, and, less commonly, renal tuberculosis. Cortical nephrocalcinosis is less common and is usually seen in oxalosis and dystrophic calcifications associated with acute cortical necrosis of hemodynamic origin (following shock).

## SPECIFIC TYPES OF RENAL STONES

## HYPERCALCIURIA CALCULI

Hypercalciuria is the most common metabolic abnormality detected in children with stones, causing mainly the formation of calcium oxalate stones and to a lesser extent calcium phosphate stones or a mixture of the two.[17] Before development of kidney stones, hypercalciuria can manifest as frequency-dysuria syndrome with or without microscopic or gross hematuria.[35] In a prospective study

---

### KEY POINTS

- Radiolucent stones that cannot be detected by plain x-ray are:
  - Uric acid stones
  - Cystine stones
  - Indinavir stones
- Ultrasound can detect radiolucent stones

---

### KEY POINTS

- When investigating children with urolithiasis, the use of CT should be minimized because of exposure to radiation.
- Urinary tract ultrasound is a preferred option for evaluation of most patients, because it does not involve harmful ionizing radiation.

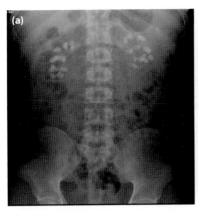
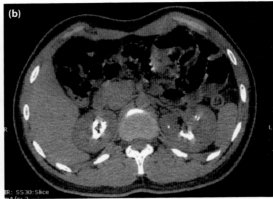

Figure 51.4 Nephrocalcinosis in a patient with renal tubular acidosis-1 (RTA-1; distal RTA) seen in **(a)** plain radiograph and **(b)** computed axial tomography scan of the abdomen. Nephrocalcinosis is predominantly affecting medullary regions.

## KEY POINTS

- Medullary calcification is common in:
  - Renal tubular acidosis (RTA-1 or distal RTA)
  - Hypercalciuria
  - Hyperparathyroidism
  - Hypervitaminosis D
  - Hyperuricemia
  - Sickle cell–associated pyramidal calcification
  - Medullary sponge kidney
  - Milk-alkali syndrome
  - Renal tuberculosis-dystrophic calcification
  - Other causes of papillary necrosis
- Cortical calcifications are common in:
  - Cortical necrosis (hemodynamic) dystrophic calcification
  - Oxalosis

of 83 children referred for unexplained hematuria without proteinuria or previous kidney stones, 26% of children had hypercalciuria.[36] In this subset of children with hematuria and hypercalciuria, Garcia et al.[37] found persistent hematuria in 29% and persistent hypercalciuria in 70% at 1 year follow-up. At 2 and 3 years of follow-up, they found persistent hematuria in 38% and 61% had persistent hypercalciuria, with 17% developing kidney stones.[37] Similarly, in a prospective study by the Southwest Pediatric Nephrology Study Group, 13% of children with hypercalciuria and hematuria developed kidney stones within 1 to 4 years of follow-up.[24]

Hypercalciuria can result from genetic or acquired causes (Table 51.6).[30] The gastrointestinal tract, bone, and kidneys play major roles in calcium metabolism under the influence of diet, fluid and electrolyte homeostasis, parathyroid hormone, calcitonin, and vitamin D metabolites. Calcium reabsorption in the renal tubules is increased by parathyroid hormone, volume contraction, alkalosis, and thiazide diuretics and decreased by volume expansion, hypercalcemia, acidosis, phosphate depletion, and loop diuretics. Thus, increased calcium excretion in the urine can occur from (1)

Table 51.6 Causes of hypercalciuria in children

**Alimentary Hypercalciuria (Absorptive Hypercalciuria)**
- Idiopathic
- Increased vitamin D intake
- Increased (supplemental) calcium intake

**Renal Hypercalciuria (Reabsorptive Hypercalciuria)**
- Impaired renal calcium reabsorption
  - Idiopathic
  - Distal renal tubular acidosis
  - Dent disease
  - Bartter syndrome
  - Familial hypomagnesemia with hypercalciuria
  - Familial hypercalciuria
  - Use of loop diuretics (furosemide)
  - Abnormalities in parathyroid calcium sensing receptor
  - High dietary salt intake
  - Low dietary potassium intake
- Bone resorption (may be associated with hypercalcemia)
  - Immobilization
  - Hyperparathyroidism
  - Corticosteroid use
  - Neoplasms
- Renal tubular phosphate leak
- Increased vitamin D synthesis (may be associated with hypercalcemia)
  - Sarcoidosis
  - Neoplasms
- Idiopathic

increased intestinal calcium absorption (idiopathic, vitamin D excess, increased enteral intake), (2) impaired renal tubular calcium reabsorption (idiopathic, distal RTA, Dent disease, Bartter syndrome, familial hypomagnesemia and hypercalciuria, abnormalities in calcium sensing receptor, loop diuretics), (3) bone resorption (immobilization, hyperparathyroidism, steroid use, neoplasms), (4) renal tubular phosphate leak, (5) increased 1,25 dihydroxy vitamin D synthesis (sarcoidosis, neoplasms, idiopathic), (6) decreased 1,25-$(OH)_2$-D-24 hydroxylase (CYP24A1) deficiency, and (7) overly high dietary salt intake and potassium intake that is too low.[30,38–40]

Although idiopathic hypercalciuria remains the most common form of hypercalciuria, a systematic search for secondary causes of hypercalciuria should be made when clinically or biochemically suspected *(vide infra)*. Idiopathic hypercalciuria has been attributed to either a defect in renal tubular reabsorption of calcium (renal hypercalciuria) or enhanced absorption by the gastrointestinal tract (absorptive hypercalciuria). An oral calcium loading test was popular in the past to differentiate between these two forms of idiopathic hypercalciuria.[41] However, the current belief is that absorptive and renal forms of hypercalciuria may represent a continuum spectrum of a single disease, and the oral loading test to differentiate between the two entities is no longer used clinically. Aladjem et al.[42] reevaluated calcium loading tests after an interval of 3 to 7 years in children who were initially diagnosed as having absorptive or renal hypercalciuria and found a different result in more than half of the children studied. On the other hand, they found a strong relationship between urinary sodium and calcium excretion and suggested a detrimental role for dietary sodium in idiopathic hypercalciuria. This clinical observation has been reported by other investigators, who also have observed an inverse effect of dietary potassium on urinary calcium excretion, that is, high dietary potassium intake decreases urinary calcium excretion by an unknown mechanism (Figure 51.5).[12]

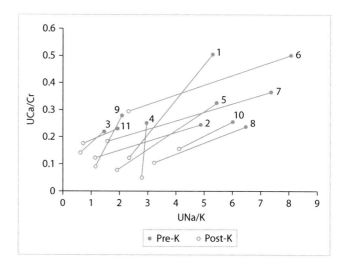

Figure 51.5 Effect of potassium therapy in 11 children with idiopathic hypercalciuria on their urine sodium-to-potassium and urine calcium-to-creatinine ratios. (Reproduced with permission from Osorio AV, Alon US. The relationship between urinary calcium, sodium, and potassium excretion and the role of potassium in treating idiopathic hypercalciuria. Pediatrics. 1997;100:675–81.)

sodium and potassium intake should be made based on urinary excretion and measurement of serum phosphorus and tubular phosphate reabsorption per glomerular filtration rate (TP/GFR) should be obtained. An increased phosphate loss in urine stimulates synthesis of 1,25$(OH)_2$ vitamin D and causes secondary hypercalciuria from increased gastrointestinal absorption of calcium. Children who are immobilized or on long-term steroid therapy can have hypercalciuria associated with or without hypercalcemia.

One of the greatest risk factors for pediatric stone formation is a low urinary flow rate.[13,16] Therefore, management of all patients with urolithiasis starts with the recommendation to maintain a high oral fluid intake. A good way to monitor compliance is to assess urine specific gravity during clinic visits. Most pediatric urologists and pediatric nephrologists recommend maintaining the specific gravity at or below 1.010.[17] Unfortunately, adherence with generalized recommendations such as "have a high fluid

> **KEY POINTS**
>
> - Idiopathic hypercalciuria remains the most common form of hypercalciuria in children.
> - Urine sodium and potassium, reflecting their dietary intake, affect urine calcium in opposing directions. Sodium increases and potassium decreases urinary calcium excretion.

Whenever hypercalciuria is detected as a risk factor for urolithiasis in a child, a secondary cause should be considered because successful correction of hypercalciuria in such cases depends on eradication of the primary cause.[43] An elevated serum calcium level should lead to evaluation for parathyroid hormone and 1,25$(OH)_2$ vitamin D. In the presence of normal serum calcium concentration, estimates of dietary

> **KEY POINTS**
>
> - A good way to advise on the recommended additional fluid intake is by calculating the difference between the desired urine output of 24 mL/kg/24 h and the actual 24-hour urine volume.
> - In hypercalciuric patients, the urine sodium-to-potassium ratio should be less than 2.5.
> - The addition of amiloride to thiazide diuretics protects against hypokalemia and, by itself, further decreases urine calcium.

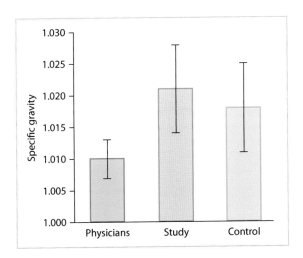

Figure 51.6 Mean (± standard deviation) urine specific gravity recommended by physicians versus readings in children with urolithiasis and control children. (Reproduced with permission from: Alon US, Zimmerman H, Alon M. Evaluation and treatment of pediatric idiopathic urolithiasis: revisited. Pediatr Nephrol. 2004;19:516–20.)

intake" or "make sure the urine looks like water" is quite poor (Figure 51.6). A more precise way of recommending high fluid intake is based on the goal of having urine flow of at least 1 mL/kg/h. Knowledge of a child's weight and urine volume during 24-hour urine collection can indicate what additional fluid intake is required to achieve the goal. For instance, in a 40-kg child with a goal of 960 mL/24 h, if 24-hour urine collection had a volume of 660 mL, the family can be advised on the need of additional daily fluid intake of 300 mL. It is important that the child also stays hydrated during the night.

When idiopathic hypercalciuria is confirmed, the next step is to assess whether dietary manipulation can normalize calcium excretion. We recommend a diet of recommended dietary allowance (RDA) for protein and calcium that is not excessive in salt (2.0 to 2.4 g sodium per day) and supplemented with at least the RDA of five servings of fruits and vegetables (3.0 to 3.5 g potassium per day). Indeed, only a minority of children in the United States adhere to the RDA of fruit and vegetable intake.[44] Compliance with these dietary recommendations can be assessed by measuring the urine sodium-to-potassium ratio, which should be less than 2.5. If, in 4 to 6 weeks, hypercalciuria persists, treatment with potassium citrate at 0.5 to 1.5 mEq of potassium/kg/day is recommended. If the child does not tolerate potassium citrate or fails to correct hypercalciuria, a thiazide diuretic can be added.[17] Another potential reason, although not yet fully substantiated, to convert from potassium citrate to thiazides is in patients developing highly alkaline urine, which by itself may promote calcium phosphate stones.[45] Chlorothiazide 15 to 25 mg/kg/day or hydrochlorothiazide 1.5 to 2.5 mg/kg/day can be used. In contrast to the latter two that need to be given on a twice-daily schedule to achieve maximum anticalciuric effect, chlorthalidone, a

longer acting agent, can be given as a single daily dose of 0.5 to 1 mg/kg/day.[46] Children on long-term thiazide diuretics will need to be monitored for dyselectrolytemia, hyperlipidemia, and hyperglycemia. The addition of amiloride might further enhance the anticalciuric effect and protect from hypokalemia.[47] Dietary restriction of calcium is not recommended, because it puts the growing child at risk for negative calcium balance and poor bone mineralization. It also may increase urinary excretion of oxalate from increased gastrointestinal absorption of oxalate resulting from decreased luminal availability of calcium to bind with it. For the same reasons, drugs such as sodium cellulose phosphate, acting by complexing intestinal calcium, are not used in children. Neutral phosphate can be used in children with hypercalciuria secondary to tubular phosphate leak. In children with hypercalciuria secondary to RTA, potassium citrate is the drug of choice for treatment of hypercalciuria. At times, this may need to be supplemented by sodium bicarbonate and calcium-sparing diuretics.

In recent years, more attention has been given to the combination of hypercalciuria, stone formation, osteoporosis, and fractures described in both adults and children.[48-50] In some cases this "syndrome" can be due to an identifiable genetic mutation.[51] A decrease in bone mineral density has been reported in 30% to 42.6% of children with idiopathic hypercalciuria.[52-54] Schwaderer et al.[55] showed that the dietary recommendations alone do not alter the natural history of lumbar bone mineral density, and therapy with potassium citrate is beneficial in children with hypercalciuria. Recently bisphosphonates have been demonstrated to improve bone density and lower urine calcium levels in hypercalciuric children with decreased bone density who were resistant to traditional therapy.[50]

## KEY POINTS

- Some hypercalciuric patients also may have osteopenia.
- Treatment of the hypercalciuria in these patients may improve their bone mineral status.

## HYPOCITRATURIA CALCULI

A decrease in urinary citrate excretion is an important factor in the genesis of urolithiasis, particularly in the form of calcium oxalate stones. Hypocitraturia can be either idiopathic, secondary to systemic acidosis or hypokalemia, or associated with various bowel diseases. Systemic acidosis and hypokalemia are believed to impair citrate synthesis and increase renal resorption, resulting in hypocitraturia. Thus, a finding of decreased urinary citrate excretion should alert the clinician to the possibility of distal or incomplete RTA, and evaluation of (urine-blood) $pCO_2$ following oral acetazolamide should be done.[56] In addition, a subtle renal acidification defect can occur secondary to renal tubular injury from chronic hypercalciuria and urolithiasis.[57] Naturally, in patients with acidosis or hypokalemia the electrolyte abnormalities should be corrected. Potassium citrate is the rational drug of choice in children with reduced urinary citrate excretion, as well as in those with hypercalciuria and hyperuricosuria, with close monitoring of urine pH. A diet rich in fruits and vegetables is recommended to enhance urine potassium and consequently citrate excretion (Figure 51.7).[39]

Because of some conflicting data about the normative values of urine citrate we evaluated a healthy school-aged population and found the 5th percentile at 180 mg citrate per gram of creatinine for both genders.[58] Furthermore, to find out why some hypercalciuric children develop stones and others do not, we compared their urine calcium-to-citrate ratio and found it to be higher in the stone-forming group (Figure 51.8). Further analysis has shown that the calcium-to-citrate ratio less than 0.33 decreases the risk for stone formation. This parameter has the advantage of being independent of the accuracy of urine collection, and its utility as both risk indicator and treatment goal was recently confirmed in studies in adults and children.[59,60] Interestingly, fruits rich in either potassium, such as melon, or citrate, such as lemon and orange, improve urine citrate excretion.[61,62]

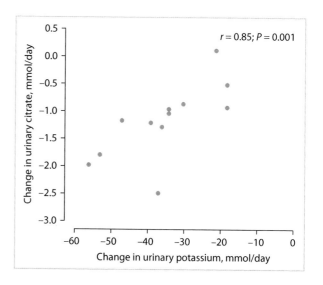

Figure 51.7 Effect of change in urine potassium excretion on urine citrate excretion. (Reproduced with permission from: Meschi T, Maggiore U, Fiaccadori E, et al. The effect of fruits and vegetables on urinary stone risk factors. Kidney Int. 2004;66:2402–10.)

## HYPEROXALURIA CALCULI

Under normal circumstances the majority of oxalate that appears in the urine is derived from endogenous production with almost equal contribution from ascorbic acid metabolism and glyoxylate metabolism. Only 10% to 15% of urinary oxalate is believed to originate from the diet. Mild hyperoxaluria can be either idiopathic or secondary to enteric hyperoxaluria from fat malabsorption. Mild hyperoxaluria can be observed in adolescents who develop food fads rich in vegetables (with high oxalate content), high in vitamin C, or poor in pyridoxine (which leads to build-up of glyoxylate). In enteric hyperoxaluria, excess fat in the gastrointestinal

---

**KEY POINTS**

The calcium-to-citrate ratio is a good indicator of the patient's risk for stone formation and a ratio of less than 0.33 mg/mg can serve as a therapeutic goal.

---

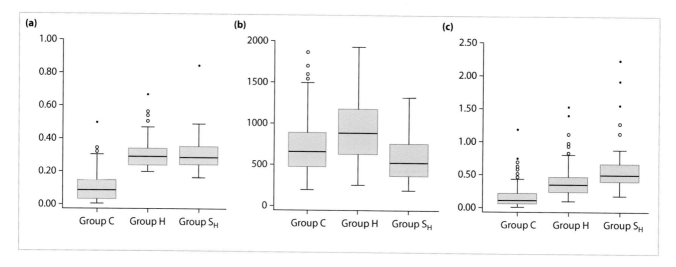

Figure 51.8 Box plot distribution of **(a)** urine calcium-to-creatinine, **(b)** citrate-to-creatinine, and **(C)** calcium-to-citrate in groups C (controls), H (hypercalciuric children with no stones), and S_H (hypercalciuric stone formers). (Reproduced with permission from: Srivastava T, Winston MJ, Auron A, Alon US. Urine calcium/citrate ratio in children with hypercalciuric stones. Pediatr Res. 2009;66:85–90.)

lumen binds to luminal calcium, which makes the latter unavailable to bind dietary oxalate, leading to increased gastrointestinal absorption of oxalate. Absence of the anaerobic intestinal oxalate-degrading bacterium *Oxalobacter formigenes* also may play a role in some cases of secondary hyperoxaluria, as has been shown in cystic fibrosis patients, in whom the development of renal stones is quite common.[63]

Moderate-to-severe hyperoxaluria is observed in primary hyperoxaluria type I and type II. In type I, the more prevalent form, the genetic mutation is in alanine:glyoxylate aminotransferase, resulting in increased urinary excretion of oxalate, glyoxlic acid, and glycolic acid. Once renal failure has developed, this leads to recurrent urolithiasis, nephrocalcinosis, renal failure, and systemic oxalate deposition (oxalosis). In type II, a rare entity, the defect is in the D-glycerate dehydrogenase enzyme, resulting in increased urinary excretion of oxalate and L-glycerate.

In children with hyperoxaluria-associated urolithiasis, a low-oxalate diet is recommended (Table 51.7). In cases of secondary hyperoxaluria resulting from fat malabsorption, a fat-restricted diet supplemented by increased calcium intake is also recommended. Most individuals with inflammatory bowel disease also have low urine citrate levels, so potassium citrate can be added as well. In primary hyperoxaluria, a trial of treatment with pyridoxine is warranted. Reduction of oxalate production by pyridoxine is effective in some children with primary hyperoxaluria in reducing the urinary excretion of oxalate. Recent studies show that only those with certain mutations will benefit from pyridoxine therapy.[64,65] The starting dose is 10 mg/day and may be increased gradually to 100 mg/day. Magnesium, citrate, pyrophosphate, and thiazide diuretics in combination also can be used in children with primary hyperoxaluria. In severe cases with systemic oxalosis, dialysis and liver-kidney transplantation may be required.

### KEY POINTS

- Inflammatory bowel disease, ileostomy, and fat malabsorption predispose to uric acid and oxalate stone resulting from:
  - Chronic volume contraction
  - Bicarbonate loss and need to produce very acidic urine (low pH)
  - Low urinary citrate and magnesium
- In steatorrhea, excess fat in stool binds calcium (saponification), leaving an abundance of oxalate in the gut to be absorbed.

## URIC ACID CALCULI

Uric acid stones account for 2% to 4% of urolithiasis in children. Contrary to calcium stones, uric acid stones are radiolucent. The excretion of uric acid is found to be increased in some children with hypercalciuria, and thus may serve

as nidus for development of calcium oxalate and phosphate stones. In children older than 2 years of age, the normal uric acid excreted per glomerular filtration rate (GFR) value is less than 0.56 mg/dL (Uric acid/GFR = $U_{uric\ acid} \times S_{creatinine}/U_{creatinine}$).[66] In addition, Matos et al.[67] published age-related nomograms of ratios of random urine uric acid to creatinine, which are higher in infancy and decrease as the child grows older (Figure 51.9).[67]

An increased urinary uric acid excretion may result from increased glomerular load of uric acid (from excessive dietary purine intake, hematologic or myeloproliferative disorders, or metabolic errors such as Lesch-Nyhan syndrome, glycogen storage disease type 1, etc.) or from isolated or generalized tubular defects. In a child with uric acid stones and hyperuricemia, an evaluation for purine salvage enzymes, hypoxanthine guanine phosphoribosyl transferase (HPRT), and phosphoribosyl pyrophosphate synthetase (PRPS) should be made.[68] Complete HPRT deficiency results in Lesch-Nyhan syndrome, in which the afflicted males have severe neurologic abnormalities in addition to recurrent uric acid calculi.

Urolithiasis associated with increased urine uric acid in the face of low or normal serum uric acid can occur from a primary tubular defect in uric acid handling by the kidney (such as in hereditary renal hypouricemia, hereditary hypouricemia with hypercalciuria and osteoporosis), secondary generalized tubular disorders, or iatrogenic administration of various uricosuric drugs (see Table 51.1).

In a significant number of patients with uric acid urolithiasis, urinary uric acid excretion may be normal. The culprit in these cases is persistent low urinary pH. Urine pH plays an important role in uric acid urolithiasis because uric acid crystals are poorly soluble in acidic urine and precipitate easily. Whereas at urine pH of 6.5, uric acid solubility is 1200 mg/L, it decreases to 200 mg/L at pH of 5.3. This is clinically best exemplified by development of uric acid urolithiasis in children on ketogenic diets for intractable seizures. Despite normal urinary uric acid excretion, the systemic acidosis leads to a constantly low urine pH and hypocitraturia. This is further worsened by poor fluid intake and prolonged immobilization, which lead to stone formation.[26] Interestingly, recent studies found an association between uric acid stones and overweight and insulin resistance causing low urine pH as a result of decreased ammonia production.[69] The therapy for uric acid calculi in most patients includes efforts to alkalinize the urine to a pH of 6.5 to 7.0 with potassium citrate and to maintain a high urine flow rate. A diet low in purine is recommended. This includes restriction of red meat, fish, fowl, coffee, cocoa, chocolate, cakes with a high yeast content ("Danish" for instance), and sardines (Table 51.7). In cases of increased uric acid production treatment with allopurinol may be necessary.

## 2,8-DIHYDROXYADENINE CALCULI

Deficiency in adenine phosphoribosyl transferase (APRT) is an autosomal recessive disorder leading to formation of

Table 51.7 Dietary considerations in children with urolithiasis

| HIGH POTASSIUM | HIGH OXALATE | HIGH PURINES |
|---|---|---|
| Fruits and fruit juices | Beets | Alcohol |
|   Apricots | Berries: blackberries, blueberries, | Asparagus |
|   Avocado |   strawberries, raspberries, currants, | Cauliflower |
|   Banana |   gooseberries | Chickoo |
|   Cantaloupe | Celery | Custard apple |
|   Grapefruit juice | Chocolate | Dry beans (lentils, lima and kidney |
|   Honeydew | Cocoa |   beans) |
|   Kiwi | Cranberry juice | Fish: Anchovies, sardines (canned), |
|   Nectarine | Dried figs |   herring, mackerel, cod, halibut, tuna, |
|   Orange | Gelatin |   carp |
|   Orange juice | Grape juice | Gravies |
|   Pear | Green beans | Meat extracts: Bouillon, broth, |
|   Prune juice | Green onions |   consommé, stock |
|   Raisins | Grits | Meat: Beef, pork, lamb, poultry |
|   Tangerine juice | Leafy greens: Collard greens, dandelion | Mushrooms |
|   Tomato juice |   greens, Swiss chard, spinach, escarole, | Organ meats: Kidney, liver, pancreas, |
|   V-8 juice |   mustard greens, sorrel, kale, rhubarb |   brain, heart |
| Vegetables | Leeks | Peas |
|   Broccoli | Nuts | Pulses |
|   Brussel sprouts | Okra | Shell fish |
|   Carrots | Pepper | Spinach |
|   Corn on cob | Summer squash | Sweet breads |
|   Lettuce, romaine and butterhead | Sweet potatoes | Tea and coffee |
|   Mushrooms | Tea | |
|   Potato | Tofu (bean curd) | |
|   Squash | | |
|   Succotash | | |
|   Tomato | | |
| Dairy products | | |
|   Cottage cheese | | |
|   Ice cream | | |
|   Milk | | |
|   Yoghurt | | |

excessive 2,8-dihydroxy adenine. These calculi are hard to distinguish from uric acid stones, and specialized chemical analysis is required to distinguish between the two. These children generally have normal levels of uric acid in the serum and urine. At times a clue to diagnosis is brownish crystals on the baby's diaper. The suspicion is that 2,8-dihydroxyadenine urolithiasis is underreported because most of these patients are incorrectly suspected of having uric acid lithiasis and respond to allopurinol (which eliminates the lithogenic 2,8-dihydroxyadenine from the urine). Thus, the correct diagnosis is often missed. The importance of correct diagnosis relies on the fact that alkalization of urine indicated for uric acid stones decreases the solubility of 2,8-dihydroxyadenine and thus increases the risk for urolithiasis. A low-purine diet is also recommended. Thus, presentation with a uric acid–like stone without increases in serum or urine uric acid excretion, or presence of other factors predisposing to uric acid calculi formation, may require evaluation for a 2,8-dihydroxyadenine stone.

### KEY POINTS

- Uric acid stones can be formed as a result of either excessive amounts of uric acid in the urine, low urine pH, or both.
- Preventive intervention includes urine alkalinization.

## XANTHINE CALCULI

Xanthine stones occur primarily from a deficiency in the enzyme xanthine dehydrogenase and secondarily from

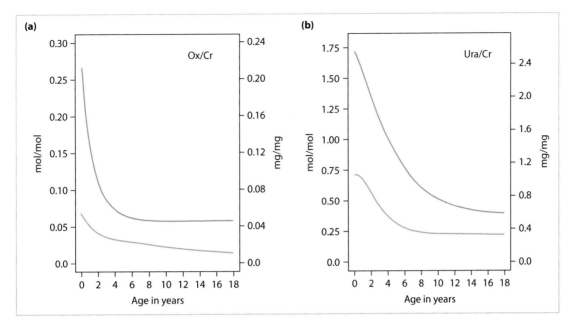

Figure 51.9 The 5th and 95th percentiles of urinary **(a)** oxalate-to-creatinine and **(b)** uric acid–to-creatinine ratios in normal children. (Reproduced with permission from: Matos V, Van Melle G, Werner D, et al. Urinary oxalate and urate to creatinine ratios in a healthy pediatric population. Am J Kidney Dis. 1999;34:e.1-e6.6.)

allopurinol therapy, which inhibits the enzyme. In hereditary xanthinuria, the enzyme deficiency results in an inability to degrade hypoxanthine and xanthine to uric acid. Uric acid is virtually undetectable in plasma and urine on a purine-free diet and is replaced in the urine by xanthine and to a lesser extent hypoxanthine in the ratio of 3:1 to 4:1. Xanthine calculi should be suspected when orange-brown sediment is noted in the urine. Xanthine stones are radiolucent.

There is no specific therapy for xanthine stones other than increased fluid intake. Special attention should be given to maintain dilute urine during the night. In cases of secondary xanthine stones due to allopurinol therapy, as in children with Lesch-Nyhan syndrome, consideration should be given to lowering the dose of allopurinol to allow the highest tolerated concentration of uric acid that can be controlled by concomitant urinary alkalinization and lessening the xanthine load (as xanthine solubility is almost unaffected by urine alkalinity).

## CYSTINE CALCULI

Cystinuria is an autosomal recessive disorder characterized by increased urinary excretion of cystine and other dibasic amino acids: ornithine, lysine, and arginine. Children with cystinuria are classified as type A, B, or AB based on the genetic mutation and the severity of urinary cystine excretion.[70,71] Children with type A have a mutation in gene *SLC3A1*, with homozygous children having a urine cystine excretion in the range of 2000 to 5000 μmol/gCr (molecular weight of cystine, 240) and heterozygous children having a cystine excretion in the range of 25 to 125 μmol/gCr. In type

B the mutation is in gene *SLC7A*, with homozygous children having a urine cystine excretion similar to that of type A, but heterozygous children have a cystine excretion in the range of 100 to 1000 μmol/gCr; the excretion is lower in the mixed form type AB, in which the child has one disease-causing mutation in each gene *SLC3A1* and *SLC7A9*.

Cystinuria accounts for 2% to 4% of children with kidney stones in developed countries. A higher incidence may be encountered in areas endemic for consanguinity. Cystine stones are usually, but not always, radiopaque because of presence of sulfur ions and occasionally may have a component of or serve as a nidus for a calcium oxalate stone. One study showed that cystinuria can be associated with hypercalciuria (18%), hyperuricosuria (22%), and hypocitraturia (44%) probably caused by renal tubular acidification defect.[72] Cystine crystals appear as flat, hexagonal, and colorless (see Figure 51.1) and should be searched for in concentrated acidic urine. Normal individuals excrete less than 60 mg of cystine per 1.73 m² of body surface area per day, whereas patients who are homozygous for cystinuria often have excretion rates greater than 400 mg/1.73 m²/day. Patients with nonspecific proximal renal tubular aminoaciduria may excrete as much as 200 mg of cystine/1.73 m²/day. The solubility of cystine in urine is approximately 250 mg/L up to pH 7.0 and rises sharply with higher pH, up to 500 mg/L or more above pH 7.5.[73]

The medical therapy includes high fluid intake, diet, urinary alkalization, and medications.[74,75] The treatment goal in this condition is to maintain a high fluid intake of 1.5 to 2.0 L/m²/24 h to maintain a urinary cystine concentration of less than 300 mg/L. The fluid intake should be distributed throughout the day and night. More than in any other stone disease, nocturnal diuresis is of crucial importance. Patients should ideally drink a large amount of water before going to sleep and get up at least once at night to void and have additional water intake. Furthermore, the urine needs to be alkalinized to a pH of 7.5. To attain a urinary pH of 7.5, the daily alkali dose of sodium bicarbonate or potassium citrate can reach 3 to 4 mEq/kg/day. Patients should be instructed to monitor their urinary pH and to maintain pH between 7.0 and 8.0. Because cystine excretion correlates with dietary sodium intake, a low-salt diet is indicated combined with high fruit juice (mostly citrus) intake. The latter contain citric acid and potassium, thus increasing both diuresis and alkali load. The diet should be normal RDA for protein, and patients should avoid excessive protein intake because the precursor for cystine is the methionine amino acid in dietary proteins.

In children in whom hydration, decreased salt intake, and urinary alkalinization have failed, D-penicillamine, or α-mercaptopropionylglycine (tiopronin, Thiola) may be used. Both these compounds are sulfhydryls that cleave cystine into two cysteine moieties to form mixed disulfides, which are 50 times more soluble than cystine. Tiopronin, (Thiola) forms a mixed disulfide of Thiola-cysteine, which is then excreted. D-penicillamine is administered at a dose of 20 to 50 mg/kg/day in divided doses, with half of the daily dose taken at bedtime because urinary cystine concentration is maximal during the night. The dose for α-mercaptopropinyl glycine (Thiola) is 15 mg/kg/day. The therapy should be supplemented with pyridoxine hydrochloride (vitamin $B_6$) 25 to 50 mg/day because of the antipyridoxine effect of the drug. The adverse effects of D-penicillamine include skin rash, fever, lymphadenopathy, and loss of taste. Proteinuria may develop after several months of treatment and may progress to nephrotic syndrome, which improves on discontinuation of therapy. Because of the potential for serious toxic effects associated with its long-term use, it is recommended to either discontinue therapy or maintain only the bedtime dose as prophylaxis when calculi are no longer present. Captopril, which is a sulfhydryl agent, has been used with mixed results in cystinuria. The surgical therapy includes lithotomy with or without chemolysis with N-acetylcysteine, D-penicillamine, Thiola or tromethamine under the direction of the urologist.

## INFECTION CALCULI

Infection-related stones constitute approximately 2% to 3% of the stones in children and are more common in young children. "Infection stone," "infection-induced stones," and "triple-phosphates stones" are all synonymous terms that refer to magnesium ammonium phosphate or struvite ($MgNH_4 PO_4 \cdot 6H_2O$) and carbonate apatite ($Ca_{10}[PO_4]_6CO_3$) stones. The formation of struvite stones requires an alkaline urinary pH, which is provided by breakdown of urea by uropathogens, such as *Proteus* and *Staphylococcus aureus*, and less commonly *Klebsiella, Serratia, Pseudomonas,* and *Staphylococcus epidermis*, which produce urease.

Abnormalities of the genitourinary tract, especially the presence of obstruction, predispose to the formation of infected stones. Infection with the previously mentioned organisms sometimes produces a soft radiolucent mucoid substance called a *matrix concretion* that may calcify rapidly into a radiopaque stone and account for some of the rapid formation of struvite stones seen in clinical practice. These stones can completely fill and form a cast of the pelvicalyceal system and are known as *staghorn calculi*. These staghorn calculi have the potential of causing severe urinary obstruction, pyelonephritis, and urosepsis. One of the essential management strategies in infection-related stones is to sterilize the urinary tract. As with any other infected foreign body, surgical removal of the offending agent may become necessary to sterilize the biologic system. Staghorn calculi in children invariably must be removed and, rarely, nephrectomy may be required. In some selected cases, irrigation with hemiacridin or buffered citrate to dissolve struvite stones has been used. Acetohydroxaminic acid is a urease inhibitor that has been used to reduce production of urinary ammonia and carbon dioxide to decrease struvite stone formation, but does not dissolve the struvite stones once they are formed. This has been used effectively in adults but has been limited by its psychoneurologic and musculointegumentary side effects, and, therefore not yet been approved for use in children.[76] With improved management of both pediatric obstructive uropathy and UTIs, infection-related stones are rarely seen today in industrialized countries.

## IDIOPATHIC CALCULI

In a number of children in whom a stone is not retrieved, routine urine chemistry analysis may be normal. In such cases an investigation for less common causes such as hypomagnesemia should be done. If still normal, we recommend as first step only nonpharmacologic interventions, including high fluid intake and an appropriate diet (see later). On rare occasions, the addition of potassium citrate is needed. We believe

---

### KEY POINTS

Therapy of cysteine stones is complex and can be frustrating because of stone recurrence. Principles include:

- Adequate hydration and urine volume
- Alkalinizing urine with oral bicarbonate ( maintain pH 7 to 8)
- Citrate fruit supplement
- Low dietary salt
- Avoid excessive dietary protein
- D-penicillamine
- Tiopronin, Thiola
- Captopril
- Cystine stones are resistant to ESWL
- Surgical removal, such as endourologic basketing or lithotomy may be necessary

that this is due to the fact that although each of the individual biochemical variables, such as calcium, uric acid, oxalate, and citrate, still may be within the normal range, under certain condition their product(s) may exceed supersaturation.

# MEDICAL MANAGEMENT OF UROLITHIASIS

Renal colic requires symptomatic treatment with quick pain control (narcotic analgesics), hydration (oral or parenteral flow rate equaling 1.5 to 2.0 times maintenance), and prophylactic antibiotics (after appropriate cultures have been obtained). Children need to be admitted to the hospital if they have intractable vomiting, intractable pain, UTI with obstruction, single kidney, or transplanted kidney. After resolution of renal colic, a course of expectant observation may be recommended for small (<4 mm) distal ureter or nonobstructed renal stones while urine is strained for stone retrieval. Stones 4 mm or greater in diameter rarely pass spontaneously and most of the time require surgical intervention.[77] In adults, combination treatment with nifedipine and corticosteroids, and more recently nonsteroidal anti-inflammatories combined with $\alpha_1$ blockers, may enhance stone expulsion.[49,78] In cases of stones causing intractable pain, large obstructing stones, or anuria (solitarily functioning kidney or bilateral stones), urgent surgical treatment is necessary.

One of the greatest risk factors for pediatric urinary stone formation is a low urinary flow rate. A high fluid intake is critical in preventing supersaturation of the urine regardless of the cause of urolithiasis. Children with urolithiasis have a lower diagnostic 24-hour urine volume than do normal children.[16] Furthermore, global warming and other conditions of hot ambience may result in insufficient urine output in spite of adequate fluid intake.[79] We recommend that children drink enough fluids to have urine that has no color to it. We advise the family to prepare daily, in advance, the fluids the child needs to consume with an optional reward system. As discussed earlier, minimal recommended fluid intake can be "tailored" for each patient based on weight and 24-hour urine volume. This amount should be further increased during outdoor activities in hot days.

---

### KEY POINT

Higher fluid intake is required during outdoor activities in hot days. The rule of thumb is that "the urine should look like water."

---

Based on epidemiologic observations there is no doubt that diet plays a role in urolithiasis.[1] Robertson et al.[4] showed the increased consumption of animal protein in Leeds, UK correlated with increased incidence of calcium oxalate stone in the population. Borghi et al.[80] showed that in men with recurrent calcium oxalate stones and hypercalciuria, restricted intake of animal protein (54 g/day) and salt

(50 mmol/day), combined with a normal calcium intake (30 mmol/day), provides greater protection than the traditional low-calcium diet (10 mmol/day). Curhan et al.[81] showed that high intake of phytate, present in fruits, vegetables, and whole grains, lowered the risk for kidney stones in younger women. Shuster et al.[82] showed that patients who consumed more than 160 mL of phosphoric acid containing soft drinks at the time of diagnosis of a stone had a significantly higher recurrence-free interval if the soda was discontinued. The association between consumption of sugar-sweetened soda and higher risk for stone formation was recently confirmed by Ferraro et al.[83] Thus, it appears that the more we deviate from a traditional balanced diet with normal intake of protein, salt, fruits, and vegetables and supplement them with rich fast foods and artificial drinks, the more we increase our risk for urolithiasis. Therefore, a diet with RDA protein and calcium intake, low in sodium and oxalate, and rich in potassium is recommended for children with hypercalciuria and idiopathic stones. In those with absorptive oxaluria, a low-oxalate, low-fat, and high-calcium diet is recommended and in those with hyperuricosuria, a diet low in purines.[49] In adults, higher dietary magnesium intake was found to have a beneficial effect in preventing stone formation.[38]

# SURGERY IN MANAGEMENT OF URINARY CALCULI

A surgical approach may be necessary in children with obstructive or infected urolithiasis. The factors that must be taken into account when selecting the choice of surgical therapy for urolithiasis depends on the size of the calculus, its location and composition, and the associated urinary tract anatomy. The surgical approach to urolithiasis may consist of extracorporeal shock wave lithotripsy (ESWL), percutaneous nephrolithotomy (PCNL), endoscopic basket extraction (Figure 51.10), open surgical approach or a combination of these different techniques.[84]

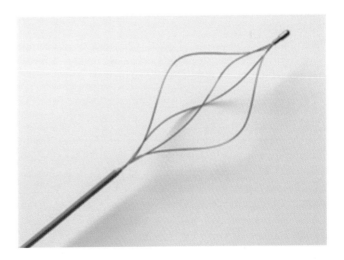

Figure 51.10 Uroendoscopic basket used to extract ureteric stones by ureteroscopy.

ESWL is frequently used in children with urolithiasis. Urolithiasis from uric acid and calcium oxalate dihydrate calculi is most responsive to ESWL; calcium oxalate monohydrate, struvite, and brushite are more difficult to fragment, whereas cystine calculi are resistant to ESWL. ESWL has a good success rate and is applicable in almost 80% of the pediatric stones. Its role may be still limited in children with large calculi, lower pole stones, and stones in anatomically abnormal urinary tract.[85] ESWL is safe and effective, with very little difference in success rates among different lithotriptors. Although renal blood flow is reduced transiently following ESWL, no significant decreases in mean ipsilateral and total glomerular filtration rate, or long-term lesions on dimercaptsuccinic acid (DMSA) renal scans have been identified in children undergoing ESWL.[86,87] The common side effects observed with ESWL are renal or perinephric hematoma, post-treatment flank pain, gross hematuria, and trauma to extrarenal tissues lying in the blast path, such as skin bruising at the entry site of the shock wave, and pulmonary impacts (infiltrates, contusion, and hemoptysis).

Percutaneous nephrolithotomy can be used alone or in combination with other surgical techniques in management of urolithiasis. It is especially useful in children with a large stone burden, orthopedic rods for spine stabilization, or a history of renal surgery. A percutaneous access to the renal pelvis is established, and a rigid or flexible nephroscope is used to manipulate the calculi. Currently available nephroscopes can accommodate laser, electrohydraulic, or ultrasonic probes; grasping forceps; basket extractors; or a combination. The calculi can then be broken down and extracted. The procedure carries the risk for significant blood loss requiring transfusion and possible urosepsis. Similarly, endoscopic procedures using ureteroscopes and cystoscopes can be used to remove a calculus using basket retrieval, grasping forceps, electrohydraulic, or ultrasonic or laser lithotripsy. Open surgery is required for calculi that are not amenable to ESWL, PCNL, or endoscopic techniques. In recent years with improved imaging techniques and pediatric-dedicated instrumentation, there has been a rise in use of endoscopic extraction and percutaneous approach and decrease in ESWL, with open surgery being extremely rarely used.[88] In children with severe stone burden, complex urinary anatomy, or previous surgical procedures, a combination of these techniques may be used together or in succession.

## OUTCOME

The literature suggests that 50% of adults will have a recurrence within 10 years, depending on the type of urolithiasis.[49] Recent reports indicate higher risk for ESRD in adults with urolithiasis.[89,90] Noe,[91] on follow-up of 27 of 44 children with hypercalciuric stones, found that 9 (33%) developed a recurrence 3 to 15 years after the initial episode (mean 7.2).[91] There was a significant association with a positive family history of stones in first-degree relatives. Hypercalciuria was the main risk factor for recurrence of stones with or

without structural abnormality. In a randomized controlled study, Soygur et al.[92] have shown that 60 mEq/day of potassium citrate given to adults with calcium oxalate stones after ESWL significantly reduced the recurrence rate. Thus, the benefits of potassium citrate and thiazide therapy have to be weighed against the risk of long-term use of these medications, especially in children presenting with a first-time idiopathic stone. Thus, we emphasize the need to develop healthy eating and drinking habits in all children with a stone and consider drug therapy only in children in whom we can identify an underlying metabolic disorder or children who develop recurrent stones.

## SUMMARY

There is a general agreement on the worldwide increase in incidence of pediatric urolithiasis. Whereas part of this increase may be due to improved diagnostic techniques, other reasons are environmental, mostly changes in dietary habits and climate conditions. The most common causes of pediatric urolithiasis include insufficient fluid intake and hypercalciuria, followed by hypocitraturia. The best diagnostic tool is noncontrast CT, but because of the involved radiation its use should be limited and instead urinary tract ultrasound used. The 24-hour urine collection biochemistry analysis continues to be the gold standard for diagnosis and the intervention based on it (at times assisted by blood chemistry findings). High fluid intake is the universal treatment for all types of kidney stones and should be part of public health policy. Similarly, public education about the opposing roles of dietary sodium and potassium in calcium stone formation should be promoted. If nonpharmacologic intervention does not correct the urine biochemical abnormalities, pharmacologic intervention is indicated. The latter is often the case in patients with noncalcium stones.

## ACKNOWLEDGMENTS

This work was supported by the Sam and Helen Kaplan Research Fund in Pediatric Nephrology. We thank Ms. Regina Johnson for her excellent administrative assistance.

## REFERENCES

1. Trinchieri A. Epidemiology of urolithiasis. Arch Ital Urol Androl. 1996;68:203–49.
2. Monk RD, Bushinsky DA. Nephrolithiasis and nephrocalcinosis. In: Johnson RJ, Feehally J, editors. Comprehensive Clinical Nephrology, 2nd ed. New York: Mosby; 2003. p 731–44.

3. Hamm LL, Alpern RJ. Regulation of acid-base balance, citrate, and urine pH. In: Coe FL, Favus MS, Pak CYC, et al., editors. Kidney Stones: Medical and Surgical Management. Philadelphia: Lippincott-Raven; 1996. p 289–302.

4. Robertson WG, Peacock M. The pattern of urinary stone disease in Leeds and in the United Kingdom in relation to animal protein intake during the period 1960-1980. Urol Int. 1982;37:394–9.

5. Better OS, Shabtai M, Kedar S, et al. Increased incidence of nephrolithiasis in lifeguards in Israel. Adv Exp Med Biol. 1980;128:467–72.

6. Lattimer JK, Hubbard M. Pediatric urologic admissions. J Urol. 1951:66:289–93.

7. Bass HN, Emanuel B. Nephrolithiasis in childhood. J Urol. 1966;95:749–53.

8. Troup CW, Lawnicki CC, Bourne RB, Hodgson NB. Renal calculus in children. J Urol. 1972;107:306–7.

9. Malek RS, Kelalis PP. Pediatric nephrolithiasis. J Urol. 1975;113:545–51.

10. Stapleton FB, McKay CP, Noe HN. Urolithiasis in children: The role of hypercalciuria. Pediatr Ann. 1987;16:980–1, 984–92.

11. Milliner DS, Murphy ME. Urolithiasis in pediatric patients. Mayo Clin Proc. 1993;68:241–8.

12. Osorio AV, Alon US. The relationship between urinary calcium, sodium, and potassium excretion and the role of potassium in treating idiopathic hypercalciuria. Pediatrics. 1997;100:675–81.

13. Penido MG, Srivastava T, Alon US. Pediatric primary urolithiasis: 12-year experience at a Midwestern Children's Hospital. J Urol. 2013;189:1493–7.

14. Routh JC, Graham DA, Nelson CP. Epidemiological trends in pediatric urolithiasis at United States freestanding pediatric hospitals. J Urol. 2010;184:1100–4.

15. Sas DJ, Hulsey TC, Shatat IF, Orak JK. Increasing incidence of kidney stones in children evaluated in the emergency department. J Pediatr. 2010;157:132–7.

16. Miller LA, Stapleton FB. Urinary volume in children with urolithiasis. J Urol. 1989;141:918–20.

17. Alon US, Zimmerman H, Alon M. Evaluation and treatment of pediatric idiopathic urolithiasis revisited. Pediatr Nephrol. 2004;19:516–20.

18. Farell G, Huang E, Kim SY, et al. Modulation of proliferating renal epithelial cell affinity of calcium oxalate monohydrate crystals. J Am Soc Nephrol. 2004;15:3052–62.

19. Ciftcioglu N, Bjorklund M, Kuorikoski K, et al. Nanobacteria: An infectious cause for kidney stone formation. Kidney Int. 1999;56:1893–8.

20. Adachi J, Kumar C, Zhang Y, et al. The human urinary proteome contains more than 1500 proteins, including a large proportion of membrane proteins. Genome Biol. 2006;7:R80.

21. Doyle IR, Ryall RL, Marshall VR. Inclusion of proteins into calcium oxalate crystals precipitated from human urine: A highly selective phenomenon. Clin Chem. 1991;37:1589–94.

22. Grover PK, Thurgood LA, Fleming DE, et al. Intracrystalline urinary proteins facilitate degradation and dissolution of calcium oxalate crystals in cultured renal cells. Am J Physiol Renal Physiol. 2008;294:F355–61.

23. Yamate T, Kohri K, Umekawa T, et al. The effect of osteopontin on the adhesion of calcium oxalate crystals to Madin-Darby canine kidney cells. Eur Urol. 1996;30:388–93.

24. Stapleton FB. Idiopathic hypercalciuria: Association with isolated hematuria and risk for urolithiasis in children. The Southwest Pediatric Nephrology Study Group. Kidney Int. 1990;37:807–11.

25. Tekin A, Tekgul S, Atsu N, et al. A study of the etiology of idiopathic calcium urolithiasis in children: Hypocitruria is the most important risk factor. J Urol. 2000;164:162–5.

26. Kielb S, Koo HP, Bloom DA, Faerber GJ. Nephrolithiasis associated with the ketogenic diet. J Urol. 2000;164:464–6.

27. Barroso U, Jednak R, Fleming P et al. Bladder calculi in children who perform clean intermittent catheterization. BJU Int 2000;85:879-84.

28. Mathoera RB, Kok DJ, Nijman RJ. Bladder calculi in augmentation cystoplasty in children. Urology 2000;56:482–7.

29. Silver RI, Gros DA, Jeffs RD, Gearhart JP. Urolithiasis in the exstrophy-epispadias complex. J Urol 1997;158:1322-6.

30. Gambaro G, Vezzoli G, Casari G, et al. Genetics of hypercalciuria and calcium nephrolithias: From the rare monogenic to the common polygenic forms. Am J Kidney Dis. 2004;44:963–86.

31. Richmond W, Colgan G, Simon S, et al. Random urine calcium/osmolality in the assessment of calciuria in children with decreased muscle mass. Clin Nephrol. 2005;64:264–70.

32. Roth CS, Bowyer BA, Berquist TH. Utility of the plain abdominal radiograph for diagnosing ureteral calculi. Ann Emerg Med. 1985;14:311–5.

33. Fielding JR, Steele G, Fox LA et al. Spiral computerized tomography in the evaluation of acute flank pain: A replacement for excretory urography. J Urol. 1997;157:2071–3.

34. Sinclair D, Wilson S, Toi A, Greenspan L. The evaluation of suspected renal colic: Ultrasound scan versus excretory urography. Ann Emerg Med. 1989;18:556–9.

35. Alon U, Warady BA, Hellerstein S. Hypercalciuria in the frequency-dysuria syndrome of childhood. J Pediatr. 1990;116:103–5.

36. Stapleton FB, Roy S 3rd, Noe HN, Jerkins G. Hypercalciuria in children with hematuria. N Engl J Med. 1984;310:1345–8.

37. Garcia CD, Miller LA, Stapleton FB. Natural history of hematuria associated with hypercalciuria in children. Am J Dis Child. 1991;145:1204–7.

38. Taylor EN, Stampfer, MJ, Curhan GC. Dietary factors and the risk of incident kidney stones in men: Insights after 14 years of follow-up. J Am Soc Nephrol. 2004;15:3325–32.

39. Meschi T, Maggiore U, Fiaccadori E et al. The effect of fruits and vegetables on urinary stone risk factors. Kidney Int. 2004;66:2402–10.

40. Nesterova G, Malicdan MC, Yasuda K, et al. 1,25-(OH)2D-24 hydroxylase (CYP24A1) deficiency as a cause of nephrolithiasis. Clin J Am Soc Nephrol. 2013;8:649–57.

41. Coe FL, Favus MJ, Crockett T, et al. Effects of low-calcium diet on urine calcium excretion, parathyroid function and serum 1,25(OH)2D3 levels in patients with idiopathic hypercalciuria and in normal subjects. Am J Med. 1982;72:25–32.

42. Aladjem M, Barr J, Lahat E, Bistritzer T. Renal and absorptive hypercalciuria: A metabolic disturbance with varying and interchanging modes of expression. Pediatrics. 1996;97:216–9.

43. Srivastava T, Alon US. Pathophysiology of hypercalciuria in children. Pediatr Nephrol. 2007;22:1659–73.

44. Muñoz KA, Krebs-Smith SM, Ballard-Barbash R, Cleveland LE. Food intakes of US children and adolescents compared with recommendations. Pediatrics. 1997;100:323–9.

45. Parks JH, Worcester EM, Coe FL, et al. Clinical implications of abundant calcium phosphate in routinely analyzed kidney stone. Kidney Int. 2004;66:777–85.

46. Wolfgram DF, Gundu V, Astor BC, et al. Hydrochlorothiazide compared to chlorthalidone in reduction of urinary calcium in patients with kidney stones. Urolithiasis. 2013;41:315–22.

47. Alon U, Costanzo L, Chan JCM. Additive hypocalciuric effects of amiloride and hydrochlorothiazide in patients treated with calcitrol. Miner Electrolyte Metab. 1984;10:379–86.

48. Vescini F, Buffa A, La Manna G, et al. Long-term potassium citrate therapy and bone mineral density in idiopathic calcium stone formers. J Endocrinol Invest. 2005;28:218–22.

49. Xu H, Zisman AL, Coe FL, et al. Kidney stones: An update on current pharmacological management and future directions. Expert Opin Pharmacother. 2013;14:435–47.

50. Freundlich M, Alon US. Bisphosphonates in children with hypercalciuria and reduced bone mineral density. Pediatr Nephrol. 2008;23:2215–20.

51. Thorleifsson G, Holm H, Edvardsson V, et al. Sequence variants in the CLDN14 gene associate with kidney stones and bone mineral density. Nat Genet. 2009;41:926–30.

52. García-Nieto V, Ferrández C, Monge M, et al. Bone mineral density in pediatric patients with idiopathic hypercalciuria. Pediatr Nephrol. 1997;11:578–83.

53. Penido MG, Lima EM, Marino VS, et al. Bone alterations in children with idiopathic hypercalciuria at the time of diagnosis. Pediatr Nephrol. 2003;18:133–9

54. Schwaderer AL, Cronin R, Mahan JD, Bates CM. Low bone density in children with hypercalciuria and/or nephrolithiasis. Pediatr Nephrol. 2008;23:2209–14.

55. Schwaderer AL, Srivastava T, Schueller L, et al. Dietary modifications alone do not improve bone mineral density in children with idiopathic hypercalciuria. Clin Nephrol. 2011;76:341–7.

56. Alon U, Hellerstein S, Warady BA. Oral acetazolamide in the assessment of (urine-blood) pCO2. Pediatr Nephrol. 1991;5:307–11.

57. Bonilla-Felix M, Villegas-Medina O, Vehaskari VM. Renal acidification in children with idiopathic hypercalciuria. J Pediatr. 1994;124:529–34.

58. Srivastava T, Winston MJ, Auron A, et al. Urine calcium/citrate ratio in children with hypercalciuric stones. Pediatr Res. 2009;66:85–90.

59. Arrabal-Polo MA, Arrabal-Martin M, Arias-Santiago S, et al. Importance of citrate and the calcium: Citrate ratio in patients with calcium renal lithiasis and severe lithogenesis. BJU Int. 2013;111:622–7.

60. MacDougall L, Taheri S, Crofton P. Biochemical risk factors for stone formation in a Scottish paediatric hospital population. Ann Clin Biochem. 2010;47:125–30.

61. Baia Lda C, Baxmann AC, Moreira SR, et al. Noncitrus alkaline fruit: A dietary alternative for the treatment of hypocitraturic stone formers. J Endourol. 2012;26:1221–6.

62. Penniston KL, Steele TH, Nakada SY. Lemonade therapy increases urinary citrate and urine volumes in patients with recurrent calcium oxalate stone formation. Urology. 2007;70:856–60.

63. Sidhu H, Hoppe B, Hesse A, et al. Absence of Oxalobacter formigenes in cystic fibrosis patients: A risk factor for hyperoxaluria. Lancet. 1998;352:1026–9.

64. Monico CG, Olson JB, Milliner DS. Determinants of pyridoxine responsiveness in primary hyperoxaluria type I. Pediatr Res. 2004:55:576A

65. Van Woerden CS, Groothoff JW, Wijburg FA, et al. Clinical implications of mutations analysis in primary hyperoxaluria type 1. Kidney Int. 2004;66:746–52.

66. Stapleton FB, Nash DA. A screening test for hyperuricosuria. J Pediatr. 1983102:88–90.

67. Matos V, Van Melle G, Werner D, et al. Urinary oxalate and urate to creatinine ratios in a healthy pediatric population. Am J Kidney Dis. 1999;34:e6.

68. Cameron JS, Moro F, Simmonds HA. Gout, uric acid and purine metabolism in paediatric nephrology. Pediatr Nephrol. 1993;7:105–18.

69. Maalouf NM, Sakhaee K, Parks JH, et al. Association of urinary pH with body weight in nephrolithiasis. Kidney Int. 2004;65:1422–5.

70. Dello-Strologo L, Pras E, Pontesilli C, et al. Comparison between *SLC3A1* and *SLC7A9* cystinuria patients and carriers: A need for a new classification. J Am Soc Nephrol. 2002;13:2547–53.

71. Font-Llitjós M, Jiménez-Vidal M, Bisceglia L, et al. New insights into cystinuria: 40 new mutations, genotype-phenotype correlation, and digenic inheritance causing partial phenotype. J Med Genet. 2005;42:58–68.

72. Sakhaee K, Poindexter JR, Pak CY. The spectrum of metabolic abnormalities in patients with cystine nephrolithiasis. J Urol. 1989;141:89–21.

73. Joly D, Rieu P, Mejean A, et al. Treatment of cystinuria. Pediatr Nephrol. 1999;13:945–50.

74. Claes DJ, Jackson E. Cystinuria: Mechanisms and management. Pediatr Nephrol. 2012;27:2031–8.

75. Chillarón J, Font-Llitjós M, Fort J, Zorzano A, et al. Pathophysiology and treatment of cystinuria. Nat Rev Nephrol. 2010;6:424–34.

76. Griffith DP, Gleeson MJ, Lee H, et al. Randomized, double-blind trial of Lithostat (acetohydroxamic acid) in the palliative treatment of infection-induced urinary calculi. Eur Urol. 1991;20:243–7.

77. Van Savage JG, Palanca LG, Andersen RD, et al. Treatment of distal ureteral stones in children: Similarities to the American Urological Association guidelines in adults. J Urol. 2000;164:1089–93.

78. Porpiglia F, Destefanis P, Fiori C, et al. Effectiveness of nifedipine and deflazacort in the management of distal ureter stones. Urology. 2000;56:579–2.

79. Masterson JH, Jourdain VJ, Collard DA, et al. Changes in urine parameters after desert exposure: Assessment of stone risk in United States Marines transiently exposed to a desert environment. J Urol. 2013;189:165–70.

80. Borghi L, Schianchi T, Meschi T, et al. Comparison of two diets for the prevention of recurrent stones in idiopathic hypercalciuria. N Engl J Med. 2002;346:77–84.

81. Curhan GC, Willett WC, Knight EL, et al. Dietary factors and the risk of incident kidney stones in younger women (Nurses Health Study II). J Am Soc Nephrol. 2003;14:698–91.

82. Shuster J, Jenkins A, Logan C, et al. Soft drink consumption and urinary stone recurrence: A randomized prevention trial. J Clin Epidemiol. 1992;45:911–6.

83. Ferraro PM, Taylor EN, Gambaro G, et al. Soda and other beverages and the risk of kidney stones. Clin J Am Soc Nephrol. 2013;8:1389–95.

84. Lottmann H, Gagnadoux MF, Daudon M. Urolithiasis in children. In: Gearhart JP, Rink RC, Mouriquano PDE, editors. Pediatric Urology. Philadelphia: WB Saunders; 2001. p 828–59.

85. Esen T, Krautschick A, Alken P. Treatment update on pediatric urolithiasis. World J Urol. 1997;15:195-202.

86. Goel MC, Baserge NS, Babu RV, et al. Pediatric kidney: Functional outcome after extracorporeal shock wave lithotripsy. J Urol. 1996;155:2044–6.

87. Lottmann HB, Archambaud F, Hellal B, et al. 99mTechnetium-dimercapto-succinic acid renal scan in the evaluation of potential long-term renal parenchymal damage associated with extracorporeal shock wave lithotripsy in children. J Urol. 1998;159:521–4.

88. Salerno A, Nappo SG, Matarazzo E, et al. Treatment of pediatric renal stones in a Western country: A changing pattern. J Pediatr Surg. 2013;48:835–9.

89. El-Zoghby ZM, Lieske JC, Foley RN, et al. Urolithiasis and the risk of ESRD. Clin J Am Soc Nephrol. 2012;7:1409–15.

90. Alexander RT, Hemmelgarn BR, Wiebe N, et al. Kidney stones and kidney function loss: A cohort study. BMJ. 2012;345:e5287.

91. Noe HN. Hypercalciuria and pediatric stone recurrences with and without structural abnormalities. J Urol. 2000;164:1094–6.

92. Soygur T, Akbay A, Kupeli S. Effect of potassium citrate therapy on stone recurrence and residual fragments after shockwave lithotripsy in lower caliceal calcium oxalate urolithiasis: A randomized controlled trial. J Endourol. 2002;16:149–52.

## REVIEW QUESTIONS

1. The greatest risk factor for pediatric stone formation is:
   a. Hypercalciuria
   b. Low urine flow
   c. Hypocitraturia
   d. Hyperoxaluria

2. A child with body weight of 50 kg has a 24-hour urine volume of 700 mL. The additional daily fluid intake recommended for this child will be:
   a. 300 mL
   b. 400 mL
   c. 500 mL
   d. 600 mL

3. In a teenager with idiopathic hypercalciuria, dietary intervention will include:
   a. Sodium intake of 2000 to 2300 and potassium intake of 3000 to 3500 mg/day
   b. Sodium intake of 1500 to 1800 and potassium intake of 3000 to 3500 mg/day
   c. Sodium intake of 1500 to 1800 and potassium intake of 2000 to 2500 mg/day
   d. Sodium intake of 2000 to 2300 and potassium intake of 2000 to 2500 mg/day

4. The risk in administrating potassium citrate is:
   a. Upset stomach
   b. Development of hypercholesterolemia

c. Severe diarrhea
d. Rendering the urine too alkaline
5. When employing thiazide diuretics:
   a. Sodium intake should be liberalized
   b. K-citrate should not be used concomitantly
   c. The addition of amiloride is beneficial
   d. Osteopenia may worsen
6. Numerical goals in managing children with hypercalciuria-to-hypocitraturia include:
   a. Urine calcium/citrate ratio < 0.20 and Na/K ratio < 2.5
   b. Urine calcium/citrate ratio < 0.33 and Na/K ratio < 2.5
   c. Urine calcium/citrate ratio < 0.20 and Na/K ratio < 3.5
   d. Urine calcium/citrate ratio < 0.33 and Na/K ratio < 3.5
7. Gastrointestinal issues causing hypocitraturia are usually associated with:
   a. Severe constipation
   b. Fat malabsorption
   c. Gastroesophageal reflux
   d. Chronic diarrhea
8. Mild absorptive hyperoxaluria is best treated by:
   a. Dietary oxalate restriction
   b. Administration of *Oxalobacter formigenes*
   c. Dietary calcium supplementation
   d. Avoidance of food high in fat

9. High incidence of uric acid stones in obese population is due to:
   a. Diet rich in purines
   b. Diet rich in salt
   c. Decreased ammonia production
   d. Insufficient fluid intake
10. To protect against stone formation in children on ketogenic diets, it is advisable to give:
    a. Potassium citrate
    b. Thiazide diuretics
    c. Allopurinol
    d. Magnesium oxide

## ANSWER KEY

1. b
2. c
3. a
4. d
5. c
6. b
7. d
8. c
9. c
10. a

# Voiding disorders

## HANS G. POHL

Derangements in the normal pattern of micturition result in a variety of urinary tract symptoms and morbidity. Such voiding disorders range from mild manifestations that represent no more than a social nuisance to severe dysfunctional elimination associated with recurrent cystitis, acute pyelonephritis, or both; hydronephrosis; and vesicoureteral reflux (VUR). Voiding disorders in children result from immature bladder function, abnormal voiding habits, and urinary sphincter dysfunction. Recurrent urinary tract infections (UTIs) and upper urinary tract changes resulting from voiding dysfunction, are generally seen in severe sphincter dysfunction associated with high bladder pressure generated during voiding, incomplete bladder emptying, functional bladder outlet obstruction, or a combination of these. Rarely, anatomic causes of incontinence are encountered from conditions such as spina bifida, posterior urethral valve, and prune belly syndrome that can affect the bladder, the urinary sphincter, or both. Diet and social factors also influence toileting behavior and need to be addressed early in the management of these patients.

## NORMAL VOIDING

A normal voiding cycle is a two-phase process, consisting of low-pressure and adequate volume bladder filling, followed by complete evacuation of the bladder.[1] Both of these phases of the voiding cycle are coordinated and active processes.

Bladder filling requires inhibition of bladder contraction and increased tone of the urinary sphincter complex. As the bladder approaches fullness, tension receptors in the bladder wall trigger afferent nerves that send signals of the need to void. Voluntary voiding involves inhibition of sphincter contractions and coordinated contraction of the bladder smooth muscle.

In the neonate, bladder filling is followed by reflexive emptying (voiding reflex). This reflexive micturition cycle is controlled by the sacral spinal cord and occurs approximately hourly. After 6 months of age, the urinary volumes increase and the frequency of voiding decreases as the control of voiding shifts from the sacral cord to the pontine voiding center, thus establishing the spino-bulbo-spinal reflex pathway.[2,3]

Around the age of 2 years, the child develops conscious sensation of bladder fullness and has urge incontinence. Between 2 and 4 years of age, the child acquires voluntary control of bowel and bladder function in the following sequence: (1) nocturnal bowel control, (2) daytime bowel control, (3) daytime bladder control, and (4) nocturnal bladder control.

A majority of children demonstrate an adult voiding pattern by 4 years of age. The timing of this sequence is influenced by ethnic, cultural, economic, and individual family differences. In the United States, the mean age at which daytime urinary control is achieved is 2 to 3 years but may vary from 1 to 5 years.[4] Of children 4 to 9 years of age, 5% to 10% may experience at least some daytime wetting.[4] In general, most school-aged children void between four and six times daily.[4]

Many functional and anatomic disturbances of voiding manifest as wetting. Thus, we have organized the discussion of these entities by the likelihood of renal damage associated with each (Table 52.1). In this classification, conditions such as daytime frequency syndrome, giggle incontinence, and overactive bladder (OAB) that are not associated with upper urinary tract injury, do not require extensive imaging or intensive follow-up. Alternatively, voiding disorders such as dysfunctional elimination, Hinman syndrome, posterior urethral valve (PUV), and neurospinal dysraphisms may cause deterioration of renal functions by virtue of high-pressure voiding and UTI. Three miscellaneous conditions—cerebral palsy (CP), attention deficit/hyperactivity disorder, and hypercalciuria—are addressed as well.

## EPIDEMIOLOGY

Urinary incontinence is frustrating for parents, socially ostracizing to patients and, and often regarded as a clinical nuisance by many physicians. It is estimated that approximately 417,000 visits to pediatrician's offices are made annually for incontinence, with primary nocturnal enuresis (PNE) representing 38% of these cases. Of such children, 75% are evaluated between 3 and 10 years of age, and 15% to 20% are between 11 and 17 years of age.[5]

The rate of outpatient visits for PNE in both the commercially insured and Medicaid populations has more than doubled from approximately 100 per 100,000 children to 283 per 100,000 children in the 6-year period from 1994 to 2000.[5] Whether there is a true increase in the prevalence of childhood incontinence or merely an increased awareness of the need to treat has led to increased referrals is unclear. Urinary incontinence in children must be evaluated in the context of the child's age, because attainment of daytime and nighttime urinary control follows a predictable maturational process. For instance, urinary incontinence is quite a normal phenomenon in children under the age of 3 years.

Table 52.1 Clinical classification of voiding disorders in children

**Low Risk for Upper Urinary Tract Deterioration**
Daytime frequency syndrome
Postvoid dribbling
Giggle incontinence
Stress urinary incontinence
Primary nocturnal enuresis
Paradoxical incontinence or ectopic ureter in girls
Sensory deficient bladder
Overactive bladder

**High Risk for Upper Urinary Tract Deterioration**
Dysfunctional elimination
Non-neurogenic neuropathic bladder or Hinman syndrome
Posterior urethral valve
Neurospinal dysraphism

**Miscellaneous Causes**
Cerebral palsy
Attention deficit/hyperactivity disorder
Hypercalciuria

## DISORDERS WITH LOW RISK FOR UPPER URINARY TRACT DETERIORATION

## DAYTIME FREQUENCY SYNDROME

Daytime frequency syndrome (DFS) consists of acute-onset urinary urgency and frequency, with or without rare episodes of incontinence and without any definable clinical cause. DFS primarily affects boys 4 to 8 years old (mean, 4.5 years) and is more prevalent in the spring and fall. No certain cause for the syndrome has been established, although some authors postulate that DFS is caused by psychosocial stress with seasonal variation.[6–10] DFS is characterized by urinary frequency without dysuria that occurs every 10 to 20 minutes during the daytime but abates completely during sleep. Nocturnal enuresis (NE) is not a feature of DFS. Evaluation of the patient is by history and physical examination, with a normal urinalysis and a negative urine culture. DFS is a self-limiting disorder and requires support and reassurance. Resolution of symptoms is common without any specific therapy and can occur in 2 days to 16 months, with an average of 2.5 months.[6,11]

## POSTVOID DRIBBLING

Postvoid dribbling or vaginal voiding occurs in prepubertal girls who are very thin or obese. In both cases an abnormal position precludes the girl from adequately opening her legs, thus causing vaginal trapping of urine. Once voiding concludes, the pooled urine drains shortly after assuming an upright posture. The diagnosis may be based on history alone, with dribbling occurring shortly after voiding. Occasionally, perineal itching suggests yeast infections. The itching is usually caused by chemical irritation and does not need be treated with antifungals.

The physical examination is usually normal, or may reveal labial adherence or labiovulvar erythema. Radiographic evaluation is not warranted. Treatment consists of having the girl sit on the toilet facing the wall (backward), with the legs spread apart. If the patient is unable or unwilling to do this, a stool or seat adaptor can be used, although these are usually cumbersome. If labial adherence is present, precisely applied topical estrogen (conjugated estrogen [Premarin] ointment, 0.625 mg) applied twice daily for no longer than 6 weeks is usually curative. Concerns regarding the potential long-term risk for cancer has significantly curtailed its use by many. Instead, application of betamethasone 0.05% ointment can be offered to lyse the labial adherence. Rarely does labial adherence require surgical lysis.

In males, urethral pooling, usually in a congenital or acquired urethral diverticulum, may cause postvoid dribbling. The physical examination is normal or may show ventral penile swelling, especially following voiding. In most circumstances, the child has previously undergone a hypospadias repair. The treatment is surgical.

## GIGGLE INCONTINENCE

Giggle incontinence, or enuresis risoria, is a disorder characterized by complete bladder emptying with giggling, laughter, or exertion. This condition may be related to cataplexy, a part of narcoleptic syndrome complex. Genetically, giggle incontinence has been linked to human leukocyte antigen (HLA) DR2 and has a strong familial predisposition.[12,13] The condition occurs primarily in peripubertal girls, is rarely seen in boys, and can persist into adulthood.[13,14] The patient is dry during day and night but experiences daytime bladder emptying associated with giggling or laughing.

Characteristic history alone is sufficient for making the diagnosis of giggle incontinence. Physical examination and urinalysis are normal in most cases. Urodynamic

and radiographic evaluation are not warranted. Frequent voiding, especially before social engagements, can be adequate treatment. Anticholinergics or Kegel exercises for strengthening pelvic floor are usually not helpful. However, methylphenidate has been shown to decrease frequency of the episodes with as-needed or continuous usage.[13] Conditioning therapy with low-voltage electric shocks to the back of the hand also has been shown to be effective.[15]

## STRESS URINARY INCONTINENCE

Stress urinary incontinence is the loss of urine with physical activity, coughing, or sneezing. This occurs most commonly in adolescent and young adult female athletes. Nygaard et al.[16] studied 156 nulliparous college varsity athletes with a mean age of 19.9 years. The prevalence of incontinence while participating in their sports was 28%. Of these females, 40% had noted incontinence in high school and 17% in junior high school.[16,17]

The diagnosis of stress incontinence is made by history. Physical examination and urinalysis are usually normal. Radiographic examination is not warranted, unless evidence of spina bifida occulta exists on physical examination (e.g., hair tuft, lipoma, asymmetric gluteal crease). In these cases an MRI of the spine should be obtained to exclude spinal cord tethering.

---

### KEY POINT

Abnormal sacral or gluteal examination should always prompt radiographic examination for spinal dysraphism abnormality.

---

## PRIMARY NOCTURNAL ENURESIS

Primary nocturnal enuresis (PNE) is defined as bedwetting in an individual who has never been dry at night. When the child begins wetting the bed after a period of nighttime continence has been achieved, enuresis is termed as being secondary.[18] PNE is usually monosymptomatic and is not associated with daytime symptoms. Although NE is considered normal in infants, society expects night dryness by 5 years of age. NE affects approximately 15% of 5-year-old children, but prevalence diminishes gradually to only 3% of adolescents.[19,20] A familial form of the disease, characterized by an increased incidence of PNE in children of enuretic parents is well known.[21]

### Pathogenesis

Pathogenesis of PNE is unclear, but dysfunction of the bladder, kidneys, and central nervous system has been implicated. Urodynamic evaluation of enuretic children during waking and sleep has shown that many children with PNE have reduced bladder capacity and demonstrate overactivity, like the infantile bladder.[18] One criticism of many of these studies has been the possible inclusion of children with daytime symptoms. One study demonstrated that the incidence of bladder overactivity might be only 16% in pure monosymptomatic enuretics.[18] Nevertheless, it appears that children with enuresis may be a heterogeneous group, with some displaying reduced functional bladder capacity only during sleep. Other children with monosymptomatic enuresis have bladder overactivity during the day and at night. These patients manage to compensate during wakeful states and do not have daytime wetting. At least one study has challenged the dictum that enuresis is characterized by complete evacuation of the bladder by demonstrating elevated postvoid residual urine measurements (>10% of bladder volume) and abnormal bursts of electromyography activity suggesting sphincter dyssynergia.[22]

Urine production usually decreases at night under control of the circadian rhythm of secretion of antidiuretic hormone (ADH).[23] Loss of the normal nighttime production of ADH results in polyuria that can exceed the functional capacity of the bladder and result in enuresis. Rittig and colleagues have done much of the work on ADH mediation of enuresis, demonstrating that nocturnal urine production was significantly greater than daytime urine production in some enuretic children.[24] This finding was explained when significantly lower nocturnal levels of ADH were demonstrated in concert with large volumes of dilute urine in enuretic children.[25] Recently, aquaporin channels, ADH-responsive transmembrane proteins responsible for urinary concentration, have been implicated in the pathophysiology of enuresis.[26]

A maturational delay in the ability to sense bladder filling and inhibit bladder contraction until wakefulness has also been implicated as a causative factor in enuresis.[27,28] There are mixed reports about a sleep arousal and developmental delay in enuretics. Some authors claim that enuretics are more difficult to arouse. However, the asymptomatic siblings of such patients have been noted to be equally as hard to awaken.[29-32]

## Treatment

Treatment of NE is divided into three categories: observation, behavioral, and pharmacologic. Observation is sufficient if the wetting does not cause a major social or family disruption, especially since PNE has an annual spontaneous resolution rate of 15%. Behavioral modification or conditioning therapy in the form of an enuresis alarm requires significant motivation of the parents and child and continued use for up to 6 months. This is, however, the most effective form of treatment available, with permanent cures occurring in over 90% in well motivated families. Relapse rate can be 25% to 30% after short-term use of the alarm for 6 to 8 weeks.[33,34] Pharmacotherapy for PNE is discussed in detail later in this chapter.

## PARADOXICAL INCONTINENCE

Paradoxical incontinence is continuous dribbling despite a normal voiding pattern. This phenomenon is exclusively seen in girls and is caused by an ectopic ureteral insertion distal to the external urinary sphincter complex, with the most common ectopic ureteral site being the urethra (35%), vaginal vestibule (34%), and vagina (25%).[35] Although boys also may have distally inserting ectopic ureters, the insertion site (e.g., seminal vesicles, vas deferens) is always proximal to the external urinary sphincter and thus incontinence is prevented.[36,37]

The physical examination should include inspecting the girl's perineum with her in the frog-legged position with the labia spread. With patience, urine often can be seen pooling in the vaginal vestibule. Radiologic investigation typically relies on identifying the ectopic ureter or the renal unit it subtends. Renal bladder ultrasound, voiding cystourethrogram, intravenous pyelogram, and computed axial tomography have been used to identify the real unit responsible for the incontinence. However, the renal unit attached to such an ectopic ureter is invariably dysplastic and often poorly visualized by traditional imaging, particularly because hydronephrosis is seldom, if ever, seen. Pattaras et al.[38] reported on a small cohort of girls with paradoxical incontinence from ectopic ureters. Nuclear renal scintigraphy with technetium-99m dimercaptosuccinic acid (DMSA)

---

### KEY POINTS

- Some patients with NE have reduced bladder capacity or infantile (overactive) pattern on urodynamic studies.
- Loss of nocturnal ADH circadian rhythm can be seen in some as a cause of NE.
- Maturational delay and sleep arousal disorders have been implicated in some.

---

### KEY POINTS

- Ectopic ureter insertion causes paradoxical incontinence in females because the ureter inserts distal to the external urinary sphincter.
- Most renal units associated with an ectopically inserted ureter are very dysplastic, contributing little to total renal function.
- DMSA renal scans are the best means of identifying the dysplastic renal unit associated with an ectopic ureter.

reliably detected and localized the hypoplastic ectopic kidneys and poorly functioning upper pole moieties in each case. Thus, once the clinical presentation suggests paradoxical incontinence from an ectopic ureter, nuclear renal scintigraphy should be considered during the initial radiologic evaluation.[38–40]

## SENSORY DEFICIENT BLADDER

Young girls and occasionally boys will avoid urinating for an extended period. Typically, the patient will awaken, eat, and go to school without voiding. The first void often occurs mid-day or even after school, with the patient often rushing to the toilet. They may wet themselves on the way to the toilet or be damp already. The clinician makes the diagnosis by asking the following three questions: (1) Does the child urinate on awakening in the morning? (2) Does the child use the toilet at school? (3) How many times does the child void during a typical day?

The patient's symptoms consist of dysuria, urgency with a full bladder, bedwetting, urinary dribbling, or a combination of these. These children may present with a UTI or for workup of a fever and abdominal pain. Physical examination may be normal or demonstrate a palpable bladder. Urinalysis is likely to show bacteriuria, and urine culture may be positive. A prevoid and postvoid renal bladder ultrasound should be done to evaluate postvoid residual. The infection should be treated and antibiotic prophylaxis continued if there have been multiple UTIs and until effective frequent bladder emptying is achieved.

> ## KEY POINTS
>
> - Patients with sensory deficit bladders usually hold urine for long periods and have urinary urgency and dribbling as common symptoms
> - These patients are prone to getting UTIs.

## OVERACTIVE BLADDER

Overactive bladder (OAB) with its many synonyms (bladder instability, urge syndrome, hyperactive bladder, persistent infantile bladder, detrusor hypertonia), is the most common voiding dysfunction of childhood. Its occurrence peaks between 5 and 7 years of life, and it has an incidence of 57.4%, with a female preponderance (60.1% in females and 38.9% in males).[41] The cause of this disorder is thought to be delayed functional development of cortical inhibitory control over the voiding reflex mediated through the reticulospinal pathways or in the inhibition center of the cerebral cortex.[42–45] In response to the urge to urinate, the child learns to contract the external urinary sphincter to suppress the bladder contraction and delay voiding. In some circumstances, the child can be seen running to the toilet in response to the urgency, and incontinence occurs when the toilet is not reached in time. Other children are able to remain dry if they concentrate on their bladders but are often wet at play or when absorbed in activity of interest. Holding maneuvers (leg crossing, squatting, Vincent curtsey) are a common observation by parents and are the child's attempt to suppress the bladder contraction by exerting pressure on the external urinary sphincter.[46]

Sphincter tightening and holding maneuvers result in increased bladder muscle stretch because contraction occurs against a fixed resistance. The OAB is associated with vesicoureteral reflux in 20% to 50% of children. In such circumstances, management of VUR should include addressing the OAB as a clinical issue. Otherwise, spontaneous resolution of the VUR may be impeded and recurrent UTIs may occur.[6,47–49]

Although imaging is not warranted in the majority of children with OAB, those who are resistant to conservative management may benefit from prevoid and postvoid renal-bladder ultrasound and an assessment of postvoid residual urine volume. The sonogram can provide information regarding upper urinary tract dilatation, bladder wall thickening, and the child's ability to empty the bladder. Voiding cystourethrography and urodynamics are recommended only if febrile UTIs have been present, or evidence of urinary tract decompensation has been documented sonographically.[50,51] Frequently, urodynamic findings include reduced functional bladder capacity with uninhibited bladder contractions.[45]

> ## KEY POINTS
>
> - OAB is the most common voiding dysfunction in children.
> - VUR is seen in in 20% to 50% of children with OAB. If untreated, OAB impedes spontaneous resolution of VUR.
> - Imaging is not necessary initially, but should be considered when conservative measures fail.
> - Initial management includes timed voiding, treatment of constipation, anticholinergic medication, and antibiotic prophylaxis for those with a history of frequent UTIs.

Conservative management of the OAB consists of timed voiding, anticholinergic therapy, prophylactic antibiotics, and treatment of any underlying constipation.[49,50,52–56] The success of timed voiding depends on the child's motivation to urinate before a spontaneous bladder contraction. If this schedule would require the child to void at a socially unacceptable frequency, anticholinergic medication should be considered. When used appropriately, anticholinergic medications offer a reasonable degree of success. These measures, in combination with elimination of caffeine, result in elimination of symptoms in 87% of children treated conservatively.[50] The child's parents must understand that treatment is a long-term process, taking an average of 2.7 years, with a range from 0.2 to 6.6 years. Because UTI may promote bladder instability, any active UTI should be treated with appropriate antibiotics. The patient should then be placed on prophylaxis with trimethoprim-sulfamethoxazole (TMP-SMX) or nitrofurantoin until a normal voiding pattern has been established.

## DISORDERS WITH HIGH RISK FOR UPPER URINARY TRACT DETERIORATION

### Dysfunctional elimination syndrome

Dysfunctional elimination syndrome (DES) encompasses constipation, urge incontinence, voiding postponement, infrequent voiding, and urinary retention that develop from a learned response to bladder overactivity.[57-59] In an effort to avoid incontinence, the patient contracts the sphincter complex, adopts postures, or both, which effectively suppresses the urinary or fecal urgency temporarily.

In its mildest form, DES is characterized by infrequent bowel movements, hard stools requiring straining, voiding postponement, and a strong or "staccato" stream that results in daytime urinary incontinence, fecal incontinence, or both. More severe forms of DES may manifest with incontinence, UTIs, bladder wall changes (distention, thickening, trabeculations, or reduced bladder contractility), VUR, and hydronephrosis.[44,49,60-62]

There is a close relationship between VUR and dysfunctional elimination. VUR can be identified in 30% to 50% of patients with DES.[49,52,63] However, this association may be biased because the majority of patients included in the studies presented with recurrent UTIs, a group known to have a high prevalence of VUR (30% to 35%). Koff et al.[49] found that among 143 patients felt to have primary VUR, 43% were identified as having significant bowel and bladder disturbances. In the children with VUR and dysfunctional elimination, breakthrough UTIs occurred in 82%; in 18% of children with VUR, no evidence of dysfunctional elimination had breakthrough UTIs.[57] These data demonstrate the influence that dysfunctional elimination has in the pathogenesis of UTI and underscores the notion that VUR itself is not a risk factor for UTI. Several studies have reported improved resolution rate of VUR in children who also were provided therapy for coexisting dysfunctional elimination, in addition to standard antimicrobial prophylaxis. Conversely, failure to address dysfunctional elimination results in a higher failure rate following antireflux procedures.[49,53,56,57] Although many children with VUR do not have abnormal voiding patterns on urodynamic investigation, and most children with DES do not have VUR, it is recommended that children with recurrent UTIs and VUR be screened for dysfunctional elimination as part of the initial evaluation.

DES is clinically suspected from the presenting history of the patient. Frequently, obesity (in as many as 30%) and psychosocial stressors (in as many as 40%) coexist with DES and should be addressed concurrently.[64] The physical examination is usually normal, but it also may reveal a palpable bladder and possibly palpable stool in the colon. An abdominal radiograph may demonstrate fecal retention. Renal and bladder ultrasound should be used to screen for increased postvoid residual urine volumes. A voiding cystourethrogram is not warranted unless documented febrile UTIs have occurred and VUR is suspected.[51] The use of noninvasive urodynamic studies combining uroflowmetry and patch electrodemyography has gained popularity among some who rely on flow patterns to select individualized treatment approaches. Staccato voiding is the most frequently seen pattern (58%), followed by interrupted and mixed patterns (19% and 10%, respectively).[65]

Treatment should first address the bowel dysfunction using cleansing with oral laxatives and enemas, if needed. A maintenance program should involve increasing the daily dietary fiber intake as well as by supplementation with a goal of a daily bowel movement. Behavioral modification should also focus on retraining urinary elimination to ensure regular and complete evacuation of the bladder. Children with bladder instability can be treated with anticholinergics, such as oxybutynin, hyoscyamine, or tolterodine, with the caveat that treatment of constipation must be addressed concurrently. If urodynamic evidence demonstrates staccato voiding, biofeedback treatments aimed at relaxation of the pelvic floor during voiding have demonstrated normalization of flow patterns in 96%.[66]

## NON-NEUROGENIC NEUROGENIC BLADDER (HINMAN SYNDROME)

Non-neurogenic neurogenic bladder represents extreme voiding dysfunction involving the lower urinary tract and affecting the upper tracts in the absence of any neurologic dysfunction.[60] Hinman syndrome constitutes functional bladder outlet obstruction resulting from a learned discoordination between bladder contraction and sphincter relaxation. The majority of patients are young males who have day and night wetting associated with chronic urinary retention, fecal retention and soiling, recurrent UTIs, and impaired renal function.[60] In addition to the clinical presentation, one also may elicit a social history significant for divorced, domineering parents; parental alcoholism; and drug, sex, or generalized abuse. Physical examination, as in DES, may demonstrate only fecal or urinary retention, and the neurologic examination is entirely normal. The diagnosis is often suggested when evidence of hydronephrosis is seen on a sonogram obtained during the evaluation for suspected DES. Some patients may present with manifestations of advanced renal dysfunction and complications from it. Voiding cystourethrography often shows a dilated, trabeculated bladder with VUR. An MRI should be obtained to exclude spina bifida occulta. These boys should be referred for urodynamic studies. Because many boys ultimately require intensive bladder retraining with biofeedback, it is practical to place a suprapubic cystostomy tube under anesthesia through which urodynamic studies and multiple biofeedback sessions can be performed without the need for repeated catheterizations. Botulinum toxin injection of the external sphincter has been performed successfully when biofeedback has failed.[67,68]

## POSTERIOR URETHRAL VALVE

Young[69] described three variations of congenital urethral membranes in 1915, a nomenclature that persists to date. Of these, only two are truly associated with urinary obstruction and are of clinical relevance. A type I valve, which represents anomalous insertion of the mesonephric duct into the fetal cloaca, is found cystoscopically between the prostatic urethra and external urinary sphincter and accounts for 95% of clinical cases.[70] The less common (5%) type III valve represents incomplete dissolution of the urogenital membrane and is encountered within the membranous urethra beyond the external sphincter.[71] Currently, most cases of PUV are diagnosed antenatally by ultrasonography. The characteristic imaging findings in such fetuses consist of bilateral severe hydronephrosis, bladder distention, bladder wall thickening, perinephric urinoma or ascites, and amniotic fluid abnormalities are seen in a male fetus.[72]

Despite endoscopic ablation of the valve in the newborn period, up to 50% of these boys will have incontinence well past toilet training, possibly because of associated primary bladder dysfunction.[73] Urodynamic assessment has shown changing patterns of bladder dysfunction with overactivity predominating in childhood leading to myogenic failure in adolescence.[74] Unfortunately, bladder dysfunction appears to correlate with deterioration in renal function through as yet unclear mechanisms.[73] Ultimately, most boys can achieve continence through institution of clean intermittent catheterization, anticholinergic medication, or both or surgical reconstruction of the urinary tract. Urodynamic studies should be performed to guide therapy, with the goal of ensuring low-pressure bladder filling and complete and regular evacuation of urine.

---

### KEY POINTS

- Hinman syndrome, which is a discoordination between the detrusor contraction and sphincter relaxation, is initially managed through biofeedback.
- Bladder dysfunction from PUV is not static. Whereas detrusor overactivity predominates in childhood, myogenic failure is seen in adolescence.

---

## NEUROSPINAL DYSRAPHISMS

Myelomeningocele accounts for 90% of all spinal dysraphic states, and it affects the lumbar, sacral, thoracic, and cervical spine, in decreasing prevalence.[75] An effective physical examination in patients with myelodysplasia would include palpation of the abdomen for bladder distention and fecal retention. In addition, urinary sphincter tone can be estimated based on inspection of the anal sphincter for laxity and reflexive contraction. Because the level of the lesion does not predict the type or degree of lower urinary tract dysfunction, neurologic and urodynamic examination of these patients is crucial.

Urodynamic studies immediately following newborn closure of the spinal defect and later have shown three main categories of prevalent bladder function: (1) a coordinated bladder and sphincter (19%), (2) discoordination with or without bladder overactivity (45%), and (3) complete paralysis (36%).[76–78] These patterns are not fixed and can change over time, resulting in varying patterns of bladder dysfunction.

Renal bladder sonography may show a dilated bladder with bladder wall thickening and dilated upper urinary tracts. Voiding cystourethrography reveals a trabeculated bladder, and VUR may be present. Magnetic resonance imaging (MRI) is the test of choice for anatomic detail of the spinal cord.[79] MRI is used to evaluate tethering of the spinal cord, syrinx or hydromyelia, increased intracranial pressure secondary to ventriculoperitoneal shunt malfunction, and partial herniation of the brainstem and cerebellum. Radiologic evaluation is repeated any time there is a change in neurologic, orthopedic, or urodynamic assessment.

Treatments are aimed at preserving nephron function and facilitating low-pressure voiding. Clean intermittent catheterization (CIC) alone or in combination with anticholinergics is used to keep the intravesical pressure less than 40 cm $H_2O$.[80–82] Rarely, a vesicostomy must be performed when the above therapies are not sufficient in adequately decompressing the bladder.[83,84]

## MISCELLANEOUS CAUSES

### CEREBRAL PALSY

Cerebral palsy (CP) a nonprogressive perinatal brain injury, is characterized by neuromuscular disability, specific symptoms complex, or cerebral dysfunction. Its incidence—currently 1.5 per 1000 live births—is increasing as smaller, younger premature infants are surviving.[85] Incontinence in children with CP is related to the degree to which the physical disability impairs reaching the toilet in time. Continence often develops at an age later than expected. If dryness is not achieved by late childhood or early puberty in a child who is physically capable and who appears trainable, further evaluation by urodynamic testing is recommended.[86] The most common clinically relevant urologic findings are exaggerated sacral reflexes, detrusor overactivity, and detrusor-sphincter dyssynergia.[87] Radiographic evaluation is not generally necessary.[88] Anticholinergics are able to provide relief of uninhibited bladder contractions in most patients with these problems. If the child has a large volume of postvoid residual urine, CIC should be advocated.

### ATTENTION DEFICIT/HYPERACTIVITY DISORDER

Children with attention deficit/hyperactivity disorder (ADHD) have a greater risk for daytime (ninefold) and nighttime (threefold) enuresis than age-matched controls.[89] The risk for daytime enuresis appears to increase with age, whereas the risk for nighttime enuresis lessens as children get older.[89] Some improvement in wetting has been demonstrated following the use of methylphenidate.[90]

---

### KEY POINTS

- Most infants with neurogenic bladder have detrusor overactivity; the next most common pattern is detrusor hyporeflexia.
- Children with CP might be incontinent as a result of their physical limitation because they cannot reach the toilet in time. It might also result from bladder overactivity and detrusor-sphincter discoordination.

---

### HYPERCALCIURIA

Idiopathic hypercalciuria has been identified in 20% to 30% of children with hematuria, dysuria, frequency-urgency syndrome, or voiding dysfunction.[91–93] It is postulated that the high concentrations of calcium in the urine irritates the bladder, causing involuntary incontinence. Although most nephrologists accept the definition of hypercalciuria as urinary calcium excretion greater than 4 mg/kg/day in children with urolithiasis, some have recommended that urinary calcium excretion greater than 2 mg/kg/day be the considered the threshold for defining hypercalciuria in children with enuresis or dysuria.[92,94] Successful treatment of the hypercalciuria can result in reduction of urinary symptoms and wetting in these patients.[94,95] Treatment is based on dietary measures aimed at decreased salt and oxalate intake and increased dietary fluid intake. Dietary calcium intake is generally not curtailed, because it is important in maintaining proper bone health in a developing child. Thiazide diuretics are helpful in reducing hypercalciuria when dietary measures fail.

## EVALUATION

### HISTORY

The diagnosis of childhood voiding disorders is made primarily by history and physical examination. Radiologic, laboratory, and complex urodynamic evaluation are rarely required but may be considered in circumstances when the clinical manifestations include UTI (febrile and afebrile), when physical examination suggests neurologic dysfunction, or when simple behavioral change or pharmacotherapy has been unsuccessful.

#### Elimination diary

Obtaining an accurate history of incontinence is of paramount importance and may be sufficient to arrive at a diagnosis. An assessment of the onset, pattern, severity, and circumstances surrounding the incontinence episodes should be noted. The interview should include the child also, depending on the child's age and maturity level.

We have found it useful to provide families with a questionnaire in advance of the initial evaluation, such that observations can be made before arriving at the clinic (Figure 52.1). These surveys document the degree to which wetting occurs during the day and night, the pattern of urinary and fecal elimination, specific behavioral patterns that can be observed in conjunction with wetting, drinking habits, and whether a UTI has coexisted with the wetting disturbance. Additionally, parents are requested to record the number of times the child voids or exhibits wetting during a 2-day interval (Table 52.2) Armed with this preliminary information, one can then obtain a more detailed history that focuses on pertinent positive observations.

#### Primary versus secondary disorder

Whether the voiding disorder is of new onset (secondary) or whether the child has never been completely continent since toilet-training was completed (primary) should be

Last name ☐ ID # ☐

First name ☐

Date of visit

Date of birth

1. Is your child toilet (potty) trained? O Yes O No
2. At what age was he/she toilet trained? ☐ Years

*Questions about your child's wetting.*

3. Does your child wet himself/herself during the day? O Yes O No
4. If yes, how often might your child wet himself/herself?
   ☐ Once a day ☐ Every other day ☐ Once a week ☐ Not sure
   ☐ Two or more times a day ☐ Twice a week ☐ Once every two weeks
5. Does your child wet the bed at night? O Yes O No
6. If yes, how often does your child wet the bed at night?
   ☐ Every night ☐ Twice a week ☐ Once every two weeks
   ☐ Every other night ☐ Once a week

*Questions about your child's urinating habits.*

7. Does he/she need to be reminded to urinate? O Yes O No
8. Does your child urinate soon after waking up? O Yes O No
9. Does he/she urinate at school? O Yes O No
10. Does your child urinate after coming home from school? O Yes O No
11. Does your child urinate just before bedtime? O Yes O No
12. Does your child squat, cross his/her leg, squirm or wiggle "before a leak"? O Yes O No
13. When your child wets does he/she have no idea that it happened? O Yes O No

*Questions about your child's drink habits.*

14. Does your child drink with meals? O Yes O No
15. What does your child drink? ☐ Water ☐ Juice ☐ Milk ☐ Caffeinated (Coke, Pepsi, Chocolate, Coffee)
16. How many cups of fluid does your child drink each day?
   ☐ 1–3 cups ☐ 4–6 cups ☐ 7–10 cups ☐ Not sure

Last Name ☐ First Name ☐

*Questions about your child's bowel movements.*

17. Are your child's underpants stained with feces? O Yes O No
18. If yes, how often might this happen?
   ☐ Once a day ☐ Every other day ☐ Once a week ☐ Not sure
   ☐ Two or more times a day ☐ Twice a week ☐ Once every two weeks
19. How often does your child usually have a bowel movement?
   ☐ Once a day ☐ Every other day ☐ Every 3 days ☐ Every 4 or more days ☐ Not sure
20. Does your child need reminding to have a BM? O Yes O No

*Questions about your child's urinary tract infections.*

21. Has your child had a urinary infection treated in the last 12 months? O Yes O No
22. How was the specimen collected?
   ☐ Bag ☐ Clean void, midstream ☐ Catheter ☐ Not sure
23. How many infections has your child been treated for in the last 12 months? ☐ Times
24. Which symptoms did he/she have with the infection?
   Wetting? O Yes O No
   Painful urination? O Yes O No
   Fever? O Yes O No
   Foul smelling urine? O Yes O No
   Frequent urination? O Yes O No
   Nausea/vomiting? O Yes O No
   Increased urge to void? O Yes O No
25. Did the infection occur while your child was on an antibiotic? O Yes O No
26. If yes, what antibiotic was he/she taking when the infection occured?
   ☐

What methods have you used to stop the bedwetting?

☐ Rewards Yes ☐ Rewards No ☐ Punishments Yes ☐ Punishments No ☐ Ditropan (oxybutynin) ☐ DDAVP pills ☐ DDAVP nasal spray ☐ Imipramine ☐ Nighttime waking ☐ Other...

Figure 52.1 Voiding questionnaire.

determined. This distinction is critical because secondary wetting disturbances are more likely associated with an identifiable abnormality in contrast to children who present with primary incontinence. For example, diabetes insipidus or diabetes mellitus, PUV, and tethered spinal cord all may manifest with a history of secondary daytime or nighttime incontinence.[96–98] Exceptions to this rule do occur, however. For instance, continuous dribbling of urine in some girls as a consequence of an ectopic ureter ending periurethrally may result in what appears as a primary incontinence, because these patients are never reported to be completely dry.

## Bladder capacity estimation

Expected bladder capacity can be estimated based on the interval between voids and the maximal voided volumes that have been recorded on the elimination diary. Expected bladder capacity should be compared with calculated estimates of bladder capacity based on age, using the following formulas[99]:

$$\text{Bladder capacity (ounces) less than 2 years} = [2 \times \text{age (years)}] + 2$$

$$\text{Bladder capacity (ounces) 2 to 13 years} = (\text{age [years]}/2) + 6$$

Table 52.2 Voiding diary

**Patient: Please fill out this diary for your child. Keep the diary for at least 3 days (*2 weekend days and at least 1 school day*). Record every time your child uses the bathroom, has wetting accidents, and has bowel movements. Also, please record activity and fluid intake.**

| DATE/TIME | Urinated/ Peed | Wetting accidents | Describe accident (Soaked/ Damp) | Activity at time of accident (School/Sleep) | Fluid intake (Type/Amount) | Bowel movement (Hard/Soft/ Loose) |
|---|---|---|---|---|---|---|
| | | | | | | |
| | | | | | | |
| | | | | | | |
| | | | | | | |
| | | | | | | |

## Urinary stream

The characteristics of the urinary stream and events immediately before and following should be noted. Children with sensory deficient bladders do not recognize bladder filling and will typically wet themselves without recognition, often described as "sitting in their own urine." By comparison, the child with urgency frequency is seen to cross the legs, squirm, grab the genitalia, or sit on one heel to inhibit the detrusor contraction. A weak urinary stream in a boy may reflect a PUV, and staccato voiding in either gender may occur because of poor relaxation of the external urinary sphincter. Upward deflection of the urinary stream, a phenomenon seen almost exclusively in circumcised boys, occurs because of meatal stenosis. However, meatal stenosis is not the cause of voiding dysfunction or enuresis. Finally, postvoid dribbling may represent release of urine pooled in the vagina on standing in girls or from a urethral diverticulum in boys, particularly those with a history of urethral trauma or surgery.

## Bowel function

Constipation, usually from idiopathic causes, is known to occur in as many as 10% of school-aged children.[58,99] Constipation has been associated with UTIs, urgency-frequency syndrome, urinary retention, incontinence, and upper urinary tract deterioration in children.[58,100,101] Significant improvement in voiding symptoms and diminished frequency of recurrent UTIs in children following specific treatment of constipation only is well documented. For this reason, it is important to inquire regarding the consistency and frequency of bowel movements, fecal incontinence, and whether prior therapy for encopresis or constipation has been attempted. However, because parents may not accurately know the bowel habits of their older children, it is often helpful to include children in the interview by specifically asking them whether any bowel movements passed are hard, painful, or associated with blood. Dietary factors may influence fecal consistency, and thus elimination, so a detailed dietary history should be obtained. This history should explore concomitant medication use that may predispose to constipation, such as anticholinergics, anticonvulsants, antacids, oral iron, and psychotherapeutics.

## PHYSICAL EXAMINATION

A comprehensive physical examination is warranted in every child with voiding dysfunction, which is most often normal. The examination should include a review of the abdomen, genitalia, perineum, anus, lower back, and lower extremity neurologic status. Palpation of the abdomen should be performed with attention to identifying constipation, which would be suggested by fullness in the lower quadrant or rectum. A palpably distended urinary bladder, particularly shortly after the child has voided, may indicate more severe voiding disturbance such as those caused by neurologic conditions, PUV, or pelvic malignancies.

In boys, when meatal stenosis is suspected, the urethral meatus should be inspected by carefully trying to spread the meatus open. If urethral mucosa is seen to evert from the meatus, the diagnosis of stenosis can be excluded. To confirm meatal stenosis, the child may be observed voiding. Typically the urinary stream is deflected upward in meatal stenosis, and to direct the stream into the toilet, the boy must aim the penis downward at an acute angle. In girls, a bifid clitoris or a urethral meatus that is patulous anteriorly is diagnostic for epispadias. An ectopic ureter to the periurethral area is suggested by continuous pooling of urine in the vaginal vault.

Rectal examination is typically not warranted in most patients with wetting. However, boys with new onset or secondary voiding dysfunction who complain of the need to strain to void, weak stream, hesitancy, or both, should be examined rectally because these symptoms are associated with prostatic rhabdomyosarcoma. In girls, rhabdomyosarcoma manifests more commonly as a vaginal introitus mass rather than with voiding complaints. Inspection of the lower back may disclose evidence of spinal dysraphism (see later). Finally, a neurologic examination of the lower extremities also may suggest spinal cord abnormalities if loss of or asymmetric strength, coordination, or both are seen.

## INVESTIGATIONS

In the vast majority of cases, urinalysis with a dipstick and microscopic examination provides important information regarding UTI and some metabolic disorders. When a negative dipstick analysis is combined with negative urine microscopy, infection can be excluded reliably and a formal urine culture is not warranted.[102,103] Dipstick analysis for urinary protein, glucose, and specific gravity is helpful to screen for causes of polyuria, such as diabetes mellitus or insipidus (nephrogenic or central). Generally, a urine specific gravity measurement of 1.022 or greater, in the absence of proteinuria or glucosuria, indicates adequate concentrating ability. Lower urine specific gravity measurements that are associated with polydipsia and polyuria should be further evaluated to exclude diabetes insipidus.

## Imaging studies

Most voiding disorders can be accurately diagnosed by clinical history only, and imaging studies are rarely necessary. Prevoid and postvoid renal-bladder ultrasonography (RBUS) is warranted to assess bladder emptying and evaluate for hydronephrosis in patients with voiding abnormalities, especially if these are present in association with febrile UTI. Hydronephrosis may suggest the presence of other anatomic abnormalities, such as VUR or PUV, which can contribute to the risk for upper urinary tract deterioration in presence of infection. In the absence of a history of febrile UTI, children do not need to have VCUG, unless other risk factors for VUR, such as a family history of reflux, are present. The advent of office-based RBUS has led some to perform this test in all children presenting with urinary incontinence. However, few children demonstrate such inefficient emptying to justify this practice.

A plain radiograph of the abdomen is helpful in demonstrating increased fecal load in children who are suspected of having constipation but do not yield reliable information on questioning. Additionally, the radiograph also screens for occult spinal dysraphism, a rare but well-recognized cause of secondary wetting and bowel disturbances.

## Screening for occult dysraphism

Rarely, unrecognized spina bifida associated with spinal cord tethering or spinal cord tumors may cause elimination disorders. Patients known to be at risk for spinal cord tethering include those with imperforate anus or VATER syndrome (vertebral defects, imperforate anus, tracheoesophageal fistula, and radial and renal dysplasia) (up to 45%), and cloacal exstrophy (up to 100%).[105–108] These patients are easily identified, but many more subtle cases of spinal cord tethering occur in the context of spina bifida occulta.

The radiographic appearance of occult spinal dysraphisms may not be visible until after 5 to 7 years of age when ossification is complete.[109] This finding can be observed in as many as 30% of normal men and 17% of normal women. When spina bifida occulta occurs as a bony abnormality and without cutaneous manifestations, it is considered a normal variant without clinical consequence. MRI examination of the spine is not warranted in such individuals. When cutaneous manifestations, such as a dimple or hair patch, are seen in a child with voiding dysfunction, an MRI should be performed.

Any child with secondary day and night wetting, new-onset constipation or encopresis, or a significant delay in toilet training should be evaluated for occult spinal disorders. Neurologic evaluation and examination of the back for skin dimpling, hair tufts, accessory skin tags or tails, and pigmentation should be undertaken in an effort to identify spinal dysraphism. In children with gait disturbances, the relative symmetry of the gluteal muscles also should be evaluated. Finally, sensation and tone of the anal sphincter can be used as a proxy for urethral sphincter function.

## Urodynamic studies

Urodynamic studies are usually recommended only for children with significant urinary, fecal, or both elimination problems, a diagnosed PUV, or Hinman syndrome. These patients are at risk for upper tract deterioration and may be found to have hydronephrosis, renal cortical scarring, or both on presentation. The data collected from urodynamic studies should be compared with values from normal children.[110] Noninvasive urodynamic studies, which comprise uroflowmetry with patch electromyography, have been advocated by some to select children for more rigorous treatment by biofeedback or those more likely to benefit from α-adrenergic therapy.[65]

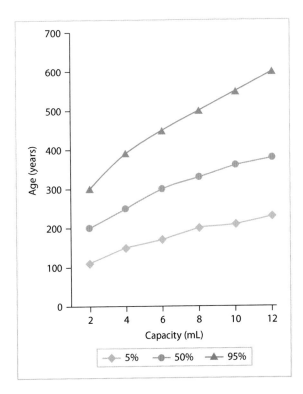

Figure 52.2 Nonlinear curve showing relationship between age (years) and bladder capacity (milliliters). (Adapted from: Kaefer M, Zurakowski D, Bauer SB, et al. Estimating normal bladder capacity in children. J Urol. 1997;158:2261–4.)

## THERAPEUTIC APPROACHES

In most cases, simple behavioral modification is sufficient to improve the incontinence. Surgery is rarely necessary and is performed only for severe cases of dysfunctional elimination that are recalcitrant to conventional behavioral modification or when signs of upper urinary tract changes are present. In some children, pharmacotherapy is used as an adjunct to behavioral modification.

## Timed and double voiding

The establishment of regular elimination habits is of paramount importance, particularly among children who are infrequent voiders and in those whose incontinence is not associated with frequency. The child should be encouraged to void as frequently as necessary to prevent wetting, based on the patterns recorded in a voiding diary. Because many of these children do not sense the need to void at lower volumes, voiding on a schedule can be associated with well-defined events throughout the day, such as waking, before meals, and before bedtime. Multialarm wristwatches are also helpful as auditory cues for timing of urination.

Older children may have large-capacity bladders, high postvoid residual urine volumes, and double or repeat voiding may be necessary. For instance, this "yo-yo" pattern may be observed especially in children with prune belly syndrome, bilateral high-grade VUR, and Hinman syndrome, in whom the upper urinary tract is highly compliant.

Initiation of double voiding can obviate the need for clean intermittent catheterization (CIC). These children should be reevaluated by RBUS after institution of double voiding to ensure that hydronephrosis is improving. Persistent or progressive hydronephrosis and UTI reflect poor compliance with these measures and demonstrate the need for more intense therapy with CIC.

## Enuresis (wetting) alarms

Enuresis alarms worn during the day by children with daytime wetting have been reported to result in appropriate behavior modification, achieving a success rate of over 60%. Unfortunately, use of enuresis alarms during the day is more cumbersome than multialarm watches that can provide similar benefit.

## Bowel program

In children with associated constipation, a bowel program should be instituted to ensure that the rectum remains empty of stool.[59] Various treatment modalities can be tailored to the severity of constipation. Increasing fiber and liquid intake, bulking agents, stool softeners, and laxatives can be tried first (Table 52.3) Suppositories, enemas, disimpaction, or a combination of these may be necessary. The recommended daily amount of fiber can be calculated using the formula:

Grams of fiber needed per day (20 g maximum) = Age (Years) + 5

For milder cases, dietary modification, fiber supplementation, or both may follow an initial bowel clean-out using laxatives. Severe constipation may require initial manual

Table 52.3 Fecal elimination programs

| | Minimal dose | Maximal dose |
| --- | --- | --- |
| **Bulking Agents** | | |
| Fiber* | Age (yr) + 5 (g) per day | 20 g/day |
| FiberCon | 1 cap (6–12 yr) or 2 caps (≥12 yr) daily | 1 cap tid (6–12 yr), 2 caps tid (≥12 yr) |
| Metamucil wafers | 1 wafer bid (6–12 yr) | 2 wafers tid (>12 yr) |
| Senokot | 1 tablet or teaspoon daily | 3 tablets or teaspoons daily |
| Citrucel | 7.5 mL in 8 oz water daily (6–12 yr) | 7.5 mL in 8 oz water tid (6–12 yr) |
| | 15 mL in 8 oz water daily (>12 yr) | 15 mL in 8 oz water tid (>12 yr) |
| **Stool Softeners** | | |
| Mineral oil | 1 mL/kg daily | 2.5 mL/kg bid |
| Lactulose | 1 mL/kg daily | 1 mL/kg tid |
| Colace | 20 mg/day (3–6 yr), 40 mg/day (7–12), or 50 mg/day (>12 yr) divided bid or tid | 60 mg/day (3–6 yr), 120 mg/day (7–12), or 200 mg/day (>12 yr) divided bid or tid |
| **Laxatives** | | |
| Milk of Magnesia† | 1 mL/kg daily | 1 mL/kg tid |
| Magnesium citrate† | 1 oz/yr of age (<6 yr) | 1 bottle (>6 yr) |
| Castor oil | 2.5 mL daily | 50 mL daily (for adults) |
| GoLYTELY | 8-oz glass q20min until rectal effluent is clear | 100 mL/kg or 4 L in adult-size teenagers |
| MiraLAX‡ | 5 mL in 40 oz water daily | 17 g (1 heaping tablespoon in 8 oz water daily (adult dose, may be reduced in children) |
| **Suppositories** | | |
| Glycerin | 1 per rectum daily to qod | 1 per rectum bid |
| Dulcolax | ½ to 1 per rectum daily (not for chronic use) | 1 per rectum bid |
| **Enemas** | | |
| Fleet phosphate§ | 1 pediatric dose daily | 1 pediatric dose bid |
| Tap water¶ | 100–250 mL enema daily | 100–250 mL enema bid |
| Milk of Magnesia | 1:1 milk to magnesia (30–150 mL) daily | 1:1 milk to magnesia (30–150 mL) tid |
| Fleet mineral oil | ½ dose daily | 1 enema daily |

bid, twice per day; qid, every other day; tid, three times per day.
* Dietary texts provide tables with the amount of fiber (in grams) in various foods.
† May result in hypermagnesemia.
‡ Advantage is no taste; safety undetermined in children; preliminary reports suggest safe in children older than 2 years of age for 6-month period.
§ May result in hyperphosphatemia.
¶ May result in hyponatremia.

disimpaction and rectal clean-out using enemas, followed by administration of laxatives, such as MiraLAX, magnesium citrate, or polyethylene glycol-electrolyte solution (GoLYTELY). In these circumstances, abdominal films obtained before and during therapy are helpful in demonstrating the fecal load. Once the clean-out phase has been completed, a maintenance phase lasting as long as 1 year should be continued with daily oral laxatives. Failure to continue these measures often results in recurrent constipation.[59]

## Biofeedback techniques

Biofeedback techniques rely on combining Kegel exercises to strengthen pelvic floor, along with urodynamic studies and positive reinforcement. Biofeedback has been used successfully to treat children with urinary and bowel elimination problems, recurrent UTI, and VUR, particularly when the underlying abnormality during voiding is a nonrelaxing pelvic floor.[111-123]

In general, after a complete urodynamic evaluation is performed, the child's perineal muscular activity is monitored during filling and voiding by an electromyographic electrode. The urodynamic equipment displays pelvic floor contraction as visual or auditory cues that the child can control. The goal is to teach the child to relax the sphincter complex completely during voiding.

McKenna et al.[121] recognized the difficulty to maintain a child's focus during these arduous biofeedback sessions. They devised a computer game that the child controls with perineal muscular activity. Using this method, they reported effective treatment of voiding dysfunction in 41 children with various forms of dysfunctional elimination habits. Overall, 90% to 100% of patients improved in all categories. Of the group, 52% of cases of nocturnal enuresis, 61% of diurnal enuresis, 33% of constipation and 73% of encopresis were completely cured.

## Pharmacologic therapy

Pharmacotherapy is reserved for voiding disorders associated with UTI or when significant social embarrassment is perceived. (Table 52.4). Any child with coexisting constipation should begin a bowel program before institution of any medication with anticholinergic effects, because these impair colonic motility as well. Anticholinergic and α-adrenergic medication may be contraindicated in

Table 52.4 Pharmacologic therapies available for treatment of daytime voiding disorders

| Type (Brand Name) | Minimal dosage | Maximal dosage | Long-acting dosage |
|---|---|---|---|
| **Anticholinergic** | | | |
| Propantheline (Pro-Banthine) | 0.5 mg/kg bid | 0.5 mg/kg qid | |
| Oxybutynin (Ditropan) | 0.2 mg/kg bid | 0.2 ml/kg qid | Ditropan XL 5-20 mg daily |
| Hyoscyamine (Levsin) | 0.03 mg/kg bid | 0.1 mL/kg qid | Levsin timecap 1–2 bid |
| **α-Adrenergic Agonist** | | | |
| Phenylephrine (Entex) | 0.5 mg/kg bid | 1 mg/kg tid | Entex LA 1 tab bid |
| Pseudoephedrine (Sudafed) | 30 mg qid (6–12 yr) | 60 mg qid (>12 yr) | Sudafed 12-hr cap bid |
| Ephedrine | 1 mg/kg/day qid | 3 mg/kg/day qid | |
| **α-Adrenergic Blockade** | | | |
| Prazosin (Minipress) | 0.05 mg/kg bid | 0.1 mg/kg tid | |
| Doxazosin mesylate (Cardura) | 0.5 mg/kg at bedtime | 8 mg at bedtime | |
| Terazosin (Hytrin) | 0.5 mg/kg at bedtime | 10 mg at bedtime | |
| **Smooth Muscle Relaxant** | | | |
| Flavoxate (Urispas) | 3 mg/kg bid | 3 mg/kg tid | |
| *Tricyclic Antidepressant* | | | |
| Imipramine (Tofranil) | 0.7 mg/kg bid | 1.2 mg/kg tid | |
| **Central Nervous System Stimulant** | | | |
| Methyphenidate (Ritalin) | 5 mg before social event | 10 mg before social event | Ritalin SR 20 mg daily |
| Dextroamphetamine | NR | | |
| Amphetamine (Adderall) | | | |
| **Antibacterial Prophylaxis** | | | |
| Nitrofurantoin (Macrodantin) | 1–2 mg/kg at bedtime | | |
| Trimethoprim-sulfamethoxazole (Septra, Bactrim, Sulfatrim) | 0.5 mg/kg at bedtime | | |
| Trimethoprim | 0.5 mg/kg at bedtime | | |
| Sulfisoxazole (Gantrisin) | 50 mg/kg at bedtime | | |

bid, twice daily; NR, not recommended; qid, four times daily; tid, three times daily.

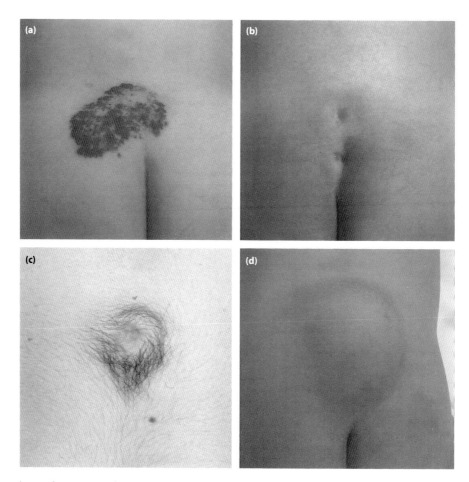

Figure 52.3 External manifestations of spinal dysraphism. (a) Hemangioma. (b) Sacral dimple. (c) Diastematomyelia. (d) Lipoma. (Photographs courtesy of John Myseros, MD, Division of Neurosurgery, Children's National Medical Center, Washington, D.C.)

children with closed-angle glaucoma or cardiac disease. Therefore, consultation with the appropriate specialist should precede their use.

## ANTICHOLINERGIC AGENTS

Anticholinergic and musculotropic medications inhibit or reduce bladder overactivity. These medications increase the threshold potential for involuntary smooth muscle cell contraction, which translates into a greater volume of urine required before the bladder contracts. The side effects of anticholinergic medications include dry mouth, facial flushing, and constipation, and, in hot climates, hyperpyrexia may occur. If blurred vision or hallucinations occur, it is recommended that the dose be decreased.

## α-ADRENERGIC STIMULANTS

α-Adrenergic agonists may be used to increase outlet resistance in patients with stress urinary incontinence. However, true stress urinary incontinence is unusual in a neurologically intact child and is customarily found in association with an anatomic abnormality of the bladder neck, such as epispadias or urogenital sinus abnormality. Teenage girls engaged in high-impact sports also have been found at risk for stress urinary incontinence.

## TRICYCLIC ANTIDEPRESSANTS

Imipramine has been the most widely used tricyclic antidepressant in children, particularly in the treatment of NE. Some have reported efficacy of this class for treatment of daytime incontinence, as well. It has a dual mechanism of action, with anticholinergic effects causing detrusor muscle relaxation and α-adrenergic effects causing increased sphincter muscle activity. Tricyclics should be used only in older children and adolescents because of their relatively long half-life and risk for side effects. Anticholinergics remain the first-line therapy for daytime incontinence from detrusor overactivity, but tricyclics may be added in incrementally greater doses for refractory cases. Children who require high doses of tricyclics should be monitored for cardiac conduction defects and arrhythmias with electrocardiography.

## α-ADRENERGIC BLOCKADE

The well-documented clinical efficacy of α-adrenergic blockade to improve urinary flow and decrease postvoid residual urine volumes in men with benign prostatic hypertrophy (BPH) has led some pediatric urologists to evaluate its utility in reducing functional outlet obstruction in children with enuresis.

The rationale for the use of α-adrenergic blockade in BPH relies on evidence of α-adrenergic receptors localized to the smooth muscle cells of the bladder outlet in both genders and especially to the prostatic tissue in males. However, in childhood enuresis associated with poor bladder emptying, it is generally believed that diminished flow results from incomplete relaxation of the external urinary sphincter and not as a result of increased tone of the bladder neck or prostatic tissues. Despite this apparent conflict, results of clinical studies using α-blocker therapy show promise.[124–126]

Three nonrandomized cohort studies of a total of 88 children have demonstrated statistically significant improvements in urinary flow rate and postvoid residual urine volumes that have resulted in cessation of or diminished enuretic episodes in approximately 80% of children treated with doxazosin (0.5 to 1 mg orally).[124–126] A major criticism of these studies has been the lack of standardized follow-up among the three studies and inclusion of varied causes of enuresis, although all children had evidence of poor bladder emptying. Side effects, related to postural hypotension, are diminished by administration just before bedtime.

## CENTRAL NERVOUS SYSTEM STIMULANTS

Central nervous system stimulants, such as methylphenidate (Ritalin), have been used successfully to treat giggle incontinence. Children with ADHD and enuresis also have been found with diminished incontinence following institution of methylphenidate. The mechanism of action is unknown.

## TREATMENT FOR PRIMARY NOCTURNAL ENURESIS

Pharmacologic therapy relies on improving functional bladder capacity through anticholinergic effects (oxybutynin, imipramine) or by diminishing nocturnal urine volume (vasopressin, desmopressin acetate [DDAVP]). Imipramine has been the first medication used to treat enuresis. It relies on antispasmodic effects on the bladder and stimulatory effects on the sphincter. Some data also suggest that imipramine may exert central effects that alter arousal, thus facilitating that the child awaken from sleep before enuresis occurs. Initial response rates to imipramine are approximately 50% but long-term cure rates, once the drug is discontinued, are poor (only 25%).[127]

Oxybutynin, a potent anticholinergic, may be helpful in the management of NE associated with bladder overactivity. Its efficacy as a single drug used to treat enuresis is approximately 10% to 50%.[128] One study evaluated combination therapy with imipramine and oxybutynin. Although the combination proved more efficacious in short-term results than either drug alone (90% achieved dryness), lasting results were seen in only 40% after the treatment was discontinued.[128]

A more direct approach to enuresis appears to be improving the kidney's concentrating ability during sleep through the use of vasopressin (DDAVP). The reported response rate to vasopressin is 40% to 70%.[129,130] The relapse rate on discontinuation is high, with only 30% of responders maintaining continence at 1 year.[131] Vasopressin can be administered intranasally as a spray as well as an orally administered tablet.

Functional bladder capacity remains an important feature in the pathogenesis of enuresis and, if unaddressed, is likely to be associated with treatment failure. In fact, several studies have shown that functional bladder capacity is a strong predictor of response to desmopressin.[132–134] One study correlated a bladder volume and wall thickness index to the response from desmopressin and found a statistically greater likelihood of resolution when DDAVP was prescribed to children with normal bladder volume and bladder wall thickness.[135] Enuretic children with reduced bladder volume and thick bladder wall and those with large bladder volumes and thin walls had a suboptimal response to oral desmopressin.[135]

## ANTIBIOTICS

Symptomatic UTI should be treated with appropriate antibiotic therapy. Prophylactic antibiotics should be considered in children with voiding disorders who have recurrent infection, because chronic inflammation may perpetuate bladder instability. TMP-SMX, nitrofurantoin, and TMP alone have been used successfully as prophylaxis. On occasion, two antibiotics are required to adequately prevent recurrent UTI.[136]

## CLEAN INTERMITTENT CATHETERIZATION

CIC is recommended in children who demonstrate persistently elevated postvoid residual urine volumes despite adherence to timed voiding and double voiding regimens and therapy for constipation. Although children are likely to develop bacteriuria with CIC, studies have demonstrated improved continence and diminished risk for pyelonephritis and upper urinary tract deterioration.[137] CIC should be performed at 3- to 4-hour intervals. So long as complete bladder emptying is achieved regularly, bacteriuria remains clinically insignificant in the majority of these children. The use of sterile catheters is unnecessary, and prophylactic antibiotics are not recommended unless the patient has been diagnosed with VUR. In such circumstances, every effort should be made to maintain sterile urine with daily antibiotic prophylaxis. Anticholinergic medication also may be used if evidence of bladder overactivity has been found.

## ENDOSCOPY AND PROCEDURES TO REDUCE BLADDER OUTLET RESISTANCE

Historically, cystourethroscopy with urethral dilation has been used in some patients with dysfunctional voiding, based on the rationale that bladder outlet obstruction was the risk factor leading to recurrent UTIs in such girls.[138] In most treatment protocols, the urethra was dilated to 28 to 32 Fr, followed by prolonged antibiotic prophylaxis. Unfortunately, no objective clinical evidence exists that urethral dilation itself, in the absence of antibiotic prophylaxis, ever diminished the risk for UTIs.[138] This should be of no surprise, because the underlying problem in some girls with recurrent UTIs is nonrelaxation of the external urinary sphincter during voiding that is untreated by dilatation. Therefore, the abnormal voiding pattern recurs after the procedure, as does the risk for UTI.

When behavioral modification and biofeedback techniques have failed to produce sphincter relaxation during voiding, a novel surgical option has been employed to temporarily paralyze the external urinary sphincter by endoscopic injection of botulinum-A toxin. Sphincter paralysis lasts between 2 and 9 months, during which the child learns to void without tightening his or her sphincter. As a result of improved bladder emptying, continence improves.[139]

## SURGERY

Surgical interventions are rarely used anymore for incontinence related to dysfunctional elimination states. Perhaps the only indication would be very high postvoid residual urine volumes associated with upper tract deterioration, which cannot be managed by CIC, and in a patient in whom future fertility is not a concern. In those circumstances, one might consider a bladder neck incision or a Y-V plasty.

Neurologic and anatomic causes of incontinence require surgical intervention to promote continence when timed voiding and CIC have been unable to provide relief. Urodynamic studies are often helpful in determining the type of procedure to perform, such as augmentation cystoplasty, Young-Dees-Leadbetter bladder neck reconstruction, Mitrofanoff procedure, sling cystourethropexy or placement of artificial sphincter device. A pediatric urologist with experience in such matters should perform the evaluation of the child with severe voiding problems that have an anatomic cause.

## SUMMARY

Incontinence, though acceptable in young children, becomes increasingly bothersome as children mature into school age. The symptom itself encompasses many disorders, both functional and anatomic. For most children who wet, a detailed history and physical examination will usually determine the type of wetting disorder and suggest an appropriate treatment course. For these children, simple behavioral modification, such as the use of a timed voiding schedule and dietary modification (which also may include the use of laxatives) can significantly diminish the number of wetting episodes and prevent UTI, when coexistent. When wetting presents with UTI and fever, radiologic evaluation should be performed and any underlying severe functional or anatomic abnormality rapidly addressed to prevent upper urinary tract deterioration.

## REFERENCES

1. Hjälmås K. Urodynamics in normal infants and children. Scand J Urol Nephrol Suppl. 1988;114:20–7.
2. Rushton HG. Wetting and functional voiding disorders. Urol Clin North Am. 1995;22:75–93.
3. Stein Z, Susser M. Social factors in the development of sphincter control. Dev Med Child Neurol. 1967;9:692–706.
4. Bloom DA, Seeley WW, Ritchey ML, McGuire EJ. Toilet habits and continence in children: An opportunity sampling in search of normal parameters. J Urol. 1993;149:1087–90.
5. Jones EA. Urinary incontinence in children. In: Litwin MS, Saigal CS, editors. Urologic Diseases in America. Washington, D.C.: US Government Printing Office; 2004. p. 137.
6. Koff SA, Byard MA. The daytime urinary frequency syndrome of childhood. J Urol. 1988;140:1280–1.
7. Bass LW. Pollakiuria, extraordinary daytime urinary frequency: Experience in a pediatric practice. Pediatrics. 1991;87:735–7.
8. Leung AK, Robson WL. Daytime urinary frequency in children. BMJ. 1988;297:1047.
9. Robson WL, Leung AK, Gangemi DJ. Daytime urinary frequency. Clin Pediatr (Phila). 1994;33:381.
10. Watemberg N, Shalev H. Daytime urinary frequency in children. Clin Pediatr (Phila). 1994;33:50–3.
11. Zoubek J, Bloom DA, Sedman AB. Extraordinary urinary frequency. Pediatrics. 1990;85:1112–4.
12. Parkes JD, Lock CB. Genetic factors in sleep disorders. J Neurol Neurosurg Psychiatry. 1989;Suppl:101–8.
13. Sher PK, Reinberg Y. Successful treatment of giggle incontinence with methylphenidate. J Urol. 1996;156:656–8.
14. Mackeith RC. Micturition induced by giggling. Guys Hosp Rep. 1964;113:250–60.
15. Elzinga-Plomp A, Boemers TM, Messer AP, et al. Treatment of enuresis risoria in children by self-administered electric and imaginary shock. Br J Urol. 1995;76:775–8.
16. Nygaard IE, Thompson FL, Svengalis SL, et al. Urinary incontinence in elite nulliparous athletes. Obstet Gynecol. 1994;84:183–7.
17. Nygaard IE, Glowacki C, Saltzman CL. Relationship between foot flexibility and urinary incontinence in nulliparous varsity athletes. Obst Gynecol. 1996;87:1049–51.
18. Norgaard JP, Hansen JH, Wildschiotz G, et al. Sleep cystometries in children with nocturnal enuresis. J Urol. 1989;141:1156–9.
19. Forsythe WI, Redmond A. Enuresis and spontaneous cure rate: Study of 1129 enuretis. Arch Dis Child. 1974;49:259–63.

20. Hellstrom AL, Hanson E, Hansson S, et al. Micturition habits and incontinence in 7-year-old Swedish school entrants. Eur J Pediatr. 1990;149:434–7.

21. Bakwin H. Enuresis in children. J Pediatr. 1961;58:806–19.

22. Hagstroem S, Kamperis K, Rittig S, et al. Monosymptomatic nocturnal enuresis is associated with abnormal nocturnal bladder emptying. J Urol. 2004;171:2562–6; discussion 6.

23. George CP, Messerli FH, Genest J, et al. Diurnal variation of plasma vasopressin in man. J Clin Endocrinol Metab. 1975;41:332–8.

24. Rittig S, Knudsen UB, Nørgaard JP, Pedersen EB, Djurhuus JC. Abnormal diurnal rhythm of plasma vasopressin and urinary output in patients with enuresis. Am J Physiol. 1989 Apr;256(4 Pt 2):F664-71.

25. Frokiaer J, Nielsen S. Do aquaporins have a role in nocturnal enuresis? Scand J Urol Nephrol Suppl. 1997;183:31–2.

26. Norgaard JP, Hansen JH, Nielsen JB, et al. Nocturnal studies in enuretics: A polygraphic study of sleep-EEG and bladder activity. Scand J Urol Nephrol Suppl. 1989;125:73–8.

27. Koff SA. Why is desmopressin sometimes ineffective at curing bedwetting? Scand J Urol Nephrol Suppl. 1995;173:103–8.

28. Boyd MM. The depth of sleep in enuretic schoolchildren and in non-enuretic controls. J Psychosom Res. 1960;4:274–81.

29. Kales A, Kales JD. Sleep disorders: Recent findings in the diagnosis and treatment of disturbed sleep. N Engl J Med. 1974;290:487–99.

30. Wolfish N. Sleep arousal function in enuretic males. Scand J Urol Nephrol Suppl. 1999;202:24–6.

31. Wolfish NM. Sleep/arousal and enuresis subtypes. J Urol. 2001;166:2444–7.

32. Houts AC. Behavioural treatment for enuresis. Scand J Urol Nephrol Suppl. 1995;173:83–6; discussion 7.

33. Monda JM, Husmann DA. Primary nocturnal enuresis: A comparison among observation, imipramine, desmopressin acetate and bed-wetting alarm systems. J Urol. 1995;154:745–8.

34. Ellerker AG. The extravesical ectopic ureter. Br J Surg. 1958;45:344–53.

35. Bukowski TP, Lewis AG, Reeves D, et al. Epididymitis in older boys: Dysfunctional voiding as an etiology. J Urol. 1995;154:762–5.

36. Umeyama T, Kawamura T, Hasegawa A, Ogawa O. Ectopic ureter presenting with epididymitis in childhood: Report of 5 cases. J Urol. 1985;134:131–3.

37. Pattaras JG, Rushton HG, Majd M. The role of 99mtechnetium dimercapto-succinic acid renal scans in the evaluation of occult ectopic ureters in girls with paradoxical incontinence. J Urol. 1999;162:821–5.

38. Braverman RM, Lebowitz RL. Occult ectopic ureter in girls with urinary incontinence: Diagnosis by using CT. AJR Am J Roentgenol. 1991;156:365–6.

39. Bozorgi F, Connolly LP, Bauer SB, et al. Hypoplastic dysplastic kidney with a vaginal ectopic ureter identified by technetium-99m-DMSA scintigraphy. J Nucl Med. 1998;39:113–5.

40. Ruarte AC, Podesta ML, Medel R. Detrusor aftercontractions in children with normal urinary tracts. BJU Int. 2002;90:286–93.

41. Koff SA, Solomon MH, Lane GA, Lieding KG. Urodynamic studies in anesthetized children. J Urol. 1980;123:61-–3.

42. Nash DF. The development of micturition control with special reference to enuresis. Ann R Coll Surg Engl. 1949;5:318–44, illust.

43. Lapides J, Diokno AC. Persistence of the infant bladder as a cause for urinary infection in girls. Trans Am Assoc Genitourin Surg. 1969;61:51–6.

44. Bauer SB, Retik AB, Colodny AH, et al. The unstable bladder in childhood. Urol Clin North Am. 1980;7:321–36.

45. Vincent SA. Postural control of urinary incontinence: The curtsy sign. Lancet. 1966;2:631–2.

46. Upadhyay J, Bolduc S, Bagli DJ, et al. Use of the dysfunctional voiding symptom score to predict resolution of vesicoureteral reflux in children with voiding dysfunction. J Urol. 2003;169:1842–6; discussion 6; author reply 6.

47. Chandra M, Saharia R, Hill V, Shi Q. Prevalence of diurnal voiding symptoms and difficult arousal from sleep in children with nocturnal enuresis. J Urol. 2004;172:311–6.

48. Koff SA, Lapides J, Piazza DH. Association of urinary tract infection and reflux with uninhibited bladder contractions and voluntary sphincteric obstruction. J Urol. 1979;122:373–6.

49. Curran MJ, Kaefer M, Peters C, et al. The overactive bladder in childhood: Long-term results with conservative management. J Urol. 2000;163:574–7.

50. Parekh DJ, Pope JCt, Adams MC, Brock JW, 3rd. The use of radiography, urodynamic studies and cystoscopy in the evaluation of voiding dysfunction. J Urol. 2001;165:215–8.

51. Homsy YL. Dysfunctional voiding syndromes and vesicoureteral reflux. Pediatr Nephrol. 1994;8:116–21.

52. Homsy YL, Nsouli I, Hamburger B, et al. Effects of oxybutynin on vesicoureteral reflux in children. J Urol. 1985;134:1168–71.

53. Koff SA, Murtagh D. The uninhibited bladder in children: Effect of treatment on vesicoureteral reflux resolution. Contrib Nephrol. 1984;39:211–20.

54. Scholtmeijer RJ, van Mastrigt R. The effect of oxyphenonium bromide and oxybutynin hydrochloride on detrusor contractility and reflux in children with vesicoureteral reflux and detrusor instability. J Urol. 1991;146:660–2.

55. Seruca H. Vesicoureteral reflux and voiding dysfunction: A prospective study. J Urol. 1989;142:494–8; discussion 501.

56. Koff SA, Wagner TT, Jayanthi VR. The relationship among dysfunctional elimination syndromes, primary vesicoureteral reflux and urinary tract infections in children. J Urol. 1998;160:1019–22.

57. O'Regan S, Yazbeck S, Schick E. Constipation, bladder instability, urinary tract infection syndrome. Clin Nephrol. 1985;23:152–4.

58. Yazbeck S, Schick E, O'Regan S. Relevance of constipation to enuresis, urinary tract infection and reflux: A review. Eur Urol. 1987;13:318–21.

59. Hinman F, Jr. Nonneurogenic neurogenic bladder (the Hinman syndrome): 15 years later. J Urol. 1986;136:769–77.

60. Van Gool J, Tanagho EA. External sphincter activity and recurrent urinary tract infection in girls. Urology. 1977;10:348–53.

61. Snodgrass W. Relationship of voiding dysfunction to urinary tract infection and vesicoureteral reflux in children. Urology. 1991;38:341–4.

62. Mayo ME, Burns MW. Urodynamic studies in children who wet. Br J Urol. 1990;65:641–5.

63. Oliver JL, Campigotto MJ, Coplen DE, et al. Psychosocial comorbidities and obesity are associated with lower urinary tract symptoms in children with voiding dysfunction. J Urol. 2013;190:1511–5.

64. Wenske S, Combs AJ, Van Batavia JP, Glassberg KI. Can staccato and interrupted/fractionated uroflow patterns alone correctly identify the underlying lower urinary tract condition? J Urol. 2012;187:2188–93.

65. Wenske S, Van Batavia JP, Combs AJ, Glassberg KI. Analysis of uroflow patterns in children with dysfunctional voiding. J Pediatr Urol. 2014;10:240–4.

66. Wein AJ. Emerging role of botulinum toxin in the treatment of neurogenic and non-neurogenic voiding dysfunction. J Urol. 2003;170:1044.

67. Smith CP, Somogyi GT, Chancellor MB. Emerging role of botulinum toxin in the treatment of neurogenic and non-neurogenic voiding dysfunction. Curr Urol Rep. 2002;3:382–7.

68. Young HH. Strictures of the prostatico-membranous urethra: Newer methods in the management of difficult lesions. Ann Surg. 1936;104:267–78.

69. Robertson WB, Hayes JA. Congenital diaphragmatic obstruction of the male posterior urethra. Br J Urol. 1969;41:592–8.

70. Rosenfeld B, Greenfield SP, Springate JE, Feld LG. Type III posterior urethral valves: Presentation and management. J Pediatr Surg. 1994;29:81–5.

71. Greenfield SP. Posterior urethral valves: New concepts. J Urol. 1997;157:996–7.

72. Parkhouse HF, Barratt TM, Dillon MJ, et al. Long-term outcome of boys with posterior urethral valves. Br J Urol. 1988;62:59–62.

73. Holmdahl G. Bladder dysfunction in boys with posterior urethral valves. Scand J Urol Nephrol Suppl. 1997;188:1–36.

74. Bauer SB, Labib KB, Dieppa RA, Retik AB. Urodynamic evaluation of boy with myelodysplasia and incontinence. Urology. 1977;10:354–62.

75. Bauer SB, Hallett M, Khoshbin S, et al. Predictive value of urodynamic evaluation in newborns with myelodysplasia. JAMA. 1984;252:650–2.

76. Lais A, Kasabian NG, Dyro FM, et al. The neurosurgical implications of continuous neurourological surveillance of children with myelodysplasia. J Urol. 1993;150:1879–83.

77. Sidi AA, Dykstra DD, Gonzalez R. The value of urodynamic testing in the management of neonates with myelodysplasia: A prospective study. J Urol. 1986;135:90–3.

78. Just M, Schwarz M, Ludwig B, et al. Cerebral and spinal MR-findings in patients with postrepair myelomeningocele. Pediatr Radiol. 1990;20:262–6.

79. Edelstein RA, Bauer SB, Kelly MD, et al. The long-term urological response of neonates with myelodysplasia treated proactively with intermittent catheterization and anticholinergic therapy. J Urol. 1995;154:1500–4.

80. Geraniotis E, Koff SA, Enrile B. The prophylactic use of clean intermittent catheterization in the treatment of infants and young children with myelomeningocele and neurogenic bladder dysfunction. J Urol. 1988;139:85–6.

81. Kasabian NG, Bauer SB, Dyro FM, et al. The prophylactic value of clean intermittent catheterization and anticholinergic medication in newborns and infants with myelodysplasia at risk of developing urinary tract deterioration. Am J Dis Child. 1992;146:840–3.

82. Duckett JW, Jr. Cutaneous vesicostomy in childhood: The Blocksom technique. Urol Clin North Am. 1974;1:485–95.

83. Mandell J, Bauer SB, Colodny AH, Retik AB. Cutaneous vesicostomy in infancy. J Urol. 1981;126:92–3.

84. Kuban KC, Leviton A. Cerebral palsy. N Engl J Med. 1994;330:188–95.

85. Murphy KP, Molnar GE, Lankasky K. Medical and functional status of adults with cerebral palsy. Dev Med Child Neurol. 1995;37:1075–84.

86. Decter RM, Bauer SB, Khoshbin S, et al. Urodynamic assessment of children with cerebral palsy. J Urol. 1987;138:1110–2.

87. Brodak PP, Scherz HC, Packer MG, Kaplan GW. Is urinary tract screening necessary for patients with cerebral palsy? J Urol. 1994;152:1586–7.

88. Robson WL, Jackson HP, Blackhurst D, Leung AK. Enuresis in children with attention-deficit hyperactivity disorder. South Med J. 1997;90:503–5.

89. Diamond IR, Tannock R, Schachar RJ. Response to methylphenidate in children with ADHD and

comorbid anxiety. J Am Acad Child Adolesc Psychiatry 1999;38:402–9.

90. Alon US, Berenbom A. Idiopathic hypercalciuria of childhood: 4- to 11-year outcome. Pediatr Nephrol. 2000;14:1011–5.

91. Heiliczer JD, Canonigo BB, Bishof NA, Moore ES. Noncalculi urinary tract disorders secondary to idiopathic hypercalciuria in children. Pediatr Clin North Am. 1987;34:711–8.

92. Parekh DJ, Pope JI, Adams MC, Brock JW, 3rd. The role of hypercalciuria in a subgroup of dysfunctional voiding syndromes of childhood. J Urol. 2000;164:1008–10.

93. Vachvanichsanong P, Malagon M, Moore ES. Urinary incontinence due to idiopathic hypercalciuria in children. J Urol. 1994;152:1226–8.

94. Stapleton FB. What is the appropriate evaluation and therapy for children with hypercalciuria and hematuria? Semin Nephrol. 1998;18:359–60.

95. Bomalaski MD, Anema JG, Coplen DE, et al. Delayed presentation of posterior urethral valves: A not so benign condition. J Urol. 1999;162:2130–2.

96. Ritchey ML, Sinha A, DiPietro MA, et al. Significance of spina bifida occulta in children with diurnal enuresis. J Urol. 1994;152:815–8.

97. Pippi Salle JL, Capolicchio G, Houle AM, et al. Magnetic resonance imaging in children with voiding dysfunction: Is it indicated? J Urol. 1998;160:1080–3.

98. Kaefer M, Zurakowski D, Bauer SB, et al. Estimating normal bladder capacity in children. J Urol. 1997;158:2261-4.

99. Guerrero RA, Cavender CP. Constipation: Physical and psychological sequelae. Pediatr Ann. 1999;28:312–6.

100. Blethyn AJ, Verrier Jones K, Newcombe R, et al. Radiological assessment of constipation. Arch Dis Child. 1995;73:532–3.

101. Dohil R, Roberts E, Jones KV, Jenkins HR. Constipation and reversible urinary tract abnormalities. Arch Dis Child. 1994;70:56–7.

102. Bolann BJ, Sandberg S, Digranes A. Implications of probability analysis for interpreting results of leukocyte esterase and nitrite test strips. Clin Chem. 1989;35:1663–8.

103. Pezzlo M. Detection of urinary tract infections by rapid methods. Clin Microbiol Rev. 1988;1:268–80.

104. Parrott TS. Urologic implications of imperforate anus. Urology. 1977;10:407–13.

105. Greenfield SP, Fera M. Urodynamic evaluation of the patient with an imperforate anus: A prospective study. J Urol. 1991;146:539–41.

106. Mathews R, Jeffs RD, Reiner WG, et al. Cloacal exstrophy: Improving the quality of life—The Johns Hopkins experience. J Urol. 1998;160:2452–6.

107. Khoury AE, Hendrick EB, McLorie GA, et al. Occult spinal dysraphism: Clinical and urodynamic

108. Sutow WW, Pryde AW. Incidence of spina bifida occulta in relation to age. AMA J Dis Child. 1956;91:211–7.

109. Wen JG, Tong EC. Cystometry in infants and children with no apparent voiding symptoms. Br J Urol. 1998;81:468–73.

110. Chin-Peuckert L, Salle JL. A modified biofeedback program for children with detrusor-sphincter dyssynergia: 5-year experience. J Urol. 2001;166:1470–5.

111. Combs AJ, Glassberg AD, Gerdes D, Horowitz M. Biofeedback therapy for children with dysfunctional voiding. Urology. 1998;52:312–5.

112. De Paepe H, Hoebeke P, Renson C, et al. Pelvic-floor therapy in girls with recurrent urinary tract infections and dysfunctional voiding. Br J Urol. 1998;81(Suppl 3):109–13.

113. De Paepe H, Renson C, Van Laecke E, et al. Pelvic-floor therapy and toilet training in young children with dysfunctional voiding and obstipation. BJU Int. 2000;85:889–93.

114. De Paepe H, Renson C, Hoebeke P, et al. The role of pelvic-floor therapy in the treatment of lower urinary tract dysfunctions in children. Scand J Urol Nephrol. 2002;36:260–7.

115. Duel BP. Biofeedback therapy and dysfunctional voiding in children. Curr Urol Rep. 2003;4:142–5.

116. Glazier DB, Ankem MK, Ferlise V, et al. Utility of biofeedback for the daytime syndrome of urinary frequency and urgency of childhood. Urology. 2001;57:791–3; discussion 3–4.

117. Herndon CD, Decambre M, McKenna PH. Interactive computer games for treatment of pelvic floor dysfunction. J Urol. 2001;166:1893–8.

118. Hoebeke P, Vande Walle J, Theunis M, et al. Outpatient pelvic-floor therapy in girls with daytime incontinence and dysfunctional voiding. Urology. 1996;48:923–7.

119. Kjolseth D, Knudsen LM, Madsen B, et al. Urodynamic biofeedback training for children with bladder-sphincter dyscoordination during voiding. Neurourol Urodyn. 1993;12:211–21.

120. McKenna PH, Herndon CD, Connery S, Ferrer FA. Pelvic floor muscle retraining for pediatric voiding dysfunction using interactive computer games. J Urol. 1999;162:1056–62; discussion 62–3.

121. Wennergren H, Oberg B. Pelvic floor exercises for children: A method of treating dysfunctional voiding. Br J Urol. 1995;76:9–15.

122. Sugar EC, Firlit CF. Urodynamic biofeedback: A new therapeutic approach for childhood incontinence/infection (vesical voluntary sphincter dyssynergia). J Urol. 1982;128:1253–8.

outcome after division of the filum terminale. J Urol. 1990;144:426–8; discussion 8–9, 43–4.

123. Austin PF, Homsy YL, Masel JL, et al. Alpha-Adrenergic blockade in children with neuropathic and nonneuropathic voiding dysfunction. J Urol 1999;162:1064–7.

124. Cain MP, Wu SD, Austin PF, et al. Alpha blocker therapy for children with dysfunctional voiding and urinary retention. J Urol. 2003;170:1514–5; discussion 6–7.

125. Yang SS, Wang CC, Chen YT. Effectiveness of alpha1-adrenergic blockers in boys with low urinary flow rate and urinary incontinence. J Formos Med Assoc. 2003;102:551–5.

126. Blackwell B, Currah, J. The psychopharmacology of nocturnal enuresis. In: Kolvin IM, Mackeith RC, Meadow SR, editors. Bladder Control and Enuresis. Philadelphia: JB Lippincott; 1973.

127. Kaneko K, Fujinaga S, Ohtomo Y, et al. Combined pharmacotherapy for nocturnal enuresis. Pediatr Nephrol. 2001;16:662–4.

128. Klauber GT. Clinical efficacy and safety of desmopressin in the treatment of nocturnal enuresis. J Pediatr. 1989;114:719–22.

129. Wille S. Comparison of desmopressin and enuresis alarm for nocturnal enuresis. Arch Dis Child. 1986;61:30–3.

130. Hjalmas K, Hanson E, Hellstrom AL, et al. Long-term treatment with desmopressin in children with primary monosymptomatic nocturnal enuresis: An open multicentre study. Swedish Enuresis Trial (SWEET) Group. Br J Urol. 1998;82:704–9.

131. Eller DA, Austin PF, Tanguay S, Homsy YL. Daytime functional bladder capacity as a predictor of response to desmopressin in monosymptomatic nocturnal enuresis. Eur Urol. 1998;33(Suppl 3):25–9.

132. Rushton HG, Belman AB, Zaontz MR, et al. The influence of small functional bladder capacity and other predictors on the response to desmopressin in the management of monosymptomatic nocturnal enuresis. J Urol. 1996;156:651–5.

133. Watanabe H, Kawauchi A, Kitamori T, Azuma Y. Treatment system for nocturnal enuresis according to an original classification system. Eur Urol. 1994;25:43–50.

134. Yeung CK, Sreedhar B, Leung VT, Metreweli C. Ultrasound bladder measurements in patients with primary nocturnal enuresis: A urodynamic and treatment outcome correlation. J Urol. 2004;171:2589–94.

135. Smith EM, Elder JS. Double antimicrobial prophylaxis in girls with breakthrough UTI. Urology. 1994;43:708--12.

136. Pohl HG, Bauer SB, Borer JG, et al. The outcome of voiding dysfunction managed with clean intermittent catheterization in neurologically and anatomically normal children. BJU Int. 2002;89:923–7.

137. Tanagho EA, Miller ER, Lyon RP, Fisher R. Spastic striated external sphincter and urinary tract infection in girls. Br J Urol. 1971;43:69–82.

138. Steinhardt GF, Naseer S, Cruz OA. Botulinum toxin: Novel treatment for dramatic urethral dilatation associated with dysfunctional voiding. J Urol. 1997;158:190–1.

## REVIEW QUESTIONS

1. A 2-year-old girl is expected to begin toilet training in which of the following sequences:
   a. Daytime bowel, daytime bladder, nocturnal bladder, nocturnal bowel
   b. Nocturnal bowel, daytime bowel, daytime bladder, nocturnal bladder
   c. Daytime bladder, nocturnal bladder, nocturnal bowel, daytime bowel
   d. Nocturnal bladder, nocturnal bowel, daytime bowel, daytime bladder

2. A 6-year-old boy is referred shortly after the beginning of second grade with new-onset urinary frequency occurring every 15 minutes. He does not have nocturnal enuresis and has not had daytime wetting. He has never had a urinary tract infection and was completely asymptomatic before the school year began. His physical examination is normal. Your treatment recommendations include:
   a. Reassurance
   b. Renal bladder sonography with prevoid and postvoid views of the bladder to investigate whether he is retaining urine
   c. An MRI of the sacral spine
   d. Anticholinergic medication

3. A 7-year-old obese girl presents with daytime incontinence lasting over a year. She has been evaluated with multiple urine cultures and only mixed bacterial growth found. She denies urgency to void, voids approximately five times daily, and never wets the bed. Her mother states that her underpants are sporadically wet, with wetting occurring shortly after the girl voids. Her physical examination is normal. Your treatment recommendations include:
   a. Renal bladder sonography with prevoid and postvoid views of the bladder to investigate whether she is retaining urine
   b. An MRI of the sacral spine
   c. Anticholinergic medication
   d. Reassurance and encouragement to void with her legs widely spaced

4. An 8-year-old girl presents with incontinence occurring when she laughs hard. Her physical examination, urinalysis, and remainder of her history are normal. You diagnose giggle incontinence and offer a prescription for:
   a. Amitriptyline
   b. Oxybutynin
   c. Vasopressin
   d. Methylphenidate

5. A 9-year-old boy presents with nighttime wetting. He has never been completely dry at night and wets the bed approximately three nights of the week. His father had the same problem until the age of 13 years. A review of the boy's voiding patterns shows that he is dry during the day, denies urgency, and has normal bowel movements. He is interested in becoming dry soon because he is planning to join the Boy Scouts. Your treatment recommendations include:
   a. Nothing, because he will grow out of it around 13 years of age, just like his father
   b. Oxybutynin and a bowel program
   c. Vasopressin
   d. Amitriptyline

6. A 9-year-old boy presents with nighttime wetting. He has never been completely dry at night and wets the bed approximately three nights out of the week. His father suffered from the same problem until the age of 13 years. A review of the boy's voiding patterns shows that he occasionally has episodes of mild incontinence during the day preceded by the need to void and has bowel movements every several days. He is interested in becoming dry soon because he is planning to join the Boy Scouts. Your treatment recommendations include:
   a. Nothing as he will grow out of it around 13 years of age, just like his father.
   b. Oxybutynin and a bowel program
   c. Vasopressin
   d. Amitriptyline

7. A 6-year-old girl has never been completely dry. Despite that she has no symptoms other than persistently damp underpants, her pediatrician has evaluated her for suspected UTIs. Each urine culture has demonstrated either no growth or fewer than 10,000 CFU/mL of mixed growth. She was toilet trained at 23 months of age. She voids five times during the day, with normal sensation to void before and no evidence of urgency. Her panties are always wet, day and night. She does not wake up to urinate in the middle of the night. Your initial recommendation includes:
   a. Timed voiding to make certain that she is not in overflow incontinence
   b. A renal-bladder sonogram
   c. A KUB examination

d. Renal scan
e. A VCUG

8. A 6-year-old girl presents with a history of five culture-proved urinary tract infections. She has never had fever with them. Instead, the cultures are obtained because of her chronic urinary incontinence. She wets most every day, generally beginning around midday and into the afternoons. Her incontinence is never preceded by a sense of urgency. She will generally stay dry throughout the night, wakes around 7 am, but doesn't void until around lunchtime. She might void once more before bedtime. Which condition is she likely to have?
   a. Paradoxical incontinence
   b. Sensory deficient bladder
   c. Detrusor overactivity
   d. Primary nocturnal enuresis

9. A 4-year-old girl presents with a history of three culture-proved febrile urinary tract infections. Her only medications include MiraLAX for chronic constipation, though she takes it rarely and complains of abdominal pain. She is frequently wet during the day, and her incontinence is preceded by urgency. Your initial recommendations include:
   a. Timed voiding and better adherence to her bowel program
   b. Oxybutynin and a bowel program
   c. Trimethoprim-sulfamethoxazole nightly
   d. Renal bladder sonogram with prevoid and postvoid views and a contrast voiding cystourethrogram, and trimethoprim-sulfamethoxazole, nightly

10. A 5-year-old girl is diagnosed with dysfunctional voiding syndrome after an evaluation for wetting, constipation, and recurrent febrile UTIs. A VCUG was negative. Your treatment recommendation includes:
    a. Timed voiding
    b. Timed voiding, bladder program
    c. Timed voiding, bladder program, anticholinergics
    d. Timed voiding, bladder program, antibiotic prophylaxis

11. Identify the incorrect statement regarding voiding abnormalities.
    a. Hinman syndrome, which is a discoordination between the detrusor contraction and sphincter relaxation, is initially managed by injecting Botox (botulinum toxin) into the sphincter.
    b. Bladder dysfunction from posterior urethral valve is not static. Whereas detrusor overactivity predominates in childhood, myogenic failure is seen in adolescence.
    c. Most infants with neurogenic bladder have complete paralysis of detrusor function.
    d. Children with cerebral palsy are incontinent only as a result of their physical limitation, because they cannot reach the toilet in time.

## ANSWER KEY

1. b
2. a
3. d
4. d
5. c
6. b
7. d
8. b
9. d
10. d
11. b

# Research tools

# 53

# Applied clinical biostatistics

SHAMIR TUCHMAN

The practicing pediatric nephrologist requires a basic and usable knowledge of how to assess and interpret the medical literature as it relates to the care of children with renal disease. The use of evidence-based approaches in making treatment decisions requires a fundamental understanding of epidemiologic principles and biostatistical methods. This chapter will provide an overview of the epidemiologic and biostatistical concepts that are meant to aid the practicing pediatric nephrologist in critically evaluating the medical literature.

## STUDY DESIGN

Clinical research studies can be categorized into several different categories and subcategories, depending on the design and the prospective or retrospective nature of data collection. For convenience, the two broad categories for study designs that are most applicable to nephrology research are *observational* and *interventional* studies. A summary of these different study designs and their associated features is shown in Table 53.1.

## INTERVENTIONAL STUDIES

In the context of clinical nephrology, interventional studies refer to clinical trials of investigational diagnostic or treatment interventions for renal disease. Interventional studies differ from observational studies in that treatment and treatment assignments to individual study subjects are preplanned, based on either random allocation or another assignment model. Randomized, double-blind, clinical trials in which treatment allocation is random and neither study subjects nor investigators know in advance who is receiving the study intervention are often referenced as the gold standard for study design. The advantages and disadvantages of such a study design are listed in Table 53.2.

In the context of interventional studies, one subgroup of this study design merits special mention. A *crossover interventional study* is one in which study subjects both act as the controls and receive the interventional treatment at different study points. The benefit of using this approach is that it improves the efficiency of the study design because the same power may be achieved to assess the effect of the intervention with a smaller sample size and hence less cost. Furthermore, using each of the study subjects as his or her own control minimizes the variation that occurs among study subjects. This helps achieve the same level of precision for estimating the effect of a treatment using fewer subjects. The limitations of using a crossover study design include their (1) increased complexity, (2) suitability only in disease conditions that are chronic and for which treatment provides a short-term effect but not a cure, (3) increased length of time that each study subject must remain in the study, and (4) the occurrence of carryover effects of the study intervention that may continue into the control study period, biasing the results toward the null hypothesis (e.g., no effect of intervention). In these situations, a wash-out period is used before crossing subjects over from intervention to control to ensure these effects have dissipated. In some instances, interventional studies with a crossover design are prone to bias when there exists a significant interaction based on the time a subject spends in the study. In these situations, data obtained after the crossover of patients may not be usable without introducing bias into the study results and analysis.

Table 53.1 Hierarchy of study design for making causal inferences

| Study design | Description | Advantages | Disadvantages |
| --- | --- | --- | --- |
| Intervention | • Clinical trials; gold-standard to test interventions<br>• Preplanned study subject allocation | • Best for making causal inferences<br>• Best controls for confounding | • Expensive and time-consuming<br>• Restricted generalizability |
| Cohort | • Often prospective<br>• Study population followed over time for disease development | • Able to make causal inferences because exposure precedes disease development<br>• Study several diseases concurrently | • Expensive and time-consuming<br>• Impractical for studying disease with long time horizon<br>• Poor for rare diseases<br>• Exposures may change over time |
| Case-control | • Often retrospective<br>• Diseased and control subjects identified *a priori*<br>• Exposures determined retrospectively for cases and controls | • Less expensive<br>• Exposures studied simultaneously<br>• Ideal for rare diseases<br>• Requires smaller sample sizes | • Cannot demonstrate causality<br>• Only studies one disease<br>• Can only approximate relative risk<br>• Prone to bias in sampling and data collection |
| Ecologic | • Population based association study<br>• Data not collected at individual level<br>• Tracks trends in disease and exposure | • Quick and inexpensive<br>• Makes use of preexisting databases | • Poor for proving causality<br>• Hypothesis "generating"<br>• No individual level exposure data collected |
| Case report | • Report of an "interesting" patient or series of patients with unique presentations or clinical course | • Often first clue to association between exposure and disease | • No statistical method for making associations<br>• Speculative in nature |

# OBSERVATIONAL STUDIES

Observational studies rely on data collection in which treatment decisions are not tied to the study itself and no intervention is made to try to modify the course of the disease. Observational studies can be further sub-categorized into ecologic, cross-sectional, case-control, and cohort studies.

# Ecologic studies

Ecologic studies are observational studies in which individual-level data are lacking and thus comparisons are made at the population level. Ecologic studies often make use of generally available data sets that do not identify individuals and make associations between potential exposures and the occurrence of disease in a population

Table 53.2 Advantages and disadvantages of a randomized controlled study design

| Advantages | Disadvantages |
| --- | --- |
| 1. Ability to make causal inferences or concrete conclusions about the effectiveness of clinical interventions (e.g., medications) because of the exposure preceding the effect.<br>2. Limit the effects of confounding factors that can be balanced between treatment groups if known and likely will be balanced as a result of randomization if unknown.<br>3. Improve efficiency of the study by increasing power by ensuring sufficient numbers of subjects in treatment and control groups. | 1. Expensive and time-consuming.<br>2. Not well suited for studying effects that take a long time to develop.<br>3. Difficult to use in studying treatment for rare diseases when large recruitment populations may be needed.<br>4. May limit the study population to certain sexes, ages, or races, which may limit the generalizability of results.<br>5. Ethical considerations limit the use of certain exposures or medications with adverse effects deemed too serious to offset any potential benefit to study subjects. |

or subpopulation. Therefore, they are relatively poor studies for making causal associations between exposure and disease and help generate hypotheses that can later be tested using cohort, case-control, or clinical trials. Cross-sectional studies are observational studies that collect data on entire groups of people (e.g., target population) at one point in time. Cross-sectional studies are well-equipped to define the prevalence of a disease state or exposure in a particular population. Therefore, cross-sectional studies are often able to quantify the absolute risk and odds ratio of developing a disease given a particular exposure of interest in a population.

## Case-control studies

Case-control studies are usually retrospective and involve identifying groups of individuals with and without disease in a population and then retrospectively determining their exposure history of interest. Case-control studies are often less expensive and quicker to conduct than cohort studies because no prospective follow-up time is needed. They are good for studying diseases that develop over a long period and allow clinicians to look at multiple exposures that may lead to the disease. They are also superior at studying rare diseases and can usually answer the research question with smaller sample sizes and thus are less expensive. The disadvantages of case-control studies are that (1) they cannot determine causality because they do not relate the time sequence of exposure to disease, (2) they can investigate only one disease at a time, and (3) because there is no time lapse in the study, they often have difficulty in providing accurate estimates of relative risk.

Case-control studies are prone to bias in both sampling of the populations and ascertainment of exposure data. In addition, the method by which controls are selected for case-control studies may introduce a source of bias into the results. Ideally, controls (1) should be free of disease at the time of selection and ideally not have had the disease under study in the past, (2) should be drawn from the same population in which cases occur, and (3) should have the same baseline potential of developing disease as the cases. As an example, a case-control study of a disease that disproportionally occurs in women should draw its controls from a population that has the same gender distribution as that from which cases are sampled. Not to do so would introduce bias into the results.

On the other end of the spectrum, it is also possible to select controls that are too similar to cases in some unmeasured risk factor for disease occurrence. When this occurs, controls are said to be *over-matched*. As an example, in an effort to match for environmental exposures, using siblings of cases of disease as controls when the disease in question has a potential genetic predisposition may introduce bias into the results. A special type of case-control study is known as a *nested* case-control study. This is essentially a case-control study conducted in a population under investigation as a cohort study. A disease of interest is identified and exposure data already collected as part of the cohort study analyzed for its association with the disease.

## Cohort studies

In cohort studies, subjects are followed over time for the occurrence of disease, with exposure data of interest often collected prospectively to determine its ultimate association with a disease. In the most basic example, two study populations are selected that differ in one or more particular exposure or risk factor from each other. Each study group is followed over time for the development of the disease of interest. In this way, the incidence of disease can be ascertained for each group and the associated risk of each exposure variable quantified. In large populations a representative but random sample of study subjects is used because of feasibility and cost considerations. All study subjects are free of the disease of interest on entering into a prospective cohort study.

One of the advantages of a cohort study is that there is a clear occurrence of relevant exposures before disease occurrence, which is essential in determining causality. Also, cohort studies, if of sufficient size and comprehensive in data collection, can determine relevant risk factors in the occurrence of multiple diseases. Cohort studies have limitations in that (1) they are not ideal for studying rare diseases or those that have a long time horizon for development, (2) they are prone to changes in exposures if the studies are long, (3) study subjects may diverge from their typical behavior or exposure pattern by simply knowing these are being monitored in the study, and (4) withdrawals from the study may bias the results if it is directly related to disease occurrence or exposures. Although many cohort studies are prospective, *retrospective* cohort studies may trace exposures predating study entry by participants and thereby ultimately save time and resources in coming to definitive conclusions. This can be done assuming the retrospective data are collected in their entirety.

## Meta-analysis

The challenge for a diligent practitioner is to synthesize, compare, and contrast the totality of differing types of studies when examining the association between a risk factor and outcome and coming to a conclusion regarding the nature of an association or lack thereof. In doing so, the practitioner must take into account the size, quality, and design of each study. Traditionally, this has been done using a qualitative or *ad hoc* approach. However, there are quantitative methodologies used to combine the results of several similar but not necessarily identical studies examining the association between an exposure and disease. This type of study design is known as a meta-analysis.

Meta-analysis has two general goals. The first is to assess the consistency of the exposure-outcome association across different studies. The second is to attempt to generate a composite estimate of this association combining the results of different studies. This improves the power to detect a significant association because it increases the sample size by combining studies. As a result, the confidence interval for an exposure-outcome association narrows, giving a more precise estimate of the association. This can be done by pooling study estimates or in certain cases pooling the raw data to generate a new estimate with a larger sample size. This process is fraught with potential pitfalls, not the least of which is forcing data together from studies that may have had different designs, definitions of the exposure and outcome, and divergent populations studied. This introduces bias into the meta-analysis and must be taken into account.

Before a meta-analysis can be properly conducted, a systematic review of the literature is required. This is a protocolized critical review of all the literature existing on a specified exposure and outcome association. This may include formal journal publications, conference proceedings, and published reviews on a designated topic often identified through journal database searches. The systematic review evaluates each study for its power, design, sources of bias, and generalizability of results in establishing the quality of the study. This is taken into account when deciding which studies to include in the meta-analysis and further taken into account (especially the size of the study population) in the actual meta-analysis when determining a summary estimate of the size and direction of an association.

Focusing on the quality of study to be included in a meta-analysis is inescapable and a central factor in deciding which studies are to be included. Assessing the quality of a study in terms of how it answers the hypothesis of the meta-analysis is also known as the *internal validity*. In this regard, studies are assessed based on (1) their design, with those with interventions (e.g., randomized clinical trials) being generally most desirable; (2) analytic approach ensuring that the authors appropriately controlled for confounding aspects and tested for interactions among risk factors; and (3) how the study was conducted in terms of issues such as selection of controls and incomplete data collection or follow-up (quality of data). Finally, studies also may be judged for their inclusion based on the generalizability of the results and application to different populations or settings. This concept is also often referred to as the *external validity*. In determining a summary estimate of an association between an exposure and disease, estimates of the association between exposure and outcome from separate studies in a meta-analysis must be pooled. If patient-level data are available, the raw data may be combined to give a single pooled estimate. Typically, this is not the case and study investigators must use methods in which a weight score is assigned to each study included. In combining these studies into one pooled estimate (e.g., relative risk), study investigators may use weights based on both the size of a study population and quality of the study design and conduct. Weighting based on study size is relatively straightforward. However, placing

a quantitative estimate on study quality is much more complex. Furthermore, it is rare for any two individual studies to be exactly alike. Therefore, a meta-analytical approach also must account for the heterogeneity among the studies included. Finally, an important overarching limitation in the use of meta-analysis is publication bias. This may result from studies that were not submitted or were not accepted for publication because of an absence of a statistically significant association between an exposure and disease, as a result of small sample size, or because an association was revealed that was the opposite of what was expected. In general, publication bias will tend to bias the pooled estimate away from the null. The degree and importance of this bias on the overall results depend on several factors. The first is the size of pooled risk estimate from the meta-analysis. As an example, a relative risk that has a narrow confidence interval based on studies included with large sample sizes is unlikely to be affected significantly by unpublished studies that had relatively small sample sizes even if the risk estimates in these studies were opposite to those derived from the meta-analysis. Also, a meta-analysis that shows a strong association (e.g., high relative risk) between exposure and outcome is unlikely to be affected to the point of nonsignificance by unpublished studies documenting an opposite relationship or no relationship (e.g., negative studies). Finally, if only studies that did not show a statistically significant association are excluded from publication, but studies showing an opposite or protective effect of exposure are published and included in the meta-analysis, then the overall pooled estimate of effect is unlikely to change significantly by the inclusion of non–statistically significant results.

One tool by which study investigators can try to estimate the potential for publication bias is the *funnel plot*. A funnel plot is a graph of the log of the effect estimate (e.g., odds ratio or relative risk) on the $y$-axis against the inverse of the standard error (e.g., sample size estimate) on the $x$-axis. Funnel plots that are symmetric with points on either side of the zero association on the $y$-axis as well as points close to the zero line are usually interpreted as having minimal associated publication bias.

## BIAS

Bias represents uncontrolled and unmeasured features of data that may result in changes in study results or its conclusions. Bias affects the internal validity of a study and may lead to incorrect conclusions about the nature, size, and degree of relationship between an exposure and disease. Bias may occur as a consequence of a systematic error in the study design, the way in which data were collected, or how the data were analyzed. There are several different categories of bias based on the specifics of the study design and conduct. A summary of these categories and associated types of bias is shown Table 53.3.

Selection bias occurs when subjects who volunteer or are selected to participate in a study are in some way different in

Table 53.3 Types of bias in study design and execution

| Type of bias | Description |
|---|---|
| **Selection** | • Selected or volunteer subjects differ in characteristics that may be associated with disease from the general or control population<br>• Most commonly affects case-control or retrospective cohort studies<br>• Dealt with effectively when randomization is used, such as in randomized controlled trials |
| **Information** | |
| Recall bias | • Subjects recall exposure histories more clearly should they have the outcome or disease under study |
| Reporting bias | • Subjects may be hesitant to report events or exposures that are personally embarrassing or may affect their standing in the study |
| Observer bias | • Study staff charged with documenting observations or examination findings do so with preconceived notions of what those results should reveal |
| Follow-up bias | • Study subjects who drop out of a study may have inherent differences in comparison to the general populations under study |
| Hawthorne effect | • In prospective studies, patients under surveillance for the occurrence of disease or exposure of interest modify their behavior because of participation in the study |
| Surveillance (detection) bias | • Investigators following subjects prospectively for the occurrence of disease may follow those with a suspected risk factor more closely and/or for a longer period |
| **Misclassification** | |
| Random | • Inaccuracy in measurement is thought to have occurred to an equal degree in all study groups |
| Differential | • Errors in measurement or classification of disease occur preferentially in one or more study groups<br>• Blinding of study subjects, investigators, or both when possible can mitigate misclassification bias |

characteristics from the general population at risk for a the disease. This occurs particularly if these differences, which are often unmeasured, are associated with the occurrence of the disease under study. Selection bias is of particular concern in case-control and retrospective cohort studies. Selection bias does not typically occur in randomized controlled trials, in which randomization prevents systematic errors in selection, or in prospective cohort studies, in which the study population is chosen without regard to prior exposure history.

Information bias occurs when data gathering in a study is done incorrectly or inconsistently and affects the conclusions rendered. Examples of information bias include interviewer bias in which the person collecting the data from study subjects may influence the responses given or the structure of interview. Recall bias is a related phenomenon in which study subjects may recall exposure histories more clearly should they have the outcome or disease under study. Contrary to this, study subjects may be hesitant to report events or exposures that are personally embarrassing or that may affect their standing in the study. This is known as reporting bias. Observer bias may occur when study staff, charged with documenting observations or clinical findings, proceed with preconceived notions of what those results should look like.

Dealing with missing or incomplete observations also can be a significant challenge in collecting data. The way in which study subjects or patients may drop out of a study may be grounded in inherent differences among populations under study. Should this be the case, this would introduce follow-up bias to the study results. In prospective studies, patients under surveillance for the occurrence of disease or exposure of interest may modify their behavior, simply by the mere fact that they are being followed by study investigators. If this modification in their behavior introduces changes in the occurrence of disease or degree of exposure, this may bias study conclusions. This is known as the *Hawthorne effect*. Finally, study investigators following subjects prospectively for the occurrence of disease may follow those with a suspected risk factor more closely or for a longer time, potentially increasing the chances of detection. This is known as surveillance or detection bias.

## Misclassification bias

In addition to sources of bias associated with gathering information in a study, bias may stem from the manner in which data are subsequently analyzed. One example of this concept is misclassification bias, wherein exposure or disease classification is flawed because of either inaccurate measurement of exposure or diagnosis of disease. If the inaccuracy in measurement is thought to have occurred to an equal degree in all study groups, this is known as *random misclassification*. In this situation, the error in measurement may not necessarily adversely affect the study conclusions, because it has occurred to an equal degree among all participants. However, if errors in measurement or classification of disease occur preferentially in one or more study groups, this represents *differential misclassification* and may indeed distort study results toward a greater or lesser association between exposure and disease. Use of blinding of the study participants, investigators, or both can help mitigate differential misclassification.

## BIOSTATISTICAL METHODS

In clinical research, in addition to the method in which a study was designed and conducted, the methodology and assumptions made in data analysis can have an impact on the ultimate conclusions of a study. The following section will present and discuss methods of data analysis commonly employed in epidemiologic studies, including regression analysis, assessment of risk, survival analysis, and receiver operating characteristic (ROC) curves. In addition, potential pitfalls associated with data analysis will be discussed.

## REGRESSION ANALYSIS

### Linear regression analysis

In its most basic form, a regression line represents a best fit line drawn through multiple data points that minimizes the sum of the squared distance ($d_i$) between all the sample points and the line (Figure 53.1). For a scatter plot of data associating a dependent (outcome) variable $y$ with an independent variable $x$, the regression line is defined by the equation:

$$y = \alpha + \beta x \tag{53.1}$$

In this example, $\alpha$ represents the value of $y$ where the independent variable is 0 (e.g., the line contacts the $y$-axis). $\beta$ represents the slope of this line and is positive when there is a positive relationship between $x$ and $y$, and $\beta$ takes on a negative value when there is an inverse relationship between $x$ and $y$. $\beta$ is 0 when there is no relationship between the independent and dependent variables.

Multivariate linear regression extends this methodology to include the relationship between one dependent variable and multiple independent variables. Multivariate linear regression serves to explain the variability in values of the $y$ variable based on its relationship to multiple dependent variables *(x1, x2, …. xi)*. In this way, we are able to determine the independent effect of a variable *xi* in relation to other variables that affect $y$. In essence, multivariate linear regression isolates the effect of each independent variable on $y$, holding the other independent variables constant. Multivariate linear regression is expressed by the equation:

$$y = \alpha + \beta_1(x_1) + \beta_2(x_2) + \beta_3(x_3) + \cdots + \beta_i(x_i). \tag{53.2}$$

In Equation 53.2, $\beta$ represents the unique relationship of each independent variable with the dependent or outcome variable. As an example, in examining the factors (independent variables) that affect systolic blood pressure in children, one may hypothesize that body mass index (BMI), the daily sodium content in milligrams of their diet, a family history of hypertension, the amount of daily aerobic exercise, age, and gender may affect the ultimate systolic blood pressures. In this case, the regression equation would be written as:

Systolic blood pressure (mm Hg) = $\alpha + \beta_1$ (BMI) + $\beta_2$ (daily sodium intake in milligrams) + $\beta_3$ (family history of hypertension) + $\beta_4$ (amount of daily aerobic exercise in minutes) + $\beta_5$ (age in years) + $\beta_6$ (male or female)

$$\tag{53.3}$$

In this hypothetical regression, one would expect the $\beta$-coefficients, $\beta_1, \beta_2, \beta_3, \beta_5,$ and $\beta_6$ to take on positive values as children with higher BMI, higher daily sodium intake, having a family history of hypertension, are older, and are male are likely to have a higher systolic blood pressure. Conversely, $\beta_4$ is likely to take on a negative value because children who get more exercise may have lower systolic blood pressure (e.g., inverse relationship). Each $\beta$-coefficient in a regression is associated with a $P$ value, which tells the reader whether that particular independent variable is significantly associated with the outcome variable adjusted for all the other independent variables in the regression. A $P$ value less than 0.05 gives some sense of the strength of the relationship between the dependent and independent variable. For example, a $P$ value of 0.001

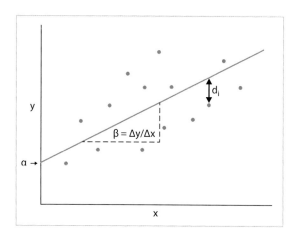

Figure 53.1 Fitted regression line for scatter plot of $y$ over $x$. $\alpha - y$: intercept where fitted regression line contacts the $y$-axis. Value of $y$ when $x = 0$. $\beta$: *slope of the fitted regression line; di: distance from each data point to fitted regression line.*

is more significant than a *P* value of 0.01, but both have a significant representation because of being less than 0.05.

## Logistic regression analysis

Multivariate logistic regression follows the same principles as multivariate linear regression, the only difference is that the outcome variable is coded as a categorical (e.g., yes/no) variable. As in linear regression, independent variables can be either linear or categorical.

## CONFOUNDING AND INTERACTION

A confounding variable is significantly associated with both the exposure and disease, but does not occur as a result of either. In this way, a confounding variable is able to partially or wholly explain the relationship between an exposure risk factor and disease occurrence. Therefore, the independent effect of the exposure as a risk factor for disease occurrence is lessened or sometimes negated, if the confounding variable is taken into consideration. Confounders are often intermediates in the pathway from a risk variable to the occurrence of disease. As an example, adolescent age is a risk factor for increased car accidents. However, adolescents are also more likely to text while driving, which increases the chances of a collision. Therefore, cell phone texting during driving confounds the relationship between the adolescent age group and traffic accidents.

Conversely, an interaction variable is one that modifies the relationship between exposure and disease, without explaining why the relationship exists. Unlike confounders, interaction variables are not on the pathophysiologic pathway between exposure and disease. As an example, smoking has a strong causal association with the development of lung cancer. In males, this association may be stronger than in females for the same number of cigarette pack-years smoked. Therefore, gender serves as an interaction variable for the relationship between smoking and lung cancer.

## RISK ASSESSMENT

At its most basic level, relative risk compares the risk for developing disease between a group of people with and without a potential exposure. Risk is determined by the probability of developing disease, given the presence or absence of a risk factor. It is estimated by using the incidence of disease development in a group having the risk factor or exposure of interest. In Table 53.4, a 2 × 2 table in which disease and exposure status are known for a population, relative risk is calculated as the incidence of disease occurrence among those exposed: $a/(a + b)$ divided by the incidence of disease among those without the exposure: $c/(c + d)$.

$$\text{Relative risk (RR)} = [a/(a + b)]/[c/(c + d)] \quad (35.4)$$

A relative risk that equals 1 suggests that there is no effect of the risk factor of interest on disease. Risk factors with

Table 53.4  2 × 2 table of exposure and disease status in a case-control study

| Exposure | Disease status | | Total |
|---|---|---|---|
| | Disease | No disease | |
| Exposed | a | b | a + b |
| Unexposed | c | d | c + d |
| Total | a + c | b + d | n |

relative risk values greater than 1 suggest increased risk for disease development, and those between 0 and 1 suggest protection against disease occurrence.

A separate but related measure to relative risk is the odds ratio. Unlike relative risk, which expresses the probability of developing disease given the presence or absence of a risk factor, the odds ratio estimates the number of those with disease divided by those without disease for each exposure group. Looking at Table 53.4, this calculates to $a/b$ for those with exposure and $c/d$ for those without the exposure. The odds ratio then becomes $a/b$ divided by $c/d$.

$$\text{Odds ratio (OR)} = (a/b)/(c/d) = ad/bc \quad (53.5)$$

In case-control studies, relative risk is difficult to ascertain and the odds ratio is the only measure that can be calculated. The odds ratio often can be a good approximation of the relative risk, assuming that the disease under study is rare. In this situation, $(a + b)$ is approximately equal to $b$ and $(c + d)$ is approximately equal to $d$ so that the equation for relative risk looks identical to that for the odds ratio.

## SURVIVAL ANALYSIS

In cohort studies or clinical trials, researchers want to get a sense of the occurrence of an outcome (e.g., death or disease) as a function of time in the study. To do this, an approach that estimates the probability of survival for two or more groups that differ in a particular exposure or intervention are compared. In its simplest form, this constitutes a life table that tracks the proportion of people still surviving (or disease free) at consecutive time points through the length of the study. In survival analysis, study subjects are censored when the event of interest occurs (e.g., death or disease). From that point onward, those subjects are not used in calculating the probability of survival at further time points in the cohort. The estimated cumulative survival probabilities at each time point in the study can be then plotted on the *y*-axis against time on the *x*-axis to give a survivor function or plot. As an example, Figure 53.2 shows a life-table survival plot of the cumulative survival probability of disease occurrence for a cohort followed for 10 years. Each study subject is screened for the occurrence of disease at yearly intervals. For the sake of simplicity, assume 100% retention in the study so that no study subjects get censored out of the study unless they develop the disease of interest and no

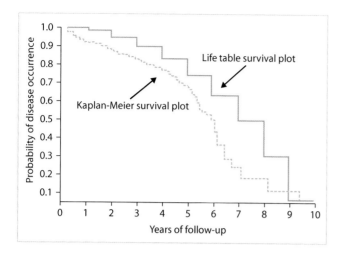

Figure 53.2 Survival plot of disease occurrence over time using life table and Kaplan-Meier methodologies. y-axis, probability of disease occurrence; x-axis, follow-up time in years; _____, life table methodology survival plot; ........, Kaplan-Meier methodology survival plot.

subjects die during the study period. At each time point, a progressively smaller proportion of the study population is free of disease. Because subjects are evaluated only on a yearly basis for disease, the probability of being free of disease at intermediate time points is assumed to be the same as the probability during the last year of evaluation. As can be seen in Figure 53.2, the theoretical disease in question will affect almost all individuals at the end of 10 years of follow-up. Actually, this is rarely the situation. In addition, many study subjects may be censored out of a cohort study for reasons other than the development of the end point of interest. Dealing with these individuals often means making the assumption that they left the study at the mid-point of each time interval. This method for dealing with those who left the study for reasons other than disease occurrence is valid only if censoring occurs uniformly through each study interval and the risk for disease (or death) at any time is uniform throughout the whole study period. Using this step-wise approach to survival analysis often leads to over-estimation of survival probabilities at a time point between study intervals. Progressively shortening the time intervals in which the population is assessed for the outcome may help mitigate some of these limitations. A method of doing just this is exemplified by the Kaplan-Meier approach to survival analysis. In the Kaplan-Meier approach, study time intervals are defined based on the time point at which a subject develops disease. This leads to a survival plot with the most possible time intervals of the shortest duration and helps minimize the problems with how to deal with the data from study withdrawals. The Kaplan-Meier approach maximizes the data that can be used to construct the survival plot. As shown in Figure 53.2, the time intervals between end points vary depending on disease occurrence and are shorter. As a result, the survival probability plot takes on a more linear appearance. This increases the power for

detecting differences in two survival plots in a population separated by an exposure of interest. Several methodologies are used to compare survival plots between two study populations. These include the Mantel-Haenszel methods, the log-rank test, and the weighted log-rank tests. Implicit in these methods is the assumption that the probability of a study outcome (e.g., events) remains constant within the time interval between events. This is known as the proportional hazards assumption.

## RECEIVER OPERATING CHARACTERISTIC CURVES AND TEST STATISTICS

Assessing the value of clinical and laboratory variables is germane to arriving at a diagnoses in patients. Therefore, understanding the ability of a clinical or laboratory test to either confirm or rule out a diagnosis is very important for practitioners. Epidemiologic assessments help evaluate the reliability and usefulness of tests used to diagnose disease. In a population of patients known to have or not have a disease of interest, each is administered a diagnostic test to detect disease. In this situation, there are four potential outcomes. The test can correctly identify patients with the disease of interest, or true positives (TPs); the test can correctly rule out the presence of disease in those who are disease free, or true negatives (TNs). The test can be positive in those who really do not have disease, or false positive (FP), and the test can incorrectly clear patients of disease when they indeed have it, or false negative (FN). A simple 2 × 2 table, as shown in Table 53.5, is able to neatly express each of the scenarios. From these four outcomes, we are able to calculate the performance characteristics of each test. The first is the ability of a test to correctly identify persons with disease when they have it. This probability is known as sensitivity and is calculated as $a/(a + c)$.

$$\text{Sensitivity} = \text{TP}/(\text{TP} + \text{FN}) = a/(a + c) \quad (53.6)$$

Conversely, the probability of a test to be negative when a patient does not have disease is known as the specificity and is calculated as $b/(b + d)$.

$$\text{Specificity} = \text{TN}/(\text{TN} + \text{FP}) = d/(b + d) \quad (53.7)$$

At times, what practitioners really wish to know is the likelihood that a patient has a disease if the ordered test comes

Table 53.5 2 × 2 table of exposure and disease status in a case-control study

| | Disease status | | |
|---|---|---|---|
| Test result | Disease | No disease | Total |
| Positive | True positive (TP) a | False positive (FP) b | a + b |
| Negative | False negative (FN) c | True negative (TN) d | c + d |
| Total | a + c | b + d | n |

back positive or, alternatively, can be reassured that he or she does not have the disease if a test comes back negative. These test statistics are known as the positive predictive value and negative predictive value, respectively. They are expressed by the equations $a/(a + b)$ and $d/(c + d)$ respectively.

$$\text{Positive predictive value (PPV)} = \text{TP/(TP + FP)} = a/(a + b)$$
$$(53.8)$$

$$\text{Negative predictive value (NPV)} = \text{TN/(TN + FN)} = d/(c + d)$$
$$(53.9)$$

In evaluating the usefulness of a new diagnostic test in a population, these test metrics are often compared to the performance of a known and well-used test already in clinical use. Both positive and negative predictive values are affected by the prevalence of a disease state in the population, even though the sensitivity and specificity of a test will not change. If we try to compare the performance of several tests at once, one metric that may be used is the likelihood ratio. The likelihood ratio is calculated as the sensitivity of a test divided by (1 – specificity). An increase in sensitivity or specificity may increase the likelihood ratio of a test. A useful plot that compares the performance of two or more diagnostic tests for disease is called the ROC plot.

An example of such a plot is shown in Figure 53.3. Consider three different diagnostic tests $a$, $b$, and $c$ for a disease $y$. Test $c$ has a sensitivity and specificity that when added together always equal 1. Therefore, when the sensitivity is 100%, the specificity is 0% and vice versa. Such a test has no discriminative value in diagnosing disease. Tests $a$ and $b$, respectively, have proportionally higher sensitivities for a given specificity. Depending on the goals of the test (e.g., ruling in or ruling out disease), one may think test $a$ or $b$ may outperform the other. However, combining the two tests together as a composite may give the ideal diagnostic test for the disease $y$. A theoretically perfect diagnostic test

$x$ would have 100% sensitivity or specificity at all times. A composite measure of how well a test performs can be estimated by the area under the ROC curve (AUC). Tests with a larger AUC that approaches the AUC of a perfect test tend to be better. Therefore, the AUC offers a convenient way of comparing two or more diagnostic tests.

## SUMMARY

Modern research publications require an increasingly greater understanding of many principles of epidemiology and biostatistics. The practicing pediatric nephrologist should be well versed in many of these concepts to properly interpret both the relevance and quality of studies as applicable to their own patients. This chapter has introduced some of the basic concepts of study design, limitations, and analytical approaches used in epidemiology.

## BIBLIOGRAPHY

1. Woodward M. Epidemiology: Study Design and Data Analysis, ed 2. Boca Raton, FL: Chapman & Hall/CRC Press; 2005.
2. Moore DS, McCabe GP. Introduction to the Practice of Statistics, ed 2. New York: W.H. Freeman; 1993.
3. Gordis L. Epidemiology, ed 3. Philadelphia: Elsevier Saunders, 2004.
4. Hennekens CH, Buring JE, Mayrent SL. Epidemiology in Medicine. Philadelphia: Lippincott Williams & Wilkins; 1987.
5. Friis RH, Sellers TA. Epidemiology for Public Health Practice. Gaithersburg, MD: Aspen Publishers; 1996.

## REVIEW QUESTIONS

1. You conducted a hypothetical observational study examining the clinical factors associated with the decline in estimated glomerular filtration rate (eGFR) in children with hypothetical inherited glomerulonephritis. The primary outcome of the study was the absolute change in eGFR after 1 year of observation. Hypothetically speaking, no patients were treated with any antiprogression medications during the study period. At the end of the study period, you analyze the data and produce a multilinear regression model of the outcome variable (absolute change in eGFR) and the potential significant covariates that you first tested using univariate models. The regression output is shown below. Please discuss the results of the regression in terms of the association and direction of effect of each covariate. For the sake of simplicity, assume that there were no significant interactions in this regression

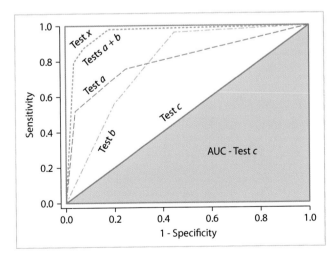

Figure 53.3 Receiver operating characteristic plot comparing tests **(a)** and **(b)**. AUC, area under the curve; Test x, theoretically perfect discriminatory test; Test c, test without discriminatory ability.

model. All covariates were measured only once at the entry into the study. Gender was coded as 1 for male and 2 for female. U p/c is the urine protein-to-creatinine ratio on a first morning specimen.

| Covariate | β-Coefficient | P Value | 95% Confidence interval | |
|---|---|---|---|---|
| Age (yr) | 6.625 | 0.024 | 0.762, | 14.012 |
| Gender | –6.761 | 0.003 | –8.682, | –4.839 |
| Systolic BP | 2.322 | 0.041 | 0.157, | 4.487 |
| Diastolic BP | 5.208 | 0.109 | –1.638, | 12.054 |
| U p/c | 8.312 | 0.0001 | 7.926, | 8.698 |
| Constant(α) | 3.224 | 0.000 | 1.471, | 4.977 |

**Answer:**
This regression analysis reveals that age, gender, systolic blood pressure, and a first morning urine protein-to-creatinine ratio are all significant determinants of the change (e.g., decline) in eGFR. Based on a nonsignificant P value, diastolic blood pressure was not found to be a determinant of change in eGFR in the multivariate models despite being significant in univariate analyses. There may be two potential reasons for this. The first is that diastolic blood pressure is intimately related to systolic blood pressure. Because they often run together (e.g., co-linear), placing both in the model may make one insignificant when adjusted for the other. The additional possibility is that there was not sufficient *power* in the study to detect a significant effect of diastolic blood pressure on eGFR. Although not provided, if there were insufficient numbers of patients in the study to perform a regression with five covariates, the diastolic blood pressure may have been affected by this. In looking at the remaining determinants, age, systolic blood pressure, and the first morning urine protein-to-creatinine ratio, all had positive and statistically significant β-coefficients in the regression. These data suggest that there is a direct relationship with these variables and eGFR in that older children with higher systolic blood pressures and higher urine protein-to-creatinine ratios had a higher absolute change in the eGFR over the year of the study. Conversely, gender had a negative association with eGFR, implying that females have a lesser change in eGFR (e.g., protective effect). Furthermore, looking at the P values and confidence intervals associated with the regression show that the strength of the association is strongest between the first morning urine protein-to-creatinine ratio and the eGFR. This can be inferred because of the narrow confidence interval and very low associated P values.

2. Given the results of the multivariate regression in Question 1, write the regression equation associated with this study.

**Answer:**
The variability in eGFR = 3.224 + 6.625*(age) + (–6.761)*(gender) + 2.322*(systolic BP) + 5.208*(diastolic BP) + 8.312*(U p/c)

3. You wish to evaluate two different diagnostic laboratory tests in terms of their ability to reliably identify disease in your population of patients. In attempting to do so, you administer the two diagnostic tests (a) and (b) to a study population of 100 subjects in which the presence or absence of disease has been confirmed using a gold-standard methodology. After performing both tests in your population, you are able to construct the following 2 × 2 tables.

**Test (a):**

| Test (a) results | Disease status | | |
|---|---|---|---|
| | Present | Absent | Total |
| Positive | 22 | 7 | 29 |
| Negative | 3 | 68 | 71 |
| | 25 | 75 | 100 |

**Test (b):**

| Test (b) Results | Disease Status | | |
|---|---|---|---|
| | Present | Absent | Total |
| *Positive | 18 | 2 | 20 |
| Negative | 7 | 73 | 80 |
| | 25 | 75 | 100 |

Calculate the sensitivity, specificity, positive predictive values, and negative predictive values for each test.

**Test (a):**
Sensitivity = TP/(TP + FN) = 22/22 + 3 = 0.88 × 100 = 88%

Specificity = TN/(TN + FP) = 68/68 + 7 = 0.91 × 100 = 91%

Positive predictive value (PPV) = TP/(TP + FP) = 22/22 + 7 = 0.76 × 100 = 76%

Negative predictive value (NPV) = TN/(TN + FN) = 68/68 + 3 = 0.96 × 100 = 96%

**Test (b):**

Sensitivity = TP/(TP + FN) = 18/18 + 7 = 0.72 × 100 = 72%

Specificity = TN/(TN + FP) = 73/73 + 2 = 0.97 × 100 = 97%

Positive predictive value (PPV) = TP/(TP + FP) = 18/18 + 2 = 0.90 × 100 = 90%

Negative predictive value (NPV) = TN/(TN + FN) = 73/73 + 7 = 0.91 × 100 = 91%

4. Compare the two diagnostic tests in question 3 in terms of their performance at both ruling in and ruling out disease in the population.

**Answer:**
One way to compare the performance of these two tests in this population is to calculate the likelihood ratios for each test.

For test (a): Likelihood ratio (a) = sensitivity/(1-specificity) = 0.88/(1 − 0.91) = 9.8
For test (b): Likelihood ratio (a) = sensitivity/(1-specificity) = 0.72/(1 − 0.97) = 24

In this scenario, test (b) has a higher likelihood ratio mostly because of its high specificity. However, the choice of which test is most favorable in this example hinges primarily on the characteristics of the disease under study. Should the disease in this example be serious and potentially fatal if undetected and/or curable on detection, test (a) may be preferable because of its higher sensitivity. This is due to the lower rate of false-negative results associated with test (a). A false-negative result in this scenario would have serious consequences for the health of this population because of disease severity. However, in a situation in which a disease is relatively mild and not associated with significant morbidity and mortality and/or further testing associated with a positive test result is both expensive and associated with its own risks, then test (b) may be preferable. This is because of its lower rate of false-positive test results (e.g., higher specificity).

5. You have conducted a case-control study examining whether maternal exposure to drug $x$ during pregnancy is associated with the development of hypertension in children younger than 10 years of age. In performing this study, you retrospectively collect data on a group of children diagnosed with hypertension with age- and gender-matched controls sampled from the same general population. You retrospectively collect exposure data from the mothers of these children to drug $x$ during pregnancy. From your data, you are able to construct the following 2 × 2 table:

| | Hypertension status | | |
|---|---|---|---|
| Exposure history | Hypertensive | Normotensive | Total |
| Exposed | 20 | 25 | 45 |
| Unexposed | 5 | 50 | 55 |
| | 25 | 75 | 100 |

Calculate the odds of developing hypertension with exposure relative to not being exposed. How does this metric relate to the calculation of a relative risk?

**Answer:**
This question is asking for a calculation of the odds ratio from this case-control study. The odds ratio (OR) is calculated from the number of those with disease divided by those without disease for each exposure group. In this question this becomes:

$$OR = ad/bc = 20 \times 50/5 \times 25 = 1000/125 = 8.$$

In the situation in which a case-control study is examining a relatively rare disease, the odds ratio can be a good approximation of the relative risk. However, in this scenario in which hypertension is hypothetically present in 25% of the population, the relative risk for disease associated with exposure $x$ is difficult to estimate.

# Index

Note: Illustrations are indicated by page numbers followed by *f*; boxes, *b*; and tables, *t*.